Acce

The *British National Formulary* (BNF) and *B* updated monthly online via MedicinesComplete, ensuring healthcare professionals always have the latest prescribing advice **DCU**

You can be alerted to all the latest updates by signing up to the BNF eNewsletter at www.pharmpress.com/bnfalerts.asp.

Withdrawn from stock

ONLINE

 MedicinesComplete

BNF on MedicinesComplete
Access BNF and *BNF for Children* on MedicinesComplete and receive the very latest drug information through monthly online updates.

BNF on FormularyComplete

BNF on FormularyComplete
Create, edit and manage your own local formulary content built upon the trusted prescribing advice of the BNF and *BNF for Children*.

BNF on Evidence Search
Search the BNF and *BNF for Children* alongside other authoritative clinical and non-clinical evidence and best practice at http://evidence.nhs.uk from NICE.

MOBILE

BNF app – Stay up to date anywhere with the BNF app available for iOS, Android and Blackberry.

BNF eBook – Available to download on the iBookstore, Amazon and other suppliers.

PRINT

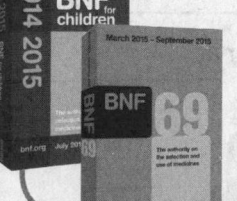

BNF subscription – if you prefer to access BNF in print, take advantage of our subscription option. We will send you the new BNF as soon as the book is published. One or two year packages (including or excluding BNFC) are available. Discounted pricing is also available on bulk sales.

If you are entitled to a free NHS copy of BNF, please note: the free print version is now distributed by NICE annually in September, instead of every six months. To buy your copy/ies of BNF 69 (March) direct, go to **www.pharmpress.com/bnf**.

How to purchase

Purchase direct from Pharmaceutical Press by visiting **www.pharmpress.com/bnf**

For enquiries about the BNF or BNFC in print, contact **direct@macmillan.co.uk**
Tel: **+44 (0) 1256 302 699**

For enquiries concerning MedicinesComplete, BNF on FormularyComplete, or bulk orders of the print edition, contact **pharmpress@rpharms.com**
Tel: **+44 (0) 20 7572 2266**

Download mobile apps by visiting your appropriate app store. Available for iOS, Android and Blackberry

For pricing information please visit the website at **www.pharmpress.com/bnf**

For international sales contact your local sales agent. Contact details at **www.pharmpress.com/agents**

Stay up to date – sign up to the BNF eNewsletter at **www.pharmpress.com/bnfalerts.asp**

British
National
Formulary

BNF 69

March 2015 –
September 2015

ROYAL
PHARMACEUTICAL
SOCIETY

Published jointly by
BMJ Group
Tavistock Square, London WC1H 9JP, UK
and
Pharmaceutical Press
Pharmaceutical Press is the publishing division of the
Royal Pharmaceutical Society
1 Lambeth High Street, London, SE1 7JN, UK

Copyright © BMJ Group and the Royal Pharmaceutical
Society of Great Britain 2015

ISBN: 978 0 85711 156 2

ISSN: 0260-535X

Printed by GGP Media GmbH, Pössneck, Germany

Typeset by Data Standards Ltd.

A catalogue record for this book is available from the
British Library.

Paper copies may be obtained through any bookseller or
direct from:
Pharmaceutical Press
c/o Macmillan Distribution (MDL)
Brunel Rd
Houndmills
Basingstoke
RG21 6XS
UK
Tel: +44 (0) 1256 302 699
Fax: +44 (0) 1256 812 521
direct@macmillan.co.uk
www.pharmpress.com

For all bulk orders of more than 20 copies:
Tel: +44 (0) 207 572 2266
pharmpress@rpharms.com

The BNF is available online through MedicinesComplete and as mobile apps; a PDA version is also available. In addition, BNF content can be integrated into a
local formulary by using BNF on FormularyComplete;
see bnf.org for details.

The BNF is also available on www.evidence.nhs.uk and
the NICE BNF smartphone app can be downloaded with
a NHS Athens password in England, Scotland, and
Wales; for technical support, email:
contactus@evidence.nhs.uk.

Distribution of printed BNFs
In **England**, NICE purchases print editions of the BNF
(September editions only) for distribution within the
NHS. For details of who is eligible to receive a copy
and further contact details, please refer to the NICE
website:
www.nice.org.uk/mpc/BritishNationalFormulary.jsp.

In **Scotland**, email:
nss.psd-bnf@nhs.net

In **Wales**, contact NHS Wales Shared Services Partnership—Contractor Services:
Tel: 01792 607420

In **Northern Ireland**, email:
ni.bnf@hscni.net

The BNF is designed as a digest for rapid reference
and it may not always include all the information
necessary for prescribing and dispensing. Also, less
detail is given on areas such as obstetrics, malignant
disease, and anaesthesia since it is expected that
those undertaking treatment will have specialist
knowledge and access to specialist literature. *BNF
for Children* should be consulted for detailed information on the use of medicines in children. The BNF
should be interpreted in the light of professional
knowledge and supplemented as necessary by specialised publications and by reference to the product
literature. Information is also available from medicines information services (see inside front cover).

Pharmaid
Numerous requests have been received from developing countries for BNFs. The Pharmaid scheme of
the Commonwealth Pharmacists Association will
dispatch old BNFs to Commonwealth countries.
BNFs will be collected from certain community
pharmacies in November. For further details check
the health press or email:
admin@commonwealthpharmacy.org

Preface

The BNF is a joint publication of the British Medical Association and the Royal Pharmaceutical Society. It is published under the authority of a Joint Formulary Committee which comprises representatives of the two professional bodies, the UK Health Departments, the Medicines and Healthcare products Regulatory Agency, and a national guideline producer. The Dental Advisory Group oversees the preparation of advice on the drug management of dental and oral conditions; the Group includes representatives of the British Dental Association and a representative from the UK Health Departments. The Nurse Prescribers' Advisory Group advises on the content relevant to nurses and includes representatives from different parts of the nursing community and from the UK Health Departments.

The BNF aims to provide prescribers, pharmacists, and other healthcare professionals with sound up-to-date information about the use of medicines.

The BNF includes key information on the selection, prescribing, dispensing and administration of medicines. Medicines generally prescribed in the UK are covered and those considered less suitable for prescribing are clearly identified. Little or no information is included on medicines promoted for purchase by the public.

Information on drugs is drawn from the manufacturers' product literature, medical and pharmaceutical literature, UK health departments, regulatory authorities, and professional bodies. Advice is constructed from clinical literature and reflects, as far as possible, an evaluation of the evidence from diverse sources. The BNF also takes account of authoritative national guidelines and emerging safety concerns. In addition, the editorial team receives advice on all therapeutic areas from expert clinicians; this ensures that the BNF's recommendations are relevant to practice.

The BNF is designed as a digest for rapid reference and it may not always include all the information necessary for prescribing and dispensing. Also, less detail is given on areas such as obstetrics, malignant disease, and anaesthesia since it is expected that those undertaking treatment will have specialist knowledge and access to specialist literature. BNF for Children should be consulted for detailed information on the use of medicines in children. The BNF should be interpreted in the light of professional knowledge and supplemented as necessary by specialised publications and by reference to the product literature. Information is also available from medicines information services (see inside front cover).

It is **important** to use the most recent BNF information for making clinical decisions. The print edition of the BNF is updated in March and September each year. Monthly updates are provided online via Medicines-Complete and the NHS Evidence portal. The more important changes for this edition are listed on p. xvii; changes listed online are cumulative (from one print edition to the next), and can be printed off each month to show the main changes since the last print edition as an aide memoire for those using print copies.

The BNF Publications website (bnf.org) includes additional information of relevance to healthcare professionals. Other digital formats of the BNF—including versions for mobile devices and integration into local formularies—are also available.

The BNF welcomes comments from healthcare professionals. Comments and constructive criticism should be sent to:
British National Formulary,
Royal Pharmaceutical Society,
1 Lambeth High Street, London SE1 7JN.
editor@bnf.org

The contact email for manufacturers or pharmaceutical companies wishing to contact BNF Publications is manufacturerinfo@bnf.org

Contents

General information and changes

Acknowledgements

The Joint Formulary Committee is grateful to individuals and organisations that have provided advice and information to the BNF.

The principal contributors for this edition were:

K.W. Ah-See, M.N. Badminton, A.K. Bahl, P.R.J. Barnes, D. Bilton, S.L. Bloom, M.F. Bultitude, I.F. Burgess, D.J. Burn, C.E. Dearden, D.W. Denning, R. Dinwiddie, P.N. Durrington, D.A.C. Elliman, P. Emery, M.D. Feher, B.G. Gazzard, A.M. Geretti, N.J.L. Gittoes, P.J. Goadsby, M. Gupta, T.L. Hawkins, B.G. Higgins, S.P. Higgins, S.H.D. Jackson, A. Jones, D.M. Keeling, J.R. Kirwan, P.G. Kopelman, T.H. Lee, A. Lekkas, D.N.J. Lockwood, A.M. Lovering, M.G. Lucas, L. Luzzatto, P.D. Mason, D.A. McArthur, K.E.L. McColl, L.M. Melvin, E. Miller, R.M. Mirakian, P. Morrison, S.M.S. Nasser, C. Nelson-Piercy, J.M. Neuberger, D.J. Nutt, L.P. Ormerod, R. Patel, W.J. Penny, A.B. Provan, M.M. Ramsay, A.S.C. Rice, D.J. Rowbotham, J.W. Sander, J.A.T. Sandoe, M. Schacter, G.J. Shortland, S.E. Slater, J. Soar, S.C.E. Sporton, M.D. Stewart, A.M. Szarewski, S. Thomas, J.P. Thompson, R.P. Walt, A.D. Weeks, A. Wilcock, A.P.R. Wilson, M.M. Yaqoob.

Expert advice on the management of oral and dental conditions was kindly provided by M. Addy, P. Coulthard, A. Crighton, M.A.O, Lewis, J.G. Meechan, N.D. Röbb, C. Scully, R.A. Seymour, R. Welbury, and J.M. Zakrzewska. S. Kaur provided valuable advice on dental prescribing policy.

Members of the British Association of Dermatologists' Therapy & Guidelines Subcommittee, D.A. Buckley, E. Duarte Williamson, M. Griffiths, J. Hughes, T. Leslie, N.J. Levell, E. Mallon, A.J. McDonagh, P. McHenry, I. Nasr, C. Saunders, V. Swale, A. Brain (Secretariat), and M.F. Mohd Mustapa (Secretariat) have provided valuable advice.

Members of the Advisory Committee on Malaria Prevention, R.H. Behrens, D. Bell, P.L. Chiodini, V. Field, F. Genasi, L. Goodyer, A. Green, J. Jones, G. Kassianos, D.G. Lalloo, D. Patel, H. Patel, M. Powell, D.V. Shingadia, N.O. Subair, C.J.M. Whitty, M. Blaze (Secretariat), and V. Smith (Secretariat) have provided valuable advice.

The UK Ophthalmic Pharmacy Group have also provided valuable advice.

The Joint British Societies' Coronary Risk Prediction Charts have been reproduced with the kind permission of P.N. Durrington.

The MHRA have provided valuable assistance.

Correspondents in the pharmaceutical industry have provided information on new products and commented on products in the BNF.

Numerous doctors, pharmacists, nurses, and others have sent comments and suggestions.

BNF interactions are provided by C.L. Preston, K. Begum, E.E. Crehan, S.L. Jones, S.Z. Khan, D.M. McGuirk, and H.K. Sandhu.

The BNF has valuable access to the *Martindale* data banks by courtesy of A. Brayfield and staff.

F. Gibson and staff provided valuable technical assistance.

E. Laughton and P.D. Lee provided considerable assistance during the production of this edition of the BNF.

BNF Staff

Managing Director, Pharmaceutical Press
Alina Lourie *B.Ed, MSc*

BNF Director
Karen Baxter *BSc, MSc, MRPharmS*

Senior Medical Adviser
Derek G. Waller *BSc, MB, BS, DM, FRCP*

Lead Editors
Bryony Jordan *BSc, DipPharmPract, MRPharmS*
John Martin *BPharm, PhD, MRPharmS*
Rachel S.M. Ryan *BPharm, MRPharmS*
Shama M.S. Wagle *BPharm, DipPharmPract, MRPharmS*

Senior Clinical Writers
Sejal Amin *BPharm, MSc*
Manjula Halai *BScChem, MPharm* (acting Project Manager)
Kate Towers *BPharm* (AU), *GCClinPharm* (acting Digital Product Manager)

Clinical Writers
Joyce Donnelly *MPharm, MRPharmS*
Kristina Fowlie *MPharm, CertPharmPract, MRPharmS*
Belén Granell Villén *BSc, DipClinPharm*
Angela M.G. McFarlane *BSc, DipClinPharm*
Sarah Mohamad *MPharm, MRPharmS*
Katie L. Page *MPharm, MRPharmS*
Heenaben Patel *MPharm, DipClinPharm, MRPharmS*
Roushin Patel *MPharm*
Dominique Shakir *MPharm, MRPharmS, IP, PGDip*
Anna Sparshatt *MPharm, CertPharmPract, CertPsychTherap*

Editorial Assistants
Rhiannon Howe *BMedSc*
Elizabeth King

Senior BNF Administrator
Heidi Homar *BA*

Clinical Decision Support Product Manager
Ferenc P. Wórum *MD* (HU), *MSc*

Operations Manager
Linda Paulus *MA*

Joint Formulary Committee 2014–2015

Chair

Derek G. Waller
BSc, MB BS, DM, FRCP

Deputy Chair

Alison Blenkinsopp
BPharm, PhD, FRPharmS, OBE

Committee Members

Julie Beynon
MB ChB, FRCA, FFPM

Carmel M. Darcy
BSc, MSc, IP, MPSNI, MRPharmS

Sue Faulding
BPharm, MSc, FRPharmS

Matt Griffiths
BA, FAETC, RGN, Cert A&E, NISP

Tracy Hall
BSc, MSc, Cert N, Dip N, RGN, DN

W. Moira Kinnear
BSc, MSc, MRPharmS

Mark P. Lythgoe
MB BS, MRPharmS

Louise Picton
BSc, DipCommPharm, MSc, MRPharmS

Michael J. Stewart
MB ChB, MD, FRCP(Ed), FRCP

Esther Wong
BSc, MPharm, MSc, DipEthics, DipPharmPract, IP, MRPharmS

Executive Secretary

Heidi Homar
BA

Dental Advisory Group 2014–2015

Chair

Sarah Manton
BDS, FDSRCS Ed, FHEA, PhD

Committee Members

Christine Arnold
BDS, DDPHRCS, MCDH

Karen Baxter
BSc, MSc, MRPharmS

Andrew K. Brewer
BSc, BchD

Barry Cockcroft
BDS, FDSRCS (Eng)

Lesley P. Longman
BSc, BDS, FDSRCS Ed, PhD

John Martin
BPharm, PhD, MRPharmS

Michelle Moffat
BDS, MFDS RCS Ed, M Paed Dent RCPS, FDS (Paed Dent) RCS Ed

Sarah Mohamad
MPharm, MRPharmS

Martin H. Thornhill
BDS, MBBS, MSc, FDSRCS (Edin), FDSRCS (Eng), FDSRCSI, PhD

Secretary

Arianne J. Matlin
MA, MSc, PhD

Executive Secretary

Heidi Homar
BA

> **Advice on dental practice**
> The **British Dental Association** has contributed to the advice on medicines for dental practice through its representatives on the Dental Advisory Group.

Nurse Prescribers' Advisory Group 2014–2015

Chair

Molly Courtenay
PhD, MSc, Cert Ed, BSc, RGN

Committee Members

Karen Baxter
BSc, MSc, MRPharmS

Penny M. Franklin
RN, RCN, RSCPHN(HV), MA, PGCE

Belén Granell Villen
BSc, PGDipClinPharm

Tracy Hall
BSc, MSc, RGN, DN, Dip N, Cert N

Jill Hill
BSc, RGN

Bryony Jordan
BSc, DipPharmPract, MRPharmS

Joan Myers
MSc, BSc, RGN, RSCN, Dip DN

Kathy Radley
BSc, RGN

Jill M. Shearer
BSc, RGN, RM

Vicky Vidler
MA, RGN, RSCN

John Wright

Executive Secretary

Heidi Homar
BA

How the BNF is constructed

The BNF is unique in bringing together authoritative, independent guidance on best practice with clinically validated drug information, enabling healthcare professionals to select safe and effective medicines for individual patients.

Information in the BNF has been validated against emerging evidence, best-practice guidelines, and advice from a network of clinical experts.

Hundreds of changes are made between print editions, and are published monthly online. The most clinically significant changes are listed at the front of each edition (p. xvii).

Joint Formulary Committee

The Joint Formulary Committee (JFC) is responsible for the content of the BNF. The JFC includes doctors appointed by the BMJ Group, pharmacists appointed by the Royal Pharmaceutical Society, and representatives from the Medicines and Healthcare products Regulatory Agency (MHRA), the UK Health Departments, and a national guideline producer. The JFC decides on matters of policy and reviews amendments to the BNF in the light of new evidence and expert advice.

Dental Advisory Group

The Dental Advisory Group oversees the preparation of advice on the drug management of dental and oral conditions; the group includes representatives from the British Dental Association and a representative from the UK Health Departments.

Editorial team

BNF clinical writers have all worked as pharmacists and have a sound understanding of how drugs are used in clinical practice. Each clinical writer is responsible for editing, maintaining, and updating specific chapters of the BNF. During the publication cycle the clinical writers review information in the BNF against a variety of sources (see below).

Amendments to the text are drafted when the clinical writers are satisfied that any new information is reliable and relevant. The draft amendments are passed to expert advisers for comment and then presented to the Joint Formulary Committee for consideration. Additionally, sections are regularly chosen from every chapter for thorough review. These planned reviews aim to verify all the information in the selected sections and to draft any amendments to reflect the current best practice.

Clinical writers prepare the text for publication and undertake a number of checks on the knowledge at various stages of the production.

Expert advisers

The BNF uses about 60 expert clinical advisers (including doctors, pharmacists, nurses, and dentists) throughout the UK to help with the clinical content. The role of these expert advisers is to review existing text and to comment on amendments drafted by the clinical writers. These clinical experts help to ensure that the BNF remains reliable by:

- commenting on the relevance of the text in the context of best clinical practice in the UK;

- checking draft amendments for appropriate interpretation of any new evidence;

- providing expert opinion in areas of controversy or when reliable evidence is lacking;

- advising on areas where the BNF diverges from summaries of product characteristics;

- providing independent advice on drug interactions, prescribing in hepatic impairment, renal impairment, pregnancy, breast-feeding, children, the elderly, palliative care, and the emergency treatment of poisoning.

In addition to consulting with regular advisers, the BNF calls on other clinical specialists for specific developments when particular expertise is required.

The BNF also works closely with a number of expert bodies that produce clinical guidelines. Drafts or pre-publication copies of guidelines are routinely received for comment and for assimilation into the BNF.

Sources of BNF information

The BNF uses a variety of sources for its information; the main ones are shown below.

Summaries of product characteristics The BNF receives summaries of product characteristics (SPCs) of all new products as well as revised SPCs for existing products. The SPCs are the principal source of product information and are carefully processed, despite the ever-increasing volume of information being issued by the pharmaceutical industry. Such processing involves:

- verifying the approved names of all relevant ingredients including 'non-active' ingredients (the BNF is committed to using approved names and descriptions as laid down by the Human Medicines Regulations 2012);

- comparing the indications, cautions, contra-indications, and side-effects with similar existing drugs. Where these are different from the expected pattern, justification is sought for their inclusion or exclusion;

- seeking independent data on the use of drugs in pregnancy and breast-feeding;

- incorporating the information into the BNF using established criteria for the presentation and inclusion of the data;

- checking interpretation of the information by a second clinical writer before submitting to a lead editor; changes relating to doses receive an extra check;

- identifying potential clinical problems or omissions and seeking further information from manufacturers or from expert advisers;

- careful validation of any areas of divergence of the BNF from the SPC before discussion by the Committee (in the light of supporting evidence);

- constructing, with the help of expert advisers, a comment on the role of the drug in the context of similar drugs.

Much of this processing is applicable to the following sources as well.

Expert advisers   The role of expert clinical advisers in providing the appropriate clinical context for all BNF information is discussed above.

Literature   Clinical writers monitor core medical and pharmaceutical journals. Research papers and reviews relating to drug therapy are carefully processed. When a difference between the advice in the BNF and the paper is noted, the new information is assessed for reliability and relevance to UK clinical practice. If necessary, new text is drafted and discussed with expert advisers and the Joint Formulary Committee. The BNF enjoys a close working relationship with a number of national information providers.

Systematic reviews   The BNF has access to various databases of systematic reviews (including the Cochrane Library and various web-based resources). These are used for answering specific queries, for reviewing existing text, and for constructing new text. Clinical writers receive training in critical appraisal, literature evaluation, and search strategies. Reviews published in Clinical Evidence are used to validate BNF advice.

Consensus guidelines   The advice in the BNF is checked against consensus guidelines produced by expert bodies. A number of bodies make drafts or pre-publication copies of the guidelines available to the BNF; it is therefore possible to ensure that a consistent message is disseminated. The BNF routinely processes guidelines from the National Institute for Health and Care Excellence (NICE), the Scottish Medicines Consortium (SMC), and the Scottish Intercollegiate Guidelines Network (SIGN).

Reference sources   Textbooks and reference sources are used to provide background information for the review of existing text or for the construction of new text. The BNF team works closely with the editorial team that produces *Martindale: The Complete Drug Reference*. The BNF has access to *Martindale* information resources and each team keeps the other informed of significant developments and shifts in the trends of drug usage.

Statutory information   The BNF routinely processes relevant information from various Government bodies including Statutory Instruments and regulations affecting the Prescription only Medicines Order. Official compendia such as the British Pharmacopoeia and its addenda are processed routinely to ensure that the BNF complies with the relevant sections of the Human Medicines Regulations 2012.

The BNF maintains close links with the Home Office (in relation to controlled drug regulations) and the Medicines and Healthcare products Regulatory Agency (including the British Pharmacopoeia Commission). Safety warnings issued by the Commission on Human Medicines (CHM) and guidelines on drug use issued by the UK health departments are processed as a matter of routine.

Relevant professional statements issued by the Royal Pharmaceutical Society are included in the BNF as are guidelines from bodies such as the Royal College of General Practitioners.

The BNF reflects information from the Drug Tariff, the Scottish Drug Tariff, and the Northern Ireland Drug Tariff.

Pricing information   NHS Prescription Services (from the NHS Business Services Authority) provides information on prices of medicinal products and appliances in the BNF.

Comments from readers   Readers of the BNF are invited to send in comments. Numerous letters and emails are received by the BNF team. Such feedback helps to ensure that the BNF provides practical and clinically relevant information. Many changes in the presentation and scope of the BNF have resulted from comments sent in by users.

Comments from industry   Close scrutiny of the BNF by the manufacturers provides an additional check and allows them an opportunity to raise issues about the BNF's presentation of the role of various drugs; this is yet another check on the balance of the BNF's advice. All comments are looked at with care and, where necessary, additional information and expert advice are sought.

Virtual user groups   The BNF has set up virtual user groups across various healthcare professions (e.g. doctors, pharmacists, nurses, dentists). The aim of these groups will be to provide feedback to the editors and publishers to ensure that BNF publications continue to serve the needs of its users.

Market research   Market research is conducted at regular intervals to gather feedback on specific areas of development, such as drug interactions or changes to the way information is presented in digital formats.

> The BNF is an independent professional publication that is kept up-to-date and addresses the day-to-day prescribing information needs of healthcare professionals. Use of this resource throughout the health service helps to ensure that medicines are used safely, effectively, and appropriately.

How to use the BNF

In order to achieve the safe, effective, and appropriate use of medicines, healthcare professionals must be able to use the BNF effectively, and keep up to date with significant changes in the BNF that are relevant to their clinical practice. *How to Use the BNF* is aimed as a quick refresher for all healthcare professionals involved with prescribing, monitoring, supplying, and administering medicines, and as a learning aid for students training to join these professions. While *How to Use the BNF* is linked to the main elements of rational prescribing, the generic structure of this section means that it can be adapted for teaching and learning in different clinical settings.

Structure of the BNF

The Contents list (on p. iv) shows that information in the BNF is divided into:

- *How the BNF is Constructed* (p. ix);
- *Changes* (p. xvii);
- *Guidance on Prescribing* (p. 1), which provides practical information on many aspects of prescribing from writing a prescription to prescribing in palliative care;
- *Emergency Treatment of Poisoning* (p. 33), which provides an overview on the management of acute poisoning;
- *Classified notes on clinical conditions, drugs, and preparations*, these notes are divided into 15 chapters, each of which is related to a particular system of the body (e.g. chapter 2, Cardiovascular System) or to an aspect of medical care (e.g. chapter 5, Infections). Each chapter is further divided into classified sections. Each section usually begins with *prescribing notes* followed by relevant drug *monographs* and *preparations* (see fig. 1). Drugs are classified in a section according to their pharmacology and therapeutic use;
- *Appendices and Indices*, includes 5 Appendices (providing information on drug interactions, Borderline substances, cautionary and advisory labels for dispensed medicines, intravenous additives, and wound management), the Dental Practitioners' Formulary, the Nurse Prescribers' Formulary, Non-medical Prescribing, Index of Manufacturers, and the main Index. The information in the Appendices should be used in conjunction with relevant information in the chapters.

Finding information in the BNF

The BNF includes a number of aids to help access relevant information:

- *Index*, where entries are included in alphabetical order of non-proprietary drug names, proprietary drug names, clinical conditions, and prescribing topics. A specific entry for 'Dental Prescribing' brings together topics of relevance to dentists. The page reference to the drug monograph is shown in **bold** type. References to drugs in Appendices 1 and 3 are not included in the main Index;
- *Contents* (p. iv), provides a hierarchy of how information in the BNF is organised;

- The beginning of each chapter includes *a classified hierarchy* of how information is organised in that chapter;
- *Running heads*, located next to the page number on the top of each page, show the section of the BNF that is being used;
- *Thumbnails*, on the outer edge of each page, show the chapter of the BNF that is being used;
- *Cross-references*, lead to additional relevant information in other parts of the BNF.

Finding dental information in the BNF

Extra signposts have been added to help access dental information in the BNF:

- *Prescribing in Dental Practice* (p. 27), includes a contents list dedicated to drugs and topics of relevance to dentists, together with cross-references to the prescribing notes in the appropriate sections of the BNF. For example, a review of this list shows that information on the local treatment of oral infections is located in chapter 12 (Ear, Nose, and Oropharynx) while information on the systemic treatment of these infections is found in chapter 5 (Infections). This section also includes advice on Medical Emergencies in Dental Practice (p. 27) and Medical Problems in Dental Practice (p. 29). Guidance on the prevention of endocarditis and advice on the management of anticoagulated patients undergoing dental surgery can also be found here;
- *Side-headings*, in the prescribing notes, side-headings facilitate the identification of advice on oral conditions (e.g. Dental and Orofacial Pain, p. 278);
- *Dental prescribing on NHS*, in the body of the BNF, preparations that can be prescribed using NHS form FP10D (GP14 in Scotland, WP10D in Wales) can be identified by means of a note headed 'Dental prescribing on NHS' (e.g. Aciclovir Tablets, p. 432).

Identifying effective drug treatments

The prescribing notes in the BNF provide an overview of the drug management of common conditions and facilitate rapid appraisal of treatment options (e.g. hypertension, p. 108). For ease of use, information on the management of certain conditions has been tabulated (e.g. acute asthma, p. 185). Information is also provided on the prevention of disease (e.g. malaria prophylaxis for travellers, p. 445).

Advice issued by the National Institute for Health and Clinical Excellence (NICE) is integrated within the BNF prescribing notes if appropriate. Summaries of NICE technology appraisals, and relevant short guidelines, are included in blue panels. The BNF also includes advice issued by the Scottish Medicines Consortium (SMC) when a medicine is restricted or not recommended for use within NHS Scotland.

In order to select safe and effective medicines for individual patients, information in the prescribing notes must be used in conjunction with other prescribing details about the drugs and knowledge of the patient's medical and drug history.

A brief description of the clinical uses of a drug can usually be found in the Indications section of its monograph (e.g. bendroflumethiazide, p. 87); a cross-reference is provided to any indications for that drug that are covered in other sections of the BNF.

The symbol ◢ is used to denote preparations that are considered by the Joint Formulary Committee to be less suitable for prescribing. Although such preparations may not be considered as drugs of first choice, their use may be justifiable in certain circumstances.

Drug management of medical emergencies

Guidance on the drug management of medical emergencies can be found in the relevant BNF chapters (e.g. treatment of anaphylaxis is included in section 3.4.3); advice on the management of medical emergencies in dental practice can be found in Prescribing in Dental Practice, p. 27. A summary of drug doses used for Medical Emergencies in the Community can be found in the glossy pages at the back of the BNF. An algorithm for Adult Advanced Life Support can also be found within these pages.

Figure 1 Illustrates the typical layout of a drug monograph and preparation records in the BNF

 DRUG NAME ◢ ←

Indications details of clinical uses

Cautions details of precautions required and also any monitoring required
  Counselling Verbal explanation to the patient of specific details of the drug treatment (e.g. posture when taking a medicine)

Contra-indications circumstances when a drug should be avoided

Hepatic impairment advice on the use of a drug in hepatic impairment

Renal impairment advice on the use of a drug in renal impairment

Pregnancy advice on the use of a drug during pregnancy

Breast-feeding advice on the use of a drug during breast-feeding

Side-effects very common (greater than 1 in 10) and common (1 in 100 to 1 in 10); *less commonly* (1 in 1000 to 1 in 100); *rarely* (1 in 10 000 to 1 in 1000); *very rarely* (less than 1 in 10 000); also reported, frequency not known

Dose
• Dose and frequency of administration (max. dose); CHILD and ELDERLY details of dose for specific age group
• By alternative route, dose and frequency

¹**Approved Name** (Non-proprietary) PoM ←
  Pharmaceutical form, sugar-free, active ingredient mg/mL, net price, pack size = basic NHS price. Label: (as in Appendix 3)
  1. Exceptions to the prescribing status are indicated by a note or footnote.

Proprietary Name (Manufacturer) PoM NHS ←
  Pharmaceutical form, colour, coating, active ingredient and amount in dosage form, net price, pack size = basic NHS price. Label: (as in Appendix 3)
  Excipients include clinically important excipients
  Electrolytes clinically significant quantities of electrolytes
  Note Specific notes about the product e.g. handling

Preparations

Preparations are included under a non-proprietary title, if they are marketed under such a title, if they are not otherwise prescribable under the NHS, or if they may be prepared extemporaneously.

Drugs

Drugs appear under pharmacopoeial or other non-proprietary titles. When there is an *appropriate current monograph* (Human Medicines Regulations 2012) preference is given to a name at the head of that monograph; otherwise a British Approved Name (BAN), if available, is used.

The symbol ◢ is used to denote those preparations that are considered by the Joint Formulary Committee to be less suitable for prescribing. Although such preparations may not be considered as drugs of first choice, their use may be justifiable in certain circumstances.

Prescription-only medicines PoM

This symbol has been placed against those preparations that are available only on a prescription issued by an appropriate practitioner. For more detailed information see *Medicines, Ethics and Practice*, London, Pharmaceutical Press (always consult latest edition).

The symbols CD2 CD3 CD4-1 CD4-2 indicate that the preparations are subject to the prescription requirements of the Misuse of Drugs Act. For regulations governing prescriptions for such preparations see Controlled Drugs and Drug Dependence.

Preparations not available for NHS prescription NHS

This symbol has been placed against those preparations included in the BNF that are not prescribable under the NHS. Those prescribable only for specific disorders have a footnote specifying the condition(s) for which the preparation remains available. Some preparations which are not *prescribable* by brand name under the NHS may nevertheless be *dispensed* using the brand name providing that the prescription shows an appropriate non-proprietary name.

Prices

Prices have been calculated from the basic cost used in pricing NHS prescriptions, see also Prices in the BNF for details.

Minimising harm in patients with co-morbidities

The drug chosen to treat a particular condition should have minimal detrimental effects on the patient's other diseases and minimise the patient's susceptibility to adverse effects. To achieve this, the *Cautions*, *Contra-indications*, and *Side-effects* of the relevant drug should be reviewed, and can usually be found in the drug monograph. However, if a class of drugs (e.g. tetracyclines, p. 380) share the same cautions, contra-indications, and side-effects, these are amalgamated in the prescribing notes while those unique to a particular drug in that class are included in its individual drug monograph. Occasionally, the cautions, contra-indications, and side-effects may be included within a preparation record if they are specific to that preparation or if the preparation is not accompanied by a monograph.

The information under Cautions can be used to assess the risks of using a drug in a patient who has co-morbidities that are also included in the Cautions for that drug—if a safer alternative cannot be found, the drug may be prescribed while monitoring the patient for adverse-effects or deterioration in the co-morbidity. Contra-indications are far more restrictive than Cautions and mean that the drug should be avoided in a patient with a condition that is contra-indicated.

The impact that potential side-effects may have on a patient's quality of life should also be assessed. For instance, in a patient who has difficulty sleeping, it may be preferable to avoid a drug that frequently causes insomnia. The prescribing notes in the BNF may highlight important safety concerns and differences between drugs in their ability to cause certain side-effects.

Prescribing for patients with hepatic or renal impairment

Drug selection should aim to minimise the potential for drug accumulation, adverse drug reactions, and exacerbation of pre-existing hepatic or renal disease. If it is necessary to prescribe drugs whose effect is altered by hepatic or renal disease, appropriate drug dose adjustments should be made, and patients should be monitored adequately. The general principles for prescribing are outlined under *Prescribing in Hepatic Impairment* (p. 17) and *Prescribing in Renal Impairment* (p. 17). Information about drugs that should be avoided or used with caution in hepatic disease or renal impairment can be found in drug monographs under *Hepatic Impairment* and *Renal Impairment* (e.g. fluconazole, p. 412). However, if a class of drugs (e.g. tetracyclines, p. 380) share the same recommendations for use in hepatic disease or renal impairment, this advice is presented in the prescribing notes under *Hepatic Impairment* and *Renal Impairment* and any advice that is unique to a particular drug in that class is included in its individual drug monograph.

Prescribing for patients who are pregnant or breast-feeding

Drug selection should aim to minimise harm to the fetus, nursing infant, and mother. The infant should be monitored for potential side-effects of drugs used by the mother during pregnancy or breast-feeding. The general principles for prescribing are outlined under *Prescribing in Pregnancy* (p. 19) and *Prescribing in Breast-feeding*

(p. 19). The prescribing notes in the BNF chapters provide guidance on the drug treatment of common conditions that can occur during pregnancy and breast-feeding (e.g. asthma, p. 186). Information about the use of specific drugs during pregnancy and breast-feeding can be found in their drug monographs under *Pregnancy* and *Breast-feeding* (e.g. fluconazole, p. 412). However, if a class of drugs (e.g. tetracyclines, p. 380) share the same recommendations for use during pregnancy or breast-feeding, this advice is amalgamated in the prescribing notes under *Pregnancy* and *Breast-feeding* while any advice that is unique to a particular drug in that class is included in its individual drug monograph.

Minimising drug interactions

Drug selection should aim to minimise drug interactions. If it is necessary to prescribe a potentially serious combination of drugs, patients should be monitored appropriately. The mechanisms underlying drug interactions are explained in Appendix 1 (p. 898).

Details of drug interactions can be found in Appendix 1 of the BNF (p. 899). Drugs and their interactions are listed in alphabetical order of the non-proprietary drug name, and cross-references to drug classes are provided where appropriate. Each drug or drug class is listed twice: in the alphabetical list and also against the drug or class with which it interacts. The symbol • is placed against interactions that are potentially serious and where combined administration of drugs should be avoided (or only undertaken with caution and appropriate monitoring). Interactions that have no symbol do not usually have serious consequences.

If a drug or drug class has interactions, a cross reference to where these can be found in Appendix 1 is provided under the Cautions of the drug monograph or prescribing notes.

Prescribing for the elderly

General guidance on prescribing for the elderly can be found on p. 25.

Prescribing for children

General guidance on prescribing for children can be found on p. 15. For detailed advice on medicines used in children, consult *BNF for Children*.

Selecting the dose

The drug dose is usually located in the *Dose* section of the drug monograph or preparation record. The dose of a drug may vary according to different indications and routes of administration. If no indication is given by the dose, then that dose can be used for the conditions specified in the Indications section of that drug monograph, but not for the conditions cross-referring to other sections of the BNF. The dose is located within the preparation record when the dose varies according to different formulations of that drug (e.g. amphotericin, p. 416) or when a preparation has a dose different to that in its monograph (e.g. *Sporanox®* liquid, p. 414). Occasionally, drug doses may be included in the prescribing notes for practical reasons (e.g. doses of drugs in *Helicobacter pylori* eradication regimens, p. 51). The right dose should be selected for the right indication, route of administration, and preparation.

Doses are either expressed in terms of a definite frequency (e.g. 1 g 4 times daily) or in the total daily dose format (e.g. 6 g daily in 3 divided doses); the total daily dose should be divided into individual doses (in the second example, the patient should receive 2 g 3 times daily).

The doses of some drugs may need to be adjusted if their effects are altered by concomitant use with other drugs, or in patients with hepatic or renal impairment (see Minimising Drug Interactions, and Prescribing for Patients with Hepatic or Renal Impairment).

Doses for specific patient groups (e.g. the elderly) may be included if they are different to the standard dose. Doses for children can be identified by the terms NEONATE, INFANT, and CHILD, and will vary according to their age or body-weight.

Conversions for imperial to metric measures can be found in the glossy pages at the back of the BNF.

Selecting a suitable preparation

Patients should be prescribed a preparation that complements their daily routine, and that provides the right dose of drug for the right indication and route of administration.

In the BNF, preparations usually follow immediately after the monograph for the drug which is their main ingredient. The preparation record (see fig. 1) provides information on the type of formulation (e.g. tablet), the amount of active drug in a solid dosage form, and the concentration of active drug in a liquid dosage form. The legal status is shown for prescription only medicines and controlled drugs; any exception to the legal status is shown by a Note immediately after the preparation record or a footnote. If a proprietary preparation has a distinct colour, coating, scoring, or flavour, this is shown in the preparation record. If a proprietary preparation includes excipients usually specified in the BNF (see p. 2), these are shown in the *Excipients* statement, and if it contains clinically significant quantities of electrolytes, these are usually shown in the *Electrolytes* statement.

Branded oral liquid preparations that do not contain fructose, glucose, or sucrose are described as 'sugar-free' in the BNF. Preparations containing hydrogenated glucose syrup, mannitol, maltitol, sorbitol, or xylitol are also marked 'sugar-free' since there is evidence that they do not cause dental caries. Patients receiving medicines containing cariogenic sugars should be advised of appropriate dental hygiene measures to prevent caries. Sugar-free preparations should be used whenever possible.

Where a drug has several preparations, those of a similar type may be grouped together under a heading (e.g. 'Modified-release' for theophylline preparations, p. 195). Where there is good evidence to show that the preparations for a particular drug are not interchangeable, this is stated in a Note either in the Dose section of the monograph or by the group of preparations affected. When the dose of a drug varies according to different formulations of that drug, the right dose should be prescribed for the preparation selected.

In the case of compound preparations, the prescribing information of all constituents should be taken into account for prescribing.

Writing prescriptions

Guidance is provided on writing prescriptions that will help to reduce medication errors, see p. 5. Prescription requirements for controlled drugs are also specified on p. 8.

Administering drugs

If a drug can be given parenterally or by more than one route, the Dose section in the monograph or preparation record provides basic information on the route of administration. Further information on administration may be found in the monograph or preparation record, often as a Note or Counselling advice. If a class of drugs (e.g. topical corticosteroids, p. 803) share the same administration advice, this may be presented in the prescribing notes.

Appendix 4 (p. 1071) provides practical information on the preparation of intravenous drug infusions, including compatibility of drugs with standard intravenous infusion fluids, method of dilution or reconstitution, and administration rates.

Advising patients

The prescriber and the patient should agree on the health outcomes that the patient desires and on the strategy for achieving them (see Taking Medicines to Best Effect, p. 1). Taking the time to explain to the patient (and carers) the rationale and the potential adverse effects of treatment may improve adherence. For some medicines there is a special need for counselling (e.g. appropriate posture during administration of doxycycline); this is shown in *Counselling* statements, usually in the Cautions or Dose section of a monograph, or within a preparation record if it is specific to that preparation.

Patients should be advised if treatment is likely to affect their ability to drive or operate machinery.

Cautionary and advisory labels that pharmacists are recommended to add when dispensing are included in the preparation record (see fig. 1). Details of these labels can be found in Appendix 3 (p. 1054); a list of products and their labels is included in alphabetical order of the non-proprietary and proprietary drug names.

Monitoring drug treatment

Patients should be monitored to ensure they are achieving the expected benefits from drug treatment without any unwanted side-effects. The prescribing notes or the Cautions in the drug monograph specify any special monitoring requirements. Further information on monitoring the plasma concentration of drugs with a narrow therapeutic index can be found as a Note under the Dose section of the drug monograph.

Identifying and reporting adverse drug reactions

Clinically relevant *Side-effects* for most drugs are included in the monographs. However, if a class of drugs (e.g. tetracyclines, p. 380) share the same side-effects, these are presented in the prescribing notes while those unique to a particular drug in that class are included in its individual drug monograph. Occasionally, side-effects may be included within a preparation record if they are specific to that preparation or if the preparation is not accompanied by a monograph.

Side-effects are generally listed in order of frequency and arranged broadly by body systems. Occasionally a rare side-effect might be listed first if it is considered to be particularly important because of its seriousness. The frequency of side-effects is described in fig. 1.

An exhaustive list of side-effects is not included for drugs that are used by specialists (e.g. cytotoxic drugs and drugs used in anaesthesia). Recognising that hypersensitivity reactions can occur with virtually all medicines, this effect is generally not listed, unless the drug carries an increased risk of such reactions. The BNF also omits effects that are likely to have little clinical consequence (e.g. transient increase in liver enzymes).

The prescribing notes in the BNF may highlight important safety concerns and differences between drugs in their ability to cause certain side-effects. Safety warnings issued by the Commission on Human Medicines (CHM) or Medicines and Healthcare products Regulatory Agency (MHRA) can also be found here or in the drug monographs.

Adverse Reactions to Drugs (p. 12) provides advice on preventing adverse drug reactions, and guidance on reporting adverse drug reactions to the MHRA. The black triangle symbol ▼ identifies those preparations in the BNF that require additional monitoring by the European Medicines Agency.

Finding significant changes in the BNF

The print edition of the BNF is published in March and September each year, and monthly updates are provided online via MedicinesComplete and the NHS Evidence portal. The BNF includes lists of changes that are relevant to clinical practice:

- *Changes* (p. xvii), provides a list of significant changes, dose changes, classification changes, new names, and new preparations that have been incorporated into the BNF, as well as a list of preparations that have been discontinued and removed from the BNF. For ease of identification, the margins of these pages are marked in blue. Changes listed online are cumulative (from one print edition to the next), and can be printed off each month to show the main changes since the last print edition as an aide memoire for those using print copies;

- *Changes to the Dental Practitioners' Formulary* (p. 1110), these are located at the end of the Dental List;

- *E-newsletter*, the BNF & BNFC e-newsletter service is available free of charge. It alerts healthcare professionals to details of significant changes in the clinical content of these publications and to the way that this information is delivered. Newsletters also review clinical case studies and provide tips on using these publications effectively. To sign up for e-newsletters go to bnf.org/newsletter. To visit the e-newsletter archive, go to www.bnf.org/bnf/org_450066.htm

- An e-learning programme developed in collaboration with the Centre for Pharmacy Postgraduate Education (CPPE), enables pharmacists to identify and assess how significant changes in the BNF affect their clinical practice. The module can be found at www.cppe.ac.uk.

So many changes are made for each update of the BNF, that not all of them can be accommodated in the *Changes* section. We encourage healthcare professionals to review regularly the prescribing information on drugs that they encounter frequently.

Nutrition

Appendix 2 (p. 1017) includes tables of ACBS-approved enteral feeds and nutritional supplements based on their energy and protein content. There are separate tables for specialised formulae for specific clinical conditions. Classified sections on foods for special diets and nutritional supplements for metabolic diseases are also included.

Wound dressings

A table on wound dressings in Appendix 5 (p. 1081) allows an appropriate dressing to be selected based on the appearance and condition of the wound. Further information about the dressing can be found by following the cross-reference to the relevant classified section in the Appendix. In section (A5.2) advanced wound contact dressings have been classified in order of increasing absorbency.

Unlicensed medicines

The BNF includes unlicensed use of medicines when the clinical need cannot be met by licensed medicines; such use should be supported by appropriate evidence and experience. When the BNF recommends an unlicensed medicine or the 'off-label' use of a licensed medicine, this is shown in the appropriate place by '[unlicensed]'.

Prices in the BNF

Basic NHS **net prices** are given in the BNF to provide an indication of relative cost. Where there is a choice of suitable preparations for a particular disease or condition the relative cost may be used in making a selection. Cost-effective prescribing must, however, take into account other factors (such as dose frequency and duration of treatment) that affect the total cost. The use of more expensive drugs is justified if it will result in better treatment of the patient, or a reduction of the length of an illness, or the time spent in hospital. We regularly update prices using the Drug Tariff and proprietary price information published by the NHS dictionary of medicines and devices (dm+d, www.dmd.nhs.uk). The weekly updated dm+d data (including prices) can be accessed using the dm+d browser of the NHS Business Services Authority (www.ppa.org.uk/systems/pcddbrowserv2_3new/browser.jsp).

Prices have generally been calculated from the net cost used in pricing NHS prescriptions in December 2014 for non-proprietary and proprietary preparations. Prices generally reflect whole dispensing packs; prices for injections are stated per ampoule, vial, or syringe. Prices for extemporaneously prepared preparations are not provided in the BNF as prices vary between different manufacturers. In Appendix 5 prices stated are per dressing or bandage.

BNF prices are not suitable for quoting to patients seeking private prescriptions or contemplating over-the-counter purchases because they do not take into account VAT, professional fees, and other overheads.

A fuller explanation of costs to the NHS may be obtained from the Drug Tariff. Separate drug tariffs are applicable to England and Wales (www.ppa.org.uk/ppa/edt_intro.htm), Scotland (www.isdscotland.org/Health-Topics/Prescribing-and-Medicines/Scottish-Drug-Tariff/), and Northern Ireland (www.dhsspsni.gov.uk/pas-tariff); prices in the different tariffs may vary.

Extra resources on the BNF website

The BNF website (bnf.org) provides additional resources such as an archive of the e-newsletter and policies.

Using other sources for medicines information

The BNF is designed as a digest for rapid reference. Less detail is given on areas such as obstetrics, malignant disease, and anaesthesia since it is expected that those undertaking treatment will have specialist knowledge and access to specialist literature. *BNF for Children* should be consulted for detailed information on the use of medicines in children. The BNF should be interpreted in the light of professional knowledge and supplemented as necessary by specialised publications and by reference to the product literature. Information is also available from medicines information services (see inside front cover).

Changes

Monthly updates are provided online via Medicines-Complete and the NHS Evidence portal. The changes listed below are cumulative (from one print edition to the next).

Significant changes

Significant changes have been made in the following sections for BNF 69:

Sodium oxybate: change to schedule under the Misuse of Drugs Regulations 2001 (and subsequent amendments), see *Xyrem*® and Controlled Drugs and Drug Dependence

Drugs and driving: new legal offence expected to come into force on 2nd March 2015, see Drugs and Driving, p. 3

Lubiprostone for treating chronic idiopathic constipation [NICE guidance], section 1.6.7

Atrial fibrillation: NICE clinical guideline 180, section 2.3.1

Concomitant use of drugs affecting the renin-angiotensin system [MHRA advice], section 2.5.5

Intravenous nicardipine for the treatment of acute life-threatening hypertension and postoperative hypertension, section 2.6.2

Ivabradine: risk of bradycardia [MHRA advice], section 2.6.3

Prasugrel with percutaneous coronary intervention for treating acute coronary syndromes [NICE guidance], section 2.9

Lipid Modification—cardiovascular risk assessment and the modification of blood lipids for the primary and secondary prevention of cardiovascular disease [NICE guidance] and Joint British Societies' consensus recommendations for the prevention of cardiovascular disease (JBS3) 2014, section 2.12

Nalmefene for reducing alcohol consumption in people with alcohol dependence [NICE guidance], section 4.10.1

Malaria prophylaxis recommendations for specific countries [update], section 5.4.1

Canagliflozin in combination therapy for treating type 2 diabetes [NICE guidance], section 6.1.2.3

Denosumab: osteonecrosis of the jaw and hypocalcaemia [MHRA advice], section 6.6.2

Dabrafenib for treating unresectable or metastatic BRAF V600 mutation-positive melanoma [NICE guidance], section 8.1.5

Imatinib for the adjuvant treatment of gastro-intestinal stromal tumours [NICE guidance], section 8.1.5

Ipilimumab for previously untreated advanced (unresectable or metastatic) melanoma [NICE guidance], section 8.1.5

Ponatinib: risk of vascular occlusive events [MHRA/CHM advice], section 8.1.5

Dimethyl fumarate for treating relapsing-remitting multiple sclerosis [NICE guidance], section 8.2.4

Lenalidomide for treating myelodysplastic syndromes associated with an isolated deletion 5q cytogenetic abnormality [NICE guidance], section 8.2.4

Enzalutamide for metastatic hormone-relapsed prostate cancer previously treated with a docetaxel-containing regimen [NICE guidance], section 8.3.4.2

The license suspension for the tetrastarches *Volulyte*® and *Voluven*® has been lifted, and both products have been re-introduced into the market following a recent European regulatory review, see section 9.2.2.2

Chlorhexidine solutions: risk of chemical burns in pre-term neonates, section 13.11.2

Varicella-zoster vaccine (*Zostavax*®), updated 2014-15 immunisation programme for prevention of herpes zoster, section 14.4

Pertussis vaccine [change to *Boostrix-IPV*® for immunisation of pregnant women], section 14.4

Dose changes

Changes in dose statements introduced into BNF 69:

Acipimox, p. 181

Atorvastatin, p. 175

Co-careldopa, p. 331

Ironorm® Drops, p. 661

Methadone [opioid dependence], p. 346

Pentasa® [dose for acute attack], p. 64

Ponatinib [initial dose with potent CYP3A4 inhibitors], p. 618

Propiverine hydrochloride, p. 565

Sodium clodronate [dose in renal impairment], p. 527

Sodium oxybate [concomitant use with valproate], p. 230

Zopiclone, p. 229

Classification changes

Classification changes have been made in the following sections for BNF 69:

New names

Name changes introduced into BNF 69:

Deleted preparations

Preparations discontinued during the compilation of BNF 69:

ACWY Vax®

Amifostine

Caprin® 300 mg tablets [75 mg tablets still available]

Carbo-Dome®

Cilazapril

Dexamethasone injection 4 mg/mL [other strengths available]

Ethyol®

Glucophage® oral powder

Isogel®

Probenecid

Rhinolast®

Rivotril® tablets [generic still available]

Testosterone implant

Vascace®

Vectavir®

Viroflu®

Vistide®

Zerolatum® *Plus*

New preparations

New preparations included in the relevant sections of BNF 69:

Anoro Ellipta® [umeclidinium with vilanterol], p. 196

Cometriq® [cabozantinib], p. 613

Daklinza® [daclatasvir], p. 439

Deltyba® [delamanid], p. 401

Entyvio® [vedolizumab], p. 69

Fomicyt® [fosfomycin], p. 390

Gazyvaro®, p. 638

Glytrin spray® [glyceryl trinitrate], p. 130

Granupas® [aminosalicylic acid], p. 400

Imbruvica® [ibrutinib], p. 616

Incruse Ellipta® [umeclidinium], p. 194

Infanrix®-*IPV+Hib* [Diphtheria, Tetanus, Pertussis (Acellular, Component), Poliomyelitis (Inactivated) and Haemophilus Type b Conjugate Vaccine (Adsorbed)], p. 849

InVita D3® [colecalciferol], p. 705

Isradipine [new generic], p. 136

Jardiance® [empagliflozin], p. 482

Latuda® [lurasidone hydrochloride], p. 244

Nicardipine injection [new generic], p. 137

Olena® [fluoxetine], p. 262

Olysio® [simeprevir], p. 439

Optaflu® [seasonal influenza vaccine], p. 856

Plegridy® [peginterferon beta-1a], p. 641

Sirturo® [bedaquiline], p. 400

Striverdi Respimat® [olodaterol], p. 190

Sylvant® [siltuximab], p. 649

Treclin® [tretinoin with clindamycin], p. 822

Triumeq® [abacavir with lamivudine and dolutegravir], p. 421

Tybost® [cobicistat], p. 431

Veletri® [epoprostenol], p. 152

Vibativ® [telavancin], p. 393

Vitaros® [alprostadil], p. 570

Vokanamet® [canagliflozin with metformin], p. 481

Volulyte® [tetrastarch]; re-introduced, p. 687

Voluven® [tetrastarch]; re-introduced, p. 687

Xultophy® [liraglutide with insulin degludec], p. 483

Zedbac® [azithromycin intravenous infusion], p. 387

Zydelig® [idelalisib], p. 616

Guidance on prescribing

General guidance

Medicines should be prescribed only when they are necessary, and in all cases the benefit of administering the medicine should be considered in relation to the risk involved. This is particularly important during pregnancy, when the risk to both mother and fetus must be considered (for further details see Prescribing in Pregnancy, p. 19).

It is important to discuss treatment options carefully with the patient to ensure that the patient is content to take the medicine as prescribed (see also Taking Medicines to Best Effect, below). In particular, the patient should be helped to distinguish the adverse effects of prescribed drugs from the effects of the medical disorder. When the beneficial effects of the medicine are likely to be delayed, the patient should be advised of this.

Taking medicines to best effect Difficulties in adherence to drug treatment occur regardless of age. Factors contributing to poor compliance with prescribed medicines include:

* prescription not collected or not dispensed;
* purpose of medicine not clear;
* perceived lack of efficacy;
* real or perceived adverse effects;
* patients' perception of the risk and severity of side-effects may differ from that of the prescriber;
* instructions for administration not clear;
* physical difficulty in taking medicines (e.g. swallowing the medicine, handling small tablets, or opening medicine containers);
* unattractive formulation (e.g. unpleasant taste);
* complicated regimen.

The prescriber and the patient should agree on the health outcomes that the patient desires and on the strategy for achieving them ('concordance'). The prescriber should be sensitive to religious, cultural, and personal beliefs that can affect a patient's acceptance of medicines.

Taking the time to explain to the patient (and relatives) the rationale and the potential adverse effects of treatment may improve adherence. Reinforcement and elaboration of the physician's instructions by the pharmacist and other members of the healthcare team also helps. Advising the patient of the possibility of alternative treatments may encourage the patient to seek advice rather than merely abandon unacceptable treatment.

Simplifying the drug regimen may help; the need for frequent administration may reduce adherence, although there appears to be little difference in adherence between once-daily and twice-daily administration. Combination products reduce the number of drugs taken but at the expense of the ability to titrate individual doses.

Biosimilar medicines A biosimilar medicine is a new biological product that is similar to a medicine that has already been authorised to be marketed (the biolo-gical reference medicine) in the European Union. The active substance of a biosimilar medicine is similar, but not identical, to the biological reference medicine. Biological products are different from standard chemical products in terms of their complexity and although theoretically there should be no important differences between the biosimilar and the biological reference medicine in terms of safety or efficacy, when prescribing biological products, it is good practice to use the brand name. This will ensure that substitution of a biosimilar medicine does not occur when the medicine is dispensed.

Biosimilar medicines have black triangle status (▼, see p. 12) at the time of initial marketing. It is important to report suspected adverse reactions to biosimilar medicines using the Yellow Card Scheme (p. 12). For biosimilar medicines, adverse reaction reports should clearly state the brand name and the batch number of the suspected medicine.

Complementary and alternative medicine An increasing amount of information on complementary and alternative medicine is becoming available. The scope of the BNF is restricted to the discussion of conventional medicines but reference is made to complementary treatments if they affect conventional therapy (e.g. interactions with St John's wort—see Appendix 1). Further information on herbal medicines is available at www.mhra.gov.uk.

Abbreviation of titles In general, titles of drugs and preparations should be written *in full*. Unofficial abbreviations should not be used as they may be misinterpreted.

Non-proprietary titles Where non-proprietary ('generic') titles are given, they should be used in prescribing. This will enable any suitable product to be dispensed, thereby saving delay to the patient and sometimes expense to the health service. The only exception is where there is a demonstrable difference in clinical effect between each manufacturer's version of the formulation, making it important that the patient should always receive the same brand; in such cases, the brand name or the manufacturer should be stated. Non-proprietary titles should **not** be invented for the purposes of prescribing generically since this can lead to confusion, particularly in the case of compound and modified-release preparations.

Titles used as headings for monographs may be used freely in the United Kingdom but in other countries may be subject to restriction.

Many of the non-proprietary titles used in this book are titles of monographs in the European Pharmacopoeia, British Pharmacopoeia, or British Pharmaceutical Codex 1973. In such cases the preparations must comply with the standard (if any) in the appropriate publication, as required by the Human Medicines Regulations 2012.

General guidance

Proprietary titles   Names followed by the symbol® are or have been used as proprietary names in the United Kingdom. These names may in general be applied only to products supplied by the owners of the trade marks.

Marketing authorisation and BNF advice   In general the *doses, indications, cautions, contra-indications,* and *side-effects* in the BNF reflect those in the manufacturers' data sheets or Summaries of Product Characteristics (SPCs) which, in turn, reflect those in the corresponding marketing authorisations (formerly known as Product Licences). The BNF does not generally include proprietary medicines that are not supported by a valid Summary of Product Characteristics or when the marketing authorisation holder has not been able to supply essential information. When a preparation is available from more than one manufacturer, the BNF reflects advice that is the most clinically relevant regardless of any variation in the marketing authorisations. Unlicensed products can be obtained from 'special-order' manufacturers or specialist importing companies, see p. 1124.

Where an unlicensed drug is included in the BNF, this is indicated in square brackets after the entry. When the BNF suggests a use (or route) that is outside the licensed indication of a product ('off-label' use), this too is indicated. Unlicensed use of medicines becomes necessary if the clinical need cannot be met by licensed medicines; such use should be supported by appropriate evidence and experience.

The doses stated in the BNF are intended for general guidance and represent, unless otherwise stated, the usual range of doses that are generally regarded as being suitable for adults.

> **Prescribing unlicensed medicines**
>
> Prescribing medicines outside the recommendations of their marketing authorisation alters (and probably increases) the prescriber's professional responsibility and potential liability. The prescriber should be able to justify and feel competent in using such medicines, and also inform the patient or the patient's carer that the prescribed medicine is unlicensed.

Oral syringes   An **oral syringe** is supplied when oral liquid medicines are prescribed in doses other than multiples of 5 mL. The oral syringe is marked in 0.5-mL divisions from 1 to 5 mL to measure doses of less than 5 mL (other sizes of oral syringe may also be available). It is provided with an adaptor and an instruction leaflet. The *5-mL spoon* is used for doses of 5 mL (or multiples thereof).

> **Important**
>
> To avoid inadvertent intravenous administration of oral liquid medicines, only an appropriate **oral** or **enteral syringe** should be used to measure an oral liquid medicine (if a medicine spoon or graduated measure cannot be used); these syringes should **not** be compatible with intravenous or other parenteral devices. Oral or enteral syringes should be clearly labelled 'Oral' or 'Enteral' in a large font size; it is the healthcare practitioner's responsibility to label the syringe with this information if the manufacturer has not done so.

Excipients   Branded oral liquid preparations that do not contain *fructose, glucose,* or *sucrose* are described as 'sugar-free' in the BNF. Preparations containing hydrogenated glucose syrup, mannitol, maltitol, sorbitol, or xylitol are also marked 'sugar-free' since there is evidence that they do not cause dental caries. Patients receiving medicines containing cariogenic sugars should be advised of appropriate dental hygiene measures to prevent caries. Sugar-free preparations should be used whenever possible.

Where information on the presence of *aspartame, gluten, sulfites, tartrazine, arachis (peanut) oil* or *sesame oil* is available, this is indicated in the BNF against the relevant preparation.

Information is provided on *selected excipients* in skin preparations (section 13.1.3), in vaccines (section 14.1), and on *selected preservatives* and *excipients* in eye drops and injections.

The presence of *benzyl alcohol* and *polyoxyl castor oil* (polyethoxylated castor oil) in injections is indicated in the BNF. Benzyl alcohol has been associated with a fatal toxic syndrome in preterm neonates, and therefore, parenteral preparations containing the preservative should not be used in neonates. Polyoxyl castor oils, used as vehicles in intravenous injections, have been associated with severe anaphylactoid reactions.

The presence of *propylene glycol* in oral or parenteral medicines is indicated in the BNF; it can cause adverse effects if its elimination is impaired, e.g. in renal failure, in neonates and young children, and in slow metabolisers of the substance. It may interact with disulfiram and metronidazole.

The *lactose* content in most medicines is too small to cause problems in most lactose-intolerant patients. However in severe lactose intolerance, the lactose content should be determined before prescribing. The amount of lactose varies according to manufacturer, product, formulation, and strength.

> **Important**
>
> In the absence of information on excipients in the BNF and in the product literature (available at www.medicines.org.uk/emc), contact the manufacturer (see Index of Manufacturers) if it is essential to check details.

Extemporaneous preparation   A product should be dispensed extemporaneously only when no product with a marketing authorisation is available.

The BP direction that a preparation must be *freshly prepared* indicates that it must be made not more than 24 hours before it is issued for use. The direction that a preparation should be *recently prepared* indicates that deterioration is likely if the preparation is stored for longer than about 4 weeks at 15–25° C.

The term **water** used without qualification means either potable water freshly drawn direct from the public supply and suitable for drinking or freshly boiled and cooled purified water. The latter should be used if the public supply is from a local storage tank or if the potable water is unsuitable for a particular preparation (Water for injections, section 9.2.2).

Drugs and driving Prescribers and other healthcare professionals should advise patients if treatment is likely to affect their ability to perform skilled tasks (e.g. driving). This applies especially to drugs with sedative effects; patients should be warned that these effects are increased by alcohol. General information about a patient's fitness to drive is available from the Driver and Vehicle Licensing Agency at www.dvla.gov.uk.

A new offence of driving, attempting to drive, or being in charge of a vehicle, with certain specified controlled drugs in excess of specified limits, is expected to come into force on 2nd March 2015. This offence is an addition to the existing rules on drug impaired driving and fitness to drive (see above), and applies to two groups of drugs—commonly abused drugs, including cannabis, cocaine, and ketamine, and drugs used mainly for medical reasons, such as opioids and benzodiazepines. Amfetamines are also expected to be added to the legislation later in 2015. Anyone found to have any of the drugs (including related drugs, for example, apomorphine) above specified limits in their blood will be guilty of an offence, whether their driving was impaired or not. This also includes prescribed drugs which metabolise to those included in the offence, for example, selegiline. However, the legislation provides a statutory "medical defence" for patients taking drugs for medical reasons in accordance with instructions, *if their driving was not impaired* — it continues to be an offence to drive if actually impaired. Patients should therefore be advised to continue taking their medicines as prescribed, and when driving, to carry suitable evidence that the drug was prescribed, or sold, to treat a medical or dental problem, and that it was taken according to the instructions given by the prescriber, or information provided with the medicine (e.g. a repeat prescription form or the medicine's patient information leaflet). Further information is available from the Department for Transport at www.gov.uk/government/collections/drug-driving

Patents In the BNF, certain drugs have been included notwithstanding the existence of actual or potential patent rights. In so far as such substances are protected by Letters Patent, their inclusion in this Formulary neither conveys, nor implies, licence to manufacture.

Health and safety When handling chemical or biological materials particular attention should be given to the possibility of allergy, fire, explosion, radiation, or poisoning. Substances such as corticosteroids, some antimicrobials, phenothiazines, and many cytotoxics, are irritant or very potent and should be handled with caution. Contact with the skin and inhalation of dust should be avoided.

Safety in the home Patients must be warned to keep all medicines out of the reach of children. All solid dose and all oral and external liquid preparations must be dispensed in a reclosable *child-resistant container* unless:

- the medicine is in an original pack or patient pack such as to make this inadvisable;
- the patient will have difficulty in opening a child-resistant container;
- a specific request is made that the product shall not be dispensed in a child-resistant container;
- no suitable child-resistant container exists for a particular liquid preparation.

All patients should be advised to dispose of *unwanted medicines* by returning them to a supplier for destruction.

Labelling of prescribed medicines There is a legal requirement for the following to appear on the label of any prescribed medicine:

- name of the patient;
- name and address of the person dispensing the medicine;
- date of dispensing;
- name of the medicine;
- directions for use of the medicine;
- precautions relating to the use of the medicine.

The Royal Pharmaceutical Society recommends that the following also appears on the label:

- the words 'Keep out of the sight and reach of children';
- where applicable, the words 'Use this medicine only on your skin'.

A pharmacist can exercise professional skill and judgement to amend or include more appropriate wording for the name of the medicine, the directions for use, or the precautions relating to the use of the medicine.

> **Non-proprietary names of compound preparations**
>
> Non-proprietary names of **compound preparations** which appear in the BNF are those that have been compiled by the British Pharmacopoeia Commission or another recognised body; whenever possible they reflect the names of the active ingredients.
>
> Prescribers should avoid creating their own compound names for the purposes of generic prescribing; such names do not have an approved definition and can be misinterpreted.
>
> Special care should be taken to avoid errors when prescribing compound preparations; in particular the hyphen in the prefix 'co-' should be retained.
>
> Special care should also be taken to avoid creating generic names for **modified-release** preparations where the use of these names could lead to confusion between formulations with different lengths of action.

EEA and Swiss prescriptions Pharmacists can dispense prescriptions issued by doctors and dentists from the European Economic Area (EEA) or Switzerland (except prescriptions for controlled drugs in Schedules 1, 2, or 3, or for drugs without a UK marketing authorisation). Prescriptions should be written in ink or otherwise so as to be indelible, should be dated, should state the name of the patient, should state the address of the prescriber, should contain particulars indicating whether the prescriber is a doctor or dentist, and should be signed by the prescriber.

Security and validity of prescriptions The Councils of the British Medical Association and the Royal Pharmaceutical Society have issued a joint statement on the security and validity of prescriptions.

In particular, prescription forms should:

- not be left unattended at reception desks;
- not be left in a car where they may be visible; and

- when not in use, be kept in a locked drawer within the surgery and at home.

Where there is any doubt about the authenticity of a prescription, the pharmacist should contact the prescriber. If this is done by telephone, the number should be obtained from the directory rather than relying on the information on the prescription form, which may be false.

Patient group direction (PGD)   In most cases, the most appropriate clinical care will be provided on an individual basis by a prescriber to a specific individual patient. However, a Patient Group Direction for supply and administration of medicines by other healthcare professionals can be used where it would benefit patient care without compromising safety.

A Patient Group Direction is a written direction relating to the supply and administration (or administration only) of a licensed prescription-only medicine (including some Controlled Drugs in specific circumstances) by certain classes of healthcare professionals; the Direction is signed by a doctor (or dentist) and by a pharmacist. Further information on Patient Group Directions is available in Health Service Circular HSC 2000/026 (England), HDL (2001) 7 (Scotland), and WHC (2000) 116 (Wales); see also the Human Medicines Regulations 2012.

NICE and Scottish Medicines Consortium   Advice issued by the National Institute for Health and Care Excellence (NICE) is included in the BNF when relevant. The BNF also includes advice issued by the Scottish Medicines Consortium (SMC) when a medicine is restricted or not recommended for use within NHS Scotland. If advice within a NICE Single Technology Appraisal differs from SMC advice, the Scottish Executive expects NHS Boards within NHS Scotland to comply with the SMC advice. Details of the advice together with updates can be obtained from www.nice.org.uk and from www.scottishmedicines.org.uk.

Prescription writing

Prescriptions[1] should be written legibly in ink or otherwise so as to be indelible[2], should be dated, should state the name and address of the patient, the address of the prescriber, an indication of the type of prescriber, and should be signed in ink by the prescriber[3]. The age and the date of birth of the patient should preferably be stated, and it is a legal requirement in the case of prescription-only medicines to state the age for children under 12 years.

The following should be noted:

(a) The strength or quantity to be contained in capsules, lozenges, tablets etc. should be stated by the prescriber. In particular, strength of liquid preparations should be clearly stated (e.g. 125 mg/5 mL).

(b) The unnecessary use of decimal points should be avoided, e.g. 3 mg, not 3.0 mg.

Quantities of 1 gram or more should be written as 1 g etc.

Quantities less than 1 gram should be written in milligrams, e.g. 500 mg, not 0.5 g.

Quantities less than 1 mg should be written in micrograms, e.g. 100 micrograms, not 0.1 mg.

When decimals are unavoidable a zero should be written in front of the decimal point where there is no other figure, e.g. 0.5 mL, not .5 mL.

Use of the decimal point is acceptable to express a range, e.g. 0.5 to 1 g.

(c) 'Micrograms' and 'nanograms' should **not** be abbreviated. Similarly 'units' should **not** be abbreviated.

(d) The term 'millilitre' (ml or mL)[4] is used in medicine and pharmacy, and cubic centimetre, c.c., or cm^3 should not be used.

(e) Dose and dose frequency should be stated; in the case of preparations to be taken 'as required' a **minimum dose interval** should be specified.

When doses other than multiples of 5 mL are prescribed for *oral liquid preparations* the dose-volume will be provided by means of an **oral syringe**, see p. 2 (except for preparations intended to be measured with a pipette).

Suitable quantities:

Elixirs, Linctuses, and Paediatric Mixtures (5-mL dose), 50, 100, or 150 mL

Adult Mixtures (10-mL dose), 200 or 300 mL

Ear Drops, Eye drops, and Nasal Drops, 10 mL (or the manufacturer's pack)

Eye Lotions, Gargles, and Mouthwashes, 200 mL

(f) For suitable quantities of dermatological preparations, see section 13.1.2.

(g) The names of drugs and preparations should be written clearly and **not** abbreviated, using approved titles **only** (see also advice in box on p. 3 to **avoid** creating generic titles for modified-release preparations).

(h) The quantity to be supplied may be stated by indicating the number of days of treatment required in the box provided on NHS forms. In most cases the exact amount will be supplied. This does not apply to items directed to be used as required—if the dose and frequency are not given then the quantity to be supplied needs to be stated.

When several items are ordered on one form the box can be marked with the number of days of treatment provided the quantity is added for any item for which the amount cannot be calculated.

(i) Although directions should preferably be in **English without abbreviation**, it is recognised that some Latin abbreviations are used (for details see Inside Back Cover).

For a sample prescription, see below.

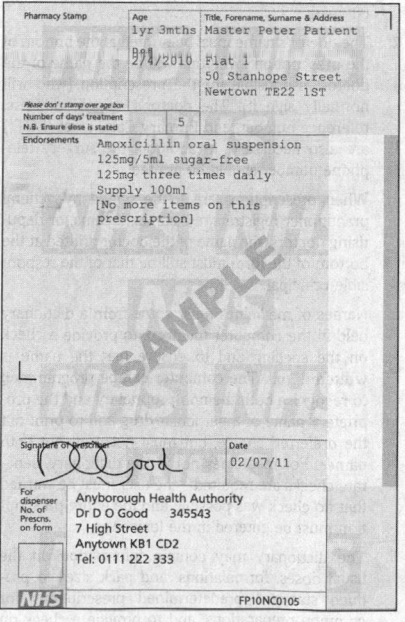

---

1. These recommendations are acceptable for **prescription-only medicines** (PoM). For items marked CD1, CD2, CD3, CD4-1, and CD4-2 see also Controlled Drugs and Drug Dependence, p. 8.
2. It is permissible to issue carbon copies of NHS prescriptions as long as they are signed in ink.
3. Computer-generated facsimile signatures do not meet the legal requirement.
4. The use of capital 'L' in mL is a printing convention throughout the BNF; both 'mL' and 'ml' are recognised SI abbreviations.

Prescribing by dentists Until new prescribing arrangements are in place for NHS prescriptions, dentists should use form FP10D (GP14 in Scotland, WP10D in Wales) to prescribe only those items listed in the Dental Practitioners' Formulary. The Human Medicines Regulations 2012 does not set any limitations upon the number and variety of substances which the dentist may administer to patients in the surgery or may order by private prescription—provided the relevant legal requirements are observed the dentist may use or order whatever is required for the clinical situation. There is no statutory requirement for the dentist to communicate with a patient's medical practitioner when prescribing for dental use. There are, however, occasions when this would be in the patient's interest and such communication is to be encouraged. For legal requirements relating to prescriptions for Controlled Drugs, see p. 8.

Computer-issued prescriptions

For computer-issued prescriptions the following advice, based on the recommendations of the Joint GP Information Technology Committee, should also be noted:

1. The computer must print out the date, the patient's surname, one forename, other initials, and address, and may also print out the patient's title and date of birth. The age of children under 12 years and of adults over 60 years must be printed in the box available; the age of children under 5 years should be printed in years and months. A facility may also exist to print out the age of patients between 12 and 60 years.

2. The doctor's name must be printed at the bottom of the prescription form; this will be the name of the doctor responsible for the prescription (who will normally sign it). The doctor's surgery address, reference number, and Primary Care Trust (PCT[1]) are also necessary. In addition, the surgery telephone number should be printed.

3. When prescriptions are to be signed by general practitioner registrars, assistants, locums, or deputising doctors, the name of the doctor printed at the bottom of the form must still be that of the responsible principal.

4. Names of medicines must come from a dictionary held in the computer memory, to provide a check on the spelling and to ensure that the name is written in full. The computer can be programmed to recognise both the non-proprietary and the proprietary name of a particular drug and to print out the preferred choice, but must not print out both names. For medicines not in the dictionary, separate checks are required—the user must be warned that no check was possible and the entire prescription must be entered in the lexicon.

5. The dictionary may contain information on the usual doses, formulations, and pack sizes to produce standard predetermined prescriptions for common preparations, and to provide a check on the validity of an individual prescription on entry.

6. The prescription must be printed in English without abbreviation; information may be entered or stored in abbreviated form. The dose must be in numbers, the frequency in words, and the quantity in numbers in brackets, thus: 40 mg four times daily (112). It must also be possible to prescribe by indicating the length of treatment required, see (h) above.

7. The BNF recommendations should be followed as in (a), (b), (c), (d), and (e) above.

8. Checks may be incorporated to ensure that all the information required for dispensing a particular drug has been filled in. For instructions such as 'as directed' and 'when required', the maximum daily dose should normally be specified.

9. Numbers and codes used in the system for organising and retrieving data must never appear on the form.

10. Supplementary warnings or advice should be written in full, should not interfere with the clarity of the prescription itself, and should be in line with any warnings or advice in the BNF; numerical codes should not be used.

11. A mechanism (such as printing a series of non-specific characters) should be incorporated to cancel out unused space, or wording such as 'no more items on this prescription' may be added after the last item. Otherwise the doctor should delete the space manually.

12. To avoid forgery the computer may print on the form the number of items to be dispensed (somewhere separate from the box for the pharmacist). The number of items per form need be limited only by the ability of the printer to produce clear and well-demarcated instructions with sufficient space for each item and a spacer line before each fresh item.

13. Handwritten alterations should only be made in exceptional circumstances—it is preferable to print out a new prescription. Any alterations must be made in the doctor's own handwriting and countersigned; computer records should be updated to fully reflect any alteration. Prescriptions for drugs used for contraceptive purposes (but which are not promoted as contraceptives) may need to be marked in handwriting with the symbol ♀ (or endorsed in another way to indicate that the item is prescribed for contraceptive purposes).

14. Prescriptions for controlled drugs can be printed from the computer, but the prescriber's signature must be handwritten[2].

15. The strip of paper on the side of the FP10SS[3] may be used for various purposes but care should be taken to avoid including confidential information. It may be advisable for the patient's name to appear at the top, but this should be preceded by 'confidential'.

16. In rural dispensing practices prescription requests (or details of medicines dispensed) will normally be entered in one surgery. The prescriptions (or dispensed medicines) may then need to be delivered to another surgery or location; if possible the computer should hold up to 10 alternatives.

17. Prescription forms that are reprinted or issued as a duplicate should be labelled clearly as such.

---

1. Health Board in Scotland, Local Health Board in Wales.

2. See Controlled Drugs and Drug Dependence p. 8; the prescriber may use a date stamp.

3. GP10SS in Scotland, WP10SS in Wales.

Emergency supply of medicines

Emergency supply requested by member of the public

Pharmacists are sometimes called upon by members of the public to make an emergency supply of medicines. The Human Medicines Regulations 2012 allows exemptions from the Prescription Only requirements for emergency supply to be made by a person lawfully conducting a retail pharmacy business provided:

(a) that the pharmacist has interviewed the person requesting the prescription-only medicine and is satisfied:

  (i) that there is immediate need for the prescription-only medicine and that it is impracticable in the circumstances to obtain a prescription without undue delay;

  (ii) that treatment with the prescription-only medicine has on a previous occasion been prescribed for the person requesting it;

  (iii) as to the dose that it would be appropriate for the person to take;

(b) that no greater quantity shall be supplied than will provide 5 days' treatment of phenobarbital, phenobarbital sodium, or Controlled Drugs in Schedules 4 or 5,[1] or 30 days' treatment for other prescription-only medicines, except when the prescription-only medicine is:

  (i) insulin, an ointment or cream, or a preparation for the relief of asthma in an aerosol dispenser when the smallest pack can be supplied;

  (ii) an oral contraceptive when a full cycle may be supplied;

  (iii) an antibiotic in liquid form for oral administration when the smallest quantity that will provide a full course of treatment can be supplied;

(c) that an entry shall be made by the pharmacist in the prescription book stating:

  (i) the date of supply;

  (ii) the name, quantity and, where appropriate, the pharmaceutical form and strength;

  (iii) the name and address of the patient;

  (iv) the nature of the emergency;

(d) that the container or package must be labelled to show:

  (i) the date of supply;

  (ii) the name, quantity and, where appropriate, the pharmaceutical form and strength;

  (iii) the name of the patient;

  (iv) the name and address of the pharmacy;

  (v) the words 'Emergency supply';

  (vi) the words 'Keep out of the reach of children' (or similar warning);

(e) that the prescription-only medicine is not a substance specifically excluded from the emergency supply provision, and does not contain a Controlled Drug specified in Schedules 1, 2, or 3 to the Misuse of Drugs Regulations 2001 except for phenobarbital or phenobarbital sodium for the treatment of epilepsy: for details see *Medicines, Ethics and Practice*, London, Pharmaceutical Press (always consult latest edition).[1]

Emergency supply requested by prescriber

Emergency supply of a prescription-only medicine may also be made at the request of a doctor, a dentist, a supplementary prescriber, a community practitioner nurse prescriber, a nurse, pharmacist, or optometrist independent prescriber, or a doctor or dentist from the European Economic Area or Switzerland, provided:

(a) that the pharmacist is satisfied that the prescriber by reason of some emergency is unable to furnish a prescription immediately;

(b) that the prescriber has undertaken to furnish a prescription within 72 hours;

(c) that the medicine is supplied in accordance with the directions of the prescriber requesting it;

(d) that the medicine is not a Controlled Drug specified in Schedules 1, 2, or 3 to the Misuse of Drugs Regulations 2001 except for phenobarbital or phenobarbital sodium for the treatment of epilepsy: for details see *Medicines, Ethics and Practice*, London, Pharmaceutical Press (always consult latest edition);[1]

(e) that an entry shall be made in the prescription book stating:

  (i) the date of supply;

  (ii) the name, quantity and, where appropriate, the pharmaceutical form and strength;

  (iii) the name and address of the practitioner requesting the emergency supply;

  (iv) the name and address of the patient;

  (v) the date on the prescription;

  (vi) when the prescription is received the entry should be amended to include the date on which it is received.

Royal Pharmaceutical Society's guidelines

1. The pharmacist should consider the medical consequences of *not* supplying a medicine in an emergency.

2. If the pharmacist is unable to make an emergency supply of a medicine the pharmacist should advise the patient how to obtain essential medical care.

For conditions that apply to supplies made at the request of a patient see *Medicines, Ethics and Practice*, London Pharmaceutical Press, (always consult latest edition).

---

1. Doctors or dentists from the European Economic Area and Switzerland, or their patients, cannot request an emergency supply of Controlled Drugs in Schedules 1, 2, or 3, or drugs that do not have a UK marketing authorisation.

Controlled Drugs and drug dependence

The Misuse of Drugs Act, 1971 prohibits certain activities in relation to 'Controlled Drugs', in particular their manufacture, supply, and possession. The penalties applicable to offences involving the different drugs are graded broadly according to the *harmfulness attributable to a drug when it is misused* and for this purpose the drugs are defined in the following three classes:

Class A includes: alfentanil, cocaine, diamorphine (heroin), dipipanone, lysergide (LSD), methadone, methylenedioxymethamfetamine (MDMA, 'ecstasy'), morphine, opium, pethidine, phencyclidine, remifentanil, and class B substances when prepared for injection

Class B includes: oral amfetamines, barbiturates, cannabis, cannabis resin, codeine, ethylmorphine, glutethimide, ketamine, nabilone, pentazocine, phenmetrazine, and pholcodine

Class C includes: certain drugs related to the amfetamines such as benzfetamine and chlorphentermine, buprenorphine, diethylpropion, mazindol, meprobamate, pemoline, pipradrol, most benzodiazepines, tramadol, zaleplon, zolpidem, zopiclone, androgenic and anabolic steroids, clenbuterol, chorionic gonadotrophin (HCG), non-human chorionic gonadotrophin, somatotropin, somatrem, and somatropin

The Misuse of Drugs Regulations 2001 (and subsequent amendments) define the classes of person who are authorised to supply and possess controlled drugs while acting in their professional capacities and lay down the conditions under which these activities may be carried out. In the regulations drugs are divided into five schedules each specifying the requirements governing such activities as import, export, production, supply, possession, prescribing, and record keeping which apply to them.

Schedule 1 includes drugs such as lysergide which is not used medicinally. Possession and supply are prohibited except in accordance with Home Office authority.

Schedule 2 includes drugs such as diamorphine (heroin), morphine, nabilone, remifentanil, pethidine, secobarbital, glutethimide, the amfetamines, sodium oxybate, and cocaine and are subject to the full controlled drug requirements relating to prescriptions, safe custody (except for secobarbital), the need to keep registers, etc. (unless exempted in Schedule 5).

Schedule 3 includes the barbiturates (except secobarbital, now Schedule 2), buprenorphine, diethylpropion, mazindol, meprobamate, midazolam, pentazocine, phentermine, temazepam, and tramadol. They are subject to the special prescription requirements (except for temazepam) and to the safe custody requirements (except for any 5,5 disubstituted barbituric acid (e.g. phenobarbital), mazindol, meprobamate, midazolam, pentazocine, phentermine, tramadol, or any stereoisomeric form or salts of the above). Records in registers do not need to be kept (although there are requirements for the retention of invoices for 2 years).

Schedule 4 includes in Part I benzodiazepines (except temazepam and midazolam, which are in Schedule 3), zaleplon, zolpidem, and zopiclone which are subject to minimal control. Part II includes androgenic and anabolic steroids, clenbuterol, chorionic gonadotrophin (HCG), non-human chorionic gonadotrophin, somatotropin, somatrem, and somatropin. Controlled drug prescription requirements do not apply and Schedule 4 Controlled Drugs are not subject to safe custody requirements.

Schedule 5 includes those preparations which, because of their strength, are exempt from virtually all Controlled Drug requirements other than retention of invoices for two years.

Prescriptions Preparations in Schedules 1, 2, 3, and 4 of the Misuse of Drugs Regulations 2001 (and subsequent amendments) are identified throughout the BNF using the following symbols:

- CD1 for preparations in Schedule 1;
- CD2 for preparations in Schedule 2;
- CD3 for preparations in Schedule 3;
- CD4-1 for preparations in Schedule 4 (Part I);
- CD4-2 for preparations in Schedule 4 (Part II).

The principal legal requirements relating to medical prescriptions are listed below (see also Department of Health Guidance, p. 9).

Prescription requirements

Prescriptions for Controlled Drugs that are subject to prescription requirements[1] must be indelible,[2] and must be *signed* by the prescriber, *be dated,* and specify the prescriber's *address*. The prescription must always state:

- the name and address of the patient;
- in the case of a preparation, the form[3] and where appropriate the strength[4] of the preparation;
- for liquids, the total volume in millilitres (in both words and figures) of the preparation to be supplied; for dosage units, the number (in both words and figures) of dosage units to be supplied; in any other case, the total quantity (in both words and figures) of the Controlled Drug to be supplied;
- the dose;[5]
- the words 'for dental treatment only' if issued by a dentist.

A pharmacist is **not** allowed to dispense a Controlled Drug unless all the information required by law is given on the prescription. In the case of a prescription for a Controlled Drug in Schedule 2 or 3, a pharmacist can amend the prescription if it specifies the total quantity

1. All preparations in Schedules 2 and 3, except temazepam.
2. A machine-written prescription is acceptable. The prescriber's signature must be handwritten.
3. The dosage form (e.g. tablets) must be included on a Controlled Drugs prescription irrespective of whether it is implicit in the proprietary name (e.g. *MST Continus*) or whether only one form is available.
4. When more than one strength of a preparation exists the strength required must be specified.
5. The instruction 'one as directed' constitutes a dose but 'as directed' does not.

only in words or in figures or if it contains minor typographical errors, provided that such amendments are indelible and clearly attributable to the pharmacist. Failure to comply with the regulations concerning the writing of prescriptions will result in inconvenience to patients and delay in supplying the necessary medicine. A prescription for a Controlled Drug in Schedules 2, 3, or 4 is valid for 28 days from the date stated thereon.[1]

Instalments and 'repeats'

A prescription may order a Controlled Drug to be dispensed by instalments; the amount of instalments and the intervals to be observed must be specified.[2]

Instalment prescriptions must be dispensed in accordance with the directions in the prescription. However, the Home Office has approved specific wording which may be included in an instalment prescription to cover certain situations; for example, if a pharmacy is closed on the day when an instalment is due. For details, see *Medicines, Ethics and Practice*, London, Pharmaceutical Press (always consult latest edition) or see *Drug Misuse and Dependence: UK Guidelines on Clinical Management* (2007), available at www.nta.nhs.uk/uploads/clinical_guidelines_2007.pdf.

Prescriptions ordering 'repeats' on the same form are **not** permitted for Controlled Drugs in Schedules 2 or 3.

Private prescriptions

Private prescriptions for Controlled Drugs in Schedules 2 and 3 must be written on specially designated forms provided by Primary Care Trusts in England, Health Boards in Scotland, Local Health Boards in Wales, or the Northern Ireland Central Services Agency; in addition, prescriptions must specify the *prescriber's identification number*. Prescriptions to be supplied by a pharmacist in hospital are exempt from the requirements for private prescriptions.

Department of Health guidance

Guidance (June 2006) issued by the Department of Health in England on prescribing and dispensing of Controlled Drugs requires:

- in general, prescriptions for Controlled Drugs in Schedules 2, 3, and 4 to be limited to a supply of up to 30 days' treatment; exceptionally, to cover a justifiable clinical need and after consideration of any risk, a prescription can be issued for a longer period, but the reasons for the decision should be recorded on the patient's notes;

- the patient's identifier to be shown on NHS and private prescriptions for Controlled Drugs in Schedules 2 and 3.

Further information is available at www.gov.uk/dh.

---

1. The prescriber may forward-date the prescription; the start date may also be specified in the body of the prescription.
2. A total of 14 days' treatment by instalment of any drug listed in Schedule 2 of the Misuse of Drugs Regulations, buprenorphine, and diazepam may be prescribed in England. In *England*, forms FP10(MDA) (blue) and FP10H (MDA) (blue) should be used. In *Scotland*, forms GP10 (peach), HBP (blue), or HBPA (pink) should be used. In *Wales* a total of 14 days' treatment by instalment of any drug listed in Schedules 2–5 of the Misuse of Drugs Regulations may be prescribed. In Wales, form WP10(MDA) or form WP10HP(AD) should be used.

For a sample prescription, see below.

Dependence and misuse

The most serious drugs of addiction are **cocaine**, **diamorphine** (heroin), **morphine**, and the **synthetic opioids**. For arrangements for prescribing of diamorphine, dipipanone, or cocaine for addicts, see p. 11.

Despite marked reduction in the prescribing of **amfetamines**, there is concern that abuse of illicit amfetamine and related compounds is widespread.

Benzodiazepines are commonly misused. However, the misuse of **barbiturates** is now uncommon, in line with declining medicinal use and consequent availability.

Cannabis (Indian hemp) has no approved medicinal use and cannot be prescribed by doctors. Its use is illegal but widespread. Cannabis is a mild hallucinogen seldom accompanied by a desire to increase the dose; withdrawal symptoms are unusual. However, cannabis extract is licensed as a medicinal product, see p. 748. **Lysergide** (lysergic acid diethylamide, LSD) is a much more potent hallucinogen; its use can lead to severe psychotic states which can be life-threatening.

There are concerns over increases in the availability and misuse of other drugs with variously combined hallucinogenic, anaesthetic, or sedative properties. These include ketamine and gamma-hydroxybutyrate (sodium oxybate, GHB).

Supervised consumption

Individuals prescribed opioid substitution therapy (section 4.10.3) can take their daily dose under the supervision of a doctor, nurse, or pharmacist during the dose stabilisation phase (usually the first 3 months of treatment), after a relapse or period of instability, or if there is a significant increase in the dose of methadone. Supervised consumption should continue (in accordance with local protocols) until the prescriber is confident that the patient is compliant with their treatment.

Controlled Drugs and drug dependence *(side tab)*

Prescribing drugs likely to cause dependence or misuse The prescriber has three main responsibilities:

- To avoid creating dependence by introducing drugs to patients without sufficient reason. In this context, the proper use of the morphine-like drugs is well understood. The dangers of other Controlled Drugs are less clear because recognition of dependence is not easy and its effects, and those of withdrawal, are less obvious.

- To see that the patient does not gradually increase the dose of a drug, given for good medical reasons, to the point where dependence becomes more likely. This tendency is seen especially with hypnotics and anxiolytics (for CSM advice see section 4.1). The prescriber should keep a close eye on the amount prescribed to prevent patients from accumulating stocks. A minimal amount should be prescribed in the first instance, or when seeing a new patient for the first time.

- To avoid being used as an unwitting source of supply for addicts. Methods include visiting more than one doctor, fabricating stories, and forging prescriptions.

Patients under temporary care should be given only small supplies of drugs unless they present an unequivocal letter from their own doctor. Doctors should also remember that their own patients may be attempting to collect prescriptions from other prescribers, especially in hospitals. It is sensible to reduce dosages steadily or to issue weekly or even daily prescriptions for small amounts if it is apparent that dependence is occurring.

The stealing and misuse of prescription forms could be minimised by the following precautions:

- do not leave unattended if called away from the consulting room or at reception desks; do not leave in a car where they may be visible; when not in use, keep in a locked drawer within the surgery and at home;

- draw a diagonal line across the blank part of the form under the prescription;

- write the quantity in words and figures when prescribing drugs prone to abuse; this is obligatory for controlled drugs (see Prescriptions, above);

- alterations are best avoided but if any are made they should be clear and unambiguous; add initials against altered items;

- if prescriptions are left for collection they should be left in a safe place in a sealed envelope.

Travelling abroad Prescribed drugs listed in Schedule 4 Part II (CD Anab) and Schedule 5 of the Misuse of Drugs Regulations 2001 are not subject to export or import licensing. However, patients intending to travel abroad for more than 3 months carrying any amount of drugs listed in Schedules 2, 3, or 4 Part I (CD Benz) will require a personal export/import licence. Further details can be obtained at www.gov.uk/controlled-drugs-licences-fees-and-returns, or from the Home Office by contacting licensing_enquiry.aadu@homeoffice.gsi.gov.uk (in cases of emergency, telephone (020) 7035 6330).

Applications must be supported by a covering letter from the prescriber and should give details of:

- the patient's name and address;
- the quantities of drugs to be carried;
- the strength and form in which the drugs will be dispensed;
- the country or countries of destination;
- the dates of travel to and from the United Kingdom.

Applications for licences should be sent to the Home Office, Drugs Licensing & Compliance Unit, Fry Building, 2 Marsham Street, London, SW1P 4DF. Alternatively, completed application forms can be emailed to dlcucommsofficer@homeoffice.gsi.gov.uk with a copy of the covering letter from the prescriber as a pdf. A minimum of two weeks should be allowed for processing the application.

Patients travelling for less than 3 months do not require a personal export/import licence for carrying Controlled Drugs, but are advised to carry a letter from the prescribing doctor. Those travelling for more than 3 months are advised to make arrangements to have their medication prescribed by a practitioner in the country they are visiting.

Doctors who want to take Controlled Drugs abroad while accompanying patients may similarly be issued with licences. Licences are not normally issued to doctors who want to take Controlled Drugs abroad solely in case a family emergency should arise.

Personal export/import licences do not have any legal status outside the UK and are issued only to comply with the Misuse of Drugs Act and to facilitate passage through UK Customs and Excise control. For clearance in the country to be visited it is necessary to approach that country's consulate in the UK.

Notification of patients receiving structured drug treatment for substance dependence

In **England**, doctors should report cases where they are providing structured drug treatment for substance dependence to their local National Drug Treatment Monitoring System (NDTMS) Team. General information about NDTMS can be found at www.nta.nhs.uk/ndtms.aspx.

Enquiries about NDTMS, and how to submit data, should initially be directed to:

Malcom Roxburgh
NTA Information Manager
Tel: (020) 7972 1964
malcolm.roxburgh@nta-nhs.org.uk

In **Scotland**, doctors should report cases to the Substance Misuse Programme (SMP).

Tel: (0131) 275 6348

In **Northern Ireland**, the Misuse of Drugs (Notification of and Supply to Addicts) (Northern Ireland) Regulations 1973 require doctors to send particulars of persons whom they consider to be addicted to certain controlled drugs to the Chief Medical Officer of the Department of Health and Social Services. The Northern Ireland contacts are:

Medical contact:

Dr Ian McMaster
C3 Castle Buildings
Belfast, BT4 3FQ
Tel: (028) 9052 2421
Fax: (028) 9052 0718
ian.mcmaster@dhsspsni.gov.uk

Administrative contact:

Public Health Information & Research Branch
Annex 2
Castle Building
Belfast, BT4 3SQ
Tel: (028) 9052 2520

Public Health Information & Research Branch also maintains the Northern Ireland Drug Misuse Database (NIDMD) which collects detailed information on those presenting for treatment, on drugs misused and injecting behaviour; participation is not a statutory requirement.

In **Wales**, doctors should report cases where they are providing structured drug treatment for substance dependence on the Welsh National Database for Substance Misuse; enquiries should be directed to: substance.misuse-queries@wales.nhs.uk

Prescribing of diamorphine (heroin), dipipanone, and cocaine for addicts

The Misuse of Drugs (Supply to Addicts) Regulations 1997 require that only medical practitioners who hold a special licence issued by the Home Secretary may prescribe, administer, or supply diamorphine, dipipanone (*Diconal®*), or cocaine in the treatment of drug addiction; other practitioners must refer any addict who requires these drugs to a treatment centre. Whenever possible the addict will be introduced by a member of staff from the treatment centre to a pharmacist whose agreement has been obtained and whose pharmacy is conveniently sited for the patient. Prescriptions for weekly supplies will be sent to the pharmacy by post and will be dispensed on a daily basis as indicated by the doctor. If any alterations of the arrangements are requested by the addict, the portion of the prescription affected must be represcribed and not merely altered.

General practitioners and other doctors do not require a special licence for prescribing diamorphine, dipipanone, and cocaine for patients (including addicts) for *relieving pain* from organic disease or injury.

For guidance on prescription writing, see p. 8.

Adverse reactions to drugs

Adverse reactions to drugs

Any drug may produce unwanted or unexpected adverse reactions. Rapid detection and recording of adverse drug reactions is of vital importance so that unrecognised hazards are identified promptly and appropriate regulatory action is taken to ensure that medicines are used safely. Healthcare professionals and coroners (see also Self-reporting below) are urged to report suspected adverse drug reactions directly to the Medicines and Healthcare products Regulatory Agency (MHRA) through the Yellow Card Scheme using the electronic form at www.mhra.gov.uk/yellowcard. Alternatively, prepaid Yellow Cards for reporting are available from the address below and are also bound in this book (inside back cover).

Send Yellow Cards to:

FREEPOST YELLOW CARD
(No other address details required)
Tel: 0800 731 6789

Suspected adverse drug reactions to *any* therapeutic agent should be reported, including drugs (*self-medication* as well as those *prescribed*), blood products, vaccines, radiographic contrast media, complementary and herbal products. For biosimilar medicines and vaccines, adverse reaction reports should clearly state the brand name and the batch number of the suspected medicine or vaccine.

Suspected adverse drug reactions should be reported through the Yellow Card Scheme at www.mhra.gov.uk/yellowcard. Yellow Cards can be used for reporting suspected adverse drug reactions to medicines, vaccines, herbal or complementary products, whether self-medicated or prescribed. This includes suspected adverse drug reactions associated with misuse, overdose, medication errors or from use of unlicensed and off-label medicines.

Spontaneous reporting is particularly valuable for recognising possible new hazards rapidly. An adverse reaction should be reported even if it is not certain that the drug has caused it, or if the reaction is well recognised, or if other drugs have been given at the same time. Reports of overdoses (deliberate or accidental) can complicate the assessment of adverse drug reactions, but provide important information on the potential toxicity of drugs.

A freephone service is available to all parts of the UK for advice and information on suspected adverse drug reactions; contact the National Yellow Card Information Service at the MHRA on 0800 731 6789. Outside office hours a telephone-answering machine will take messages.

The following Yellow Card Centres can be contacted for further information:

Yellow Card Centre
Northwest
2nd Floor
70 Pembroke Place
Liverpool L69 3GF
Tel: (0151) 794 8122

Yellow Card Centre Wales
Cardiff University
Department of Pharmacology, Therapeutics and Toxicology
Heath Park
Cardiff CF14 4XN
Tel: (029) 2074 4181

Yellow Card Centre
Northern & Yorkshire
Wolfson Unit
Claremont Place
Newcastle upon
Tyne NE2 4HH
Tel: (0191) 260 6182

Yellow Card Centre
Scotland
CARDS, Royal Infirmary
of Edinburgh
51 Little France Crescent
Old Dalkeith Road
Edinburgh EH16 4SA
Tel: (0131) 242 2919
YCCScotland@luht.scot.nhs.uk

Yellow Card Centre West
Midlands
City Hospital
Dudley Road
Birmingham B18 7QH
Tel: (0121) 507 5672

The MHRA's database facilitates the monitoring of adverse drug reactions.

More detailed information on reporting and a list of products currently under additional monitoring can be found on the MHRA website: www.mhra.gov.uk.

MHRA Drug Safety Update
Drug Safety Update is a monthly newsletter from the MHRA and the Commission on Human Medicines (CHM); it is available at www.mhra.gov.uk/drugsafetyupdate.

Self-reporting   Patients and their carers can also report suspected adverse drug reactions to the MHRA. Reports can be submitted directly to the MHRA through the Yellow Card Scheme using the electronic form at www.mhra.gov.uk/yellowcard, by telephone on 0808 100 3352, or by downloading the Yellow Card form from www.mhra.gov.uk. Alternatively, patient Yellow Cards are available from pharmacies and GP surgeries. Information for patients about the Yellow Card Scheme is available in other languages at www.mhra.gov.uk/yellowcard.

Prescription-event monitoring   In addition to the MHRA's Yellow Card Scheme, an independent scheme monitors the safety of new medicines using a different approach. The Drug Safety Research Unit identifies patients who have been prescribed selected new medicines and collects data on clinical events in these patients. The data are submitted on a voluntary basis by general practitioners on green forms. More information about the scheme and the Unit's educational material is available from www.dsru.org.

Newer drugs and vaccines   Only limited information is available from clinical trials on the safety of new medicines. Further understanding about the safety of medicines depends on the availability of information from routine clinical practice.

The black triangle symbol (▼) identifies newly licensed medicines that require additional monitoring by the European Medicines Agency. Such medicines include new active substances, biosimilar medicines, and medicines that the European Medicines Agency consider require additional monitoring. The black triangle symbol also appears in the Patient Information Leaflets for relevant medicines, with a brief explanation of what it means. Products usually retain a black triangle for 5 years, but this can be extended if required.

Spontaneous reporting is particularly valuable for recognising possible new hazards rapidly. For medicines showing the black triangle symbol, the MHRA asks that **all** suspected reactions (including those considered not to be serious) are reported through the Yellow Card Scheme. An adverse reaction should be reported even if it is not certain that the drug has caused it, or if the reaction is well recognised, or if other drugs have been given at the same time.

Established drugs and vaccines   Healthcare professionals and coroners are asked to report all suspected reactions to established drugs (including over-the-counter, herbal, and unlicensed medicines and medicines used off-label) and vaccines that are **serious, medically significant, or result in harm**. Serious reactions include those that are fatal, life-threatening, disabling, incapacitating, or which result in or prolong hospitalisation, or a congenital abnormality; they should be reported even if the effect is well recognised. Examples include anaphylaxis, blood disorders, endocrine disturbances, effects on fertility, haemorrhage from any site, renal impairment, jaundice, ophthalmic disorders, severe CNS effects, severe skin reactions, reactions in pregnant women, and any drug interactions. Reports of serious adverse reactions are required to enable comparison with other drugs of a similar class. Reports of overdoses (deliberate or accidental) can complicate the assessment of adverse drug reactions, but provide important information on the potential toxicity of drugs.

For established drugs there is no need to report well-known, relatively minor side-effects, such as dry mouth with tricyclic antidepressants or constipation with opioids.

Medication errors   Adverse drug reactions where harm occurs as a result of a medication error are reportable as a Yellow Card or through the local risk management systems into the National Reporting and Learning System (NRLS). If reported to the NRLS, these will be shared with the MHRA. If the NRLS is not available and harm occurs, report using a Yellow Card.

Adverse reactions to medical devices   Suspected adverse reactions to medical devices including dental or surgical materials, intra-uterine devices, and contact lens fluids should be reported. Information on reporting these can be found at: www.mhra.gov.uk.

Side-effects in the BNF   The BNF includes clinically relevant side-effects for most drugs; an exhaustive list is not included for drugs that are used by specialists (e.g. cytotoxic drugs and drugs used in anaesthesia). Where causality has not been established, side-effects in the manufacturers' literature may be omitted from the BNF.

Recognising that hypersensitivity reactions can occur with virtually all medicines, this effect is not generally listed, unless the drug carries an increased risk of such reactions. The BNF also omits effects that are likely to have little clinical consequence (e.g. transient increase in liver enzymes).

Side-effects are generally listed in order of frequency and arranged broadly by body systems. Occasionally a rare side-effect might be listed first if it is considered to be particularly important because of its seriousness.

In the product literature the frequency of side-effects is generally described as follows:

Very common	greater than 1 in 10
Common	1 in 100 to 1 in 10
Uncommon ['less commonly' in BNF]	1 in 1000 to 1 in 100
Rare	1 in 10 000 to 1 in 1000
Very rare	less than 1 in 10 000

Special problems

Delayed drug effects   Some reactions (e.g. cancers, chloroquine retinopathy, and retroperitoneal fibrosis) may become manifest months or years after exposure. Any suspicion of such an association should be reported directly to the MHRA through the Yellow Card Scheme.

The elderly   Particular vigilance is required to identify adverse reactions in the elderly.

Congenital abnormalities   When an infant is born with a congenital abnormality or there is a malformed aborted fetus doctors are asked to consider whether this might be an adverse reaction to a drug and to report all drugs (including self-medication) taken during pregnancy.

Children   Particular vigilance is required to identify and report adverse reactions in children, including those resulting from the unlicensed use of medicines; **all** suspected reactions should be reported directly to the MHRA through the Yellow Card Scheme (see also Adverse Drug Reactions in Children, p. 15).

Prevention of adverse reactions

Adverse reactions may be prevented as follows:

- never use any drug unless there is a good indication. If the patient is pregnant do not use a drug unless the need for it is imperative;

- allergy and idiosyncrasy are important causes of adverse drug reactions. Ask if the patient had previous reactions;

- ask if the patient is already taking other drugs *including self-medication drugs, health supplements, complementary and alternative therapies*; interactions may occur;

- age and hepatic or renal disease may alter the metabolism or excretion of drugs, so that much smaller doses may be needed. Genetic factors may also be responsible for variations in metabolism, notably of isoniazid and the tricyclic antidepressants;

- prescribe as few drugs as possible and give very clear instructions to the elderly or any patient likely to misunderstand complicated instructions;

- whenever possible use a familiar drug; with a new drug, be particularly alert for adverse reactions or unexpected events;

- warn the patient if serious adverse reactions are liable to occur.

Oral side-effects of drugs

Drug-induced disorders of the mouth may be due to a local action on the mouth or to a systemic effect manifested by oral changes. In the latter case urgent

Adverse reactions to drugs

Adverse reactions to drugs

referral to the patient's medical practitioner may be necessary.

Oral mucosa

Medicaments left in contact with or applied directly to the oral mucosa can lead to inflammation or ulceration; the possibility of allergy should also be borne in mind.

Aspirin tablets allowed to dissolve in the sulcus for the treatment of toothache can lead to a white patch followed by ulceration.

Flavouring agents, particularly **essential oils**, may sensitise the skin, but mucosal swelling is not usually prominent.

The oral mucosa is particularly vulnerable to ulceration in patients treated with cytotoxic drugs, e.g. **methotrexate**. Other drugs capable of causing oral ulceration include **ACE inhibitors, gold, nicorandil, NSAIDs, pancreatin, penicillamine, proguanil,** and **protease inhibitors**.

Erythema multiforme or Stevens-Johnson syndrome may follow the use of a wide range of drugs including **antibacterials, antiretrovirals, sulfonamide derivatives,** and **anticonvulsants**; the oral mucosa may be extensively ulcerated, with characteristic target lesions on the skin. Oral lesions of toxic epidermal necrolysis have been reported with a similar range of drugs.

Lichenoid eruptions are associated with **ACE inhibitors, NSAIDs, methyldopa, chloroquine, oral antidiabetics, thiazide diuretics,** and **gold**.

Candidiasis can complicate treatment with **antibacterials** and **immunosuppressants** and is an occasional side-effect of **corticosteroid inhalers**, see also p. 200.

Teeth and Jaw

Brown staining of the teeth frequently follows the use of **chlorhexidine** mouthwash, spray or gel, but can readily be removed by polishing. **Iron** salts in liquid form can stain the enamel black. Superficial staining has been reported rarely with **co-amoxiclav** suspension.

Intrinsic staining of the teeth is most commonly caused by **tetracyclines**. They will affect the teeth if given at any time from about the fourth month *in utero* until the age of twelve years; they are contra-indicated during pregnancy, in breast-feeding women, and in children under 12 years. All tetracyclines can cause permanent, unsightly staining in children, the colour varying from yellow to grey.

Excessive ingestion of **fluoride** leads to *dental fluorosis* with mottling of the enamel and areas of hypoplasia or pitting; fluoride supplements occasionally cause mild mottling (white patches) if the dose is too large for the child's age (taking into account the fluoride content of the local drinking water and of toothpaste).

The risk of *osteonecrosis of the jaw* is substantially greater for patients receiving intravenous bisphosphonates in the treatment of cancer than for patients receiving oral bisphosphonates for osteoporosis or Paget's disease. All patients receiving bisphosphonates should have a dental check-up (and any necessary remedial work should be performed) before bisphosphonate treatment, or as soon as possible after starting treatment, see also Bisphosphonates: Osteonecrosis of the Jaw, p. 524. For cancer patients taking bevacizumab or sunitinib, see also MHRA/CHM advice (Bevacizumab and sunitinib: risk of osteonecrosis of the jaw), p. 595.

Periodontium

Gingival overgrowth (gingival hyperplasia) is a side-effect of **phenytoin** and sometimes of **ciclosporin** or of **nifedipine** (and some other calcium-channel blockers).

Thrombocytopenia may be drug related and may cause bleeding at the gingival margins, which may be spontaneous or may follow mild trauma (such as toothbrushing).

Salivary glands

The most common effect that drugs have on the salivary glands is to *reduce flow* (xerostomia). Patients with a persistently dry mouth may have poor oral hygiene; they are at an increased risk of dental caries and oral infections (particularly candidiasis). Many drugs have been implicated in xerostomia, particularly **antimuscarinics** (anticholinergics), **antidepressants** (including tricyclic antidepressants, and selective serotonin reuptake inhibitors), **alpha-blockers, antihistamines, antipsychotics, baclofen, bupropion, clonidine,** $5HT_1$ **agonists, opioids,** and **tizanidine**. Excessive use of **diuretics** can also result in xerostomia.

Some drugs (e.g. clozapine, neostigmine) can *increase saliva production* but this is rarely a problem unless the patient has associated difficulty in swallowing.

Pain in the salivary glands has been reported with some **antihypertensives** (e.g. clonidine, methyldopa) and with **vinca alkaloids**.

Swelling of the salivary glands can occur with **iodides, antithyroid drugs, phenothiazines,** and **sulfonamides**.

Taste

There can be *decreased* taste acuity or *alteration* in taste sensation. Many drugs are implicated, including **amiodarone, calcitonin, ACE inhibitors, carbimazole, clarithromycin, gold, griseofulvin, lithium salts, metformin, metronidazole, penicillamine, phenindione, propafenone, protease inhibitors, terbinafine,** and **zopiclone**.

Defective medicines

During the manufacture or distribution of a medicine an error or accident may occur whereby the finished product does not conform to its specification. While such a defect may impair the therapeutic effect of the product and could adversely affect the health of a patient, it should **not** be confused with an Adverse Drug Reaction where the product conforms to its specification.

The Defective Medicines Report Centre assists with the investigation of problems arising from licensed medicinal products thought to be defective and co-ordinates any necessary protective action. Reports on suspect defective medicinal products should include the brand or the non-proprietary name, the name of the manufacturer or supplier, the strength and dosage form of the product, the product licence number, the batch number or numbers of the product, the nature of the defect, and an account of any action already taken in consequence. The Centre can be contacted at:

The Defective Medicines Report Centre
Medicines and Healthcare products Regulatory Agency
151 Buckingham Palace Road
London, SW1W 9SZ
Tel: (020) 3080 6588
info@mhra.gsi.gov.uk

Prescribing for children

> For detailed advice on medicines used for children, consult *BNF for Children*

Children, and particularly neonates, differ from adults in their response to drugs. Special care is needed in the neonatal period (first 28 days of life) and doses should always be calculated with care. At this age, the risk of toxicity is increased by reduced drug clearance and differing target organ sensitivity.

Whenever possible, intramuscular injections should be **avoided** in children because they are painful.

Where possible, medicines for children should be prescribed within the terms of the marketing authorisation (product licence). However, many children may require medicines not specifically licensed for paediatric use.

Although medicines cannot be promoted outside the limits of the licence, the Human Medicines Regulations 2012 does not prohibit the use of unlicensed medicines. It is recognised that the informed use of unlicensed medicines or of licensed medicines for unlicensed applications ('off-label' use) is often necessary in paediatric practice.

Adverse drug reactions in children   Suspected adverse drug reactions in children and young adults under 18 years should be reported through the Yellow Card Scheme (see p. 12). Yellow cards can be used for reporting suspected adverse drug reactions to medicines, vaccines, herbal or complementary products, whether self-medicated or prescribed. This includes suspected adverse drug reactions associated with misuse, overdose, medication errors or from use of unlicensed and off-label medicines.

Report all suspected adverse drug reactions that are:

- **serious, medically significant or result in harm**. Serious events are fatal, life-threatening, a congenital abnormality, disabling or incapacitating, or resulting in hospitalisation;

- associated with **newer drugs and vaccines (▼)**; the most up to date list of black triangle medicines is available at: www.mhra.gov.uk/blacktriangle

If in doubt whether to report a suspected adverse drug reaction, please complete a Yellow Card.

The identification and reporting of adverse reactions to drugs in children and neonates is particularly important because:

- the action of the drug and its pharmacokinetics in children (especially in the very young) may be different from that in adults;

- drugs may not have been extensively tested in children;

- many drugs are not specifically licensed for use in children and are used either 'off-label' or as unlicensed products;

- drugs may affect the way a child grows and develops or may cause delayed adverse reactions which do not occur in adults;

- suitable formulations may not be available to allow precise dosing in children or they may contain excipients that should be used with caution in children;

- the nature and course of illnesses and adverse drug reactions may differ between adults and children.

Even if reported through the British Paediatric Surveillance Unit's Orange Card Scheme, any identified suspected adverse drug reactions should also be submitted to the Yellow Card Scheme.

Adverse drug reactions where harm occurs as a result of a medication error are reportable as a Yellow Card or through the local risk management systems into the National Reporting and Learning System (NRLS). If reported to the NRLS, these will be shared with the MHRA. If the NRLS is not available and harm occurs, report using a Yellow Card.

Prescription writing   Prescriptions should be written according to the guidelines in Prescription Writing (p. 5) Inclusion of age is a legal requirement in the case of prescription-only medicines for children under 12 years of age, but it is preferable to state the age for **all** prescriptions for children.

It is particularly important to state the strengths of capsules or tablets. Although liquid preparations are particularly suitable for children, they may contain sugar which encourages dental decay. Sugar-free medicines are preferred for long-term treatment.

Many children are able to swallow tablets or capsules and may prefer a solid dose form; involving the child and parents in choosing the formulation is helpful.

When a prescription for a liquid oral preparation is written and the dose ordered is smaller than 5 mL an **oral syringe** will be supplied (for details, see p. 2). Parents should be advised not to add any medicines to the infant's feed, since the drug may interact with the milk or other liquid in it; moreover the ingested dosage may be reduced if the child does not drink all the contents.

Parents must be warned to keep **all** medicines out of reach of children, see Safety in the Home, p. 3.

Rare paediatric conditions

Information on substances such as *biotin* and *sodium benzoate* used in rare metabolic conditions is included in *BNF for Children*; further information can be obtained from:

Alder Hey Children's Hospital
Drug Information Centre
Liverpool L12 2AP
Tel: (0151) 252 5381

Great Ormond Street Hospital for Children
Pharmacy
Great Ormond St
London WC1N 3JH
Tel: (020) 7405 9200

Dosage in children

Children's doses in the BNF are stated in the individual drug entries or a cross-reference is provided to *BNF for Children*.

Prescribing for children

Doses are generally based on body-weight (in kilograms) or the following age ranges:

first month (neonate)

up to 1 year (infant)

1–6 years

6–12 years

Dose calculation   Many children's doses are standardised by **weight** (and therefore require multiplying by the body-weight in kilograms to determine the child's dose); occasionally, the doses have been standardised by **body surface area** (in m^2). These methods should be used rather than attempting to calculate a child's dose on the basis of doses used in adults.

For most drugs the adult maximum dose should not be exceeded. For example if the dose is stated as 8 mg/kg (max. 300 mg), a child weighing 10 kg should receive 80 mg but a child weighing 40 kg should receive 300 mg (rather than 320 mg).

Young children may require a higher dose per kilogram than adults because of their higher metabolic rates. Other problems need to be considered. For example, calculation by body-weight in the overweight child may result in much higher doses being administered than necessary; in such cases, dose should be calculated from an ideal weight, related to height and age (see inside back cover).

Body surface area (BSA) estimates are sometimes preferable to body-weight for calculation of paediatric doses since many physiological phenomena correlate better with body surface area. Body surface area can be estimated from weight. For more information, refer to *BNF for Children*.

Where the dose for children is not stated, prescribers should consult *BNF for Children* or seek advice from a medicines information centre.

Dose frequency   Antibacterials are generally given at regular intervals throughout the day. Some flexibility should be allowed in children to avoid waking them during the night. For example, the night-time dose may be given at the child's bedtime.

Where new or potentially toxic drugs are used, the manufacturers' recommended doses should be carefully followed.

Prescribing in hepatic impairment

Liver disease may alter the response to drugs in several ways as indicated below, and drug prescribing should be kept to a minimum in all patients with severe liver disease. The main problems occur in patients with jaundice, ascites, or evidence of encephalopathy.

Impaired drug metabolism Metabolism by the liver is the main route of elimination for many drugs, but hepatic reserve is large and liver disease has to be severe before important changes in drug metabolism occur. Routine liver-function tests are a poor guide to the capacity of the liver to metabolise drugs, and in the individual patient it is not possible to predict the extent to which the metabolism of a particular drug may be impaired.

A few drugs, e.g. rifampicin and fusidic acid, are excreted in the bile unchanged and can accumulate in patients with intrahepatic or extrahepatic obstructive jaundice.

Hypoproteinaemia The hypoalbuminaemia in severe liver disease is associated with reduced protein binding and increased toxicity of some highly protein-bound drugs such as phenytoin and prednisolone.

Reduced clotting Reduced hepatic synthesis of blood-clotting factors, indicated by a prolonged prothrombin time, increases the sensitivity to oral anticoagulants such as warfarin and phenindione.

Hepatic encephalopathy In severe liver disease many drugs can further impair cerebral function and may precipitate hepatic encephalopathy. These include all sedative drugs, opioid analgesics, those diuretics that produce hypokalaemia, and drugs that cause constipation.

Fluid overload Oedema and ascites in chronic liver disease can be exacerbated by drugs that give rise to fluid retention, e.g. NSAIDs and corticosteroids.

Hepatotoxic drugs Hepatotoxicity is either dose-related or unpredictable (idiosyncratic). Drugs that cause dose-related toxicity may do so at lower doses in the presence of hepatic impairment than in individuals with normal liver function, and some drugs that produce reactions of the idiosyncratic kind do so more frequently in patients with liver disease. These drugs should be avoided or used very carefully in patients with liver disease.

Where care is needed when prescribing in hepatic impairment, this is indicated under the relevant drug in the BNF.

Prescribing in renal impairment

The use of drugs in patients with reduced renal function can give rise to problems for several reasons:

- reduced renal excretion of a drug or its metabolites may cause toxicity;
- sensitivity to some drugs is increased even if elimination is unimpaired;
- many side-effects are tolerated poorly by patients with renal impairment;
- some drugs are not effective when renal function is reduced.

Many of these problems can be avoided by reducing the dose or by using alternative drugs.

Principles of dose adjustment in renal impairment

The level of renal function below which the dose of a drug must be reduced depends on the proportion of the drug eliminated by renal excretion and its toxicity.

For many drugs with only minor or no dose-related side-effects very precise modification of the dose regimen is unnecessary and a simple scheme for dose reduction is sufficient.

For more toxic drugs with a small safety margin or patients at extremes of weight, dose regimens based on creatinine clearance (see below for details) should be used. When both efficacy and toxicity are closely related to plasma-drug concentration, recommended regimens should be regarded only as a guide to initial treatment; subsequent doses must be adjusted according to clinical response and plasma-drug concentration.

Renal function declines with age; many elderly patients have renal impairment but, because of reduced muscle mass, this may not be indicated by a raised serum creatinine. It is wise to assume at least mild impairment of renal function when prescribing for the elderly.

The total daily maintenance dose of a drug can be reduced either by reducing the size of the individual doses or by increasing the interval between doses. For some drugs, although the size of the maintenance dose is reduced it is important to give a loading dose if an immediate effect is required. This is because it takes about five times the half-life of the drug to achieve steady-state plasma concentrations. Because the plasma half-life of drugs excreted by the kidney is prolonged in renal impairment it can take many doses for the reduced dosage to achieve a therapeutic plasma concentration. The loading dose should usually be the same size as the initial dose for a patient with normal renal function.

Nephrotoxic drugs should, if possible, be avoided in patients with renal disease because the consequences of nephrotoxicity are likely to be more serious when renal reserve is already reduced.

Dose recommendations are based on the severity of renal impairment.

Renal function is measured either in terms of estimated **glomerular filtration rate** (eGFR) calculated from a formula derived from the Modification of Diet in Renal

Disease study ('MDRD formula' that uses serum creatinine, age, sex, and race (for Afro-Caribbean patients)) or it can be expressed as **creatinine clearance** (best derived from a 24-hour urine collection but often calculated from the Cockcroft and Gault formula (CG).

Cockcroft and Gault formula

$$\text{Estimated Creatinine Clearance in mL/minute} = \frac{(140 - \text{Age}) \times \text{Weight} \times \text{Constant}}{\text{Serum creatinine}}$$

Age in years
Weight in kilograms; use ideal body-weight
Serum creatinine in micromol/litre
Constant = 1.23 for men; 1.04 for women

The serum-creatinine concentration is sometimes used instead as a measure of renal function but it is only a **rough guide** to drug dosing.

Important

Renal function in adults is increasingly being reported on the basis of estimated glomerular filtration rate (eGFR) normalised to a body surface area of 1.73 m^2 and derived from the Modification of Diet in Renal Disease (MDRD) formula. However, published information on the effects of renal impairment on drug elimination is usually stated in terms of creatinine clearance as a surrogate for glomerular filtration rate (GFR).

The information on dosage adjustment in the BNF is expressed in terms of eGFR, rather than creatinine clearance, for most drugs (see exceptions below: Toxic Drugs and Patients at Extremes of Weight). Although the two measures of renal function are not interchangeable, in practice, for most drugs and for most patients (over 18 years) of average build and height, eGFR (MDRD 'formula') can be used to determine dosage adjustments in place of creatinine clearance. An individual's absolute glomerular filtration rate can be calculated from the eGFR as follows:

GFR $_{\text{Absolute}}$ = eGFR × (individual's body surface area/1.73)

Toxic drugs For potentially toxic drugs with a small safety margin, creatinine clearance (calculated from the Cockcroft and Gault formula) should be used to adjust drug dosages in addition to plasma-drug concentration and clinical response.

Patients at extremes of weight In patients at both extremes of weight (BMI of less than 18.5 kg/m^2 or greater than 30 kg/m^2) the absolute glomerular filtration rate or creatinine clearance (calculated from the Cockcroft and Gault formula) should be used to adjust drug dosages.

In the BNF, values for eGFR, creatinine clearance (for toxic drugs), or another measure of renal function are included where possible. However, where such values are not available, the BNF reflects the terms used in the published information.

Chronic kidney disease in adults: UK guidelines for identification, management and referral (March 2006) define renal function as follows:

Degree of impairment	eGFR mL/minute/1.73 m^2
Normal - Stage 1	More than 90 (with other evidence of kidney damage)
Mild - Stage 2	60–89 (with other evidence of kidney damage)
Moderate[1] - Stage 3	30–59
Severe - Stage 4	15–29
Established renal failure - Stage 5	Less than 15

1. NICE clinical guideline 73 (September 2008)—Chronic kidney disease: Stage 3A eGFR 45–59, Stage 3B eGFR 30–44

Dialysis

For prescribing in patients on continuous ambulatory peritoneal dialysis (CAPD) or haemodialysis, consult specialist literature.

Drug prescribing should be kept to the minimum in all patients with severe renal disease.

If even mild renal impairment is considered likely on clinical grounds, renal function should be checked before prescribing **any** drug which requires dose modification.

Where care is needed when prescribing in renal impairment, this is indicated under the relevant drug in the BNF.

Prescribing in pregnancy

Drugs can have harmful effects on the embryo or fetus at any time during pregnancy. It is important to bear this in mind when prescribing for a woman of *childbearing age* or for men *trying* to *father* a child.

During the *first trimester* drugs can produce congenital malformations (teratogenesis), and the period of greatest risk is from the third to the eleventh week of pregnancy.

During the *second* and *third trimesters* drugs can affect the growth or functional development of the fetus, or they can have toxic effects on fetal tissues.

Drugs given shortly before term or during labour can have adverse effects on labour or on the neonate after delivery.

Not all the damaging effects of intrauterine exposure to drugs are obvious at birth, some may only manifest later in life. Such late-onset effects include malignancy, e.g. adenocarcinoma of the vagina after puberty in females exposed to diethylstilbestrol in the womb, and adverse effects on intellectual, social, and functional development.

The BNF identifies drugs which:

- may have harmful effects in pregnancy and indicates the trimester of risk
- are not known to be harmful in pregnancy

The information is based on human data, but information from *animal* studies has been included for some drugs when its omission might be misleading.

Where care is needed when prescribing in pregnancy, this is indicated under the relevant drug in the BNF.

> **Important**
> Drugs should be prescribed in pregnancy only if the expected benefit to the mother is thought to be greater than the risk to the fetus, and all drugs should be avoided if possible during the first trimester. Drugs which have been extensively used in pregnancy and appear to be usually safe should be prescribed in preference to new or untried drugs; and the smallest effective dose should be used.
> Few drugs have been shown conclusively to be teratogenic in humans, but no drug is safe beyond all doubt in early pregnancy. Screening procedures are available when there is a known risk of certain defects.
> **Absence of information does not imply safety.**
> It should be noted that the BNF provides independent advice and may not always agree with the product literature.
> Information on drugs and pregnancy is also available from the UK Teratology Information Service. www. uktis.org
>
> Tel: 0844 892 0909 (09.00–17:00 Monday to Friday; urgent enquiries only outside these hours).

Prescribing in breast-feeding

Breast-feeding is beneficial; the immunological and nutritional value of breast milk to the infant is greater than that of formula feeds.

Although there is concern that drugs taken by the mother might affect the infant, there is very little information on this. In the absence of evidence of an effect, the potential for harm to the infant can be inferred from:

- the amount of drug or active metabolite of the drug delivered to the infant (dependent on the pharmacokinetic characteristics of the drug in the mother);
- the efficiency of absorption, distribution, and elimination of the drug by the infant (infant pharmacokinetics);
- the nature of the effect of the drug on the infant (pharmacodynamic properties of the drug in the infant).

The amount of drug transferred in breast milk is rarely sufficient to produce a discernible effect on the infant. This applies particularly to drugs that are poorly absorbed and need to be given parenterally. However, there is a theoretical possibility that a small amount of drug present in breast milk can induce a hypersensitivity reaction.

A clinical effect can occur in the infant if a pharmacologically significant quantity of the drug is present in milk. For some drugs (e.g. fluvastatin), the ratio between the concentration in milk and that in maternal plasma

may be high enough to expose the infant to adverse effects. Some infants, such as those born prematurely or who have jaundice, are at a slightly higher risk of toxicity.

Some drugs inhibit the infant's sucking reflex (e.g. phenobarbital) while others can affect lactation (e.g. bromocriptine).

The BNF identifies drugs:

- that should be used with caution or are contraindicated in breast-feeding;
- that can be given to the mother during breast-feeding because they are present in milk in amounts which are too small to be harmful to the infant;
- that might be present in milk in significant amount but are not known to be harmful.

Where care is needed when prescribing in breast-feeding, this is indicated under the relevant drug in the BNF.

> **Important**
> For many drugs insufficient evidence is available to provide guidance and it is advisable to administer only essential drugs to a mother during breast-feeding. Because of the inadequacy of information on drugs in breast-feeding, absence of information does not imply safety.

Prescribing in palliative care

Palliative care is an approach that improves the quality of life of patients and their families facing life-threatening illness, through the prevention and relief of suffering by means of early identification and impeccable assessment and treatment of pain and other problems, physical, psychosocial, and spiritual. Careful assessment of symptoms and needs of the patient should be undertaken by a multidisciplinary team.

Specialist palliative care is available in most areas as day hospice care, home-care teams (often known as Macmillan teams), in-patient hospice care, and hospital teams. Many acute hospitals and teaching centres now have consultative, hospital-based teams.

Hospice care of terminally ill patients has shown the importance of symptom control and psychosocial support of the patient and family. Families should be included in the care of the patient if they wish.

Many patients wish to remain at home with their families. Although some families may at first be afraid of caring for the patient at home, support can be provided by community nursing services, social services, voluntary agencies and hospices together with the general practitioner. The family may be reassured by the knowledge that the patient will be admitted to a hospital or hospice if the family cannot cope.

Drug treatment   The number of drugs should be as few as possible, for even the taking of medicine may be an effort. Oral medication is usually satisfactory unless there is severe nausea and vomiting, dysphagia, weakness, or coma, when parenteral medication may be necessary.

Pain

Pain management in palliative care is focused on achieving control of pain by administering the right drug in the right dose at the right time. Analgesics can be divided into three broad classes: non-opioid (paracetamol, NSAID), opioid (e.g. codeine 'weak', morphine 'strong') and adjuvant (e.g. antidepressants, antiepileptics). Drugs from the different classes are used alone or in combination according to the type of pain and response to treatment. Analgesics are more effective in preventing pain than in the relief of established pain; it is important that they are given regularly.

Paracetamol (p. 281) or a **NSAID** (p. 716) given regularly will often be sufficient to manage mild pain. If non-opioid analgesics alone are not sufficient, then an opioid analgesic alone or in combination with a non-opioid analgesic at an adequate dosage, may be helpful in the control of moderate pain. **Codeine** (p. 286) or **tramadol** (p. 295) can be considered for moderate pain. If these preparations do not control the pain then **morphine** (p. 291) is the most useful opioid analgesic. Alternatives to morphine, including transdermal **buprenorphine** (p. 285), transdermal **fentanyl** (p. 288), **hydromorphone** (p. 290), **methadone** (p. 291), or **oxycodone** (p. 293), should be initiated by those with experience in palliative care. Initiation of an opioid analgesic should not be delayed by concern over a theoretical likelihood of psychological dependence (addiction).

Bone metastases   In addition to the above approach, radiotherapy, **bisphosphonates** (p. 523),

and radioactive isotopes of **strontium** (p. 530) (*Metastron*® available from GE Healthcare) may be useful for pain due to bone metastases.

Neuropathic pain   Patients with **neuropathic pain** (p. 296) may benefit from a trial of a tricyclic antidepressant. An antiepileptic may be added or substituted if pain persists; **gabapentin** and **pregabalin** (p. 309) are licensed for neuropathic pain. Ketamine is sometimes used under specialist supervision for neuropathic pain that responds poorly to opioid analgesics. Pain due to nerve compression may be reduced by a corticosteroid such as dexamethasone 8mg daily, which reduces oedema around the tumour, thus reducing compression. Nerve blocks or regional anaesthesia techniques (including the use of epidural and intrathecal catheters) can be considered when pain is localised to a specific area.

Pain management with opioids

Oral route   Treatment with morphine is given by mouth as immediate-release or modified-release preparations. During the titration phase the initial dose is based on the previous medication used, the severity of the pain, and other factors such as presence of renal impairment, increasing age, or frailty. Recommended starting doses vary but, generally, a starting dose between 20–30 mg daily is safe for opioid-naïve patients and 40–60 mg daily for patients being switched from a regular weak opioid. The dose is given either as an immediate-release preparation 4-hourly or as a modified-release preparation 12-hourly, in addition to rescue doses.

If pain occurs between regular doses of morphine ('breakthrough pain'), an additional dose ('rescue dose') of immediate-release morphine should be given. An additional dose should also be given 30 minutes before an activity that causes pain, such as wound dressing. The standard dose of a strong opioid for breakthrough pain is usually one-tenth to one-sixth of the regular 24-hour dose, repeated every 2–4 hours as required (up to hourly may be needed if pain is severe or in the last days of life). Review pain management if rescue analgesic is required frequently (twice daily or more). Each patient should be assessed on an individual basis. Formulations of fentanyl that are administered nasally, buccally or sublingually are also licensed for breakthrough pain.

When adjusting the dose of morphine, the number of rescue doses required and the response to them should be taken into account; increments of morphine should not exceed one-third to one-half of the total daily dose every 24 hours. Thereafter, the dose should be adjusted with careful assessment of the pain, and the use of adjuvant analgesics should also be considered. Upward titration of the dose of morphine stops when either the pain is relieved or unacceptable adverse effects occur, after which it is necessary to consider alternative measures.

Morphine immediate-release 30 mg 4-hourly (or modified-release 100 mg 12-hourly) is usually adequate for most patients; some patients require morphine immediate-release up to 200 mg 4-hourly (or modified-release 600 mg 12-hourly), occasionally more is needed.

Once their pain is controlled, patients started on 4-hourly immediate-release morphine can be transferred to the same total 24-hour dose of morphine given as the modified-release preparation for 12-hourly or 24-hourly administration. The first dose of the modified-release preparation is given with, or within 4 hours of, the last dose of the immediate-release preparation. For preparations suitable for 12-hourly or 24-hourly administration see modified-release preparations under Morphine, p. 291. Increments should be made to the dose, not to the frequency of administration. The patient must be monitored closely for efficacy and side-effects, particularly constipation, and nausea and vomiting. A suitable laxative (p. 69) should be prescribed routinely.

Oxycodone, (p. 293) can be used in patients who require an opioid but cannot tolerate morphine. If the patient is already receiving an opioid, oxycodone should be started at a dose equivalent to the current analgesic (see below). Oxycodone immediate-release preparations can be given for breakthrough pain.

Equivalent doses of opioid analgesics

This is only an **approximate** guide (doses may not correspond with those given in clinical practice); patients should be carefully monitored after any change in medication and dose titration may be required

Analgesic	Route	Dose
Codeine	PO	100 mg
Diamorphine	IM, IV, SC	3 mg
Dihydrocodeine	PO	100 mg
Hydromorphone	PO	2 mg
Morphine	PO	10 mg
Morphine	IM, IV, SC	5 mg
Oxycodone	PO	6.6 mg
Tramadol	PO	100 mg

PO = by mouth; IM = intramuscular, IV = intravenous, SC = subcutaneous

Parenteral route The equivalent parenteral dose of morphine (subcutaneous, intramuscular, or intravenous) is about half of the oral dose. If the patient becomes unable to swallow, generally morphine is administered as a continuous subcutaneous infusion (for details, see Continuous Subcutaneous Infusions below). Diamorphine is sometimes preferred, because being more soluble, it can be given in a smaller volume. The equivalent subcutaneous dose of diamorphine is about one-third of the oral dose of morphine.

If the patient can resume taking medicines by mouth, then oral morphine may be substituted for subcutaneous infusion of morphine or diamorphine, see table above of approximate equivalent doses of morphine and diamorphine. The infusion is discontinued when the first oral dose of morphine is given.

Rectal route Morphine is also available for rectal administration as suppositories; alternatively oxycodone suppositories can be obtained on special order.

Transdermal route Transdermal preparations of fentanyl and buprenorphine are available (section 4.7.2); they are not suitable for acute pain or in patients whose analgesic requirements are changing rapidly because the long time to steady state prevents rapid titration of the dose. Prescribers should ensure that they

are familiar with the correct use of transdermal preparations, see under buprenorphine (p. 285) and fentanyl (p. 288) (inappropriate use has caused fatalities). Immediate-release morphine can be given for breakthrough pain.

The following 24-hour oral doses of morphine are considered to be *approximately* equivalent to the buprenorphine and fentanyl patches shown, however when switching due to possible opioid-induced hyperalgesia, reduce the calculated equivalent dose of the new opioid by one-quarter to one-half.

Buprenorphine patches are *approximately* equivalent to the following 24-hour doses of oral morphine

morphine salt 12 mg daily	≡	BuTrans® '5' patch	7-day patches
morphine salt 24 mg daily	≡	BuTrans® '10' patch	7-day patches
morphine salt 48 mg daily	≡	BuTrans® '20' patch	7-day patches
morphine salt 84 mg daily	≡	Transtec® '35' patch	4-day patches
morphine salt 126 mg daily	≡	Transtec® '52.5' patch	4-day patches
morphine salt 168 mg daily	≡	Transtec® '70' patch	4-day patches

Note Conversion ratios vary and these figures are a guide only. Morphine equivalences for transdermal opioid preparations have been approximated to allow comparison with available preparations of oral morphine

72-hour Fentanyl patches are *approximately* equivalent to the following 24-hour doses of oral morphine

morphine salt 30 mg daily	≡	fentanyl '12' patch
morphine salt 60 mg daily	≡	fentanyl '25' patch
morphine salt 120 mg daily	≡	fentanyl '50' patch
morphine salt 180 mg daily	≡	fentanyl '75' patch
morphine salt 240 mg daily	≡	fentanyl '100' patch

Note Fentanyl equivalences in this table are for patients on well-tolerated opioid therapy for long periods; for patients who are opioid naive or who have been stable on oral morphine or other immediate release opioid for only several weeks, see Transdermal Route above, and section 4.7.2. Conversion ratios vary and these figures are a guide only. Morphine equivalences for transdermal opioid preparations have been approximated to allow comparison with available preparations of oral morphine

Symptom control

Unlicensed indications or routes
Several recommendations in this section involve unlicensed indications or routes.

Anorexia Anorexia may be helped by prednisolone 15–30 mg daily or dexamethasone 2–4 mg daily.

Bowel colic and excessive respiratory secretions Bowel colic and excessive respiratory secretions may be reduced by a subcutaneous injection of hyoscine hydrobromide 400 micrograms, hyoscine butylbromide 20 mg, or glycopyrronium 200 micrograms. These antimuscarinics are generally given every 4 hours when required, but hourly use is occasionally necessary, particularly in excessive respiratory secretions. If symptoms persist, they can be given regularly via a continuous infusion device, see p. 23. Care is required to avoid the discomfort of dry mouth.

Capillary bleeding   Capillary bleeding can be treated with tranexamic acid (section 2.11) by mouth; treatment is usually discontinued one week after the bleeding has stopped, or, if necessary, it can be continued at a reduced dose. Alternatively, gauze soaked in tranexamic acid 100 mg/mL or adrenaline (epinephrine) solution 1 mg/mL (1 in 1000) can be applied to the affected area.

Vitamin K may be useful for the treatment and prevention of bleeding associated with prolonged clotting in liver disease. In severe chronic cholestasis, absorption of vitamin K may be impaired; either parenteral or water-soluble oral vitamin K should be considered (section 9.6.6).

Constipation   Constipation is a common cause of distress and is almost invariable after administration of an opioid analgesic. It should be prevented if possible by the regular administration of laxatives; a faecal softener with a peristaltic stimulant (e.g. co-danthramer) or lactulose solution with a senna preparation should be used (section 1.6.2 and section 1.6.3). Methylnaltrexone (section 1.6.6) is licensed for the treatment of opioid-induced constipation.

Convulsions   Patients with cerebral tumours or uraemia may be susceptible to convulsions. Prophylactic treatment with phenytoin or carbamazepine (section 4.8.1) should be considered. When oral medication is no longer possible, diazepam 10 mg given rectally (as a solution) (section 4.8.2), or phenobarbital 50–200 mg twice daily given by injection, can be continued as prophylaxis. For the use of midazolam by subcutaneous infusion using a continuous infusion device, see below.

Dry mouth   Dry mouth may be relieved by good mouth care and measures such as chewing sugar-free gum, sucking ice or pineapple chunks, or the use of artificial saliva (section 12.3.5); dry mouth associated with candidiasis can be treated by oral preparations of nystatin or miconazole (section 12.3.2); alternatively, fluconazole can be given by mouth (section 5.2.1). Dry mouth may be caused by certain medications including opioids, antimuscarinic drugs (e.g. hyoscine), antidepressants and some antiemetics; if possible, an alternative preparation should be considered.

Dysphagia   A corticosteroid such as dexamethasone 8 mg daily may help, temporarily, if there is an obstruction due to tumour. See also Dry Mouth above.

Dyspnoea   Breathlessness at rest may be relieved by regular oral morphine in carefully titrated doses, starting at 5 mg every 4 hours. Diazepam 5–10 mg daily may be helpful for dyspnoea associated with anxiety. A corticosteroid, such as dexamethasone 4–8 mg daily, may also be helpful if there is bronchospasm or partial obstruction.

Fungating tumours   Fungating tumours can be treated by regular dressing and antibacterial drugs; systemic treatment with metronidazole (section 5.1.11) is often required to reduce malodour but topical metronidazole (section 13.10.1.2) is also used.

Gastro-intestinal pain   The pain of bowel colic may be reduced by loperamide 2–4 mg 4 times daily. Hyoscine hydrobromide (section 4.6) may also be helpful, given sublingually at a dose of 300 micrograms 3 times daily as *Kwells*® tablets. Subcutaneous injections of hyoscine butylbromide, hyoscine hydrobromide, and glycopyrronium can also be used to treat bowel colic (see above). For doses by continuous subcutaneous infusion, see p. 23.

Gastric distension pain due to pressure on the stomach may be helped by a preparation incorporating an antacid with an antiflatulent (section 1.1.1) and a prokinetic such as domperidone 10 mg 3 times daily before meals.

Hiccup   Hiccup due to gastric distension may be helped by a preparation incorporating an antacid with an antiflatulent (section 1.1.1). If this fails, metoclopramide 10 mg every 6 to 8 hours by mouth or by subcutaneous or intramuscular injection can be added; if this also fails, baclofen 5 mg twice daily, or nifedipine 10 mg three times daily, or chlorpromazine (section 4.2.1) can be tried.

Hypercalcaemia   see section 9.5.1.2

Insomnia   Patients with advanced cancer may not sleep because of discomfort, cramps, night sweats, joint stiffness, or fear. There should be appropriate treatment of these problems before hypnotics are used. Benzodiazepines, such as temazepam (section 4.1.1), may be useful.

Intractable cough   Intractable cough may be relieved by moist inhalations or by regular administration of oral morphine in an initial dose of 5 mg every 4 hours. Methadone linctus should be avoided because it has a long duration of action and tends to accumulate.

Muscle spasm   The pain of muscle spasm can be helped by a muscle relaxant such as diazepam 5–10 mg daily or baclofen 5–10 mg 3 times daily.

Nausea and vomiting   Nausea and vomiting are common in patients with advanced cancer. Ideally, the cause should be determined before treatment with an antiemetic (section 4.6) is started. A prokinetic antiemetic may be a preferred choice for first-line therapy.

Nausea and vomiting may occur with opioid therapy particularly in the initial stages but can be prevented by giving an antiemetic such as haloperidol or metoclopramide. An antiemetic is usually necessary only for the first 4 or 5 days and therefore combined preparations containing an opioid with an antiemetic are not recommended because they lead to unnecessary antiemetic therapy (and associated side-effects when used long-term).

Metoclopramide has a prokinetic action and is used in a dose of 10 mg 3 times daily by mouth for nausea and vomiting associated with gastritis, gastric stasis, and functional bowel obstruction. Drugs with antimuscarinic effects antagonise prokinetic drugs and, if possible, should not be used concurrently.

Haloperidol is used by mouth in an initial dose of 1.5 mg once or twice daily (can be increased if necessary to 5–10 mg daily in divided doses) for most metabolic causes of vomiting (e.g. hypercalcaemia, renal failure).

Cyclizine is given in a dose of 50 mg up to 3 times daily by mouth. It is used for nausea and vomiting due to mechanical bowel obstruction, raised intracranial pressure, and motion sickness.

Levomepromazine is used as an antiemetic; it is given by mouth or by subcutaneous injection in an initial dose of 6 mg or 6.25 mg at bedtime, titrated if necessary to 12.5–25 mg twice daily (6-mg tablets available from 'special-order' manufacturers or specialist importing companies, see p. 1124). For the dose by subcutaneous infusion, see below. Dexamethasone 8–16 mg daily by mouth can be used as an adjunct.

Antiemetic therapy should be reviewed every 24 hours; it may be necessary to substitute the antiemetic or to add another one.

For the administration of antiemetics by subcutaneous infusion using a continuous infusion device, see below.

For the treatment of nausea and vomiting associated with cancer chemotherapy, see section 8.1.

Pruritus Pruritus, even when associated with obstructive jaundice, often responds to simple measures such as application of emollients (section 13.2.1). In the case of obstructive jaundice, further measures include administration of colestyramine (section 1.9.2).

Raised intracranial pressure Headache due to raised intracranial pressure often responds to a high dose of a corticosteroid, such as dexamethasone 16 mg daily for 4 to 5 days, subsequently reduced to 4–6 mg daily if possible; dexamethasone should be given before 6 p.m. to reduce the risk of insomnia.

Restlessness and confusion Restlessness and confusion may require treatment with an antipsychotic, e.g. haloperidol 2 mg by mouth or 2.5 mg by subcutaneous injection, or levomepromazine 6 mg by mouth or 6.25 mg by subcutaneous injection, both repeated every 2 hours if required. The dose and frequency is adjusted according to the level of patient distress and the response. A regular maintenance dose should also be considered, given twice daily either by mouth or by subcutaneous injection; alternatively use a continuous infusion device, see below.

Levomepromazine is licensed to treat pain in palliative care—this use is reserved for distressed patients with severe pain unresponsive to other measures (seek specialist advice).

Continuous subcutaneous infusions

Although drugs can usually be administered *by mouth* to control the symptoms of advanced cancer, the parenteral route may sometimes be necessary. Repeated administration of *intramuscular injections* can be difficult in a cachectic patient. This has led to the use of portable continuous infusion devices, such as syringe drivers, to give a *continuous subcutaneous infusion*, which can provide good control of symptoms with little discomfort or inconvenience to the patient.

> **Syringe driver rate settings**
> Staff using syringe drivers should be **adequately trained** and different rate settings should be **clearly identified** and **differentiated**; incorrect use of syringe drivers is a common cause of medication errors.

Indications for the **parenteral route** are:

- the patient is unable to take medicines by mouth owing to *nausea and vomiting, dysphagia, severe weakness,* or *coma;*

- there is *malignant bowel obstruction* in patients for whom further surgery is inappropriate (avoiding the need for an intravenous infusion or for insertion of a nasogastric tube);

- occasionally when the patient *does not wish* to take regular medication by mouth.

Bowel colic and excessive respiratory secretions Hyoscine hydrobromide effectively reduces respiratory secretions and bowel colic and is sedative (but occasionally causes paradoxical agitation); it is given in a *subcutaneous infusion dose* of 1.2–2 mg/24 hours.

Hyoscine butylbromide is used for bowel colic and for excessive respiratory secretions, and is less sedative than hyoscine hydrobromide. Hyoscine butylbromide is given in a *subcutaneous infusion dose* of 60–300 mg/24 hours for bowel colic and 20–120 mg/24 hours for excessive respiratory secretions (**important:** these doses of *hyoscine butylbromide* must not be confused with the much lower dose of *hyoscine hydrobromide,* above).

Glycopyrronium 0.6–1.2 mg/24 hours by subcutaneous infusion may also be used to treat bowel colic or excessive respiratory secretions.

Confusion and restlessness Haloperidol has little sedative effect; it is given in a *subcutaneous infusion dose* of 5–15 mg/24 hours.

Levomepromazine has a sedative effect; it is given in an initial *subcutaneous infusion dose* of 12.5–50 mg/24 hours, titrated according to response (doses greater than 100 mg/24 hours should be given under specialist supervision).

Midazolam is a sedative and an antiepileptic that may be used in addition to an antipsychotic drug in a very restless patient; it is given in an initial *subcutaneous infusion dose* of 10–20 mg/24 hours, titrated according to response (usual dose 20–60 mg/24 hours). Midazolam is also used for myoclonus.

Convulsions If a patient has previously been receiving an antiepileptic drug *or* has a primary or secondary cerebral tumour *or* is at risk of convulsion (e.g. owing to uraemia) antiepileptic medication should not be stopped. Midazolam is the benzodiazepine antiepileptic of choice for *continuous subcutaneous infusion,* and it is given initially in a dose of 20–40 mg/24 hours.

> **Prescribing of midazolam in palliative care**
> The use of high-strength midazolam (5 mg/mL in 2 mL and 10 mL ampoules, or 2 mg/mL in 5 mL ampoules) should be considered in palliative care and other situations where a higher strength may be more appropriate to administer the prescribed dose, and where the risk of overdosage has been assessed. It is advised that flumazenil (section 15.1.7) is available when midazolam is used, to reverse the effects if necessary.

Nausea and vomiting Haloperidol is given in a *subcutaneous infusion dose* of 2.5–10 mg/24 hours.

Prescribing in palliative care

Levomepromazine is given in a *subcutaneous infusion dose* of 5–25 mg/24 hours but sedation can limit the dose.

Cyclizine is particularly likely to precipitate if mixed with diamorphine or other drugs (see under Mixing and Compatibility, below); it is given in a *subcutaneous infusion dose* of 150 mg/24 hours.

Metoclopramide can cause skin reactions; it is given in a *subcutaneous infusion dose* of 30–100 mg/24 hours.

Octreotide (section 8.3.4.3), which stimulates water and electrolyte absorption and inhibits water secretion in the small bowel, can be used by subcutaneous infusion in a dose of 250–500 micrograms/24 hours to reduce intestinal secretions and to reduce vomiting due to bowel obstruction. Doses of 750 micrograms/24 hours, and occasionally higher, are sometimes required.

Pain control Diamorphine is the preferred opioid since its high solubility permits a large dose to be given in a small volume (see under Mixing and Compatibility, below). The table below shows approximate equivalent doses of morphine and diamorphine.

Mixing and compatibility The general principle that injections should be given into separate sites (and should not be mixed) does not apply to the use of syringe drivers in palliative care. Provided that there is evidence of compatibility, selected injections can be mixed in syringe drivers. Not all types of medication can be used in a subcutaneous infusion. In particular, chlorpromazine, prochlorperazine, and diazepam are **contra-indicated** as they cause skin reactions at the injection site; to a lesser extent cyclizine and levomepromazine also sometimes cause local irritation.

In theory injections dissolved in water for injections are more likely to be associated with pain (possibly owing to their hypotonicity). The use of physiological saline (sodium chloride 0.9%) however increases the likelihood of precipitation when more than one drug is used; moreover subcutaneous infusion rates are so slow (0.1–0.3 mL/hour) that pain is not usually a problem when water is used as a diluent.

Diamorphine can be given by subcutaneous infusion in a strength of up to 250 mg/mL; up to a strength of 40 mg/mL either *water for injections* or *physiological saline* (sodium chloride 0.9%) is a suitable diluent—above that strength only *water for injections* is used (to avoid precipitation).

The following can be mixed with *diamorphine*:

Cyclizine[1]	Hyoscine hydrobromide
Dexamethasone[2]	Levomepromazine
Haloperidol[3]	Metoclopramide[4]
Hyoscine butylbromide	Midazolam

Subcutaneous infusion solution should be monitored regularly both to check for precipitation (and discolora-

tion) and to ensure that the infusion is running at the correct rate.

Problems encountered with syringe drivers The following are problems that may be encountered with syringe drivers and the action that should be taken:

- if the subcutaneous infusion runs *too quickly* check the rate setting and the calculation;

- if the subcutaneous infusion runs *too slowly* check the start button, the battery, the syringe driver, the cannula, and make sure that the injection site is not inflamed;

- if there is an *injection site reaction* make sure that the site does not need to be changed—firmness or swelling at the site of injection is not in itself an indication for change, but pain or obvious inflammation is.

Equivalent doses of morphine sulfate and diamorphine hydrochloride given over 24 hours

These equivalences are *approximate only* and should be adjusted according to response

MORPHINE		PARENTERAL DIAMORPHINE
Oral morphine sulfate	Subcutaneous infusion of morphine sulfate	Subcutaneous infusion of diamorphine hydrochloride
over 24 hours	over 24 hours	over 24 hours
30 mg	15 mg	10 mg
60 mg	30 mg	20 mg
90 mg	45 mg	30 mg
120 mg	60 mg	40 mg
180 mg	90 mg	60 mg
240 mg	120 mg	80 mg
360 mg	180 mg	120 mg
480 mg	240 mg	160 mg
600 mg	300 mg	200 mg
780 mg	390 mg	260 mg
960 mg	480 mg	320 mg
1200 mg	600 mg	400 mg

If breakthrough pain occurs give a subcutaneous (preferable) or intramuscular injection equivalent to one-tenth to one-sixth of the total 24-hour subcutaneous infusion dose. It is kinder to give an intermittent bolus injection *subcutaneously*—absorption is smoother so that the risk of adverse effects at peak absorption is avoided (an even better method is to use a subcutaneous butterfly needle).
To minimise the risk of infection no individual subcutaneous infusion solution should be used for longer than 24 hours.

---

1. Cyclizine may precipitate at concentrations above 10 mg/mL *or* in the presence of sodium chloride 0.9% *or* as the concentration of diamorphine relative to cyclizine increases; mixtures of diamorphine and cyclizine are also likely to precipitate after 24 hours.
2. Special care is needed to avoid precipitation of dexamethasone when preparing it.
3. Mixtures of haloperidol and diamorphine are likely to precipitate after 24 hours if haloperidol concentration is above 2 mg/mL.
4. Under some conditions infusions containing metoclopramide become discoloured; such solutions should be discarded.

Prescribing for the elderly

Old people, especially the very old, require special care and consideration from prescribers. *Medicines for Older People*, a component document of the National Service Framework for Older People,[1] describes how to maximise the benefits of medicines and how to avoid excessive, inappropriate, or inadequate consumption of medicines by older people.

Appropriate prescribing   Elderly patients often receive multiple drugs for their multiple diseases. This greatly increases the risk of drug interactions as well as adverse reactions, and may affect compliance (see Taking medicines to best effect under General guidance). The balance of benefit and harm of some medicines may be altered in the elderly. Therefore, elderly patients' medicines should be reviewed regularly and medicines which are not of benefit should be stopped.

Non-pharmacological measures may be more appropriate for symptoms such as headache, sleeplessness, and lightheadedness when associated with social stress as in widowhood, loneliness, and family dispersal.

In some cases prophylactic drugs are inappropriate if they are likely to complicate existing treatment or introduce unnecessary side-effects, especially in elderly patients with poor prognosis or with poor overall health. However, elderly patients should not be denied medicines which may help them, such as anticoagulants or antiplatelet drugs for atrial fibrillation, antihypertensives, statins, and drugs for osteoporosis.

Form of medicine   Frail elderly patients may have difficulty swallowing tablets; if left in the mouth, ulceration may develop. They should always be encouraged to take their tablets or capsules with enough fluid, and whilst in an upright position to avoid the possibility of oesophageal ulceration. It can be helpful to discuss with the patient the possibility of taking the drug as a liquid if available.

Manifestations of ageing   In the very old, manifestations of normal ageing may be mistaken for disease and lead to inappropriate prescribing. In addition, age-related muscle weakness and difficulty in maintaining balance should not be confused with neurological disease. Disorders such as lightheadedness not associated with postural or postprandial hypotension are unlikely to be helped by drugs.

Sensitivity   The nervous system of elderly patients is more sensitive to many commonly used drugs, such as opioid analgesics, benzodiazepines, antipsychotics, and antiparkinsonian drugs, all of which must be used with caution. Similarly, other organs may also be more susceptible to the effects of drugs such as antihypertensives and NSAIDs.

Pharmacokinetics

Pharmacokinetic changes can markedly increase the tissue concentration of a drug in the elderly, especially in debilitated patients.

The most important effect of age is reduced renal clearance. Many aged patients thus *excrete drugs slowly*,

and are *highly susceptible to nephrotoxic drugs*. Acute illness can lead to rapid reduction in renal clearance, especially if accompanied by dehydration. Hence, a patient stabilised on a drug with a narrow margin between the therapeutic and the toxic dose (e.g. digoxin) can rapidly develop adverse effects in the aftermath of a myocardial infarction or a respiratory-tract infection. The hepatic metabolism of lipid soluble drugs is reduced in elderly patients because there is a reduction in liver volume. This is important for drugs with a narrow therapeutic window.

Adverse reactions

Adverse reactions often present in the elderly in a vague and non-specific fashion. *Confusion* is often the presenting symptom (caused by almost any of the commonly used drugs). Other common manifestations are *constipation* (with antimuscarinics and many tranquillisers) and postural *hypotension* and *falls* (with diuretics and many psychotropics).

Hypnotics   Many hypnotics with long half-lives have serious hangover effects, including drowsiness, unsteady gait, slurred speech, and confusion. Hypnotics with short half-lives should be used but they too can present problems (section 4.1.1). Short courses of hypnotics are occasionally useful for helping a patient through an acute illness or some other crisis but every effort must be made to avoid dependence. Benzodiazepines impair balance, which can result in falls.

Diuretics   Diuretics are overprescribed in old age and should **not** be used on a long-term basis to treat simple gravitational oedema which will usually respond to increased movement, raising the legs, and support stockings. A few days of diuretic treatment may speed the clearing of the oedema but it should rarely need continued drug therapy.

NSAIDs   Bleeding associated with aspirin and other NSAIDs is more common in the elderly who are more likely to have a fatal or serious outcome. NSAIDs are also a special hazard in patients with cardiac disease or renal impairment which may again place older patients at particular risk.

Owing to the *increased susceptibility of the elderly* to the *side-effects of NSAIDs* the following recommendations are made:

- for *osteoarthritis, soft-tissue lesions*, and *back pain*, first try measures such as weight reduction (if obese), warmth, exercise, and use of a walking stick;

- for *osteoarthritis, soft-tissue lesions, back pain*, and *pain in rheumatoid arthritis*, paracetamol should be used first and can often provide adequate pain relief;

- alternatively, a low-dose NSAID (e.g. ibuprofen up to 1.2 g daily) may be given;

- for pain relief when either drug is inadequate, paracetamol in a full dose plus a low-dose NSAID may be given;

- if necessary, the NSAID dose can be increased or an opioid analgesic given with paracetamol;

- do not give two NSAIDs at the same time.

---

1. Department of Health. National Service Framework for Older People. London: Department of Health, March 2001.

For advice on prophylaxis of NSAID-induced peptic ulcers if continued NSAID treatment is necessary, see section 1.3.

Other drugs   Other drugs which commonly cause adverse reactions are *antiparkinsonian drugs, antihypertensives, psychotropics,* and *digoxin.* The usual maintenance dose of digoxin in very old patients is 125 micrograms daily (62.5 micrograms in those with renal disease); lower doses are often inadequate but toxicity is common in those given 250 micrograms daily.

Drug-induced blood disorders are much more common in the elderly. Therefore drugs with a tendency to cause bone marrow depression (e.g. *co-trimoxazole, mianserin*) should be avoided unless there is no acceptable alternative.

The elderly generally require a lower maintenance dose of *warfarin* than younger adults; once again, the outcome of bleeding tends to be more serious.

Guidelines

Always consider whether a drug is indicated at all.

Limit range   It is a sensible policy to prescribe from a limited range of drugs and to be thoroughly familiar with their effects in the elderly.

Reduce dose   Dosage should generally be substantially lower than for younger patients and it is common to start with about 50% of the adult dose. Some drugs (e.g. long-acting antidiabetic drugs such as glibenclamide) should be avoided altogether.

Review regularly   Review repeat prescriptions regularly. In many patients it may be possible to stop some drugs, provided that clinical progress is monitored. It may be necessary to reduce the dose of some drugs as renal function declines.

Simplify regimens   Elderly patients benefit from simple treatment regimens. Only drugs with a clear indication should be prescribed and whenever possible given once or twice daily. In particular, regimens which call for a confusing array of dosage intervals should be avoided.

Explain clearly   Write full instructions on every prescription (*including* repeat prescriptions) so that containers can be properly labelled with full directions. Avoid imprecisions like 'as directed'. Child-resistant containers may be unsuitable.

Repeats and disposal   Instruct patients what to do when drugs run out, and also how to dispose of any that are no longer necessary. Try to prescribe matching quantities.

If these guidelines are followed most elderly people will cope adequately with their own medicines. If not then it is essential to enrol the help of a third party, usually a relative or a friend.

Prescribing in dental practice

The following is a list of topics of particular relevance to dentists.

> Advice on the drug management of dental and oral conditions has been integrated into the BNF. For ease of access, guidance on such conditions is usually identified by means of a relevant heading (e.g. Dental and Orofacial Pain) in the appropriate sections of the BNF. For guidance on finding dental information in the BNF see How to Use the BNF, p. xi.

Medical emergencies in dental practice

This section provides guidelines on the management of the more common medical emergencies which may arise in dental practice. Dentists and their staff should be familiar with standard resuscitation procedures, but in all circumstances it is advisable to summon medical assistance as soon as possible. For an **algorithm** of the procedure for **cardiopulmonary resuscitation**, see inside back cover.

> **The drugs referred to in this section include:**
> Adrenaline Injection (Epinephrine Injection), adrenaline 1 in 1000, (adrenaline 1 mg/mL as acid tartrate), 1-mL amps
> Aspirin Dispersible Tablets 300 mg
> Glucagon Injection, glucagon (as hydrochloride), 1-unit vial (with solvent)
> Glucose (for administration by mouth)
> Glyceryl Trinitrate Spray
> Midazolam Oromucosal Solution, midazolam 5 mg/mL
> Oxygen
> Salbutamol Aerosol Inhalation, salbutamol 100 micrograms/metered inhalation

Adrenal insufficiency

Adrenal insufficiency **may** follow prolonged therapy with corticosteroids and can persist for years after stopping. A patient with adrenal insufficiency may become hypotensive under the stress of a dental visit (important: see also p. 495 for details of corticosteroid cover before dental surgical procedures under general anaesthesia).

Management

- Lay the patient flat
- Give **oxygen** (see section 3.6)
- Transfer patient urgently to hospital

Anaphylaxis

A severe allergic reaction may follow oral or parenteral administration of a drug. Anaphylactic reactions in dentistry may follow the administration of a drug or contact with substances such as latex in surgical gloves. In general, the more rapid the onset of the reaction the more profound it tends to be. Symptoms may develop within minutes and rapid treatment is essential.

Anaphylactic reactions may also be associated with *additives* and *excipients* in foods and medicines (see Excipients, p. 2). Refined arachis (peanut) oil, which may be present in some medicinal products, is unlikely to cause an allergic reaction—nevertheless it is wise to check the full formula of preparations which may contain allergens (including those for topical application, particularly if they are intended for use in the mouth or for application to the nasal mucosa).

Symptoms and signs

- Paraesthesia, flushing, and swelling of face
- Generalised itching, especially of hands and feet

Prescribing in dental practice

- Bronchospasm and laryngospasm (with wheezing and difficulty in breathing)
- Rapid weak pulse together with fall in blood pressure and pallor; finally cardiac arrest

Management

First-line treatment includes securing the airway, restoration of blood pressure (laying the patient flat and raising the feet, or in the recovery position if unconscious or nauseous and at risk of vomiting), and administration of **adrenaline** (epinephrine) injection (section 3.4.3). This is given **intramuscularly** in a dose of 500 micrograms (0.5 mL adrenaline injection 1 in 1000); a dose of 300 micrograms (0.3 mL adrenaline injection 1 in 1000) may be appropriate for *immediate self-administration*. The dose is repeated if necessary at 5-minute intervals according to blood pressure, pulse, and respiratory function. **Oxygen** administration is also of primary importance (see section 3.6). Arrangements should be made to transfer the patient to hospital urgently.

> For further details on the management of anaphylaxis including details of paediatric doses of adrenaline, see p. 213

Asthma

Patients with asthma may have an attack while at the dental surgery. Most attacks will respond to 2 puffs of the patient's short-acting beta$_2$ agonist inhaler such as **salbutamol** 100 micrograms/puff; further puffs are required if the patient does not respond rapidly. If the patient is unable to use the inhaler effectively, further puffs should be given through a large-volume spacer device (or, if not available, through a plastic or paper cup with a hole in the bottom for the inhaler mouthpiece). If the response remains unsatisfactory, or if further deterioration occurs, then the patient should be transferred urgently to hospital. Whilst awaiting transfer, **oxygen** (section 3.6) should be given with salbutamol 5 mg or terbutaline 10 mg by nebuliser; if a nebuliser is unavailable, then 2–10 puffs of salbutamol 100 micrograms/metered inhalation should be given (preferably a large-volume spacer), and repeated every 10–20 minutes if necessary. If asthma is part of a more generalised anaphylactic reaction, an intramuscular injection of **adrenaline** (as detailed under Anaphylaxis above) should be given.

For a table describing the management of acute asthma, see p. 185

Patients with severe chronic asthma or whose asthma has deteriorated previously during a dental procedure may require an increase in their prophylactic medication before a dental procedure. This should be discussed with the patient's medical practitioner and may include increasing the dose of inhaled or oral corticosteroid.

Cardiac emergencies

If there is a history of *angina* the patient will probably carry **glyceryl trinitrate** spray or tablets (or isosorbide dinitrate tablets) and should be allowed to use them. Hospital admission is not necessary if symptoms are mild and resolve rapidly with the patient's own medication. See also Coronary Artery Disease on p. 30.

Arrhythmias may lead to a sudden reduction in cardiac output with loss of consciousness. Medical assistance should be summoned. For advice on pacemaker interference, see also Pacemakers, p. 30.

The pain of *myocardial infarction* is similar to that of angina but generally more severe and more prolonged. For general advice see also Coronary Artery Disease on p. 30

Symptoms and signs of myocardial infarction

- Progressive onset of severe, crushing pain across front of chest; pain may radiate towards the shoulder and down arm, or into neck and jaw
- Skin becomes pale and clammy
- Nausea and vomiting are common
- Pulse may be weak and blood pressure may fall
- Breathlessness

Initial management of myocardial infarction

Call immediately for medical assistance and an ambulance, as appropriate.

Allow the patient to rest in the position that feels most comfortable; in the presence of breathlessness this is likely to be sitting position, whereas the syncopal patient should be laid flat; often an intermediate position (dictated by the patient) will be most appropriate. **Oxygen** may be administered (see section 3.6).

Sublingual glyceryl trinitrate may relieve pain. Intramuscular injection of drugs should be avoided because absorption may be too slow (particularly when cardiac output is reduced) and pain relief is inadequate. Intramuscular injection also increases the risk of local bleeding into the muscle if the patient is given a thrombolytic drug.

Reassure the patient as much as possible to relieve further anxiety. If available, aspirin in a single dose of 300 mg should be given. A note (to say that aspirin has been given) should be sent with the patient to the hospital. For further details on the initial management of myocardial infarction, see p. 167.

If the patient collapses and loses consciousness attempt standard resuscitation measures. For an **algorithm** of the procedure for **cardiopulmonary resuscitation**, see inside back cover.

Epileptic seizures

Patients with epilepsy must continue with their normal dosage of anticonvulsant drugs when attending for dental treatment. It is not uncommon for epileptic patients not to volunteer the information that they are epileptic but there should be little difficulty in recognising a tonic-clonic (grand mal) seizure.

Symptoms and signs

- There may be a brief warning (but variable)
- Sudden loss of consciousness, the patient becomes rigid, falls, may give a cry, and becomes cyanotic (tonic phase)
- After 30 seconds, there are jerking movements of the limbs; the tongue may be bitten (clonic phase)
- There may be frothing from mouth and urinary incontinence
- The seizure typically lasts a few minutes; the patient may then become flaccid but remain unconscious. After a variable time the patient regains consciousness but may remain confused for a while

Management

During a convulsion try to ensure that the patient is not at risk from injury but make no attempt to put anything in the mouth or between the teeth (in mistaken belief that this will protect the tongue). Give **oxygen** (section 3.6) to support respiration if necessary.

Do not attempt to restrain convulsive movements.

After convulsive movements have subsided place the patient in the coma (recovery) position and check the airway.

After the convulsion the patient may be confused ('post-ictal confusion') and may need reassurance and sympathy. The patient should not be sent home until fully recovered. Seek medical attention or transfer the patient to hospital if it was the first episode of epilepsy, or if the convulsion was atypical, prolonged (or repeated), or if injury occurred.

Medication should only be given if convulsive seizures are prolonged (convulsive movements lasting 5 minutes or longer) or repeated rapidly.

Midazolam oromucosal solution can be given by the buccal route in adults as a single dose of 10 mg [unlicensed]. For further details on the management of status epilepticus, including details of paediatric doses of midazolam, see p. 322.

Focal seizures similarly need very little active management (in an automatism only a minimum amount of restraint should be applied to prevent injury). Again, the patient should be observed until post-ictal confusion has completely resolved.

Hypoglycaemia

Insulin-treated diabetic patients attending for dental treatment under local anaesthesia should inject insulin and eat meals as normal. If food is omitted the blood glucose will fall to an abnormally low level (hypoglycaemia). Patients can often recognise the symptoms themselves and this state responds to sugar in water or a few lumps of sugar. Children may not have such prominent changes but may appear unduly lethargic.

Symptoms and signs

- Shaking and trembling
- Sweating
- 'Pins and needles' in lips and tongue
- Hunger
- Palpitation
- Headache (occasionally)
- Double vision
- Difficulty in concentration
- Slurring of speech
- Confusion
- Change of behaviour; truculence
- Convulsions
- Unconsciousness

Management

Initially glucose 10–20 g is given by mouth either in liquid form or as granulated sugar or sugar lumps. Approximately 10 g of glucose is available from non-diet versions of *Lucozade*® *Energy Original* 55 mL, *Coca-Cola*® 100 mL, *Ribena*® *Blackcurrant* 19 mL (to be

diluted), 2 teaspoons sugar, and also from 3 sugar lumps[1]. If necessary this may be repeated in 10–15 minutes.

If glucose cannot be given by mouth, if it is ineffective, or if the hypoglycaemia causes unconsciousness, **glucagon** 1 mg (1 unit) should be given by intramuscular (or subcutaneous) injection; a child under 8 years or of body-weight under 25 kg should be given 500 micrograms. Once the patient regains consciousness oral glucose should be administered as above. If glucagon is ineffective or contra-indicated, the patient should be transferred urgently to hospital. The patient must also be admitted to hospital if hypoglycaemia is caused by an oral antidiabetic drug.

Syncope

Insufficient blood supply to the brain results in loss of consciousness. The commonest cause is a vasovagal attack or simple faint (syncope) due to emotional stress.

Symptoms and signs

- Patient feels faint
- Low blood pressure
- Pallor and sweating
- Yawning and slow pulse
- Nausea and vomiting
- Dilated pupils
- Muscular twitching

Management

- Lay the patient as flat as is reasonably comfortable and, in the absence of associated breathlessness, raise the legs to improve cerebral circulation
- Loosen any tight clothing around the neck
- Once consciousness is regained, give sugar in water or a cup of sweet tea

Other possible causes

Postural hypotension can be a consequence of rising abruptly or of standing upright for too long; antihypertensive drugs predispose to this. When rising, susceptible patients should take their time. Management is as for a vasovagal attack.

Under stressful circumstances, some patients hyperventilate. This gives rise to feelings of faintness but does not usually result in syncope. In most cases reassurance is all that is necessary; rebreathing from cupped hands or a bag may be helpful but calls for careful supervision.

Adrenal insufficiency or arrhythmias are other possible causes of syncope, see p. 27 and p. 30 .

Medical problems in dental practice

Individuals presenting at the dental surgery may also suffer from an unrelated medical condition; this may require modification to the management of their dental condition. If the patient has systemic disease or is taking other medication, the matter may need to be discussed with the patient's general practitioner or hospital consultant.

1. Proprietary products of quick-acting carbohydrate (e.g. GlucoGel®, Dextrogel®, GSF-Syrup®, Rapilose® gel) are available on prescription for the patient to keep to hand in case of hypoglycaemia

For advice on adrenal insufficiency, anaphylaxis, asthma, cardiac emergencies, epileptic seizures, hypoglycaemia and syncope see under Medical Emergencies in Dental Practice.

Allergy

Patients should be asked about any history of allergy; those with a history of atopic allergy (asthma, eczema, hay fever, etc.) are at special risk. Those with a history of a severe allergy or of anaphylactic reactions are at high risk—it is essential to confirm that they are not allergic to any medication, or to any dental materials or equipment (including latex gloves). See also Anaphylaxis on p. 27.

Arrhythmias

Patients, especially those who suffer from heart failure or who have sustained a myocardial infarction, may have irregular cardiac rhythm. Atrial fibrillation is a common arrhythmia even in patients with normal hearts and is of little concern except that dentists should be aware that such patients may be receiving anticoagulant therapy. The patient's medical practitioner should be asked whether any special precautions are necessary. Premedication (e.g. with temazepam) may be useful in some instances for very anxious patients.

See also Cardiac emergencies, p. 28 and Dental Anaesthesia, p. 891.

Cardiac prostheses

For an account of the risk of infective endocarditis in patients with prosthetic heart valves, see Infective Endocarditis, below. For advice on patients receiving anticoagulants, see Thromboembolic disease, below.

Coronary artery disease

Patients are vulnerable for at least 4 weeks following a myocardial infarction or following any sudden increase in the symptoms of angina. It would be advisable to check with the patient's medical practitioner before commencing treatment. See also Cardiac Emergencies on p. 28.

Treatment with low-dose aspirin (75 mg daily), clopidogrel, or dipyridamole should not be stopped routinely nor should the dose be altered before dental procedures.

A Working Party of the British Society for Antimicrobial Chemotherapy has not recommended antibiotic prophylaxis for patients following coronary artery bypass surgery.

Cyanotic heart disease

Patients with cyanotic heart disease are at risk in the dental chair, particularly if they have pulmonary hypertension. In such patients a syncopal reaction increases the shunt away from the lungs, causing more hypoxia which worsens the syncopal reaction—a vicious circle that may prove fatal. The advice of the cardiologist should be sought on any patient with congenital cyanotic heart disease. Treatment in hospital is more appropriate for some patients with this condition.

Hypertension

Patients with hypertension are likely to be receiving antihypertensive drugs such as those described in section 2.5. Their blood pressure may fall dangerously low

under general anaesthesia, see also under Dental Anaesthesia on p. 891.

Immunosuppression and indwelling intraperitoneal catheters

See Table 2, section 5.1

Infective endocarditis

While almost any dental procedure can cause bacteraemia, there is no clear association with the development of infective endocarditis. Routine daily activities such as tooth brushing also produce a bacteraemia and may present a greater risk of infective endocarditis than a single dental procedure.

Antibacterial prophylaxis and chlorhexidine mouthwash are **not** recommended for the prevention of endocarditis in patients undergoing dental procedures. Such prophylaxis may expose patients to the adverse effects of antimicrobials when the evidence of benefit has not been proven.

Reduction of oral bacteraemia   Patients at risk of endocarditis[1] should be advised to maintain the highest possible standards of oral hygiene in order to reduce the:

● need for dental extractions or other surgery;

● chances of severe bacteraemia if dental surgery is needed;

● possibility of 'spontaneous' bacteraemia.

Postoperative care   Patients at risk of endocarditis[1] should be warned to report to the doctor or dentist any unexplained illness that develops after dental treatment. Any infection in patients at risk of endocarditis[1] should be investigated promptly and treated appropriately to reduce the risk of endocarditis.

Patients on anticoagulant therapy   For general advice on dental surgery in patients receiving oral anticoagulant therapy see Thromboembolic Disease, below.

Joint prostheses

See Table 2, section 5.1

Pacemakers

Pacemakers prevent asystole or severe bradycardia. Some ultrasonic scalers, electronic apex locators, electro-analgesic devices, and electrocautery devices interfere with the normal function of pacemakers (including shielded pacemakers) and should not be used. The manufacturer's literature should be consulted whenever possible. If severe bradycardia occurs in a patient fitted with a pacemaker, electrical equipment should be switched off and the patient placed supine with the legs elevated. If the patient loses consciousness and the pulse remains slow or is absent, cardiopulmonary resuscitation (see inside back cover) may be needed. Call immediately for medical assistance and an ambulance, as appropriate.

---

1. Patients at risk of endocarditis include those with valve replacement, acquired valvular heart disease with stenosis or regurgitation, structural congenital heart disease (including surgically corrected or palliated structural conditions, but excluding isolated atrial septal defect, fully repaired ventricular septal defect, fully repaired patent ductus arteriosus, and closure devices considered to be endothelialised), hypertrophic cardiomyopathy, or a previous episode of infective endocarditis

A Working Party of the British Society for Antimicrobial Chemotherapy does not recommend antibacterial prophylaxis for patients with pacemakers.

Thromboembolic disease

Patients receiving a **heparin** or an oral anticoagulant such as **warfarin**, **acenocoumarol** (nicoumalone), **phenindione**, **apixaban**, **dabigatran etexilate**, or **rivaroxaban** may be liable to excessive bleeding after extraction of teeth or other dental surgery. Often dental surgery can be delayed until the anticoagulant therapy has been completed.

For a patient requiring long-term therapy with warfarin, the patient's medical practitioner should be consulted and the International Normalised Ratio (INR) should be assessed 72 hours before the dental procedure. This allows sufficient time for dose modification if necessary. In those with an unstable INR (including those who require weekly monitoring of their INR, or those who have had some INR measurements greater than 4.0 in the last 2 months), the INR should be assessed within 24 hours of the dental procedure. Patients requiring minor dental procedures (including extractions) who have an INR below 4.0 may continue warfarin without dose adjustment. There is no need to check the INR for a patient requiring a non-invasive dental procedure.

If it is necessary to remove several teeth, a single extraction should be done first; if this goes well further teeth may be extracted at subsequent visits (two or three at a time). Measures should be taken to minimise bleeding during and after the procedure. This includes the use of sutures and a haemostatic such as oxidised cellulose, collagen sponge or resorbable gelatin sponge. Scaling and root planing should initially be restricted to a limited area to assess the potential for bleeding.

For a patient on long-term warfarin, the advice of the clinician responsible for the patient's anticoagulation should be sought if:

- the INR is unstable, or if the INR is greater than 4.0;
- the patient has thrombocytopenia, haemophilia, or other disorders of haemostasis, or suffers from liver impairment, alcoholism, or renal failure;
- the patient is receiving antiplatelet drugs, cytotoxic drugs or radiotherapy.

Intramuscular injections are *contra-indicated* in patients taking anticoagulants with an INR above the therapeutic range, and in those with any disorder of haemostasis. In patients taking anticoagulants who have a stable INR within the therapeutic range, intramuscular injections should be avoided if possible; if an intramuscular injection is necessary, the patient should be informed of the increased risk of localised bleeding and monitored carefully.

A local anaesthetic containing a vasoconstrictor should be given by infiltration, or by intraligamentary or mental nerve injection if possible. If regional nerve blocks cannot be avoided the local anaesthetic should be given cautiously using an aspirating syringe.

Drugs which have potentially serious interactions with anticoagulants include aspirin and other NSAIDs, carbamazepine, imidazole and triazole antifungals (including miconazole), erythromycin, clarithromycin, and metronidazole; for details of these and other interactions with anticoagulants, see Appendix 1 (dabigatran etexilate, heparins, phenindione, rivaroxaban, and coumarins).

Although studies have failed to demonstrate an interaction, common experience in anticoagulant clinics is that the INR can be altered following a course of an oral broad-spectrum antibiotic, such as ampicillin or amoxicillin.

Information on the treatment of patients who take anticoagulants is available at www.npsa.nhs.uk/patientsafety/alerts-and-directives/alerts/anticoagulant.

Liver disease

Liver disease may alter the response to drugs and drug prescribing should be kept to a minimum in patients with severe liver disease. Problems are likely mainly in patients with *jaundice*, *ascites*, or evidence of *encephalopathy*.

For guidance on prescribing for patients with hepatic impairment, see p. 17. Where care is needed when prescribing in hepatic impairment, this is indicated under the relevant drug in the BNF.

Renal impairment

The use of drugs in patients with reduced renal function can give rise to many problems. Many of these problems can be avoided by reducing the dose or by using alternative drugs.

Special care is required in renal transplantation and immunosuppressed patients; if necessary such patients should be referred to specialists.

For guidance on prescribing in patients with renal impairment, see p. 17. Where care is needed when prescribing in renal impairment, this is indicated under the relevant drug in the BNF.

Pregnancy

Drugs taken during pregnancy can be harmful to the fetus and should be prescribed only if the expected benefit to the mother is thought to be greater than the risk to the fetus; all drugs should be avoided if possible during the first trimester.

For guidance on prescribing in pregnancy, see p. 19. Where care is needed when prescribing in pregnancy, this is indicated under the relevant drug in the BNF.

Breast-feeding

Some drugs taken by the mother whilst breast-feeding can be transferred to the breast milk, and may affect the infant.

For guidance on prescribing in breast-feeding, see p. 19. Where care is needed when prescribing in breast-feeding, this is indicated under the relevant drug in the BNF.

Prescribing in dental practice

Drugs and sport

UK Anti-Doping, the national body responsible for the UK's anti-doping policy, advises that athletes are personally responsible should a prohibited substance be detected in their body. An advice card listing examples of permitted and prohibited substances is available from:

UK Anti-Doping
Oceanic House
1a Cockspur Street
London SW1Y 5BG
Tel: (020) 7766 7350
information@ukad.org.uk
www.ukad.org.uk

> **General Medical Council's advice**
> Doctors who prescribe or collude in the provision of drugs or treatment with the intention of improperly enhancing an individual's performance in sport contravene the GMC's guidance, and such actions would usually raise a question of a doctor's continued registration. This does not preclude the provision of any care or treatment where the doctor's intention is to protect or improve the patient's health.

Emergency treatment of poisoning

These notes provide only an overview of the treatment of poisoning, and it is strongly recommended that either **TOXBASE** or the **UK National Poisons Information Service** (see below) be consulted when there is doubt about the degree of risk or about management.

Hospital admission Patients who have features of poisoning should generally be admitted to hospital. Patients who have taken poisons with delayed action should also be admitted, even if they appear well. Delayed-action poisons include aspirin, iron, paracetamol, tricyclic antidepressants, and co-phenotrope (diphenoxylate with atropine, *Lomotil*®); the effects of modified-release preparations are also delayed. A note of all relevant information, including what treatment has been given, should accompany the patient to hospital.

Further information and advice

TOXBASE, the primary clinical toxicology database of the National Poisons Information Service, is available on the internet to registered users at www.toxbase.org (a backup site is available at www.toxbasebackup.org if the main site cannot be accessed). It provides information about routine diagnosis, treatment, and management of patients exposed to drugs, household products, and industrial and agricultural chemicals.

Specialist information and advice on the treatment of poisoning is available day and night from the **UK National Poisons Information Service** on the following number:
Tel: 0844 892 0111

Advice on laboratory analytical services can be obtained from TOXBASE or from the National Poisons Information Service.

Help with identifying capsules or tablets may be available from a regional medicines information centre (see inside front cover) or (out of hours) from the National Poisons Information Service.

General care

It is often impossible to establish with certainty the identity of the poison and the size of the dose. This is not usually important because only a few poisons (such as opioids, paracetamol, and iron) have specific antidotes; few patients require active removal of the poison. In most patients, treatment is directed at managing symptoms as they arise. Nevertheless, knowledge of the type and timing of poisoning can help in anticipating the course of events. All relevant information should be sought from the poisoned individual and from carers or parents. However, such information should be interpreted with care because it may not be complete or entirely reliable. Sometimes symptoms arise from other illnesses and patients should be assessed carefully. Accidents may involve domestic and industrial products (the contents of which are not generally known). The **National Poisons Information Service** should be consulted when there is doubt about any aspect of suspected poisoning.

Respiration

Respiration is often impaired in unconscious patients. An obstructed airway requires immediate attention. In the absence of trauma, the airway should be opened with simple measures such as chin lift or jaw thrust. An oropharyngeal or nasopharyngeal airway may be useful in patients with reduced consciousness to prevent obstruction, provided ventilation is adequate. Intubation and ventilation should be considered in patients whose airway cannot be protected or who have respiratory acidosis because of inadequate ventilation; such patients should be monitored in a critical care area.

Most poisons that impair consciousness also depress respiration. Assisted ventilation (either mouth-to-mouth or using a bag-valve-mask device) may be needed. Oxygen is not a substitute for adequate ventilation, although it should be given in the highest concentration possible in poisoning with carbon monoxide and irritant gases.

Blood pressure

Hypotension is common in severe poisoning with central nervous system depressants. A systolic blood pressure of less than 70 mmHg may lead to irreversible brain damage or renal tubular necrosis. Hypotension should be corrected initially by raising the foot of the bed and administration of an infusion of either sodium chloride or a colloid. Vasoconstrictor sympathomimetics (section 2.7.2) are rarely required and their use may be discussed with the National Poisons Information Service.

Fluid depletion without hypotension is common after prolonged coma and after aspirin poisoning due to vomiting, sweating, and hyperpnoea.

Hypertension, often transient, occurs less frequently than hypotension in poisoning; it may be associated with sympathomimetic drugs such as amfetamines, phencyclidine, and cocaine.

Heart

Cardiac conduction defects and arrhythmias can occur in acute poisoning, notably with tricyclic antidepressants, some antipsychotics, and some antihistamines. Arrhythmias often respond to correction of underlying hypoxia, acidosis, or other biochemical abnormalities, but ventricular arrhythmias that cause serious hypotension require treatment (section 2.3.1). If the QT interval is prolonged, specialist advice should be sought because the use of some anti-arrhythmic drugs may be inappropriate. Supraventricular arrhythmias are seldom life-threatening and drug treatment is best withheld until the patient reaches hospital.

Body temperature

Hypothermia may develop in patients of any age who have been deeply unconscious for some hours, particularly following overdose with barbiturates or phenothiazines. It may be missed unless core temperature is measured using a low-reading rectal thermometer or by

Emergency treatment of poisoning

some other means. Hypothermia should be managed by prevention of further heat loss and appropriate rewarming as clinically indicated.

Hyperthermia can develop in patients taking CNS stimulants; children and the elderly are also at risk when taking therapeutic doses of drugs with antimuscarinic properties. Hyperthermia is initially managed by removing all unnecessary clothing and using a fan. Sponging with tepid water will promote evaporation. Advice should be sought from the National Poisons Information Service on the management of severe hyperthermia resulting from conditions such as the serotonin syndrome.

Both hypothermia and hyperthermia require urgent hospitalisation for assessment and supportive treatment.

Convulsions

Single short-lived convulsions (lasting less than 5 minutes) do not require treatment. If convulsions are protracted or recur frequently, lorazepam 4 mg or diazepam (preferably as emulsion) 10 mg should be given by slow intravenous injection into a large vein (section 4.8.2). Benzodiazepines should not be given by the intramuscular route for convulsions. If the intravenous route is not readily available, midazolam oromucosal solution [unlicensed use in adults and children under 3 months] can be given by the buccal route or diazepam can be administered as a rectal solution (section 4.8.2).

Methaemoglobinaemia

Drug- or chemical-induced methaemoglobinaemia should be treated with methylthioninium chloride if the methaemoglobin concentration is 30% or higher, or if symptoms of tissue hypoxia are present despite oxygen therapy. Methylthioninium chloride reduces the ferric iron of methaemoglobin back to the ferrous iron of haemoglobin; in high doses, methylthioninium can itself cause methaemoglobinaemia.

◢ METHYLTHIONINIUM CHLORIDE

(Methylene blue)

Indications drug- or chemical-induced methaemoglobinaemia

Cautions children under 3 months more susceptible to methaemoglobinaemia from high doses of methylthioninium; G6PD deficiency (seek advice from National Poisons Information Service); chlorate poisoning (reduces efficacy of methylthioninium); methaemoglobinaemia due to treatment of cyanide poisoning with sodium nitrite (seek advice from National Poisons Information Service); pulse oximetry may give false estimation of oxygen saturation; **interactions:** Appendix 1 (methylthioninium)

Renal impairment use with caution in severe impairment (dose reduction may be required)

Pregnancy no information available, but risk to fetus of untreated methaemoglobinaemia likely to be significantly higher than risk of treatment

Breast-feeding manufacturer advises avoid breast-feeding for up to 6 days after administration—no information available

Side-effects nausea, vomiting, abdominal pain, hyperbilirubinaemia (in infants), chest pain, arrhythmia, hypertension, hypotension, dyspnoea, tachypnoea, headache, dizziness, tremor, confusion, anxiety, agitation, fever, haemolytic anaemia, methaemoglobinaemia, blue-green discoloration of urine, faeces, and skin, mydriasis, sweating

Dose

By slow intravenous injection over 5 minutes, ADULT and CHILD over 3 months, 1–2 mg/kg, repeated after 30–60 minutes if necessary; seek advice from National Poisons Information Service if further repeat doses required (max. cumulative dose per course 7 mg/kg, or if aniline- or dapsone-induced methaemoglobinaemia, 4 mg/kg); CHILD under 3 months, seek advice from National Poisons Information Service

Proveblue® (Martindale) PoM
Injection, methylthioninium chloride 5 mg/mL, net price 10-mL amp = £39.38

Removal and elimination

Prevention of absorption

Given by mouth, **activated charcoal** can bind many poisons in the gastro-intestinal system, thereby reducing their absorption. The **sooner** it is given the **more effective** it is, but it may still be effective up to 1 hour after ingestion of the poison—longer in the case of modified-release preparations or of drugs with antimuscarinic (anticholinergic) properties. It is particularly useful for the prevention of absorption of poisons that are toxic in small amounts, such as antidepressants.

For the use of charcoal in active elimination techniques, see below.

Active elimination techniques

Repeated doses of **activated charcoal** by mouth *enhance the elimination* of some drugs after they have been absorbed; repeated doses are given after overdosage with:

Carbamazepine

Dapsone

Phenobarbital

Quinine

Theophylline

The usual dose of activated charcoal in adults and children over 12 years of age is 50 g initially then 50 g every 4 hours. Vomiting should be treated (e.g. with an antiemetic drug) since it may reduce the efficacy of charcoal treatment. In cases of intolerance, the dose may be reduced and the frequency increased (e.g. 25 g every 2 hours *or* 12.5 g every hour) but this may compromise efficacy.

In children under 12 years of age, activated charcoal is given in a dose of 1 g/kg (max. 50 g) every 4 hours; the dose may be reduced and the frequency increased if not tolerated.

Other techniques intended to enhance the elimination of poisons after absorption are only practicable in hospital and are only suitable for a small number of severely poisoned patients. Moreover, they only apply to a limited number of poisons. Examples include:

- haemodialysis for ethylene glycol, lithium, methanol, phenobarbital, salicylates, and sodium valproate;

- alkalinisation of the urine for salicylates.

Removal from the gastro-intestinal tract

Gastric lavage is rarely required; for substances that cannot be removed effectively by other means (e.g. iron), it should be considered only if a life-threatening amount has been ingested within the previous hour. It should be carried out only if the airway can be protected adequately. Gastric lavage is contra-indicated if a corrosive substance or a petroleum distillate has been ingested, but it may occasionally be considered in patients who have ingested drugs that are not adsorbed by charcoal, such as iron or lithium. Induction of *emesis* (e.g. with ipecacuanha) is **not** recommended because there is no evidence that it affects absorption and it may increase the risk of aspiration.

Whole bowel irrigation (by means of a bowel cleansing preparation) has been used in poisoning with certain modified-release or enteric-coated formulations, in severe poisoning with iron and lithium salts, and if illicit drugs are carried in the gastro-intestinal tract ('body-packing'). However, it is not clear that the procedure improves outcome and advice should be sought from the National Poisons Information Service.

▮ CHARCOAL, ACTIVATED

Indications   reduction of absorption of poisons in the gastro-intestinal system; see also active elimination techniques, above

Cautions   drowsy or comatose patient (risk of aspiration—ensure airway protected); reduced gastro-intestinal motility (risk of obstruction); **not** for poisoning with petroleum distillates, corrosive substances, alcohols, malathion, cyanides, and metal salts including iron and lithium salts

Side-effects   black stools

Dose

• Reduction of absorption, ADULT and CHILD over 12 years, 50 g; CHILD under 12 years, 1 g/kg (max. 50 g)

• Active elimination, see notes above
 Note   Activated charcoal doses in BNF may differ from those in product literature. Suspension or reconstituted powder may be mixed with soft drinks (e.g. caffeine-free diet cola) or fruit juices to mask the taste

Actidose-Aqua® Advance (Alliance)
 Oral suspension, activated charcoal 1.04 g/5 mL, net price 50-g pack (240 mL) = £12.89

Carbomix® (Beacon)
 Granules, activated charcoal, net price 50-g pack = £11.90

Charcodote® (TEVA UK)
 Oral suspension, activated charcoal 1 g/5 mL, net price 50-g pack = £11.88

Specific drugs

Alcohol

Acute intoxication with alcohol (ethanol) is common in adults but also occurs in children. The features include ataxia, dysarthria, nystagmus, and drowsiness, which may progress to coma, with hypotension and acidosis. Aspiration of vomit is a special hazard and hypoglycaemia may occur in children and some adults. Patients are managed supportively, with particular attention to maintaining a clear airway and measures to reduce the risk of aspiration of gastric contents. The blood glucose is measured and glucose given if indicated.

> The **National Poisons Information Service** (Tel: 0844 892 0111) will provide specialist advice on all aspects of poisoning day and night

Analgesics (non-opioid)

Aspirin   The main features of salicylate poisoning are hyperventilation, tinnitus, deafness, vasodilatation, and sweating. Coma is uncommon but indicates very severe poisoning. The associated acid-base disturbances are complex.

Treatment must be in hospital, where plasma salicylate, pH, and electrolytes can be measured; absorption of aspirin may be slow and the plasma-salicylate concentration may continue to rise for several hours, requiring repeated measurement. Plasma-salicylate concentration may not correlate with clinical severity in the young and the elderly, and clinical and biochemical assessment is necessary. Generally, the clinical severity of poisoning is less below a plasma-salicylate concentration of 500 mg/litre (3.6 mmol/litre), unless there is evidence of metabolic acidosis. Activated charcoal can be given within 1 hour of ingesting more than 125 mg/kg of aspirin. Fluid losses should be replaced and intravenous sodium bicarbonate may be given (ensuring plasma-potassium concentration is within the reference range) to enhance urinary salicylate excretion (optimum urinary pH 7.5–8.5).

Plasma-potassium concentration should be corrected before giving sodium bicarbonate as hypokalaemia may complicate alkalinisation of the urine.

Haemodialysis is the treatment of choice for severe salicylate poisoning and should be considered when the plasma-salicylate concentration exceeds 700 mg/litre (5.1 mmol/litre) or in the presence of severe metabolic acidosis.

NSAIDs   Mefenamic acid has important consequences in overdosage because it can cause convulsions, which if prolonged or recurrent require treatment, see p. 34.

Overdosage with ibuprofen may cause nausea, vomiting, epigastric pain, and tinnitus, but more serious toxicity is very uncommon. Activated charcoal followed by symptomatic measures are indicated if more than 100 mg/kg has been ingested within the preceding hour.

Paracetamol

> In cases of **intravenous paracetamol** poisoning contact the National Poisons Information Service for advice on risk assessment and management.

Toxic doses of paracetamol may cause severe hepatocellular necrosis and, much less frequently, renal tubular necrosis. Nausea and vomiting, the only early features of poisoning, usually settle within 24 hours. Persistence beyond this time, often associated with the onset of right subcostal pain and tenderness, usually indicates development of hepatic necrosis. Liver damage is maximal 3–4 days after paracetamol overdose and may lead to encephalopathy, haemorrhage, hypoglycaemia, cerebral oedema, and death. Therefore, despite a lack of significant early symptoms, patients who have taken an overdose of paracetamol should be transferred to hospital urgently.

To avoid underestimating the potentially toxic paracetamol dose ingested by obese patients who weigh more than 110 kg, use a body-weight of 110 kg (rather than their actual body-weight) when calculating the total dose of paracetamol ingested (in mg/kg).

Acetylcysteine protects the liver if infused up to, and possibly beyond, 24 hours of ingesting paracetamol. It is most effective if given within 8 hours of ingestion, after which effectiveness declines. Very rarely, giving acetylcysteine by mouth [unlicensed route] is an alternative if intravenous access is not possible—contact the National Poisons Information Service for advice.

Neonates less than 45 weeks corrected gestational age may be more susceptible to paracetamol-induced liver toxicity, therefore, treatment with acetylcysteine should be considered in all paracetamol overdoses, and advice should be sought from the National Poisons Information Service.

Acute overdose Hepatotoxicity may occur after a single ingestion of more than 150 mg/kg paracetamol taken in less than 1 hour. Rarely, hepatotoxicity may develop with single ingestions as low as 75 mg/kg of paracetamol taken in less than 1 hour. Patients who have ingested 75 mg/kg or more of paracetamol in less than 1 hour should be referred to hospital. Administra-

tion of activated charcoal should be considered if paracetamol in excess of 150 mg/kg is thought to have been ingested within the previous hour.

Patients at risk of liver damage and, therefore, requiring acetylcysteine, can be identified from a single measurement of the plasma-paracetamol concentration, related to the time from ingestion, provided this time interval is not less than 4 hours; earlier samples may be misleading. The concentration is plotted on a paracetamol treatment graph, with a reference line ('treatment line') joining plots of 100 mg/litre (0.66 mmol/litre) at 4 hours and 3.13 mg/litre (0.02 mmol/litre) at 24 hours (see p. 36). Acetylcysteine treatment should commence immediately in patients:

- whose plasma-paracetamol concentration falls on or above the *treatment line* on the paracetamol treatment graph (see p. 36);

- who present 8–24 hours after taking an acute overdose of more than 150 mg/kg of paracetamol, even if the plasma-paracetamol concentration is not yet available; acetylcysteine can be discontinued if the plasma-paracetamol concentration is later reported to be below the *treatment line* on the paracetamol treatment graph (see p. 36), provided that the patient is asymptomatic and liver function tests, serum creatinine and INR are normal.

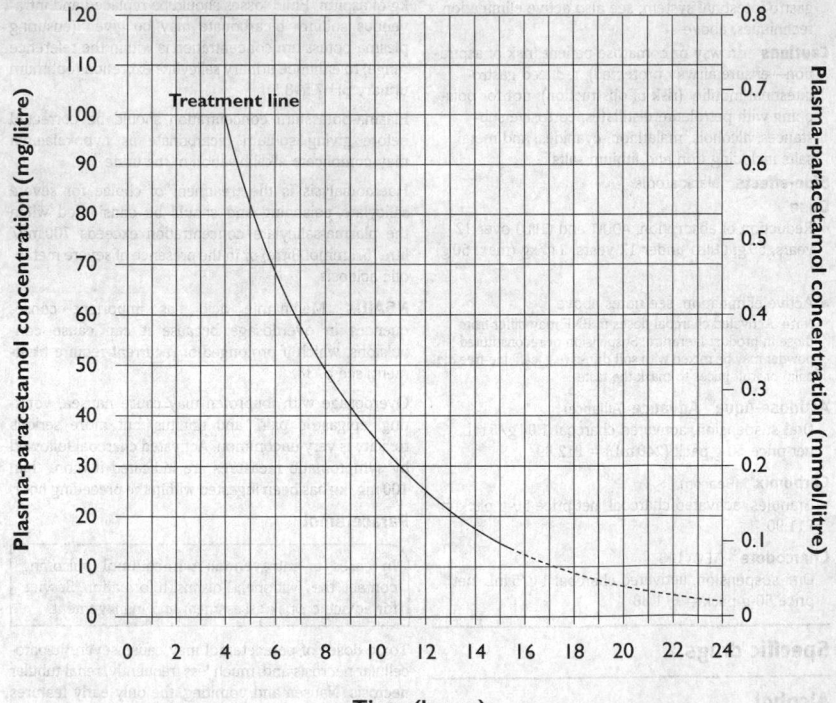

Patients whose plasma-paracetamol concentrations are on or above the **treatment line** should be treated with acetylcysteine by intravenous infusion.

The prognostic accuracy after 15 hours is uncertain, but a plasma-paracetamol concentration on or above the treatment line should be regarded as carrying a serious risk of liver damage.

Graph reproduced courtesy of Medicines and Healthcare products Regulatory Agency

The prognostic accuracy of a plasma-paracetamol concentration taken after 15 hours is uncertain, but a concentration on or above the *treatment line* on the paracetamol treatment graph (see p. 36) should be regarded as carrying a serious risk of liver damage. If more than 15 hours have elapsed since ingestion, or there is doubt about appropriate management, advice should be sought from the National Poisons Information Service.

'Staggered' overdose, uncertain time of overdose, or therapeutic excess A 'staggered' overdose involves ingestion of a potentially toxic dose of paracetamol over more than one hour, with the possible intention of causing self-harm. Therapeutic excess is the inadvertent ingestion of a potentially toxic dose of paracetamol during its clinical use. The paracetamol treatment graph is unreliable if a 'staggered' overdose is taken, if there is uncertainty about the time of the overdose, or if there is therapeutic excess. In these cases, patients who have taken more than 150 mg/kg of paracetamol in any 24-hour period are at risk of toxicity and should be commenced on acetylcysteine immediately, unless it is more than 24 hours since the last ingestion, the patient is asymptomatic, the plasma-paracetamol concentration is undetectable, and liver function tests, serum creatinine and INR are normal.

Rarely, toxicity can occur with paracetamol doses between 75–150 mg/kg in any 24-hour period; clinical judgement of the individual case is necessary to determine whether to treat those who have ingested this amount of paracetamol. For small adults, this may be within the licensed dose, but ingestion of a licensed dose of paracetamol is not considered an overdose.

Although there is some evidence suggesting that factors such as the use of liver enzyme-inducing drugs (e.g. carbamazepine, efavirenz, nevirapine, phenobarbital, phenytoin, primidone, rifabutin, rifampicin, St John's wort), chronic alcoholism, and starvation may increase the risk of hepatotoxicity, the CHM has advised that these should no longer be used in the assessment of paracetamol toxicity.

Significant toxicity is unlikely if, 24 hours or longer after the last paracetamol ingestion, the patient is asymptomatic, the plasma-paracetamol concentration is undetectable, and liver function tests, serum creatinine and INR are normal. Patients with clinical features of hepatic injury such as jaundice or hepatic tenderness should be treated urgently with acetylcysteine. If there is uncertainty about a patient's risk of toxicity after paracetamol overdose, treatment with acetylcysteine should be commenced. Advice should be sought from the National Poisons Information Service whenever necessary.

Acetylcysteine dose and administration For paracetamol overdosage, acetylcysteine is given in a total dose that is divided into 3 consecutive intravenous infusions over a total of 21 hours. The tables below include the dose of acetylcysteine, for adults and children of body-weight 40 kg and over, in terms of the volume of Acetylcysteine Concentrate for Intravenous Infusion required for each of the 3 infusions. The requisite dose of acetylcysteine is added to Glucose Intravenous Infusion 5%.

> **Note** Glucose Intravenous Infusion 5% is the preferred fluid; Sodium Chloride Intravenous Infusion 0.9% is an alternative if Glucose Intravenous Infusion 5% is unsuitable

First infusion (based on an acetylcysteine dose of approx. 150 mg/kg)—add requisite volume of Acetylcysteine Concentrate for Intravenous Infusion to 200 mL Glucose Intravenous Infusion 5%; infuse over 1 hour.

Body-weight	Volume of Acetylcysteine Concentrate for Intravenous Infusion 200 mg/mL required to prepare first infusion
40–49 kg	34 mL
50–59 kg	42 mL
60–69 kg	49 mL
70–79 kg	57 mL
80–89 kg	64 mL
90–99 kg	72 mL
100–109 kg	79 mL
≥110 kg	83 mL (max. dose)

Second infusion (based on an acetylcysteine dose of approx. 50 mg/kg; start immediately after completion of first infusion)—add requisite volume of Acetylcysteine Concentrate for Intravenous Infusion to 500 mL Glucose Intravenous Infusion 5%; infuse over 4 hours.

Body-weight	Volume of Acetylcysteine Concentrate for Intravenous Infusion 200 mg/mL required to prepare second infusion
40–49 kg	12 mL
50–59 kg	14 mL
60–69 kg	17 mL
70–79 kg	19 mL
80–89 kg	22 mL
90–99 kg	24 mL
100–109 kg	27 mL
≥110 kg	28 mL (max. dose)

Third infusion (based on an acetylcysteine dose of approx. 100 mg/kg; start immediately after completion of second infusion)—add requisite volume of Acetylcysteine Concentrate for Intravenous Infusion to 1 litre Glucose Intravenous Infusion 5%; infuse over 16 hours

Body-weight	Volume of Acetylcysteine Concentrate for Intravenous Infusion 200 mg/mL required to prepare third infusion
40–49 kg	23 mL
50–59 kg	28 mL
60–69 kg	33 mL
70–79 kg	38 mL
80–89 kg	43 mL
90–99 kg	48 mL
100–109 kg	53 mL
≥110 kg	55 mL (max. dose)

> The **National Poisons Information Service** (Tel: 0844 892 0111) will provide specialist advice on all aspects of poisoning day and night

Emergency treatment of poisoning

ACETYLCYSTEINE

Indications paracetamol overdosage, see notes above

Cautions atopy; asthma (see Side-effects below but do not delay acetylcysteine treatment); acetylcysteine may slightly increase INR and prothrombin time

Side-effects hypersensitivity-like reactions managed by reducing infusion rate or suspending until reaction settled (rash also managed by giving antihistamine; acute asthma managed by giving nebulised short-acting beta$_2$agonist)—contact the National Poisons Information Service if reaction severe; slight increase in INR and prothrombin time

Dose

* By intravenous infusion, ADULT and CHILD body-weight over 40 kg, see Acetylcysteine Dose and Administration in notes above; CHILD body-weight under 20 kg, initially 150 mg/kg in 3 mL/kg glucose 5% and given over 1 hour, followed by 50 mg/kg in 7 mL/kg glucose 5% and given over 4 hours, then 100 mg/kg in 14 mL/kg glucose 5% and given over 16 hours; CHILD body-weight 20–40 kg, initially 150 mg/kg in 100 mL glucose 5% and given over 1 hour, followed by 50 mg/kg in 250 mL glucose 5% and given over 4 hours, then 100 mg/kg in 500 mL glucose 5% and given over 16 hours

    Note Glucose 5% is preferred infusion fluid; sodium chloride 0.9% is an alternative if glucose 5% unsuitable

Acetylcysteine (Non-proprietary) [PoM]

Concentrate for intravenous infusion, acetylcysteine 200 mg/mL, net price 10-mL amp = £1.96

Parvolex® (Phoenix) [PoM]

Concentrate for intravenous infusion, acetylcysteine 200 mg/mL, net price 10-mL amp = £2.25

Electrolytes Na$^+$ 14 mmol/10-mL amp

Analgesics (opioid)

Opioids (narcotic analgesics) cause coma, respiratory depression, and pinpoint pupils. The specific antidote **naloxone** is indicated if there is coma or bradypnoea. Since naloxone has a shorter duration of action than many opioids, close monitoring and repeated injections are necessary according to the respiratory rate and depth of coma. When repeated administration of naloxone is required, it can be given by continuous intravenous infusion instead and the rate of infusion adjusted according to vital signs. The effects of some opioids, such as buprenorphine, are only partially reversed by naloxone. Dextropropoxyphene and methadone have very long durations of action; patients may need to be monitored for long periods following large overdoses.

Naloxone reverses the opioid effects of dextropropoxyphene; the long duration of action of dextropropoxyphene calls for prolonged monitoring and further doses of naloxone may be required. Norpropoxyphene, a metabolite of dextropropoxyphene, also has cardiotoxic effects which may require treatment with **sodium bicarbonate**, or **magnesium sulfate**, or both; arrhythmias may occur for up to 12 hours.

NALOXONE HYDROCHLORIDE

Indications overdosage with opioids; reversal of postoperative respiratory depression and reversal of neonatal respiratory and CNS depression resulting from opioid administration to mother during labour (section 15.1.7)

Cautions physical dependence on opioids; cardiac irritability; naloxone is short-acting, see notes above

Pregnancy section 15.1.7

Breast-feeding section 15.1.7

Side-effects section 15.1.7

Dose

* By intravenous injection, 400 micrograms; if no response after 1 minute, give 800 micrograms, and if still no response after another 1 minute, repeat dose of 800 micrograms; if still no response, give 2 mg (4 mg may be required in a seriously poisoned patient), then review diagnosis; further doses may be required if respiratory function deteriorates; CHILD under 12 years 100 micrograms/kg (max 2 mg); if no response, repeat at intervals of 1 minute to a total max. 2 mg, then review diagnosis; further doses may be required if respiratory function deteriorates

* By subcutaneous *or* intramuscular injection, ADULT and CHILD dose as for intravenous injection but use only if intravenous route not feasible (onset of action slower); for intramuscular injection in a *non-medical setting*, see under preparations

* By continuous intravenous infusion using an infusion pump, ADULT and CHILD, rate adjusted according to response (initially, rate may be set at 60% of the initial resuscitative *intravenous injection* dose per hour)

    Note The initial resuscitative *intravenous injection* dose is that which maintained satisfactory ventilation for at least 15 minutes

Important Doses used in acute opioid overdosage may not be appropriate for the management of opioid-induced respiratory depression and sedation in those receiving palliative care and in chronic opioid use; see also section 15.1.7 for management of postoperative respiratory depression

[1]**Naloxone** (Non-proprietary) [PoM]

Injection, naloxone hydrochloride 20 micrograms/mL, net price 2-mL amp = £5.50; 400 micrograms/mL, 1-mL amp = £4.10; 1 mg/mL, 2-mL prefilled syringe = £16.50

[1]**Minijet® Naloxone** (UCB Pharma) [PoM]

Injection, naloxone hydrochloride 400 micrograms/mL, net price 1-mL disposable syringe = £20.40, 2-mL disposable syringe = £12.96, 5-mL disposable syringe = £20.40

[1]**Prenoxad®** (Martindale) [PoM]

Injection, naloxone hydrochloride 1 mg/mL, net price 2-mL prefilled syringe = £18.00

Electrolytes Na$^+$ < 0.5 mmol/syringe

Dose by intramuscular injection (into deltoid region or anterolateral thigh) in a *non-medical setting*, ADULT 400 micrograms repeated at intervals of 2–3 minutes (in subsequent resuscitation cycles if patient not breathing normally) until consciousness regained, breathing normally, medical assistance available, or contents of syringe used up

Antidepressants

Tricyclic and related antidepressants Tricyclic and related antidepressants cause dry mouth, coma of varying degree, hypotension, hypothermia, hyperreflexia, extensor plantar responses, convulsions, respiratory failure, cardiac conduction defects, and arrhythmias. Dilated pupils and urinary retention also occur. Metabolic acidosis may complicate severe poisoning; delirium with confusion, agitation, and visual and auditory hallucinations are common during recovery.

---

1. [PoM] restriction does not apply where administration is for saving life in emergency

Assessment in hospital is strongly advised in case of poisoning by *tricyclic and related antidepressants* but symptomatic treatment can be given before transfer. Supportive measures to ensure a clear airway and adequate ventilation during transfer are mandatory. Intravenous lorazepam or intravenous diazepam (preferably in emulsion form) may be required to treat convulsions. Activated charcoal given within 1 hour of the overdose reduces absorption of the drug. Although arrhythmias are worrying, some will respond to correction of hypoxia and acidosis. The use of anti-arrhythmic drugs is best avoided, but intravenous infusion of sodium bicarbonate can arrest arrhythmias or prevent them in those with an extended QRS duration. Diazepam given by mouth is usually adequate to sedate delirious patients but large doses may be required.

Selective serotonin re-uptake inhibitors (SSRIs)

Symptoms of poisoning by selective serotonin re-uptake inhibitors include nausea, vomiting, agitation, tremor, nystagmus, drowsiness, and sinus tachycardia; convulsions may occur. Rarely, severe poisoning results in the serotonin syndrome, with marked neuropsychiatric effects, neuromuscular hyperactivity, and autonomic instability: hyperthermia, rhabdomyolysis, renal failure, and coagulopathies may develop.

Management of SSRI poisoning is supportive. Activated charcoal given within 1 hour of the overdose reduces absorption of the drug. Convulsions can be treated with lorazepam, diazepam, or midazolam oromucosal solution [unlicensed use in adults and children under 3 months] (see p. 34). Contact the National Poisons Information Service for the management of hyperthermia or the serotonin syndrome.

> The **National Poisons Information Service** (Tel: 0844 892 0111) will provide specialist advice on all aspects of poisoning day and night

Antimalarials

Overdosage with quinine, chloroquine, or hydroxychloroquine is extremely hazardous and difficult to treat. Urgent advice from the National Poisons Information Service is essential. Life-threatening features include arrhythmias (which can have a very rapid onset) and convulsions (which can be intractable).

Beta-blockers

Therapeutic overdosages with beta-blockers may cause lightheadedness, dizziness, and possibly syncope as a result of bradycardia and hypotension; heart failure may be precipitated or exacerbated. These complications are most likely in patients with conduction system disorders or impaired myocardial function. Bradycardia is the most common arrhythmia caused by beta-blockers, but sotalol may induce ventricular tachyarrhythmias (sometimes of the torsade de pointes type). The effects of massive overdosage can vary from one beta-blocker to another; propranolol overdosage in particular may cause coma and convulsions.

Acute massive overdosage must be managed in hospital and expert advice should be obtained. Maintenance of a clear airway and adequate ventilation is mandatory. An intravenous injection of atropine is required to treat bradycardia (3 mg for an adult, 40 micrograms/kg (max. 3 mg) for a child). Cardiogenic shock unresponsive to atropine is probably best treated with an intravenous injection of glucagon 2–10 mg (CHILD 50–150 micrograms/kg, max. 10 mg) [unlicensed indication and dose] in glucose 5% (with precautions to protect the airway in case of vomiting) followed by an intravenous infusion of 50 micrograms/kg/hour. If glucagon is not available, intravenous isoprenaline (available from 'special-order' manufacturers or specialist importing companies, see p. 1124) is an alternative. A cardiac pacemaker can be used to increase the heart rate.

Calcium-channel blockers

Features of calcium-channel blocker poisoning include nausea, vomiting, dizziness, agitation, confusion, and coma in severe poisoning. Metabolic acidosis and hyperglycaemia may occur. Verapamil and diltiazem have a profound cardiac depressant effect causing hypotension and arrhythmias, including complete heart block and asystole. The dihydropyridine calcium-channel blockers cause severe hypotension secondary to profound peripheral vasodilatation.

Activated charcoal should be considered if the patient presents within 1 hour of overdosage with a calcium-channel blocker; repeated doses of activated charcoal are considered if a modified-release preparation is involved. In patients with significant features of poisoning, calcium chloride or calcium gluconate (section 9.5.1.1) is given by injection; atropine is given to correct symptomatic bradycardia. In severe cases, an insulin and glucose infusion may be required in the management of hypotension and myocardial failure. For the management of hypotension, the choice of inotropic sympathomimetic depends on whether hypotension is secondary to vasodilatation or to myocardial depression—advice should be sought from the National Poisons Information Service (p. 33).

Hypnotics and anxiolytics

Benzodiazepines Benzodiazepines taken alone cause drowsiness, ataxia, dysarthria, nystagmus, and occasionally respiratory depression, and coma. Activated charcoal can be given within 1 hour of ingesting a significant quantity of benzodiazepine, provided the patient is awake and the airway is protected. Benzodiazepines potentiate the effects of other central nervous system depressants taken concomitantly. Use of the benzodiazepine antagonist flumazenil [unlicensed indication] can be hazardous, particularly in mixed overdoses involving tricyclic antidepressants or in benzodiazepine-dependent patients. Flumazenil may prevent the need for ventilation, particularly in patients with severe respiratory disorders; it should be used on expert advice only and not as a diagnostic test in patients with a reduced level of consciousness.

Iron salts

Iron poisoning in childhood is usually accidental. The symptoms are nausea, vomiting, abdominal pain, diarrhoea, haematemesis, and rectal bleeding. Hypotension and hepatocellular necrosis can occur later. Coma, shock, and metabolic acidosis indicate severe poisoning.

Advice should be sought from the National Poisons Information Service if a significant quantity of iron has been ingested within the previous hour.

Mortality is reduced by intensive and specific therapy with **desferrioxamine**, which chelates iron. The serum-iron concentration is measured as an emergency and intravenous desferrioxamine given to chelate absorbed iron in excess of the expected iron binding capacity. In **severe toxicity** intravenous desferrioxamine should be given *immediately* without waiting for the result of the serum-iron measurement.

DESFERRIOXAMINE MESILATE

(Deferoxamine Mesilate)

Indications iron poisoning; chronic iron overload (section 9.1.3)

Cautions section 9.1.3

Renal impairment section 9.1.3

Pregnancy section 9.1.3

Breast-feeding section 9.1.3

Side-effects section 9.1.3

Dose

- By continuous intravenous infusion, ADULT and CHILD up to 15 mg/kg/hour, reduced after 4–6 hours; max. 80 mg/kg in 24 hours (in severe cases, higher doses on advice from the National Poisons Information Service)

◢**Preparations**

Section 9.1.3

Lithium

Most cases of lithium intoxication occur as a complication of long-term therapy and are caused by reduced excretion of the drug because of a variety of factors including dehydration, deterioration of renal function, infections, and co-administration of diuretics or NSAIDs (or other drugs that interact). Acute deliberate overdoses may also occur with delayed onset of symptoms (12 hours or more) owing to slow entry of lithium into the tissues and continuing absorption from modified-release formulations.

The early clinical features are non-specific and may include apathy and restlessness which could be confused with mental changes arising from the patient's depressive illness. Vomiting, diarrhoea, ataxia, weakness, dysarthria, muscle twitching, and tremor may follow. Severe poisoning is associated with convulsions, coma, renal failure, electrolyte imbalance, dehydration, and hypotension.

Therapeutic serum-lithium concentrations are within the range of 0.4–1 mmol/litre; concentrations in excess of 2 mmol/litre are usually associated with serious toxicity and such cases may need treatment with haemodialysis if neurological symptoms or renal failure are present. In acute overdosage much higher serum-lithium concentrations may be present without features of toxicity and all that is usually necessary is to take measures to increase urine output (e.g. by increasing fluid intake but avoiding diuretics). Otherwise, treatment is supportive with special regard to electrolyte balance, renal function, and control of convulsions. Gastric lavage may be considered if it can be performed within 1 hour of ingesting significant quantities of lithium. Whole-bowel irrigation should be considered for significant ingestion, but advice should be sought from the National Poisons Information Service, p. 33.

Phenothiazines and related drugs

Phenothiazines cause less depression of consciousness and respiration than other sedatives. Hypotension, hypothermia, sinus tachycardia, and arrhythmias may complicate poisoning. Dystonic reactions can occur with therapeutic doses (particularly with prochlorperazine and trifluoperazine), and convulsions may occur in severe cases. Arrhythmias may respond to correction of hypoxia, acidosis, and other biochemical abnormalities, but specialist advice should be sought if arrhythmias result from a prolonged QT interval; the use of some anti-arrhythmic drugs can worsen such arrhythmias. Dystonic reactions are rapidly abolished by injection of drugs such as procyclidine (section 4.9.2) or diazepam (section 4.8.2, emulsion preferred).

Second-generation antipsychotic drugs

Features of poisoning by second-generation antipsychotic drugs (section 4.2.1) include drowsiness, convulsions, extrapyramidal symptoms, hypotension, and ECG abnormalities (including prolongation of the QT interval). Management is supportive. Activated charcoal can be given within 1 hour of ingesting a significant quantity of a second-generation antipsychotic drug.

Stimulants

Amfetamines Amfetamines cause wakefulness, excessive activity, paranoia, hallucinations, and hypertension followed by exhaustion, convulsions, hyperthermia, and coma. The early stages can be controlled by diazepam or lorazepam; advice should be sought from the National Poisons Information Service (p. 33) on the management of hypertension. Later, tepid sponging, anticonvulsants, and artificial respiration may be needed.

Cocaine Cocaine stimulates the central nervous system, causing agitation, dilated pupils, tachycardia, hypertension, hallucinations, hyperthermia, hypertonia, and hyperreflexia; cardiac effects include chest pain, myocardial infarction, and arrhythmias.

Initial treatment of cocaine poisoning involves intravenous administration of diazepam to control agitation and cooling measures for hyperthermia (see Body temperature, p. 33); hypertension and cardiac effects require specific treatment and expert advice should be sought.

Ecstasy Ecstasy (methylenedioxymethamfetamine, MDMA) may cause severe reactions, even at doses that were previously tolerated. The most serious effects are delirium, coma, convulsions, ventricular arrhythmias, hyperthermia, rhabdomyolysis, acute renal failure, acute hepatitis, disseminated intravascular coagulation, adult respiratory distress syndrome, hyperreflexia, hypotension and intracerebral haemorrhage; hyponatraemia has also been associated with ecstasy use.

Treatment of methylenedioxymethamfetamine poisoning is supportive, with diazepam to control severe agitation or persistent convulsions and close monitoring including ECG. Self-induced water intoxication should be considered in patients with ecstasy poisoning.

'Liquid ecstasy' is a term used for sodium oxybate (gamma-hydroxybutyrate, GHB), which is a sedative.

Theophylline

Theophylline and related drugs are often prescribed as modified-release formulations and toxicity can therefore be delayed. They cause vomiting (which may be severe and intractable), agitation, restlessness, dilated pupils, sinus tachycardia, and hyperglycaemia. More serious effects are haematemesis, convulsions, and supraventricular and ventricular arrhythmias. Severe hypokalaemia may develop rapidly.

Repeated doses of activated charcoal can be used to eliminate theophylline even if more than 1 hour has elapsed after ingestion and especially if a modified-release preparation has been taken (see also under Active Elimination Techniques, p. 34). Ondansetron (section 4.6) may be effective for severe vomiting that is resistant to other antiemetics [unlicensed indication]. Hypokalaemia is corrected by intravenous infusion of potassium chloride (section 9.2.2.1) and may be so severe as to require 60 mmol/hour (high doses require ECG monitoring). Convulsions should be controlled by intravenous administration of lorazepam or diazepam (see Convulsions, p. 34). Sedation with diazepam may be necessary in agitated patients.

Provided the patient does **not** suffer from asthma, a short-acting beta-blocker (section 2.4) can be administered intravenously to reverse severe tachycardia, hypokalaemia, and hyperglycaemia.

Other poisons

Consult either the National Poisons Information Service day and night or TOXBASE, see p. 33.

> The **National Poisons Information Service** (Tel: 0844 892 0111) will provide specialist advice on all aspects of poisoning day and night

Cyanides

Oxygen should be administered to patients with cyanide poisoning. The choice of antidote depends on the severity of poisoning, certainty of diagnosis, and the cause. Dicobalt edetate is the antidote of choice when there is a strong clinical suspicion of severe cyanide poisoning. **Dicobalt edetate** itself is toxic, associated with anaphylactoid reactions, and is potentially fatal if administered in the absence of cyanide poisoning. A regimen of **sodium nitrite** followed by **sodium thiosulfate** is an alternative if dicobalt edetate is not available.

Hydroxocobalamin (*Cyanokit*®—no other preparation of hydroxocobalamin is suitable) can be considered for use in victims of smoke inhalation who show signs of significant cyanide poisoning.

◼ DICOBALT EDETATE

Indications severe poisoning with cyanides
Cautions owing to toxicity to be used only for definite cyanide poisoning when patient tending to lose, or has lost, consciousness; **not** to be used as a precautionary measure
Side-effects hypotension, tachycardia, and vomiting; anaphylactoid reactions including facial and laryngeal oedema and cardiac abnormalities

Dose
- By intravenous injection, ADULT 300 mg over 1 minute (5 minutes if condition less serious) followed immediately by 50 mL of glucose intravenous infusion 50%; if response inadequate a second dose of both may be given, but risk of cobalt toxicity; CHILD consult the National Poisons Information Service

¹**Dicobalt Edetate** (Non-proprietary) PoM
Injection, dicobalt edetate 15 mg/mL, net price 20-mL (300-mg) amp = £16.99

◼ HYDROXOCOBALAMIN

Indications poisoning with cyanides (see notes above)
Side-effects gastro-intestinal disturbances, transient hypertension, peripheral oedema, dyspnoea, throat disorders, hot flush, dizziness, headache, restlessness, memory impairment, red coloration of urine, lymphocytopenia, eye disorders, pustular rashes, pruritus, reversible red coloration of skin and mucous membranes

Dose
- By intravenous infusion, ADULT 5 g over 15 minutes; a second dose of 5 g can be given over 15 minutes–2 hours depending on severity of poisoning and patient stability; CHILD under 18 years with body-weight 5 kg and over, 70 mg/kg (max. 5 g) over 15 minutes; a second dose of 70 mg/kg (max. 5 g) can be given over 15 minutes–2 hours depending on severity of poisoning and patient stability

Cyanokit® (Swedish Orphan) PoM
Intravenous infusion, powder for reconstitution, hydroxocobalamin, net price 5-g vial = £772.00
Note Deep red colour of hydroxocobalamin may interfere with laboratory tests (see Side-effects, above) and haemodialysis

◼ SODIUM NITRITE

Indications poisoning with cyanides (used in conjunction with sodium thiosulfate)
Side-effects flushing and headache due to vasodilatation

Dose
- By intravenous injection over 5–20 minutes (as sodium nitrite injection 30 mg/mL), 300 mg; CHILD 4–10 mg/kg (max. 300 mg)

¹**Sodium Nitrite** PoM
Injection, sodium nitrite 3% (30 mg/mL) in water for injections
Available from 'special-order' manufacturers or specialist importing companies, see p. 1124

◼ SODIUM THIOSULFATE

Indications in conjunction with sodium nitrite for cyanide poisoning

Dose
- By intravenous injection over 10 minutes (as sodium thiosulfate injection 500 mg/mL), 12.5 g; dose may be repeated in severe cyanide poisoning if dicobalt edetate not available; CHILD 400 mg/kg (max. 12.5 g); dose may be repeated in severe cyanide poisoning if dicobalt edetate not available

---

1. PoM restriction does not apply where administration is for saving life in emergency

Emergency treatment of poisoning

Emergency treatment of poisoning

[1]**Sodium Thiosulfate** PoM
Injection, sodium thiosulfate 50% (500 mg/mL) in water for injections
Available from 'special-order' manufacturers or specialist importing companies, see p. 1124

Ethylene glycol and methanol

Fomepizole (available from 'special-order' manufacturers or specialist importing companies, see p. 1124) is the treatment of choice for ethylene glycol and methanol (methyl alcohol) poisoning. If necessary, **ethanol** (by mouth or by intravenous infusion) can be used, but with caution. Advice on the treatment of ethylene glycol and methanol poisoning should be obtained from the National Poisons Information Service. It is important to start antidote treatment promptly in cases of suspected poisoning with these agents.

Heavy metals

Heavy metal antidotes include succimer (DMSA) [unlicensed], unithiol (DMPS) [unlicensed], sodium calcium edetate [unlicensed], and dimercaprol. Dimercaprol in the management of heavy metal poisoning has been superseded by other chelating agents. In all cases of heavy metal poisoning, the advice of the National Poisons Information Service should be sought.

Noxious gases

Carbon monoxide   Carbon monoxide poisoning is usually due to inhalation of smoke, car exhaust, or fumes caused by blocked flues or incomplete combustion of fuel gases in confined spaces.

Immediate treatment of carbon monoxide poisoning is essential. The person should be moved to fresh air, the airway cleared, and high-flow **oxygen** 100% administered through a tight-fitting mask with an inflated face seal. Artificial respiration should be given as necessary and continued until adequate spontaneous breathing starts, or stopped only after persistent and efficient treatment of cardiac arrest has failed. The patient should be admitted to hospital because complications may arise after a delay of hours or days. Cerebral oedema may occur in severe poisoning and is treated with an intravenous infusion of mannitol (section 2.2.5). Referral for hyperbaric oxygen treatment should be discussed with the National Poisons Information Service if the patient is pregnant or in cases of severe poisoning, such as if the patient is or has been unconscious, or has psychiatric or neurological features other than a headache, or has myocardial ischaemia or an arrhythmia, or has a blood carboxyhaemoglobin concentration of more than 20%.

Sulfur dioxide, chlorine, phosgene, ammonia   All of these gases can cause upper respiratory tract and conjunctival irritation. Pulmonary oedema, with severe breathlessness and cyanosis may develop suddenly up to 36 hours after exposure. Death may occur. Patients are kept under observation and those who develop pulmonary oedema are given oxygen. Assisted ventilation may be necessary in the most serious cases.

1. PoM restriction does not apply where administration is for saving life in emergency

CS Spray

CS spray, which is used for riot control, irritates the eyes (hence 'tear gas') and the respiratory tract; symptoms normally settle spontaneously within 15 minutes. If symptoms persist, the patient should be removed to a well-ventilated area, and the exposed skin washed with soap and water after removal of contaminated clothing. Contact lenses should be removed and rigid ones washed (soft ones should be discarded). Eye symptoms should be treated by irrigating the eyes with physiological saline (or water if saline is not available) and advice sought from an ophthalmologist. Patients with features of severe poisoning, particularly respiratory complications, should be admitted to hospital for symptomatic treatment.

Nerve agents

Treatment of nerve agent poisoning is similar to organophosphorus insecticide poisoning (see below), but advice must be sought from the National Poisons Information Service. The risk of cross-contamination is significant; adequate decontamination and protective clothing for healthcare personnel are essential. In emergencies involving the release of nerve agents, kits ('NAAS pods') containing **pralidoxime** can be obtained through the Ambulance Service from the National Blood Service (or the Welsh Blood Service in South Wales or designated hospital pharmacies in Northern Ireland and Scotland—see TOXBASE for list of designated centres).

> The **National Poisons Information Service** (Tel: 0844 892 0111) will provide specialist advice on all aspects of poisoning day and night

Pesticides

Organophosphorus insecticides   Organophosphorus insecticides are usually supplied as powders or dissolved in organic solvents. All are absorbed through the bronchi and intact skin as well as through the gut and inhibit cholinesterase activity, thereby prolonging and intensifying the effects of acetylcholine. Toxicity between different compounds varies considerably, and onset may be delayed after skin exposure.

Anxiety, restlessness, dizziness, headache, miosis, nausea, hypersalivation, vomiting, abdominal colic, diarrhoea, bradycardia, and sweating are common features of organophosphorus poisoning. Muscle weakness and fasciculation may develop and progress to generalised flaccid paralysis, including the ocular and respiratory muscles. Convulsions, coma, pulmonary oedema with copious bronchial secretions, hypoxia, and arrhythmias occur in severe cases. Hyperglycaemia and glycosuria without ketonuria may also be present.

Further absorption of the organophosphorus insecticide should be prevented by moving the patient to fresh air, removing soiled clothing, and washing contaminated skin. In severe poisoning it is vital to ensure a clear airway, frequent removal of bronchial secretions, and adequate ventilation and oxygenation; gastric lavage may be considered provided that the airway is protected. **Atropine** will reverse the muscarinic effects of acetylcholine and is given by intravenous injection in a dose of 2 mg (20 micrograms/kg (max. 2 mg) in a child) as atropine sulfate every 5 to 10 minutes (according to the severity of poisoning) until the skin becomes flushed and dry, the pupils dilate, and bradycardia is abolished.

Pralidoxime chloride, a cholinesterase reactivator, is used as an adjunct to atropine in moderate or severe poisoning. It improves muscle tone within 30 minutes of administration. Pralidoxime chloride is continued until the patient has not required atropine for 12 hours. Pralidoxime chloride can be obtained from designated centres, the names of which are held by the National Poisons Information Service (see p. 33).

PRALIDOXIME CHLORIDE

Indications adjunct to atropine in the treatment of poisoning by organophosphorus insecticide or nerve agent

Cautions myasthenia gravis

Contra-indications poisoning with carbamates or with organophosphorus compounds without anti-cholinesterase activity

Renal impairment use with caution

Side-effects drowsiness, dizziness, disturbances of vision, nausea, tachycardia, headache, hyperventilation, and muscular weakness

Dose

• By intravenous infusion, ADULT and CHILD initially 30 mg/kg over 20 minutes, followed by 8 mg/kg/hour; usual max. 12 g in 24 hours

Note The loading dose may be administered by intravenous injection (diluted to a concentration of 50 mg/mL with water for injections) over at least 5 minutes if pulmonary oedema is present or if it is not practical to administer an intravenous infusion; pralidoxime chloride doses in BNF may differ from those in product literature

¹Pralidoxime chloride (PoM)
Injection, powder for reconstitution, pralidoxime chloride 1 g/vial
Available as *Protopam*® (from designated centres for organophosphorus insecticide poisoning or from the National Blood Service (or Welsh Ambulance Services for Mid West and South East Wales)—see TOXBASE for list of designated centres)

Snake bites and animal stings

Snake bites Envenoming from snake bite is uncommon in the UK. Many exotic snakes are kept, some illegally, but the only indigenous venomous snake is the adder (*Vipera berus*). The bite may cause local and systemic effects. Local effects include pain, swelling, bruising, and tender enlargement of regional lymph nodes. Systemic effects include early anaphylactic symptoms (transient hypotension with syncope, angioedema, urticaria, abdominal colic, diarrhoea, and vomiting), with later persistent or recurrent hypotension, ECG abnormalities, spontaneous systemic bleeding, coagulopathy, adult respiratory distress syndrome, and acute renal failure. Fatal envenoming is rare but the potential for severe envenoming must not be underestimated.

Early anaphylactic symptoms should be treated with **adrenaline (epinephrine)** (section 3.4.3). Indications for antivenom treatment include *systemic envenoming*, especially hypotension (see above), ECG abnormalities, vomiting, haemostatic abnormalities, and marked local envenoming such that after bites on the hand or foot, swelling extends beyond the wrist or ankle within 4 hours of the bite. For both **adults** and **children**, the contents of one vial (10 mL) of **European viper venom**

antiserum (to order, email immform@dh.gsi.gov.uk) is given *by intravenous injection* over 10–15 minutes or *by intravenous infusion* over 30 minutes after diluting in sodium chloride 0.9% (use 5 mL diluent/kg bodyweight). The dose can be repeated after 1–2 hours if symptoms of *systemic envenoming* persist. However, for those patients who present with clinical features of *severe envenoming* (e.g. shock, ECG abnormalities, or local swelling that has advanced from the foot to above the knee or from the hand to above the elbow within 2 hours of the bite), an initial dose of 2 vials (20 mL) of the antiserum is recommended; if symptoms of *systemic envenoming* persist contact the National Poisons Information Service. Adrenaline (epinephrine) injection must be immediately to hand for treatment of anaphylactic reactions to the antivenom (for the management of anaphylaxis, see section 3.4.3).

Antivenom is available for bites by certain foreign snakes and spiders, stings by scorpions and fish. For information on identification, management, and for supply in an emergency, telephone the National Poisons Information Service. Whenever possible the TOXBASE entry should be read, and relevant information collected, before telephoning the National Poisons Information Service (see p. 33).

Insect stings Stings from ants, wasps, hornets, and bees cause local pain and swelling but seldom cause severe direct toxicity unless many stings are inflicted at the same time. If the sting is in the mouth or on the tongue local swelling may threaten the upper airway. The stings from these insects are usually treated by cleaning the area with a topical antiseptic. Bee stings should be removed as quickly as possible. Anaphylactic reactions require immediate treatment with intramuscular **adrenaline (epinephrine)**; self-administered intramuscular adrenaline (e.g. *EpiPen*®) is the best first-aid treatment for patients with severe hypersensitivity. An inhaled bronchodilator should be used for asthmatic reactions. For the management of anaphylaxis, see section 3.4.3. A short course of an **oral antihistamine** or a **topical corticosteroid** may help to reduce inflammation and relieve itching. A vaccine containing extracts of bee and wasp venom can be used to reduce the risk of anaphylaxis and systemic reactions in patients with systemic hypersensitivity to bee or wasp stings (section 3.4.2).

Marine stings The severe pain of weeverfish (*Trachinus vipera*) and Portuguese man-o'-war stings can be relieved by immersing the stung area immediately in uncomfortably hot, but not scalding, water (not more than 45°C). People stung by jellyfish and Portuguese man-o'-war around the UK coast should be removed from the sea as soon as possible. Adherent tentacles should be lifted off carefully (wearing gloves or using tweezers) or washed off with seawater. Alcoholic solutions, including suntan lotions, should **not** be applied because they can cause further discharge of stinging hairs. Ice packs can be used to reduce pain.

---

1. (PoM) restriction does not apply where administration is for saving life in emergency

1 Gastro-intestinal system

This chapter also includes advice on the drug management of the following:

Clostridium difficile infection, p. 62
constipation, p. 69
Crohn's disease, p. 61
diverticular disease, p. 62
food allergy, p. 69
Helicobacter pylori infection, p. 50
irritable bowel syndrome, p. 62
NSAID-associated ulcers, p. 51
ulcerative colitis, p. 61

1.1 Dyspepsia and gastro-oesophageal reflux disease

1.1.1 Antacids and simeticone

1.1.2 Compound alginates and proprietary indigestion preparations

Dyspepsia

Dyspepsia covers upper abdominal pain, fullness, early satiety, bloating, and nausea. It can occur with gastric and duodenal ulceration (section 1.3) and gastric cancer but most commonly it is of uncertain origin.

Urgent endoscopic investigation is required if dyspepsia is accompanied by 'alarm features' (e.g. bleeding, dysphagia, recurrent vomiting, or weight loss). Urgent investigation should also be considered for patients over 55 years with unexplained, recent-onset dyspepsia that has not responded to treatment.

Patients with dyspepsia should be advised about life-style changes (see Gastro-oesophageal reflux disease, below). Some medications may cause dyspepsia—these should be stopped, if possible. Antacids may provide some symptomatic relief.

If symptoms persist in *uninvestigated dyspepsia*, treatment involves a **proton pump inhibitor** (section 1.3.5) for up to 4 weeks. A proton pump inhibitor can be used intermittently to control symptoms long term. Patients with uninvestigated dyspepsia, who do not respond to an initial trial with a proton pump inhibitor, should be tested for *Helicobacter pylori* and given eradication therapy (section 1.3) if *H. pylori* is present. Alternatively, particularly in populations where *H. pylori* infection is more likely, the 'test and treat' strategy for *H. pylori* can be used before a trial with a proton pump inhibitor.

If *H. pylori* is present in patients with *functional (investigated, non-ulcer) dyspepsia*, eradication therapy should be provided. If symptoms persist, treatment with either a **proton pump inhibitor** (section 1.3.5) or a **histamine H₂-receptor antagonist** (section 1.3.1) can be given for 4 weeks. These antisecretory drugs can be used intermittently to control symptoms long term. However, most patients with functional dyspepsia do not benefit symptomatically from *H. pylori* eradication therapy or antisecretory drugs.

Gastro-oesophageal reflux disease

Gastro-oesophageal reflux disease (including non-erosive gastro-oesophageal reflux and erosive oesophagitis) is associated with heartburn, acid regurgitation, and sometimes, difficulty in swallowing (dysphagia); oesophageal inflammation (oesophagitis), ulceration, and stricture formation may occur and there is an association with asthma.

The management of gastro-oesophageal reflux disease includes drug treatment, lifestyle changes and, in some cases, surgery. Initial treatment is guided by the severity of symptoms and treatment is then adjusted according to response. The extent of healing depends on the severity of the disease, the treatment chosen, and the duration of therapy.

Patients with gastro-oesophageal reflux disease should be advised about lifestyle changes (avoidance of excess alcohol and of aggravating foods such as fats); other measures include weight reduction, smoking cessation, and raising the head of the bed.

For *mild symptoms* of gastro-oesophageal reflux disease, initial management may include the use of **antacids** and **alginates**. Alginate-containing antacids can form a 'raft' that floats on the surface of the stomach contents to reduce reflux and protect the oesophageal mucosa. **Histamine H₂-receptor antagonists** (section 1.3.1) may relieve symptoms and permit reduction in antacid consumption. However, **proton pump inhibitors** (section 1.3.5) provide more effective relief of symptoms than H₂-receptor antagonists. When symptoms abate, treatment is titrated down to a level which maintains remission (e.g. by giving treatment intermittently).

For *severe symptoms* of gastro-oesophageal reflux disease or for patients with a proven or severe pathology (e.g. *oesophagitis, oesophageal ulceration, oesophagopharyngeal reflux, Barrett's oesophagus*), initial management involves the use of a **proton pump inhibitor** (section 1.3.5); patients need to be reassessed if symptoms persist despite treatment for 4–6 weeks with a proton pump inhibitor. When symptoms abate, treatment is titrated down to a level which maintains remission (e.g. by reducing the dose of the proton pump inhibitor or by giving it intermittently, or by substituting treatment with a histamine H₂-receptor antagonist). However, for endoscopically confirmed *erosive, ulcerative*, or *stricturing* disease, or *Barrett's oesophagus*, treatment with a proton pump inhibitor usually needs to be maintained at the minimum effective dose.

Pregnancy If dietary and lifestyle changes (see notes above) fail to control gastro-oesophageal reflux disease in pregnancy, an antacid (section 1.1.1) or an alginate (section 1.1.2) can be used. If this is ineffective, ranitidine (section 1.3.1) can be tried. Omeprazole (section 1.3.5) is reserved for women with severe or complicated reflux disease.

Children Gastro-oesophageal reflux disease is common in infancy but most symptoms resolve without treatment between 12 and 18 months of age. In infants, mild or moderate reflux without complications can be managed initially by changing the frequency and volume of feed; a feed thickener or thickened formula feed can be used (with advice of a dietitian—see Appendix 2 for suitable products). If necessary, a suitable alginate-containing preparation can be used instead of thickened feeds. For older children, life-style changes similar to those for adults (see above) may be helpful followed if necessary by treatment with an alginate-containing preparation.

Children who do not respond to these measures or who have problems such as respiratory disorders or suspected oesophagitis need to be referred to hospital; an H₂-receptor antagonist (section 1.3.1) may be needed to reduce acid secretion. If the oesophagitis is resistant to H₂-receptor blockade, the proton pump inhibitor omeprazole (section 1.3.5) can be tried.

1.1.1 Antacids and simeticone

Antacids (usually containing aluminium or magnesium compounds) can often relieve symptoms in *ulcer dyspepsia* and in *non-erosive gastro-oesophageal reflux* (see also section 1.1); they are also sometimes used in functional (non-ulcer) dyspepsia but the evidence of benefit is uncertain. Antacids are best given when symptoms occur or are expected, usually between meals and at bedtime, 4 or more times daily; additional doses may be required up to once an hour. Conventional doses e.g. 10 mL 3 or 4 times daily of liquid magnesium–aluminium antacids promote ulcer healing, but less well than antisecretory drugs (section 1.3); proof of a relationship between healing and neutralising capacity is lacking. Liquid preparations are more effective than tablet preparations.

Aluminium- and **magnesium-containing** antacids (e.g. aluminium hydroxide, and magnesium carbonate, hydroxide and trisilicate), being relatively insoluble in water, are long-acting if retained in the stomach. They are suitable for most antacid purposes. Magnesium-containing antacids tend to be laxative whereas aluminium-containing antacids may be constipating; antacids containing both magnesium and aluminium may reduce these colonic side-effects. Aluminium accumulation does not appear to be a risk if renal function is normal.

The acid-neutralising capacity of preparations that contain more than one antacid may be the same as simpler preparations. Complexes such as **hydrotalcite** confer no special advantage.

Sodium bicarbonate should no longer be prescribed alone for the relief of dyspepsia but it is present as an ingredient in many indigestion remedies. However, it retains a place in the management of urinary-tract disorders (section 7.4.3) and acidosis (section 9.2.1.3 and section 9.2.2). Sodium bicarbonate should be avoided in patients on salt-restricted diets.

Bismuth-containing antacids (unless chelates) are not recommended because absorbed bismuth can be neurotoxic, causing encephalopathy; they tend to be constipating. **Calcium-containing** antacids (section 1.1.2) can induce rebound acid secretion: with modest doses the clinical significance is doubtful, but prolonged high doses also cause hypercalcaemia and alkalosis, and can precipitate the milk-alkali syndrome.

Simeticone (activated dimeticone) is added to an antacid as an antifoaming agent to relieve flatulence. These preparations may be useful for the relief of hiccup in palliative care. **Alginates**, added as protectants, may be useful in gastro-oesophageal reflux disease (section 1.1 and section 1.1.2). The amount of additional ingredient or antacid in individual preparations varies widely, as does their sodium content, so that preparations may not be freely interchangeable.

See also section 1.3 for drugs used in the treatment of peptic ulceration.

Hepatic impairment In patients with fluid retention, avoid antacids containing large amounts of sodium. Avoid antacids that cause constipation because this can precipitate coma. Avoid antacids containing magnesium salts in hepatic coma if there is a risk of renal failure.

Renal impairment In patients with fluid retention, avoid antacids containing large amounts of sodium. There is a risk of accumulation and aluminium toxicity with antacids containing aluminium salts. Absorption of aluminium from aluminium salts is increased by citrates, which are contained in many effervescent preparations (such as effervescent analgesics). Antacids containing magnesium salts should be avoided or used at a reduced dose because there is an increased risk of toxicity.

Interactions Antacids should preferably not be taken at the same time as other drugs since they may impair absorption. Antacids may also damage enteric coatings designed to prevent dissolution in the stomach. See also Appendix 1 (antacids, calcium salts).

> **Low Na$^+$**
> The words 'low Na$^+$' added after some preparations indicate a sodium content of less than 1 mmol per tablet or 10-mL dose.

Aluminium- and magnesium-containing antacids

◢ ALUMINIUM HYDROXIDE

Indications dyspepsia; hyperphosphataemia (section 9.5.2.2)

Cautions see notes above; **interactions**: Appendix 1 (antacids)

Contra-indications hypophosphataemia; neonates and infants

Hepatic impairment see notes above

Renal impairment see notes above

Side-effects see notes above

◢ **Aluminium-only preparations**

Alu-Cap$^®$ (Meda)
Capsules, green/red, dried aluminium hydroxide 475 mg (low Na$^+$). Net price 120-cap pack = £13.71
Dose antacid, 1 capsule 4 times daily and at bedtime; CHILD not recommended for antacid therapy

◢ **Co-magaldrox**
Co-magaldrox is a mixture of aluminium hydroxide and magnesium hydroxide; the proportions are expressed in the form x/y where x and y are the strengths in milligrams per unit dose of magnesium hydroxide and aluminium hydroxide respectively

Maalox$^®$ (Sanofi-Aventis)
Suspension, sugar-free, co-magaldrox 195/220 (magnesium hydroxide 195 mg, dried aluminium hydroxide 220 mg/5 mL (low Na$^+$)). Net price 500 mL = £3.35
Dose ADULT and CHILD over 14 years, 10–20 mL 20–60 minutes after meals and at bedtime or when required

Mucogel$^®$ (Chemidex)
Suspension, sugar-free, co-magaldrox 195/220 (magnesium hydroxide 195 mg, dried aluminium hydroxide 220 mg/5 mL (low Na$^+$)). Net price 500 mL = £2.99
Dose ADULT and CHILD over 12 years, 10–20 mL 3 times daily, 20–60 minutes after meals, and at bedtime or when required

◢ MAGNESIUM CARBONATE

Indications dyspepsia

Cautions see notes above; **interactions**: Appendix 1 (antacids)

Contra-indications hypophosphataemia

Hepatic impairment see notes above

Renal impairment see notes above; magnesium carbonate mixture has a high sodium content

Side-effects diarrhoea; belching due to liberated carbon dioxide

Aromatic Magnesium Carbonate Mixture, BP
(Aromatic Magnesium Carbonate Oral Suspension)
Oral suspension, light magnesium carbonate 3%, sodium bicarbonate 5%, in a suitable vehicle containing aromatic cardamom tincture. Contains about 6 mmol Na$^+$/10 mL. Net price 200 mL = 66p
Dose 10 mL 3 times daily in water

For **preparations** also containing aluminium, see above and section 1.1.2.

◢ MAGNESIUM TRISILICATE

Indications dyspepsia

Cautions see notes above; **interactions**: Appendix 1 (antacids)

Contra-indications see under Magnesium Carbonate

Hepatic impairment see notes above

Renal impairment see notes above; magnesium trisilicate mixture has a high sodium content

Side-effects diarrhoea, belching due to liberated carbon dioxide; silica-based renal stones reported on long-term treatment

Magnesium Trisilicate Tablets, Compound, BP
Tablets, magnesium trisilicate 250 mg, dried aluminium hydroxide 120 mg
Dose 1–2 tablets chewed when required

Magnesium Trisilicate Mixture, BP
(Magnesium Trisilicate Oral Suspension)
Oral suspension, 5% each of magnesium trisilicate, light magnesium carbonate, and sodium bicarbonate in a suitable vehicle with a peppermint flavour. Contains about 6 mmol Na$^+$/10 mL
Dose 10–20 mL in water 3 times daily or as required; CHILD 5–12 years, 5–10 mL in water 3 times daily or as required

For **preparations** also containing aluminium, see above and section 1.1.2.

Aluminium-magnesium complexes

HYDROTALCITE

Aluminium magnesium carbonate hydroxide hydrate

Indications dyspepsia

Cautions see notes above; **interactions**: Appendix 1 (antacids)

Hepatic impairment see notes above

Renal impairment see notes above

Side-effects see notes above

◀**With simeticone**

Altacite Plus® see below

Antacid preparations containing simeticone

Altacite Plus® (Peckforton)

Suspension, sugar-free, co-simalcite 125/500 (simeticone 125 mg, hydrotalcite 500 mg)/5 mL (low Na⁺). Net price 500 mL = £3.20

Dose 10 mL between meals and at bedtime when required; CHILD 8–12 years 5 mL between meals and at bedtime when required

Maalox Plus® (Sanofi-Aventis)

Suspension, sugar-free, dried aluminium hydroxide 220 mg, simeticone 25 mg, magnesium hydroxide 195 mg/5 mL (low Na⁺). Net price 500 mL = £3.90

Dose 5–10 mL 4 times daily (after meals and at bedtime) or when required; CHILD under 12 years see *BNF for Children*

Simeticone alone

Simeticone (activated dimeticone) is an antifoaming agent. It is licensed for infantile colic but evidence of benefit is uncertain.

Dentinox® (DDD)

Colic drops (= emulsion), simeticone 21 mg/2.5-mL dose. Net price 100 mL = £1.73

Dose colic or wind pains, NEONATE and INFANT 2.5 mL with or after each feed (max. 6 doses in 24 hours); may be added to bottle feed

Note The brand name *Dentinox®* is also used for other preparations including teething gel

Infacol® (Forest)

Liquid, sugar-free, simeticone 40 mg/mL (low Na⁺). Net price 50 mL = £2.71. Counselling, use of dropper

Dose colic or wind pains, NEONATE and INFANT 0.5–1 mL before feeds

1.1.2 Compound alginates and proprietary indigestion preparations

Alginate taken in combination with an antacid increases the viscosity of stomach contents and can protect the oesophageal mucosa from acid reflux. Some alginate-containing preparations form a viscous gel ('raft') that floats on the surface of the stomach contents, thereby reducing symptoms of reflux.

Antacids may damage enteric coatings designed to prevent dissolution in the stomach. For **interactions**, see Appendix 1 (antacids, calcium salts).

Alginate raft-forming oral suspensions

The following preparations contain sodium alginate, sodium bicarbonate, and calcium carbonate in a suitable flavoured vehicle, and conform to the specification for Alginate Raft-forming Oral Suspension, BP.

Acidex® (Pinewood)

Liquid, sugar-free, sodium alginate 250 mg, sodium bicarbonate 133.5 mg, calcium carbonate 80 mg/5 mL. Contains about 3 mmol Na⁺/5 mL. Net price 500 mL (aniseed- or peppermint-flavour) = £2.50

Dose 10–20 mL after meals and at bedtime; CHILD 6–12 years 5–10 mL after meals and at bedtime

Gaviscon® (Reckitt Benckiser)

Suspension, sugar-free, aniseed- or peppermint flavour, sodium alginate 250 mg, sodium bicarbonate 133.5 mg, calcium carbonate 80 mg/5 mL. Contains 3.1 mmol Na⁺/5 mL. Net price 300 mL = £4.20, 600 mL = £6.89

Dose 10–20 mL after meals and at bedtime; CHILD 6–12 years 5–10 mL after meals and at bedtime

Peptac® (TEVA UK)

Suspension, sugar-free, sodium bicarbonate 133.5 mg, sodium alginate 250 mg, calcium carbonate 80 mg/5 mL. Contains 3.1 mmol Na⁺/5 mL. Net price 500 mL (aniseed- or peppermint-flavoured) = £1.95

Dose 10–20 mL after meals and at bedtime; CHILD 6–12 years 5–10 mL after meals and at bedtime

Other compound alginate preparations

Gastrocote® (Actavis)

Tablets, alginic acid 200 mg, dried aluminium hydroxide 80 mg, magnesium trisilicate 40 mg, sodium bicarbonate 70 mg. Contains about 1 mmol Na⁺/tablet. Net price 100-tab pack = £3.51

Cautions diabetes mellitus (high sugar content)

Dose ADULT and CHILD over 6 years, 1–2 tablets chewed 4 times daily (after meals and at bedtime)

Liquid, sugar-free, peach-coloured, dried aluminium hydroxide 80 mg, magnesium trisilicate 40 mg, sodium alginate 220 mg, sodium bicarbonate 70 mg/5 mL. Contains 2.13 mmol Na⁺/5 mL. Net price 500 mL = £2.67

Dose 5–15 mL 4 times daily (after meals and at bedtime); CHILD 6–12 years, 5–10 mL 4 times daily (after meals and at bedtime)

Gaviscon® Advance (Reckitt Benckiser)

Chewable tablets, sugar-free, sodium alginate 500 mg, potassium bicarbonate 100 mg. Contains 2.25 mmol Na⁺, 1 mmol K⁺/tablet. Net price 60-tab pack (peppermint-flavoured) = £3.07

Excipients include aspartame (section 9.4.1)

Dose ADULT and CHILD over 12 years, 1–2 tablets to be chewed after meals and at bedtime; CHILD 6–12 years, 1 tablet to be chewed after meals and at bedtime (under medical advice only)

Suspension, sugar-free, aniseed- or peppermint flavour, sodium alginate 500 mg, potassium bicarbonate 100 mg/5 mL. Contains 2.3 mmol Na⁺, 1 mmol K⁺/5 mL, net price 250 mL = £2.56, 500 mL = £5.12

Dose ADULT and CHILD over 12 years, 5–10 mL after meals and at bedtime; CHILD 2–12 years, 2.5–5 mL after meals and at bedtime (under medical advice only)

1 Gastro-intestinal system

Gaviscon Infant® (Reckitt Benckiser)

Oral powder, sugar-free, sodium alginate 225 mg, magnesium alginate 87.5 mg, with colloidal silica and mannitol/dose. Contains 0.92 mmol Na⁺/dose. Net price 30 doses = £3.69

Dose INFANT body-weight under 4.5 kg, 1 'dose' mixed with feeds (or water in breast-fed infants) when required (max. 6 times in 24 hours); body-weight over 4.5 kg, 2 'doses' mixed with feeds (or water in breast-fed infants) when required (max. 6 times in 24 hours); CHILD 2 'doses' in water after each meal (max. 6 times in 24 hours)

Note Not to be used in preterm neonates, or where excessive water loss likely (e.g. fever, diarrhoea, vomiting, high room temperature), or if intestinal obstruction. Not to be used with other preparations containing thickening agents

Important Each half of the dual-sachet is identified as 'one dose'. To avoid errors prescribe with directions in terms of 'dose'

1.2 Antispasmodics and other drugs altering gut motility

Drugs in this section include antimuscarinic compounds and drugs believed to be direct relaxants of intestinal smooth muscle. The smooth muscle relaxant properties of antimuscarinic and other antispasmodic drugs may be useful in *irritable bowel syndrome* and in *diverticular disease*.

Antimuscarinics

Antimuscarinics (formerly termed 'anticholinergics') reduce intestinal motility. They are used for the management of *irritable bowel syndrome* and *diverticular disease*. However, their value has not been established and response varies. Other indications for antimuscarinic drugs include arrhythmias (section 2.3.1), asthma and airways disease (section 3.1.2), motion sickness (section 4.6), parkinsonism (section 4.9.2), urinary incontinence (section 7.4.2), mydriasis and cycloplegia (section 11.5), premedication (section 15.1.3) and as an antidote to organophosphorus poisoning (p. 42).

Antimuscarinics that are used for gastro-intestinal smooth muscle spasm include the tertiary amines **atropine sulfate** and **dicycloverine hydrochloride** and the quaternary ammonium compounds **propantheline bromide** and **hyoscine butylbromide**. The quaternary ammonium compounds are less lipid soluble than atropine and are less likely to cross the blood–brain barrier; they are also less well absorbed from the gastro-intestinal tract.

Dicycloverine hydrochloride has a much less marked antimuscarinic action than atropine and may also have some direct action on smooth muscle. Hyoscine butylbromide is advocated as a gastro-intestinal antispasmodic, but it is poorly absorbed; the injection is useful in endoscopy and radiology. Atropine and the belladonna alkaloids are outmoded treatments, any clinical virtues being outweighed by atropinic side-effects.

Cautions Antimuscarinics should be used with caution in Down's syndrome, in children and in the elderly; they should also be used with caution in gastro-oesophageal reflux disease, diarrhoea, ulcerative colitis, autonomic neuropathy, acute myocardial infarction, hypertension, conditions characterised by tachycardia (including hyperthyroidism, cardiac insufficiency, car-

diac surgery), pyrexia, and in individuals susceptible to angle-closure glaucoma. **Interactions:** Appendix 1 (antimuscarinics).

Contra-indications Antimuscarinics are contra-indicated in myasthenia gravis (but may be used to decrease muscarinic side-effects of anticholinesterases—section 10.2.1), paralytic ileus, pyloric stenosis, toxic megacolon, and prostatic enlargement.

Side-effects Side-effects of antimuscarinics include constipation, transient bradycardia (followed by tachycardia, palpitation and arrhythmias), reduced bronchial secretions, urinary urgency and retention, dilatation of the pupils with loss of accommodation, photophobia, dry mouth, flushing and dryness of the skin. Side-effects that occur occasionally include confusion (particularly in the elderly), nausea, vomiting, and giddiness; very rarely, angle-closure glaucoma may occur.

ATROPINE SULFATE

Indications symptomatic relief of gastro-intestinal disorders characterised by smooth muscle spasm; mydriasis and cycloplegia (section 11.5); premedication (section 15.1.3); see also notes above

Cautions see notes above

Contra-indications see notes above

Pregnancy manufacturer advises caution

Breast-feeding small amount present in milk—manufacturer advises caution; may suppress lactation

Side-effects see notes above

Dose
- 0.6–1.2 mg at night

Atropine (Non-proprietary) PoM

Tablets, atropine sulfate 600 micrograms. Net price 28-tab pack = £25.64

DICYCLOVERINE HYDROCHLORIDE
(Dicyclomine hydrochloride)

Indications symptomatic relief of gastro-intestinal disorders characterised by smooth muscle spasm

Cautions see notes above

Contra-indications see notes above; also infants under 6 months

Pregnancy not known to be harmful; manufacturer advises use only if essential

Breast-feeding avoid—present in milk; apnoea reported in infant

Side-effects see notes above

Dose
- 10–20 mg 3 times daily; INFANT 6–24 months 5–10 mg 3–4 times daily, 15 minutes before feeds; CHILD 2–12 years 10 mg 3 times daily

Dicycloverine (Non-proprietary) PoM

Tablets, dicycloverine hydrochloride 10 mg, net price 100-tab pack = £75.93; 20 mg, 84-tab pack = £80.15

Syrup, dicycloverine hydrochloride 10 mg/5 mL, net price 120 mL = £75.13

Note Dicycloverine hydrochloride can be sold to the public provided that max. single dose is 10 mg and max. daily dose is 60 mg

◢Compound preparations

Kolanticon® (Peckforton)

Gel, sugar-free, dicycloverine hydrochloride 2.5 mg, dried aluminium hydroxide 200 mg, light magnesium oxide 100 mg, simeticone 20 mg/5 mL, net price 200 mL = £2.21, 500 mL = £3.94

Dose ADULT and CHILD over 12 years, 10–20 mL every 4 hours when required

◼ HYOSCINE BUTYLBROMIDE

Indications symptomatic relief of gastro-intestinal or genito-urinary disorders characterised by smooth muscle spasm; bowel colic and excessive respiratory secretions (see Prescribing in Palliative Care, p. 23)

Cautions see notes above

Contra-indications see notes above

Pregnancy manufacturer advises avoid

Breast-feeding amount too small to be harmful

Side-effects see notes above

Dose

- By mouth (but poorly absorbed, see notes above), smooth muscle spasm, 20 mg 4 times daily; CHILD 6–12 years, 10 mg 3 times daily

  Irritable bowel syndrome, 10 mg 3 times daily, increased if required up to 20 mg 4 times daily

- By intramuscular *or* slow intravenous injection, acute spasm and spasm in diagnostic procedures, 20 mg repeated after 30 minutes if necessary (may be repeated more frequently in endoscopy), max. 100 mg daily; CHILD 2–18 years see *BNF for Children*

Buscopan® (Boehringer Ingelheim) [PoM]

Tablets, coated, hyoscine butylbromide 10 mg, net price 56-tab pack = £3.00

Note Hyoscine butylbromide tablets can be sold to the public for medically confirmed irritable bowel syndrome, provided single dose does not exceed 20 mg, daily dose does not exceed 80 mg, and pack does not contain a total of more than 240 mg

Injection, hyoscine butylbromide 20 mg/mL, net price 1-mL amp = 29p

◼ PROPANTHELINE BROMIDE

Indications symptomatic relief of gastro-intestinal disorders characterised by smooth muscle spasm; urinary frequency (section 7.4.2); gustatory sweating (section 6.1.5)

Cautions see notes above

Contra-indications see notes above

Hepatic impairment manufacturer advises caution

Renal impairment manufacturer advises caution

Pregnancy manufacturer advises avoid unless essential

Breast-feeding may suppress lactation

Side-effects see notes above

Dose

- ADULT and CHILD over 12 years, 15 mg 3 times daily at least 1 hour before meals and 30 mg at night, max. 120 mg daily

Pro-Banthine® (Archimedes) [PoM]

Tablets, pink, s/c, propantheline bromide 15 mg, net price 112-tab pack = £20.74. Label: 23

Other antispasmodics

Alverine, **mebeverine**, and **peppermint oil** are believed to be direct relaxants of intestinal smooth muscle and may relieve pain in *irritable bowel syndrome* and *diverticular disease*. They have no serious adverse effects but, like all antispasmodics, should be avoided in paralytic ileus. Peppermint oil occasionally causes heartburn.

◼ ALVERINE CITRATE

Indications adjunct in gastro-intestinal disorders characterised by smooth muscle spasm; dysmenorrhoea

Contra-indications paralytic ileus

Pregnancy use with caution

Breast-feeding manufacturer advises avoid—limited information available

Side-effects nausea; dyspnoea; headache, dizziness; pruritus, rash; hepatitis also reported

Dose

- ADULT and CHILD over 12 years, 60–120 mg 1–3 times daily

Spasmonal® (Meda)

Capsules, alverine citrate 60 mg (blue/grey), net price 100-cap pack = £16.45; 120 mg (*Spasmonal® Forte*, blue/grey), 60-cap pack = £19.42

◼ MEBEVERINE HYDROCHLORIDE

Indications adjunct in gastro-intestinal disorders characterised by smooth muscle spasm

Contra-indications paralytic ileus

Pregnancy not known to be harmful—manufacturers advise avoid

Breast-feeding manufacturers advise avoid—no information available

Side-effects allergic reactions (including rash, urticaria, angioedema) reported

Dose

- ADULT and CHILD over 10 years 135–150 mg 3 times daily preferably 20 minutes before meals; CHILD under 10 years see *BNF for Children*

[1]**Mebeverine Hydrochloride** (Non-proprietary) [PoM]

Tablets, mebeverine hydrochloride 135 mg, net price 100-tab pack = £15.69. Counselling, administration

Oral suspension, mebeverine hydrochloride (as mebeverine embonate) 50 mg/5 mL, net price 300 mL = £143.43. Counselling, administration

Colofac® (Abbott Healthcare) [PoM]

Tablets, s/c, mebeverine hydrochloride 135 mg, net price 100-tab pack = £7.52. Counselling, administration

---

1. Mebeverine hydrochloride can be sold to the public for symptomatic relief of irritable bowel syndrome provided that max. single dose is 135 mg and max. daily dose is 405 mg; for uses other than symptomatic relief of irritable bowel syndrome provided that max. single dose is 100 mg and max. daily dose is 300 mg

1   **Gastro-intestinal system**

◢**Modified release**

Colofac® MR (Abbott Healthcare) (PoM)

Capsules, m/r, mebeverine hydrochloride 200 mg, net price 60-cap pack = £6.92. Label: 25

Dose irritable bowel syndrome, 1 capsule twice daily; CHILD 12–18 years see *BNF for Children*

◢**Compound preparations**

Fybogel® Mebeverine (Reckitt Benckiser)

Granules, buff, effervescent, ispaghula husk 3.5 g, mebeverine hydrochloride 135 mg/sachet, net price 10 sachets = £3.75. Label: 13, 22, counselling, see below

Excipients include aspartame (section 9.4.1)

Electrolytes K⁺ 7 mmol/sachet

Dose irritable bowel syndrome, ADULT and CHILD over 12 years, 1 sachet in water, morning and evening 30 minutes before food; an additional sachet may also be taken before the midday meal if necessary

Counselling Preparations that swell in contact with liquid should always be carefully swallowed with water and should not be taken immediately before going to bed

▌ PEPPERMINT OIL

Indications relief of abdominal colic and distension, particularly in irritable bowel syndrome

Cautions sensitivity to menthol

Pregnancy not known to be harmful

Breast-feeding significant levels of menthol in breast milk unlikely

Side-effects heartburn, perianal irritation; rarely, allergic reactions (including rash, headache, bradycardia, muscle tremor, ataxia)

Local irritation Capsules should not be broken or chewed because peppermint oil may irritate mouth or oesophagus

Dose
● See preparations

Colpermin® (McNeil)

Capsules, m/r, e/c, light blue/dark blue, blue band, peppermint oil 0.2 mL. Net price 100-cap pack = £12.05. Label: 5, 22, 25

Excipients include arachis (peanut) oil

Dose ADULT and CHILD over 15 years, 1–2 capsules, swallowed whole with water, 3 times daily for up to 3 months if necessary

Mintec® (Almirall)

Capsules, e/c, green/ivory, peppermint oil 0.2 mL. Net price 84-cap pack = £7.04. Label: 5, 22, 25

Dose ADULT over 18 years, 1–2 capsules swallowed whole with water, 3 times daily before meals for up to 2–3 months if necessary

1.3 Antisecretory drugs and mucosal protectants

Peptic ulceration commonly involves the stomach, duodenum, and lower oesophagus; after gastric surgery it involves the gastro-enterostomy stoma.

Healing can be promoted by general measures, stopping smoking and taking antacids and by antisecretory drug treatment, but relapse is common when treatment ceases. Nearly all duodenal ulcers and most gastric ulcers not associated with NSAIDs are caused by *Helicobacter pylori*.

The management of *H. pylori* infection and of NSAID-associated ulcers is discussed below.

Helicobacter pylori infection

Eradication of *Helicobacter pylori* reduces recurrence of gastric and duodenal ulcers and the risk of rebleeding. It also causes regression of most localised gastric mucosa-associated lymphoid-tissue (MALT) lymphomas. The presence of *H. pylori* should be confirmed before starting eradication treatment. Acid inhibition combined with antibacterial treatment is highly effective in the eradication of *H. pylori*; reinfection is rare. Antibiotic-associated colitis is an uncommon risk.

For initial treatment, a one-week triple-therapy regimen that comprises a proton pump inhibitor, clarithromycin, and *either* amoxicillin *or* metronidazole can be used. However, if a patient has been treated with metronidazole for other infections, a regimen containing a proton pump inhibitor, amoxicillin and clarithromycin is preferred for initial therapy. If a patient has been treated with a macrolide for other infections, a regimen containing a proton pump inhibitor, amoxicillin and metronidazole is preferred for initial therapy. These regimens eradicate *H. pylori* in about 85% of cases. There is usually no need to continue antisecretory treatment (with a proton pump inhibitor or H₂-receptor antagonist), however, if the ulcer is large, or complicated by haemorrhage or perforation, then antisecretory treatment is continued for a further 3 weeks. Treatment failure usually indicates antibacterial resistance or poor compliance. Resistance to amoxicillin is rare. However, resistance to clarithromycin and metronidazole is common and can develop during treatment.

Two-week triple-therapy regimens offer the possibility of higher eradication rates compared to one-week regimens, but adverse effects are common and poor compliance is likely to offset any possible gain.

Two-week dual-therapy regimens using a proton pump inhibitor and a single antibacterial are licensed, but produce low rates of *H. pylori* eradication and are **not** recommended.

Tinidazole is also used occasionally for *H. pylori* eradication as an alternative to metronidazole; tinidazole should be combined with antisecretory drugs and other antibacterials.

Routine retesting, to confirm eradication, is not necessary unless the patient has gastric MALT lymphoma or complicated *H. pylori* associated peptic ulcer.

A two-week regimen comprising a proton pump inhibitor (e.g. omeprazole 20 mg twice daily) *plus* tripotassium dicitratobismuthate 120 mg four times daily, *plus* tetracycline 500 mg four times daily, *plus* metronidazole 400–500 mg three times daily can be used for eradication failure. Alternatively, the patient can be referred for endoscopy and treatment based on the results of culture and sensitivity testing.

For the role of *H. pylori* eradication therapy in patients starting or taking a NSAID, see NSAID-associated Ulcers, p. 51. For *H. pylori* eradication in patients with dyspepsia, see also section 1.1.

Recommended regimens for *Helicobacter pylori* eradication in adults

Acid suppressant	Antibacterial			Price for 7-day course
	Amoxicillin	Clarithromycin	Metronidazole	
Esomeprazole 20 mg twice daily	1 g twice daily	500 mg twice daily	—	£6.63
	—	250 mg twice daily	400 mg twice daily	£4.30
Lansoprazole 30 mg twice daily	1 g twice daily	500 mg twice daily	—	£5.52
	1 g twice daily	—	400 mg twice daily	£3.70
	—	250 mg twice daily	400 mg twice daily	£3.19
Omeprazole 20 mg twice daily	1 g twice daily	500 mg twice daily	—	£5.36
	500 mg 3 times daily	—	400 mg 3 times daily	£3.40
	—	250 mg twice daily	400 mg twice daily	£3.03
Pantoprazole 40 mg twice daily	1 g twice daily	500 mg twice daily	—	£5.48
	—	250 mg twice daily	400 mg twice daily	£3.15
Rabeprazole 20 mg twice daily	1 g twice daily	500 mg twice daily	—	£6.04
	—	250 mg twice daily	400 mg twice daily	£3.71

Test for *Helicobacter pylori*

^{13}C-Urea breath test kits are available for the diagnosis of gastro-duodenal infection with *Helicobacter pylori*. The test involves collection of breath samples before and after ingestion of an oral solution of ^{13}C-urea; the samples are sent for analysis by an appropriate laboratory. The test should not be performed within 4 weeks of treatment with an antibacterial or within 2 weeks of treatment with an antisecretory drug. A specific ^{13}C-urea breath test kit for children is available (*Helicobacter Test INFAI for children of the age 3–11*®). However, the appropriateness of testing for *H. pylori* infection in children has not been established.

diabact UBT® (Seahorse) [PoM]
Tablets, ^{13}C-urea 50 mg, net price 1 kit (including 1 tablet, 4 breath-sample containers, straws) = £21.25 (analysis included), 10-kit pack (hosp. only) = £74.50 (analysis not included)

Helicobacter Test INFAI® (Infai) [PoM]
Oral powder, ^{13}C-urea 75 mg, net price 1 kit (including 4 breath-sample containers, straws) = £19.75 (spectrometric analysis included), 1 kit (including 2 breath bags) = £19.20 (spectroscopic analysis not included), 50-test set = £855.00 (spectrometric analysis included); 45 mg (*Helicobacter Test INFAI for children of the age 3–11*®), 1 kit (including 4 breath-sample containers, straws) = £19.20 (spectrometric analysis included)

Pylobactell® (Torbet) [PoM]
Soluble tablets, ^{13}C-urea 100 mg, net price 1 kit (including 6 breath-sample containers, 30-mL mixing and administration vial, straws) = £20.75 (analysis included)

NSAID-associated ulcers

Gastro-intestinal bleeding and ulceration can occur with NSAID use (section 10.1.1). The risk of serious upper gastro-intestinal side-effects varies between individual NSAIDs (see NSAIDs and Gastro-intestinal Events, p. 718). Whenever possible, the NSAID should be **withdrawn** if an ulcer occurs.

Patients at high risk of developing gastro-intestinal complications with a NSAID include those aged over 65 years, those with a history of peptic ulcer disease or serious gastro-intestinal complication, those taking other medicines that increase the risk of gastro-intestinal side-effects, or those with serious co-morbidity (e.g. cardiovascular disease, diabetes, renal or hepatic impairment). In those at risk of ulceration, a proton pump inhibitor can be considered for protection against gastric and duodenal ulcers associated with non-selective NSAIDs; a H_2-receptor antagonist such as ranitidine given at twice the usual dose or misoprostol are alternatives. Colic and diarrhoea may limit the dose of misoprostol. A combination of a cyclo-oxygenase-2 selective inhibitor with a proton pump inhibitor may be more appropriate for those with a history of upper gastro-intestinal bleeding or 3 or more risk factors for gastro-intestinal ulceration, but see NSAIDs and Cardiovascular Events, p. 717.

NSAID use and *H. pylori* infection are independent risk factors for gastro-intestinal bleeding and ulceration. In patients already taking a NSAID, eradication of *H. pylori* is unlikely to reduce the risk of NSAID-induced bleeding or ulceration. However, in patients with dyspepsia or a history of gastric or duodenal ulcer, who are *H. pylori* positive, and who are about to start long-term treatment with a non-selective NSAID, eradication of *H. pylori* may reduce the overall risk of ulceration.

In a patient who has developed an ulcer, if the *NSAID can be discontinued*, a proton pump inhibitor usually produces the most rapid healing; alternatively, the ulcer can be treated with a H_2-receptor antagonist or misoprostol. On healing, patients should be tested for *H. pylori* and given eradication therapy if *H. pylori* is present (see also Test for *Helicobacter pylori*, p. 51).

If *treatment with a non-selective NSAID needs to continue*, the following options are suitable:

- Treat ulcer with a proton pump inhibitor and on healing continue the proton pump inhibitor (dose not normally reduced because asymptomatic ulcer recurrence may occur);

- Treat ulcer with a proton pump inhibitor and on healing switch to misoprostol for maintenance therapy (colic and diarrhoea may limit the dose of misoprostol);

Gastro-intestinal system

1

- Treat ulcer with a proton pump inhibitor and switch non-selective NSAID to a cyclo-oxygenase-2 selective inhibitor, but see NSAIDs and Cardiovascular Events, p. 717; on healing, continuation of the proton pump inhibitor in patients with a history of upper gastro-intestinal bleeding may provide further protection against recurrence.

If *treatment with a cyclo-oxygenase-2 selective inhibitor needs to continue*, treat ulcer with a proton pump inhibitor; on healing continuation of the proton pump inhibitor in patients with a history of upper gastro-intestinal bleeding may provide further protection against recurrence.

1.3.1 H₂-receptor antagonists

Histamine H₂-receptor antagonists heal *gastric and duodenal ulcers* by reducing gastric acid output as a result of histamine H₂-receptor blockade; they are also used to relieve symptoms of *gastro-oesophageal reflux disease* (section 1.1). H₂-receptor antagonists should not normally be used for *Zollinger-Ellison syndrome* because proton pump inhibitors (section 1.3.5) are more effective.

Maintenance treatment with low doses for the prevention of peptic ulcer disease has largely been replaced in *Helicobacter pylori* positive patients by eradication regimens (section 1.3).

H₂-receptor antagonists are used for the treatment of *functional dyspepsia* (section 1.1). H₂-receptor antagonists may be used for the treatment of *uninvestigated dyspepsia* in patients without alarm features.

H₂-receptor antagonist therapy can promote healing of *NSAID-associated ulcers* (particularly duodenal) (section 1.3).

Treatment with a H₂-receptor antagonist has not been shown to be beneficial in haematemesis and melaena, but prophylactic use reduces the frequency of bleeding from *gastroduodenal erosions in hepatic coma*, and possibly in other conditions requiring intensive care. H₂-receptor antagonists also reduce the risk of *acid aspiration* in obstetric patients at delivery (Mendelson's syndrome).

Cautions H₂-receptor antagonists might mask symptoms of gastric cancer; particular care is required in patients presenting with 'alarm features' (see p. 44), in such cases gastric malignancy should be ruled out before treatment.

Side-effects Side-effects of the H₂-receptor antagonists include diarrhoea, headache, and dizziness. Rash (including erythema multiforme and toxic epidermal necrolysis) occurs less frequently. Other side-effects reported rarely or very rarely include hepatitis, cholestatic jaundice, bradycardia, psychiatric reactions (including confusion, depression, and hallucinations) particularly in the elderly or the very ill, blood disorders (including leucopenia, thrombocytopenia, and pancytopenia), arthralgia, and myalgia. Gynaecomastia and impotence occur occasionally with cimetidine and there are isolated reports with the other H₂-receptor antagonists.

▮ CIMETIDINE

Indications benign gastric and duodenal ulceration, stomal ulcer, reflux oesophagitis, other conditions where gastric acid reduction is beneficial (see notes above and section 1.9.4)

Cautions see notes above; **interactions:** Appendix 1 (histamine H₂-antagonists) and notes above

Hepatic impairment increased risk of confusion; reduce dose

Renal impairment reduce dose; 200 mg 4 times daily if eGFR 30–50 mL/minute/1.73 m²; 200 mg 3 times daily if eGFR 15–30 mL/minute/1.73 m²; 200 mg twice daily if eGFR less than 15 mL/minute/1.73 m²; occasional risk of confusion

Pregnancy manufacturer advises avoid unless essential

Breast-feeding significant amount present in milk— not known to be harmful but manufacturer advises avoid

Side-effects see notes above; also malaise; *less commonly* tachycardia; *rarely* interstitial nephritis; *very rarely* pancreatitis, galactorrhoea, vasculitis, alopecia

Dose

- 400 mg twice daily (with breakfast and at night) *or* 800 mg at night (benign gastric and duodenal ulceration) for at least 4 weeks (6 weeks in gastric ulceration, 8 weeks in NSAID-associated ulceration); when necessary the dose may be increased to 400 mg 4 times daily; INFANT under 1 year 20 mg/kg daily in divided doses has been used; CHILD 1–12 years, 25–30 mg/kg daily in divided doses; max. 400 mg 4 times daily

Maintenance, 400 mg at night *or* 400 mg morning and night

- Reflux oesophagitis, 400 mg 4 times daily for 4–8 weeks

- Prophylaxis of stress ulceration, 200–400 mg every 4–6 hours

- Gastric acid reduction (prophylaxis of acid aspiration; do not use syrup), obstetrics 400 mg at start of labour, then up to 400 mg every 4 hours if required (max. 2.4 g daily); surgical procedures 400 mg 90–120 minutes before induction of general anaesthesia

- Short-bowel syndrome, 400 mg twice daily (with breakfast and at bedtime) adjusted according to response

- To reduce degradation of pancreatic enzyme supplements, 0.8–1.6 g daily in 4 divided doses 1–1½ hours before meals

¹Cimetidine (Non-proprietary) ⒫ⓞⓜ

Tablets, cimetidine 200 mg, net price 60-tab pack = £5.26; 400 mg, 60-tab pack = £1.91; 800 mg, 30-tab pack = £9.88

Oral solution, cimetidine 200 mg/5 mL, net price 300 mL = £14.28

Excipients may include propylene glycol (see Excipients, p. 2)

___

1. Cimetidine can be sold to the public for adults and children over 16 years (provided packs do not contain more than 2 weeks' supply) for the short-term symptomatic relief of heartburn, dyspepsia, and hyperacidity (max. single dose 200 mg, max. daily dose 800 mg), and for the prophylactic management of nocturnal heartburn (single night-time dose 100 mg)

Tagamet® (Chemidex) [PoM]

Tablets, all green, f/c, cimetidine 200 mg, net price 120-tab pack = £19.58; 400 mg, 60-tab pack = £22.62; 800 mg, 30-tab pack = £22.62

Syrup, orange, cimetidine 200 mg/5 mL. Net price 600 mL = £28.49

Excipients include propylene glycol 10%, (see Excipients, p. 2)

FAMOTIDINE

Indications see under Dose

Cautions see notes above; **interactions:** Appendix 1 (histamine H$_2$-antagonists) and notes above

Renal impairment use normal dose every 36–48 hours or use half normal dose if eGFR less than 50 mL/minute/1.73 m^2; seizures reported very rarely

Pregnancy manufacturer advises avoid unless potential benefit outweighs risk

Breast-feeding present in milk—not known to be harmful but manufacturer advises avoid

Side-effects see notes above; also constipation; *less commonly* dry mouth, nausea, vomiting, flatulence, taste disorders, anorexia, fatigue; *very rarely* chest tightness, interstitial pneumonia, seizures, paraesthesia

Dose

- Benign gastric and duodenal ulceration, treatment, 40 mg at night for 4–8 weeks; maintenance (duodenal ulceration), 20 mg at night
- Reflux oesophagitis, 20–40 mg twice daily for 6–12 weeks; maintenance, 20 mg twice daily
- CHILD not recommended

[1]**Famotidine** (Non-proprietary) [PoM]

Tablets, famotidine 20 mg, net price 28-tab pack = £21.57; 40 mg, 28-tab pack = £38.22

NIZATIDINE

Indications see under Dose

Cautions see notes above; also avoid rapid intravenous injection (risk of arrhythmias and postural hypotension); **interactions:** Appendix 1 (histamine H$_2$-antagonists) and notes above

Hepatic impairment manufacturer advises caution

Renal impairment use half normal dose if eGFR 20–50 mL/minute/1.73 m^2; use one-quarter normal dose if eGFR less than 20 mL/minute/1.73 m^2

Pregnancy manufacturer advises avoid unless essential

Breast-feeding amount too small to be harmful

Side-effects see notes above; also sweating; *rarely* nausea, fever, vasculitis, hyperuricaemia

Dose

- Benign gastric, duodenal or NSAID-associated ulceration, treatment, 300 mg in the evening *or* 150 mg twice daily for 4–8 weeks; maintenance, 150 mg at night
- Gastro-oesophageal reflux disease, 150–300 mg twice daily for up to 12 weeks
- CHILD not recommended

[2]**Nizatidine** (Non-proprietary) [PoM]

Capsules, nizatidine 150 mg, net price 30-cap pack = £6.49; 300 mg, 30-cap pack = £15.32

RANITIDINE

Indications see under Dose, other conditions where reduction of gastric acidity is beneficial (see notes above and section 1.9.4)

Cautions see notes above; **interactions:** Appendix 1 (histamine H$_2$-antagonists) and notes above

Renal impairment use half normal dose if eGFR less than 50 mL/minute/1.73 m^2

Pregnancy manufacturer advises avoid unless essential, but not known to be harmful

Breast-feeding significant amount present in milk, but not known to be harmful

Side-effects see notes above; *less commonly* blurred vision; also reported pancreatitis, involuntary movement disorders, interstitial nephritis, alopecia

Dose

- By mouth, benign gastric and duodenal ulceration, chronic episodic dyspepsia, ADULT and CHILD over 12 years, 150 mg twice daily *or* 300 mg at night for 4–8 weeks in benign gastric and duodenal ulceration, up to 6 weeks in chronic episodic dyspepsia, and up to 8 weeks in NSAID-associated ulceration (in duodenal ulcer 300 mg can be given twice daily for 4 weeks to achieve a higher healing rate); CHILD 3–12 years, (benign gastric and duodenal ulceration) 2–4 mg/kg (max. 150 mg) twice daily for 4–8 weeks

Prophylaxis of NSAID-associated gastric or duodenal ulcer [unlicensed dose], ADULT and CHILD over 12 years, 300 mg twice daily

Gastro-oesophageal reflux disease, ADULT and CHILD over 12 years, 150 mg twice daily *or* 300 mg at night for up to 8 weeks or if necessary 12 weeks (moderate to severe, 600 mg daily in 2–4 divided doses for up to 12 weeks); long-term treatment of healed gastro-oesophageal reflux disease, 150 mg twice daily; CHILD 3–12 years, 2.5–5 mg/kg (max. 300 mg) twice daily

Gastric acid reduction (prophylaxis of acid aspiration) in obstetrics, ADULT and CHILD over 12 years, by mouth, 150 mg at onset of labour, then every 6 hours; surgical procedures, by intramuscular *or* slow intravenous injection, 50 mg 45–60 minutes before induction of anaesthesia (intravenous injection diluted to 20 mL and given over at least 2 minutes), or by mouth, 150 mg 2 hours before induction of anaesthesia and also when possible on the preceding evening

- By intramuscular injection, 50 mg every 6–8 hours
- By slow intravenous injection, ADULT and CHILD over 12 years, 50 mg diluted to 20 mL and given over at least 2 minutes; may be repeated every 6–8 hours
- Prophylaxis of stress ulceration [unlicensed dose], ADULT and CHILD over 12 years, by slow intravenous injection over at least 2 minutes, 50 mg diluted to 20 mL every 8 hours (may be changed to 150 mg twice daily by mouth when oral feeding commences)

---

1. Famotidine can be sold to the public for adults and children over 16 years (provided packs do not contain more than 2 weeks' supply) for the short-term symptomatic relief of heartburn, dyspepsia, and hyperacidity, and for the prevention of these symptoms when associated with consumption of food or drink including when they cause sleep disturbance (max. single dose 10 mg, max. daily dose 20 mg)

2. Nizatidine can be sold to the public for the prevention and treatment of symptoms of food-related heartburn and meal-induced indigestion in adults and children over 16 years; max. single dose 75 mg, max. daily dose 150 mg for max. 14 days

1 Gastro-intestinal system

Gastro-intestinal system 1

Ranitidine (Non-proprietary) [PoM]
Tablets, ranitidine (as hydrochloride) 150 mg, net price 60-tab pack = £1.76; 300 mg, 30-tab pack = £2.02
Brands include *Ranitic*®
Effervescent tablets, ranitidine (as hydrochloride) 150 mg, net price 60-tab pack = £31.04; 300 mg, 30-tab pack = £31.04. Label: 13
Excipients may include sodium (check with supplier)
Oral solution, ranitidine (as hydrochloride) 75 mg/5 mL, net price 100 mL = £2.75, 300 mL = £7.75
Excipients may include alcohol (check with supplier)
Note Sugar-free versions are available and can be ordered by specifying 'sugar-free' on the prescription
Note Ranitidine can be sold to the public for adults and children over 16 years (provided packs do not contain more than 2 weeks' supply) for the short-term symptomatic relief of heartburn, dyspepsia, and hyperacidity, and for the prevention of these symptoms when associated with consumption of food or drink (max. single dose 75 mg, max. daily dose 300 mg)

Injection, ranitidine (as hydrochloride) 25 mg/mL, net price 2-mL amp = 54p

Zantac® (GSK) [PoM]
Tablets, f/c, ranitidine (as hydrochloride) 150 mg, net price 60-tab pack = £1.30; 300 mg, 30-tab pack = £1.30
Syrup, sugar-free, ranitidine (as hydrochloride) 75 mg/5 mL, net price 300 mL = £20.76
Excipients include alcohol 8%
Injection, ranitidine (as hydrochloride) 25 mg/mL, net price 2-mL amp = 56p

1.3.2 Selective antimuscarinics

Pirenzepine is a selective antimuscarinic drug which was used for the treatment of gastric and duodenal ulcers. It has been discontinued.

1.3.3 Chelates and complexes

Tripotassium dicitratobismuthate is a bismuth chelate effective in healing gastric and duodenal ulcers. For the role of tripotassium dicitratobismuthate in a *Helicobacter pylori* eradication regimen for those who have not responded to first-line regimens, see section 1.3.

The bismuth content of tripotassium dicitratobismuthate is low but absorption has been reported; encephalopathy (described with older high-dose bismuth preparations) has not been reported.

Sucralfate may act by protecting the mucosa from acid-pepsin attack in gastric and duodenal ulcers. It is a complex of aluminium hydroxide and sulfated sucrose but has minimal antacid properties. It should be used with caution in patients under intensive care (**important:** reports of bezoar formation, see Bezoar Formation below)

TRIPOTASSIUM DICITRATOBISMUTHATE

Indications benign gastric and duodenal ulceration; see also *Helicobacter pylori* infection, section 1.3

Cautions see notes above; **interactions:** Appendix 1 (tripotassium dicitratobismuthate)

Renal impairment avoid in severe impairment
Pregnancy manufacturer advises avoid on theoretical grounds
Breast-feeding no information available
Side-effects may darken tongue and blacken faeces; *less commonly* nausea, vomiting, diarrhoea, constipation, rash, and pruritus reported

De-Noltab® (Astellas)
Tablets, f/c, tripotassium dicitratobismuthate 120 mg, net price 112-tab pack = £5.09. Counselling, see below
Electrolytes K⁺ 2 mmol/tablet

$Electrolytes$ K$^+$ 2 mmol/tablet
Dose 2 tablets twice daily *or* 1 tablet 4 times daily; taken for 28 days followed by further 28 days if necessary; maintenance not indicated but course may be repeated after interval of 1 month; CHILD not recommended
Counselling To be swallowed with half a glass of water; twice-daily dosage to be taken 30 minutes before breakfast and main evening meal; four-times-daily dosage to be taken as follows: one dose 30 minutes before breakfast, midday meal and main evening meal, and one dose 2 hours after main evening meal; milk should not be drunk by itself during treatment but small quantities may be taken in tea or coffee or on cereal; antacids, fruit, or fruit juice should not be taken half an hour before or after a dose; may darken tongue and blacken faeces

SUCRALFATE

Indications see under Dose

Cautions administration of sucralfate and enteral feeds should be separated by 1 hour; **interactions:** Appendix 1 (sucralfate)
Bezoar formation Following reports of bezoar formation associated with sucralfate, caution is advised in seriously ill patients, especially those receiving concomitant enteral feeds or those with predisposing conditions such as delayed gastric emptying

Renal impairment use with caution; aluminium is absorbed and may accumulate

Pregnancy no evidence of harm; absorption from gastro-intestinal tract negligible

Breast-feeding amount probably too small to be harmful

Side-effects constipation; *less frequently* diarrhoea, nausea, indigestion, flatulence, gastric discomfort, back pain, dizziness, headache, drowsiness, bezoar formation (see above), dry mouth and rash

Dose
• Benign gastric and duodenal ulceration and chronic gastritis, ADULT and CHILD over 15 years, 2 g twice daily (on rising and at bedtime) *or* 1 g 4 times daily 1 hour before meals and at bedtime, taken for 4–6 weeks or in resistant cases up to 12 weeks; max. 8 g daily
• Prophylaxis of stress ulceration, ADULT and CHILD over 15 years, 1 g 6 times daily; max. 8 g daily
• CHILD under 15 years see *BNF for Children*

Antepsin® (Chugai) [PoM]
Tablets, scored, sucralfate 1 g, net price 50-tab pack = £6.36. Label: 5
Note Crushed tablets may be dispersed in water
Suspension, sucralfate, 1 g/5 mL, net price 250 mL (aniseed- and caramel-flavoured) = £6.36. Label: 5

1.3.4 Prostaglandin analogues

Misoprostol, a synthetic prostaglandin analogue has antisecretory and protective properties, promoting healing of *gastric and duodenal ulcers*. It can prevent NSAID-associated ulcers, its use being most appropriate for the frail or very elderly from whom NSAIDs cannot be withdrawn.

For comment on the use of misoprostol to induce abortion or labour [unlicensed indications], see section 7.1.1.

MISOPROSTOL

Indications   see notes above and under Dose

Cautions   inflammatory bowel disease; conditions where hypotension might precipitate severe complications (e.g. cerebrovascular disease, cardiovascular disease)

Contra-indications   planning pregnancy (**important:** see Women of Childbearing Age, and also Pregnancy, below)

Women of childbearing age Manufacturer advises that misoprostol should not be used in women of childbearing age unless pregnancy has been excluded. In such patients it is advised that misoprostol should only be used if the patient takes *effective contraceptive measures* and has been advised of the *risks of taking misoprostol if pregnant*.

Pregnancy   avoid—potent uterine stimulant (has been used to induce abortion); teratogenic risk in first trimester; **important:** see also Women of Childbearing Age, above

Breast-feeding   present in milk, but amount probably too small to be harmful

Side-effects   diarrhoea (may occasionally be severe and require withdrawal, reduced by giving single doses not exceeding 200 micrograms and by avoiding magnesium-containing antacids); also reported: abdominal pain, dyspepsia, flatulence, nausea and vomiting, abnormal vaginal bleeding (including intermenstrual bleeding, menorrhagia, and postmenopausal bleeding), rashes, dizziness

Dose

* Benign gastric and duodenal ulceration and NSAID-associated ulceration, ADULT over 18 years, 800 micrograms daily (in 2–4 divided doses) with breakfast (or main meals) and at bedtime; treatment should be continued for at least 4 weeks and may be continued for up to 8 weeks if required

* Prophylaxis of NSAID-induced gastric and duodenal ulcer, ADULT over 18 years, 200 micrograms 4 times daily (if not tolerated, reduced to 200 micrograms 2–3 times daily, but less effective)

Cytotec® (Pharmacia) [PoM]
Tablets, scored, misoprostol 200 micrograms, net price 60-tab pack = £10.03. Label: 21

◢With diclofenac or naproxen
Section 10.1.1

1.3.5   Proton pump inhibitors

Proton pump inhibitors inhibit gastric acid secretion by blocking the hydrogen-potassium adenosine triphosphatase enzyme system (the 'proton pump') of the gastric parietal cell. Proton pump inhibitors are effective short-term treatments for *gastric* and *duodenal ulcers*; they are also used in combination with antibacterials for the eradication of *Helicobacter pylori* (see p. 51 for

specific regimens). Following endoscopic treatment of severe peptic ulcer bleeding, an intravenous, high-dose proton pump inhibitor reduces the risk of rebleeding and the need for surgery. Proton pump inhibitors can be used for the treatment of *dyspepsia* and *gastro-oesophageal reflux disease* (section 1.1).

Proton pump inhibitors are also used for the prevention and treatment of NSAID-associated ulcers (see p. 51). In patients who need to continue NSAID treatment after an ulcer has healed, the dose of proton pump inhibitor should normally not be reduced because asymptomatic ulcer deterioration may occur.

A proton pump inhibitor can be used to reduce the degradation of pancreatic enzyme supplements (section 1.9.4) in patients with cystic fibrosis. They can also be used to control excessive secretion of gastric acid in *Zollinger–Ellison syndrome*; high doses are often required.

Cautions   Proton pump inhibitors may mask the symptoms of gastric cancer; particular care is required in those presenting with 'alarm features' (see p. 44), in such cases gastric malignancy should be ruled out before treatment. Patients at risk of osteoporosis should maintain an adequate intake of calcium and vitamin D, and, if necessary, receive other preventative therapy (see section 6.6). Measurement of serum-magnesium concentrations should be considered before and during prolonged treatment with a proton pump inhibitor, especially when used with other drugs that cause hypomagnesaemia or with digoxin. A proton pump inhibitor should be prescribed for appropriate indications at the lowest effective dose for the shortest period; the need for long-term treatment should be reviewed periodically.

Side-effects   Side-effects of the proton pump inhibitors include gastro-intestinal disturbances (including nausea, vomiting, abdominal pain, flatulence, diarrhoea, constipation), and headache. Less frequent side-effects include dry mouth, peripheral oedema, dizziness, sleep disturbances, fatigue, paraesthesia, arthralgia, myalgia, rash, and pruritus. Other side-effects reported rarely or very rarely include taste disturbance, stomatitis, hepatitis, jaundice, hypersensitivity reactions (including anaphylaxis, bronchospasm), fever, depression, hallucinations, confusion, gynaecomastia, interstitial nephritis, hyponatraemia, hypomagnesaemia (usually after 1 year of treatment, but sometimes after 3 months of treatment), blood disorders (including leucopenia, leucocytosis, pancytopenia, thrombocytopenia), visual disturbances, sweating, photosensitivity, alopecia, Stevens-Johnson syndrome, and toxic epidermal necrolysis. By decreasing gastric acidity, proton pump inhibitors may increase the risk of gastro-intestinal infections (including *Clostridium difficile* infection). Proton pump inhibitors can increase the risk of fractures, particularly when used at high doses for over a year in the elderly.

Rebound acid hypersecretion and protracted dyspepsia may occur after stopping prolonged treatment with a proton pump inhibitor.

ESOMEPRAZOLE

Indications   see under Dose

Cautions   see notes above; interactions: Appendix 1 (proton pump inhibitors)

Hepatic impairment   in severe hepatic impairment max. 20 mg daily (CHILD 1–12 years max. 10 mg daily);

for severe peptic ulcer bleeding in severe hepatic impairment, initial intravenous infusion of 80 mg, then by continuous intravenous infusion, 4 mg/hour for 72 hours

Renal impairment   manufacturer advises caution in severe renal insufficiency

Pregnancy   manufacturer advises caution—no information available

Breast-feeding   manufacturer advises avoid—no information available

Side-effects   see notes above

Dose

- By mouth duodenal ulcer associated with *Helicobacter pylori*, see eradication regimens on p. 51

  NSAID-associated gastric ulcer, ADULT over 18 years, 20 mg once daily for 4–8 weeks; prophylaxis in patients with an increased risk of gastroduodenal complications who require continued NSAID treatment, 20 mg daily

  Gastro-oesophageal reflux disease (in the presence of erosive reflux oesophagitis), ADULT and CHILD over 12 years, 40 mg once daily for 4 weeks, continued for further 4 weeks if not fully healed or symptoms persist; maintenance 20 mg daily; CHILD 1–12 years, body-weight 10–20 kg, 10 mg once daily for 8 weeks; body-weight over 20 kg, 10–20 mg once daily for 8 weeks

  Symptomatic treatment of gastro-oesophageal reflux disease (in the absence of oesophagitis), ADULT and CHILD over 12 years, 20 mg once daily for up to 4 weeks, then 20 mg daily when required; CHILD 1–12 years, body-weight over 10 kg, 10 mg once daily for up to 8 weeks

  Zollinger–Ellison syndrome, ADULT over 18 years, initially 40 mg twice daily, adjusted according to response; usual range 80–160 mg daily (above 80 mg in 2 divided doses)

- By intravenous injection over at least 3 minutes *or* by intravenous infusion, ADULT over 18 years, gastro-oesophageal reflux disease, 40 mg once daily; symptomatic reflux disease without oesophagitis, treatment of NSAID-associated gastric ulcer, prevention of NSAID-associated gastric or duodenal ulcer, 20 mg daily; continue until oral administration possible

- Severe peptic ulcer bleeding (following endoscopic treatment), ADULT over 18 years, initial intravenous infusion of 80 mg over 30 minutes, then by continuous intravenous infusion 8 mg/hour for 72 hours, then by mouth 40 mg once daily for 4 weeks

Esomeprazole (Non-proprietary) PoM

Capsules, enclosing e/c pellets, esomeprazole (as magnesium salt) 20 mg, net price 28-cap pack = £3.40; 40 mg, 28-cap pack = £3.96. Counselling, administration

Brands include *Emozul®*

Counselling Do not chew or crush capsules; swallow whole *or* mix capsule contents in water and drink within 30 minutes; for administration through a gastric tube, consult product literature

Tablets, e/c, esomeprazole (as magnesium salt) 20 mg, net price 28-tab pack = £3.51; 40 mg, 28-tab pack = £4.39. Counselling, administration

Counselling Do not chew or crush tablets; swallow whole *or* disperse in water and drink within 30 minutes; for administration through a gastric tube, consult product literature

Injection, powder for reconstitution, esomeprazole (as sodium salt), net price 40-mg vial = £3.10

Nexium® (AstraZeneca) PoM

Tablets, e/c, f/c, esomeprazole (as magnesium trihydrate) 20 mg (light pink), net price 28-tab pack = £18.50; 40 mg (pink), 28-tab pack = £25.19. Counselling, administration

Counselling Do not chew or crush tablets; swallow whole *or* disperse in water and drink within 30 minutes; for administration through a gastric tube, consult product literature

Granules, yellow, e/c, esomeprazole (as magnesium trihydrate) 10 mg/sachet, net price 28-sachet pack = £25.19. Label: 25, counselling, administration

Counselling Disperse the contents of each sachet in approx. 15 mL water. Stir and leave to thicken for a few minutes; stir again before administration and use within 30 minutes; rinse container with 15 mL water to obtain full dose; for administration through a gastric tube, consult product literature

Injection, powder for reconstitution, esomeprazole (as sodium salt), net price 40-mg vial = £4.25

◢**With naproxen**

Section 10.1.1

LANSOPRAZOLE

Indications   see under Dose

Cautions   see notes above; **interactions**: Appendix 1 (proton pump inhibitors)

Hepatic impairment   use half normal dose in moderate to severe liver disease

Pregnancy   manufacturer advises avoid

Breast-feeding   avoid—present in milk in *animal* studies

Side-effects   see notes above; also glossitis, pancreatitis, anorexia, restlessness, tremor, impotence, petechiae, and purpura; *very rarely* colitis, raised serum cholesterol or triglycerides

Dose

- Benign gastric ulcer, 30 mg daily in the morning for 8 weeks

- Duodenal ulcer, 30 mg daily in the morning for 4 weeks; maintenance 15 mg daily

- NSAID-associated duodenal or gastric ulcer, 30 mg once daily for 4 weeks, continued for further 4 weeks if not fully healed; prophylaxis, 15–30 mg once daily

- Eradication of *Helicobacter pylori* associated with duodenal ulcer or ulcer-like dyspepsia, see eradication regimens on p. 51

- Zollinger-Ellison syndrome (and other hypersecretory conditions), initially 60 mg once daily adjusted according to response; daily doses of 120 mg or more given in two divided doses

- Gastro-oesophageal reflux disease, 30 mg daily in the morning for 4 weeks, continued for further 4 weeks if not fully healed; maintenance 15–30 mg daily

- Acid-related dyspepsia, 15–30 mg daily in the morning for 2–4 weeks

- CHILD under 18 years see *BNF for Children*

Note Lansoprazole doses in BNF may differ from those in product literature

Lansoprazole (Non-proprietary) PoM

Capsules, enclosing e/c granules, lansoprazole 15 mg, net price 28-cap pack = £1.18; 30 mg, 28-cap pack = £1.67. Label: 5, 22, 25

Dental prescribing on NHS Lansoprazole capsules may be prescribed

Zoton® (Pfizer) PoM

FasTab® (= orodispersible tablet), lansoprazole 15 mg, net price 28-tab pack = £2.99; 30 mg, 28-tab pack = £5.50. Label: 5, 22, counselling, administration

Excipients include aspartame (section 9.4.1)

Counselling Tablets should be placed on the tongue, allowed to disperse and swallowed, or may be swallowed whole with a glass of water. Alternatively, tablets can be dispersed in a small amount of water and administered by an oral syringe or nasogastric tube

OMEPRAZOLE

Indications see under Dose

Cautions see notes above; **interactions**: Appendix 1 (proton pump inhibitors)

Hepatic impairment not more than 20 mg daily should be needed

Pregnancy not known to be harmful

Breast-feeding present in milk but not known to be harmful

Side-effects see notes above; also agitation and impotence

Dose

- By mouth, benign gastric and duodenal ulcers, 20 mg once daily for 4 weeks in duodenal ulceration or 8 weeks in gastric ulceration; in severe or recurrent cases increase to 40 mg daily; prevention of relapse in gastric ulcer, 20 mg once daily, increased to 40 mg once daily if necessary; prevention of relapse in duodenal ulcer, 20 mg once daily (range 10–40 mg daily)

NSAID-associated duodenal or gastric ulcer and gastroduodenal erosions, 20 mg once daily for 4 weeks, continued for further 4 weeks if not fully healed; prophylaxis in patients with a history of NSAID-associated duodenal or gastric ulcers, gastroduodenal lesions, or dyspeptic symptoms who require continued NSAID treatment, 20 mg once daily

Duodenal or benign gastric ulcer associated with *Helicobacter pylori*, see eradication regimens on p. 51

Zollinger–Ellison syndrome, initially 60 mg once daily; usual range 20–120 mg daily (above 80 mg in 2 divided doses)

Gastro-oesophageal reflux disease, 20 mg once daily for 4 weeks, continued for further 4–8 weeks if not fully healed; 40 mg once daily has been given for 8 weeks in gastro-oesophageal reflux disease refractory to other treatment; maintenance 20 mg once daily

Acid reflux disease (long-term management), 10 mg daily increasing to 20 mg once daily if symptoms return

Acid-related dyspepsia, 10–20 mg once daily for 2–4 weeks according to response

Severe ulcerating reflux oesophagitis, CHILD over 1 year, body-weight 10–20 kg, 10 mg once daily increased if necessary to 20 mg once daily for 4–12 weeks; body-weight over 20 kg, 20 mg once daily increased if necessary to 40 mg once daily for 4–12 weeks; to be initiated by hospital paediatrician

- By intravenous injection over 5 minutes or by intravenous infusion over 20–30 minutes, treatment and prevention of benign gastric ulcers, duodenal ulcers, or NSAID-associated ulcers, gastro-oesophageal reflux disease, 40 mg once daily until oral administration possible

Zollinger-Ellison syndrome, initially 60 mg once daily, adjusted according to response; daily doses above 60 mg given in 2 divided doses

- Major peptic ulcer bleeding (following endoscopic treatment) [unlicensed indication], initial intravenous infusion of 80 mg over 40–60 minutes, then by continuous intravenous infusion, 8 mg/hour for 72 hours (then change to oral therapy)

Counselling Swallow whole, or disperse *MUPS*® tablets in water, or mix capsule contents or *MUPS*® tablets with fruit juice or yoghurt. Preparations consisting of an e/c tablet within a capsule should **not** be opened

Omeprazole (Non-proprietary) PoM

Capsules, enclosing e/c granules, omeprazole 10 mg, net price 28-cap pack = £1.25; 20 mg, 28-cap pack = £1.24; 40 mg, 7-cap pack = £1.18, 28-cap pack = £4.98. Counselling, administration

Dental prescribing on NHS Gastro-resistant omeprazole capsules may be prescribed

Capsules, enclosing e/c tablet, omeprazole 10 mg, net price 28-cap pack = £1.04; 20 mg, 28-cap pack = £1.04. Counselling, administration

Brands include *Mepradec*®

Dental prescribing on NHS Gastro-resistant omeprazole capsules may be prescribed

[1]Tablets, e/c, omeprazole 10 mg, net price 28-tab pack = £7.90; 20 mg, 28-tab pack = £7.11; 40 mg, 7-tab pack = £5.36. Label: 25

Intravenous infusion, powder for reconstitution, omeprazole (as sodium salt), net price 40-mg vial = £4.16

Losec® (AstraZeneca) PoM

MUPS® (multiple-unit pellet system = dispersible tablets), f/c, omeprazole 10 mg (light pink), net price 28-tab pack = £7.75; 20 mg (pink), 28-tab pack = £11.60; 40 mg (red-brown), 7-tab pack = £5.80. Counselling, administration

Capsules, enclosing e/c granules, omeprazole 10 mg (pink), net price 28-cap pack = £9.30; 20 mg (pink/brown), 28-cap pack = £13.92; 40 mg (brown), 7-cap pack = £6.96. Counselling, administration

Intravenous infusion, powder for reconstitution, omeprazole (as sodium salt), net price 40-mg vial = £6.50

Injection, powder for reconstitution, omeprazole (as sodium salt), net price 40-mg vial (with solvent) = £6.49

◢With ketoprofen

Section 10.1.1

PANTOPRAZOLE

Indications see under Dose

Cautions see notes above; **interactions**: Appendix 1 (proton pump inhibitors)

Hepatic impairment max. 20 mg daily in severe impairment and cirrhosis—monitor liver function (discontinue if deterioration)

Renal impairment max. oral dose 40 mg daily

Pregnancy manufacturer advises avoid unless potential benefit outweighs risk—fetotoxic in *animals*

---

1. Omeprazole 10 mg tablets can be sold to the public for the short-term relief of reflux-like symptoms (eg heartburn) in adults over 18 years, max. daily dose 20 mg for max. 4 weeks, and a pack size of 28 tablets

1

Gastro-intestinal system

Breast-feeding manufacturer advises avoid unless potential benefit outweighs risk—small amount present in milk

Side-effects see notes above; also hyperlipidaemia, weight changes

Dose

- By mouth, benign gastric ulcer, ADULT over 18 years, 40 mg daily for 8 weeks; in severe cases increase up to 80 mg daily

  Duodenal ulcer, ADULT over 18 years, 40 mg daily for 4 weeks; in severe cases increase up to 80 mg daily

  Duodenal or benign gastric ulcer associated with *Helicobacter pylori*, see eradication regimens on p. 51

  Prophylaxis of NSAID-associated gastric or duodenal ulcer in patients with an increased risk of gastroduodenal complications who require continued NSAID treatment, ADULT over 18 years, 20 mg daily

  Gastro-oesophageal reflux disease, ADULT and CHILD over 12 years, 20–80 mg daily in the morning for 4 weeks, continued for further 4 weeks if not fully healed; maintenance 20 mg daily, increased to 40 mg daily if symptoms return

  Zollinger–Ellison syndrome (and other hypersecretory conditions), ADULT over 18 years, initially 80 mg once daily adjusted according to response (ELDERLY max. 40 mg daily); daily doses above 80 mg given in 2 divided doses

- By intravenous injection over at least 2 minutes *or* by intravenous infusion, ADULT over 18 years, duodenal ulcer, gastric ulcer, and gastro-oesophageal reflux, 40 mg daily until oral administration can be resumed

  Zollinger–Ellison syndrome (and other hypersecretory conditions), ADULT over 18 years, initially 80 mg (160 mg if rapid acid control required) then 80 mg once daily adjusted according to response; daily doses above 80 mg given in 2 divided doses

Pantoprazole (Non-proprietary) ⒫ᴏᴹ

Tablets, e/c, pantoprazole 20 mg, net price 28-tab pack = £1.21; 40 mg, 28-tab pack = £1.57. Label: 25

Note Pantoprazole 20 mg tablets can be sold to the public for the short-term treatment of reflux symptoms (e.g. heartburn) in adults over 18 years, max. daily dose 20 mg for max. 4 weeks

Injection, powder for reconstitution, pantoprazole (as sodium salt), net price 40-mg vial = £4.65

Protium® (Takeda) ⒫ᴏᴹ

Injection, powder for reconstitution, pantoprazole (as sodium salt), net price 40-mg vial = £5.11

RABEPRAZOLE SODIUM

Indications see under Dose

Cautions see notes above; **interactions:** Appendix 1 (proton pump inhibitors)

Hepatic impairment manufacturer advises caution in severe hepatic dysfunction

Pregnancy manufacturer advises avoid—no information available

Breast-feeding manufacturer advises avoid—no information available

Side-effects see notes above; also cough, influenza-like syndrome, and rhinitis; *less commonly* chest pain and nervousness; *rarely* anorexia and weight gain

Dose

- Benign gastric ulcer, 20 mg daily in the morning for 8 weeks

- Duodenal ulcer, 20 mg daily in the morning for 4 weeks

- Duodenal and benign gastric ulcer associated with *Helicobacter pylori*, see eradication regimens on p. 51

- Gastro-oesophageal reflux disease, 20 mg once daily for 4–8 weeks; maintenance 10–20 mg daily; symptomatic treatment in the absence of oesophagitis, 10 mg daily for up to 4 weeks, then 10 mg daily when required

- Zollinger–Ellison syndrome, initially 60 mg once daily adjusted according to response (max. 120 mg daily); doses above 100 mg daily given in 2 divided doses

- CHILD not recommended

Rabeprazole (Non-proprietary) ⒫ᴏᴹ

Tablets, e/c, rabeprazole sodium 10 mg, net price 28-tab pack = £2.55; 20 mg, 28-tab pack = £3.29. Label: 25

Pariet® (Janssen, Eisai) ⒫ᴏᴹ

Tablets, e/c, rabeprazole sodium 10 mg (pink), net price 28-tab pack = £5.78; 20 mg (yellow), 28-tab pack = £11.34. Label: 25

1.4 Acute diarrhoea

1.4.1 Adsorbents and bulk-forming drugs
1.4.2 Antimotility drugs
1.4.3 Enkephalinase inhibitors

The priority in acute diarrhoea, as in gastro-enteritis, is the prevention or reversal of fluid and electrolyte depletion. This is particularly important in infants and in frail and elderly patients. For details of **oral rehydration preparations**, see section 9.2.1.2. Severe depletion of fluid and electrolytes requires immediate admission to hospital and urgent replacement.

Antimotility drugs (section 1.4.2) relieve symptoms of acute diarrhoea. They are used in the management of uncomplicated acute diarrhoea in adults; fluid and electrolyte replacement may be necessary in case of dehydration. However, antimotility drugs are **not** recommended for acute diarrhoea in young children.

Racecadotril (section 1.4.3) is licensed, as an adjunct to rehydration, for the symptomatic treatment of uncomplicated acute diarrhoea.

Antispasmodics (section 1.2) are occasionally of value in treating abdominal cramp associated with diarrhoea but they should **not** be used for primary treatment. Antispasmodics and antiemetics should be **avoided** in young children with gastro-enteritis because they are rarely effective and have troublesome side-effects.

Antibacterial drugs are generally unnecessary in simple gastro-enteritis because the complaint usually resolves quickly without them, and infective diarrhoeas in the UK often have a viral cause. Systemic bacterial infection does, however, need appropriate systemic treatment; for drugs used in campylobacter enteritis, shigellosis, and salmonellosis, see Table 1, section 5.1. **Ciprofloxacin** is occasionally used for prophylaxis against travellers' diarrhoea, but routine use is **not** recommended. Lactobacillus preparations have not been shown to be effective.

Colestyramine (section 1.9.2), binds unabsorbed bile salts and provides symptomatic relief of diarrhoea following ileal disease or resection.

1.4.1   Adsorbents and bulk-forming drugs

Adsorbents such as kaolin are **not** recommended for *acute diarrhoeas*. Bulk-forming drugs, such as ispaghula, methylcellulose, and sterculia (section 1.6.1) are useful in controlling diarrhoea associated with diverticular disease.

◢ KAOLIN, LIGHT ◢

Indications   diarrhoea but see notes above
Cautions   interactions: Appendix 1 (kaolin)

Kaolin Mixture, BP ◢
(Kaolin Oral Suspension)
Oral suspension, light kaolin or light kaolin (natural) 20%, light magnesium carbonate 5%, sodium bicarbonate 5% in a suitable vehicle with a peppermint flavour.
Dose 10–20 mL every 4 hours

1.4.2   Antimotility drugs

Antimotility drugs prolong the duration of intestinal transit by binding to opioid receptors in the gastro-intestinal tract. Loperamide does not cross the blood-brain barrier readily. Antimotility drugs have a role in the management of uncomplicated *acute diarrhoea* in adults but not in young children; see also section 1.4. However, in severe cases, fluid and electrolyte replacement (section 9.2.1.2) are of primary importance.

For comments on the role of antimotility drugs in *chronic bowel disorders* see section 1.5. For their role in *stoma care* see section 1.8.

Loperamide can be used for faecal incontinence [unlicensed indication] after the underlying cause of incontinence has been addressed.

◢ CODEINE PHOSPHATE

Indications   see notes above; cough suppression (section 3.9.1); pain (section 4.7.2)
Cautions   section 4.7.2; tolerance and dependence may occur with prolonged use; **interactions:** Appendix 1 (opioid analgesics)
Contra-indications   section 4.7.2; also conditions where inhibition of peristalsis should be avoided, where abdominal distension develops, or in acute diarrhoeal conditions such as acute ulcerative colitis or antibiotic-associated colitis
Hepatic impairment   section 4.7.2
Renal impairment   section 4.7.2
Pregnancy   section 4.7.2
Breast-feeding   section 4.7.2
Side-effects   section 4.7.2
Dose
• Acute diarrhoea, ADULT and CHILD over 12 years, 30 mg 3–4 times daily (range 15–60 mg)

◢ **Preparations**
Section 4.7.2

◢ CO-PHENOTROPE

A mixture of diphenoxylate hydrochloride and atropine sulfate in the mass proportions 100 parts to 1 part respectively

Indications   adjunct to rehydration in acute diarrhoea (but see notes above); control of faecal consistency after colostomy or ileostomy (section 1.8)
Cautions   section 4.7.2; also young children are particularly susceptible to **overdosage** and symptoms may be delayed and observation is needed for at least 48 hours after ingestion; presence of subclinical doses of atropine may give rise to atropine side-effects in susceptible individuals or in overdosage (section 1.2); **interactions:** Appendix 1 (antimuscarinics, opioid analgesics)
Contra-indications   section 4.7.2 and also see under Antimuscarinics (section 1.2)
Hepatic impairment   section 4.7.2; also avoid in jaundice
Renal impairment   section 4.7.2
Pregnancy   section 4.7.2 and also see under Atropine Sulfate (section 1.2)
Breast-feeding   may be present in milk
Side-effects   section 4.7.2 and also see under Antimuscarinics (section 1.2); also abdominal pain, anorexia, and fever
Dose
• See preparations

Co-phenotrope (Non-proprietary) PoM
Tablets, co-phenotrope 2.5/0.025 (diphenoxylate hydrochloride 2.5 mg, atropine sulfate 25 micrograms), net price 100 = £10.74
Brands include *Lomotil*®
Dose initially 4 tablets, followed by 2 tablets every 6 hours until diarrhoea controlled; CHILD under 4 years see *BNF for Children*, 4–9 years 1 tablet 3 times daily, 9–12 years 1 tablet 4 times daily, 12–16 years 2 tablets 3 times daily, but see also notes above
Note Co-phenotrope 2.5/0.025 can be sold to the public for adults and children over 16 years (provided packs do not contain more than 20 tablets) as an adjunct to rehydration in acute diarrhoea (max. daily dose 10 tablets)

◢ LOPERAMIDE HYDROCHLORIDE

Indications   symptomatic treatment of acute diarrhoea; adjunct to rehydration in acute diarrhoea in adults and children over 4 years (but see notes above); chronic diarrhoea in adults only
Cautions   see notes above; **interactions:** Appendix 1 (loperamide)
Contra-indications   conditions where inhibition of peristalsis should be avoided, where abdominal distension develops, or in conditions such as active ulcerative colitis or antibiotic-associated colitis
Hepatic impairment   risk of accumulation—manufacturer advises caution
Pregnancy   manufacturers advise avoid—no information available
Breast-feeding   amount probably too small to be harmful
Side-effects   nausea, flatulence, headache, dizziness; *less commonly* dyspepsia, vomiting, abdominal pain, dry mouth, drowsiness, rash (rarely Stevens-Johnson syndrome, toxic epidermal necrolysis); *rarely* paralytic ileus, fatigue, hypertonia, urinary retention

1   Gastro-intestinal system

Dose

- Acute diarrhoea, 4 mg initially followed by 2 mg after each loose stool for up to 5 days; usual dose 6–8 mg daily; max. 16 mg daily; CHILD under 4 years not recommended; 4–8 years, 1 mg 3–4 times daily for up to 3 days only; 8–12 years, 2 mg 4 times daily for up to 5 days
- Chronic diarrhoea in adults, initially, 4–8 mg daily in divided doses, subsequently adjusted according to response and given in 2 divided doses for maintenance; max. 16 mg daily; CHILD under 18 years see BNF for Children
- Faecal incontinence [unlicensed indication], initially 500 micrograms daily, adjusted according to response; max. 16 mg daily in divided doses

Loperamide (Non-proprietary) ▣PoM

Capsules, loperamide hydrochloride 2 mg, net price 30-cap pack = £2.72

Tablets, loperamide hydrochloride 2 mg, net price 30-tab pack = £2.15

Brands include Norimode®

Note Loperamide can be sold to the public, provided it is licensed and labelled for the treatment of acute diarrhoea in adults and children over 12 years of age, or for acute diarrhoea associated with irritable bowel syndrome (after initial diagnosis by a doctor) in adults over 18 years of age

Imodium® (Janssen) ▣PoM

Syrup, sugar-free, red, loperamide hydrochloride 1 mg/5 mL. Net price 100 mL = £1.17

◢Compound preparations

Imodium® Plus (McNeil)

Caplets (= tablets), loperamide hydrochloride 2 mg, simeticone 125 mg, net price 6-tab pack = £2.27, 12-tab pack = £3.58

Dose acute diarrhoea with abdominal colic, initially 2 caplets (CHILD 12–18 years 1 caplet) then 1 caplet after each loose stool; max. 4 caplets daily for up to 2 days; CHILD under 12 years not recommended

◤ MORPHINE

Indications see notes above; cough in terminal disease (section 3.9.1); pain (section 4.7.2)

Cautions see notes above and under Morphine Salts (section 4.7.2)

Contra-indications see notes above and under Morphine Salts (section 4.7.2)

Hepatic impairment section 4.7.2

Renal impairment section 4.7.2

Pregnancy section 4.7.2

Breast-feeding see under Morphine Salts (section 4.7.2)

Side-effects see notes above and under Morphine Salts (section 4.7.2); sedation and the risk of dependence are greater

Dose

- See preparation

Kaolin and Morphine Mixture, BP ◢

(Kaolin and Morphine Oral Suspension)

Oral suspension, light kaolin or light kaolin (natural) 20%, sodium bicarbonate 5%, and chloroform and morphine tincture 4% in a suitable vehicle. Contains anhydrous morphine 550–800 micrograms/10 mL.

Dose ADULT and CHILD over 12 years, 10 mL every 6 hours in water

1.4.3 Enkephalinase inhibitors

Racecadotril is a pro-drug of thiorphan. Thiorphan is an enkephalinase inhibitor that inhibits the breakdown of endogenous opioids, thereby reducing intestinal secretions. Racecadotril is licensed, as an adjunct to rehydration, for the symptomatic treatment of uncomplicated acute diarrhoea; it should only be used in children over 3 months of age when usual supportive measures, including oral rehydration, are insufficient to control the condition. Racecadotril does not affect the duration of intestinal transit.

The Scottish Medicines Consortium, p. 4 has advised (July 2014) that racecadotril (Hidrasec®) is **not** recommended for use within NHS Scotland for the treatment of acute diarrhoea in children because there is insufficient evidence that it improves the recovery rate.

◤ RACECADOTRIL

Indications see notes above

Hepatic impairment manufacturer advises caution in adults and to avoid in children

Renal impairment manufacturer advises caution in adults and to avoid in children

Pregnancy manufacturer advises avoid—no information available

Breast-feeding manufacturer advises avoid—no information available

Side-effects headache; less commonly rash

Dose

- ADULT over 18 years, 100 mg initially, then 100 mg 3 times daily (preferably before food) until diarrhoea stops; max. duration of treatment 7 days; CHILD 3 months–18 years, body-weight less than 9 kg, 10 mg 3 times daily until diarrhoea stops (max. duration of treatment 7 days); body-weight 9–13 kg, 20 mg 3 times daily until diarrhoea stops (max. duration of treatment 7 days); body-weight 13–27 kg, 30 mg 3 times daily until diarrhoea stops (max. duration of treatment 7 days); body-weight over 27 kg, 60 mg 3 times daily until diarrhoea stops (max. duration of treatment 7 days)

Hidrasec® (Abbott Healthcare) ▣PoM

Capsules, ivory, racecadotril 100 mg, net price 20-cap pack = £8.42

Granules, racecadotril 10 mg/sachet, net price 20-sachet pack = £8.42; 30 mg/sachet, 20-sachet pack = £8.42. Counselling, administration

Excipients include sucrose 970 mg/10 mg sachet (2.9 g/30 mg sachet)

Counselling granules may be added to food or mixed with water or bottle feeds and then taken immediately

1.5 Chronic bowel disorders

Once tumours are ruled out individual symptoms of chronic bowel disorders need specific treatment including dietary manipulation as well as drug treatment and the maintenance of a liberal fluid intake.

Inflammatory bowel disease

Chronic inflammatory bowel diseases include *ulcerative colitis* and *Crohn's disease*. Effective management requires drug therapy, attention to nutrition, and in severe or chronic active disease, surgery.

Aminosalicylates (balsalazide, mesalazine, olsalazine, and sulfasalazine), **corticosteroids** (hydrocortisone, beclometasone, budesonide, and prednisolone), and **drugs that affect the immune response** are used in the treatment of inflammatory bowel disease.

Treatment of acute ulcerative colitis and Crohn's disease Acute mild to moderate disease affecting the rectum (proctitis) or the recto-sigmoid is treated initially with local application of an aminosalicylate (section 1.5.1); alternatively, a local corticosteroid can be used but it is less effective. A combination of a local aminosalicylate and a local corticosteroid can be used for proctitis that does not respond to a local aminosalicylate alone. Foam preparations and suppositories are especially useful when patients have difficulty retaining liquid enemas.

Diffuse inflammatory bowel disease or disease that does not respond to local therapy requires oral treatment. Mild disease affecting the proximal colon can be treated with an oral aminosalicylate alone; a combination of a local and an oral aminosalicylate can be used in proctitis or distal colitis. Refractory or moderate inflammatory bowel disease usually requires adjunctive use of an oral corticosteroid such as **prednisolone** (section 1.5.2) for 4–8 weeks. Modified-release **budesonide** is licensed for Crohn's disease affecting the ileum and the ascending colon; it causes fewer systemic side-effects than oral prednisolone but may be less effective. **Beclometasone dipropionate** by mouth is licensed as an adjunct to mesalazine for mild to moderate ulcerative colitis, but it is not known whether it is as effective as other corticosteroids.

Severe inflammatory bowel disease or disease that is not responding to an oral corticosteroid requires hospital admission and treatment with an intravenous corticosteroid (such as hydrocortisone or methylprednisolone, section 6.3.2); other therapy may include intravenous fluid and electrolyte replacement, and possibly parenteral nutrition. Specialist supervision is required for patients who fail to respond adequately to these measures. Patients with severe ulcerative colitis that has not responded to intravenous corticosteroids, may benefit from a short course of intravenous **ciclosporin** [unlicensed indication] (section 1.5.3). Patients with unresponsive or chronically active Crohn's disease may benefit from **azathioprine** (section 1.5.3), **mercaptopurine** (section 1.5.3) [unlicensed indication], or once-weekly **methotrexate** (section 1.5.3) [unlicensed indication]; these drugs have a slower onset of action.

Infliximab (section 1.5.3) is licensed for the management of severe active Crohn's disease and severe ulcerative colitis in patients whose condition has not responded adequately to treatment with a corticosteroid and a conventional drug that affects the immune response, or who are intolerant of them.

NICE guidance
Infliximab and adalimumab for Crohn's disease (May 2010)

Infliximab or adalimumab is recommended for the treatment of severe active Crohn's disease that has not responded to conventional therapy (including corticosteroids and other drugs affecting the immune response) or when conventional therapy cannot be used because of intolerance or contraindications; infliximab can also be used in a similar way in children over 6 years of age. In adults over 18 years of age, infliximab is recommended for the treatment of fistulating Crohn's disease that has not responded to conventional therapy (including antibacterials, drainage, and other drugs affecting the immune response) or when conventional therapy cannot be used because of intolerance or contraindications.

Infliximab or adalimumab should be given as a planned course of treatment for 12 months or until treatment failure, whichever is shorter. Treatment should be continued beyond 12 months only if there is evidence of active disease—in these cases the need for treatment should be reviewed at least annually. If the disease relapses after stopping treatment, adalimumab or infliximab can be restarted [but see Hypersensitivity Reactions under Infliximab, p. 67].

www.nice.org.uk/TA187

NICE guidance
Infliximab for subacute manifestations of ulcerative colitis (April 2008)

Infliximab is **not** recommended for the treatment of subacute manifestations of moderate to severe active ulcerative colitis that would normally be managed in an outpatient setting.

www.nice.org.uk/TA140

NICE guidance
Infliximab for acute exacerbations of ulcerative colitis (December 2008)

Infliximab is recommended as an option for the treatment of acute exacerbations of severe ulcerative colitis when treatment with ciclosporin is contra-indicated or inappropriate.

www.nice.org.uk/TA163

Adalimumab (section 1.5.3) is licensed for the treatment of severe active Crohn's disease and severe ulcerative colitis in patients whose condition has not responded adequately to treatment with a corticosteroid and a conventional drug that affects the immune response, or who are intolerant of them. For inducing remission, adalimumab can be used in combination with a corticosteroid, but it may be given alone if a corticosteroid is inappropriate or is not tolerated. Adalimumab may also be used for Crohn's disease in patients who have relapsed while taking infliximab or who cannot tolerate infliximab because of hypersensitivity reactions.

Golimumab (section 1.5.3) is licensed for the treatment of severe ulcerative colitis in patients whose condition has not responded adequately to conventional therapy, or who are intolerant of it.

1 Gastro-intestinal system

Vedolizumab (section 1.5.3) is licensed for the treatment of moderate to severe active Crohn's disease and ulcerative colitis in patients who have had an inadequate response with, lost response to, or are intolerant to either conventional therapy or a tumour necrosis factor alpha inhibitor.

Maintenance of remission of acute ulcerative colitis and Crohn's disease

Smoking cessation (section 4.10.2) reduces the risk of relapse in Crohn's disease and should be encouraged. Aminosalicylates are efficacious in the maintenance of remission of ulcerative colitis, but there is no evidence of efficacy in the maintenance of remission of Crohn's disease. Corticosteroids are not suitable for maintenance treatment because of their side-effects. In resistant or frequently relapsing cases either azathioprine (section 1.5.3) or mercaptopurine (section 1.5.3) [unlicensed indication], given under close supervision may be helpful. Methotrexate (section 1.5.3) is tried in Crohn's disease if azathioprine or mercaptopurine cannot be used [unlicensed indication]. Maintenance therapy with infliximab should be considered for patients with Crohn's disease or ulcerative colitis who respond to the initial induction course of infliximab; fixed-interval dosing is superior to intermittent dosing. Adalimumab is licensed for maintenance therapy in Crohn's disease and ulcerative colitis. Golimumab is licensed for maintenance therapy in ulcerative colitis.

Fistulating Crohn's disease

Treatment may not be necessary for simple, asymptomatic perianal fistulas. Metronidazole (section 5.1.11) or ciprofloxacin (section 5.1.12) can improve symptoms of fistulating Crohn's disease but complete healing occurs rarely [unlicensed indication]. Metronidazole by mouth is used at a dose of 10–20 mg/kg daily in divided doses (usual dose 400–500 mg 3 times daily); it is usually given for 1 month but no longer than 3 months because of concerns about peripheral neuropathy. Ciprofloxacin by mouth is given at a dose of 500 mg twice daily. Other antibacterials should be given if specifically indicated (e.g. sepsis associated with fistulas and perianal disease) and for managing bacterial overgrowth in the small bowel. Fistulas may also require surgical exploration and local drainage.

Either azathioprine or mercaptopurine is used as a second-line treatment for fistulating Crohn's disease and continued for maintenance [unlicensed indication]. Infliximab is used for fistulating Crohn's disease refractory to conventional treatments; fixed-interval dosing is superior to intermittent dosing. Maintenance therapy with infliximab should be considered for patients who respond to the initial induction course of infliximab. Adalimumab can be used if there is intolerance to infliximab [unlicensed indication]

Adjunctive treatment of inflammatory bowel disease

Due attention should be paid to diet; high-fibre or low-residue diets should be used as appropriate.

Antimotility drugs such as codeine and loperamide, and antispasmodic drugs may precipitate paralytic ileus and megacolon in active ulcerative colitis; treatment of the inflammation is more logical. An osmotic laxative, such as a macrogol, may be required in proctitis (section 1.6.4). Diarrhoea resulting from the loss of bile-salt absorption (e.g. in terminal ileal disease or bowel resection) may improve with colestyramine (section 1.9.2), which binds bile salts.

Clostridium difficile infection

Clostridium difficile infection is caused by colonisation of the colon with Clostridium difficile and production of toxin. It often follows antibiotic therapy and is usually of acute onset, but may become chronic. It is a particular hazard of ampicillin, amoxicillin, co-amoxiclav, second- and third-generation cephalosporins, clindamycin, and quinolones, but few antibiotics are free of this side-effect. Treatment options include metronidazole, vancomycin, and fidaxomicin (see table 1, section 5.1).

Diverticular disease

Diverticular disease is treated with a high-fibre diet, bran supplements, and bulk-forming drugs (section 1.6.1). Antispasmodics may provide symptomatic relief when colic is a problem (section 1.2). Antibacterials are used only when the diverticula in the intestinal wall become infected. Antimotility drugs which slow intestinal motility, e.g. codeine, diphenoxylate, and loperamide could possibly exacerbate the symptoms of diverticular disease and are contra-indicated.

Irritable bowel syndrome

Irritable bowel syndrome can present with pain, constipation, or diarrhoea. In some patients there may be important psychological aggravating factors which respond to reassurance and possibly specific treatment e.g. with an antidepressant.

The fibre intake of patients with irritable bowel syndrome should be reviewed. If an increase in dietary fibre is required, soluble fibre (e.g. ispaghula husk, sterculia, or oats) is recommended; insoluble fibre (e.g. bran) may exacerbate symptoms and its use should be discouraged. A laxative (section 1.6) can be used to treat constipation. An osmotic laxative, such as a macrogol, is preferred; lactulose may cause bloating. Linaclotide (section 1.6.7) is licensed for the treatment of moderate to severe irritable bowel syndrome associated with constipation. Stimulant laxatives should be avoided or used only occasionally. Loperamide (section 1.4.2) may relieve diarrhoea and antispasmodic drugs (section 1.2) may relieve pain. Opioids with a central action, such as codeine, are better avoided because of the risk of dependence.

A tricyclic antidepressant (section 4.3.1) can be used for abdominal pain or discomfort [unlicensed indication] in patients who have not responded to laxatives, loperamide, or antispasmodics. Low doses of a tricyclic antidepressant are used (e.g. amitriptyline, initially 5–10 mg each night, increased if necessary in steps of 10 mg at intervals of at least 2 weeks to max. 30 mg each night). A selective serotonin reuptake inhibitor (section 4.3.3) may be considered in those who do not respond to a tricyclic antidepressant [unlicensed indication].

Malabsorption syndromes

Individual conditions need specific management and also general nutritional consideration. Coeliac disease (gluten enteropathy) usually needs a gluten-free diet and pancreatic insufficiency needs pancreatin supplements (section 1.9.4)

For further information on foods for special diets (ACBS), see Appendix 2.

1.5.1 Aminosalicylates

Sulfasalazine is a combination of 5-aminosalicylic acid ('5-ASA') and sulfapyridine; sulfapyridine acts only as a carrier to the colonic site of action but still causes side-effects. In the newer aminosalicylates, **mesalazine** (5-aminosalicylic acid), **balsalazide** (a prodrug of 5-amino-salicylic acid) and **olsalazine** (a dimer of 5-aminosali-cylic acid which cleaves in the lower bowel), the sulfo-namide-related side-effects of sulfasalazine are avoided, but 5-aminosalicylic acid alone can still cause side-effects including blood disorders (see recommendation below) and lupus-like syndrome also seen with sulfasa-lazine.

Cautions   Renal function should be monitored before starting an oral aminosalicylate, at 3 months of treat-ment, and then annually during treatment (more fre-quently in renal impairment). Blood disorders can occur with aminosalicylates (see recommendation below).

> ### Blood disorders
>
> Patients receiving aminosalicylates should be advised to report any unexplained bleeding, bruising, purpura, sore throat, fever or malaise that occurs during treatment. A blood count should be per-formed and the drug stopped immediately if there is suspicion of a blood dyscrasia.

Contra-indications   Aminosalicylates should be avoided in salicylate hypersensitivity.

Side-effects   Side-effects of the aminosalicylates include diarrhoea, nausea, vomiting, abdominal pain, exacerbation of symptoms of colitis, headache, hyper-sensitivity reactions (including rash and urticaria); side-effects that occur rarely include acute pancreatitis, hepatitis, myocarditis, pericarditis, lung disorders (including eosinophilia and fibrosing alveolitis), periph-eral neuropathy, blood disorders (including agranulo-cytosis, aplastic anaemia, leucopenia, methaemoglobin-aemia, neutropenia, and thrombocytopenia—see also recommendation above), renal dysfunction (interstitial nephritis, nephrotic syndrome), myalgia, arthralgia, skin reactions (including lupus erythematosus-like syndrome, Stevens-Johnson syndrome), alopecia.

BALSALAZIDE SODIUM

Indications   treatment of mild to moderate ulcerative colitis and maintenance of remission

Cautions   see notes above; also history of asthma
  Blood disorders See recommendation above

Contra-indications   see notes above

Hepatic impairment   avoid in severe impairment

Renal impairment   manufacturer advises avoid in moderate to severe impairment

Pregnancy   manufacturer advises avoid

Breast-feeding   monitor infant for diarrhoea

Side-effects   see notes above; also cholelithiasis

Dose
- Acute attack, 2.25 g 3 times daily until remission occurs or for up to max. 12 weeks
- Maintenance, 1.5 g twice daily, adjusted according to response (max. 6 g daily)
- CHILD under 18 years see *BNF for Children*

Colazide® (Almirall) [PoM]
Capsules, beige, balsalazide sodium 750 mg. Net price 130-cap pack = £30.42. Label: 21, 25, counsel-ling, blood disorder symptoms (see recommendation above)

MESALAZINE

Indications   treatment of mild to moderate ulcerative colitis and maintenance of remission; see also under preparations

Cautions   see notes above; elderly
  Blood disorders See recommendation above

Contra-indications   see notes above

Hepatic impairment   avoid in severe impairment

Renal impairment   use with caution; avoid if eGFR less than 20 mL/minute/1.73 m^2

Pregnancy   negligible quantities cross placenta

Breast-feeding   diarrhoea reported but negligible amounts detected in breast milk; monitor infant for diarrhoea

Side-effects   see notes above

Dose
- See under preparations, below
  Note There is no evidence to show that any one oral preparation of mesalazine is more effective than another; however, the delivery characteristics of oral mesalazine preparations may vary. If it is necessary to switch a patient to a different brand of mesalazine, the patient should be advised to report any changes in symptoms

Asacol® (Warner Chilcott) [PoM]
Foam enema, mesalazine 1 g/metered application, net price 14-application canister with disposable applicators and plastic bags = £26.72. Counselling, blood disorder symptoms (see recommendation above)
  Excipients include disodium edetate, hydroxybenzoates (parabens), polysorbate 20, sodium metabisulfite
  Dose acute attack affecting the rectosigmoid region, 1 metered application (mesalazine 1 g) into the rectum daily for 4–6 weeks; acute attack affecting the descending colon, 2 metered applications (mesalazine 2 g) once daily for 4–6 weeks; CHILD 12–18 years, see *BNF for Children*
Suppositories, mesalazine 250 mg, net price 20-sup-pos pack = £4.82; 500 mg, 10-suppos pack = £4.82. Counselling, blood disorder symptoms (see recom-mendation above)
  Dose acute attack or maintenance, by rectum 0.75–1.5 g daily in divided doses, with last dose at bedtime; CHILD 12–18 years, see *BNF for Children*

Asacol® MR (Warner Chilcott) [PoM]
Tablets, red, e/c, mesalazine 400 mg, net price 90-tab pack = £29.41, 120-tab pack = £39.21. Label: 5, 25, counselling, blood disorder symptoms (see recommendation above)
  Dose ulcerative colitis, acute attack, 2.4 g daily in divided doses; maintenance of remission of ulcerative colitis and Crohn's ileo-colitis, 1.2–2.4 g daily in divided doses; CHILD 12–18 years, see *BNF for Children*

Tablets, red-brown, e/c, mesalazine 800 mg, net price 180-tab pack = £117.62. Label: 5, 25, counsel-ling, blood disorder symptoms (see recommendation above)
  Dose ADULT over 18 years, ulcerative colitis, acute attack, 2.4–4.8 g daily in divided doses; maintenance of remission of ulcerative colitis, up to 2.4 g once daily or in divided doses; maintenance of remission of Crohn's ileo-colitis, up to 2.4 g daily in divided doses
  Note Preparations that lower stool pH (e.g. lactulose) may prevent release of mesalazine

1   Gastro-intestinal system

1 Gastro-intestinal system

Ipocol® (Sandoz) [PoM]

Tablets, e/c, mesalazine 400 mg, net price 120-tab pack = £17.68. Label: 5, 25, counselling, blood disorder symptoms (see recommendation above)

Dose acute attack, 2.4 g daily in divided doses; maintenance, 1.2–2.4 g daily in divided doses; CHILD 6–18 years, see *BNF for Children*

Note Preparations that lower stool pH (e.g. lactulose) may prevent release of mesalazine

Mezavant® XL (Shire) [PoM]

Tablets, m/r, red-brown, e/c, mesalazine 1.2 g, net price 60-tab pack = £62.44. Label: 21, 25, counselling, blood disorder symptoms (see recommendations above)

Dose ADULT over 18 years, acute attack, 2.4 g once daily, increase if necessary to 4.8 g once daily (review treatment at 8 weeks); maintenance, 2.4 g once daily

Octasa® (Tillotts) [PoM]

Tablets, m/r, red-brown, e/c, mesalazine 400 mg, net price 90-tab pack = £19.50, 120-tab pack = £26.00; 800 mg, 90-tab pack = £47.50, 180-tab pack = £95.00. Label: 25, counselling, blood disorder symptoms (see recommendations above)

Dose ulcerative colitis, acute attack, 2.4–4.8 g once daily or in divided doses (dose over 2.4 g daily in divided doses only); maintenance of remission of ulcerative colitis and Crohn's ileo-colitis, 1.2–2.4 g once daily or in divided doses; CHILD 6–18 years, see *BNF for Children*

Pentasa® (Ferring) [PoM]

Tablets, m/r, mesalazine 500 mg (grey, scored), net price 100-tab pack = £30.74; 1 g, 60-tab pack = £36.89. Counselling, administration, see dose, blood disorder symptoms (see recommendation above)

Dose acute attack, up to 4 g once daily or in 2–3 divided doses; maintenance, 2 g once daily; tablets may be dispersed in water, but should not be crushed or chewed; CHILD 5–18 years see *BNF for Children*

Granules, m/r, pale grey-brown, mesalazine 1 g/sachet, net price 50-sachet pack = £30.74; 2 g/sachet, 60-sachet pack = £73.78. Counselling, administration, see dose, blood disorder symptoms (see recommendation above)

Dose acute attack, up to 4 g once daily or in 2–4 divided doses; maintenance, 2 g once daily; granules should be placed on tongue and washed down with water or orange juice without chewing; CHILD 5–18 years see *BNF for Children*

Retention enema, mesalazine 1 g in 100-mL pack. Net price 7 enemas = £17.73. Counselling, blood disorder symptoms (see recommendation above)

Dose by rectum ADULT and CHILD over 12 years, 1 enema at bedtime

Suppositories, mesalazine 1 g. Net price 28-suppos pack = £40.01. Counselling, blood disorder symptoms (see recommendation above)

Dose by rectum ulcerative proctitis, ADULT and CHILD over 15 years, acute attack, 1 g daily for 2–4 weeks; maintenance, 1 g daily; CHILD 12–15 years see *BNF for Children*

Salofalk® (Dr Falk) [PoM]

Tablets, e/c, yellow, mesalazine 250 mg, net price 100-tab pack = £16.19; 500 mg, 100-tab pack = £32.38. Label: 5, 25, counselling, blood disorder symptoms (see recommendation above)

Dose acute attack, 0.5–1 g 3 times daily; maintenance, 500 mg three times daily; CHILD 5–18 years see *BNF for Children*

Granules, m/r, grey, e/c, vanilla-flavoured, mesalazine 500 mg/sachet, net price 100-sachet pack = £28.74; 1 g/sachet, 50-sachet pack = £28.74; 1.5 g/sachet, 60-sachet pack = £48.85; 3 g/sachet, 60-sachet pack = £97.70. Label: 25, counselling, admin-

istration, see dose, blood disorder symptoms (see recommendation above)

Excipients include aspartame (section 9.4.1)

Dose acute attack, 1.5–3 g once daily (preferably in the morning) or 0.5–1 g 3 times daily; maintenance, 500 mg 3 times daily; CHILD 5–18 years see *BNF for Children*

Counselling granules should be placed on tongue and washed down with water without chewing

Note Preparations that lower stool pH (e.g. lactulose) may prevent release of mesalazine

Suppositories, mesalazine 500 mg. Net price 30-suppos pack = £14.81. Counselling, blood disorder symptoms (see recommendation above)

Dose ADULT and CHILD over 15 years, acute attack, by rectum, 0.5–1 g 2–3 times daily adjusted according to response; CHILD 12–15 years see *BNF for Children*

Enema, mesalazine 2 g in 59-mL pack. Net price 7 enemas = £29.92. Counselling, blood disorder symptoms (see recommendation above)

Dose acute attack or maintenance, by rectum, 2 g daily at bedtime; CHILD 12–18 years see *BNF for Children*

Rectal foam, mesalazine 1 g/metered application, net price 14-application canister with disposable applicators and plastic bags = £30.17. Counselling, blood disorder symptoms (see recommendation above)

Excipients include cetostearyl alcohol, disodium edetate, polysorbate 60, propylene glycol, sodium metabisulfite

Dose mild ulcerative colitis affecting sigmoid colon and rectum, ADULT and CHILD over 12 years, 2 metered applications (mesalazine 2 g) into the rectum at bedtime or in 2 divided doses

---

OLSALAZINE SODIUM

Indications treatment of mild ulcerative colitis and maintenance of remission

Cautions see notes above

  Blood disorders See recommendation above

Contra-indications see notes above

Renal impairment use with caution; manufacturer advises avoid in significant impairment

Pregnancy manufacturer advises avoid unless potential benefit outweighs risk

Breast-feeding monitor infant for diarrhoea

Side-effects see notes above; watery diarrhoea common; also reported, tachycardia, palpitation, pyrexia, blurred vision, and photosensitivity

Dose

- ADULT and CHILD over 12 years, acute attack, 1 g daily in divided doses after meals increased if necessary over 1 week to max. 3 g daily (max. single dose 1 g); maintenance, 500 mg twice daily after meals
- CHILD under 12 years see *BNF for Children*

Dipentum® (UCB Pharma) [PoM]

Capsules, brown, olsalazine sodium 250 mg. Net price 112-cap pack = £19.77. Label: 21, counselling, blood disorder symptoms (see recommendation above)

Tablets, yellow, scored, olsalazine sodium 500 mg. Net price 60-tab pack = £21.18. Label: 21, counselling, blood disorder symptoms (see recommendation above)

SULFASALAZINE

(Sulphasalazine)

Indications treatment of mild to moderate and severe ulcerative colitis and maintenance of remission; active Crohn's disease; rheumatoid arthritis (section 10.1.3)

Cautions see notes above; also history of allergy or asthma; G6PD deficiency (section 9.1.5); slow acetylator status; risk of haematological and hepatic toxicity (differential white cell, red cell, and platelet counts initially and at monthly intervals for first 3 months; liver function tests at monthly intervals for first 3 months); maintain adequate fluid intake; upper gastro-intestinal side-effects common over 4 g daily; acute porphyria (section 9.8.2); **interactions:** Appendix 1 (sulfasalazine)

Blood disorders See recommendation above

Contra-indications see notes above; also sulfonamide hypersensitivity; child under 2 years of age

Hepatic impairment use with caution

Renal impairment risk of toxicity, including crystalluria, in moderate impairment—ensure high fluid intake; avoid in severe impairment

Pregnancy theoretical risk of neonatal haemolysis in third trimester; adequate folate supplements should be given to mother

Breast-feeding small amounts in milk (1 report of bloody diarrhoea); theoretical risk of neonatal haemolysis especially in G6PD-deficient infants

Side-effects see notes above; also cough, insomnia, dizziness, fever, blood disorders (including Heinz body anaemia, megaloblastic anaemia), proteinuria, tinnitus, stomatitis, taste disturbances, and pruritus; *less commonly* dyspnoea, depression, convulsions, vasculitis, and alopecia; also reported loss of appetite, hypersensitivity reactions (including exfoliative dermatitis, epidermal necrolysis, photosensitivity, anaphylaxis, serum sickness), ataxia, hallucinations, aseptic meningitis, oligospermia, crystalluria, disturbances of smell, and parotitis; yellow-orange discoloration of skin, urine, and other body fluids; some soft contact lenses may be stained

Dose
- By mouth, acute attack 1–2 g 4 times daily (but see **cautions**) until remission occurs (if necessary corticosteroids may also be given), reducing to a maintenance dose of 500 mg 4 times daily; CHILD 2–12 years see *BNF for Children*
- By rectum, in suppositories, alone or in conjunction with oral treatment 0.5–1 g morning and night after a bowel movement; CHILD 5–12 years see *BNF for Children*

Sulfasalazine (Non-proprietary) PoM
Tablets, sulfasalazine 500 mg, net price 112 = £5.93. Label: 14, counselling, blood disorder symptoms (see recommendation above), contact lenses may be stained

Tablets, e/c, sulfasalazine 500 mg. Net price 112-tab pack = £12.64. Label: 5, 14, 25, counselling, blood disorder symptoms (see recommendation above), contact lenses may be stained

Brands include *Sulazine EC*

Suspension, sulfasalazine 250 mg/5 mL, net price 500 mL = £39.75. Label: 14, counselling, blood disorder symptoms (see recommendation above), contact lenses may be stained

Excipients may include alcohol

Note Sugar-free versions are available and can be ordered by specifying 'sugar-free' on the prescription

Salazopyrin (Pharmacia) PoM
Tablets, yellow, scored, sulfasalazine 500 mg, net price 112-tab pack = £6.97. Label: 14, counselling, blood disorder symptoms (see recommendation above), contact lenses may be stained

EN-Tabs® (= tablets e/c), yellow, f/c, sulfasalazine 500 mg, net price 112-tab pack = £8.43. Label: 5, 14, 25, counselling, blood disorder symptoms (see recommendation above), contact lenses may be stained

Suppositories, yellow, sulfasalazine 500 mg, net price 10-suppos pack = £3.30. Label: 14, counselling, blood disorder symptoms (see recommendation above), contact lenses may be stained

1.5.2 Corticosteroids

For the role of corticosteroids in acute ulcerative colitis and Crohn's disease, see Inflammatory Bowel Disease, p. 61.

BECLOMETASONE DIPROPIONATE

Indications adjunct to aminosalicylates in acute mild to moderate ulcerative colitis; asthma (section 3.2); allergic and vasomotor rhinitis (section 12.2.1); oral ulceration [unlicensed indication] (section 12.3.1)

Cautions section 6.3.2; **interactions:** Appendix 1 (corticosteroids)

Contra-indications section 6.3.2

Hepatic impairment manufacturer advises avoid in severe impairment—no information available

Pregnancy section 6.3.2

Breast-feeding section 6.3.2

Side-effects section 6.3.2; also nausea, constipation, headache, and drowsiness

Dose
- 5 mg in the morning; max. duration of treatment 4 weeks; CHILD safety and efficacy not established

Clipper® (Chiesi) PoM
Tablets, m/r, ivory, beclometasone dipropionate 5 mg, net price 30-tab pack = £56.56. Label: 25

BUDESONIDE

Indications see preparations

Cautions section 6.3.2; for autoimmune hepatitis, monitor liver function tests every 2 weeks for 1 month, then at least every 3 months; **interactions:** Appendix 1 (corticosteroids)

Contra-indications section 6.3.2

Hepatic impairment section 6.3.2

Pregnancy section 6.3.2

Breast-feeding section 6.3.2

Side-effects section 6.3.2

Dose
- See preparations

Budenofalk® (Dr Falk) PoM
Capsules, pink, enclosing e/c granules, budesonide 3 mg, net price 100-cap pack = £75.05. Label: 5, 10, steroid card, 22, 25

Dose mild to moderate Crohn's disease affecting the ileum or ascending colon, chronic diarrhoea due to collagenous colitis, ADULT over 18 years, 3 mg 3 times daily for up to 8 weeks; reduce dose for the last 2 weeks of treatment (see also section 6.3.2); CHILD 12–18 years see *BNF for Children*

Autoimmune hepatitis, ADULT over 18 years, induction of remission, 3 mg 3 times daily; maintenance, 3 mg twice daily

1 Gastro-intestinal system

Granules, e/c, budesonide 9 mg/sachet, net price 60-sachet pack (lemon-flavoured) = £135.00. Label: 5, 10, steroid card, 22, 25, counselling, administration

Dose mild to moderate Crohn's disease affecting the ileum or ascending colon, collagenous colitis, ADULT over 18 years, 9 mg in the morning for up to 8 weeks; reduce dose for the last 2 weeks of treatment (see also section 6.3.2)

Counselling Granules should be placed on tongue and washed down with water without chewing

Rectal foam, budesonide 2 mg/metered application, net price 14-application canister with disposable applicators and plastic bags = £57.11

Excipients include cetyl alcohol, disodium edetate, propylene glycol, sorbic acid

Dose ulcerative colitis affecting sigmoid colon and rectum, by rectum, ADULT over 18 years, 1 metered application (budesonide 2 mg) once daily for up to 8 weeks

Entocort® (AstraZeneca) [PoM]

CR Capsules, grey/pink, enclosing e/c, m/r granules, budesonide 3 mg, net price 100-cap pack = £99.00. Label: 5, 10, steroid card, 25

Note Dispense in original container (contains desiccant)

Dose mild to moderate Crohn's disease affecting the ileum or ascending colon, 9 mg once daily in the morning for up to 8 weeks; reduce dose for the last 2–4 weeks of treatment (see also section 6.3.2); CHILD 12–18 years see *BNF for Children*

Enema, budesonide 2 mg/100 mL when dispersible tablet reconstituted in isotonic saline vehicle, net price pack of 7 dispersible tablets and bottles of vehicle = £39.60

Dose ulcerative colitis involving rectal and recto-sigmoid disease, by rectum, 1 enema at bedtime for 4 weeks; CHILD 12–18 years see *BNF for Children*

▌ HYDROCORTISONE

Indications ulcerative colitis, proctitis, proctosigmoiditis

Cautions section 6.3.2; systemic absorption may occur; prolonged use should be avoided

Contra-indications intestinal obstruction, bowel perforation, recent intestinal anastomoses, extensive fistulas; untreated infection

Side-effects section 6.3.2; also local irritation

Dose
- By rectum see preparations

Colifoam® (Meda) [PoM]

Foam in aerosol pack, hydrocortisone acetate 10%, net price 14-application canister with applicator = £9.33

Excipients include cetyl alcohol, hydroxybenzoates (parabens), propylene glycol

Dose initially 1 metered application (125 mg hydrocortisone acetate) inserted into the rectum once or twice daily for 2–3 weeks, then once on alternate days; CHILD 2–18 years see *BNF for Children*

▌ PREDNISOLONE

Indications ulcerative colitis, and Crohn's disease; other indications, see section 6.3.2, see also preparations

Cautions section 6.3.2; systemic absorption may occur with rectal preparations; prolonged use should be avoided

Contra-indications section 6.3.2; intestinal obstruction, bowel perforation, recent intestinal anastomoses, extensive fistulas; untreated infection

Hepatic impairment section 6.3.2

Renal impairment section 6.3.2

Pregnancy section 6.3.2

Breast-feeding section 6.3.2

Side-effects section 6.3.2

Dose
- By mouth, initially 20–40 mg daily (up to 60 mg daily in some cases), preferably taken in the morning after breakfast; continued until remission occurs, followed by reducing doses
- By rectum, see preparations

▌ Oral preparations

Section 6.3.2

▌ Rectal preparations

Prednisolone (Non-proprietary) [PoM]

Rectal foam in aerosol pack, prednisolone 20 mg (as metasulfobenzoate sodium)/metered application, net price 14-application canister with disposable applicators = £68.00

Dose proctitis and distal ulcerative colitis, 1 metered application (20 mg prednisolone) inserted into the rectum once or twice daily for 2 weeks, continued for further 2 weeks if good response; CHILD 12–18 years see *BNF for Children*

Predsol® (RPH) [PoM]

Retention enema, prednisolone 20 mg (as sodium phosphate) in 100-mL single-dose disposable packs fitted with a nozzle. Net price 7 = £7.50

Dose rectal and rectosigmoidal ulcerative colitis and Crohn's disease, by rectum, initially 20 mg at bedtime for 2–4 weeks, continued if good response; CHILD not recommended

Suppositories, prednisolone 5 mg (as sodium phosphate). Net price 10 = £1.35

Dose ADULT and CHILD proctitis and rectal complications of Crohn's disease, by rectum, 5 mg inserted night and morning after a bowel movement

1.5.3 ▌ Drugs affecting the immune response

For the role of **azathioprine**, **ciclosporin**, **mercaptopurine**, and **methotrexate** in the treatment of inflammatory bowel disease, see p. 61.

Folic acid (section 9.1.2) should be given to reduce the possibility of methotrexate toxicity [unlicensed indication]. Folic acid is usually given at a dose of 5 mg once weekly on a different day to the methotrexate; alternative regimens may be used in some settings.

▌ AZATHIOPRINE

Indications see under Inflammatory Bowel Disease, p. 61; autoimmune conditions and prophylaxis of transplant rejection (section 8.2.1); rheumatoid arthritis (section 10.1.3); severe refractory eczema (section 13.5.3)

Cautions section 8.2.1

Contra-indications section 8.2.1

Hepatic impairment section 8.2.1

Renal impairment section 8.2.1

Pregnancy section 8.2.1

Breast-feeding section 8.2.1

Side-effects section 8.2.1

Dose
- Severe acute Crohn's disease, maintenance of remission of Crohn's disease or ulcerative colitis, ADULT over 18 years, by mouth, 2–2.5 mg/kg daily; some patients may respond to lower doses

▌ Preparations

Section 8.2.1

CICLOSPORIN
(Cyclosporin)

Indications   severe acute ulcerative colitis refractory to corticosteroid treatment [unlicensed indication]; transplantation and graft-versus-host disease, nephrotic syndrome (section 8.2.2); rheumatoid arthritis (section 10.1.3); atopic dermatitis and psoriasis (section 13.5.3)

Cautions   section 8.2.2

Hepatic impairment   section 8.2.2

Renal impairment   section 8.2.2

Pregnancy   see Immunosuppressant therapy, p. 628

Breast-feeding   section 8.2.2

Side-effects   section 8.2.2

Dose

- By continuous intravenous infusion, ADULT over 18 years, 2 mg/kg daily over 24 hours; dose adjusted according to blood-ciclosporin concentration and response

◢**Preparations**
Section 8.2.2

MERCAPTOPURINE
(6-Mercaptopurine)

Indications   see under Inflammatory Bowel disease, p. 61; acute leukaemias and chronic myeloid leukaemia (section 8.1.3)

Cautions   section 8.1.3

Hepatic impairment   section 8.1.3

Renal impairment   section 8.1.3

Pregnancy   section 8.1.3

Breast-feeding   section 8.1.3

Side-effects   section 8.1.3

Dose

- Severe acute Crohn's disease, maintenance of remission of Crohn's disease or ulcerative colitis [unlicensed indications], ADULT over 18 years, by mouth, 1–1.5 mg/kg daily; some patients may respond to lower doses

◢**Preparations**
Section 8.1.3

METHOTREXATE

Indications   see under Inflammatory Bowel Disease, p. 61; malignant disease (section 8.1.3); rheumatoid arthritis (section 10.1.3); psoriasis (section 13.5.3)

Cautions   section 10.1.3

Contra-indications   section 10.1.3

Hepatic impairment   section 10.1.3

Renal impairment   section 10.1.3

Pregnancy   section 10.1.3

Breast-feeding   section 10.1.3

Side-effects   section 10.1.3

Dose

- By intramuscular injection, severe Crohn's disease [unlicensed indication], ADULT over 18 years, induction of remission, 25 mg once weekly; maintenance, 15 mg once weekly
- By mouth, maintenance of remission of severe

Crohn's disease [unlicensed indication], ADULT over 18 years, 10–25 mg once weekly

> **Important**
> Note that the above dose is a **weekly** dose. To avoid error with low-dose methotrexate, it is recommended that:
> - the patient is carefully advised of the **dose and frequency** and the **reason** for taking methotrexate and any other prescribed medicine (e.g. folic acid);
> - only one strength of methotrexate tablet (usually 2.5 mg) is prescribed and dispensed;
> - the prescription and the dispensing label clearly show the dose and frequency of methotrexate administration;
> - the patient is warned to report immediately the onset of any feature of blood disorders (e.g. sore throat, bruising, and mouth ulcers), liver toxicity (e.g. nausea, vomiting, abdominal discomfort, and dark urine), and respiratory effects (e.g. shortness of breath).

◢**Preparations**
Section 10.1.3

Cytokine modulators

Infliximab, **adalimumab**, and **golimumab** are monoclonal antibodies which inhibit the pro-inflammatory cytokine, tumour necrosis factor alpha. They should be used under specialist supervision. Adequate resuscitation facilities must be available when infliximab is used.

ADALIMUMAB

Indications   see under Inflammatory Bowel Disease, p. 61; ankylosing spondylitis, psoriatic arthritis, rheumatoid arthritis, juvenile idiopathic arthritis (section 10.1.3); psoriasis (section 13.5.3)

Cautions   section 10.1.3, p. 737
   Important See section 10.1.3, p. 737 for information on tuberculosis and blood disorders

Contra-indications   section 10.1.3, p. 737

Pregnancy   section 10.1.3, p. 737

Breast-feeding   section 10.1.3, p. 737

Side-effects   section 10.1.3, p. 737

Dose

- By subcutaneous injection, severe active Crohn's disease, ADULT over 18 years, initially 80 mg, then 40 mg 2 weeks after initial dose or accelerated regimen, initially 160 mg (alternatively can be given as divided injections over 2 days), then 80 mg 2 weeks after initial dose; maintenance, 40 mg on alternate weeks, increased if necessary to 40 mg weekly; review treatment if no response within 12 weeks of initial dose; CHILD 6–18 years, see *BNF for Children*

Severe active ulcerative colitis, ADULT over 18 years, initially 160 mg (alternatively can be given as divided injections over 2 days), then 80 mg 2 weeks after initial dose; maintenance, 40 mg on alternate weeks, increased if necessary to 40 mg weekly; review treatment if no response within 8 weeks of initial dose

Note Max. 40 mg administered at a single site

◢**Preparations**
Section 10.1.3

INFLIXIMAB

Indications   see under Inflammatory Bowel Disease, p. 61; ankylosing spondylitis, rheumatoid arthritis (section 10.1.3); psoriasis (section 13.5.3)

1

Gastro-intestinal system

Cautions see section 10.1.3, p. 740; also history of dysplasia or colon carcinoma

Hypersensitivity reactions Risk of delayed hypersensitivity if drug-free interval exceeds 16 weeks

Important See section 10.1.3, p. 740 for information on tuberculosis, blood disorders, and hypersensitivity reactions

Contra-indications see section 10.1.3, p. 740

Pregnancy section 10.1.3, p. 740

Breast-feeding section 10.1.3, p. 740

Side-effects see section 10.1.3, p. 740; also hepatosplenic T-cell lymphoma

Dose

- By intravenous infusion, severe active Crohn's disease, ADULT over 18 years, initially 5 mg/kg, then 5 mg/kg 2 weeks after initial dose; then if the condition has responded, maintenance 5 mg/kg 6 weeks after initial dose, then 5 mg/kg every 8 weeks; CHILD 6–18 years, see *BNF for Children*

Fistulating Crohn's disease, ADULT over 18 years, initially 5 mg/kg, then 5 mg/kg 2 weeks and 6 weeks after initial dose, then if condition has responded, consult product literature for guidance on further doses; CHILD under 18 years, see *BNF for Children*

Severe active ulcerative colitis, ADULT over 18 years, initially 5 mg/kg, then 5 mg/kg 2 weeks and 6 weeks after initial dose, then 5 mg/kg every 8 weeks; discontinue if no response 14 weeks after initial dose; CHILD 6–18 years, see *BNF for Children*

◢**Preparations**
Section 10.1.3

▎GOLIMUMAB

Indications see under Inflammatory Bowel Disease, p. 61; ankylosing spondylitis, psoriatic arthritis, rheumatoid arthritis (section 10.1.3)

Cautions section 10.1.3, p. 740; also risk factors for dysplasia or carcinoma of the colon—screen for dysplasia regularly

Important See section 10.1.3, p. 740 for information on tuberculosis and blood disorders

Contra-indications section 10.1.3, p. 740

Hepatic impairment section 10.1.3, p. 740

Pregnancy section 10.1.3, p. 740

Breast-feeding section 10.1.3, p. 740

Side-effects section 10.1.3, p. 740

Dose

- By subcutaneous injection, ADULT over 18 years, initially 200 mg, then 100 mg 2 weeks after initial dose; maintenance, 50 mg every 4 weeks (100 mg every 4 weeks if body-weight over 80 kg); review treatment if no response after 4 doses

Note For doses requiring multiple injections, each injection should be administered at a different site

Missed dose If dose administered more than 2 weeks late, subsequent doses should be administered on the new monthly due date

◢**Preparations**
Section 10.1.3

Vedolizumab

Vedolizumab is a monoclonal antibody that binds specifically to the $\alpha_4\beta_7$ integrin, which is preferentially expressed on gut homing T helper lymphocytes; it should be used under specialist supervision. Prescribers should be aware of the potential increased risk of opportunistic infections, including progressive multifocal leukoencephalopathy (PML), or infections for which the gut is a defensive barrier.

▎VEDOLIZUMAB

Indications see under Inflammatory Bowel Disease, p. 61

Cautions controlled chronic severe infection; history of recurring severe infection; monitor closely for infection before, during and after treatment—potential increased risk of opportunistic infection (see also Tuberculosis below); monitor for new onset or worsening neurological signs and symptoms (withhold treatment if progressive multifocal leukoencephalopathy (PML) is suspected); patients should be brought up to date with current immunisation schedule (section 14.1) before initiating treatment; previous treatment with rituximab or natalizumab (wait at least 12 weeks between natalizumab use and initiation of vedolizumab unless potential benefit outweighs risk); **interactions:** Appendix 1 (vedolizumab)

Tuberculosis Patients must be screened for tuberculosis before starting treatment; if latent tuberculosis is diagnosed, appropriate treatment must be initiated prior to vedolizumab treatment; if tuberculosis is diagnosed during treatment, discontinue vedolizumab until infection is resolved

Infusion-related reactions Infusion-related and hypersensitivity reactions have been reported. Patients should be observed continuously during each infusion for signs and symptoms of acute hypersensitivity reactions; they should also be observed for 2 hours after the initial two infusions, and for 1 hour after subsequent infusions. Discontinue treatment if a severe infusion-related or other severe reaction occurs and initiate appropriate treatment (e.g. adrenaline and antihistamines); if a mild to moderate infusion-related reaction occurs, interrupt infusion or reduce infusion rate and initiate appropriate treatment (if reaction subsides the infusion may be continued)—consider pretreatment with an antihistamine, hydrocortisone, and/or paracetamol prior to subsequent infusions in patients who experience mild to moderate infusion-related reactions

Alert card Patients should be provided with a patient alert card and a patient information leaflet

Contra-indications severe active infection (see also Cautions)ts

Pregnancy manufacturer advises use only if potential benefit outweighs risk; effective contraception required during and for at least 18 weeks after treatment

Breast-feeding manufacturer advises avoid—present in milk in *animal* studies

Side-effects nausea, dyspepsia, constipation, flatulence, hypertension, oropharyngeal pain, nasal congestion, cough, headache, paraesthesia, malaise, pyrexia, infections (including gastroenteritis, upper respiratory tract infection, pharyngitis), arthralgia, muscle spasms, back pain, muscular weakness, rash, pruritus, eczema, erythema, night sweats, acne; *less commonly* vulvovaginal candidiasis, oral candidiasis, folliculitis, infusion-related reactions (see Cautions); *also reported* dizziness, tuberculosis, salmonella sepsis, listeria meningitis

Dose

- By intravenous infusion over 30 minutes, moderate to severe active ulcerative colitis, ADULT over 18 years, initially 300 mg, repeated 2 weeks and 6 weeks after initial dose, then every 8 weeks thereafter (if treatment is interrupted or response decreases, dosing frequency may be increased—consult product literature); review treatment if no response within 10 weeks of initial dose

- By intravenous infusion over 30 minutes, moderate to severe active Crohn's disease, ADULT over 18 years, initially 300 mg, repeated 2 weeks and 6 weeks after initial dose, then every 8 weeks thereafter—if no response is observed, an additional dose of 300 mg may be given 10 weeks after initial dose; if treatment is interrupted or response decreases, dosing frequency may be increased—consult product literature; review treatment if no response within 14 weeks of initial dose

Entyvio® (Takeda) ▼ PoM
Concentrate for intravenous infusion, powder for reconstitution, vedolizumab, net price 300-mg vial = £2050.00. Alert card and patient information leaflet

1.5.4 Food allergy

Allergy with classical symptoms of vomiting, colic and diarrhoea caused by specific foods such as shellfish should be managed by strict avoidance. The condition should be distinguished from symptoms of occasional food intolerance in those with irritable bowel syndrome. **Sodium cromoglicate** may be helpful as an adjunct to dietary avoidance.

SODIUM CROMOGLICATE
(Sodium cromoglycate)

Indications   food allergy (in conjunction with dietary restriction); asthma (section 3.3.1); allergic conjunctivitis (section 11.4.2); allergic rhinitis (section 12.2.1)
Pregnancy   not known to be harmful
Breast-feeding   unlikely to be present in milk
Side-effects   occasional nausea, rashes, and joint pain
Dose
- 200 mg 4 times daily before meals; may be increased if necessary after 2–3 weeks to a max. of 40 mg/kg daily and then reduced according to response; CHILD 2–14 years 100 mg 4 times daily before meals; may be increased if necessary after 2–3 weeks to a max. of 40 mg/kg daily and then reduced according to response
Counselling   Capsules may be swallowed whole or the contents dissolved in hot water and diluted with cold water before taking

Nalcrom® (Sanofi-Aventis) PoM
Capsules, sodium cromoglicate 100 mg. Net price 100-cap pack = £41.14. Label: 22, counselling, see dose above

1.6 Laxatives

Before prescribing laxatives it is important to be sure that the patient *is* constipated and that the constipation is *not* secondary to an underlying undiagnosed complaint.

It is also important for those who complain of constipation to understand that bowel habit can vary considerably in frequency without doing harm. Some people tend to consider themselves constipated if they do not have a bowel movement each day. A useful definition of constipation is the passage of hard stools less frequently than the patient's own normal pattern and this can be explained to the patient.

Misconceptions about bowel habits have led to excessive laxative use. Abuse may lead to hypokalaemia.

Thus, laxatives should generally be **avoided** except where straining will exacerbate a condition (such as angina) or increase the risk of rectal bleeding as in haemorrhoids. Laxatives are also of value in *drug-induced constipation*, for the expulsion of *parasites* after anthelmintic treatment, and to clear the alimentary tract before *surgery and radiological procedures*. Prolonged treatment of constipation is sometimes necessary.

For the role of laxatives in the treatment of irritable bowel syndrome, see p. 62. For the prevention of opioid-induced constipation in palliative care, see p. 22.

Children   Laxatives should be prescribed by a healthcare professional experienced in the management of constipation in children. Delays of greater than 3 days between stools may increase the likelihood of pain on passing hard stools leading to anal fissure, anal spasm and eventually to a learned response to avoid defaecation.

In *infants*, increased intake of fluids, particularly fruit juice containing sorbitol (e.g. prune, pear, or apple), may be sufficient to soften the stool. In infants under 1 year of age with mild constipation, **lactulose** (section 1.6.4) can be used to soften the stool; either an oral preparation containing **macrogols** or, rarely, **glycerol** suppositories can be used to clear faecal impaction. The infant should be referred to a hospital paediatric specialist if these measures fail.

The diet of *children over 1 year of age* should be reviewed to ensure that it includes an adequate intake of fibre and fluid. An osmotic laxative containing **macrogols** (section 1.6.4) can also be used, particularly in children with chronic constipation; **lactulose** is an alternative in children who cannot tolerate a macrogol. If there is an inadequate response to the osmotic laxative, a **stimulant laxative** (section 1.6.2) can be added.

Treatment of faecal impaction may initially increase symptoms of soiling and abdominal pain. In children over 1 year of age with faecal impaction, an oral preparation containing **macrogols** (section 1.6.4) is used to clear faecal mass and to establish and maintain soft well-formed stools. If disimpaction does not occur after 2 weeks, a **stimulant laxative** (section 1.6.2) can be added. If the impacted mass is not expelled following treatment with macrogols and a stimulant laxative, a **sodium citrate** enema can be administered. Although rectal administration of laxatives may be effective, this route is frequently distressing for the child and may lead to persistence of withholding. A **phosphate enema** may be administered under specialist supervision if disimpaction does not occur after a sodium citrate enema; a **bowel cleansing preparation** (section 1.6.5) is an alternative. Manual evacuation under anaesthetic may be necessary if disimpaction does not occur after oral and rectal treatment, or if the child is afraid.

Long-term regular use of laxatives is essential to maintain well-formed stools and prevent recurrence of faecal impaction; intermittent use may provoke relapses. In children with chronic constipation, laxatives should be continued for several weeks after a regular pattern of bowel movements or toilet training is established. The dose of laxatives should then be tapered gradually, over a period of months, according to response. Some children may require laxative therapy for several years.

> For children with chronic constipation, it may be necessary to exceed the licensed doses of some laxatives. Parents and carers of children should be advised to adjust the dose of laxative in order to establish a regular pattern of bowel movements in which stools are soft, well-formed, and passed without discomfort.
>
> Laxatives should be administered at a time that produces an effect that is likely to fit in with the child's toilet routine.

Pregnancy If dietary and lifestyle changes fail to control constipation in pregnancy, moderate doses of poorly absorbed laxatives may be used. A bulk-forming laxative should be tried first. An osmotic laxative, such as lactulose, can also be used. Bisacodyl or senna may be suitable, if a stimulant effect is necessary.

> The laxatives that follow have been divided into 5 main groups (sections 1.6.1–1.6.5). This simple classification disguises the fact that some laxatives have a complex action.

1.6.1 Bulk-forming laxatives

Bulk-forming laxatives relieve constipation by increasing faecal mass which stimulates peristalsis; patients should be advised that the full effect may take some days to develop.

Bulk-forming laxatives are of particular value in those with small hard stools, but should not be required unless fibre cannot be increased in the diet. A balanced diet, including adequate fluid intake and fibre is of value in preventing constipation.

Bulk-forming laxatives can be used in the management of patients with *colostomy, ileostomy, haemorrhoids, anal fissure, chronic diarrhoea associated with diverticular disease, irritable bowel syndrome*, and as adjuncts in *ulcerative colitis* (section 1.5). Adequate fluid intake must be maintained to avoid intestinal obstruction. Unprocessed wheat **bran**, taken with food or fruit juice, is a most effective bulk-forming preparation. Finely ground bran, though more palatable, has poorer water-retaining properties, but can be taken as bran bread or biscuits in appropriately increased quantities. Oat bran is also used.

Methylcellulose, **ispaghula**, and **sterculia** are useful in patients who cannot tolerate bran. Methylcellulose also acts as a faecal softener.

ISPAGHULA HUSK

Indications see notes above

Cautions adequate fluid intake should be maintained to avoid intestinal obstruction—it may be necessary to supervise elderly or debilitated patients or those with intestinal narrowing or decreased motility

Contra-indications difficulty in swallowing, intestinal obstruction, colonic atony, faecal impaction

Side-effects flatulence, abdominal distension, gastro-intestinal obstruction or impaction; hypersensitivity reported

Dose

● See preparations below

   Counselling Preparations that swell in contact with liquid should always be carefully swallowed with water and should not be taken immediately before going to bed

Fybogel® (Reckitt Benckiser)
   Granules, buff, effervescent, sugar- and gluten-free, ispaghula husk 3.5 g/sachet (low Na$^+$), net price 30 sachets (plain, lemon, or orange flavour) = £2.20. Label: 13, counselling, see above
   Excipients include aspartame 16 mg/sachet (see section 9.4.1)
   Dose 1 sachet or 2 level 5-mL spoonfuls in water twice daily preferably after meals; CHILD (but see section 1.6) 6–12 years ½–1 level 5-mL spoonful in water twice daily, preferably after meals

Ispagel Orange® (LPC)
   Granules, beige, effervescent, sugar- and gluten-free, ispaghula husk 3.5 g/sachet, net price 30 sachets = £1.69. Label: 13, counselling, see above
   Excipients include aspartame (see section 9.4.1)
   Dose 1 sachet in water 1–3 times daily, preferably after meals; CHILD (but see section 1.6) 6–12 years see *BNF for Children*

Regulan® (Procter & Gamble)
   Powder, beige, sugar- and gluten-free, ispaghula husk 3.4 g/5.85-g sachet (orange or lemon/lime flavour). Net price 30 sachets = £2.44. Label: 13, counselling, see above
   Excipients include aspartame (see section 9.4.1)
   Dose 1 sachet in 150 mL water 1–3 times daily, preferably after meals; CHILD (but see section 1.6) 6–12 years ½–1 level 5-mL spoonful in water 1–3 times daily, preferably after meals

METHYLCELLULOSE

Indications see notes above

Cautions see under Ispaghula Husk

Contra-indications see under Ispaghula Husk; also infective bowel disease

Side-effects see under Ispaghula Husk

Dose

● See preparations below

   Counselling Preparations that swell in contact with liquid should always be carefully swallowed with water and should not be taken immediately before going to bed

Celevac® (AMCo)
   Tablets, pink, scored, methylcellulose '450' 500 mg, net price 112-tab pack = £3.22. Counselling, see above and dose
   Dose constipation and diarrhoea, 3–6 tablets twice daily; in constipation the dose should be taken with at least 300 mL liquid; in diarrhoea, ileostomy, and colostomy control, avoid liquid intake for 30 minutes before and after dose; CHILD 7–12 years see *BNF for Children*

STERCULIA

Indications see notes above

Cautions see under Ispaghula Husk

Contra-indications see under Ispaghula Husk

Pregnancy manufacturer of *Normacol Plus*® advises avoid

Breast-feeding manufacturer of *Normacol Plus*® advises avoid

Side-effects   see under Ispaghula Husk

Dose

- See under preparations below

   Counselling Preparations that swell in contact with liquid should always be carefully swallowed with water and should not be taken immediately before going to bed

Normacol® (Norgine)

Granules, coated, gluten-free, sterculia 62%. Net price 500 g = £6.85; 60 × 7-g sachets = £5.77. Label: 25, 27, counselling, see above

Dose 1–2 heaped 5-mL spoonfuls, or the contents of 1–2 sachets, washed down without chewing with plenty of liquid once or twice daily after meals; CHILD (but see section 1.6) 6–12 years half adult dose

Normacol Plus® (Norgine)

Granules, brown, coated, gluten-free, sterculia 62%, frangula (standardised) 8%. Net price 500 g = £7.32; 60 × 7 g sachets = £6.16. Label: 25, 27, counselling, see above

Dose constipation and after haemorrhoidectomy, 1–2 heaped 5-mL spoonfuls or the contents of 1–2 sachets washed down without chewing with plenty of liquid once or twice daily after meals; CHILD 6–12 years see *BNF for Children*

1.6.2 Stimulant laxatives

Stimulant laxatives include **bisacodyl**, **sodium picosulfate**, and members of the **anthraquinone** group, **senna** and **dantron**. The indications for dantron are limited (see below) by its potential carcinogenicity (based on *rodent* carcinogenicity studies) and evidence of genotoxicity. Powerful stimulants such as **cascara** (an anthraquinone) and **castor oil** are obsolete. **Docusate sodium** probably acts both as a stimulant and as a softening agent.

Stimulant laxatives increase intestinal motility and often cause abdominal cramp; they should be avoided in intestinal obstruction. Excessive use of stimulant laxatives can cause diarrhoea and related effects such as hypokalaemia; however, prolonged use may be justifiable in some circumstances (see section 1.6 for the use of stimulant laxatives in children).

Glycerol suppositories act as a rectal stimulant by virtue of the mildly irritant action of glycerol.

The **parasympathomimetics** bethanechol, neostigmine, and pyridostigmine (see section 7.4.1 and section 10.2.1) enhance parasympathetic activity in the gut and increase intestinal motility. They are rarely used for their gastro-intestinal effects. Organic obstruction of the gut must first be excluded and they should not be used shortly after bowel anastomosis.

◢ BISACODYL

Indications   see under Dose

Cautions   see notes above

Contra-indications   see notes above, acute surgical abdominal conditions, acute inflammatory bowel disease, severe dehydration

Pregnancy   see Pregnancy, p. 70

Side-effects   see notes above; nausea and vomiting; colitis also reported; *suppositories*, local irritation

Dose

- Constipation, by mouth, 5–10 mg at night, increased if necessary to max. 20 mg at night; CHILD (but see

section 1.6) 4–18 years 5–20 mg once daily, adjusted according to response

By rectum in suppositories, 10 mg in the morning; CHILD (but see section 1.6) 2–18 years 5–10 mg once daily, adjusted according to response

- Before radiological procedures and surgery, by mouth, 10 mg in the morning and 10 mg in the evening on the day before procedure, and by rectum in suppositories, 10 mg 1–2 hours before procedure the following day; CHILD 4–18 years see *BNF for Children*

Note tablets act in 10–12 hours; suppositories act in 20–60 minutes

Bisacodyl (Non-proprietary)

Tablets, e/c, bisacodyl 5 mg. Net price 100 = £3.43. Label: 5, 25

Suppositories, bisacodyl 10 mg. Net price 12 = £3.53

Paediatric suppositories, bisacodyl 5 mg. Net price 5 = 99p

Note The brand name *Dulcolax®* ⓈⒽⓈ (Boehringer Ingelheim) is used for bisacodyl tablets, net price 10-tab pack = 74p; suppositories (10 mg), 10 = £1.57; paediatric suppositories (5 mg), 5 = 94p

The brand name *Dulcolax® Pico Liquid* is used for sodium picosulfate elixir

◢ DANTRON

(Danthron)

Indications   only for constipation in terminally ill patients of all ages

Cautions   see notes above; *rodent* studies indicate potential carcinogenic risk; avoid prolonged contact with skin (as in incontinent patients or infants wearing nappies)—risk of irritation and excoriation

Contra-indications   See notes above

Pregnancy   manufacturers of co-danthramer and co-danthrusate advise avoid—no information available

Breast-feeding   manufacturers of co-danthramer and co-danthrusate advise avoid—limited information available

Side-effects   see notes above; urine may be coloured red

Dose

- See under preparations

◢With poloxamer '188' (as co-danthramer)

Note Co-danthramer suspension 5 mL = one co-danthramer capsule, but strong co-danthramer suspension 5 mL = two strong co-danthramer capsules

Co-danthramer (Non-proprietary) ⒫ⓄⓂ

Capsules, co-danthramer 25/200 (dantron 25 mg, poloxamer '188' 200 mg). Net price 60-cap pack = £12.86. Label: 14, (urine red)

Dose 1–2 capsules at bedtime; CHILD 1 capsule at bedtime (restricted indications, see notes above)

Strong capsules, co-danthramer 37.5/500 (dantron 37.5 mg, poloxamer '188' 500 mg). Net price 60-cap pack = £15.55. Label: 14, (urine red)

Dose ADULT and CHILD over 12 years, 1–2 capsules at bedtime (restricted indications, see notes above)

Suspension, co-danthramer 25/200 in 5 mL (dantron 25 mg, poloxamer '188' 200 mg/5 mL). Net price 300 mL = £109.15. Label: 14, (urine red)

Note Sugar-free versions are available and can be ordered by specifying 'sugar-free' on the prescription

Brands include *Danlax®*

Dose 5–10 mL at night; CHILD 2.5–5 mL (restricted indications, see notes above)

Strong suspension, co-danthramer 75/1000 in 5 mL (dantron 75 mg, poloxamer '188' 1 g/5 mL). Net price 300 mL = £266.08. Label: 14, (urine red)

Note Sugar-free versions are available and can be ordered by specifying 'sugar-free' on the prescription

Dose ADULT and CHILD over 12 years, 5 mL at night (restricted indications, see notes above)

◀ **With docusate sodium (as co-danthrusate)**

Co-danthrusate (Non-proprietary) PoM

Capsules, co-danthrusate 50/60 (dantron 50 mg, docusate sodium 60 mg). Net price 63-cap pack = £42.50. Label: 14, (urine red)

Brands include *Normax*® JHS

Dose 1–3 capsules at night; CHILD 6–12 years 1 capsule at night (restricted indications, see notes above)

Suspension, yellow, co-danthrusate 50/60 (dantron 50 mg, docusate sodium 60 mg/5 mL). Net price 200 mL = £89.92. Label: 14, (urine red)

Brands include *Normax*®

Dose 5–15 mL at night; CHILD 6–12 years 5 mL at night (restricted indications, see notes above)

■ DOCUSATE SODIUM
(Dioctyl sodium sulphosuccinate)

Indications constipation, adjunct in abdominal radiological procedures

Cautions see notes above; do not give with liquid paraffin; rectal preparations not indicated if haemorrhoids or anal fissure

Contra-indications see notes above

Pregnancy not known to be harmful—manufacturer advises caution

Breast-feeding present in milk following oral administration—manufacturer advises caution; rectal administration not known to be harmful

Side-effects see notes above; also rash

Dose

• By mouth, chronic constipation, up to 500 mg daily in divided doses; CHILD (but see section 1.6) 6 months–2 years 12.5 mg 3 times daily, adjusted according to response (use paediatric solution); 2–12 years 12.5–25 mg 3 times daily, adjusted according to response (use paediatric oral solution)

Note Oral preparations act within 1–2 days

With barium meal, ADULT and CHILD over 12 years, 400 mg

Dioctyl® (UCB Pharma)

Capsules, yellow/white, docusate sodium 100 mg, net price 30-cap pack = £2.09, 100-cap pack = £6.98

Docusol® (Typharm)

Adult oral solution, sugar-free, docusate sodium 50 mg/5 mL, net price 300 mL = £5.49

Paediatric oral solution, sugar-free, docusate sodium 12.5 mg/5 mL, net price 300 mL = £5.29

◀ **Rectal preparations**

Norgalax Micro-enema® (Norgine)

Enema, docusate sodium 120 mg in 10-g single-dose disposable packs. Net price 10-g unit = 66p

Dose ADULT and CHILD (but see section 1.6) over 12 years, 10-g unit

■ GLYCEROL
(Glycerin)

Indications constipation

Dose

• See below

Glycerol Suppositories, BP
(Glycerin Suppositories)

Suppositories, gelatin 140 mg, glycerol 700 mg, purified water to 1 g, net price 12 = 88p (1 g), £1.08 (2 g), £1.72 (4 g)

Dose 1 suppository moistened with water before use, when required. The usual sizes are for INFANT under 1 year, small (1-g mould), CHILD 1–12 years medium (2-g mould), ADULT and CHILD over 12 years, large (4-g mould)

■ SENNA

Indications constipation

Cautions see above

Contra-indications see notes above

Pregnancy see Pregnancy, p. 70

Breast-feeding not known to be harmful

Side-effects see notes above

Dose

• See under preparations

Note Acts in 8–12 hours

Senna (Non-proprietary)

Tablets, total sennosides (calculated as sennoside B) 7.5 mg. Net price 60 = £7.12

Brands include *Senokot*® JHS

Dose 2–4 tablets, usually at night; initial dose should be low then gradually increased; CHILD (but see section 1.6) 2–6 years see *BNF for Children*; 6–18 years 1–4 tablets once daily, adjusted according to response

Note Lower dose on packs on sale to the public

Manevac® (HFA Healthcare)

Granules, coated, senna fruit 12.4%, ispaghula 54.2%, net price 400 g = £9.25. Label: 25, counselling, administration

Excipients include sucrose 800 mg per level 5-mL spoonful of granules

Dose ADULT and CHILD over 12 years, 1–2 level 5-mL spoonfuls at night with at least 150 mL water, fruit juice, milk or warm drink

Counselling Preparations that swell in contact with liquid should always be carefully swallowed with water or appropriate fluid and should not be taken immediately before going to bed

Senokot® (Reckitt Benckiser)

Tablets JHS, see above

Syrup, sugar-free, brown, total sennosides (calculated as sennoside B) 7.5 mg/5 mL, net price 500 mL = £2.69

Dose 10–20 mL, usually at bedtime; CHILD (but see section 1.6) 1 month–2 years see *BNF for Children*, 2–4 years 2.5–10 mL once daily, adjusted according to response; 4–18 years 2.5–20 mL once daily, adjusted according to response

Note Lower dose on packs on sale to the public

■ SODIUM PICOSULFATE
(Sodium picosulphate)

Indications constipation; bowel evacuation before abdominal radiological and endoscopic procedures on the colon, and surgery (section 1.6.5); acts within 6–12 hours

Cautions see notes above; active inflammatory bowel disease (avoid if fulminant)

Contra-indications see notes above; severe dehydration

Pregnancy see Pregnancy, p. 70

Breast-feeding not known to be present in milk but manufacturer advises avoid unless potential benefit outweighs risk

Side-effects see notes above; also nausea and vomiting

Dose

- 5–10 mg at night; CHILD (but see section 1.6) 1 month–4 years 2.5–10 mg once daily, adjusted according to response; 4–18 years 2.5–20 mg once daily, adjusted according to response

  Note Sodium picosulfate doses in BNF may differ from those in product literature

Sodium Picosulfate (Non-proprietary)

Elixir, sodium picosulfate 5 mg/5 mL, net price 100 mL = £2.14

Note The brand name *Dulcolax®* Pico Liquid (Boehringer Ingelheim) is used for sodium picosulfate elixir 5 mg/5 mL

◢**Bowel cleansing preparations**
Section 1.6.5

Other stimulant laxatives

Unstandardised preparations of cascara, frangula, rhubarb, and senna should be **avoided** as their laxative action is unpredictable. Aloes, colocynth, and jalap should be **avoided** as they have a drastic purgative action.

1.6.3 Faecal softeners

Liquid paraffin, the traditional lubricant, has disadvantages (see below). Bulk laxatives (section 1.6.1) and non-ionic surfactant 'wetting' agents e.g. docusate sodium (section 1.6.2) also have softening properties. Such drugs are useful for oral administration in the management of haemorrhoids and anal fissure; glycerol (section 1.6.2) is useful for rectal use.

Enemas containing **arachis oil** (ground-nut oil, peanut oil) lubricate and soften impacted faeces and promote a bowel movement.

◢ ARACHIS OIL

Indications see notes above

Dose

- See below

Arachis Oil Enema (Non-proprietary)

Enema, arachis (peanut) oil in 130-mL single-dose disposable packs. Net price 130 mL = £7.98

Dose to soften impacted faeces, 130 mL; the enema should be warmed before use; CHILD (but see section 1.6) under 3 years not recommended; over 3 years reduce adult dose in proportion to body-weight (medical supervision only), see *BNF for Children*

◢ LIQUID PARAFFIN

Indications constipation

Cautions avoid prolonged use; contra-indicated in children under 3 years

Side-effects anal seepage of paraffin and consequent anal irritation after prolonged use, granulomatous reactions caused by absorption of small quantities of liquid paraffin (especially from the emulsion), lipoid pneumonia, and interference with the absorption of fat-soluble vitamins

Dose

- See under preparation

Liquid Paraffin Oral Emulsion, BP

Oral emulsion, liquid paraffin 5 mL, vanillin 5 mg, chloroform 0.025 mL, benzoic acid solution 0.2 mL, methylcellulose-20 200 mg, saccharin sodium 500 micrograms, water to 10 mL

Dose ADULT over 18 years, 10–30 mL at night when required

Counselling Should not be taken immediately before going to bed

1.6.4 Osmotic laxatives

Osmotic laxatives increase the amount of water in the large bowel, either by drawing fluid from the body into the bowel or by retaining the fluid they were administered with.

Lactulose is a semi-synthetic disaccharide which is not absorbed from the gastro-intestinal tract. It produces an osmotic diarrhoea of low faecal pH, and discourages the proliferation of ammonia-producing organisms. It is therefore useful in the treatment of *hepatic encephalopathy*.

Macrogols are inert polymers of ethylene glycol which sequester fluid in the bowel; giving fluid with macrogols may reduce the dehydrating effect sometimes seen with osmotic laxatives.

Saline purgatives such as **magnesium hydroxide** are commonly abused but are satisfactory for occasional use; adequate fluid intake should be maintained. **Magnesium salts** are useful where rapid bowel evacuation is required. **Sodium salts** should be avoided as they may give rise to sodium and water retention in susceptible individuals. **Phosphate enemas** are useful in bowel clearance before radiology, endoscopy, and surgery.

◢ LACTULOSE

Indications constipation (may take up to 48 hours to act), hepatic encephalopathy (portal systemic encephalopathy)

Cautions lactose intolerance; **interactions:** Appendix 1 (lactulose)

Contra-indications galactosaemia, intestinal obstruction

Pregnancy not known to be harmful; see also Pregnancy, p. 70

Side-effects nausea (can be reduced by administration with water, fruit juice or with meals), vomiting, flatulence, cramps, and abdominal discomfort

Dose

- See under preparations below

Lactulose (Non-proprietary)

Solution, lactulose 3.1–3.7 g/5 mL with other ketoses. Net price 300-mL = £1.95, 500-mL = £3.25, 10 × 15 mL sachet pack = £2.50

Brands include *Duphalac®* [JHS], *Lactugal®*, *Laevolac®*

Dose constipation, initially 15 mL twice daily, adjusted according to response; CHILD (but see section 1.6) under 1 year 2.5 mL twice daily, adjusted according to response; 1–5 years 2.5–10 mL twice daily, adjusted according to response; 5–18 years 5–20 mL twice daily, adjusted according to response

Hepatic encephalopathy, 30–50 mL 3 times daily, subsequently adjusted to produce 2–3 soft stools daily; CHILD 12–18 years see *BNF for Children*

Note Lactulose doses in BNF may differ from those in product literature

1 Gastro-intestinal system

Gastro-intestinal system

1

▎ MACROGOLS

(Polyethylene glycols)

Indications   see preparations below

Cautions   discontinue if symptoms of fluid and electrolyte disturbance; see also preparations below; **interactions**: Appendix 1 (macrogols)

Contra-indications   intestinal perforation or obstruction, paralytic ileus, severe inflammatory conditions of the intestinal tract (such as Crohn's disease, ulcerative colitis, and toxic megacolon), see also preparations below

Pregnancy   limited data, but manufacturer advises that it can be used

Breast-feeding   manufacturer advises that it can be used

Side-effects   abdominal distension and pain, nausea, flatulence

Dose
● See preparations below

Macrogol Oral Powder, Compound (Non-proprietary)

Oral powder, macrogol '3350' (polyethylene glycol '3350') 13.125 g, sodium bicarbonate 178.5 mg, sodium chloride 350.7 mg, potassium chloride 46.6 mg/sachet, net price 20-sachet pack = £4.45, 30-sachet pack = £8.87. Label: 13, counselling, administration
Brands include *Laxido® Orange, Molaxole®*

Cautions   patients with cardiovascular impairment should not take more than 2 sachets in any 1 hour

Dose   chronic constipation, ADULT and CHILD over 12 years, 1–3 sachets daily in divided doses usually for up to 2 weeks; maintenance, 1–2 sachets daily

Faecal impaction, ADULT and CHILD over 12 years, 4 sachets on first day, then increased in steps of 2 sachets daily to max. 8 sachets daily; total daily dose to be drunk within a 6 hour period. After disimpaction, switch to maintenance laxative therapy if required

Counselling   Contents of each sachet to be dissolved in half a glass (approx. 125 mL) of water; after reconstitution the solution should be kept in a refrigerator and discarded if unused after 6 hours

Movicol® (Norgine)

Oral powder, macrogol '3350' (polyethylene glycol '3350') 13.125 g, sodium bicarbonate 178.5 mg, sodium chloride 350.7 mg, potassium chloride 46.6 mg/sachet, net price 20-sachet pack (lime and lemon flavour) = £4.45, 30-sachet pack (lime- and lemon- or chocolate- or plain-flavoured) = £6.68, 50-sachet pack (lime- and lemon- or plain-flavoured) = £11.13. Label: 13, counselling, administration
Note   Amount of potassium chloride varies according to flavour of *Movicol®* as follows: plain-flavour (sugar-free) = 50.2 mg/sachet; lime and lemon flavour = 46.6 mg/sachet; chocolate flavour = 31.7 mg/sachet. 1 sachet when reconstituted with 125 mL water provides K^+ 5.4 mmol/litre

Cautions   patients with cardiovascular impairment should not take more than 2 sachets in any 1 hour

Dose   chronic constipation, ADULT and CHILD over 12 years, 1–3 sachets daily in divided doses usually for up to 2 weeks; maintenance, 1–2 sachets daily

Faecal impaction, ADULT and CHILD over 12 years, 4 sachets on first day, then increased in steps of 2 sachets daily to max. 8 sachets daily; total daily dose to be drunk within a 6 hour period. After disimpaction, switch to maintenance laxative therapy if required

Counselling   Contents of each sachet to be dissolved in half a glass (approx. 125 mL) of water; after reconstitution the solution should be kept in a refrigerator and discarded if unused after 6 hours

Oral concentrate, macrogol '3350' (polyethylene glycol '3350') 13.125 g, sodium bicarbonate 178.5 mg, sodium chloride 350.7 mg, potassium chloride 46.6 mg/25 mL, net price 500 mL (orange-flavoured) = £4.45. Label: 13, counselling, administration
Note   25 mL of oral concentrate when diluted with 100 mL water provides K^+ 5.4 mmol/litre

Dose   chronic constipation, ADULT and CHILD over 12 years, 25 mL 1–3 times daily usually for up to 2 weeks; maintenance, 25 mL 1–2 times daily

Counselling   25 mL of oral concentrate to be diluted with half a glass (approx. 100 mL) of water. After dilution the solution should be discarded if unused after 24 hours

Movicol®-Half (Norgine)

Oral powder, sugar-free, macrogol '3350' (polyethylene glycol '3350') 6.563 g, sodium bicarbonate 89.3 mg, sodium chloride 175.4 mg, potassium chloride 23.3 mg/sachet, net price 20-sachet pack (lime and lemon flavour) = £2.92, 30-sachet pack = £4.38. Label: 13, counselling, administration

Cautions   patients with cardiovascular impairment should not take more than 4 sachets in any 1 hour

Dose   chronic constipation, ADULT and CHILD over 12 years, 2–6 sachets daily in divided doses usually for up to 2 weeks; maintenance, 2–4 sachets daily

Faecal impaction, ADULT and CHILD over 12 years, 8 sachets on first day, then increased in steps of 4 sachets daily to max. 16 sachets daily; total daily dose to be drunk within a 6 hour period. After disimpaction, switch to maintenance laxative therapy if required

Counselling   Contents of each sachet to be dissolved in quarter of a glass (approx. 60–65 mL) of water; after reconstitution the solution should be kept in a refrigerator and discarded if unused after 6 hours

Movicol® Paediatric (Norgine) ℞oM

Oral powder, macrogol '3350' (polyethylene glycol '3350') 6.563 g, sodium bicarbonate 89.3 mg, sodium chloride 175.4 mg, potassium chloride 25.1 mg/sachet, net price 30-sachet pack (chocolate- or plain-flavoured) = £4.38. Label: 13, counselling, administration
Note   Amount of potassium chloride varies according to flavour of *Movicol® Paediatric* as follows: chocolate flavour = 15.9 mg/sachet; plain flavour (sugar-free) = 25.1 mg/sachet. 1 sachet when reconstituted with 62.5 mL water provides K^+ 5.4 mmol/litre

Cautions   *with high doses,* impaired gag reflex, reflux oesophagitis, impaired consciousness

Contra-indications   cardiovascular impairment; renal impairment

Dose   chronic constipation and prevention of faecal impaction, CHILD under 2 years see *BNF for Children*; 2–6 years 1 sachet daily, adjusted according to response (max. 4 sachets daily); 6–12 years 2 sachets daily, adjusted according to response (max. 4 sachets daily)

Faecal impaction, CHILD under 5 years see *BNF for Children*; 5–12 years 4 sachets on first day then increased in steps of 2 sachets daily to 12 sachets daily (taken in divided doses over 12 hours each day until impaction resolves). After disimpaction, switch to maintenance laxative therapy

Counselling   Contents of each sachet to be dissolved in quarter of a glass (approx. 60–65 mL) of water; after reconstitution the solution should be kept in a refrigerator and discarded if unused after 24 hours

▎ MAGNESIUM SALTS

Indications   see under preparations below

Cautions   elderly and debilitated; see also notes above; **interactions**: Appendix 1 (antacids)

Contra-indications   acute gastro-intestinal conditions

Hepatic impairment   avoid in hepatic coma if risk of renal failure

Renal impairment   avoid or reduce dose; increased risk of toxicity

Side-effects   colic

Dose

- See preparations

◢ Magnesium hydroxide

Magnesium Hydroxide Mixture, BP

Aqueous suspension containing about 8% hydrated magnesium oxide. Do not store in cold place

Dose constipation, 30–45 mL with water at bedtime when required; CHILD 3–12 years, 5–10 mL with water at bedtime when required

◢ Magnesium hydroxide with liquid paraffin

Liquid Paraffin and Magnesium Hydroxide Oral Emulsion, BP ◢

Oral emulsion, 25% liquid paraffin in aqueous suspension containing 6% hydrated magnesium oxide

Dose constipation, 5–20 mL when required

Note Liquid paraffin and magnesium hydroxide preparations on sale to the public include: *Milpar*® ᴶᴴˢ

◢ Magnesium sulfate

Magnesium Sulfate

Dose rapid bowel evacuation (acts in 2–4 hours) 5–10 g in a glass of water preferably before breakfast

Note Magnesium sulfate is on sale to the public as Epsom Salts

◢ Bowel cleansing preparations

Section 1.6.5

◢ PHOSPHATES (RECTAL)

Indications   rectal use in constipation; bowel evacuation before abdominal radiological procedures, endoscopy, and surgery

Cautions   elderly and debilitated, electrolyte disturbances, congestive heart failure, ascites, uncontrolled hypertension, maintain adequate hydration

Contra-indications   acute gastro-intestinal conditions (including gastro-intestinal obstruction, inflammatory bowel disease, and conditions associated with increased colonic absorption)

Renal impairment   use with caution

Side-effects   local irritation, electrolyte disturbances

Dose

- See under preparations

Fleet® Ready-to-use Enema (Casen-Fleet)

Enema, sodium acid phosphate 21.4 g, sodium phosphate 9.4 g/118 mL, net price 133-mL pack (delivers 118 mL dose) with standard tube = 68p

Dose ADULT and CHILD (but see section 1.6) over 12 years, 118 mL; CHILD 3–12 years, on doctor's advice only (under 3 years not recommended)

Phosphates Enema BP Formula B

Enema, sodium dihydrogen phosphate dihydrate 12.8 g, disodium phosphate dodecahydrate 10.24 g, purified water, freshly boiled and cooled, to 128 mL. Net price 128 mL with standard tube = £2.98, with long rectal tube = £17.93

Dose 128 mL; CHILD (but see section 1.6) over 3 years, reduced according to body weight see *BNF for Children*

◢ SODIUM CITRATE (RECTAL)

Indications   rectal use in constipation

Cautions   elderly and debilitated; see also notes above

Contra-indications   acute gastro-intestinal conditions

Dose

- See under preparations

Micolette Micro-enema® (Pinewood)

Enema, sodium citrate 450 mg, sodium lauryl sulfoacetate 45 mg, glycerol 625 mg, together with potassium sorbate and sorbitol in a viscous solution, in 5-mL single-dose disposable packs with nozzle. Net price 5 mL = 41p

Dose ADULT and CHILD over 3 years, 5–10 mL (but see section 1.6)

Micralax Micro-enema® (RPH)

Enema, sodium citrate 450 mg, sodium alkylsulfoacetate 45 mg, sorbic acid 5 mg, together with glycerol and sorbitol in a viscous solution in 5-mL single-dose disposable packs with nozzle. Net price 5 mL = 41p

Dose ADULT and CHILD over 3 years, 5 mL (but see section 1.6)

Relaxit Micro-enema® (Crawford)

Enema, sodium citrate 450 mg, sodium lauryl sulfate 75 mg, sorbic acid 5 mg, together with glycerol and sorbitol in a viscous solution in 5-mL single-dose disposable packs with nozzle. Net price 5 mL = 43p

Dose ADULT and CHILD (but see section 1.6) 5 mL (insert only half nozzle length in child under 3 years)

1.6.5   Bowel cleansing preparations

Bowel cleansing preparations are used before colonic surgery, colonoscopy, or radiological examination to ensure the bowel is free of solid contents. They are **not** treatments for constipation.

Cautions   Bowel cleansing preparations should be used with caution in patients with fluid and electrolyte disturbances. Renal function should be measured before starting treatment in patients at risk of fluid and electrolyte disturbances. Hypovolaemia should be corrected before administration of bowel cleansing preparations. Adequate hydration should be maintained during treatment. Bowel cleansing preparations should be used with caution in colitis (avoid if acute severe colitis), in children, in the elderly, and in those who are debilitated. They should also be used with caution in patients with an impaired gag reflex or possibility of regurgitation or aspiration.

Other oral drugs should not be taken one hour before or after administration of bowel cleansing preparations because absorption may be impaired. Consider withholding ACE inhibitors, angiotensin-II receptor antagonists, and NSAIDs on the day that bowel cleansing preparations are given and for up to 72 hours after the procedure. Also consider withholding diuretics on the day that bowel cleansing preparations are given. See also Combined Hormonal Contraceptives (section 7.3.1) and Oral Progestogen-only Contraceptives (section 7.3.2.1).

Contra-indications   Bowel cleansing preparations are contra-indicated in patients with gastro-intestinal obstruction or perforation, gastric retention, acute severe colitis, or toxic megacolon.

1

Gastro-intestinal system

Side-effects Side-effects of bowel cleansing preparations include nausea, vomiting, abdominal pain (usually transient—reduced by taking more slowly), and abdominal distension. Less frequent side-effects include headache, dizziness, dehydration, and electrolyte disturbances.

◼ MACROGOLS

Indications   see notes above

Cautions   see notes above; also heart failure; **interactions**: Appendix 1 (macrogols)

Contra-indications   see notes above

Pregnancy   manufacturers advise use only if essential—no information available

Breast-feeding   manufacturers advise use only if essential—no information available

Side-effects   see notes above; also fatigue, sleep disturbances, and anal discomfort

Dose
• See preparations

Klean-Prep® (Norgine)

Oral powder, sugar-free, macrogol '3350' (polyethylene glycol '3350') 59 g, anhydrous sodium sulfate 5.685 g, sodium bicarbonate 1.685 g, sodium chloride 1.465 g, potassium chloride 743 mg/sachet, net price 4 sachets = £9.07. Label: 10, patient information leaflet, 13, counselling

Excipients   include aspartame (section 9.4.1)

Electrolytes   1 sachet when reconstituted with 1 litre of water provides Na$^+$ 125 mmol, K$^+$ 10 mmol, Cl$^-$ 35 mmol, HCO$_3^-$ 20 mmol

Dose   bowel evacuation before surgery, colonoscopy, or radiological examination, 2 litres of reconstituted solution on the evening before procedure and 2 litres of reconstituted solution on the morning of procedure; alternatively, a glass (approx. 250 mL) of reconstituted solution every 10–15 minutes, or by nasogastric tube 20–30 mL/minute, starting on the day before procedure until 4 litres have been consumed. Treatment can be stopped if bowel motions become watery and clear; CHILD 12–18 years see BNF for Children

Counselling   1 sachet should be reconstituted with 1 litre of water. Flavouring such as clear fruit cordials may be added if required. Solid food should not be taken for at least 2 hours before starting treatment. After reconstitution the solution should be kept in a refrigerator and discarded if unused after 24 hours

Moviprep® (Norgine)

Oral powder, lemon- or orange-flavoured, Sachet A (containing macrogol '3350' (polyethylene glycol '3350') 100 g, anhydrous sodium sulphate 7.5 g, sodium chloride 2.691 g, potassium chloride 1.015 g) and Sachet B (containing ascorbic acid 4.7 g, sodium ascorbate 5.9 g), net price 4-sachet pack (2 each of sachet A and B) = £9.87. Label: 10, patient information leaflet, 13, counselling, see below

Excipients   include aspartame (section 9.4.1)

Electrolytes   1 pair of sachets (A+B) when reconstituted with 1 litre of water provides Na$^+$ 181.6 mmol (Na$^+$ 56.2 mmol absorbable), K$^+$ 14.2 mmol, Cl$^-$ 59.8 mmol

Contra-indications   G6PD deficiency

Renal impairment   caution if eGFR less than 30 mL/minute/1.73 m^2

Dose   bowel evacuation for surgery, colonoscopy or radiological examination, ADULT over 18 years, 1 litre of reconstituted solution on the evening before procedure and 1 litre of reconstituted solution early on the morning of procedure; alternatively, 2 litres of reconstituted solution on the evening before procedure; treatment should be completed at least 1 hour before colonoscopy

Counselling   One pair of sachets (A and B) should be reconstituted in 1 litre of water and taken over 1–2 hours.

Solid food should not be taken during treatment until procedure completed. 1 litre of other clear fluid should also be taken during treatment. Treatment can be stopped if bowel motions become watery and clear

◼ MAGNESIUM CITRATE

Reconstitution of a sachet containing 11.57 g magnesium carbonate and 17.79 g anhydrous citric acid produces a solution containing magnesium citrate

Indications   see preparations

Cautions   see notes above

Contra-indications   see notes above

Hepatic impairment   avoid in hepatic coma if risk of renal failure

Renal impairment   avoid if eGFR less than 30 mL/minute/1.73 m^2—risk of hypermagnesaemia

Pregnancy   caution

Breast-feeding   caution

Side-effects   see notes above

Dose
• See preparations

Citramag® (Sanochemia)

Oral powder, sugar-free, effervescent, magnesium carbonate 11.57 g, anhydrous citric acid 17.79 g/sachet, net price 10-sachet pack (lemon and lime flavour) = £18.92. Label: 10, patient information leaflet, 13, counselling, see below

Electrolytes   Mg^{2+} 118 mmol/sachet

Dose   bowel evacuation for surgery, colonoscopy or radiological examination, on day before procedure, 1 sachet at 8 a.m. and 1 sachet between 2 and 4 p.m.; CHILD 5–10 years one-third adult dose; over 10 years and frail ELDERLY one-half adult dose

Counselling   One sachet should be reconstituted with 200 mL of hot water; the solution should be allowed to cool for approx. 30 minutes before drinking. Low residue or fluid only diet (e.g. water, fruit squash, clear soup, black tea or coffee) recommended before procedure (according to prescriber's advice) and copious intake of clear fluids recommended until procedure

◼ PHOSPHATES (ORAL)

Indications   see preparations

Cautions   see notes above; also cardiac disease (avoid in congestive cardiac failure)

Contra-indications   see notes above; also ascites; congestive cardiac failure

Hepatic impairment   use with caution in cirrhosis; avoid in ascites

Renal impairment   avoid if eGFR less than 60 mL/minute/1.73 m^2

Pregnancy   caution

Breast-feeding   caution

Side-effects   see notes above; also chest pain, arrhythmias, asthenia, and renal failure

Dose
• See preparations

OsmoPrep® (TMC)

Tablets, monobasic sodium phosphate monohydrate 1.102 g, disodium phosphate 398 mg, net price 32-tab pack = £8.50. Label: 10, patient information leaflet, counselling, see below

Electrolytes   Na$^+$ 13.6 mmol, Mg^{2+} 0.34 mmol, phosphate 10.8 mmol/tablet

Dose   bowel evacuation before diagnostic procedure, ADULT over 18 years, 4 tablets every 15 minutes until a total of 20 tablets have been consumed on the evening before procedure, then on the next day (starting 3–5 hours before procedure) 4 tablets every 15 minutes until a total of 12 tablets have been consumed; do not repeat course within 7 days

Counselling On the day before procedure, a light, low-fibre breakfast may be consumed in the morning, clear liquid diet recommended after 12 noon. Each dose of 4 tablets to be taken with 250 mL clear liquid. Copious intake of water or other clear liquids recommended during treatment

Fleet Phospho-soda® (Casen-Fleet)

Oral solution, sugar-free, sodium dihydrogen phosphate dihydrate 24.4 g, disodium phosphate dodecahydrate 10.8 g/45 mL. Net price 2 × 45-mL bottles = £4.79. Label: 10, patient information leaflet, counselling

Electrolytes Na⁺ 217 mmol, phosphate 186 mmol/45 mL

Dose bowel evacuation before colonic surgery, colonoscopy or radiological examination, ADULT over 18 years, 45 mL diluted with half a glass (120 mL) of cold water, followed by one full glass (240 mL) of cold water

Timing of doses is dependent on the time of the procedure

For morning procedure, first dose should be taken at 7 a.m. and second at 7 p.m. on day before the procedure

For afternoon procedure, first dose should be taken at 7 p.m. on day before and second dose at 7 a.m. on day of the procedure

Acts within half to 6 hours of first dose

Counselling Intake of solid food should be stopped for at least 6 hours before starting treatment and until procedure completed. Copious intake of water or other clear fluids (e.g. clear soup, strained fruit juice without pulp, black tea or coffee) recommended until midnight before morning procedure and until 8 a.m. before afternoon procedure. At least one glass (approx 240 mL) of water or other clear fluid should also be taken immediately before each dose

---

■ SODIUM PICOSULFATE WITH MAGNESIUM CITRATE

Indications see preparations

Cautions see notes above; also recent gastro-intestinal surgery; cardiac disease (avoid in congestive cardiac failure)

Contra-indications see notes above; also gastro-intestinal ulceration; ascites; congestive cardiac failure

Hepatic impairment avoid in hepatic coma if risk of renal failure

Renal impairment avoid if eGFR less than 30 mL/minute/1.73 m² — risk of hypermagnesaemia

Pregnancy caution

Breast-feeding caution

Side-effects see notes above; also anal discomfort, sleep disturbances, fatigue, and rash

Dose
• See preparations

CitraFleet® (Casen-Fleet)

Oral powder, sodium picosulfate 10 mg/sachet, with magnesium citrate, net price 2-sachet pack (lemon-flavoured) = £3.25. Label: 10, patient information leaflet, 13, counselling, see below

Electrolytes K⁺ 5 mmol, Mg²⁺ 86 mmol/sachet

Dose bowel evacuation on day before radiological examination, endoscopy, or surgery, ADULT over 18 years, 1 sachet before 8 a.m. then 1 sachet 6–8 hours later

Acts within 3 hours of first dose

Counselling One sachet should be reconstituted with 150 mL (approx. half a glass) of cold water; patients should be warned that heat is generated during reconstitution and that the solution should be allowed to cool before drinking. Low residue diet recommended on the day before procedure and copious intake of water or other clear fluids recommended during treatment

Picolax® (Ferring)

Oral powder, sugar-free, sodium picosulfate 10 mg/sachet, with magnesium citrate, net price 20-sachet pack = £33.90. Label: 10, patient information leaflet, 13, counselling, see below

Electrolytes K⁺ 5 mmol, Mg²⁺ 87 mmol/sachet

Dose bowel evacuation on day before radiological procedure, endoscopy, or surgery, ADULT and CHILD over 9 years, 1 sachet before 8 a.m. then 1 sachet 6–8 hours later; CHILD 1–2 years, quarter sachet before 8 a.m. then quarter sachet 6–8 hours later; 2–4 years, half sachet before 8 a.m. then half sachet 6–8 hours later; 4–9 years, 1 sachet before 8 a.m. then half sachet 6–8 hours later

Acts within 3 hours of first dose

Counselling One sachet should be reconstituted with 150 mL (approx. half a glass) of cold water; patients should be warned that heat is generated during reconstitution and that the solution should be allowed to cool before drinking. Low residue diet recommended on the day before procedure and copious intake of water or other clear fluids recommended during treatment

---

▌1.6.6 Peripheral opioid-receptor antagonists

Methylnaltrexone is a peripherally acting opioid-receptor antagonist that is licensed for the treatment of opioid-induced constipation in patients receiving palliative care, when response to other laxatives is inadequate; it should be used as an adjunct to existing laxative therapy. Methylnaltrexone does not alter the central analgesic effect of opioids. For the prevention of opioid-induced constipation in palliative care, see p. 22.

■ METHYLNALTREXONE BROMIDE

Indications opioid-induced constipation in terminally ill patients, when response to other laxatives is inadequate

Cautions diverticular disease; faecal impaction; patients with colostomy or peritoneal catheter

Contra-indications gastro-intestinal obstruction; acute surgical abdominal conditions

Hepatic impairment manufacturer advises avoid in severe hepatic impairment — no information available

Renal impairment if eGFR less than 30 mL/minute/1.73 m², reduce dose as follows: body-weight under 62 kg, 75 micrograms/kg on alternate days; body-weight 62–114 kg, 8 mg on alternate days; body-weight over 114 kg, 75 micrograms/kg on alternate days

Pregnancy toxicity at high doses in *animal* studies — manufacturer advises avoid unless essential

Breast-feeding manufacturer advises use only if potential benefit outweighs risk — present in milk in *animal* studies

Side-effects abdominal pain, nausea, diarrhoea, flatulence; dizziness; injection site reactions, hyperhidrosis; also reported gastro-intestinal perforation

Dose
• By subcutaneous injection, ADULT over 18 years, body-weight under 38 kg, 150 micrograms/kg on alternate days; body-weight 38–62 kg, 8 mg on alternate days; body-weight 62–114 kg, 12 mg on alternate days; body-weight over 114 kg, 150 micrograms/kg on alternate days; may be given less frequently depending on response; 2 consecutive doses may be given 24 hours apart if no response to treatment on the preceding day; rotate sites of injection; max. duration of treatment 4 months

Note May act within 30–60 minutes

Relistor® (Wyeth) (PoM)
Injection, methylnaltrexone bromide 20 mg/mL, net price 0.6-mL vial = £21.05, 7-vial pack (with syringes and needles) = £147.35

1.6.7 Other drugs used in constipation

Linaclotide is a guanylate cyclase-C receptor agonist that is licensed for the treatment of moderate to severe irritable bowel syndrome associated with constipation. It increases intestinal fluid secretion and transit, and decreases visceral pain. It is metabolised within the gastro-intestinal tract and is virtually undetectable in the plasma after therapeutic doses. The *Scottish Medicines Consortium* (p. 4) has advised (May 2013) that linaclotide (*Constella®*) is accepted for restricted use within NHS Scotland for moderate to severe irritable bowel syndrome in patients whose condition has not responded adequately to all other treatments, or who are intolerant of them. For other treatments used in irritable bowel syndrome see section 1.5.

Lubiprostone is a chloride-channel activator that acts in the gut to increase intestinal fluid secretion, which increases motility. It is licensed for the treatment of chronic idiopathic constipation in adults whose condition has not responded adequately to lifestyle changes (including dietary changes). The *Scottish Medicines Consortium* (p. 4) has advised (July 2014) that lubiprostone (*Amitiza®*) is **not** recommended for use within NHS Scotland.

NICE guidance
Lubiprostone for treating chronic idiopathic constipation (July 2014)

Lubiprostone is recommended as an option for treating chronic idiopathic constipation for adults in whom treatment with at least 2 laxatives from different classes, at the highest tolerated recommended doses for at least 6 months, has failed to provide adequate relief and for whom invasive treatment for constipation is being considered. If treatment with lubiprostone is not effective after 2 weeks, the patient should be re-examined and the benefit of continuing treatment reconsidered.

Lubiprostone should only be prescribed by a clinician with experience of treating chronic idiopathic constipation, after careful review of the patient's previous courses of laxative treatments.
www.nice.org.uk/TA318

Prucalopride is a selective serotonin 5HT₄-receptor agonist with prokinetic properties. It is licensed for the treatment of chronic constipation in women, when other laxatives have failed to provide an adequate response. Headache and gastro-intestinal symptoms (including abdominal pain, nausea, and diarrhoea) are the most frequent side-effects. The side-effects generally occur at the start of treatment and are usually transient. The *Scottish Medicines Consortium* (p. 4) has advised (November 2010) that prucalopride (*Resolor®*) is **not** recommended for use within NHS Scotland because weaknesses in the clinical data prevent an assessment of its efficacy in the target population.

NICE guidance
Prucalopride for the treatment of chronic constipation in women (December 2010)

Prucalopride is recommended as an option for the treatment of chronic constipation in women for whom treatment with at least 2 laxatives from different classes, at the highest tolerated recommended doses for at least 6 months, has failed to provide adequate relief and invasive treatment for constipation is being considered. If treatment with prucalopride is not effective after 4 weeks, the patient should be re-examined and the benefit of continuing treatment reconsidered.

Prucalopride should only be prescribed by a clinician with experience of treating chronic constipation, after careful review of the patient's previous courses of laxative treatments.
www.nice.org.uk/TA211

LINACLOTIDE

Indications moderate to severe irritable bowel syndrome with constipation

Cautions predisposition to fluid and electrolyte disturbances

Contra-indications gastro-intestinal obstruction; inflammatory bowel disease

Pregnancy manufacturer advises avoid

Breast-feeding unlikely to be present in milk in significant amounts, but manufacturer advises avoid

Side-effects diarrhoea (if severe or prolonged, consider suspending treatment), flatulence, abdominal pain or distension, dizziness; *less commonly* decreased appetite, hypokalaemia, dehydration, orthostatic hypotension

Dose
• ADULT over 18 years, 290 micrograms once daily; review treatment if no response after 4 weeks

Constella® (Almirall) ▼ (PoM)
Capsules, linaclotide 290 micrograms, net price 28-cap pack = £37.56. Label: 22
Note Dispense in original container (contains desiccant); discard any capsules remaining 18 weeks after opening

LUBIPROSTONE

Indications chronic idiopathic constipation when response to lifestyle changes (including diet) is inadequate

Contra-indications gastro-intestinal obstruction

Hepatic impairment initially 24 micrograms once daily in moderate to severe impairment; if tolerated, and if necessary, increased to 24 micrograms twice daily

Pregnancy manufacturer advises avoid—toxicity in *animal* studies

Breast-feeding manufacturer advises avoid

Side-effects nausea, diarrhoea, abdominal pain, dyspepsia, flatulence, palpitation, oedema, hot flush, dyspnoea, headache, dizziness, hyperhidrosis; *less commonly* vomiting, chest pain, syncope, muscle spasm; also reported tachycardia, influenza-like symptoms, rash

Dose
• ADULT over 18 years, 24 micrograms twice daily for 2 weeks

Amitiza® (Sucampo) [PoM]

Capsules, amber, lubiprostone 24 micrograms, net price 28-cap pack = £29.68, 56-cap pack = £53.48. Label: 21

Note Dispense in original container; discard any capsules remaining 4 weeks after opening

◼ PRUCALOPRIDE

Indications chronic constipation in women when other laxatives fail to provide an adequate response

Cautions history of arrhythmias or ischaemic heart disease; concomitant use with drugs that prolong QT interval; severe, unstable chronic illness

Contra-indications intestinal perforation or obstruction; severe inflammatory conditions of the intestinal tract (such as Crohn's disease, ulcerative colitis, and toxic megacolon)

Hepatic impairment in severe impairment, initially 1 mg once daily, increased if necessary to 2 mg once daily

Renal impairment max. 1 mg daily if eGFR less than 30 mL/minute/1.73 m²

Pregnancy manufacturer advises avoid and recommends effective contraception during treatment

Breast-feeding manufacturer advises avoid—present in milk

Side-effects nausea, vomiting, abdominal pain, dyspepsia, flatulence, diarrhoea, rectal bleeding; headache, dizziness, fatigue; polyuria; *less commonly* anorexia, palpitation, tremor, and fever

Dose

- ADULT over 18 years, 2 mg once daily; ELDERLY over 65 years, initially 1 mg once daily, increased if necessary to 2 mg once daily

Note Review treatment if no response after 4 weeks

Resolor® (Shire) [PoM]

Tablets, f/c, prucalopride (as succinate) 1 mg (white), net price 28-tab pack = £38.69; 2 mg (pink), 28-tab pack = £59.52

1.7   Local preparations for anal and rectal disorders

1.7.1   Soothing haemorrhoidal preparations

1.7.2   Compound haemorrhoidal preparations with corticosteroids

1.7.3   Rectal sclerosants

1.7.4   Management of anal fissures

Anal and perianal pruritus, soreness, and excoriation are best treated by application of bland ointments and suppositories (section 1.7.1). These conditions occur commonly in patients suffering from haemorrhoids, fistulas, and proctitis. Cleansing with attention to any minor faecal soiling, adjustment of the diet to avoid hard stools, the use of bulk-forming materials such as bran (section 1.6.1) and a high residue diet are helpful. In proctitis these measures may supplement treatment with corticosteroids or sulfasalazine (see section 1.5).

When necessary, topical preparations containing **local anaesthetics** (section 1.7.1) or **corticosteroids** (section 1.7.2) are used, provided perianal thrush has been excluded. Perianal thrush is treated with a topical antifungal preparation (section 13.10.2).

For the management of *anal fissures*, see section 1.7.4.

1.7.1   Soothing haemorrhoidal preparations

Soothing preparations containing mild astringents such as bismuth subgallate, zinc oxide, and hamamelis may give symptomatic relief in haemorrhoids. Many proprietary preparations also contain lubricants, vasoconstrictors, or mild antiseptics.

Local anaesthetics are used to relieve pain associated with *haemorrhoids* and *pruritus ani* but good evidence is lacking. Lidocaine ointment (section 15.2) is used before emptying the bowel to relieve pain associated with *anal fissure*. Alternative local anaesthetics include tetracaine, cinchocaine (dibucaine), and pramocaine (pramoxine), but they are more irritant. Local anaesthetic ointments can be absorbed through the rectal mucosa therefore excessive application should be **avoided**, particularly in infants and children. Preparations containing local anaesthetics should be used for short periods only (no longer than a few days) since they may cause sensitisation of the anal skin.

1.7.2   Compound haemorrhoidal preparations with corticosteroids

Corticosteroids are often combined with local anaesthetics and soothing agents in preparations for haemorrhoids. They are suitable for occasional short-term use after exclusion of infections, such as herpes simplex; prolonged use can cause atrophy of the anal skin. See section 13.4 for general comments on topical corticosteroids and section 1.7.1 for comment on local anaesthetics.

Children Haemorrhoids in children are rare. Treatment is usually symptomatic and the use of a locally applied cream is appropriate for short periods; however, local anaesthetics can cause stinging initially and this may aggravate the child's fear of defaecation.

Anugesic-HC® (Pfizer) [PoM]

Cream, benzyl benzoate 1.2%, bismuth oxide 0.875%, hydrocortisone acetate 0.5%, Peru balsam 1.85%, pramocaine hydrochloride 1%, zinc oxide 12.35%. Net price 30 g (with rectal nozzle) = £3.71

Dose apply night and morning and after a bowel movement; do not use for longer than 7 days; CHILD not recommended

Suppositories, buff, benzyl benzoate 33 mg, bismuth oxide 24 mg, bismuth subgallate 59 mg, hydrocortisone acetate 5 mg, Peru balsam 49 mg, pramocaine hydrochloride 27 mg, zinc oxide 296 mg, net price 12 = £2.69

Dose insert 1 suppository night and morning and after a bowel movement; do not use for longer than 7 days; CHILD not recommended

Anusol-HC® (McNeil) [PoM]

Ointment, benzyl benzoate 1.25%, bismuth oxide 0.875%, bismuth subgallate 2.25%, hydrocortisone acetate 0.25%, Peru balsam 1.875%, zinc oxide 10.75%. Net price 30 g (with rectal nozzle) = £2.49

Dose apply night and morning and after a bowel movement; do not use for longer than 7 days; CHILD not recommended

Note A proprietary brand (*Anusol Plus HC*® ointment) is on sale to the public

Suppositories, benzyl benzoate 33 mg, bismuth oxide 24 mg, bismuth subgallate 59 mg, hydrocortisone acetate 10 mg, Peru balsam 49 mg, zinc oxide 296 mg. Net price 12 = £1.74

Dose insert 1 suppository night and morning and after a bowel movement; do not use for longer than 7 days; CHILD not recommended

Note A proprietary brand (*Anusol Plus HC*®) suppositories) is on sale to the public

Perinal® (Dermal)

Spray application, hydrocortisone 0.2%, lidocaine hydrochloride 1%. Net price 30-mL pack = £6.11

Dose ADULT and CHILD over 14 years, spray once over the affected area up to 3 times daily; do not use for longer than 7 days without medical advice; CHILD under 14 years on medical advice only

Proctofoam HC® (Meda) [PoM]

Foam in aerosol pack, hydrocortisone acetate 1%, pramocaine hydrochloride 1%. Net price 21.2-g pack (approx. 40 applications) with applicator = £6.07

Dose haemorrhoids and proctitis, 1 applicatorful (4–6 mg hydrocortisone acetate, 4–6 mg pramocaine hydrochloride) by rectum 2–3 times daily and after each bowel movement (max. 4 times daily); do not use for longer than 7 days; CHILD not recommended

Proctosedyl® (Sanofi-Aventis) [PoM]

Ointment, cinchocaine (dibucaine) hydrochloride 0.5%, hydrocortisone 0.5%. Net price 30 g = £10.34 (with cannula)

Dose apply morning and night and after a bowel movement, externally or by rectum; do not use for longer than 7 days

Suppositories, cinchocaine (dibucaine) hydrochloride 5 mg, hydrocortisone 5 mg. Net price 12 = £5.08

Dose insert 1 suppository night and morning and after a bowel movement; do not use for longer than 7 days

Scheriproct® (Bayer) [PoM]

Ointment, cinchocaine (dibucaine) hydrochloride 0.5%, prednisolone hexanoate 0.19%. Net price 30 g = £2.94

Dose apply twice daily for 5–7 days (3–4 times daily on 1st day if necessary), then once daily for a few days after symptoms have cleared

Suppositories, cinchocaine (dibucaine) hydrochloride 1 mg, prednisolone hexanoate 1.3 mg. Net price 12 = £1.38

Dose insert 1 suppository daily after a bowel movement, for 5–7 days (in severe cases initially 2–3 times daily)

Ultraproct® (Meadow) [PoM]

Ointment, cinchocaine (dibucaine) hydrochloride 0.5%, fluocortolone caproate 0.095%, fluocortolone pivalate 0.092%, net price 30 g (with rectal nozzle) = £4.57

Dose apply twice daily for 5–7 days (3–4 times daily on 1st day if necessary), then once daily for a few days after symptoms have cleared

Suppositories, cinchocaine (dibucaine) hydrochloride 1 mg, fluocortolone caproate 630 micrograms, fluocortolone pivalate 610 micrograms, net price 12 = £2.15

Dose insert 1 suppository daily after a bowel movement, for 5–7 days (in severe cases initially 2–3 times daily) then 1 suppository every other day for 1 week

Uniroid-HC® (Chemidex) [PoM]

Ointment, cinchocaine (dibucaine) hydrochloride 0.5%, hydrocortisone 0.5%. Net price 30 g (with applicator) = £4.23

Dose ADULT and CHILD over 12 years, apply twice daily and after a bowel movement, externally or by rectum; do not use for longer than 7 days; CHILD under 12 years on medical advice only

Suppositories, cinchocaine (dibucaine) hydrochloride 5 mg, hydrocortisone 5 mg. Net price 12 = £1.91

Dose ADULT and CHILD over 12 years, insert 1 suppository twice daily and after a bowel movement; do not use for longer than 7 days

Xyloproct® (AstraZeneca) [PoM]

Ointment (water-miscible), aluminium acetate 3.5%, hydrocortisone acetate 0.275%, lidocaine 5%, zinc oxide 18%, net price 20 g (with applicator) = £4.19

Dose apply several times daily; short-term use only

1.7.3 Rectal sclerosants

Oily phenol injection is used to inject haemorrhoids particularly when unprolapsed.

PHENOL

Indications see notes above

Side-effects irritation, tissue necrosis

Oily Phenol Injection, BP [PoM]

phenol 5% in a suitable fixed oil. Net price 5-mL amp = £4.79

Dose 2–3 mL into the submucosal layer at the base of the pile; several injections may be given at different sites, max. total injected 10 mL at any one time

1.7.4 Management of anal fissures

The management of *anal fissures* requires stool softening by increasing dietary fibre in the form of bran or by using a bulk-forming laxative. Short-term use of local anaesthetic preparations may help (section 1.7.1). If these measures are inadequate, the patient should be referred for specialist treatment in hospital. The use of a topical nitrate (e.g. glyceryl trinitrate 0.4% ointment) may be considered. Before considering surgery, topical diltiazem 2% may be used twice daily [unlicensed indication] in patients with chronic anal fissures unresponsive to topical nitrates.

The *Scottish Medicines Consortium* (p. 4) has advised (January 2008) that glyceryl trinitrate 0.4% ointment (*Rectogesic*®) is **not** recommended for use within NHS Scotland for the relief of pain associated with chronic anal fissure.

GLYCERYL TRINITRATE

Indications anal fissure; angina, left ventricular failure (section 2.6.1); extravasation (section 10.3)

Cautions section 2.6.1

Contra-indications section 2.6.1

Hepatic impairment section 2.6.1

Renal impairment section 2.6.1

Pregnancy section 2.6.1

Breast-feeding section 2.6.1

Side-effects section 2.6.1; also diarrhoea, burning, itching, and rectal bleeding

Dose
- See preparations

Rectogesic® (ProStrakan) [PoM]
Rectal ointment, glyceryl trinitrate 0.4%, net price 30 g = £39.30

Excipients include lanolin, propylene glycol

Dose ADULT over 18 years, apply 2.5 cm of ointment to anal canal every 12 hours until pain stops; max. duration of use 8 weeks

Note 2.5 cm of ointment contains glyceryl trinitrate 1.5 mg; discard tube 8 weeks after first opening

1.8 Stoma care

Prescribing for patients with stoma calls for special care. The following is a brief account of some of the main points to be borne in mind.

Enteric-coated and *modified-release* preparations are **unsuitable**, particularly in patients with an ileostomy, as there may not be sufficient release of the active ingredient.

Laxatives Enemas and washouts should **not** be prescribed for patients with an ileostomy as they may cause rapid and severe loss of water and electrolytes.

Colostomy patients may suffer from constipation and whenever possible should be treated by increasing fluid intake or dietary fibre. **Bulk-forming drugs** (section 1.6.1) should be tried. If they are insufficient, as small a dose as possible of senna (section 1.6.2) should be used.

Antidiarrhoeals Drugs such as **loperamide**, **codeine phosphate**, or **co-phenotrope** (diphenoxylate with atropine) are effective. Bulk-forming drugs (section 1.6.1) may be tried but it is often difficult to adjust the dose appropriately.

Antibacterials should **not** be given for an episode of acute diarrhoea.

Antacids The tendency to diarrhoea from magnesium salts or constipation from aluminium salts may be increased in these patients.

Diuretics Diuretics should be used with caution in patients with an ileostomy as they may become excessively dehydrated and potassium depletion may easily occur. It is usually advisable to use a **potassium-sparing** diuretic (see section 2.2.3).

Digoxin Patients with a stoma are particularly susceptible to hypokalaemia if on digoxin therapy and potassium supplements or a potassium-sparing diuretic may be advisable (for comment see section 9.2.1.1).

Potassium supplements Liquid formulations are preferred to modified-release formulations (see above).

Analgesics Opioid analgesics (see section 4.7.2) may cause troublesome constipation in colostomy patients. When a non-opioid analgesic is required **paracetamol** is usually suitable but anti-inflammatory analgesics may cause gastric irritation and bleeding.

Iron preparations Iron preparations may cause loose stools and sore skin in these patients. If this is troublesome and if iron is definitely indicated an intramuscular iron preparation (see section 9.1.1.2) should

be used. Modified-release preparations should be **avoided** for the reasons given above.

Care of stoma Patients are usually given advice about the use of *cleansing agents*, *protective creams*, *lotions*, *deodorants*, or *sealants* whilst in hospital, either by the surgeon or by stoma care nurses. Voluntary organisations offer help and support to patients with stoma.

1.9 Drugs affecting intestinal secretions

1.9.1	**Drugs affecting biliary composition and flow**
1.9.2	**Bile acid sequestrants**
1.9.3	**Aprotinin**
1.9.4	**Pancreatin**

1.9.1 Drugs affecting biliary composition and flow

The use of laparoscopic cholecystectomy and of endoscopic biliary techniques has limited the place of the bile acid **ursodeoxycholic acid** in gallstone disease. Ursodeoxycholic acid is suitable for patients with unimpaired gall bladder function, small or medium-sized radiolucent stones, and whose mild symptoms are not amenable to other treatment; it should be used cautiously in those with liver disease (but see below). Patients should be given dietary advice (including avoidance of excessive cholesterol and calories) and they require radiological monitoring. Long-term prophylaxis may be needed after complete dissolution of the gallstones has been confirmed because they may recur in up to 25% of patients within one year of stopping treatment.

Ursodeoxycholic acid is also used in primary biliary cirrhosis; liver tests improve in most patients but the effect on overall survival is uncertain.

URSODEOXYCHOLIC ACID

Indications see under Dose and under preparations

Cautions see notes above; in primary biliary cirrhosis, monitor liver function every 4 weeks for 3 months, then every 3 months; **interactions**: Appendix 1 (bile acids)

Contra-indications radio-opaque stones, non-functioning gall bladder, acute inflammation of the gall bladder, frequent episodes of biliary colic, inflammatory diseases and other conditions of the small intestine, colon and liver which interfere with enterohepatic circulation of bile salts

Hepatic impairment avoid in chronic liver disease (but used in primary biliary cirrhosis)

Pregnancy no evidence of harm but manufacturer advises avoid

Breast-feeding not known to be harmful but manufacturer advises avoid

Side-effects diarrhoea; *very rarely* abdominal pain, gallstone calcification, urticaria; *also reported* nausea, vomiting, pruritus

Dose
- Dissolution of gallstones, 8–12 mg/kg daily as a single dose at bedtime *or* in two divided doses, for up to 2

1 Gastro-intestinal system

years; treatment is continued for 3–4 months after stones dissolve

• Primary biliary cirrhosis, 12–16 mg/kg daily in 3 divided doses for 3 months, then 12–16 mg/kg once daily at bedtime

Ursodeoxycholic Acid (Non-proprietary) PoM

Tablets, ursodeoxycholic acid 150 mg, net price 60-tab pack = £16.72; 300 mg, 60-tab pack = £38.86. Label: 21

Capsules, ursodeoxycholic acid 250 mg, net price 60-cap pack = £25.29. Label: 21

Destolit® (Norgine) PoM

Tablets, scored, ursodeoxycholic acid 150 mg, net price 60-tab pack = £18.39. Label: 21

Ursofalk® (Dr Falk) PoM

Capsules, ursodeoxycholic acid 250 mg, net price 60-cap pack = £30.17, 100-cap pack = £31.88. Label: 21

Tablets, f/c, scored, ursodeoxycholic acid 500 mg, net price 100-tab pack = £80.00. Label: 21

Suspension, sugar-free, ursodeoxycholic acid 250 mg/5 mL, net price 250 mL = £26.98. Label: 21

Ursogal® (Galen) PoM

Tablets, scored, ursodeoxycholic acid 150 mg, net price 60-tab pack = £14.49. Label: 21

Capsules, ursodeoxycholic acid 250 mg, net price 60-cap pack = £25.93. Label: 21

Other preparations for biliary disorders

A **terpene** mixture (*Rowachol*®) raises biliary cholesterol solubility. It is not considered to be a useful adjunct.

Rowachol® (Rowa) PoM ◢

Capsules, green, e/c, borneol 5 mg, camphene 5 mg, cineole 2 mg, menthol 32 mg, menthone 6 mg, pinene 17 mg in olive oil. Net price 50-cap pack = £7.35. Label: 22

Dose 1–2 capsules 3 times daily before food (but see notes above)

1.9.2 Bile acid sequestrants

Colestyramine is an anion-exchange resin that is not absorbed from the gastro-intestinal tract. It relieves diarrhoea and pruritus by forming an insoluble complex with bile acids in the intestine. Colestyramine can interfere with the absorption of a number of drugs. Colestyramine is also used in hypercholesterolaemia (section 2.12).

COLESTYRAMINE

(Cholestyramine)

Indications   pruritus associated with partial biliary obstruction and primary biliary cirrhosis; diarrhoea associated with Crohn's disease, ileal resection, vagotomy, diabetic vagal neuropathy, and radiation; hypercholesterolaemia (section 2.12)

Cautions   section 2.12

Contra-indications   section 2.12

Pregnancy   section 2.12

Breast-feeding   section 2.12

Side-effects   section 2.12

Dose

• Pruritus, 4–8 g daily in a suitable liquid; CHILD 1–18 years see *BNF for Children*

• Diarrhoea, initially 4 g daily increased by 4 g at weekly intervals to 12–24 g daily in a suitable liquid in 1–4 divided doses, then adjusted as required; max. 36 g daily; CHILD 1–18 years see *BNF for Children*

Counselling Other drugs should be taken at least 1 hour before or 4–6 hours after colestyramine to reduce possible interference with absorption

Note The contents of each sachet should be mixed with at least 150 mL of water or other suitable liquid such as fruit juice, skimmed milk, thin soups, and pulpy fruits with a high moisture content

◢Preparations

Section 2.12

1.9.3 Aprotinin

Aprotinin is no longer used for the treatment of acute pancreatitis.

1.9.4 Pancreatin

Supplements of pancreatin are given by mouth to compensate for reduced or absent exocrine secretion in cystic fibrosis, and following pancreatectomy, gastrectomy, or chronic pancreatitis. They assist the digestion of starch, fat, and protein. Pancreatin may also be necessary if a tumour (e.g. pancreatic cancer) obstructs outflow from the pancreas.

Pancreatin is inactivated by gastric acid therefore pancreatin preparations are best taken with food (or immediately before or after food). Gastric acid secretion may be reduced by giving cimetidine or ranitidine an hour beforehand (section 1.3). Concurrent use of antacids also reduces gastric acidity. Enteric-coated preparations deliver a higher enzyme concentration in the duodenum (provided the capsule contents are swallowed whole without chewing). Higher-strength preparations are also available (**important:** see advice below).

Since pancreatin is also inactivated by heat, excessive heat should be avoided if preparations are mixed with liquids or food; the resulting mixtures should not be kept for more than one hour.

Dosage is adjusted according to size, number, and consistency of stools, so that the patient thrives; extra allowance will be needed if snacks are taken between meals.

Pancreatin can irritate the perioral skin and buccal mucosa if retained in the mouth, and excessive doses can cause perianal irritation. The most frequent side-effects are gastro-intestinal, including nausea, vomiting, and abdominal discomfort; hyperuricaemia and hyperuricosuria have been associated with very high doses. Hypersensitivity reactions occur occasionally and may affect those handling the powder.

PANCREATIN

Indications   see above

Cautions   see above and (for higher-strength preparations) see below

Pregnancy   not known to be harmful

Side-effects   see above and (for higher-strength preparations) see below

Dose

• See preparations

Creon® 10 000 (Abbott Healthcare)

Capsules, brown/clear, enclosing buff-coloured e/c granules of pancreatin (pork), providing: protease 600 units, lipase 10 000 units, amylase 8000 units. Net price 100-cap pack = £12.93. Counselling, see dose

Dose ADULT and CHILD initially 1–2 capsules with each meal either taken whole or contents mixed with acidic fluid or soft food (then swallowed immediately without chewing)

Creon® Micro (Abbott Healthcare)

Gastro-resistant granules, brown, pancreatin (pork), providing: protease 200 units, lipase 5000 units, amylase 3600 units per 100 mg, net price 20 g = £31.50 Counselling, see dose

Dose ADULT and CHILD initially 100 mg with each meal either taken whole or mixed with acidic fluid or soft food (then swallowed immediately without chewing)

Pancrex® (Essential)

Granules, pancreatin (pork), providing minimum of: protease 300 units, lipase 5000 units, amylase 4000 units/g. Net price 300 g = £57.00. Label: 25, counselling, see dose

Dose ADULT and CHILD 5–10 g just before meals washed down or mixed with a little milk or water

Pancrex V® (Essential)

Capsules, pancreatin (pork), providing minimum of: protease 430 units, lipase 8000 units, amylase 9000 units. Net price 300-cap pack = £53.20. Counselling, see dose

Dose ADULT and CHILD over 1 year 2–6 capsules with each meal, swallowed whole or sprinkled on food; INFANT up to 1 year contents of 1–2 capsules mixed with feeds

Capsules '125', pancreatin (pork), providing minimum of: protease 160 units, lipase 2950 units, amylase 3300 units, net price 300-cap pack = £42.07. Counselling, see dose

Dose NEONATE contents of 1–2 capsules mixed with feeds

Tablets, e/c, pancreatin (pork), providing minimum of: protease 110 units, lipase 1900 units, amylase 1700 units. Net price 300-tab pack = £38.79. Label: 5, 25, counselling, see dose

Dose ADULT and CHILD 5–15 tablets before each meal

Tablets forte, e/c, pancreatin (pork), providing minimum of: protease 330 units, lipase 5600 units, amylase 5000 units. Net price 300-tab pack = £48.11. Label: 5, 25, counselling, see dose

Dose ADULT and CHILD 6–10 tablets before each meal

Powder, pancreatin (pork), providing minimum of: protease 1400 units, lipase 25 000 units, amylase 30 000 units/g. Net price 300 g = £58.88. Counselling, see dose

Dose ADULT and CHILD over 1 month, 0.5–2 g before each meal, washed down or mixed with liquid; NEONATE 250–500 mg with each feed

◢ Higher-strength preparations

The high-strength pancreatin preparations *Nutrizym 22®* and *Pancrease HL®* have been associated with the development of large bowel strictures (fibrosing colonopathy) in children with cystic fibrosis aged between 2 and 13 years. No association was found with *Creon® 25 000* and *Creon® 40 000*. The following is recommended:

• *Pancrease HL®* and *Nutrizym 22®* should not be used in children aged 15 years or less with cystic fibrosis;

• the total dose of pancreatic enzyme supplements used in patients with cystic fibrosis should not usually exceed 10 000 units of lipase per kg body-weight daily;

• if a patient on any pancreatin preparation develops new abdominal symptoms (or any change in existing abdominal symptoms) the patient should be reviewed to exclude the possibility of colonic damage.

Possible risk factors are gender (boys at greater risk than girls), more severe cystic fibrosis, and concomitant use of laxatives. The peak age for developing fibrosing colonopathy is between 2 and 8 years.

Counselling It is important to ensure adequate hydration at all times in patients receiving higher-strength pancreatin preparations.

Creon® 25 000 (Abbott Healthcare) PoM

Capsules, orange/clear, enclosing brown-coloured e/c pellets of pancreatin (pork), providing: protease (total) 1000 units, lipase 25 000 units, amylase 18 000 units, net price 100-cap pack = £28.25. Counselling, see above and under dose

Dose ADULT and CHILD initially 1–2 capsules with meals either taken whole or contents mixed with acidic fluid or soft food (then swallowed immediately without chewing)

Creon® 40 000 (Abbott Healthcare) PoM

Capsules, brown/clear, enclosing brown-coloured e/c granules of pancreatin (pork), providing: protease (total) 1600 units, lipase 40 000 units, amylase 25 000 units, net price 100-cap pack = £41.80. Counselling, see above and under dose

Dose ADULT and CHILD initially 1–2 capsules with meals either taken whole or contents mixed with acidic fluid or soft food (then swallowed immediately without chewing)

Nutrizym 22® (Merck Serono) PoM

Capsules, red/yellow, enclosing e/c minitablets of pancreatin (pork), providing minimum of: protease 1100 units, lipase 22 000 units, amylase 19 800 units. Net price 100-cap pack = £33.33. Counselling, see above and under dose

Dose ADULT and CHILD over 15 years, 1–2 capsules with meals and 1 capsule with snacks, swallowed whole or contents taken with water or mixed with soft food (then swallowed immediately without chewing)

Pancrease HL® (Janssen) PoM

Capsules, enclosing light brown e/c minitablets of pancreatin (pork), providing minimum of: protease 1250 units, lipase 25 000 units, amylase 22 500 units. Net price 100 = £40.38. Counselling, see above and under dose

Dose ADULT and CHILD over 15 years, 1–2 capsules during each meal and 1 capsule with snacks swallowed whole or contents mixed with slightly acidic liquid or soft food (then swallowed immediately without chewing)

2 Cardiovascular system

This chapter also includes advice on the drug management of the following:

angina, p. 165
arrhythmias, p. 93
cardiovascular disease risk, p. 108 and p. 172
heart failure, p. 118
hypertension, p. 108
myocardial infarction, p. 165
phaeochromocytoma, p. 118
stroke, p. 161

2.1 Positive inotropic drugs

2.1.1 Cardiac glycosides
2.1.2 Phosphodiesterase type-3 inhibitors

Positive inotropic drugs increase the force of contraction of the myocardium; for sympathomimetics with inotropic activity see section 2.7.1.

2.1.1 Cardiac glycosides

Digoxin is a cardiac glycoside that increases the force of myocardial contraction and reduces conductivity within the atrioventricular (AV) node.

Digoxin is most useful for controlling ventricular response in persistent and permanent atrial fibrillation and atrial flutter (section 2.3.1). For reference to the role of digoxin in heart failure, see section 2.5.5.

For management of atrial fibrillation the maintenance dose of digoxin can usually be determined by the ventricular rate at rest, which should not usually be allowed to fall persistently below 60 beats per minute.

Digoxin is now rarely used for rapid control of heart rate (see section 2.3 for the management of supraventricular arrhythmias). Even with intravenous administration, response may take many hours; persistence of tachycardia is therefore not an indication for exceeding the recommended dose. The intramuscular route is **not** recommended.

In patients with heart failure who are in sinus rhythm a loading dose is not required, and a satisfactory plasma-digoxin concentration can be achieved over a period of about a week.

Digoxin has a long half-life and maintenance doses need to be given only once daily (although higher doses may be divided to avoid nausea); renal function is the most important determinant of digoxin dosage.

Unwanted effects depend both on the concentration of digoxin in the plasma and on the sensitivity of the conducting system or of the myocardium, which is often increased in heart disease. It can sometimes be difficult to distinguish between toxic effects and clinical deterioration because symptoms of both are similar. The plasma concentration alone cannot indicate toxicity reliably, but the likelihood of toxicity increases progressively through the range 1.5 to 3 micrograms/litre for digoxin. Digoxin should be used with special care in the elderly, who may be particularly susceptible to digitalis toxicity.

Regular monitoring of plasma-digoxin concentration during maintenance treatment is not necessary unless problems are suspected. Hypokalaemia predisposes the patient to digitalis toxicity; it is managed by giving a potassium-sparing diuretic or, if necessary, potassium supplementation.

If toxicity occurs, digoxin should be withdrawn; serious manifestations require urgent specialist management. **Digoxin-specific antibody fragments** are available for reversal of life-threatening overdosage (see Digoxin-specific Antibody, below).

▌ DIGOXIN

Indications   heart failure (see also section 2.5.5), supraventricular arrhythmias (particularly atrial fibrillation and atrial flutter; see also section 2.3.2)

Cautions   recent myocardial infarction; sick sinus syndrome; thyroid disease; reduce dose in the elderly; severe respiratory disease; hypokalaemia, hypomagnesaemia, hypercalcaemia, and hypoxia (risk of digitalis toxicity); monitor serum electrolytes and renal function; avoid rapid intravenous administration (risk of hypertension and reduced coronary flow); **interactions:** Appendix 1 (cardiac glycosides)

Contra-indications   intermittent complete heart block, second degree AV block; supraventricular arrhythmias associated with accessory conducting pathways e.g. Wolff-Parkinson-White syndrome; ventricular tachycardia or fibrillation; hypertrophic cardiomyopathy (unless concomitant atrial fibrillation and heart failure—but use with caution); myocarditis; constrictive pericarditis (unless to control atrial fibrillation or improve systolic dysfunction—but use with caution)

Renal impairment   reduce dose and monitor plasma-digoxin concentration; toxicity increased by electrolyte disturbances

Pregnancy   may need dosage adjustment

Breast-feeding   amount too small to be harmful

Side-effects   see notes above; also nausea, vomiting, diarrhoea; arrhythmias, conduction disturbances; dizziness; blurred or yellow vision; rash, eosinophilia; *less commonly* depression; *very rarely* anorexia, intestinal ischaemia and necrosis, psychosis, apathy, confusion, headache, fatigue, weakness, gynaecomastia on long-term use, and thrombocytopenia

Dose

- Rapid digitalisation, for atrial fibrillation or flutter, by mouth, 0.75–1.5 mg over 24 hours in divided doses
- Maintenance, for atrial fibrillation or flutter, by mouth, according to renal function and initial loading dose; usual range 125–250 micrograms daily
- Heart failure (for patients in sinus rhythm), by mouth, 62.5–125 micrograms once daily
- Emergency loading dose, for atrial fibrillation or flutter, by intravenous infusion (but rarely necessary), 0.75–1 mg over at least 2 hours (see also Cautions) then maintenance dose by mouth on the following day

Note The above doses may need to be reduced if digoxin (or another cardiac glycoside) has been given in the preceding 2 weeks. When switching from intravenous to oral route may need to increase dose by 20–33% to maintain the same plasma-digoxin concentration. Digoxin doses in the BNF may differ from those in product literature. For plasma concentration monitoring, blood should be taken at least 6 hours after a dose

Digoxin (Non-proprietary) PoM
 Tablets, digoxin 62.5 micrograms, net price 28-tab pack = £1.48; 125 micrograms, 28-tab pack = £1.08; 250 micrograms, 28-tab pack = £1.01
 Injection, digoxin 250 micrograms/mL, net price 2-mL amp = 70p
 Paediatric injection, digoxin 100 micrograms/mL
 Available from 'special-order' manufacturers or specialist importing companies, see p. 1124

Lanoxin® (Aspen) PoM
 Tablets, digoxin 125 micrograms, net price 500-tab pack = £8.09; 250 micrograms (scored), 500-tab pack = £8.09
 Injection, digoxin 250 micrograms/mL, net price 2-mL amp = 66p

Lanoxin-PG® (Aspen) PoM
 Tablets, blue, digoxin 62.5 micrograms, net price 500-tab pack = £8.09
 Elixir, yellow, digoxin 50 micrograms/mL. Do not dilute, measure with pipette. Net price 60 mL = £5.35. Counselling, use of pipette

Digoxin-specific antibody

Serious cases of digoxin toxicity should be discussed with the National Poisons Information Service, p. 33. **Digoxin-specific antibody fragments** are indicated for the treatment of known or strongly suspected life-threatening digoxin toxicity associated with ventricular arrhythmias or bradyarrhythmias unresponsive to atropine and when measures beyond the withdrawal of digoxin and correction of any electrolyte abnormalities are considered necessary (see also notes above).

DigiFab® (BTG) ▼ PoM
 Intravenous infusion, powder for reconstitution, digoxin-specific antibody fragments (F(ab)), net price 40-mg vial = £750.00 (hosp. only)
 Dose consult product literature

2.1.2 Phosphodiesterase type-3 inhibitors

Enoximone and milrinone are phosphodiesterase type-3 inhibitors that exert most of their effect on the myocardium. Sustained haemodynamic benefit has been observed after administration, but there is no evidence of any beneficial effect on survival.

ENOXIMONE

Indications congestive heart failure where cardiac output reduced and filling pressures increased

Cautions heart failure associated with hypertrophic cardiomyopathy, stenotic or obstructive valvular disease or other outlet obstruction; monitor blood pressure, heart rate, ECG, central venous pressure, fluid and electrolyte status, renal function, platelet count, hepatic enzymes; avoid extravasation; **interactions:** Appendix 1 (phosphodiesterase type-3 inhibitors)

Hepatic impairment dose reduction may be required

Renal impairment consider dose reduction

Pregnancy manufacturer advises use only if potential benefit outweighs risk

Breast-feeding manufacturer advises caution—no information available

Side-effects ectopic beats; less frequently ventricular tachycardia or supraventricular arrhythmias (more likely in patients with pre-existing arrhythmias); hypotension; also headache, insomnia, nausea and vomiting, diarrhoea; occasionally, chills, oliguria, fever, urinary retention; upper and lower limb pain

Dose
- By slow intravenous injection (rate not exceeding 12.5 mg/minute), diluted before use, initially 0.5–1 mg/kg, then 500 micrograms/kg every 30 minutes until satisfactory response or total of 3 mg/kg given; maintenance, initial dose of up to 3 mg/kg may be repeated every 3–6 hours as required
- By intravenous infusion, initially 90 micrograms/kg/ minute over 10–30 minutes, followed by continuous or intermittent infusion of 5–20 micrograms/kg/ minute

  Total dose over 24 hours should not usually exceed 24 mg/kg

Perfan® (INCA-Pharm) [PoM]
Injection, enoximone 5 mg/mL. For dilution before use. Net price 20-mL amp = £15.02
Excipients include alcohol, propylene glycol
Note Plastic apparatus should be used; crystal formation if glass used

MILRINONE

Indications short-term treatment of severe congestive heart failure unresponsive to conventional maintenance therapy (not immediately after myocardial infarction); acute heart failure, including low output states following heart surgery

Cautions see under Enoximone; also correct hypokalaemia; **interactions:** Appendix 1 (phosphodiesterase type-3 inhibitors)

Contra-indications severe hypovolaemia

Renal impairment reduce dose and monitor response if eGFR less than 50 mL/minute/1.73 m²—consult product literature for details

Pregnancy manufacturer advises use only if potential benefit outweighs risk

Breast-feeding manufacturer advises avoid—no information available

Side-effects ectopic beats, ventricular tachycardia, supraventricular arrhythmias (more likely in patients with pre-existing arrhythmias), hypotension; headache; *less commonly* ventricular fibrillation, chest pain, tremor, hypokalaemia, thrombocytopenia; *very rarely* bronchospasm, anaphylaxis, and rash

Dose
- By intravenous injection over 10 minutes, either undiluted or diluted before use, 50 micrograms/kg followed by intravenous infusion at a rate of 375–750 nanograms/kg/minute, usually for up to 12 hours following surgery or for 48–72 hours in congestive heart failure; max. daily dose 1.13 mg/kg

Primacor® (Sanofi-Aventis) [PoM]
Injection, milrinone (as lactate) 1 mg/mL, net price 10-mL amp = £19.91

2.2 Diuretics

2.2.1 Thiazides and related diuretics
2.2.2 Loop diuretics
2.2.3 Potassium-sparing diuretics and aldosterone antagonists
2.2.4 Potassium-sparing diuretics with other diuretics
2.2.5 Osmotic diuretics
2.2.6 Mercurial diuretics
2.2.7 Carbonic anhydrase inhibitors
2.2.8 Diuretics with potassium

Thiazides (section 2.2.1) are used to relieve oedema due to chronic heart failure (section 2.5.5) and, in lower doses, to reduce blood pressure.

Loop diuretics (section 2.2.2) are used in pulmonary oedema due to left ventricular failure and in patients with chronic heart failure (section 2.5.5).

Combination diuretic therapy may be effective in patients with oedema resistant to treatment with one diuretic. Vigorous diuresis, particularly with loop diuretics, may induce acute hypotension; rapid reduction of plasma volume should be avoided.

Elderly Lower initial doses of diuretics should be used in the elderly because they are particularly susceptible to the side-effects. The dose should then be adjusted according to renal function. Diuretics should not be used continuously on a long-term basis to treat simple gravitational oedema (which will usually respond to increased movement, raising the legs, and support stockings).

Potassium loss Hypokalaemia can occur with both thiazide and loop diuretics. The risk of hypokalaemia depends on the duration of action as well as the potency and is thus greater with thiazides than with an equipotent dose of a loop diuretic.

Hypokalaemia is dangerous in severe cardiovascular disease and in patients also being treated with cardiac glycosides. Often the use of potassium-sparing diuretics (section 2.2.3) avoids the need to take potassium supplements.

Cardiovascular system

In hepatic failure, hypokalaemia caused by diuretics can precipitate encephalopathy, particularly in alcoholic cirrhosis; diuretics can also increase the risk of hypomagnesaemia in alcoholic cirrhosis, leading to arrhythmias. Spironolactone, a potassium-sparing diuretic (section 2.2.3), is chosen for oedema arising from cirrhosis of the liver.

Potassium supplements or potassium-sparing diuretics are seldom necessary when thiazides are used in the routine treatment of hypertension (see also section 9.2.1.1).

2.2.1 Thiazides and related diuretics

Thiazides and related compounds are moderately potent diuretics; they inhibit sodium reabsorption at the beginning of the distal convoluted tubule. They act within 1 to 2 hours of oral administration and most have a duration of action of 12 to 24 hours; they are usually administered early in the day so that the diuresis does not interfere with sleep.

In the management of *hypertension* a low dose of a thiazide produces a maximal or near-maximal blood pressure lowering effect, with very little biochemical disturbance. Higher doses cause more marked changes in plasma potassium, sodium, uric acid, glucose, and lipids, with little advantage in blood pressure control. **Chlortalidone** and **indapamide** are the preferred diuretics in the management of hypertension (see section 2.5).

For reference to the use of thiazides in chronic heart failure see section 2.5.5.

Bendroflumethiazide can be used for mild or moderate heart failure; it is licensed for the treatment of hypertension but is no longer considered the first-line diuretic for this indication (see section 2.5), although patients with stable and controlled blood pressure currently taking bendroflumethiazide can continue treatment.

Chlortalidone, a thiazide-related compound, has a longer duration of action than the thiazides and may be given on alternate days to control oedema. It is also useful if acute retention is liable to be precipitated by a more rapid diuresis or if patients dislike the altered pattern of micturition caused by other diuretics.

Xipamide and indapamide are chemically related to chlortalidone. Indapamide is claimed to lower blood pressure with less metabolic disturbance, particularly less aggravation of diabetes mellitus.

Metolazone is particularly effective when combined with a loop diuretic (even in renal failure); profound diuresis can occur and the patient should therefore be monitored carefully.

The thiazide diuretics benzthiazide, clopamide, cyclopenthiazide, hydrochlorothiazide, and hydroflumethiazide do not offer any significant advantage over other thiazides and related diuretics.

Cautions See also section 2.2. Thiazides and related diuretics can exacerbate diabetes, gout, and systemic lupus erythematosus. Electrolytes should be monitored, particularly with high doses, long-term use, or in renal impairment. Thiazides and related diuretics should also be used with caution in nephrotic syndrome, hyperaldosteronism, and malnourishment; **interactions:** Appendix 1 (diuretics)

Contra-indications Thiazides and related diuretics should be avoided in refractory hypokalaemia, hyponatraemia and hypercalcaemia, symptomatic hyperuricaemia, and Addison's disease.

Hepatic impairment Thiazides and related diuretics should be used with caution in mild to moderate impairment and avoided in severe liver disease. Hypokalaemia may precipitate coma, although hypokalaemia can be prevented by using a potassium-sparing diuretic. There is an increased risk of hypomagnesaemia in alcoholic cirrhosis.

Renal impairment Thiazides and related diuretics are ineffective if eGFR is less than 30 mL/minute/$1.73 m^2$ and should be avoided; metolazone remains effective but with a risk of excessive diuresis.

Pregnancy Thiazides and related diuretics should not be used to treat gestational hypertension. They may cause neonatal thrombocytopenia, bone marrow suppression, jaundice, electrolyte disturbances, and hypoglycaemia; placental perfusion may also be reduced. Stimulation of labour, uterine inertia, and meconium staining have also been reported.

Breast-feeding The amount of bendroflumethiazide, chlortalidone, cyclopenthiazide, and metolazone present in milk is too small to be harmful; large doses may suppress lactation. For indapamide and xipamide see individual drugs.

Side-effects Side-effects of thiazides and related diuretics include mild gastro-intestinal disturbances, postural hypotension, altered plasma-lipid concentrations, metabolic and electrolyte disturbances including hypokalaemia (see also notes above), hyponatraemia, hypomagnesaemia, hypercalcaemia, hyperglycaemia, hypochloraemic alkalosis, hyperuricaemia, and gout. Less common side-effects include blood disorders such as agranulocytosis, leucopenia, and thrombocytopenia, and impotence. Pancreatitis, intrahepatic cholestasis, cardiac arrhythmias, headache, dizziness, paraesthesia, visual disturbances, and hypersensitivity reactions (including pneumonitis, pulmonary oedema, photosensitivity, and severe skin reactions) have also been reported.

BENDROFLUMETHIAZIDE
(Bendrofluazide)

Indications oedema, hypertension (see also notes above)

Cautions see above

Contra-indications see notes above

Hepatic impairment see notes above

Renal impairment see notes above

Pregnancy see notes above

Breast-feeding see notes above

Side-effects see notes above

Dose
- Oedema, initially 5–10 mg daily in the morning *or* on alternate days; maintenance 5–10 mg 1–3 times weekly
- Hypertension, 2.5 mg daily in the morning; higher doses rarely necessary (see notes above)

2 Cardiovascular system

Bendroflumethiazide (Non-proprietary) POM
Tablets, bendroflumethiazide 2.5 mg, net price 28 = 86p; 5 mg, 28 = 89p
Brands include *Aprinox*®, *Neo-Naclex*®

CHLORTALIDONE
(Chlorthalidone)

Indications ascites due to cirrhosis in stable patients (under close supervision), oedema due to nephrotic syndrome, hypertension (see also notes above), mild to moderate chronic heart failure; diabetes insipidus (see section 6.5.2)

Cautions see notes above

Contra-indications see notes above

Hepatic impairment see notes above

Renal impairment see notes above

Pregnancy see notes above

Breast-feeding see notes above

Side-effects see notes above; also *rarely* jaundice and allergic interstitial nephritis

Dose
- Oedema, up to 50 mg daily
- Hypertension, 25 mg daily in the morning, increased to 50 mg daily if necessary (but see notes above)
- Heart failure, 25–50 mg daily in the morning, increased if necessary to 100–200 mg daily (reduce to lowest effective dose for maintenance)

Hygroton® (Alliance) POM
Tablets, yellow, scored, chlortalidone 50 mg, net price 28-tab pack = £1.64
Note May be difficult to obtain

CYCLOPENTHIAZIDE

Indications oedema, hypertension (see also notes above); heart failure

Cautions see notes above

Contra-indications see notes above

Hepatic impairment see notes above

Renal impairment see notes above

Pregnancy see notes above

Breast-feeding see notes above

Side-effects see notes above; also *rarely* depression

Dose
- Heart failure, 250–500 micrograms daily in the morning increased if necessary to 1 mg daily (reduce to lowest effective dose for maintenance)
- Hypertension, initially 250 micrograms daily in the morning, increased if necessary to 500 micrograms daily (but see notes above)
- Oedema, up to 500 micrograms daily for a short period

Navidrex® (AMCo) POM
Tablets, scored, cyclopenthiazide 500 micrograms, net price 28-tab pack = £1.27
Excipients include gluten
Note May be difficult to obtain

INDAPAMIDE

Indications essential hypertension

Cautions see notes above; also acute porphyria (section 9.8.2)

Contra-indications see notes above; also hypersensitivity to sulfonamides

Hepatic impairment see notes above

Renal impairment see notes above

Pregnancy see notes above

Breast-feeding present in milk—manufacturer advises avoid

Side-effects see notes above; also palpitation, diuresis with doses above 2.5 mg daily

Dose
- 2.5 mg daily in the morning

Indapamide (Non-proprietary) POM
Tablets, s/c, indapamide 2.5 mg, net price 28-tab pack £1.88, 56-tab pack = £2.61

Natrilix® (Servier) POM
Tablets, f/c, indapamide 2.5 mg. Net price 30-tab pack = £3.40, 60-tab pack = £6.80

◢**Modified release**
Ethibide XL® (Genus) POM
Tablets, m/r, indapamide 1.5 mg, net price 30-tab pack = £4.05. Label: 25
Dose hypertension, 1 tablet daily, preferably in the morning

Natrilix SR® (Servier) POM
Tablets, m/r, indapamide 1.5 mg, net price 30-tab pack = £3.40. Label: 25
Dose hypertension, 1 tablet daily, preferably in the morning

Tensaid XL® (Generics) POM
Tablets, m/r, f/c, indapamide 1.5 mg, net price 30-tab pack = £3.40. Label: 25
Dose hypertension, 1 tablet daily, preferably in the morning

METOLAZONE

Indications oedema, hypertension (see also notes above)

Cautions see notes above; also acute porphyria (section 9.8.2)

Contra-indications see notes above

Hepatic impairment see notes above

Renal impairment see notes above

Pregnancy see notes above

Breast-feeding see notes above

Side-effects see notes above; also chills, chest pain

Dose
- Oedema, 5–10 mg daily in the morning, increased if necessary to 20 mg daily in resistant oedema, max. 80 mg daily
- Hypertension, initially 5 mg daily in the morning; maintenance 5 mg on alternate days

Metolazone (Non-proprietary) POM
Tablets, metolazone 2.5 mg and 5 mg
Available from 'special-order' manufacturers or specialist-importing companies, see p. 1124

XIPAMIDE

Indications oedema, hypertension (see also notes above)

Cautions see notes above; also acute porphyria (section 9.8.2)

Contra-indications see notes above

Hepatic impairment see notes above

Renal impairment see notes above
Pregnancy see notes above
Breast-feeding no information available
Side-effects see notes above
Dose

- Oedema, initially 40 mg daily in the morning, increased to 80 mg in resistant cases; maintenance 20 mg in the morning
- Hypertension, 20 mg daily in the morning

Diurexan® (Meda) (PoM)
Tablets, scored, xipamide 20 mg, net price 140-tab pack = £19.46

2.2.2 Loop diuretics

Loop diuretics are used in pulmonary oedema due to left ventricular failure; intravenous administration produces relief of breathlessness and reduces pre-load sooner than would be expected from the time of onset of diuresis. Loop diuretics are also used in patients with chronic heart failure. Diuretic-resistant oedema (except lymphoedema and oedema due to peripheral venous stasis or calcium-channel blockers) can be treated with a loop diuretic combined with a thiazide or related diuretic (e.g. bendroflumethiazide 5–10 mg daily or metolazone 5–20 mg daily).

If necessary, a loop diuretic can be added to antihypertensive treatment to achieve better control of blood pressure in those with resistant hypertension, or in patients with impaired renal function or heart failure.

Loop diuretics inhibit reabsorption from the ascending limb of the loop of Henlé in the renal tubule and are powerful diuretics.

Furosemide and **bumetanide** are similar in activity; both act within 1 hour of oral administration and diuresis is complete within 6 hours so that, if necessary, they can be given twice in one day without interfering with sleep. Following intravenous administration they have a peak effect within 30 minutes. The diuresis associated with these drugs is dose related.

Torasemide has properties similar to those of furosemide and bumetanide, and is indicated for oedema and for hypertension.

Cautions Hypovolaemia and hypotension should be corrected before initiation of treatment with loop diuretics; electrolytes should be monitored during treatment (see also Potassium Loss, section 2.2). Loop diuretics can exacerbate diabetes (but hyperglycaemia is less likely than with thiazides) and gout. If there is an enlarged prostate, urinary retention can occur, although this is less likely if small doses and less potent diuretics are used initially; an adequate urinary output should be established before initiating treatment; **interactions:** Appendix 1 (diuretics).

Contra-indications Loop diuretics should be avoided in severe hypokalaemia, severe hyponatraemia, anuria, comatose and precomatose states associated with liver cirrhosis, and in renal failure due to nephrotoxic or hepatotoxic drugs.

Hepatic impairment Hypokalaemia induced by loop diuretics may precipitate hepatic encephalopathy and coma—potassium-sparing diuretics can be used to prevent this.

Renal impairment High doses of loop diuretics may occasionally be needed; high doses or rapid intravenous administration can cause tinnitus and deafness; high doses of bumetanide can also cause musculoskeletal pain.

Pregnancy Furosemide and bumetanide should not be used to treat gestational hypertension because of the maternal hypovolaemia associated with this condition.

Side-effects Side-effects of loop diuretics include mild gastro-intestinal disturbances, pancreatitis, hepatic encephalopathy, postural hypotension, temporary increase in serum-cholesterol and triglyceride concentration, hyperglycaemia (less common than with thiazides), acute urinary retention, electrolyte disturbances (including hyponatraemia, hypokalaemia (see section 2.2), hypocalcaemia, hypochloraemia, and hypomagnesaemia), metabolic alkalosis, blood disorders (including bone-marrow depression, thrombocytopenia, and leucopenia), hyperuricaemia, visual disturbances, tinnitus and deafness (usually with high parenteral doses and rapid administration, and in renal impairment), and hypersensitivity reactions (including rash, photosensitivity, and pruritus).

BUMETANIDE

Indications oedema (see notes above)
Cautions see notes above
Contra-indications see notes above
Hepatic impairment see notes above
Renal impairment see notes above
Pregnancy see notes above
Breast-feeding no information available; may inhibit lactation
Side-effects see notes above; also gynaecomastia, breast pain, musculoskeletal pain (associated with high doses in renal failure)
Dose

- By mouth, 1 mg in the morning, repeated after 6–8 hours if necessary; severe cases, 5 mg daily increased by 5 mg every 12–24 hours according to response; ELDERLY, 500 micrograms daily may be sufficient
- By intravenous injection, 1–2 mg, repeated after 20 minutes if necessary; ELDERLY, 500 micrograms daily may be sufficient
- By intravenous infusion, 2–5 mg over 30–60 minutes; ELDERLY, 500 micrograms daily may be sufficient
- By intramuscular injection, 1 mg initially then adjusted according to response; ELDERLY, 500 micrograms daily may be sufficient

Bumetanide (Non-proprietary) (PoM)
Tablets, bumetanide 1 mg, net price 28-tab pack = £1.37; 5 mg, 28-tab pack = £6.94
Oral liquid, bumetanide 1 mg/5 mL, net price 150 mL = £128.00
Injection, bumetanide 500 micrograms/mL, net price 4-mL amp = £1.79

FUROSEMIDE
(Frusemide)

Indications oedema (see notes above); resistant hypertension (see notes above)
Cautions see notes above; also hypoproteinaemia may reduce diuretic effect and increase risk of side-effects; hepatorenal syndrome; intravenous administration rate should not usually exceed 4 mg/minute,

however single doses of up to 80 mg may be administered more rapidly

Contra-indications   see notes above

Hepatic impairment   see notes above

Renal impairment   see notes above; also lower rate of infusion may be necessary

Pregnancy   see notes above

Breast-feeding   amount too small to be harmful; may inhibit lactation

Side-effects   see notes above; also intrahepatic cholestasis and gout

Dose

* By mouth, oedema, initially 40 mg in the morning; maintenance 20–40 mg daily; CHILD under 18 years see *BNF for Children*
  Resistant oedema, 80–120 mg daily
  Resistant hypertension, 40–80 mg daily
* By intramuscular injection *or* slow intravenous injection (rate of administration, see Cautions above), initially 20–50 mg, increased if necessary in steps of 20 mg not less than every 2 hours; doses greater than 50 mg by intravenous infusion only; max. 1.5 g daily; CHILD under 18 years see *BNF for Children*

Furosemide (Non-proprietary) ▣ⓄⓂ
Tablets, furosemide 20 mg, net price 28 = 97p; 40 mg, 28 = 88p; 500 mg, 28 = £18.04
Brands include *Rusyde*®
Oral solution, sugar-free, furosemide, net price 20 mg/5 mL, 150 mL = £14.46; 40 mg/5 mL, 150 mL = £18.66; 50 mg/5 mL, 150 mL = £20.17
Brands include *Frusol*® (contains alcohol 10%)
Injection, furosemide 10 mg/mL, net price 2-mL amp = 35p, 5-mL amp = 32p, 25-mL amp = £2.50

Lasix® (Sanofi-Aventis) ▣ⓄⓂ
Injection, furosemide 10 mg/mL, net price 2-mL amp = 75p
Note Large-volume furosemide injections also available; brands include *Minijet*®

▌TORASEMIDE

Indications   oedema (see notes above), hypertension

Cautions   see notes above

Contra-indications   see notes above

Hepatic impairment   see notes above

Renal impairment   see notes above

Pregnancy   manufacturer advises avoid—toxicity in *animal* studies

Breast-feeding   manufacturer advises avoid—no information available

Side-effects   see notes above; also dry mouth; *rarely* limb paraesthesia

Dose

* Oedema, 5 mg once daily, preferably in the morning, increased if required to 20 mg once daily; usual max. 40 mg daily
* Hypertension, 2.5 mg daily, increased if necessary to 5 mg once daily

Torasemide (Non-proprietary) ▣ⓄⓂ
Tablets, torasemide 5 mg, net price 28-tab pack = £14.47; 10 mg, 28-tab pack = £18.67

Torem® (Meda) ▣ⓄⓂ
Tablets, torasemide 2.5 mg, net price 28-tab pack = £3.78; 5 mg (scored), 28-tab pack = £5.53; 10 mg (scored), 28-tab pack = £8.14

2.2.3   Potassium-sparing diuretics and aldosterone antagonists

Amiloride and **triamterene** on their own are weak diuretics. They cause retention of potassium and are therefore given with thiazide or loop diuretics as a more effective alternative to potassium supplements. See section 2.2.4 for compound preparations with thiazides or loop diuretics.

Potassium supplements must **not** be given with potassium-sparing diuretics. Administration of a potassium-sparing diuretic to a patient receiving an ACE inhibitor or an angiotensin-II receptor antagonist can also cause severe hyperkalaemia (see also Concomitant Use Of Drugs Affecting the Renin-angiotensin System, p. 120).

▌AMILORIDE HYDROCHLORIDE

Indications   oedema; potassium conservation when used as an adjunct to thiazide or loop diuretics for hypertension, congestive heart failure, or hepatic cirrhosis with ascites

Cautions   monitor electrolytes; diabetes mellitus; elderly; **interactions:** Appendix 1 (diuretics)

Contra-indications   hyperkalaemia; anuria; Addison's disease

Renal impairment   monitor plasma-potassium concentration (high risk of hyperkalaemia in renal impairment); manufacturers advise avoid in severe impairment

Pregnancy   not used to treat gestational hypertension

Breast-feeding   manufacturer advises avoid—no information available

Side-effects   abdominal pain, gastro-intestinal bleeding, dry mouth, thirst, diarrhoea, constipation, anorexia, jaundice, dyspepsia, flatulence, vomiting, nausea, angina, arrhythmias, palpitation, postural hypotension, dyspnoea, cough, nasal congestion, confusion, headache, insomnia, weakness, tremor, agitation, dizziness, malaise, paraesthesia, encephalopathy, urinary disturbances, sexual dysfunction, hyperkalaemia, muscle cramp, arthralgia, visual disturbance, raised intra-ocular pressure, tinnitus, alopecia, pruritus, rash

Dose

* Used alone, initially 10 mg daily *or* 5 mg twice daily, adjusted according to response; max. 20 mg daily
* With other diuretics, congestive heart failure and hypertension, initially 5–10 mg daily; cirrhosis with ascites, initially 5 mg daily

Amiloride (Non-proprietary) ▣ⓄⓂ
Tablets, amiloride hydrochloride 5 mg, net price 28-tab pack = £11.20
Oral solution, sugar-free, amiloride hydrochloride 5 mg/5 mL, net price 150 mL = £39.73
Brands include *Amilamont*® (Excipients include propylene glycol, see Excipients, p. 2)

◀Compound preparations with thiazide or loop diuretics
Section 2.2.4

◼ TRIAMTERENE

Indications oedema, potassium conservation with thiazide and loop diuretics

Cautions see under Amiloride Hydrochloride; also gout; may cause blue fluorescence of urine

Contra-indications see under Amiloride Hydro-chloride

Hepatic impairment use with caution; avoid in progressive impairment

Renal impairment monitor plasma-potassium concentration (high risk of hyperkalaemia in renal impairment); avoid in progressive impairment

Pregnancy not used to treat gestational hypertension; avoid unless essential

Breast-feeding present in milk—manufacturer advises avoid

Side-effects nausea, vomiting, diarrhoea, hyperkalaemia; *less commonly* dry mouth, headache, hyperuricaemia, rash; *rarely* megaloblastic anaemia, pancytopenia, photosensitivity, serum-sickness; *very rarely* triamterene found in kidney stones, renal failure (reversible on discontinuation); *also reported* jaundice, slight decrease in blood pressure, malaise

Dose
- Initially 150–250 mg daily, reducing to alternate days after 1 week; taken in divided doses after breakfast and lunch; lower initial dose when given with other diuretics

  Counselling Urine may look slightly blue in some lights

Triamterene (Non-proprietary) ꜰᴏᴍ
   Capsules, triamterene 50 mg, net price 30-cap pack = £19.95. Label: 14, (see above), 21

◢**Compound preparations with thiazides or loop diuretics**
Section 2.2.4

Aldosterone antagonists

Spironolactone potentiates thiazide or loop diuretics by antagonising aldosterone; it is a potassium-sparing diuretic. Spironolactone is of value in the treatment of oedema and ascites caused by cirrhosis of the liver; furosemide (section 2.2.2) can be used as an adjunct. Low doses of spironolactone are beneficial in moderate to severe heart failure, see section 2.5.5, and when used in resistant hypertension [unlicensed indication], see section 2.5.

Spironolactone is also used in primary hyperaldosteronism (Conn's syndrome). It is given before surgery or if surgery is not appropriate, in the lowest effective dose for maintenance.

Eplerenone is licensed for use as an adjunct in left ventricular dysfunction with evidence of heart failure after a myocardial infarction (see also section 2.5.5 and section 2.10.1); it is also licensed as an adjunct in chronic mild heart failure with left ventricular systolic dysfunction.

Potassium supplements must **not** be given with aldosterone antagonists.

◼ EPLERENONE

Indications adjunct in stable patients with left ventricular ejection fraction ≤ 40% with evidence of heart failure, following myocardial infarction (start therapy within 3–14 days of event); adjunct in chronic mild heart failure with left ventricular ejection fraction ≤ 30%

Cautions measure plasma-potassium concentration before treatment, during initiation, and when dose changed; elderly; **interactions:** Appendix 1 (diuretics)

Contra-indications hyperkalaemia; concomitant use of potassium-sparing diuretics or potassium supplements

Hepatic impairment avoid in severe impairment

Renal impairment increased risk of hyperkalaemia—close monitoring required; initially 25 mg on alternate days if eGFR 30–60 mL/minute/1.73 m², adjust dose according to serum-potassium concentration—consult product literature; avoid if eGFR less than 30 mL/minute/1.73 m²

Pregnancy manufacturer advises caution—no information available

Breast-feeding manufacturer advises use only if potential benefit outweighs risk

Side-effects diarrhoea, constipation, nausea, hypotension, cough, dizziness, syncope, azotaemia, hyperkalaemia, renal impairment, muscle spasm, musculoskeletal pain, rash, pruritus; *less commonly* flatulence, vomiting, cholecystitis, tachycardia, atrial fibrillation, postural hypotension, arterial thrombosis, dyslipidaemia, pharyngitis, headache, insomnia, hypoaesthesia, hypothyroidism, hyperglycaemia, gynaecomastia, pyelonephritis, epidermal growth factor receptor decreased, hyponatraemia, dehydration, eosinophilia, malaise, back pain, sweating; *also reported* angioedema

Dose
- Initially 25 mg once daily, increased within 4 weeks to 50 mg once daily; CHILD not recommended

Inspra® (Pfizer) ꜰᴏᴍ
   Tablets, yellow, f/c, eplerenone 25 mg, net price 28-tab pack = £42.72; 50 mg, 28-tab pack = £42.72

◼ SPIRONOLACTONE

Indications oedema and ascites in cirrhosis of the liver; malignant ascites; nephrotic syndrome; oedema in congestive heart failure; moderate to severe heart failure (adjunct—see also section 2.5.5); resistant hypertension [unlicensed indication] (adjunct—see also section 2.5); treatment of primary hyperaldosteronism

Cautions potential metabolic products carcinogenic in *rodents*; elderly; monitor electrolytes—discontinue if hyperkalaemia occurs (in *severe heart failure* monitor potassium and creatinine 1 week after initiation and after any dose increase, monthly for first 3 months, then every 3 months for 1 year, and then every 6 months); acute porphyria (section 9.8.2); **interactions:** Appendix 1 (diuretics)

Contra-indications hyperkalaemia; anuria; Addison's disease

Renal impairment monitor plasma-potassium concentration (high risk of hyperkalaemia in renal impairment); avoid in acute renal insufficiency or severe impairment

Pregnancy use only if potential benefit outweighs risk—feminisation of male fetus in *animal* studies

Breast-feeding metabolites present in milk, but amount probably too small to be harmful

2

Cardiovascular system

Side-effects gastro-intestinal disturbances, hepato-toxicity, malaise, confusion, drowsiness, dizziness, gynaecomastia, benign breast tumour, breast pain, menstrual disturbances, changes in libido, hypertrichosis, electrolyte disturbances including hyperkalaemia (discontinue) and hyponatraemia, acute renal failure, hyperuricaemia, leucopenia, agranulocytosis, thrombocytopenia, leg cramps, alopecia, rash, Stevens-Johnson syndrome

Dose
- Oedema and ascites in cirrhosis of the liver, 100–400 mg daily, adjusted according to response
- Malignant ascites, initially 100–200 mg daily, increased to 400 mg daily if required; maintenance dose adjusted according to response
- Nephrotic syndrome, 100–200 mg daily
- Oedema in congestive heart failure, initially 100 mg (range 25–200 mg) daily in single or divided doses; maintenance dose adjusted according to response
- Moderate to severe heart failure (adjunct), initially 25 mg once daily, increased according to response to max. 50 mg once daily (see section 2.5.5)
- Resistant hypertension (adjunct), 25 mg once daily [unlicensed indication] (see section 2.5)
- Primary hyperaldosteronism in patients awaiting surgery, 100–400 mg daily; long-term maintenance if surgery inappropriate, use lowest effective dose
- CHILD under 18 years see *BNF for Children*

Spironolactone (Non-proprietary) [PoM]
Tablets, spironolactone 25 mg, net price 28 = £1.55; 50 mg, 28 = £1.97; 100 mg, 28 = £2.43. Label: 21
Oral suspensions, spironolactone 5 mg/5 mL, 10 mg/5 mL, 25 mg/5 mL, 50 mg/5 mL, and 100 mg/5 mL. Label: 21
Available from 'special-order' manufacturers or specialist importing companies, see p. 1124

Aldactone® (Pharmacia) [PoM]
Tablets, f/c, spironolactone 25 mg (buff), net price 100-tab pack = £8.89; 50 mg (white), 100-tab pack = £17.78; 100 mg (buff), 28-tab pack = £9.96. Label: 21

◢**With thiazides or loop diuretics**
Section 2.2.4

2.2.4 Potassium-sparing diuretics with other diuretics

Although it is preferable to prescribe thiazides (section 2.2.1) and potassium-sparing diuretics (section 2.2.3) separately, the use of fixed combinations may be justified if compliance is a problem. Potassium-sparing diuretics are not usually necessary in the routine treatment of hypertension, unless hypokalaemia develops. For **interactions**, see Appendix 1 (diuretics).

◢**Amiloride with thiazides**
Co-amilozide (Non-proprietary) [PoM]
Tablets, co-amilozide 2.5/25 (amiloride hydrochloride 2.5 mg, hydrochlorothiazide 25 mg), net price 28-tab pack = £5.95
Brands include *Moduret 25*®
Dose hypertension, initially 1 tablet daily, increased if necessary to max. 2 tablets daily
Congestive heart failure, initially 1 tablet daily, increased if necessary to max. 4 tablets daily; reduce for maintenance if possible

Oedema and ascites in cirrhosis of the liver, initially 2 tablets daily, increased if necessary to max. 4 tablets daily; reduce for maintenance if possible
Tablets, co-amilozide 5/50 (amiloride hydrochloride 5 mg, hydrochlorothiazide 50 mg), net price 28 = £1.18
Brands include *Moduretic*®
Dose hypertension, initially ½ tablet daily, increased if necessary to max. 1 tablet daily
Congestive heart failure, initially ½ tablet daily, increased if necessary to max. 2 tablets daily; reduce for maintenance if possible
Oedema and ascites in cirrhosis of the liver, initially 1 tablet daily, increased if necessary to max. 2 tablets daily; reduce for maintenance if possible

Navispare® (AMCo) [PoM]
Tablets, f/c, orange, amiloride hydrochloride 2.5 mg, cyclopenthiazide 250 micrograms, net price 28-tab pack = £3.24
Excipients include gluten
Dose hypertension, 1–2 tablets in the morning

◢**Amiloride with loop diuretics**
Co-amilofruse (Non-proprietary) [PoM]
Tablets, co-amilofruse 2.5/20 (amiloride hydrochloride 2.5 mg, furosemide 20 mg), net price 28-tab pack = £2.67, 56-tab pack = £1.95
Brands include *Frumil LS*®
Dose oedema, 1–2 tablets in the morning
Tablets, co-amilofruse 5/40 (amiloride hydrochloride 5 mg, furosemide 40 mg), net price 28-tab pack = £2.63, 56-tab pack = £2.50
Brands include *Frumil*®
Dose oedema, 1–2 tablets in the morning
Tablets, co-amilofruse 10/80 (amiloride hydrochloride 10 mg, furosemide 80 mg), net price 28-tab pack = £17.30
Dose oedema, 1 tablet in the morning

Amiloride with bumetanide (Non-proprietary) [PoM]
Tablets, amiloride hydrochloride 5 mg, bumetanide 1 mg, net price 28-tab pack = £30.30
Dose oedema, 1–2 tablets daily

◢**Triamterene with thiazides**
Counselling Urine may look slightly blue in some lights

Co-triamterzide (Non-proprietary) [PoM]
Tablets, co-triamterzide 50/25 (triamterene 50 mg, hydrochlorothiazide 25 mg), net price 30-tab pack = 95p. Label: 14, (see above), 21
Brands include *Triam-Co*®
Dose hypertension, 1 tablet daily after breakfast, increased if necessary, max. 4 daily
Oedema, 2 tablets daily (1 after breakfast and 1 after midday meal) increased to 3 daily if necessary (2 after breakfast and 1 after midday meal); usual maintenance in oedema, 1 daily or 2 on alternate days; max. 4 daily

Dyazide® (AMCo) [PoM]
Tablets, peach, scored, co-triamterzide 50/25 (triamterene 50 mg, hydrochlorothiazide 25 mg), net price 30-tab pack = 95p. Label: 14, (see above), 21
Dose hypertension, 1 tablet daily after breakfast, increased if necessary, max. 4 daily
Oedema, 2 tablets daily (1 after breakfast and 1 after midday meal) increased to 3 daily if necessary (2 after breakfast and 1 after midday meal); usual maintenance in oedema, 1 daily or 2 on alternate days; max. 4 daily

Cardiovascular system

2

Kalspare® (DHP Healthcare) ℞
Tablets, orange, f/c, scored, triamterene 50 mg, chlortalidone 50 mg, net price 28-tab pack = £9.90. Label: 14, (see above), 21
Dose hypertension, oedema, 1–2 tablets in the morning

◢**Triamterene with loop diuretics**
Counselling Urine may look slightly blue in some lights

Frusene® (Orion) ℞
Tablets, yellow, scored, triamterene 50 mg, furosemide 40 mg, net price 56-tab pack = £4.34. Label: 14, (see above)
Dose oedema, ½–2 tablets daily in the morning

◢**Spironolactone with thiazides**
Co-flumactone (Non-proprietary) ℞ ◢
Tablets, co-flumactone 25/25 (hydroflumethiazide 25 mg, spironolactone 25 mg), net price 100-tab pack = £20.23
Brands include *Aldactide 25*®
Dose congestive heart failure, initially 4 tablets daily; range 1–8 tablets daily (but not recommended because spironolactone generally given in lower dose)
Tablets, co-flumactone 50/50 (hydroflumethiazide 50 mg, spironolactone 50 mg), net price 28-tab pack = £10.70
Brands include *Aldactide 50*®
Dose congestive heart failure, initially 2 tablets daily; range 1–4 tablets daily (but not recommended because spironolactone generally given in lower dose)

◢**Spironolactone with loop diuretics**
Lasilactone® (Sanofi-Aventis) ℞
Capsules, blue/white, spironolactone 50 mg, furosemide 20 mg, net price 28-cap pack = £7.97
Dose resistant oedema, 1–4 capsules daily

2.2.5 Osmotic diuretics

Mannitol is an osmotic diuretic that can be used to treat cerebral oedema and raised intra-ocular pressure.

◢ MANNITOL

Indications see notes above; glaucoma (section 11.6)
Cautions extravasation causes inflammation and thrombophlebitis; monitor fluid and electrolyte balance, serum osmolality, and pulmonary and renal function; assess cardiac function before and during treatment; **interactions**: Appendix 1 (mannitol)
Contra-indications severe cardiac failure; severe pulmonary oedema; intracranial bleeding (except during craniotomy); anuria; severe dehydration
Renal impairment use with caution in severe impairment
Pregnancy manufacturer advises avoid unless essential—no information available
Breast-feeding manufacturer advises avoid unless essential—no information available
Side-effects *less commonly* hypotension, thrombophlebitis, fluid and electrolyte imbalance; *rarely* dry mouth, thirst, nausea, vomiting, oedema, raised intracranial pressure, arrhythmia, hypertension, pulmonary oedema, chest pain, headache, convulsions, dizziness, chills, fever, urinary retention, focal osmotic nephrosis, dehydration, cramp, blurred vision, rhinitis, skin necrosis, and hypersensitivity reactions (including urticaria and anaphylaxis); *very rarely* congestive heart failure and acute renal failure

Dose
- Cerebral oedema and raised intra-ocular pressure, by intravenous infusion over 30–60 minutes, 0.25–2 g/kg repeated if necessary 1–2 times after 4–8 hours
Note For mannitol 20%, an in-line filter is recommended (15-micron filters have been used)

Mannitol (Baxter) ℞
Intravenous infusion, mannitol 10%, net price 500-mL *Viaflo*® bag = £3.20; 20%, net price 250-mL *Viaflex*® bag = £3.78, 500-mL *Viaflex*® bag = £5.80

2.2.6 Mercurial diuretics

Mercurial diuretics are effective but are now almost never used because of their nephrotoxicity.

2.2.7 Carbonic anhydrase inhibitors

The carbonic anhydrase inhibitor **acetazolamide** is a weak diuretic and is little used for its diuretic effect. It is used for prophylaxis against mountain sickness [unlicensed indication] but is not a substitute for acclimatisation.

Acetazolamide and eye drops of dorzolamide and brinzolamide inhibit the formation of aqueous humour and are used in glaucoma (section 11.6).

2.2.8 Diuretics with potassium

Many patients on diuretics do not need potassium supplements (section 9.2.1.1). For many of those who do, the amount of potassium in combined preparations may not be enough, and for this reason their use is to be discouraged.

Diuretics with potassium and potassium-sparing diuretics should **not** usually be given together.
Counselling Modified-release potassium tablets should be swallowed whole with plenty of fluid during meals while sitting or standing

Diumide-K Continus® (Teofarma) ℞ ◢
Tablets, white/orange, f/c, furosemide 40 mg, potassium 8 mmol for modified release, net price 30-tab pack = £3.00. Label: 25, 27, counselling, see above

2.3 Anti-arrhythmic drugs

2.3.1 Management of arrhythmias
2.3.2 Drugs for arrhythmias

2.3.1 Management of arrhythmias

Management of an arrhythmia requires precise diagnosis of the type of arrhythmia, and electrocardiography is essential; underlying causes such as heart failure require appropriate treatment.

Ectopic beats If ectopic beats are spontaneous and the patient has a normal heart, treatment is rarely required and reassurance to the patient will often suffice. If they are particularly troublesome, beta-blockers are sometimes effective and may be safer than other suppressant drugs.

2   Cardiovascular system

Atrial fibrillation Treatment of patients with atrial fibrillation aims to reduce symptoms and prevent complications, especially stroke. All patients with atrial fibrillation should be assessed for their risk of stroke and thromboembolism (see below). Atrial fibrillation can be managed by either controlling the ventricular rate ('rate control') or by attempting to restore and maintain sinus rhythm ('rhythm control'). At any stage if treatment fails to control symptoms, or, if symptoms reoccur after cardioversion and specialised management is required, referral should be made within 4 weeks. If drug treatment fails to control the symptoms of atrial fibrillation or is unsuitable, ablation strategies can be considered. Review anticoagulation, stroke, and bleeding risk at least annually in all patients with atrial fibrillation.

Acute presentation

All patients with life-threatening haemodynamic instability caused by new-onset atrial fibrillation should undergo emergency electrical cardioversion without delaying to achieve anticoagulation. In patients presenting acutely but without life-threatening haemodynamic instability, rate or rhythm control can be offered if the onset of arrhythmia is less than 48 hours; rate control is preferred if onset is more than 48 hours or uncertain. Consideration of pharmacological or electrical cardioversion should be based on clinical circumstances. If pharmacological cardioversion has been agreed, intravenous amiodarone, or alternatively flecainide, can be used (amiodarone is preferred if there is structural heart disease). If urgent rate control is required, a beta-blocker or verapamil can be given intravenously.

Cardioversion

Sinus rhythm can be restored by electrical cardioversion, or pharmacological cardioversion with an oral or intravenous antiarrhythmic drug e.g. flecainide or amiodarone. If atrial fibrillation has been present for more than 48 hours, electrical cardioversion is preferred and should not be attempted until the patient has been fully anticoagulated (section 2.8.2) for at least 3 weeks; if this is not possible, parenteral anticoagulation (section 2.8.1) should be commenced, and a left atrial thrombus ruled out immediately before cardioversion; oral anticoagulation should be given after cardioversion and continued for at least 4 weeks; prior to cardioversion, offer rate control as appropriate.

Drug treatment

Rate control is the preferred first-line drug treatment strategy for atrial fibrillation except in patients with new-onset atrial fibrillation, heart failure secondary to atrial fibrillation, atrial flutter suitable for an ablation strategy, atrial fibrillation with a reversible cause, or if rhythm control is more suitable based on clinical judgement. Ventricular rate can be controlled with a standard beta-blocker (not sotalol) (section 2.4) or a rate-limiting calcium channel blocker such as diltiazem [unlicensed indication], or verapamil as monotherapy. Choice of drug should be based on individual symptoms, heart rate, comorbidities, and patient preference. Digoxin is usually only effective for controlling the ventricular rate at rest, and should therefore only be used as monotherapy in predominantly sedentary patients with non-paroxysmal atrial fibrillation. When a single drug fails to adequately control the ventricular rate, a combination of two drugs including a beta-blocker, digoxin, or diltiazem can be used. If symptoms are not controlled with a combination of two drugs, a rhythm-control strategy

should be considered. If ventricular function is diminished, the combination of a beta-blocker (that is licensed for use in heart failure) and digoxin is preferred (see section 2.5.5, and **interactions**: Appendix 1 (cardiac glycosides)). Digoxin is also used when atrial fibrillation is accompanied by congestive heart failure.

If drug treatment is required to maintain sinus rhythm ('rhythm control') post-cardioversion, a standard beta-blocker is used. If a standard beta-blocker is not appropriate or is ineffective, consider an oral anti-arrhythmic drug such as sotalol (section 2.4), flecainide, propafenone, or amiodarone; dronedarone may be considered in paroxysmal or persistent atrial fibrillation (see NICE guidance). If necessary, amiodarone can be started 4 weeks before and continuing for up to 12 months after electrical cardioversion to increase success of the procedure, and to maintain sinus rhythm. Flecainide or propafenone should not be given when there is known ischaemic or structural heart disease. Consider amiodarone in patients with left ventricular impairment and heart failure.

Paroxysmal atrial fibrillation

In symptomatic paroxysmal atrial fibrillation, ventricular rhythm is controlled with a standard beta-blocker. Alternatively, if symptoms persist or a standard beta-blocker is not appropriate, an oral anti-arrhythmic drug such as dronedarone (see NICE guidance), sotalol, flecainide, propafenone, or amiodarone can be given (see also Paroxysmal Supraventricular Tachycardia below, and Supraventricular Arrhythmias). In selected patients with infrequent episodes of symptomatic paroxysmal atrial fibrillation, sinus rhythm can be restored using the 'pill-in-the-pocket' approach; this involves the patient taking oral flecainide or propafenone to self-treat an episode of atrial fibrillation when it occurs.

Stroke prevention

All patients with atrial fibrillation should be assessed for their risk of stroke and the need for thromboprophylaxis; this needs to be balanced with the patient's risk of bleeding; a NICE[1] guideline recommends using the CHA_2DS_2-VASc assessment tool for stroke risk and the HAS-BLED tool for bleeding risk prior to and during anticoagulation. Risk factors for stroke taken into account by CHA_2DS_2-VASc include prior ischaemic stroke, transient ischaemic attacks, or thromboembolic events, heart failure, left ventricular systolic dysfunction, vascular disease, diabetes, hypertension, females, and patients over 65 years. Patients with a very low risk of stroke (CHA_2DS_2-VASc score of 0 for men or 1 for women) do not require an antithrombotic for stroke prevention. Parenteral anticoagulation should be offered to patients with new-onset atrial fibrillation who are receiving subtherapeutic or no anticoagulation therapy until assessment is made, and appropriate anticoagulation is started. Oral anticoagulation should be offered to patients with confirmed diagnosis of atrial fibrillation in whom sinus rhythm has not been successfully restored within 48 hours of onset, patients who have had, or are at high risk of recurrence of atrial fibrillation such as those with structural heart disease, prolonged history of atrial fibrillation (more than 12 months), a history of failed attempts at cardioversion, and patients whom the risk of stroke outweighs the risk of bleeding. Anticoagulation treatment should not be withheld solely because of the risk of falls, and choice of

---

1. NICE clinical guideline 180 (June 2014). Atrial fibrillation: The management of atrial fibrillation

treatment should be based on clinical features and patient preferences. Oral anticoagulation may be with a vitamin K antagonist (e.g warfarin, or in non-valvular atrial fibrillation with apixaban, dabigatran etexilate, or rivaroxaban (section 2.8.2). Anticoagulants are also indicated during cardioversion procedures (see above). Aspirin (section 2.9) is less effective than warfarin at preventing emboli; the modest benefit is offset by the risk of bleeding, and aspirin should not be offered as monotherapy solely for stroke prevention in atrial fibrillation. If anticoagulant treatment is contraindicated or not tolerated, left atrial appendage occlusion can be considered.

Atrial flutter   Like atrial fibrillation, treatment options for atrial flutter involve either controlling the ventricular rate or attempting to restore and maintain sinus rhythm. However, atrial flutter generally responds less well to drug treatment than atrial fibrillation.

Control of the ventricular rate is usually an interim measure pending restoration of sinus rhythm. Ventricular rate can be controlled by administration of a beta-blocker (section 2.4), diltiazem [unlicensed indication], or verapamil (section 2.6.2); an intravenous beta-blocker or verapamil is preferred for rapid control. Digoxin (section 2.1.1) can be added if rate control remains inadequate, and may be particularly useful in those with heart failure.

Conversion to sinus rhythm can be achieved by electrical cardioversion (by cardiac pacing or direct current), pharmacological cardioversion, or catheter ablation. If the duration of atrial flutter is unknown, or it has lasted for over 48 hours, cardioversion should not be attempted until the patient has been fully anticoagulated (see section 2.8.2) for at least 3 weeks; if this is not possible, parenteral anticoagulation (section 2.8.1) should be commenced and a left atrial thrombus ruled out immediately before cardioversion; oral anticoagulation should be given after cardioversion and continued for at least 4 weeks.

Direct current cardioversion is usually the treatment of choice when rapid conversion to sinus rhythm is necessary (e.g. when atrial flutter is associated with haemodynamic compromise); catheter ablation is preferred for the treatment of recurrent atrial flutter. There is a limited role for anti-arrhythmic drugs as their use is not always successful. Flecainide or propafenone can slow atrial flutter, resulting in 1:1 conduction to the ventricles, and should therefore be prescribed in conjunction with a ventricular rate controlling drug such as a beta-blocker, diltiazem [unlicensed indication], or verapamil. Amiodarone can be used when other drug treatments are contra-indicated or ineffective.

All patients should be assessed for their risk of stroke and the need for thromboprophylaxis; the choice of anticoagulant is based on the same criteria as for atrial fibrillation (see notes above).

Paroxysmal supraventricular tachycardia   This will often terminate spontaneously or with reflex vagal stimulation such as a Valsalva manoeuvre, immersing the face in ice-cold water, or carotid sinus massage; such manoeuvres should be performed with ECG monitoring.

If the effects of reflex vagal stimulation are transient or ineffective, or if the arrhythmia is causing severe symptoms, intravenous adenosine (section 2.3.2) should be given. If adenosine is ineffective or contra-indicated,

intravenous verapamil (section 2.6.2) is an alternative, but it should be avoided in patients recently treated with beta-blockers (see p. 139).

Failure to terminate paroxysmal supraventricular tachycardia with reflex vagal stimulation or drug treatment may suggest an arrhythmia of atrial origin, such as focal atrial tachycardia or atrial flutter.

Treatment with direct current cardioversion is needed in haemodynamically unstable patients or when the above measures have failed to restore sinus rhythm (and an alternative diagnosis has not been found).

Recurrent episodes of paroxysmal supraventricular tachycardia can be treated by catheter ablation, or prevented with drugs such as diltiazem, verapamil, beta-blockers including sotalol (section 2.4), flecainide, or propafenone (section 2.3.2).

Arrhythmias after myocardial infarction   In patients with a paroxysmal tachycardia or rapid irregularity of the pulse it is best not to administer an anti-arrhythmic until an ECG record has been obtained. Bradycardia, particularly if complicated by hypotension, should be treated with 500 micrograms of atropine sulfate given intravenously; the dose may be repeated every 3–5 minutes if necessary up to a maximum total dose of 3 mg. If there is a risk of asystole, or if the patient is unstable and has failed to respond to atropine, adrenaline should be given by intravenous infusion in a dose of 2–10 micrograms/minute, adjusted according to response.

For further advice, refer to the most recent recommendations of the Resuscitation Council (UK) available at www.resus.org.uk.

Ventricular tachycardia   Pulseless ventricular tachycardia or ventricular fibrillation should be treated with immediate defibrillation (see Cardiopulmonary Resuscitation, section 2.7.3).

Patients with unstable sustained ventricular tachycardia, who continue to deteriorate with signs of hypotension or reduced cardiac output, should receive direct current cardioversion to restore sinus rhythm. If this fails, intravenous amiodarone (section 2.3.2) should be administered and direct current cardioversion repeated.

Patients with sustained ventricular tachycardia who are haemodynamically stable can be treated with intravenous anti-arrhythmic drugs. Amiodarone is the preferred drug. Flecainide, propafenone (section 2.3.2), and, although less effective, lidocaine (section 2.3.2) have all been used. If sinus rhythm is not restored, direct current cardioversion or pacing should be considered. Catheter ablation is an alternative if cessation of the arrhythmia is not urgent. Non-sustained ventricular tachycardia can be treated with a beta-blocker (section 2.4).

All patients presenting with ventricular tachycardia should be referred to a specialist. Following restoration of sinus rhythm, patients who remain at high risk of cardiac arrest will require maintenance therapy. Most patients will be treated with an implantable cardioverter defibrillator. Beta-blockers or sotalol (in place of a standard beta-blocker), or amiodarone (in combination with a standard beta-blocker), can be used in addition to the device in some patients; alternatively, they can be used alone when use of an implantable cardioverter defibrillator is not appropriate.

2 Cardiovascular system

Torsade de pointes is a form of ventricular tachycardia associated with a long QT syndrome (usually drug-induced, but other factors including hypokalaemia, severe bradycardia, and genetic predisposition are also implicated). Episodes are usually self-limiting, but are frequently recurrent and can cause impairment or loss of consciousness. If not controlled, the arrhythmia can progress to ventricular fibrillation and sometimes death. Intravenous infusion of magnesium sulfate (section 9.5.1.3) is usually effective. A beta-blocker (but not sotalol) and atrial (or ventricular) pacing can be considered. Anti-arrhythmics can further prolong the QT interval, thus worsening the condition.

2.3.2 Drugs for arrhythmias

Anti-arrhythmic drugs can be classified clinically into those that act on supraventricular arrhythmias (e.g. verapamil), those that act on both supraventricular and ventricular arrhythmias (e.g. amiodarone), and those that act on ventricular arrhythmias (e.g. lidocaine).

Anti-arrhythmic drugs can also be classified according to their effects on the electrical behaviour of myocardial cells during activity (the Vaughan Williams classification) although this classification is of less clinical significance:

> Class I: membrane stabilising drugs (e.g. lidocaine, flecainide)
>
> Class II: beta-blockers
>
> Class III: amiodarone; sotalol (also Class II)
>
> Class IV: calcium-channel blockers (includes verapamil but not dihydropyridines)

Cautions The negative inotropic effects of anti-arrhythmic drugs tend to be additive. Therefore special care should be taken if two or more are used, especially if myocardial function is impaired. Most drugs that are effective in countering arrhythmias can also provoke them in some circumstances; moreover, hypokalaemia enhances the arrhythmogenic (pro-arrhythmic) effect of many drugs.

Supraventricular arrhythmias

Adenosine is usually the treatment of choice for terminating paroxysmal supraventricular tachycardia. As it has a very short duration of action (half-life only about 8 to 10 seconds, but prolonged in those taking dipyridamole), most side-effects are short lived. Unlike verapamil, adenosine can be used after a beta-blocker. Verapamil may be preferable to adenosine in asthma.

Dronedarone is a multi-channel blocking anti-arrhythmic drug; it is licensed for the maintenance of sinus rhythm after cardioversion in clinically stable patients with paroxysmal or persistent atrial fibrillation, when alternative treatments are unsuitable; dronedarone should be initiated and monitored under specialist supervision.

NICE guidance
Dronedarone for the treatment of non-permanent atrial fibrillation (December 2012)

Dronedarone is an option for the maintenance of sinus rhythm after successful cardioversion in paroxysmal or persistent atrial fibrillation which is not controlled by first-line therapy (usually including beta-blockers), **and** after alternative options have been considered in patients:

- who have at least 1 of the following cardiovascular risk factors: hypertension requiring drugs of at least 2 different classes, diabetes mellitus, previous transient ischaemic attack, stroke or systemic embolism, left atrial diameter of 50 mm or greater, or age 70 years or older **and**
- who do not have left ventricular systolic dysfunction nor a history of, or current, heart failure

Patients who do not meet the above criteria who are currently receiving dronedarone should have the option to continue treatment until they and their clinicians consider it appropriate to stop.

www.nice.org.uk/TA197

Oral administration of a **cardiac glycoside** (such as digoxin, section 2.1.1) slows the ventricular response in cases of atrial fibrillation and atrial flutter. However, intravenous infusion of digoxin is rarely effective for rapid control of ventricular rate. Cardiac glycosides are contra-indicated in supraventricular arrhythmias associated with accessory conducting pathways (e.g. Wolff-Parkinson-White syndrome).

Verapamil (section 2.6.2) is usually effective for supraventricular tachycardias. An initial intravenous dose (**important**: serious beta-blocker interaction hazard, see p. 139) may be followed by oral treatment; hypotension may occur with large doses. It should not be used for tachyarrhythmias where the QRS complex is wide (i.e. broad complex) unless a supraventricular origin has been established beyond reasonable doubt. It is also contra-indicated in atrial fibrillation or atrial flutter associated with accessory conducting pathways (e.g. Wolff-Parkinson-White syndrome). It should not be used in children with arrhythmias without specialist advice; some supraventricular arrhythmias in childhood can be accelerated by verapamil with dangerous consequences.

Intravenous administration of a **beta-blocker** (section 2.4) such as esmolol or propranolol, can achieve rapid control of the ventricular rate.

Drugs for both supraventricular and ventricular arrhythmias include **amiodarone, beta-blockers** (see p. 102), **disopyramide, flecainide, procainamide** (available from 'special-order' manufacturers or specialist importing companies, see p. 1124), and **propafenone**, see below under Supraventricular and Ventricular Arrhythmias.

▶ ADENOSINE

Indications rapid reversion to sinus rhythm of paroxysmal supraventricular tachycardias, including those associated with accessory conducting pathways (e.g. Wolff-Parkinson-White syndrome); aid to diagnosis of broad or narrow complex supraventricular tachycardias; in conjunction with radionuclide myocardial perfusion imaging in patients who cannot exercise adequately or for whom exercise is inappropriate

Cautions monitor ECG and have resuscitation facilities available; atrial fibrillation or flutter with accessory pathway (conduction down anomalous pathway may increase); first-degree AV block; bundle branch block; QT-interval prolongation; left main coronary artery stenosis; uncorrected hypovolaemia; stenotic valvular heart disease; left to right shunt; pericarditis; pericardial effusion; autonomic dysfunction; stenotic carotid artery disease with cerebrovascular insufficiency; recent myocardial infarction; severe heart failure; heart transplant (see below); **interactions:** Appendix 1 (adenosine)

Contra-indications second- or third-degree AV block and sick sinus syndrome (unless pacemaker fitted); long QT syndrome; severe hypotension; decompensated heart failure; chronic obstructive lung disease (including asthma)

Pregnancy large doses may produce fetal toxicity; manufacturer advises use only if potential benefit outweighs risk

Breast-feeding no information available—unlikely to be present in milk owing to short half-life

Side-effects nausea, arrhythmia (discontinue if asystole or severe bradycardia occur), sinus pause, AV block, flushing, angina (discontinue), dizziness, dyspnoea, headache, apprehension; *less commonly* metallic taste, palpitation, hyperventilation, weakness, blurred vision, sweating; *very rarely* transient worsening of intracranial hypertension, bronchospasm, injection-site reactions; *also reported* vomiting, syncope, hypotension (discontinue if severe), cardiac arrest, respiratory failure (discontinue), convulsions

Dose
- By rapid intravenous injection into central or large peripheral vein, 6 mg over 2 seconds with cardiac monitoring; if necessary followed by 12 mg after 1–2 minutes, and then by 12 mg after a further 1–2 minutes; increments should not be given if high level AV block develops at any particular dose

 Important Patients with a **heart transplant** are very sensitive to effects of adenosine and should receive initial dose of 3 mg over 2 seconds, followed if necessary by 6 mg after 1–2 minutes, and then by 12 mg after a further 1–2 minutes.

 Also, if essential to give with dipyridamole reduce adenosine dose to a quarter of the usual dose

 Note Adenosine doses in the BNF may differ from those in product literature

- By intravenous infusion in conjunction with radionuclide myocardial perfusion imaging—consult product literature

Adenosine (Non-proprietary) (PoM)
 Injection, adenosine 3 mg/mL, net price 2-mL vial = £4.45 (hosp. only)
 Intravenous infusion, adenosine 3 mg/mL, net price 10-mL vial = £11.67 (hosp. only)

Adenocor® (Sanofi-Aventis) (PoM)
 Injection, adenosine 3 mg/mL, net price 2-mL vial = £4.99 (hosp. only)
 Electrolytes Na⁺ 0.15 mmol/mL

Adenoscan® (Sanofi-Aventis) (PoM)
 Intravenous infusion, adenosine 3 mg/mL, net price 10-mL vial = £14.26 (hosp. only)
 Electrolytes Na⁺ 0.15 mmol/mL

◼ DRONEDARONE

Indications see notes above

Cautions monitor liver function (see Hepatic Disorders below); monitor for heart failure (see Heart

Failure below); perform ECG at least every 6 months—consider discontinuation if atrial fibrillation reoccurs; coronary artery disease; correct hypokalaemia and hypomagnesaemia before starting and during treatment; measure serum creatinine before treatment and 7 days after initiation—if raised, measure again after a further 7 days and consider discontinuation if creatinine continues to rise; **interactions:** Appendix 1 (dronedarone)

 Hepatic disorders Liver injury, including life-threatening acute liver failure reported rarely; monitor liver function before treatment, 1 week and 1 month after initiation of treatment, then monthly for 6 months, then every 3 months for 6 months and periodically thereafter—discontinue treatment if 2 consecutive alanine aminotransferase concentrations exceed 3 times upper limit of normal. Patients or their carers should be told how to recognise signs of liver disorder and advised to seek prompt medical attention if symptoms such as abdominal pain, anorexia, nausea, vomiting, fever, malaise, itching, dark urine, or jaundice develop

 Heart failure New-onset or worsening heart failure reported; patients or their carers should be told how to recognise signs of heart failure and advised to seek prompt medical attention if symptoms such as weight gain, dependent oedema, or dyspnoea develop or worsen; if heart failure or left ventricular systolic dysfunction develops, discontinue treatment

Contra-indications liver or lung toxicity associated with previous amiodarone use; second- or third-degree AV block, complete bundle branch block, distal block, sinus node dysfunction, atrial conduction defects, or sick sinus syndrome (unless pacemaker fitted); permanent atrial fibrillation; bradycardia; prolonged QT interval; existing or previous heart failure or left ventricular systolic dysfunction (see also Heart Failure above); haemodynamically unstable patients

Hepatic impairment avoid in severe impairment; see also Hepatic Disorders above

Renal impairment avoid if eGFR less than 30 mL/minute/1.73 m²

Pregnancy manufacturer advises avoid—toxicity in *animal* studies

Breast-feeding manufacturer advises avoid—present in milk in *animal* studies

Side-effects gastro-intestinal disturbances, QT-interval prolongation, bradycardia, heart failure (see also Heart Failure above), malaise, rash, pruritus, raised serum creatinine; *less commonly* taste disturbance, interstitial lung disease including pneumonitis and pulmonary fibrosis (investigate if symptoms such as dyspnoea or dry cough develop and discontinue treatment if confirmed), erythema, eczema, dermatitis, photosensitivity; *rarely* liver injury (including life-threatening acute liver failure—see also Hepatic Disorders above)

Dose
- ADULT over 18 years, 400 mg twice daily

Multaq® (Sanofi-Aventis) ▼ (PoM)
 Tablets, f/c, dronedarone (as hydrochloride) 400 mg, net price 20-tab pack = £22.50, 60-tab pack = £67.50. Label: 21, counselling, hepatic disorders, heart failure

Supraventricular and ventricular arrhythmias

Amiodarone is used in the treatment of arrhythmias, particularly when other drugs are ineffective or contra-indicated. It can be used for paroxysmal supraventricular, nodal and ventricular tachycardias, atrial fibrillation and flutter, and ventricular fibrillation. It can also be used for tachyarrhythmias associated with Wolff-Parkinson-White syndrome. It should be initiated only under hospital or specialist supervision. Amiodarone may be given by intravenous infusion as well as by mouth, and has the advantage of causing little or no myocardial depression. Unlike oral amiodarone, intravenous amiodarone acts relatively rapidly.

Intravenous injection of amiodarone can be used in cardiopulmonary resuscitation for ventricular fibrillation or pulseless tachycardia unresponsive to other interventions (section 2.7.3).

Amiodarone has a very long half-life (extending to several weeks) and only needs to be given once daily (but high doses can cause nausea unless divided). Many weeks or months may be required to achieve steady-state plasma-amiodarone concentration; this is particularly important when drug interactions are likely (see also Appendix 1).

Most patients taking amiodarone develop corneal microdeposits (reversible on withdrawal of treatment); these rarely interfere with vision, but drivers may be dazzled by headlights at night. However, if vision is impaired or if optic neuritis or optic neuropathy occur, amiodarone must be stopped to prevent blindness and expert advice sought. Because of the possibility of phototoxic reactions, patients should be advised to shield the skin from light during treatment and for several months after discontinuing amiodarone; a wide-spectrum sunscreen (section 13.8.1) to protect against both long-wave ultraviolet and visible light should be used.

Amiodarone contains iodine and can cause disorders of thyroid function; both hypothyroidism and hyperthyroidism may occur. Clinical assessment alone is unreliable, and laboratory tests should be performed before treatment and every 6 months. Thyroxine (T4) may be raised in the absence of hyperthyroidism; therefore tri-iodothyronine (T3), T4, and thyroid-stimulating hormone (thyrotrophin, TSH) should all be measured. A raised T3 and T4 with a very low or undetectable TSH concentration suggests the development of thyrotoxicosis. The thyrotoxicosis may be very refractory, and amiodarone should usually be withdrawn at least temporarily to help achieve control; treatment with carbimazole may be required. Hypothyroidism can be treated with replacement therapy without withdrawing amiodarone if it is essential; careful supervision is required.

Pneumonitis should always be suspected if new or progressive shortness of breath or cough develops in a patient taking amiodarone. Fresh neurological symptoms should raise the possibility of peripheral neuropathy.

Amiodarone is also associated with hepatotoxicity and treatment should be discontinued if severe liver function abnormalities or clinical signs of liver disease develop.

Beta-blockers act as anti-arrhythmic drugs principally by attenuating the effects of the sympathetic system on automaticity and conductivity within the heart, for details see section 2.4. For special reference to the role of sotalol in ventricular arrhythmias, see p. 102.

Disopyramide can be given by intravenous injection to control arrhythmias after myocardial infarction (including those not responding to lidocaine), but it impairs cardiac contractility. Oral administration of disopyramide is useful, but it has an antimuscarinic effect

which limits its use in patients susceptible to angle-closure glaucoma or with prostatic hyperplasia.

Flecainide belongs to the same general class as lidocaine and may be of value for serious symptomatic ventricular arrhythmias. It may also be indicated for junctional re-entry tachycardias and for paroxysmal atrial fibrillation. However, it can precipitate serious arrhythmias in a small minority of patients (including those with otherwise normal hearts).

Propafenone is used for the prophylaxis and treatment of ventricular arrhythmias and also for some supraventricular arrhythmias. It has complex mechanisms of action, including weak beta-blocking activity (therefore caution is needed in obstructive airways disease—contra-indicated if severe).

Drugs for supraventricular arrhythmias include **adenosine**, **cardiac glycosides**, and **verapamil**; see above under Supraventricular Arrhythmias. Drugs for ventricular arrhythmias include **lidocaine**; see under Ventricular Arrhythmias, p. 100.

Mexiletine and procainamide are both available from 'special-order' manufacturers or specialist importing companies, see p. 1124. Mexiletine can be used for life-threatening ventricular arrhythmias; procainamide is given by intravenous injection to control ventricular arrhythmias.

◼ AMIODARONE HYDROCHLORIDE

Indications   see notes above (should be initiated in hospital or under specialist supervision)

Cautions   liver-function and thyroid-function tests required before treatment and then every 6 months (see notes above for tests of thyroid function); hypokalaemia (measure serum-potassium concentration before treatment); chest x-ray required before treatment; heart failure; elderly; severe bradycardia and conduction disturbances in excessive dosage; intravenous use may cause moderate and transient fall in blood pressure (circulatory collapse precipitated by rapid administration or overdosage) or severe hepatocellular toxicity (monitor transaminases closely); administration by central venous catheter recommended if repeated or continuous infusion required—infusion via peripheral veins may cause pain and inflammation; ECG monitoring and resuscitation facilities must be available during intravenous use; acute porphyria (section 9.8.2); extreme caution or avoid concomitant use of drugs that prolong QT interval; **interactions**: Appendix 1 (amiodarone)

Contra-indications   (except in cardiac arrest) sinus bradycardia, sino-atrial heart block; unless pacemaker fitted avoid in severe conduction disturbances or sinus node disease; thyroid dysfunction; iodine sensitivity; avoid *intravenous use* in severe respiratory failure, circulatory collapse, or severe arterial hypotension; avoid bolus injection in congestive heart failure or cardiomyopathy

Pregnancy   possible risk of neonatal goitre; use only if no alternative

Breast-feeding   avoid; present in milk in significant amounts; theoretical risk of neonatal hypothyroidism from release of iodine

Side-effects   nausea, vomiting, taste disturbances, raised serum transaminases (may require dose reduction or withdrawal if accompanied by acute liver disorders), jaundice; bradycardia (see Cautions);

pulmonary toxicity (including pneumonitis and fibrosis); tremor, sleep disorders; hypothyroidism, hyperthyroidism; reversible corneal microdeposits (sometimes with night glare); phototoxicity, persistent slate-grey skin discoloration (see also notes above), injection-site reactions; *less commonly* onset or worsening of arrhythmia, conduction disturbances (see Cautions), peripheral neuropathy and myopathy (usually reversible on withdrawal); *very rarely* chronic liver disease including cirrhosis, sinus arrest, bronchospasm (in patients with severe respiratory failure), ataxia, benign intracranial hypertension, headache, vertigo, epididymo-orchitis, impotence, haemolytic or aplastic anaemia, thrombocytopenia, rash (including exfoliative dermatitis), hypersensitivity including vasculitis, alopecia, impaired vision due to optic neuritis or optic neuropathy (including blindness), anaphylaxis on rapid injection, also hypotension, respiratory distress syndrome, sweating, and hot flushes

Dose
- By mouth, 200 mg 3 times daily for 1 week reduced to 200 mg twice daily for a further week; maintenance, usually 200 mg daily or the minimum required to control the arrhythmia
- By intravenous infusion (see Cautions above), initially 5 mg/kg over 20–120 minutes with ECG monitoring; subsequent infusion given if necessary according to response up to max. 1.2 g in 24 hours
- Ventricular fibrillation or pulseless ventricular tachycardia refractory to defibrillation, section 2.7.3

Amiodarone (Non-proprietary) (PoM)
Tablets, amiodarone hydrochloride 100 mg, net price 28-tab pack = £1.23; 200 mg, 28-tab pack = £2.00. Label: 11
Injection, amiodarone hydrochloride 30 mg/mL, net price 10-mL prefilled syringe = £13.50
Excipients may include benzyl alcohol (avoid in neonates unless no safer alternative available, see Excipients, p. 2)
Sterile concentrate, amiodarone hydrochloride 50 mg/mL, net price 3-mL amp = £1.33, 6-mL amp = £2.86. For dilution and use as an infusion
Excipients may include benzyl alcohol (avoid in neonates unless no safer alternative available, see Excipients, p. 2)

Cordarone X® (Sanofi-Aventis) (PoM)
Tablets, scored, amiodarone hydrochloride 100 mg, net price 28-tab pack = £4.28; 200 mg, 28-tab pack = £6.99. Label: 11
Sterile concentrate, amiodarone hydrochloride 50 mg/mL, net price 3-mL amp = £1.60. For dilution and use as an infusion
Excipients include benzyl alcohol (avoid in neonates unless no safer alternative available, see Excipients, p. 2)

◢ DISOPYRAMIDE

Indications prevention and treatment of ventricular and supraventricular arrhythmias, including after myocardial infarction; maintenance of sinus rhythm after cardioversion

Cautions monitor for hypotension, hypoglycaemia, ventricular tachycardia, ventricular fibrillation or torsade de pointes (discontinue if occur); monitor serum potassium; atrial flutter or atrial tachycardia with partial block, structural heart disease, heart failure (avoid if severe); prostatic enlargement; susceptibility to angle-closure glaucoma; myasthenia gravis;

elderly; avoid in acute porphyria (section 9.8.2); **interactions**: Appendix 1 (disopyramide)

Contra-indications second- and third-degree AV block or bifascicular block (unless pacemaker fitted), bundle-branch block associated with first-degree AV block; severe sinus node dysfunction; severe heart failure (unless secondary to arrhythmia)

Hepatic impairment half-life prolonged—may need dose reduction; avoid modified-release preparation

Renal impairment reduce dose by increasing dose interval; adjust according to response; avoid modified-release preparation

Pregnancy manufacturer advises use only if potential benefit outweighs risk; may induce labour if used in third trimester

Breast-feeding present in milk—use only if essential and monitor infant for antimuscarinic effects

Side-effects ventricular tachycardia, ventricular fibrillation or torsade de pointes (usually associated with prolongation of QRS complex or QT interval—see Cautions above), myocardial depression, hypotension, AV block; antimuscarinic effects include dry mouth, blurred vision, urinary retention, and very rarely angle-closure glaucoma; gastro-intestinal irritation; psychosis, cholestatic jaundice, hypoglycaemia also reported (see Cautions above)

Dose
- By mouth, 300–800 mg daily in divided doses
- By slow intravenous injection, 2 mg/kg over at least 5 minutes to a max. of 150 mg, with ECG monitoring, followed immediately *either* by 200 mg by mouth, then 200 mg every 8 hours for 24 hours *or* 400 micrograms/kg/hour by intravenous infusion; max. 300 mg in first hour and 800 mg daily

Disopyramide (Non-proprietary) (PoM)
Capsules, disopyramide (as phosphate) 100 mg, net price 84 = £21.83; 150 mg, 84 = £18.76

Rythmodan® (Sanofi-Aventis) (PoM)
Capsules, disopyramide 100 mg (green/beige), net price 84-cap pack = £14.14; 150 mg, 84-cap pack = £18.76
Injection, disopyramide (as phosphate) 10 mg/mL, net price 5-mL amp = £2.61

◢ Modified release
Rythmodan Retard® (Sanofi-Aventis) (PoM)
Tablets, m/r, scored, f/c, disopyramide (as phosphate) 250 mg, net price 60-tab pack = £32.08. Label: 25
Dose 250–375 mg every 12 hours

◢ FLECAINIDE ACETATE

Indications *capsules, tablets, and injection:* AV nodal reciprocating tachycardia, arrhythmias associated with accessory conducting pathways (e.g. Wolff-Parkinson-White syndrome), disabling symptoms of paroxysmal atrial fibrillation in patients without left ventricular dysfunction (arrhythmias of recent onset will respond more readily)

Immediate-release tablets only: symptomatic sustained ventricular tachycardia, disabling symptoms of premature ventricular contractions or non-sustained ventricular tachycardia in patients resistant to or intolerant of other therapy

Injection only: ventricular tachyarrhythmias resistant to other treatment

2 Cardiovascular system

Cautions patients with pacemakers (especially those who may be pacemaker dependent because stimulation threshold may rise appreciably); atrial fibrillation following heart surgery; elderly (accumulation may occur); ECG monitoring and resuscitation facilities must be available during intravenous use; **interactions**: Appendix 1 (flecainide)

Contra-indications heart failure; abnormal left ventricular function; history of myocardial infarction and either asymptomatic ventricular ectopics or asymptomatic non-sustained ventricular tachycardia; long-standing atrial fibrillation where conversion to sinus rhythm not attempted; haemodynamically significant valvular heart disease; avoid in sinus node dysfunction, atrial conduction defects, second-degree or greater AV block, bundle branch block or distal block unless pacing rescue available

Hepatic impairment avoid (or reduce dose) in severe liver disease

Renal impairment reduce initial oral dose to max. 100 mg daily or reduce intravenous dose by 50%, if eGFR less than 35 mL/minute/1.73 m^2

Pregnancy used in pregnancy to treat maternal and fetal arrhythmias in specialist centres; toxicity reported in *animal* studies; infant hyperbilirubinaemia also reported

Breast-feeding significant amount present in milk but not known to be harmful

Side-effects oedema, pro-arrhythmic effects; dyspnoea; dizziness, asthenia, fatigue, fever; visual disturbances; *rarely* pneumonitis, hallucinations, depression, confusion, amnesia, dyskinesia, convulsions, peripheral neuropathy; *also reported* gastrointestinal disturbances, anorexia, hepatic dysfunction, flushing, syncope, drowsiness, tremor, vertigo, headache, anxiety, insomnia, ataxia, paraesthesia, anaemia, leucopenia, thrombocytopenia, corneal deposits, tinnitus, increased antinuclear antibodies, hypersensitivity reactions (including rash, urticaria, and photosensitivity), increased sweating

Dose
- By mouth (initiated under direction of hospital consultant), ventricular arrhythmias, initially 100 mg twice daily (max. 400 mg daily usually reserved for rapid control or in heavily built patients), reduced after 3–5 days to the lowest dose that controls arrhythmia

  Supraventricular arrhythmias, 50 mg twice daily, increased if required to max. 300 mg daily
- By slow intravenous injection (in hospital), 2 mg/kg over 10–30 minutes, max. 150 mg, with ECG monitoring; followed if required by infusion at a rate of 1.5 mg/kg/hour for 1 hour, subsequently reduced to 100–250 micrograms/kg/hour for up to 24 hours; max. cumulative dose in first 24 hours, 600 mg; transfer to *oral* treatment, as above

Flecainide (Non-proprietary) [PoM]
Tablets, flecainide acetate 50 mg, net price 60-tab pack = £3.55; 100 mg, 60-tab pack = £5.11

Tambocor® (Meda) [PoM]
Tablets, flecainide acetate 50 mg, net price 60-tab pack = £11.57; 100 mg (scored), 60-tab pack = £16.53

Injection, flecainide acetate 10 mg/mL, net price 15-mL amp = £4.40

◢Modified release
Tambocor® XL (Meda) [PoM]
Capsules, m/r, grey/pink, flecainide acetate 200 mg, net price 30-cap pack = £14.77. Label: 25
Dose supraventricular arrhythmias, 200 mg once daily
Note Not to be used to control arrhythmias in acute situations; patients stabilised on 200 mg daily immediate-release flecainide may be transferred to *Tambocor® XL*

PROPAFENONE HYDROCHLORIDE

Indications ventricular arrhythmias; paroxysmal supraventricular tachyarrhythmias which include paroxysmal atrial flutter or fibrillation and paroxysmal re-entrant tachycardias involving the AV node or accessory pathway, where standard therapy ineffective or contra-indicated

Cautions heart failure; elderly; pacemaker patients; potential for conversion of paroxysmal atrial fibrillation to atrial flutter with 2:1 or 1:1 conduction block; great caution in obstructive airways disease owing to beta-blocking activity (contra-indicated if severe); **interactions**: Appendix 1 (propafenone)
Driving May affect performance of skilled tasks e.g. driving

Contra-indications uncontrolled congestive heart failure with left ventricular ejection fraction less than 35%, cardiogenic shock (except arrhythmia induced), myocardial infarction within last 3 months, severe bradycardia, Brugada syndrome, electrolyte disturbances, severe obstructive pulmonary disease, marked hypotension; myasthenia gravis; unless adequately paced avoid in sinus node dysfunction, atrial conduction defects, second degree or greater AV block, bundle branch block or distal block

Pregnancy use only if potential benefit outweighs risk
Breast-feeding use with caution—present in milk
Side-effects abdominal pain, nausea, vomiting, diarrhoea, constipation, dry mouth, taste disturbance, sino-atrial, atrioventricular, or intraventricular blocks, bradycardia, tachycardia, palpitation, chest pain, dyspnoea, dizziness, malaise, anxiety, sleep disorders, headache, blurred vision; *less commonly* abdominal distension, flatulence, anorexia, pro-arrhythmic effects, hypotension, syncope, ataxia, paraesthesia, erectile dysfunction, thrombocytopenia, vertigo, rash; *also reported* jaundice, cholestasis, hepatitis, convulsions, confusion, restlessness, extrapyramidal symptoms, reduced sperm count (reversible on withdrawal), agranulocytosis, leucopenia, granulocytopenia, lupus erythematosus-like syndrome

Dose
- ADULT over 18 years, initially 150 mg 3 times daily after food under direct hospital supervision with ECG monitoring and blood pressure control (if QRS interval prolonged by more than 20%, reduce dose or discontinue until ECG returns to normal limits); may be increased at intervals of at least 3 days (ELDERLY at least 5 days) to 300 mg twice daily and, if necessary, to max. 300 mg 3 times daily; body-weight under 70 kg, reduce total daily dose

Arythmol® (Abbott Healthcare) [PoM]
Tablets, f/c, propafenone hydrochloride 150 mg, net price 90-tab pack = £7.37; 300 mg, 60-tab pack = £9.34. Label: 21, 25, counselling, driving

Ventricular arrhythmias

Intravenous **lidocaine** can be used for the treatment of ventricular tachycardia in haemodynamically stable patients (section 2.3.1), and ventricular fibrillation and pulseless ventricular tachycardia in cardiac arrest refractory to defibrillation (section 2.7.3), however it is no longer the anti-arrhythmic drug of first choice.

Drugs for both supraventricular and ventricular arrhythmias include **amiodarone, beta-blockers, disopyramide, flecainide, procainamide** (available from 'special-order' manufacturers or specialist importing companies, see p. 1124), and **propafenone**, see above under Supraventricular and Ventricular Arrhythmias.

Mexiletine is available from 'special-order' manufacturers or specialist importing companies (see p. 1124) for treatment of life-threatening ventricular arrhythmias.

LIDOCAINE HYDROCHLORIDE
(Lignocaine hydrochloride)

Indications ventricular arrhythmias, especially after myocardial infarction; eye (section 11.7); local anaesthesia (section 15.2)

Cautions lower doses in congestive cardiac failure and following cardiac surgery; monitor ECG and have resuscitation facilities available; elderly; acute porphyria (consider infusion with glucose for its anti-porphyrinogenic effects); **interactions:** Appendix 1 (lidocaine)

Contra-indications sino-atrial disorders, all grades of atrioventricular block, severe myocardial depression

Hepatic impairment caution—increased risk of side-effects

Renal impairment possible accumulation of lidocaine and active metabolite; caution in severe impairment

Pregnancy crosses the placenta but not known to be harmful in *animal* studies—use if benefit outweighs risk

Breast-feeding present in milk but amount too small to be harmful

Side-effects dizziness, paraesthesia, or drowsiness (particularly if injection too rapid); other CNS effects include confusion, respiratory depression and convulsions; hypotension and bradycardia (may lead to cardiac arrest); *rarely* hypersensitivity reactions including anaphylaxis

Dose

- By intravenous injection, in patients without gross circulatory impairment, 100 mg as a bolus over a few minutes (50 mg in lighter patients or those whose circulation is severely impaired), followed immediately by infusion of 4 mg/minute for 30 minutes, 2 mg/minute for 2 hours, then 1 mg/minute; reduce concentration further if infusion continued beyond 24 hours (ECG monitoring and specialist advice for infusion)

  Note Following *intravenous injection* lidocaine has a short duration of action (lasting for 15–20 minutes). If an *intravenous infusion* is not immediately available the initial *intravenous injection* of 50–100 mg can be repeated if necessary once or twice at intervals of not less than 10 minutes

Lidocaine (Non-proprietary) [PoM]

Injection 1%, lidocaine hydrochloride 10 mg/mL, net price 2-mL amp = 28p; 5-mL amp = 27p; 10-mL amp = 42p; 20-mL amp = 79p

Injection 2%, lidocaine hydrochloride 20 mg/mL, net price 2-mL amp = 31p; 5-mL amp = 32p; 10-mL amp = 60p; 20-mL amp = 85p

Infusion, lidocaine hydrochloride 0.1% (1 mg/mL) and 0.2% (2 mg/mL) in glucose intravenous infusion 5%. 500-mL containers

Minijet® Lignocaine (UCB Pharma) [PoM]

Injection, lidocaine hydrochloride 1% (10 mg/mL), net price 10-mL disposable syringe = £8.48; 2% (20 mg/mL), 5-mL disposable syringe = £8.18

2.4 Beta-adrenoceptor blocking drugs

Beta-adrenoceptor blocking drugs (beta-blockers) block the beta-adrenoceptors in the heart, peripheral vasculature, bronchi, pancreas, and liver.

Many beta-blockers are now available and in general they are all equally effective. There are, however, differences between them, which may affect choice in treating particular diseases or individual patients.

Intrinsic sympathomimetic activity (ISA, partial agonist activity) represents the capacity of beta-blockers to stimulate as well as to block adrenergic receptors. **Oxprenolol, pindolol, acebutolol,** and **celiprolol** have intrinsic sympathomimetic activity; they tend to cause less bradycardia than the other beta-blockers and may also cause less coldness of the extremities.

Some beta-blockers are lipid soluble and some are water soluble. **Atenolol, celiprolol, nadolol,** and **sotalol** are the most water-soluble; they are less likely to enter the brain, and may therefore cause less sleep disturbance and nightmares. Water-soluble beta-blockers are excreted by the kidneys and dosage reduction is often necessary in renal impairment.

Beta-blockers with a relatively short duration of action have to be given two or three times daily. Many of these are, however, available in modified-release formulations so that administration once daily is adequate for hypertension. For angina twice-daily treatment may sometimes be needed even with a modified-release formulation. Some beta-blockers, such as atenolol, bisoprolol, celiprolol, and nadolol, have an intrinsically longer duration of action and need to be given only once daily.

Beta-blockers slow the heart and can depress the myocardium; they are contra-indicated in patients with second- or third-degree heart block. Beta-blockers should also be avoided in patients with worsening unstable heart failure; care is required when initiating a beta-blocker in those with stable heart failure (see also section 2.5.5). **Sotalol** may prolong the QT interval, and it occasionally causes life-threatening ventricular arrhythmias (**important:** particular care is required to avoid hypokalaemia in patients taking sotalol).

Labetalol, celiprolol, carvedilol, and **nebivolol** are beta-blockers that have, in addition, an arteriolar vasodilating action, by diverse mechanisms, and thus lower peripheral resistance. There is no evidence that these drugs have important advantages over other beta-blockers in the treatment of hypertension.

Beta-blockers can precipitate bronchospasm and should therefore usually be avoided in patients with a history of asthma. When there is no suitable alternative, it may be necessary for a patient with well-controlled asthma, or chronic obstructive pulmonary disease (without significant reversible airways obstruction), to receive treatment with a beta-blocker for a co-existing condition (e.g. heart failure or following myocardial infarction). In this situation, a cardioselective beta-blocker should be selected and initiated at a low dose by a specialist; the patient should be closely monitored for adverse effects.

2 Cardiovascular system

Atenolol, bisoprolol, metoprolol, nebivolol, and (to a lesser extent) acebutolol, have less effect on the beta$_2$ (bronchial) receptors and are, therefore, relatively *cardioselective*, but they are not *cardiospecific*. They have a lesser effect on airways resistance but are not free of this side-effect.

Beta-blockers are also associated with fatigue, coldness of the extremities (may be less common with those with ISA, see above), and sleep disturbances with nightmares (may be less common with the water-soluble beta-blockers, see above).

Beta-blockers can affect carbohydrate metabolism, causing hypoglycaemia or hyperglycaemia in patients with or without diabetes; they can also interfere with metabolic and autonomic responses to hypoglycaemia, thereby masking symptoms such as tachycardia. However, beta-blockers are not contra-indicated in diabetes, although the cardioselective beta-blockers (see above) may be preferred. Beta-blockers should be avoided altogether in those with frequent episodes of hypoglycaemia. Beta-blockers, especially when combined with a thiazide diuretic, should be avoided for the routine treatment of uncomplicated hypertension in patients with diabetes or in those at high risk of developing diabetes.

Pregnancy   Beta-blockers may cause intra-uterine growth restriction, neonatal hypoglycaemia, and bradycardia; the risk is greater in severe hypertension. The use of labetalol in maternal hypertension is not known to be harmful, except possibly in the first trimester. Information on the safety of carvedilol during pregnancy is lacking. If beta-blockers are used close to delivery, infants should be monitored for signs of beta-blockade (and alpha-blockade with labetalol or carvedilol). For the treatment of hypertension in pregnancy, see section 2.5.

Breast-feeding   Infants should be monitored as there is a risk of possible toxicity due to beta-blockade (and alpha-blockade with labetalol or carvedilol), but the amount of most beta-blockers present in milk is too small to affect infants. Acebutolol, atenolol, nadolol, and sotalol are present in milk in greater amounts than other beta-blockers. The manufacturers of celiprolol, esmolol, nebivolol, and timolol advise avoidance if breast-feeding.

Hypertension   The mode of action of beta-blockers in hypertension is not understood, but they reduce cardiac output, alter baroceptor reflex sensitivity, and block peripheral adrenoceptors. Some beta-blockers depress plasma renin secretion. It is possible that a central effect may also partly explain their mode of action.

Beta-blockers are effective for reducing blood pressure but other antihypertensives (section 2.5) are usually more effective for reducing the incidence of stroke, myocardial infarction, and cardiovascular mortality, especially in the elderly. Other antihypertensives are therefore preferred for routine initial treatment of uncomplicated hypertension.

In general, the dose of a beta-blocker does not have to be high; for example, atenolol is given in a dose of 25–50 mg daily and it is rarely necessary to increase the dose to 100 mg.

Beta-blockers can be used to control the pulse rate in patients with *phaeochromocytoma* (section 2.5.4). However, they should never be used alone as beta-blockade without concurrent alpha-blockade may lead to a hypertensive crisis. For this reason phenoxybenzamine should always be used together with the beta-blocker.

Angina   By reducing cardiac work beta-blockers improve exercise tolerance and relieve symptoms in patients with *angina* (for further details on the management of stable angina and acute coronary syndromes, see section 2.10.1). As with hypertension there is no good evidence of the superiority of any one drug, although occasionally a patient will respond better to one beta-blocker than to another. There is some evidence that sudden withdrawal may cause an exacerbation of angina and therefore gradual reduction of dose is preferable when beta-blockers are to be stopped. There is a risk of precipitating heart failure when beta-blockers and verapamil are used together in established ischaemic heart disease (**important**: see p. 139).

Myocardial infarction   For advice on the management of ST-segment elevation myocardial infarction and non-ST-segment elevation myocardial infarction, see section 2.10.1. Several studies have shown that some beta-blockers can reduce the recurrence rate of *myocardial infarction*. However, uncontrolled heart failure, hypotension, bradyarrhythmias, and obstructive airways disease render beta-blockers unsuitable in some patients following a myocardial infarction. **Atenolol** and **metoprolol** may reduce early mortality after intravenous and subsequent oral administration in the acute phase, while **acebutolol**, **metoprolol**, **propranolol**, and **timolol** have protective value when started in the early convalescent phase. The evidence relating to other beta-blockers is less convincing; some have not been tested in trials of secondary prevention. Sudden cessation of a beta-blocker can cause a rebound worsening of myocardial ischaemia.

Arrhythmias   Beta-blockers act as *anti-arrhythmic drugs* principally by attenuating the effects of the sympathetic system on automaticity and conductivity within the heart. They can be used in conjunction with digoxin to control the ventricular response in atrial fibrillation, especially in patients with thyrotoxicosis. Beta-blockers are also useful in the management of supraventricular tachycardias, and are used to control those following myocardial infarction (see above).

Esmolol is a relatively cardioselective beta-blocker with a very short duration of action, used intravenously for the short-term treatment of supraventricular arrhythmias, sinus tachycardia, or hypertension, particularly in the peri-operative period. It may also be used in other situations, such as acute myocardial infarction, when sustained beta-blockade might be hazardous.

Sotalol, a non-cardioselective beta-blocker with additional class III anti-arrhythmic activity, is used for prophylaxis in paroxysmal supraventricular arrhythmias. It also suppresses ventricular ectopic beats and non-sustained ventricular tachycardia. It has been shown to be more effective than lidocaine in the termination of spontaneous sustained ventricular tachycardia due to coronary disease or cardiomyopathy. However, it may induce torsade de pointes in susceptible patients.

Heart failure   Beta-blockers may produce benefit in heart failure by blocking sympathetic activity. **Bisoprolol** and **carvedilol** reduce mortality in any grade of stable heart failure; **nebivolol** is licensed for stable mild to moderate heart failure in patients over 70 years. Treatment should be initiated by those experienced in the management of heart failure (section 2.5.5).

Thyrotoxicosis   Beta-blockers are used in pre-operative preparation for thyroidectomy. Administration of propranolol can reverse clinical symptoms of *thyrotoxicosis* within 4 days. Routine tests of increased thyroid function remain unaltered. The thyroid gland is rendered less vascular thus making surgery easier (section 6.2.2).

Other uses   Beta-blockers have been used to alleviate some symptoms of *anxiety*; probably patients with palpitation, tremor, and tachycardia respond best (see also section 4.1.2 and section 4.9.3). Beta-blockers are also used in the *prophylaxis of migraine* (section 4.7.4.2). Betaxolol, carteolol, levobunolol, and timolol are used topically in *glaucoma* (section 11.6).

▉ PROPRANOLOL HYDROCHLORIDE

Indications   see under Dose

Cautions   see notes above; also avoid abrupt withdrawal especially in ischaemic heart disease; first-degree AV block; portal hypertension (risk of deterioration in liver function); diabetes; history of obstructive airways disease (introduce cautiously and monitor lung function—see notes above); myasthenia gravis; symptoms of hypoglycaemia and thyrotoxicosis may be masked (also see notes above); psoriasis; history of hypersensitivity—may increase sensitivity to allergens and result in more serious hypersensitivity response, also may reduce response to adrenaline (epinephrine) (see also section 3.4.3); **interactions:** Appendix 1 (beta-blockers), **important:** verapamil interaction, see also p. 139

Contra-indications   asthma (but see notes above), uncontrolled heart failure, Prinzmetal's angina, marked bradycardia, hypotension, sick sinus syndrome, second- or third- degree AV block, cardiogenic shock, metabolic acidosis, severe peripheral arterial disease; phaeochromocytoma (apart from specific use with alpha-blockers, see also notes above)

Bronchospasm Beta-blockers, including those considered to be cardioselective, should usually be avoided in patients with a history of asthma or bronchospasm. However, when there is no alternative, a cardioselective beta-blocker can be given to these patients with caution and under specialist supervision.

Hepatic impairment   reduce oral dose

Renal impairment   manufacturer advises caution—dose reduction may be required

Pregnancy   see notes above

Breast-feeding   see notes above

Side-effects   see notes above; also gastro-intestinal disturbances; bradycardia, heart failure, hypotension, conduction disorders, peripheral vasoconstriction (including exacerbation of intermittent claudication and Raynaud's phenomenon); bronchospasm (see above), dyspnoea; headache, fatigue, sleep disturbances, paraesthesia, dizziness, vertigo, psychoses; sexual dysfunction; purpura, thrombocytopenia; visual disturbances; exacerbation of psoriasis, alopecia; *rarely* rashes and dry eyes (reversible on withdrawal); **overdosage:** see Emergency Treatment of Poisoning, p. 39

Dose

● By mouth, hypertension, initially 80 mg twice daily, increased at weekly intervals as required; maintenance 160–320 mg daily

Prophylaxis of variceal bleeding in portal hypertension, initially 40 mg twice daily, increased to 80 mg twice daily according to heart rate; max. 160 mg twice daily

Phaeochromocytoma (only with an alpha-blocker), 60 mg daily for 3 days before surgery *or* 30 mg daily in patients unsuitable for surgery

Angina, initially 40 mg 2–3 times daily; maintenance 120–240 mg daily

Arrhythmias, hypertrophic cardiomyopathy, anxiety tachycardia, and thyrotoxicosis (adjunct), 10–40 mg 3–4 times daily

Anxiety with symptoms such as palpitation, sweating, tremor, 40 mg once daily, increased to 40 mg 3 times daily if necessary

Prophylaxis after myocardial infarction, 40 mg 4 times daily for 2–3 days, then 80 mg twice daily, beginning 5 to 21 days after infarction

Essential tremor, initially 40 mg 2–3 times daily; maintenance 80–160 mg daily

Migraine prophylaxis, 80–240 mg daily in divided doses

● By intravenous injection, arrhythmias and thyrotoxic crisis, 1 mg over 1 minute; if necessary repeat at 2-minute intervals; max. total dose 10 mg (5 mg in anaesthesia)

Note Excessive bradycardia can be countered with intravenous injection of atropine sulfate 0.6–2.4 mg in divided doses of 600 micrograms; for **overdosage** see Emergency Treatment of Poisoning, p. 39

Propranolol (Non-proprietary) ▣PoM▣

Tablets, propranolol hydrochloride 10 mg, net price 28 = £2.55; 40 mg, 28 = £2.33; 80 mg, 56 = £4.99; 160 mg, 56 = £5.63. Label: 8
Brands include *Angilol*®

Oral solution, propranolol hydrochloride 5 mg/5 mL, net price 150 mL = £12.50; 10 mg/5 mL, 150 mL = £16.45; 40 mg/5 mL, 150 mL = £31.50; 50 mg/5 mL, 150 mL = £19.98. Label: 8
Brands include *Syprol*®

Injection, propranolol hydrochloride 1 mg/mL
Available from 'special-order' manufacturers or specialist importing companies, see p. 1124

◢**Modified release**

Note Modified-release preparations can be used for once daily administration

Propranolol m/r preparations ▣PoM▣

Capsules, m/r, propranolol hydrochloride 80 mg. Label: 8, 25
Brands include *Bedranol SR*®, *Half Beta Prograne*®

Capsules, m/r, propranolol hydrochloride 160 mg. Label: 8, 25
Brands include *Bedranol SR*®, *Beta Prograne*®, *Slo-Pro*®

▉ ACEBUTOLOL

Indications   see under Dose

Cautions   see under Propranolol Hydrochloride

Contra-indications   see under Propranolol Hydrochloride

Renal impairment   halve dose if eGFR 25–50 mL/minute/1.73 m², use quarter dose if eGFR less than 25 mL/minute/1.73 m², do not administer more than once daily

Pregnancy   see notes above

Breast-feeding   see notes above

Side-effects   see under Propranolol Hydrochloride

Cardiovascular system 2

Dose
- Hypertension, initially 400 mg once daily *or* 200 mg twice daily, increased after 2 weeks to 400 mg twice daily if necessary; up to 1.2 g daily has been used
- Angina, initially 400 mg once daily *or* 200 mg twice daily; 300 mg 3 times daily in severe angina; up to 1.2 g daily has been used
- Arrhythmias, 0.4–1.2 g daily in 2–3 divided doses

Sectral® (Sanofi-Aventis) [PoM]
Capsules, acebutolol (as hydrochloride) 100 mg (buff/white), net price 84-cap pack = £14.97; 200 mg (buff/pink), 56-cap pack = £19.18. Label: 8
Tablets, f/c, acebutolol 400 mg (as hydrochloride), net price 28-tab pack = £18.62. Label: 8

ATENOLOL

Indications   see under Dose

Cautions   see under Propranolol Hydrochloride

Contra-indications   see under Propranolol Hydrochloride

Renal impairment   max. 50 mg daily (10 mg on alternate days *intravenously*) if eGFR 15–35 mL/minute/1.73 m^2; max. 25 mg daily or 50 mg on alternate days (10 mg every 4 days *intravenously*) if eGFR less than 15 mL/minute/1.73 m^2

Pregnancy   see notes above

Breast-feeding   see notes above

Side-effects   see under Propranolol Hydrochloride

Dose
- By mouth, hypertension, 25–50 mg daily (higher doses rarely necessary)
  Angina, 100 mg daily in 1 or 2 doses
  Arrhythmias, 50–100 mg daily
  Migraine prophylaxis [unlicensed], 50–200 mg daily in divided doses
- By intravenous injection, arrhythmias, 2.5 mg at a rate of 1 mg/minute, repeated at 5-minute intervals to a max. of 10 mg
  Note Excessive bradycardia can be countered with intravenous injection of atropine sulfate 0.6–2.4 mg in divided doses of 600 micrograms; for **overdosage** see Emergency Treatment of Poisoning, p. 39
- By intravenous infusion, arrhythmias, 150 micrograms/kg over 20 minutes, repeated every 12 hours if required
  Early intervention within 12 hours of myocardial infarction (section 2.10.1), by intravenous injection over 5 minutes, 5 mg, then by mouth, 50 mg after 15 minutes, 50 mg after 12 hours, then 100 mg daily

Atenolol (Non-proprietary) [PoM]
Tablets, atenolol 25 mg, net price 28-tab pack = 91p; 50 mg, 28-tab pack = 95p; 100 mg, 28-tab pack = £1.03. Label: 8

Tenormin® (AstraZeneca) [PoM]
LS tablets, orange, f/c, scored, atenolol 50 mg, net price 28-tab pack = £5.11. Label: 8
Tablets, orange, f/c, scored, atenolol 100 mg, net price 28-tab pack = £6.49. Label: 8
Syrup, sugar-free, atenolol 25 mg/5 mL, net price 300 mL = £13.55. Label: 8
Injection, atenolol 500 micrograms/mL, net price 10-mL amp = £3.45. (hosp. only)

◢ With diuretic

Co-tenidone (Non-proprietary) [PoM]
Tablets, co-tenidone 50/12.5 (atenolol 50 mg, chlortalidone 12.5 mg), net price 28-tab pack = £2.33; co-tenidone 100/25 (atenolol 100 mg, chlortalidone 25 mg), 28-tab pack = £2.47. Label: 8
Dose hypertension, 1 tablet daily (but see also under Dose above)

Kalten® (BPC 100) [PoM]
Capsules, red/ivory, atenolol 50 mg, amiloride hydrochloride 2.5 mg, hydrochlorothiazide 25 mg, net price 28-cap pack = £10.58. Label: 8
Dose hypertension, 1 capsule daily

Tenoret 50® (AstraZeneca) [PoM]
Tablets, brown, f/c, co-tenidone 50/12.5 (atenolol 50 mg, chlortalidone 12.5 mg), net price 28-tab pack = £5.18. Label: 8
Dose hypertension, 1 tablet daily

Tenoretic® (AstraZeneca) [PoM]
Tablets, brown, f/c, co-tenidone 100/25 (atenolol 100 mg, chlortalidone 25 mg), net price 28-tab pack = £5.18. Label: 8
Dose hypertension, 1 tablet daily (but see also under Dose above)

◢ With calcium-channel blocker

Note Only indicated when calcium-channel blocker or beta-blocker alone proves inadequate. For prescribing information on nifedipine see section 2.6.2

Beta-Adalat® (Bayer) [PoM]
Capsules, reddish-brown, atenolol 50 mg, nifedipine 20 mg (m/r), net price 28-cap pack = £9.00. Label: 8, 25
Dose hypertension, 1 capsule daily, increased if necessary to twice daily; ELDERLY, 1 daily
Angina, 1 capsule twice daily

Tenif® (AstraZeneca) [PoM]
Capsules, reddish-brown, atenolol 50 mg, nifedipine 20 mg (m/r), net price 28-cap pack = £12.76. Label: 8, 25
Dose hypertension, 1 capsule daily, increased if necessary to twice daily; ELDERLY, 1 daily
Angina, 1 capsule twice daily

BISOPROLOL FUMARATE

Indications   see under Dose

Cautions   see under Propranolol Hydrochloride; ensure heart failure not worsening before increasing dose

Contra-indications   see under Propranolol Hydrochloride; also acute or decompensated heart failure requiring intravenous inotropes; sino-atrial block

Hepatic impairment   max. 10 mg daily in severe impairment

Renal impairment   reduce dose if eGFR less than 20 mL/minute/1.73 m^2 (max. 10 mg daily)

Pregnancy   see notes above

Breast-feeding   see notes above

Side-effects   see under Propranolol Hydrochloride; also *less commonly* depression, muscle weakness, and cramp; *rarely* hypertriglyceridaemia, syncope, and hearing impairment; *very rarely* conjunctivitis

Dose
- Hypertension and angina, usually 10 mg once daily (5 mg may be adequate in some patients); max. 20 mg daily

- Adjunct in heart failure (section 2.5.5), initially 1.25 mg once daily (in the morning) for 1 week then, if well tolerated, increased to 2.5 mg once daily for 1 week, then 3.75 mg once daily for 1 week, then 5 mg once daily for 4 weeks, then 7.5 mg once daily for 4 weeks, then 10 mg once daily; max. 10 mg daily

Bisoprolol Fumarate (Non-proprietary) PoM

Tablets, bisoprolol fumarate 5 mg, net price 28-tab pack = 99p; 10 mg, 28-tab pack = £1.05. Label: 8

Cardicor® (Merck Serono) PoM

Tablets, f/c, bisoprolol fumarate 1.25 mg (white), net price 28-tab pack = £2.35; 2.5 mg (scored, white), 28-tab pack = £2.35; 3.75 mg (scored, off-white), 28-tab pack = £4.90; 5 mg (scored, light yellow), 28-tab pack = £5.90; 7.5 mg (scored, yellow), 28-tab pack = £5.90; 10 mg (scored, orange), 28-tab pack = £5.90. Label: 8

CARVEDILOL

Indications hypertension; angina; adjunct to diuretics, digoxin, or ACE inhibitors in symptomatic chronic heart failure

Cautions see under Propranolol Hydrochloride; monitor renal function during dose titration in patients with heart failure who also have renal impairment, low blood pressure, ischaemic heart disease, or diffuse vascular disease

Contra-indications see under Propranolol Hydrochloride; acute or decompensated heart failure requiring intravenous inotropes

Hepatic impairment avoid

Pregnancy see notes above

Breast-feeding see notes above

Side-effects postural hypotension, dizziness, headache, fatigue, gastro-intestinal disturbances, bradycardia; occasionally diminished peripheral circulation, peripheral oedema and painful extremities, dry mouth, dry eyes, eye irritation or disturbed vision, impotence, disturbances of micturition, influenza-like symptoms; rarely angina, AV block, exacerbation of intermittent claudication or Raynaud's phenomenon; allergic skin reactions, exacerbation of psoriasis, nasal stuffiness, wheezing, depressed mood, sleep disturbances, paraesthesia, heart failure, changes in liver enzymes, thrombocytopenia, leucopenia also reported

Dose

- Hypertension, initially 12.5 mg once daily, increased after 2 days to usual dose of 25 mg once daily; if necessary may be further increased at intervals of at least 2 weeks to max. 50 mg daily in single or divided doses; ELDERLY initial dose of 12.5 mg daily may provide satisfactory control
- Angina, initially 12.5 mg twice daily, increased after 2 days to 25 mg twice daily
- Adjunct in heart failure (section 2.5.5) initially 3.125 mg twice daily (with food), dose increased at intervals of at least 2 weeks to 6.25 mg twice daily, then to 12.5 mg twice daily, then to 25 mg twice daily; increase to highest dose tolerated, max. 25 mg twice daily in patients with severe heart failure or body-weight less than 85 kg and 50 mg twice daily in patients over 85 kg

Carvedilol (Non-proprietary) PoM

Tablets, carvedilol 3.125 mg, net price 28-tab pack = £1.44; 6.25 mg, 28-tab pack = £1.52; 12.5 mg, 28-tab pack = £1.55; 25 mg, 28-tab pack = £1.52. Label: 8

CELIPROLOL HYDROCHLORIDE

Indications mild to moderate hypertension

Cautions see under Propranolol Hydrochloride

Contra-indications see under Propranolol Hydrochloride

Hepatic impairment consider dose reduction

Renal impairment reduce dose by half if eGFR 15–40 mL/minute/1.73 m^2; avoid if eGFR less than 15 mL/minute/1.73 m^2

Pregnancy see notes above

Breast-feeding see notes above

Side-effects see under Propranolol Hydrochloride; also hot flushes; rarely depression, pneumonitis

Dose

- 200 mg once daily in the morning, increased to 400 mg once daily if necessary

Celiprolol (Non-proprietary) PoM

Tablets, celiprolol hydrochloride 200 mg, net price 28-tab pack = £3.65; 400 mg, 28-tab pack = £10.71. Label: 8, 22

Celectol® (Zentiva) PoM

Tablets, f/c, scored, celiprolol hydrochloride 200 mg, net price 28-tab pack = £19.83; 400 mg, 28-tab pack = £39.65. Label: 8, 22

ESMOLOL HYDROCHLORIDE

Indications short-term treatment of supraventricular arrhythmias (including atrial fibrillation, atrial flutter, sinus tachycardia); tachycardia and hypertension in peri-operative period

Cautions see under Propranolol Hydrochloride

Contra-indications see under Propranolol Hydrochloride

Renal impairment manufacturer advises caution

Pregnancy see notes above

Breast-feeding see notes above

Side-effects see under Propranolol Hydrochloride; also on infusion venous irritation and thrombophlebitis

Dose

- By intravenous infusion, usually within range 50–200 micrograms/kg/minute (consult product literature for details of dose titration and doses during peri-operative period)

Brevibloc® (Baxter) PoM

Injection, esmolol hydrochloride 10 mg/mL, net price 10-mL vial = £7.79, 250-mL infusion bag = £89.69

LABETALOL HYDROCHLORIDE

Indications hypertension (including hypertension in pregnancy, hypertension with angina, and hypertension following acute myocardial infarction); hypertensive crises (see section 2.5); controlled hypotension in anaesthesia

Cautions see under Propranolol Hydrochloride; interferes with laboratory tests for catecholamines; liver damage (see below)

Liver damage Severe hepatocellular damage reported after both short-term and long-term treatment. Appropriate laboratory testing needed at first symptom of liver dysfunction and if laboratory evidence of damage (or if jaundice) labetalol should be stopped and not restarted

2 Cardiovascular system

Contra-indications see under Propranolol Hydrochloride

Hepatic impairment avoid—severe hepatocellular injury reported

Renal impairment dose reduction may be required

Pregnancy see notes above

Breast-feeding see notes above

Side-effects postural hypotension (avoid upright position during and for 3 hours after intravenous administration), tiredness, weakness, headache, rashes, scalp tingling, difficulty in micturition, epigastric pain, nausea, vomiting; liver damage (see above); rarely lichenoid rash

Dose

- By mouth, initially 100 mg (50 mg in elderly) twice daily with food, increased at intervals of 14 days to usual dose of 200 mg twice daily; up to 800 mg daily in 2 divided doses (3–4 divided doses if higher); max. 2.4 g daily

- By intravenous injection, 50 mg over at least 1 minute, repeated after 5 minutes if necessary; max. total dose 200 mg

  Note Excessive bradycardia can be countered with intravenous injection of atropine sulfate 0.6–2.4 mg in divided doses of 600 micrograms; for **overdosage** see Emergency Treatment of Poisoning, p. 39

- By intravenous infusion, 2 mg/minute until satisfactory response then discontinue; usual total dose 50–200 mg, (**not** recommended for phaeochromocytoma, see under Phaeochromocytoma, section 2.5.4)

  Hypertension of pregnancy, 20 mg/hour, doubled every 30 minutes; usual max. 160 mg/hour

  Hypertension following myocardial infarction, 15 mg/hour, gradually increased to max. 120 mg/hour

Labetalol Hydrochloride (Non-proprietary) (PoM)

Tablets, f/c, labetalol hydrochloride 100 mg, net price, 56 = £6.92; 200 mg, 56 = £9.67; 400 mg, 56 = £23.14. Label: 8, 21

Injection, labetalol hydrochloride 5 mg/mL, net price 20-mL amp = £4.91

Trandate® (PharSafer) (PoM)

Tablets, all orange, f/c, labetalol hydrochloride 50 mg, net price 56-tab pack = £3.79; 100 mg, 56-tab pack = £4.64; 200 mg, 56-tab pack = £7.41; 400 mg, 56-tab pack = £10.15.Label: 8, 21

◢ METOPROLOL TARTRATE

Indications see under Dose

Cautions see under Propranolol Hydrochloride

Contra-indications see under Propranolol Hydrochloride

Hepatic impairment reduce dose in severe impairment

Pregnancy see notes above

Breast-feeding see notes above

Side-effects see under Propranolol Hydrochloride

Dose

- By mouth, hypertension, initially 100 mg daily, increased if necessary to 200 mg daily in 1–2 divided doses; max. 400 mg daily (but high doses rarely necessary)

  Angina, 50–100 mg 2–3 times daily

  Arrhythmias, usually 50 mg 2–3 times daily; up to 300 mg daily in divided doses if necessary

  Migraine prophylaxis, 100–200 mg daily in divided doses

  Hyperthyroidism (adjunct), 50 mg 4 times daily

- By intravenous injection, arrhythmias, up to 5 mg at rate 1–2 mg/minute, repeated after 5 minutes if necessary, total dose 10–15 mg

  Note Excessive bradycardia can be countered with intravenous injection of atropine sulfate 0.6–2.4 mg in divided doses of 600 micrograms; for **overdosage** see Emergency Treatment of Poisoning, p. 39

  In surgery, by slow intravenous injection 2–4 mg at induction or to control arrhythmias developing during anaesthesia; 2-mg doses may be repeated to a max. of 10 mg

  Early intervention within 12 hours of infarction, by intravenous injection 5 mg every 2 minutes to a max. of 15 mg, followed after 15 minutes by 50 mg by mouth every 6 hours for 48 hours; maintenance 200 mg daily in divided doses

Metoprolol Tartrate (Non-proprietary) (PoM)

Tablets, metoprolol tartrate 50 mg, net price 28 = £1.03, 56 = £1.80; 100 mg, 28 = £1.17, 56 = £1.90. Label: 8

Betaloc® (AstraZeneca) (PoM)

Injection, metoprolol tartrate 1 mg/mL, net price 5-mL amp = £1.00

Lopresor® (Recordati) (PoM)

Tablets, f/c, scored, metoprolol tartrate 50 mg (pink), net price 56-tab pack = £2.57; 100 mg (blue), 56-tab pack = £6.68. Label: 8

◢ Modified release

Lopresor SR® (Recordati) (PoM)

Tablets, m/r, yellow, f/c, metoprolol tartrate 200 mg, net price 28-tab pack = £9.80. Label: 8, 25

Dose hypertension, 200 mg daily; angina, 200–400 mg daily; migraine prophylaxis, 200 mg daily

---

◢ NADOLOL

Indications see under Dose

Cautions see under Propranolol Hydrochloride

Contra-indications see under Propranolol Hydrochloride

Hepatic impairment manufacturer advises caution

Renal impairment increase dosage interval if eGFR less than 50 mL/minute/1.73 m^2

Pregnancy see notes above

Breast-feeding see notes above

Side-effects see under Propranolol Hydrochloride

Dose

- Hypertension, initially 80 mg once daily, increased in increments of up to 80 mg at weekly intervals if required; max. 240 mg daily (higher doses rarely necessary)

- Angina, initially 40 mg once daily, increased at weekly intervals if required; usual max. 160 mg daily (rarely up to 240 mg may be required)

- Arrhythmias, initially 40 mg once daily, increased at weekly intervals up to 160 mg if required; reduce to 40 mg if bradycardia occurs

- Migraine prophylaxis, initially 40 mg once daily, increased in 40 mg increments at weekly intervals according to response; usual maintenance dose 80–160 mg once daily

- Thyrotoxicosis (adjunct), 80–160 mg once daily

Corgard® (Sanofi-Aventis) [PoM]

Tablets, blue, scored, nadolol 80 mg, net price 28-tab pack = £5.00. Label: 8

NEBIVOLOL

Indications essential hypertension; adjunct in stable mild to moderate heart failure in patients over 70 years

Cautions see under Propranolol Hydrochloride

Contra-indications see under Propranolol Hydrochloride; also acute or decompensated heart failure requiring intravenous inotropes

Hepatic impairment no information available—manufacturer advises avoid

Renal impairment for *hypertension*, initially 2.5 mg once daily, increased to 5 mg once daily if required; for *heart failure*, manufacturer advises avoid if serum creatinine greater than 250 micromol/litre

Pregnancy see notes above

Breast-feeding see notes above

Side-effects see under Propranolol Hydrochloride; also oedema and depression

Dose

• Hypertension, 5 mg daily; ELDERLY initially 2.5 mg daily, increased if necessary to 5 mg daily

• Adjunct in heart failure (section 2.5.5), initially 1.25 mg once daily, then if tolerated increased at intervals of 1–2 weeks to 2.5 mg once daily, then to 5 mg once daily, then to max. 10 mg once daily

Nebivolol (Non-proprietary) [PoM]

Tablets, nebivolol (as hydrochloride) 5 mg, net price 28-tab pack = £1.56. Label: 8

Nebilet® (Menarini) [PoM]

Tablets, scored, nebivolol (as hydrochloride) 5 mg, net price 28-tab pack = £9.23. Label: 8

Note Also available as *Hypoloc*®

OXPRENOLOL HYDROCHLORIDE

Indications see under Dose

Cautions see under Propranolol Hydrochloride

Contra-indications see under Propranolol Hydrochloride

Hepatic impairment reduce dose

Pregnancy see notes above

Breast-feeding see notes above

Side-effects see under Propranolol Hydrochloride

Dose

• Hypertension, 80–160 mg daily in 2–3 divided doses, increased as required; max. 320 mg daily

• Angina, 80–160 mg daily in 2–3 divided doses; max. 320 mg daily

• Arrhythmias, 40–240 mg daily in 2–3 divided doses; max. 240 mg daily

• Anxiety symptoms (short-term use), 40–80 mg daily in 1–2 divided doses

Oxprenolol (Non-proprietary) [PoM]

Tablets, coated, oxprenolol hydrochloride 20 mg, net price 56 = £5.37; 40 mg, 56 = £7.22; 80 mg, 56 = £11.70; 160 mg, 20 = £2.36. Label: 8

◢ **Modified release**

Slow-Trasicor® (AMCo) [PoM]

Tablets, m/r, f/c, oxprenolol hydrochloride 160 mg, net price 28-tab pack = £7.96. Label: 8, 25

Dose hypertension, angina, initially 160 mg once daily; if necessary may be increased to max. 320 mg daily

PINDOLOL

Indications see under Dose

Cautions see under Propranolol Hydrochloride

Contra-indications see under Propranolol Hydrochloride

Renal impairment may adversely affect renal function in severe impairment—manufacturer advises avoid

Pregnancy see notes above

Breast-feeding see notes above

Side-effects see under Propranolol Hydrochloride

Dose

• Hypertension, initially 5 mg 2–3 times daily *or* 15 mg once daily, increased as required at weekly intervals; usual maintenance 15–30 mg daily; max. 45 mg daily

• Angina, 2.5–5 mg up to 3 times daily

Pindolol (Non-proprietary) [PoM]

Tablets, pindolol 5 mg, net price 100-tab pack = £8.22. Label: 8

Visken® (AMCo) [PoM]

Tablets, scored, pindolol 5 mg, net price 56-tab pack = £5.85; 15 mg, 28-tab pack = £10.55. Label: 8

◢ **With diuretic**

Viskaldix® (AMCo) [PoM]

Tablets, scored, pindolol 10 mg, clopamide 5 mg, net price 28-tab pack = £6.70. Label: 8

Dose hypertension, 1 tablet daily in the morning, increased if necessary after 2–3 weeks to 2 tablets once daily; max. 3 tablets daily

SOTALOL HYDROCHLORIDE

Indications life-threatening arrhythmias including ventricular tachyarrhythmias; symptomatic non-sustained ventricular tachyarrhythmias; prophylaxis of paroxysmal atrial tachycardia or fibrillation, paroxysmal AV re-entrant tachycardias (both nodal and involving accessory pathways), and paroxysmal supraventricular tachycardia after cardiac surgery; maintenance of sinus rhythm following cardioversion of atrial fibrillation or flutter

Cautions see under Propranolol Hydrochloride; correct hypokalaemia, hypomagnesaemia, or other electrolyte disturbances; severe or prolonged diarrhoea; extreme caution or avoid concomitant use of drugs that prolong QT interval

Contra-indications see under Propranolol Hydrochloride; congenital or acquired long QT syndrome; torsade de pointes; renal failure

Renal impairment use half normal dose if eGFR 30–60 mL/minute/1.73 m^2; use one-quarter normal dose if eGFR 10–30 mL/minute/1.73 m^2; avoid if eGFR less than 10 mL/minute/1.73 m^2

Pregnancy see notes above

Breast-feeding see notes above

Side-effects see under Propranolol Hydrochloride; arrhythmogenic (pro-arrhythmic) effect (torsade de pointes—increased risk in women)

Cardiovascular system 2

Dose

- By mouth with ECG monitoring and measurement of corrected QT interval, arrhythmias, initially 80 mg daily in 1–2 divided doses increased gradually at intervals of 2–3 days to usual dose of 160–320 mg daily in 2 divided doses; higher doses of 480–640 mg daily for life-threatening ventricular arrhythmias under specialist supervision

Sotalol (Non-proprietary) PoM
Tablets, sotalol hydrochloride 40 mg, net price 28 = £1.28; 80 mg, 28 = £1.46; 160 mg, 28 = £5.86. Label: 8

Beta-Cardone® (PharSafer) PoM
Tablets, scored, sotalol hydrochloride 40 mg (green), net price 56-tab pack = £1.29; 80 mg (pink), 56-tab pack = £1.91; 200 mg, 28-tab pack = £2.40. Label: 8

Sotacor® (Bristol-Myers Squibb) PoM
Tablets, scored, sotalol hydrochloride 80 mg, net price 30-tab pack = £3.28. Label: 8

TIMOLOL MALEATE

Indications see under Dose; glaucoma (section 11.6)
Cautions see under Propranolol Hydrochloride
Contra-indications see under Propranolol Hydrochloride
Hepatic impairment dose reduction may be necessary
Renal impairment manufacturer advises caution—dose reduction may be required
Pregnancy see notes above
Breast-feeding see notes above
Side-effects see under Propranolol Hydrochloride

Dose

- Hypertension, initially 10 mg daily in 1–2 divided doses; gradually increased if necessary to max. 60 mg daily, usual maintenance dose 10–30 mg daily (doses above 30 mg daily given in divided doses)
- Angina, initially 5 mg twice daily increased if necessary by 10 mg daily every 3–4 days; max. 30 mg twice daily
- Prophylaxis after myocardial infarction, initially 5 mg twice daily, increased after 2 days to 10 mg twice daily if tolerated
- Migraine prophylaxis, 10–20 mg daily in 1–2 divided doses

Timolol (Non-proprietary) PoM
Tablets, timolol maleate 10 mg, net price 30-tab pack = £6.52. Label: 8

◀ **With diuretic**

Timolol with amiloride and hydrochlorothiazide
(Non-proprietary) PoM
Tablets, scored, timolol maleate 10 mg, amiloride hydrochloride 2.5 mg, hydrochlorothiazide 25 mg, net price 28-tab pack = £29.87. Label: 8
Dose hypertension, 1–2 tablets daily

Prestim® (Meda) PoM
Tablets, scored, timolol maleate 10 mg, bendroflumethiazide 2.5 mg, net price 30-tab pack = £3.49. Label: 8
Dose hypertension, 1–2 tablets daily; max. 4 daily

2.5 Hypertension and heart failure

2.5.1	Vasodilator antihypertensive drugs
2.5.2	Centrally acting antihypertensive drugs
2.5.3	Adrenergic neurone blocking drugs
2.5.4	Alpha-adrenoceptor blocking drugs
2.5.5	Drugs affecting the renin-angiotensin system

Hypertension Lowering raised blood pressure decreases the risk of stroke, coronary events, heart failure, and renal impairment. Advice on antihypertensive therapy in this section takes into account the recommendations of NICE clinical guidance 127 (August 2011), Hypertension—Clinical management of primary hypertension in adults.

Possible causes of hypertension (e.g. renal disease, endocrine causes), contributory factors, risk factors, and the presence of any complications of hypertension, such as left ventricular hypertrophy, should be established. Patients should be given advice on lifestyle changes to reduce blood pressure or cardiovascular risk; these include smoking cessation, weight reduction, reduction of excessive intake of alcohol and caffeine, reduction of dietary salt, reduction of total and saturated fat, increasing exercise, and increasing fruit and vegetable intake.

Thresholds and targets for treatment Patients presenting with a blood pressure of 140/90 mmHg or higher when measured in a clinic setting, should be offered ambulatory blood pressure monitoring (or home blood pressure monitoring if ambulatory blood pressure monitoring is unsuitable) to confirm the diagnosis and stage of hypertension.

Stage 1 hypertension:

- Clinic blood pressure 140/90 mmHg or higher, *and* ambulatory daytime average or home blood pressure average 135/85 mmHg or higher
- Treat patients under 80 years who have stage 1 hypertension and target-organ damage (e.g. left ventricular hypertrophy, chronic kidney disease, hypertensive retinopathy), cardiovascular disease, renal disease, diabetes, or a 10 year cardiovascular risk $\geq 20\%$; in the absence of these conditions, advise lifestyle changes and review annually. For patients under 40 years with stage 1 hypertension but **no** overt target-organ damage, cardiovascular disease, renal disease, or diabetes, consider seeking specialist advice for evaluation of secondary causes of hypertension

Stage 2 hypertension:

- Clinic blood pressure 160/100 mmHg or higher, *and* ambulatory daytime average or home blood pressure average 150/95 mmHg or higher
- Treat all patients who have stage 2 hypertension, regardless of age

Severe hypertension:

- Clinic systolic blood pressure ≥ 180 mmHg *or* clinic diastolic blood pressure ≥ 110 mmHg; treat promptly—see Hypertensive Crises, p. 110

A target clinic blood pressure below 140/90 mmHg is suggested for patients under 80 years; a target ambulatory or home blood pressure average (during the patient's waking hours) of below 135/85 mmHg is suggested for patients under 80 years; see also Hypertension in the Elderly, below. A target clinic blood pressure below 130/80 mmHg should be considered for those with established atherosclerotic cardiovascular disease, or diabetes in the presence of kidney, eye, or cerebrovascular disease. In some individuals it may not be possible to reduce blood pressure below the suggested targets despite the use of appropriate therapy.

Drug treatment of hypertension   A single antihypertensive drug is often inadequate in the management of hypertension, and additional antihypertensive drugs are usually added in a step-wise manner until control is achieved. Unless it is necessary to lower the blood pressure urgently (see Hypertensive Crises, below), an interval of at least 4 weeks should be allowed to determine response; clinicians should ensure antihypertensive drugs are titrated to the optimum or maximum tolerated dose at each step of treatment. Response to drug treatment may be affected by age and ethnicity.

Patients under 55 years:

Step 1

- **ACE inhibitor** (section 2.5.5.1); if not tolerated, offer an **angiotensin-II receptor antagonist** (section 2.5.5.2). If both ACE inhibitors and angiotensin-II receptor antagonists are contra-indicated or not tolerated, consider a **beta-blocker** (section 2.4); beta-blockers, especially when combined with a thiazide diuretic, should be avoided for the routine treatment of uncomplicated hypertension in patients with diabetes or at high risk of developing diabetes

Step 2

- ACE inhibitor or angiotensin-II receptor antagonist in combination with a **calcium-channel blocker** (section 2.6.2). If a calcium-channel blocker is not tolerated or if there is evidence of, or a high risk of, heart failure, give a **thiazide-related diuretic** (e.g. chlortalidone or indapamide) (section 2.2.1). If a beta-blocker was given at Step 1, add a calcium-channel blocker in preference to a thiazide-related diuretic (see Step 1 above)

Step 3

- ACE inhibitor or angiotensin-II receptor antagonist in combination with a calcium-channel blocker *and* a thiazide-related diuretic

Step 4 (resistant hypertension)

- Consider seeking specialist advice

- Add low-dose **spironolactone** (section 2.2.3) [unlicensed indication], *or* use high-dose thiazide-related diuretic if plasma-potassium concentration above 4.5 mmol/litre

- Monitor renal function and electrolytes

- If additional diuretic therapy is contra-indicated, ineffective, or not tolerated, consider an **alpha-blocker** (section 2.5.4) *or* a beta-blocker

Patients over 55 years, and patients of any age who are of African or Caribbean family origin:

Step 1

- Calcium-channel blocker; if not tolerated or if there is evidence of, or a high risk of, heart failure, give a thiazide-related diuretic (e.g. chlortalidone or indapamide)

Step 2

- Calcium-channel blocker *or* thiazide-related diuretic in combination with an ACE inhibitor or angiotensin-II receptor antagonist (an angiotensin-II receptor antagonist in combination with a calcium-channel blocker is preferred in patients of African or Caribbean family origin)

Steps 3 and 4

- Treat as for patients under 55 years (see above)

Other measures to reduce cardiovascular risk
Aspirin (section 2.9) in a dose of 75 mg daily reduces the risk of cardiovascular events and myocardial infarction. Unduly high blood pressure must be controlled before aspirin is given. Unless contra-indicated, aspirin is recommended for all patients with established cardiovascular disease. Use of aspirin in primary prevention, in those with or without diabetes, is of unproven benefit (see also section 2.9). For the role of aspirin in the prevention of stroke in patients with atrial fibrillation, see section 2.3.1

Statins are also of benefit in cardiovascular disease or in those who are at high risk of developing cardiovascular disease (section 2.12).

Hypertension in the elderly   Benefit from antihypertensive therapy is evident up to at least 80 years of age, but it is probably inappropriate to apply a strict age limit when deciding on drug therapy. Patients who reach 80 years of age while taking antihypertensive drugs should continue treatment, provided that it continues to be of benefit and does not cause significant side-effects. If patients are aged over 80 years when diagnosed with stage 1 hypertension, the decision to treat should be based on the presence of other co-morbidities; patients with stage 2 hypertension should be treated as for patients over 55 years (see above). A target clinic blood pressure below 150/90 mmHg is suggested for patients over 80 years; the suggested target ambulatory or home blood pressure average (during the patient's waking hours) is below 145/85 mmHg.

Isolated systolic hypertension   Isolated systolic hypertension (systolic pressure $\geq$ 160 mmHg, diastolic pressure < 90 mmHg) is common in patients over 60 years, and is associated with an increased cardiovascular disease risk; it should be treated as for patients with both a raised systolic and diastolic blood pressure (see above). Patients with severe postural hypotension should be referred to a specialist.

Hypertension in diabetes   For patients with diabetes, a target clinic blood pressure below 140/80 mmHg is suggested (below 130/80 mmHg is advised if kidney, eye, or cerebrovascular disease are also present). However, in some individuals, it may not be possible to achieve this level of control despite appropriate therapy. Most patients require a combination of antihypertensive drugs.

2

Cardiovascular system

2 Cardiovascular system

Hypertension is common in type 2 diabetes, and anti-hypertensive treatment prevents macrovascular and microvascular complications. In type 1 diabetes, hypertension usually indicates the presence of diabetic nephropathy. An ACE inhibitor (or an angiotensin-II receptor antagonist) may have a specific role in the management of diabetic nephropathy (section 6.1.5); in patients with type 2 diabetes, an ACE inhibitor (or an angiotensin-II receptor antagonist) can delay progression of microalbuminuria to nephropathy.

Hypertension in renal disease A target clinic blood pressure below 140/90 mmHg is suggested (below 130/80 mmHg is advised in patients with chronic kidney disease and diabetes, or if proteinuria exceeds 1 g in 24 hours). An ACE inhibitor (or an angiotensin-II receptor antagonist) should be considered for patients with proteinuria; however, ACE inhibitors should be used with caution in renal impairment, see section 2.5.5.1. Thiazide diuretics may be ineffective and high doses of loop diuretics may be required.

Hypertension in pregnancy Hypertensive complications in pregnancy can be hazardous for both the mother and the fetus, and are associated with a significant risk of morbidity and mortality; complications can occur in pregnant women with pre-existing chronic hypertension, or in those who develop hypertension in the latter half of pregnancy.

Labetalol (section 2.4) is widely used for treating hypertension in pregnancy. **Methyldopa** (section 2.5.2) is considered safe for use in pregnancy. Modified-release preparations of **nifedipine** [unlicensed] are also used, but see section 2.6.2 (p. 137) for warnings on use during pregnancy.

The following advice takes into account the recommendations of NICE Clinical Guideline 107 (August 2010), Hypertension in Pregnancy.

Pregnant women with chronic hypertension who are already receiving antihypertensive treatment should have their drug therapy reviewed. In uncomplicated chronic hypertension, a target blood pressure of <150/100 mmHg is recommended; women with target-organ damage as a result of chronic hypertension, and in women with chronic hypertension who have given birth, a target blood pressure of <140/90 mmHg is advised. Long-term antihypertensive treatment should be reviewed 2 weeks following the birth. Women managed with methyldopa during pregnancy should discontinue treatment and restart their original antihypertensive medication within 2 days of the birth.

Pregnant women are at high risk of developing pre-eclampsia if they have chronic kidney disease, diabetes mellitus, autoimmune disease, chronic hypertension, or if they have had hypertension during a previous pregnancy; these women are advised to take **aspirin** (section 2.9) in a dose of 75 mg once daily [unlicensed indication] from week 12 of pregnancy until the baby is born. Women with more than one moderate risk factor (first pregnancy, aged ≥40 years, pregnancy interval >10 years, BMI ≥35 kg/m^2 at first visit, multiple pregnancy, or family history of pre-eclampsia) for developing pre-eclampsia are also advised to take aspirin 75 mg once daily [unlicensed indication] from week 12 of pregnancy until the baby is born.

Women with pre-eclampsia or gestational hypertension who present with a blood pressure over 150/100 mmHg, should receive initial treatment with

oral labetalol to achieve a target blood pressure of <150 mmHg systolic, and diastolic 80–100 mmHg. If labetalol is unsuitable, methyldopa or modified-release nifedipine may be considered. Women with gestational hypertension or pre-eclampsia who have been managed with methyldopa during pregnancy should discontinue treatment within 2 days of the birth. Women with a blood pressure of ≥160/110 mmHg who require critical care during pregnancy or after birth should receive immediate treatment with either oral or intravenous labetalol, intravenous hydralazine (section 2.5.1), or oral modified-release nifedipine to achieve a target blood pressure of <150 mmHg systolic, and diastolic 80–100 mmHg.

For use of magnesium sulfate in pre-eclampsia and eclampsia, see section 9.5.1.3.

Hypertensive crises If blood pressure is reduced too quickly in the management of hypertensive crises, there is a risk of reduced organ perfusion leading to cerebral infarction, blindness, deterioration in renal function, and myocardial ischaemia.

A *hypertensive emergency* is defined as severe hypertension with acute damage to the target organs (e.g. signs of papilloedema or retinal haemorrhage, or the presence of clinical conditions such as acute coronary syndromes, acute aortic dissection, acute pulmonary oedema, hypertensive encephalopathy, acute cerebral infarction, intracerebral or subarachnoid haemorrhage, eclampsia, or rapidly progressing renal failure); prompt treatment with intravenous antihypertensive therapy is generally required. Over the first few minutes or within 2 hours, blood pressure should be reduced by 20–25%. When intravenous therapy is indicated, treatment options include sodium nitroprusside [unlicensed] (section 2.5.1), nicardipine (section 2.6.2), labetalol (section 2.4), glyceryl trinitrate (section 2.6.1), phentolamine (section 2.5.4), hydralazine (section 2.5.1), or esmolol (section 2.4); choice of drug is dependent on concomitant conditions and clinical status of the patient.

Severe hypertension (blood pressure ≥180/110 mmHg) without acute target-organ damage is defined as a *hypertensive urgency*; blood pressure should be reduced gradually over 24–48 hours with oral antihypertensive therapy, such as labetalol, or the calcium-channel blockers (section 2.6.2) amlodipine or felodipine. Use of sublingual nifedipine is not recommended.

For advice on short-term management of hypertensive episodes in phaeochromocytoma, see under Phaeochromocytoma, section 2.5.4.

2.5.1 Vasodilator antihypertensive drugs

Vasodilators have a potent hypotensive effect, especially when used in combination with a beta-blocker and a thiazide. **Important:** for a warning on the hazards of a very rapid fall in blood pressure, see Hypertensive crises, above.

Hydralazine is given by mouth as an adjunct to other antihypertensives for the treatment of resistant hypertension but is rarely used; when used alone it causes tachycardia and fluid retention. The incidence of side-effects is lower if the dose is kept below 100 mg daily, but systemic lupus erythematosus should be suspected if there is unexplained weight loss, arthritis, or any other unexplained ill health.

Sodium nitroprusside [unlicensed] is given by intravenous infusion to control severe hypertensive emergencies when parenteral treatment is necessary.

Minoxidil should be reserved for the treatment of severe hypertension resistant to other drugs. Vasodilatation is accompanied by increased cardiac output and tachycardia and the patients develop fluid retention. For this reason the addition of a beta-blocker and a diuretic (usually furosemide, in high dosage) are mandatory. Hypertrichosis is troublesome and renders this drug unsuitable for women.

Prazosin, **doxazosin**, and **terazosin** (section 2.5.4) have alpha-blocking and vasodilator properties.

Ambrisentan, **bosentan**, **iloprost**, **macitentan**, **sildenafil**, and **tadalafil** are licensed for the treatment of pulmonary arterial hypertension and should be used under specialist supervision. **Epoprostenol** (section 2.8.1) can be used in patients with primary pulmonary hypertension resistant to other treatments. Bosentan is also licensed to reduce the number of new digital ulcers in patients with systemic sclerosis and ongoing digital ulcer disease. **Riociguat** is licensed for the treatment of pulmonary arterial hypertension and chronic thromboembolic pulmonary hypertension; it should be used under specialist supervision.

Sitaxentan has been withdrawn from the market because the benefit of treatment does not outweigh the risk of severe hepatotoxicity.

The *Scottish Medicines Consortium* (p. 4) has advised (November 2005) that iloprost (*Ventavis*®) is accepted for restricted use within NHS Scotland in patients in whom bosentan is ineffective or not tolerated, and should only be prescribed by specialists in the Scottish Pulmonary Vascular Unit.

The *Scottish Medicines Consortium* (p. 4) has advised (October 2008) that ambrisentan (*Volibris*®) should be prescribed only by specialists in the Scottish Pulmonary Vascular Unit or other similar specialists.

The *Scottish Medicines Consortium* (p. 4) has advised (January 2010 and February 2011) that sildenafil tablets (*Revatio*®) should be initiated only by specialists in the Scottish Pulmonary Vascular Unit or other similar specialists and that sildenafil injection (*Revatio*®) should be prescribed only on the advice of specialists in the Scottish Pulmonary Vascular Unit or the Scottish Adult Congenital Cardiac Service.

The *Scottish Medicines Consortium* (p. 4) has advised (June 2012) that tadalafil (*Adcirca*®) should be initiated only by specialists in the Scottish Pulmonary Vascular Unit or other similar specialists.

The *Scottish Medicines Consortium* (p. 4) has advised (March 2014) that macitentan (*Opsumit*®) should be initiated and prescribed only by specialists in the Scottish Pulmonary Vascular Unit or other similar specialists.

AMBRISENTAN

Indications   pulmonary arterial hypertension

Cautions   not to be initiated in significant anaemia; monitor haemoglobin concentration or haematocrit after 1 month and 3 months of starting treatment, and periodically thereafter (reduce dose or discontinue treatment if significant decrease in haemoglobin concentration or haematocrit observed); monitor liver function before treatment, and monthly thereafter—discontinue if liver enzymes raised significantly or if symptoms of liver impairment develop; **interactions:** Appendix 1 (ambrisentan)

Contra-indications   idiopathic pulmonary fibrosis

Hepatic impairment   avoid in severe impairment

Renal impairment   use with caution if eGFR less than 30 mL/minute/1.73 m^2

Pregnancy   avoid (teratogenic in *animal* studies); exclude pregnancy before treatment and ensure effective contraception during treatment; monthly pregnancy tests advised

Breast-feeding   manufacturer advises avoid—no information available

Side-effects   abdominal pain, constipation, diarrhoea, nausea, vomiting, palpitation, flushing, hypotension, peripheral oedema, chest pain, heart failure, upper respiratory-tract disorders, dyspnoea, epistaxis, headache, dizziness, malaise, anaemia; *less commonly* hepatic injury, autoimmune hepatitis, syncope

Dose
* ADULT over 18 years, 5 mg once daily, increased if necessary to 10 mg once daily

Note Max. 5 mg daily with concomitant ciclosporin

Volibris® (GSK) ▼ PoM
  Tablets, f/c, ambrisentan 5 mg (pale pink), net price 30-tab pack = £1618.08; 10 mg (dark pink), 30-tab pack = £1618.08

BOSENTAN

Indications   pulmonary arterial hypertension; systemic sclerosis with ongoing digital ulcer disease (to reduce number of new digital ulcers)

Cautions   not to be initiated if systemic systolic blood pressure is below 85 mmHg; monitor haemoglobin before and during treatment (monthly for first 4 months, then 3-monthly); avoid abrupt withdrawal; monitor liver function before treatment, at monthly intervals during treatment, and 2 weeks after dose increase (reduce dose or suspend treatment if liver enzymes raised significantly)—discontinue if symptoms of liver impairment; **interactions:** Appendix 1 (bosentan)

Contra-indications   acute porphyria (section 9.8.2)

Hepatic impairment   avoid in moderate and severe impairment

Pregnancy   avoid (teratogenic in *animal* studies); effective contraception required during administration (hormonal contraception not considered effective); monthly pregnancy tests advised

Breast-feeding   manufacturer advises avoid—no information available

Side-effects   diarrhoea, gastro-oesophageal reflux, flushing, hypotension, palpitation, oedema, syncope, headache, anaemia; *less commonly* thrombocytopenia, neutropenia, leucopenia; *rarely* liver cirrhosis, liver failure (see cautions above)

Dose
* Pulmonary arterial hypertension, initially 62.5 mg twice daily increased after 4 weeks to 125 mg twice daily; max. 250 mg twice daily; CHILD under 18 years see *BNF for Children*

2 **Cardiovascular system**

Cardiovascular system

2

- Systemic sclerosis with ongoing digital ulcer disease, initially 62.5 mg twice daily increased after 4 weeks to 125 mg twice daily

Tracleer® (Actelion) [PoM]
Tablets, f/c, orange, bosentan (as monohydrate) 62.5 mg, net price 56-tab pack = £1510.21; 125 mg, 56-tab pack = £1510.21

HYDRALAZINE HYDROCHLORIDE

Indications moderate to severe hypertension (adjunct); heart failure (with long-acting nitrate, but see section 2.5.5); hypertensive emergencies (including during pregnancy) (see section 2.5)

Cautions coronary artery disease (may provoke angina, avoid after myocardial infarction until stabilised), cerebrovascular disease; occasionally blood pressure reduction too rapid even with low parenteral doses; manufacturer advises test for antinuclear factor and for proteinuria every 6 months and check acetylator status before increasing dose above 100 mg daily, but evidence of clinical value unsatisfactory; **interactions:** Appendix 1 (hydralazine)

Contra-indications idiopathic systemic lupus erythematosus, severe tachycardia, high output heart failure, myocardial insufficiency due to mechanical obstruction, cor pulmonale, dissecting aortic aneurysm; acute porphyria (section 9.8.2)

Hepatic impairment reduce dose

Renal impairment reduce dose if eGFR less than 30 mL/minute/1.73 m²

Pregnancy neonatal thrombocytopenia reported, but risk should be balanced against risk of uncontrolled maternal hypertension; manufacturer advises avoid before third trimester

Breast-feeding present in milk but not known to be harmful; monitor infant

Side-effects tachycardia, palpitation, flushing, hypotension, fluid retention, gastro-intestinal disturbances; headache, dizziness; systemic lupus erythematosus-like syndrome after long-term therapy with over 100 mg daily (or less in women and in slow acetylator individuals) (see also notes above); rarely rashes, fever, peripheral neuritis, polyneuritis, paraesthesia, arthralgia, myalgia, increased lacrimation, nasal congestion, dyspnoea, agitation, anxiety, anorexia; blood disorders (including leucopenia, thrombocytopenia, haemolytic anaemia), abnormal liver function, jaundice, raised plasma creatinine, proteinuria and haematuria reported

Dose
- By mouth, hypertension, 25 mg twice daily, increased to usual max. 50 mg twice daily (see notes above) Heart failure (initiated in hospital) 25 mg 3–4 times daily, increased every 2 days if necessary; usual maintenance dose 50–75 mg 4 times daily
- By slow intravenous injection, hypertensive emergencies and hypertension with renal complications, 5–10 mg diluted with 10 mL sodium chloride 0.9%; may be repeated after 20–30 minutes (see Cautions)
- By intravenous infusion, hypertensive emergencies and hypertension with renal complications, initially 200–300 micrograms/minute; maintenance usually 50–150 micrograms/minute

Hydralazine (Non-proprietary) [PoM]
Tablets, hydralazine hydrochloride 25 mg, net price 56 = £10.28; 50 mg, 56 = £18.47

Apresoline® (AMCo) [PoM]
Tablets, yellow, s/c, hydralazine hydrochloride 25 mg, net price 84-tab pack = £3.38
Excipients include propylene glycol (see Excipients, p. 2)
Injection, powder for reconstitution, hydralazine hydrochloride, net price 20-mg amp = £2.22

ILOPROST

Indications idiopathic or familial pulmonary arterial hypertension

Cautions unstable pulmonary hypertension with advanced right heart failure; hypotension (do not initiate if systolic blood pressure below 85 mmHg); acute pulmonary infection; chronic obstructive pulmonary disease; severe asthma; to minimise accidental exposure use only with nebulisers listed under *Ventavis®* preparation in a well ventilated room; **interactions:** Appendix 1 (iloprost)

Contra-indications unstable angina; within 6 months of myocardial infarction; decompensated cardiac failure (unless under close medical supervision); severe arrhythmias; congenital or acquired heart-valve defects; within 3 months of cerebrovascular events; pulmonary veno-occlusive disease; conditions which increase risk of bleeding

Hepatic impairment elimination reduced—initially 2.5 micrograms at intervals of 3–4 hours (max. 6 times daily), adjusted according to response (consult product literature)

Pregnancy use if potential benefit outweighs risk

Breast-feeding manufacturer advises avoid—no information available

Side-effects nausea, vomiting, diarrhoea, oral irritation, haemorrhage, hypotension, chest pain, dyspnoea, cough, headache, throat or jaw pain, rash; *also reported* taste disturbance, bronchospasm, wheezing, thrombocytopenia

Dose
- By inhalation of nebulised solution, initial dose 2.5 micrograms increased to 5 micrograms for second dose, if tolerated maintain at 5 micrograms 6–9 times daily according to response; reduce to 2.5 micrograms 6–9 times daily if higher dose not tolerated; CHILD 8–18 years see *BNF for Children*

Ventavis® (Bayer) [PoM]
Nebuliser solution, iloprost (as trometamol) 10 micrograms/mL, net price 30 × 1-mL (10 microgram) unit-dose vials = £400.19, 168 × 1-mL = £2241.08. For use with *HaloLite®* [NHS], *I-Neb AAD®* [NHS], *Prodose®* [NHS], or *Venta-Neb®* [NHS] nebuliser
Note Delivery characteristics of nebuliser devices may vary—only switch devices under medical supervision

MACITENTAN

Indications pulmonary arterial hypertension

Cautions patients over 75 years; pulmonary veno-occlusive disease; monitor liver function before treatment, then monthly thereafter (discontinue if unexplained persistent raised serum transaminases or signs of hepatic injury—can restart on advice on hepatologist if liver function tests return to normal and no hepatic injury); monitor haemoglobin concentration before treatment and then as indicated; **interactions:** Appendix 1 (macitentan)
Hepatotoxicty Patients should be told how to recognise

signs of liver disorder and advised to seek immediate medical attention if symptoms such as dark urine, nausea, vomiting, fatigue, abdominal pain, or pruritus develop

Contra-indications   severe anaemia

Hepatic impairment   do not initiate if serum transaminases exceed 3 times upper limit of normal; avoid in moderate and severe impairment

Renal impairment   consider monitoring blood pressure (risk of hypotension); manufacturer advises caution in severe impairment and avoid in patients undergoing dialysis (no information available)

Pregnancy   toxicity in *animal* studies; manufacturer advises exclude pregnancy before treatment and ensure effective contraception during and for one month after stopping treatment; monthly pregnancy tests advised

Breast-feeding   manufacturer advises avoid—present in milk in *animal* studies

Side-effects   hypotension, upper respiratory-tract disorders, bronchitis, headache, urinary-tract infection, anaemia; *also reported* leucopenia, thrombocytopenia

Dose

- ADULT over 18 years, 10 mg once daily

Opsumit® (Actelion) ▼ PoM
Tablets, f/c, macitentan 10 mg, net price 30-tab pack = £2306.00. Counselling, hepatotoxicity, patient card

---

▮ MINOXIDIL

Indications   severe hypertension, in addition to a diuretic and a beta-blocker

Cautions   see notes above; angina; after myocardial infarction (until stabilised); acute porphyria (section 9.8.2); **interactions**: Appendix 1 (vasodilator antihypertensives)

Contra-indications   phaeochromocytoma

Renal impairment   use with caution in significant impairment

Pregnancy   avoid—possible toxicity including reduced placental perfusion; neonatal hirsutism reported

Breast-feeding   present in milk but not known to be harmful

Side-effects   sodium and water retention; weight gain, peripheral oedema, tachycardia, hypertrichosis; reversible rise in creatinine and blood urea nitrogen; occasionally, gastro-intestinal disturbances, breast tenderness, rashes

Dose

- Initially 5 mg (ELDERLY, 2.5 mg) daily, in 1–2 divided doses, increased in steps of 5–10 mg at intervals of at least 3 days; max. 100 mg daily (seldom necessary to exceed 50 mg daily)

Loniten® (Pharmacia) PoM
Tablets, scored, minoxidil 2.5 mg, net price 60-tab pack = £8.88; 5 mg, 60-tab pack = £15.83; 10 mg, 60-tab pack = £30.68

▮ RIOCIGUAT

Indications   chronic thromboembolic pulmonary hypertension that is recurrent or persistent following surgery, or is inoperable; monotherapy or in combination with an endothelin receptor antagonist for idiopathic or hereditary pulmonary arterial hypertension, or pulmonary arterial hypertension associated with connective tissue disease

Cautions   hypotension (do not initiate if systolic blood pressure below 95 mmHg); hypovolaemia; severe left ventricular outflow obstruction; autonomic dysfunction; smoking cessation advised (response possibly reduced); dose adjustment may be necessary if smoking started or stopped during treatment; elderly (risk of hypotension); **interactions**: Appendix 1 (riociguat)

Contra-indications   pulmonary veno-occlusive disease; history of serious haemoptysis; previous bronchial artery embolisation

Hepatic impairment   titrate dose cautiously in moderate impairment; manufacturer advises avoid in severe impairment—no information available

Renal impairment   titrate dose cautiously—risk of hypotension; manufacturer advises avoid if eGFR less than 30 mL/minute/1.73m²—limited information available

Pregnancy   avoid—toxicity in *animal* studies; effective contraception required during treatment; monthly pregnancy tests advised

Breast-feeding   manufacturer advises avoid—present in milk in *animal* studies

Side-effects   nausea, vomiting, diarrhoea, constipation, dyspepsia, gastro-oesophageal reflux, gastritis, dysphagia, peripheral oedema, palpitation, hypotension, haemoptysis, epistaxis, nasal congestion, dizziness, headache, anaemia; *less commonly* pulmonary haemorrhage

Dose

- ADULT over 18 years, initially 1 mg three times daily for 2 weeks, increased in steps of 0.5 mg three times daily every 2 weeks up to max. 2.5 mg three times daily if systolic blood pressure ≥ 95 mmHg and no signs of hypotension; if treatment interrupted for 3 or more days, restart at 1 mg three times daily for 2 weeks and titrate as before

Note During titration, reduce dose by 0.5 mg three times daily if systolic blood pressure falls below 95 mmHg and patient shows signs of hypotension

Adempas® (Bayer) ▼ PoM
Tablets, f/c, riociguat 0.5 mg (white), net price 42-tab pack = £997.36, 84-tab pack = £1994.72; 1 mg (pale yellow), 42-tab pack = £997.36, 84-tab pack = £1994.72; 1.5mg (yellow-orange), 42-tab pack = £997.36, 84-tab pack = £1994.72; 2 mg (pale orange), 42-tab pack = £997.36, 84-tab pack = £1994.72; 2.5 mg (red-orange), 42-tab pack = £997.36, 84-tab pack = £1994.72

▮ SILDENAFIL

Indications   pulmonary arterial hypertension; erectile dysfunction (section 7.4.5)

Cautions   hypotension (avoid if systolic blood pressure below 90 mmHg); intravascular volume depletion; left ventricular outflow obstruction; cardiovascular disease; autonomic dysfunction; pulmonary veno-occlusive disease; anatomical deformation of the penis, predisposition to priapism; bleeding disorders or active peptic ulceration; consider gradual withdrawal; **interactions**: Appendix 1 (sildenafil)

Contra-indications   recent history of stroke or myocardial infarction, history of non-arteritic anterior ischaemic optic neuropathy; hereditary degenerative

2 Cardiovascular system

retinal disorders; sickle-cell anaemia; avoid concomitant use of nitrates

Hepatic impairment for *pulmonary hypertension*, if usual dose not tolerated, reduce *oral* dose to 20 mg twice daily, or reduce *intravenous* dose to 10 mg twice daily; manufacturer advises avoid in severe impairment

Renal impairment for *pulmonary hypertension*, if usual dose not tolerated, reduce *oral* dose to 20 mg twice daily, or reduce *intravenous* dose to 10 mg twice daily

Pregnancy use only if potential benefit outweighs risk—no evidence of harm in *animal* studies

Breast-feeding manufacturer advises avoid—no information available

Side-effects diarrhoea, dyspepsia, gastritis, abdominal distension, gastro-oesophageal reflux, haemorrhoids, dry mouth, flushing, oedema, bronchitis, cough, headache, migraine, night sweats, paraesthesia, insomnia, anxiety, tremor, vertigo, fever, influenza-like symptoms, anaemia, back and limb pain, myalgia, visual disturbances, retinal haemorrhage, photophobia, painful red eyes, nasal congestion, epistaxis, cellulitis, alopecia; *less commonly* gynaecomastia, priapism, haematuria, penile haemorrhage; *also reported* rash, retinal vascular occlusion, non-arteritic anterior ischaemic optic neuropathy (discontinue if sudden visual impairment occurs), and sudden hearing loss (advise patient to seek medical help)

Dose
- By mouth, 20 mg 3 times daily; CHILD under 18 years see *BNF for Children*
- By intravenous injection, when oral route not appropriate, 10 mg three times daily

Revatio® (Pfizer) [PoM]
Tablets, f/c, sildenafil (as citrate), 20 mg, net price 90-tab pack = £446.33

Oral suspension, sildenafil (as citrate) 10 mg/mL when reconstituted with water, net price 112-mL = £186.75

Injection, sildenafil (as citrate), 800 micrograms/mL, net price 20-mL vial = £45.28

◢**Preparations for erectile dysfunction**
Section 7.4.5

SODIUM NITROPRUSSIDE

Indications hypertensive emergencies (see section 2.5); controlled hypotension in anaesthesia; acute or chronic heart failure

Cautions hypothyroidism, hyponatraemia, ischaemic heart disease, impaired cerebral circulation, elderly; hypothermia; monitor blood pressure (including intra-arterial blood pressure) and blood-cyanide concentration, and if treatment exceeds 3 days, also blood-thiocyanate concentration; avoid sudden withdrawal—terminate infusion over 15–30 minutes; protect infusion from light; **interactions:** Appendix 1 (sodium nitroprusside)

Contra-indications severe vitamin B_{12} deficiency; Leber's optic atrophy; compensatory hypertension

Hepatic impairment use with caution; avoid in hepatic failure—cyanide or thiocyanate metabolites may accumulate

Renal impairment avoid prolonged use—cyanide or thiocyanate metabolites may accumulate

Pregnancy avoid prolonged use—potential for accumulation of cyanide in fetus

Breast-feeding no information available; caution advised due to thiocyanate metabolite

Side-effects associated with over rapid reduction in blood pressure (reduce infusion rate): headache, dizziness, nausea, retching, abdominal pain, perspiration, palpitation, anxiety, retrosternal discomfort; occasionally reduced platelet count, acute transient phlebitis

Cyanide Side-effects caused by excessive plasma concentration of the cyanide metabolite include tachycardia, sweating, hyperventilation, arrhythmias, marked metabolic acidosis (discontinue and give antidote, see p. 41)

Dose
- Hypertensive emergencies, by intravenous infusion, initially 0.5–1.5 micrograms/kg/minute, then increased in steps of 500 nanograms/kg/minute every 5 minutes within range 0.5–8 micrograms/kg/minute (lower doses if already receiving other antihypertensives); stop if response unsatisfactory with max. dose in 10 minutes
  Note Lower initial dose of 300 nanograms/kg/minute has been used
- Maintenance of blood pressure at 30–40% lower than pretreatment diastolic blood pressure, 20–400 micrograms/minute (lower doses for patients being treated with other antihypertensives)
- Controlled hypotension in surgery, by intravenous infusion, max. 1.5 micrograms/kg/minute
- Heart failure, by intravenous infusion, initially 10–15 micrograms/minute, increased every 5–10 minutes as necessary; usual range 10–200 micrograms/minute normally for max. 3 days

Sodium Nitroprusside (Non-proprietary) [PoM]
Intravenous infusion, powder for reconstitution, sodium nitroprusside 10 mg/mL
Available from 'special-order' manufacturers or specialist importing companies, see p. 1124

TADALAFIL

Indications pulmonary arterial hypertension; benign prostatic hypertrophy (section 7.4.5); erectile dysfunction (section 7.4.5)

Cautions hypotension (avoid if systolic blood pressure below 90 mmHg); aortic and mitral valve disease; pericardial constriction; congestive cardiomyopathy; left ventricular dysfunction; life-threatening arrhythmias; coronary artery disease; uncontrolled hypertension; pulmonary veno-occlusive disease; predisposition to priapism; anatomical deformation of the penis; hereditary degenerative retinal disorders; **interactions:** Appendix 1 (tadalafil)

Contra-indications acute myocardial infarction in past 90 days; history of non-arteritic anterior ischaemic optic neuropathy; avoid concomitant use of nitrates

Hepatic impairment initially 20 mg once daily in mild to moderate impairment; avoid in severe impairment

Renal impairment initially 20 mg once daily in mild to moderate impairment, increased to 40 mg once daily if tolerated; avoid in severe impairment

Pregnancy manufacturer advises avoid

Breast-feeding manufacturer advises avoid—present in milk in *animal* studies

Side-effects nausea, vomiting, dyspepsia, gastro-oesophageal reflux, chest pain, palpitation, flushing, hypotension, nasopharyngitis, epistaxis, headache, myalgia, back and limb pain, increased uterine bleeding, blurred vision, facial oedema, rash; *less commonly* tachycardia, hypertension, seizures, amnesia, priapism, hyperhidrosis; *also reported* unstable angina, arrhythmia, myocardial infarction, stroke, hearing loss, non-arteritic anterior ischaemic optic neuropathy, retinal vascular occlusion, visual field defect, Stevens-Johnson syndrome

Dose

- ADULT over 18 years, 40 mg once daily

Adcirca® (Lilly) PoM

Tablets, f/c, tadalafil 20 mg (orange), net price 56-tab pack = £491.22

2.5.2 Centrally acting antihypertensive drugs

Methyldopa is a centrally acting antihypertensive; it may be used for the management of hypertension in pregnancy. Side-effects are minimised if the daily dose is kept below 1 g.

Clonidine has the disadvantage that sudden withdrawal of treatment may cause severe rebound hypertension.

Moxonidine, a centrally acting drug, is licensed for mild to moderate essential hypertension. It may have a role when thiazides, calcium-channel blockers, ACE inhibitors, and beta-blockers are not appropriate or have failed to control blood pressure.

CLONIDINE HYDROCHLORIDE

Indications hypertension; migraine (section 4.7.4.2); Tourette syndrome [unlicensed] (section 4.9.3); menopausal flushing (section 6.4.1.1); sedation [unlicensed] (section 15.1.4.4)

Cautions must be withdrawn gradually to avoid severe rebound hypertension; mild to moderate bradyarrhythmia; constipation; polyneuropathy; Raynaud's syndrome or other occlusive peripheral vascular disease; history of depression; **interactions:** Appendix 1 (clonidine)

Driving Drowsiness may affect performance of skilled tasks (e.g. driving); effects of alcohol may be enhanced

Contra-indications severe bradyarrhythmia secondary to second- or third-degree AV block or sick sinus syndrome

Renal impairment use with caution

Pregnancy may lower fetal heart rate, but risk should be balanced against risk of uncontrolled maternal hypertension; avoid intravenous injection

Breast-feeding avoid—present in milk

Side-effects constipation, nausea, dry mouth, vomiting, salivary gland pain, postural hypotension, dizziness, sleep disturbances, headache, malaise, drowsiness, depression, sexual dysfunction, *less commonly* bradycardia, Raynaud's syndrome, delusion, hallucination, paraesthesia, pruritus, rash, urticaria; *rarely* colonic pseudo-obstruction, AV block, gynaecomastia, decreased lacrimation, nasal dryness, alopecia; *also reported* hepatitis, fluid retention, bradyarrhythmia, confusion, impaired visual accommodation

Dose

- By mouth, 50–100 micrograms 3 times daily, increased every second or third day; usual max. dose 1.2 mg daily

Catapres® (Boehringer Ingelheim) PoM

Tablets, scored, clonidine hydrochloride 100 micrograms, net price 100-tab pack = £8.04. Label: 3, 8

Dixarit® PoM

Section 4.7.4.2

METHYLDOPA

Indications hypertension

Cautions monitor blood counts and liver-function before treatment and at intervals during first 6–12 weeks or if unexplained fever occurs; history of depression; positive direct Coombs' test in up to 20% of patients (may affect blood cross-matching); interference with laboratory tests; **interactions:** Appendix 1 (methyldopa)

Driving Drowsiness may affect performance of skilled tasks (e.g. driving); effects of alcohol may be enhanced

Contra-indications depression, phaeochromocytoma; acute porphyria (section 9.8.2)

Hepatic impairment manufacturer advises caution in history of liver disease; avoid in active liver disease

Renal impairment start with small dose; increased sensitivity to hypotensive and sedative effect

Pregnancy not known to be harmful

Breast-feeding amount too small to be harmful

Side-effects gastro-intestinal disturbances, dry mouth, stomatitis, sialadenitis; bradycardia, exacerbation of angina, postural hypotension, oedema; sedation, headache, dizziness, asthenia, myalgia, arthralgia, paraesthesia, nightmares, mild psychosis, depression, impaired mental acuity, parkinsonism, Bell's palsy; hepatitis, jaundice; pancreatitis; haemolytic anaemia; bone-marrow depression, leucopenia, thrombocytopenia, eosinophilia; hypersensitivity reactions including lupus erythematosus-like syndrome, drug fever, myocarditis, pericarditis; rashes (including toxic epidermal necrolysis); nasal congestion, failure of ejaculation, impotence, decreased libido, gynaecomastia, hyperprolactinaemia, amenorrhoea

Dose

- Initially 250 mg 2–3 times daily, increased gradually at intervals of at least 2 days, max. 3 g daily; ELDERLY initially 125 mg twice daily, increased gradually, max. 2 g daily

Methyldopa (Non-proprietary) PoM

Tablets, coated, methyldopa (anhydrous) 125 mg, net price 56-tab pack = £91.85; 250 mg, 56-tab pack = £6.33; 500 mg, 56-tab pack = £9.84. Label: 3, 8

Aldomet® (Aspen) PoM

Tablets, all yellow, f/c, methyldopa (anhydrous) 250 mg, net price 60 = £6.15; 500 mg, 30 = £4.55. Label: 3, 8

MOXONIDINE

Indications mild to moderate essential hypertension

Cautions avoid abrupt withdrawal (if concomitant treatment with beta-blocker has to be stopped, discontinue beta-blocker first, then moxonidine after a few days); severe coronary artery disease; unstable angina; first-degree AV block; moderate heart failure; **interactions:** see Appendix 1 (moxonidine)

Contra-indications conduction disorders (sick sinus syndrome, sino-atrial block, second- or third-degree AV block); bradycardia; severe heart failure

2 Cardiovascular system

2 Cardiovascular system

Renal impairment max. single dose 200 micrograms and max. daily dose 400 micrograms if eGFR 30–60 mL/minute/1.73 m²; avoid if eGFR less than 30 mL/minute/1.73 m²

Pregnancy manufacturer advises avoid—no information available

Breast-feeding present in milk—manufacturer advises avoid

Side-effects dry mouth, diarrhoea, nausea, vomiting, dyspepsia, dizziness, somnolence, insomnia, back pain, rash, pruritus; *less commonly* bradycardia, tinnitus, angioedema, oedema, nervousness, neck pain

Dose

- 200 micrograms once daily in the morning, increased if necessary after 3 weeks to 400 micrograms daily in 1–2 divided doses; max. 600 micrograms daily in 2 divided doses (max. single dose 400 micrograms)

Moxonidine (Non-proprietary) PoM
Tablets, f/c, moxonidine 200 micrograms, net price 28-tab pack = £2.42; 300 micrograms, net price 28-tab pack = £2.61; 400 micrograms, net price 28-tab pack = £2.70. Label: 3

Physiotens® (Abbott Healthcare) PoM
Tablets, f/c, moxonidine 200 micrograms (pink), net price 28-tab pack = £9.72; 300 micrograms (red), 28-tab pack = £11.49; 400 micrograms (red), 28-tab pack = £13.26. Label: 3

2.5.3 Adrenergic neurone blocking drugs

Adrenergic neurone blocking drugs prevent the release of noradrenaline from postganglionic adrenergic neurones. These drugs do not control supine blood pressure and may cause postural hypotension. For this reason they have largely fallen from use, but may be necessary with other therapy in resistant hypertension.

Guanethidine, which also depletes the nerve endings of noradrenaline, is licensed for rapid control of blood pressure, however alternative treatments are preferred (see section 2.5).

GUANETHIDINE MONOSULFATE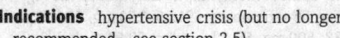

Indications hypertensive crisis (but no longer recommended—see section 2.5)

Cautions coronary or cerebral arteriosclerosis, asthma, history of peptic ulceration; **interactions:** Appendix 1 (adrenergic neurone blockers)

Contra-indications phaeochromocytoma, heart failure

Renal impairment reduce dose if eGFR 40–65 mL/minute/1.73 m²; avoid if eGFR less than 40 mL/minute/1.73 m²

Pregnancy postural hypotension and reduced utero-placental perfusion; should not be used to treat hypertension in pregnancy

Side-effects postural hypotension, failure of ejaculation, fluid retention, nasal congestion, headache, diarrhoea, drowsiness

Dose

- By intramuscular injection, 10–20 mg, repeated after 3 hours if required

Guanethidine Monosulfate (Non-proprietary) PoM ▨
Injection, guanethidine monosulfate 10 mg/mL, net price 1-mL amp = £44.83

2.5.4 Alpha-adrenoceptor blocking drugs

Prazosin has post-synaptic alpha-blocking and vasodilator properties and rarely causes tachycardia. It may, however, reduce blood pressure rapidly after the first dose and should be introduced with caution. **Doxazosin**, **indoramin**, and **terazosin** have properties similar to those of prazosin.

Alpha-blockers can be used with other antihypertensive drugs in the treatment of resistant hypertension (section 2.5).

Prostatic hyperplasia Alfuzosin, doxazosin, indoramin, prazosin, tamsulosin, and terazosin are indicated for benign prostatic hyperplasia (section 7.4.1).

DOXAZOSIN

Indications hypertension (see notes above); benign prostatic hyperplasia (section 7.4.1)

Cautions care with initial dose (postural hypotension); pulmonary oedema due to aortic or mitral stenosis; cataract surgery (risk of intra-operative floppy iris syndrome); heart failure; **interactions:** Appendix 1 (alpha-blockers)

    Driving May affect performance of skilled tasks e.g. driving

Contra-indications history of postural hypotension; monotherapy in overflow bladder or anuria

Hepatic impairment use with caution; manufacturer advises avoid in severe impairment—no information available

Pregnancy no evidence of teratogenicity; manufacturers advise use only when potential benefit outweighs risk

Breast-feeding accumulates in milk—manufacturer advises avoid

Side-effects see section 7.4.1; also dyspnoea, coughing; fatigue, vertigo, paraesthesia, sleep disturbance, anxiety; influenza-like symptoms; back pain, myalgia; *less commonly* weight changes, angina, myocardial infarction, hypoaesthesia, tremor, agitation, micturition disturbance, epistaxis, arthralgia, tinnitus, and gout; *very rarely* cholestasis, hepatitis, jaundice, bradycardia, arrhythmias, bronchospasm, hot flushes, gynaecomastia, abnormal ejaculation, leucopenia, thrombocytopenia, and alopecia

Dose

- Hypertension, 1 mg daily, increased after 1–2 weeks to 2 mg once daily, and thereafter to 4 mg once daily, if necessary; max. 16 mg daily

Doxazosin (Non-proprietary) PoM
Tablets, doxazosin (as mesilate) 1 mg, net price 28-tab pack = 92p; 2 mg, 28-tab pack = 94p; 4 mg, 28-tab pack = £1.10. Counselling, initial dose, driving
Brands include *Doxadura®*

Cardura® (Pfizer) PoM
Tablets, doxazosin (as mesilate) 1 mg, net price 28-tab pack = £10.56; 2 mg, 28-tab pack = £14.08. Counselling, initial dose, driving

◢ **Modified-release**

Doxazosin (Non-proprietary) PoM
Tablets, m/r, doxazosin (as mesilate) 4 mg, net price 28-tab pack = £5.00. Label: 25, counselling, initial dose, driving
Brands include *Doxadura® XL, Doxzogen® XL, Raporsin® XL, Slocinx® XL*
Dose hypertension, benign prostatic hyperplasia, 4 mg once daily, increased to 8 mg once daily after 4 weeks if necessary

Cardura® XL (Pfizer) PoM
Tablets, m/r, doxazosin (as mesilate) 4 mg, net price 28-tab pack = £5.00; 8 mg, 28-tab pack = £9.98. Label: 25, counselling, driving, initial dose
Dose hypertension, benign prostatic hyperplasia, 4 mg once daily, increased to 8 mg once daily after 4 weeks if necessary

---

◼ INDORAMIN

Indications hypertension (see notes above); benign prostatic hyperplasia (section 7.4.1)

Cautions avoid alcohol (enhances rate and extent of absorption); control incipient heart failure before initiating indoramin; elderly; Parkinson's disease (extrapyramidal disorders reported); epilepsy (convulsions in *animal* studies); history of depression; cataract surgery (risk of intra-operative floppy iris syndrome); **interactions**: Appendix 1 (alpha-blockers)
Driving Drowsiness may affect performance of skilled tasks (e.g. driving); effects of alcohol may be enhanced

Contra-indications established heart failure

Hepatic impairment manufacturer advises caution

Renal impairment manufacturer advises caution

Pregnancy no evidence of teratogenicity; manufacturers advise use only when potential benefit outweighs risk

Breast-feeding no information available

Side-effects see section 7.4.1; also sedation; *less commonly* fatigue, weight gain, failure of ejaculation; also reported extrapyramidal disorders, urinary frequency, and incontinence

Dose
● Hypertension, initially 25 mg twice daily, increased by 25–50 mg daily at intervals of 2 weeks; max. daily dose 200 mg in 2–3 divided doses

Indoramin (Non-proprietary) PoM
Tablets, indoramin (as hydrochloride) 25 mg, net price 84-tab pack = £60.26. Label: 2

Doralese® PoM
Section 7.4.1 (prostatic hyperplasia)

◼ PRAZOSIN

Indications hypertension (see notes above); congestive heart failure (but see section 2.5.5); Raynaud's syndrome (see also section 2.6.4); benign prostatic hyperplasia (section 7.4.1)

Cautions first dose may cause collapse due to hypotension (therefore should be taken on retiring to bed); elderly; cataract surgery (risk of intra-operative floppy iris syndrome); **interactions**: Appendix 1 (alpha-blockers)
Driving May affect performance of skilled tasks e.g. driving

Contra-indications not recommended for congestive heart failure due to mechanical obstruction (e.g. aortic stenosis)

Hepatic impairment initially 500 micrograms daily; increased with caution

Renal impairment initially 500 micrograms daily in moderate to severe impairment; increased with caution

Pregnancy no evidence of teratogenicity; manufacturers advise use only when potential benefit outweighs risk

Breast-feeding amount probably too small to be harmful

Side-effects see section 7.4.1; also dyspnoea; nervousness; urinary frequency; *less commonly* insomnia, paraesthesia, sweating, arthralgia, eye disorders, tinnitus, and epistaxis; *rarely* pancreatitis, flushing, vasculitis, bradycardia, hallucinations, worsening of narcolepsy, gynaecomastia, urinary incontinence, and alopecia

Dose
● Hypertension (see notes above), 500 micrograms 2–3 times daily for 3–7 days, the initial dose on retiring to bed at night (to avoid collapse, see Cautions); increased to 1 mg 2–3 times daily for a further 3–7 days; further increased if necessary to max. 20 mg daily in divided doses

● Congestive heart failure (but see section 2.5.5), 500 micrograms 2–4 times daily (initial dose at bedtime, see above), increasing to 4 mg daily in divided doses; maintenance 4–20 mg daily in divided doses (but rarely used)

● Raynaud's syndrome (but efficacy not established, see section 2.6.4), initially 500 micrograms twice daily (initial dose at bedtime, see above) increased, if necessary, after 3–7 days to usual maintenance 1–2 mg twice daily

Prazosin (Non-proprietary) PoM
Tablets, prazosin (as hydrochloride) 500 micrograms, net price 56-tab pack = £2.51; 1 mg, 56-tab pack = £3.23; 2 mg, 56-tab pack = £4.39; 5 mg, 56-tab pack = £8.75. Counselling, initial dose, driving

Hypovase® (Pfizer) PoM
Tablets, prazosin (as hydrochloride) 500 micrograms, net price 60-tab pack = £2.69; 1 mg, scored, 60-tab pack = £3.46. Counselling, initial dose, driving

---

◼ TERAZOSIN

Indications mild to moderate hypertension (see notes above); benign prostatic hyperplasia (section 7.4.1)

Cautions first dose may cause collapse due to hypotension (within 30–90 minutes, therefore should be taken on retiring to bed) (may also occur with rapid dose increase); cataract surgery (risk of intra-operative floppy iris syndrome); **interactions**: Appendix 1 (alpha-blockers)
Driving May affect performance of skilled tasks e.g. driving

Pregnancy no evidence of teratogenicity; manufacturers advise use only when potential benefit outweighs risk

Breast-feeding no information available

Side-effects see section 7.4.1; *also reported* weight gain, dyspnoea, paraesthesia, nervousness, decreased libido, thrombocytopenia, back pain, and pain in extremities

Dose
● Hypertension, 1 mg at bedtime (compliance with bedtime dose important, see Cautions); dose doubled after 7 days if necessary; usual maintenance dose 2–10 mg once daily; more than 20 mg daily rarely improves efficacy

2 Cardiovascular system

Terazosin (Non-proprietary) [PoM]

Tablets, terazosin (as hydrochloride) 2 mg, net price 28-tab pack = £2.44; 5 mg, 28-tab pack = £2.76; 10 mg, 28-tab pack = £8.04. Counselling, initial dose, driving

Hytrin® (AMCo) [PoM]

Tablets, terazosin (as hydrochloride) 2 mg (yellow), net price 28-tab pack = £2.20; 5 mg (tan), 28-tab pack = £4.13; 10 mg (blue), 28-tab pack = £8.24; starter pack (for hypertension) of 7 × 1-mg tabs with 21 × 2-mg tabs = £10.97. Counselling, initial dose, driving

Phaeochromocytoma

Long-term management of phaeochromocytoma involves surgery. However, surgery should not take place until there is adequate blockade of both alpha- and beta-adrenoceptors; the optimal choice of drug therapy remains unclear. Alpha-blockers are used in the short-term management of hypertensive episodes in phaeochromocytoma. Once alpha blockade is established, tachycardia can be controlled by the cautious addition of a beta-blocker (section 2.4); a cardioselective beta-blocker is preferred.

Phenoxybenzamine, a powerful alpha-blocker, is effective in the management of phaeochromocytoma but it has many side-effects. **Phentolamine** is a short-acting alpha-blocker used mainly during surgery of phaeochromocytoma; its use for the diagnosis of phaeochromocytoma has been superseded by measurement of catecholamines in blood and urine.

Metirosine (available from 'special-order' manufacturers or specialist importing companies, see p. 1124) inhibits the enzyme tyrosine hydroxylase, and hence the synthesis of catecholamines. It is rarely used in the pre-operative management of phaeochromocytoma, and long term in patients unsuitable for surgery; an alpha-adrenoceptor blocking drug may also be required. Metirosine should **not** be used to treat essential hypertension.

▌ PHENOXYBENZAMINE HYDROCHLORIDE

Indications hypertensive episodes in phaeochromocytoma

Cautions elderly; congestive heart failure; severe ischaemic heart disease (see also Contra-indications); cerebrovascular disease (avoid if history of cerebrovascular accident); monitor blood pressure regularly during infusion; carcinogenic in *animals*; avoid in acute porphyria (section 9.8.2); avoid extravasation (irritant to tissues)

Contra-indications history of cerebrovascular accident; during recovery period after myocardial infarction (usually 3–4 weeks); avoid infusion in hypovolaemia

Renal impairment use with caution

Pregnancy hypotension may occur in newborn

Breast-feeding may be present in milk

Side-effects postural hypotension with dizziness and marked compensatory tachycardia, lassitude, nasal congestion, miosis, inhibition of ejaculation; rarely gastro-intestinal disturbances; decreased sweating and dry mouth after intravenous infusion; idiosyncratic profound hypotension within few minutes of

starting infusion; convulsions following rapid intravenous infusion also reported

Dose

- See under preparations

Phenoxybenzamine (Non-proprietary) [PoM]

Capsules, phenoxybenzamine hydrochloride 10 mg, net price 30-cap pack = £32.87

Dose by mouth, phaeochromocytoma, intially 10 mg daily, increased by 10 mg daily until hypertension controlled or treatment not tolerated; usual dose 1–2 mg/kg daily in 2 divided doses

Injection concentrate, phenoxybenzamine hydrochloride 50 mg/mL. To be diluted before use, net price 2-mL amp = £57.14 (hosp. only)

Dose by intravenous infusion (preferably through large vein), adjunct in severe shock (but rarely used) and phaeochromocytoma, 1 mg/kg daily over at least 2 hours; do not repeat within 24 hours (intensive care facilities needed)

Caution Owing to risk of contact sensitisation healthcare professionals should avoid contamination of hands

▌ PHENTOLAMINE MESILATE

Indications hypertensive episodes due to phaeochromocytoma e.g. during surgery; diagnosis of phaeochromocytoma (but see notes above)

Cautions monitor blood pressure (avoid in hypotension), heart rate; gastritis, peptic ulcer; elderly; **interactions:** Appendix 1 (alpha-blockers)

Contra-indications hypotension; history of myocardial infarction; coronary insufficiency, angina, or other evidence of coronary artery disease

Renal impairment manufacturer advises caution—no information available

Pregnancy use with caution—may cause marked decrease in maternal blood pressure with resulting fetal anoxia

Breast-feeding manufacturer advises avoid—no information available

Side-effects postural hypotension, tachycardia, dizziness, flushing; nausea and vomiting, diarrhoea, nasal congestion; also acute or prolonged hypotension, angina, chest pain, arrhythmias

Dose

- Hypertensive episodes, by intravenous injection, 2–5 mg repeated if necessary
- Diagnosis of phaeochromocytoma, consult product literature

Phentolamine (Non-proprietary) [PoM]

Injection, phentolamine mesilate 10 mg/mL

Available from 'special-order' manufacturers or specialist importing companies, see p. 1124

2.5.5 Drugs affecting the renin-angiotensin system

2.5.5.1	Angiotensin-converting enzyme inhibitors
2.5.5.2	Angiotensin-II receptor antagonists
2.5.5.3	Renin inhibitors

Heart failure

Drug treatment of heart failure associated with a reduced left ventricular ejection fraction (left ventricular systolic dysfunction) is covered below; optimal management of heart failure with a preserved left ventricular ejection fraction has not been established.

The treatment of chronic heart failure aims to relieve symptoms, improve exercise tolerance, reduce the incidence of acute exacerbations, and reduce mortality. An **ACE inhibitor**, titrated to a 'target dose' (or the maximum tolerated dose if lower), together with a **beta-blocker**, form the basis of treatment for all patients with heart failure due to left ventricular systolic dysfunction.

An ACE inhibitor (section 2.5.5.1) is generally advised for patients with asymptomatic left ventricular systolic dysfunction or symptomatic heart failure. An **angiotensin-II receptor antagonist** (section 2.5.5.2) may be a useful alternative for patients who, because of side-effects such as cough, cannot tolerate ACE inhibitors; a relatively high dose of the angiotensin-II receptor antagonist may be required to produce benefit. Candesartan or valsartan may be given under specialist supervision as adjuncts to an ACE inhibitor in the the treatment of heart failure when other treatments are unsuitable; the concomitant use of this combination, together with an aldosterone antagonist or a potassium-sparing diuretic is not recommended (see also Concomitant Use of Drugs Affecting The Renin-angiotensin System, p. 120).

The beta-blockers bisoprolol and carvedilol (section 2.4) are of value in any grade of stable heart failure due to left ventricular systolic dysfunction; nebivolol (section 2.4) is licensed for stable mild to moderate heart failure in patients over 70 years. Beta-blocker treatment should be started by those experienced in the management of heart failure, at a very low dose and titrated very slowly over a period of weeks or months. Symptoms may deteriorate initially, calling for adjustment of concomitant therapy.

The aldosterone antagonist **spironolactone** can be added to an ACE inhibitor and a beta-blocker in patients who continue to remain symptomatic (particularly in those with moderate to severe heart failure); low doses of spironolactone (section 2.2.3, p. 91) reduce symptoms and mortality in these patients. If spironolactone cannot be used, **eplerenone** (section 2.2.3) may be considered for the management of heart failure after an acute myocardial infarction with evidence of left ventricular systolic dysfunction, or for chronic mild heart failure with left ventricular systolic dysfunction. Close monitoring of serum creatinine, eGFR, and potassium is necessary, particularly following any change in treatment or any change in the patient's clinical condition.

Patients who cannot tolerate an ACE inhibitor or an angiotensin-II receptor antagonist, or in whom they are contra-indicated, may be given **isosorbide dinitrate** (section 2.6.1) with **hydralazine** (section 2.5.1), but this combination may be poorly tolerated. The combination of isosorbide dinitrate and hydralazine may be considered in addition to standard therapy with an ACE inhibitor and a beta-blocker in patients who continue to remain symptomatic (particularly in patients of African or Caribbean origin who have moderate to severe heart failure).

Digoxin (section 2.1.1) improves symptoms of heart failure and exercise tolerance and reduces hospitalisation due to acute exacerbations but it does not reduce mortality. Digoxin is reserved for patients with worsening or severe heart failure due to left ventricular systolic dysfunction who remain symptomatic despite treatment

with an ACE inhibitor and a beta-blocker in combination with either an aldosterone antagonist, candesartan, or isosorbide dinitrate with hydralazine.

Patients with fluid overload should also receive either a loop or a thiazide diuretic (with salt or fluid restriction where appropriate). A **thiazide diuretic** (section 2.2.1) may be of benefit in patients with mild heart failure and good renal function; however, thiazide diuretics are ineffective in patients with poor renal function (eGFR less than $30 \, \text{mL/minute}/1.73 \, \text{m}^2$, see Renal Impairment, section 2.2.1) and a **loop diuretic** (section 2.2.2) is preferred. If diuresis with a single diuretic is insufficient, a combination of a loop diuretic and a thiazide diuretic may be tried; addition of metolazone (section 2.2.1) may also be considered but the resulting diuresis may be profound and care is needed to avoid potentially dangerous electrolyte disturbances.

2.5.5.1   Angiotensin-converting enzyme inhibitors

Angiotensin-converting enzyme inhibitors (ACE inhibitors) inhibit the conversion of angiotensin I to angiotensin II. They have many uses and are generally well tolerated. The main indications of ACE inhibitors are shown below.

Heart failure   ACE inhibitors are used in all grades of heart failure, usually combined with a beta-blocker (section 2.5.5). Potassium supplements and potassium-sparing diuretics should be discontinued before introducing an ACE inhibitor because of the risk of hyperkalaemia. However, a low dose of spironolactone may be beneficial in severe heart failure (section 2.5.5) and can be used with an ACE inhibitor provided serum potassium is monitored carefully. Profound first-dose hypotension may occur when ACE inhibitors are introduced to patients with heart failure who are already taking a high dose of a loop diuretic (e.g. furosemide 80 mg daily or more). Temporary withdrawal of the loop diuretic reduces the risk, but may cause severe rebound pulmonary oedema. Therefore, for patients on high doses of loop diuretics, the ACE inhibitor may need to be initiated under specialist supervision, see below. An ACE inhibitor can be initiated in the community in patients who are receiving a low dose of a diuretic or who are not otherwise at risk of serious hypotension; nevertheless, care is required and a very low dose of the ACE inhibitor is given initially. For comment on the use of an ACE inhibitor with other drugs affecting the renin-angiotensin system, see Concomitant Use of Drugs Affecting The Renin-angiotensin System, p. 120.

Hypertension   An ACE inhibitor may be the most appropriate initial drug for hypertension in younger Caucasian patients; Afro-Caribbean patients, those aged over 55 years, and those with primary aldosteronism respond less well (see section 2.5). ACE inhibitors are particularly indicated for hypertension in patients with type 1 diabetes with nephropathy (see also section 6.1.5). They may reduce blood pressure very rapidly in some patients particularly in those receiving diuretic therapy (see Cautions, below); the first dose should preferably be given at bedtime.

Diabetic nephropathy   For comment on the role of ACE inhibitors in the management of diabetic nephropathy, see section 6.1.5.

Prophylaxis of cardiovascular events ACE inhibitors are used in the early and long-term management of patients who have had a myocardial infarction, see section 2.10.1. ACE inhibitors may also have a role in preventing cardiovascular events.

Initiation under specialist supervision ACE inhibitors should be initiated under specialist supervision and with careful clinical monitoring in those with severe heart failure or in those:

- receiving multiple or high-dose diuretic therapy (e.g. more than 80 mg of furosemide daily or its equivalent);

- receiving concomitant angiotensin-II receptor antagonist or aliskiren;

- with hypovolaemia;

- with hyponatraemia (plasma-sodium concentration below 130 mmol/litre);

- with hypotension (systolic blood pressure below 90 mmHg);

- with unstable heart failure;

- receiving high-dose vasodilator therapy;

- known renovascular disease.

Renal effects Renal function and electrolytes should be checked before starting ACE inhibitors (or increasing the dose) and monitored during treatment (more frequently if features mentioned below present); hyperkalaemia and other side-effects of ACE inhibitors are more common in those with impaired renal function and the dose may need to be reduced (see Renal impairment below and under individual drugs). Although ACE inhibitors now have a specialised role in some forms of renal disease, including chronic kidney disease, they also occasionally cause impairment of renal function which may progress and become severe in other circumstances (at particular risk are the elderly). A specialist should be involved if renal function is significantly reduced as a result of treatment with an ACE inhibitor.

Concomitant treatment with NSAIDs increases the risk of renal damage, and potassium-sparing diuretics (or potassium-containing salt substitutes) increase the risk of hyperkalaemia.

In patients with severe bilateral renal artery stenosis (or severe stenosis of the artery supplying a single functioning kidney), ACE inhibitors reduce or abolish glomerular filtration and are likely to cause severe and progressive renal failure. They are therefore not recommended in patients known to have these forms of critical renovascular disease.

ACE inhibitor treatment is unlikely to have an adverse effect on overall renal function in patients with severe unilateral renal artery stenosis and a normal contralateral kidney, but glomerular filtration is likely to be reduced (or even abolished) in the affected kidney and the long-term consequences are unknown.

ACE inhibitors are therefore best avoided in patients with known or suspected renovascular disease, unless the blood pressure cannot be controlled by other drugs. If ACE inhibitors are used, they should be initiated only under specialist supervision and renal function should be monitored regularly.

ACE inhibitors should also be used with particular caution in patients who may have undiagnosed and clinically silent renovascular disease. This includes patients with peripheral vascular disease or those with severe generalised atherosclerosis.

Cautions ACE inhibitors need to be initiated with care in patients receiving diuretics (**important:** see Concomitant diuretics, below); first doses can cause hypotension especially in patients taking high doses of diuretics, on a low-sodium diet, on dialysis, dehydrated, or with heart failure (see above). They should also be used with caution in peripheral vascular disease or generalised atherosclerosis owing to risk of clinically silent renovascular disease; for use in pre-existing renovascular disease, see Renal Effects above. The risk of agranulocytosis is possibly increased in collagen vascular disease (blood counts recommended). ACE inhibitors should be used with care in patients with severe or symptomatic aortic stenosis (risk of hypotension) and in hypertrophic cardiomyopathy. They should also be used with care (or avoided) in those with a history of idiopathic or hereditary angioedema. If jaundice or marked elevations of hepatic enzymes occur during treatment then the ACE inhibitor should be discontinued—risk of hepatic necrosis (see also Hepatic impairment, below). **Interactions:** Appendix 1 (ACE inhibitors).

Anaphylactoid reactions To prevent anaphylactoid reactions, ACE inhibitors should be avoided during dialysis with high-flux polyacrylonitrile membranes and during low-density lipoprotein apheresis with dextran sulfate; they should also be withheld before desensitisation with wasp or bee venom.

Concomitant diuretics ACE inhibitors can cause a very rapid fall in blood pressure in volume-depleted patients; treatment should therefore be initiated with very low doses. If the dose of diuretic is greater than 80 mg furosemide or equivalent, the ACE inhibitor should be initiated under close supervision and in some patients the diuretic dose may need to be reduced or the diuretic discontinued at least 24 hours beforehand (may not be possible in heart failure—risk of pulmonary oedema). If high-dose diuretic therapy cannot be stopped, close observation is recommended after administration of the first dose of ACE inhibitor, for at least 2 hours or until the blood pressure has stabilised.

Concomitant use of drugs affecting the renin-angiotensin system Combination therapy with two drugs affecting the renin-angiotensin system (ACE inhibitors, angiotensin-II receptor antagonists, and aliskiren) is not recommended due to an increased risk of hyperkalaemia, hypotension, and renal impairment, compared to use of a single drug. Patients with diabetic nephropathy are particularly susceptible to developing hyperkalaemia and should not be given an ACE inhibitor with an angiotensin-II receptor antagonist. There is some evidence that the benefits of combination use of an ACE inhibitor with candesartan or valsartan may outweigh the risks in selected patients with heart failure for whom other treatments are unsuitable, however, the concomitant use of this combination, together with an aldosterone antagonist or a potassium-sparing diuretic is not recommended.

For patients currently taking combination therapy, the need for continued combined therapy should be reviewed. If combination therapy is considered essential, it should be carried out under specialist supervision, with close monitoring of blood pressure, renal function, and electrolytes (particularly potassium); monitoring should be considered at the start of treatment, then monthly, and also after any change in dose or during intercurrent illness.

Contra-indications ACE inhibitors are contra-indicated in patients with hypersensitivity to ACE inhibitors (including angioedema). The combination of an ACE inhibitor with aliskiren is contra-indicated in those with diabetes mellitus or if eGFR is less than 60 mL/minute/1.73m^2.

Hepatic impairment Use of prodrugs such as enalapril, fosinopril, imidapril, moexipril, perindopril, quinapril, ramipril, and trandolapril requires close monitoring in patients with impaired liver function

Renal impairment ACE inhibitors should be used with caution and the response monitored (see Renal effects above); hyperkalaemia and other side effects more common; the dose may need to be reduced, see individual drugs.

Pregnancy ACE inhibitors should be avoided in pregnancy unless essential. They may adversely affect fetal and neonatal blood pressure control and renal function; skull defects and oligohydramnios have also been reported.

Breast-feeding Information on the use of ACE inhibitors in breast-feeding is limited. Fosinopril, imidapril, lisinopril, moexipril, perindopril, ramipril, and trandolapril are not recommended; alternative treatment options, with better established safety information during breast-feeding, are available. Captopril, enalapril, and quinapril should be avoided in the first few weeks after delivery, particularly in preterm infants, due to the risk of profound neonatal hypotension; if essential, they may be used in mothers breast-feeding older infants—the infant's blood pressure should be monitored.

Side-effects ACE inhibitors can cause profound hypotension (see Cautions) and renal impairment (see Renal effects above), and a persistent dry cough. They can also cause angioedema (onset may be delayed; higher incidence reported in Afro-Caribbean patients), rash (which may be associated with pruritus and urticaria), pancreatitis, and upper respiratory-tract symptoms such as sinusitis, rhinitis, and sore throat. Gastrointestinal effects reported with ACE inhibitors include nausea, vomiting, dyspepsia, diarrhoea, constipation, and abdominal pain. Altered liver function tests, cholestatic jaundice, hepatitis, fulminant hepatic necrosis, and hepatic failure have been reported—discontinue if marked elevation of hepatic enzymes or jaundice. Hyperkalaemia, hypoglycaemia, and blood disorders including thrombocytopenia, leucopenia, neutropenia, and haemolytic anaemia have also been reported. Other reported side-effects include headache, dizziness, fatigue, malaise, taste disturbance, paraesthesia, bronchospasm, fever, serositis, vasculitis, myalgia, arthralgia, positive antinuclear antibody, raised erythrocyte sedimentation rate, eosinophilia, leucocytosis, and photosensitivity.

Combination products Products incorporating an ACE inhibitor with a thiazide diuretic or a calcium-channel blocker are available for the management of hypertension. Use of these combination products should be reserved for patients whose blood pressure has not responded adequately to a single antihypertensive drug and who have been stabilised on the individual components of the combination in the same proportions.

CAPTOPRIL

Indications essential hypertension; chronic heart failure (adjunct—see section 2.5.5); following myocardial infarction, see dose below; diabetic nephropathy in type 1 diabetes

Cautions see notes above

Contra-indications see notes above

Renal impairment see notes above; reduce dose; max. initial dose 50 mg if eGFR above 40 mL/minute/1.73m^2; max. initial dose 25 mg daily (do not exceed 100 mg daily) if eGFR 20–40 mL/minute/1.73 m^2; max. initial dose 12.5 mg daily (do not exceed 75 mg daily) if eGFR 10–20 mL/minute/1.73 m^2; max. initial dose 6.25 mg daily (do not exceed 37.5 mg daily) if eGFR less than 10 mL/minute/1.73 m^2

Pregnancy see notes above

Breast-feeding see notes above

Side-effects see notes above; also dry mouth, dyspnoea, sleep disorder, alopecia; *less commonly* tachycardia, palpitation, arrhythmia, angina, pallor, flushing, Raynaud's syndrome; *rarely* stomatitis, anorexia; *very rarely* glossitis, peptic ulcer, syncope, cerebrovascular events, cardiac arrest, cardiogenic shock, allergic alveolitis, eosinophilic pneumonia, confusion, depression, impotence, gynaecomastia, hyponatraemia, blurred vision, photosensitivity, Stevens-Johnson syndrome

Dose
- Hypertension, initially 12.5–25 mg twice daily; ELDERLY intially 6.25 mg twice daily; in volume depletion (see Concomitant diuretics), cardiac decompensation, or renovascular hypertension, initially 6.25–12.5 mg as a single dose preferably under close medical supervision, then twice daily; increased if necessary at intervals of at least 2 weeks up to max. 150 mg daily in 2 divided doses (max. 100 mg daily in 1–2 divided doses in volume depletion, cardiac decompensation, or renovascular hypertension); once-daily dosing may be appropriate if other concomitant antihypertensive drugs taken
- Heart failure (adjunct), initially 6.25–12.5 mg 2–3 times daily under close medical supervision (see notes above), increased gradually at intervals of at least 2 weeks up to max. 150 mg daily in divided doses if tolerated
- Short-term treatment within 24 hours of onset of myocardial infarction in clinically stable patients, initially 6.25 mg, then 12.5 mg after 2 hours, followed by 25 mg 12 hours later; if tolerated, continue at 50 mg twice daily for 4 weeks
- Prophylaxis of symptomatic heart failure after myocardial infarction in clinically stable patients with asymptomatic left ventricular dysfunction, initially 6.25 mg once daily, starting 3–16 days after infarction under close medical supervision, then 12.5 mg 3 times daily for 2 days, then 25 mg 3 times daily if tolerated; increase gradually to 75–150 mg daily in 2–3 divided doses if tolerated
- Diabetic nephropathy, 75–100 mg daily in divided doses

Captopril (Non-proprietary) [PoM]
Tablets, captopril 12.5 mg, net price 56-tab pack = £2.44; 25 mg, 56-tab pack = £1.48; 50 mg, 56-tab pack = £2.47
Brands include *Ecopace®*, *Kaplon®*

Capoten® (Squibb) [PoM]
Tablets, scored, captopril 25 mg, net price 28-tab pack = £5.26

Noyada® (Martindale) [PoM]
Oral solution, captopril 5 mg/5 mL, net price 100 mL = £98.21; 25 mg/5 mL, 100 mL = £108.94
Electrolytes Na⁺ approx. 77 micromol/5 mL

◢ **With diuretic**

Note For mild to moderate hypertension in patients stabilised on the individual components in the same proportions. For prescribing information on thiazides, see section 2.2.1

Co-zidocapt (Non-proprietary) [PoM]
Tablets, co-zidocapt 12.5/25 (hydrochlorothiazide 12.5 mg, captopril 25 mg), net price 28-tab pack = £14.10
Brands include *Capto-co®*

Tablets, co-zidocapt 25/50 (hydrochlorothiazide 25 mg, captopril 50 mg), net price 28-tab pack = £14.00
Brands include *Capto-co®*

Capozide® (Squibb) [PoM]
Tablets, scored, co-zidocapt 25/50 (hydrochlorothiazide 25 mg, captopril 50 mg), net price 30-tab pack = £7.52

ENALAPRIL MALEATE

Indications hypertension; symptomatic heart failure (adjunct—see section 2.5.5); prevention of symptomatic heart failure in patients with asymptomatic left ventricular dysfunction

Cautions see notes above

Contra-indications see notes above

Hepatic impairment see notes above

Renal impairment see notes above; max. initial dose 2.5 mg daily if eGFR less than 30 mL/minute/1.73 m²

Pregnancy see notes above

Breast-feeding see notes above

Side-effects see notes above; also dyspnoea; depression, asthenia; blurred vision; *less commonly* dry mouth, peptic ulcer, anorexia, ileus; arrhythmias, palpitation, flushing; confusion, nervousness, drowsiness, insomnia, vertigo; impotence; muscle cramps; tinnitus; alopecia, sweating; hyponatraemia; *rarely* stomatitis, glossitis, Raynaud's syndrome, pulmonary infiltrates, allergic alveolitis, dream abnormalities, gynaecomastia, Stevens-Johnson syndrome, toxic epidermal necrolysis, exfoliative dermatitis, pemphigus; *very rarely* gastro-intestinal angioedema

Dose

• Hypertension, used alone, initially 5 mg once daily; if used in addition to diuretic (see notes above), or in renal impairment, lower initial doses may be required; usual maintenance dose 20 mg once daily; max. 40 mg once daily

• Heart failure (adjunct), asymptomatic left ventricular dysfunction, initially 2.5 mg once daily under close medical supervision (see notes above), increased gradually over 2–4 weeks to 10–20 mg twice daily if tolerated

Enalapril Maleate (Non-proprietary) [PoM]
Tablets, enalapril maleate 2.5 mg, net price 28-tab pack = £1.16; 5 mg, 28-tab pack = £1.02; 10 mg, 28-tab pack = £1.05; 20 mg, 28-tab pack = £1.16
Brands include *Ednyt®*

Innovace® (MSD) [PoM]
Tablets, enalapril maleate 2.5 mg, net price 28-tab pack = £5.35; 5 mg (scored), 28-tab pack = £7.51; 10 mg (red), 28-tab pack = £10.53; 20 mg (peach), 28-tab pack = £12.51

◢ **With diuretic**

Note For mild to moderate hypertension in patients stabilised on the individual components in the same proportions. For prescribing information on thiazides, see section 2.2.1

Innozide® (MSD) [PoM]
Tablets, yellow, scored, enalapril maleate 20 mg, hydrochlorothiazide 12.5 mg, net price 28-tab pack = £13.90
Note Non-proprietary tablets containing enalapril maleate (20 mg) and hydrochlorothiazide (12.5 mg) are available

FOSINOPRIL SODIUM

Indications hypertension; congestive heart failure (adjunct—see section 2.5.5)

Cautions see notes above

Contra-indications see notes above

Hepatic impairment see notes above

Renal impairment see notes above

Pregnancy see notes above

Breast-feeding see notes above

Side-effects see notes above; chest pain; musculoskeletal pain

Dose

• Hypertension, initially 10 mg daily, increased if necessary after 4 weeks; usual dose range 10–40 mg (doses over 40 mg not shown to increase efficacy); if used in addition to diuretic see notes above

• Heart failure (adjunct), initially 10 mg once daily under close medical supervision (see notes above), increased gradually to 40 mg once daily if tolerated

Fosinopril sodium (Non-proprietary) [PoM]
Tablets, fosinopril sodium 10 mg, net price 28-tab pack = £1.92; 20 mg, 28-tab pack = £2.48

IMIDAPRIL HYDROCHLORIDE

Indications essential hypertension

Cautions see notes above

Contra-indications see notes above

Hepatic impairment see notes above

Renal impairment see notes above; initial dose 2.5 mg daily if eGFR 30–80 mL/minute/1.73 m²; avoid if eGFR less than 30 mL/minute/1.73 m²

Pregnancy see notes above

Breast-feeding see notes above

Side-effects see notes above; dry mouth, glossitis, ileus; bronchitis, dyspnoea; sleep disturbances, depression, confusion, blurred vision, tinnitus, impotence

Dose

• Initially 5 mg daily before food; if used in addition to diuretic (see notes above), in elderly, in patients with heart failure, angina or cerebrovascular disease, or in renal or hepatic impairment, initially 2.5 mg daily; if necessary increase dose at intervals of at least 3 weeks; usual maintenance dose 10 mg once daily; max. 20 mg daily (elderly, 10 mg daily)

Tanatril® (Chiesi) [PoM]
Tablets, scored, imidapril hydrochloride 5 mg, net price 28-tab pack = £6.40; 10 mg, 28-tab pack = £7.22; 20 mg, 28-tab pack = £8.67

LISINOPRIL

Indications hypertension (but see notes above); symptomatic heart failure (adjunct—see section 2.5.5); short-term treatment following myocardial infarction in haemodynamically stable patients; renal complications of diabetes mellitus

Cautions see notes above

Contra-indications see notes above

Renal impairment see notes above; max. initial doses 5–10 mg daily if eGFR 30–80 mL/minute/1.73 m² (max. 40 mg daily); 2.5–5 mg daily if eGFR 10–30 mL/minute/1.73 m² (max. 40 mg daily); 2.5 mg daily if eGFR less than 10 mL/minute/1.73 m²

Pregnancy see notes above

Breast-feeding see notes above

Side-effects see notes above; also *less commonly* tachycardia, palpitation, cerebrovascular accident, myocardial infarction, Raynaud's syndrome, confusion, mood changes, vertigo, sleep disturbances, asthenia, impotence; *rarely* dry mouth, gynaecomastia, alopecia, psoriasis; *very rarely* allergic alveolitis, pulmonary infiltrates, profuse sweating, pemphigus, Stevens-Johnson syndrome, and toxic epidermal necrolysis

Dose

- Hypertension, initially 10 mg once daily; if used in addition to diuretic (see notes above) or in cardiac decompensation or in volume depletion, initially 2.5–5 mg once daily; usual maintenance dose 20 mg once daily; max. 80 mg once daily
- Heart failure (adjunct), initially 2.5 mg once daily under close medical supervision (see notes above); increased in steps no greater than 10 mg at intervals of at least 2 weeks up to max. 35 mg once daily if tolerated
- Prophylaxis after myocardial infarction, systolic blood pressure over 120 mmHg, 5 mg within 24 hours, followed by further 5 mg 24 hours later, then 10 mg after a further 24 hours, and continuing with 10 mg once daily for 6 weeks (or continued if heart failure); systolic blood pressure 100–120 mmHg, initially 2.5 mg once daily, increased to maintenance dose of 5 mg once daily

  Note Should not be started after myocardial infarction if systolic blood pressure less than 100 mmHg; temporarily reduce maintenance dose to 5 mg and if necessary 2.5 mg daily if systolic blood pressure 100 mmHg or less during treatment; withdraw if prolonged hypotension occurs (systolic blood pressure less than 90 mmHg for more than 1 hour)
- Renal complications of diabetes mellitus, initially 2.5–5 mg once daily adjusted according to response; usual dose range 10–20 mg once daily

Lisinopril (Non-proprietary) ⓟₒₘ

Tablets, lisinopril (as dihydrate) 2.5 mg, net price 28-tab pack = 96p; 5 mg, 28-tab pack = 99p; 10 mg, 28-tab pack = £1.01; 20 mg, 28-tab pack = £1.11

Zestril® (AstraZeneca) ⓟₒₘ

Tablets, lisinopril (as dihydrate) 5 mg (pink), net price = 28-tab pack = £4.71; 10 mg (pink), 28-tab pack = £7.38; 20 mg (pink), 28-tab pack = £6.51

◢With diuretic

Note For mild to moderate hypertension in patients stabilised on the individual components in the same proportions. For prescribing information on thiazides, see section 2.2.1

Carace Plus® (MSD) ⓟₒₘ

Carace 20 Plus tablets, yellow, scored, lisinopril 20 mg, hydrochlorothiazide 12.5 mg, net price 28-tab pack = £11.43

Zestoretic® (AstraZeneca) ⓟₒₘ

Zestoretic 10 tablets, peach, lisinopril (as dihydrate) 10 mg, hydrochlorothiazide 12.5 mg, net price 28-tab pack = £6.81

Zestoretic 20 tablets, lisinopril (as dihydrate) 20 mg, hydrochlorothiazide 12.5 mg, net price 28-tab pack = £11.52

MOEXIPRIL HYDROCHLORIDE

Indications essential hypertension

Cautions see notes above; also significant mitral valve stenosis

Contra-indications see notes above

Hepatic impairment see notes above; initial dose 3.75 mg once daily

Renal impairment see notes above; if eGFR less than 40 mL/minute/1.73 m², initial dose 3.75 mg once daily titrated to max. 15 mg once daily

Pregnancy see notes above

Breast-feeding see notes above

Side-effects see notes above; also arrhythmias, tachycardia, palpitation, angina, syncope, flushing, cerebrovascular accident, myocardial infarction, dyspnoea, appetite and weight changes, dry mouth, confusion, depression, numbness, drowsiness, sleep disturbance, impotence, hyperuricaemia, blurred vision, tinnitus, sweating, pemphigus, Stevens-Johnson syndrome, toxic epidermal necrolysis, alopecia

Dose

- Monotherapy, initially 7.5 mg once daily adjusted according to response; usual range 7.5–15 mg once daily (max. 30 mg once daily); if used in addition to diuretic (see notes above), with nifedipine or other antihypertensive drug, or in elderly, initially 3.75 mg once daily

Perdix® (UCB Pharma) ⓟₒₘ

Tablets, f/c, pink, scored, moexipril hydrochloride 7.5 mg, net price 28-tab pack = £6.04; 15 mg, 28-tab pack = £6.96

PERINDOPRIL ERBUMINE

Indications hypertension (but see notes above); symptomatic heart failure (adjunct—see section 2.5.5); prophylaxis of cardiac events following myocardial infarction or revascularisation in stable coronary artery disease

Cautions see notes above

Contra-indications see notes above

Hepatic impairment see notes above

Renal impairment see notes above; max. initial dose 2 mg once daily if eGFR 30–60 mL/minute/1.73 m²; 2 mg once daily on alternate days if eGFR 15–30 mL/minute/1.73 m²

Pregnancy see notes above

Breast-feeding see notes above

Side-effects see notes above; also asthenia, mood and sleep disturbances

Dose

- Hypertension, initially 4 mg once daily in the morning for 1 month, subsequently adjusted according to

response; if used in addition to diuretic (see notes above), in elderly, in renal impairment, in cardiac decompensation, or in volume depletion, initially 2 mg once daily; max. 8 mg daily
- Heart failure (adjunct), initially 2 mg once daily in the morning under close medical supervision (see notes above), increased after at least 2 weeks to max. 4 mg once daily if tolerated
- Following myocardial infarction or revascularisation, initially 4 mg once daily in the morning increased after 2 weeks to 8 mg once daily if tolerated; ELDERLY 2 mg once daily for 1 week, then 4 mg once daily for 1 week, thereafter increased to 8 mg once daily if tolerated

Perindopril (Non-proprietary) PoM
Tablets, perindopril erbumine (= *tert*-butylamine) 2 mg, net price 30-tab pack = £1.34; 4 mg, 30-tab pack = £1.58; 8 mg, 30-tab pack = £1.69. Label: 22

PERINDOPRIL ARGININE

Indications see under Perindopril Erbumine and notes above
Cautions see notes above
Contra-indications see notes above
Hepatic impairment see notes above
Renal impairment see notes above; max. initial dose 2.5 mg once daily if eGFR 30–60 mL/minute/1.73 m^2; 2.5 mg once daily on alternate days if eGFR 15–30 mL/minute/1.73 m^2
Pregnancy see notes above
Breast-feeding see notes above
Side-effects see under Perindopril Erbumine and notes above
Dose
- Hypertension, initially 5 mg once daily in the morning for 1 month, subsequently adjusted according to response; if used in addition to diuretic (see notes above), in elderly, in renal impairment, in cardiac decompensation, or in volume depletion, initially 2.5 mg once daily; max. 10 mg daily
- Heart failure (adjunct), initially 2.5 mg once daily in the morning under close medical supervision (see notes above), increased after 2 weeks to max. 5 mg once daily if tolerated
- Following myocardial infarction or revascularisation, initially 5 mg once daily in the morning increased after 2 weeks to 10 mg once daily if tolerated; ELDERLY 2.5 mg once daily for 1 week, then 5 mg once daily for 1 week, thereafter increased to 10 mg once daily if tolerated

Coversyl® **Arginine** (Servier) PoM
Tablets, f/c, perindopril arginine 2.5 mg (white), net price 30-tab pack = £4.43; 5 mg (light green, scored), 30-tab pack = £6.28; 10 mg (green), 30-tab pack = £10.65. Label: 22

◢**Perindopril arginine with diuretic**
Note For hypertension not adequately controlled by perindopril alone. For prescribing information on indapamide, see section 2.2.1

Coversyl® **Arginine Plus** (Servier) PoM
Tablets, f/c, perindopril arginine 5 mg, indapamide 1.25 mg, net price 30-tab pack = £9.51. Label: 22

QUINAPRIL

Indications essential hypertension; congestive heart failure (adjunct—see section 2.5.5)
Cautions see notes above
Contra-indications see notes above
Hepatic impairment see notes above
Renal impairment see notes above; max. initial dose 2.5 mg once daily if eGFR less than 40 mL/minute/1.73 m^2
Pregnancy see notes above
Breast-feeding see notes above
Side-effects see notes above; asthenia, chest pain, oedema, flatulence, nervousness, depression, insomnia, blurred vision, impotence, and back pain
Dose
- Hypertension, initially 10 mg once daily; with a diuretic (see notes above), in elderly, or in renal impairment initially 2.5 mg daily; usual maintenance dose 20–40 mg daily in single or 2 divided doses; up to 80 mg daily has been given
- Heart failure (adjunct), initial dose 2.5 mg daily under close medical supervision (see notes above), increased gradually to 10–20 mg daily in 1–2 divided doses if tolerated; max. 40 mg daily

Quinapril (Non-proprietary) PoM
Tablets, quinapril (as hydrochloride) 5 mg, net price 28-tab pack = £8.27; 10 mg, 28-tab pack = £8.23; 20 mg, 28-tab pack = £1.87; 40 mg, 28-tab pack = £2.39
Brands include *Quinil*®

Accupro® (Pfizer) PoM
Tablets, f/c, quinapril (as hydrochloride) 5 mg (brown), net price 28-tab pack = £8.60; 10 mg (brown), 28-tab pack = £8.60; 20 mg (brown), 28-tab pack = £10.79; 40 mg (red-brown), 28-tab pack = £9.75

◢**With diuretic**
Note For hypertension in patients stabilised on the individual components in the same proportions. For prescribing information on thiazides, see section 2.2.1

Accuretic® (Pfizer) PoM
Tablets, pink, f/c, scored, quinapril (as hydrochloride) 10 mg, hydrochlorothiazide 12.5 mg, net price 28-tab pack = £11.75

RAMIPRIL

Indications hypertension; symptomatic heart failure (adjunct—see section 2.5.5); following myocardial infarction in patients with clinical evidence of heart failure; prevention of cardiovascular events in patients with atherosclerotic cardiovascular disease or with diabetes mellitus and at least one additional risk factor for cardiovascular disease; nephropathy (consult product literature)
Cautions see notes above
Contra-indications see notes above
Hepatic impairment max. daily dose 2.5 mg; see also notes above
Renal impairment see notes above; max. daily dose 5 mg if eGFR 30–60 mL/minute/1.73 m^2; max. initial dose 1.25 mg once daily (do not exceed 5 mg daily) if eGFR less than 30 mL/minute/1.73 m^2
Pregnancy see notes above
Breast-feeding see notes above

Side-effects see notes above; also stomatitis, syncope, dyspnoea, bronchitis, muscle cramps; *less commonly* dry mouth, arrhythmias, tachycardia, palpitations, angina, chest pain, myocardial infarction, peripheral oedema, flushing, loss of appetite, nervousness, depression, anxiety, impotence, decreased libido, visual disturbances, sweating; *rarely* confusion, tremor, conjunctivitis, impaired hearing, tinnitus, onycholysis; *also reported* cerebrovascular accident, precipitation or exacerbation of Raynaud's syndrome, sleep disturbance, gynaecomastia, hyponatraemia, skin reactions including erythema multiforme, pemphigoid exanthema, Stevens-Johnson syndrome, and toxic epidermal necrolysis, alopecia

Dose

• Hypertension, initially 1.25–2.5 mg once daily, increased at intervals of 2–4 weeks to max. 10 mg once daily; if used in addition to diuretic see notes above

• Heart failure (adjunct), initially 1.25 mg once daily under close medical supervision (see notes above), increased gradually at intervals of 1–2 weeks to max. 10 mg daily if tolerated (preferably taken in 2 divided doses)

• Prophylaxis after myocardial infarction (started at least 48 hours after infarction), initially 2.5 mg twice daily, increased after 3 days to 5 mg twice daily

Note If initial 2.5-mg dose not tolerated, give 1.25 mg twice daily for 2 days before increasing to 2.5 mg twice daily, then 5 mg twice daily; withdraw if dose cannot be increased to 2.5 mg twice daily

• Prophylaxis of cardiovascular events, initially 2.5 mg once daily, increased after 1–2 weeks to 5 mg once daily, then increased after a further 2–3 weeks to 10 mg once daily

• Nephropathy, initially 1.25 mg once daily, increased after 2 weeks to 2.5 mg once daily, then increased after a further 2 weeks to 5 mg once daily if tolerated

Ramipril (Non-proprietary) ℞

Capsules, ramipril 1.25 mg, net price 28-cap pack = £1.08; 2.5 mg, 28-cap pack = £1.15; 5 mg, 28-cap pack = £1.22; 10 mg, 28-cap pack = £1.31

Tablets, ramipril 1.25 mg, net price 28-tab pack = £1.25; 2.5 mg, 28-tab pack = £1.13; 5 mg, 28-tab pack = £1.21; 10 mg, 28-tab pack = £1.40

Oral solution, ramipril 2.5 mg/5 mL, net price 150 mL = £94.40

Tritace® (Sanofi-Aventis) ℞

Tablets, scored, ramipril 1.25 mg (white), net price 28-tab pack = £5.09; 2.5 mg (yellow), 28-tab pack = £7.22; 5 mg (red), 28-tab pack = £10.05; 10 mg (white), 28-tab pack = £13.68

Titration pack, tablets, 35-day starter pack of ramipril 7 × 2.5 mg with 21 × 5 mg and 7 × 10 mg, net price = £13.00

◢**With calcium-channel blocker**

Note For hypertension in patients stabilised on the individual components in the same proportions. For prescribing information on felodipine, see section 2.6.2

Triapin® (Sanofi-Aventis) ℞

Triapin® tablets, f/c, brown, ramipril 5 mg, felodipine 5 mg (m/r), net price 28-tab pack = £16.13. Label: 25

Triapin mite® tablets, f/c, orange, ramipril 2.5 mg, felodipine 2.5 mg (m/r), net price 28-tab pack = £24.55. Label: 25

◢ **TRANDOLAPRIL**

Indications mild to moderate hypertension; following myocardial infarction in patients with left ventricular dysfunction

Cautions see notes above

Contra-indications see notes above

Hepatic impairment see notes above

Renal impairment see notes above; max. 2 mg daily if eGFR less than 10 mL/minute/1.73 m²

Pregnancy see notes above

Breast-feeding see notes above

Side-effects see notes above; also ileus, dry mouth; tachycardia, palpitation, arrhythmias, angina, transient ischaemic attacks, cerebral haemorrhage, myocardial infarction, syncope; dyspnoea, bronchitis; asthenia, nervousness, sleep disturbances; hot flushes; alopecia, sweating, skin reactions including Stevens-Johnson syndrome, toxic epidermal necrolysis, and psoriasis-like efflorescence

Dose

• Hypertension, initially 500 micrograms once daily, increased at intervals of 2–4 weeks; usual range 1–2 mg once daily; max. 4 mg daily; if used in addition to diuretic see notes above

• Prophylaxis after myocardial infarction (starting as early as 3 days after infarction), initially 500 micrograms once daily, gradually increased to max. 4 mg once daily

Note If symptomatic hypotension develops during titration, do not increase dose further; if possible, reduce dose of any adjunctive treatment and if this is not effective or feasible, reduce dose of trandolapril

Trandolapril (Non-proprietary) ℞

Capsules, trandolapril 500 micrograms, net price 14-cap pack = £1.74; 1 mg, 28-cap pack = £17.32; 2 mg, 28-cap pack = £1.96; 4 mg, 28-cap pack = £12.38

2.5.5.2 Angiotensin-II receptor antagonists

Azilsartan, candesartan, eprosartan, irbesartan, losartan, olmesartan, telmisartan, and **valsartan** are angiotensin-II receptor antagonists with many properties similar to those of the ACE inhibitors. However, unlike ACE inhibitors, they do not inhibit the breakdown of bradykinin and other kinins, and thus are less likely to cause the persistent dry cough which can complicate ACE inhibitor therapy. They are therefore a useful alternative for patients who have to discontinue an ACE inhibitor because of persistent cough.

An angiotensin-II receptor antagonist may be used as an alternative to an ACE inhibitor in the management of heart failure (section 2.5.5) or diabetic nephropathy (section 6.1.5). Candesartan and valsartan are also licensed as adjuncts to ACE inhibitors under specialist supervision, in the management of heart failure when other treatments are unsuitable, but see also Concomitant Use Of Drugs Affecting The Renin-angiotensin System, p. 120.

Cautions Angiotensin-II receptor antagonists should be used with caution in renal artery stenosis (see also Renal Effects under ACE Inhibitors, section 2.5.5.1). Monitoring of plasma-potassium concentration is advised, particularly in the elderly and in patients with renal impairment; lower initial doses may be appropriate in these patients. Angiotensin-II receptor antagonists should be used with caution in aortic or mitral valve stenosis and in hypertrophic cardiomyopathy. Those with primary aldosteronism, and Afro-Caribbean patients (particularly those with left ventricular hypertrophy), may not benefit from an angiotensin-II receptor antagonist. **Interactions:** see Concomitant Use Of Drugs Affecting The Renin-angiotensin System, p. 120 and Appendix 1 (angiotensin-II receptor antagonists).

Contra-indications   The combination of an angiotensin-II receptor antagonist with aliskiren is contra-indicated in those with diabetes mellitus or if eGFR is less than 60 mL/minute/1.73m^2.

Pregnancy   Angiotensin-II receptor antagonists should be avoided in pregnancy unless essential. They may adversely affect fetal and neonatal blood pressure control and renal function; skull defects and oligohydramnios have also been reported.

Breast-feeding   Information on the use of angiotensin-II receptor antagonists in breast-feeding is limited. They are not recommended in breast-feeding and alternative treatment options, with better established safety information during breast-feeding, are available.

Side-effects   Side-effects are usually mild. Symptomatic hypotension including dizziness may occur, particularly in patients with intravascular volume depletion (e.g. those taking high-dose diuretics). Hyperkalaemia occurs occasionally; angioedema has also been reported with some angiotensin-II receptor antagonists.

◤ AZILSARTAN MEDOXOMIL

Indications   hypertension (see also notes above)

Cautions   see notes above; heart failure

Contra-indications   see notes above

Hepatic impairment   manufacturer advises monitor closely and consider initial dose of 20 mg in mild to moderate impairment (limited information available), and to avoid in severe impairment (no information available)

Renal impairment   manufacturer advises caution in severe impairment—no information available

Pregnancy   see notes above

Breast-feeding   see notes above

Side-effects   see notes above; also diarrhoea, raised creatine kinase; *less commonly* peripheral oedema, malaise, raised creatinine, hyperuricaemia

Dose

- Initially 40 mg once daily, increased if necessary to max. 80 mg once daily (in intravascular volume depletion or in ELDERLY over 75 years, consider initial dose of 20 mg once daily); CHILD not recommended

Edarbi® (Takeda) ▼ PoM

Tablets, azilsartan medoxomil (as potassium salt) 20 mg, net price 28-tab pack = £16.80; 40 mg, 28-tab pack = £16.80; 80 mg, 28-tab pack = £19.95

◤ CANDESARTAN CILEXETIL

Indications   hypertension; heart failure with impaired left ventricular systolic function in conjunction with an ACE inhibitor (under specialist supervision), or when ACE inhibitors are not tolerated (see also section 2.5.5)

Cautions   see notes above

Contra-indications   see notes above; cholestasis

Hepatic impairment   initially 4 mg once daily in mild or moderate impairment; avoid in severe impairment

Renal impairment   initially 4 mg daily; use with caution if eGFR less than 15 mL/minute/1.73m^2—limited experience

Pregnancy   see notes above

Breast-feeding   see notes above

Side-effects   see notes above; also vertigo, headache; *very rarely* nausea, hepatitis, cough, blood disorders, hyponatraemia, back pain, arthralgia, myalgia, rash, urticaria, pruritus

Dose

- Hypertension, initially 8 mg (intravascular volume depletion 4 mg) once daily, increased if necessary at intervals of 4 weeks to max. 32 mg once daily; usual maintenance dose 8 mg once daily
- Heart failure, initially 4 mg once daily, increased at intervals of at least 2 weeks to 'target' dose of 32 mg once daily or to max. tolerated dose

Candesartan Cilexetil (Non-proprietary) PoM

Tablets, candesartan cilexetil 2 mg, net price 7-tab pack = £1.90; 4 mg, 7-tab pack = 86p, 28-tab pack = £1.10; 8 mg, 28-tab pack = £1.44; 16 mg, 28-tab pack = £1.79; 32 mg, 28-tab pack = £2.45

Amias® (Takeda) PoM

Tablets, candesartan cilexetil 2 mg (white), net price 7-tab pack = £3.58; 4 mg (white, scored), 7-tab pack = £3.88, 28-tab pack = £9.78; 8 mg (pink, scored), 28-tab pack = £9.89; 16 mg (pink, scored), 28-tab pack = £12.72; 32 mg (pink, scored), 28-tab pack = £16.13

◤ EPROSARTAN

Indications   hypertension (see also notes above)

Cautions   see notes above

Contra-indications   see notes above

Hepatic impairment   halve initial dose in mild or moderate liver disease; avoid if severe

Renal impairment   halve initial dose if eGFR less than 60 mL/minute/1.73 m^2

Pregnancy   see notes above

Breast-feeding   see notes above

Side-effects   see notes above; also flatulence, hypertriglyceridaemia, arthralgia, rhinitis; *rarely* headache, asthenia, anaemia, hypersensitivity reactions (including rash, pruritus, urticaria); *very rarely* nausea

Dose

- 600 mg once daily (elderly over 75 years, initially 300 mg once daily); if necessary increased after 2–3 weeks to 800 mg once daily

Teveten® (Abbott Healthcare) PoM

Tablets, f/c, eprosartan (as mesilate) 300 mg, net price 28-tab pack = £7.31; 600 mg, 28-tab pack = £14.31. Label: 21

◤ IRBESARTAN

Indications   hypertension; renal disease in hypertensive type 2 diabetes mellitus (see also notes above)

Cautions   see notes above

Contra-indications   see notes above

Pregnancy   see notes above

Breast-feeding   see notes above

Side-effects   see notes above; also nausea, vomiting; fatigue; musculoskeletal pain; *less commonly* diarrhoea, dyspepsia, flushing, tachycardia, chest pain, cough, and sexual dysfunction; *rarely* rash, urticaria; *very rarely* headache, myalgia, arthralgia, tinnitus, taste disturbance, hepatitis, renal dysfunction, and cutaneous vasculitis

Dose
- Hypertension, initially 150 mg once daily, increased if necessary to 300 mg once daily (in haemodialysis or in ELDERLY over 75 years, initial dose of 75 mg once daily may be used); CHILD not recommended
- Renal disease in hypertensive type 2 diabetes mellitus, initially 150 mg once daily, increased to 300 mg once daily if tolerated (in haemodialysis or in ELDERLY over 75 years, consider initial dose of 75 mg once daily); CHILD not recommended

Irbesartan (Non-proprietary) [PoM]
Tablets, irbesartan 75 mg, net price 28-tab pack = £1.43; 150 mg, 28-tab pack = £1.67; 300 mg, 28-tab pack = £2.49
Brands include *Sabervel*®

Aprovel® (Bristol-Myers Squibb, Sanofi-Aventis) [PoM]
Tablets, f/c, irbesartan 75 mg, net price 28-tab pack = £9.69; 150 mg, 28-tab pack = £11.84; 300 mg, 28-tab pack = £15.93

◢**With diuretic**
Note For hypertension not adequately controlled with irbesartan alone. For prescribing information on thiazides, see section 2.2.1

Irbesartan with hydrochlorothiazide (Non-proprietary) [PoM]
Tablets, irbesartan 150 mg, hydrochlorothiazide 12.5 mg, net price 28-tab pack = £9.32; irbesartan 300 mg, hydrochlorothiazide 12.5 mg, 28-tab pack = £12.17; irbesartan 300mg, hydrochlorothiazide 25mg, 28-tab pack = £11.32

CoAprovel® (Bristol-Myers Squibb, Sanofi-Aventis) [PoM]
Tablets, f/c, irbesartan 150 mg, hydrochlorothiazide 12.5 mg (peach), net price 28-tab pack = £11.84; irbesartan 300 mg, hydrochlorothiazide 12.5 mg (peach), 28-tab pack = £15.93; irbesartan 300 mg, hydrochlorothiazide 25 mg (pink), 28-tab pack = £15.93

▮ LOSARTAN POTASSIUM

Indications hypertension (including reduction of stroke risk in hypertension with left ventricular hypertrophy); chronic heart failure when ACE inhibitors are unsuitable or contra-indicated; diabetic nephropathy in type 2 diabetes mellitus (see also notes above)

Cautions see notes above; severe heart failure

Contra-indications see notes above

Hepatic impairment consider dose reduction in mild to moderate impairment; manufacturer advises avoid in severe impairment—no information available

Pregnancy see notes above

Breast-feeding see notes above

Side-effects see notes above; vertigo; *less commonly* gastro-intestinal disturbances, angina, palpitation, oedema, dyspnoea, headache, sleep disorders, malaise, urticaria, pruritus, rash; *rarely* hepatitis, atrial fibrillation, cerebrovascular accident, syncope, paraesthesia; also reported pancreatitis, anaphylaxis, cough, depression, erectile dysfunction, anaemia, thrombocytopenia, hyponatraemia, arthralgia, myalgia, renal impairment, rhabdomyolysis, tinnitus,

photosensitivity, and vasculitis (including Henoch-Schönlein purpura)

Dose
- Hypertension, diabetic nephropathy in type 2 diabetes mellitus, usually 50 mg once daily (intravascular volume depletion, initially 25 mg once daily); if necessary increased after several weeks to 100 mg once daily; ELDERLY over 75 years initially 25 mg daily
- Chronic heart failure, initially 12.5 mg once daily, increased at weekly intervals to max. 150 mg once daily if tolerated

Losartan Potassium (Non-proprietary) [PoM]
Tablets, losartan potassium 12.5 mg, net price 28-tab pack = £5.15; 25 mg, 28-tab pack = £1.18; 50 mg, 28-tab pack = £1.29; 100 mg, 28-tab pack = £1.40

Cozaar® (MSD) [PoM]
Tablets, f/c, losartan potassium 12.5 mg (blue), net price 28-tab pack = £8.09; 25 mg (white), net price 28-tab pack = £16.18; 50 mg (white, scored), 28-tab pack = £12.80; 100 mg (white), 28-tab pack = £16.18
Oral suspension, losartan potassium 12.5 mg/5 mL when reconstituted with solvent provided, net price 200-mL (berry-citrus flavour) = £53.68

◢**With diuretic**
Note For hypertension not adequately controlled with losartan alone. For prescribing information on thiazides, see section 2.2.1

Losartan potassium with hydrochlorothiazide (Non-proprietary) [PoM]
Tablets, losartan potassium 100 mg, hydrochlorothiazide 25 mg, net price 28-tab pack = £1.93

Cozaar-Comp® (MSD) [PoM]
Tablets 50/12.5, yellow, f/c, losartan potassium 50 mg, hydrochlorothiazide 12.5 mg, net price 28-tab pack = £12.80
Tablets 100/12.5, white, f/c, losartan potassium 100 mg, hydrochlorothiazide 12.5 mg, net price 28-tab pack = £16.18
Tablets 100/25, yellow, f/c, losartan potassium 100 mg, hydrochlorothiazide 25 mg, net price 28-tab pack = £16.18

▮ OLMESARTAN MEDOXOMIL

Indications hypertension (see also notes above)

Cautions see notes above

Contra-indications see notes above; biliary obstruction

Hepatic impairment dose should not exceed 20 mg daily in moderate impairment; manufacturer advises avoid in severe impairment—no information available

Renal impairment max. 20 mg daily if eGFR 20–60 mL/minute/1.73 m^2; avoid if eGFR less than 20 mL/minute/1.73 m^2

Pregnancy see notes above

Breast-feeding see notes above

Side-effects see notes above; also gastro-intestinal disturbances; chest pain, peripheral oedema, hyper-triglyceridaemia; fatigue; influenza-like symptoms, cough, pharyngitis, rhinitis; urinary-tract infection; haematuria, hyperuricaemia; arthritis, musculo-skeletal pain; *less commonly* angina, vertigo, rash; *very rarely* headache, thrombocytopenia, myalgia, pruritus, urticaria

2

Cardiovascular system

Dose
- Initially 10 mg once daily; if necessary increased to 20 mg once daily; max. 40 mg daily

Olmetec® (Daiichi Sankyo) [PoM]
Tablets, f/c, olmesartan medoxomil 10 mg, net price 28-tab pack = £10.95; 20 mg, 28-tab pack = £12.95; 40 mg, 28-tab pack = £17.50

◢**With calcium-channel blocker**

Note For hypertension in patients stabilised on the individual components in the same proportions. For prescribing information on amlodipine, see section 2.6.2

Sevikar® (Daiichi Sankyo) [PoM]
Tablets 20/5, white, f/c, olmesartan medoxomil 20 mg, amlodipine (as besilate) 5 mg, net price 28-tab pack = £16.95

Tablets 40/5, ivory, f/c, olmesartan medoxomil 40 mg, amlodipine (as besilate) 5 mg, net price 28-tab pack = £16.95

Tablets 40/10, brownish-red, f/c, olmesartan medoxomil 40 mg, amlodipine (as besilate) 10 mg, net price 28-tab pack = £16.95

◢**With calcium-channel blocker and diuretic**

Note For hypertension in patients stabilised on the individual components in the same proportions, or for hypertension not adequately controlled with olmesartan and amlodipine. For prescribing information on amlodipine, see section 2.6.2; for prescribing information on thiazides, see section 2.2.1

Sevikar HCT® (Daiichi Sankyo) [PoM]
Tablets 20/5/12.5, light orange, f/c, olmesartan medoxomil 20 mg, amlodipine (as besilate) 5 mg, hydrochlorothiazide 12.5 mg, net price 28-tab pack = £16.95

Tablets 40/5/12.5, light yellow, f/c, olmesartan medoxomil 40 mg, amlodipine (as besilate) 5 mg, hydrochlorothiazide 12.5 mg, net price 28-tab pack = £16.95

Tablets 40/10/12.5, greyish-red, f/c, olmesartan medoxomil 40 mg, amlodipine (as besilate) 10 mg, hydrochlorothiazide 12.5 mg, net price 28-tab pack = £16.95

Tablets 40/5/25, light yellow, f/c, olmesartan medoxomil 40 mg, amlodipine (as besilate) 5 mg, hydrochlorothiazide 25 mg, net price 28-tab pack = £16.95

Tablets 40/10/25, greyish-red, f/c, olmesartan medoxomil 40 mg, amlodipine (as besilate) 10 mg, hydrochlorothiazide 25 mg, net price 28-tab pack = £16.95

◢**With diuretic**

Note For hypertension not adequately controlled with olmesartan alone. For prescribing information on thiazides, see section 2.2.1

Olmetec Plus® (Daiichi Sankyo) [PoM]
Tablets, f/c, olmesartan medoxomil 20 mg, hydro-chlorothiazide 12.5 mg (red-yellow), net price 28-tab pack = £12.95; olmesartan medoxomil 20 mg, hydrochlorothiazide 25 mg (pink), 28-tab pack = £12.95; olmesartan medoxomil 40 mg, hydrochloro-thiazide 12.5 mg (red-yellow), 28-tab pack = £17.50

◢ **TELMISARTAN**

Indications hypertension (see also notes above); prevention of cardiovascular events in patients with established atherosclerotic cardiovascular disease, or type 2 diabetes mellitus with target-organ damage

Cautions see notes above
Contra-indications see notes above
Hepatic impairment 20–40 mg once daily in mild or moderate impairment; avoid in severe impairment or biliary obstruction
Renal impairment manufacturer advises initial dose of 20 mg once daily in severe impairment
Pregnancy see notes above
Breast-feeding see notes above
Side-effects see notes above; also gastro-intestinal disturbances; chest pain; influenza-like symptoms including pharyngitis and sinusitis; urinary-tract infection; arthralgia, myalgia, back pain, leg cramps; eczema; *less commonly* dry mouth, flatulence, anxiety, vertigo, tendinitis-like symptoms, abnormal vision, increased sweating; *rarely* bradycardia, tachycardia, dyspnoea, insomnia, depression, blood disorders, increase in uric acid, eosinophilia, rash, and pruritus; syncope and asthenia also reported

Dose
- Hypertension, usually 40 mg once daily (but 20 mg may be sufficient), increased if necessary after at least 4 weeks, to max. 80 mg once daily
- Prevention of cardiovascular events, 80 mg once daily

Micardis® (Boehringer Ingelheim) ▼ [PoM]
Tablets, telmisartan 20 mg, net price 28-tab pack = £11.10; 40 mg, 28-tab pack = £13.61; 80 mg, 28-tab pack = £17.00

◢**With diuretic**

Note For patients with hypertension not adequately controlled by telmisartan alone. For prescribing information on thiazides, see section 2.2.1

Micardis Plus® (Boehringer Ingelheim) [PoM]
Tablets 40/12.5, red/white, telmisartan 40 mg, hydrochlorothiazide 12.5 mg, net price 28-tab pack = £13.61

Tablets 80/12.5, red/white, telmisartan 80 mg, hydrochlorothiazide 12.5 mg, net price 28-tab pack = £17.00

Tablets 80/25, yellow/white, telmisartan 80 mg, hydrochlorothiazide 25 mg, net price 28-tab pack = £17.00

◢ **VALSARTAN**

Indications hypertension; heart failure when ACE inhibitors cannot be used, or in conjunction with an ACE inhibitor (under specialist supervision) when a beta-blocker cannot be used (see also section 2.5.5); myocardial infarction with left ventricular failure or left ventricular systolic dysfunction (adjunct—see section 2.5.5 and section 2.10.1)

Cautions see notes above
Contra-indications see notes above; biliary cirrhosis; cholestasis
Hepatic impairment max. dose 80 mg daily in mild to moderate impairment; avoid if severe
Renal impairment use with caution if eGFR less than 10 mL/minute/1.73 m^2—no information available
Pregnancy see notes above
Breast-feeding see notes above
Side-effects see notes above; renal impairment; *less commonly* gastro-intestinal disturbance, syncope, fatigue, cough, headache, acute renal failure; neutro-penia, thrombocytopenia, myalgia, and hypersensi-

Cardiovascular system

2

tivity reactions (including rash, pruritus, vasculitis, and serum sickness) also reported

Dose

- Hypertension, usually 80 mg once daily (initially 40 mg once daily in intravascular volume depletion); if necessary increased at intervals of 4 weeks up to max. 320 mg daily
- Heart failure, initially 40 mg twice daily increased at intervals of at least 2 weeks up to max. 160 mg twice daily
- Myocardial infarction, initially 20 mg twice daily increased over several weeks to 160 mg twice daily if tolerated

Valsartan (Non-proprietary) ▼ PoM

Tablets, valsartan 40 mg, net price 7-tab pack = £2.92; 80 mg, 28-tab pack = £13.97; 160 mg, 28-tab pack = £18.41; 320 mg, 28-tab pack = £15.44

Diovan® (Novartis) ▼ PoM

Capsules, valsartan 40 mg (grey), net price 28-cap pack = £13.97; 80 mg (grey/pink), 28-cap pack = £13.97; 160 mg (dark grey/pink), 28-cap pack = £18.41

Tablets, f/c, valsartan 40 mg (yellow, scored), net price 7-tab pack = £3.49; 320 mg (dark grey-violet), 28-tab pack = £20.23

◢**With diuretic**

Note For hypertension not adequately controlled by valsartan alone. For prescribing information on thiazides, see section 2.2.1

Valsartan with hydrochlorothiazide (Non-proprietary) PoM

Tablets 80/12.5, valsartan 80 mg, hydrochlorothiazide 12.5 mg, net price 28-tab pack = £8.97

Tablets 160/12.5, valsartan 160 mg, hydrochlorothiazide 12.5 mg, net price 28-tab pack = £2.67

Tablets 160/25, valsartan 160 mg, hydrochlorothiazide 25 mg, net price 28-tab pack = £11.87

Co-Diovan® (Novartis) PoM

Tablets 80/12.5, orange, f/c, valsartan 80 mg, hydrochlorothiazide 12.5 mg, net price 28-tab pack = £13.97

Tablets 160/12.5, red, f/c, valsartan 160 mg, hydrochlorothiazide 12.5 mg, net price 28-tab pack = £18.41

Tablets 160/25, brown-orange, f/c, valsartan 160 mg, hydrochlorothiazide 25 mg, net price 28-tab pack = £18.41

◢**With amlodipine**

Section 2.6.2

2.5.5.3 Renin inhibitors

Renin inhibitors inhibit renin directly; renin converts angiotensinogen to angiotensin I. **Aliskiren** is licensed for the treatment of hypertension, either alone or in combination with other antihypertensives. Combination treatment with an ACE inhibitor or an angiotensin-II receptor antagonist is contra-indicated in patients with diabetes mellitus or if eGFR is less than 60 mL/minute/ $1.73m^2$; in all other patients, combination treatment with an ACE inhibitor or an angiotensin-II receptor antagonist is not recommended (see also Concomitant Use Of Drugs Affecting The Renin-angiotensin System, p. 120). The *Scottish Medicines Consortium* (p. 4) has

advised (January 2010) that aliskiren (*Rasilez*®) is **not** recommended for use within NHS Scotland.

◼ ALISKIREN

Indications essential hypertension

Cautions see notes above; patients taking concomitant diuretics, on a low-sodium diet, or who are dehydrated (first doses may cause hypotension—initiate with care); renal artery stenosis; patients at risk of renal impairment; diabetes mellitus; monitor glucose tolerance and renal function; moderate to severe heart failure; history of angioedema (avoid in hereditary or idiopathic angioedema); **interactions:** Appendix 1 (aliskiren)

Contra-indications see notes above

Renal impairment see notes above; caution in renal artery stenosis—no information available; avoid if eGFR less than 30 mL/minute/$1.73m^2$—no information available; monitor plasma-potassium concentration

Pregnancy manufacturer advises avoid—no information available; other drugs acting on the renin-angiotensin system have been associated with fetal malformations and neonatal death

Breast-feeding present in milk in *animal* studies—manufacturer advises avoid

Side-effects diarrhoea, dizziness, hyperkalaemia, arthralgia; *less commonly* hypotension, palpitation, peripheral oedema, acute renal failure (reversible on discontinuation of treatment), anaemia, rash (including Stevens-Johnson syndrome and toxic epidermal necrolysis); *rarely* angioedema

Dose

- ADULT over 18 years, 150 mg once daily, increased if necessary to 300 mg once daily

Rasilez® (Novartis) PoM

Tablets, f/c, aliskiren (as hemifumarate) 150 mg (pink), net price 28-tab pack = £23.76; 300 mg (red), net price 28-tab pack = £28.56. Label: 21

2.6 **Nitrates, calcium-channel blockers, and other antianginal drugs**

2.6.1   Nitrates

2.6.2   Calcium-channel blockers

2.6.3   Other antianginal drugs

2.6.4   Peripheral vasodilators and related drugs

Nitrates, calcium-channel blockers, and potassium-channel activators have vasodilating effects. Vasodilators can act in heart failure by arteriolar dilatation which reduces both peripheral vascular resistance and left ventricular pressure during systole resulting in improved cardiac output. They can also cause venous dilatation which results in dilatation of capacitance vessels, increase of venous pooling, and diminution of venous return to the heart (decreasing left ventricular end-diastolic pressure).

For details on the management of stable angina and acute coronary syndromes, see section 2.10.1.

2 **Cardiovascular system**

2 Cardiovascular system

2.6.1 Nitrates

Nitrates have a useful role in *angina* (for details on the management of stable and unstable angina, see section 2.10.1). Although they are potent coronary vasodilators, their principal benefit follows from a reduction in venous return which reduces left ventricular work. Unwanted effects such as flushing, headache, and postural hypotension may limit therapy, especially when angina is severe or when patients are unusually sensitive to the effects of nitrates.

Sublingual **glyceryl trinitrate** is one of the most effective drugs for providing rapid symptomatic relief of angina, but its effect lasts only for 20 to 30 minutes; the 300-microgram tablet is often appropriate when glyceryl trinitrate is first used. The *aerosol spray* provides an alternative method of rapid relief of symptoms for those who find difficulty in dissolving sublingual preparations. Duration of action may be prolonged by *transdermal* preparations (but tolerance may develop, see below).

Isosorbide dinitrate is active *sublingually* and is a more stable preparation for those who only require nitrates infrequently. It is also effective by mouth for prophylaxis; although the effect is slower in onset, it may persist for several hours. Duration of action of up to 12 hours is claimed for *modified-release* preparations. The activity of isosorbide dinitrate may depend on the production of active metabolites, the most important of which is isosorbide mononitrate. **Isosorbide mononitrate** itself is also licensed for angina prophylaxis; modified-release formulations (for once daily administration) are available.

Glyceryl trinitrate or isosorbide dinitrate may be tried by *intravenous injection* when the sublingual form is ineffective in patients with chest pain due to myocardial infarction or severe ischaemia. Intravenous injections are also useful in the treatment of congestive heart failure.

Tolerance Many patients on long-acting or transdermal nitrates rapidly develop tolerance (with reduced therapeutic effects). Reduction of blood-nitrate concentrations to low levels for 4 to 12 hours each day usually maintains effectiveness in such patients. If tolerance is suspected during the use of transdermal patches they should be left off for 8–12 hours (usually overnight) in each 24 hours; in the case of modified-release tablets of isosorbide dinitrate (and conventional formulations of isosorbide mononitrate), the second of the two daily doses should be given after about 8 hours rather than after 12 hours. Conventional formulations of isosorbide mononitrate should not usually be given more than twice daily unless small doses are used; modified-release formulations of isosorbide mononitrate should only be given once daily, and used in this way do not produce tolerance.

GLYCERYL TRINITRATE

Indications anal fissure (section 1.7.4); extravasation (section 10.3)
Sublingual: prophylaxis and treatment of angina
Injection: control of hypertension and myocardial ischaemia during and after cardiac surgery; induction of controlled hypotension during surgery; congestive heart failure; unstable angina

Transdermal: see under preparations below
Cautions hypothyroidism; malnutrition; hypothermia; recent history of myocardial infarction; heart failure due to obstruction; hypoxaemia or other ventilation and perfusion abnormalities; susceptibility to angle-closure glaucoma; metal-containing transdermal systems should be removed before magnetic resonance imaging procedures, cardioversion, or diathermy; avoid abrupt withdrawal; monitor blood pressure and heart rate during intravenous infusion; tolerance (see notes above); **interactions:** Appendix 1 (nitrates)
Contra-indications hypersensitivity to nitrates; hypotensive conditions and hypovolaemia; hypertrophic cardiomyopathy; aortic stenosis; cardiac tamponade; constrictive pericarditis; mitral stenosis; toxic pulmonary oedema; raised intracranial pressure due to cerebral haemorrhage or head trauma; marked anaemia
Hepatic impairment caution in severe impairment
Renal impairment manufacturers advise use with caution in severe impairment
Pregnancy not known to be harmful
Breast-feeding no information available—manufacturers advise use only if potential benefit outweighs risk
Side-effects postural hypotension, tachycardia (but paradoxical bradycardia also reported); throbbing headache, dizziness; *less commonly* nausea, vomiting, heartburn, flushing, syncope, temporary hypoxaemia, rash, application site reactions with transdermal patches; *very rarely* angle-closure glaucoma
Injection Specific side-effects following injection (particularly if given too rapidly) include severe hypotension, diaphoresis, apprehension, restlessness, muscle twitching, retrosternal discomfort, palpitation, abdominal pain; prolonged administration has been associated with methaemoglobinaemia
Dose
- Sublingually, 0.3–1 mg, repeated as required; see also under preparations
- By intravenous infusion, 10–200 micrograms/minute, adjusted according to response; max. 400 micrograms/minute; consult product literature for recommended starting doses specific to indication
- By transdermal application, see under preparations

◢ Short-acting tablets and sprays

Glyceryl Trinitrate (Non-proprietary)
Sublingual tablets, glyceryl trinitrate 300 micrograms, net price 100 = £2.71; 500 micrograms, 100 = £2.03; 600 micrograms, 100 = £13.11. Label: 16
Note Glyceryl trinitrate tablets should be supplied in glass containers of not more than 100 tablets, closed with a foil-lined cap, and containing no cotton wool wadding; they should be discarded after 8 weeks in use

Aerosol spray, glyceryl trinitrate 400 micrograms/metered dose, net price 200-dose unit = £3.29
Dose treatment or prophylaxis of angina, spray 1–2 doses under tongue and then close mouth

Coro-Nitro Pump Spray® (Ayrton Saunders)
Aerosol spray, glyceryl trinitrate 400 micrograms/metered dose, net price 200-dose unit = £1.25
Dose treatment or prophylaxis of angina, spray 1–2 doses under tongue and then close mouth

Glytrin Spray® (Aspire)
Aerosol spray, glyceryl trinitrate 400 micrograms/metered dose, net price 200-dose unit = £3.44
Dose treatment or prophylaxis of angina, spray 1–2 doses under tongue and then close mouth
Cautions flammable

GTN 300 mcg (Martindale)
Sublingual tablets, glyceryl trinitrate 300 micrograms, net price 100 = £2.71. Label: 16

Nitrolingual Pumpspray® (Merck Serono)
Aerosol spray, glyceryl trinitrate 400 micrograms/
metered dose, net price 180-dose unit = £3.10, 200-
dose unit = £3.44
Dose treatment or prophylaxis of angina, spray 1–2 doses
under tongue and then close mouth

Nitromin® (Egis)
Aerosol spray, glyceryl trinitrate 400 micrograms/
metered dose, net price 180-dose unit = £2.63, 200-
dose unit = £2.71
Dose treatment or prophylaxis of angina, spray 1–2 doses
under tongue and then close mouth

◢**Parenteral preparations**
Note Glass or polyethylene apparatus is preferable; loss of
potency will occur if PVC is used

Glyceryl Trinitrate (Non-proprietary) [PoM]
Injection, glyceryl trinitrate 1 mg/mL. To be diluted
before use or given undiluted with syringe pump.
Net price 50-mL vial = £15.90
Injection, glyceryl trinitrate 5 mg/mL. To be diluted
before use. Net price 5-mL amp = £6.49; 10-mL
amp = £12.98
Excipients may include ethanol, propylene glycol (see
Excipients, p. 2)

Nitrocine® (UCB Pharma) [PoM]
Injection, glyceryl trinitrate 1 mg/mL. To be diluted
before use or given undiluted with syringe pump.
Net price 10-mL amp = £5.88
Excipients Include propylene glycol (see Excipients, p. 2)

Nitronal® (Merck Serono) [PoM]
Injection, glyceryl trinitrate 1 mg/mL. To be diluted
before use or given undiluted with syringe pump.
Net price 5-mL vial = £1.80; 50-mL vial = £14.76

◢**Transdermal preparations**
Deponit® (UCB Pharma)
Patches, self-adhesive, transparent, glyceryl trinitrate, '5' patch (releasing approx. 5 mg/24 hours
when in contact with skin), net price 28 = £12.77;
'10' patch (releasing approx.10 mg/24 hours), 28 =
£14.06
Dose prophylaxis of angina, apply one '5' or one '10'
patch to lateral chest wall, upper arm, thigh, abdomen, or
shoulder; increase to two '10' patches every 24 hours if
necessary; replace every 24 hours, siting replacement
patch on different area; see also notes above (Tolerance)

Minitran® (Meda)
Patches, self-adhesive, transparent, glyceryl trinitrate, '5' patch (releasing approx. 5 mg/24 hours
when in contact with skin), net price 30 = £11.62;
'10' patch (releasing approx. 10 mg/24 hours), 30 =
£12.87; '15' patch (releasing approx. 15 mg/24
hours), 30 = £14.19
Dose prophylaxis of angina, apply one '5' patch to chest
or upper arm; replace every 24 hours, siting replacement
patch on different area; adjust dose according to response;
see also notes above (Tolerance)
Maintenance of venous patency ('5' patch only), consult
product literature

Nitro-Dur® (MSD)
Patches, self-adhesive, buff, glyceryl trinitrate,
'0.2 mg/h' patch (releasing approx. 5 mg/24 hours
when in contact with skin), net price 28 = £10.59;
'0.4 mg/h' patch (releasing approx. 10 mg/24 hours),
28 = £11.72; '0.6 mg/h' patch (releasing approx.15
mg/24 hours), 28 = £12.90
Dose prophylaxis of angina, apply one '0.2 mg/h' patch to
chest or outer upper arm; replace every 24 hours, siting
replacement patch on different area: adjust dose according
to response; max. 15 mg in 24 hours; see also notes above
(Tolerance)

Percutol® (Aspire)
Ointment, glyceryl trinitrate 2%, net price 60 g =
£79.00. Counselling, see administration below
Excipients include wool fat
Dose prophylaxis of angina, usual dose 1–2 inches of
ointment measured on to *Applirule®*, and applied (usually
to chest, arm, or thigh) without rubbing in and secured
with surgical tape, every 3–4 hours as required; to
determine dose, ½ inch on first day then increased by
½ inch/day until headache occurs, then reduced by ½ inch
Note Approx. 800 micrograms/hour absorbed from 1 inch
of ointment

Transiderm-Nitro® (Novartis)
Patches, self-adhesive, pink, glyceryl trinitrate, '5'
patch (releasing approx. 5 mg/24 hours when in
contact with skin), net price 28 = £17.05; '10' patch
(releasing approx. 10 mg/24 hours), 28 = £18.74
Dose prophylaxis of angina, apply one '5' or one '10'
patch to lateral chest wall; replace every 24 hours, siting
replacement patch on different area; max. two '10' patches
daily; see also notes above (Tolerance)
Prophylaxis of phlebitis and extravasation ('5' patch only),
consult product literature

◼ **ISOSORBIDE DINITRATE**

Indications prophylaxis and treatment of angina; left
ventricular failure
Cautions see under Glyceryl Trinitrate
Contra-indications see under Glyceryl Trinitrate
Hepatic impairment see under Glyceryl Trinitrate
Renal impairment see under Glyceryl Trinitrate
Pregnancy may cross placenta—manufacturers
advise avoid unless potential benefit outweighs risk
Breast-feeding see under Glyceryl Trinitrate
Side-effects see under Glyceryl Trinitrate
Dose
● By mouth, daily in divided doses, angina 30–120 mg,
left ventricular failure 40–160 mg, up to 240 mg if
required
● By intravenous infusion, 2–10 mg/hour; higher doses
up to 20 mg/hour may be required

◢**Short-acting tablets and sprays**
Isosorbide Dinitrate (Non-proprietary)
Tablets, isosorbide dinitrate 10 mg, net price 56-tab
pack = £13.41; 20 mg, 56-tab pack = £14.38

Angitak® (LPC)
Aerosol spray, isosorbide dinitrate 1.25 mg/metered
dose, net price 200-dose unit = £4.51
Dose treatment or prophylaxis of angina, spray 1–3 doses
under tongue whilst holding breath; allow 30 second
interval between each dose

2 Cardiovascular system

◢Modified-release preparations

Isoket Retard® (UCB Pharma)

Retard-20 tablets, m/r, scored, isosorbide dinitrate 20 mg, net price 56-tab pack = £2.58. Label: 25

Retard-40 tablets, m/r, scored, isosorbide dinitrate 40 mg, net price 56-tab pack = £6.36. Label: 25

Dose prophylaxis of angina, 40 mg daily in 1–2 divided doses, increased if necessary to 60–80 mg daily in 2–3 divided doses

◢Parenteral preparations

Isoket® (UCB Pharma) PoM

Injection 0.1%, isosorbide dinitrate 1 mg/mL. To be diluted before use. Net price 10-mL amp = £2.69

Note Glass or polyethylene infusion apparatus is preferable; loss of potency if PVC used

■ ISOSORBIDE MONONITRATE

Indications prophylaxis of angina; adjunct in congestive heart failure

Cautions see under Glyceryl Trinitrate

Contra-indications see under Glyceryl Trinitrate

Hepatic impairment see under Glyceryl Trinitrate

Renal impairment see under Glyceryl Trinitrate

Pregnancy manufacturers advise avoid unless potential benefit outweighs risk

Breast-feeding see under Glyceryl Trinitrate

Side-effects see under Glyceryl Trinitrate

Dose

● Initially 20 mg 2–3 times daily *or* 40 mg twice daily (10 mg twice daily in those who have not previously received nitrates); up to 120 mg daily in divided doses if required

Isosorbide Mononitrate (Non-proprietary)

Tablets, isosorbide mononitrate 10 mg, net price 56 = £5.69; 20 mg, 56 = £6.92; 40 mg, 56 = £8.38. Label: 25

Note May be difficult to obtain

Ismo® (Durbin)

Ismo 10 tablets, isosorbide mononitrate 10 mg, net price 60-tab pack = £3.31. Label: 25

Ismo 20 tablets, scored, isosorbide mononitrate 20 mg, net price 60-tab pack = £4.85. Label: 25

Note May be difficult to obtain

◢Modified release

Chemydur® **60XL** (AMCo)

Tablets, m/r, scored, ivory, isosorbide mononitrate 60 mg, net price 28-tab pack = £3.49. Label: 25

Dose prophylaxis of angina, 1 tablet in the morning (half a tablet for 2–4 days to minimise possibility of headache), increased if necessary to 2 tablets

Elantan LA® (UCB Pharma)

Elantan LA 25 capsules, m/r, brown/white, enclosing white micropellets, isosorbide mononitrate 25 mg, net price 28-cap pack = £3.40. Label: 25

Dose prophylaxis of angina, 1 capsule in the morning, increased if necessary to 2 capsules

Elantan LA 50 capsules, m/r, brown/pink, enclosing white micropellets, isosorbide mononitrate 50 mg, net price 28-cap pack = £3.69. Label: 25

Dose prophylaxis of angina, 1 capsule daily in the morning, increased if necessary to 2 capsules

Imdur® (AstraZeneca)

Durules® (= tablets m/r), yellow, f/c, scored, isosorbide mononitrate 60 mg, net price 28-tab pack = £10.50. Label: 25

Dose prophylaxis of angina, 1 tablet in the morning (half a tablet if headache occurs), increased to 2 tablets in the morning if required

Isib 60XL® (Ranbaxy)

Tablets, m/r, scored, yellow, isosorbide mononitrate 60 mg, net price 28-tab pack = £8.15. Label: 25

Dose prophylaxis of angina, 1 tablet in the morning (half a tablet for 2–4 days if headache occurs), increased if necessary to 2 tablets

Note Also available as Cibral 60XL®, Xismox 60XL®

Ismo Retard® (Durbin)

Tablets, m/r, s/c, isosorbide mononitrate 40 mg, net price 30-tab pack = £10.71. Label: 25

Dose prophylaxis of angina, 1 tablet daily in morning

Isodur® (Galen)

Isodur 25XL capsules, m/r, brown/white, isosorbide mononitrate 25 mg, net price 28-cap pack = £4.63. Label: 25

Isodur 50XL capsules, m/r, brown/red, isosorbide mononitrate 50 mg, net price 28-cap pack = £6.45. Label: 25

Dose prophylaxis of angina, 25–50 mg daily in the morning, increased if necessary to 50–100 mg once daily

Isotard® (ProStrakan)

Isotard 25XL tablets, m/r, ivory, isosorbide mononitrate 25 mg, net price 28-tab pack = £6.75. Label: 25

Isotard 40XL tablets, m/r, ivory, isosorbide mononitrate 40 mg, net price 28-tab pack = £6.75. Label: 25

Isotard 50XL tablets, m/r, ivory, isosorbide mononitrate 50 mg, net price 28-tab pack = £6.75. Label: 25

Isotard 60XL tablets, m/r, ivory, isosorbide mononitrate 60 mg, net price 28-tab pack = £5.75. Label: 25

Dose prophylaxis of angina, 25–60 mg daily in the morning (if headache occurs with 60-mg tablet, half a 60-mg tablet may be given for 2–4 days), increased if necessary to 50–120 mg daily

Modisal XL® (Sandoz)

Tablets, m/r, ivory, isosorbide mononitrate 60 mg, net price 28-tab pack = £11.14. Label: 25

Dose prophylaxis of angina, 1 tablet daily in the morning (half a tablet for first 2–4 days to minimise possibility of headache), increased if necessary to 2 tablets once daily

Monomax® (Chiesi)

Monomax® SR capsules, m/r, isosorbide mononitrate 40 mg, net price 28-cap pack = £6.52; 60 mg, 28-cap pack = £8.86. Label: 25

Dose prophylaxis of angina, 40–60 mg daily in the morning, increased if necessary to 120 mg daily

Monomax® XL tablets, m/r, isosorbide mononitrate 60 mg, net price 28-tab pack = £5.25. Label: 25

Dose prophylaxis of angina, 1 tablet in the morning (half a tablet for first 2–4 days to minimise possibility of headache), increased if necessary to 2 tablets

Monomil XL® (TEVA UK)

Tablets, m/r, isosorbide mononitrate 60 mg, net price 28-tab pack = £3.49. Label: 25

Dose prophylaxis of angina, 1 tablet daily in the morning (half a tablet daily for first 2–4 days to minimise possibility of headache), increased if necessary to 2 tablets once daily

Monosorb XL 60® (Dexcel)

Tablets, m/r, f/c, isosorbide mononitrate 60 mg, net price 28-tab pack = £15.35. Label: 25

Dose prophylaxis of angina, 1 tablet daily in the morning (half a tablet for first 2–4 days to minimise possibility of headache), increased if necessary to 2 tablets

Zemon® (Neolab)

Zemon 40XL tablets, m/r, ivory, isosorbide mononitrate 40 mg, net price 28-tab pack = £14.25. Label: 25

Zemon 60XL tablets, scored, m/r, ivory, isosorbide mononitrate 60 mg, net price 28-tab pack = £11.14. Label: 25

Dose prophylaxis of angina, 40–60 mg daily in the morning (half a 60-mg tablet may be given for 2–4 days to minimise possibility of headache), increased if necessary to 80–120 mg once daily

2.6.2 Calcium-channel blockers

Calcium-channel blockers (less correctly called 'calcium-antagonists') interfere with the inward displacement of calcium ions through the slow channels of active cell membranes. They influence the myocardial cells, the cells within the specialised conducting system of the heart, and the cells of vascular smooth muscle. Thus, myocardial contractility may be reduced, the formation and propagation of electrical impulses within the heart may be depressed, and coronary or systemic vascular tone may be diminished.

Calcium-channel blockers differ in their predilection for the various possible sites of action and, therefore, their therapeutic effects are disparate, with much greater variation than those of beta-blockers. There are important differences between verapamil, diltiazem, and the dihydropyridine calcium-channel blockers (amlodipine, felodipine, lacidipine, lercanidipine, nicardipine, nifedipine, and nimodipine). Verapamil and diltiazem should usually be **avoided** in heart failure because they may further depress cardiac function and cause clinically significant deterioration.

Verapamil is used for the treatment of angina (section 2.10.1), hypertension (section 2.5), and arrhythmias (section 2.3.2). It is a highly negatively inotropic calcium channel-blocker and it reduces cardiac output, slows the heart rate, and may impair atrioventricular conduction. It may precipitate heart failure, exacerbate conduction disorders, and cause hypotension at high doses and should **not** be used with beta-blockers (see p. 139). Constipation is the most common side-effect.

Nifedipine relaxes vascular smooth muscle and dilates coronary and peripheral arteries. It has more influence on vessels and less on the myocardium than does verapamil, and unlike verapamil has no anti-arrhythmic activity. It rarely precipitates heart failure because any negative inotropic effect is offset by a reduction in left ventricular work. Short-acting formulations of nifedipine are not recommended for angina or long-term management of hypertension; their use may be associated with large variations in blood pressure and reflex tachycardia. **Nicardipine** has similar effects to those of nifedipine and may produce less reduction of myocardial contractility. **Amlodipine** and **felodipine** also resemble nifedipine and nicardipine in their effects and do not reduce myocardial contractility and they do not produce clinical deterioration in heart failure. They have a longer duration of action and can be given once daily.

Nifedipine, nicardipine, amlodipine, and felodipine are used for the treatment of angina (section 2.10.1) or hypertension. All are valuable in forms of angina associated with coronary vasospasm. Side-effects associated with vasodilation such as flushing and headache (which become less obtrusive after a few days), and ankle swelling (which may respond only partially to diuretics) are common.

Intravenous nicardipine is licensed for the treatment of acute life-threatening hypertension, for example in the event of malignant arterial hypertension or hypertensive encephalopathy; aortic dissection, when a short-acting beta-blocker is not suitable, or in combination with a beta-blocker when beta-blockade alone is not effective; severe pre-eclampsia, when other intravenous antihypertensives are not recommended or are contra-indicated; and for treatment of postoperative hypertension. It should only be administered under the supervision of a specialist and in a hospital or intensive care setting in which patients can be closely monitored.

Isradipine, **lacidipine**, and **lercanidipine** have similar effects to those of nifedipine and nicardipine; they are indicated for hypertension only.

Nimodipine is related to nifedipine but the smooth muscle relaxant effect preferentially acts on cerebral arteries. Its use is confined to prevention and treatment of vascular spasm following aneurysmal subarachnoid haemorrhage.

Diltiazem is effective in most forms of angina (section 2.10.1); the longer-acting formulation is also used for hypertension. It may be used in patients for whom beta-blockers are contra-indicated or ineffective. It has a less negative inotropic effect than verapamil and significant myocardial depression occurs rarely. Nevertheless because of the risk of bradycardia it should be used with caution in association with beta-blockers.

Unstable angina Calcium-channel blockers do not reduce the risk of myocardial infarction in unstable angina. The use of diltiazem or verapamil should be reserved for patients resistant to treatment with beta-blockers.

Withdrawal There is some evidence that sudden withdrawal of calcium-channel blockers may be associated with an exacerbation of angina.

AMLODIPINE

Indications hypertension, prophylaxis of angina

Cautions interactions: Appendix 1 (calcium-channel blockers)

Contra-indications cardiogenic shock, unstable angina, significant aortic stenosis

Hepatic impairment may need dose reduction—half-life prolonged

Pregnancy no information available—manufacturer advises avoid, but risk to fetus should be balanced against risk of uncontrolled maternal hypertension

Breast-feeding manufacturer advises avoid—no information available

Side-effects abdominal pain, nausea; palpitation, flushing, oedema; headache, dizziness, sleep disturbances, fatigue; *less commonly* gastro-intestinal disturbances, dry mouth, taste disturbances, hypotension, syncope, chest pain, dyspnoea, rhinitis, mood changes, asthenia, tremor, paraesthesia, urinary disturbances, impotence, gynaecomastia, weight changes, myalgia, muscle cramps, back pain, arthralgia, visual disturbances, tinnitus, pruritus, rashes (including isolated reports of erythema multiforme), sweating, alopecia, purpura, and skin discoloration; *very rarely* gastritis, pancreatitis, hepatitis, jaundice, cholestasis, gingival hyperplasia, myocardial infarction, arrhythmias, tachycardia, vasculitis, coughing, peripheral neuropathy, hyperglycaemia, thrombocytopenia, angioedema, and urticaria; **overdosage**, see Emergency Treatment of Poisoning, p. 39

Dose

- Hypertension or angina, initially 5 mg once daily; max. 10 mg once daily

Note Tablets from various suppliers may contain different salts (e.g. amlodipine besilate, amlodipine maleate, and amlodipine mesilate) but the strength is expressed in terms of amlodipine (base); tablets containing different salts are considered interchangeable

Amlodipine (Non-proprietary) ℗ᴼᴹ

Tablets, amlodipine (as maleate or as mesilate) 5 mg, net price 28-tab pack = £1.00; 10 mg, 28-tab pack = £1.03
Brands include *Amlostin*®

Istin® (Pfizer) ℗ᴼᴹ

Tablets, amlodipine (as besilate) 5 mg, net price 28-tab pack = £11.08; 10 mg, 28-tab pack = £16.55

◢ With valsartan

Note For hypertension in patients stabilised on the individual components in the same proportions. For prescribing information on valsartan, see section 2.5.5.2

Exforge® (Novartis) ℗ᴼᴹ

Tablets 5/80, f/c, dark yellow, amlodipine 5 mg, valsartan 80 mg, net price 28-tab pack = £16.76
Tablets 5/160, f/c, dark yellow, amlodipine 5 mg, valsartan 160 mg, net price 28-tab pack = £22.09
Tablets 10/160, f/c, light yellow, amlodipine 10 mg, valsartan 160 mg, net price 28-tab pack = £22.09

◼ DILTIAZEM HYDROCHLORIDE

Indications prophylaxis and treatment of angina; hypertension

Cautions heart failure or significantly impaired left ventricular function, bradycardia (avoid if severe), first degree AV block, or prolonged PR interval; **interactions:** Appendix 1 (calcium-channel blockers)

Contra-indications severe bradycardia, left ventricular failure with pulmonary congestion, second- or third-degree AV block (unless pacemaker fitted), sick sinus syndrome; acute porphyria (section 9.8.2)

Hepatic impairment reduce dose

Renal impairment start with smaller dose

Pregnancy avoid

Breast-feeding significant amount present in milk—no evidence of harm but avoid unless no safer alternative

Side-effects bradycardia, sino-atrial block, AV block, palpitation, dizziness, hypotension, malaise, asthenia, headache, hot flushes, gastro-intestinal disturbances, oedema (notably of ankles); rarely rashes (including erythema multiforme and exfoliative dermatitis), photosensitivity; hepatitis, gynaecomastia, gum hyperplasia, extrapyramidal symptoms, depression reported; **overdosage**, see Emergency Treatment of Poisoning, p. 39

Dose

- Angina, 60 mg 3 times daily (elderly initially twice daily); increased if necessary to 360 mg daily
- Longer-acting formulations, see under preparations below

◢ Standard formulations

Note These formulations are licensed as generics and there is no requirement for brand name dispensing. Although their means of formulation has called for the strict designation 'modified-release' their duration of action corresponds to that of tablets requiring administration 3 times daily

Diltiazem (Non-proprietary) ℗ᴼᴹ

Tablets, m/r (but see note above), diltiazem hydrochloride 60 mg, net price 84 = £18.39. Label: 25

Tildiem® (Sanofi-Aventis) ℗ᴼᴹ

Tablets, m/r (but see note above), off-white, diltiazem hydrochloride 60 mg, net price 90-tab pack = £7.96. Label: 25

◢ Longer-acting formulations

Note Different versions of modified-release preparations containing more than 60 mg diltiazem hydrochloride may not have the same clinical effect. To avoid confusion between these different formulations of diltiazem, prescribers should specify the brand to be dispensed

Adizem-SR® (Napp) ℗ᴼᴹ

Capsules, m/r, diltiazem hydrochloride 90 mg (white), net price 56-cap pack = £8.50; 120 mg (brown/white), 56-cap pack = £9.45; 180 mg (brown/white), 56-cap pack = £14.15. Label: 25
Tablets, m/r, f/c, scored, diltiazem hydrochloride 120 mg, net price 56-tab pack = £14.72. Label: 25
Dose mild to moderate hypertension, usually 120 mg twice daily (dose form not appropriate for initial dose titration)
Angina, initially 90 mg twice daily (elderly, dose form not appropriate for initial dose titration); increased to 180 mg twice daily if required

Adizem-XL® (Napp) ℗ᴼᴹ

Capsules, m/r, diltiazem hydrochloride 120 mg (pink/blue), net price 28-cap pack = £9.14; 180 mg (dark pink/blue), 28-cap pack = £10.37; 200 mg (brown), 28-cap pack = £6.30; 240 mg (red/blue), 28-cap pack = £11.52; 300 mg (maroon/blue), 28-cap pack = £9.14. Label: 25
Dose angina and mild to moderate hypertension, initially 240 mg once daily, increased if necessary to 300 mg once daily; in elderly and in hepatic or renal impairment, initially 120 mg daily

Angitil SR® (Chiesi) ℗ᴼᴹ

Capsules, m/r, diltiazem hydrochloride 90 mg (white), net price 56-cap pack = £7.03; 120 mg (brown), 56-cap pack = £6.91; 180 mg (brown), 56-cap pack = £13.27. Label: 25
Dose angina and mild to moderate hypertension, initially 90 mg twice daily; increased if necessary to 120 mg or 180 mg twice daily

Angitil XL® (Chiesi) ℗ᴼᴹ

Capsules, m/r, diltiazem hydrochloride 240 mg (white), net price 28-cap pack = £7.94; 300 mg (yellow), 28-cap pack = £6.98. Label: 25
Dose angina and mild to moderate hypertension, initially 240 mg once daily (in hepatic and renal impairment, dose form not appropriate for initial dose titration); increased if necessary to 300 mg once daily

Dilcardia SR® (Generics) [PoM]

Capsules, m/r, diltiazem hydrochloride 60 mg (pink/white), net price 56-cap pack = £6.03; 90 mg (pink/yellow), 56-cap pack = £9.61; 120 mg (pink/orange), 56-cap pack = £10.69. Label: 25

Dose angina and mild to moderate hypertension, initially 90 mg twice daily; increased if necessary to 180 mg twice daily; ELDERLY and in hepatic or renal impairment, initially 60 mg twice daily, max. 90 mg twice daily

Dilzem SR® (TEVA UK) [PoM]

Capsules, m/r, all beige, diltiazem hydrochloride 60 mg, net price 56-cap pack = £6.04; 90 mg, 56-cap pack = £11.29; 120 mg, 56-cap pack = £12.89. Label: 25

Dose angina and mild to moderate hypertension, initially 90 mg twice daily (elderly 60 mg twice daily); up to 180 mg twice daily may be required

Dilzem XL® (TEVA UK) [PoM]

Capsules, m/r, diltiazem hydrochloride 120 mg, net price 28-cap pack = £7.78; 180 mg, 28-cap pack = £11.55; 240 mg, 28-cap pack = £11.03. Label: 25

Dose angina and mild to moderate hypertension, initially 180 mg once daily (elderly and in hepatic and renal impairment, 120 mg once daily); if necessary may be increased to 360 mg once daily

Slozem® (Merck Serono) [PoM]

Capsules, m/r, diltiazem hydrochloride 120 mg (pink/clear), net price 28-cap pack = £7.00; 180 mg (pink/clear), 28-cap pack = £7.80; 240 mg (red/clear), 28-cap pack = £8.20; 300 mg (red/white), 28-cap pack = £8.50. Label: 25

Dose angina and mild to moderate hypertension, initially 240 mg once daily (elderly and in hepatic and renal impairment, 120 mg once daily); if necessary may be increased to 360 mg once daily

Tildiem LA® (Sanofi-Aventis) [PoM]

Capsules, m/r, diltiazem hydrochloride 200 mg (pink/grey, containing white pellets), net price 28-cap pack = £6.27; 300 mg (white/yellow, containing white pellets), 28-cap pack = £9.01. Label: 25

Dose angina and mild to moderate hypertension, initially 200 mg once daily before or with food, increased if necessary to 300–400 mg daily, max. 500 mg daily; ELDERLY and in hepatic or renal impairment, initially 200 mg daily, increased if necessary to 300 mg daily

Tildiem Retard® (Sanofi-Aventis) [PoM]

Tablets, m/r, diltiazem hydrochloride 90 mg, net price 56-tab pack = £7.27; 120 mg, 56-tab pack = £7.15. Label: 25

Counselling Tablet membrane may pass through gastrointestinal tract unchanged, but being porous has no effect on efficacy

Dose mild to moderate hypertension, initially 90 mg or 120 mg twice daily; increased if necessary to 360 mg daily in divided doses; ELDERLY and in hepatic or renal impairment, initially 120 mg once daily; increased if necessary to 120 mg twice daily

Angina, initially 90 mg or 120 mg twice daily; increased if necessary to 480 mg daily in divided doses; ELDERLY and in hepatic or renal impairment, dose form not appropriate for initial titration; up to 120 mg twice daily may be required

Viazem XL® (Genus) [PoM]

Capsules, m/r, diltiazem hydrochloride 120 mg (lavender), net price 28-cap pack = £6.60; 180 mg (white/blue-green), 28-cap pack = £7.36; 240 mg (blue-green/lavender), 28-cap pack = £7.74; 300 mg (white/lavender), 28-cap pack = £8.03; 360 mg (blue-green), 28-cap pack = £13.85. Label: 25

Dose angina and mild to moderate hypertension, initially 180 mg once daily, adjusted according to response to 240 mg once daily, max. 360 mg once daily; ELDERLY and in hepatic or renal impairment, initially 120 mg once daily, adjusted according to response

Zemtard® (Galen) [PoM]

Zemtard 120XL capsules, m/r, brown/orange, diltiazem hydrochloride 120 mg, net price 28-cap pack = £5.19. Label: 25

Zemtard 180XL capsules, m/r, grey/pink, diltiazem hydrochloride 180 mg, net price 28-cap pack = £5.27 Label: 25

Zemtard 240XL capsules, m/r, blue, diltiazem hydrochloride 240 mg, net price 28-cap pack = £5.36. Label: 25

Zemtard 300XL capsules, m/r, white/blue, diltiazem hydrochloride 300 mg, net price 28-cap pack = £5.70. Label: 25

Dose angina and mild to moderate hypertension, 180–300 mg once daily, increased if necessary to 360 mg once daily in hypertension and to 480 mg once daily in angina; ELDERLY and in hepatic or renal impairment, initially 120 mg once daily

FELODIPINE

Indications hypertension, prophylaxis of angina

Cautions withdraw if ischaemic pain occurs or existing pain worsens shortly after initiating treatment or if cardiogenic shock develops; severe left ventricular dysfunction; predisposition to tachycardia; **interactions**: Appendix 1 (calcium-channel blockers)

Contra-indications unstable angina, uncontrolled heart failure; significant cardiac valvular obstruction (e.g. aortic stenosis); cardiac outflow obstruction; within 1 month of myocardial infarction

Hepatic impairment dose reduction may be required

Pregnancy avoid; toxicity in *animal* studies; may inhibit labour

Breast-feeding present in milk but amount probably too small to be harmful

Side-effects flushing, peripheral oedema, headache; *less commonly* nausea, abdominal pain, palpitation, tachycardia, dizziness, paraesthesia, malaise, rash, pruritus; *rarely* vomiting, syncope, impotence, arthralgia, myalgia; *very rarely* gum hyperplasia, urinary frequency, leucocytoclastic vasculitis, photosensitivity; **overdosage**, see Emergency Treatment of Poisoning, p. 39

Dose

- Hypertension, initially 5 mg (ELDERLY 2.5 mg) daily in the morning; usual maintenance 5–10 mg once daily; doses above 20 mg daily rarely needed
- Angina, initially 5 mg (ELDERLY 2.5 mg) daily in the morning, increased if necessary to 10 mg once daily

Felodipine (Non-proprietary) [PoM]

Tablets, m/r, felodipine 2.5 mg, net price 28-tab pack = £6.31; 5 mg, 28-tab pack = £4.21; 10 mg, 28-tab pack = £5.66, 30-tab pack = £6.99. Label: 25

Brands include Cardioplen XL®, Felogen XL®, Felotens XL®, Keloc SR®, Neofel XL®, Parmid XL®, Vascalpha®

Plendil® (AstraZeneca) [PoM]

Tablets, m/r, f/c, felodipine 2.5 mg (yellow), net price 28-tab pack = £6.31; 5 mg (pink), 28-tab pack = £4.21; 10 mg (red-brown), 28-tab pack = £5.66. Label: 25

◢**With ramipril**

Section 2.5.5.1

ISRADIPINE

Indications hypertension

Cautions sick sinus syndrome (if pacemaker not fitted); severe aortic stentosis; poor cardiac reserve;

2 Cardiovascular system

chronic heart failure; **interactions:** Appendix 1 (calcium-channel blockers)

Contra-indications   cardiogenic shock; during or within 1 month of myocardial infarction; unstable angina; acute porphyria (section 9.8.2)

Hepatic impairment   1.25 mg twice daily, increased if necessary after 3–4 weeks according to response; maintenance dose of 2.5 mg or 5 mg once daily may be sufficient

Renal impairment   use with caution

Pregnancy   may inhibit labour; risk to fetus should be balanced against risk of uncontrolled maternal hypertension

Breast-feeding   manufacturer advises avoid—present in milk in *animal* studies

Side-effects   abdominal discomfort; tachycardia, palpitation, flushing, peripheral oedema; dyspnoea; headache, fatigue, dizziness; polyuria; rash; *less commonly* hypotension, weight gain; *very rarely* vomiting, nausea, gum hyperplasia, anorexia, drowsiness, arrhythmia, bradycardia, heart failure, cough, depression, paraesthesia, anxiety, erectile dysfunction, blood disorders (such as thrombocytopenia, leucopenia, anaemia), arthralgia, visual disturbance, hypersensitivity reactions; hepatitis and gynaecomastia also reported; **overdosage,** see Emergency Treatment of Poisoning, p. 39

Dose

- 2.5 mg twice daily, increased if necessary after 3–4 weeks to 5 mg twice daily (exceptionally up to 10 mg twice daily); ELDERLY 1.25 mg twice daily, increased if necessary after 3–4 weeks according to response; maintenance dose of 2.5 mg or 5 mg once daily may be sufficient

Isradipine (Sandoz) PoM
Tablets, yellow, scored, isradipine 2.5 mg, net price 56-tab pack = £211.01

▮ LACIDIPINE

Indications   hypertension

Cautions   cardiac conduction abnormalities; poor cardiac reserve; **interactions:** Appendix 1 (calcium-channel blockers)

Contra-indications   cardiogenic shock, unstable angina, aortic stenosis; avoid within 1 month of myocardial infarction; acute porphyria (section 9.8.2)

Hepatic impairment   antihypertensive effect possibly increased

Pregnancy   manufacturer advises avoid; may inhibit labour

Breast-feeding   manufacturer advises avoid—no information available

Side-effects   flushing, palpitation, oedema; headache, dizziness; *rarely* gastro-intestinal disturbances, gum hyperplasia, aggravation of angina, mood disturbances, asthenia, polyuria, muscle cramps, skin rash (including pruritus and erythema); **overdosage,** see Emergency Treatment of Poisoning, p. 39

Dose

- Initially 2 mg as a single daily dose, preferably in the morning; increased after 3–4 weeks to 4 mg daily, then if necessary to 6 mg daily

Motens® (GSK) PoM
Tablets, both f/c, lacidipine 2 mg, net price 28-tab pack = £2.95; 4 mg (scored), 28-tab pack = £3.10

▮ LERCANIDIPINE HYDROCHLORIDE

Indications   mild to moderate hypertension

Cautions   left ventricular dysfunction; sick sinus syndrome (if pacemaker not fitted); **interactions:** Appendix 1 (calcium-channel blockers)

Contra-indications   aortic stenosis; unstable angina; uncontrolled heart failure; within 1 month of myocardial infarction; acute porphyria (section 9.8.2)

Hepatic impairment   avoid in severe disease

Renal impairment   avoid if eGFR less than 30 mL/minute/1.73 m^2

Pregnancy   manufacturer advises avoid—no information available

Breast-feeding   manufacturer advises avoid

Side-effects   *less commonly* flushing, peripheral oedema, palpitation, tachycardia, headache, dizziness; *rarely* gastro-intestinal disturbances, angina, asthenia, drowsiness, polyuria, myalgia, rash; *very rarely* gingival hyperplasia, myocardial infarction, hypotension; **overdosage,** see Emergency Treatment of Poisoning, p. 39

Dose

- Initially 10 mg once daily; increased, if necessary, after at least 2 weeks to 20 mg daily

Lercanidipine Hydrochloride (Non-proprietary) PoM
Tablets, lercanidipine hydrochloride 10 mg, net price 28-tab pack = £1.63; 20 mg, 28-tab pack = £2.09. Label: 22

Zanidip® (Recordati) PoM
Tablets, f/c, lercanidipine hydrochloride 10 mg (yellow), net price 28-tab pack = £5.70; 20 mg (pink), 28-tab pack = £10.82. Label: 22

▮ NICARDIPINE HYDROCHLORIDE

Indications   see notes above and section 2.5; see also under dose and preparations

Cautions   withdraw if ischaemic pain occurs or existing pain worsens within 30 minutes of initiating treatment or increasing dose; systemic hypotension and reflex tachycardia with rapid reduction of blood pressure may occur—during intravenous use consider stopping infusion or decreasing dose by half; congestive heart failure; significantly impaired left ventricular function; pulmonary oedema; portal hypertension; elevated intracranial pressure; stroke; elderly; monitor blood pressure and heart rate at least every 5 minutes during intravenous infusion, and then until stable, and continue monitoring for at least 12 hours after end of infusion; **interactions:** Appendix 1 (calcium-channel blockers)

Contra-indications   cardiogenic shock; compensatory hypertension; advanced aortic stenosis; unstable or acute attacks of angina; avoid within 1 month of myocardial infarction for oral route and avoid within 8 days of myocardial infarction for intravenous route; acute porphyria (section 9.8.2)

Hepatic impairment   use *oral* treatment with caution—consider using lowest initial dose and extending dosing interval according to individual response; use *intravenous* treatment with caution—use lower initial dose (see Dose below)

Renal impairment   consider using lowest initial *oral* dose and extending dosing interval according to individual response; use *intravenous* treatment with caution—use lower initial dose (see Dose below)

Pregnancy for treatment of acute life-threatening hypertension only; may inhibit labour, not to be used in multiple pregnancy (twins or more) unless there is no other acceptable alternative; toxicity in *animal* studies; risk of severe maternal hypotension and fatal foetal hypoxia—avoid excessive decrease in blood pressure

Breast-feeding manufacturer advises avoid—present in breast milk

Side-effects nausea, vomiting; dizziness, headache; peripheral oedema, palpitations, tachycardia, hypotension; flushing; also reported gastro-intestinal disturbances, gingival hyperplasia, paralytic ileus, atrioventricular block, dyspnoea, pulmonary oedema, drowsiness, insomnia, depression, tinnitus, paraesthesia, frequency of micturition, impotence, pruritus, rashes, and thrombocytopenia; **overdosage**, see Emergency Treatment of Poisoning, p. 39

Dose

- Prophylaxis of angina, mild to moderate hypertension, ADULT over 18 years, by mouth, initially 20 mg 3 times daily, increased, after at least three days, to 30 mg 3 times daily (usual range 60–120 mg daily)

- Acute life-threatening hypertension, postoperative hypertension, (specialist use only), ADULT over 18 years, by continuous intravenous infusion, initially 3–5 mg/hour for 15 minutes, increased according to response by 0.5–1 mg every 15 minutes (max. rate 15 mg/hour); reduce dose gradually when target blood pressure achieved, usual maintenance dose 2–4 mg/hour; ELDERLY and in hepatic or renal impairment, initially 1–5 mg/hour, increased or decreased by 500 micrograms/hour after 30 minutes, depending on response (max. rate 15 mg/hour); CHILD under 18 years see *BNF for Children*

- Acute life-threatening hypertension in pregnancy, (specialist use only), ADULT over 18 years, by continuous intravenous infusion, initially 1–5 mg/hour, increased or decreased by 500 micrograms/hour after 30 minutes, depending on response; usual max. 4 mg/hour in treatment of pre-eclampsia (max. rate 15 mg/hour)

Nicardipine (Non-proprietary) [PoM]
Capsules, nicardipine hydrochloride 20 mg, net price 56-cap pack = £6.00; 30 mg, 56-cap pack = £6.28

Nicardipine (AMCo) [PoM]
Injection, nicardipine hydrochloride 1 mg/mL, net price 10-mL amp = £10.00

Cardene® (Astellas) [PoM]
Capsules, nicardipine hydrochloride 20 mg (blue/white), net price 56-cap pack = £6.00; 30 mg (blue/pale blue), 56-cap pack = £6.96

◢ **Modified release**

Cardene SR® (Astellas) [PoM]
Capsules, m/r, nicardipine hydrochloride 30 mg, net price 56-cap pack = £7.15; 45 mg (blue), 56-cap pack = £10.40. Label: 25
Dose mild to moderate hypertension, initially 30 mg twice daily; usual effective dose 45 mg twice daily (range 30–60 mg twice daily)

◢ **NIFEDIPINE**

Indications prophylaxis of angina; hypertension; Raynaud's phenomenon; premature labour (section 7.1.3)

Cautions see notes above; also withdraw if ischaemic pain occurs or existing pain worsens shortly after initiating treatment; poor cardiac reserve; heart failure or significantly impaired left ventricular function (heart failure deterioration observed); severe hypotension; elderly; diabetes mellitus; **interactions**: Appendix 1 (calcium-channel blockers)

Contra-indications cardiogenic shock; advanced aortic stenosis; within 1 month of myocardial infarction; unstable or acute attacks of angina

Hepatic impairment dose reduction may be required in severe liver disease

Pregnancy may inhibit labour; manufacturer advises avoid before week 20; risk to fetus should be balanced against risk of uncontrolled maternal hypertension; use only if other treatment options are not indicated or have failed

Breast-feeding amount too small to be harmful but manufacturers advise avoid

Side-effects gastro-intestinal disturbance; hypotension, oedema, vasodilatation, palpitation; headache, dizziness, lethargy, asthenia; *less commonly* tachycardia, syncope, chills, nasal congestion, dyspnoea, anxiety, sleep disturbance, vertigo, migraine, paraesthesia, tremor, polyuria, dysuria, nocturia, erectile dysfunction, epistaxis, myalgia, joint swelling, visual disturbance, sweating, hypersensitivity reactions (including angioedema, jaundice, pruritus, urticaria, and rash); *rarely* anorexia, gum hyperplasia, mood disturbances, hyperglycaemia, male infertility, purpura, and photosensitivity reactions; also reported dysphagia, intestinal obstruction, intestinal ulcer, bezoar formation (with some modified-release preparations), gynaecomastia, agranulocytosis, and anaphylaxis; **overdosage**, see Emergency Treatment of Poisoning, p. 39

Dose

- See preparations below

Nifedipine (Non-proprietary) [PoM]
Capsules, nifedipine 5 mg, net price 84-cap pack = £15.87; 10 mg, 84-cap pack = £7.72
Dose angina prophylaxis (but not recommended, see notes above) and Raynaud's phenomenon, initially 5 mg 3 times daily, adjusted according to response to 20 mg 3 times daily
Hypertension, not recommended therefore no dose stated

Adalat® (Bayer) [PoM]
Capsules, orange, nifedipine 5 mg, net price 90-cap pack = £5.73; 10 mg, 90-cap pack = £7.30
Dose angina prophylaxis (but not recommended, see notes above) and Raynaud's phenomenon, initially 5 mg 3 times daily, adjusted according to response to max. 20 mg 3 times daily
Hypertension, not recommended therefore no dose stated

◢ **Modified release**
Note Different versions of modified-release preparations may not have the same clinical effect. To avoid confusion between these different formulations of nifedipine, prescribers should specify the brand to be dispensed. Modified-release formulations may not be suitable for dose titration in hepatic disease

Adalat® **LA** (Bayer) [PoM]
LA 20 tablets, m/r, f/c, pink, nifedipine 20 mg, net price 28-tab pack = £5.27. Label: 25
LA 30 tablets, m/r, f/c, pink, nifedipine 30 mg, net price 28-tab pack = £6.85. Label: 25

2 Cardiovascular system

LA 60 tablets, m/r, f/c, pink, nifedipine 60 mg, net price 28-tab pack = £9.03. Label: 25

Counselling Tablet membrane may pass through gastro-intestinal tract unchanged, but being porous has no effect on efficacy

Cautions dose form not appropriate for use in hepatic impairment or where there is a history of oesophageal or gastro-intestinal obstruction, decreased lumen diameter of the gastro-intestinal tract, or inflammatory bowel disease (including Crohn's disease)

Dose hypertension, 20–30 mg once daily, increased if necessary to max. 90 mg once daily

Angina prophylaxis, 30 mg once daily, increased if necessary to max. 90 mg once daily

Adalat® Retard (Bayer) [PoM]

Retard 10 tablets, m/r, f/c, grey-pink, nifedipine 10 mg, net price 56-tab pack = £7.34. Label: 25

Retard 20 tablets, m/r, f/c, grey-pink, nifedipine 20 mg, net price 56-tab pack = £8.81. Label: 25

Dose hypertension and angina prophylaxis, 10 mg twice daily, adjusted according to response to 40 mg twice daily

Adipine® MR (Chiesi) [PoM]

Tablets, m/r, nifedipine 10 mg (pink), net price 56-tab pack = £3.73; 20 mg (pink), 56-tab pack = £5.21. Label: 25

Dose hypertension and angina prophylaxis, 10 mg twice daily, adjusted according to response to 40 mg twice daily

Adipine® XL (Chiesi) [PoM]

Tablets, m/r, red, nifedipine 30 mg, net price 28-tab pack = £4.70; 60 mg, 28-tab pack = £7.10. Label: 25

Dose hypertension and angina prophylaxis, 30 mg once daily, increased if necessary; max. 90 mg once daily

Coracten SR® (UCB Pharma) [PoM]

Capsules, m/r, nifedipine 10 mg (grey/pink, enclosing yellow pellets), net price 60-cap pack = £3.90; 20 mg (pink/brown, enclosing yellow pellets), 60-cap pack = £5.41. Label: 25

Dose hypertension and angina prophylaxis, initially 10 mg twice daily, increased if necessary to max. 40 mg twice daily

Coracten XL® (UCB Pharma) [PoM]

Capsules, m/r, nifedipine 30 mg (brown), net price 28-cap pack = £4.89; 60 mg (orange), 28-cap pack = £7.34. Label: 25

Dose hypertension and angina prophylaxis, 30 mg once daily, increased if necessary; max. 90 mg once daily

Fortipine LA 40® (AMCo) [PoM]

Tablets, m/r, red, nifedipine 40 mg, net price 30-tab pack = £14.40. Label: 21, 25

Dose hypertension and angina prophylaxis, 40 mg once daily, increased if necessary to 80 mg daily in 1–2 divided doses

Nifedipress® MR (Dexcel) [PoM]

Tablets, m/r, pink, nifedipine 10 mg, net price 56-tab pack = £9.23; 20 mg, 56-tab pack = £10.06. Label: 25

Dose hypertension and angina prophylaxis, initially 10 mg twice daily adjusted according to response to 40 mg twice daily

Note Also available as *Calchan® MR*, *Kentipine® MR*

Tensipine MR® (Genus) [PoM]

Tablets, m/r, pink-grey, nifedipine 10 mg, net price 56-tab pack = £4.30; 20 mg, 56-tab pack = £5.49. Label: 25

Dose hypertension and angina prophylaxis, initially 10 mg twice daily adjusted according to response to 40 mg twice daily

Valni XL® (Zentiva) [PoM]

Tablets, m/r, red, nifedipine 30 mg, net price 28-tab pack = £7.29; 60 mg, 28-tab pack = £9.14. Label: 25

Cautions dose form not appropriate for use in hepatic impairment, or where there is a history of oesophageal or gastro-intestinal obstruction, decreased lumen diameter of the gastro-intestinal tract, inflammatory bowel disease, or ileostomy after proctocolectomy

Dose severe hypertension and prophylaxis of angina, 30 mg once daily, increased if necessary to max. 90 mg once daily

◀ **With atenolol**

Section 2.4

▌ NIMODIPINE

Indications prevention and treatment of ischaemic neurological deficits following aneurysmal subarachnoid haemorrhage

Cautions cerebral oedema or severely raised intracranial pressure; hypotension; avoid concomitant administration of nimodipine tablets and infusion, other calcium-channel blockers, or beta-blockers; concomitant nephrotoxic drugs; **interactions:** Appendix 1 (calcium-channel blockers, alcohol (infusion only))

Contra-indications within 1 month of myocardial infarction; unstable angina; acute porphyria (section 9.8.2)

Hepatic impairment elimination reduced in cirrhosis—monitor blood pressure

Renal impairment manufacturer advises monitor renal function closely with intravenous administration

Pregnancy manufacturer advises use only if potential benefit outweighs risk

Breast-feeding manufacturer advises avoid—present in milk

Side-effects hypotension, variation in heart-rate, flushing, headache, gastro-intestinal disorders, nausea, sweating and feeling of warmth; thrombocytopenia and ileus reported; **overdosage**, see Emergency Treatment of Poisoning, p. 39

Dose

● Prevention, by mouth, 60 mg every 4 hours, starting within 4 days of aneurysmal subarachnoid haemorrhage and continued for 21 days

● Treatment, by intravenous infusion via central catheter, initially 1 mg/hour (up to 500 micrograms/hour if body-weight less than 70 kg or if blood pressure unstable), increased after 2 hours to 2 mg/hour if no severe fall in blood pressure; continue for at least 5 days (max. 14 days); if surgical intervention during treatment, continue for at least 5 days after surgery; max. total duration of nimodipine use 21 days

Nimotop® (Bayer) [PoM]

Tablets, yellow, f/c, nimodipine 30 mg, net price 100-tab pack = £40.00

Intravenous infusion, nimodipine 200 micrograms/mL; also contains ethanol 20% and macrogol '400' 17%. Net price 50-mL vial (with polyethylene infusion catheter) = £13.60

Note Polyethylene, polypropylene, or glass apparatus should be used; PVC should be avoided

▌ VERAPAMIL HYDROCHLORIDE

Indications see under Dose and preparations

Cautions first-degree AV block; acute phase of myocardial infarction (avoid if bradycardia, hypotension, left ventricular failure); patients taking beta-blockers (**important**: see below); **interactions**: Appendix 1 (calcium-channel blockers)

Verapamil and beta-blockers Verapamil injection should not be given to patients recently treated with beta-blockers because of the risk of hypotension and asystole. The suggestion that when verapamil injection has been given first, an interval of 30 minutes before giving a beta-blocker is sufficient has not been confirmed.

It may also be hazardous to give verapamil and a beta-blocker together by mouth (should only be contemplated if myocardial function well preserved).

Contra-indications   hypotension, bradycardia, second- and third-degree AV block, sick sinus syndrome, cardiogenic shock, sino-atrial block; history of heart failure or significantly impaired left ventricular function, even if controlled by therapy; atrial flutter or fibrillation associated with accessory conducting pathways (e.g. Wolff-Parkinson-White syndrome); acute porphyria (section 9.8.2)

Hepatic impairment   oral dose may need to be reduced

Pregnancy   may reduce uterine blood flow with fetal hypoxia; manufacturer advises avoid in first trimester unless absolutely necessary; may inhibit labour

Breast-feeding   amount too small to be harmful

Side-effects   constipation; less commonly nausea, vomiting, flushing, headache, dizziness, fatigue, ankle oedema; rarely allergic reactions (erythema, pruritus, urticaria, angioedema, Stevens-Johnson syndrome); myalgia, arthralgia, paraesthesia, erythromelalgia; increased prolactin concentration; rarely gynaecomastia and gingival hyperplasia after long-term treatment; after intravenous administration or high doses, hypotension, heart failure, bradycardia, heart block, and asystole; **overdosage**, see Emergency Treatment of Poisoning, p. 39

Dose

• By mouth, supraventricular arrhythmias (but see also Contra-indications), 40–120 mg 3 times daily

  Angina, 80–120 mg 3 times daily

  Hypertension, 240–480 mg daily in 2–3 divided doses

  Prophylaxis of cluster headache [unlicensed] (under specialist supervision), 240–960 mg daily in 3–4 divided doses

• By slow intravenous injection over 2 minutes (3 minutes in elderly), supraventricular arrhythmias (but see also Contra-indications), 5–10 mg (preferably with ECG monitoring); in paroxysmal tachyarrhythmias a further 5 mg after 5–10 minutes if required

Verapamil (Non-proprietary) [PoM]

Tablets, coated, verapamil hydrochloride 40 mg, net price 84-tab pack = £2.07; 80 mg, 84-tab pack = £2.44; 120 mg, 28-tab pack = £1.82; 160 mg, 56-tab pack = £28.20

Oral solution, verapamil hydrochloride 40 mg/5 mL, net price 150 mL = £36.90

Brands include *Zolvera*®

Cordilox® (Dexcel) [PoM]

Tablets, yellow, f/c, verapamil hydrochloride 40 mg, net price 84-tab pack = £1.50; 80 mg, 84-tab pack = £2.05; 120 mg, 28-tab pack = £1.15; 160 mg, 56-tab pack = £2.80

Injection, verapamil hydrochloride 2.5 mg/mL, net price 2-mL amp = £1.11

Securon® (Abbott Healthcare) [PoM]

Injection, verapamil hydrochloride 2.5 mg/mL, net price 2-mL amp = £1.08

◢**Modified release**

Half Securon SR® (Abbott Healthcare) [PoM]

Tablets, m/r, f/c, verapamil hydrochloride 120 mg, net price 28-tab pack = £7.71. Label: 25

Dose see *Securon SR*®

Securon SR® (Abbott Healthcare) [PoM]

Tablets, m/r, pale green, f/c, scored, verapamil hydrochloride 240 mg, net price 28-tab pack = £5.55. Label: 25

Dose hypertension, 240 mg daily (new patients initially 120 mg), increased if necessary to max. 480 mg daily (doses above 240 mg daily as 2 divided doses)

Angina, 240 mg twice daily (may sometimes be reduced to once daily)

Prophylaxis after myocardial infarction where beta-blockers not appropriate (started at least 1 week after infarction), 360 mg daily in divided doses, given as 240 mg in the morning and 120 mg in the evening *or* 120 mg 3 times daily

Univer® (TEVA UK) [PoM]

Capsules, m/r, verapamil hydrochloride 120 mg (yellow/dark blue), net price 28-cap pack = £4.86; 180 mg (yellow), 56-cap pack = £11.38; 240 mg (yellow/dark blue), 28-cap pack = £7.67. Label: 25

Excipients include propylene glycol (see Excipients, p. 2)

Dose hypertension, 240 mg daily, max. 480 mg daily (new patients, initial dose 120 mg); angina, 360 mg daily, max. 480 mg daily

Verapress MR® (Dexcel) [PoM]

Tablets, m/r, pale green, f/c, verapamil hydrochloride 240 mg, net price 28-tab pack = £9.90. Label: 25

Dose hypertension, 1 tablet daily, increased to twice daily if necessary; angina, 1 tablet twice daily (may sometimes be reduced to once daily)

Note Also available as *Cordilox*® *MR*

Vertab® **SR 240** (Chiesi) [PoM]

Tablets, m/r, pale green, f/c, scored, verapamil hydrochloride 240 mg, net price 28-tab pack = £5.45. Label: 25

Dose mild to moderate hypertension, 240 mg daily, increased to twice daily if necessary; angina, 240 mg twice daily (may sometimes be reduced to once daily)

2.6.3   Other antianginal drugs

Nicorandil, a potassium-channel activator with a nitrate component, has both arterial and venous vasodilating properties and is licensed for the prevention and long-term treatment of angina (section 2.10.1). Nicorandil has similar efficacy to other antianginal drugs in controlling symptoms; it may produce additional symptomatic benefit in combination with other antianginal drugs [unlicensed indication].

Ivabradine lowers the heart rate by its action on the sinus node. It is licensed for the treatment of angina in patients who are in normal sinus rhythm in combination with a beta-blocker, or when beta-blockers are contra-indicated or not tolerated. Ivabradine, in combination with standard therapy including a beta-blocker (unless contra-indicated or not tolerated), is also licensed for mild to severe chronic heart failure in patients who are in sinus rhythm. The *Scottish Medicines Consortium* (p. 4) has advised (September 2012) that ivabradine (*Procoralan*®) is accepted for restricted use within NHS Scotland in accordance with its licensed indication for heart failure only if resting heart rate remains ≥ 75 beats per minute despite optimal standard therapy.

2   **Cardiovascular system**

2 Cardiovascular system

Ranolazine is licensed as adjunctive therapy in patients who are inadequately controlled or intolerant of first-line antianginal drugs. The *Scottish Medicines Consortium* (p. 4) has advised (October 2012) that ranolazine (*Ranexa*®) is **not** recommended for use within NHS Scotland.

IVABRADINE

Indications   treatment of angina in patients in normal sinus rhythm (see notes above); mild to severe chronic heart failure (see notes above)

Cautions   monitor for atrial fibrillation or other arrhythmias (treatment ineffective); monitor for bradycardia, especially after any dose increase, and discontinue if resting heart rate persistently below 50 beats per minute or continued symptoms of bradycardia despite dose reduction; intraventricular conduction defects; hypotension (avoid if severe); retinitis pigmentosa; elderly; **interactions**: Appendix 1 (ivabradine)

Contra-indications   *for angina*, do not initiate if heart rate below 60 beats per minute; *for heart failure*, do not initiate if heart rate below 75 beats per minute; unstable or acute heart failure; cardiogenic shock; acute myocardial infarction; unstable angina; immediately after cerebrovascular accident; sick-sinus syndrome; sino-atrial block; patients dependent on pacemaker; second- and third-degree heart block; congenital QT syndrome

Hepatic impairment   manufacturer advises caution in moderate impairment; avoid in severe impairment

Renal impairment   manufacturer advises use with caution if eGFR less than 15 mL/minute/1.73 m^2—no information available

Pregnancy   manufacturer advises avoid—toxicity in *animal* studies

Breast-feeding   present in milk in *animal* studies—manufacturer advises avoid

Side-effects   bradycardia, first-degree heart block, ventricular extrasystoles, headache, dizziness, visual disturbances including phosphenes and blurred vision; *less commonly* nausea, constipation, diarrhoea, palpitations, supraventricular extrasystoles, dyspnoea, angioedema, vertigo, muscle cramps, eosinophilia, hyperuricaemia, raised plasma-creatinine concentration, rash; *very rarely* atrial fibrillation, second- and third-degree heart block, sick sinus syndrome

Dose
- Angina, initially 5 mg twice daily, increased if necessary after 3–4 weeks to 7.5 mg twice daily (if not tolerated reduce dose to 2.5–5 mg twice daily); ELDERLY initially 2.5 mg twice daily
- Heart failure, initially 5 mg twice daily, increased if necessary after 2 weeks to 7.5 mg twice daily (if not tolerated reduce dose to 2.5 mg twice daily)

Note Heart rate at rest should not be allowed to fall below 50 beats per minute

Procoralan® (Servier) PoM
Tablets, pink, f/c, ivabradine (as hydrochloride) 5 mg (scored), net price 56-tab pack = £40.17; 7.5 mg, 56-tab pack = £40.17

NICORANDIL

Indications   prophylaxis and treatment of stable angina (including risk reduction of acute coronary syndromes in patients at high risk)

Cautions   hypovolaemia; low systolic blood pressure; acute pulmonary oedema; acute myocardial infarction with acute left ventricular failure and low filling pressures; **interactions**: Appendix 1 (nicorandil)

Driving Patients should be warned not to drive or operate machinery until it is established that their performance is unimpaired

Contra-indications   cardiogenic shock; left ventricular failure with low filling pressures; hypotension

Pregnancy   manufacturer advises use only if potential benefit outweighs risk—no information available

Breast-feeding   no information available—manufacturer advises avoid

Side-effects   nausea, vomiting, rectal bleeding, cutaneous vasodilation with flushing, increase in heart rate (at high doses), dizziness, headache (especially on initiation, usually transitory), weakness; *less commonly* oral ulceration, hypotension, myalgia, angioedema; *rarely* intestinal ulceration, anal ulceration, abdominal pain, hepatitis, cholestasis, jaundice, skin ulceration, rash, pruritus

Dose
- Initially 10 mg twice daily (if susceptible to headache 5 mg twice daily); usual dose 10–20 mg twice daily; up to 30 mg twice daily may be used

Nicorandil (Non-proprietary) PoM
Tablets, nicorandil 10 mg, net price 60-tab pack = £3.97; 20 mg, 60-tab pack = £7.94

Ikorel® (Zentiva) PoM
Tablets, scored, nicorandil 10 mg, net price 60-tab pack = £7.71; 20 mg, 60-tab pack = £14.64

RANOLAZINE

Indications   as adjunctive therapy in the treatment of stable angina in patients inadequately controlled or intolerant of first-line antianginal therapies

Cautions   moderate to severe congestive heart failure; QT interval prolongation; elderly; body-weight less than 60 kg; **interactions**: Appendix 1 (ranolazine)

Hepatic impairment   use with caution in mild impairment; avoid in moderate and severe impairment

Renal impairment   use with caution if eGFR 30–80 mL/minute/1.73 m^2; avoid if eGFR less than 30 mL/minute/1.73 m^2

Pregnancy manufacturer advises avoid unless essential—no information available

Breast-feeding manufacturer advises avoid—no information available

Side-effects constipation, nausea, vomiting, dizziness, headache, asthenia; *less commonly* abdominal pain, weight loss, dry mouth, dyspepsia, flatulence, hot flush, hypotension, syncope, prolonged QT interval, peripheral oedema, dysponea, cough, epistaxis, lethargy, hypoaesthesia, drowsiness, tremor, anxiety, confusion, hallucination, insomnia, anorexia, dysuria, haematuria, chromaturia, dehydration, pain in extremities, muscle cramp, joint swelling, visual disturbance, tinnitus, pruritus, sweating; *rarely* pancreatitis, erosive duodenitis, cold extremities, throat tightness, angioedema, amnesia, loss of consciousness, erectile dysfunction, renal failure, parosmia, impaired hearing, allergic dermatitis, urticaria, rash

Dose

- ADULT over 18 years, initially 375 mg twice daily, increased after 2–4 weeks to 500 mg twice daily and then adjusted according to response to max. 750 mg twice daily (reduce dose to 375–500 mg twice daily if not tolerated)

Ranexa® (Menarini) ▼ PoM

Tablets, m/r, ranolazine 375 mg (blue), net price 60-tab pack = £48.98; 500 mg (orange), 60-tab pack = £48.98; 750 mg (green), 60-tab pack = £48.98. Label: 25, patient alert card

2.6.4 Peripheral vasodilators and related drugs

Peripheral vascular disease can be either occlusive (e.g. *intermittent claudication*) in which occlusion of the peripheral arteries is caused by atherosclerosis, or vasospastic (e.g. *Raynaud's syndrome*).

Peripheral arterial occlusive disease is associated with an increased risk of cardiovascular events; this risk is reduced by measures such as smoking cessation (section 4.10.2), effective control of blood pressure (section 2.5), regulating blood lipids (section 2.12), optimising glycaemic control in diabetes (section 6.1), taking aspirin in a dose of 75 mg daily (section 2.9), and possibly weight reduction in obesity (section 4.5). Exercise training can improve symptoms of intermittent claudication; revascularisation procedures may be appropriate.

> **NICE guidance**
> **Cilostazol, naftidrofuryl oxalate, pentoxifylline and inositol nicotinate for the treatment of intermittent claudication in people with peripheral arterial disease (May 2011)**
>
> Naftidrofuryl oxalate is an option for the treatment of intermittent claudication in patients with peripheral arterial disease in whom vasodilator therapy is considered appropriate.
>
> Cilostazol, pentoxifylline, and inositol nicotinate are not recommended for the treatment of intermittent claudication in patients with peripheral arterial disease; patients currently receiving these treatments should have the option to continue until they and their clinician consider it appropriate to stop.
> www.nice.org.uk/TA223

Naftidrofuryl can alleviate symptoms of intermittent claudication and improve pain-free walking distance in moderate disease. Patients taking naftidrofuryl should be assessed for improvement after 3–6 months.

Cilostazol is licensed for use in intermittent claudication to improve walking distance in patients without peripheral tissue necrosis who do not have pain at rest; use is restricted to second-line treatment where lifestyle modifications and other appropriate interventions have failed to improve symptoms. Cilostazol should be initiated by those experienced in the management of intermittent claudication. Patients receiving cilostazol should be assessed for improvement after 3 months; consider discontinuation of treatment if there is no clinically relevant improvement in walking distance. The *Scottish Medicines Consortium* (p. 4) has advised (October 2005) that cilostazol is not recommended for the treatment of intermittent claudication within NHS Scotland.

Inositol nicotinate and pentoxifylline are not established as being effective for the treatment of intermittent claudication.

Management of *Raynaud's syndrome* includes avoidance of exposure to cold and stopping smoking. More severe symptoms may require vasodilator treatment, which is most often successful in primary Raynaud's syndrome. **Nifedipine** (section 2.6.2) is useful for reducing the frequency and severity of vasospastic attacks. Alternatively, **naftidrofuryl** may produce symptomatic improvement; **inositol nicotinate** (a nicotinic acid derivative) may also be considered. Pentoxifylline, prazosin, and moxisylyte are not established as being effective for the treatment of Raynaud's syndrome.

Vasodilator therapy is not established as being effective for *chilblains* (section 13.13).

CILOSTAZOL

Indications intermittent claudication in patients without rest pain and no peripheral tissue necrosis (but see notes above)

Cautions atrial or ventricular ectopy, atrial fibrillation, atrial flutter (contra-indicated if severe); stable coronary disease; diabetes mellitus (higher risk of intraocular bleeding); surgery; concomitant drugs that increase risk of bleeding (contra-indicated with concomitant use of 2 or more antiplatelets or anticoagulants); interactions: Appendix 1 (cilostazol)

Blood disorders Patients should be advised to report any unexplained bleeding, bruising, sore throat, or fever. A blood count should be performed and the drug stopped immediately if there is suspicion of a blood dyscrasia

Contra-indications predisposition to bleeding (e.g. active peptic ulcer, haemorrhagic stroke in previous 6 months, proliferative diabetic retinopathy, poorly controlled hypertension); history of severe tachyarrhythmia; prolongation of QT interval; unstable angina; myocardial infarction in previous 6 months; coronary intervention in previous 6 months; congestive heart failure

Hepatic impairment avoid in moderate or severe liver disease

Renal impairment avoid if eGFR less than 25 mL/minute/1.73 m^2

Pregnancy avoid—toxicity in *animal* studies

Breast-feeding present in milk in *animal* studies—manufacturer advises avoid

2 Cardiovascular system

2 Cardiovascular system

Side-effects diarrhoea, nausea, vomiting, dyspepsia, flatulence, abdominal pain, anorexia, tachycardia, palpitation, angina, arrhythmia, oedema, rhinitis, pharyngitis, dizziness, headache, malaise, rash, pruritus, ecchymosis; *less commonly* gastritis, myocardial infarction, congestive heart failure, postural hypotension, dyspnoea, pneumonia, cough, insomnia, abnormal dreams, anxiety, hyperglycaemia, diabetes mellitus, anaemia, haemorrhage, myalgia; *rarely* increased urinary frequency, bleeding disorders, thrombocythaemia, renal impairment; *also reported* hypertension, pyrexia, hot flushes, thrombocytopenia, agranulocytosis, leucopenia, pancytopenia, aplastic anemia, hepatitis, conjunctivitis, tinnitus, Stevens-Johnson syndrome, toxic epidermal necrolysis

Dose
- 100 mg twice daily 30 minutes before food

Note Reduce dose to 50 mg twice daily with concomitant use of potent inhibitors of cytochrome P450 enzymes CYP3A4 (e.g. clarithromycin, itraconazole, protease inhibitors) or CYP2C19, or with erythromycin or omeprazole

Pletal® (Otsuka) ▼ PoM
Tablets, cilostazol 50 mg, net price 56-tab pack = £35.31; 100 mg, 56-tab pack = £33.37. Counselling, blood disorders, see above

INOSITOL NICOTINATE

Indications peripheral vascular disease (but see notes above); hyperlipidaemia (section 2.12)

Cautions cerebrovascular insufficiency, unstable angina

Contra-indications recent myocardial infarction, acute phase of a cerebrovascular accident

Pregnancy no information available—manufacturer advises avoid unless potential benefit outweighs risk

Side-effects nausea, vomiting, hypotension, flushing, syncope, oedema, headache, dizziness, paraesthesia, rash

Dose
- 3 g daily in 2–3 divided doses; max. 4 g daily

Hexopal® (Genus)
Tablets, scored, inositol nicotinate 500 mg, net price 100 = £30.76
Tablets forte, scored, inositol nicotinate 750 mg, net price 112-tab pack = £51.03

MOXISYLYTE
(Thymoxamine)

Indications primary Raynaud's syndrome (short-term treatment)

Cautions diabetes mellitus

Contra-indications active liver disease

Pregnancy manufacturer advises avoid

Side-effects nausea, diarrhoea, flushing, headache, dizziness; hepatic reactions including cholestatic jaundice and hepatitis reported to CSM

Dose
- Initially 40 mg 4 times daily, increased to 80 mg 4 times daily if poor initial response; discontinue after 2 weeks if no response

Opilon® (Archimedes) PoM
Tablets, yellow, f/c, moxisylyte 40 mg (as hydrochloride), net price 112-tab pack = £90.22. Label: 21

NAFTIDROFURYL OXALATE

Indications see under Dose

Side-effects nausea, epigastric pain, rash, hepatitis, hepatic failure

Dose
- Peripheral vascular disease (see notes above), 100–200 mg 3 times daily
- Cerebral vascular disease, 100 mg 3 times daily

Naftidrofuryl (Non-proprietary) PoM
Capsules = naftidrofuryl oxalate 100 mg, net price 84-cap pack = £6.27. Label: 25, 27

Praxilene® (Merck Serono) PoM
Capsules, pink, naftidrofuryl oxalate 100 mg, net price 84-cap pack = £8.10. Label: 25, 27

PENTOXIFYLLINE
(Oxpentifylline)

Indications peripheral vascular disease (but see notes above); venous leg ulcers [unlicensed indication] (Appendix A5.8.7)

Cautions hypotension, coronary artery disease; avoid in acute porphyria (section 9.8.2); **interactions:** Appendix 1 (pentoxifylline)

Contra-indications cerebral haemorrhage, extensive retinal haemorrhage, acute myocardial infarction, severe cardiac arrhythmias

Hepatic impairment manufacturer advises reduce dose in severe impairment

Renal impairment reduce dose by 30–50% if eGFR less than 30 mL/minute/1.73 m^2

Pregnancy manufacturer advises avoid—no information available

Breast-feeding present in milk—manufacturer advises use only if potential benefit outweighs risk

Side-effects nausea, vomiting, diarrhoea, dizziness, agitation, sleep disturbances, headache; *rarely* angina, hypotension; *very rarely* bleeding; *also reported* intrahepatic cholestasis, tachycardia, flushing, thrombocytopenia

Dose
- 400 mg 2–3 times daily

Trental® (Sanofi-Aventis) PoM
Tablets, m/r, pink, s/c, pentoxifylline 400 mg, net price 90-tab pack = £19.39. Label: 21, 25

Other preparations used in peripheral vascular disease

Rutosides (oxerutins, *Paroven®*) are not vasodilators and are not generally regarded as effective preparations as capillary sealants or for the treatment of cramps; side-effects include headache, flushing, rashes, mild gastro-intestinal disturbances.

Paroven® (Novartis Consumer Health)
Capsules, yellow, oxerutins 250 mg, net price 120-cap pack = £16.81
Dose relief of symptoms of oedema associated with chronic venous insufficiency, 500 mg twice daily

2.7 Sympathomimetics

2.7.1 Inotropic sympathomimetics
2.7.2 Vasoconstrictor sympathomimetics
2.7.3 Cardiopulmonary resuscitation

The properties of sympathomimetics vary according to whether they act on alpha or on beta adrenergic receptors. Adrenaline (epinephrine) (section 2.7.3) acts on both alpha and beta receptors and increases both heart rate and contractility (beta$_1$ effects); it can cause peripheral vasodilation (a beta$_2$ effect) or vasoconstriction (an alpha effect).

2.7.1 Inotropic sympathomimetics

The cardiac stimulants **dobutamine** and **dopamine** act on beta$_1$ receptors in cardiac muscle, and increase contractility with little effect on rate.

Dopexamine acts on beta$_2$ receptors in cardiac muscle to produce its positive inotropic effect; and on peripheral dopamine receptors to increase renal perfusion; it is reported not to induce vasoconstriction.

Isoprenaline injection is available from 'special-order' manufacturers or specialist importing companies, see p. 1124.

Shock Shock is a medical emergency associated with a high mortality. The underlying causes of shock such as haemorrhage, sepsis, or myocardial insufficiency should be corrected. The profound hypotension of shock must be treated promptly to prevent tissue hypoxia and organ failure. Volume replacement is essential to correct the hypovolaemia associated with haemorrhage and sepsis but may be detrimental in cardiogenic shock. Depending on haemodynamic status, cardiac output may be improved by the use of sympathomimetic inotropes such as adrenaline (epinephrine), dobutamine or dopamine (see notes above). In septic shock, when fluid replacement and inotropic support fail to maintain blood pressure, the vasoconstrictor noradrenaline (norepinephrine) (section 2.7.2) may be considered. In cardiogenic shock peripheral resistance is frequently high and to raise it further may worsen myocardial performance and exacerbate tissue ischaemia.

The use of sympathomimetic inotropes and vasoconstrictors should preferably be confined to the intensive care setting and undertaken with invasive haemodynamic monitoring.

For advice on the management of anaphylactic shock, see section 3.4.3.

DOBUTAMINE

Indications inotropic support in infarction, cardiac surgery, cardiomyopathies, septic shock, cardiogenic shock, and during positive end expiratory pressure ventilation; cardiac stress testing (consult product literature)

Cautions arrhythmias; occlusive vascular disease; ischaemic heart disease; acute myocardial infarction; acute heart failure; severe hypotension; extreme caution or avoid in marked obstruction of cardiac ejection (such as idiopathic hypertrophic subaortic stenosis); tachycardia; correct hypovolaemia, metabolic acidosis, hypoxia, and hypercapnia before starting and during treatment; monitor serum-potassium concentration; tolerance may develop with continuous infusions longer than 72 hours; hyperthyroidism; diabetes mellitus; susceptibility to angle-closure glaucoma; elderly; extravasation may cause tissue necrosis; **interactions**: Appendix 1 (sympathomimetics)

Contra-indications phaeochromocytoma

Pregnancy no evidence of harm in *animal* studies—manufacturers advise use only if potential benefit outweighs risk

Breast-feeding manufacturers advise avoid—no information available

Side-effects nausea, hypotension, hypertension (marked increase in systolic blood pressure indicates overdose), arrhythmias, tachycardia, palpitation, chest pain, dyspnoea, bronchospasm, headache, fever, eosinophilia, reduced platelet aggregation (on prolonged use), rash, phlebitis; *rarely* psychosis; *very rarely* bradycardia, cardiac arrest, AV block, myocardial infarction, coronary artery spasm, hypokalaemia, angle-closure glaucoma, petechial bleeding; *also reported* vomiting, cerebral haemorrhage, pulmonary oedema, anxiety, paraesthesia, tremor, myoclonic spasm, increased urinary urgency, pruritus of scalp

Dose
• By intravenous infusion, usual dose 2.5–10 micrograms/kg/minute, adjusted according to response; dose range 0.5–40 micrograms/kg/minute has been used

Dobutamine (Non-proprietary) PoM
Injection, dobutamine (as hydrochloride) 5 mg/mL. To be diluted before use or given undiluted with syringe pump. Net price 50-mL vial = £7.50
Excipients may include sulfites
Concentrate for intravenous infusion, dobutamine (as hydrochloride) 12.5 mg/mL. To be diluted before use. Net price 20-mL amp = £5.20
Excipients may include sulfites

DOPAMINE HYDROCHLORIDE

Indications cardiogenic shock in infarction or cardiac surgery

Cautions correct hypovolaemia; low dose in shock due to acute myocardial infarction—see notes above; hyperthyroidism; **interactions**: Appendix 1 (sympathomimetics)

Contra-indications tachyarrhythmia, phaeochromocytoma

Pregnancy manufacturer advises use only if potential benefit outweighs risk

Side-effects nausea, vomiting, chest pain, palpitation, tachycardia, vasoconstriction, hypotension, dyspnoea, headache; *less commonly* bradycardia, hypertension, gangrene, mydriasis; *rarely* fatal ventricular arrhythmias

Dose
• By intravenous infusion, 2–5 micrograms/kg/minute initially (see notes above)

2 Cardiovascular system

2 Cardiovascular system

Dopamine (Non-proprietary) PoM

Concentrate for intravenous infusion, dopamine hydrochloride 40 mg/mL, net price 5-mL amp = £3.88; 160 mg/mL, 5-mL amp = £3.40. To be diluted before use

Intravenous infusion, dopamine hydrochloride 1.6 mg/mL in glucose 5% intravenous infusion Available from 'special-order manufacturers or specialist importing companies', see p. 1124

DOPEXAMINE HYDROCHLORIDE

Indications inotropic support and vasodilator in exacerbations of chronic heart failure and in heart failure associated with cardiac surgery

Cautions myocardial infarction, recent angina, hypo-kalaemia, hyperglycaemia; correct hypovolaemia before starting and during treatment, monitor blood pressure, pulse, plasma potassium, and blood glucose; hyperthyroidism; avoid abrupt withdrawal; **interactions**: Appendix 1 (sympathomimetics)

Contra-indications left ventricular outlet obstruction such as hypertrophic cardiomyopathy or aortic stenosis; phaeochromocytoma, thrombocytopenia

Pregnancy no information available—manufacturer advises avoid

Side-effects nausea, vomiting; tachycardia, bradycardia, arrhythmias, angina, myocardial infarction; tremor, headache; dyspnoea; reversible thrombocytopenia; sweating

Dose

- By intravenous infusion into central or large peripheral vein, 500 nanograms/kg/minute, may be increased to 1 microgram/kg/minute and further increased up to 6 micrograms/kg/minute in increments of 0.5–1 microgram/kg/minute at intervals of not less than 15 minutes

Dopacard® (TEVA UK) PoM

Concentrate for intravenous infusion, dopexamine hydrochloride 10 mg/mL (1%). To be diluted before use. Net price 5-mL amp = £25.20

Note Contact with metal in infusion apparatus should be minimised

2.7.2 Vasoconstrictor sympathomimetics

Vasoconstrictor sympathomimetics raise blood pressure transiently by acting on alpha-adrenergic receptors to constrict peripheral vessels. They are sometimes used as an emergency method of elevating blood pressure where other measures have failed (see also section 2.7.1).

The danger of vasoconstrictors is that although they raise blood pressure they also reduce perfusion of vital organs such as the kidney.

Spinal and epidural anaesthesia may result in sympathetic block with resultant hypotension. Management may include intravenous fluids (which are usually given prophylactically), oxygen (section 3.6), elevation of the legs, and injection of a pressor drug such as ephedrine. As well as constricting peripheral vessels **ephedrine** also accelerates the heart rate (by acting on beta receptors). Use is made of this dual action of ephedrine to manage associated bradycardia (although intravenous injection of atropine sulfate 400 to 600 micrograms may also be required if bradycardia persists).

EPHEDRINE HYDROCHLORIDE

Indications see under Dose

Cautions hyperthyroidism, diabetes mellitus, ischaemic heart disease, hypertension, susceptibility to angle-closure glaucoma, elderly; may cause acute urine retention in prostatic hypertrophy; **interactions**: Appendix 1 (sympathomimetics)

Renal impairment use with caution

Pregnancy increased fetal heart rate reported with parenteral ephedrine

Breast-feeding irritability and disturbed sleep reported

Side-effects nausea, vomiting, anorexia; tachycardia (sometimes bradycardia), arrhythmias, anginal pain, vasoconstriction with hypertension, vasodilation with hypotension, dizziness and flushing; dyspnoea; headache, anxiety, restlessness, confusion, psychoses, insomnia, tremor; difficulty in micturition, urine retention; sweating, hypersalivation; changes in blood-glucose concentration; *very rarely* angle-closure glaucoma

Dose

- Reversal of hypotension from spinal or epidural anaesthesia, by slow intravenous injection of a solution containing ephedrine hydrochloride 3 mg/mL, 3–6 mg (max. 9 mg) repeated every 3–4 minutes according to response to max. 30 mg

Ephedrine Hydrochloride (Non-proprietary) PoM

Injection, ephedrine hydrochloride 3 mg/mL, net price 10-mL amp = £6.34; 30 mg/mL, net price 1-mL amp = 41p

METARAMINOL

Indications acute hypotension (see notes above); priapism (section 7.4.5) [unlicensed indication]

Cautions see under Noradrenaline; longer duration of action than noradrenaline (norepinephrine), see below; cirrhosis

Hypertensive response Metaraminol has a longer duration of action than noradrenaline, and an excessive vasopressor response may cause a prolonged rise in blood pressure

Contra-indications see under Noradrenaline

Pregnancy may reduce placental perfusion—manufacturer advises use only if potential benefit outweighs risk

Breast-feeding manufacturer advises caution—no information available

Side-effects see under Noradrenaline; also tachycardia; fatal ventricular arrhythmia reported in Laennec's cirrhosis

Dose

- By intravenous infusion, 15–100 mg, adjusted according to response
- In emergency, by intravenous injection, 0.5–5 mg then by intravenous infusion, 15–100 mg, adjusted according to response

Metaraminol (Non-proprietary) PoM

Injection, metaraminol 10 mg (as tartrate)/mL Available from 'special-order' manufacturers or specialist importing companies, see p. 1124

NORADRENALINE/NOREPINEPHRINE

Indications see under dose

Cautions coronary, mesenteric, or peripheral vascular thrombosis; following myocardial infarction, Prinzmetal's variant angina, hyperthyroidism, diabetes mellitus; hypoxia or hypercapnia; uncorrected hypovolaemia; elderly; extravasation at injection site may cause necrosis; **interactions:** Appendix 1 (sympathomimetics)

Contra-indications hypertension (monitor blood pressure and rate of flow frequently)

Pregnancy avoid—may reduce placental perfusion

Side-effects anorexia, nausea, vomiting, hypoxia, arrhythmias, peripheral ischaemia, palpitation, hypertension, bradycardia, tachycardia, dyspnoea, headache, insomnia, confusion, anxiety, psychosis, weakness, tremor, urinary retention, angle-closure glaucoma

Dose

- Acute hypotension, by intravenous infusion, via central venous catheter, of a solution containing noradrenaline 40 micrograms (base)/mL at an initial rate of 0.16–0.33 mL/minute, adjusted according to response

Note 1 mg of noradrenaline base is equivalent to 2 mg of noradrenaline acid tartrate. Dose expressed as the base

Noradrenaline/Norepinephrine (Non-proprietary) ⓘⓞⓜ
Injection, noradrenaline base 1 mg/mL (as noradrenaline acid tartrate 2 mg/mL). For dilution before use. Net price 2-mL amp = £2.20, 4-mL amp = £4.40, 20-mL amp = £6.35

Note For a period of time, preparations on the UK market may be described as *either* noradrenaline base or noradrenaline acid tartrate; doses above are expressed as the base

---

PHENYLEPHRINE HYDROCHLORIDE

Indications acute hypotension (see notes above); priapism (section 7.4.5) [unlicensed indication]

Cautions see under Noradrenaline; longer duration of action than noradrenaline (norepinephrine), see below; coronary disease

Hypertensive response Phenylephrine has a longer duration of action than noradrenaline, and an excessive vasopressor response may cause a prolonged rise in blood pressure

Contra-indications see under Noradrenaline; severe hyperthyroidism

Pregnancy avoid if possible; malformations reported following use in first trimester; fetal hypoxia and bradycardia reported in late pregnancy and labour

Side-effects see under Noradrenaline; also tachycardia or reflex bradycardia

Dose

- By subcutaneous *or* intramuscular injection, 2–5 mg, followed if necessary after at least 15 minutes by further doses of 1–10 mg
- By slow intravenous injection of a 1 mg/mL solution, 100–500 micrograms repeated as necessary after at least 15 minutes
- By intravenous infusion, initial rate up to 180 micrograms/minute reduced to 30–60 micrograms/minute according to response

Phenylephrine (Non-proprietary) ⓘⓞⓜ
Injection, phenylephrine hydrochloride 10 mg/mL (1%), net price 1-mL amp = £9.91

2.7.3 Cardiopulmonary resuscitation

The algorithm for cardiopulmonary resuscitation (see inside back cover) reflects the most recent recommen-

dations of the Resuscitation Council (UK). These guidelines are available at www.resus.org.uk.

Cardiac arrest can be associated with ventricular fibrillation, pulseless ventricular tachycardia, asystole, and pulseless electrical activity (electromechanical dissociation). **Adrenaline (epinephrine)** 1 in 10 000 (100 micrograms/mL) is recommended in a dose of 1 mg (10 mL) by intravenous injection repeated every 3–5 minutes if necessary. Administration through a central line results in a faster response than peripheral administration, however placement of a central line must not interfere with chest compressions; drugs administered peripherally must be followed by a flush of at least 20 mL Sodium Chloride 0.9% injection to aid entry into the central circulation. Intravenous injection of **amiodarone** 300 mg (from a prefilled syringe *or* diluted in 20 mL Glucose 5%) should be considered after adrenaline to treat ventricular fibrillation or pulseless ventricular tachycardia in cardiac arrest refractory to defibrillation. An additional dose of amiodarone 150 mg can be given by intravenous injection if necessary, followed by an intravenous infusion of amiodarone 900 mg over 24 hours. **Lidocaine**, in a dose of 1 mg/kg, is an alternative if amiodarone is not available; a total dose of 3 mg/kg lidocaine should not be exceeded during the first hour. **Atropine** is no longer recommended in the treatment of asystole or pulseless electrical activity.

During cardiopulmonary arrest if intravenous access cannot be obtained, the intraosseous route can be used instead. Drug administration via the endotracheal route is no longer recommended.

For the management of acute anaphylaxis see section 3.4.3.

ADRENALINE/EPINEPHRINE

Indications see notes above

Cautions ischaemic heart disease, severe angina, obstructive cardiomyopathy, hypertension, arrhythmias, cerebrovascular disease, occlusive vascular disease, arteriosclerosis, monitor blood pressure and ECG; cor pulmonale; organic brain damage, psychoneurosis; hyperreflexia; diabetes mellitus, hyperthyroidism, phaeochromocytoma; prostate disorders; hypokalaemia, hypercalcaemia; susceptibility to angle-closure glaucoma; elderly; **interactions:** Appendix 1 (sympathomimetics)

Renal impairment manufacturers advise use with caution in severe impairment

Pregnancy may reduce placental perfusion and cause tachycardia, cardiac irregularities, and extrasystoles in fetus; can delay second stage of labour; manufacturers advise use only if benefit outweighs risk

Breast-feeding present in milk but unlikely to be harmful as poor oral bioavailability

Side-effects nausea, vomiting, dry mouth, anorexia, hypersalivation; arrhythmias, tachycardia, angina, myocardial infarction, pallor, palpitation, cold extremities, hypertension (risk of cerebral haemorrhage); dyspnoea, pulmonary oedema (on excessive dosage or extreme sensitivity); anxiety, tremor, restlessness, headache, insomnia, confusion, weakness, dizziness, psychosis; hyperglycaemia; urinary retention, difficulty in micturition; metabolic acidosis; hypokalaemia; tissue necrosis at injection site and of extremities, bowel, liver and kidneys; mydriasis, angle-closure glaucoma, sweating

2   Cardiovascular system

Dose
• See notes above

Adrenaline/Epinephrine 1 in 10 000, Dilute (Non-proprietary) [PoM]
    Injection, adrenaline (as acid tartrate) 100 micrograms/mL. 10-mL amp.
    Excipients   may include sulfites
    Brands include *Minijet® Adrenaline*

2.8 Anticoagulants and protamine

2.8.1   Parenteral anticoagulants
2.8.2   Oral anticoagulants
2.8.3   Protamine sulfate

The main use of anticoagulants is to prevent thrombus formation or extension of an existing thrombus in the slower-moving venous side of the circulation, where the thrombus consists of a fibrin web enmeshed with platelets and red cells.

Anticoagulants are of less use in preventing thrombus formation in arteries, for in faster-flowing vessels thrombi are composed mainly of platelets with little fibrin.

For the uses of anticoagulants see Parenteral anticoagulants, below and Oral anticoagulants, p. 152

Venous thromboembolism

Venous thromboembolism includes deep-vein thrombosis and pulmonary embolism, and occurs as a result of thrombus formation in a vein.

Prophylaxis of venous thromboembolism   All patients admitted to hospital should undergo a risk assessment for venous thromboembolism on admission. Patients considered to be at high risk include those anticipated to have a substantial reduction in mobility, those with obesity, malignant disease, history of venous thromboembolism, thrombophilic disorder, or patients over 60 years. Patients with risk factors for bleeding (e.g. acute stroke, thrombocytopenia, acquired or untreated inherited bleeding disorders) should only receive pharmacological prophylaxis when the risk of bleeding does not outweigh the risk of venous thromboembolism. A NICE Guideline[1] provides a full list of risk factors, and gives recommendations for prophylaxis. A venous thromboembolism risk assessment checklist is also available from the Department of Health (www.gov.uk/dh).

Patients scheduled for surgery should be offered mechanical prophylaxis (e.g. anti-embolism stockings) on admission if appropriate; prophylaxis should continue until the patient is sufficiently mobile. Choice of mechanical prophylaxis will depend on factors such as the type of surgery, suitability for the patient, and their condition.

Patients undergoing general or orthopaedic surgery, who are considered to be at high risk of venous thromboembolism (see above), should be offered pharmacological prophylaxis. Choice of prophylaxis will depend on the type of surgery, suitability for the patient, and local policy. A low molecular weight heparin is suitable in all types of general and orthopaedic surgery; unfrac-

1. NICE clinical guideline 92 (January 2010). Venous thromboembolism: reducing the risk

tionated heparin is preferred for patients in renal failure. Fondaparinux is an option for patients undergoing hip or knee replacement surgery, hip fracture surgery, gastro-intestinal, bariatric, or day surgery procedures. The oral anticoagulants apixaban, dabigatran etexilate, and rivaroxaban are indicated for thromboprophylaxis following hip or knee replacement surgery (see section 2.8.2). Pharmacological prophylaxis in general surgery should usually continue for 5–7 days, or until sufficient mobility has been re-established. Pharmacological prophylaxis should be extended to 28 days after major cancer surgery in the abdomen or pelvis. Hip or knee replacement surgery, and hip fracture surgery, require an extended duration of pharmacological prophylaxis, depending on the preparation used (consult product literature).

General medical patients who are considered to be at high risk of venous thromboembolism (see above) should be offered pharmacological prophylaxis on admission. Choice of prophylaxis will depend on the medical condition, suitability for the patient, and local policy. Patients should receive either a low molecular weight heparin, unfractionated heparin (if patient in renal failure), or fondaparinux. Prophylaxis should continue until the patient is no longer considered to be at significant risk of venous thromboembolism. Mechanical prophylaxis (e.g. anti-embolism stockings) can be offered to medical patients in whom pharmacological prophylaxis is contra-indicated, and continued until the patient is sufficiently mobile.

2.8.1   Parenteral anticoagulants

Heparin

Heparin initiates anticoagulation rapidly but has a short duration of action. It is often referred to as '**standard**' or '**unfractionated heparin**' to distinguish it from the **low molecular weight heparins** (see p. 148), which have a longer duration of action. Although a low molecular weight heparin is generally preferred for routine use, unfractionated heparin can be used in those at high risk of bleeding because its effect can be terminated rapidly by stopping the infusion.

Treatment   For the initial treatment of deep-vein thrombosis and pulmonary embolism a low molecular weight heparin is used; alternatively, unfractionated heparin is given as an intravenous loading dose, followed by continuous intravenous infusion (using an infusion pump) or (for deep-vein thrombosis only) by intermittent subcutaneous injection. Intermittent intravenous injection of unfractionated heparin is no longer recommended. An oral anticoagulant (usually warfarin, section 2.8.2) is started at the same time as unfractionated or low molecular weight heparin (the heparin needs to be continued for at least 5 days and until the INR is ≥2 for at least 24 hours). Laboratory monitoring for unfractionated heparin, preferably on a daily basis, is essential; determination of the activated partial thromboplastin time (APTT) is the most widely used measure (for unfractionated heparin). A low molecular weight heparin or, in some circumstances, unfractionated heparin is also used in regimens for the management of myocardial infarction and unstable angina (section 2.10.1).

Prophylaxis For details on the use of heparins in the prophylaxis of venous thromboembolism see section 2.8.

Pregnancy Heparins are used for the management of venous thromboembolism in pregnancy because they do not cross the placenta. Low molecular weight heparins are preferred because they have a lower risk of osteoporosis and of heparin-induced thrombocytopenia. Low molecular weight heparins are eliminated more rapidly in pregnancy, requiring alteration of the dosage regimen for drugs such as dalteparin, enoxaparin, and tinzaparin; see also under individual drugs. Treatment should be stopped at the onset of labour and advice sought from a specialist on continuing therapy after birth.

Extracorporeal circuits Unfractionated heparin is also used in the maintenance of extracorporeal circuits in cardiopulmonary bypass and haemodialysis.

Haemorrhage If haemorrhage occurs it is usually sufficient to withdraw unfractionated or low molecular weight heparin, but if rapid reversal of the effects of the heparin is required, protamine sulfate (section 2.8.3) is a specific antidote (but only partially reverses the effects of low molecular weight heparins).

◼ HEPARIN

Indications see under Dose

Cautions see notes above; also elderly; concomitant use of drugs that increase risk of bleeding; **interactions**: Appendix 1 (heparin)

Heparin-induced thrombocytopenia Clinically important heparin-induced thrombocytopenia is immune-mediated and does not usually develop until after 5–10 days; it can be complicated by thrombosis. Platelet counts should be measured just before treatment with unfractionated or low molecular weight heparin, and regular monitoring of platelet counts may be required if given for longer than 4 days[1]. Signs of heparin-induced thrombocytopenia include a 30% reduction of platelet count, thrombosis, or skin allergy. If heparin-induced thrombocytopenia is strongly suspected or confirmed, the heparin should be **stopped** and an alternative anticoagulant, such as argatroban or danaparoid, should be given. Ensure platelet counts return to normal range in those who require warfarin

Hyperkalaemia Inhibition of aldosterone secretion by unfractionated or low molecular weight heparin can result in hyperkalaemia; patients with diabetes mellitus, chronic renal failure, acidosis, raised plasma potassium or those taking potassium-sparing drugs seem to be more susceptible. The risk appears to increase with duration of therapy, and plasma-potassium concentration should be measured in patients at risk of hyperkalaemia before starting the heparin and monitored regularly thereafter, particularly if treatment is to be continued for longer than 7 days

Contra-indications haemophilia and other haemorrhagic disorders, thrombocytopenia (including history of heparin-induced thrombocytopenia), recent cerebral haemorrhage, severe hypertension; peptic ulcer; after major trauma or recent surgery to eye or nervous system; acute bacterial endocarditis; spinal or epidural anaesthesia with treatment doses of unfractionated or low molecular weight heparin; hypersensitivity to unfractionated or low molecular weight heparin

Hepatic impairment risk of bleeding increased—reduce dose or avoid in severe impairment (including oesophageal varices)

Renal impairment risk of bleeding increased in severe impairment—dose may need to be reduced

Pregnancy does not cross the placenta; maternal osteoporosis reported after prolonged use; multidose vials may contain benzyl alcohol—some manufacturers advise avoid; see also notes above

Breast-feeding not excreted into milk due to high molecular weight

Side-effects haemorrhage (see notes above), thrombocytopenia (see Cautions), *rarely* rebound hyperlipidaemia following unfractionated heparin withdrawal, priapism, hyperkalaemia (see Cautions), osteoporosis (risk lower with low molecular weight heparins), alopecia on prolonged use, injection-site reactions, skin necrosis, and hypersensitivity reactions (including urticaria, angioedema, and anaphylaxis)

Dose

- Treatment of pulmonary embolism, unstable angina, and acute peripheral arterial occlusion, by intravenous injection, loading dose of 5000 units *or* 75 units/kg (10 000 units in severe pulmonary embolism), followed by continuous intravenous infusion of 18 units/kg/hour (laboratory monitoring essential—preferably on a daily basis, and dose adjusted accordingly); CHILD under 18 years see *BNF for Children*

- Treatment of deep-vein thrombosis, by intravenous injection, loading dose of 5000 units *or* 75 units/kg, followed by continuous intravenous infusion of 18 units/kg/hour *or* by subcutaneous injection of 15 000 units every 12 hours (laboratory monitoring essential—preferably on a daily basis, and dose adjusted accordingly); CHILD under 18 years see *BNF for Children*

- Thromboprophylaxis in medical patients (see also notes above), by subcutaneous injection, 5000 units every 8–12 hours

- Thrombophylaxis in surgical patients (see also notes above), by subcutaneous injection, 5000 units 2 hours before surgery, then every 8–12 hours

- Thromboprophylaxis during pregnancy, (but see notes above), by subcutaneous injection, 5000–10 000 units every 12 hours (with monitoring); **important**: prevention of prosthetic heart-valve thrombosis in pregnancy calls for **specialist management**

- Haemodialysis by intravenous injection initially 1000–5000 units, followed by continuous intravenous infusion of 250–1000 units/hour

- Myocardial infarction, see section 2.10.1

- Prevention of clotting in extracorporeal circuits, consult product literature

> Doses above take into account the guidelines of the British Society for Haematology; for doses of the low molecular weight heparins, see p. 148

Heparin Sodium (Non-proprietary) PoM

Injection, heparin sodium 1000 units/mL, net price 1-mL amp = £1.49, 5-mL amp = £3.75, 5-mL vial = £1.53, 10-mL amp = £6.46, 20-mL amp = £4.75; 5000 units/mL, 1-mL amp = £2.90, 5-mL amp = £7.58, 5-mL vial = £6.31; 25 000 units/mL, 0.2-mL amp = £3.74, 1-mL amp = £7.70, 5-mL vial = £11.11

Excipients may contain benzyl alcohol (avoid in neonates, see Excipients, p. 2)

---

1. See the British Society for Haematology's Guidelines on the diagnosis and management of heparin-induced thrombocytopenia: second edition. *Br J Haematol* 2012; **159**: 528–540

Heparin Calcium (Non-proprietary) PoM
Injection, heparin calcium 25 000 units/mL, net price 0.2-mL amp = £3.91

Low molecular weight heparins

Low molecular weight heparins (**dalteparin**, **enoxaparin**, and **tinzaparin**) are usually preferred over unfractionated heparin in the *prevention* of venous thromboembolism because they are as effective and they have a lower risk of heparin-induced thrombocytopenia; see Prophylaxis of Venous Thromboembolism, p. 146. The standard prophylactic regimen does not require anticoagulant monitoring. The duration of action of low molecular weight heparin is longer than that of unfractionated heparin and *once-daily subcutaneous* administration is possible for some indications, making them convenient to use.

Low molecular weight heparins are generally preferred over unfractionated heparin in the *treatment* of deep-vein thrombosis and pulmonary embolism (see also Treatment, above), and are also used in the treatment of myocardial infarction (section 2.10.1), unstable coronary artery disease (section 2.10.1) and for the prevention of clotting in extracorporeal circuits.

Dalteparin is also licensed for the extended treatment and prophylaxis of venous thromboembolism in patients with solid tumours; treatment is recommended for a duration of 6 months. The *Scottish Medicines Consortium* (p. 4) has advised (February 2011) that dalteparin (*Fragmin®*) is accepted for restricted use within NHS Scotland as extended treatment of symptomatic venous thromboembolism and prevention of its recurrence in patients with solid tumours; treatment should be initiated by healthcare professionals experienced in the treatment of venous thromboembolism.

Routine monitoring of anti-Factor Xa activity is not usually required during treatment with low molecular weight heparins, but may be necessary in patients at increased risk of bleeding (e.g. in renal impairment and those who are underweight or overweight).

Haemorrhage See under Heparin.

Pregnancy See under Heparin.

DALTEPARIN SODIUM

Indications see notes above and under preparations

Cautions see under Heparin and notes above

Contra-indications see under Heparin

Hepatic impairment dose reduction may be required in severe impairment

Renal impairment risk of bleeding may be increased—dose reduction, and monitoring of anti-Factor Xa, may be required; use of unfractionated heparin may be preferable

Pregnancy not known to be harmful; multidose vial contains benzyl alcohol—manufacturer advises avoid; see also Pregnancy, p. 147

Breast-feeding no information available

Side-effects see under Heparin

Dose
• See under preparations below

Fragmin® (Pfizer) ▼ PoM
Injection (single-dose syringe), dalteparin sodium 12 500 units/mL, net price 2500-unit (0.2-mL) syringe = £1.86; 25 000 units/mL, 5000-unit (0.2-mL) syringe = £2.82, 7500-unit (0.3-mL) syringe = £4.23, 10 000-unit (0.4-mL) syringe = £5.65, 12 500-unit (0.5-mL) syringe = £7.06, 15 000-unit (0.6-mL) syringe = £8.47, 18 000-unit (0.72-mL) syringe = £10.16

Dose prophylaxis of deep-vein thrombosis, in surgical patients, by subcutaneous injection, moderate risk, 2500 units 1–2 hours before surgery then 2500 units every 24 hours; high risk, 2500 units 1–2 hours before surgery, then 2500 units 8–12 hours later (*or* 5000 units on the evening before surgery), then 5000 units on the following evening), then 5000 units every 24 hours

Prophylaxis of deep-vein thrombosis in medical patients, by subcutaneous injection, 5000 units every 24 hours

Treatment of deep-vein thrombosis and of pulmonary embolism, by subcutaneous injection, as a single daily dose, ADULT body-weight under 46 kg, 7500 units daily; body-weight 46–56 kg, 10 000 units daily; body-weight 57–68 kg, 12 500 units daily; body-weight 69–82 kg, 15 000 units daily; body-weight 83 kg and over, 18 000 units daily, with oral anticoagulant treatment until adequate oral anticoagulation established; monitoring of anti-Factor Xa not usually required; for patients at increased risk of haemorrhage, see below

Treatment of venous thromboembolism in pregnancy [unlicensed indication], by subcutaneous injection, early pregnancy body-weight under 50 kg, 5000 units twice daily; body-weight 50–70 kg, 6000 units twice daily; body-weight 70–90 kg, 8000 units twice daily; body-weight over 90 kg, 10 000 units twice daily

Extended treatment and prophylaxis of venous thromboembolism in patients with solid tumours, by subcutaneous injection, once daily for 30 days, ADULT body-weight 40–45 kg, 7500 units daily; body-weight 46–56 kg, 10 000 units daily; body-weight 57–68 kg, 12 500 units daily; body-weight 69–82 kg, 15 000 units daily; body-weight 83 kg and over, 18 000 units daily; *then* once daily for a further 5 months, by subcutaneous injection, ADULT body-weight 40–56 kg, 7500 units daily; body-weight 57–68 kg, 10 000 units daily; body-weight 69–82 kg, 12 500 units daily; body-weight 83–98 kg, 15 000 units daily; body-weight 99 kg and over, 18 000 units daily; interrupt treatment or reduce dose in chemotherapy-induced thrombocytopenia—consult product literature

Injection, dalteparin sodium 2500 units/mL (for subcutaneous or intravenous use), net price 4-mL (10 000-unit) amp = £5.12; 10 000-units/mL (for subcutaneous or intravenous use), 1-mL (10 000-unit) amp = £5.12; 25 000 units/mL (for subcutaneous use only), 4-mL (100 000-unit) vial = £48.66

Excipients include benzyl alcohol (in 100 000-unit/4 mL multidose vial) (avoid in neonates, see Excipients, p. 2)

Dose treatment of deep-vein thrombosis and of pulmonary embolism, by subcutaneous injection, 200 units/kg (max. 18 000 units) as a single daily dose (*or* 100 units/kg twice daily if increased risk of haemorrhage) until adequate oral anticoagulation established

Note For monitoring, blood should be taken 3–4 hours after a dose (recommended plasma concentration of anti-Factor Xa 0.5–1 unit/mL); monitoring not required for once-daily treatment regimen and not generally necessary for twice-daily regimen

Unstable coronary artery disease, by subcutaneous injection, 120 units/kg every 12 hours (max. 10 000 units twice daily) for 5–8 days

Prevention of clotting in extracorporeal circuits, consult product literature

Injection (graduated syringe), dalteparin sodium 10 000 units/mL, net price 1-mL (10 000-unit) syringe = £5.65

Dose unstable coronary artery disease (including non-ST-segment-elevation myocardial infarction), by subcutaneous injection, 120 units/kg every 12 hours (max. 10 000 units twice daily) for up to 8 days; beyond 8 days (if awaiting angiography or revascularisation) women body-weight less than 80 kg and men less than 70 kg, 5000 units every 12 hours, women body-weight greater than 80 kg and men greater than 70 kg, 7500 units every 12 hours, until day of procedure (max. 45 days)

ENOXAPARIN SODIUM

Indications   see notes above and under preparations

Cautions   see under Heparin and notes above; low body-weight (increased risk of bleeding)

Contra-indications   see under Heparin

Hepatic impairment   manufacturer advises caution—no information available

Renal impairment   risk of bleeding increased; reduce dose if eGFR less than 30 mL/minute/1.73 m^2—consult product literature for details; monitoring of anti-factor Xa may be required; use of unfractionated heparin may be preferable

Pregnancy   not known to be harmful; see also Pregnancy, p. 147

Breast-feeding   manufacturer advises avoid—no information available

Side-effects   see under Heparin

Dose

● See under preparation below

Clexane® (Sanofi-Aventis) [PoM]

Injection, enoxaparin sodium 100 mg/mL, net price 20-mg (0.2-mL, 2000-units) syringe = £2.27, 40-mg (0.4-mL, 4000-units) syringe = £3.03, 60-mg (0.6-mL, 6000-units) syringe = £4.57, 80-mg (0.8-mL, 8000-units) syringe = £6.49, 100-mg (1-mL, 10 000-units) syringe = £8.03; 300 mg (3-mL, 30 000-units) vial (*Clexane® Multidose*) = £21.33; 150 mg/mL (*Clexane® Forte*), 120-mg (0.8-mL, 12 000-units) syringe = £9.77, 150-mg (1-mL, 15 000-units) syringe = £11.10

Excipients include benzyl alcohol (in 300 mg multidose vials) (avoid in neonates, see Excipients, p. 2)

Dose prophylaxis of deep-vein thrombosis especially in surgical patients, by subcutaneous injection, *moderate risk*, 20 mg (2000 units) approx. 2 hours before surgery then 20 mg (2000 units) every 24 hours; *high risk* (e.g. orthopaedic surgery), 40 mg (4000 units) 12 hours before surgery then 40 mg (4000 units) every 24 hours

Prophylaxis of deep-vein thrombosis in medical patients, by subcutaneous injection, 40 mg (4000 units) every 24 hours

Treatment of deep-vein thrombosis or pulmonary embolism, by subcutaneous injection, 1.5 mg/kg (150 units/kg) every 24 hours until adequate oral anticoagulation established

Treatment of acute ST-segment elevation myocardial infarction, ADULT under 75 years, by intravenous injection, 30 mg (3000 units) followed by subcutaneous injection, 1 mg/kg (100 units/kg), then by subcutaneous injection, 1 mg/kg every 12 hours for up to 8 days (max. 100 mg (10 000 units) for first two subcutaneous doses only); ELDERLY over 75 years, by subcutaneous injection *only*, 750 micrograms/kg (75 units/kg) every 12 hours (max. 75 mg (7500 units) for first two doses only); patients undergoing percutaneous coronary intervention, additional dose, by intravenous injection, 300 micrograms/kg (30 units/kg) at time of procedure if last subcutaneous dose given more than 8 hours previously

Note When administered in conjunction with a thrombolytic, enoxaparin should be given between 15 minutes before and 30 minutes after the start of thrombolytic therapy

Unstable angina and non-ST-segment-elevation myocardial infarction, by subcutaneous injection, 1 mg/kg (100 units/kg) every 12 hours usually for 2–8 days (minimum 2 days)

Prevention of clotting in extracorporeal circuits, consult product literature

Treatment of venous thromboembolism in pregnancy [unlicensed indication], by subcutaneous injection, early pregnancy body-weight under 50 kg, 40 mg (4000 units) twice daily; body-weight 50–70 kg, 60 mg (6000 units) twice daily; body-weight 70–90 kg, 80 mg (8000 units) twice daily; body-weight over 90 kg, 100 mg (10 000 units) twice daily

TINZAPARIN SODIUM

Indications   see notes above and under preparations

Cautions   see under Heparin and notes above

Contra-indications   see under Heparin

Hepatic impairment   manufacturer advises avoid in severe impairment

Renal impairment   risk of bleeding may be increased; monitoring of anti-Factor Xa may be required if eGFR less than 30 mL/minute/1.73 m^2; dose reduction may be required if eGFR less than 20 mL/minute/1.73 m^2; unfractionated heparin may be preferable

Pregnancy   not known to be harmful; vials contain benzyl alcohol—manufacturer advises avoid; see also Pregnancy, p. 147

Breast-feeding   manufacturer advises avoid—no information available

Side-effects   see under Heparin; also *less commonly* headache

Dose

● See under preparations below

Innohep® (LEO) [PoM]

Injection, tinzaparin sodium 10 000 units/mL, net price 2500-unit (0.25-mL) syringe = £1.98, 3500-unit (0.35-mL) syringe = £2.77, 4500-unit (0.45-mL) syringe = £3.56, 20 000-unit (2-mL) vial = £10.57

Excipients include benzyl alcohol (in vial) (avoid in neonates, see Excipients, p. 2)

Dose prophylaxis of deep-vein thrombosis, by subcutaneous injection, general surgery, 3500 units 2 hours before surgery, then 3500 units every 24 hours; orthopaedic surgery, 50 units/kg 2 hours before surgery, then 50 units/kg every 24 hours *or* 4500 units 12 hours before surgery, then 4500 units every 24 hours

Prevention of clotting in extracorporeal circuits, consult product literature

Injection, tinzaparin sodium 20 000 units/mL, net price 0.5-mL (10 000-unit) syringe = £5.95, 0.7-mL (14 000-unit) syringe = £8.34, 0.9-mL (18 000-unit) syringe = £10.71, 2-mL (40 000-unit) vial = £34.20

Excipients include benzyl alcohol (in vial) (avoid in neonates, see Excipients, p. 2), sulfites (in 20 000 units/mL vial and syringe)

Dose treatment of deep-vein thrombosis and of pulmonary embolism, by subcutaneous injection, 175 units/kg once daily until adequate oral anticoagulation established

Treatment of venous thromboembolism in pregnancy [unlicensed indication], by subcutaneous injection, 175 units/kg once daily (based on early pregnancy body-weight)

Note Treatment regimens do not require anticoagulation monitoring

Heparinoids

Danaparoid is a heparinoid used for prophylaxis of deep-vein thrombosis in patients undergoing general or orthopaedic surgery. Providing there is no evidence of cross-reactivity, it also has a role in patients who develop heparin-induced thrombocytopenia.

2 Cardiovascular system

DANAPAROID SODIUM

Indications prevention of deep-vein thrombosis in general or orthopaedic surgery; thromboembolic disease in patients with history of heparin-induced thrombocytopenia

Cautions recent bleeding or risk of bleeding; concomitant use of drugs that increase risk of bleeding; antibodies to heparins (risk of antibody-induced thrombocytopenia); body-weight over 90 kg (monitor anti factor Xa activity); **interactions**: Appendix 1 (danaparoid)

Contra-indications haemophilia and other haemorrhagic disorders, thrombocytopenia (unless patient has heparin-induced thrombocytopenia), recent cerebral haemorrhage, severe hypertension, active peptic ulcer (unless this is the reason for operation), diabetic retinopathy, acute bacterial endocarditis, spinal or epidural anaesthesia with treatment doses of danaparoid

Hepatic impairment caution in moderate impairment (increased risk of bleeding); avoid in severe impairment unless patient has heparin-induced thrombocytopenia and no alternative available

Renal impairment caution in moderate impairment; increased risk of bleeding (monitor anti-Factor Xa activity); avoid in severe impairment unless patient has heparin-induced thrombocytopenia and no alternative available

Pregnancy manufacturer advises avoid—limited information available but not known to be harmful

Breast-feeding amount probably too small to be harmful but manufacturer advises avoid

Side-effects bleeding; hypersensitivity reactions (including rash)

Dose

- Prevention of deep-vein thrombosis, by subcutaneous injection, 750 units twice daily for 7–10 days; initiate treatment before operation (with last preoperative dose 1–4 hours before surgery)
- Thromboembolic disease in patients with history of heparin-induced thrombocytopenia, by intravenous injection, 2500 units (1250 units if body-weight under 55 kg, 3750 units if over 90 kg), followed by intravenous infusion of 400 units/hour for 2 hours, then 300 units/hour for 2 hours, then 200 units/hour for 5 days

Organan® (MSD) [PoM]
Injection, danaparoid sodium 1250 units/mL, net price 0.6-mL amp (750 units) = £26.67

Argatroban

Argatroban monohydrate, a direct thrombin inhibitor, is licensed for anticoagulation in patients with heparin-induced thrombocytopenia type II who require parenteral antithrombotic treatment. The dose of argatroban is adjusted according to activated partial thromboplastin time (APTT). An oral anticoagulant can be given with argatroban, but it should only be started once thrombocytopenia has substantially resolved.

ARGATROBAN MONOHYDRATE

Indications see notes above

Cautions risk of bleeding including severe hypertension, diabetic retinopathy, spinal anaesthesia, major surgery (especially of brain, spinal cord, or eye), immediately after lumbar puncture, bleeding disorders, and gastro-intestinal ulceration; concomitant use of drugs that increase risk of bleeding; determine activated partial thromboplastin time 2 hours after start of treatment, then 2 or 4 hours after infusion rate altered (consult product literature), and at least once daily thereafter; **interactions**: Appendix 1 (argatroban)

Hepatic impairment reduce initial dose to 500 nanograms/kg/minute in moderate impairment; avoid in severe impairment *or* in patients with hepatic impairment undergoing percutaneous coronary intervention

Pregnancy manufacturer advises avoid unless essential—limited information available

Breast-feeding avoid—no information available

Side-effects nausea, haemorrhage, purpura; *less commonly* hiccups, vomiting, constipation, diarrhoea, gastritis, hepatic failure, hepatomegaly, hyperbilirubinaemia, tachycardia, hypertension, hypotension, dizziness, syncope, headache, fever, malaise, hypoglycaemia, hyponatraemia, renal impairment, muscle weakness, myalgia, visual disturbance, deafness, rash, sweating, alopecia

Dose

- ADULT over 18 years, by continuous intravenous infusion, initially 2 micrograms/kg/minute, adjusted according to activated partial thromboplastin time, up to max. 10 micrograms/kg/minute; max. duration of treatment 14 days

  Note For dose in cardiac surgery, percutaneous coronary intervention, or critically ill patients, consult product literature

  Note When initiating concomitant warfarin treatment, argatroban dose should be temporarily reduced to 2 micrograms/kg/minute and INR measured after 4–6 hours; warfarin should be initiated at intended maintenance dose (do not give loading dose of warfarin); consult product literature for further details

Exembol® (Mitsubishi) [PoM]
Concentrate for intravenous infusion, argatroban monohydrate 100 mg/mL, net price 2.5-mL vial = £248.50
Note Contains ethanol

Hirudins

Bivalirudin, a hirudin analogue, is a thrombin inhibitor which is licensed for unstable angina or non-ST-segment elevation myocardial infarction in patients planned for urgent or early intervention, and as an anticoagulant for patients undergoing percutaneous coronary intervention (including patients with ST-segment elevation myocardial infarction undergoing primary percutaneous coronary intervention—see also section 2.10.1); bivalirudin should be administered in combination with aspirin and clopidogrel. The *Scottish Medicines Consortium* (p. 4) has advised (November 2008) that bivalirudin (*Angiox*®) is accepted for restricted use within NHS Scotland for patients with acute coronary syndromes planned for urgent or early intervention who would have been considered for treatment with unfractionated heparin in combination with a glycoprotein IIb/IIIa inhibitor; it should not be used as an alternative to heparin alone. The *Scottish Medicines Consortium* (p. 4) has advised (August 2010) that bivalirudin (*Angiox*®) is accepted for restricted use within NHS Scotland as an anticoagulant in patients undergoing percutaneous coronary intervention who would have been considered for treatment with unfractionated heparin in combination with a glycoprotein IIb/IIIa inhibitor; it should not be used as an alternative to heparin alone.

> **NICE guidance**
> **Bivalirudin for the treatment of ST-segment elevation myocardial infarction (July 2011)**
> Bivalirudin in combination with aspirin and clopidogrel is recommended for the treatment of adults with ST-segment elevation myocardial infarction undergoing primary percutaneous coronary intervention.
> www.nice.org.uk/TA230

BIVALIRUDIN

Indications unstable angina or non-ST-segment elevation myocardial infarction in patients planned for urgent or early intervention; anticoagulation for patients undergoing percutaneous coronary intervention (including patients with ST-segment elevation myocardial infarction undergoing primary percutaneous coronary intervention)

Cautions previous exposure to lepirudin (theoretical risk from lepirudin antibodies); brachytherapy procedures; concomitant use of drugs that increase risk of bleeding; **interactions**: Appendix 1 (bivalirudin)

Contra-indications severe hypertension; subacute bacterial endocarditis; active bleeding; bleeding disorders

Renal impairment for *percutaneous coronary intervention*, reduce rate of infusion to 1.4 mg/kg/hour if eGFR 30–60 mL/minute/1.73 m^2 and monitor blood clotting parameters; for *acute coronary syndromes* and *percutaneous coronary intervention*, avoid if eGFR less than 30 mL/minute/1.73 m^2

Pregnancy manufacturer advises avoid unless potential benefit outweighs risk—no information available

Breast-feeding manufacturer advises caution—no information available

Side-effects bleeding (discontinue), ecchymosis; *less commonly* nausea, hypotension, allergic reactions (including isolated reports of anaphylaxis), headache, thrombocytopenia, anaemia; *rarely* vomiting, thrombosis, bradycardia, tachycardia, dyspnoea, back pain

Dose
- Unstable angina or non-ST-segment elevation myocardial infarction (in addition to aspirin and clopidogrel), initially by intravenous injection, 100 micrograms/kg then by intravenous infusion 250 micrograms/kg/hour (for up to 72 hours in medically managed patients); patients proceeding to percutaneous coronary intervention or coronary artery bypass surgery *without* cardiopulmonary bypass, additional bolus dose by intravenous injection 500 micrograms/kg, then by intravenous infusion 1.75 mg/kg/hour for duration of procedure; following percutaneous coronary intervention, reduce infusion rate to 250 micrograms/kg/hour for 4–12 hours as necessary; patients proceeding to coronary artery bypass surgery *with* cardiopulmonary bypass, discontinue intravenous infusion 1 hour before procedure and treat with unfractionated heparin
- Anticoagulation in patients undergoing percutaneous coronary intervention (in addition to aspirin and clopidogrel), initially by intravenous injection, 750 micrograms/kg followed immediately by intravenous

infusion 1.75 mg/kg/hour during procedure and for up to 4 hours after procedure; a reduced infusion rate of 250 micrograms/kg/hour may be continued for a further 4–12 hours if necessary

Angiox® (The Medicines Company) [PoM]
Injection, powder for reconstitution, bivalirudin, net price 250-mg vial = £310.00

Heparin flushes

The use of heparin flushes should be kept to a minimum. For maintaining patency of peripheral venous catheters, sodium chloride injection 0.9% is as effective as heparin flushes. The role of heparin flushes in maintaining patency of arterial and central venous catheters is unclear.

Heparin Sodium (Non-proprietary) [PoM]
Solution, heparin sodium 10 units/mL, net price 5-mL amp = £1.50; 100 units/mL, 2-mL amp = £1.57
Excipients may include benzyl alcohol (avoid in neonates, see Excipients, p. 2)
Dose to maintain patency of catheters, cannulas, etc. 10–200 units flushed through every 4–8 hours. Not for therapeutic use

Epoprostenol

Epoprostenol (prostacyclin) can be given to inhibit platelet aggregation during renal dialysis when heparins are unsuitable or contra-indicated. It is also licensed for the treatment of primary pulmonary hypertension resistant to other treatment, usually with oral anticoagulation; it should be initiated by specialists in pulmonary hypertension. Epoprostenol is a potent vasodilator. It has a short half-life of approximately 3 minutes and therefore it must be administered by continuous intravenous infusion.

EPOPROSTENOL

Indications see notes above

Cautions anticoagulant monitoring required when given with anticoagulants; haemorrhagic diathesis; concomitant use of drugs that increase risk of bleeding; dose titration for pulmonary hypertension should be in hospital (risk of pulmonary oedema); extreme caution in coronary artery disease; pulmonary veno-occlusive disease; avoid abrupt withdrawal when used for primary pulmonary hypertension (risk of rebound pulmonary hypertension); reconstituted solution highly alkaline—avoid extravasation (irritant to tissues)

Contra-indications severe left ventricular dysfunction

Pregnancy use if potential benefit outweighs risk

Breast-feeding manufacturer advises avoid—no information available

Side-effects nausea, vomiting, diarrhoea, abdominal pain, bleeding, bradycardia, tachycardia, hypotension, flushing, chest pain, anxiety, headache, sepsis, thrombocytopenia, jaw pain, arthralgia, rash; *less commonly* dry mouth, sweating; *very rarely* pallor, agitation, malaise, hyperthyroidism; *also reported* pulmonary oedema (avoid chronic use if occurs during dose titration), hyperglycaemia

Dose
- See product literature

Flolan® (GSK) [PoM]

Infusion, powder for reconstitution, epoprostenol (as sodium salt), net price 500-microgram vial (with diluent) = £22.22; 1.5-mg vial (with diluent) = £44.76

Veletri® (Actelion) [PoM]

Infusion, powder for reconstitution, epoprostenol (as sodium salt), net price 500-microgram vial = £24.44; 1.5-mg vial = £44.24

Fondaparinux

Fondaparinux sodium is a synthetic pentasaccharide that inhibits activated factor X.

For details on the use of fondaparinux in the prophylaxis of venous thromboembolism, see section 2.8, p. 146.

◼ FONDAPARINUX SODIUM

Indications   prophylaxis of venous thromboembolism in medical patients immobilised because of acute illness, and patients undergoing major orthopaedic surgery of the hip or leg, or abdominal surgery; treatment of deep-vein thrombosis, superficial-vein thrombosis, and pulmonary embolism; treatment of unstable angina or non-ST-segment elevation myocardial infarction; treatment of ST-segment elevation myocardial infarction

Cautions   bleeding disorders, active gastro-intestinal ulcer disease; recent intracranial haemorrhage; brain, spinal, or ophthalmic surgery; spinal or epidural anaesthesia (risk of spinal haematoma—avoid if using treatment doses); risk of catheter thrombus during percutaneous coronary intervention; low body-weight; elderly patients; concomitant use of drugs that increase risk of bleeding; **interactions**: Appendix 1 (fondaparinux)

Contra-indications   active bleeding; bacterial endocarditis

Hepatic impairment   caution in severe impairment (increased risk of bleeding)

Renal impairment   increased risk of bleeding; for *treatment of acute coronary syndromes* avoid if eGFR less than 20 mL/minute/1.73 m^2; for *treatment of venous thromboembolism* use with caution if eGFR 30–50 mL/minute/1.73 m^2, avoid if eGFR less than 30 mL/minute/1.73 m^2; for *prophylaxis of venous thromboembolism* and *treatment of superficial-vein thrombosis* reduce dose to 1.5 mg daily if eGFR 20–50 mL/minute/1.73 m^2, avoid if eGFR less than 20 mL/minute/1.73 m^2

Pregnancy   manufacturer advises avoid unless potential benefit outweighs possible risk—no information available

Breast-feeding   present in milk in *animal* studies—manufacturer advises avoid

Side-effects   bleeding, purpura, anaemia; *less commonly* gastro-intestinal disturbances, oedema, hepatic impairment, chest pain, dyspnoea, thrombocytopenia, thrombocythaemia, rash, pruritus; *rarely* hypotension, flushing, cough, vertigo, dizziness, anxiety, drowsiness, confusion, headache, hypokalaemia, hyperbilirubinaemia, injection-site reactions; also reported atrial fibrillation, tachycardia, and pyrexia

Dose

* Prophylaxis of venous thromboembolism after surgery, by subcutaneous injection, 2.5 mg 6 hours after surgery then 2.5 mg once daily; CHILD under 17 years not recommended

* Prophylaxis of venous thromboembolism in medical patients, by subcutaneous injection, 2.5 mg once daily; CHILD under 17 years not recommended

* Treatment of superficial-vein thrombosis, by subcutaneous injection, ADULT body-weight over 50 kg, 2.5 mg once daily for at least 30 days (max. 45 days if high risk of thromboembolic complications); treatment should be stopped 24 hours before surgery and restarted at least 6 hours post operatively; CHILD under 17 years not recommended

* Unstable angina and non-ST-segment elevation myocardial infarction, by subcutaneous injection, 2.5 mg once daily for up to 8 days (or until hospital discharge if sooner); treatment should be stopped 24 hours before coronary artery bypass graft surgery (where possible) and restarted 48 hours post operatively; CHILD under 17 years not recommended

* ST-segment elevation myocardial infarction, initially by intravenous injection or infusion, 2.5 mg for first day, thereafter by subcutaneous injection 2.5 mg once daily for up to 8 days (or until hospital discharge if sooner); treatment should be stopped 24 hours before coronary artery bypass graft surgery (where possible) and restarted 48 hours post operatively; CHILD under 17 years not recommended

* Treatment of deep-vein thrombosis and of pulmonary embolism, by subcutaneous injection, ADULT body-weight under 50 kg, 5 mg every 24 hours; body-weight 50–100 kg, 7.5 mg every 24 hours; body-weight over 100 kg, 10 mg every 24 hours; CHILD under 17 years not recommended

Note An oral anticoagulant (usually warfarin, section 2.8.2) is started at the same time as fondaparinux (fondaparinux should be continued for at least 5 days and until INR ≥ 2 for at least 24 hours)

Arixtra® (GSK) ▼ [PoM]

Injection, fondaparinux sodium 5 mg/mL, net price 0.3-mL (1.5-mg) prefilled syringe = £6.28; 0.5-mL (2.5-mg) prefilled syringe = £6.28

Injection, fondaparinux sodium 12.5 mg/mL, net price 0.4-mL (5-mg) prefilled syringe = £11.65, 0.6-mL (7.5-mg) prefilled syringe = £11.65, 0.8-mL (10-mg) prefilled syringe = £11.65

2.8.2 Oral anticoagulants

Coumarins and phenindione

The oral anticoagulants **warfarin**, **acenocoumarol** and **phenindione**, antagonise the effects of vitamin K, and take at least 48 to 72 hours for the anticoagulant effect to develop fully; warfarin is the drug of choice. If an immediate effect is required, unfractionated or low molecular weight heparin must be given concomitantly.

Uses   Indications for these oral anticoagulants include *deep-vein thrombosis, pulmonary embolism, atrial fibrillation* in those who are at risk of embolisation (see also section 2.3.1), and *mechanical prosthetic heart valves* (to prevent emboli developing on the valves).

These oral anticoagulants should not be used in cerebral artery thrombosis or peripheral artery occlusion as first-line therapy; aspirin is more appropriate for reduction of risk in transient ischaemic attacks (see p. 161). Unfractionated or a low molecular weight heparin (section 2.8.1) is usually preferred for the prophylaxis of venous thromboembolism in patients undergoing surgery; alternatively, warfarin can be continued in selected patients currently taking long-term warfarin and who are at high risk of thromboembolism (seek expert advice).

Dose   The base-line prothrombin time should be determined but the initial dose should not be delayed whilst awaiting the result.

For patients who require rapid anticoagulation the usual adult induction dose of warfarin is 5–10 mg on the first day (elderly patients should receive a lower induction dose); subsequent doses depend upon the prothrombin time, reported as INR (international normalised ratio). For patients who do not require rapid anticoagulation, a lower loading dose can be used over 3–4 weeks. The daily maintenance dose of warfarin is usually 3–9 mg (taken at the **same time** each day).

Target INR   The following indications and target INRs[1] for warfarin take into account recommendations of the British Society for Haematology[2]:

INR 2.5 for:

- treatment of deep-vein thrombosis or pulmonary embolism (including those associated with antiphospholipid syndrome or for recurrence in patients no longer receiving warfarin)

- atrial fibrillation (see also section 2.3.1)

- cardioversion—target INR should be achieved at least 3 weeks before cardioversion and anticoagulation should continue for at least 4 weeks after the procedure (higher target values, such as an INR of 3, can be used for up to 4 weeks before the procedure to avoid cancellations due to low INR)

- dilated cardiomyopathy

- mitral stenosis or regurgitation in patients with either atrial fibrillation, a history of systemic embolism, a left atrial thrombus, or an enlarged left atrium

- bioprosthetic heart valves in the mitral position (treat for 3 months), or in patients with a history of systemic embolism (treat for at least 3 months), or with a left atrial thrombus at surgery (treat until clot resolves), or with other risk factors (e.g. atrial fibrillation or a low ventricular ejection fraction)

- acute arterial embolism requiring embolectomy (consider long-term treatment)

- myocardial infarction (see also section 2.10.1);

INR 3.5 for:

- recurrent deep-vein thrombosis or pulmonary embolism in patients currently receiving anticoagulation and with an INR above 2;

Mechanical prosthetic heart valves:

- the recommended target INR depends on the type and location of the valve, and patient-related risk factors

- consider increasing the INR target or adding an antiplatelet drug, if an embolic event occurs whilst anticoagulated at the target INR.

Duration   The risks of thromboembolism recurrence and anticoagulant-related bleeding should be considered when deciding the duration of anticoagulation.

The following durations of warfarin for the treatment of deep-vein thrombosis and pulmonary embolism reflect the recommendations of the British Society for Haematology[2]:

- 6 weeks for isolated calf-vein deep-vein thrombosis

- 3 months for venous thromboembolism provoked by surgery or other transient risk factor (e.g. combined oral contraceptive use, pregnancy, plaster cast)

- *at least* 3 months for unprovoked proximal deep-vein thrombosis or pulmonary embolism; long-term anticoagulation may be required.

Monitoring   It is essential that the INR be determined daily or on alternate days in early days of treatment, *then* at longer intervals (depending on response[3]) *then* up to every 12 weeks.

Haemorrhage   The main adverse effect of all oral anticoagulants is haemorrhage. Checking the INR and omitting doses when appropriate is essential; if the anticoagulant is stopped but not reversed, the INR should be measured 2–3 days later to ensure that it is falling. The cause of an elevated INR should be investigated. The following recommendations (which take into account the recommendations of the British Society for Haematology[2]) are based on the result of the INR and whether there is major or minor bleeding; the recommendations apply to patients taking warfarin:

- Major bleeding—stop warfarin; give phytomenadione (vitamin K₁) 5 mg by slow intravenous injection; give dried prothrombin complex (factors II, VII, IX, and X—section 2.11) 25–50 units/kg (if dried prothrombin complex unavailable, fresh frozen plasma 15 mL/kg can be given but is less effective); recombinant factor VIIa is not recommended for emergency anticoagulation reversal

- INR > 8.0, minor bleeding—stop warfarin; give phytomenadione (vitamin K₁) 1–3 mg by slow intravenous injection; repeat dose of phytomenadione if INR still too high after 24 hours; restart warfarin when INR <5.0

- INR > 8.0, no bleeding—stop warfarin; give phytomenadione (vitamin K₁) 1–5 mg by mouth using the intravenous preparation orally [unlicensed use]; repeat dose of phytomenadione if INR still too high after 24 hours; restart warfarin when INR <5.0

- INR 5.0–8.0, minor bleeding—stop warfarin; give phytomenadione (vitamin K₁) 1–3 mg by slow intravenous injection; restart warfarin when INR <5.0

- INR 5.0–8.0, no bleeding—withhold 1 or 2 doses of warfarin and reduce subsequent maintenance dose

- Unexpected bleeding at therapeutic levels—always investigate possibility of underlying cause e.g. unsuspected renal or gastro-intestinal tract pathology

---

1. An INR which is within 0.5 units of the target value is generally satisfactory; larger deviations require dosage adjustment. Target values (rather than ranges) are now recommended.
2. Guidelines on Oral Anticoagulation with Warfarin—fourth edition. *Br J Haematol* 2011; **154**: 311–324

3. Change in patient's clinical condition, particularly associated with liver disease, intercurrent illness, or drug administration, necessitates more frequent testing. See also **interactions**, Appendix 1 (coumarins). Major changes in diet (especially involving salads and vegetables) and in alcohol consumption may also affect warfarin control.

2

Cardiovascular system

Peri-operative anticoagulation Warfarin should usually be stopped 5 days before elective surgery; phytomenadione (vitamin K$_1$) 1–5 mg by mouth (using the intravenous preparation orally [unlicensed use]) should be given the day before surgery if the INR is ≥1.5. If haemostasis is adequate, warfarin can be resumed at the normal maintenance dose on the evening of surgery or the next day.

Patients stopping warfarin prior to surgery who are considered to be at high risk of thromboembolism (e.g. those with a venous thromboembolic event within the last 3 months, atrial fibrillation with previous stroke or transient ischaemic attack, or mitral mechanical heart valve) may require interim therapy ('bridging') with a low molecular weight heparin (using treatment dose). The low molecular weight heparin should be stopped at least 24 hours before surgery; if the surgery carries a high risk of bleeding, the low molecular weight heparin should not be restarted until at least 48 hours after surgery.

Patients on warfarin who require emergency surgery that can be delayed for 6–12 hours can be given intravenous phytomenadione (vitamin K$_1$) 5 mg to reverse the anticoagulant effect. If surgery cannot be delayed, dried prothrombin complex (e.g. 25 units/kg) can be given in addition to intravenous phytomenadione (vitamin K$_1$) and the INR checked before surgery.

Combined anticoagulant and antiplatelet therapy Existing antiplatelet therapy following an acute coronary syndrome or percutaneous coronary intervention should be continued for the necessary duration according to the indication being treated (see section 2.9). The addition of warfarin, when indicated (e.g. for venous thromboembolism or atrial fibrillation) should be considered following an assessment of the patient's risk of bleeding and discussion with a cardiologist. The duration of treatment with dual therapy (e.g. aspirin and warfarin) or triple therapy (e.g. aspirin with clopidogrel and warfarin) should be kept to a minimum where possible. The risk of bleeding with aspirin and warfarin dual therapy is lower than with clopidogrel and warfarin. Depending on the indications being treated and the patient's risk of thromboembolism, it may be possible to withhold antiplatelet therapy until warfarin therapy is complete, or vice versa (on specialist advice) in order to reduce the length of time on dual or triple therapy.

Hepatic impairment Acenocoumarol should be used with caution in mild to moderate impairment; warfarin, acenocoumarol, and phenindione should be avoided in severe impairment, especially if prothrombin time is already prolonged.

Renal impairment Warfarin, acenocoumarol, and phenindione should be used with caution in mild to moderate impairment. In severe impairment, monitor INR more frequently with warfarin, and avoid acenocoumarol and phenindione.

Pregnancy Warfarin, acenocoumarol, and phenindione are teratogenic and should not be given in the first trimester of pregnancy. Women of child-bearing age should be warned of this danger since stopping these drugs before the sixth week of gestation may largely avoid the risk of fetal abnormality. These oral anticoagulants cross the placenta with risk of congenital malformations, and placental, fetal, or neonatal haemorrhage, especially during the last few weeks of pregnancy and at delivery. Therefore, if at all possible, they should

be avoided in pregnancy, especially in the first and third trimesters. Difficult decisions may have to be made, particularly in women with prosthetic heart valves, atrial fibrillation, or with a history of recurrent venous thrombosis or pulmonary embolism.

Breast-feeding With warfarin, acenocoumarol, and phenindione there is a risk of haemorrhage which is increased by vitamin-K deficiency. Warfarin is not present in milk in significant amounts, and appears safe, but phenindione should be avoided; the manufacturer of acenocoumarol recommends prophylactic vitamin K for the infant (consult product literature).

Treatment booklets Anticoagulant treatment booklets should be issued to all patients; these booklets include advice for patients on anticoagulant treatment, an alert card to be carried by the patient at all times, and a section for recording of INR results and dosage information. In **England, Wales**, and **Northern Ireland**, they are available for purchase from:

3M Security Print and Systems Limited
Gorse Street, Chadderton
Oldham
OL9 9QH
Tel: 0845 610 1112

GP practices can obtain supplies through their Local Area Team stores. NHS Trusts can order supplies from www.nhsforms.co.uk or by emailing nhsforms@mmm.com.

In **Scotland**, treatment booklets and starter information packs can be obtained by emailing stockorders.dppas@theapsgroup.com or by fax on (0131) 6299 967

Electronic copies of the booklets and further advice are also available at www.npsa.nhs.uk/nrls/alerts-and-directives/alerts/anticoagulant.

WARFARIN SODIUM

Indications prophylaxis of embolisation in rheumatic heart disease and atrial fibrillation; prophylaxis after insertion of prosthetic heart valve; prophylaxis and treatment of venous thrombosis and pulmonary embolism; transient ischaemic attacks

Cautions see notes above; also conditions in which risk of bleeding is increased, e.g. history of gastro-intestinal bleeding, peptic ulcer, recent surgery, recent ischaemic stroke, postpartum (delay warfarin until risk of haemorrhage is low—usually 5–7 days after delivery), bacterial endocarditis (use only if warfarin otherwise indicated); uncontrolled hypertension; concomitant use of drugs that increase risk of bleeding; avoid cranberry juice; **interactions:** Appendix 1 (coumarins)

Contra-indications haemorrhagic stroke; significant bleeding; avoid use within 48 hours postpartum

Hepatic impairment see notes above

Renal impairment see notes above

Pregnancy see notes above

Breast-feeding see notes above

Side-effects haemorrhage—see notes above; also nausea, vomiting, diarrhoea, jaundice, hepatic dysfunction, pancreatitis, pyrexia, alopecia, purpura, rash, 'purple toes', skin necrosis (increased risk in patients with protein C or protein S deficiency)

Dose

- See notes above

Warfarin (Non-proprietary) [PoM]

Tablets, warfarin sodium 500 micrograms (white), net price 28-tab pack = £1.49; 1 mg (brown), 28-tab pack = £1.00; 3 mg (blue), 28-tab pack = £1.03; 5 mg (pink), 28-tab pack = £1.05. Label: 10, anti-coagulant card

Brands include Marevan®

Oral suspension, warfarin sodium 1 mg/mL, net price 150 mL = £90.00. Label: 10, anticoagulant card

Note Sugar-free versions are available and can be ordered by specifying 'sugar-free' on the prescription

▌ACENOCOUMAROL

(Nicoumalone)

Indications see under Warfarin Sodium

Cautions see under Warfarin Sodium; also patients over 65 years

Contra-indications see under Warfarin Sodium

Hepatic impairment see notes above

Renal impairment see notes above

Pregnancy see notes above

Breast-feeding see notes above

Side-effects see under Warfarin Sodium; also rarely anorexia; very rarely vasculitis

Dose

- Initially 2–4 mg once daily for 2 days; alternatively, 6 mg on first day, 4 mg on second day; maintenance dose usually 1–8 mg daily (taken at same time of day) adjusted according to response

Note Lower doses may be required in patients over 65 years, liver disease, severe heart failure with hepatic congestion, and malnutrition

Sinthrome® (Novartis) [PoM]

Tablets, acenocoumarol 1 mg, net price 100-tab pack = £4.62. Label: 10, anticoagulant card

▌PHENINDIONE

Indications prophylaxis of embolisation in rheumatic heart disease and atrial fibrillation; prophylaxis after insertion of prosthetic heart valve; prophylaxis and treatment of venous thrombosis and pulmonary embolism

Cautions see under Warfarin Sodium; **interactions:** Appendix 1 (phenindione)

Contra-indications see under Warfarin Sodium

Hepatic impairment see notes above

Renal impairment see notes above

Pregnancy see notes above

Breast-feeding see notes above

Side-effects see under Warfarin Sodium; also hypersensitivity reactions including exfoliative dermatitis, exanthema, fever, leucopenia, agranulocytosis, eosinophilia, and renal damage; micro-adenopathy and urine coloured pink or orange

Dose

- 200 mg on day 1; 100 mg on day 2, then adjusted according to response; maintenance dose usually 50–150 mg daily

Phenindione (Non-proprietary) [PoM]

Tablets, phenindione 10 mg, net price 28-tab pack = £79.01; 25 mg, 28-tab pack = £99.89; 50 mg, 28-tab pack = £51.84. Label: 10, anticoagulant card, 14, (urine pink or orange)

Dabigatran etexilate

Dabigatran etexilate, a direct thrombin inhibitor, is given orally for prophylaxis of venous thromboembolism in adults after total hip replacement or total knee replacement surgery—see Prophylaxis of Venous Thromboembolism, p. 146; it is also licensed for the treatment of deep-vein thrombosis and pulmonary embolism, and prophylaxis of recurrent deep-vein thrombosis and pulmonary embolism in adults. Duration of treatment should be determined by balancing the benefit of treatment with the bleeding risk; shorter duration of treatment (at least 3 months) should be based on transient risk factors i.e recent surgery, trauma, immobilisation, and longer duration of treatment should be based on permanent risk factors, or idiopathic deep-vein thrombosis or pulmonary embolism. Dabigatran etexilate is also licensed for the prevention of stroke and systemic embolism in patients with non-valvular atrial fibrillation and with one or more risk factors such as previous stroke or transient ischaemic attack, symptomatic heart failure, age ≥ 75 years, diabetes mellitus, or hypertension. Dabigatran etexilate has a rapid onset of action and does not require routine anticoagulant monitoring (INR tests are unreliable in patients taking dabigatran etexilate). The most common side-effect is haemorrhage and patients should be monitored for signs of bleeding or anaemia; treatment should be stopped if severe bleeding occurs.

> **NICE guidance**
> **Dabigatran etexilate for the prevention of venous thromboembolism after hip or knee replacement surgery in adults (September 2008)**
>
> Dabigatran etexilate is an option for the prophylaxis of venous thromboembolism in adults after total hip replacement or total knee replacement surgery.
> www.nice.org.uk/TA157

> **NICE guidance**
> **Dabigatran etexilate for the prevention of stroke and systemic embolism in atrial fibrillation (March 2012)**
>
> Dabigatran etexilate is an option for the prevention of stroke and systemic embolism in patients with non-valvular atrial fibrillation and with one or more of the following risk factors:
>
> - previous stroke, transient ischaemic attack, or systemic embolism
> - left ventricular ejection fraction < 40%
> - symptomatic heart failure
> - age ≥ 75 years
> - age ≥ 65 years in patients with diabetes mellitus, coronary artery disease, or hypertension
>
> The risks and benefits of dabigatran compared to warfarin should be discussed with the patient.
> www.nice.org.uk/TA249

2

Cardiovascular system

Cardiovascular system

2

■ DABIGATRAN ETEXILATE

Indications   see notes above

Cautions   see notes above; also elderly; body-weight less than 50 kg; anaesthesia with postoperative indwelling epidural catheter (risk of paralysis—give initial dose at least 2 hours after catheter removal and monitor neurological signs); bacterial endocarditis; bleeding disorders; thrombocytopenia; recent biopsy or major trauma; oesophagitis, gastritis, gastro-oesophageal reflux; assess renal function (manufacturer recommends Cockroft and Gault formula to calculate creatinine clearance) before treatment in all patients and at least annually in elderly and patients with renal impairment; concomitant use of drugs that increase risk of bleeding; **interactions**: Appendix 1 (dabigatran)

Contra-indications   active bleeding; significant risk of major bleeding (e.g. recent gastro-intestinal ulcer, oesophageal varices, recent brain, spine, or ophthalmic surgery, recent intracranial haemorrhage, malignant neoplasms, vascular aneurysm); do not use as anticoagulant for prosthetic heart valve

Hepatic impairment   avoid in severe liver disease, especially if prothrombin time already prolonged

Renal impairment   avoid if creatinine clearance less than 30 mL/minute; for *prophylaxis of venous thromboembolism following knee or hip replacement surgery,* reduce initial dose to 75 mg and subsequent doses to 150 mg once daily if creatinine clearance 30–50 mL/ minute; reduce dose to 75 mg once daily if creatinine clearance 30–50 mL/minute and patient receiving concomitant treatment with verapamil; for *treatment of deep-vein thrombosis and pulmonary embolism, prophylaxis of recurrent deep-vein thrombosis and pulmonary embolism, prophylaxis of stroke and systemic embolism in non-valvular atrial fibrillation,* consider reduced dose of 110 mg twice daily if creatinine clearance 30–50 mL/minute, based on individual assessment of thromboembolic risk and risk of bleeding; monitor renal function at least annually (manufacturer recommends Cockroft and Gault formula to calculate creatinine clearance)

Pregnancy   manufacturer advises avoid unless essential—toxicity in *animal* studies

Breast-feeding   manufacturer advises avoid—no information available

Side-effects   nausea, dyspepsia, diarrhoea, abdominal pain, anaemia, haemorrhage—see notes above; *less commonly* hepatobiliary disorders, vomiting, dysphagia, gastro-intestinal ulcer, gastro-oesophageal reflux, oesophagitis, thrombocytopenia

Dose

• Prophylaxis of venous thromboembolism following total knee replacement surgery, ADULT over 18 years, 110 mg (ELDERLY over 75 years, 75 mg) 1–4 hours after surgery, followed 12–24 hours later by 220 mg (ELDERLY over 75 years or patient receiving concomitant treatment with amiodarone or verapamil, 150 mg) once daily for 9 days

• Prophylaxis of venous thromboembolism following total hip replacement surgery, ADULT over 18 years, 110 mg (ELDERLY over 75 years, 75 mg) 1–4 hours after surgery, followed 12–24 hours later by 220 mg (ELDERLY over 75 years or patient receiving concomitant treatment with amiodarone or verapamil, 150 mg) once daily for 27–34 days

• Treatment of deep-vein thrombosis and pulmonary embolism, and prophylaxis of recurrent deep-vein thrombosis and pulmonary embolism (see notes above), ADULT over 18 years, 150 mg (ELDERLY over 80 years or receiving concomitant treatment with verapamil, 110 mg) twice daily, following at least 5 days treatment with a parenteral anticoagulant. (Lower dose of 110 mg twice daily may be considered for patients aged 75–80 years, or with moderate renal impairment, or at increased risk of bleeding)

• Prophylaxis of stroke and systemic embolism in non-valvular atrial fibrillation (see notes above), ADULT over 18 years, 150 mg (ELDERLY over 80 years, or receiving concomitant treatment with verapamil, 110 mg) twice daily. (Lower dose of 110 mg twice daily may be considered for patients aged 75–80 years, or with moderate renal impairment, or at increased risk of bleeding)

Note For information on changing from, or to, other anticoagulants, consult product literature

Note When given concomitantly with amiodarone or verapamil, doses should be taken at the same time

Pradaxa® (Boehringer Ingelheim) ▢PoM▢
   Capsules, blue/ivory, dabigatran etexilate (as mesilate) 75 mg, net price 10-cap pack = £10.98, 60-cap pack = £65.90; 110 mg 10-cap pack = £10.98, 60-cap pack = £65.90; 150 mg, 60-cap pack = £65.90. Label: 25

Apixaban

Apixaban, a direct inhibitor of activated factor X (factor Xa), is given orally for the prophylaxis of venous thromboembolism in adults after hip or knee replacement surgery—see Prophylaxis of Venous Thromboembolism, p. 146. It is also licensed for the treatment of deep-vein thrombosis and pulmonary embolism, and prophylaxis of recurrent deep-vein thrombosis and pulmonary embolism, although, it should not be used as an alternative to unfractionated heparin in pulmonary embolism in patients with haemodynamic instability, or who may receive thrombolysis or pulmonary embolectomy. Duration of treatment should be determined by balancing the benefit of treatment with the bleeding risk; shorter duration of treatment (at least 3 months) should be based on transient risk factors i.e recent surgery, trauma, immobilisation. Apixaban is also licensed for the prophylaxis of stroke and systemic embolism in patients with non-valvular atrial fibrillation and at least one risk factor such as previous stroke or transient ischaemic attack, symptomatic heart failure, diabetes mellitus, hypertension, or age ≥ 75 years. Apixaban does not require routine anticoagulant monitoring (INR tests are unreliable in patients taking apixaban). Haemorrhage is a common side-effect and patients should be monitored for signs of bleeding or anaemia; treatment should be stopped if severe bleeding occurs.

> **NICE guidance**
> **Apixaban for the prevention of venous thromboembolism after total hip or knee replacement in adults (January 2012)**
> Apixaban is an option for the prevention of venous thromboembolism in adults after elective hip or knee replacement surgery.
> www.nice.org.uk/TA245

APIXABAN

Indications see notes above

Cautions see notes above; also risk of bleeding; concomitant use of drugs that increase risk of bleeding; prosthetic heart valve (efficacy not established); anaesthesia with postoperative indwelling epidural catheter (risk of paralysis—monitor neurological signs and wait 20–30 hours after apixaban dose before removing catheter and do not give next dose until at least 5 hours after catheter removal); **interactions**: Appendix 1 (apixaban)

Contra-indications active bleeding; significant risk of major bleeding (e.g. recent gastro-intestinal ulcer, oesophageal varices, recent brain, spine, or ophthalmic surgery, recent intracranial haemorrhage, malignant neoplasms, vascular aneurysm)

Hepatic impairment avoid in severe impairment and in hepatic disease associated with coagulopathy

Renal impairment *for prophylaxis of venous thromboembolism following knee or hip replacement surgery, prophylaxis of recurrent deep-vein thrombosis or pulmonary embolism, and treatment of deep-vein thrombosis or pulmonary embolism,* use with caution if creatinine clearance 15–29 mL/minute; *for prophylaxis of stroke and systemic embolism in atrial fibrillation,* reduce dose to 2.5 mg twice daily if creatinine clearance 15–29 mL/minute, or if serum-creatinine ≥ 133 micromol/litre and age ≥ 80 years or body-weight ≤ 60kg; manufacturer advises avoid if creatinine clearance less than 15 mL/minute—no information available

Pregnancy manufacturer advises avoid—no information available

Breast-feeding manufacturer advises avoid—present in milk in *animal* studies

Side-effects nausea, haemorrhage (see notes above), bruising, anaemia; *less commonly* hypotension, thrombocytopenia, rash

Dose

- Prophylaxis of venous thromboembolism following knee replacement surgery, ADULT over 18 years, 2.5 mg twice daily for 10–14 days, starting 12–24 hours after surgery
- Prophylaxis of venous thromboembolism following hip replacement surgery, ADULT over 18 years, 2.5 mg twice daily for 32–38 days, starting 12–24 hours after surgery
- Treatment of deep-vein thrombosis or pulmonary embolism, ADULT over 18 years, initial treatment 10 mg twice daily for 7 days, then 5 mg twice daily for continued treatment (see notes above)
- Prophylaxis of recurrent deep-vein thrombosis or pulmonary embolism, ADULT over 18 years, 2.5 mg

twice daily (following completion of 6 months anticoagulant treatment)
- Prophylaxis of stroke and systemic embolism in non-valvular atrial fibrillation (see notes above), ADULT over 18 years, 5 mg (ELDERLY over 80 years with body-weight ≤ 60 kg, 2.5 mg) twice daily

Note For information on changing from, or to, other anticoagulants, consult product literature

Eliquis® (Bristol-Myers Squibb) ▼ PoM
Tablets, yellow, f/c, apixaban 2.5 mg, net price 10-tab pack = £10.98, 20-tab pack = £21.96, 60-tab pack = £65.90; 5 mg, 56-tab pack = £61.50

Rivaroxaban

Rivaroxaban, a direct inhibitor of activated factor X (factor Xa), is given orally for prophylaxis of venous thromboembolism in adults after hip or knee replacement surgery—see Prophylaxis of Venous Thromboembolism, p. 146; it is given for the treatment of deep-vein thrombosis and pulmonary embolism, and prophylaxis of recurrent deep-vein thrombosis and pulmonary embolism, although it should not be used as an alternative to unfractionated heparin in pulmonary embolism in patients with haemodynamic instability, or who may receive thrombolysis or pulmonary embolectomy. Rivaroxaban is also licensed for the prophylaxis of stroke and systemic embolism in patients with non-valvular atrial fibrillation and with at least one of the following risk factors: congestive heart failure, hypertension, previous stroke or transient ischaemic attack, age ≥ 75 years, or diabetes mellitus. Low-dose rivaroxaban, in combination with aspirin alone or aspirin and clopidogrel, is licensed for the prevention of atherothrombotic events following an acute coronary syndrome with elevated cardiac biomarkers, see section 2.10.1. Treatment should be started as soon as possible after the patient has been stabilised following the acute coronary event, at the earliest 24 hours after admission to hospital, and at the time when parenteral anticoagulation therapy would normally be discontinued; the usual duration of treatment is 12 months. Rivaroxaban does not require routine anticoagulant monitoring (INR tests are unreliable in patients taking rivaroxaban). The common side-effects are nausea and haemorrhage, and patients should be monitored for signs of bleeding or anaemia; treatment should be stopped if severe bleeding occurs.

The *Scottish Medicines Consortium* (p. 4) has advised (January 2012) that rivaroxaban (*Xarelto*®) is accepted for restricted use within NHS Scotland for the prevention of stroke and systemic embolism in accordance with the licensed indication; use is restricted to patients with poor INR control despite compliance with coumarin anticoagulant therapy, or to patients who are allergic to, or unable to tolerate, a coumarin anticoagulant.

2 Cardiovascular system

NICE guidance
Rivaroxaban for the prevention of stroke and systemic embolism in atrial fibrillation (May 2012)

Rivaroxaban is an option for the prevention of stroke and systemic embolism in accordance with its licensed indication (see notes above). The risks and benefits of rivaroxaban compared with warfarin should be discussed with the patient.

www.nice.org.uk/TA256

NICE guidance
Rivaroxaban for the treatment of deep-vein thrombosis and prevention of recurrent deep-vein thrombosis and pulmonary embolism (July 2012)

Rivaroxaban is an option for the treatment of deep-vein thrombosis and prevention of recurrent deep-vein thombosis and pulmonary embolism in adults after diagnosis of acute deep-vein thrombosis.

www.nice.org.uk/TA261

NICE guidance
Rivaroxaban for treating pulmonary embolism and preventing recurrent venous thromboembolism (June 2013)

Rivaroxaban is an option for treating pulmonary embolism and preventing recurrent deep-vein thrombosis and pulmonary embolism in adults.

www.nice.org.uk/TA287

▌RIVAROXABAN

Indications see notes above

Cautions see notes above; also risk of bleeding; concomitant use of drugs that increase risk of bleeding; severe hypertension; prosthetic heart valve (efficacy not established); vascular retinopathy; anaesthesia with postoperative indwelling epidural catheter (risk of paralysis—monitor neurological signs and wait at least 18 hours after rivaroxaban dose before removing catheter and do not give next dose until at least 6 hours after catheter removal); bronchiectasis; **interactions**: Appendix 1 (rivaroxaban)

Contra-indications active bleeding; significant risk of major bleeding (e.g. recent gastro-intestinal ulcer, oesophageal varices, recent brain, spine, or ophthalmic surgery, recent intracranial haemorrhage, malignant neoplasms, vascular aneurysm); in *acute coronary syndrome*—previous stroke or transient ischaemic attack

Hepatic impairment avoid in liver disease with coagulopathy

Renal impairment *for prophylaxis of venous thromboembolism following knee or hip replacement surgery and prophylaxis of atherothrombotic events in acute coronary syndrome,* use with caution if creatinine clearance 15–29 mL/minute; *for treatment of deep-vein thrombosis or pulmonary embolism and prophylaxis of recurrent deep-vein thrombosis and pulmonary embolism,* initially 15 mg twice daily for 21 days, then 20 mg once daily (but consider reducing to 15 mg once daily if risk of bleeding outweighs risk of recurrent deep-vein thrombosis or pulmonary embolism) if creatinine clearance 15–49 mL/minute; *for prophylaxis of stroke*

and systemic embolism in atrial fibrillation, reduce dose to 15 mg once daily if creatinine clearance 15–49 mL/minute; use with caution if concomitant use of drugs that increase plasma-rivaroxaban concentration (consult product literature); avoid if creatinine clearance less than 15 mL/minute; manufacturer recommends Cockroft and Gault formula to calculate creatinine clearance

Pregnancy manufacturer advises avoid—toxicity in *animal* studies

Breast-feeding manufacturer advises avoid—present in milk in *animal* studies

Side-effects nausea, vomiting, diarrhoea, constipation, dyspepsia, abdominal pain, hypotension, dizziness, headache, renal impairment, haemorrhage (see notes above), pain in extremities, pruritus, rash; *less commonly* dry mouth, thrombocythaemia, tachycardia, syncope, angioedema, malaise; *rarely* jaundice, oedema

Dose
- Prophylaxis of venous thromboembolism following knee replacement surgery, ADULT over 18 years, 10 mg once daily for 2 weeks starting 6–10 hours after surgery
- Prophylaxis of venous thromboembolism following hip replacement surgery, ADULT over 18 years, 10 mg once daily for 5 weeks starting 6–10 hours after surgery
- Treatment of deep-vein thrombosis or pulmonary embolism, ADULT over 18 years, initial treatment 15 mg twice daily with food for 21 days, then for continued treatment and prophylaxis of recurrent deep-vein thrombosis and pulmonary embolism, 20 mg once daily with food
- Prophylaxis of stroke and systemic embolism in non-valvular atrial fibrillation (see notes above), ADULT over 18 years, 20 mg once daily with food
- Prophylaxis of atherothrombotic events in acute coronary syndrome (with aspirin alone *or* aspirin and clopidogrel) (see notes above, section 2.9, and section 2.10.1), ADULT over 18 years, 2.5 mg twice daily; usual duration 12 months

Note For information on changing from, or to, other anticoagulants, consult product literature

Xarelto® (Bayer) ▼ PoM
Tablets, f/c, rivaroxaban 2.5 mg (light yellow), net price 56-tab pack = £58.80; 10 mg (light red), 10-tab pack = £21.00, 30-tab pack = £63.00, 100-tab pack = £210.00; 15 mg (red), 14-tab pack = £29.40, 28-tab pack = £58.80, 42-tab pack = £88.20, 100-tab pack = £210.00; 20 mg (brown-red), 28-tab pack = £58.80, 100-tab pack = £210.00
Note Tablets may be crushed and mixed with water or apple puree just before administration

2.8.3 Protamine sulfate

Protamine sulfate is used to treat overdosage of unfractionated or low molecular weight heparin. The long half-life of low molecular weight heparins should be taken into consideration when determining the dose of protamine sulfate; the effects of low molecular weight heparins can persist for up to 24 hours after administration. Excessive doses of protamine sulfate can have an anticoagulant effect.

◢ PROTAMINE SULFATE

Indications see above

Cautions see above; also monitor activated partial thromboplastin time or other appropriate blood clotting parameters; increased risk of allergic reaction to protamine (including previous treatment with protamine or protamine insulin, allergy to fish, men who are infertile or who have had a vasectomy)

Side-effects nausea, vomiting, lassitude, flushing, hypotension, hypertension, bradycardia, dyspnoea, rebound bleeding, back pain; hypersensitivity reactions (including angioedema, anaphylaxis) and pulmonary oedema reported

Dose
- Overdosage with intravenous injection of unfractionated heparin, by intravenous injection (rate not exceeding 5 mg/minute), 1 mg neutralises 80–100 units heparin when given within 15 minutes of heparin; if longer than 15 minutes since heparin, less protamine required (consult product literature for details) as heparin rapidly excreted; max. 50 mg
- Overdosage with intravenous infusion of unfractionated heparin, by intravenous injection (rate not exceeding 5 mg/minute), 25–50 mg once heparin infusion stopped
- Overdosage with subcutaneous injection of unfractionated heparin, 1 mg neutralises 100 units heparin; give 25–50 mg by intravenous injection (rate not exceeding 5 mg/minute) then any remaining dose given by intravenous infusion over 8–16 hours; max. total dose 50 mg
- Overdosage with subcutaneous injection of low molecular weight heparin, by intermittent intravenous injection (rate not exceeding 5 mg/minute) or by continuous intravenous infusion, 1 mg **neutralises** approx. 100 units low molecular weight heparin (consult product literature of low molecular weight heparin for details); max. 50 mg

Protamine Sulfate (Non-proprietary) ꜰᴏᴍ
Injection, protamine sulfate 10 mg/mL, net price 5-mL amp = £1.14, 10-mL amp = £3.96

2.9 Antiplatelet drugs

Antiplatelet drugs decrease platelet aggregation and inhibit thrombus formation in the arterial circulation, because in faster-flowing vessels, thrombi are composed mainly of platelets with little fibrin.

Use of **aspirin** in primary prevention of cardiovascular events, in patients with or without diabetes, is of unproven benefit. Long-term use of aspirin, in a dose of 75 mg daily, is of benefit in established cardiovascular disease (secondary prevention); unduly high blood pressure must be controlled before aspirin is given. If the patient is at a high risk of gastro-intestinal bleeding, a proton pump inhibitor (section 1.3.5) can be added.

Aspirin in a dose of 75–300 mg daily is given following coronary bypass surgery. For details on the use of aspirin in atrial fibrillation see section 2.3.1; for intermittent claudication see section 2.6.4; for stable angina and acute coronary syndromes see section 2.10.1; for use following placement of coronary stents see below; for use in stroke see also below.

Clopidogrel is licensed for the prevention of atherothrombotic events in patients with a history of symptomatic ischaemic disease. Clopidogrel, in combination with low-dose aspirin, is also licensed for acute coronary syndrome without ST-segment elevation (section 2.10.1); in these circumstances the combination is given for up to 12 months (most benefit occurs during the first 3 months; there is no evidence of benefit beyond 12 months). Clopidogrel, in combination with low-dose aspirin, is also licensed for acute myocardial infarction with ST-segment elevation (section 2.10.1); the combination is licensed for at least 4 weeks, but the optimum treatment duration has not been established. In patients undergoing percutaneous coronary intervention, clopidogrel is used as an adjunct with aspirin (see also below). Patients, who are not already taking clopidogrel, should receive a 300 mg loading dose prior to the procedure; alternatively, a 600 mg [unlicensed] loading dose may produce a greater and more rapid inhibition of platelet aggregation.

Clopidogrel is also licensed, in combination with low-dose aspirin, for the prevention of atherothrombotic and thromboembolic events in patients with atrial fibrillation (and at least one risk factor for a vascular event), and for whom warfarin is unsuitable.

Use of clopidogrel with aspirin increases the risk of bleeding. Clopidogrel monotherapy may be an alternative when aspirin is contra-indicated, for example in those with aspirin hypersensitivity, or when aspirin is not tolerated despite the addition of a proton pump inhibitor (see also NICE guidance, below).

For details on the use of clopidogrel in stroke, see below.

The *Scottish Medicines Consortium* (p. 4) has advised (February 2004) that clopidogrel be accepted for restricted use for the treatment of confirmed acute coronary syndrome (without ST-segment elevation), in combination with aspirin. Clopidogrel should be initiated in hospital inpatients only. The *Scottish Medicines Consortium* has also advised (July 2007) that clopidogrel be accepted for restricted use for patients with ST-segment elevation acute myocardial infarction in combination with aspirin; treatment with clopidogrel is restricted to 4 weeks only.

Dipyridamole is used by mouth as an adjunct to oral anticoagulation for prophylaxis of thromboembolism associated with prosthetic heart valves. Modified-release preparations are licensed for secondary prevention of ischaemic stroke and transient ischaemic attacks (see also Long-term Management, under Ischaemic Stroke, below).

2 Cardiovascular system

Cardiovascular system

2

NICE guidance
Clopidogrel and modified-release dipyridamole in the prevention of occlusive vascular events (December 2010)

The guidance applies to patients who have had an occlusive vascular event, or who have established peripheral arterial disease. The guidance does **not** apply to patients who have had, or are at risk of, stroke associated with atrial fibrillation, or who need prophylaxis for occlusive events following coronary revascularisation or carotid artery procedures.

Clopidogrel monotherapy is recommended as an option to prevent occlusive vascular events in patients who have had:

- an ischaemic stroke, or who have peripheral arterial disease or multivascular disease, **or**
- a myocardial infarction, only if aspirin is contra-indicated or not tolerated.

Modified-release dipyridamole, in combination with aspirin, is recommended as an option to prevent occlusive vascular events in patients who have had:

- a transient ischaemic attack, **or**
- an ischaemic stroke, only if clopidogrel is contra-indicated or not tolerated.

Modified-release dipyridamole monotherapy is recommended as an option to prevent occlusive vascular events in patients who have had:

- an ischaemic stroke, only if aspirin and clopidogrel are contra-indicated or not tolerated, **or**
- a transient ischaemic attack, only if aspirin is contra-indicated or not tolerated.

www.nice.org.uk/TA210

NICE guidance
Ticagrelor for the treatment of acute coronary syndromes (October 2011)

Ticagrelor, in combination with low-dose aspirin, is recommended for up to 12 months as a treatment option in adults with acute coronary syndromes, that is, people:

- with ST-segment elevation myocardial infarction—defined as ST elevation or new left bundle branch block on electrocardiogram—that cardiologists intend to treat with primary percutaneous coronary intervention, **or**
- with non-ST-segment elevation myocardial infarction (NSTEMI), **or**
- admitted to hospital with unstable angina—defined as ST or T wave changes on electrocardiogram suggestive of ischaemia plus one of the characteristics defined below. Before ticagrelor is continued beyond the initial treatment, the diagnosis of unstable angina should first be confirmed, ideally by a cardiologist. Characteristics to be used in defining treatment with ticagrelor for unstable angina are:

  - age 60 years or older;
  - previous myocardial infarction or previous coronary artery bypass grafting;
  - coronary artery disease with stenosis of 50% or more in at least two vessels;
  - previous ischaemic stroke;
  - previous transient ischaemic attack, carotid stenosis of at least 50%, or cerebral revascularisation;
  - diabetes mellitus;
  - peripheral arterial disease, **or**
  - chronic renal dysfunction (creatinine clearance less than 60 mL/minute/1.73 m^2).

www.nice.org.uk/TA236

Prasugrel, in combination with aspirin, is licensed for the prevention of atherothrombotic events in patients with acute coronary syndrome undergoing percutaneous coronary intervention (section 2.10.1); the combination is usually given for up to 12 months.

The *Scottish Medicines Consortium* (p. 4) has advised (August 2009) that prasugrel (*Efient®*), in combination with aspirin, be accepted for restricted use within NHS Scotland for the prevention of atherothrombotic events in patients with acute coronary syndrome undergoing percutaneous coronary intervention who are eligible to receive the 10 mg dose of prasugrel.

NICE guidance
Prasugrel with percutaneous coronary intervention for treating acute coronary syndromes (July 2014)

Prasugrel 10 mg in combination with aspirin is recommended as an option, within its marketing authorisation, for preventing atherothrombotic events in adults with acute coronary syndrome (unstable angina (UA), non-ST segment elevation myocardial infarction (NSTEMI) or ST segment elevation myocardial infarction (STEMI)) having primary or delayed percutaneous coronary intervention.

www.nice.org.uk/TA317

Ticagrelor, in combination with aspirin, is licensed for the prevention of atherothrombotic events in patients with acute coronary syndrome; the combination is usually given for up to 12 months.

Antiplatelet drugs and coronary stents Patients selected for percutaneous coronary intervention, with the placement of a coronary stent, will require dual antiplatelet therapy with aspirin and either clopidogrel, prasugrel, or ticagrelor. Aspirin therapy should continue indefinitely. Clopidogrel is recommended for 1 month following elective percutaneous coronary intervention with placement of a bare-metal stent, and for 12 months if percutaneous coronary intervention with placement of a bare-metal stent was for an acute coronary syndrome; clopidogrel should be given for 12 months following placement of a drug-eluting stent. Clopidogrel should not be discontinued prematurely in patients with a drug-eluting stent—there is an increased risk of stent thrombosis as a result of the eluted drug slowing the re-endothelialisation process. Patients considered to be at high risk of developing late stent thrombosis with a drug-eluting stent may require a longer duration of treatment with clopidogrel. Prasugrel or ticagrelor are alternatives to clopidogrel in certain patients undergoing percutaneous coronary intervention (see notes above).

Glycoprotein IIb/IIIa inhibitors Glycoprotein IIb/IIIa inhibitors prevent platelet aggregation by blocking the binding of fibrinogen to receptors on platelets. **Abciximab** is a monoclonal antibody which binds to glycoprotein IIb/IIIa receptors and to other related sites; it is licensed as an adjunct to unfractionated heparin and aspirin for the prevention of ischaemic complications in high-risk patients undergoing percutaneous transluminal coronary intervention. Abciximab should be used once only (to avoid additional risk of thrombocytopenia). **Eptifibatide** (in combination with unfractionated heparin and aspirin) and **tirofiban** (in combination with unfractionated heparin, aspirin, and clopidogrel) also inhibit glycoprotein IIb/IIIa receptors; they are licensed for use to prevent early myocardial infarction in patients with unstable angina or non-ST-segment-elevation myocardial infarction (section 2.10.1). Tirofiban is also licensed for use in combination with unfractionated heparin, aspirin, and clopidogrel, for the reduction of major cardiovascular events in patients with ST-segment elevation myocardial infarction intended for primary percutaneous coronary intervention. Abciximab, eptifibatide and tirofiban should be used by specialists only.

For use of epoprostenol, see section 2.8.1.

Management of stroke

Stroke is associated with a significant risk of morbidity and mortality. Patients presenting with acute symptoms should be immediately transferred to hospital for accurate diagnosis of stroke type, and urgent initiation of appropriate treatment; patients should be managed by a specialist multidisciplinary stroke team.

The following notes give an overview of the initial and long-term management of transient ischaemic attack, ischaemic stroke, and intracerebral haemorrhage.

Transient ischaemic attack

Patients suspected of having a transient ischaemic attack should immediately receive aspirin 300 mg once daily (patients with aspirin hypersensitivity, or those intolerant of aspirin despite the addition of a proton pump inhibitor, should receive clopidogrel 75 mg once daily [unlicensed use] as an alternative). Following a confirmed diagnosis, patients should receive treatment for secondary prevention (see Long-term Management, under Ischaemic Stroke, below).

Ischaemic stroke

Initial management Alteplase (section 2.10.2) is recommended in the treatment of acute ischaemic stroke if it can be administered within 4.5 hours of symptom onset; it should be given by medical staff experienced in the administration of thrombolytics and the treatment of acute stroke, preferably within a specialist stroke centre. Treatment with aspirin 300 mg once daily for 14 days should be initiated 24 hours after thrombolysis (or as soon as possible within 48 hours of symptom onset in patients not receiving thrombolysis); patients with aspirin hypersensitivity, or those intolerant of aspirin despite the addition of a proton pump inhibitor, should receive clopidogrel 75 mg once daily [unlicensed use] as an alternative.

Anticoagulants are not recommended as an alternative to antiplatelet drugs in acute ischaemic stroke in patients who are in sinus rhythm. However, parenteral anticoagulants (section 2.8.1) may be indicated in patients who are symptomatic of, or at high risk of developing, deep vein thrombosis or pulmonary embolism; warfarin should not be commenced in the acute phase of ischaemic stroke.

Anticoagulants (section 2.8.2) should be considered after cardio-embolic ischaemic stroke in patients with atrial fibrillation, however patients presenting with atrial fibrillation following a disabling ischaemic stroke should receive aspirin 300 mg once daily for 14 days, before

being considered for anticoagulant treatment. Patients already receiving anticoagulation for a prosthetic heart valve who experience a disabling ischaemic stroke and are at significant risk of haemorrhagic transformation, should have their anticoagulant treatment stopped for 7 days and substituted with aspirin 300 mg once daily.

Treatment of hypertension in the acute phase of ischaemic stroke can result in reduced cerebral perfusion, and should therefore only be instituted in the event of a hypertensive emergency (see section 2.5), or in those patients considered for thrombolysis.

Long-term management Patients should receive long-term treatment following a transient ischaemic attack or an ischaemic stroke to reduce the risk of further cardiovascular events.

Following a *transient ischaemic attack*, long-term treatment with modified-release dipyridamole 200 mg twice daily in combination with aspirin 75 mg once daily is recommended. If patients are intolerant of aspirin, or it is contra-indicated, then modified-release dipyridamole alone is recommended; If patients are intolerant of dipyridamole, or it is contra-indicated, then aspirin alone is recommended. Patients who are intolerant of both aspirin and dipyridamole should receive clopidogrel alone [unlicensed use].

Following an *ischaemic stroke* (not associated with atrial fibrillation—see below), clopidogrel 75 mg once daily is recommended as long-term treatment. If clopidogrel is contra-indicated or not tolerated, patients should receive modified-release dipyridamole 200 mg twice daily in combination with aspirin 75 mg once daily; if both aspirin and clopidogrel are contra-indicated or not tolerated, then modified-release dipyridamole alone is recommended; if both dipyridamole and clopidogrel are contra-indicated or not tolerated, then aspirin alone is recommended.

Patients with stroke associated with atrial fibrillation should be reviewed for long-term treatment with warfarin or an alternative anticoagulant (see Initial Management under Ischaemic Stroke, above, and section 2.3).

Anticoagulants are not routinely recommended in the long-term prevention of recurrent stroke, except in patients with atrial fibrillation (section 2.3).

A statin (section 2.12) should be initiated 48 hours after stroke symptom onset, irrespective of the patient's serum-cholesterol concentration.

Following the acute phase of ischaemic stroke, blood pressure should be measured and treatment initiated to achieve a target blood pressure of <130/80 mmHg (see section 2.5). Beta-blockers should not be used in the management of hypertension following a stroke, unless they are indicated for a co-existing condition.

All patients should be advised to make lifestyle modifications that include beneficial changes to diet, exercise, weight, alcohol intake, and smoking.

Intracerebral haemorrhage

Initial management Surgical intervention may be required following intracerebral haemorrhage to remove the haematoma and relieve intracranial pressure. Patients taking anticoagulants should have this treatment stopped and reversed (see section 2.8.2); anticoagulant therapy has, however, been used in patients with intracerebral haemorrhage who are symptomatic of deep vein thrombosis or pulmonary embo-

2 Cardiovascular system

lism; placement of a caval filter is an alternative in this situation.

Long-term management   Aspirin therapy should only be given to patients at a high risk of a cardiac ischaemic event. Anticoagulant therapy is not recommended following an intracerebral haemorrhage, even in those with atrial fibrillation, unless the patient is at very high risk of an ischaemic stroke or cardiac ischaemic events; advice from a specialist should be sought in this situation. Blood pressure should be measured and treatment initiated where appropriate (see section 2.5), taking care to avoid hypoperfusion. Statins should be avoided following intracerebral haemorrhage, however they can be used with caution when the risk of a vascular event outweighs the risk of further haemorrhage.

◢ ABCIXIMAB

Indications   prevention of ischaemic cardiac complications in patients undergoing percutaneous coronary intervention; short-term prevention of myocardial infarction in patients with unstable angina not responding to conventional treatment and who are scheduled for percutaneous coronary intervention (use under specialist supervision)

Cautions   measure baseline prothrombin time, activated clotting time, activated partial thromboplastin time, platelet count, haemoglobin and haematocrit; monitor haemoglobin and haematocrit 12 hours and 24 hours after start of treatment and platelet count 2–4 hours and 24 hours after start of treatment; concomitant use of drugs that increase risk of bleeding; discontinue if uncontrollable serious bleeding occurs or emergency cardiac surgery needed; consult product literature for details of procedures to minimise bleeding; elderly

Contra-indications   active internal bleeding; major surgery, intracranial or intraspinal surgery or trauma within last 2 months; stroke within last 2 years; intracranial neoplasm, arteriovenous malformation or aneurysm, severe hypertension, haemorrhagic diathesis, thrombocytopenia, vasculitis, hypertensive retinopathy

Hepatic impairment   avoid in severe liver disease—increased risk of bleeding

Renal impairment   caution in severe impairment—increased risk of bleeding

Pregnancy   manufacturer advises use only if potential benefit outweighs risk—no information available

Breast-feeding   manufacturer advises avoid—no information available

Side-effects   bleeding manifestations; nausea, vomiting, hypotension, bradycardia, chest pain, back pain, headache, fever, puncture site pain, thrombocytopenia; *rarely* cardiac tamponade, adult respiratory distress, hypersensitivity reactions

Dose

● ADULT initially by intravenous injection over 1 minute, 250 micrograms/kg, then by intravenous infusion, 125 nanograms/kg/minute (max. 10 micrograms/minute); for prevention of ischaemic complications start 10–60 minutes before percutaneous coronary intervention and continue infusion for 12 hours; for unstable angina start up to 24 hours before possible percutaneous coronary intervention and continue infusion for 12 hours after intervention

ReoPro® (Lilly) [PoM]
Injection, abciximab 2 mg/mL, net price 5-mL vial = £250.24

◢ ASPIRIN (antiplatelet)
(Acetylsalicylic Acid)

Indications   secondary prevention of thrombotic cerebrovascular or cardiovascular disease, and following by-pass surgery (see also section 2.10.1 and notes above)

Cautions   asthma; uncontrolled hypertension; previous peptic ulceration (but manufacturers may advise avoidance of low-dose aspirin in history of peptic ulceration); concomitant use of drugs that increase risk of bleeding; G6PD deficiency (section 9.1.5); dehydration; elderly; **interactions:** Appendix 1 (aspirin)

Contra-indications   use other than as an antiplatelet in children and adolescents under 16 years (Reye's syndrome, section 4.7.1); active peptic ulceration; haemophilia and other bleeding disorders
Hypersensitivity   Aspirin and other NSAIDs are **contraindicated** in history of hypersensitivity to aspirin or any other NSAID—which includes those in whom attacks of asthma, angioedema, urticaria, or rhinitis have been precipitated by aspirin or any other NSAID

Hepatic impairment   avoid in severe impairment—increased risk of gastro-intestinal bleeding

Renal impairment   use with caution; avoid in severe impairment; sodium and water retention; deterioration in renal function; increased risk of gastro-intestinal bleeding

Pregnancy   use with caution during third trimester; impaired platelet function and risk of haemorrhage; delayed onset and increased duration of labour with increased blood loss; avoid analgesic doses if possible in last few weeks (low doses probably not harmful); with high doses, closure of fetal ductus arteriosus *in utero* and possibly persistent pulmonary hypertension of newborn; kernicterus in jaundiced neonates

Breast-feeding   avoid—possible risk of Reye's syndrome; regular use of high doses could impair platelet function and produce hypoprothrombinaemia in infant if neonatal vitamin K stores low

Side-effects   bronchospasm; gastro-intestinal irritation, gastro-intestinal haemorrhage (occasionally major), also other haemorrhage (e.g. subconjunctival)

Dose

● See notes above

[1]Aspirin (Non-proprietary) [PoM]
Dispersible tablets, aspirin 75 mg, net price 28 = 84p; 300 mg, see section 4.7.1. Label: 13, 21, 32
Tablets, e/c, aspirin 75 mg, net price 28-tab pack = 87p; 56-tab pack = £1.58; 300 mg, see section 4.7.1. Label: 5, 25, 32
Brands include *Micropirin®, Caprin®*

Nu-Seals® Aspirin (Alliance) [PoM]
Tablets, e/c, aspirin 75 mg, net price 56-tab pack = £3.12; 300 mg, see section 4.7.1. Label: 5, 25, 32
Note Tablets may be chewed at diagnosis for rapid absorption

◢With dipyridamole
See under Dipyridamole, p. 163

---

1. Aspirin tablets 75 mg may be sold to the public in packs of up to 100 tablets; for details relating to other strengths see section 4.7.1 and *Medicines, Ethics and Practice*, London, Pharmaceutical Press (always consult latest edition)

2 Cardiovascular system

CLOPIDOGREL

Indications prevention of atherothrombotic events in peripheral arterial disease, or within 35 days of myocardial infarction, or within 6 months of ischaemic stroke; prevention of artherothrombotic events in acute coronary syndrome without ST-segment elevation (given with aspirin—see notes above) and in acute myocardial infarction with ST-segment elevation (given with aspirin—see notes above); prevention of atherothrombotic and thromboembolic events in patients with atrial fibrillation (given with aspirin—see notes above) and for whom warfarin is unsuitable

Cautions patients at risk of increased bleeding from trauma, surgery, or other pathological conditions; concomitant use of drugs that increase risk of bleeding; discontinue 7 days before elective surgery if antiplatelet effect not desirable; history of hypersensitivity reactions to thienopyridines (e.g. prasugrel); **interactions:** Appendix 1 (clopidogrel)

Contra-indications active bleeding

Hepatic Impairment manufacturer advises caution (risk of bleeding); avoid in severe impairment

Renal impairment manufacturer advises caution

Pregnancy manufacturer advises avoid—no information available

Breast-feeding manufacturer advises avoid

Side-effects dyspepsia, abdominal pain, diarrhoea; bleeding disorders (including gastro-intestinal and intracranial); *less commonly* nausea, vomiting, gastritis, flatulence, constipation, gastric and duodenal ulcers, headache, dizziness, paraesthesia, leucopenia, decreased platelets (very rarely severe thrombocytopenia), eosinophilia, rash, and pruritus; *rarely* vertigo; *very rarely* colitis, pancreatitis, hepatitis, acute liver failure, vasculitis, confusion, hallucinations, taste disturbance, stomatitis, bronchospasm, interstitial pneumonitis, eosinophilic pneumonia, blood disorders (including thrombocytopenic purpura, agranulocytosis, pancytopenia, acquired haemophilia), and hypersensitivity-like reactions (including fever, glomerulonephritis, arthralgia, Stevens-Johnson syndrome, toxic epidermal necrolysis, lichen planus)

Dose
- Prevention of atherothrombotic events in peripheral arterial disease or after myocardial infarction or ischaemic stroke, 75 mg once daily
- Acute coronary syndrome (without ST-segment elevation), initially 300 mg then 75 mg daily (with aspirin—see notes above)
- Acute myocardial infarction (with ST-segment elevation), initially 300 mg then 75 mg daily (with aspirin—see notes above); initial dose omitted if patient over 75 years
- Prevention of atherothrombotic and thromboembolic events in patients with atrial fibrillation (with aspirin—see notes above), 75 mg once daily

Clopidogrel (Non-proprietary) ▣ PoM
Tablets, clopidogrel (as besilate or hydrochloride) 75 mg, net price 28-tab pack = £1.88, 30-tab pack = £1.83
Brands include *Grepid®*

Plavix® (Sanofi-Aventis) ▣ PoM
Tablets, pink, f/c, clopidogrel (as hydrogen sulfate) 75 mg, net price 30-tab pack = £35.64; 300 mg, 30-tab pack = £142.54

DIPYRIDAMOLE

Indications see notes above and under Dose

Cautions rapidly worsening angina, aortic stenosis, recent myocardial infarction, left ventricular outflow obstruction, heart failure; may exacerbate migraine; hypotension; myasthenia gravis (risk of exacerbation); coagulation disorders; concomitant use of drugs that increase risk of bleeding; **interactions:** Appendix 1 (dipyridamole)

Pregnancy not known to be harmful

Breast-feeding manufacturers advise use only if essential—small amount present in milk

Side-effects gastro-intestinal effects, dizziness, myalgia, throbbing headache, hypotension, hot flushes and tachycardia; worsening symptoms of coronary heart disease; hypersensitivity reactions such as rash, urticaria, severe bronchospasm and angioedema; increased bleeding during or after surgery; thrombocytopenia reported

Dose
- By mouth, 300–600 mg daily in 3–4 divided doses Modified-release preparations, see under preparation below
- By intravenous injection, diagnostic only, consult product literature

Dipyridamole (Non-proprietary) ▣ PoM
Tablets, coated, dipyridamole 25 mg, net price 84 = £8.56; 100 mg, 84 = £3.70. Label: 22
Oral suspension, dipyridamole 50 mg/5 mL, net price 150 mL = £40.64

Persantin® (Boehringer Ingelheim) ▣ PoM
Tablets, s/c, dipyridamole 100 mg, net price 84-tab pack = £6.30. Label: 22
Injection, dipyridamole 5 mg/mL, net price 2-mL amp = 16p

◢ **Modified release**

Persantin® Retard (Boehringer Ingelheim) ▣ PoM
Capsules, m/r, red/orange containing yellow pellets, dipyridamole 200 mg, net price 60-cap pack = £10.06. Label: 21, 25
Dose secondary prevention of ischaemic stroke and transient ischaemic attacks (used alone or with aspirin), adjunct to oral anticoagulation for prophylaxis of thromboembolism associated with prosthetic heart valves, 200 mg twice daily preferably with food
Note Dispense in original container (pack contains a desiccant) and discard any capsules remaining 6 weeks after opening

◢ **With aspirin**

For prescribing information on aspirin, see under Aspirin, p. 162

Asasantin® Retard (Boehringer Ingelheim) ▣ PoM
Capsules, red/ivory, aspirin 25 mg, dipyridamole 200 mg (m/r), net price 60-cap pack = £9.84. Label: 21, 25, 32
Dose secondary prevention of ischaemic stroke and transient ischaemic attacks, 1 capsule twice daily
Note Dispense in original container (pack contains a desiccant) and discard any capsules remaining 6 weeks after opening

EPTIFIBATIDE

Indications in combination with aspirin and unfractionated heparin for the prevention of early myocardial infarction in patients with unstable angina or non-ST-segment-elevation myocardial infarction and with last episode of chest pain within 24 hours (use under specialist supervision)

Cautions risk of bleeding, concomitant drugs that increase risk of bleeding—discontinue immediately if uncontrolled serious bleeding; measure baseline prothrombin time, activated partial thromboplastin time, platelet count, haemoglobin, haematocrit and serum creatinine; monitor haemoglobin, haematocrit and platelets within 6 hours after start of treatment then at least once daily; discontinue if thrombolytic therapy, intra-aortic balloon pump or emergency cardiac surgery necessary

Contra-indications abnormal bleeding within 30 days, major surgery or severe trauma within 6 weeks, stroke within last 30 days or any history of haemorrhagic stroke, intracranial disease (aneurysm, neoplasm or arteriovenous malformation), severe hypertension, haemorrhagic diathesis, increased prothrombin time or INR, thrombocytopenia

Hepatic impairment avoid in severe liver disease—increased risk of bleeding

Renal impairment reduce infusion to 1 microgram/kg/minute if eGFR 30–50 mL/minute/1.73 m²; avoid if eGFR less than 30 mL/minute/1.73 m²

Pregnancy manufacturer advises use only if potential benefit outweighs risk—no information available

Breast-feeding manufacturer advises avoid—no information available

Side-effects bleeding manifestations; *very rarely* anaphylaxis and rash

Dose
● Initially by intravenous injection, 180 micrograms/kg, then by intravenous infusion, 2 micrograms/kg/minute for up to 72 hours (up to 96 hours if percutaneous coronary intervention during treatment)

Integrilin® (GSK) PoM
Injection, eptifibatide 2 mg/mL, net price 10-mL (20-mg) vial = £13.61
Infusion, eptifibatide 750 micrograms/mL, net price 100-mL (75-mg) vial = £42.79

PRASUGREL

Indications in combination with aspirin for the prevention of atherothrombotic events in patients with acute coronary syndrome undergoing percutaneous coronary intervention

Cautions patients at increased risk of bleeding (e.g. from recent trauma, surgery, gastro-intestinal bleeding, or active peptic ulcer disease); concomitant use of drugs that increase risk of bleeding; discontinue at least 7 days before elective surgery if antiplatelet effect not desirable; elderly; body-weight less than 60 kg; history of hypersensitivity reactions to thienopyridines (e.g. clopidogrel); **interactions:** Appendix 1 (prasugrel)

Contra-indications active bleeding; history of stroke or transient ischaemic attack

Hepatic impairment use with caution in moderate impairment—increased risk of bleeding; avoid in severe impairment

Renal impairment use with caution—increased risk of bleeding

Pregnancy manufacturer advises use only if potential benefit outweighs risk

Breast-feeding manufacturer advises avoid—no information available

Side-effects haemorrhage (including gastro-intestinal and intracranial), haematoma, haematuria, anaemia, rash; *less commonly* hypersensitivity reactions including angioedema; *rarely* thrombocytopenia; *also reported* thrombotic thrombocytopenic purpura

Dose
● ADULT over 18 years, (with aspirin—see notes above) initially 60 mg as a single dose then body-weight over 60 kg, 10 mg once daily *or* body-weight under 60 kg or ELDERLY over 75 years, 5 mg once daily
Note Patients undergoing coronary angiography within 48 hours of admission for unstable angina or NSTEMI should be given the initial 60-mg dose at the time of percutaneous coronary intervention to minimise the risk of bleeding

Efient® (Lilly) PoM
Tablets, f/c, prasugrel (as hydrochloride) 5 mg (yellow), net price 28-tab pack = £47.56; 10 mg (beige), 28-tab pack = £47.56

TICAGRELOR

Indications in combination with aspirin for the prevention of atherothrombotic events in patients with acute coronary syndrome

Cautions patients at increased risk of bleeding (e.g. from recent trauma, surgery, gastro-intestinal bleeding, or coagulation disorders); concomitant use of drugs that increase risk of bleeding; discontinue 7 days before elective surgery if antiplatelet effect not desirable; bradycardia, sick sinus syndrome, or second- or third-degree AV block (unless pacemaker fitted); asthma or chronic obstructive pulmonary disease; history of hyperuricaemia; monitor renal function 1 month after initiation

Contra-indications active bleeding; history of intracranial haemorrhage

Hepatic impairment avoid in moderate or severe impairment—no information available

Pregnancy manufacturer advises avoid—toxicity in *animal* studies

Breast-feeding manufacturer advises avoid—present in milk in *animal* studies

Side-effects dyspnoea, haemorrhage, bruising; *less commonly* nausea, vomiting, diarrhoea, abdominal pain, dyspepsia, gastritis, dizziness, headache, rash, pruritus; *rarely* constipation, paraesthesia, confusion, hyperuricaemia, raised serum creatinine, vertigo

Dose
● ADULT over 18 years, (with aspirin—see notes above) initially 180 mg as a single dose, then 90 mg twice daily

Brilique® (AstraZeneca) PoM
Tablets, yellow, f/c, ticagrelor 90 mg, net price 56-tab pack = £54.60

TIROFIBAN

Indications in combination with unfractionated heparin, aspirin, and clopidogrel for prevention of early myocardial infarction in patients with unstable angina or non-ST-segment-elevation myocardial infarction (NSTEMI) and with last episode of chest pain within 12 hours (use under specialist supervision); in combination with unfractionated heparin, aspirin, and clopidogrel for reduction of major cardiovascular events in patients with ST-segment elevation myo-

Cardiovascular system

2

cardial infarction (STEMI) intended for primary per-cutaneous coronary intervention (PCI) (use under specialist supervision)

Cautions   major surgery or severe trauma within 3 months (avoid if within 6 weeks); traumatic or pro-tracted cardiopulmonary resuscitation, organ biopsy or lithotripsy within last 2 weeks; risk of bleeding including active peptic ulcer within 3 months, uncontrolled severe hypertension, acute pericarditis, aortic dissection, haemorrhagic retinopathy, vasculitis, haematuria, faecal occult blood, elderly, low body-weight; severe heart failure, cardiogenic shock, anaemia; puncture of non-compressible vessel within 24 hours; concomitant drugs that increase risk of bleeding (including within 48 hours of thrombolytic administration); monitor platelet count, haemoglobin and haematocrit before treatment, 2–6 hours after start of treatment and then at least once daily; dis-continue if thrombolytic therapy, intra-aortic balloon pump or emergency cardiac surgery necessary; dis-continue immediately if serious or uncontrollable bleeding occurs; **interactions:** Appendix 1 (tirofiban)

Contra-indications   abnormal bleeding within 30 days; stroke within 30 days or any history of hae-morrhagic stroke, intracranial disease (aneurysm, neoplasm or arteriovenous malformation); severe hypertension; increased prothrombin time or INR; thrombocytopenia

Hepatic impairment   caution in mild to moderate liver disease; avoid in severe liver disease—increased risk of bleeding

Renal impairment   increased risk of bleeding; monitor carefully if eGFR less than 60 mL/minute/1.73 m²; use half normal dose if eGFR less than 30 mL/min-ute/1.73 m²

Pregnancy   manufacturer advises use only if potential benefit outweighs risk—no information available

Breast-feeding   manufacturer advises avoid—no information available

Side-effects   nausea, headache, fever, bleeding man-ifestations, reversible thrombocytopenia

Dose

• Unstable angina or NSTEMI with angiography planned for 4–48 hours after diagnosis, by intra-venous infusion, initially 400 nanograms/kg/minute for 30 minutes, then 100 nanograms/kg/minute for at least 48 hours (continue during and for 12–24 hours after percutaneous coronary intervention); max. duration of treatment 108 hours

• Unstable angina or NSTEMI with angiography *within* 4 hours of diagnosis *or* STEMI intended for primary PCI, by intravenous injection, 25 micrograms/kg given over 3 minutes at start of percutaneous coron-ary intervention, then by intravenous infusion, 150 nanograms/kg/minute for 12–24 hours; max. duration of treatment 48 hours

Aggrastat® (Correvio) [PoM]
Concentrate for intravenous infusion, tirofiban (as hydrochloride) 250 micrograms/mL. For dilution before use, net price 50-mL (12.5-mg) vial = £146.11
Electrolytes Na⁺ <0.5 mmol/mL

Intravenous infusion, tirofiban (as hydrochloride) 50 micrograms/mL, net price 250-mL *Intravia®* bag = £160.72
Electrolytes Na⁺ <0.5 mmol/mL

2.10 Stable angina, acute coronary syndromes, and fibrinolysis

2.10.1   Management of stable angina and acute coronary syndromes
2.10.2   Fibrinolytic drugs

2.10.1 Management of stable angina and acute coronary syndromes

Stable angina

It is important to distinguish stable angina from unstable angina. *Stable angina* usually results from atherosclerotic plaques in the coronary arteries that restrict blood flow and oxygen supply to the heart; it is often precipitated by exertion and relieved by rest. Treatment involves management of acute anginal pain, and long-term management to prevent angina attacks and to reduce the risk of cardiovascular events.

Management of stable angina

Acute attacks of stable angina should be managed with sublingual **glyceryl trinitrate** (section 2.6.1); sublingual glyceryl trinitrate can also be taken immediately before performing activities that are known to bring on an attack. If attacks occur more than twice a week, regular drug therapy is required and should be introduced in a step-wise manner according to response.

Patients with stable angina should be given a beta-blocker (section 2.4) or a calcium-channel blocker (section 2.6.2). In those with left-ventricular dysfunction, beta-blocker treatment should be started at a very low dose and titrated very slowly over a period of weeks or months (section 2.5.5); the rate-limiting calcium-channel blockers, diltiazem and verapamil, are contra-indicated in patients with left-ventricular dysfunction because they may precipitate heart failure. If a beta-blocker or a calcium-channel blocker alone fails to control symptoms adequately, a combination of a beta-blocker and a dihydropyridine calcium-channel blocker (e.g. amlodipine, felodipine, modified-release nifedipine) should be used; if this combination is not appropriate due to intolerance of, or contra-indication to, *either* beta-blockers *or* calcium-channel blockers, addition of a long-acting **nitrate** (section 2.6.1), **ivabra-dine**, **nicorandil**, or **ranolazine** (section 2.6.3) can be considered.

For those patients in whom both beta-blockers *and* calcium-channel blockers are not tolerated or are con-tra-indicated, monotherapy with a long-acting nitrate, ivabradine, nicorandil, or ranolazine should be considered.

Response to treatment should be assessed every 2–4 weeks after initiating or changing drug therapy; the drug should be titrated (according to symptom control) to the maximum tolerated dose. Consider referring the patient to a specialist if a combination of two drugs fails to control symptoms. Addition of a third antianginal drug should only be considered if symptom control is not achieved with two drugs and the patient is either due to

2 Cardiovascular system

undergo a revascularisation procedure, or a revascularisation procedure is considered inappropriate. See section 2.9 for the use of antiplatelet drugs in patients undergoing coronary stenting.

For long-term prevention of cardiovascular events, see Prevention of cardiovascular events, below.

Acute coronary syndromes

Acute coronary syndromes encompass a spectrum of conditions which include unstable angina, and myocardial infarction with or without ST-segment elevation. Patients with different acute coronary syndromes may present similarly; definitive diagnosis is made on the basis of clinical presentation, ECG changes, and measurement of biochemical cardiac markers.

Unstable angina and non-ST-segment elevation myocardial infarction (NSTEMI) are related acute coronary syndromes that fall between the classifications of stable angina and ST-segment elevation myocardial infarction (STEMI). They usually occur as a result of atheromatous plaque rupture, and are often characterised by stable angina that suddenly worsens, recurring or prolonged angina at rest, or new onset of severe angina. Patients with unstable angina have no evidence of myocardial necrosis, whereas in NSTEMI, myocardial necrosis (less significant than with STEMI) will be evident. There is a risk of progression to STEMI or sudden death, particularly in patients who experience pain at rest.

ST-segment elevation myocardial infarction (STEMI) is an acute coronary syndrome where atheromatous plaque rupture leads to thrombosis and myocardial ischaemia, with irreversible necrosis of the heart muscle, often leading to long-term complications. STEMI can also occasionally occur as a result of coronary spasm or embolism, arteritis, spontaneous thrombosis, or sudden severe elevation in blood pressure.

Management of unstable angina and non-ST-segment elevation myocardial infarction (NSTEMI)

These conditions are managed similarly; the aims of management are to provide supportive care and pain relief during the acute attack and to prevent further cardiac events and death. For advice on the management of patients with acute ST-segment elevation myocardial infarction (STEMI), see below.

Initial management Oxygen (section 3.6) should be administered if there is evidence of hypoxia, pulmonary oedema, or continuing myocardial ischaemia; hyperoxia should be avoided and particular care is required in patients with chronic obstructive airways disease.

Nitrates (section 2.6.1) are used to relieve ischaemic pain. If sublingual glyceryl trinitrate is not effective, intravenous or buccal glyceryl trinitrate or intravenous isosorbide dinitrate is given. If pain continues, **diamorphine** or **morphine** (section 4.7.2) can be given by slow intravenous injection; an antiemetic such as metoclopramide should also be given (section 4.6).

Aspirin (chewed or dispersed in water) is given for its antiplatelet effect in a dose of 300 mg (section 2.9). If aspirin is given before arrival at hospital, a note saying that it has been given should be sent with the patient. **Clopidogrel** in a dose of 300 mg (or 600 mg [unlicensed] if used prior to percutaneous coronary intervention) should also be given (see section 2.9). **Prasugrel**, in a dose of 60 mg, is an alternative to clopidogrel in certain patients undergoing percutaneous coronary intervention (see NICE guidance, p. 160). **Ticagrelor**, in a dose of 180 mg, is also an alternative to clopidogrel (see NICE guidance, p. 160). Patients should also receive either **unfractionated heparin**, a low molecular weight heparin, or **fondaparinux** (section 2.8.1).

Patients without contra-indications should receive beta-blockers (section 2.4) which should be continued indefinitely. In patients with left ventricular dysfunction and in whom beta-blockers are inappropriate, **diltiazem** or **verapamil** can be given (section 2.6.2).

The glycoprotein IIb/IIIa inhibitors **eptifibatide** (in combination with unfractionated heparin and aspirin) and **tirofiban** (in combination with unfractionated heparin, aspirin, and clopidogrel) (section 2.9) can be used for unstable angina or for NSTEMI in patients at a high risk of either myocardial infarction or death.

In intermediate- and high-risk patients, abciximab or eptifibatide (in combination with unfractionated heparin and aspirin), or tirofiban (in combination with unfractionated heparin, aspirin, and clopidogrel) can also be used in patients undergoing percutaneous coronary intervention, to reduce the immediate risk of vascular occlusion. In intermediate- and high-risk patients in whom early intervention is planned, bivalirudin (section 2.8.1) can be considered as an alternative to the combination of a glyocprotein IIb/IIIa inhibitor plus a heparin.

Revascularisation procedures are often appropriate for patients with unstable angina or NSTEMI; see section 2.9 for the use of antiplatelet drugs in patients undergoing coronary stenting.

Long-term management The need for long-term angina treatment or for coronary angiography should be assessed. Most patients will require standard angina treatment (see management of stable angina, above) to prevent recurrence of symptoms.

Prevention of cardiovascular events Patients with stable angina, unstable angina, or NSTEMI should be given advice and treatments to reduce their cardiovascular risk. The importance of life-style changes, especially stopping smoking, should be emphasised. **Aspirin** should be given indefinitely in a dose of 75 mg daily. Antihypertensive treatment should be initiated if appropriate (see section 2.5), and a **statin** (section 2.12) should also be given.

In patients with stable angina, addition of an **ACE inhibitor** (section 2.5.5.1) should be considered for patients with diabetes (and should be continued if indicated for a co-morbidity).

In patients with unstable angina or NSTEMI, clopidogrel (section 2.9) is given, in combination with aspirin, for up to 12 months—most benefit occurs during the first 3 months. Prasugrel or ticagrelor are alternatives to clopidogrel in certain patients (see section 2.9). An ACE inhibitor should also be given.

Low-dose rivaroxaban (section 2.8.2), in combination with aspirin alone *or* aspirin and clopidogrel, is licensed for the prevention of atherothrombotic events following an acute coronary syndrome with elevated cardiac biomarkers. Treatment should be started as soon as possible after the patient has been stabilised following the acute coronary event, at the earliest 24 hours after admission to hospital, and at the time when parenteral anticoagulation therapy would normally be discontinued; the usual duration of treatment is 12 months.

Management of ST-segment elevation myocardial infarction (STEMI)

> Local guidelines for the management of myocardial infarction should be followed where they exist

These notes give an overview of the initial and long-term management of myocardial infarction with ST-segment elevation (STEMI). For advice on the management of non-ST-segment elevation myocardial infarction (NSTEMI) and unstable angina, see above. The aims of management of STEMI are to provide supportive care and pain relief, to promote reperfusion and to reduce mortality. Oxygen, nitrates, and diamorphine or morphine can provide initial support and pain relief; aspirin and percutaneous coronary intervention or thrombolytics promote reperfusion; anticoagulants help to reduce re-occlusion and systemic embolisation; long-term use of aspirin, beta-blockers, ACE inhibitors, and statins help to reduce mortality further.

Initial management **Oxygen** (section 3.6) should be administered if there is evidence of hypoxia, pulmonary oedema, or continuing myocardial ischaemia; hyperoxia should be avoided and particular care is required in patients with chronic obstructive airways disease.

The pain (and anxiety) of myocardial infarction is managed with slow intravenous injection of **diamorphine** or **morphine** (section 4.7.2); an antiemetic such as metoclopramide (or, if left ventricular function is not compromised, cyclizine) by intravenous injection should also be given (section 4.6).

Aspirin (chewed or dispersed in water) is given for its antiplatelet effect (section 2.9); a dose of 300 mg is suitable. If aspirin is given before arrival at hospital, a note saying that it has been given should be sent with the patient. **Clopidogrel**, in a dose of 300 mg (or 600 mg [unlicensed] if used prior to percutaneous coronary intervention), should also be given (section 2.9). **Prasugrel**, in a dose of 60 mg, is an alternative to clopidogrel in certain patients undergoing percutaneous coronary intervention (see NICE guidance, p. 160). **Ticagrelor**, in a dose of 180 mg, is also an alternative to clopidogrel (see NICE guidance, p. 160).

Patency of the occluded artery can be restored by percutaneous coronary intervention or by giving a **thrombolytic drug** (section 2.10.2), unless contra-indicated. Percutaneous coronary intervention is the preferred method; a **glycoprotein IIb/IIIa inhibitor** (section 2.9) can be used to reduce the risk of immediate vascular occlusion in intermediate- and high-risk patients. Patients undergoing percutaneous coronary intervention should also receive either unfractionated heparin or a low molecular weight heparin (e.g. enoxaparin); **bivalirudin** (section 2.8.1) is an alternative to the combination of a glycoprotein IIb/IIIa inhibitor plus a heparin (see also NICE guidance, p. 151). In patients who cannot be offered percutaneous coronary intervention within 90 minutes of diagnosis, a thrombolytic drug should be administered along with either unfractionated heparin (for maximum 2 days), a low molecular weight

heparin (e.g. enoxaparin), or fondaparinux. See section 2.9 for the use of antiplatelet drugs in patients undergoing coronary stenting.

Patients who do not receive reperfusion therapy (with percutaneous coronary intervention or a thrombolytic) should be treated with either fondaparinux, enoxaparin, or unfractionated heparin. Prescribers should consult product literature and local protocols (where they exist) for details of anticoagulant dose and duration.

Nitrates (section 2.6.1) are used to relieve ischaemic pain. If sublingual glyceryl trinitrate is not effective, intravenous glyceryl trinitrate or isosorbide dinitrate is given.

Early administration of some **beta-blockers** (section 2.4) has been shown to be of benefit and should be given to patients without contra-indications.

ACE inhibitors (section 2.5.5.1), and angiotensin-II receptor antagonists (section 2.5.5.2) if an ACE inhibitor cannot be used, are also of benefit to patients who have no contra-indications; in hypertensive and normotensive patients treatment with an ACE inhibitor, or an angiotensin-II receptor antagonist, can be started within 24 hours of the myocardial infarction and continued for at least 5–6 weeks (see below for long-term treatment).

All patients should be closely monitored for hyperglycaemia; those with diabetes or raised blood-glucose concentration should receive **insulin**.

Long-term management Long-term management following STEMI involves the use of several drugs which should ideally be started before the patient is discharged from hospital.

Aspirin (section 2.9) should be given to all patients, unless contra-indicated, at a dose of 75 mg daily. The addition of **clopidogrel** (section 2.9) has been shown to reduce morbidity and mortality. Prasugrel or ticagrelor are alternatives to clopidogrel in certain patients (see section 2.9). For those intolerant of clopidogrel, and who are at low risk of bleeding, the combination of **warfarin** (section 2.8.2) and aspirin should be considered. In those intolerant of both aspirin and clopidogrel, warfarin alone can be used. Warfarin should be continued for those who are already being treated for another indication, such as atrial fibrillation, with the addition of aspirin if there is a low risk of bleeding (see also section 2.8.2, p. 154). The combination of aspirin with clopidogrel or warfarin increases the risk of bleeding. Low-dose rivaroxaban (section 2.8.2), in combination with aspirin alone *or* aspirin and clopidogrel, is licensed for the prevention of atherothrombotic events following STEMI, also see notes above. See section 2.9 for details of antiplatelet drug duration following coronary stenting.

Beta-blockers (section 2.4) should be given to all patients in whom they are not contra-indicated. Acebutolol, metoprolol, propranolol, and timolol are suitable; for patients with left ventricular dysfunction, carvedilol, bisoprolol, or long-acting metoprolol may be appropriate (section 2.5.5).

Diltiazem [unlicensed] or **verapamil** (section 2.6.2) can be considered if a beta-blocker cannot be used; however, they are contra-indicated in those with left ventricular dysfunction. Other calcium-channel blockers have no place in routine long-term management after a myocardial infarction.

An **ACE inhibitor** (section 2.5.5.1) should be considered for all patients, especially those with evidence of left ventricular dysfunction. If an ACE inhibitor cannot be used, an angiotensin-II receptor antagonist may be used for patients with heart failure. A relatively high dose of either the ACE inhibitor or angiotensin-II receptor antagonist may be required to produce benefit.

Nitrates (section 2.6.1) are used for patients with angina.

Eplerenone (section 2.2.3) is licensed for use following a myocardial infarction in those with left ventricular dysfunction and evidence of heart failure.

For the role of **statins** in preventing recurrent cardiovascular events, see section 2.12.

2.10.2 Fibrinolytic drugs

Fibrinolytic drugs act as thrombolytics by activating plasminogen to form plasmin, which degrades fibrin and so breaks up thrombi.

The value of thrombolytic drugs for the treatment of *myocardial infarction* has been established (section 2.10.1). **Streptokinase** and **alteplase** have been shown to reduce mortality. **Reteplase** and **tenecteplase** are also licensed for acute myocardial infarction. Thrombolytic drugs are indicated for any patient with acute myocardial infarction for whom the benefit is likely to outweigh the risk of treatment. Trials have shown that the benefit is greatest in those with ECG changes that include ST segment elevation (especially in those with anterior infarction) and in patients with bundle branch block. Patients should not be denied thrombolytic treatment on account of age alone because mortality in the elderly is high and the reduction in mortality is the same as in younger patients. Alteplase should be given within 6–12 hours of symptom onset, reteplase and streptokinase within 12 hours of symptom onset, but ideally all should be given within 1 hour; use after 12 hours requires specialist advice. Tenecteplase should be given as early as possible and usually within 6 hours of symptom onset.

Alteplase, streptokinase, and **urokinase** can be used for other thromboembolic disorders such as deep-vein thrombosis and pulmonary embolism. Alteplase is also used for acute ischaemic stroke (see section 2.9).

Urokinase is also licensed to restore the patency of occluded intravenous catheters and cannulas blocked with fibrin clots.

Cautions   Thrombolytic drugs should be used with caution if there is a risk of bleeding including that from venepuncture or invasive procedures. They should also be used with caution in external chest compression, elderly, hypertension, conditions in which thrombolysis might give rise to embolic complications such as enlarged left atrium with atrial fibrillation (risk of dissolution of clot and subsequent embolisation), and recent or concurrent use of drugs that increase the risk of bleeding.

Contra-indications   Thrombolytic drugs are contra-indicated in recent haemorrhage, trauma, or surgery (including dental extraction), coagulation defects, bleeding diatheses, aortic dissection, aneurysm, coma, history of cerebrovascular disease especially recent events or with any residual disability, recent symptoms of possible peptic ulceration, heavy vaginal bleeding,

severe hypertension, active pulmonary disease with cavitation, acute pancreatitis, pericarditis, bacterial endocarditis, and oesophageal varices; also in the case of streptokinase, previous allergic reactions to either streptokinase or anistreplase (no longer available).

Prolonged persistence of antibodies to streptokinase and anistreplase (no longer available) can reduce the effectiveness of subsequent treatment; therefore, streptokinase should not be used again beyond 4 days of first administration of either streptokinase or anistreplase.

Hepatic impairment   Thrombolytic drugs should be avoided in severe hepatic impairment as there is an increased risk of bleeding.

Pregnancy   Thrombolytic drugs can possibly lead to premature separation of the placenta in the first 18 weeks of pregnancy. There is also a risk of maternal haemorrhage throughout pregnancy and post-partum, and also a theoretical risk of fetal haemorrhage throughout pregnancy.

Side-effects   Side-effects of thrombolytics are mainly nausea and vomiting and bleeding. When thrombolytics are used in myocardial infarction, reperfusion arrhythmias and recurrent ischaemia and angina may occur. Reperfusion may also cause cerebral and pulmonary oedema. Hypotension can also occur and can usually be controlled by elevating the patient's legs, or by reducing the rate of infusion or stopping it temporarily. Back pain, fever, and convulsions have been reported. Bleeding is usually limited to the site of injection, but intracerebral haemorrhage or bleeding from other sites can occur. Serious bleeding calls for discontinuation of the thrombolytic and may require administration of coagulation factors and antifibrinolytic drugs (e.g. tranexamic acid). Rarely further embolism may occur (either due to clots that break away from the original thrombus or to cholesterol crystal emboli). Thrombolytics can cause allergic reactions (including rash, flushing and uveitis) and anaphylaxis has been reported (for details of management see Allergic Emergencies, section 3.4.3). Guillain-Barré syndrome has been reported rarely after streptokinase treatment.

> **NICE guidance**
> **Alteplase for the treatment of acute ischaemic stroke (September 2012)**
> Alteplase is recommended for the treatment of acute ischaemic stroke in adults in accordance with its licensed indication if:
> - treatment is started as early as possible within 4.5 hours of onset of stroke symptoms, *and*
> - intracranial haemorrhage has been excluded by appropriate imaging techniques
>
> www.nice.org.uk/TA264

◢ ALTEPLASE

(rt-PA, tissue-type plasminogen activator)

Indications   acute myocardial infarction (see notes above and section 2.10.1); pulmonary embolism; acute ischaemic stroke (treatment under specialist neurology physician **only**); thrombolytic treatment of occluded central venous access devices (including those used for haemodialysis)

Cautions   see notes above; *in acute stroke*, monitor for intracranial haemorrhage, monitor blood pressure

2 Cardiovascular system

(antihypertensive recommended if systolic above 180 mmHg or diastolic above 105 mmHg)

Contra-indications see notes above; hypersensitivity to gentamicin (residue from manufacturing process); *in acute stroke*, convulsion accompanying stroke, severe stroke, history of stroke in patients with diabetes, stroke in last 3 months, hypoglycaemia, hyperglycaemia

Hepatic impairment see notes above

Pregnancy see notes above

Side-effects see notes above; also risk of cerebral bleeding increased in acute stroke

Dose

● See under preparations below

Actilyse® (Boehringer Ingelheim) PoM

Injection, powder for reconstitution, alteplase 10 mg (5.8 million units)/vial, net price per vial (with diluent) = £144.00; 20 mg (11.6 million units)/vial (with diluent and transfer device) = £216.00; 50 mg (29 million units)/vial (with diluent and transfer device) = £360.00

Dose myocardial infarction, accelerated regimen (initiated within 6 hours of symptom onset), 15 mg by intravenous injection, followed by intravenous infusion of 50 mg over 30 minutes, then 35 mg over 60 minutes (total dose 100 mg over 90 minutes); in patients less than 65 kg, 15 mg by intravenous injection, followed by intravenous infusion of 0.75 mg/kg over 30 minutes, then 0.5 mg/kg over 60 minutes (max. total dose 100 mg over 90 minutes)

Myocardial infarction, initiated within 6–12 hours of symptom onset, 10 mg by intravenous injection, followed by intravenous infusion of 50 mg over 60 minutes, then 4 infusions each of 10 mg over 30 minutes (total dose 100 mg over 3 hours; max. 1.5 mg/kg in patients less than 65 kg)

Pulmonary embolism, 10 mg by intravenous injection over 1–2 minutes, followed by intravenous infusion of 90 mg over 2 hours; max. 1.5 mg/kg in patients less than 65 kg

Acute stroke (treatment **must** begin within 4.5 hours of symptom onset), by intravenous administration over 60 minutes, 900 micrograms/kg (max. 90 mg); initial 10% of dose by intravenous injection, remainder by intravenous infusion; ELDERLY over 80 years not recommended

Actilyse Cathflo® (Boehringer Ingelheim) PoM

Injection, powder for reconstitution, alteplase 2 mg (1.16 million units)/vial, net price per vial (with diluent) = £45.00

Dose thrombolytic treatment of occluded central venous access devices, consult product literature

RETEPLASE

Indications acute myocardial infarction (see notes above and section 2.10.1)

Cautions see notes above

Contra-indications see notes above

Hepatic impairment see notes above

Pregnancy see notes above

Breast-feeding manufacturer advises avoid breast-feeding for 24 hours after dose (express and discard milk during this time)

Side-effects see notes above

Dose

● By intravenous injection (initiated within 12 hours of symptom onset), 10 units over not more than 2 minutes, followed after 30 minutes by a further 10 units

Rapilysin® (Actavis) PoM

Injection, powder for reconstitution, reteplase 10 units/vial, net price pack of 2 vials (with 2 prefilled syringes of diluent and transfer device) = £566.00

STREPTOKINASE

Indications acute myocardial infarction (see notes above and section 2.10.1); deep-vein thrombosis, pulmonary embolism, acute arterial thromboembolism, and central retinal venous or arterial thrombosis

Cautions see notes above

Contra-indications see notes above

Hepatic impairment see notes above

Pregnancy see notes above

Side-effects see notes above

Dose

● Myocardial infarction (initiated within 12 hours of symptom onset), by intravenous infusion, 1.5 million units over 60 minutes

● Deep-vein thrombosis, pulmonary embolism, acute arterial thromboembolism, central retinal venous or arterial thrombosis, by intravenous infusion, 250 000 units over 30 minutes, then 100 000 units every hour for up to 12–72 hours according to condition with monitoring of clotting parameters (consult product literature)

Streptase® (CSL Behring) PoM

Injection, powder for reconstitution, streptokinase, net price 250 000-unit vial = £13.52; 1.5 million-unit vial = £70.92 (hosp. only)

TENECTEPLASE

Indications acute myocardial infarction (see notes above and section 2.10.1)

Cautions see notes above

Contra-indications see notes above

Hepatic impairment see notes above

Pregnancy see notes above

Breast-feeding manufacturer advises avoid breast-feeding for 24 hours after dose (express and discard milk during this time)

Side-effects see notes above

Dose

● By intravenous injection over 10 seconds (initiated within 6 hours of symptom onset), 30–50 mg according to body-weight—consult product literature; max. 50 mg

Metalyse® (Boehringer Ingelheim) PoM

Injection, powder for reconstitution, tenecteplase, net price 40-mg (8000-unit) vial = £502.25; 50-mg (10 000-unit) vial = £502.25 (both with prefilled syringe of water for injection)

UROKINASE

Indications thromboembolic occlusive vascular disease including deep-vein thrombosis, pulmonary embolism, and occlusive peripheral arterial disease; occluded arteriovenous haemodialysis shunts, and intravenous catheters and cannulas blocked by fibrin clots

Cautions see notes above

Contra-indications see notes above

Hepatic impairment dose reduction may be required; see also notes above

Renal impairment dose reduction may be required

Pregnancy see notes above

2 Cardiovascular system

Breast-feeding manufacturer advises avoid—no information available

Side-effects see notes above

Dose

- See under preparations below

Urokinase (Non-proprietary) PoM

Injection, powder for reconstitution, urokinase, net price 10 000-unit vial = £33.79; 50 000-unit vial = £69.70; 100 000-unit vial = £106.17; 250 000-unit vial = £185.65; 500 000-unit vial = £365.00

Dose deep-vein thrombosis, by intravenous infusion, initially 4400 units/kg over 10–20 minutes, followed by 100 000 units/hour for 2–3 days

Pulmonary embolism, by intravenous infusion, initially 4400 units/kg over 10–20 minutes, followed by 4400 units/kg/hour for 12 hours

Occlusive peripheral arterial disease, consult product literature

Occluded central venous catheters, by injection directly into catheter, dissolve in sodium chloride 0.9% to a concentration of 5000 units/mL; use a volume sufficient to fill the catheter lumen; leave for 20–60 minutes then aspirate the lysate; repeat if necessary

Occluded arteriovenous haemodialysis shunts, consult product literature

Syner-KINASE® (Syner-Med) PoM

Injection, powder for reconstitution, urokinase, net price 10 000-unit vial = £35.95; 25 000-unit vial = £45.95; 100 000-unit vial = £112.95

Dose deep-vein thrombosis, by intravenous infusion, initially 4400 units/kg in 15 mL sodium chloride 0.9% over 10 minutes, followed by 4400 units/kg/hour for 12–24 hours

Pulmonary embolism, by intravenous infusion, initially 4400 units/kg in 15 mL sodium chloride 0.9% over 10 minutes, followed by 4400 units/kg/hour for 12 hours *or* by injection into pulmonary artery, initially 15 000 units/kg, subsequent doses adjusted according to response; max. 3 doses in 24 hours

Occlusive peripheral arterial disease, consult product literature

Occluded catheters and cannulas, by injection directly into catheter or cannula, 5000–25 000 units dissolved in suitable volume of sodium chloride 0.9% to fill the catheter or cannula lumen; leave for 20–60 minutes then aspirate the lysate; repeat if necessary

2.11 Antifibrinolytic drugs and haemostatics

Fibrin dissolution can be impaired by the administration of **tranexamic acid**, which inhibits fibrinolysis. It can be used to prevent bleeding or to treat bleeding associated with excessive fibrinolysis (e.g. in surgery, dental extraction, obstetric disorders, and traumatic hyphaema) and in the management of menorrhagia. Tranexamic acid may also be used in hereditary angioedema, epistaxis, and in thrombolytic overdose.

Desmopressin (section 6.5.2) is used in the management of mild to moderate haemophilia and von Willebrand's disease. It is also used for fibrinolytic response testing.

Etamsylate reduces capillary bleeding in the presence of a normal number of platelets; it does not act by fibrin stabilisation, but probably by correcting abnormal adhesion. Etamsylate is less effective than other treatments in the management of heavy menstrual bleeding and its use is no longer recommended.

ETAMSYLATE
(Ethamsylate)

Indications short-term blood loss in menorrhagia

Cautions exclude structural or histological causes of menorrhagia, or fibroids causing distortion of the uterine cavity, before initiating treatment

Contra-indications acute porphyria (see section 9.8.2)

Breast-feeding present in milk—manufacturer advises avoid

Side-effects nausea, vomiting, diarrhoea, fever (discontinue treatment), headache, rashes

Dose

- 500 mg 4 times daily during menstruation

Dicynene® (Sanofi-Aventis) PoM

Tablets, scored, etamsylate 500 mg, net price 100-tab pack = £8.44

Excipients include sulfites

TRANEXAMIC ACID

Indications see notes above

Cautions massive haematuria (avoid if risk of ureteric obstruction); irregular menstrual bleeding (exclude structural or histological causes of menorrhagia, or fibroids causing distortion of the uterine cavity, before initiating treatment); patients receiving oral contraceptives (increased risk of thrombosis); regular liver function tests in long-term treatment of hereditary angioedema

Contra-indications thromboembolic disease; fibrinolytic conditions following disseminated intravascular coagulation (unless predominant activation of fibrinolytic system with severe bleeding); history of convulsions

Renal impairment reduce dose—consult product literature for details

Pregnancy no evidence of teratogenicity in *animal* studies; manufacturer advises use only if potential benefit outweighs risk—crosses the placenta

Breast-feeding small amount present in milk—antifibrinolytic effect in infant unlikely

Side-effects nausea, vomiting, diarrhoea (reduce dose); *less commonly* dermatitis; *rarely* thromboembolic events, visual disturbances including impairment of colour vision (discontinue); *also reported* malaise and hypotension on rapid intravenous injection, convulsions (usually with high doses)

Dose

- By mouth, local fibrinolysis, 1–1.5 g (*or* 15–25 mg/kg) 2–3 times daily

  Menorrhagia (initiated when menstruation has started), 1 g 3 times daily for up to 4 days; max. 4 g daily

  Hereditary angioedema, 1–1.5 g 2–3 times daily

  Epistaxis, 1 g 3 times daily for 7 days

- By slow intravenous injection (rate not exceeding 100 mg/minute), local fibrinolysis, 0.5–1 g 2–3 times daily

  General fibrinolysis, 1 g (*or* 15 mg/kg) every 6–8 hours

- By continuous intravenous infusion, local fibrinolysis [unlicensed route], following initial treatment by intravenous injection, 25–50 mg/kg over 24 hours

Tranexamic acid (Non-proprietary) PoM

Tablets, tranexamic acid 500 mg, net price 60-tab pack = £7.17

Injection, tranexamic acid 100 mg/mL, net price 5-mL amp = £1.50 (hosp. only)

Cyklokapron® (Meda) PoM

Tablets, f/c, scored, tranexamic acid 500 mg, net price 60-tab pack = £14.30

Cyklokapron® (Pfizer) PoM

Injection, tranexamic acid 100 mg/mL, net price 5-mL amp = £1.55

Blood-related products

▮ DRIED PROTHROMBIN COMPLEX
(Human Prothrombin Complex)

Dried prothrombin complex is prepared from human plasma by a suitable fractionation technique, and contains factor IX, together with variable amounts of factors II, VII, and X

Indications treatment and peri-operative prophylaxis of haemorrhage in patients with congenital deficiency of factors II, VII, IX, or X if purified specific coagulation factors not available; treatment and peri-operative prophylaxis of haemorrhage in patients with acquired deficiency of factors II, VII, IX, or X (e.g. during warfarin treatment—see section 2.8.2)

Cautions risk of thrombosis; disseminated intravascular coagulation; history of myocardial infarction or coronary heart disease; postoperative use

Contra-indications angina; recent myocardial infarction (except in life-threatening haemorrhage following overdosage of oral anticoagulants, and before induction of fibrinolytic therapy); history of heparin-induced thrombocytopenia

Hepatic impairment monitor closely (risk of thromoembolic complications)

Side-effects thrombotic events (including disseminated intravascular coagulation); *rarely* headache; *very rarely* pyrexia, antibody formation, hypersensitivity reactions (including anaphylaxis); nephrotic syndrome also reported

Available from CSL Behring (*Beriplex*® *P/N*), Octapharma (*Octaplex*®)

▮ FACTOR VIIa (RECOMBINANT)
Eptacog alfa (activated)

Indications treatment and prophylaxis of haemorrhage in patients with haemophilia A or B with inhibitors to factors VIII or IX, acquired haemophilia, factor VII deficiency, or Glanzmann's thrombasthenia

Cautions risk of thrombosis or disseminated intravascular coagulation

Side-effects *less commonly* fever, venous thromboembolic events (including deep vein thrombosis and pulmonary embolism), rash; *rarely* nausea, angina, headache, arterial thrombotic events (including myocardial infarction and cerebrovascular accident), coagulation disorders; *also reported* flushing, angioedema, anaphylaxis

Available from Novo Nordisk (*NovoSeven*®)

▮ FACTOR VIII FRACTION, DRIED
(Human Coagulation Factor VIII, Dried)

Dried factor VIII fraction is prepared from human plasma by a suitable fractionation technique; it may also contain varying amounts of von Willebrand factor

Indications treatment and prophylaxis of haemorrhage in congenital factor VIII deficiency (haemophilia A), acquired factor VIII deficiency, von Willebrand's disease

Cautions monitor for development of factor VIII inhibitors; intravascular haemolysis after large or frequently repeated doses in patients with blood groups A, B, or AB—less likely with high potency concentrates

Side-effects gastro-intestinal disturbances, taste disturbances; flushing, palpitation; dyspnoea, coughing; headache, dizziness, paraesthesia, drowsiness; blurred vision; antibody formation; hypersensitivity reactions including hypotension, angioedema, chills, fever, urticaria, and anaphylaxis

Available from Biotest UK (*Haemoctin*®), CSL Behring (*Haemate*® *P*), BPL (*Optivate*®, High Purity Factor VIII and von Willebrand factor concentrate; *8Y*®), Grifols (*Alphanate*®; *Fanhdi*®), Octapharma (*Octanate*®; *Wilate*®); *Haemoctin*®, *Optivate*®, *Fanhdi*®, and *Octanate*® are not indicated for use in von Willebrand's disease

Note Preparation of recombinant human coagulation factor VIII (octocog alfa) available from CSL Behring (*Helixate*® *NexGen*), Baxter (*Advate*®), Bayer (*Kogenate*® *Bayer*); preparation of recombinant human coagulation factor VIII (moroctocog alfa) available from Wyeth (*ReFacto AF*®); octocog alfa and moroctocog alfa are not indicated for use in von Willebrand's disease

▮ FACTOR VIII INHIBITOR BYPASSING FRACTION

Preparations with factor VIII inhibitor bypassing activity are prepared from human plasma

Indications treatment and prophylaxis of haemorrhage in patients with congenital factor VIII deficiency (haemophilia A) and factor VIII inhibitors; treatment of haemorrhage in non-haemophiliac patients with acquired factor VIII inhibitors

Contra-indications disseminated intravascular coagulation

Side-effects thrombosis, disseminated intravascular coagulation, myocardial infarction; paraesthesia; pyrexia; hypersensitivity reactions including hypotension, flushing, urticaria, rash, and anaphylaxis

Available from Baxter (*FEIBA*®)

▮ FACTOR IX FRACTION, DRIED

Dried factor IX fraction is prepared from human plasma by a suitable fractionation technique; it may also contain clotting factors II, VII, and X

Indications treatment and prophylaxis of haemorrhage in congenital factor IX deficiency (haemophilia B)

Cautions risk of thrombosis—principally with former low purity products

Contra-indications disseminated intravascular coagulation

Side-effects gastro-intestinal disturbances; headache, dizziness; allergic reactions, including chills, fever

2 Cardiovascular system

Available from CSL Behring (*Mononine*®), BPL (*Replenine*®-*VF*, Dried Factor IX Fraction), Grifols (*AlphaNine*®), Biotest UK (*Haemonine*®)

Note Preparation of recombinant coagulation factor IX (nonacog alfa) available from Pfizer (*BeneFIX*®)

■ FACTOR XIII FRACTION, DRIED

(Human Fibrin-stabilising Factor, Dried)

Indications congenital factor XIII deficiency

Side-effects rarely, allergic reactions and fever

Available from CSL Behring (*Fibrogammin*® P)

■ FIBRINOGEN, DRIED

(Human Fibrinogen)

Fibrinogen is prepared from human plasma

Indications treatment of haemorrhage in congenital hypofibrinogenaemia or afibrinogenaemia

Cautions risk of thrombosis

Pregnancy manufacturer advises not known to be harmful—no information available

Breast-feeding manufacturer advises avoid—no information available

Side-effects *rarely* fever, allergic reactions; *very rarely* thromboembolic events (including myocardial infarction and pulmonary embolism)

Available from CSL Behring (*Riastap*®)

■ FRESH FROZEN PLASMA

Fresh frozen plasma is prepared from the supernatant liquid obtained by centrifugation of one donation of whole blood

Indications to replace coagulation factors or other plasma proteins where their concentration or functional activity is critically reduced

Cautions need for compatibility; cardiac decompensation; pulmonary oedema; severe protein S deficiency (avoid products with low protein S activity e.g. *OctaplasLG*®)

Contra-indications avoid use as a volume expander; IgA deficiency with confirmed antibodies to IgA

Side-effects nausea, rash, pruritus; *less commonly* vomiting, oedema; *rarely* tachycardia, agitation, allergic reactions (including chills, fever, bronchospasm, cardiorespiratory collapse); *very rarely* arrhythmia, thromboembolism, hypertension

Available from Regional Blood Transfusion Services

Note A preparation of solvent/detergent treated human plasma (frozen) from pooled donors is available from Octapharma (*OctaplasLG*®)

■ PROTEIN C CONCENTRATE

Protein C is prepared from human plasma

Indications congenital protein C deficiency

Cautions hypersensitivity to heparins

Side-effects *very rarely* fever, bleeding, dizziness, and hypersensitivity reactions

Available from Baxter (*Ceprotin*®)

2.12 Lipid-regulating drugs

Primary and secondary prevention of cardiovascular disease Preventative measures should be taken in individuals with a high risk of developing cardiovascular disease (primary prevention) and to prevent recurrence of events in those with established cardiovascular disease (secondary prevention).

Primary prevention Individuals at high risk of developing cardiovascular disease include those who have diabetes mellitus, chronic kidney disease (eGFR < 60 mL/minute/1.73m²) and/or albuminuria, and those with familial hypercholesterolaemia. The risk also increases with age; those aged 85 years and over are at particularly high risk, especially if they smoke or have hypertension. Preventative measures are also required for other individuals who are considered to be at high risk of developing atherosclerotic cardiovascular disease based on risk estimated using risk calculators (see below); those with a 10-year risk of cardiovascular disease of 10% or more stand to benefit most from drug treatment. Patients with a 10-year cardiovascular risk of less than 10% may benefit from an assessment of their lifetime risk (using the JBS3 tool, see below), discussion on the impact of lifestyle interventions and, if necessary, drug therapy.

Risk calculators Risk assessment calculators are recommended by both NICE[1] and JBS3.[2] They should not be used in patients at high cardiovascular risk. Both calculators are unsuitable for assessing risk in those aged 85 years and over, and NICE advises against using a risk assessment tool in those with type 1 diabetes mellitus.

The QRISK®2 risk calculator (www.qrisk.org/) is recommended by NICE Clinical Guideline181[1], and the JBS3 risk calculator (www.jbs3risk.com/pages/risk_calculator.htm) is endorsed by JBS3.[2] Both tools assess cardiovascular risk—coronary heart disease (angina and myocardial infarction), stroke, and transient ischaemic attack, on the basis of lipid profile, systolic blood pressure, gender, age, ethnicity, smoking status, BMI, chronic kidney disease, diabetes mellitus, atrial fibrillation, treated hypertension, rheumatoid arthritis, or a family history of premature cardiovascular disease. Risk assessment tools underestimate risk in patients with additional risk due to existing conditions or medication, such as:

- serious mental disorder
- autoimmune disorders such as systemic lupus erythematosus and other systemic inflammatory disorders
- antiretroviral treatment
- medication causing dyslipidaemia as a side-effect e.g. antipsychotics, corticosteroids, or immunosuppressants
- triglyceride concentration > 4.5 mmol/litre

Cardiovascular disease risk is also underestimated in those who are already taking antihypertensive or lipid-regulating drugs, and in those who have recently stopped smoking. Severe obesity (BMI > 40 kg/m²) also increases cardiovascular risk; the need for further treatment of risk factors in patients below the cardiovascular risk threshold for treatment should be based on clinical judgement.

1. NICE clinical guideline 181 (July 2014). Lipid Modification—Cardiovascular risk assessment and the modification of blood lipids for the primary and secondary prevention of cardiovascular disease
2. Joint British Societies' consensus recommendations for the prevention of cardiovascular disease (JBS3) 2014

Reduction in low-density lipoprotein cholesterol

Dose (mg/day)	5	10	20	40	80
Atorvastatin	–	37%[1]	43%[2]	49%[2]	55%[2]
Fluvastatin	–	–	21%[3]	27%[3]	33%[1]
Pravastatin	–	20%[3]	24%[3]	29%[3]	–
Rosuvastatin	38%[1]	43%[2]	48%[2]	53%[2]	–
Simvastatin	–	27%[3]	32%[1]	37%[1]	42%[2,4]

1. 31%–40%: medium intensity
2. Above 40%: high intensity
3. 20%–30%: low intensity
4. Advice from the MHRA: there is an increased risk of myopathy associated with high-dose (80 mg) simvastatin. The 80 mg dose should be considered only in patients with severe hypercholesterolaemia and high risk of cardiovascular complications who have not achieved their treatment goals on lower doses, when the benefits are expected to outweigh the potential risks

Preventative measures for primary prevention All patients at high risk of cardiovascular disease should be advised to make lifestyle modifications that include beneficial changes to diet, exercise, weight management, alcohol consumption, and smoking cessation.

Offer a statin as first-line drug treatment if lifestyle modifications are inappropriate or ineffective (see also Statins for the Prevention of Cardiovascular Disease below). Lipid-regulating drug treatment must be combined with advice on diet and lifestyle measures, and where appropriate, treatment of comorbidities and secondary causes of dyslipidaemia.

Secondary prevention Statins should be offered to all patients, including the elderly, with cardiovascular disease such as those with coronary heart disease (including history of angina or acute myocardial infarction), occlusive arterial disease (including peripheral vascular disease, non-haemorrhagic stroke, or transient ischaemic attacks).

Preventative measures for secondary prevention Patients should be advised to make lifestyle modifications that include beneficial changes to diet, exercise, weight management, alcohol consumption, and smoking cessation, however, initiation of lipid-regulating drug treatment should not be delayed to manage modifiable risk factors, and must be combined with advice on diet and lifestyle measures, and where appropriate, treatment of comorbidities and secondary causes of dyslipidaemia.

Statins for the prevention of cardiovascular disease A statin (see p. 174) reduces the risk of cardiovascular disease events, and is the drug of first choice for primary and secondary prevention of cardiovascular disease.

Before starting treatment with statins, at least one full lipid profile (non-fasting) should be measured, including total cholesterol, HDL-cholesterol, non-HDL-cholesterol (calculated as total cholesterol minus HDL-cholesterol), and triglyceride concentrations. HbA_{1c}, thyroid-stimulating hormone, and renal and hepatic function should also be assessed. Secondary causes of dyslipidaemia should be addressed; these include uncontrolled diabetes mellitus, hepatic disease, nephrotic syndrome, and excessive alcohol consumption. Patients with hypothyroidism should receive adequate thyroid replacement therapy (before assessing the requirement for lipid-regulating treatment if for primary prevention) because correcting hypothyroidism itself may resolve

the lipid abnormality. Untreated hypothyroidism increases the risk of myositis with lipid-regulating drugs.

For the purpose of reducing cardiovascular risk, NICE Clinical Guideline 181[1] defines statins by the percentage reduction in LDL-cholesterol they achieve, see table above.

For *primary prevention*, NICE Clinical Guideline 181 recommends that atorvastatin, a high-intensity statin (when prescribed at a dose of at least 20 mg/day), should be offered to those with a 10-year risk of cardiovascular disease of 10% or more; patients aged 85 years and over may benefit from atorvastatin to reduce the risk of non-fatal myocardial infarction. For *secondary prevention*, atorvastatin is also recommended. See Atorvastatin p. 175 for recommended doses. Patients taking a low- or medium-intensity statin should discuss the benefits and risks of switching to a high intensity statin at their next medication review.

A statin should be considered for *all* adults with type 1 diabetes mellitus, particularly those aged 40 years and over, or who have had diabetes for more than 10 years, or who have established nephropathy, or other risk factors for cardiovascular disease. JBS3 recommendations[2] in diabetes mellitus differ in certain respects from NICE Clinical Guideline 181[1]—see JBS3 recommendations for further details. In type 2 diabetes, assess level of risk using the risk calculator and treat for primary prevention if necessary.

Total cholesterol, HDL-cholesterol, and non-HDL cholesterol concentrations should be checked 3 months after starting treatment with a high intensity statin. NICE Clinical Guideline 181 recommends aiming for a reduction in non-HDL cholesterol concentration greater than 40%; JBS3 recommends a target non-HDL cholesterol concentration below 2.5 mmol/litre. If these are not achieved, ensure lifestyle modifications are optimised and consider increasing the dose of the statin if started on less than atorvastatin 80 mg and the patient is judged to be at higher risk because of comorbidities, risk score or, using clinical judgement.

Specialist advice should be sought about treatment options for patients at high risk of cardiovascular disease or those with existing cardiovascular disease, who are intolerant of three different statins.

Fibrates should not be routinely used for primary or secondary prevention. **Nicotinic acid, bile acid**

1. NICE clinical guideline 181 (July 2014). Lipid Modification—Cardiovascular risk assessment and the modification of blood lipids for the primary and secondary prevention of cardiovascular disease
2. Joint British Societies' consensus recommendations for the prevention of cardiovascular disease (JBS3) 2014

sequestrants, and **omega-3 fatty acid compounds** are not recommended for primary or secondary prevention.

Hypercholesterolaemia, hypertriglyceridaemia, and familial hypercholesterolaemia

A statin is also the drug of first choice for treating hypercholesterolaemia and moderate hypertriglyceridaemia. Severe hyperlipidaemia not adequately controlled with a maximal dose of a statin may require the use of an additional lipid-regulating drug such as **ezetimibe**; such treatment should generally be supervised by a specialist.

A number of conditions, some familial, are characterised by very high LDL-cholesterol concentration, high triglyceride concentration, or both. **Fenofibrate** may be added to statin therapy if triglycerides remain high even after the LDL-cholesterol concentration has been reduced adequately; nicotinic acid may also be used to further lower triglyceride or LDL-cholesterol concentration.

Combination of a statin with a fibrate or with nicotinic acid carries an increased risk of side-effects (including rhabdomyolysis—see Muscle Effects, p. 175) and should be used under specialist supervision; monitoring of liver function and creatine kinase should also be considered. The concomitant administration of gemfibrozil with a statin increases the risk of rhabdomyolysis considerably—this combination should **not** be used.

A statin is recommended for all patients with familial hypercholesterolaemia. A 'high-intensity' statin (as defined in NICE Clinical Guideline 71[1] e.g. rosuvastatin (initiated by a specialist) or atorvastatin) should be considered in order to achieve the recommended reduction in LDL-cholesterol concentration of greater than 50% from baseline; a 'high-intensity' statin is one that produces a greater LDL-cholesterol reduction than simvastatin 40 mg. Patients with heterozygous familial hypercholesterolaemia who have contra-indications to, or are intolerant of, statins should receive ezetimibe. The combination of a statin and ezetimibe can be considered if a statin alone fails to provide adequate control (or if intolerance limits dose titration), and when a switch to an alternative statin is being considered. Patients for whom statins and ezetimibe are inappropriate, should be referred to a specialist for the consideration of treatment with a bile acid sequestrant, nicotinic acid, or a fibrate.

The prescribing of drug therapy in homozygous familial hypercholesterolaemia should be undertaken in a specialist centre. **Lomitapide** is licensed as an adjunct to dietary measures and other lipid-regulating drugs for the treatment of homozygous familial hypercholesterolaemia.

Statins

The statins (**atorvastatin**, **fluvastatin**, **pravastatin**, **rosuvastatin**, and **simvastatin**) competitively inhibit 3-hydroxy-3-methylglutaryl coenzyme A (HMG CoA) reductase, an enzyme involved in cholesterol synthesis, especially in the liver. Statins are more effective than other lipid-regulating drugs at lowering LDL-cholesterol concentration but they are less effective than the fibrates in reducing triglyceride concentration. However, statins reduce cardiovascular disease events and total mortality irrespective of the initial cholesterol concentration.

Statins are used for the primary and secondary prevention of cardiovascular disease (see p. 172).

Cautions See Lipid-regulating drugs, p. 173 for details of the management of hypothyroidism and the monitoring recommended before starting treatment with a statin.

Statins should be used with caution in those with a history of liver disease or with a high alcohol intake—see also Hepatic impairment, below. There is little information available on a rational approach to liver-function monitoring; however, a NICE guideline[2] suggests that liver enzymes should be measured before treatment, and repeated within 3 months and at 12 months of starting treatment, unless indicated at other times by signs or symptoms suggestive of hepatotoxicity. Those with serum transaminases that are raised, but less than 3 times the upper limit of the reference range, should **not** be routinely excluded from statin therapy. Those with serum transaminases of more than 3 times the upper limit of the reference range should discontinue statin therapy.

Statins should be used with caution in those with risk factors for myopathy or rhabdomyolysis (see Muscle Effects below); patients should be advised to report unexplained muscle pain. Before initiation of statin treatment, creatine kinase concentration should be measured in patients who have had persistent, generalised, unexplained muscle pain (whether associated or not with previous lipid-regulating drugs); if the concentration is more than 5 times the upper limit of normal, a repeat measurement should be taken after 7 days. If the repeat concentration remains above 5 times the upper limit, statin treatment should not be started; if concentrations are still raised but less than 5 times the upper limit, the statin should be started at a lower dose.

Patients at high risk of diabetes mellitus should have fasting blood-glucose concentration or HbA$_{1C}$ checked before starting statin treatment, and then repeated after 3 months (see Side-effects). **Interactions:** Appendix 1 (statins).

Hepatic impairment Statins should be used with caution in those with a history of liver disease and avoided in active liver disease or when there are unexplained persistent elevations in serum transaminases.

Pregnancy Statins should be avoided in pregnancy (discontinue 3 months before attempting to conceive) as congenital anomalies have been reported and the decreased synthesis of cholesterol possibly affects fetal development. Adequate contraception is required during treatment and for 1 month afterwards.

Breast-feeding The manufacturers of atorvastatin, fluvastatin, rosuvastatin, and simvastatin advise avoiding use in mothers who are breast-feeding as there is no information available. The manufacturers of pravastatin advise against use in breast-feeding mothers as a small amount of drug is present in breast milk.

Side-effects The statins have been associated with myalgia, myopathy, myositis, and rhabdomyolysis (see Muscle Effects below). Statins can alter liver function tests, and rarely cause hepatitis and jaundice; pancreatitis and hepatic failure have been reported very rarely. Other side-effects include gastro-intestinal disturbances,

---

1. NICE Clinical Guideline 71 (August 2008). Identification and management of familial hypercholesterolaemia

2. NICE clinical guideline 181 (July 2014). Lipid Modification—Cardiovascular risk assessment and the modification of blood lipids for the primary and secondary prevention of cardiovascular disease

sleep disturbance, headache, dizziness, depression, paraesthesia, asthenia, peripheral neuropathy, amnesia, fatigue, sexual dysfunction, thrombocytopenia, arthralgia, visual disturbance, alopecia, and hypersensitivity reactions (including rash, pruritus, urticaria, and very rarely lupus erythematosus-like reactions). In very rare cases, statins can cause interstitial lung disease; if patients develop symptoms such as dyspnoea, cough, and weight loss, they should seek medical attention. Statins can cause hyperglycaemia and may be associated with the development of diabetes mellitus, particularly in those already at risk of the condition; statins should not be discontinued if there is an increase in the blood-glucose concentration or HbA$_{1c}$ as the benefits continue to outweigh the risks.

Muscle effects The risk of myopathy, myositis, and rhabdomyolysis associated with statin use is rare. Although myalgia has been reported commonly in patients receiving statins, muscle toxicity truly attributable to statin use is rare. Muscle toxicity can occur with all statins, however the likelihood increases with higher doses and in certain patients (see below). Statins should be used with caution in patients at increased risk of muscle toxicity, including those with a personal or family history of muscular disorders, previous history of muscular toxicity, a high alcohol intake, renal impairment, hypothyroidism, and in the elderly. There is an increased incidence of myopathy if a statin is given at a high dose, or if it is given with a fibrate (the combination of a statin and gemfibrozil should preferably be avoided), with lipid-lowering doses of nicotinic acid, with fusidic acid (risk of rhabdomyolysis—the combination of a statin and fusidic acid should be avoided; temporarily discontinue statin and restart 7 days after last fusidic acid dose), or with drugs that increase the plasma-statin concentration, such as macrolide antibiotics, imidazole and triazole antifungals, and ciclosporin—see **interactions:** Appendix 1 (statins); close monitoring of liver function and, if muscular symptoms occur, of creatine kinase is necessary. In patients at increased risk of muscle effects, a statin should not usually be started if the baseline creatine kinase concentration is more than 5 times the upper limit of normal (some patients may present with an extremely elevated baseline creatine kinase concentration, for example because of a physical occupation or rigorous exercise—specialist advice should be sought regarding consideration of statin therapy in these patients).

If muscular symptoms or raised creatine kinase occur during treatment, other possible causes (e.g. rigorous physical activity, hypothyroidism, infection, recent trauma, and drug or alcohol addiction) should be excluded before statin therapy is implicated, particularly if statin treatment has previously been tolerated for more than 3 months. When a statin is suspected to be the cause of myopathy, and creatine kinase concentration is markedly elevated (more than 5 times upper limit of normal), or if muscular symptoms are severe, treatment should be discontinued. If symptoms resolve and creatine kinase concentrations return to normal, the statin should be reintroduced at a lower dose and the patient monitored closely; an alternative statin should be prescribed if unacceptable side-effects are experienced with a particular statin. Statins should not be discontinued in the event of small, asymptomatic elevations of creatine kinase. Routine monitoring of creatine kinase is unnecessary in asymptomatic patients.

Counselling Advise patient to report promptly unexplained muscle pain, tenderness, or weakness.

ATORVASTATIN

Indications primary hypercholesterolaemia, heterozygous familial hypercholesterolaemia, homozygous familial hypercholesterolaemia or combined (mixed) hyperlipidaemia in patients who have not responded adequately to diet and other appropriate measures; primary prevention of cardiovascular events in patients at high risk of a first cardiovascular event; secondary prevention of cardiovascular events [unlicensed]

Cautions see notes above; also haemorrhagic stroke

Hepatic impairment see notes above

Renal impairment in chronic kidney disease, for primary and secondary prevention of cardiovascular events [unlicensed starting dose in *primary* prevention; unlicensed in *secondary* prevention], initially 20 mg once daily, increased if necessary (on specialist advice if eGFR < 30 mL/minute/1.73m^2); max. 80 mg once daily

Pregnancy see notes above

Breast-feeding see notes above

Side-effects see notes above; also nasopharyngitis; epistaxis, pharyngeolaryngeal pain, back pain, hyperglycaemia; *less commonly* blurred vision, pyrexia, anorexia, malaise, chest pain, weight gain, hypoglycaemia, tinnitus, peripheral oedema, neck pain; *rarely* cholestasis, Stevens-Johnson syndrome, toxic epidermal necrolysis; *very rarely* gynaecomastia, hearing loss

Dose
- Primary hypercholesterolaemia and combined hyperlipidaemia, ADULT over 18 years, usually 10 mg once daily; if necessary, may be increased at intervals of at least 4 weeks to max. 80 mg once daily
- Familial hypercholesterolaemia, ADULT over 18 years, initially 10 mg daily, increased at intervals of at least 4 weeks to 40 mg once daily; if necessary, further increased to max. 80 mg once daily (or 40 mg once daily combined with anion-exchange resin in heterozygous familial hypercholesterolaemia)
- Primary prevention of cardiovascular events, ADULT over 18 years, 20 mg once daily increased if necessary (see Lipid-Regulating Drugs) [unlicensed starting dose]
- Secondary prevention of cardiovascular events [unlicensed], ADULT over 18 years, 80 mg once daily
- CHILD under 18 years see *BNF for Children*

Note Max. 10 mg daily with concomitant ciclosporin, or tipranavir combined with ritonavir (see also Appendix 1)

Atorvastatin (Non-proprietary) ℗⊙ℳ
Tablets, atorvastatin (as calcium trihydrate) 10 mg, net price 28-tab pack = £1.19; 20 mg, 28-tab pack = £1.45; 40 mg, 28-tab pack = £1.67; 80 mg, 28-tab pack = £2.68. Counselling, muscle effects, see notes above

Lipitor® (Pfizer) ℗⊙ℳ
Chewable tablets ▼, atorvastatin (as calcium trihydrate) 10 mg, net price 30-tab pack = £13.80; 20 mg, 30-tab pack = £26.40. Label: 24, counselling, muscle effects, see notes above

Tablets, all f/c, atorvastatin (as calcium trihydrate) 10 mg, net price 28-tab pack = £13.00; 20 mg, 28-tab pack = £24.64; 40 mg 28-tab pack = £24.64; 80 mg, 28-tab pack = £28.21. Counselling, muscle effects, see notes above

FLUVASTATIN

Note The *Scottish Medicines Consortium* (p. 4) has advised (February 2004) that fluvastatin is accepted for restricted use for the secondary prevention of coronary events after percutaneous coronary angioplasty; if the patient has previously been receiving another statin, then there is no need to change the statin

Indications adjunct to diet in primary hypercholesterolaemia or combined (mixed) hyperlipidaemia (types IIa and IIb); prevention of coronary events after percutaneous coronary intervention

Cautions see notes above

Hepatic impairment see notes above

Renal impairment manufacturer advises doses above 40 mg daily should be initiated with caution if eGFR less than 30 mL/minute/1.73 m^2

Pregnancy see notes above

Breast-feeding see notes above

Side-effects see notes above; also *very rarely* vasculitis

Dose

- Hypercholesterolaemia or combined hyperlipidaemia, initially 20–40 mg daily in the evening, adjusted at intervals of at least 4 weeks; up to 80 mg daily (given in 2 divided doses) may be required; CHILD under 18 years see *BNF for Children*
- Following percutaneous coronary intervention, 80 mg daily

Fluvastatin (Non-proprietary) ℗ₒₘ

Capsules, fluvastatin (as sodium salt) 20 mg, net price 28-cap pack = £2.41; 40 mg, 28-cap pack = £2.48. Counselling, muscle effects, see notes above

Lescol® (Novartis) ℗ₒₘ

Capsules, fluvastatin (as sodium salt) 20 mg (brown/yellow), net price 28-cap pack = £15.26; 40 mg (brown/orange), 28-cap pack = £15.26, 56-cap pack = £30.53. Counselling, muscle effects, see notes above

◢**Modified release**

Fluvastatin (Non-proprietary) ℗ₒₘ

Tablets, m/r, fluvastatin (as sodium salt) 80 mg, net price 28-tab pack = £19.20. Label: 25, counselling, muscle effects, see notes above
Brands include *Dorisin®XL, Luvinsta® XL, Pinmactil®, Stefluvin® XL*
Dose 80 mg once daily (dose form not appropriate for initial dose titration)

Lescol® XL (Novartis) ℗ₒₘ

Tablets, m/r, yellow, fluvastatin (as sodium salt) 80 mg, net price 28-tab pack = £19.20. Label: 25, counselling, muscle effects, see notes above
Dose 80 mg once daily (dose form not appropriate for initial dose titration)

PRAVASTATIN SODIUM

Indications adjunct to diet for primary hypercholesterolaemia or combined (mixed) hyperlipidaemias in patients who have not responded adequately to dietary control; adjunct to diet to prevent cardiovascular events in patients with hypercholesterolaemia; prevention of cardiovascular events in patients with previous myocardial infarction or unstable angina; reduction of hyperlipidaemia in patients receiving immunosuppressive therapy following solid-organ transplantation

Cautions see notes above

Hepatic impairment see notes above

Renal impairment manufacturer advises initial dose of 10 mg once daily in moderate to severe impairment

Pregnancy see notes above

Breast-feeding see notes above

Side-effects see notes above; *less commonly* abnormal urination (including dysuria, nocturia and frequency); *very rarely* fulminant hepatic necrosis

Dose

- Hypercholesterolaemia or combined hyperlipidaemias, 10–40 mg once daily at night, adjusted at

intervals of at least 4 weeks; CHILD under 18 years see *BNF for Children*
- Familial hypercholesterolaemia, CHILD under 18 years see *BNF for Children*
- Prevention of cardiovascular events, 40 mg once daily at night
- Post-transplantation hyperlipidaemia, initially 20 mg once daily at night, increased if necessary (under close medical supervision) to max. 40 mg once daily at night

Pravastatin (Non-proprietary) ℗ₒₘ

Tablets, pravastatin sodium 10 mg, net price 28-tab pack = £1.43; 20 mg, 28-tab pack = £1.65; 40 mg, 28-tab pack = £2.00. Counselling, muscle effects, see notes above

Lipostat® (Squibb) ℗ₒₘ

Tablets, all yellow, pravastatin sodium 10 mg, net price 28-tab pack = £14.18; 20 mg, 28-tab pack = £26.01; 40 mg, 28-tab pack = £26.01. Counselling, muscle effects, see notes above

ROSUVASTATIN

Indications primary hypercholesterolaemia (type IIa including heterozygous familial hypercholesterolaemia), mixed dyslipidaemia (type IIb), or homozygous familial hypercholesterolaemia in patients who have not responded adequately to diet and other appropriate measures; prevention of cardiovascular events in patients at high risk of a first cardiovascular event

Cautions see notes above; patients of Asian origin (see under Dose); patients with risk factors for myopathy or rhabdomyolysis, including personal or family history of muscular disorders or toxicity (see under Dose)

Hepatic impairment see notes above

Renal impairment initially 5 mg once daily (do not exceed 20 mg daily) if eGFR 30–60 mL/minute/1.73 m^2; avoid if eGFR less than 30 mL/minute/1.73 m^2

Pregnancy see notes above

Breast-feeding see notes above

Side-effects see notes above; also proteinuria; *very rarely* gynaecomastia, haematuria; *also reported* oedema, Stevens-Johnson syndrome

Dose

- Hypercholesterolaemia, initially 5–10 mg once daily increased if necessary at intervals of at least 4 weeks to 20 mg once daily, increased after further 4 weeks to 40 mg daily only in severe hypercholesterolaemia with high cardiovascular risk and under specialist supervision; ELDERLY over 70 years, initially 5 mg once daily; patient of ASIAN origin or with risk factors for myopathy or rhabdomyolysis, initially 5 mg once daily increased if necessary to max. 20 mg daily; CHILD under 18 years see *BNF for Children*
- Prevention of cardiovascular events, 20 mg once daily; ELDERLY over 70 years, patient of ASIAN origin or with risk factors for myopathy or rhabdomyolysis, initially 5 mg once daily increased if necessary to max. 20 mg daily

Note Initially 5 mg once daily with concomitant fibrate increased if necessary to max. 20 mg daily. For dose adjustments with concomitant atazanavir, clopidogrel, darunavir, dronedarone, eltrombopag, ezetimibe, itraconazole, lopinavir, or tipranavir, consult product literature

(sidebar) **2** **Cardiovascular system**

Crestor® (AstraZeneca) [PoM]

Tablets, f/c, rosuvastatin (as calcium salt) 5 mg (yellow), net price 28-tab pack = £18.03; 10 mg (pink), 28-tab pack = £18.03; 20 mg (pink), 28-tab pack = £26.02; 40 mg (pink), 28-tab pack = £29.69. Counselling, muscle effects, see notes above

---

■ SIMVASTATIN

Indications primary hypercholesterolaemia, homozygous familial hypercholesterolaemia or combined (mixed) hyperlipidaemia in patients who have not responded adequately to diet and other appropriate measures; prevention of cardiovascular events in patients with atherosclerotic cardiovascular disease or diabetes mellitus

Cautions see notes above; also 80-mg dose only for those with severe hypercholesterolaemia and at high risk of cardiovascular complications

Hepatic impairment see notes above

Renal impairment doses above 10 mg daily should be used with caution if eGFR less than 30 mL/minute/1.73 m²

Pregnancy see notes above

Breast-feeding see notes above

Side-effects see notes above; also *rarely* anaemia; *also reported* tendinopathy

Dose

*   Primary hypercholesterolaemia, combined hyperlipidaemia, 10–20 mg daily at night, adjusted at intervals of at least 4 weeks; max. 80 mg once daily at night; CHILD under 18 years see *BNF for Children*
*   Homozygous familial hypercholesterolaemia, initially 40 mg daily at night, adjusted at intervals of at least 4 weeks; max. 80 mg once daily at night
*   Heterozygous familial hypercholesterolaemia, CHILD under 18 years see *BNF for Children*
*   Prevention of cardiovascular events, initially 20–40 mg once daily at night, adjusted at intervals of at least 4 weeks; max. 80 mg once daily at night

Note 10 mg daily with concomitant bezafibrate or ciprofibrate (see also Appendix 1). Max. 20 mg daily with concomitant amiodarone, verapamil, diltiazem, amlodipine, or ranolazine. Max. 40 mg daily with concomitant lomitapide

¹Simvastatin (Non-proprietary) [PoM]

Tablets, simvastatin 10 mg, net price 28-tab pack = 90p, 20 mg, 28-tab pack = 98p; 40 mg, 28-tab pack = £1.23; 80 mg, 28-tab pack = £1.81. Counselling, muscle effects, see notes above
Brands include *Simvador®*

Oral suspension, simvastatin 20 mg/5 mL, net price 150 mL = £117.41, 40 mg/5 mL, 150 mL = £179.36. Counselling, muscle effects, see notes above
Excipients may include propylene glycol

¹Zocor® (MSD) [PoM]

Tablets, all f/c, simvastatin 10 mg (peach), net price 28-tab pack = £18.03; 20 mg (tan), 28-tab pack = £29.69; 40 mg (red), 28-tab pack = £29.69; 80 mg (red), 28-tab pack = £29.69. Counselling, muscle effects, see notes above

1. Simvastatin 10 mg tablets can be sold to the public to reduce risk of first coronary event in individuals at moderate risk of coronary heart disease (approx. 10–15% risk of major event in 10 years), max. daily dose 10 mg and pack size of 28 tablets; treatment should form part of a programme to reduce risk of coronary heart disease

■ With ezetimibe

Note For homozygous familial hypercholesterolaemia, primary hypercholesterolaemia, and mixed hyperlipidaemia in patients stabilised on the individual components in the same proportions, or for patients not adequately controlled by statin alone. For prescribing information on ezetimibe, see Ezetimibe

Inegy® (MSD) [PoM]

Tablets, simvastatin 20 mg, ezetimibe 10 mg, net price 28-tab pack = £33.42; simvastatin 40 mg, ezetimibe 10 mg, 28-tab pack = £38.98; simvastatin 80 mg, ezetimibe 10 mg, 28-tab pack = £41.21. Counselling, muscle effects, see notes above

---

Bile acid sequestrants

Colesevelam, **colestipol**, and **colestyramine** are bile acid sequestrants used in the management of hypercholesterolaemia. They act by binding bile acids, preventing their reabsorption; this promotes hepatic conversion of cholesterol into bile acids; the resultant increased LDL-receptor activity of liver cells increases the clearance of LDL-cholesterol from the plasma. Bile acid sequestrants effectively reduce LDL-cholesterol but can aggravate hypertriglyceridaemia. Treatment with bile acid sequestrants may be appropriate under specialist supervision if statins and ezetimibe are inappropriate, and when LDL-cholesterol is severely raised, for example in familial hypercholesterolaemia.

Cautions Bile acid sequestrants interfere with the absorption of fat-soluble vitamins; supplements of vitamins A, D, K, and folic acid may be required when treatment is prolonged. **Interactions:** Appendix 1 (bile acid sequestrants)

Pregnancy and breast-feeding Bile acid sequestrants should be used with caution as although the drugs are not absorbed, they may cause fat-soluble vitamin deficiency on prolonged use.

Side-effects As bile acid sequestrants are not absorbed, gastro-intestinal side-effects predominate. Constipation is common, but diarrhoea has occurred, as have nausea, vomiting, and gastro-intestinal discomfort. Hypertriglyceridaemia may be aggravated. An increased bleeding tendency has been reported due to hypoprothrombinaemia associated with vitamin K deficiency.

Counselling Other drugs should be taken at least 1 hour before (4 hours before colesevelam), or 4–6 hours after bile acid sequestrants to reduce possible interference with absorption. Colesevelam can be taken at the same time as a statin or ezetimibe.

■ COLESEVELAM HYDROCHLORIDE

Indications primary hypercholesterolaemia as an adjunct to dietary measures, either alone or with a statin; primary and familial hypercholesterolaemia, in combination with ezetimibe, either with or without a statin

Cautions see notes above; also gastro-intestinal motility disorders, major gastro-intestinal surgery, inflammatory bowel disease; patients receiving ciclosporin should have their blood-ciclosporin concentration monitored before, during, and after treatment with colesevelam; **interactions:** Appendix 1 (colesevelam)

Contra-indications bowel or biliary obstruction

Hepatic impairment manufacturer advises caution

Pregnancy see notes above
Breast-feeding see notes above
Side-effects see notes above; also headache; myalgia
Dose
- Monotherapy, 3.75 g daily in 1–2 divided doses; max. 4.375 g daily
- Combination therapy with a statin, or ezetimibe, or both, 2.5–3.75 g daily in 1–2 divided doses

Cholestagel® (Genzyme) ▼ [PoM]
Tablets, f/c, colesevelam hydrochloride 625 mg, net price 180-cap pack = £96.10. Label: 21, counselling, avoid other drugs at same time (see notes above)

▮ COLESTYRAMINE
(Cholestyramine)

Indications hyperlipidaemias, particularly type IIa, in patients who have not responded adequately to diet and other appropriate measures; primary prevention of coronary heart disease in men aged 35–59 years with primary hypercholesterolaemia who have not responded to diet and other appropriate measures; pruritus associated with partial biliary obstruction and primary biliary cirrhosis (section 1.9.2); diarrhoeal disorders (section 1.9.2)

Cautions see notes above; **interactions**: Appendix 1 (colestyramine)
Contra-indications complete biliary obstruction (not likely to be effective)
Pregnancy see notes above
Breast-feeding see notes above
Side-effects see notes above; intestinal obstruction reported rarely and hyperchloraemic acidosis reported on prolonged use
Dose
- Lipid reduction, initially 4 g daily increased by 4 g at weekly intervals to 12–24 g daily in 1–4 divided doses, then adjusted as required; max. 36 g daily
- Pruritus, see section 1.9.2
- Diarrhoeal disorders, see section 1.9.2
- CHILD 6–12 years, see *BNF for Children*
Note The contents of each sachet should be mixed with at least 150 mL of water or other suitable liquid such as fruit juice, skimmed milk, thin soups, and pulpy fruits with a high moisture content

Colestyramine (Non-proprietary) [PoM]
Powder, sugar-free, colestyramine (anhydrous) 4 g/sachet, net price 50-sachet pack = £31.85. Label: 13, counselling, avoid other drugs at same time (see notes above)
Excipients may include aspartame (see section 9.4.1)

Questran® (Bristol-Myers Squibb) [PoM]
Powder, colestyramine (anhydrous) 4 g/sachet, net price 50-sachet pack = £10.76. Label: 13, counselling, avoid other drugs at same time (see notes above)
Excipients include sucrose 3.79 g/sachet

Questran Light® (Bristol-Myers Squibb) [PoM]
Powder, sugar-free, colestyramine (anhydrous) 4 g/sachet, net price 50-sachet pack = £16.15. Label: 13, counselling, avoid other drugs at same time (see notes above)
Excipients include aspartame (see section 9.4.1)

▮ COLESTIPOL HYDROCHLORIDE

Indications hyperlipidaemias, particularly type IIa, in patients who have not responded adequately to diet and other appropriate measures
Cautions see notes above; **interactions**: Appendix 1 (colestipol)
Pregnancy see notes above
Breast-feeding see notes above
Side-effects see notes above
Dose
- Initially 5 g 1–2 times daily in liquid increased if necessary in 5-g increments at intervals of 1 month to max. 30 g daily (in 1–2 divided doses)
Note the contents of each sachet should be mixed with at least 100 mL of water or other suitable liquid such as fruit juice or skimmed milk; alternatively it can be mixed with thin soups, cereals, yoghurt, or pulpy fruits ensuring at least 100 mL of liquid is provided

Colestid® (Pharmacia) [PoM]
Granules, yellow, colestipol hydrochloride 5 g/sachet, net price 30 sachets = £15.05. Label: 13, counselling, avoid other drugs at same time (see notes above)
Colestid Orange, granules, yellow/orange, colestipol hydrochloride 5 g/sachet, with aspartame, net price 30 sachets = £15.05. Label: 13, counselling, avoid other drugs at same time (see notes above)

Ezetimibe

Ezetimibe inhibits the intestinal absorption of cholesterol and, if used alone, has a modest effect on lowering LDL-cholesterol, with little effect on other lipoproteins. It is licensed as an adjunct to dietary manipulation in patients with primary hypercholesterolaemia in combination with a statin or alone (if a statin is inappropriate), in patients with homozygous familial hypercholesterolaemia in combination with a statin, and in patients with homozygous familial sitosterolaemia (phytosterolaemia). If ezetimibe is used in combination with a statin, there is an increased risk of rhabdomyolysis (see also Muscle Effects, p. 175)

> **NICE guidance**
> **Ezetimibe for the treatment of primary hypercholesterolaemia (November 2007)**
> Ezetimibe, used in accordance with the licensed indications for *Ezetrol®*, is an option for the treatment of adults with primary hypercholesterolaemia.
> www.nice.org.uk/TA132

▮ EZETIMIBE

Indications adjunct to dietary measures and statin treatment in primary hypercholesterolaemia and homozygous familial hypercholesterolaemia (ezetimibe alone in primary hypercholesterolaemia if statin inappropriate or not tolerated); adjunct to dietary measures in homozygous sitosterolaemia
Cautions interactions: Appendix 1 (ezetimibe)
Hepatic impairment avoid in moderate and severe impairment—may accumulate
Pregnancy manufacturer advises use only if potential benefit outweighs risk—no information available
Breast-feeding manufacturer advises avoid—present in milk in *animal* studies

Side-effects gastro-intestinal disturbances; headache, fatigue; myalgia; *rarely* arthralgia, hypersensitivity reactions (including rash, angioedema, and anaphylaxis), hepatitis; *very rarely* pancreatitis, cholelithiasis, cholecystitis, thrombocytopenia, raised creatine kinase, myopathy, and rhabdomyolysis

Dose

• ADULT and CHILD over 10 years, 10 mg once daily

Ezetrol® (MSD) PoM

Tablets, ezetimibe 10 mg, net price 28-tab pack = £26.31

◢**With simvastatin**

See under Simvastatin

Fibrates

Bezafibrate, ciprofibrate, fenofibrate, and **gemfibrozil** act mainly by decreasing serum triglycerides; they have variable effects on LDL-cholesterol. Fibrates are mainly used in those whose serum-triglyceride concentration is greater than 10 mmol/litre or in those who cannot tolerate a statin (specialist use).

Fibrates can cause a myositis-like syndrome, especially if renal function is impaired. Also, combination of a fibrate with a statin increases the risk of muscle effects (especially rhabdomyolysis) and should be used with caution (see Muscle Effects, p. 175) and monitoring of liver function and creatine kinase should be considered; gemfibrozil and statins should **not** be used concomitantly.

◢ **BEZAFIBRATE**

Indications adjunct to diet and other appropriate measures in mixed hyperlipidaemia if statin contra-indicated or not tolerated, or in severe hypertriglyceridaemia; also see notes above

Cautions correct hypothyroidism before initiating treatment (see p. 173); **interactions:** Appendix 1 (fibrates)

Contra-indications hypoalbuminaemia; gall bladder disease; nephrotic syndrome; photosensitivity to fibrates

Hepatic impairment avoid in severe liver disease

Renal impairment reduce dose to 400 mg daily if eGFR 40–60 mL/minute/1.73 m²; reduce dose to 200 mg every 1–2 days if eGFR 15–40 mL/minute/1.73 m²; avoid *immediate-release* preparations if eGFR less than 15 mL/minute/1.73 m²; avoid *modified-release* preparations if eGFR less than 60 mL/minute/1.73 m²

Myotoxicity Special care needed in patients with renal disease, as progressive increases in serum creatinine concentration or failure to follow dosage guidelines may result in myotoxicity (rhabdomyolysis); discontinue if myotoxicity suspected or creatine kinase concentration increases significantly

Pregnancy manufacturers advise avoid—no information available

Breast-feeding manufacturer advises avoid—no information available

Side-effects abdominal distension, diarrhoea, nausea, anorexia; *less commonly* cholestasis, dizziness, headache, renal failure, erectile dysfunction, myotoxicity (with myasthenia, myalgia, or very rarely rhabdomyolysis)—special risk in renal impairment (see Myotoxicity above), urticaria, pruritus, rash, photosensitivity reactions, alopecia; *rarely* pancreatitis,

peripheral neuropathy; *very rarely* gallstones, interstitial lung disease, anaemia, leucopenia, pancytopenia, increased platelet count, thrombocytopenic purpura, Stevens-Johnson syndrome, toxic epidermal necrolysis

Dose

• See preparations below

Bezafibrate (Non-proprietary) PoM

Tablets, bezafibrate 200 mg, net price 100-tab pack = £6.10. Label: 21

Dose 200 mg 3 times daily; CHILD over 10 years, see *BNF for Children*

Bezalip® (Actavis) PoM

Tablets, f/c, bezafibrate 200 mg, net price 100-tab pack = £8.63. Label: 21

Dose 200 mg 3 times daily; CHILD over 10 years, see *BNF for Children*

◢**Modified release**

Bezafibrate (Non-proprietary) PoM

Tablets, m/r, bezafibrate 400 mg, net price 28-tab pack = £3.25. Label: 21, 25

Brands include *Fibrazate® XL*

Dose 400 mg once daily (dose form not appropriate in patients with renal impairment)

Bezalip® Mono (Actavis) PoM

Tablets, m/r, f/c, bezafibrate 400 mg, net price 30-tab pack = £7.63. Label: 21, 25

Dose 400 mg once daily (dose form not appropriate in patients with renal impairment)

◢ **CIPROFIBRATE**

Indications adjunct to diet and other appropriate measures in mixed hyperlipidaemia if statin contra-indicated or not tolerated, or in severe hypertriglyceridaemia; also see notes above

Cautions see under Bezafibrate; also liver function tests recommended every 3 months for first year (discontinue treatment if significantly raised)

Contra-indications see under Bezafibrate

Hepatic impairment use with caution in mild to moderate impairment; avoid in severe impairment

Renal impairment reduce dose to 100 mg on alternate days in moderate impairment; avoid in severe impairment; see also Myotoxicity under Bezafibrate

Pregnancy manufacturers advise avoid—toxicity in *animal* studies

Breast-feeding manufacturer advises avoid—present in milk in *animal* studies

Side-effects see under Bezafibrate; *also reported* pneumonitis, pulmonary fibrosis

Dose

• 100 mg daily

Ciprofibrate (Non-proprietary) PoM

Tablets, ciprofibrate 100 mg, net price 28-tab pack = £106.64

◢ **FENOFIBRATE**

Indications adjunct to diet and other appropriate measures in mixed hyperlipidaemia if statin contra-indicated or not tolerated, or in severe hypertriglyceridaemia; adjunct to statin in mixed hyperlipidaemia if triglycerides and HDL-cholesterol inadequately controlled in patients at high cardiovascular risk; also see notes above

Cautions see under Bezafibrate; liver function tests recommended every 3 months for first year (discontinue treatment if significantly raised)

Contra-indications gall bladder disease; pancreatitis (unless due to severe hypertriglyceridaemia); photosensitivity to ketoprofen

Hepatic impairment avoid

Renal impairment reduce dose to 134 mg daily if eGFR less than 60 mL/minute/1.73 m^2; reduce dose to 67 mg daily if eGFR less than 20 mL/minute/1.73 m^2; avoid if eGFR less than 15 mL/minute/1.73 m^2; see also Myotoxicity under Bezafibrate

Pregnancy avoid—embryotoxicity in *animal* studies

Breast-feeding manufacturers advise avoid—no information available

Side-effects see under Bezafibrate; also *less commonly* pancreatitis, pulmonary embolism; *rarely* hepatitis; *also reported* interstitial pneumopathies

Dose
* See preparations below

Fenofibrate (Non-proprietary) PoM

Capsules, fenofibrate (micronised) 67 mg, net price 90-cap pack = £20.13. Label: 21

Dose initially 3 capsules daily, increased if necessary to 4 capsules daily (max. 3 capsules daily with concomitant statin); CHILD under 18 years see *BNF for Children*

Capsules, fenofibrate (micronised) 200 mg, net price 28-cap pack = £4.41. Label: 21

Dose 1 capsule daily (dose form not appropriate for children or in renal impairment)

Capsules, fenofibrate (micronised) 267 mg, net price 28-cap pack = £5.44. Label: 21

Dose 1 capsule daily (dose form not appropriate for initial dose titration, with concomitant statin, for children, or in renal impairment)

Lipantil® (Abbott Healthcare) PoM

Lipantil® Micro 67 capsules, yellow, fenofibrate (micronised) 67 mg, net price 90-cap pack = £23.30. Label: 21

Dose initially 3 capsules daily, increased if necessary to 4 capsules daily (max. 3 capsules daily with concomitant statin); CHILD under 18 years see *BNF for Children*

Lipantil® Micro 200 capsules, orange, fenofibrate (micronised) 200 mg, net price 28-cap pack = £14.23. Label: 21

Dose initially 1 capsule daily (dose form not appropriate for children or in renal impairment)

Lipantil® Micro 267 capsules, orange/cream, fenofibrate (micronised) 267 mg, net price 28-cap pack = £21.75. Label: 21

Dose 1 capsule daily (dose form not appropriate for initial dose titration, with concomitant statin, for children, or in renal impairment)

Supralip® 160 (Abbott Healthcare) PoM

Tablets, f/c, fenofibrate (micronised) 160 mg, net price 28-tab pack = £6.69. Label: 21

Dose 160 mg daily (dose form not appropriate for children or in renal impairment)

◢ GEMFIBROZIL

Indications adjunct to diet and other appropriate measures in mixed hyperlipidaemia or primary hypercholesterolaemia if statin contra-indicated or not tolerated, or in severe hypertriglyceridaemia; adjunct to diet and other appropriate measures in primary prevention of cardiovascular disease in men with hyperlipidaemias if statin contra-indicated or not tolerated; also see notes above

Cautions monitor blood counts for first year; monitor liver-function (discontinue treatment if abnormalities persist); preferably avoid use with statins (high risk of rhabdomyolysis); correct hypothyroidism before initiating treatment (see p. 173); elderly; **interactions:** Appendix 1 (fibrates)

Contra-indications history of gall-bladder or biliary-tract disease including gallstones; photosensitivity to fibrates

Hepatic impairment avoid

Renal impairment initially 900 mg daily if eGFR 30–80 mL/minute/1.73 m^2; avoid if eGFR less than 30 mL/minute/1.73 m^2; see also Myotoxicity under Bezafibrate

Pregnancy manufacturers advise avoid unless essential—toxicity in *animal* studies

Breast-feeding manufacturer advises avoid—no information available

Side-effects dyspepsia, diarrhoea, constipation, nausea, vomiting, abdominal pain, flatulence, headache, fatigue, vertigo, eczema, rash; *less commonly* atrial fibrillation; *rarely* pancreatitis, appendicitis, disturbances in hepatic function including hepatitis and cholestatic jaundice, angioedema, dizziness, paraesthesia, depression, drowsiness, sexual dysfunction, thrombocytopenia, anaemia, leucopenia, eosinophilia, bone-marrow suppression, myalgia, myopathy, myasthenia, myositis accompanied by increase in creatine kinase (discontinue if raised significantly), blurred vision, pruritus, urticaria, exfoliative dermatitis, alopecia, photosensitivity

Dose
* 1.2 g daily, usually in 2 divided doses; range 0.9–1.2 g daily; CHILD not recommended

Gemfibrozil (Non-proprietary) PoM

Capsules, gemfibrozil 300 mg, net price 112-cap pack = £35.57. Label: 22

Tablets, gemfibrozil 600 mg, net price 30-tab pack = £16.23, 56-tab pack = £34.89. Label: 22

Lopid® (Pfizer) PoM

'300' capsules, white/maroon, gemfibrozil 300 mg, net price 100-cap pack = £31.76. Label: 22

'600' tablets, f/c, gemfibrozil 600 mg, net price 56-tab pack = £35.57. Label: 22

Lomitapide

Lomitapide, an inhibitor of microsomal triglyceride transfer protein (MTP), reduces lipoprotein secretion and circulating concentrations of lipoprotein-borne lipids such as cholesterol and triglycerides. Lomitapide is licensed for the treatment of homozygous familial hypercholesterolaemia and should be used under specialist supervision. Lomitapide can interfere with the absorption of fat-soluble nutrients and supplementation of vitamin E and fatty acids is required.

◢ LOMITAPIDE

Indications adjunct to dietary measures and other lipid-regulating drugs with or without low-density lipoprotein apheresis in homozygous familial hypercholesterolaemia (see notes above)

Cautions see notes above; patients over 65 years; monitor liver function tests before treatment, then at least monthly and before each dose increase for first year, then at least every 3 months and before each dose increase thereafter; screen for hepatic steatosis and fibrosis before treatment, then annually thereafter; concomitant use of hepatotoxic drugs; **interactions:** Appendix 1 (lomitapide)

Contra-indications significant or chronic bowel disease

Hepatic impairment reduce dose if serum transaminases raised during treatment (consult product literature); max. 40 mg daily in mild impairment; avoid in moderate to severe impairment, or if unexplained persistent abnormal liver function tests

Renal impairment max. 40 mg daily in end-stage renal disease

Pregnancy avoid—teratogenicity and embryotoxicity in *animal* studies; manufacturer advises exclude pregnancy before treatment and ensure effective contraception used

Breast-feeding manufacturer advises avoid—no information available

Side-effects hepatic steatosis, hepatomegaly, raised serum transaminases (see Hepatic Impairment), diarrhoea, constipation, nausea, vomiting, dyspepsia, gastro-oesophageal reflux disease, abdominal pain, bloating, flatulence, eructation, tenesmus, haemorrhoids, gastroenteritis, appetite changes, weight loss, dizziness, headache, migraine, malaise, hypokalaemia, neutropenia, leucopenia, muscle spasms, ecchymosis, erythematous rash; *less commonly* dry mouth, haematemesis, gastro-intestinal haemorrhage, hyperbilirubinaemia, chest pain, drowsiness, paraesthesia, vertigo, pyrexia, haematuria, anaemia, proteinuria, arthralgia, myalgia, pain in extremities, joint swelling, abnormal gait, eye swelling, dry skin, sweating

Dose
- ADULT over 18 years, initially 5 mg once daily at least 2 hours after evening meal, increased if necessary after 2 weeks to 10 mg once daily, then increased after at least 4 weeks to 20 mg once daily, then in steps of 20 mg daily at intervals of at least 4 weeks up to max. 60 mg once daily

    Note With concomitant weak inhibitors of cytochrome P450 enzyme CYP3A4 (e.g. cimetidine, ranolazine, and fosaprepitant), reduce lomitapide dose to 5 mg once daily (if taking less than 40 mg once daily), or to 10 mg once daily (if taking 40–60 mg once daily), then adjust as necessary

Lojuxta (Aegerion) ▼ PoM
Capsules, lomitapide (as mesilate) 5 mg (orange), net price 28-cap pack = £17765.00; 10 mg (orange-white), 28-cap pack = £17765.00; 20 mg (white), 28-cap price = £17765.00

Nicotinic acid group

The value of **nicotinic acid** is limited by its side-effects, especially vasodilatation. In doses of 1.5 to 3 g daily it lowers both cholesterol and triglyceride concentrations by inhibiting synthesis; it also increases HDL-cholesterol. Nicotinic acid is used by specialists in combination with a statin if the statin alone cannot adequately control dyslipidaemia (raised LDL-cholesterol, triglyceridaemia, and low HDL-cholesterol).

Acipimox is indicated as an adjunct or alternative treatment in hypertriglyceridaemia with or without hypercholesterolaemia in patients who have not responded adequately to lifestyle changes and other lipid-regulating drugs. Acipimox seems to have fewer

side-effects than nicotinic acid but may be less effective in its lipid-regulating capabilities.

ACIPIMOX

Indications adjunct or alternative treatment in hyperlipidaemias of types IIb and IV in patients who have not responded adequately to other lipid-regulating drugs such as a statin or fibrate, and lifestyle changes (including diet, excercise, and weight reduction)

Cautions monitor hepatic and renal function

Contra-indications peptic ulcer

Renal impairment reduce dose to 250 mg 1–2 times daily if eGFR 30–60 mL/minute/1.73 m²; avoid if eGFR less than 30 mL/minute/1.73 m²

Pregnancy manufacturer advises avoid—no information available

Breast-feeding manufacturer advises avoid—no information available

Side-effects dyspepsia, flushing, abdominal pain, headache, malaise, urticaria; *less commonly* nausea, bronchospasm, myositis, myalgia, arthralgia, anaphylactoid reaction, pruritus, rash, erythema; *also reported* diarrhoea, vasodilatation, dry eyes

Dose
- 250 mg 2–3 times daily

Olbetam® (Pharmacia) PoM
Capsules, brown/pink, acipimox 250 mg, net price 90-cap pack = £46.33. Label: 21

NICOTINIC ACID

Indications adjunct to statin in dyslipidaemia or used alone if statin not tolerated (see also p. 172)

Cautions unstable angina, acute myocardial infarction, diabetes mellitus, gout, history of peptic ulceration; **interactions:** Appendix 1 (nicotinic acid)

Contra-indications arterial bleeding; active peptic ulcer disease

Hepatic impairment manufacturer advises monitor liver function in mild to moderate impairment and avoid in severe impairment; discontinue if severe abnormalities in liver function tests

Renal impairment manufacturer advises use with caution—no information available

Pregnancy no information available—manufacturer advises avoid unless potential benefit outweighs risk

Breast-feeding present in milk—avoid

Side-effects diarrhoea, nausea, vomiting, abdominal pain, dyspepsia; flushing; pruritus; rash; *less commonly* tachycardia, palpitation, shortness of breath, peripheral oedema, headache, dizziness, increase in uric acid, hypophosphataemia, prolonged prothrombin time, and reduced platelet count; *rarely* hypotension, syncope, rhinitis, insomnia, reduced glucose tolerance, myalgia, myopathy, myasthenia; *very rarely* anorexia, rhabdomyolysis, visual disturbance, and jaundice also reported

Note Prostaglandin-mediated symptoms (such as flushing) can be reduced by low initial doses taken with meals or, if patient taking aspirin, aspirin dose should be taken 30 minutes before nicotinic acid

Dose
- See under preparation

◢ **Modified release**

Niaspan® PoM

Tablets, m/r, nicotinic acid 500 mg; 750 mg; 1 g
Available from 'special-order' manufacturers or specialist importing companies, see p. 1124

Omega-3 fatty acid compounds

There is no evidence that omega-3 fatty acid compounds reduce the risk of cardiovascular disease.

The *Scottish Medicines Consortium* (p. 4) has advised (November 2002) that omega-3-acid ethyl esters are **not** recommended for use within NHS Scotland for the treatment of hypertriglyceridaemia.

OMEGA-3-ACID ETHYL ESTERS

Indications adjunct to diet and statin in type IIb or III hypertriglyceridaemia; adjunct to diet in type IV hypertriglyceridaemia; adjunct in secondary prevention in those who have had a myocardial infarction in the preceding 3 months

Cautions haemorrhagic disorders, anticoagulant treatment (bleeding time increased)

Hepatic impairment monitor liver function

Pregnancy manufacturers advise use only if potential benefit outweighs risk—no information available

Breast-feeding manufacturers advise avoid—no information available

Side-effects dyspepsia, nausea; *less commonly* taste disturbances, abdominal pain, gastritis, dizziness; *rarely* hepatic disorders, headache, hyperglycaemia, acne, rash; *very rarely* gastro-intestinal haemorrhage, hypotension, nasal dryness, urticaria, and increased white cell count

Dose

● See under preparations below

Omacor® (Abbott Healthcare)

Capsules, 1 g of omega-3-acid ethyl esters 90 containing eicosapentaenoic acid 460 mg and docosahexaenoic acid 380 mg, net price 28-cap pack = £14.24, 100-cap pack = £50.84. Label: 21
Dose hypertriglyceridaemia, initially 2 capsules daily with food, increased if necessary to 4 capsules daily
Secondary prevention after myocardial infarction, 1 capsule daily with food

Prestylon® (TEVA UK)

Capsules, 1 g of omega-3-acid ethyl esters 90 containing eicosapentaenoic acid 460 mg and docosahexaenoic acid 380 mg, net price 28-cap pack = £10.68, 100-cap pack = £38.13. Label: 21
Dose hypertriglyceridaemia, initially 2 capsules daily with food, increased if necessary to 4 capsules daily
Secondary prevention after myocardial infarction, 1 capsule daily with food

OMEGA-3-MARINE TRIGLYCERIDES

Indications adjunct in the reduction of plasma triglycerides in severe hypertriglyceridaemia

Cautions haemorrhagic disorders, anticoagulant treatment; aspirin-sensitive asthma; type 2 diabetes

Side-effects occasional nausea and belching

Dose

● See under preparations below

Maxepa® (Seven Seas)

Capsules, 1 g concentrated fish oils containing eicosapentaenoic acid 170 mg, docosahexaenoic acid 115 mg, net price 200-cap pack = £29.28. Label: 21
Dose 5 capsules twice daily with food
Liquid, golden-coloured, concentrated fish oils containing approx. eicosapentaenoic acid 157 mg, docosahexaenoic acid 106 mg/1 mL, net price 150 mL = £21.59. Label: 21
Dose 5 mL twice daily with food

2.13 Local sclerosants

Sodium tetradecyl sulfate is used in sclerotherapy of spider veins and varicose veins, and phenol is used in haemorrhoids (section 1.7.3).

SODIUM TETRADECYL SULFATE

Indications sclerotherapy of reticular veins and spider veins in legs and varicose veins

Cautions arterial disease; asymptomatic patent foramen ovale (use smaller volumes and avoid Valsalva manoeuvre immediately after administration); history of migraine (use smaller volumes); extravasation may cause necrosis of tissues; test dose recommended before each treatment; resuscitation facilities must be available; venous insufficiency with lymphoedema (pain and inflammation may worsen)

Contra-indications inability to walk; high risk of thromboembolism; recent acute superficial thrombophlebitis, deep vein thrombosis, or pulmonary embolism; recent surgery; varicose veins caused by tumours (unless tumour removed); uncontrolled diabetes mellitus, hyperthyroidism, asthma, neoplasm, blood disorders, respiratory or skin disease; significant valvular incompetence in deep veins; occlusive arterial disease; phlebitis; acute infection; symptomatic patent foramen ovale (if administered as foam)

Pregnancy avoid unless benefits outweigh risks—no information available

Breast-feeding use with caution—no information available

Side-effects superficial thrombophlebitis, phlebitis, telangiectatic matting, skin discoloration, local pain and burning; *less commonly* deep-vein thrombosis, scotoma; *rarely* vasovagal reactions, chest pain, cough, shortness of breath, headache, migraine, paraesthesia; *very rarely* nausea, vomiting, diarrhoea, swollen tongue, dry mouth, transient ischaemic attack, stroke, palpitation, pulmonary embolism, vasculitis, circulatory collapse, weakness, fever, hot flushes, hypersensitivity reactions (including anaphylaxis), sloughing and necrosis of skin and tissues

Dose

● Consult product literature

Fibrovein® (STD Pharmaceutical) PoM

Injection, sodium tetradecyl sulfate 0.2%, net price 5-mL vial = £7.00; 0.5%, 2-mL amp = £3.60; 1%, 2-mL amp = £4.30; 3%, 2-mL amp = £6.40, 5-mL vial = £15.85
Excipients include benzyl alcohol (see Excipients, p. 2)

3 Respiratory system

This chapter also includes advice on the drug management of the following:
- severe acute asthma, p. 186
- anaphylaxis, p. 213
- angioedema, p. 215
- chronic asthma, p. 184
- chronic obstructive pulmonary disease, p. 186
- croup, p. 188

3.1 Bronchodilators

3.1.1	**Adrenoceptor agonists**
3.1.2	**Antimuscarinic bronchodilators**
3.1.3	**Theophylline**
3.1.4	**Compound bronchodilator preparations**
3.1.5	**Peak flow meters, inhaler devices and nebulisers**

Asthma

Drugs used in the management of asthma include beta$_2$ agonists (section 3.1.1), antimuscarinic bronchodilators (section 3.1.2), theophylline (section 3.1.3), corticosteroids (section 3.2), cromoglicate and nedocromil (section 3.3.1), leukotriene receptor antagonists (section 3.3.2), and, in specialist centres, omalizumab (section 3.4.2).

For tables outlining the management of chronic and acute asthma, see p. 184 and p. 185. For advice on the management of medical emergencies in dental practice, see p. 28.

Administration of drugs for asthma

Inhalation This route delivers the drug directly to the airways; the dose required is smaller than when given by mouth and side-effects are reduced. See also Inhaler devices, section 3.1.5.

Solutions for nebulisation are available for use in severe acute asthma. They are administered over 5–10 minutes from a nebuliser, usually driven by oxygen in hospital. See also Nebulisers, section 3.1.5.

Oral The oral route is used when administration by inhalation is not possible. Systemic side-effects occur more frequently when a drug is given orally rather than by inhalation. Drugs given by mouth for the treatment of asthma include beta$_2$ agonists, corticosteroids, theophylline, and leukotriene receptor antagonists.

Parenteral Drugs such as beta$_2$ agonists, corticosteroids, and aminophylline can be given by injection in acute severe asthma when administration by nebulisation is inadequate or inappropriate. If the patient is being treated in the community, urgent transfer to hospital should be arranged.

Respiratory system · 3

Management of chronic asthma

Important Start at **step most appropriate** to initial severity; before initiating a new drug consider whether diagnosis is correct, check compliance and inhaler technique, and eliminate trigger factors for acute exacerbations

Adult and Child over 5 years	**Child under 5 years[4]**
Step 1: occasional relief bronchodilator Inhaled short-acting beta$_2$ agonist as required (up to once daily) **Note** Move to step 2 if needed more than twice a week, or if night-time symptoms at least once a week, or if exacerbation in the last 2 years	**Step 1: occasional relief bronchodilator** Short-acting beta$_2$ agonist as required (not more than once daily) **Note** Preferably by inhalation (less effective and more side-effects when given by mouth) Move to step 2 if needed more than twice a week, or if night-time symptoms at least once a week, or if exacerbation in the last 2 years
Step 2: regular inhaled preventer therapy Inhaled short-acting beta$_2$ agonist as required *plus* Regular standard-dose[1] inhaled corticosteroid (alternatives[2] are considerably less effective)	**Step 2: regular preventer therapy** Inhaled short-acting beta$_2$ agonist as required *plus* *Either* regular standard-dose[1] inhaled corticosteroid *Or* (if inhaled corticosteroid cannot be used) leukotriene receptor antagonist
Step 3: inhaled corticosteroid + long-acting inhaled beta$_2$ agonist Inhaled short-acting beta$_2$ agonist as required *plus* Regular standard-dose[1] inhaled corticosteroid *plus* Regular inhaled long-acting beta$_2$ agonist (salmeterol *or* formoterol) *If asthma not controlled* Increase dose of inhaled corticosteroid to upper end of standard dose range[1] *and* *Either* stop long-acting beta$_2$ agonist if of no benefit *Or* continue long-acting beta$_2$ agonist if of some benefit *If asthma still not controlled and long-acting beta$_2$ agonist stopped, add one of* Leukotriene receptor antagonist Modified-release oral theophylline Modified-release oral beta$_2$ agonist; CHILD under 12 years not recommended	**Step 3: add-on therapy** **Child under 2 years:** Refer to respiratory paediatrician **Child 2–5 years:** Inhaled short-acting beta$_2$ agonist as required *plus* Regular inhaled corticosteroid in standard dose[1] *plus* Leukotriene receptor antagonist
	Step 4: persistent poor control Refer to respiratory paediatrician
	Stepping down Regularly review need for treatment
Step 4: high-dose inhaled corticosteroid + regular bronchodilators Inhaled short-acting beta$_2$ agonist as required *with* Regular high-dose[3] inhaled corticosteroid *plus* Inhaled long-acting beta$_2$ agonist *plus* In adults 6-week sequential therapeutic trial of one or more of Leukotriene receptor antagonist Modified-release oral theophylline Modified-release oral beta$_2$ agonist	1. Standard-dose inhaled corticosteroids **Beclometasone dipropionate** or **budesonide** 100–400 micrograms twice daily; CHILD under 12 years 100–200 micrograms twice daily **Fluticasone propionate** 50–200 micrograms twice daily; CHILD 4–12 years 50–100 micrograms twice daily **Mometasone furoate** 400 micrograms as a single dose in the evening or in 2 divided doses; CHILD under 12 years not recommended **Note** Dose adjustments may be required for some inhaler devices, see under individual preparations, section 3.2 2. Alternatives to inhaled corticosteroid are leukotriene receptor antagonists, theophylline, inhaled cromoglicate, or inhaled nedocromil 3. High-dose inhaled corticosteroids **Beclometasone dipropionate** or **budesonide** 0.4–1 mg twice daily; CHILD 5–12 years 200–400 micrograms twice daily **Fluticasone propionate** 200–500 micrograms twice daily; CHILD 5–12 years 100–200 micrograms twice daily **Mometasone furoate** 400 micrograms twice daily; CHILD under 12 years not recommended **Note** Dose adjustments may be required for some inhaler devices, see under individual preparations, section 3.2. Failure to achieve control with these doses is unusual, see also Side-effects of Inhaled Corticosteroids, section 3.2
Step 5: regular corticosteroid tablets Refer to a respiratory specialist Inhaled short-acting beta$_2$ agonist as required *with* Regular high-dose[3] inhaled corticosteroid *and* One or more long-acting bronchodilators (see step 4) *plus* Regular prednisolone tablets (as single daily dose) **Note** In addition to regular prednisolone, continue high-dose inhaled corticosteroid (in exceptional cases may exceed licensed doses); these patients should normally be referred to an asthma clinic	
Stepping down Review treatment every 3 months; if control achieved, stepwise reduction may be possible; reduce dose of *inhaled* corticosteroid slowly (consider reduction every 3 months, decreasing dose by up to 50% each time)	4. Lung-function measurements cannot be used to guide management in those under 5 years

Advice on the management of chronic asthma is based on the recommendations of the British Thoracic Society and Scottish Intercollegiate Guidelines Network (updated January 2012); updates available at www.brit-thoracic.org.uk

Management of acute asthma

> **Important**　Patients with severe or life-threatening acute asthma may not be distressed and may not have all of these abnormalities; the presence of any should alert the doctor. Regard each emergency consultation as being for **severe acute asthma** until shown otherwise

Moderate acute asthma	Severe acute asthma	Life-threatening acute asthma
• Able to talk • Respiration (breaths/minute) < 25; CHILD 2–5 years ≤ 40, 5–12 years ≤ 30 • Pulse (beats/minute) < 110; CHILD 2–5 years ≤ 140, 5–12 years ≤ 125 • Arterial oxygen saturation ≥ 92% • Peak flow > 50% of predicted or best; CHILD 5–12 years ≥ 50% *Treat at home or in surgery and assess response to treatment*	• Cannot complete sentences in one breath; CHILD too breathless to talk or feed • Respiration (breaths/minute) ≥ 25; CHILD 2–5 years > 40; 5–12 years > 30 • Pulse (beats/minute) ≥ 110; CHILD 2–5 years > 140; 5–12 years > 125 • Arterial oxygen saturation ≥ 92%; CHILD under 12 years < 92% • Peak flow 33–50% of predicted or best; CHILD 5–12 years 33–50% *Start treatment below and send immediately to hospital*	• Silent chest, feeble respiratory effort, cyanosis • Hypotension, bradycardia, arrhythmia, exhaustion, agitation (in children), or reduced level of consciousness • Arterial oxygen saturation < 92% • Peak flow < 33% of predicted or best; CHILD 5–12 years < 33% *Start treatment below and send immediately to hospital; consult with senior medical staff and refer to intensive care*
Treatment • Inhaled **short-acting beta₂ agonist** via a large-volume spacer or oxygen-driven nebuliser (if available); give 2–10 puffs of **salbutamol** 100 micrograms/metered inhalation each inhaled separately, and repeat at 10–20 minute intervals if necessary *or* give nebulised **salbutamol** 5 mg (CHILD under 5 years 2.5 mg, 5–12 years 2.5–5 mg) or **terbutaline** 10 mg (CHILD under 5 years 5 mg, 5–12 years 5–10 mg), and repeat at 20–30 minute intervals if necessary • **Prednisolone** 40–50 mg by mouth for at least 5 days; CHILD 1–2 mg/kg (max. 40 mg) for up to 3 days, or longer if necessary; if the child has been taking an oral corticosteroid for more than a few days, give prednisolone 2 mg/kg (max. 60 mg) *Monitor response for 15–30 minutes* *If response is poor or a relapse occurs in 3–4 hours, send immediately to hospital for assessment and further treatment*	**Treatment** • High-flow **oxygen** (if available) • Inhaled **short-acting beta₂ agonist** via a large-volume spacer or oxygen-driven nebuliser (if available) as for moderate acute asthma • **Prednisolone** by mouth as for moderate acute asthma *or* intravenous **hydrocortisone** (preferably as sodium succinate) 100 mg every 6 hours until conversion to oral prednisolone is possible; CHILD 4 mg/kg (max. 100 mg) (alternatively, if weight unavailable, CHILD under 2 years 25 mg, 2–5 years 50 mg, 5–12 years 100 mg) *Monitor response for 15–30 minutes* *If response is poor:* • Inhaled **ipratropium bromide** via oxygen-driven nebuliser (if available) 500 micrograms every 4–6 hours (CHILD under 12 years 250 micrograms repeated every 20–30 minutes for the first 2 hours, then every 4–6 hours as necessary) *Refer those who fail to respond and require ventilatory support to an intensive care or high-dependency unit* • Consider intravenous **beta₂ agonist**, **aminophylline** (p. 195), or **magnesium sulfate** [unlicensed indication] (p. 186) only after consultation with senior medical staff	**Treatment** • High-flow **oxygen** (if available) • **Short-acting beta₂ agonist** via oxygen-driven nebuliser (if available); give **salbutamol** 5 mg (CHILD under 5 years 2.5 mg, 5–12 years 2.5–5 mg) or **terbutaline** 10 mg (CHILD under 5 years 5 mg, 5–12 years 5–10 mg), and repeat at 20–30 minute intervals or as necessary; reserve intravenous beta₂ agonists for those in whom inhaled therapy cannot be used reliably • **Prednisolone** by mouth as for moderate acute asthma *or* intravenous **hydrocortisone** as for severe acute asthma • Inhaled **ipratropium bromide** via oxygen-driven nebuliser (if available) as for severe acute asthma *Monitor response for 15–30 minutes* *If response is poor:* • Consider intravenous **aminophylline** (p. 195) or **magnesium sulfate** [unlicensed indication] (p. 186) only after consultation with senior medical staff

Follow up in all cases

Monitor symptoms and peak flow. Set up asthma action plan and check inhaler technique

Review by general practitioner or appropriate primary care health professional within 48 hours, see also p. 186

Advice on the management of acute asthma is based on the recommendations of the British Thoracic Society and Scottish Intercollegiate Guidelines Network (updated January 2012); updates available at www.brit-thoracic.org.uk

3 Respiratory system

Pregnancy and breast-feeding

It is particularly important that asthma should be well controlled during pregnancy; when this is achieved asthma has no important effects on pregnancy, labour, or on the fetus. Drugs for asthma should preferably be administered by inhalation to minimise exposure of the fetus. Inhaled drugs, theophylline, and prednisolone (see section 6.3.2) can be taken as normal during pregnancy and breast-feeding. For the use of leuko-triene receptor antagonists during pregnancy see section 3.3.2. Women planning to become pregnant should be counselled about the importance of taking their asthma medication regularly to maintain good control.

Severe acute exacerbations of asthma can have an adverse effect on pregnancy and should be treated promptly in hospital with conventional therapy, includ-ing nebulisation of a beta₂ agonist and oral or parenteral administration of a corticosteroid; prednisolone is the preferred corticosteroid for oral administration since very little of the drug reaches the fetus. Oxygen should be given immediately to maintain arterial oxygen saturation of 94–98% and prevent maternal and fetal hypoxia. An intravenous beta₂ agonist, aminophylline, or magnesium sulfate can be used during pregnancy if necessary; parenteral beta₂ agonists can affect the myo-metrium (see section 7.1.3).

Management of severe acute asthma

> **Important**
> Regard each emergency consultation as being for severe acute asthma until shown otherwise.
> Failure to respond adequately at any time requires immediate transfer to hospital.

Severe acute asthma can be fatal and **must** be treated promptly. All patients with severe acute asthma should be given high-flow **oxygen** (if available) and an inhaled **short-acting beta₂ agonist** via a large-volume spacer or nebuliser; give 2–10 puffs of **salbutamol** 100 micr-ograms/metered inhalation, each puff inhaled sepa-rately via a large-volume spacer, and repeat at 10–20 minute intervals or as necessary. If there are life-threa-tening features, give salbutamol or **terbutaline** via an oxygen-driven nebuliser every 20–30 minutes or as necessary, see p. 190 and p. 192. In all cases a systemic **corticosteroid** (section 6.3.2) should be given. For adults, give prednisolone 40–50 mg by mouth for at least 5 days, or intravenous hydrocortisone (preferably as sodium succinate) 100 mg every 6 hours until con-version to oral prednisolone is possible. For children, give prednisolone 1–2 mg/kg by mouth (max. 40 mg) for up to 3 days, or longer if necessary, or intravenous hydrocortisone (preferably as sodium succinate) 4 mg/kg (max. 100 mg) every 6 hours (alternatively, if weight unavailable, CHILD under 2 years 25 mg every 6 hours, 2–5 years 50 mg every 6 hours, 5–12 years 100 mg every 6 hours) until conversion to oral prednisolone is possible. If the child has been taking an oral corticosteroid for more than a few days, then give prednisolone 2 mg/kg (max. 60 mg). In severe or life-threatening asthma, also consider initial treatment with **ipratropium** by nebuli-ser, 500 micrograms every 4–6 hours (CHILD under 12 years 250 micrograms repeated every 20–30 minutes for the first 2 hours, then every 4–6 hours as necessary).

Most patients do not require and do not benefit from the addition of **intravenous aminophylline** or of **intra-venous beta₂ agonist**; both cause more adverse effects than nebulised beta₂ agonists. Nevertheless, an occa-sional patient who has not been taking theophylline may benefit from aminophylline infusion (see p. 195). A single dose of **magnesium sulfate injection** (see sec-tion 9.5.1.3) [unlicensed indication] 1.2–2 g (equivalent to approx. 4.8–8 mmol Mg²⁺) by intravenous infusion over 20 minutes can be used for patients with severe acute asthma, but evidence of benefit is limited.

Treatment of severe acute asthma is safer in hospital where resuscitation facilities are immediately available. Treatment should **never** be delayed for investigations, patients should **never** be sedated, and the possibility of a pneumothorax should be considered.

If the patient's condition deteriorates despite pharma-cological treatment, intermittent positive pressure ven-tilation may be needed.

For a table outlining the management of acute asthma, see p. 185.

Follow up in all cases Episodes of acute asthma should be regarded as a failure of preventative therapy. A careful history should be taken to establish the reason for the exacerbation. Inhaler technique should be checked and regular treatment should be reviewed in accordance with the Management of Chronic Asthma table, p. 184. Patients should be given a written asthma action plan aimed at preventing relapse, optimising treatment, and preventing delay in seeking assistance in future exacerbations. Follow-up within 48 hours should be arranged with the general practitioner or appropriate primary care health professional. Patients should also be reviewed by a respiratory specialist within one month of the exacerbation.

Chronic obstructive pulmonary disease

Smoking cessation (section 4.10.2) reduces the progres-sive decline in lung function in chronic obstructive pulmonary disease (COPD, chronic bronchitis, or emphysema). Infection can complicate chronic obstruc-tive pulmonary disease and may be prevented by vaccination (pneumococcal vaccine and influenza vaccine, section 14.4).

A trial of a high-dose inhaled corticosteroid or an oral corticosteroid is recommended for patients with mod-erate or severe airflow obstruction if the diagnosis is in doubt.

Symptoms of chronic obstructive pulmonary disease may be alleviated by an inhaled **short-acting beta₂ agonist** (section 3.1.1.1) or a **short-acting anti-muscarinic bronchodilator** (section 3.1.2) used as required.

When the airways obstruction is more severe, regular inhaled therapy should be used, see also Use of Inhaled Therapies in Chronic Obstructive Pulmonary Disease, p. 187. It is important to check compliance and inhaler technique before initiating a new drug.

If the Forced Expiratory Volume in 1 second (FEV₁), is 50% of predicted or more, either a long-acting anti-muscarinic bronchodilator (section 3.1.2) or a long-act-ing beta₂ agonist (section 3.1.1.1) should be used. Short-acting antimuscarinic bronchodilators should be discon-tinued when a long-acting antimuscarinic bronchodila-tor is started. A long-acting beta₂ agonist with a cortico-steroid (section 3.2) in a combination inhaler can be

Use of inhaled therapies in chronic obstructive pulmonary disease

Advice on the use of inhaled therapies in chronic obstructive pulmonary disease is based on the recommendations of the National Institute for Health and Care Excellence (2010). Management of chronic obstructive pulmonary disease in adults in primary and secondary care. London: NICE. Available from www.nice.org.uk/CG101 Reproduced with permission

3 Respiratory system

used for patients who remain symptomatic despite regular treatment with a long-acting beta₂ agonist.

If FEV₁ is less than 50% of predicted, *either* a long-acting antimuscarinic bronchodilator *or* a long-acting beta₂ agonist with a corticosteroid in a combination inhaler should be used.

In any patient who remains breathless or continues to have exacerbations, triple therapy with a long-acting beta₂ agonist and a corticosteroid in a combination inhaler *plus* a long-acting antimuscarinic bronchodilator should be used.

If an inhaled corticosteroid is not appropriate, a long-acting antimuscarinic bronchodilator can be used with a long-acting beta₂ agonist.

If symptoms persist or if the patient is unable to use an inhaler, oral modified-release **aminophylline** or **theophylline** (section 3.1.3) can be used.

Indacaterol (section 3.1.1.1) is a long-acting beta₂ agonist licensed for the maintenance treatment of chronic obstructive pulmonary disease.

In patients with severe chronic obstructive pulmonary disease associated with chronic bronchitis and a history of frequent exacerbations, **roflumilast** (section 3.3.3) is

licensed as an adjunct to existing bronchodilator treatment.

A **mucolytic** drug (section 3.7) may be considered for a patient with a chronic productive cough.

Long-term **oxygen** therapy (section 3.6) prolongs survival in patients with severe chronic obstructive pulmonary disease and hypoxaemia.

During an exacerbation of chronic obstructive pulmonary disease, bronchodilator therapy can be administered through a nebuliser if necessary and oxygen given if appropriate. **Aminophylline** can be given intravenously if response to nebulised bronchodilators is poor. A short course of **oral corticosteroid** (section 6.3.2), such as prednisolone 30 mg daily for 7–14 days, should be given if increased breathlessness interferes with daily activities. **Antibacterial** treatment (Table 1, section 5.1) is required if sputum becomes more purulent than usual, or if there are other signs of infection.

Patients who have had an episode of hypercapnic respiratory failure should be given a 24% or 28% Venturi mask and an *oxygen alert card* (see p. 188) endorsed with the oxygen saturations required during previous exacerbations. Patients and their carers should be instructed to show the card to emergency healthcare providers in the event of an exacerbation, see also section 3.6.

Oxygen alert card

Name: _____

I am at risk of type II respiratory failure with a raised CO_2 level.

Please use my ____% Venturi mask to achieve an oxygen saturation of ____% to ____% during exacerbations.

Use compressed air to drive nebulisers (with nasal oxygen at 2 litres/minute). If compressed air not available, limit oxygen-driven nebulisers to 6 minutes.

Oxygen alert card based on British Thoracic Society guideline for emergency oxygen use in adult patients (October 2008); available at www.brit-thoracic.org.uk

Croup

Mild croup is largely self-limiting, but treatment with a single dose of a corticosteroid (e.g. dexamethasone 150 micrograms/kg) by mouth may be of benefit.

More severe croup (or mild croup that might cause complications) calls for hospital admission; a single dose of a corticosteroid (e.g. dexamethasone 150 micrograms/kg or prednisolone 1–2 mg/kg by mouth, section 6.3.2) should be administered before transfer to hospital. In hospital, dexamethasone 150 micrograms/kg (by mouth or by injection) or budesonide 2 mg (by nebulisation, section 3.2) will often reduce symptoms; the dose may need to be repeated after 12 hours if necessary.

For severe croup not effectively controlled with corticosteroid treatment, nebulised adrenaline solution 1 in 1000 (1 mg/mL) should be given with close clinical monitoring in a dose of 400 micrograms/kg (max. 5 mg) repeated after 30 minutes if necessary; the effects of nebulised adrenaline last 2–3 hours and the child needs to be monitored carefully for recurrence of the obstruction.

3.1.1 Adrenoceptor agonists
(Sympathomimetics)

3.1.1.1 Selective beta₂ agonists
3.1.1.2 Other adrenoceptor agonists

The selective beta₂ agonists (selective beta₂-adrenoceptor agonists, selective beta₂ stimulants) (section 3.1.1.1) such as salbutamol or terbutaline are the safest and most effective short-acting beta₂ agonists for asthma. Less selective beta₂ agonists such as ephedrine (section 3.1.1.2) should be avoided whenever possible.

Adrenaline (epinephrine) (which has both alpha- and beta-adrenoceptor agonist properties) is used in the emergency management of allergic and anaphylactic reactions (section 3.4.3) and in the management of croup (see above).

3.1.1.1 Selective beta₂ agonists

Selective beta₂ agonists produce bronchodilation. A short-acting beta₂ agonist is used for immediate relief of asthma symptoms while some long-acting beta₂ agonists are added to an inhaled corticosteroid in patients requiring prophylactic treatment.

Management of Chronic Asthma table, see p. 184
Management of Acute Asthma table, see p. 185

Short-acting beta₂ agonists   Mild to moderate symptoms of asthma respond rapidly to the inhalation of a selective short-acting beta₂ agonist such as **salbutamol** or **terbutaline**. If beta₂ agonist inhalation is needed more often than twice a week, or if night-time symptoms occur at least once a week, or if the patient has suffered an exacerbation in the last 2 years, then prophylactic treatment should be considered using a stepped approach as outlined in the Management of Chronic Asthma table, p. 184.

A short-acting beta₂ agonist inhaled immediately before exertion reduces *exercise-induced asthma*; however, frequent exercise-induced asthma probably reflects poor overall control and calls for reassessment of asthma treatment.

Long-acting beta₂ agonists   Formoterol (eformoterol) and **salmeterol** are longer-acting beta₂ agonists which are administered by inhalation. They should be used for asthma only in patients who regularly use an inhaled corticosteroid (see CHM advice below). They have a role in the long-term control of chronic asthma (see Management of Chronic Asthma table, p. 184) and they can be useful in nocturnal asthma. Salmeterol should not be used for the relief of an asthma attack; it has a slower onset of action than salbutamol or terbutaline. Formoterol is licensed for short-term symptom relief and for the prevention of exercise-induced bronchospasm; its speed of onset of action is similar to that of salbutamol.

Combination inhalers that contain a long-acting beta₂ agonist and a corticosteroid (section 3.2) ensure that long-acting beta₂ agonists are not used without concomitant corticosteroids, but reduce the flexibility to adjust the dose of each component.

CHM advice

To ensure safe use, the CHM has advised that for the management of chronic asthma, long-acting beta₂ agonists (formoterol and salmeterol) should:

- be added only if regular use of standard-dose inhaled corticosteroids has failed to control asthma adequately;
- not be initiated in patients with rapidly deteriorating asthma;
- be introduced at a low dose and the effect properly monitored before considering dose increase;
- be discontinued in the absence of benefit;
- not be used for the relief of exercise-induced asthma symptoms unless regular inhaled corticosteroids are also used;
- be reviewed as clinically appropriate: stepping down therapy should be considered when good long-term asthma control has been achieved.

A daily dose of 24 micrograms of formoterol should be sufficient for the majority of children, particularly for younger age-groups; higher doses should be used rarely, and only when control is not maintained on the lower dose.

Patients should be advised to report any deterioration in symptoms following initiation of treatment with a long-acting beta₂ agonist, see Management of Chronic Asthma table, p. 184.

Indacaterol and **olodaterol** are long-acting beta₂ agonists licensed for chronic obstructive pulmonary disease; they are not indicated for the relief of acute bronchospasm. **Vilanterol** is a long-acting beta₂ agonist available in a combination inhaler with fluticasone furoate (see section 3.2) *or* with umeclidinium (see Anoro Ellipta®, p. 196).

The *Scottish Medicines Consortium* (p.) has advised (July 2014) that olodaterol (*Striverdi Respimat*®) is **not** recommended for use within NHS Scotland.

Inhalation *Pressurised-metered dose inhalers* are an effective and convenient method of drug administration in mild to moderate asthma. A spacer device (section 3.1.5) may improve drug delivery. At recommended inhaled doses, the duration of action of salbutamol and terbutaline is about 3 to 5 hours, and 12 hours for salmeterol and formoterol. The **dose**, the frequency, and the maximum number of inhalations in 24 hours of the beta$_2$ agonist should be **stated explicitly** to the patient. The patient should be advised to seek medical advice when the prescribed dose of beta$_2$ agonist fails to provide the usual degree of symptomatic relief because this usually indicates a worsening of the asthma and the patient may require a prophylactic drug such as an inhaled corticosteroid (see Management of Chronic Asthma table, p. 184).

Nebuliser (or respirator) solutions of salbutamol and terbutaline are used for the treatment of severe acute asthma in hospital or in general practice. Patients with a severe attack of asthma should preferably have oxygen during nebulisation since beta$_2$ agonists can increase arterial hypoxaemia. For the use of nebulisers in chronic obstructive pulmonary disease, see section 3.1.5. The dose given by nebuliser is substantially higher than that given by inhaler. Patients should therefore be warned that it is dangerous to exceed the prescribed dose and they should seek medical advice if they fail to respond to the usual dose of the respirator solution, see also section 3.1.5.

Oral Oral preparations of beta$_2$ agonists may be used by patients who cannot manage the inhaled route. They are sometimes used for children and the elderly, but inhaled beta$_2$ agonists are more effective and have fewer side-effects. The longer-acting oral preparations, including bambuterol, may be of value in nocturnal asthma but they have a limited role and inhaled long-acting beta$_2$ agonists are usually preferred.

Parenteral Salbutamol or terbutaline can be given intravenously for severe or life-threatening acute asthma; patients should be carefully monitored and the dose adjusted according to response and heart rate. The regular use of beta$_2$ agonists by the subcutaneous route is not recommended since the evidence of benefit is uncertain and it may be difficult to withdraw such treatment once started. Beta$_2$ agonists may also be given by intramuscular injection.

Children Selective beta$_2$ agonists are useful even in children under the age of 18 months. They are most effective by the inhaled route; a pressurised metered-dose inhaler should be used with a spacer device in children under 5 years (see NICE guidance, section 3.1.5). A beta$_2$ agonist may also be given by mouth but administration by inhalation is preferred; a long-acting inhaled beta$_2$ agonist may be used where appropriate (see Management of Chronic Asthma table, p. 184). In severe attacks nebulisation using a selective beta$_2$ agonist or ipratropium is advisable (see also Management of Chronic Asthma table and Management of Acute Asthma table, p. 184 and p. 185).

Cautions Beta$_2$ agonists should be used with caution in hyperthyroidism, cardiovascular disease, arrhythmias, susceptibility to QT-interval prolongation, and hypertension. Beta$_2$ agonists should be used with caution in diabetes—monitor blood glucose (risk of keto-acidosis, especially when beta$_2$ agonist given intravenously). **Interactions:** Appendix 1 (sympathomimetics, beta$_2$).

Hypokalaemia Potentially serious hypokalaemia may result from beta$_2$ agonist therapy. Particular caution is required in severe asthma, because this effect may be potentiated by concomitant treatment with theophylline and its derivatives, corticosteroids, and diuretics, and by hypoxia. Plasma-potassium concentration should therefore be monitored in severe asthma.

Side-effects Side-effects of the beta$_2$ agonists include fine tremor (particularly in the hands), nervous tension, headache, muscle cramps, and palpitation. Other side-effects include tachycardia, arrhythmias, peripheral vasodilation, myocardial ischaemia, and disturbances of sleep and behaviour. Paradoxical bronchospasm (occasionally severe), urticaria, angioedema, hypotension, and collapse have also been reported. High doses of beta$_2$ agonists are associated with hypokalaemia (see Hypokalaemia above).

BAMBUTEROL HYDROCHLORIDE

Note Bambuterol is a pro-drug of terbutaline

Indications asthma and other conditions associated with reversible airways obstruction

Cautions see notes above

Hepatic impairment avoid in severe impairment

Renal impairment reduce initial dose by half if eGFR less than 50 mL/minute/1.73m^2

Pregnancy manufacturer advises avoid—no information available; see also p. 186

Breast-feeding see p. 186

Side-effects see notes above

Dose
● 20 mg once daily at bedtime if patient has previously tolerated beta$_2$ agonists; other patients, initially 10 mg once daily at bedtime, increased if necessary after 1–2 weeks to 20 mg once daily; CHILD not recommended

Bambec® (AstraZeneca) ▼PoM
Tablets, both scored, bambuterol hydrochloride 10 mg, net price 28-tab pack = £14.46; 20 mg, 28-tab pack = £15.77

FORMOTEROL FUMARATE
(Eformoterol fumarate)

Indications reversible airways obstruction (including nocturnal asthma and prophylaxis of exercise-induced bronchospasm) in patients requiring long-term regular bronchodilator therapy, see also Management of Chronic Asthma table, p. 184; chronic obstructive pulmonary disease

Note For use in asthma only in patients who regularly use an inhaled corticosteroid, see notes above

Cautions see notes above

Pregnancy see p. 186

Breast-feeding see p. 186

Side-effects see notes above; *very rarely* QT-interval prolongation; taste disturbances, nausea, dizziness, rash, and pruritus also reported

Dose
● See under preparations below
  Counselling Advise patients not to exceed prescribed dose, and to follow manufacturer's directions; if a previously effective dose of inhaled formoterol fails to provide adequate relief, a doctor's advice should be obtained as soon as possible

Formoterol (Non-proprietary) [PoM]
Dry powder for inhalation, formoterol fumarate 12 micrograms/metered inhalation, net price 120-dose unit = £23.75. Counselling, administration
Brands include *Easyhaler®* *Formoterol*
Dose by inhalation of powder, asthma, ADULT and CHILD over 12 years, 12 micrograms twice daily, increased to 24 micrograms twice daily in more severe airways obstruction; CHILD 6–12 years, 12 micrograms twice daily
Chronic obstructive pulmonary disease, 12 micrograms twice daily

Atimos Modulite® (Chiesi) [PoM]
Aerosol inhalation, formoterol fumarate 12 micrograms/metered inhalation, net price 100-dose unit = £30.06. Counselling, administration
Dose by aerosol inhalation, asthma, ADULT and CHILD over 12 years, 12 micrograms twice daily, increased to max. 24 micrograms twice daily in more severe airways obstruction
Chronic obstructive pulmonary disease, ADULT over 18 years, 12 micrograms twice daily; for symptom relief additional doses may be taken to total max. 48 micrograms daily (max. single dose 24 micrograms)

Foradil® (Novartis) [PoM]
Dry powder for inhalation, formoterol fumarate 12 micrograms/capsule, net price 60-cap pack (with inhaler device) = £23.38. Counselling, administration
Dose by inhalation of powder, asthma, ADULT and CHILD over 12 years, 12 micrograms twice daily, increased to 24 micrograms twice daily in more severe airways obstruction; CHILD 6–12 years, 12 micrograms twice daily
Chronic obstructive pulmonary disease, 12 micrograms twice daily

Oxis® (AstraZeneca) [PoM]
Turbohaler® (= dry powder inhaler), formoterol fumarate 6 micrograms/metered inhalation, net price 60-dose unit = £24.80; 12 micrograms/metered inhalation, 60-dose unit = £24.80. Counselling, administration
Dose by inhalation of powder, chronic asthma, 6–12 micrograms 1–2 times daily; increased up to 24 micrograms twice daily if necessary; occasionally up to 72 micrograms daily may be needed (max. single dose 36 micrograms); reassess treatment if additional doses required on more than 2 days a week; CHILD 6–18 years, 6–12 micrograms 1–2 times daily; occasionally up to 48 micrograms daily may be needed (max. single dose 12 micrograms) (see also CHM advice, p. 188)
Relief of bronchospasm, ADULT and CHILD over 6 years, 6–12 micrograms
Prophylaxis of exercise-induced bronchospasm, 12 micrograms before exercise; CHILD 6–18 years, 6–12 micrograms before exercise
Chronic obstructive pulmonary disease, 12 micrograms 1–2 times daily; for symptom relief additional doses can be taken to total max. 48 micrograms daily (max. single dose 24 micrograms)

◀Compound preparations
For **compound preparations** containing formoterol, see *Flutiform®*, *Fostair®* and *Symbicort®*, section 3.2

INDACATEROL

Indications maintenance treatment of chronic obstructive pulmonary disease

Cautions see notes above; convulsive disorders

Hepatic impairment use with caution in severe impairment—no information available

Pregnancy manufacturer advises use only if potential benefit outweighs risk

Breast-feeding manufacturer advises avoid—present in milk in *animal* studies

Side-effects see notes above; also peripheral oedema, cough, oropharyngeal pain, nasopharyngitis, dizziness, sinusitis, rhinorrhoea; *less commonly* atrial fibrillation, chest pain, hyperglycaemia, paraesthesia, pruritus, rash

Dose
• By inhalation of powder, ADULT over 18 years, 150 micrograms once daily, increased to max. 300 micrograms once daily

Onbrez Breezhaler® (Novartis) [PoM]
Inhalation powder, hard capsule (for use with *Onbrez Breezhaler®* device), indacaterol (as maleate) 150 micrograms, net price 30-cap pack with *Onbrez Breezhaler®* device = £29.26; 300 micrograms, net price 30-cap pack with *Onbrez Breezhaler®* device = £29.26. Counselling, administration

OLODATEROL

Indications maintenance treatment of chronic obstructive pulmonary disease

Cautions see notes above; convulsive disorders, aneurysm

Hepatic impairment use with caution in severe impairment—no information available

Pregnancy manufacturer advises avoid—no information available

Breast-feeding manufacturer advises avoid—present in milk in *animal* studies

Side-effects see notes above; also *less commonly* nasopharyngitis, dizziness; *rarely* hypertension, arthralgia

Dose
• By inhalation, ADULT over 18 years, 5 micrograms (2 puffs) once daily

Striverdi Respimat® (Boehringer Ingelheim) ▼ [PoM]
Solution for inhalation, olodaterol (as hydrochloride) 2.5 micrograms/metered inhalation, net price 60-dose unit = £26.35. Counselling, administration

SALBUTAMOL
(Albuterol)

Indications asthma and other conditions associated with reversible airways obstruction; premature labour (section 7.1.3)

Cautions see notes above

Pregnancy see p. 186

Breast-feeding see p. 186

Side-effects see notes above; also lactic acidosis with high doses

Dose
• By mouth (but use by inhalation preferred), ADULT over 18 years, 4 mg (elderly and sensitive patients initially 2 mg) 3–4 times daily; max. single dose 8 mg (but unlikely to provide much extra benefit or to be tolerated); CHILD under 2 years see *BNF for Children*; 2–6 years 1–2 mg 3–4 times daily, 6–12 years 2 mg 3–4 times daily, 12–18 years 2–4 mg 3–4 times daily
• By subcutaneous or intramuscular injection, 500 micrograms, repeated every 4 hours if necessary
• By slow intravenous injection (but see also Management of Acute Asthma table, p. 185), (dilute to a concentration of 50 micrograms/mL), 250 micr-

ograms, repeated if necessary; CHILD under 18 years see *BNF for Children*

- By intravenous infusion (but see also Management of Acute Asthma table, p. 185), initially 5 micrograms/ minute, adjusted according to response and heart-rate usually in range 3–20 micrograms/minute, or more if necessary; CHILD under 18 years see *BNF for Children*
- By aerosol inhalation (but see also Management of Acute Asthma table, p. 185, *or* Management of Chronic Asthma table, p. 184), 100–200 micrograms (1–2 puffs); for persistent symptoms up to 4 times daily; CHILD 100 micrograms (1 puff), increased to 200 micrograms (2 puffs) if necessary; for persistent symptoms up to 4 times daily

  Prophylaxis of allergen- or exercise-induced bron-chospasm, 200 micrograms (2 puffs); CHILD 100 micr-ograms (1 puff), increased to 200 micrograms (2 puffs) if necessary
- By inhalation of powder (but see also Management of Chronic Asthma table, p. 184) see under individual preparations
- By inhalation of nebulised solution, ADULT and CHILD over 5 years 2.5–5 mg, repeated up to 4 times daily or more frequently in severe cases; CHILD under 5 years 2.5 mg, repeated up to 4 times daily or more fre-quently in severe cases; see also Management of Acute Asthma table, p. 185 and Management of Chronic Asthma table, p. 184

◢ Oral

Salbutamol (Non-proprietary) PoM

Tablets, salbutamol (as sulfate) 2 mg, net price 28-tab pack = £103.08; 4 mg, 28-tab pack = £105.52

Oral solution, salbutamol (as sulfate) 2 mg/5 mL, net price 150 mL = 72p

Brands include *Salapin* ® (sugar-free)

Ventmax ® **SR** (Chiesi) PoM

Capsules, m/r, salbutamol (as sulfate) 4 mg (green/ grey), net price 56-cap pack = £8.08; 8 mg (white), 56-cap pack = £9.69. Label: 25

Dose 8 mg twice daily; CHILD 3–12 years 4 mg twice daily

Ventolin ® (A&H) PoM

Syrup, sugar-free, salbutamol (as sulfate) 2 mg/5 mL, net price 150 mL = 72p

◢ Parenteral

Ventolin ® (A&H) PoM

Injection, salbutamol (as sulfate) 500 micrograms/ mL, net price 1-mL amp = 38p

Solution for intravenous infusion, salbutamol (as sulfate) 1 mg/mL. Dilute before use. Net price 5-mL amp = £2.48

◢ Inhalation

Counselling Advise patients not to exceed prescribed dose and to follow manufacturer's directions; if a previously effective dose of inhaled salbutamol fails to provide at least 3 hours relief, a doctor's advice should be obtained as soon as possible.

Salbutamol (Non-proprietary) PoM

Aerosol inhalation, salbutamol (as sulfate) 100 micr-ograms/metered inhalation, net price 200-dose unit = £1.50. Counselling, administration

Brands include *AirSalb* ®, *Salamol* ®

Nebuliser solution, salbutamol (as sulfate) 1 mg/mL, net price 20 × 2.5 mL (2.5 mg) = £1.91; 2 mg/mL, 20 × 2.5 mL (5 mg) = £3.82. May be diluted with sterile sodium chloride 0.9%

Brands include *Salamol Steri-Neb* ®

Airomir ® (TEVA UK) PoM

Aerosol inhalation, salbutamol (as sulfate) 100 micr-ograms/metered inhalation, net price 200-dose unit = £1.97. Counselling, administration

Autohaler (breath-actuated aerosol inhalation), sal-butamol (as sulfate) 100 micrograms/metered inha-lation, net price 200-dose unit = £6.02. Counselling, administration

Asmasal Clickhaler ® (RPH) PoM

Dry powder for inhalation, salbutamol (as sulfate) 95 micrograms/metered inhalation, net price 200-dose unit = £5.65. Counselling, administration

Dose acute bronchospasm, by inhalation of powder, ADULT and CHILD over 5 years, 1–2 puffs; for persistent symptoms up to 4 times daily (but see also Management of Chronic Asthma table, p. 184)

Prophylaxis of allergen- or exercise-induced bronchospasm, by inhalation of powder, ADULT and CHILD over 5 years, 1–2 puffs

Easyhaler ® **Salbutamol** (Orion) PoM

Dry powder for inhalation, salbutamol (as sulfate) 100 micrograms/metered inhalation, net price 200-dose unit = £3.31; 200 micrograms/metered inhala-tion, 200-dose unit = £6.63. Counselling, administra-tion

Dose acute bronchospasm, by inhalation of powder, ADULT and CHILD over 12 years, initially 100–200 micrograms, increased to 400 micrograms if necessary; max. 800 micrograms daily (but see also Management of Chronic Asthma table, p. 184); CHILD 5–12 years, 100–200 micrograms; max. 800 micrograms daily (but see also Management of Chronic Asthma table, p. 184)

Prophylaxis of allergen- or exercise-induced bronchospasm, by inhalation of powder, ADULT and CHILD over 12 years, 200 micrograms; CHILD 5–12 years, 100–200 micrograms

Pulvinal ® **Salbutamol** (Chiesi) PoM

Dry powder for inhalation, salbutamol 200 micr-ograms/metered inhalation, net price 100-dose unit = £4.85. Counselling, administration

Dose acute bronchospasm, by inhalation of powder, ADULT and CHILD over 5 years, 200 micrograms; for persistent symptoms up to 800 micrograms daily (but see also Management of Chronic Asthma table, p. 184)

Prophylaxis of allergen- or exercise- induced bronchospasm, ADULT and CHILD over 5 years, 200 micrograms

Salamol Easi-Breathe ® (TEVA UK) PoM

Aerosol inhalation, salbutamol 100 micrograms/ metered inhalation, net price 200-dose breath-actu-ated unit = £6.30. Counselling, administration

Salbulin Novolizer ® (Meda) PoM

Dry powder for inhalation, salbutamol (as sulfate) 100 micrograms/metered inhalation, net price refill-able 200-dose unit = £4.95; 200-dose refill = £2.75. Counselling, administration

Dose acute bronchospasm, by inhalation of powder, ADULT 100–200 micrograms; for persistent symptoms up to 800 micrograms daily (but see also Management of Chronic Asthma table, p. 184); CHILD 6–12 years 100–200 micrograms; for persistent symptoms up to 400 micrograms daily (but see also Management of Chronic Asthma table, p. 184)

Prophylaxis of allergen- or exercise-induced bronchospasm, by inhalation of powder, ADULT 200 micrograms; CHILD 6–12 years 100–200 micrograms

3

Respiratory system

Ventolin® (A&H) [PoM]

Accuhaler® (dry powder for inhalation), disk containing 60 blisters of salbutamol (as sulfate) 200 micrograms/blister with *Accuhaler®* device, net price = £3.00. Counselling, administration

Dose acute bronchospasm, by inhalation of powder, ADULT and CHILD over 5 years, 200 micrograms; for persistent symptoms up to 4 times daily (but see also Management of Chronic Asthma table, p. 184)

Prophylaxis of allergen- or exercise-induced bronchospasm, by inhalation of powder, ADULT and CHILD over 5 years, 200 micrograms

Evohaler® (aerosol inhalation), salbutamol (as sulfate) 100 micrograms/metered inhalation, net price 200-dose unit = £1.50. Counselling, administration

Nebules® (for use with nebuliser), salbutamol (as sulfate) 1 mg/mL, net price 20 × 2.5 mL (2.5 mg) = £1.65; 2 mg/mL, 20 × 2.5 mL (5 mg) = £2.78. May be diluted with sterile sodium chloride 0.9% if administration time in excess of 10 minutes is required

Respirator solution (for use with a nebuliser or ventilator), salbutamol (as sulfate) 5 mg/mL, net price 20 mL = £2.18 (hosp. only). May be diluted with sterile sodium chloride 0.9%

◢**Compound preparations**

For **compound preparations** containing salbutamol, see section 3.1.4

Management of Chronic Asthma table, see p. 184
Management of Acute Asthma table, see p. 185

◢ SALMETEROL

Indications reversible airways obstruction (including nocturnal asthma and prevention of exercise-induced bronchospasm) in patients requiring long-term regular bronchodilator therapy, see also Management of Chronic Asthma table, p. 184; chronic obstructive pulmonary disease

Note Not for immediate relief of acute asthma attacks; for use in asthma only in patients who regularly use an inhaled corticosteroid, see notes above

Cautions see notes above

Pregnancy see p. 186

Breast-feeding see p. 186

Side-effects see notes above; nausea, dizziness, arthralgia, and rash also reported

Dose

● By inhalation, asthma, 50 micrograms (2 puffs or 1 blister) twice daily; up to 100 micrograms (4 puffs or 2 blisters) twice daily in more severe airways obstruction; CHILD 5–12 years, 50 micrograms (2 puffs or 1 blister) twice daily

Chronic obstructive pulmonary disease 50 micrograms (2 puffs or 1 blister) twice daily

Counselling Advise patients that salmeterol should **not** be used for relief of acute attacks, not to exceed prescribed dose, and to follow manufacturer's directions; if a previously effective dose of inhaled salmeterol fails to provide adequate relief, a doctor's advice should be obtained as soon as possible

Salmeterol (Non-proprietary) [PoM]

Aerosol inhalation, salmeterol (as xinafoate) 25 micrograms/metered inhalation, net price 120-dose unit = £27.80. Counselling, administration

Brands include *Neovent®*

Serevent® (A&H) [PoM]

Accuhaler® (dry powder for inhalation), disk containing 60 blisters of salmeterol (as xinafoate) 50 micrograms/blister with *Accuhaler®* device, net price = £29.26. Counselling, administration

Evohaler® (aerosol inhalation), salmeterol (as xinafoate) 25 micrograms/metered inhalation, net price 120-dose unit = £29.26. Counselling, administration

◢**Compound preparations**

For **compound preparations** containing salmeterol, see section 3.2

◢ TERBUTALINE SULFATE

Indications asthma and other conditions associated with reversible airways obstruction; premature labour (section 7.1.3)

Cautions see notes above

Pregnancy see p. 186

Breast-feeding see p. 186

Side-effects see notes above

Dose

● By mouth (but use by inhalation preferred), initially 2.5 mg 3 times daily for 1–2 weeks, then up to 5 mg 3 times daily; CHILD 1 month–7 years 75 micrograms/kg 3 times daily; 7–15 years 2.5 mg 2–3 times daily

● By subcutaneous *or* slow intravenous injection, 250–500 micrograms up to 4 times daily; CHILD 2–15 years 10 micrograms/kg to a max. of 300 micrograms

● By continuous intravenous infusion as a solution containing 3–5 micrograms/mL, 90–300 micrograms/hour for 8–10 hours; CHILD 1 month–18 years, initially 2–4 micrograms/kg as a loading dose, then 1–10 micrograms/kg/hour according to response and heart rate (max. 300 micrograms/hour); high doses with close monitoring

● By inhalation of powder (*Turbohaler®*), ADULT and CHILD over 5 years, 500 micrograms (1 inhalation); for persistent symptoms up to 4 times daily (but see Management of Chronic Asthma table, p. 184)

● By inhalation of nebulised solution (but see also Management of Acute Asthma table, p. 185), 5–10 mg 2–4 times daily; additional doses may be necessary in severe acute asthma; CHILD under 5 years 5 mg 2–4 times daily, 5–12 years 5–10 mg 2–4 times daily [unlicensed dose]

◢**Oral and parenteral**

Bricanyl® (AstraZeneca) [PoM]

Tablets, scored, terbutaline sulfate 5 mg, net price 100-tab pack= £4.91

Syrup, sugar-free, terbutaline sulfate 1.5 mg/5 mL, net price 100 mL = £2.80

Injection, terbutaline sulfate 500 micrograms/mL, net price 1-mL amp = 43p; 5-mL amp = £1.67

◢**Inhalation**

Counselling Advise patients not to exceed prescribed dose and to follow manufacturer's directions; if a previously effective dose of inhaled terbutaline fails to provide at least 3 hours relief, a doctor's advice should be obtained as soon as possible

Bricanyl® (AstraZeneca) [PoM]

Turbohaler® (= dry powder inhaler), terbutaline sulfate 500 micrograms/metered inhalation, net price 100-dose unit = £6.92. Counselling, administration

Respules® (= single-dose units for nebulisation), terbutaline sulfate 2.5 mg/mL, net price 20 × 2-mL units (5-mg) = £5.82

3.1.1.2 Other adrenoceptor agonists

Ephedrine is less suitable and less safe for use as a bronchodilator than the selective beta$_2$ agonists, because it is more likely to cause arrhythmias and other side-effects; it should be avoided whenever possible.

Adrenaline (epinephrine) injection (1 in 1000) is used in the emergency treatment of acute allergic and anaphylactic reactions (section 3.4.3), in angioedema (section 3.4.3), and in cardiopulmonary resuscitation (section 2.7.3). Adrenaline solution (1 in 1000) is used by nebulisation in the management of severe croup (section 3.1).

EPHEDRINE HYDROCHLORIDE

Indications　reversible airways obstruction, but see notes above

Cautions　hyperthyroidism; diabetes mellitus; ischaemic heart disease; hypertension; elderly; prostatic hypertrophy (risk of acute retention); **interactions**: Appendix 1 (sympathomimetics)

Renal impairment　use with caution

Pregnancy　manufacturer advises avoid

Breast-feeding　present in milk; manufacturer advises avoid—irritability and disturbed sleep reported

Side-effects　tachycardia; anxiety, restlessness, insomnia; tremor, arrhythmias, dry mouth, and cold extremities also reported

Dose

- 15–60 mg 3 times daily; CHILD up to 1 year 7.5 mg 3 times daily, 1–5 years 15 mg 3 times daily, 6–12 years 30 mg 3 times daily

¹Ephedrine Hydrochloride (Non-proprietary) PoM
Tablets, ephedrine hydrochloride 15 mg, net price 28 = £13.47; 30 mg, 28 = £20.57

3.1.2 Antimuscarinic bronchodilators

Ipratropium can provide short-term relief in chronic asthma, but short-acting beta$_2$ agonists act more quickly and are preferred. Ipratropium by nebulisation can be added to other standard treatment in life-threatening asthma or if acute asthma fails to improve with standard therapy (see Management of Acute Asthma table, p. 185).

The aerosol inhalation of ipratropium can be used for short-term relief in mild chronic obstructive pulmonary disease in patients who are not using a long-acting antimuscarinic drug. Its maximal effect occurs 30–60 minutes after use; its duration of action is 3 to 6 hours and bronchodilation can usually be maintained with treatment 3 times a day.

Aclidinium, glycopyrronium, tiotropium, and **umeclidinium** are licensed for the maintenance treatment of patients with chronic obstructive pulmonary disease. They are not suitable for the relief of acute bronchospasm.

1. For exemptions see *Medicines, Ethics and Practice*, London, Pharmaceutical Press (always consult latest edition)

Cautions　Antimuscarinic bronchodilators should be used with caution in patients with prostatic hyperplasia, bladder outflow obstruction, and those susceptible to angle-closure glaucoma (see below); **interactions**: Appendix 1 (antimuscarinics).

Glaucoma *Acute angle-closure glaucoma* has been reported with nebulised ipratropium, particularly when given with nebulised salbutamol (and possibly other beta$_2$ agonists); care needed to protect patient's eyes from nebulised drug or from drug powder.

Side-effects　Dry mouth is the most common side-effect of antimuscarinic bronchodilators; also gastrointestinal motility disorder (including constipation and diarrhoea), cough, and headache; less commonly nausea, gastro-oesophageal reflux disease, dysphagia, tachycardia, palpitation, atrial fibrillation, throat irritation, pharyngitis, dysphonia, bronchospasm, including paradoxical bronchospasm, urinary retention, mydriasis, angle-closure glaucoma, blurred vision, and nasopharyngitis can occur. Dental caries and dry skin have occurred rarely.

ACLIDINIUM BROMIDE

Indications　maintenance treatment of chronic obstructive pulmonary disease

Cautions　see notes above; also myocardial infarction within last 6 months, unstable angina, newly diagnosed arrhythmia within last 3 months, hospitalisation with moderate or severe heart failure within last 12 months

Pregnancy　manufacturer advises use only if potential benefit outweighs risk

Breast-feeding　manufacturer advises avoid

Side-effects　see notes above; also sinusitis

Dose

- See under preparation below

Eklira Genuair® (Almirall) ▼ PoM
Inhalation powder, aclidinium bromide 375 micrograms (≡ aclidinium 322 micrograms)/inhalation (delivered dose), net price 60-dose unit = £28.60. Counselling, administration
Dose by inhalation of powder, ADULT over 18 years, 1 inhalation twice daily

GLYCOPYRRONIUM

Indications　maintenance treatment of chronic obstructive pulmonary disease; palliative care (Prescribing in Palliative Care, p. 21); hyperhidrosis (section 13.12); premedication (section 15.1.3)

Cautions　see notes above; also unstable ischaemic heart disease, left ventricular failure, arrhythmia (excluding chronic stable atrial fibrillation), history of myocardial infarction or QT-interval prolongation

Renal impairment　use with caution if eGFR less than 30 mL/minute/1.73m^2

Pregnancy　manufacturer advises use only if potential benefit outweighs risk

Breast-feeding　manufacturer advises use only if potential benefit outweighs risk

Side-effects　see notes above; also insomnia; *less commonly* malaise, hyperglycaemia, hypoaesthesia, rhinitis, epistaxis

Dose

- See under preparation below

3　Respiratory system

Seebri Breezhaler® (Novartis) ▼ PoM
Inhalation powder, hard capsule, (for use with *Seebri Breezhaler®* device), orange, glycopyrronium (as glycopyrronium bromide) 50 micrograms, net price 30-cap pack with *Seebri Breezhaler®* device = £27.50, 6-cap pack with *Seebri Breezhaler®* device = £5.50. Counselling, administration
Dose by inhalation of powder, ADULT over 18 years, 50 micrograms (1 capsule) once daily
Equivalence Each 50 microgram capsule of glycopyrronium delivers 44 micrograms of glycopyrronium

IPRATROPIUM BROMIDE

Indications reversible airways obstruction, particularly in chronic obstructive pulmonary disease; rhinitis (section 12.2.2)

Cautions see notes above; also cystic fibrosis

Pregnancy see p. 186

Breast-feeding see p. 186

Side-effects see notes above; also dizziness; *less commonly* vomiting, stomatitis, laryngospasm, pruritus

Dose
* By aerosol inhalation, 20–40 micrograms 3–4 times daily; CHILD up to 6 years 20 micrograms 3 times daily, 6–12 years 20–40 micrograms 3 times daily
* By inhalation of nebulised solution, reversible airways obstruction in chronic obstructive pulmonary disease, 250–500 micrograms 3–4 times daily

Acute bronchospasm (but see also Management of Acute Asthma table, p. 185), 500 micrograms repeated as necessary; CHILD under 5 years 125–250 micrograms, max. 1 mg daily; 6–12 years 250 micrograms, max. 1 mg daily

Counselling Advise patient not to exceed prescribed dose and to follow manufacturer's directions

Ipratropium Bromide (Non-proprietary) PoM
Nebuliser solution, ipratropium bromide 250 micrograms/mL, net price 20 × 1-mL (250-microgram) unit-dose vials = £4.39, 60 × 1-mL = £21.78; 20 × 2-mL (500-microgram) = £5.23, 60 × 2-mL = £26.97. If dilution is necessary use only sterile sodium chloride 0.9%

Atrovent® (Boehringer Ingelheim) PoM
Aerosol inhalation, ipratropium bromide 20 micrograms/metered inhalation, net price 200-dose unit = £5.56. Counselling, administration
Nebuliser solution, isotonic, ipratropium bromide 250 micrograms/mL, net price 20 × 1-mL unit-dose vials = £4.14, 60 × 1-mL vials = £12.44; 20 × 2-mL vials = £4.87, 60 × 2-mL vials = £14.59. If dilution is necessary use only sterile sodium chloride 0.9%

Ipratropium Steri-Neb® (TEVA UK) PoM
Nebuliser solution, isotonic, ipratropium bromide 250 micrograms/mL, net price 20 × 1-mL (250-microgram) unit-dose vials = £14.99; 20 × 2-mL (500-microgram) = £15.99. If dilution is necessary use only sterile sodium chloride 0.9%

Respontin® (A&H) PoM
Nebuliser solution, isotonic, ipratropium bromide 250 micrograms/mL, net price 20 × 1-mL (250-microgram) unit-dose vials = £4.78; 20 × 2-mL (500-microgram) = £5.60. If dilution is necessary use only sterile sodium chloride 0.9%

◀**Compound ipratropium preparations**
Section 3.1.4

TIOTROPIUM

Indications maintenance treatment of chronic obstructive pulmonary disease

Cautions see notes above; also cardiac rhythm disorders (with *Spiriva Respimat®*)—use *Spiriva Respimat®* only when patient unable to use *Handihaler®* device

Pregnancy manufacturer advises use only if potential benefit outweighs risk

Breast-feeding manufacturer advises avoid—no information available

Renal impairment plasma-tiotropium concentration raised; use with caution if eGFR less than 50 mL/minute/1.73 m^2

Side-effects see notes above; also taste disturbance, oropharyngeal candidiasis, dizziness, epistaxis, pruritus; *rarely* intestinal obstruction (including paralytic ileus), insomnia, sinusitis, gingivitis, glossitis, stomatitis; *also reported* dehydration, joint swelling

Dose
* See under preparations below

Spiriva® (Boehringer Ingelheim) PoM
Inhalation powder, hard capsule (for use with *HandiHaler®* device), green, tiotropium (as tiotropium bromide monohydrate) 18 micrograms, net price 30-cap pack with *HandiHaler®* device = £34.87, 30-cap refill = £33.50. Counselling, administration
Dose by inhalation of powder, ADULT over 18 years, 18 micrograms once daily
Respimat® (solution for inhalation), tiotropium (as tiotropium bromide monohydrate) 2.5 micrograms/metered inhalation, net price 60-dose unit = £33.50. Counselling, administration
Dose by inhalation, ADULT over 18 years, 5 micrograms (2 puffs) once daily
Note The *Scottish Medicines Consortium* has advised (November 2007) that *Spiriva Respimat®* is restricted for use in chronic obstructive pulmonary disease in patients who have poor manual dexterity and difficulty using the *Handihaler®* device

UMECLIDINIUM

Indications maintenance treatment of chronic obstructive pulmonary disease

Cautions see notes above; also cardiac disorders (particularly cardiac rhythm disorders)

Pregnancy manufacturer advises use only if potential benefit outweighs risk

Breast-feeding manufacturer advises avoid—no information available

Hepatic impairment use with caution in severe impairment

Side-effects see notes above; also *less commonly* arrhythmias, urinary tract infection, sinusitis, rash

Dose
* See under preparation below

Incruse Ellipta® (GSK) ▼ PoM
Inhalation powder, umeclidinium (as bromide) 55 micrograms (≡ umeclidinium bromide 65 micrograms)/inhalation (delivered dose), net price 30-dose unit = £27.50. Counselling, administration
Dose by inhalation of powder, ADULT over 18 years, 55 micrograms (1 inhalation) once daily

3.1.3 Theophylline

Theophylline is a xanthine used as a bronchodilator in *asthma* (see Management of Chronic Asthma table, p. 184) and stable *chronic obstructive pulmonary disease* (see p. 186); it is not generally effective in exacerbations of chronic obstructive pulmonary disease. Theophylline may have an additive effect when used in conjunction with small doses of beta₂ agonists; the combination may increase the risk of side-effects, including hypokalaemia (see p. 189).

Theophylline is given by injection as **aminophylline**, a mixture of theophylline with ethylenediamine, which is 20 times more soluble than theophylline alone. Aminophylline injection is needed rarely for severe acute asthma, see Management of Acute Asthma table, p. 185. It must be given by **very slow** intravenous injection (over at least 20 minutes); it is too irritant for intramuscular use. Measurement of plasma-theophylline concentration may be helpful and is **essential** if aminophylline is to be given to patients who are already taking theophylline, because serious side-effects such as convulsions and arrhythmias can occasionally precede other symptoms of toxicity.

Theophylline is metabolised in the liver. The plasma-theophylline concentration is *increased* in heart failure, hepatic impairment, viral infections, in the elderly, and by drugs that inhibit its metabolism. The plasma-theophylline concentration is *decreased* in smokers, by alcohol consumption, and by drugs that induce its metabolism. Differences in the half-life of theophylline are important because the toxic dose is close to the therapeutic dose. For **interactions:** see Appendix 1 (theophylline).

Plasma-theophylline concentration In most individuals, a plasma-theophylline concentration of 10–20 mg/litre (55–110 micromol/litre) is required for satisfactory bronchodilation, although a lower plasma-theophylline concentration may be effective. Adverse effects can occur within the range 10–20 mg/litre and both the frequency and severity increase at concentrations above 20 mg/litre.

Plasma-theophylline concentration is measured 5 days after starting oral treatment and at least 3 days after any dose adjustment. A blood sample should usually be taken 4–6 hours after an oral dose of a modified-release preparation (sampling times may vary—consult local guidelines). If aminophylline is given intravenously, a blood sample should be taken 4–6 hours after treatment.

Caffeine is a xanthine derivative used as a respiratory stimulant in *neonatal apnoea*, see *BNF for Children* section 3.5.1.

THEOPHYLLINE

Indications   reversible airways obstruction, severe acute asthma; see also Management of Chronic Asthma table p. 184 and Management of Acute Asthma table p. 185

Cautions   see notes above, also cardiac arrhythmias or other cardiac disease; hypertension; hyperthyroidism; peptic ulcer; epilepsy; elderly; fever; hypokalaemia risk, see p. 189; monitor plasma-theophylline concentration (see notes above); dose adjustment may be necessary if smoking started or stopped during treatment

Hepatic impairment   reduce dose

Pregnancy   neonatal irritability and apnoea have been reported; see also p. 186

Breast-feeding   present in milk—irritability in infant reported; modified-release preparations preferable; see also p. 186

Side-effects   nausea, vomiting, gastric irritation, diarrhoea, palpitation, tachycardia, arrhythmias, headache, CNS stimulation, insomnia, convulsions; **overdosage:** see Emergency Treatment of Poisoning, p. 41

Dose
* See under preparations below
  Note Plasma-theophylline concentration for optimum response 10–20 mg/litre (55–110 micromol/litre); narrow margin between therapeutic and toxic dose, see also notes above

◢Modified release

Note The rate of absorption from modified-release preparations can vary between brands. If a prescription for a modified-release oral theophylline preparation does not specify a brand name, the pharmacist should contact the prescriber and agree the brand to be dispensed. Additionally, it is essential that a patient discharged from hospital should be maintained on the brand on which that patient was stabilised as an in-patient.

Nuelin SA® (Meda)
SA tablets, m/r, theophylline 175 mg, net price 60-tab pack = £6.38. Label: 21, 25
Dose 175–350 mg every 12 hours; CHILD 6–12 years 175 mg every 12 hours

SA 250 tablets, m/r, scored, theophylline 250 mg, net price 60-tab pack = £8.92. Label: 21, 25
Dose 250–500 mg every 12 hours; CHILD 6–12 years 125–250 mg every 12 hours

Slo-Phyllin® (Merck Serono)
Capsules, m/r, theophylline 60 mg (white/clear, enclosing white pellets), net price 56-cap pack = £2.76; 125 mg (brown/clear, enclosing white pellets), 56-cap pack = £3.48; 250 mg (purple/clear, enclosing white pellets), 56-cap pack = £4.34. Label: 25, or counselling, see below
Dose 250–500 mg every 12 hours; CHILD 2–6 years 60–120 mg every 12 hours, 6–12 years 125–250 mg every 12 hours
Counselling Swallow whole with fluid *or* swallow enclosed granules with soft food (e.g. yoghurt)

Uniphyllin Continus® (Napp)
Tablets, m/r, theophylline 200 mg, net price 56-tab pack = £2.96; 300 mg, 56-tab pack = £4.77; 400 mg, 56-tab pack = £5.65. Label: 25
Dose 200 mg every 12 hours, increased according to response to 400 mg every 12 hours; CHILD 2–12 years, 9 mg/kg (up to 200 mg) every 12 hours; some children with chronic asthma may require 10–16 mg/kg (max. 400 mg) every 12 hours
Note May be appropriate to give larger evening or morning dose to achieve optimum therapeutic effect when symptoms most severe; in patients whose night or daytime symptoms persist despite other therapy, who are not currently receiving theophylline, total daily requirement may be added as single evening or morning dose

AMINOPHYLLINE

Note Aminophylline is a stable mixture or combination of theophylline and ethylenediamine; the ethylenediamine confers greater solubility in water

Indications   reversible airways obstruction, severe acute asthma

Cautions   see under Theophylline

Hepatic impairment   see under Theophylline

3

Respiratory system

Pregnancy   see under Theophylline

Breast-feeding   see under Theophylline

Side-effects   see under Theophylline; also allergy to ethylenediamine can cause urticaria, erythema, and exfoliative dermatitis; hypotension, arrhythmias, and convulsions especially if given rapidly by intravenous injection

Dose

- See under preparations, below

Note Plasma-theophylline concentration for optimum response 10–20 mg/litre (55–110 micromol/litre); narrow margin between therapeutic and toxic dose, see also notes above

> To avoid excessive dosage in obese patients, dose should be calculated on the basis of ideal weight for height

Aminophylline (Non-proprietary) PoM

Injection, aminophylline 25 mg/mL, net price 10-mL amp = 65p

Dose severe acute asthma or acute exacerbation of chronic obstructive pulmonary disease in patients **not** previously treated with theophylline, by slow intravenous injection over at least 20 minutes (with close monitoring), 250–500 mg (5 mg/kg), then see below; CHILD under 12 years 5 mg/kg, then see below

Severe acute asthma or acute exacerbation of chronic obstructive pulmonary disease by intravenous infusion (with close monitoring), 500–700 micrograms/kg/hour, adjusted according to plasma-theophylline concentration; ELDERLY 300 micrograms/kg/hour; CHILD under 12 years 1 mg/kg/hour, adjusted according to plasma-theophylline concentration

Note Patients taking oral theophylline or aminophylline should not normally receive a loading dose of intravenous aminophylline; plasma-theophylline concentration should be measured in all patients receiving intravenous aminophylline (see notes above)

◢**Modified release**

Note Advice about modified-release theophylline preparations (see p. 195) also applies to modified-release aminophylline preparations

Phyllocontin Continus® (Napp)

Tablets, m/r, yellow, f/c, aminophylline hydrate 225 mg, net price 56-tab pack = £2.40. Label: 25

Dose ADULT and CHILD body-weight over 40 kg initially 1 tablet twice daily, increased after 1 week to 2 tablets twice daily according to plasma-theophylline concentration

Forte tablets, m/r, yellow, f/c, aminophylline hydrate 350 mg, net price 56-tab pack = £4.22. Label: 25

Dose initially 1 tablet twice daily, increased after 1 week to 2 tablets twice daily if necessary

Note *Phyllocontin Continus® Forte* tablets are for smokers and other patients with shorter theophylline half-life (see notes above)

3.1.4   Compound bronchodilator preparations

In general, patients are best treated with single-ingredient preparations, such as a selective beta₂ agonist (section 3.1.1.1) or ipratropium bromide (section 3.1.2), so that the dose of each drug can be adjusted. This flexibility is lost with compound bronchodilator preparations. However, a combination product may be appropriate for patients stabilised on individual components in the same proportion.

For prescribing information, see under individual drugs.

Ipratropium bromide with salbutamol (Non-proprietary) PoM ◢

Nebuliser solution, ipratropium bromide 500 micrograms, salbutamol (as sulfate) 2.5 mg/2.5-mL vial, net price 60 unit-dose vials = £23.75

Brands include *Salipraneb, Ipramol*

Dose bronchospasm in chronic obstructive pulmonary disease, by inhalation of nebulised solution, ADULT and CHILD over 12 years, 1 vial (2.5 mL) 3–4 times daily

Glaucoma In addition to other potential side-effects, acute angle-closure glaucoma has been reported with nebulised ipratropium—for details, see p. 193

Anoro Ellipta® (GSK) ▼ PoM

Anoro Ellipta® 55 micrograms/ 22 micrograms, (dry powder for inhalation), umeclidinium 55 micrograms, vilanterol (as trifenatate) 22 micrograms/ inhalation (delivered dose), net price 30-dose unit = £32.50. Counselling, administration

The *Scottish Medicines Consortium* (p. 4) has advised (July 2014) that *Anoro Ellipta®* is **not** recommended for use within NHS Scottland.

Cautions see section 3.1.1.1 and section 3.1.2; also severe hepatic impairment, severe cardiovascular disease, convulsive disorders

Pregnancy manufacturer advises use only if potential benefit outweighs risk

Breast-feeding manufacturer advises avoid—no information available

Side-effects see section 3.1.1.1 and section 3.1.2; also urinary tract infection, sinusitis, oropharyngeal pain; *less commonly* rash

Dose by inhalation of powder, maintenance treatment of chronic obstructive pulmonary disease, ADULT over 18 years, 1 inhalation once daily

Combivent® (Boehringer Ingelheim) PoM ◢

Nebuliser solution, isotonic, ipratropium bromide 500 micrograms, salbutamol (as sulfate) 2.5 mg/2.5-mL vial, net price 60 unit-dose vials = £24.10

Dose bronchospasm in chronic obstructive pulmonary disease, by inhalation of nebulised solution, ADULT and CHILD over 12 years, 1 vial (2.5 mL) 3–4 times daily

Glaucoma In addition to other potential side-effects, acute angle-closure glaucoma has been reported with nebulised ipratropium—for details, see p. 193

3.1.5   Peak flow meters, inhaler devices and nebulisers

Peak flow meters

When used in addition to symptom-based monitoring, peak flow monitoring has not been proven to improve asthma control in either adults or children, however measurement of peak flow may be of benefit in adult patients who are 'poor perceivers' and hence slow to detect deterioration in their asthma, and for those with more severe asthma.

When peak flow meters are used, patients must be given clear guidelines as to the action they should take if their peak flow falls below a certain level. Patients can be encouraged to adjust some of their own treatment (within specified limits) according to changes in peak flow rate.

Peak flow charts should be issued to patients where appropriate, and are available to purchase from:

3M Security Print and Systems Limited
Gorse Street, Chadderton
Oldham
OL9 9QH
Tel: 0845 610 1112

GP practices can obtain supplies through their Area Team stores.

NHS Hospitals can order supplies from www.nhsforms.co.uk or by emailing nhsforms@mmm.com.

In Scotland, peak flow charts can be obtained by emailing stockorders.dppas@apsgroup.co.uk.

Standard Range Peak Flow Meter

Conforms to standard EN ISO 23747:2007

AirZone®, range 60–720 litres/minute, net price = £4.69, replacement mouthpiece = 38p (Clement Clarke)

Medi®, range 60–800 litres/minute, net price = £4.50 (Medicare)

MicroPeak®, range 60–900 litres/minute, net price = £6.50, replacement mouthpiece = 38p (Micro Medical)

Mini-Wright®, range 60–800 litres/minute, net price = £7.08, replacement mouthpiece = 38p (Clement Clarke)

Personal Best®, range 60–800 litres/minute, net price = £6.86 (Respironics)

Piko-1®, range 15–999 litres/minute, net price = £9.50, replacement mouthpiece = 38p (nSPIRE Health)

Pinnacle®, range 60–900 litres/minute, net price = £6.50 (Fyne Dynamics)

Pocketpeak®, range 60–800 litres/minute, net price = £6.53, replacement mouthpiece = 38p (nSPIRE Health)

Vitalograph®, range 50–800 litres/minute, net price = £4.83 (children's coloured version also available) (Vitalograph)

Low Range Peak Flow Meter

Compliant to standard EN ISO 23747:2007 except for scale range

Medi®, range 40–420 litres/minute, net price = £6.50 (Medicare)

Mini-Wright®, range 30–400 litres/minute, net price = £7.14, replacement mouthpiece = 38p (Clement Clarke)

Pocketpeak®, range 50–400 litres/minute, net price = £6.53, replacement mouthpiece = 38p (nSPIRE Health)

Drug delivery devices

Inhaler devices These include *pressurised metered-dose inhalers, breath-actuated inhalers*, and *dry powder inhalers*. Many patients can be taught to use a pressurised metered-dose inhaler effectively but some patients, particularly the elderly and children, find them difficult to use. *Spacer devices* (see below) can help such patients because they remove the need to coordinate actuation with inhalation. Dry powder inhalers may be useful in adults and children over 5 years who are unwilling or unable to use a pressurised metered-dose inhaler. Alternatively, breath-actuated inhalers are suitable for adults and older children provided they can use the device effectively.

On changing from a pressurised metered-dose inhaler to a dry powder inhaler, patients may notice a lack of sensation in the mouth and throat previously associated with each actuation. Coughing may also occur.

The patient should be instructed carefully on the use of the inhaler and it is important to check that the inhaler continues to be used correctly because inadequate inhalation technique may be mistaken for a lack of response to the drug.

> ### NICE guidance
> #### Inhaler devices for children under 5 years with chronic asthma (August 2000)
> A child's needs and likelihood of good compliance should govern the choice of inhaler and spacer device; only then should cost be considered.
> - corticosteroid and bronchodilator therapy should be delivered by pressurised metered-dose inhaler and spacer device, with a facemask if necessary;
> - if this is not effective, and depending on the child's condition, nebulised therapy may be considered and, in children over 3 years, a dry powder inhaler may also be considered [but see notes above].
>
> www.nice.org.uk/TA10

> ### NICE guidance
> #### Inhaler devices for children 5–15 years with chronic asthma (March 2002)
> A child's needs, ability to develop and maintain effective technique, and likelihood of good compliance should govern the choice of inhaler device; only then should cost be considered.
> - corticosteroid therapy should be routinely delivered by a pressurised metered-dose inhaler and spacer device;
> - for other inhaled drugs, particularly bronchodilators, a wider range of devices should be considered;
> - children and their carers should be trained in the use of the chosen device; suitability of the device should be reviewed at least annually. Inhaler technique and compliance should be monitored.
>
> www.nice.org.uk/TA38

Spacer devices Spacer devices remove the need for coordination between actuation of a pressurised metered-dose inhaler and inhalation. The spacer device reduces the velocity of the aerosol and subsequent impaction on the oropharynx and allows more time for evaporation of the propellant so that a larger proportion of the particles can be inhaled and deposited in the lungs. Spacer devices are particularly useful for patients with poor inhalation technique, for children, for patients requiring high doses of inhaled corticosteroids (see Management of Chronic Asthma table, p. 184), for nocturnal asthma, and for patients prone to candidiasis with inhaled corticosteroids. The size of the spacer is important, the larger spacers with a one-way valve (*Volumatic®*) being most effective. It is important to prescribe a spacer device that is compatible with the metered-dose inhaler, see devices below. Spacer devices should not be regarded as interchangeable; patients should be advised not to switch between spacer devices.

Use and care of spacer devices Patients should inhale from the spacer device as soon as possible after actuation because the drug aerosol is very short-lived; single-dose actuation is recommended. Tidal breathing is as effective as single breaths. The device should be cleaned once a month by washing in mild detergent and then allowed to dry in air without rinsing; the mouthpiece should be wiped clean of detergent before use. Some manufacturers recommend more frequent cleaning, but this should be avoided since any electrostatic charge may affect drug delivery. Spacer devices should be replaced every 6–12 months.

A2A Spacer® (Clement Clarke)

Spacer device, for use with all pressurised (aerosol) inhalers, net price = £4.15; with small or medium mask = £6.68

Able Spacer® (Clement Clarke)

Spacer device, small-volume device. For use with all pressurised (aerosol) inhalers, net price standard device = £4.39; with infant or child mask = £7.16

AeroChamber® Plus (GSK)

Spacer device, medium-volume device. For use with all pressurised (aerosol) inhalers, net price standard device (blue) = £4.79; with mask (blue) = £7.99; infant device (orange) with mask = £7.99; child device (yellow) with mask = £7.99

Babyhaler® (A&H) ⟨NHS⟩

Spacer device, for paediatric use with *Flixotide®*, and *Ventolin®* inhalers, net price = £11.34

Haleraid® (A&H) ⟨NHS⟩

Inhalation aid, device to place over pressurised (aerosol) inhalers to aid when strength in hands is impaired (e.g. in arthritis). For use with *Flixotide®*, *Seretide®*, *Serevent®*, and *Ventolin®* inhalers. Available as *Haleraid®-120* for 120-dose inhalers and *Haleraid®-200* for 200-dose inhalers, net price = 80p

OptiChamber® (Respironics)

Spacer device, for use with all pressurised (aerosol) inhalers, net price = £4.28

OptiChamber® Diamond (Respironics)

Spacer device, for use with all pressurised (aerosol) inhalers, net price standard device = £4.49; with small, medium, or large mask = £7.49

Pocket Chamber® (nSPIRE Health)

Spacer device, small-volume device. For use with all pressurised (aerosol) inhalers, net price = £4.18; with infant, small, medium, or large mask = £9.75

Space Chamber Plus® (Medical Developments)

Spacer device, for use with all pressurised (aerosol) inhalers, net price standard device = £4.26; compact device = £4.26

Volumatic® (A&H)

Spacer inhaler, large-volume device. For use with *Clenil Modulite®*, *Flixotide®*, *Seretide®*, *Serevent®*, and *Ventolin®* inhalers, net price = £3.81; with paediatric mask = £6.70

Vortex® (Pari)

Spacer device, medium-volume device. For use with all pressurised (aerosol) inhalers, net price with mouthpiece = £6.28; with mask for infant or child = £7.99; with adult mask = £9.97 ⟨NHS⟩

Nebulisers

> In England and Wales nebulisers and compressors are not available on the NHS (but they are free of VAT); some nebulisers (but not compressors) are available on form GP10A in Scotland (for details consult Scottish Drug Tariff).

A nebuliser converts a solution of a drug into an aerosol for inhalation. It is used to deliver higher doses of drug to the airways than is usual with standard inhalers. The main indications for use of a nebuliser are to deliver:

- a beta₂ agonist or ipratropium to a patient with an *acute exacerbation* of asthma or of chronic obstructive pulmonary disease;

- a beta₂ agonist, corticosteroid, or ipratropium on a *regular basis* to a patient with severe asthma or reversible airways obstruction when the patient is unable to use other inhalational devices;

- an antibiotic (such as colistimethate sodium) or a mucolytic to a patient with cystic fibrosis;

- budesonide or adrenaline to a child with severe croup;

- pentamidine for the prophylaxis and treatment of pneumocystis pneumonia.

The use of nebulisers in chronic persistent asthma and chronic obstructive pulmonary disease should be considered only:

- after a review of the diagnosis;

- after review of therapy (see Management of Chronic Asthma table, p. 184 and Chronic Obstructive Pulmonary Disease, p. 186) and the patient's ability to use hand-held devices;

- after increased doses of inhaled therapy from hand-held inhalers (with a spacer if necessary) have been tried for 2 weeks;

- if the patient remains breathless, despite correctly using optimal therapy

Before prescribing a nebuliser, a home trial should preferably be undertaken to monitor response for up to 2 weeks on standard treatment and up to 2 weeks on nebulised treatment. If prescribed, patients must:

- have clear instructions from a doctor, specialist nurse, physiotherapist, or pharmacist on the use of the nebuliser (including maintenance and cleaning) and on peak-flow monitoring;

- be instructed not to treat acute attacks at home without also seeking help;

- have regular follow up by a doctor, specialist nurse or physiotherapist after about 1 month and annually thereafter

The proportion of a nebuliser solution that reaches the lungs depends on the type of nebuliser and although it can be as high as 30%, it is more frequently close to 10% and sometimes below 10%. The remaining solution is left in the nebuliser as residual volume or is deposited in the mouthpiece and tubing. The extent to which the nebulised solution is deposited in the airways or alveoli depends on the droplet size, pattern of breath inhalation, and condition of the lung. Droplets with a mass median diameter of 1–5 microns are deposited in the airways and are therefore appropriate for asthma, whereas a particle size of 1–2 microns is needed for alveolar deposition of pentamidine to combat pneumocystis infection. The type of nebuliser is therefore chosen according to the deposition required and according to the viscosity of the solution.

Jet nebulisers are more widely used than ultrasonic nebulisers. Most jet nebulisers require an optimum gas flow rate of 6–8 litres/minute and in hospital can be driven by piped air or oxygen; in acute asthma the nebuliser should be driven by oxygen. Domiciliary oxygen cylinders do not provide an adequate flow rate therefore an electrical compressor is required for domiciliary use.

For patients at risk of hypercapnia, such as those with chronic obstructive pulmonary disease, oxygen can be dangerous and the nebuliser should be driven by air (see section 3.1). If oxygen is required, it should be given simultaneously by nasal cannula.

> **Tubing**
>
> The Department of Health has reminded users of the need to use the correct grade of tubing when connecting a nebuliser to a medical gas supply or compressor.

Ultrasonic nebulisers produce an aerosol by ultrasonic vibration of the drug solution and therefore do not require a gas flow; they are not suitable for the nebulisation of some drugs, such as dornase alfa and nebulised suspensions.

Nebuliser diluent

Nebulisation may be carried out using an undiluted nebuliser solution or it may require dilution beforehand. The usual diluent is sterile sodium chloride 0.9% (physiological saline).

Sodium Chloride (Non-proprietary) PoM
  Nebuliser solution, sodium chloride 0.9%, net price 20 × 2.5 mL = £20.60
  Brands include *Saline Steripoule®*, *Saline Steri-Neb®*

3.2   Corticosteroids

Corticosteroids are used for the management of reversible and irreversible airways disease. An inhaled corticosteroid used for 3–4 weeks may help to distinguish asthma from chronic obstructive pulmonary disease; clear improvement over 3–4 weeks suggests asthma.

Asthma   Corticosteroids are effective in *asthma*; they reduce airway inflammation (and hence reduce oedema and secretion of mucus into the airway).

An inhaled corticosteroid is used regularly for prophylaxis of asthma when patients require a beta$_2$ agonist more than twice a week, or if symptoms disturb sleep at least once a week, or if the patient has suffered an exacerbation in the last 2 years requiring a systemic corticosteroid (see Management of Chronic Asthma table, p. 184). *Regular use* of inhaled corticosteroids reduces the risk of exacerbation of asthma.

Current and previous smoking reduces the effectiveness of inhaled corticosteroids and higher doses may be necessary.

Corticosteroid inhalers must be used regularly for maximum benefit; alleviation of symptoms usually occurs 3 to 7 days after initiation. **Beclometasone dipropionate**, **budesonide**, **fluticasone propionate**, and **mometasone furoate** appear to be equally effective. Preparations that combine a corticosteroid with a long-acting beta$_2$ agonist may be helpful for patients stabilised on the individual components in the same proportion.

In adults using an inhaled corticosteroid and a long-acting beta$_2$ agonist for the prophylaxis of asthma, but who are poorly controlled, (see step 3 of the Management of Chronic Asthma table, p. 184) *Symbicort®* (bud-esonide with formoterol) can be used as a reliever (instead of a short-acting beta$_2$ agonist), in addition to its regular use for the prophylaxis of asthma. *Symbicort®* can also be used in this way in adults using an inhaled corticosteroid with a dose greater than beclometasone dipropionate 400 micrograms daily[1], but who are poorly controlled (see step 2 of the Management of Chronic Asthma table, p. 184). When starting this treatment, the total regular daily dose of inhaled corticosteroid should not be reduced. Patients must be carefully instructed on the appropriate dose and management of exacerbations before initiating this therapy, see *Symbicort®* p. 202. Patients using budesonide with formoterol as a reliever once a day or more should have their treatment reviewed regularly. The use of *Symbicort®* for both reliever and maintenance therapy is also used by some specialists in children 12–18 years [unlicensed]. *Fostair®* can also be used in adults as a reliever (instead of a short-acting beta$_2$ agonist) in addition to its regular use for the prophylaxis of asthma, see *Fostair®*, p. 202. It may be particularly useful for patients with poorly controlled asthma requiring reliever therapy, or for those who have had previous exacerbations of asthma which needed medical intervention. Patients requiring frequent daily use of *Fostair®* as a reliever should have their maintenance treatment reviewed. This approach has not been investigated with combination inhalers containing other corticosteroids and long-acting beta$_2$ agonists.

High doses of inhaled corticosteroid can be prescribed for patients who respond only partially to standard doses with a long-acting beta$_2$ agonist or another long-acting bronchodilator (see Management of Chronic Asthma table, p. 184). High doses should be continued only if there is clear benefit over the lower dose. The recommended maximum dose of an inhaled corticosteroid should not generally be exceeded. However, if a higher dose is required, then it should be initiated and supervised by a specialist. The use of high doses of inhaled corticosteroid can minimise the requirement for an oral corticosteroid (see also Side-effects of Inhaled Corticosteroids, p. 200).

Systemic corticosteroid therapy may be necessary during episodes of stress, such as severe infection, or if the asthma is worsening, when higher doses are needed and access of inhaled drug to small airways may be reduced; patients may need a reserve supply of corticosteroid tablets.

Chronic obstructive pulmonary disease   In *chronic obstructive pulmonary disease* inhaled corticosteroid therapy may reduce exacerbations when given in combination with an inhaled long-acting beta$_2$ agonist, see section 3.1, p. 186.

Cautions of inhaled corticosteroids

Paradoxical bronchospasm   The potential for paradoxical bronchospasm (calling for discontinuation and alternative therapy) should be borne in mind—mild bronchospasm may be prevented by inhalation of a short-acting beta$_2$ agonist beforehand (or by transfer from an aerosol inhalation to a dry powder inhalation).

CFC-free inhalers   Chlorofluorocarbon (CFC) propellants in pressurised aerosol inhalers have been replaced by hydrofluoroalkane (HFA) propellants.

---

1. For standard doses of other inhaled corticosteroids, see Management of Chronic Asthma table, p. 184.

3 Respiratory system

Doses for corticosteroid CFC-free pressurised metered-dose inhalers may be different from traditional CFC-containing inhalers and may differ between brands, see MHRA/CHM advice below.

For **interactions**: see Appendix 1 (corticosteroids)

MHRA/CHM advice (July 2008)

- Beclometasone dipropionate CFC-free pressurised metered-dose inhalers (Qvar® and Clenil Modulite®) are **not** interchangeable and should be prescribed by brand name; Qvar® has extra-fine particles, is more potent than traditional beclometasone dipropionate CFC-containing inhalers, and is approximately twice as potent as Clenil Modulite®;
- Fostair® is a combination beclometasone dipropionate and formoterol fumarate CFC-free pressurised metered-dose inhaler; Fostair® has extra-fine particles and is more potent than traditional beclometasone dipropionate CFC-free inhalers.

Side-effects of inhaled corticosteroids Inhaled corticosteroids have considerably fewer systemic effects than oral corticosteroids (section 6.3.2), but adverse effects have been reported.

High doses of inhaled corticosteroids (see Management of Chronic Asthma table, p. 184) used for prolonged periods can induce adrenal suppression. Inhaled corticosteroids have been associated with adrenal crisis and coma in children; excessive doses should be **avoided**. Consider giving a 'steroid card' (section 6.3.2) to support communication of the risks associated with treatment, and specific written advice to consider corticosteroid replacement during an episode of stress, such as severe intercurrent illness or an operation, to patients using greater than maximum licensed doses of inhaled corticosteroids. Use of other corticosteroid therapy (including topical) or concurrent use of drugs which inhibit corticosteroid metabolism should be taken into account when assessing systemic risk.

High doses of inhaled corticosteroid have been associated with lower respiratory tract infections, including pneumonia, in older patients with chronic obstructive pulmonary disease.

Bone mineral density may be reduced following long-term inhalation of higher doses of corticosteroids, predisposing patients to osteoporosis (section 6.6). It is therefore sensible to ensure that the dose of an inhaled corticosteroid is no higher than necessary to keep a patient's asthma under good control.

In children, growth restriction associated with systemic corticosteroid therapy does not seem to occur with recommended doses of inhaled therapy; although initial growth velocity may be reduced, there appears to be no effect on achieving normal adult height. However, the height and weight of children receiving prolonged treatment with inhaled corticosteroid should be monitored annually; if growth is slowed, referral to a paediatrician should be considered. Large-volume spacer devices should be used for administering inhaled corticosteroids in children under 15 years (see NICE guidance, section 3.1.5); they are also useful in older children and adults, particularly if high doses are required. Spacer devices increase airway deposition and reduce oropharyngeal deposition.

A small risk of glaucoma with prolonged high doses of inhaled corticosteroids has been reported. Hoarseness, dysphonia, throat irritation, and candidiasis of the mouth or throat may occur with inhaled corticosteroids (see Candidiasis below). Paradoxical bronchospasm has

been reported very rarely. Anxiety, depression, sleep disturbances, behavioural changes including hyperactivity, irritability, and aggression (particularly in children) have been reported; hyperglycaemia (usually only with high doses), cataracts, skin thinning and bruising have also been reported.

Candidiasis The risk of oral candidiasis can be reduced by using a spacer device with the corticosteroid inhaler; rinsing the mouth with water after inhalation of a dose may also be helpful. Antifungal oral suspension or oral gel (section 12.3.2) can be used to treat oral candidiasis without discontinuing therapy.

Oral An acute attack of asthma should be treated with a short course of an oral corticosteroid starting with a high dose, see Management of Acute Asthma table, p. 185. Patients whose asthma has deteriorated rapidly usually respond quickly to corticosteroids. The dose can usually be stopped abruptly; tapering is not needed provided that the patient receives an inhaled corticosteroid in an adequate dose (apart from those on maintenance oral corticosteroid treatment or where oral corticosteroids are required for 3 or more weeks); see also Withdrawal of Corticosteroids, section 6.3.2. In patients who have needed several courses of oral corticosteroids and in whom the possibility of a period on maintenance corticosteroids is being considered, it may be useful to taper the corticosteroid dose gradually to identify a threshold dose for asthma control. This should only be done after other standard options for controlling asthma have been tried (see the Management of Chronic Asthma table, p. 184).

In chronic asthma, when the response to other drugs has been inadequate, longer term administration of an oral corticosteroid may be necessary; in such cases high doses of an inhaled corticosteroid should be continued to minimise oral corticosteroid requirements, see Management of Chronic Asthma table, p. 184. Patients taking long-term oral corticosteroids for asthma can often be transferred to an inhaled corticosteroid but the transfer must be slow, with gradual reduction in the dose of the oral corticosteroid, and at a time when the asthma is well controlled.

During an acute exacerbation of chronic obstructive pulmonary disease, prednisolone 30 mg daily should be given for 7–14 days; treatment can be stopped abruptly. Prolonged treatment with oral prednisolone is of no benefit and maintenance treatment is not normally recommended.

An oral corticosteroid should normally be taken as a single dose in the morning to reduce the disturbance to circadian cortisol secretion. Dosage should always be titrated to the lowest dose that controls symptoms. Regular peak-flow measurements help to optimise the dose.

Parenteral For the use of hydrocortisone injection in the emergency treatment of acute severe asthma, see Management of Acute Asthma table, p. 185.

NICE guidance
Inhaled corticosteroids for the treatment of chronic asthma in children under 12 years (November 2007)

For children under 12 years with chronic asthma in whom treatment with an inhaled corticosteroid is considered appropriate, the least costly product that is suitable for an individual (taking into consideration NICE TAs 38 and 10), within its marketing authorisation is recommended.

For children under 12 years with chronic asthma in whom treatment with an inhaled corticosteroid and a long-acting beta₂ agonist is considered appropriate, the following apply:

- the use of a combination inhaler within its marketing authorisation is recommended as an option;
- the decision to use a combination inhaler or two agents in separate inhalers should be made on an individual basis, taking into consideration therapeutic need, and the likelihood of treatment adherence;
- if a combination inhaler is chosen, then the least costly inhaler that is suitable for the individual is recommended.

www.nice.org.uk/TA131

NICE guidance
Inhaled corticosteroids for the treatment of chronic asthma in adults and children over 12 years (March 2008)

For adults and children over 12 years with chronic asthma in whom treatment with an inhaled corticosteroid is considered appropriate, the least costly product that is suitable for an individual (taking into consideration NICE TAs 38 and 10), within its marketing authorisation is recommended.

For adults and children over 12 years with chronic asthma in whom treatment with an inhaled corticosteroid and a long-acting beta₂ agonist is considered appropriate, the following apply:

- the use of a combination inhaler within its marketing authorisation is recommended as an option;
- the decision to use a combination inhaler or two agents in separate inhalers should be made on an individual basis, taking into consideration therapeutic need, and the likelihood of treatment adherence;
- if a combination inhaler is chosen, then the least costly inhaler that is suitable for the individual is recommended.

www.nice.org.uk/TA138

▌ BECLOMETASONE DIPROPIONATE
(Beclomethasone Dipropionate)

Indications prophylaxis of asthma (see also Management of Chronic Asthma table, p. 184)

Cautions see notes above

Pregnancy see p. 186

Breast-feeding see p. 186

Side-effects see notes above

Dose

- By aerosol inhalation, see Management of Chronic Asthma table, p. 184 (**important:** for *Clenil Modulite*® and *Qvar*®, see under preparations)
- By inhalation of dry powder (**important:** for *Asmabec*® see under preparation), 200–400 micrograms twice daily; adjusted as necessary up to 800 micrograms twice daily; CHILD over 5 years 100–200 micrograms twice daily, adjusted as necessary

---

Beclometasone (Non-proprietary) PoM

Dry powder for inhalation, beclometasone dipropionate 100 micrograms/metered inhalation, net price 100-dose unit = £5.36; 200 micrograms/metered inhalation, 100-dose unit = £9.89, 200-dose unit = £14.93; 400 micrograms/metered inhalation, 100-dose unit = £19.61. Label: 8, counselling, administration; also 10 and steroid card with high doses

Brands include *Pulvinal*® *Beclometasone Dipropionate, Easyhaler*® *Beclometasone Dipropionate*

Asmabec Clickhaler® (RPH) PoM

Dry powder for inhalation, beclometasone dipropionate 100 micrograms/metered inhalation, net price 200-dose unit = £9.81; 250 micrograms/metered inhalation, 100-dose unit = £12.31. Label: 8, counselling, administration; also 10 and steroid card with high doses

Dose by inhalation of powder, prophylaxis of asthma, 100–400 micrograms twice daily, adjusted as necessary; max. 1 mg twice daily; CHILD 6–12 years 100–200 micrograms twice daily, adjusted as necessary

Clenil Modulite® (Chiesi) PoM

Aerosol inhalation, beclometasone dipropionate 50 micrograms/metered inhalation, net price 200-dose unit = £3.70; 100 micrograms/metered inhalation = £7.42; 200 micrograms/metered inhalation = £16.17; 250 micrograms/metered inhalation = £16.29. Label: 8, counselling, administration; also 10 and steroid card with high doses

Dose by aerosol inhalation, 200–400 micrograms twice daily, adjusted as necessary up to 1 mg twice daily; CHILD under 12 years 100–200 micrograms twice daily

Note *Clenil Modulite*® is not interchangeable with other CFC-free beclometasone dipropionate inhalers; the MHRA has advised (July 2008) that CFC-free beclometasone dipropionate inhalers should be prescribed by brand name, see p. 200

Dental prescribing on NHS *Clenil Modulite*® 50 micrograms/metered inhalation may be prescribed

Qvar® (TEVA UK) PoM

Aerosol inhalation, beclometasone dipropionate 50 micrograms/metered inhalation, net price 200-dose unit = £7.87; 100 micrograms/metered inhalation, 200-dose unit = £17.21. Label: 8, counselling, administration; also 10 and steroid card with high doses

Autohaler® (breath-actuated aerosol inhalation), beclometasone dipropionate 50 micrograms/metered inhalation, net price 200-dose unit = £7.87; 100 micrograms/metered inhalation, 200-dose unit = £17.21. Label: 8, counselling, administration; also 10 and steroid card with high doses

Easi-Breathe® (breath-actuated aerosol inhalation), beclometasone dipropionate 50 micrograms/metered inhalation, net price 200-dose = £7.74; 100 micrograms/metered inhalation, 200-dose = £16.95. Label: 8, counselling, administration; also 10 and steroid card with high doses

Dose by aerosol inhalation, prophylaxis of asthma, ADULT and CHILD over 12 years, 50–200 micrograms twice daily, increased if necessary to max. 400 micrograms twice daily

Important When switching a patient with well-controlled asthma from another corticosteroid inhaler, initially a 100-microgram metered dose of *Qvar*® should be prescribed for:

- 200–250 micrograms of beclometasone dipropionate or budesonide
- 100 micrograms of fluticasone propionate

When switching a patient with poorly controlled asthma from another corticosteroid inhaler, initially a 100-microgram metered dose of *Qvar*® should be prescribed for

3 Respiratory system

100 micrograms of beclometasone dipropionate, budesonide, or fluticasone propionate; the dose of *Qvar*® should be adjusted according to response

Note *Qvar*® is not interchangeable with other CFC-free beclometasone dipropionate inhalers; the MHRA has advised (July 2008) that beclometasone dipropionate CFC-free inhalers should be prescribed by brand name, see p. 200.

◀**Compound preparations**

For prescribing information on formoterol fumarate, see section 3.1.1.1

Fostair® (Chiesi) PoM

Aerosol inhalation, beclometasone dipropionate 100 micrograms, formoterol fumarate 6 micrograms/metered inhalation, net price 120-dose unit = £29.32. Label: 8, counselling, administration, 10, steroid card with high doses

Dose by aerosol inhalation, asthma maintenance therapy, ADULT over 18 years, 1–2 puffs twice daily; max. 4 puffs daily

Asthma, maintenance and reliever therapy (but see p. 199), ADULT over 18 years, 1 puff twice daily; for relief of symptoms, 1 puff as needed; max. 8 puffs daily

When switching patients from other beclometasone dipropionate and formoterol fumarate inhalers, *Fostair*® *100/6* can be prescribed for patients already using beclometasone dipropionate 250 micrograms in another CFC-free inhaler; the dose of *Fostair*® should be adjusted according to response

Chronic obstructive pulmonary disease with forced expiratory volume in 1 second < 50% of predicted (but see notes, p. 186), ADULT over 18 years, 2 puffs twice daily

Note The MHRA has advised (July 2008) that beclometasone dipropionate CFC-free inhalers should be prescribed by brand name, see p. 200

▌BUDESONIDE

Indications prophylaxis of asthma (see also Management of Chronic Asthma table, p. 184); croup

Cautions see notes above

Pregnancy see p. 186

Breast-feeding see p. 186

Side-effects see notes above

Dose
● See preparations below

Budesonide (Non-proprietary) PoM

Dry powder for inhalation, budesonide 100 micrograms/metered inhalation, net price 200-dose unit = £8.86; 200 micrograms/metered inhalation, 200-dose unit = £17.71; 400 micrograms/metered inhalation, 100-dose unit = £17.71. Label: 8, counselling, administration; also 10 and steroid card with high doses

Brands include *Easyhaler*® *Budesonide*

Dose by inhalation of powder, ADULT and CHILD over 12 years, 100–800 micrograms twice daily, adjusted as necessary; alternatively, in mild to moderate asthma, for patients previously stabilised on a twice daily dose, 200–400 micrograms (max. 800 micrograms) as a single dose in the evening; CHILD 6–12 years 100–400 micrograms twice daily, adjusted as necessary; alternatively, in mild to moderate asthma, for patients previously stabilised on a twice daily dose, 200–400 micrograms as a single dose in the evening

Nebuliser suspension, budesonide 250 micrograms/mL, net price 20 × 2-mL (500-microgram) unit = £26.42; 500 micrograms/mL, 20 × 2-mL (1-mg) unit = £40.00. May be diluted with sterile sodium chloride 0.9%. Label: 8, counselling, administration, 10, steroid card

Note Not suitable for use in ultrasonic nebulisers

Dose prophylaxis of asthma, by inhalation of nebulised suspension, ADULT and CHILD over 12 years, 0.25–1 mg

twice daily, adjusted according to response (usual max. 2 mg daily, but higher doses may be used in severe disease); CHILD 6 months–12 years, 125–500 micrograms twice daily, adjusted according to response (max. 2 mg daily)

Note Once daily administration may be considered in adults and children with mild to moderate stable asthma using a maintenance dose of budesonide 0.25–1 mg daily

Budelin Novolizer® (Meda) PoM

Dry powder for inhalation, budesonide 200 micrograms, net price refillable inhaler device and 100-dose cartridge = £14.86; 100-dose refill cartridge = £9.59. Label: 8, counselling, administration; also 10 and steroid card with high doses

Dose by inhalation of powder, ADULT and CHILD over 12 years, 200–800 micrograms twice daily, adjusted as necessary; alternatively, in mild to moderate asthma, for patients previously stabilised on a twice daily dose, 200–400 micrograms (max. 800 micrograms) as a single dose in the evening; CHILD 6–12 years 200–400 micrograms twice daily, adjusted as necessary; alternatively, in mild to moderate asthma, for patients previously stabilised on a twice daily dose, 200–400 micrograms as a single dose in the evening

Pulmicort® (AstraZeneca) PoM

Turbohaler® (= dry powder inhaler), budesonide 100 micrograms/metered inhalation, net price 200-dose unit = £11.84; 200 micrograms/metered inhalation, 100-dose unit = £11.84; 400 micrograms/metered inhalation, 50-dose unit = £13.86. Label: 8, counselling, administration; also 10 and steroid card with high doses

Dose by inhalation of powder, ADULT and CHILD over 12 years, 100–800 micrograms twice daily, adjusted as necessary; alternatively, in mild to moderate asthma, for patients previously stabilised on a twice daily dose, 200–400 micrograms (max. 800 micrograms) as a single dose in the evening; CHILD 5–12 years 100–400 micrograms twice daily, adjusted as necessary; alternatively, in mild to moderate asthma, for patients previously stabilised on a twice daily dose, 200–400 micrograms as a single dose in the evening

Respules® (= single-dose units for nebulisation), budesonide 250 micrograms/mL, net price 20 × 2-mL (500-microgram) unit = £26.42; 500 micrograms/mL, 20 × 2-mL (1-mg) unit = £40.00. May be diluted with sterile sodium chloride 0.9%. Label: 8, counselling, administration, 10, steroid card

Dose prophylaxis of asthma, by inhalation of nebulised suspension, ADULT and CHILD over 12 years, 1–2 mg twice daily, reduced to 0.5–1 mg twice daily; CHILD 3 months–12 years, 0.5–1 mg twice daily, reduced to 250–500 micrograms twice daily

Croup, by inhalation of nebulised suspension, CHILD over 1 month, 2 mg as a single dose (*or* as two 1-mg doses separated by 30 minutes); dose may be repeated every 12 hours until clinical improvement

Note Not suitable for use in ultrasonic nebulisers

◀**Compound preparations**

For prescribing information on formoterol fumarate, see section 3.1.1.1

Symbicort® (AstraZeneca) PoM

Symbicort 100/6 Turbohaler® (= dry powder inhaler), budesonide 100 micrograms, formoterol fumarate 6 micrograms/metered inhalation, net price 120-dose unit = £33.00. Label: 8, counselling, administration

Dose by inhalation of powder, asthma maintenance therapy, 1–2 puffs twice daily increased if necessary to max. 4 puffs twice daily, reduced to 1 puff once daily if control maintained; CHILD 6–12 years, 1–2 puffs twice daily reduced to 1 puff once daily if control maintained; 12–17 years, 1–2 puffs twice daily reduced to 1 puff once daily if control maintained

Asthma, maintenance and reliever therapy (but see p. 199), 2 puffs daily in 1–2 divided doses; for relief of symptoms,

1 puff as needed up to max. 6 puffs at a time; max. 8 puffs daily; up to 12 puffs daily can be used for a limited time but medical assessment should be considered; CHILD 12–18 years, see *BNF for Children*

Symbicort 200/6 Turbohaler® (= dry powder inhaler), budesonide 200 micrograms, formoterol fumarate 6 micrograms/metered inhalation, net price 120-dose unit = £38.00. Label: 8, counselling, administration; also 10 and steroid card with high doses

Dose by inhalation of powder, asthma maintenance therapy, 1–2 puffs twice daily increased if necessary to max. 4 puffs twice daily, reduced to 1 puff once daily if control maintained; CHILD 12–17 years 1–2 puffs twice daily reduced to 1 puff once daily if control maintained

Asthma, maintenance and reliever therapy (but see p. 199), 2 puffs daily in 1–2 divided doses, increased if necessary to 2 puffs twice daily; for relief of symptoms, 1 puff as needed up to max. 6 puffs at a time; max. 8 puffs daily; up to 12 puffs daily can be used for a limited time but medical assessment should be considered; CHILD 12–18 years, see *BNF for Children*

Chronic obstructive pulmonary disease with forced expiratory volume in 1 second <50% of predicted, 2 puffs twice daily

Symbicort 400/12 Turbohaler® (= dry powder inhaler), budesonide 400 micrograms, formoterol fumarate 12 micrograms/metered inhalation, net price 60-dose unit = £38.00. Label: 8, counselling, administration; also 10 and steroid card with high doses

Dose by inhalation of powder, asthma maintenance therapy, 1 puff twice daily increased if necessary to max. 2 puffs twice daily, reduced to 1 puff once daily if control maintained; CHILD 12–17 years 1 puff twice daily reduced to 1 puff once daily if control maintained

Chronic obstructive pulmonary disease with forced expiratory volume in 1 second <50% of predicted, 1 puff twice daily

---

◼ CICLESONIDE

Indications prophylaxis of asthma

Cautions see notes above

Pregnancy see p. 186

Breast-feeding see p. 186

Side-effects see notes above; also nausea, taste disturbance

Dose

• By aerosol inhalation, 160 micrograms daily as a single dose reduced to 80 micrograms daily if control maintained; dose may be increased to max. 320 micrograms twice daily if necessary in severe asthma [unlicensed]; CHILD 12–18 years, 160 micrograms daily as a single dose reduced to 80 micrograms daily if control maintained

Alvesco® (Takeda) ▪PoM▪
Aerosol inhalation, ciclesonide 80 micrograms/metered inhalation, net price 120-dose unit = £32.83; 160 micrograms/metered inhalation, 60-dose unit = £19.31, 120-dose unit = £38.62. Label: 8, counselling, administration

---

◼ FLUTICASONE

Indications prophylaxis of asthma (see also Management of Chronic Asthma table, p. 184)

Cautions see notes above

Pregnancy see p. 186

Breast-feeding see p. 186

Side-effects see notes above; also dyspepsia and arthralgia

Dose

• See preparations below

Flixotide® (A&H) ▪PoM▪
Accuhaler® (dry powder for inhalation), disk containing 60 blisters of fluticasone propionate 50 micrograms/blister with *Accuhaler®* device, net price = £6.38; 100 micrograms/blister with *Accuhaler®* device = £8.93; 250 micrograms/blister with *Accuhaler®* device = £21.26; 500 micrograms/blister with *Accuhaler®* device = £36.14. Label: 8, counselling, administration; also label 10 and steroid card with high doses

Note *Flixotide Accuhaler®* 250 micrograms and 500 micrograms are not indicated for children

Dose by inhalation of powder, prophylaxis of asthma, ADULT and CHILD over 16 years, 100–500 micrograms twice daily, increased according to severity of asthma; max. 1 mg twice daily (doses above 500 micrograms twice daily initiated by a specialist); CHILD 5–16 years, 50–100 micrograms twice daily adjusted as necessary; max. 200 micrograms twice daily

Evohaler® aerosol inhalation, fluticasone propionate 50 micrograms/metered inhalation, net price 120-dose unit = £5.44; 125 micrograms/metered inhalation, 120-dose unit = £21.26; 250 micrograms/metered inhalation, 120-dose unit = £36.14. Label: 8, counselling, administration; also label 10 and steroid card with high doses

Note *Flixotide Evohaler®* 125 micrograms and 250 micrograms not indicated for children

Dose by aerosol inhalation, prophylaxis of asthma, ADULT and CHILD over 16 years, 100–500 micrograms twice daily, increased according to severity of asthma; max. 1 mg twice daily; (doses above 500 micrograms twice daily initiated by a specialist); CHILD 4–16 years, 50–100 micrograms twice daily adjusted as necessary; max. 200 micrograms twice daily

Nebules® (= single-dose units for nebulisation), fluticasone propionate 250 micrograms/mL, net price 10 × 2-mL (500-microgram) unit = £9.34; 1 mg/mL, 10 × 2-mL (2-mg) unit = £37.35. May be diluted with sterile sodium chloride 0.9%. Label: 8, counselling, administration, 10, steroid card

Dose by inhalation of nebulised suspension, prophylaxis of asthma, ADULT and CHILD over 16 years, 0.5–2 mg twice daily; CHILD 4–16 years, 1 mg twice daily

Note Not suitable for use in ultrasonic nebulisers

◂Compound preparations

For prescribing information on formoterol and salmeterol, see Formoterol Fumarate and Salmeterol, section 3.1.1.1.

Flutiform® (Napp) ▼ ▪PoM▪
Flutiform® 50 micrograms/5 micrograms (aerosol inhalation), fluticasone propionate 50 micrograms, formoterol fumarate 5 micrograms/metered inhalation, net price 120-dose unit = £18.00. Label: 8, counselling, administration

Dose by aerosol inhalation, prophylaxis of asthma, ADULT and CHILD over 12 years, 2 puffs twice daily

Flutiform® 125 micrograms/5 micrograms (aerosol inhalation), fluticasone propionate 125 micrograms, formoterol fumarate 5 micrograms/metered inhalation, net price 120-dose unit = £29.26. Label: 8, counselling, administration, 10, steroid card

Dose by aerosol inhalation, prophylaxis of asthma, ADULT and CHILD over 12 years, 2 puffs twice daily

Flutiform® 250 micrograms/10 micrograms (aerosol inhalation), fluticasone propionate 250 micrograms, formoterol fumarate 10 micrograms/metered inhalation, net price 120-dose unit = £45.56. Label: 8, counselling, administration, 10, steroid card

Dose by aerosol inhalation, prophylaxis of asthma, ADULT over 18 years, 2 puffs twice daily

Respiratory system

3

Relvar Ellipta® (GSK) ▼ PoM

Relvar Ellipta® 92 micrograms/22 micrograms (dry powder for inhalation), fluticasone furoate 92 micrograms, vilanterol (as trifenatate) 22 micrograms/inhalation (delivered dose), net price 30-dose unit = £27.80. Label: 8, counselling, administration, 10, steroid card

Cautions see notes above and also section 3.1.1.1

Pregnancy manufacturer advises use only if potential benefit outweighs risk

Breast-feeding manufacturer advises avoid—no information available

Side-effects see under Fluticasone and also section 3.1.1.1; also abdominal pain, back pain

Dose by inhalation of powder, prophylaxis of asthma, ADULT and CHILD over 12 years, 1 inhalation once daily

Chronic obstructive pulmonary disease with forced expiratory volume in 1 second < 70% of predicted (but see notes, p. 186, ADULT over 18 years, 1 inhalation once daily

Important 1 inhalation (delivered dose) of fluticasone *furoate* 92 micrograms once daily is approximately equivalent to fluticasone *propionate* 250 micrograms twice daily

Note The *Scottish Medicines Consortium* (p. 4) has advised (March 2014) that fluticasone furoate/vilanterol (*Relvar Ellipta®*) is accepted for restricted use within NHS Scotland in patients with severe chronic obstructive pulmonary disease with a forced expiratory volume in 1 second (FEV₁) less than 50% of the predicted normal value

Relvar Ellipta® 184 micrograms/22 micrograms (dry powder for inhalation), fluticasone furoate 184 micrograms, vilanterol (as trifenatate) 22 micrograms/inhalation (delivered dose), net price 30-dose unit = £38.87. Label: 8, counselling, administration, 10, steroid card

Cautions see notes above and also section 3.1.1.1

Hepatic impairment avoid in moderate to severe impairment; max. dose fluticasone furoate 92 micrograms, vilanterol 22 micrograms

Pregnancy manufacturer advises use only if potential benefit outweighs risk

Breast-feeding manufacturer advises avoid—no information available

Side-effects see under Fluticasone and also section 3.1.1.1; also abdominal pain, back pain

Dose by inhalation of powder, prophylaxis of asthma, ADULT and CHILD over 12 years, 1 inhalation once daily

Important 1 inhalation (delivered dose) of fluticasone *furoate* 184 micrograms once daily is approximately equivalent to fluticasone *propionate* 500 micrograms twice daily

Seretide® (A&H) PoM

Seretide 100 Accuhaler® (dry powder for inhalation), disk containing 60 blisters of fluticasone propionate 100 micrograms, salmeterol (as xinafoate) 50 micrograms/blister with *Accuhaler®* device, net price = £18.00. Label: 8, counselling, administration

Dose by inhalation of powder, prophylaxis of asthma, ADULT and CHILD over 5 years, 1 inhalation twice daily, reduced to 1 inhalation once daily if control maintained

Seretide 250 Accuhaler® (dry powder for inhalation), disk containing 60 blisters of fluticasone propionate 250 micrograms, salmeterol (as xinafoate) 50 micrograms/blister with *Accuhaler®* device, net price = £35.00. Label: 8, counselling, administration, 10, steroid card

Dose by inhalation of powder, prophylaxis of asthma, ADULT and CHILD over 12 years, 1 inhalation twice daily

Seretide 500 Accuhaler® (dry powder for inhalation), disk containing 60 blisters of fluticasone propionate 500 micrograms, salmeterol (as xinafoate) 50 micrograms/blister with *Accuhaler®* device,

net price = £40.92. Label: 8, counselling, administration, 10, steroid card

Dose by inhalation of powder, prophylaxis of asthma, ADULT and CHILD over 12 years, 1 inhalation twice daily

Chronic obstructive pulmonary disease with forced expiratory volume in 1 second <60% of predicted (but see notes, p. 186), ADULT 1 inhalation twice daily

Note The *Scottish Medicines Consortium* has advised (December 2008) that *Seretide 500 Accuhaler®* is **not** recommended for use within NHS Scotland for chronic obstructive pulmonary disease in patients with a forced expiratory volume in 1 second (FEV₁) less than 60% and greater than 50% of the predicted normal value, with significant symptoms despite regular bronchodilator therapy, and a history of repeated exacerbations

Seretide 50 Evohaler® (aerosol inhalation), fluticasone propionate 50 micrograms, salmeterol (as xinafoate) 25 micrograms/metered inhalation, net price 120-dose unit = £18.00. Label: 8, counselling, administration

Dose by aerosol inhalation, prophylaxis of asthma, ADULT and CHILD over 5 years, 2 puffs twice daily, reduced to 2 puffs once daily if control maintained

Seretide 125 Evohaler® (aerosol inhalation), fluticasone propionate 125 micrograms, salmeterol (as xinafoate) 25 micrograms/metered inhalation, net price 120-dose unit = £35.00. Label: 8, counselling, administration, 10, steroid card

Dose by aerosol inhalation, prophylaxis of asthma, ADULT and CHILD over 12 years, 2 puffs twice daily

Seretide 250 Evohaler® (aerosol inhalation), fluticasone propionate 250 micrograms, salmeterol (as xinafoate) 25 micrograms/metered inhalation, net price 120-dose unit = £59.48. Label: 8, counselling, administration, 10, steroid card

Dose by aerosol inhalation, prophylaxis of asthma, ADULT and CHILD over 12 years, 2 puffs twice daily

▌ MOMETASONE FUROATE

Indications prophylaxis of asthma (see also Management of Chronic Asthma table, p. 184)

Cautions see notes above

Pregnancy see p. 186

Breast-feeding see p. 186

Side-effects see notes above; also headache; *less commonly* dyspepsia, weight gain, palpitation

Dose

● By inhalation of powder, ADULT and CHILD over 12 years, 400 micrograms as a single dose in the evening or in 2 divided doses, reduced to 200 micrograms once daily if control maintained; dose may be increased to max. 400 micrograms twice daily in severe asthma

Asmanex® (MSD) PoM

Twisthaler (= dry powder inhaler), mometasone furoate 200 micrograms/metered inhalation, net price 30-dose unit = £15.70, 60-dose unit = £23.54; 400 micrograms/metered inhalation, 30-dose unit = £21.78, 60-dose unit = £36.05. Label: 8, counselling, administration, 10, steroid card

Note The *Scottish Medicines Consortium* has advised (November 2003) that *Asmanex®* is restricted for use following failure of first-line inhaled corticosteroids

3.3 Cromoglicate and related therapy, leukotriene receptor antagonists, and phosphodiesterase type-4 inhibitors

3.3.1   Cromoglicate and related therapy
3.3.2   Leukotriene receptor antagonists
3.3.3   Phosphodiesterase type-4 inhibitors

3.3.1 Cromoglicate and related therapy

The mode of action of **sodium cromoglicate** and **nedocromil** is not completely understood. They may be of value in asthma with an allergic basis, but, in practice, it is difficult to predict who will benefit; they could probably be given for 4 to 6 weeks to assess response. Dose frequency is adjusted according to response but is usually 3 to 4 times a day initially; this may subsequently be reduced. Withdrawal of sodium cromoglicate or nedocromil should be done gradually over a period of one week—symptoms of asthma may recur.

In general, *prophylaxis* with sodium cromoglicate is less effective than prophylaxis with corticosteroid inhalations (see Management of Chronic Asthma table, p. 184). There is evidence of efficacy of nedocromil in children aged 5–12 years. Sodium cromoglicate and nedocromil are of no value in the treatment of acute attacks of asthma.

Sodium cromoglicate can prevent exercise-induced asthma. However, exercise-induced asthma may reflect poor overall control and the patient should be re-assessed.

Paradoxical bronchospasm If paradoxical bronchospasm occurs, a short-acting beta$_2$ agonist such as salbutamol or terbutaline (section 3.1.1.1) should be used to control symptoms; treatment with sodium cromoglicate or nedocromil should be discontinued.

Side-effects Side-effects associated with inhalation of sodium cromoglicate and nedocromil include throat irritation, cough, bronchospasm (including paradoxical bronchospasm—see above), and headache.

SODIUM CROMOGLICATE
(Sodium Cromoglycate)

Indications prophylaxis of asthma (see also Management of Chronic Asthma table, p. 184); food allergy (section 1.5.4); allergic conjunctivitis (section 11.4.2); allergic rhinitis (section 12.2.1)

Cautions see notes above; also discontinue if eosinophilic pneumonia occurs

Pregnancy see p. 186

Breast-feeding see p. 186

Side-effects see notes above; also rhinitis, eosinophilic pneumonia

Dose

• By aerosol inhalation, ADULT and CHILD over 5 years, 10 mg (2 puffs) 4 times daily, increased if necessary to 6–8 times daily; or additional dose may also be taken before exercise; maintenance, 5 mg (1 puff) 4 times daily

Intal® CFC-Free Inhaler (Sanofi-Aventis) [PoM]
Aerosol inhalation, sodium cromoglicate 5 mg/metered inhalation, net price 112-dose unit = £18.33. Label: 8, counselling, administration

NEDOCROMIL SODIUM

Indications prophylaxis of asthma (see also Management of Chronic Asthma table, p. 184)

Cautions see notes above

Pregnancy see p. 186

Breast-feeding see p. 186

Side-effects see notes above; also nausea, vomiting, dyspepsia, abdominal pain, pharyngitis; *rarely* taste disturbances

Dose

• By aerosol inhalation, ADULT and CHILD over 6 years 4 mg (2 puffs) 4 times daily, when control achieved may be possible to reduce to twice daily
 Counselling Regular use is necessary

Tilade® CFC-free Inhaler (Sanofi-Aventis) [PoM]
Aerosol inhalation, mint-flavoured, nedocromil sodium 2 mg/metered inhalation, net price 112-dose unit = £39.94. Label: 8, counselling, administration

3.3.2 Leukotriene receptor antagonists

The leukotriene receptor antagonists, **montelukast** and **zafirlukast**, block the effects of cysteinyl leukotrienes in the airways. They are effective in asthma when used alone or with an inhaled corticosteroid (see Management of Chronic Asthma table p. 184).

Montelukast has not been shown to be more effective than a standard dose of inhaled corticosteroid, but the two drugs appear to have an additive effect. The leukotriene receptor antagonists may be of benefit in exercise-induced asthma and in those with concomitant rhinitis, but they are less effective in those with severe asthma who are also receiving high doses of other drugs.

Churg-Strauss syndrome has occurred very rarely in association with the use of leukotriene receptor antagonists; in many of the reported cases the reaction followed the reduction or withdrawal of oral corticosteroid therapy. Prescribers should be alert to the development of eosinophilia, vasculitic rash, worsening pulmonary symptoms, cardiac complications, or peripheral neuropathy.

Pregnancy There is limited evidence for the safe use of leukotriene receptor antagonists during pregnancy; however, they can be taken as normal in women who have shown a significant improvement in asthma not achievable with other drugs before becoming pregnant, see also p. 186.

MONTELUKAST

Indications prophylaxis of asthma, see notes above and Management of Chronic Asthma table, p. 184; symptomatic relief of seasonal allergic rhinitis in patients with asthma

Cautions interactions: Appendix 1 (leukotriene receptor antagonists)

Respiratory system   **3**

Pregnancy manufacturer advises avoid unless essential, see also notes above

Breast-feeding manufacturer advises avoid unless essential

Side-effects abdominal pain, thirst, headache, hyperkinesia (in young children); *less commonly* dry mouth, dyspepsia, oedema, dizziness, drowsiness, malaise, sleep disturbances, sleep-walking, abnormal dreams, anxiety, agitation (including aggressive behaviour or hostility), depression, psychomotor hyperactivity (including irritability and restlessness), paraesthesia, hypoaesthesia, seizures, arthralgia, myalgia (including muscle cramps), epistaxis, bruising; *rarely* palpitation, tremor, disturbance in attention, memory impairment, increased bleeding tendency; *very rarely* hepatic eosinophilic infiltration, hepatic disorders, hallucinations, suicidal thoughts and behaviour, disorientation, Churg-Strauss syndrome (see notes above), erythema nodosum, erythema multiforme

Dose

- Prophylaxis of asthma, ADULT and CHILD over 15 years, 10 mg once daily in the evening; CHILD 6 months–6 years 4 mg once daily in the evening, 6–15 years 5 mg once daily in the evening
- Seasonal allergic rhinitis, ADULT and CHILD over 15 years, 10 mg once daily in the evening

Montelukast (Non-proprietary) [PoM]

Chewable tablets, montelukast (as sodium salt) 4 mg, net price 28-tab pack = £2.11; 5 mg, 28-tab pack = £2.23. Label: 23, 24

Excipients include aspartame (section 9.4.1)

Granules, montelukast (as sodium salt) 4 mg, net price 28-sachet pack = £4.34. Counselling, administration

Counselling Granules may be swallowed or mixed with cold, soft food (not liquid) and taken immediately

Tablets, montelukast (as sodium salt) 10 mg, net price 28-tab pack = £2.42

Singulair® (MSD) [PoM]

Chewable tablets, pink, cherry-flavoured, montelukast (as sodium salt) 4 mg, net price 28-tab pack = £25.69; 5 mg, 28-tab pack = £25.69. Label: 23, 24

Excipients include aspartame equivalent to phenylalanine 674 micrograms/4-mg tablet and 842 micrograms/5-mg tablet (section 9.4.1)

Granules, montelukast (as sodium salt) 4 mg, net price 28-sachet pack = £25.69. Counselling, administration

Counselling Granules may be swallowed or mixed with cold, soft food (not liquid) and taken immediately

Tablets, beige, f/c, montelukast (as sodium salt) 10 mg, net price 28-tab pack = £26.97

Note The *Scottish Medicines Consortium* has advised (June 2007) that *Singulair*® chewable tablets and granules are restricted for use as an alternative to low-dose inhaled corticosteroids for children 2–14 years with mild persistent asthma who have not recently had serious asthma attacks that required oral corticosteroid use and who are not capable of using inhaled corticosteroids; *Singulair*® chewable tablets and granules should be initiated by a specialist in paediatric asthma

ZAFIRLUKAST

Indications prophylaxis of asthma, see notes above and Management of Chronic Asthma table, p. 184

Cautions elderly; interactions: Appendix 1 (leukotriene receptor antagonists)

Hepatic disorders Patients or their carers should be told how to recognise development of liver disorder and advised to seek medical attention if symptoms or signs such as persistent nausea, vomiting, malaise, or jaundice develop

Hepatic impairment manufacturer advises avoid

Renal impairment manufacturer advises caution in moderate to severe impairment

Pregnancy manufacturer advises use only if potential benefit outweighs risk; see also notes above

Breast-feeding present in milk—manufacturer advises avoid

Side-effects gastro-intestinal disturbances, respiratory infections, headache, insomnia, malaise; *rarely* bleeding disorders, hypersensitivity reactions including angioedema and skin reactions, arthralgia, myalgia, hepatitis, hyperbilirubinaemia, thrombocytopenia; *very rarely* Churg-Strauss syndrome (see notes above), agranulocytosis

Dose

- ADULT and CHILD over 12 years, 20 mg twice daily

Accolate® (AstraZeneca) [PoM]

Tablets, f/c, zafirlukast 20 mg, net price 56-tab pack = £17.75. Label: 23

3.3.3 Phosphodiesterase type-4 inhibitors

Roflumilast is a phosphodiesterase type-4 inhibitor with anti-inflammatory properties; it is licensed as an adjunct to bronchodilators for the maintenance treatment of patients with severe chronic obstructive pulmonary disease associated with chronic bronchitis and a history of frequent exacerbations.

> **NICE guidance**
> **Roflumilast for the management of severe chronic obstructive pulmonary disease (January 2012)**
> Roflumilast is recommended only in the context of research as part of a clinical trial for adults with severe chronic obstructive pulmonary disease associated with chronic bronchitis with a history of frequent exacerbations as an add-on to bronchodilator treatment.
> Patients receiving roflumilast should have the option to continue treatment until they and their clinicians consider it appropriate to stop.
> www.nice.org.uk/TA244

ROFLUMILAST

Indications see notes above

Cautions monitor body-weight; latent infection (such as tuberculosis, viral hepatitis, herpes infection); history of psychiatric illness, or concomitant use of drugs likely to cause psychiatric events (discontinue if new or worsening psychiatric symptoms occur); **interactions**: Appendix 1 (roflumilast)

Contra-indications severe immunological disease; severe acute infectious disease; cancer (except basal cell carcinoma); concomitant treatment with immunosuppressive drugs (except short-term systemic corticosteroids); moderate to severe cardiac failure; history of depression associated with suicidal ideation or behaviour

Hepatic impairment caution in mild impairment; avoid in moderate to severe impairment

Pregnancy manufacturer advises avoid—toxicity in *animal* studies; women of child-bearing age should use effective contraception

Breast-feeding manufacturer advises avoid—present in milk in *animal* studies

Side-effects diarrhoea, nausea, abdominal pain, weight loss, decreased appetite, headache, insomnia; *less commonly* gastritis, vomiting, gastro-oesophageal reflux, dyspepsia, palpitation, anxiety, tremor, vertigo, dizziness, malaise, muscle spasm, myalgia, back pain, rash; *rarely* taste disturbances, haematochezia, constipation, respiratory tract infections, depression, nervousness, suicidal ideation and behaviour, gynaecomastia, raised creatine kinase, urticaria

Dose

● ADULT over 18 years, 500 micrograms once daily

Daxas® (Takeda) ▼ [PoM]

Tablets, yellow, f/c, roflumilast 500 micrograms, net price 30-tab pack = £37.71, 90-tab pack = £113.14. Counselling, patient card

Counselling Patients should be given a patient card before starting treatment and advised to record body-weight at regular intervals

3.4 Antihistamines, hyposensitisation, and allergic emergencies

3.4.1 Antihistamines
3.4.2 Allergen immunotherapy
3.4.3 Allergic emergencies

3.4.1 Antihistamines

All antihistamines are of potential value in the treatment of nasal allergies, particularly seasonal allergic rhinitis (hay fever), and they may be of some value in vasomotor rhinitis. They reduce rhinorrhoea and sneezing but are usually less effective for nasal congestion. Antihistamines are used topically in the eye (section 11.4.2), in the nose (section 12.2.1), and on the skin (section 13.3).

Oral antihistamines are also of some value in preventing urticaria and are used to treat urticarial rashes, pruritus, and insect bites and stings; they are also used in drug allergies. Injections of chlorphenamine or promethazine are used as an adjunct to adrenaline (epinephrine) in the emergency treatment of anaphylaxis and angioedema (section 3.4.3). For the use of antihistamines (including cinnarizine, cyclizine, and promethazine teoclate) in nausea and vomiting, see section 4.6. Buclizine is included as an anti-emetic in a preparation for migraine (section 4.7.4.1). For reference to the use of antihistamines for occasional insomnia, see section 4.1.1.

All older antihistamines cause sedation but **alimemazine** and **promethazine** may be more sedating whereas **chlorphenamine** and **cyclizine** (section 4.6) may be less so. This sedating activity is sometimes used to manage the pruritus associated with some allergies. There is little evidence that any one of the older, 'sedating' antihistamines is superior to another and patients vary widely in their response.

Non-sedating antihistamines such as **acrivastine, bilastine, cetirizine, desloratadine** (an active metabolite of loratadine), **fexofenadine** (an active metabolite of terfenadine), **levocetirizine** (an isomer of cetirizine), **loratadine, mizolastine**, and **rupatadine** cause less sedation and psychomotor impairment than the older antihistamines because they penetrate the blood brain barrier only to a slight extent.

Cautions and contra-indications Sedating antihistamines have significant antimuscarinic activity and they should therefore be used with caution in prostatic hypertrophy, urinary retention, susceptibility to angle-closure glaucoma, and pyloroduodenal obstruction. Caution may be required in epilepsy. Children and the elderly are more susceptible to side-effects. Many antihistamines should be avoided in acute porphyria but some are thought to be safe, see section 9.8.2. **Interactions:** Appendix 1 (antihistamines).

Hepatic impairment Sedating antihistamines should be avoided in severe liver disease—increased risk of coma.

Pregnancy Most manufacturers of antihistamines advise avoiding their use during pregnancy; however, there is no evidence of teratogenicity except for hydroxyzine where toxicity has been reported with high doses in *animal* studies. The use of sedating antihistamines in the latter part of the third trimester may cause adverse effects in neonates such as irritability, paradoxical excitability, and tremor.

Breast-feeding Most antihistamines are present in breast milk in varying amounts; although not known to be harmful, most manufacturers advise avoiding their use in mothers who are breast-feeding.

Side-effects Drowsiness is a significant side-effect with most of the older antihistamines although paradoxical stimulation may occur rarely, especially with high doses or in children and the elderly. Drowsiness may diminish after a few days of treatment and is considerably less of a problem with the newer antihistamines (see also notes above). Side-effects that are more common with the older antihistamines include headache, psychomotor impairment, and antimuscarinic effects such as urinary retention, dry mouth, blurred vision, and gastro-intestinal disturbances.

Other rare side-effects of antihistamines include hypotension, palpitation, arrhythmias, extrapyramidal effects, dizziness, confusion, depression, sleep disturbances, tremor, convulsions, hypersensitivity reactions (including bronchospasm, angioedema, and anaphylaxis, rashes, and photosensitivity reactions), blood disorders, liver dysfunction, and angle-closure glaucoma.

Non-sedating antihistamines

Driving Although drowsiness is rare, nevertheless patients should be advised that it can occur and may affect performance of skilled tasks (e.g. driving); excess alcohol should be avoided.

ACRIVASTINE

Indications symptomatic relief of allergy such as hay fever, chronic idiopathic urticaria

Cautions see notes above

Contra-indications see notes above; also hypersensitivity to triprolidine; elderly

Renal impairment avoid in severe impairment

Pregnancy see notes above
Breast-feeding see notes above
Side-effects see notes above
Dose

- ADULT and CHILD over 12 years, 8 mg 3 times daily

Acrivastine (Non-proprietary)
Capsules, acrivastine 8 mg, net price 12-cap pack = £2.75, 24-cap pack = £4.76. Counselling, driving
Brands include *Benadryl® Allergy Relief*

BILASTINE

Indications symptomatic relief of allergic rhinoconjunctivitis and urticaria
Cautions see notes above
Contra-indications see notes above
Pregnancy avoid—limited information available; see also notes above
Breast-feeding avoid—no information available; see also notes above
Side-effects headache, malaise; *less commonly* abdominal pain, diarrhoea, increased appetite, weight gain, thirst, gastritis, prolongation of the QT interval, dyspnoea, anxiety, insomnia, vertigo, dizziness, pyrexia, oral herpes, tinnitus
Dose

- ADULT and CHILD over 12 years, 20 mg once daily
Counselling Advise patient to take tablet 1 hour before or 2 hours after food or fruit juice

Ilaxten® (Menarini) ▼ PoM
Tablets, scored, bilastine 20 mg, net price 30-tab pack = £15.09. Label: 23, counselling, administration

CETIRIZINE HYDROCHLORIDE

Indications symptomatic relief of allergy such as hay fever, chronic idiopathic urticaria
Cautions see notes above
Contra-indications see notes above
Renal impairment use half normal dose if eGFR 30–50 mL/minute/1.73 m²; use half normal dose and reduce dose frequency to alternate days if eGFR 10–30 mL/minute/1.73 m²; avoid if eGFR less than 10 mL/minute/1.73 m²
Pregnancy see notes above
Breast-feeding see notes above
Side-effects see notes above
Dose

- ADULT and CHILD over 12 years, 10 mg once daily; CHILD 1–2 years see *BNF for Children*, 2–6 years 2.5 mg twice daily, 6–12 years 5 mg twice daily

Cetirizine (Non-proprietary)
Tablets, cetirizine hydrochloride 10 mg, net price 30-tab pack = £1.07. Counselling, driving
Dental prescribing on NHS Cetirizine Tablets 10 mg may be prescribed

Oral solution, cetirizine hydrochloride 5 mg/5 mL, net price 200 mL = £1.76. Counselling, driving
Note Sugar-free versions are available and can be ordered by specifying sugar-free on the prescription
Excipients may include propylene glycol (see Excipients, p. 2)
Dental prescribing on NHS Cetirizine Oral Solution 5 mg/5 mL may be prescribed

DESLORATADINE

Note Desloratadine is a metabolite of loratadine
Indications symptomatic relief of allergic rhinitis and urticaria
Cautions see notes above
Contra-indications see notes above; also hypersensitivity to loratadine
Renal impairment use with caution in severe impairment
Pregnancy see notes above
Breast-feeding see notes above
Side-effects see notes above; *rarely* myalgia; *very rarely* hallucinations
Dose

- 5 mg once daily; CHILD 1–6 years 1.25 mg once daily, 6–12 years 2.5 mg once daily

Desloratadine (Non-proprietary) PoM
Tablets, desloratadine 5 mg, net price 30-tab pack = £1.28. Counselling, driving

Neoclarityn® (MSD) PoM
Tablets, f/c, desloratadine 5 mg, net price 30-tab pack = £6.77. Counselling, driving
Oral solution, sugar-free, bubblegum-flavoured, desloratadine 2.5 mg/5 mL, net price 100 mL = £6.77; 150 mL = £10.15. Counselling, driving
Excipients include propylene glycol, sorbitol 150 mg/mL (see Excipients, p. 2)

FEXOFENADINE HYDROCHLORIDE

Note Fexofenadine is a metabolite of terfenadine
Indications see under Dose
Cautions see notes above
Contra-indications see notes above
Pregnancy see notes above
Breast-feeding see notes above
Side-effects see notes above
Dose

- Seasonal allergic rhinitis, 120 mg once daily; CHILD 6–12 years, 30 mg twice daily
- Chronic idiopathic urticaria, ADULT and CHILD over 12 years, 180 mg once daily

Fexofenadine Hydrochloride (Non-proprietary) PoM
Tablets, f/c, fexofenadine hydrochloride 120 mg, net price 30-tab pack = £3.21; 180 mg, 30-tab pack = £4.23. Label: 5, counselling, driving

Telfast® (Sanofi-Aventis) PoM
Tablets, f/c, peach, fexofenadine hydrochloride 30 mg, net price 60-tab pack = £5.46; 120 mg, 30-tab pack = £5.99; 180 mg, 30-tab pack = £7.58. Label: 5, counselling, driving

LEVOCETIRIZINE HYDROCHLORIDE

Note Levocetirizine is an isomer of cetirizine
Indications symptomatic relief of allergy such as hay fever, urticaria
Cautions see notes above
Contra-indications see notes above
Renal impairment use on alternate days if eGFR 30–50 mL/minute/1.73 m²; 5 mg every 3 days if eGFR 10–30 mL/minute/1.73 m²; avoid if eGFR less than 10 mL/minute/1.73 m²
Pregnancy see notes above
Breast-feeding see notes above

3 Respiratory system

Side-effects see notes above; *very rarely* weight gain

Dose

- ADULT and CHILD over 6 years, 5 mg once daily; CHILD under 6 years see *BNF for Children*

Levocetirizine Hydrochloride (Non-proprietary) PoM

Tablets, levocetirizine hydrochloride 5 mg, net price 30-tab pack = £3.95. Counselling, driving

Xyzal® (UCB Pharma) PoM

Tablets, f/c, levocetirizine hydrochloride 5 mg, net price 30-tab pack = £4.39. Counselling, driving

Oral solution, sugar-free, levocetirizine hydrochloride 2.5 mg/5 mL, net price 200 mL = £6.00. Counselling, driving

LORATADINE

Indications symptomatic relief of allergy such as hay fever, chronic idiopathic urticaria

Cautions see notes above

Contra-indications see notes above

Hepatic impairment reduce dose frequency to alternate days in severe impairment

Pregnancy see notes above

Breast-feeding see notes above

Side-effects see notes above

Dose

- ADULT and CHILD over 12 years 10 mg once daily; CHILD 2–12 years, body-weight under 30 kg, 5 mg once daily; body-weight over 30 kg, 10 mg once daily

Loratadine (Non-proprietary)

Tablets, loratadine 10 mg, net price 30-tab pack = £1.10. Counselling, driving

Dental prescribing on NHS Loratadine 10 mg Tablets may be prescribed

Syrup, loratadine 5 mg/5 mL, net price 100 mL = £2.25. Counselling, driving

Excipients may include propylene glycol (see Excipients, p. 2)

Dental prescribing on NHS Loratadine Syrup 5 mg/5 mL may be prescribed

MIZOLASTINE

Indications symptomatic relief of allergy such as hay fever, urticaria

Cautions see notes above

Contra-indications see notes above; also susceptibility to QT-interval prolongation (including cardiac disease and hypokalaemia)

Hepatic impairment manufacturer advises avoid in significant impairment

Pregnancy see notes above

Breast-feeding see notes above

Side-effects see notes above; weight gain; anxiety, asthenia; *less commonly* arthralgia and myalgia

Dose

- ADULT and CHILD over 12 years 10 mg once daily

Mizollen® (Sanofi-Aventis) PoM

Tablets, m/r, f/c, scored, mizolastine 10 mg, net price 30-tab pack = £6.92. Label: 25, counselling, driving

RUPATADINE

Indications symptomatic relief of allergic rhinitis, urticaria

Cautions see notes above; also susceptibility to QT-interval prolongation (including cardiac disease and hypokalaemia); elderly

Hepatic impairment manufacturer advises avoid—no information available

Renal impairment manufacturer advises avoid—no information available

Pregnancy manufacturer advises caution—limited information available; see also notes above

Breast-feeding manufacturer advises caution; see also notes above

Side-effects see notes above; also asthenia; *less commonly* pyrexia, irritability, increased appetite, arthralgia, and myalgia

Dose

- ADULT and CHILD over 12 years, 10 mg once daily

Rupafin® (GSK) ▼ PoM

Tablets, pink, rupatadine (as fumarate) 10 mg, net price 30-tab pack = £5.00. Counselling, driving

Sedating antihistamines

Driving Drowsiness may affect performance of skilled tasks (e.g. driving); sedating effects enhanced by alcohol.

ALIMEMAZINE TARTRATE
(Trimeprazine tartrate)

Indications urticaria and pruritus, premedication

Cautions see notes above; see also section 4.2.1

Contra-indications see notes above; see also section 4.2.1

Hepatic impairment see notes above

Renal impairment avoid

Pregnancy see notes above

Breast-feeding see notes above

Side-effects see notes above; see also section 4.2.1

Dose

- Urticaria and pruritus, 10 mg 2–3 times daily, in severe cases up to max. 100 mg daily has been used; ELDERLY 10 mg 1–2 times daily; CHILD under 2 years, see *BNF for Children*, 2–5 years 2.5 mg 3–4 times daily, 5–12 years 5 mg 3–4 times daily
- Premedication, CHILD 2–7 years up to 2 mg/kg 1–2 hours before operation

Alimemazine (Non-proprietary) PoM

Tablets, alimemazine tartrate 10 mg, net price 28-tab pack = £6.27. Label: 2

Oral solution, alimemazine tartrate 7.5 mg/5 mL, net price 100 mL = £14.36; 30 mg/5 mL, 100 mL = £41.88. Label: 2

CHLORPHENAMINE MALEATE
(Chlorpheniramine maleate)

Indications symptomatic relief of allergy such as hay fever, urticaria, food allergy, drug reactions; relief of itch associated with chickenpox; emergency treatment of anaphylactic reactions (section 3.4.3)

Cautions see notes above

Contra-indications see notes above

Hepatic impairment see notes above

Pregnancy see notes above

Breast-feeding see notes above

Side-effects see notes above; also exfoliative dermatitis and tinnitus reported; injections may cause transient hypotension or CNS stimulation and may be irritant

Dose

- By mouth, 4 mg every 4–6 hours, max. 24 mg daily (ELDERLY max. 12 mg daily); CHILD under 1 year see *BNF for Children*; 1–2 years 1 mg twice daily; 2–6 years 1 mg every 4–6 hours, max. 6 mg daily; 6–12 years 2 mg every 4–6 hours, max. 12 mg daily
- By intramuscular injection *or* by intravenous injection over 1 minute, 10 mg, repeated if required up to max. 4 doses in 24 hours; CHILD under 6 months 250 micrograms/kg (max. 2.5 mg); 6 months–6 years 2.5 mg; 6–12 years 5 mg; these doses may be repeated if required up to max. 4 doses in 24 hours

Chlorphenamine (Non-proprietary)

Tablets, chlorphenamine maleate 4 mg, net price 28 = 98p. Label: 2

Dental prescribing on NHS Chlorphenamine tablets may be prescribed

Oral solution, chlorphenamine maleate 2 mg/5 mL, net price 150 mL = £1.66. Label: 2

Note Sugar-free versions are available and can be ordered by specifying 'sugar-free' on the prescription

Dental prescribing on NHS Chlorphenamine oral solution may be prescribed

Injection [PoM][1], chlorphenamine maleate 10 mg/mL, net price 1-mL amp = £3.36

Piriton® (GSK Consumer Healthcare)

Tablets, yellow, scored, chlorphenamine maleate 4 mg, net price 28 = £1.62. Label: 2

Syrup, chlorphenamine maleate 2 mg/5 mL, net price 150 mL = £2.49. Label: 2

CLEMASTINE

Indications symptomatic relief of allergy such as hay fever, urticaria

Cautions see notes above

Contra-indications see notes above

Hepatic impairment see notes above

Pregnancy see notes above

Breast-feeding see notes above

Side-effects see notes above

Dose

- 1 mg twice daily, increased up to 6 mg daily if required; CHILD 1–3 years 250–500 micrograms twice daily; 3–6 years 500 micrograms twice daily; 6–12 years 0.5–1 mg twice daily

Tavegil® (Novartis Consumer Health)

Tablets, scored, clemastine (as hydrogen fumarate) 1 mg, net price 60-tab pack = £4.10. Label: 2

CYPROHEPTADINE HYDROCHLORIDE

Indications symptomatic relief of allergy such as hay fever, urticaria; pruritus

Cautions see notes above

Contra-indications see notes above

Hepatic impairment see notes above

Pregnancy see notes above

Breast-feeding see notes above

---

1. [PoM] restriction does not apply where administration is for saving life in emergency

Side-effects see notes above

Dose

- 4 mg 3 times daily; usual range 4–20 mg daily, max. 32 mg daily; CHILD 2–6 years 2 mg 2–3 times daily, max. 12 mg daily; 7–14 years 4 mg 2–3 times daily, max. 16 mg daily

Periactin® (Auden Mckenzie)

Tablets, scored, cyproheptadine hydrochloride 4 mg, net price 30-tab pack = £5.99. Label: 2

HYDROXYZINE HYDROCHLORIDE

Indications pruritus

Cautions see notes above; also susceptibility to QT-interval prolongation

Contra-indications see notes above

Hepatic impairment reduce daily dose by one-third; see also notes above

Renal impairment reduce daily dose by half

Pregnancy toxicity in *animal* studies with high doses; see also notes above

Breast-feeding manufacturer advises avoid; see also notes above

Side-effects see notes above

Dose

- Pruritus, initially 25 mg at night increased if necessary to 25 mg 3–4 times daily; CHILD 1–6 years initially 5–15 mg at night increased if necessary to 50 mg daily in 3–4 divided doses; 6–12 years initially 15–25 mg at night increased if necessary to 50–100 mg daily in 3–4 divided doses; CHILD under 1 year see *BNF for Children*

Atarax® (Alliance) [PoM]

Tablets, both f/c, hydroxyzine hydrochloride 10 mg (orange), net price 84-tab pack = £2.18; 25 mg (green), 28-tab pack = £1.22. Label: 2

Ucerax® (UCB Pharma) [PoM]

Tablets [NHS], f/c, scored, hydroxyzine hydrochloride 25 mg, net price 25-tab pack = £1.22. Label: 2

Syrup, hydroxyzine hydrochloride 10 mg/5 mL, net price 200-mL pack = £1.78. Label: 2

KETOTIFEN

Indications allergic rhinitis

Cautions see notes above

Contra-indications see notes above

Hepatic impairment see notes above

Pregnancy see notes above

Breast-feeding see notes above

Side-effects see notes above; also excitation, irritability, nervousness; *less commonly* cystitis; *rarely* weight gain; *very rarely* Stevens-Johnson syndrome

Dose

- 1 mg twice daily with food increased if necessary to 2 mg twice daily; initial treatment in readily sedated patients 0.5–1 mg at night; CHILD 3 years and over, 1 mg twice daily

Zaditen® (Swedish Orphan) [PoM]

Tablets, scored, ketotifen (as hydrogen fumarate) 1 mg, net price 60-tab pack = £7.53. Label: 2, 21

Elixir, ketotifen (as hydrogen fumarate), 1 mg/5 mL, net price 300 mL (strawberry-flavoured) = £8.91. Label: 2, 21

PROMETHAZINE HYDROCHLORIDE

Indications symptomatic relief of allergy such as hay fever and urticaria; emergency treatment of anaphylactic reactions; sedation (section 4.1.1); nausea and vomiting (section 4.6)

Cautions see notes above; avoid extravasation with intravenous injection; severe coronary artery disease

Contra-indications see notes above

Hepatic impairment see notes above

Renal impairment use with caution

Pregnancy see notes above

Breast-feeding see notes above

Side-effects see notes above; also restlessness; intramuscular injection may be painful

Dose

- By mouth, 10–20 mg 2–3 times daily; CHILD 2–5 years 5–15 mg daily in 1–2 divided doses, 5–10 years 10–25 mg daily in 1–2 divided doses
- By deep intramuscular injection, 25–50 mg; max. 100 mg; CHILD 5–10 years 6.25–12.5 mg
- By slow intravenous injection in emergencies, 25–50 mg as a solution containing 2.5 mg/mL in water for injections; max. 100 mg

Promethazine (Non-proprietary) PoM
[1]Injection, promethazine hydrochloride 25 mg/mL, net price 1-mL amp = 68p, 2-mL amp = £1.20
Excipients may include sulfites

Phenergan® (Sanofi-Aventis)
Tablets, both blue, f/c, promethazine hydrochloride 10 mg, net price 56-tab pack = £2.96; 25 mg, 56-tab pack = £4.65. Label: 2
Dental prescribing on NHS May be prescribed as Promethazine Hydrochloride Tablets 10 mg or 25 mg
Elixir, golden, promethazine hydrochloride 5 mg/5 mL, net price 100 mL = £2.85. Label: 2
Excipients include sulfites
Electrolytes Na+ 1.6 mmol/5 mL
Dental prescribing on NHS May be prescribed as Promethazine Hydrochloride Oral Solution 5 mg/5 mL
Injection PoM[1], promethazine hydrochloride 25 mg/mL, net price 1-mL amp = 67p
Excipients include sulfites

3.4.2 Allergen immunotherapy

Immunotherapy using allergen vaccines containing house dust mite, animal dander (cat or dog), or extracts of grass and tree pollen can reduce symptoms of asthma and allergic rhinoconjunctivitis. A vaccine containing extracts of wasp and bee venom is used to reduce the risk of severe anaphylaxis and systemic reactions in individuals with hypersensitivity to wasp and bee stings. An oral preparation of grass pollen extract (*Grazax*®) is also licensed for disease-modifying treatment of grass pollen-induced rhinitis and conjunctivitis. Those requiring immunotherapy must be referred to a hospital specialist for accurate diagnosis, assessment, and treatment.

1. PoM restriction does not apply where administration is for saving life in emergency

---

Desensitising vaccines

In view of concerns about the safety of desensitising vaccines, it is recommended that they are used by specialists and only for the following indications:

- seasonal allergic hay fever (caused by pollen) that has not responded to anti-allergic drugs;
- hypersensitivity to wasp and bee venoms.

Desensitising vaccines should generally be avoided or used with particular care in patients with asthma.

Desensitising vaccines should be avoided in pregnant women, in children under five years old, and in those taking beta-blockers (adrenaline may be ineffective in case of a hypersensitivity reaction), or ACE inhibitors (risk of severe anaphylactoid reactions).

Hypersensitivity reactions to immunotherapy (especially to wasp and bee venom extracts) can be life-threatening; bronchospasm usually develops within 1 hour and anaphylaxis within 30 minutes of injection. Therefore, cardiopulmonary resuscitation must be immediately available and patients need to be monitored for at least 1 hour after injection. If symptoms or signs of hypersensitivity develop (e.g. rash, urticaria, bronchospasm, faintness), **even when mild**, the patient should be observed until these have **resolved completely**.

The first dose of oral grass pollen extract (*Grazax*®) should be taken under medical supervision and the patient should be monitored for 20–30 minutes.

For details on the management of anaphylaxis, see section 3.4.3.

Each set of allergen extracts usually contains vials for the administration of graded amounts of allergen to patients undergoing hyposensitisation. Maintenance sets containing vials at the highest strength are available. Product literature must be consulted for details of allergens, vial strengths, and administration.

NICE guidance
Pharmalgen® for bee and wasp venom allergy (February 2012)
Pharmalgen® is an option for the treatment of IgE-mediated bee and wasp venom allergy in those who have had:

- a severe systemic reaction to bee or wasp venom;
- a moderate systemic reaction to bee or wasp venom and who have a raised baseline serum-tryptase concentration, a high risk of future stings, or anxiety about future stings.

Treatment with *Pharmalgen*® should be initiated and monitored in a specialist centre experienced in venom immunotherapy.
www.nice.org.uk/TA246

BEE AND WASP ALLERGEN EXTRACTS

Indications hypersensitivity to wasp or bee venom (see notes above)

Cautions see notes above and consult product literature

Contra-indications see notes above and consult product literature

Pregnancy avoid

Side-effects consult product literature

3 Respiratory system

Respiratory system (side tab) **3**

Dose

- By subcutaneous injection, consult product literature

Pharmalgen® (ALK-Abelló) PoM

Bee venom extract (*Apis mellifera*) or wasp venom extract (*Vespula* spp.), net price initial treatment set = £60.00 (bee), £60.00 (wasp); maintenance treatment set = £37.50 (bee), £37.50 (wasp)

GRASS AND TREE POLLEN EXTRACTS

Indications treatment of seasonal allergic hay fever due to grass or tree pollen in patients who have failed to respond to anti-allergy drugs (see notes above)

Cautions see notes above and consult product literature

Contra-indications see notes above and consult product literature

Pregnancy consult product literature

Side-effects see notes above and consult product literature

Dose

- See under preparations below

Pollinex® (Allergy) PoM

Grasses and rye or tree pollen extract, net price initial treatment set (3 vials) and extension course treatment (1 vial) = £450.00

Dose By subcutaneous injection, consult product literature

◢ **Grass pollen extract**

Grazax® (ALK-Abelló) PoM

Oral lyophilisates (= freeze-dried tablets), grass pollen extract 75 000 units, net price 30-tab pack = £80.12. Counselling, administration

Dose ADULT and CHILD over 5 years, 1 tablet daily; start treatment at least 4 months before start of pollen season and continue for up to 3 years

Counselling Tablets should be placed under the tongue and allowed to disperse. Advise patient not to swallow for 1 minute, or eat or drink for 5 minutes after taking the tablet

Omalizumab

Omalizumab is a monoclonal antibody that binds to immunoglobulin E (IgE). It is used as additional therapy in individuals with proven IgE-mediated sensitivity to inhaled allergens, whose severe persistent allergic asthma cannot be controlled adequately with high-dose inhaled corticosteroid together with a long-acting beta₂ agonist. Omalizumab should be initiated by physicians in specialist centres experienced in the treatment of severe persistent asthma.

Churg-Strauss syndrome has occurred rarely in patients given omalizumab; the reaction is usually associated with the reduction of oral corticosteroid therapy. Churg-Strauss syndrome can present as eosinophilia, vasculitic rash, cardiac complications, worsening pulmonary symptoms, or peripheral neuropathy. Hypersensitivity reactions can also occur immediately following treatment with omalizumab or sometimes more than 24 hours after the first injection.

For details on the management of anaphylaxis, see section 3.4.3.

The *Scottish Medicines Consortium* p. 4 has advised (May 2011) that omalizumab is accepted for restricted use within NHS Scotland as add-on therapy to improve asthma control in children (6 to 12 years), adolescents,

and adults with severe persistent allergic asthma. Omalizumab is restricted to patients who are prescribed chronic systemic corticosteroids and in whom all other treatments have failed. The response should be assessed at 16 weeks and omalizumab treatment discontinued in patients who have not shown a marked improvement in overall asthma control.

NICE guidance
Omalizumab for severe persistent allergic asthma (April 2013)

Omalizumab is recommended as an option for treating severe persistent confirmed allergic IgE-mediated asthma as an add-on to optimised standard therapy in adults and children aged 6 years and over

- who need continuous or frequent treatment with oral corticosteroids (defined as 4 or more courses in the previous year), and
- only if the manufacturer makes omalizumab available with the discount agreed in the patient access scheme.

Optimised standard therapy is defined as a full trial of and, if tolerated, documented compliance with inhaled high-dose corticosteroids, long-acting beta₂ agonists, leukotriene receptor antagonists, theophyllines, oral corticosteroids, and smoking cessation if clinically appropriate.

Patients currently receiving omalizumab whose disease does not meet the criteria should be able to continue treatment until they and their clinician consider it appropriate to stop.

www.nice.org.uk/TA278

OMALIZUMAB

Indications prophylaxis of allergic asthma (see notes above)

Cautions autoimmune disease; susceptibility to helminth infection—discontinue if infection does not respond to anthelmintic

Hepatic impairment manufacturer advises caution—no information available

Renal impairment manufacturer advises caution—no information available

Pregnancy manufacturer advises avoid unless essential

Breast-feeding manufacturer advises avoid—present in milk in *animal* studies

Side-effects abdominal pain, headache, pyrexia; *less commonly* dyspepsia, nausea, diarrhoea, weight gain, postural hypotension, flushing, pharyngitis, bronchospasm, cough, syncope, paraesthesia, dizziness, drowsiness, malaise, influenza-like illness, photosensitivity, urticaria, rash, pruritus; *rarely* laryngoedema, parasitic infection, antibody formation; *also reported* arterial thromboembolic events, Churg-Strauss syndrome (see notes above), thrombocytopenia, arthralgia, myalgia, joint swelling, alopecia, serum sickness (including fever and lymphadenopathy)

Dose

- By subcutaneous injection, ADULT and CHILD over 6 years, according to immunoglobulin E concentration and body-weight, consult product literature

Xolair® (Novartis) PoM

Injection, omalizumab 150 mg/mL, net price 0.5-mL (75-mg) prefilled syringe = £128.07; 1-mL (150-mg) prefilled syringe = £256.15

3.4.3 Allergic emergencies

Adrenaline (epinephrine) provides physiological reversal of the immediate symptoms associated with hypersensitivity reactions such as *anaphylaxis* and *angioedema*.

Anaphylaxis

Anaphylaxis is a severe, life-threatening, generalised or systemic hypersensitivity reaction. It is characterised by the rapid onset of respiratory and/or circulatory problems and is usually associated with skin and mucosal changes; prompt treatment is required. Patients with pre-existing asthma, especially poorly controlled asthma, are at particular risk of life-threatening reactions. Insect stings are a recognised risk (in particular wasp and bee stings). Latex and certain foods, including eggs, fish, cow's milk protein, peanuts, sesame, shellfish, soy, and tree nuts may also precipitate anaphylaxis. Medicinal products particularly associated with anaphylaxis include blood products, vaccines, hyposensitising (allergen) preparations, antibacterials, aspirin and other NSAIDs, and neuromuscular blocking drugs. In the case of drugs, anaphylaxis is more likely after parenteral administration; resuscitation facilities must always be available for injections associated with special risk. Anaphylactic reactions may also be associated with *additives and excipients* in foods and medicines. Refined arachis (peanut) oil, which may be present in some medicinal products, is unlikely to cause an allergic reaction—nevertheless it is wise to check the full formula of preparations which may contain allergens.

First-line treatment of anaphylaxis includes securing the airway, restoration of blood pressure (laying the patient flat and raising the legs, or in the recovery position if unconscious or nauseated and at risk of vomiting) and administration of **adrenaline** (epinephrine) injection. Adrenaline is given **intramuscularly** in a dose of 500 micrograms (0.5 mL adrenaline injection 1 in 1000); a dose of 300 micrograms (0.3 mL adrenaline injection 1 in 1000) may be appropriate for *immediate self-administration*. The dose is repeated if necessary at 5-minute intervals according to blood pressure, pulse, and respiratory function (**important: possible need for** *intravenous route* using *dilute solution*, see below). Patients receiving beta-blockers require special consideration (see under Adrenaline, p. 214). High-flow **oxygen** administration (section 3.6) and intravenous fluids (section 9.2.2) are also of primary importance. An antihistamine (e.g. **chlorphenamine**, given by slow intravenous injection or intramuscular injection in a dose of 10 mg, see p. 209) is a useful adjunctive treatment, given after adrenaline. An intravenous corticosteroid e.g. **hydrocortisone** (preferably as sodium succinate) in a dose of 200 mg (section 6.3.2) is of secondary value in the initial management of anaphylaxis because the onset of action is delayed for several hours, but should be given to prevent further deterioration in severely affected patients.

Continuing respiratory deterioration requires further treatment with **bronchodilators** including inhaled or intravenous salbutamol (see p. 190), inhaled ipratropium (see p. 194), intravenous aminophylline (see p. 195), or intravenous magnesium sulfate [unlicensed indication] (see Acute Severe Asthma, p. 186); in addition to oxygen, assisted respiration and possibly emergency tracheotomy may be necessary.

When a patient is so ill that there is doubt about the adequacy of the circulation, the initial injection of adrenaline may need to be given as a *dilute solution by the intravenous route*; for details of cautions, dose, and strength, see under Intravenous Adrenaline (Epinephrine), p. 214.

Cardiopulmonary arrest may follow an anaphylactic reaction; resuscitation should be started immediately (see p. 145).

For advice on the management of medical emergencies in dental practice, see p. 27.

On discharge, patients should be considered for further treatment with an oral antihistamine (section 3.4.1) and an oral corticosteroid (section 6.3.2) for up to 3 days to reduce the risk of further reaction. Patients should be instructed to return to hospital if symptoms recur and to contact their general practitioner for follow-up.

Patients who are suspected of having had an anaphylactic reaction should be referred to a specialist for specific allergy diagnosis. Avoidance of the allergen is the principal treatment; if appropriate, an adrenaline auto-injector should be given or a replacement supplied (see Self-administration of Adrenaline).

Intramuscular adrenaline (epinephrine)

The *intramuscular route* is the *first choice route* for the administration of adrenaline (epinephrine) in the management of anaphylaxis. Adrenaline is best given as an intramuscular injection into the anterolateral aspect of the middle third of the thigh; it has a rapid onset of action after intramuscular administration and in the shocked patient its absorption from the intramuscular site is faster and more reliable than from the subcutaneous site.

Patients with severe allergy should be instructed in the self-administration of adrenaline by intramuscular injection (for details see under Self-administration of Adrenaline (Epinephrine), below).

Prompt injection of adrenaline is of paramount importance. The following adrenaline doses are recommended for the emergency treatment of anaphylaxis by appropriately trained healthcare professionals and are based on the revised recommendations of the Working Group of the Resuscitation Council (UK).

Dose of intramuscular injection of adrenaline (epinephrine) for the emergency treatment of anaphylaxis by healthcare professionals		
Age	Dose	Volume of adrenaline **1 in 1000** (1 mg/mL)
Child under 6 years	150 micrograms	0.15 mL[1]
Child 6–12 years	300 micrograms	0.3 mL
Adult and child 12–18 years	500 micrograms	0.5 mL[2]

These doses may be repeated several times if necessary at 5-minute intervals according to blood pressure, pulse, and respiratory function.

1. Use suitable syringe for measuring small volume
2. 300 micrograms (0.3 mL) if child is small or prepubertal

Respiratory system

3

Intravenous adrenaline (epinephrine)

Intravenous adrenaline should be given only by those experienced in its use, in a setting where patients can be carefully monitored. When the patient is severely ill and there is real doubt about the adequacy of the circulation and absorption after intramuscular injection, adrenaline (epinephrine) can be given by *slow intravenous injection* in a dose of 50 micrograms (0.5 mL of the dilute 1 in 10 000 adrenaline injection) repeated according to response; if multiple doses are required, adrenaline should be given as a **slow** intravenous infusion *stopping when a response has been obtained*; children may respond to as little as 1 microgram/kg (0.01 mL/kg of the dilute 1 in 10 000 adrenaline injection) by **slow** *intravenous injection*.

Great vigilance is needed to ensure that the *correct strength* of adrenaline injection is used; anaphylactic shock kits need to make a *very clear distinction* between the 1 in 10 000 strength and the 1 in 1000 strength. It is also important that, where intramuscular injection might still succeed, time should not be wasted seeking intravenous access.

For reference to the use of the intravenous route for *cardiac resuscitation*, see section 2.7.3.

Self-administration of adrenaline (epinephrine)

Individuals at considerable risk of anaphylaxis need to carry adrenaline (epinephrine) at all times and need to be *instructed in advance* when and how to inject it. In addition, the packs need to be **clearly labelled with instructions** on how to administer adrenaline (intramuscularly, preferably at the midpoint of the outer thigh, through light clothing if necessary) so that in the case of rapid collapse someone else is able to give it. It is important to ensure individuals at risk and carers understand that:

- two injection devices should be carried at all times to treat symptoms until medical assistance is available; if, after the first injection, the individual does not start to feel better, the second injection should be given 5 to 15 minutes after the first,

- an ambulance should be called after every administration, even if symptoms improve,

- the individual should lie down with their legs raised (unless they have breathing difficulties, in which case they should sit up) and, if possible, should not be left alone.

Adrenaline for administration by intramuscular injection is available in 'auto-injectors' (e.g. *Emerade®*, *EpiPen®*, and *Jext®*), pre-assembled syringes fitted with a needle suitable for very rapid administration (if necessary by a bystander or a healthcare provider if it is the only preparation available); injection technique is device specific.

For doses of adrenaline for self-administration, see individual preparations under Adrenaline/Epinephrine (Intramuscular Injection for Self-administration, below).

■ ADRENALINE/EPINEPHRINE

Indications emergency treatment of acute anaphylaxis; angioedema; cardiopulmonary resuscitation (section 2.7.3); priapism [unlicensed] (section 7.4.5)

Cautions for cautions in non-life-threatening situations, see section 2.7.3

Interactions Severe anaphylaxis in patients taking beta-blockers may not respond to adrenaline—consider bronchodilator therapy, see intravenous salbutamol (p. 190);

adrenaline can cause severe hypertension and bradycardia in those taking non-cardioselective beta-blockers. Other **interactions**, see Appendix 1 (sympathomimetics).

Renal impairment section 2.7.3
Pregnancy section 2.7.3
Breast-feeding section 2.7.3
Side-effects section 2.7.3
Dose

- Acute anaphylaxis, by intramuscular injection (preferably midpoint in anterolateral thigh) of 1 in 1000 (1 mg/mL) solution for administration by *healthcare professionals*, see notes and table above

- Acute anaphylaxis, by intramuscular injection for *self-administration*, see under preparations

- Acute anaphylaxis when there is doubt as to the adequacy of the circulation, by slow intravenous injection of 1 in 10 000 (100 micrograms/mL) solution (extreme caution—specialist use only), see notes above

Important Intravenous route should be used with **extreme care** by specialists only, see notes above

■ Intramuscular or subcutaneous

¹Adrenaline/Epinephrine 1 in 1000 (Non-proprietary) PoM
Injection, adrenaline (as acid tartrate) 1 mg/mL, net price 0.5-mL amp = £5.06; 1-mL amp = 41p
Excipients may include sulfites

¹Minijet® Adrenaline 1 in 1000 (UCB Pharma) PoM
Injection, adrenaline (as hydrochloride) 1 in 1000 (1 mg/mL), net price 1 mL (with 25 gauge × 0.25 inch needle for subcutaneous injection) = £13.90, 1 mL (with 21 gauge × 1.5 inch needle for intramuscular injection) = £15.00 (both disposable syringes)
Excipients include sulfites

■ Intravenous

Extreme caution, see notes above

Adrenaline/Epinephrine 1 in 10 000, Dilute (Non-proprietary) PoM
Injection, adrenaline (as acid tartrate) 100 micrograms/mL, 10-mL amp, 1-mL and 10-mL prefilled syringe
Excipients may include sulfites

Minijet® Adrenaline 1 in 10 000 (UCB Pharma) PoM
Injection, adrenaline (as hydrochloride) 1 in 10 000 (100 micrograms/mL), net price 3-mL prefilled syringe = £7.54; 10-mL prefilled syringe = £6.99
Excipients include sulfites

■ Intramuscular injection for self-administration

Note Injection technique is device specific. To ensure patients receive the auto-injector device that they have been trained to use, prescribers should specify the brand to be dispensed

Emerade® (iMed) PoM
¹Emerade® 150 micrograms, (delivering a single dose of adrenaline (as tartrate) 150 micrograms), adrenaline 1 mg/mL (1 in 1000), net price 0.5-mL auto-injector device = £26.94
Excipients include sulfites
Note 0.35 mL of the solution remains in the auto-injector device after use
Dose by intramuscular injection, CHILD body-weight 15–30 kg, 150 micrograms (but on the basis of a dose of 10 micrograms/kg, 300 micrograms may be more appropriate for some children) repeated after 5–15 minutes as necessary; CHILD body-weight under 15 kg [unlicensed], 150 micrograms repeated after 5–15 minutes as necessary

---

1. PoM restriction does not apply to the intramuscular administration of up to 1 mg of adrenaline injection 1 in 1000 (1 mg/mL) for the emergency treatment of anaphylaxis

[1]Emerade® 300 micrograms, (delivering a single dose of adrenaline (as tartrate) 300 micrograms), adrenaline 1 mg/mL (1 in 1000), net price 0.5-mL auto-injector device = £26.94

Excipients include sulfites

Note 0.2 mL of the solution remains in the auto-injector device after use

Dose by intramuscular injection, ADULT and CHILD body-weight over 30 kg, 300 micrograms repeated after 5–15 minutes as necessary

[1]Emerade® 500 micrograms, (delivering a single dose of adrenaline (as tartrate) 500 micrograms), adrenaline 1 mg/mL (1 in 1000), net price 0.5-mL auto-injector device = £28.74

Excipients include sulfites

Note No solution remains in the auto-injector device after use

Dose by intramuscular injection, ADULT and CHILD over 12 years at risk of severe anaphylaxis, 500 micrograms repeated after 5–15 minutes as necessary

EpiPen® (Meda) [PoM]

Epipen® Jr Auto-injector 0.15 mg (delivering a single dose of adrenaline 150 micrograms), adrenaline 500 micrograms/mL (1 in 2000), net price 2-mL auto-injector device = £26.45, 2 × 2-mL auto-injector device = £52.90

Excipients include sulfites

Note 1.7 mL of the solution remains in the auto-injector device after use

Dose by intramuscular injection, CHILD body-weight 15–30 kg, 150 micrograms (but on the basis of a dose of 10 micrograms/kg, 300 micrograms may be more appropriate for some children) repeated after 5–15 minutes as necessary; CHILD body-weight under 15 kg [unlicensed], 150 micrograms repeated after 5–15 minutes as necessary

[1]EpiPen® Auto-injector 0.3 mg (delivering a single dose of adrenaline 300 micrograms), adrenaline 1 mg/mL (1 in 1000), net price 2-mL auto-injector device = £26.45, 2 × 2-mL auto-injector device = £52.90

Excipients include sulfites

Note 1.7 mL of the solution remains in the auto-injector device after use

Dose by intramuscular injection, ADULT and CHILD body-weight over 30 kg, 300 micrograms repeated after 5–15 minutes as necessary

Jext® (ALK-Abelló) [PoM]

[1]Jext® 150 micrograms (delivering a single dose of adrenaline (as tartrate) 150 micrograms), adrenaline 1 mg/mL (1 in 1000), net price 1.4-mL auto-injector device = £23.99

Excipients include sulfites

Note 1.25 mL of the solution remains in the auto-injector device after use

Dose by intramuscular injection, CHILD body-weight 15–30 kg, 150 micrograms (but on the basis of a dose of 10 micrograms/kg, 300 micrograms may be more appropriate for some children) repeated after 5–15 minutes as necessary; CHILD body-weight under 15 kg [unlicensed], 150 micrograms repeated after 5–15 minutes as necessary

[1]Jext® 300 micrograms (delivering a single dose of adrenaline (as tartrate) 300 micrograms), adrenaline 1 mg/mL (1 in 1000), net price 1.4-mL auto-injector device = £23.99

Excipients include sulfites

Note 1.1 mL of the solution remains in the auto-injector device after use

Dose by intramuscular injection, ADULT and CHILD body-weight over 30 kg, 300 micrograms repeated after 5–15 minutes as necessary

---

1. [PoM] restriction does not apply to the intramuscular administration of up to 1 mg of adrenaline injection 1 in 1000 (1 mg/mL) for the emergency treatment of anaphylaxis

Angioedema

Angioedema is dangerous if *laryngeal oedema* is present. In this circumstance **adrenaline (epinephrine)** injection and **oxygen** should be given as described under Anaphylaxis (see p. 213); antihistamines and corticosteroids should also be given. Tracheal intubation may be necessary.

Hereditary angioedema   The treatment of hereditary angioedema should be under specialist supervision. Unlike allergic angioedema, adrenaline, corticosteroids, and antihistamines should not be used for the treatment of acute attacks, including attacks involving laryngeal oedema, as they are ineffective and may delay appropriate treatment—intubation may be necessary. The administration of **C1-esterase inhibitor**, an endogenous complement blocker derived from human plasma, (in fresh frozen plasma or in partially purified form) can terminate acute attacks of *hereditary angioedema*; it can also be used for short-term prophylaxis before dental, medical or surgical procedures. **Conestat alfa** and **icatibant** are licensed for the treatment of acute attacks of hereditary angioedema in adults with C1-esterase inhibitor deficiency.

Tranexamic acid (section 2.11) and **danazol** (section 6.7.2) [unlicensed indication] are used for short-term and long-term prophylaxis of hereditary angioedema. Short-term prophylaxis with tranexamic acid or danazol is started several days before planned procedures (e.g. dental work) and continued for 2–5 days afterwards. Danazol should be avoided in children because of its androgenic effects.

C1-ESTERASE INHIBITOR

C1-esterase inhibitor is prepared from human plasma

Indications   see under preparations

Cautions   vaccination against hepatitis A, p. 850 and hepatitis B, p. 852 may be required

Pregnancy   manufacturer advises avoid unless essential

Side-effects   thrombosis (with high doses), headache, fever

Dose

• See under preparations

Berinert® (CSL Behring) [PoM]

Injection, powder for reconstitution, C1-esterase inhibitor, net price 500-unit vial (with solvent) = £467.50

Electrolytes Na⁺ approx. 2.1 mmol/vial

Dose by slow intravenous injection *or* intravenous infusion, acute attacks of hereditary angioedema, ADULT and CHILD 20 units/kg

Short-term prophylaxis of hereditary angioedema before dental, medical or surgical procedures, ADULT 1000 units as a single dose less than 6 hours before procedure, CHILD 15–30 units/kg (max. 1000 units) as a single dose less than 6 hours before procedure

Cinryze® (ViroPharma) ▼ [PoM]

Injection, powder for reconstitution, C1-esterase inhibitor, net price 500-unit vial (with solvent) = £668.00

Electrolytes Na⁺ approx. 0.5 mmol/vial

Dose by slow intravenous injection, acute attacks of hereditary angioedema, ADULT and CHILD over 12 years, 1000 units as a single dose; dose may be repeated if necessary

Short-term prophylaxis of hereditary angioedema before dental, medical, or surgical procedures, ADULT and CHILD over 12 years, 1000 units up to 24 hours before procedure

3 Respiratory system

Long-term prophylaxis of severe, recurrent attacks of hereditary angioedema where acute treatment is inadequate, or when oral prophylaxis is inadequate or not tolerated, ADULT and CHILD over 12 years, 1000 units every 3–4 days, interval between doses adjusted according to response

CONESTAT ALFA

Indications acute attacks of hereditary angioedema in patients with C1-esterase inhibitor deficiency

Cautions test for immunoglobulin E (IgE) antibodies against rabbit allergens before starting treatment, repeat antibody testing annually or after 10 treatments—consult product literature

Contra-indications rabbit allergy

Pregnancy use only if potential benefit outweighs risk—toxicity in *animal* studies

Breast-feeding use only if potential benefit outweighs risk—no information available

Side-effects headache; *less commonly* nausea, diarrhoea, abdominal discomfort, throat irritation, vertigo, paraesthesia, urticaria

Dose
- By slow intravenous injection over 5 minutes, ADULT over 18 years, body-weight under 84 kg, 50 units/kg as a single dose; body-weight over 84 kg, 4200 units as a single dose; dose may be repeated if necessary (max. 2 doses in 24 hours)

Ruconest® (Swedish Orphan) ▼ PoM
Injection, powder for reconstitution, conestat alfa, net price 2100-unit vial = £750.00

ICATIBANT

Indications acute attacks of hereditary angioedema in patients with C1-esterase inhibitor deficiency

Cautions ischaemic heart disease, stroke

Pregnancy manufacturer advises use only if potential benefit outweighs risk—toxicity in *animal* studies

Breast-feeding manufacturer advises avoid for 12 hours after administration

Side-effects nausea, dizziness, headache, pyrexia, injection-site reactions, rash, pruritus, erythema

Dose
- By subcutaneous injection, ADULT over 18 years, 30 mg as a single dose, repeated after 6 hours if necessary; a third dose may be given after a further 6 hours (max. 3 doses in 24 hours)

Firazyr® (Shire HGT) PoM
Injection, icatibant (as acetate) 10 mg/mL, net price 3-mL prefilled syringe = £1395.00

3.5 Respiratory stimulants and pulmonary surfactants

3.5.1 Respiratory stimulants
3.5.2 Pulmonary surfactants

3.5.1 Respiratory stimulants

Respiratory stimulants (analeptic drugs) have a limited place in the treatment of ventilatory failure in patients with chronic obstructive pulmonary disease. They are effective only when given by intravenous injection or infusion and have a short duration of action. Their use has largely been replaced by ventilatory support including nasal intermittent positive pressure ventilation. However, occasionally when ventilatory support is contra-indicated and in patients with hypercapnic respiratory failure who are becoming drowsy or comatose, respiratory stimulants in the short term may arouse patients sufficiently to co-operate and clear their secretions.

Respiratory stimulants can also be harmful in respiratory failure since they stimulate non-respiratory as well as respiratory muscles. They should only be given under **expert supervision** in hospital and must be combined with active physiotherapy. There is at present no oral respiratory stimulant available for long-term use in chronic respiratory failure.

Doxapram is given by continuous intravenous infusion. Frequent arterial blood gas and pH measurements are necessary during treatment to ensure correct dosage.

For the use of **caffeine citrate** in the management of neonatal apnoea, see *BNF for Children*.

DOXAPRAM HYDROCHLORIDE

Indications see under Dose

Cautions give with oxygen in severe irreversible airways obstruction or severely decreased lung compliance (because of increased work load of breathing); give with beta₂ agonist in bronchoconstriction; hypertension (avoid if severe), impaired cardiac reserve; phaeochromocytoma; **interactions:** Appendix 1 (doxapram)

Contra-indications severe hypertension; status asthmaticus; coronary artery disease; hyperthyroidism; epilepsy and other convulsive disorders; physical obstruction of respiratory tract; cerebral oedema, cerebrovascular accident

Hepatic impairment use with caution

Pregnancy no evidence of harm, but manufacturer advises avoid unless benefit outweighs risk

Side-effects nausea, vomiting; hypertension, tachycardia, bradycardia, extrasystoles, arrhythmias, chest pain, flushing; dyspnoea, cough, bronchospasm, laryngospasm; pyrexia, headache, dizziness, hyperactivity, confusion, hallucination, convulsions; urinary retention, incontinence, perineal warmth; muscle spasms

Dose
- Postoperative respiratory depression, by intravenous injection over at least 30 seconds, 1–1.5 mg/kg repeated if necessary after intervals of 1 hour *or* alternatively by intravenous infusion, 2–3 mg/minute adjusted according to response; CHILD not recommended
- Acute respiratory failure, by intravenous infusion, 1.5–4 mg/minute adjusted according to response (given concurrently with oxygen and whenever possible monitor with frequent measurement of blood gas tensions); CHILD not recommended

Doxapram Hydrochloride (Non-proprietary) PoM
Injection, doxapram hydrochloride 20 mg/mL, net price 5-mL amp = £6.00

3.5.2 Pulmonary surfactants

Pulmonary surfactants are used in the management of respiratory distress syndrome (hyaline membrane disease) in neonates and preterm neonates. They may also be given prophylactically to preterm neonates at risk of developing the syndrome.

Side-effects Pulmonary surfactants have been associated with intracranial haemorrhage. Bradycardia, pulmonary haemorrhage, and decreased oxygen saturation have been reported rarely; hyperoxia and obstruction of the endotracheal tube by mucous secretions have also been reported.

▌ BERACTANT

Indications (specialist use only); treatment of respiratory distress syndrome in preterm neonates over 700 g; prophylaxis of respiratory distress syndrome in preterm neonates less than 32 weeks corrected gestational age

Cautions consult product literature

Side-effects see notes above

Dose

- Treatment of respiratory distress syndrome, by endotracheal tube, phospholipid 100 mg/kg equivalent to a volume of 4 mL/kg, preferably within 8 hours of birth; dose may be repeated within 48 hours at intervals of at least 6 hours for up to 4 doses
- Prophylaxis of respiratory distress syndrome, by endotracheal tube, phospholipid 100 mg/kg equivalent to a volume of 4 mL/kg soon after birth, preferably within 15 minutes; dose may be repeated within 48 hours at intervals of at least 6 hours for up to 4 doses

Survanta® (AbbVie) ▣PoM▣
Suspension, beractant (bovine lung extract) providing phospholipid 25 mg/mL, with lipids and proteins, net price 8-mL vial = £306.43

▌ PORACTANT ALFA

Indications (specialist use only); treatment of respiratory distress syndrome in neonates over 700 g; prophylaxis of respiratory distress syndrome in preterm neonates 24–31 weeks corrected gestational age

Cautions consult product literature

Side-effects see notes above; also *rarely* hypotension

Dose

- Treatment of respiratory distress syndrome, by endotracheal tube, 100–200 mg/kg; further doses of 100 mg/kg may be repeated at intervals of 12 hours; max. total dose 300–400 mg/kg

- Prophylaxis of respiratory distress syndrome, by endotracheal tube, 100–200 mg/kg soon after birth, preferably within 15 minutes; further doses of 100 mg/kg may be repeated 6–12 hours later and after a further 12 hours if still intubated; max. total dose 300–400 mg/kg

Curosurf® (Chiesi) ▣PoM▣
Suspension, poractant alfa (porcine lung phospholipid fraction) 80 mg/mL, net price 1.5-mL vial = £281.64; 3-mL vial = £547.40

3.6 Oxygen

Oxygen should be regarded as a drug. It is prescribed for hypoxaemic patients to increase alveolar oxygen tension and decrease the work of breathing. The concentration of oxygen required depends on the condition being treated; the administration of an inappropriate concentration of oxygen can have serious or even fatal consequences.

Oxygen is probably the most common drug used in medical emergencies. It should be prescribed initially to achieve a normal or near–normal oxygen saturation; in most acutely ill patients with a normal or low arterial carbon dioxide (P_aCO_2), oxygen saturation should be 94–98% oxygen saturation. However, in some clinical situations such as cardiac arrest and carbon monoxide poisoning (see also Emergency Treatment of Poisoning, p. 42) it is more appropriate to aim for the highest possible oxygen saturation until the patient is stable. A lower target of 88–92% oxygen saturation is indicated for patients at risk of hypercapnic respiratory failure, see below.

High concentration oxygen therapy is safe in uncomplicated cases of conditions such as pneumonia, pulmonary thromboembolism, pulmonary fibrosis, shock, severe trauma, sepsis, or anaphylaxis. In such conditions low arterial oxygen (P_aO_2) is usually associated with low or normal arterial carbon dioxide (P_aCO_2), and therefore there is little risk of hypoventilation and carbon dioxide retention.

In acute severe asthma, the arterial carbon dioxide (P_aCO_2) is usually subnormal but as asthma deteriorates it may rise steeply (particularly in children). These patients usually require high concentrations of oxygen and if the arterial carbon dioxide (P_aCO_2) remains high despite other treatment, intermittent positive-pressure ventilation needs to be considered urgently.

Low concentration oxygen therapy (controlled oxygen therapy) is reserved for patients at risk of hypercapnic respiratory failure, which is more likely in those with:

- chronic obstructive pulmonary disease;
- advanced cystic fibrosis;
- severe non-cystic fibrosis bronchiectasis;
- severe kyphoscoliosis or severe ankylosing spondylitis;
- severe lung scarring caused by tuberculosis;
- musculoskeletal disorders with respiratory weakness, especially if on home ventilation;
- an overdose of opioids, benzodiazepines, or other drugs causing respiratory depression.

Until blood gases can be measured, initial oxygen should be given using a controlled concentration of 28% or less, titrated towards a target oxygen saturation of 88–92%. The aim is to provide the patient with enough oxygen to achieve an acceptable arterial oxygen tension without worsening carbon dioxide retention and respiratory acidosis. Patients may carry an *oxygen alert card*, see section 3.1.

Domiciliary oxygen Oxygen should only be prescribed for use in the home after careful evaluation in hospital by respiratory experts.

Patients should be advised of the risks of continuing to smoke when receiving oxygen therapy, including the

3

Respiratory system

Respiratory system 3

risk of fire. Smoking cessation therapy (section 4.10.2) should be recommended before home oxygen prescription.

Air travel Some patients with arterial hypoxaemia require supplementary oxygen for air travel. The patient's requirement should be discussed with the airline before travel.

Long-term oxygen therapy

Long-term administration of oxygen (usually at least 15 hours daily) prolongs survival in some patients with chronic obstructive pulmonary disease.

Assessment for long-term oxygen therapy requires measurement of arterial blood gas tensions. Measurements should be taken on 2 occasions at least 3 weeks apart to demonstrate clinical stability, and not sooner than 4 weeks after an acute exacerbation of the disease. Long-term oxygen therapy should be considered for patients with:

- chronic obstructive pulmonary disease with P_aO_2 < 7.3 kPa when breathing air during a period of clinical stability;

- chronic obstructive pulmonary disease with P_aO_2 7.3–8 kPa in the presence of secondary polycythaemia, nocturnal hypoxaemia, peripheral oedema, or evidence of pulmonary hypertension;

- severe chronic asthma with P_aO_2 < 7.3 kPa or persistent disabling breathlessness;

- interstitial lung disease with P_aO_2 < 8 kPa and in patients with P_aO_2 > 8 kPa with disabling dyspnoea;

- cystic fibrosis when P_aO_2 < 7.3 kPa or if P_aO_2 7.3–8 kPa in the presence of secondary polycythaemia, nocturnal hypoxaemia, pulmonary hypertension, or peripheral oedema;

- pulmonary hypertension, without parenchymal lung involvement when P_aO_2 < 8 kPa;

- neuromuscular or skeletal disorders, after specialist assessment;

- obstructive sleep apnoea despite continuous positive airways pressure therapy, after specialist assessment;

- pulmonary malignancy or other terminal disease with disabling dyspnoea;

- heart failure with daytime P_aO_2 < 7.3 kPa when breathing air or with nocturnal hypoxaemia;

- paediatric respiratory disease, after specialist assessment.

Increased respiratory depression is seldom a problem in patients with stable respiratory failure treated with low concentrations of oxygen although it may occur during exacerbations; patients and relatives should be warned to call for medical help if drowsiness or confusion occur.

Short-burst oxygen therapy

Oxygen is occasionally prescribed for short-burst (intermittent) use for episodes of breathlessness not relieved by other treatment in patients with severe chronic obstructive pulmonary disease, interstitial lung disease, heart failure, and in palliative care. It is important, however, that the patient does not rely on oxygen instead of obtaining medical help or taking more specific treatment. Short-burst oxygen therapy can be used

to improve exercise capacity and recovery; it should only be continued if there is proven improvement in breathlessness or exercise tolerance.

Ambulatory oxygen therapy

Ambulatory oxygen is prescribed for patients on long-term oxygen therapy who need to be away from home on a regular basis. Patients who are not on long-term oxygen therapy can be considered for ambulatory oxygen therapy if there is evidence of exercise-induced oxygen desaturation and of improvement in blood oxygen saturation and exercise capacity with oxygen. Ambulatory oxygen therapy is not recommended for patients with heart failure or those who smoke.

Oxygen therapy equipment

Under the NHS oxygen may be supplied as **oxygen cylinders**. Oxygen flow can be adjusted as the cylinders are equipped with an oxygen flow meter with 'medium' (2 litres/minute) and 'high' (4 litres/minute) settings.

Oxygen concentrators are more economical for patients who require oxygen for long periods, and in England and Wales can be ordered on the NHS on a regional tendering basis (see below). A concentrator is recommended for a patient who requires oxygen for more than 8 hours a day (or 21 cylinders per month). Exceptionally, if a higher concentration of oxygen is required the output of 2 oxygen concentrators can be combined using a 'Y' connection.

A nasal cannula is usually preferred for long-term oxygen therapy from an oxygen concentrator. It can, however, produce dermatitis and mucosal drying in sensitive individuals.

Giving oxygen by nasal cannula allows the patient to talk, eat, and drink, but the concentration of oxygen is not controlled; this may not be appropriate for acute respiratory failure. When oxygen is given through a nasal cannula at a rate of 1–2 litres/minute the inspiratory oxygen concentration is usually low, but it varies with ventilation and can be high if the patient is under-ventilating.

Arrangements for supplying oxygen

The following oxygen services may be ordered in England and Wales:

- emergency oxygen;

- short-burst (intermittent) oxygen therapy;

- long-term oxygen therapy;

- ambulatory oxygen.

The type of oxygen service (or combination of services) should be ordered on a Home Oxygen Order Form (HOOF); the amount of oxygen required (hours per day) and flow rate should be specified. The clinician will determine the appropriate equipment to be provided. Special needs or preferences should be specified on the HOOF.

The clinician should obtain the patient's consent to pass on the patient's details to the supplier, the fire brigade, and other relevant organisations. The supplier will contact the patient to make arrangements for delivery, installation, and maintenance of the equipment. The supplier will also train the patient to use the equipment.

The clinician should send the HOOF to the supplier who will continue to provide the service until a revised HOOF is received, or until notified that the patient no longer requires the home oxygen service.

East of England North East	BOC Medical
	to order:
	Tel: 0800 136 603
	Fax: 0800 169 9989
South West	Air Liquide
	to order:
	Tel: 0808 202 2229
	Fax: 0191 497 4340
London East Midlands North West	Air Liquide
	to order:
	Tel: 0500 823 773
	Fax: 0800 781 4610
Yorkshire and Humberside West Midlands Wales	Air Products
	to order:
	Tel: 0800 373 580
	Fax: 0800 214 709
South East Coast South Central	Dolby Vivisol
	to order.
	Tel: 08443 814 402
	Fax: 0800 781 4610

In **Scotland** refer the patient for assessment by a respiratory consultant. If the need for a concentrator is confirmed the consultant will arrange for the provision of a concentrator through the Common Services Agency. In **Northern Ireland** oxygen concentrators and cylinders should be prescribed on form HS21; oxygen concentrators are supplied by a local contractor. In **Scotland** and **Northern Ireland** prescriptions for oxygen cylinders and accessories can be dispensed by pharmacists contracted to provide domiciliary oxygen services.

3.7 Mucolytics

Mucolytics are prescribed to facilitate expectoration by reducing sputum viscosity. In some patients with chronic obstructive pulmonary disease and a chronic productive cough, mucolytics can reduce exacerbations; mucolytic therapy should be stopped if there is no benefit after a 4-week trial. Steam inhalation with postural drainage is effective in bronchiectasis and in some cases of chronic bronchitis.

Mucolytics should be used with caution in those with a history of peptic ulceration because they may disrupt the gastric mucosal barrier.

For reference to dornase alfa and hypertonic saline, see below.

▎CARBOCISTEINE

Indications reduction of sputum viscosity, see notes above

Cautions see notes above

Contra-indications active peptic ulceration

Pregnancy manufacturer advises avoid in first trimester

Breast-feeding no information available

Side-effects *rarely* gastro-intestinal bleeding; *also reported* Stevens-Johnson syndrome, erythema multiforme

Dose

● Initially 2.25 g daily in divided doses, then 1.5 g daily in divided doses as condition improves; CHILD 2–5

years 62.5–125 mg 4 times daily, 5–12 years 250 mg 3 times daily

Carbocisteine (Non-proprietary) [PoM]
Capsules, carbocisteine 375 mg, net price 120-cap pack = £17.70
Brands include *Mucodyne*®

Oral liquid, carbocisteine 125 mg/5 mL, net price 300 mL = £5.08; 250 mg/5 mL, 300 mL = £6.99
Brands include *Mucodyne*® *Paediatric* 125 mg/5 mL (cherry- and raspberry-flavoured) and *Mucodyne*® 250 mg/5 mL (cinnamon- and rum-flavoured)

▎ERDOSTEINE

Indications symptomatic treatment of acute exacerbations of chronic bronchitis

Cautions see notes above

Hepatic impairment manufacturer advises max. 300 mg daily in mild to moderate impairment; avoid in severe impairment

Renal impairment avoid if eGFR less than 25 mL/minute/1.73 m^2—no information available

Pregnancy manufacturer advises avoid—no information available

Breast-feeding manufacturer advises avoid—no information available

Side-effects *very rarely* nausea, vomiting, diarrhoea, abdominal pain, taste disturbance, headache, rash, and urticaria

Dose

● ADULT over 18 years, 300 mg twice daily for up to 10 days

Erdotin® (Galen) ▼ [PoM]
Capsules, yellow/green, erdosteine 300 mg, net price 20-cap pack = £4.25
Note The *Scottish Medicines Consortium* (October 2007) has advised that erdosteine (*Erdotin*®) is not recommended for the symptomatic treatment of acute exacerbations of chronic bronchitis

Dornase alfa

Dornase alfa is a genetically engineered version of a naturally occurring human enzyme which cleaves extracellular deoxyribonucleic acid (DNA). It is used in cystic fibrosis and is administered by inhalation using a jet nebuliser (section 3.1.5).

▎DORNASE ALFA

Phosphorylated glycosylated recombinant human deoxyribonuclease 1 (rhDNase)

Indications management of cystic fibrosis patients with a forced vital capacity (FVC) of greater than 40% of predicted to improve pulmonary function

Pregnancy no evidence of teratogenicity; manufacturer advises use only if potential benefit outweighs risk

Breast-feeding amount probably too small to be harmful—manufacturer advises caution

Side-effects *rarely* dyspepsia, chest pain, dysphonia, dyspnoea, pharyngitis, laryngitis, pyrexia, conjunctivitis, rhinitis, rash, urticaria

Dose

● ADULT and CHILD over 5 years, by inhalation of nebulised solution (by jet nebuliser), 2500 units (2.5 mg) once daily (patients over 21 years may benefit from twice daily dosage)

Pulmozyme® (Roche) [PoM]

Nebuliser solution, dornase alfa 1000 units (1 mg)/mL. Net price 2.5-mL (2500 units) vial = £16.55

Note For use undiluted with jet nebulisers only; ultrasonic nebulisers are unsuitable

Hypertonic sodium chloride

Nebulised hypertonic sodium chloride solution (3–7%) is used to mobilise lower respiratory tract secretions in mucous consolidation (e.g. cystic fibrosis). Nebulised hypertonic sodium chloride solution (3%) is used for mild to moderate acute viral bronchiolitis in infants.

Temporary irritation, such as coughing, hoarseness, or reversible bronchoconstriction may occur; an inhaled bronchodilator can be used before treatment with hypertonic sodium chloride to reduce the risk of these adverse effects.

MucoClear® 3% (Pari)

Nebuliser solution, sodium chloride 3%, net price 20 × 4 mL = £12.98; 60 × 4 mL = £27.00

Dose by inhalation of nebulised solution, 4 mL 2–4 times daily

MucoClear® 6% (Pari)

Nebuliser solution, sodium chloride 6%, net price 20 × 4 mL = £12.98; 60 × 4 mL = £27.00

Dose by inhalation of nebulised solution, 4 mL twice daily

Nebusal® 7% (Forest)

Nebuliser solution, sodium chloride 7%, net price 60 × 4 mL = £27.00

Dose by inhalation of nebulised solution, 4 mL up to twice daily

Ivacaftor

Ivacaftor is licensed for the treatment of cystic fibrosis in patients who have a G551D mutation in the cystic fibrosis transmembrane conductance regulator (CFTR) gene; it should be prescribed by a physician experienced in the treatment of cystic fibrosis. If the patient's genotype is unknown, a validated genotyping method should be performed to confirm the presence of the G551D mutation in at least one allele of the CFTR gene before starting treatment.

 IVACAFTOR

Indications treatment of cystic fibrosis in patients who have a G551D mutation in the CFTR gene

Cautions test liver function before treatment, every 3 months during the first year of treatment, then annually thereafter; **interactions:** Appendix 1 (ivacaftor)

Contra-indications organ transplantation (no information available); avoid grapefruit and Seville oranges

Hepatic impairment max. 150 mg once daily in moderate impairment; in severe impairment, manufacturer recommends use only if potential benefit outweighs risk—starting dose 150 mg on alternate days, dosing interval adjusted according to clinical response and tolerability

Renal impairment caution in severe impairment

Pregnancy manufacturer advises use only if potential benefit outweighs risk—no information available

Breast-feeding manufacturer advises use only if potential benefit outweighs risk—no information available

Side-effects abdominal pain, diarrhoea, oropharyngeal pain, pharyngeal oedema, headache, dizziness, upper respiratory-tract infection, rhinitis, nasopharyngitis, nasal congestion, ear discomfort, tinnitus, rash; *less commonly* vestibular disorder, gynaecomastia

Dose

● ADULT and CHILD over 6 years, 150 mg every 12 hours

Note Reduce dose to 150 mg twice a week with concomitant use of itraconazole, posaconazole, voriconazole, telithromycin, and clarithromycin; reduce dose to 150 mg once daily with concomitant use of fluconazole and erythromycin

Kalydeco® (Vertex) ▼ [PoM]

Tablets, f/c, ivacaftor 150 mg, net price 56-tab pack = £14000.00. Label: 25, counselling, administration

Counselling Tablets should be taken with fat-containing food

Mannitol

Mannitol, administered by inhalation, improves mucus clearance and is licensed for the treatment of cystic fibrosis as an add-on therapy to standard care. Patients must be assessed for bronchial hyperresponsiveness to inhaled mannitol before starting the therapeutic dose regimen; an initiation dose assessment must be carried out under medical supervision—for details of the initiation dose regimen, consult product literature.

The *Scottish Medicines Consortium*, p. 4 has advised (November 2013) that mannitol (*Bronchitol®*) is accepted for restricted use within NHS Scotland for the treatment of cystic fibrosis in adults aged 18 years and over as an add-on therapy to best standard of care. Mannitol is restricted to patients who are not currently using dornase alfa due to lack of response, intolerance, or ineligibility and have rapidly declining lung function and in whom other osmotic agents are considered unsuitable.

> **NICE guidance**
> **Mannitol dry powder for inhalation for treating cystic fibrosis (November 2012)**
> Mannitol dry powder for inhalation is recommended as an option for treating cystic fibrosis in adults:
> ● who cannot use dornase alfa (rhDNase) because of ineligibility, intolerance or inadequate response to dornase alfa (rhDNase), **and**
> ● whose lung function is rapidly declining (forced expiratory volume in 1 second decline greater than 2% annually), **and**
> ● for whom other osmotic agents are not considered appropriate.
> www.nice.org.uk/TA266

 MANNITOL

Indications see notes above

Cautions see notes above; also asthma, haemoptysis

Contra-indications bronchial hyperresponsiveness to inhaled mannitol, non-CF bronchiectasis, impaired lung function (forced expiratory volume in 1 second < 30% of predicted)

Pregnancy manufacturer advises avoid

Breast-feeding manufacturer advises avoid

Side-effects vomiting, cough, wheezing, haemoptysis, throat irritation, pharyngolaryngeal pain, headache; *less commonly* nausea, eructation, flatulence, gastro-oesophageal reflux disease, glossodynia, stomatitis, bronchospasm, dysphonia, dyspnoea, hyperventilation, pharyngitis, transient insomnia, dizziness, malaise, pyrexia, influenza-like illness, arthralgia, oral candidiasis, ear pain, rhinorrhoea, acne, pruritus, rash

Dose

- By inhalation of powder, ADULT over 18 years, initiation dose (see notes above), then 400 mg twice daily
Counselling The dose should be administered 5–15 minutes after a bronchodilator and before physiotherapy; the second daily dose should be taken 2–3 hours before bedtime

Bronchitol® (Pharmaxis) PoM
Inhalation powder, hard capsule (for use with disposable inhaler device), mannitol 40 mg, net price 280-cap pack with 2 disposable inhaler devices = £231.66; initiation dose pack, 10-cap pack with disposable inhaler device = £8.27. Counselling, administration

3.8 Aromatic inhalations

Inhalations containing volatile substances such as eucalyptus oil are traditionally used and although the vapour may contain little of the additive it encourages deliberate inspiration of warm moist air which is often comforting in bronchitis; boiling water should not be used owing to the risk of scalding. Inhalations are also used for the relief of nasal obstruction in acute rhinitis or sinusitis. Menthol and eucalyptus inhalation is used to relieve sinusitis affecting the maxillary antrum (section 12.2.2)

Children The use of strong aromatic decongestants (applied as rubs or to pillows) is not advised for infants under the age of 3 months. Carers of young infants in whom nasal obstruction with mucus is a problem can readily be taught appropriate techniques of suction aspiration but sodium chloride 0.9% given as nasal drops is preferred; administration before feeds may ease feeding difficulties caused by nasal congestion.

Benzoin Tincture, Compound, BP
(Friars' Balsam)
Tincture, balsamic acids approx. 4.5%. Label: 15
Side-effects allergic contact dermatitis
Dose add 5 mL to a pint of hot, **not** boiling, water and inhale the vapour; repeat after 4 hours if required

Menthol and Eucalyptus Inhalation, BP 1980
Inhalation, racementhol or levomenthol 2 g, eucalyptus oil 10 mL, light magnesium carbonate 7 g, water to 100 mL
Dose add one teaspoonful to a pint of hot, **not** boiling, water and inhale the vapour
Dental prescribing on the NHS Menthol and Eucalyptus Inhalation BP, 1980 may be prescribed

3.9 Cough preparations

3.9.1	Cough suppressants
3.9.2	Demulcent and expectorant cough preparations

3.9.1 Cough suppressants

Cough may be a symptom of an underlying disorder, such as asthma (section 3.1.1), gastro-oesophageal reflux disease (section 1.1), or rhinitis (section 12.2.1),

which should be addressed before prescribing cough suppressants. Cough may be a side-effect of another drug, such as an ACE inhibitor (section 2.5.5.1), or it can be associated with smoking or environmental pollutants. Cough can also have a significant habit component. When there is no identifiable cause, cough suppressants may be useful, for example if sleep is disturbed. They may cause sputum retention and this may be harmful in patients with chronic bronchitis and bronchiectasis.

Codeine may be effective but it is constipating and can cause dependence; **dextromethorphan** and **pholcodine** have fewer side-effects.

Sedating antihistamines are used as the cough suppressant component of many compound cough preparations on sale to the public; all tend to cause drowsiness which may reflect their main mode of action.

Children The use of over-the-counter cough suppressants containing codeine should be avoided in children under 18 years. Cough suppressants containing similar opioid analgesics such as dextromethorphan and pholcodine are not generally recommended in children and should be avoided in children under 6 years.

MHRA/CHM advice (March 2008 and February 2009) Over-the-counter cough and cold medicines for children
Children under 6 years should not be given over-the-counter cough and cold medicines containing the following ingredients:
- brompheniramine, chlorphenamine, diphenhydramine, doxylamine, promethazine, or triprolidine (antihistamines);
- dextromethorphan or pholcodine (cough suppressants);
- guaifenesin or ipecacuanha (expectorants);
- phenylephrine, pseudoephedrine, ephedrine, oxymetazoline, or xylometazoline (decongestants).

Over-the-counter cough and cold medicines can be considered for children aged 6–12 years after basic principles of best care have been tried, but treatment should be restricted to 5 days or less. Children should not be given more than 1 cough or cold preparation at a time because different brands may contain the same active ingredient; care should be taken to give the correct dose.

MHRA/CHM advice (October 2010) Over-the-counter codeine-containing liquid medicines for children
Children under 18 years should not use codeine-containing over-the-counter liquid medicines for cough suppression

---

CODEINE PHOSPHATE

Indications dry or painful cough; diarrhoea (section 1.4.2); pain (section 4.7.2)
Cautions see notes above and section 4.7.2
Contra-indications section 4.7.2
Hepatic impairment section 4.7.2
Renal impairment section 4.7.2
Pregnancy section 4.7.2
Breast-feeding section 4.7.2
Side-effects section 4.7.2

3   Respiratory system

Dose
- See under preparations below

Codeine Linctus, BP

Linctus (= oral solution), codeine phosphate 15 mg/5 mL, net price 100 mL = 78p (diabetic, 78p)

Brands include *Galcodine*®

Dose ADULT over 18 years 5–10 mL 3–4 times daily

Note BP directs that when Diabetic Codeine Linctus is prescribed, Codeine Linctus formulated with a vehicle appropriate for administration to diabetics, whether or not labelled 'Diabetic Codeine Linctus', shall be dispensed or supplied

◢Other preparations

Tablets, syrup, and injection section 4.7.2

PHOLCODINE

Indications dry cough

Cautions asthma; chronic, persistent, or productive cough; interactions: Appendix 1 (pholcodine)

Contra-indications chronic bronchitis, chronic obstructive pulmonary disease, bronchiectasis, patients at risk of respiratory failure

Hepatic impairment avoid

Renal impairment use with caution; avoid in severe impairment

Pregnancy manufacturer advises avoid unless potential benefit outweighs risk

Breast-feeding manufacturer advises avoid unless potential benefit outweighs risk—no information available

Side-effects nausea, vomiting, constipation, sputum retention, drowsiness, dizziness, excitation, confusion, rash

Dose
- See under preparations below

Pholcodine Linctus, BP

Linctus (= oral solution), pholcodine 5 mg/5 mL in a suitable flavoured vehicle, containing citric acid monohydrate 1%. Net price 100 mL = 52p

Brands include *Pavacol-D*® (sugar-free), *Galenphol*® (sugar-free)

Dose 5–10 mL 3–4 times daily; CHILD (but not generally recommended, see notes above) 6–12 years 2.5–5 mL

Pholcodine Linctus, Strong, BP

Linctus (= oral solution), pholcodine 10 mg/5 mL in a suitable flavoured vehicle, containing citric acid monohydrate 2%. Net price 100 mL = 44p

Brands include *Galenphol*®

Dose ADULT and CHILD over 12 years, 5 mL 3–4 times daily

Galenphol® (Thornton & Ross)

Paediatric linctus (= oral solution), orange, sugar-free, pholcodine 2 mg/5 mL. Net price 100 mL = £0.19

Dose CHILD (but not generally recommended, see notes above) 6–12 years 10 mL 3 times daily

Palliative care

Diamorphine and methadone have been used to control distressing cough in terminal lung cancer although morphine is now preferred (see Prescribing in Palliative Care p. 22). In other circumstances they are contra-indicated because they induce sputum retention and ventilatory failure as well as causing opioid dependence. Methadone linctus should be avoided because it has a long duration of action and tends to accumulate.

METHADONE HYDROCHLORIDE

Indications cough in terminal disease

Cautions section 4.7.2

Contra-indications section 4.7.2

Hepatic impairment section 4.7.2

Renal impairment section 4.7.2

Pregnancy section 4.7.2

Breast-feeding section 4.7.2

Side-effects section 4.7.2; longer-acting than morphine therefore effects may be cumulative

Dose
- See below

Methadone Linctus CD2 ◢

Linctus (= oral solution), methadone hydrochloride 2 mg/5 mL in a suitable vehicle with a tolu flavour. Label: 2

Dose 2.5–5 mL every 4–6 hours, reduced to twice daily on prolonged use

MORPHINE HYDROCHLORIDE

Indications cough in terminal disease (see also Prescribing in Palliative Care p. 22)

Cautions section 4.7.2

Contra-indications section 4.7.2

Hepatic impairment section 4.7.2

Renal impairment section 4.7.2

Pregnancy section 4.7.2

Breast-feeding section 4.7.2

Side-effects section 4.7.2

Dose
- Initially 5 mg every 4 hours

◢Preparations

Section 4.7.2

3.9.2 Demulcent and expectorant cough preparations

Demulcent cough preparations contain soothing substances such as syrup or glycerol and some patients believe that such preparations relieve a dry irritating cough. Preparations such as **simple linctus** have the advantage of being harmless and inexpensive; **paediatric simple linctus** is particularly useful in children.

Expectorants are claimed to promote expulsion of bronchial secretions, but there is no evidence that any drug can specifically facilitate expectoration.

Compound preparations are on sale to the public for the treatment of cough and colds but should not be used in children under 6 years; the rationale for some is dubious. Care should be taken to give the correct dose and to not use more than one preparation at a time, see MHRA/CHM advice, p. 221.

Simple Linctus, BP

Linctus (= oral solution), citric acid monohydrate 2.5% in a suitable vehicle with an anise flavour, net price 200 mL = 92p

Dose ADULT and CHILD over 12 years 5 mL 3–4 times daily

A sugar-free version is also available

Respiratory system

3

Simple Linctus, Paediatric, BP

Linctus (= oral solution), citric acid monohydrate 0.625% in a suitable vehicle with an anise flavour, net price 200 mL = 96p

Dose CHILD 1 month–12 years 5–10 mL 3–4 times daily

A sugar-free version is also available

3.10 Systemic nasal decongestants

Nasal decongestants for administration by mouth may not be as effective as preparations for local application (section 12.2.2) but they do not give rise to rebound nasal congestion on withdrawal. **Pseudoephedrine** is available over the counter; it has few sympathomimetic effects.

Systemic decongestants should be used with **caution** in diabetes, hypertension, hyperthyroidism, susceptibility to angle-closure glaucoma, prostatic hypertrophy, ischaemic heart disease, and should be **avoided** in patients taking monoamine oxidase inhibitors; **interactions:** Appendix 1 (sympathomimetics).

PSEUDOEPHEDRINE HYDROCHLORIDE

Indications　see notes above

Cautions　see notes above

Hepatic impairment　manufacturer advises use with caution in severe impairment

Renal impairment　use with caution in mild to moderate impairment; manufacturer advises avoid in severe impairment

Pregnancy　defective closure of the abdominal wall (gastroschisis) reported very rarely in newborns after first trimester exposure

Breast-feeding　may suppress lactation; avoid if lactation not well established or if milk production insufficient

Side-effects　nausea, vomiting, hypertension, tachycardia, headache, anxiety, restlessness, insomnia; *rarely* hallucinations, rash; *very rarely* angle-closure glaucoma; urinary retention also reported

Dose

● 60 mg 3–4 times daily; CHILD 6–12 years 30 mg 3–4 times daily

¹Galpseud® (Thornton & Ross) [PoM]

Tablets, pseudoephedrine hydrochloride 60 mg, net price 24-tab pack = £2.25

Linctus, orange, sugar-free, pseudoephedrine hydrochloride 30 mg/5 mL, net price 100 mL = 70p

¹Sudafed® (McNeil) [PoM]

Tablets, red, f/c, pseudoephedrine hydrochloride 60 mg, net price 24 = £2.12

Elixir, red, pseudoephedrine hydrochloride 30 mg/5 mL, net price 100 mL = £1.84

1. Can be sold to the public provided no more than 720 mg of pseudoephedrine salts are supplied, and ephedrine base (or salts) are not supplied at the same time; for details see *Medicines, Ethics and Practice*, London, Pharmaceutical Press (always consult latest edition)

3.11 Antifibrotics

Pirfenidone is licensed for the treatment of mild to moderate idiopathic pulmonary fibrosis; treatment should be initiated and supervised by an appropriate specialist. The exact mechanism of action of pirfenidone is not yet understood, but it is believed to slow down the progression of idiopathic pulmonary fibrosis by exerting both antifibrotic and anti-inflammatory properties.

The *Scottish Medicines Consortium*, p. 4 has advised (August 2013) that pirfenidone is accepted for restricted use within NHS Scotland for the treatment of mild to moderate idiopathic pulmonary fibrosis. Pirfenidone is restricted for use in patients with a predicted forced vital capacity less than or equal to 80%, and only whilst pirfenidone is available at the price agreed in the patient access scheme.

> **NICE guidance**
> **Pirfenidone for treating idiopathic pulmonary fibrosis (April 2013)**
> Pirfenidone is recommended as an option for treating idiopathic pulmonary fibrosis only if:
> ● the patient has a forced vital capacity (FVC) between 50% and 80% predicted, **and**
> ● the manufacturer provides pirfenidone with the discount agreed in the patient access scheme.
> Treatment should be discontinued if there is evidence of disease progression, defined as a decline in predicted FVC of 10% or more within any 12 month period.
> Patients currently receiving pirfenidone that is not recommended according to the above criteria should have the option to continue treatment until they and their clinician consider it appropriate to stop.
> www.nice.org.uk/TA282

PIRFENIDONE

Indications　see notes above

Cautions　test liver function before treatment, then at monthly intervals for the next 6 months, and then every 3 months thereafter; review if abnormal liver function tests—dose reduction, treatment interruption or discontinuation may be required (consult product literature); avoid exposure to direct sunlight and concomitant use of drugs known to cause photosensitivity—if photosensitivity reaction or rash occurs, dose adjustment or treatment interruption may be required (consult product literature); concomitant use with ciprofloxacin—reduce dose of pirfenidone to 2 capsules three times daily with high-dose ciprofloxacin (750 mg twice daily); monitor for weight loss; treatment interruption—see note below; **interactions:** Appendix 1 (pirfenidone)

Driving Dizziness or malaise may affect performance of skilled tasks (e.g. driving)

Contra-indications　cigarette smoking

Hepatic impairment　caution in mild to moderate impairment, particularly if concomitant use of CYP1A2 inhibitors; avoid in severe impairment

Renal impairment　avoid if eGFR less than 30 mL/minute/1.73m²

Pregnancy　manufacturer advises avoid—no information available

Breast-feeding　manufacturer advises avoid—no information available

Respiratory system　**3**

Respiratory system *(sidebar)*

Side-effects dyspepsia, nausea, diarrhoea, gastro-oesophageal reflux disease, vomiting, abdominal discomfort, gastritis, constipation, flatulence, (gastro-intestinal side-effects may require dose reduction or treatment interruption—consult product literature), raised hepatic enzymes, anorexia, weight loss, non-cardiac chest pain, hot flush, insomnia, dizziness, headache, somnolence, malaise, dysgeusia, upper respiratory tract infection, urinary tract infection, myalgia, arthralgia, photosensitivity reaction, rash, pruritus, erythema, dry skin; *rarely* raised bilirubin in combination with raised hepatic transaminases

Dose

- ADULT over 18 years, initially 1 capsule three times daily for 7 days, then 2 capsules three times daily for 7 days, then 3 capsules three times daily (see also Cautions, above)

  Note If treatment is interrupted for 14 consecutive days or more, the initial 2 week titration regimen should be repeated; if treatment is interrupted for less than 14 consecutive days, the dose can be resumed at the previous daily dose without titration

Esbriet® (InterMune) ▼ PoM

Capsule, blue/gold, pirfenidone 267 mg, net price 63-cap pack = £501.92, 252-cap pack = £2007.70, 270-cap pack = £2151.10. Label: 21, 25, Counselling, driving, see above

4 Central nervous system

4.1 Hypnotics and anxiolytics

Most anxiolytics ('sedatives') will induce sleep when given at night and most hypnotics will sedate when given during the day. Prescribing of these drugs is widespread but dependence (both physical and psychological) and tolerance occur. This may lead to difficulty in withdrawing the drug after the patient has been taking it regularly for more than a few weeks (see Dependence and Withdrawal, below). Hypnotics and anxiolytics should therefore be reserved for short courses to alleviate acute conditions after causal factors have been established.

Benzodiazepines are the most commonly used anxiolytics and hypnotics; they act at benzodiazepine receptors which are associated with gamma-aminobutyric acid (GABA) receptors. Older drugs such as meprobamate and barbiturates are **not** recommended—they have more side-effects and interactions than benzodiazepines and are much more dangerous in overdosage.

Paradoxical effects A paradoxical increase in hostility and aggression may be reported by patients taking benzodiazepines. The effects range from talkativeness and excitement to aggressive and antisocial acts. Adjustment of the dose (up or down) sometimes attenuates the impulses. Increased anxiety and perceptual disorders are other paradoxical effects. Increased hostility and aggression after barbiturates and alcohol usually indicates intoxication.

Driving Hypnotics and anxiolytics may impair judgement and increase reaction time, and so affect ability to drive or operate machinery; they increase the effects of alcohol. Moreover the hangover effects of a night dose may impair driving on the following day. See also Drugs and Driving under General Guidance, p. 3.

Dependence and withdrawal Withdrawal of a benzodiazepine should be gradual because abrupt withdrawal may produce confusion, toxic psychosis, convulsions, or a condition resembling delirium tremens. Abrupt withdrawal of a barbiturate is even more likely to have serious effects.

The benzodiazepine withdrawal syndrome may develop at any time up to 3 weeks after stopping a long-acting benzodiazepine, but may occur within a day in the case of a short-acting one. It is characterised by insomnia, anxiety, loss of appetite and of body-weight, tremor, perspiration, tinnitus, and perceptual disturbances. Some symptoms may be similar to the original complaint and encourage further prescribing; some symptoms may continue for weeks or months after stopping benzodiazepines.

Benzodiazepine withdrawal should be flexible and carried out at a reduction rate that is tolerable for the patient. The rate should depend on the initial dose of benzodiazepine, duration of use, and the patient's clinical response. Short-term users of benzodiazepines (2–4 weeks only) can usually taper off within 2–4 weeks. However, long-term users should be withdrawn over a much longer period of several months or more.

A suggested protocol for withdrawal for prescribed long-term benzodiazepine patients is as follows:

1. Transfer patient stepwise, one dose at a time over about a week, to an equivalent daily dose of diazepam[1] preferably taken at night

2. Reduce diazepam dose, usually by 1–2 mg every 2–4 weeks (in patients taking high doses of benzodiazepines, initially it may be appropriate to reduce the dose by up to one-tenth every 1–2 weeks). If uncomfortable withdrawal symptoms occur, maintain this dose until symptoms lessen

3. Reduce diazepam dose further, if necessary in smaller steps; steps of 500 micrograms may be appropriate towards the end of withdrawal. Then stop completely.

4. For long-term patients, the period needed for complete withdrawal may vary from several months to a year or more

Withdrawal symptoms for long-term users usually resolve within 6–18 months of the last dose. Some patients will recover more quickly, others may take longer. The addition of beta-blockers, antidepressants and antipsychotics should be **avoided** where possible. Counselling can be of considerable help both during and after the taper.

---

1. Approximate equivalent doses, diazepam 5 mg
   ≡ alprazolam 250 micrograms
   ≡ clobazam 10 mg
   ≡ clonazepam 250 micrograms
   ≡ flurazepam 7.5–15 mg
   ≡ chlordiazepoxide 12.5 mg
   ≡ loprazolam 0.5–1 mg
   ≡ lorazepam 500 micrograms
   ≡ lormetazepam 0.5–1 mg
   ≡ nitrazepam 5 mg
   ≡ oxazepam 10 mg
   ≡ temazepam 10 mg

Important: benzodiazepine indications

1. Benzodiazepines are indicated for the short-term relief (two to four weeks only) of anxiety that is severe, disabling, or causing the patient unacceptable distress, occurring alone or in association with insomnia or short-term psychosomatic, organic, or psychotic illness.

2. The use of benzodiazepines to treat short-term 'mild' anxiety is inappropriate.

3. Benzodiazepines should be used to treat insomnia only when it is severe, disabling, or causing the patient extreme distress.

4.1.1 Hypnotics

Before a hypnotic is prescribed the cause of the insomnia should be established and, where possible, underlying factors should be treated. However, it should be noted that some patients have unrealistic sleep expectations, and others understate their alcohol consumption which is often the cause of the insomnia. Short-acting hypnotics are preferable in patients with sleep onset insomnia, when sedation the following day is undesirable, or when prescribing for elderly patients (but see below). Long-acting hypnotics are indicated in patients with poor sleep maintenance (e.g. early morning waking) that causes daytime effects, when an anxiolytic effect is needed during the day, or when sedation the following day is acceptable; see also Important: Benzodiazepine Indications, above.

Transient insomnia may occur in those who normally sleep well and may be due to extraneous factors such as noise, shift work, and jet lag. If a hypnotic is indicated one that is rapidly eliminated should be chosen, and only one or two doses should be given.

Short-term insomnia is usually related to an emotional problem or serious medical illness. It may last for a few weeks and may recur; a hypnotic can be useful but should not be given for more than three weeks (preferably only one week). Intermittent use is desirable with omission of some doses. A short-acting drug is usually appropriate.

Chronic insomnia is rarely benefited by hypnotics and is sometimes due to mild dependence caused by injudicious prescribing of hypnotics. Psychiatric disorders such as anxiety, depression, and abuse of drugs and alcohol are common causes. Sleep disturbance is very common in depressive illness and early wakening is often a useful pointer. The underlying psychiatric complaint should be treated, adapting the drug regimen to alleviate insomnia. For example, clomipramine or mirtazapine prescribed for depression will also help to promote sleep if taken at night. Other causes of insomnia include daytime cat-napping and physical causes such as pain, pruritus, and dyspnoea.

Hypnotics should **not** be prescribed indiscriminately and routine prescribing is undesirable. They should be reserved for short courses in the acutely distressed. Tolerance to their effects develops within 3 to 14 days of continuous use and long-term efficacy cannot be assured. A major drawback of long-term use is that withdrawal can cause rebound insomnia and a withdrawal syndrome (section 4.1).

Where prolonged administration is unavoidable hypnotics should be discontinued as soon as feasible and the patient warned that sleep may be disturbed for a few days before normal rhythm is re-established; broken sleep with vivid dreams may persist for several weeks.

Children The prescribing of hypnotics to children, except for occasional use such as for night terrors and somnambulism (sleep-walking), is not justified.

Elderly Benzodiazepines and the Z–drugs should be avoided in the elderly, because the elderly are at greater risk of becoming ataxic and confused, leading to falls and injury.

Dental procedures Some anxious patients may benefit from the use of hypnotics such as temazepam or diazepam. Temazepam is preferred when it is important to minimise any residual effect the following day.

Benzodiazepines

Benzodiazepines used as hypnotics include **nitrazepam** and **flurazepam** which have a prolonged action and may give rise to residual effects on the following day; repeated doses tend to be cumulative.

Loprazolam, **lormetazepam**, and **temazepam** act for a shorter time and they have little or no hangover effect. Withdrawal phenomena are more common with the short-acting benzodiazepines.

If insomnia is associated with daytime anxiety then the use of a long-acting benzodiazepine anxiolytic such as **diazepam** given as a single dose at night may effectively treat both symptoms.

For general guidelines on benzodiazepine prescribing see section 4.1.2 and for benzodiazepine withdrawal see section 4.1.

Hepatic impairment Benzodiazepines can precipitate coma if used in hepatic impairment. If treatment is necessary, benzodiazepines with shorter half lives are safer, such as temazepam or oxazepam. Start with smaller initial doses or reduce dose; avoid in severe impairment.

Renal impairment Patients with renal impairment have increased cerebral sensitivity to benzodiazepines; start with small doses in severe impairment.

Pregnancy There is a risk of neonatal withdrawal symptoms when benzodiazepines are used during pregnancy. Avoid regular use and use only if there is a clear indication such as seizure control. High doses administered during late pregnancy or labour may cause neonatal hypothermia, hypotonia, and respiratory depression.

Breast-feeding Benzodiazepines are present in milk, and should be avoided if possible during breast-feeding.

◼ NITRAZEPAM

Indications insomnia (short-term use; see p. 226)
Cautions respiratory disease; muscle weakness and myasthenia gravis; history of drug or alcohol abuse; hypoalbuminaemia; marked personality disorder; reduce dose in elderly and debilitated; avoid prolonged use (and abrupt withdrawal thereafter); acute porphyria (section 9.8.2); **interactions:** Appendix 1 (anxiolytics and hypnotics)
  Driving Drowsiness may persist the next day and affect performance of skilled tasks (e.g. driving); effects of alcohol enhanced; see also Drugs and Driving, p. 3

Contra-indications respiratory depression; marked neuromuscular respiratory weakness including unstable myasthenia gravis; acute pulmonary insufficiency; sleep apnoea syndrome; not for use alone to treat depression (or anxiety associated with depression) or chronic psychosis
Hepatic impairment see notes above
Renal impairment see notes above
Pregnancy see notes above
Breast-feeding see notes above
Side-effects drowsiness and lightheadedness the next day; confusion and ataxia (especially in the elderly); amnesia may occur; dependence; see also under Diazepam (section 4.1.2); **overdosage:** see Emergency Treatment of Poisoning, p. 39
Dose
● 5–10 mg at bedtime; ELDERLY (or debilitated) 2.5–5 mg

Nitrazepam (Non-proprietary) CD4-1
  Tablets, nitrazepam 5 mg, net price 28 = £1.88. Label: 19
  Brands include *Mogadon*® JHS
  Oral suspension, nitrazepam 2.5 mg/5 mL. Net price 150 mL = £10.60. Label: 19

◼ FLURAZEPAM

Indications insomnia (short-term use; see p. 226)
Cautions see under Nitrazepam
Contra-indications see under Nitrazepam
Hepatic impairment see notes above
Renal impairment see notes above
Pregnancy see notes above
Breast-feeding see notes above
Side-effects see under Nitrazepam
Dose
● 15–30 mg at bedtime; ELDERLY (or debilitated) 15 mg; CHILD not recommended

Dalmane® (Meda) CD4-1 JHS
  Capsules, flurazepam (as hydrochloride), 15 mg (grey/yellow), net price 30-cap pack = £6.73; 30 mg (black/grey), 30-cap pack = £8.63. Label: 19

◼ LOPRAZOLAM

Indications insomnia (short-term use; see p. 226)
Cautions see under Nitrazepam
Contra-indications see under Nitrazepam
Hepatic impairment see notes above
Renal impairment see notes above
Pregnancy see notes above
Breast-feeding see notes above
Side-effects see under Nitrazepam; shorter acting
Dose
● 1 mg at bedtime, increased to 1.5 or 2 mg if required; ELDERLY (or debilitated) 0.5 or 1 mg; CHILD not recommended

Loprazolam (Non-proprietary) CD4-1
  Tablets, loprazolam 1 mg (as mesilate). Net price 28-tab pack = £18.00. Label: 19

◼ LORMETAZEPAM

Indications insomnia (short-term use; see p. 226)
Cautions see under Nitrazepam
Contra-indications see under Nitrazepam

4 Central nervous system

Central nervous system 4

Hepatic impairment see notes above
Renal impairment see notes above
Pregnancy see notes above
Breast-feeding see notes above
Side-effects see under Nitrazepam; shorter acting
Dose

- 0.5–1.5 mg at bedtime; ELDERLY (or debilitated) 500 micrograms; CHILD not recommended

Lormetazepam (Non-proprietary) CD4-1
Tablets, lormetazepam 500 micrograms, net price 30-tab pack = £28.86; 1 mg, 30-tab pack = £30.41. Label: 19

▌ TEMAZEPAM

Indications insomnia (short-term use; see p. 226); see also section 15.1.4.1 for peri-operative use
Cautions see under Nitrazepam
Contra-indications see under Nitrazepam
Hepatic impairment see notes above
Renal impairment see notes above
Pregnancy see notes above
Breast-feeding see notes above
Side-effects see under Nitrazepam; shorter acting
Dose

- 10–20 mg at bedtime, exceptional circumstances 30–40 mg; ELDERLY (or debilitated) 10 mg at bedtime, exceptional circumstances 20 mg; CHILD not recommended

Temazepam (Non-proprietary) CD3
Tablets, temazepam 10 mg, net price 28-tab pack = £19.77; 20 mg, 28-tab pack = £18.99. Label: 19
Dental prescribing on NHS Temazepam Tablets may be prescribed

Oral solution, temazepam 10 mg/5 mL, net price 300 mL = £68.79. Label: 19
Note Sugar-free versions are available and can be ordered by specifying 'sugar-free' on the prescription
Dental prescribing on NHS Temazepam Oral Solution may be prescribed

Zaleplon, zolpidem, and zopiclone

Zaleplon, zolpidem and zopiclone are non-benzodiazepine hypnotics (sometimes referred to as Z-drugs), but they act at the benzodiazepine receptor. They are not licensed for long-term use; dependence has been reported in a small number of patients. Zolpidem and zopiclone have a short duration of action; zaleplon is very short acting.

> **NICE guidance**
> **Zaleplon, zolpidem and zopiclone for the short-term management of insomnia (April 2004)**
> Zaleplon, zolpidem and zopiclone are recommended for the short-term management of severe insomnia that interferes with normal daily life, and should be prescribed for short periods of time only.
> www.nice.org.uk/TA77

▌ ZALEPLON

Indications insomnia (short-term use—up to 2 weeks)
Cautions respiratory insufficiency (avoid if severe); muscle weakness and myasthenia gravis, history of drug or alcohol abuse; depression (risk of suicidal

ideation); avoid prolonged use (risk of tolerance and withdrawal symptoms); **interactions:** Appendix 1 (anxiolytics and hypnotics)
Contra-indications sleep apnoea syndrome, marked neuromuscular respiratory weakness including unstable myasthenia gravis
Hepatic impairment can precipitate coma; reduce dose to 5 mg (avoid if severe impairment)
Renal impairment avoid in severe impairment
Pregnancy use only if necessary and restrict to occasional short-term use; risk of withdrawal symptoms in neonate if used in late pregnancy
Breast-feeding present in milk but amount probably too small to be harmful
Side-effects amnesia, paraesthesia, drowsiness; dysmenorrhea; *less commonly* nausea, anorexia, asthenia, incoordination, confusion, impaired concentration, depression, depersonalisation, dizziness, hallucinations, disturbances of smell, hearing, speech, and vision; photosensitivity; paradoxical effects (see p. 225) and sleep-walking also reported
Dose

- ADULT over 18 years, 10 mg at bedtime or after going to bed if difficulty falling asleep; ELDERLY 5 mg
Note Patients should be advised not to take a second dose during a single night

Sonata® (Meda) CD4-1
Capsules, zaleplon 5 mg (white/light brown), net price 14-cap pack = £3.12; 10 mg (white), 14-cap pack = £3.76. Label: 2

▌ ZOLPIDEM TARTRATE

Indications insomnia (short-term use—up to 4 weeks)
Cautions depression, muscle weakness and myasthenia gravis, history of drug or alcohol abuse; elderly; avoid prolonged use (and abrupt withdrawal thereafter); **interactions:** Appendix 1 (anxiolytics and hypnotics)
Driving Drowsiness may persist the next day—leave at least 8 hours between taking zolpidem and performing skilled tasks (e.g. driving, or operating machinery); effects of alcohol and other CNS depressants enhanced
Contra-indications obstructive sleep apnoea, acute or severe respiratory depression, marked neuromuscular respiratory weakness including unstable myasthenia gravis, psychotic illness
Hepatic impairment can precipitate coma; reduce dose to 5 mg (avoid if severe impairment)
Renal impairment use with caution
Pregnancy avoid regular use (risk of neonatal withdrawal symptoms); high doses during late pregnancy or labour may cause neonatal hypothermia, hypotonia, and respiratory depression
Breast-feeding small amounts present in milk—avoid
Side-effects diarrhoea, nausea, vomiting, dizziness, headache, drowsiness, hallucination, agitation, asthenia, amnesia; dependence, memory disturbances, nightmares, depression, confusion, perceptual disturbances or diplopia, tremor, ataxia, falls, skin reactions, changes in libido; paradoxical effects (see p. 225), muscular weakness, and sleep-walking also reported
Dose

- ADULT over 18 years, 10 mg at bedtime; ELDERLY (or debilitated) 5 mg at bedtime

Zolpidem (Non-proprietary) ⊂CD4-1⊃

Tablets, zolpidem tartrate 5 mg, net price 28-tab pack = £1.73; 10 mg, 28-tab pack = £1.61. Label: 19

Stilnoct® (Sanofi-Aventis) ⊂CD4-1⊃

Tablets, both f/c, zolpidem tartrate 5 mg, net price 28-tab pack = £1.10; 10 mg, 28-tab pack = £1.00. Label: 19

◼ ZOPICLONE

Indications insomnia (short-term use—up to 4 weeks)

Cautions elderly; muscle weakness; myasthenia gravis (avoid if unstable); chronic pulmonary insufficiency; history of drug abuse; psychiatric illness; avoid prolonged use (risk of tolerance and withdrawal symptoms); **interactions:** Appendix 1 (anxiolytics and hypnotics)

> **Driving** Drowsiness may persist the next day and affect performance of skilled tasks (e.g. driving); effects of alcohol enhanced

Contra-indications marked neuromuscular respiratory weakness including unstable myasthenia gravis; respiratory failure; severe sleep apnoea syndrome

Hepatic impairment reduce dose to 3.75 mg in mild to moderate impairment, dose can be increased with caution if necessary; avoid in severe impairment—can precipitate encephalopathy

Renal impairment start with reduced dose of 3.75 mg; increased cerebral sensitivity

Pregnancy not recommended (risk of neonatal withdrawal symptoms); use during late pregnancy or labour may cause neonatal hypothermia, hypotonia, and respiratory depression

Breast-feeding present in milk—avoid

Side-effects taste disturbance; *less commonly* nausea, vomiting, dizziness, drowsiness, dry mouth, headache; *rarely* amnesia, confusion, depression, hallucinations, nightmares; *very rarely* light headedness, incoordination, paradoxical effects (see p. 225) and sleep-walking also reported

Dose

● ADULT over 18 years, 7.5 mg at bedtime; ELDERLY initially 3.75 mg at bedtime increased if necessary

> **Note** In patients with chronic pulmonary insufficiency an initial dose of 3.75 mg is recommended due to an increased risk of respiratory depression

Zopiclone (Non-proprietary) ⊂CD4-1⊃

Tablets, zopiclone 3.75 mg, net price 28-tab pack = £1.50; 7.5 mg, 28-tab pack = £1.43. Label: 19

Zimovane® (Sanofi-Aventis) ⊂CD4-1⊃

Tablets, f/c, zopiclone 3.75 mg (*Zimovane®* LS), net price 28-tab pack = £2.24; 7.5 mg (scored), 28-tab pack = £3.26. Label: 19, 25

Chloral and derivatives

Chloral hydrate and derivatives were formerly popular hypnotics for children (but the use of hypnotics in children is not usually justified). There is no convincing evidence that they are particularly useful in the elderly and their role as hypnotics is now very limited.

◼ CHLORAL HYDRATE ◢

Indications insomnia (short-term use)

Cautions reduce dose in elderly and debilitated; avoid prolonged use (and abrupt withdrawal thereafter);

avoid contact with skin and mucous membranes; **interactions:** Appendix 1 (anxiolytics and hypnotics)

> **Driving** Drowsiness may persist the next day and affect performance of skilled tasks (e.g. driving); effects of alcohol enhanced

Contra-indications severe cardiac disease; gastritis; acute porphyria (section 9.8.2)

Hepatic impairment can precipitate coma; reduce dose in mild to moderate impairment; avoid in severe impairment

Renal impairment avoid in severe impairment

Pregnancy avoid

Breast-feeding risk of sedation in infant—avoid

Side-effects gastric irritation (nausea and vomiting reported), abdominal distention, flatulence, headache, tolerance, dependence, excitement, delirium (especially on abrupt withdrawal), ketonuria, and rash

Dose

● See under preparations below

Chloral Mixture, BP 2000 ᴾᵒᴹ ◢
(Chloral Oral Solution)

Mixture, chloral hydrate 500 mg/5 mL in a suitable vehicle. Label: 19, 27

> **Dose** 5–20 mL; CHILD 1–12 years 30–50 mg/kg (max. 1 g), taken well diluted with water at bedtime
> Available from 'special-order' manufacturers or specialist importing companies, see p. 1124

Chloral Elixir, Paediatric, BP 2000 ᴾᵒᴹ ◢
(Chloral Oral Solution, Paediatric)

Elixir, chloral hydrate 200 mg/5 mL (4%) in a suitable vehicle with a black currant flavour. Label: 1, 27

> **Dose** CHILD 1 month–1 year 30–50 mg/kg, taken well diluted with water at bedtime
> Available from 'special-order' manufacturers or specialist importing companies, see p. 1124

◢**Cloral betaine**

Welldorm® (Marlborough) ᴾᵒᴹ ◢

Tablets, blue-purple, f/c, cloral betaine 707 mg (≡ chloral hydrate 414 mg), net price 30-tab pack = £12.10. Label: 19, 27

> **Dose** ADULT and CHILD over 12 years, 1–2 tablets with water or milk at bedtime, max. 5 tablets (chloral hydrate 2 g) daily

Elixir, red, chloral hydrate 143.3 mg/5 mL, net price 150-mL pack = £8.70. Label: 19, 27

> **Dose** 15–45 mL (chloral hydrate 0.4–1.3 g) with water or milk, at bedtime, max. 70 mL (chloral hydrate 2 g) daily; CHILD 2–12 years, 1–1.75 mL/kg (chloral hydrate 30–50 mg/kg), max. 35 mL (chloral hydrate 1 g) daily

Clomethiazole

Clomethiazole may be a useful hypnotic for elderly patients because of its freedom from hangover but, as with all hypnotics, routine administration is undesirable and dependence occurs. It is also licensed for use in acute alcohol withdrawal, but see section 4.10.1.

◼ CLOMETHIAZOLE
(Chlormethiazole)

Indications see under Dose; alcohol withdrawal (section 4.10.1)

Cautions cardiac and respiratory disease (confusional state may indicate hypoxia), chronic pulmonary insufficiency, sleep apnoea syndrome; history of drug abuse; avoid prolonged use (and abrupt withdrawal thereafter); marked personality disorder; elderly; excessive sedation may occur (particularly with higher doses); **interactions:** Appendix 1 (anxiolytics and hypnotics)

Driving Drowsiness may persist the next day and affect performance of skilled tasks (e.g. driving); effects of alcohol enhanced

Contra-indications acute pulmonary insufficiency; alcohol-dependent patients who continue to drink

Hepatic impairment can precipitate coma; reduce dose

Renal impairment start with small doses in severe impairment; increased cerebral sensitivity

Pregnancy avoid if possible—especially during first and third trimesters

Breast-feeding use only if benefit outweighs risk—present in breast milk but effects unknown

Side-effects nasal congestion and irritation (increased nasopharyngeal and bronchial secretions), conjunctival irritation, headache; *rarely* gastro-intestinal disturbances, paradoxical excitement, confusion, dependence, rash, urticaria, bullous eruption, anaphylaxis, alterations in liver enzymes

Dose
- See preparations below

Clomethiazole (Non-proprietary) PoM

Capsules, clomethiazole base 192 mg in an oily basis, net price 60-cap pack = £15.71. Label: 19

Dose Severe insomnia in the elderly (short-term use), 1–2 capsules at bedtime

Restlessness and agitation in the elderly, 1 capsule 3 times daily

Alcohol withdrawal (but see section 4.10.1), initially 2–4 capsules, if necessary repeated after some hours; day 1 (first 24 hours), 9–12 capsules in 3–4 divided doses; day 2, 6–8 capsules in 3–4 divided doses; day 3, 4–6 capsules in 3–4 divided doses; then gradually reduced over days 4–6; total treatment for not more than 9 days; CHILD not recommended

Oral solution, clomethiazole (as edisilate) 157.5 mg/5 mL, net price 300-mL = £22.00. Label: 19

Excipients include alcohol 0.13%

Dose Severe insomnia in the elderly (short-term use), 5–10 mL at bedtime

Reslessness and agitation in the elderly, 5 mL 3 times daily

Alcohol withdrawal (but see section 4.10.1), initially 10–20 mL, if necessary repeated after some hours; day 1 (first 24 hours), 45–60 mL in 3–4 divided doses; day 2, 30–40 mL in 3–4 divided doses; day 3, 20–30 mL in 3–4 divided doses; then gradually reduced over days 4–6; total treatment for not more than 9 days; CHILD not recommended

Antihistamines

Some **antihistamines** (section 3.4.1) such as promethazine are on sale to the public for occasional insomnia; their prolonged duration of action can often cause drowsiness the following day. The sedative effect of antihistamines may diminish after a few days of continued treatment; antihistamines are associated with headache, psychomotor impairment and antimuscarinic effects.

Promethazine is also popular for use in children, but the use of hypnotics in children is not usually justified.

PROMETHAZINE HYDROCHLORIDE

Indications sedation (short-term use); allergy and urticaria (section 3.4.1); nausea and vomiting (section 4.6)

Cautions see Promethazine Hydrochloride, section 3.4.1

Contra-indications see notes in section 3.4.1

Hepatic impairment see notes in section 3.4.1

Renal impairment see Promethazine Hydrochloride, section 3.4.1

Pregnancy see notes in section 3.4.1

Breast-feeding see notes in section 3.4.1

Side-effects see Promethazine Hydrochloride, section 3.4.1

Dose
- By mouth, 25–50 mg; CHILD 2–5 years 15–20 mg, 5–10 years 20–25 mg
- By deep intramuscular injection, 25–50 mg; CHILD 5–10 years 6.25–12.5 mg

Preparations
Section 3.4.1

Alcohol

Alcohol is a poor hypnotic because the diuretic action interferes with sleep during the latter part of the night. Alcohol also disturbs sleep patterns, and so can worsen sleep disorders; **interactions:** Appendix 1 (alcohol).

Sodium oxybate

Sodium oxybate is a central nervous system depressant that is licensed for the treatment of narcolepsy with cataplexy.

SODIUM OXYBATE

Indications narcolepsy with cataplexy (under specialist supervision)

Cautions history of drug abuse or depression; epilepsy; body mass index of 40 kg/m^2 or greater (higher risk of sleep apnoea); elderly; respiratory disorders; heart failure and hypertension (high sodium content); risk of discontinuation effects including rebound cataplexy and withdrawal symptoms; **interactions:** Appendix 1 (sodium oxybate)

Driving Leave at least 6 hours between taking sodium oxybate and performing skilled tasks (e.g. driving or operating machinery); effects of alcohol and other CNS depressants enhanced

Contra-indications major depression, succinic semialdehyde dehydrogenase deficiency

Hepatic impairment halve initial dose

Renal impairment caution—contains 3.96 mmol Na$^+$/mL

Pregnancy avoid

Breast-feeding no information available

Side-effects nausea, vomiting, diarrhoea, abdominal pain, taste disturbance, anorexia, hypertension, palpitation, peripheral oedema, dyspnoea, sleep disorders (including sleep-walking and sleep paralysis), confusion, disorientation, paraesthesia, hypoaesthesia, impaired attention, depression, drowsiness, anxiety, dizziness, headache, tremor, asthenia, urinary incontinence, nocturnal enuresis, arthralgia, back pain, muscle spasm, blurred vision, nasal congestion, vertigo, sweating, rash; *less commonly* faecal incontinence, myoclonus, psychosis, paranoia, suicidal behaviour, hallucination, agitation, amnesia, restless legs syndrome; *also reported* respiratory depression, dependence, seizures, suicidal ideation, euphoria, sleep apnoea, urticaria

Dose

- ADULT over 18 years, initially 2.25 g on retiring and repeated 2.5–4 hours later, increased according to response in steps of 1.5 g daily in 2 divided doses at intervals of 1–2 weeks; max. 9 g daily in two divided doses

  Note If sodium oxybate and valproate used concomitantly, reduce initial dose of sodium oxybate to 1.8 g on retiring and repeat 2.5–4 hours later

  Note Dose titration should be repeated if restarting after interval of more than 14 days

  Counselling Dilute each dose with 60 mL water; prepare both doses before retiring. Observe the same time interval (2–3 hours) each night between the last meal and the first dose

Xyrem® (UCB Pharma) CD2

Oral solution, sugar-free, sodium oxybate 500 mg/mL, net price 180 mL (with graduated syringe) = £360.00. Label: 13, 19, counselling, administration, driving (see notes above)
Electrolytes Na+ 3.96 mmol/mL

Melatonin

Melatonin is a pineal hormone; it is licensed for the short-term treatment of insomnia in adults over 55 years. For information on the use of melatonin in children and adolescents see *BNF for Children*.

MELATONIN

Indications insomnia (short-term use)

Cautions autoimmune disease (manufacturer advises avoid—no information available); **interactions:** Appendix 1 (melatonin)

Hepatic impairment clearance reduced—avoid

Renal impairment no information available—use with caution

Pregnancy no information available—avoid

Breast-feeding present in milk—avoid

Side-effects *less commonly* abdominal pain, dyspepsia, dry mouth, mouth ulceration, nausea, weight gain, hypertension, chest pain, malaise, dizziness, restlessness, nervousness, irritability, anxiety, headache, abnormal dreams, proteinuria, glycosuria, pruritus, rash, dry skin; *rarely* thirst, flatulence, halitosis, salivation, vomiting, gastritis, hypertriglyceridaemia, angina, palpitation, syncope, hot flushes, aggression, impaired memory, restless legs syndrome, paraesthesia, mood changes, priapism, increased libido, prostatitis, polyuria, haematuria, leucopenia, thrombocytopenia, electrolyte disturbances, muscle spasm, arthritis, lacrimation, visual disturbances, nail disorder; *also reported* galactorrhoea, mouth and tongue oedema

Dose

- ADULT over 55 years, 2 mg once daily 1–2 hours before bedtime for up to 13 weeks; CHILD 1 month–18 years see *BNF for Children*

Circadin® (Flynn) PoM

Tablets, m/r, melatonin 2 mg, net price 30-tab pack = £15.39. Label: 2, 21, 25

4.1.2 Anxiolytics

Benzodiazepine anxiolytics can be effective in alleviating anxiety states. Although these drugs are sometimes prescribed for stress-related symptoms, unhappiness, or minor physical disease, their use in such conditions is inappropriate. Benzodiazepine anxiolytics should not be used as sole treatment for chronic anxiety, and they are not appropriate for treating depression or chronic psychosis. In bereavement, psychological adjustment may be inhibited by benzodiazepines. In children, anxiolytic treatment should be used only to relieve acute anxiety (and related insomnia) caused by fear (e.g. before surgery).

Anxiolytic benzodiazepine treatment should be limited to the lowest possible dose for the shortest possible time (see p. 226). Dependence is particularly likely in patients with a history of alcohol or drug abuse and in patients with marked personality disorders.

Some antidepressants (section 4.3) are licensed for use in anxiety and related disorders; see section 4.3 for a comment on their role in chronic anxiety. Some antipsychotics, in low doses, are also sometimes used in severe anxiety for their sedative action, but long-term use should be avoided because of the risk of adverse effects (section 4.2.1). The use of antihistamines (e.g. hydroxyzine) for their sedative effect in anxiety is not appropriate.

Beta-blockers (section 2.4) do not affect psychological symptoms of anxiety, such as worry, tension, and fear, but they do reduce autonomic symptoms, such as palpitation and tremor; they do not reduce non-autonomic symptoms, such as muscle tension. Beta-blockers are therefore indicated for patients with predominantly somatic symptoms; this, in turn, may prevent the onset of worry and fear.

Benzodiazepines

Benzodiazepines are indicated for the *short-term relief of severe anxiety*; long-term use should be avoided (see p. 226). Diazepam, alprazolam, chlordiazepoxide, and clobazam have a sustained action. Shorter-acting compounds such as **lorazepam** and **oxazepam** may be preferred in patients with hepatic impairment but they carry a greater risk of withdrawal symptoms.

In *panic disorders* (with or without agoraphobia) resistant to antidepressant therapy (section 4.3), a benzodiazepine (lorazepam 3–5 mg daily or clonazepam 1–2 mg daily (section 4.8.1) [both unlicensed]) may be used; alternatively, a benzodiazepine may be used as short-term adjunctive therapy at the start of antidepressant treatment to prevent the initial worsening of symptoms.

Diazepam or lorazepam are very occasionally administered intravenously for the *control of panic attacks*. This route is the most rapid but the procedure is not without risk (section 4.8.2) and should be used only when alternative measures have failed. The intramuscular route has no advantage over the oral route.

For guidelines on benzodiazepine withdrawal, see p. 226.

Hepatic impairment Benzodiazepines can precipitate coma if used in hepatic impairment. If treatment is necessary, benzodiazepines with shorter half lives are safer, such as temazepam or oxazepam. Start with smaller initial doses or reduce dose; avoid in severe impairment.

Renal impairment Patients with renal impairment have increased cerebral sensitivity to benzodiazepines; start with small doses in severe impairment.

Pregnancy There is a risk of neonatal withdrawal symptoms when benzodiazepines are used during pregnancy. Avoid regular use and use only if there is a clear indication such as seizure control. High doses administered during late pregnancy or labour may cause neonatal hypothermia, hypotonia, and respiratory depression.

Breast-feeding Benzodiazepines are present in milk, and should be avoided if possible during breast-feeding.

DIAZEPAM

Indications short-term use in anxiety or insomnia (see p. 226); life-threatening acute drug-induced dystonic reactions (see also section 4.9.2); adjunct in acute alcohol withdrawal; status epilepticus (section 4.8.2); febrile convulsions (section 4.8.3); muscle spasm (section 10.2.2); peri-operative use (section 15.1.4.1)

Cautions respiratory disease; muscle weakness and myasthenia gravis; organic brain changes; history of drug or alcohol dependence; personality disorder (within the fearful group—dependent, avoidant, obsessive-compulsive) may increase risk of dependence; reduce dose in elderly and debilitated; avoid prolonged use (and abrupt withdrawal thereafter); special precautions for intravenous injection (section 4.8.2); when given parenterally, close observation required until full recovery from sedation; **interactions:** Appendix 1 (anxiolytics and hypnotics)
Driving Drowsiness may affect performance of skilled tasks (e.g. driving); effects of alcohol enhanced; see also Drugs and Driving, p. 3

Contra-indications respiratory depression; marked neuromuscular respiratory weakness including unstable myasthenia gravis; acute pulmonary insufficiency; sleep apnoea syndrome; not for chronic psychosis; phobic or obsessional states; hyperkinesis; should not be used alone in depression or in anxiety with depression; avoid injections containing benzyl alcohol in neonates (see under preparations below)

Hepatic impairment see notes above

Renal impairment see notes above

Pregnancy see notes above

Breast-feeding see notes above

Side-effects drowsiness and lightheadedness the next day; confusion and ataxia (especially in the elderly); amnesia; dependence; paradoxical increase in aggression (see also section 4.1); muscle weakness; *occasionally:* headache, vertigo, dizziness, slurred speech, hypotension, salivation changes, gastro-intestinal disturbances, visual disturbances, dysarthria, tremor, changes in libido, gynaecomastia, incontinence, urinary retention; *rarely* apnoea, respiratory depression, blood disorders, jaundice, skin reactions; on intravenous injection, pain, thrombophlebitis; **overdosage:** see Emergency Treatment of Poisoning, p. 39

Dose
- By mouth, anxiety, 2 mg 3 times daily increased if necessary to 15–30 mg daily in divided doses; ELDERLY (or debilitated) half adult dose
  Insomnia associated with anxiety, 5–15 mg at bedtime
- By intramuscular injection *or* slow intravenous injection (into a large vein, at a rate of not more than 5 mg/minute), for severe acute anxiety, control of acute

panic attacks, and acute alcohol withdrawal, 10 mg, repeated if necessary after not less than 4 hours
Note Only use intramuscular route when oral and intravenous routes not possible
- By slow intravenous injection (into a large vein, at a rate of not more than 5 mg/minute), for acute drug-induced dystonic reactions, 5–10 mg repeated as necessary after at least 10 minutes; CHILD 1 month–12 years, 100 micrograms/kg repeated as necessary after at least 10 minutes
- By rectum as rectal solution, acute anxiety and agitation, 500 micrograms/kg repeated after 12 hours as required; ELDERLY 250 micrograms/kg; CHILD not recommended

Note Emulsion formulation preferred for intravenous injection; special precautions for intravenous injection, see section 4.8.2

Diazepam (Non-proprietary) ⒸD4-1
Tablets, diazepam 2 mg, net price 28-tab pack = 96p; 5 mg, 28-tab pack = 98p; 10 mg, 28-tab pack = £1.14. Label: 2 or 19
Brands include *Rimapam*®ᴶᴴˢ, *Tensium*®ᴶᴴˢ
Dental prescribing on NHS Diazepam Tablets may be prescribed

Oral solution, diazepam 2 mg/5 mL, net price 100-mL pack = £19.09. Label: 2 or 19
Brands include *Dialar*®ᴶᴴˢ
Dental prescribing on NHS Diazepam Oral Solution 2 mg/5 mL may be prescribed
Note Sugar-free versions are available and can be ordered by specifying 'sugar-free' on the prescription

Strong oral solution, diazepam 5 mg/5 mL, net price 100-mL pack = £55.00. ᴶᴴˢLabel: 2 or 19
Brands include *Dialar*®ᴶᴴˢ

Injection (solution), diazepam 5 mg/mL, net price 2-mL amp = 45p
Excipients may include benzyl alcohol (avoid in neonates, see Excipients, p. 2), ethanol, propylene glycol
Note Do not dilute (except for intravenous infusion, see Appendix 4)

Injection (emulsion), diazepam 5 mg/mL, net price 2-mL amp = 91p
Brands include *Diazemuls*®
Note For intravenous injection or infusion, see Appendix 4

Rectal tubes (= rectal solution), diazepam 2 mg/mL, net price 1.25-mL (2.5-mg) tube = £1.13, 2.5-mL (5-mg) tube = £1.17; 4 mg/mL, 2.5-mL (10-mg) tube = £1.47. Label: 2 or 19
Brands include *Diazepam Desitin*®, *Diazepam Rectubes*®, *Stesolid*®,

ALPRAZOLAM

Indications short-term use in anxiety (see p. 226)
Cautions see under Diazepam
Contra-indications see under Diazepam
Hepatic impairment see notes above
Renal impairment see notes above
Pregnancy see notes above
Breast-feeding see notes above
Side-effects see under Diazepam
Dose
- 250–500 micrograms 3 times daily (ELDERLY or debilitated 250 micrograms 2–3 times daily), increased if necessary to a total of 3 mg daily; CHILD not recommended

Central nervous system

4

Alprazolam (Non-proprietary) CD4-1 ᴺᴴˢ

Tablets, alprazolam 250 micrograms, net price 60-tab pack = £2.97; 500 micrograms, 60-tab pack = £5.69. Label: 2

Brands include *Xanax*® ᴺᴴˢ

CHLORDIAZEPOXIDE HYDROCHLORIDE

Indications short-term use in anxiety (see p. 226); adjunct in acute alcohol withdrawal (section 4.10.1)

Cautions see under Diazepam

Contra-indications see under Diazepam

Hepatic impairment see notes above

Renal impairment see notes above

Pregnancy see notes above

Breast-feeding see notes above

Side-effects see under Diazepam

Dose

* Anxiety, 10 mg 3 times daily increased if necessary to 60–100 mg daily in divided doses; ELDERLY (or debilitated) half adult dose; CHILD not recommended
* Treatment of alcohol withdrawal in moderate dependence, 10–30 mg 4 times daily (according to local protocol), gradually reduced over 5–7 days
* Treatment of alcohol withdrawal in severe dependence, 10–50 mg 4 times daily (with 10–40 mg as required, if necessary, for the first 2 days; max. total daily dose 250 mg) (according to local protocol), gradually reduced over 7–10 days

Chlordiazepoxide (Non-proprietary) CD4-1

Capsules, chlordiazepoxide hydrochloride 5 mg, net price 100-cap pack = £8.62; 10 mg, 100-cap pack = £15.32. Label: 2

Brands include *Librium*® ᴺᴴˢ

Chlordiazepoxide Hydrochloride (Non-proprietary) CD4-1

Tablets, chlordiazepoxide hydrochloride 5 mg, net price 100 = £20.30; 10 mg, 100 = £25.20. Label: 2

LORAZEPAM

Indications short-term use in anxiety or insomnia (see p. 226); status epilepticus (section 4.8.2); peri-operative (section 15.1.4.1)

Cautions see under Diazepam; short acting; when given parenterally, facilities for managing respiratory depression with mechanical ventilation must be available

Contra-indications see under Diazepam

Hepatic impairment see notes above

Renal impairment see notes above

Pregnancy see notes above

Breast-feeding see notes above

Side-effects see under Diazepam

Dose

* By mouth, anxiety, 1–4 mg daily in divided doses; ELDERLY (or debilitated) half adult dose

  Insomnia associated with anxiety, 1–2 mg at bedtime; CHILD not recommended
* By intramuscular *or* slow intravenous injection (into a large vein), acute panic attacks, 25–30 micrograms/kg (usual range 1.5–2.5 mg), repeated every 6 hours if necessary; CHILD not recommended

  Note Only use intramuscular route when oral and intravenous routes not possible

Lorazepam (Non-proprietary) CD4-1

Tablets, lorazepam 1 mg, net price 28-tab pack = £2.61; 2.5 mg, 28-tab pack = £3.77. Label: 2 or 19

Injection, lorazepam 4 mg/mL, net price 1-mL amp = 35p

Excipients include benzyl alcohol, propylene glycol (see Excipients, p. 2)

Brands include *Ativan*®

Note For intramuscular injection it should be diluted with an equal volume of water for injections or physiological saline (but only use when oral and intravenous routes not possible)

OXAZEPAM

Indications anxiety (short-term use; see p. 226)

Cautions see under Diazepam; short acting

Contra-indications see under Diazepam

Hepatic impairment see notes above

Renal impairment see notes above

Pregnancy see notes above

Breast-feeding see notes above

Side-effects see under Diazepam

Dose

* Anxiety, 15–30 mg (elderly or debilitated 10–20 mg) 3–4 times daily; CHILD not recommended
* Insomnia associated with anxiety, 15–25 mg (max. 50 mg) at bedtime; CHILD not recommended

Oxazepam (Non-proprietary) CD4-1

Tablets, oxazepam 10 mg, net price 28-tab pack = £1.52; 15 mg, 28-tab pack = £1.49. Label: 2

Buspirone

Buspirone is thought to act at specific serotonin ($5HT_{1A}$) receptors. Response to treatment may take up to 2 weeks. It does not alleviate the symptoms of benzodiazepine withdrawal. Therefore a patient taking a benzodiazepine still needs to have the benzodiazepine withdrawn gradually; it is advisable to do this before starting buspirone. The dependence and abuse potential of buspirone is low; it is, however, licensed for short-term use only (but specialists occasionally use it for several months).

BUSPIRONE HYDROCHLORIDE

Indications anxiety (short-term use)

Cautions does not alleviate benzodiazepine withdrawal (see notes above); **interactions:** Appendix 1 (anxiolytics and hypnotics)

Driving May affect performance of skilled tasks (e.g. driving); effects of alcohol may be enhanced

Contra-indications epilepsy; acute porphyria (section 9.8.2)

Hepatic impairment reduce dose in mild to moderate disease; avoid in severe disease

Renal impairment reduce dose; avoid if eGFR less than 20 mL/minute/1.73 m^2

Pregnancy avoid

Breast-feeding avoid

Side-effects nausea; dizziness, headache, nervousness, excitement; *rarely* dry mouth, tachycardia, palpitation, chest pain, drowsiness, confusion, seizures, fatigue, and sweating

Dose

- ADULT over 18 years, 5 mg 2–3 times daily, increased as necessary every 2–3 days; usual range 15–30 mg daily in divided doses; max. 45 mg daily

Buspirone Hydrochloride (Non-proprietary) PoM
Tablets, buspirone hydrochloride 5 mg, net price 30-tab pack = £7.93; 10 mg, 30-tab pack = £9.41. Counselling, driving

Meprobamate

Meprobamate is less effective than the benzodiazepines, more hazardous in overdosage, and can also induce dependence. It is not recommended.

> **Meprobamate**
> The European Medicines Agency has recommended (January 2012) the suspension of all marketing authorisations for meprobamate because the risks, particularly of serious CNS side-effects, outweigh the benefits.

◣ MEPROBAMATE ◢

Indications short-term use in anxiety, but see notes above

Cautions respiratory disease, muscle weakness, epilepsy (may induce seizures), history of drug or alcohol abuse, marked personality disorder; elderly and debilitated; avoid prolonged use, abrupt withdrawal (may precipitate convulsions); **interactions:** Appendix 1 (anxiolytics and hypnotics)
Driving Drowsiness may affect performance of skilled tasks (e.g. driving); effects of alcohol enhanced

Contra-indications acute pulmonary insufficiency; respiratory depression; acute porphyria (section 9.8.2)

Hepatic impairment can precipitate coma

Renal impairment start with small doses in severe impairment; increased cerebral sensitivity

Pregnancy avoid if possible

Breast-feeding avoid; concentration in milk may exceed maternal plasma concentrations fourfold and may cause drowsiness in infant

Side-effects see under Diazepam, but incidence greater and drowsiness most common side-effect; also gastro-intestinal disturbances, hypotension, paraesthesia, weakness, CNS effects including headache, paradoxical excitement, disturbances of vision; rarely agranulocytosis and rashes

Dose

- 400 mg 3–4 times daily; ELDERLY half adult dose or less; CHILD not recommended

Meprobamate (Non-proprietary) CD3 ◢
Tablets, scored, meprobamate 400 mg, net price 84-tab pack = £200.54. Label: 2

4.1.3 Barbiturates

The intermediate-acting **barbiturates** have a place only in the treatment of severe intractable insomnia in patients **already taking** barbiturates; they should be **avoided** in the elderly. Intermediate-acting barbiturate preparations containing amobarbital sodium, butobarbital, and secobarbital sodium are available on a named-patient basis.

The long-acting barbiturate phenobarbital is still sometimes of value in epilepsy (section 4.8.1) but its use as a sedative is unjustified.

The very short-acting barbiturate thiopental is used in anaesthesia (section 15.1.1).

4.2 Drugs used in psychoses and related disorders

4.2.1 Antipsychotic drugs

4.2.2 Antipsychotic depot injections

4.2.3 Drugs used for mania and hypomania

Advice of Royal College of Psychiatrists on doses of antipsychotic drugs above BNF upper limit. Unless otherwise stated, doses in the BNF are licensed doses—any higher dose is therefore **unlicensed** (for an explanation of the significance of this, see p. 2).

1. Consider alternative approaches including adjuvant therapy and newer or second-generation antipsychotic drugs such as clozapine.

2. Bear in mind risk factors, including obesity; particular caution is indicated in older patients, especially those over 70 (see p. 235).

3. Consider potential for drug interactions—see **interactions:** Appendix 1 (antipsychotics).

4. Carry out ECG to exclude untoward abnormalities such as prolonged QT interval; repeat ECG periodically and reduce dose if prolonged QT interval or other adverse cardiac abnormality develops.

5. Increase dose slowly and not more often than once weekly.

6. Carry out regular pulse, blood pressure, and temperature checks; ensure that patient maintains adequate fluid intake.

7. Consider high-dose therapy to be for limited period and review regularly; abandon if no improvement after 3 months (return to standard dosage).

Important When prescribing an antipsychotic for administration on an emergency basis, the intramuscular dose should be **lower** than the corresponding oral dose (owing to absence of first-pass effect), particularly if the patient is very active (increased blood flow to muscle considerably increases the rate of absorption). The prescription should specify the dose for **each route** and should **not** imply that the same dose can be given by mouth or by intramuscular injection. The dose of antipsychotic for emergency use should be reviewed at least **daily**.

4.2.1 Antipsychotic drugs

Antipsychotic drugs are also known as 'neuroleptics' and (misleadingly) as 'major tranquillisers'.

In the short term they are used to calm disturbed patients whatever the underlying psychopathology, which may be schizophrenia, brain damage, mania, toxic delirium, or agitated depression. Antipsychotic drugs are used to alleviate severe anxiety but this too should be a short-term measure.

Schizophrenia The aim of treatment is to alleviate the suffering of the patient (and carer) and to improve social and cognitive functioning. Many patients require life-long treatment with antipsychotic medication. Antipsychotic drugs relieve positive psychotic symptoms such as thought disorder, hallucinations, and delusions, and prevent relapse; they are usually less effective on negative symptoms such as apathy and social withdrawal. In many patients, negative symptoms persist between episodes of treated positive symptoms, but earlier treatment of psychotic illness may protect against the development of negative symptoms over time. Patients with acute schizophrenia generally respond better than those with chronic symptoms.

Long-term treatment of a patient with a definitive diagnosis of schizophrenia is usually required after the first episode of illness in order to prevent relapses. Doses that are effective in acute episodes should generally be continued as prophylaxis.

First-generation antipsychotic drugs The first-generation antipsychotic drugs act predominantly by blocking dopamine D_2 receptors in the brain. First-generation antipsychotic drugs are not selective for any of the four dopamine pathways in the brain and so can cause a range of side-effects, particularly extrapyramidal symptoms and elevated prolactin. The **phenothiazine** derivatives can be divided into 3 main groups:

> *Group 1*: chlorpromazine, levomepromazine, and promazine, generally characterised by pronounced sedative effects and moderate antimuscarinic and extrapyramidal side-effects.
>
> *Group 2*: pericyazine and pipotiazine, generally characterised by moderate sedative effects, but fewer extrapyramidal side-effects than groups 1 or 3.
>
> *Group 3*: fluphenazine, perphenazine, prochlorperazine, and trifluoperazine, generally characterised by fewer sedative and antimuscarinic effects, but more pronounced extrapyramidal side-effects than groups 1 and 2.

Butyrophenones (benperidol and haloperidol) resemble the *group 3* phenothiazines in their clinical properties. **Thioxanthenes** (flupentixol and zuclopentixol) have moderate sedative, antimuscarinic effects, and extrapyramidal effects. **Diphenylbutylpiperidines** (pimozide) and the **substituted benzamides** (sulpiride) have reduced sedative, antimuscarinic, and extrapyramidal effects.

Second-generation antipsychotic drugs The second-generation antipsychotic drugs (sometimes referred to as atypical antipsychotic drugs) act on a range of receptors in comparison to first-generation antipsychotic drugs and have more distinct clinical profiles, particularly with regard to side-effects.

Amisulpride is a selective dopamine receptor antagonist with high affinity for mesolimbic D_2 and D_3 receptors; **aripiprazole** is a dopamine D_2 partial agonist with weak $5\text{-}HT_{1a}$ partial agonism and $5\text{-}HT_{2A}$ receptor antagonism; **clozapine** is a dopamine D_1, dopamine D_2, $5\text{-}HT_{2A}$, alpha$_1$-adrenoceptor, and muscarinic-receptor antagonist; **lurasidone** is a dopamine D_2, $5\text{-}HT_{2A}$, $5\text{-}HT_7$, alpha$_{2A}$- and alpha$_{2C}$- adrenoceptor antagonist, and is a partial agonist at $5\text{-}HT_{1a}$ receptors; **olanzapine** is a dopamine D_1, D_2, D_4, $5\text{-}HT_2$, histamine-1-, and muscarinic-receptor antagonist; **paliperidone** is a metabolite of risperidone; **quetiapine** is a dopamine D_1, dopamine D_2, $5\text{-}HT_2$, alpha$_1$-adrenoceptor, and histamine-1 receptor antagonist; and **risperidone** is a dopamine D_2, $5\text{-}HT_{2A}$, alpha$_1$-adrenoceptor, and histamine-1 receptor antagonist.

Cautions Antipsychotic drugs should be used with **caution** in patients with cardiovascular disease; an ECG may be required (see individual drug monographs), particularly if physical examination identifies cardiovascular risk factors, if there is a personal history of cardiovascular disease, or if the patient is being admitted as an inpatient. Antipsychotic drugs should also be used with caution in Parkinson's disease (may be exacerbated by antipsychotics), epilepsy (and conditions predisposing to seizures), depression, myasthenia gravis, prostatic hypertrophy, or a susceptibility to angle-closure glaucoma. Caution is also required in severe respiratory disease and in patients with a history of jaundice or who have blood dyscrasias (perform blood counts if unexplained infection or fever develops). As photosensitisation may occur with higher dosages, patients should avoid direct sunlight. Patients with schizophrenia should have physical health monitoring (including cardiovascular disease risk assessment) at least once per year. **Interactions:** Appendix 1 (antipsychotics).

Contra-indications Antipsychotic drugs may be **contra-indicated** in comatose states, CNS depression, and phaeochromocytoma.

Prescribing for the elderly

The balance of risks and benefit should be considered before prescribing antipsychotic drugs for elderly patients. In elderly patients with dementia, antipsychotic drugs are associated with a small increased risk of mortality and an increased risk of stroke or transient ischaemic attack. Furthermore, elderly patients are particularly susceptible to postural hypotension and to hyper- and hypothermia in hot or cold weather.

It is recommended that:

- Antipsychotic drugs should not be used in elderly patients to treat mild to moderate psychotic symptoms.
- Initial doses of antipsychotic drugs in elderly patients should be reduced (to half the adult dose or less), taking into account factors such as the patient's weight, co-morbidity, and concomitant medication.
- Treatment should be reviewed regularly.

Driving Drowsiness may affect performance of skilled tasks (e.g. driving or operating machinery), especially at start of treatment; effects of alcohol are enhanced.

Withdrawal There is a high risk of relapse if medication is stopped after 1–2 years. Withdrawal of antipsychotic drugs after long-term therapy should always be gradual and closely monitored to avoid the risk of acute withdrawal syndromes or rapid relapse. Patients should be monitored for 2 years after withdrawal of antipsychotic medication for signs and symptoms of relapse.

Hepatic impairment All antipsychotic drugs can precipitate coma if used in hepatic impairment; phenothiazines are hepatotoxic. See also under individual drugs.

Renal impairment Start with small doses of antipsychotic drugs in severe renal impairment because of increased cerebral sensitivity. See also under individual drugs.

Pregnancy Extrapyramidal effects and withdrawal syndrome have been reported occasionally in the neonate when antipsychotic drugs are taken during the third trimester of pregnancy. Following maternal use of antipsychotic drugs in the third trimester, neonates should

Central nervous system 4

Equivalent doses of oral antipsychotics

These equivalences are intended **only** as an approximate guide; individual dosage instructions should **also** be checked; patients should be carefully monitored after **any** change in medication

Antipsychotic drug	Daily dose
Chlorpromazine	100 mg
Clozapine	50 mg
Haloperidol	2–3 mg
Pimozide	2 mg
Risperidone	0.5–1 mg
Sulpiride	200 mg
Trifluoperazine	5 mg

Important These equivalences must **not** be extrapolated beyond the maximum dose for the drug. Higher doses require careful titration in specialist units and the equivalences shown here may not be appropriate

Dosage
After an initial period of stabilisation, in most patients, the total daily oral dose can be given as a single dose. For the advice of The Royal College of Psychiatrists on doses above the BNF upper limit, see p. 234.

First-generation antipsychotic drugs

BENPERIDOL

Indications   control of deviant antisocial sexual behaviour (but see notes above)

Cautions   see notes above; also manufacturer advises regular blood counts and liver function tests during long-term treatment; risk factors for stroke

Contra-indications   see notes above

Hepatic impairment   see notes above

Renal impairment   see notes above

Pregnancy   see notes above

Breast-feeding   see notes above

Side-effects   see notes above

Dose
- 0.25–1.5 mg daily in divided doses, adjusted according to response; ELDERLY (or debilitated) initially half adult dose; CHILD not recommended

Anquil® (Archimedes) ℗oM
Tablets, scored, benperidol 250 micrograms, net price 112-tab pack = £117.31. Label: 2
Note The proprietary name Benquil® has been used for benperidol tablets

CHLORPROMAZINE HYDROCHLORIDE

Warning Owing to the risk of contact sensitisation, pharmacists, nurses, and other health workers should avoid direct contact with chlorpromazine; tablets should not be crushed and solutions should be handled with care

Indications   see under Dose; antiemetic in palliative care (section 4.6)

Cautions   see notes above; also diabetes; patients should remain supine, with blood pressure monitoring for 30 minutes after intramuscular injection; dose

adjustment may be necessary if smoking started or stopped during treatment

Contra-indications   see notes above; hypothyroidism

Hepatic impairment   see notes above

Renal impairment   see notes above

Pregnancy   see notes above

Breast-feeding   see notes above

Side-effects   see notes above; also hyperglycaemia

Dose
- By mouth, schizophrenia and other psychoses, mania, short-term adjunctive management of severe anxiety, psychomotor agitation, excitement, and violent or dangerously impulsive behaviour, initially 25 mg 3 times daily (or 75 mg at night), adjusted according to response, to usual maintenance dose of 75–300 mg daily (but up to 1 g daily may be required in psychoses); ELDERLY (or debilitated) third to half adult dose; CHILD under 18 years see BNF for Children

  Intractable hiccup, 25–50 mg 3–4 times daily
- By deep intramuscular injection, (for relief of acute symptoms but see also Cautions and Side-effects), 25–50 mg every 6–8 hours; CHILD under 18 years see BNF for Children
- By rectum in suppositories as chlorpromazine base 100 mg every 6–8 hours [unlicensed]
  Note For equivalent therapeutic effect 100 mg chlorpromazine base given rectally as a suppository ≡ 20–25 mg chlorpromazine hydrochloride by intramuscular injection ≡ 40–50 mg of chlorpromazine base or hydrochloride by mouth

Chlorpromazine (Non-proprietary) ℗oM
Tablets, chlorpromazine hydrochloride 25 mg, net price 28-tab pack = £2.50; 50 mg, 28-tab pack = £2.32; 100 mg, 28-tab pack = £2.63. Label: 2, 11
Brands include Chloractil®

Oral solution, chlorpromazine hydrochloride 25 mg/ 5 mL, net price 150 mL = £2.35; 100 mg/5 mL, 150 mL = £5.50. Label: 2, 11

Injection, chlorpromazine hydrochloride 25 mg/mL, net price 1-mL amp = 60p, 2-mL amp = 63p

Suppositories, chlorpromazine 25 mg and 100 mg. Label: 2, 11
Available from 'special-order' manufacturers or specialist importing companies, see p. 1124

Largactil® (Sanofi-Aventis) ℗oM
Injection, chlorpromazine hydrochloride 25 mg/mL, net price 2-mL amp = 75p

FLUPENTIXOL
(Flupenthixol)

Indications   schizophrenia and other psychoses, particularly with apathy and withdrawal but not mania or psychomotor hyperactivity; depression (section 4.3.4)

Cautions   see notes above; diabetes; avoid in acute porphyria (section 9.8.2)

Contra-indications   see notes above; also excitable and overactive patients

Hepatic impairment   see notes above

Renal impairment   see notes above

Pregnancy   see notes above

Breast-feeding   see notes above

Side-effects   see notes above; less sedating but extrapyramidal symptoms frequent; hyperglycaemia

Dose
- Psychosis, initially 3–9 mg twice daily adjusted according to the response; max. 18 mg daily; ELDERLY

(or debilitated) initially quarter to half adult dose; CHILD not recommended

Depixol® (Lundbeck) [PoM]
Tablets, yellow, s/c, flupentixol 3 mg (as dihydrochloride), net price 100 = £13.92. Label: 2

Fluanxol® (Lundbeck) [PoM]
Section 4.3.4 (depression)

◀**Depot preparation**
Section 4.2.2

▊ HALOPERIDOL

Indications   see under Dose; motor tics (section 4.9.3)

Cautions   see notes above; also subarachnoid haemorrhage; metabolic disturbances such as hypokalaemia, hypocalcaemia, or hypomagnesaemia; thyrotoxicosis; arteriosclerosis; dose adjustment may be necessary if smoking started or stopped during treatment; baseline ECG required before treatment—assess need for further ECGs during treatment on an individual basis

Contra-indications   see notes above; QT-interval prolongation (avoid concomitant administration of drugs that prolong QT interval); bradycardia; lesions of the basal ganglia; Parkinson's disease

Hepatic impairment   see notes above

Renal impairment   see notes above

Pregnancy   avoid unless benefits outweigh risks; see also notes above

Breast-feeding   see notes above

Side-effects   see notes above, but less sedating and fewer antimuscarinic or hypotensive symptoms; pigmentation and photosensitivity reactions rare; depression; weight loss; *less commonly* dyspnoea, oedema; *rarely* bronchospasm, hypoglycaemia, and inappropriate antidiuretic hormone secretion; hypertension, sweating, Stevens-Johnson syndrome, and toxic epidermal necrolysis also reported

Dose
* Schizophrenia, psychoses, mania and hypomania, organic brain damage (depending on symptoms), ADULT over 18 years, by mouth, *initially* 2–20 mg daily as a single dose or in divided doses, *maintenance* 1–3 mg three times daily adjusted according to response (max. 20 mg daily in divided doses); ELDERLY (or debilitated) initially half adult dose; CHILD under 18 years see *BNF for Children*
  By intramuscular injection, ADULT over 18 years, initially 2–5 mg, repeated according to response and tolerability to max. 12 mg daily; ELDERLY (or debilitated) initially half adult dose
  Note BNF doses differ from those in product literature
* Agitation and restlessness in the elderly, by mouth, initially 0.75–1.5 mg 2–3 times daily adjusted according to response if necessary
* Management of mental or behavioural problems such as aggression, hyperactivity and self-mutilation in the mentally retarded and in patients with organic brain damage (depending on symptoms), Gilles de la Tourette syndrome, severe tics, intractable hiccup, as an adjunct to short-term management of moderate to severe psychomotor agitation, excitement, and violent or dangerously impulsive behaviour, by mouth, ADULT over 18 years, *initially* 1.5–3 mg 2–3 times daily (3–5 mg 2–3 times daily in severely affected or resis-

tant patients), *maintenance* 0.5–1 mg three times daily (increased to 2–3 mg three times daily if necessary); once symptoms controlled, gradually reduce dose to the lowest effective maintenance dose; ELDERLY (or debilitated) initially half adult dose; CHILD under 18 years see *BNF for Children*
* Nausea and vomiting, see Prescribing in Palliative Care, p. 22
  By intramuscular injection, 1–2 mg

Haloperidol (Non-proprietary) [PoM]
Tablets, haloperidol 500 micrograms, net price 28-tab pack = 91p; 1.5 mg, 28-tab pack = £2.50; 5 mg, 28-tab pack = £3.26; 10 mg, 28-tab pack = £10.95; 20 mg, 28-tab pack = £20.75. Label: 2
Oral liquid, haloperidol 5 mg/5 mL, net price 100-mL pack = £6.41; 10 mg/5 mL, 100-mL pack = £7.10. Label: 2
Injection, haloperidol 5 mg/mL, net price 1-mL amp = 36p
Important When prescribing, dispensing, or administering, check that this injection is the correct preparation—this preparation is usually used in hospital for the rapid control of an *acute episode* and should **not** be confused with depot preparations which are usually used in the community or clinics for *maintenance* treatment

Dozic® (Rosemont) [PoM]
Oral liquid, sugar-free, haloperidol 5 mg/5 mL, net price 100-mL pack = £6.30. Label: 2

Haldol® (Janssen) [PoM]
Oral liquid, sugar-free, haloperidol 10 mg/5 mL, net price 100-mL pack (with pipette) = £4.45. Label: 2

Serenace® (TEVA UK) [PoM]
Capsules, green, haloperidol 500 micrograms, net price 30-cap pack = £1.18. Label: 2

◀**Depot preparation**
Section 4.2.2

▊ LEVOMEPROMAZINE
(Methotrimeprazine)

Indications   see under Dose

Cautions   see notes above; diabetes; patients receiving large initial doses should remain supine
Elderly Risk of postural hypotension; not recommended for ambulant patients over 50 years unless risk of hypotensive reaction assessed

Contra-indications   see notes above

Hepatic impairment   see notes above

Renal impairment   see notes above

Pregnancy   see notes above

Breast-feeding   see notes above

Side-effects   see notes above; occasionally raised erythrocyte sedimentation rate occurs; hyperglycaemia also reported

Dose
* Schizophrenia, by mouth initially 25–50 mg daily in divided doses increased as necessary; bedpatients initially 100–200 mg daily usually in 3 divided doses, increased if necessary to 1 g daily; ELDERLY, see Cautions
* Pain in palliative care, see p. 23
* Restlessness and confusion in palliative care, see p. 23; CHILD 1–18 years see *BNF for Children*
* Nausea and vomiting in palliative care, by mouth, see p. 22, or by subcutaneous infusion, see p. 23; CHILD 1 month–18 years see *BNF for Children*

Nozinan® (Sanofi-Aventis) [PoM]

Tablets, scored, levomepromazine maleate 25 mg, net price 84-tab pack = £20.26. Label: 2

Injection, levomepromazine hydrochloride 25 mg/mL, net price 1-mL amp = £2.01

PERICYAZINE

(Periciazine)

Indications see under Dose

Cautions see notes above

Contra-indications see notes above

Hepatic impairment see notes above

Renal impairment see notes above; avoid in renal impairment

Pregnancy see notes above

Breast-feeding see notes above

Side-effects see notes above; more sedating; hypotension common when treatment initiated; respiratory depression

Dose

* Schizophrenia and other psychoses, initially 75 mg daily in divided doses increased at weekly intervals by steps of 25 mg according to response; usual max. 300 mg daily (elderly initially 15–30 mg daily); CHILD and INFANT over 1 year (schizophrenia or behavioural disorders only), initially, 500 micrograms daily for 10-kg child, increased by 1 mg for each additional 5 kg body-weight to max. total daily dose of 10 mg; dose may be gradually increased according to response but maintenance should not exceed twice initial dose

* Short-term adjunctive management of severe anxiety, psychomotor agitation, and violent or dangerously impulsive behaviour, initially 15–30 mg (elderly 5–10 mg) daily divided into 2 doses, taking the larger dose at bedtime, adjusted according to response; CHILD not recommended

Pericyazine (Non-proprietary) [PoM]

Tablets, pericyazine 2.5 mg, net price 84-tab pack = £15.50; 10 mg, 84-tab pack = £40.00. Label: 2

Syrup, pericyazine 10 mg/5 mL, net price 100-mL pack = £46.27. Label: 2

PERPHENAZINE

Indications see under Dose; antiemetic (section 4.6)

Cautions see notes above; hypothyroidism

Contra-indications see notes above; also agitation and restlessness in the elderly

Hepatic impairment see notes above

Renal impairment see notes above

Pregnancy see notes above

Breast-feeding see notes above

Side-effects see notes above; less sedating; extrapyramidal symptoms, especially dystonia, more frequent, particularly at high dosage; rarely systemic lupus erythematosus

Dose

* Schizophrenia and other psychoses, mania, short-term adjunctive management of anxiety, severe psychomotor agitation, excitement, and violent or dangerously impulsive behaviour, initially 4 mg 3 times daily adjusted according to the response; max. 24 mg daily; ELDERLY quarter to half adult dose (but see Cautions); CHILD under 14 years not recommended

Fentazin® (AMCo) [PoM]

Tablets, s/c, perphenazine 2 mg, net price 100 = £29.09; 4 mg, 100 = £34.25. Label: 2

PIMOZIDE

Indications see under Dose

Cautions see notes above

ECG monitoring Following reports of sudden unexplained death, an ECG is recommended before treatment. It is also recommended that patients taking pimozide should have an annual ECG (if the QT interval is prolonged, treatment should be reviewed and either withdrawn or dose reduced under close supervision) and that pimozide should **not** be given with other antipsychotic drugs (including depot preparations), tricyclic antidepressants or other drugs which prolong the QT interval, such as certain antimalarials, anti-arrhythmic drugs and certain antihistamines and should **not** be given with drugs which cause electrolyte disturbances (especially diuretics)

Contra-indications see notes above; history or family history of congenital QT prolongation; history of arrhythmias

Hepatic impairment see notes above

Renal impairment see notes above

Pregnancy see notes above

Breast-feeding see notes above

Side-effects see notes above; less sedating; serious arrhythmias reported; glycosuria and, rarely, hyponatraemia reported

Dose

* Schizophrenia, ADULT and CHILD over 12 years, initially 2 mg daily, increased according to response in steps of 2–4 mg at intervals of not less than 1 week; usual dose range 2–20 mg daily; ELDERLY half usual starting dose

* Monosymptomatic hypochondriacal psychosis, paranoid psychosis, ADULT and CHILD over 12 years, initially 4 mg daily, increased according to response in steps of 2–4 mg at intervals of not less than 1 week; max. 16 mg daily; ELDERLY half usual starting dose

Orap® (Janssen) [PoM]

Tablets, scored, green, pimozide 4 mg, net price 100 = £40.31. Label: 2

PROCHLORPERAZINE

Indications see under Dose; antiemetic (section 4.6)

Cautions see notes above; also hypotension more likely after intramuscular injection

Contra-indications see notes above; children, but see section 4.6 for use as antiemetic

Hepatic impairment see notes above

Renal impairment see notes above

Pregnancy see notes above

Breast-feeding see notes above

Side-effects see notes above; less sedating; extrapyramidal symptoms, particularly dystonias, more frequent; respiratory depression may occur in susceptible patients

Dose

* By mouth, schizophrenia and other psychoses, mania, prochlorperazine maleate or mesilate, 12.5 mg twice daily for 7 days adjusted at intervals of 4–7 days to usual dose of 75–100 mg daily according to response; CHILD not recommended

Short-term adjunctive management of severe anxiety, 15–20 mg daily in divided doses; max. 40 mg daily; CHILD not recommended

Central nervous system

4

- By deep intramuscular injection, psychoses, mania, prochlorperazine mesilate 12.5–25 mg 2–3 times daily; CHILD not recommended

◢Preparations

Section 4.6

PROMAZINE HYDROCHLORIDE

Indications see under Dose

Cautions see notes above; also cerebral arterio-sclerosis

Contra-indications see notes above

Hepatic impairment see notes above

Renal impairment see notes above

Pregnancy see notes above

Breast-feeding see notes above

Side-effects see notes above; also haemolytic anaemia

Dose

- Short-term adjunctive management of psychomotor agitation, 100–200 mg 4 times daily; CHILD not recommended
- Agitation and restlessness in elderly, 25–50 mg 4 times daily

Promazine (Non-proprietary) (PoM)

Tablets, promazine hydrochloride 25 mg, net price 100 = £37.53; 50 mg, 100 = £72.67. Label: 2

Oral solution, promazine hydrochloride 25 mg/5 mL, net price 150 mL = £11.87; 50 mg/5 mL, 150 mL = £13.93. Label: 2

SULPIRIDE

Indications schizophrenia

Cautions see notes above; also excited, agitated, or aggressive patients (even low doses may aggravate symptoms)

Contra-indications see notes above

Hepatic impairment see notes above

Renal impairment see notes above

Pregnancy see notes above

Breast-feeding see notes above

Side-effects see notes above; also hepatitis

Dose

- ADULT and CHILD over 14 years, 200–400 mg twice daily; max. 800 mg daily in predominantly negative symptoms, and 2.4 g daily in mainly positive symptoms; ELDERLY, lower initial dose, increased gradually according to response

Sulpiride (Non-proprietary) (PoM)

Tablets, sulpiride 200 mg, net price 30-tab pack = £5.15, 56-tab pack = £6.46; 400 mg, 30-tab pack = £18.80. Label: 2

Dolmatil® (Sanofi-Aventis) (PoM)

Tablets, both scored, sulpiride 200 mg, net price 100-tab pack = £6.00; 400 mg (f/c), 100-tab pack = £19.00. Label: 2

Sulpor® (Rosemont) (PoM)

Oral solution, sugar-free, lemon- and aniseed-flavoured, sulpiride 200 mg/5 mL, net price 150 mL = £25.38. Label: 2

TRIFLUOPERAZINE

Indications see under Dose; antiemetic (section 4.6)

Cautions see notes above

Contra-indications see notes above

Hepatic impairment see notes above

Renal impairment see notes above

Pregnancy see notes above

Breast-feeding see notes above

Side-effects see notes above; extrapyramidal symptoms more frequent, especially at doses exceeding 6 mg daily; anorexia; muscle weakness

Dose

- Schizophrenia and other psychoses, short-term adjunctive management of psychomotor agitation, excitement, and violent or dangerously impulsive behaviour, ADULT and CHILD over 12 years, initially 5 mg twice daily, increased by 5 mg daily after 1 week, then at intervals of 3 days, according to the response; ELDERLY reduce initial dose by at least half
- Short-term adjunctive management of severe anxiety, ADULT and CHILD over 12 years, 2–4 mg daily in divided doses, increased if necessary to 6 mg daily; CHILD 3–5 years up to 1 mg daily, 6–12 years up to 4 mg daily; ELDERLY reduce initial dose by at least half

Trifluoperazine (Non-proprietary) (PoM)

Tablets, trifluoperazine (as hydrochloride) 1 mg, net price 112-tab pack = £54.00; 5 mg, 112-tab pack = £77.00. Label: 2

Oral solution, trifluoperazine (as hydrochloride) 1 mg/5 mL, net price 200-mL = £32.86; 5 mg/5 mL, 150-mL = £25.50 Label: 2

Stelazine® (AMCo) (PoM)

Tablets, both blue, f/c, trifluoperazine (as hydrochloride) 1 mg, net price 112 = £4.11; 5 mg, 112 = £5.87. Label: 2

ZUCLOPENTHIXOL

Indications schizophrenia and other psychoses

Cautions see notes above; avoid in acute porphyria (section 9.8.2)

Contra-indications see notes above; apathetic or withdrawn states

Hepatic impairment see notes above; halve dose and consider serum-level monitoring

Renal impairment see notes above; halve dose in renal failure

Pregnancy see notes above

Breast-feeding see notes above

Side-effects see notes above; urinary frequency or incontinence; weight loss (less common than weight gain)

Dose

- By mouth, initially 20–30 mg daily in divided doses, increasing to a max. of 150 mg daily if necessary; usual maintenance dose 20–50 mg daily; max. single dose 40 mg; ELDERLY (or debilitated) initially quarter to half adult dose; CHILD not recommended

Clopixol® (Lundbeck) (PoM)

Tablets, f/c, zuclopenthixol (as dihydrochloride) 2 mg (red), net price 100 = £3.14; 10 mg (light red-brown), 100 = £8.06; 25 mg (red-brown), 100 = £16.13. Label: 2

◢Depot preparation

Section 4.2.2

ZUCLOPENTHIXOL ACETATE

Indications short-term management of acute psychosis, mania, or exacerbations of chronic psychosis

4

Central nervous system

Cautions see notes above; avoid in acute porphyria (section 9.8.2)

Contra-indications see notes above

Hepatic impairment see notes above

Renal impairment see notes above

Pregnancy see notes above

Breast-feeding see notes above

Side-effects see notes above

Dose

● By deep intramuscular injection into the gluteal muscle or lateral thigh, 50–150 mg (ELDERLY 50–100 mg), repeated if necessary after 2–3 days (1 additional dose may be needed 1–2 days after the first injection); max. cumulative dose 400 mg in 2 weeks and max. 4 injections; max. duration of treatment 2 weeks—if maintenance treatment necessary change to an oral antipsychotic 2–3 days after last injection, or to a longer acting antipsychotic depot injection given concomitantly with last injection of zuclopenthixol acetate; CHILD not recommended

Clopixol Acuphase® (Lundbeck) PoM

Injection (oily), zuclopenthixol acetate 50 mg/mL, net price 1-mL amp = £4.84

Important When prescribing, dispensing, or administering, check that this is the correct preparation—this preparation is usually used in hospital for an *acute episode* and should **not** be confused with depot preparations which are usually used in the community or clinics for *maintenance* treatment

◢**Depot preparation**
Section 4.2.2

Second-generation antipsychotic drugs

◤ AMISULPRIDE

Indications schizophrenia

Cautions see notes above

Contra-indications see notes above; also prolactin-dependent tumours; pre-pubertal children

Renal impairment halve dose if eGFR 30–60 mL/minute/1.73 m^2; use one-third dose if eGFR 10–30 mL/minute/1.73 m^2; no information available if eGFR less than 10 mL/minute/1.73 m^2

Pregnancy avoid

Breast-feeding avoid—no information available

Side-effects see notes above; also anxiety; *less commonly* bradycardia

Dose

● Acute psychotic episode, 400–800 mg daily in 2 divided doses, adjusted according to response; max. 1.2 g daily; CHILD under 18 years not recommended

● Predominantly negative symptoms, 50–300 mg daily; CHILD under 18 years not recommended

Amisulpride (Non-proprietary) PoM

Tablets, amisulpride 50 mg, net price 60-tab pack = £3.60; 100 mg, 60-tab pack = £6.18; 200 mg, 60-tab pack = £10.58; 400 mg, 60-tab pack = £37.32. Label: 2

Solian® (Sanofi-Aventis) PoM

Tablets, amisulpride 50 mg, net price 60-tab pack = £22.76; 100 mg, 60-tab pack = £35.29; 200 mg, 60-tab pack = £58.99; 400 mg, 60-tab pack = £117.97. Label: 2

Solution, 100 mg/mL, net price 60 mL (caramel flavour) = £33.76. Label: 2

◤ ARIPIPRAZOLE

Indications see under Dose

Cautions see notes above; cerebrovascular disease; elderly (reduce initial dose)

Contra-indications see notes above

Hepatic impairment use with caution in severe impairment

Pregnancy see, p. 235; also use only if potential benefit outweighs risk

Breast-feeding manufacturer advises avoid—present in milk

Side-effects see notes above; hypersalivation, anxiety, drowsiness, malaise; *less commonly* depression, dry mouth; *also reported* anorexia, oropharyngeal spasm, laryngospasm, respiratory disorders (including infection), hepatitis, pancreatitis, bradycardia, pathological gambling, suicidal ideation, hyponatraemia, urinary disorders, myalgia, rhabdomyolysis, oedema, sweating, alopecia

Dose

● Schizophrenia, by mouth, ADULT over 18 years, 10–15 mg once daily, usual maintenance 15 mg once daily; max. 30 mg once daily; for dose adjustments due to concomitant use of interacting drugs, consult product literature; CHILD under 18 years see *BNF for Children*

● Treatment and recurrence prevention of mania, by mouth, ADULT over 18 years, 15 mg once daily, increased if necessary; max. 30 mg once daily; for dose adjustments due to concomitant use of interacting drugs, consult product literature; CHILD under 18 years see *BNF for Children*

● Control of agitation and disturbed behaviour in schizophrenia, by intramuscular injection, ADULT over 18 years, initially 5.25–15 mg (usual dose 9.75 mg) as a single dose followed by 5.25–15 mg after 2 hours if necessary; max. 3 injections daily; max. daily combined oral and parenteral dose 30 mg; for dose adjustments due to concomitant use of interacting drugs, consult product literature

Abilify® (Otsuka) PoM

Tablets, aripiprazole 5 mg (blue), net price 28-tab pack = £96.04; 10 mg (pink), 28-tab pack = £96.04; 15 mg (yellow), 28-tab pack = £96.04; 30 mg (pink), 28-tab pack = £192.08. Label: 2

Orodispersible tablets, aripiprazole 10 mg (pink), net price 28-tab pack = £96.04; 15 mg (yellow), 28-tab pack = £96.04. Label: 2, counselling, administration

Excipients include aspartame (section 9.4.1)

Counselling Tablets should be placed on the tongue and allowed to dissolve, or be dispersed in water and swallowed

Oral solution, aripiprazole 1 mg/mL, net price 150 mL with measuring cup = £102.90. Label: 2

Injection, aripiprazole 7.5 mg/mL, net price 1.3-mL (9.75-mg) vial = £3.43

Important When prescribing, dispensing, or administering, check that this injection is the correct preparation—this preparation is usually used in hospital for the rapid control of an *acute episode* and should **not** be confused with depot preparations which are usually used in the community or clinics for *maintenance* treatment

◢**Depot preparation**
section 4.2.2

◤ CLOZAPINE

Indications schizophrenia (including psychosis in Parkinson's disease) in patients unresponsive to, or intolerant of, conventional antipsychotic drugs

Cautions see notes above; adult over 60 years; monitor leucocyte and differential blood counts (see Agranulocytosis, below); prostatic hypertrophy, susceptibility to angle-closure glaucoma; taper off other antipsychotics before starting; close medical supervision during initiation (risk of collapse because of hypotension and convulsions); dose adjustment may be necessary if smoking started or stopped during treatment

Withdrawal On planned withdrawal reduce dose over 1–2 weeks to avoid risk of rebound psychosis. If abrupt withdrawal necessary observe patient carefully

Agranulocytosis Neutropenia and potentially fatal agranulocytosis reported. Leucocyte and differential blood counts must be normal before starting; monitor counts every week for 18 weeks then at least every 2 weeks and if clozapine continued and blood count stable after 1 year at least every 4 weeks (and 4 weeks after discontinuation); if leucocyte count below 3000/mm³ or if absolute neutrophil count below 1500/mm³ discontinue permanently and refer to haematologist. Patients who have a low white blood cell count because of benign ethnic neutropenia may be started on clozapine with the agreement of a haematologist. Avoid drugs which depress leucopoiesis; patients should report immediately symptoms of infection, especially influenza-like illness

Myocarditis and cardiomyopathy Fatal myocarditis (most commonly in first 2 months) and cardiomyopathy reported.

- Perform physical examination and take full medical history before starting
- Specialist examination required if cardiac abnormalities or history of heart disease found—clozapine initiated only in absence of severe heart disease and if benefit outweighs risk
- Persistent tachycardia especially in first 2 months should prompt observation for other indicators for myocarditis or cardiomyopathy
- If myocarditis or cardiomyopathy suspected clozapine should be stopped and patient evaluated urgently by cardiologist
- Discontinue permanently in clozapine-induced myocarditis or cardiomyopathy

Intestinal obstruction Impairment of intestinal peristalsis, including constipation, intestinal obstruction, faecal impaction, and paralytic ileus, (including fatal cases) reported. Clozapine should be used with caution in patients receiving drugs that may cause constipation (e.g. antimuscarinic drugs) or in those with a history of colonic disease or lower abdominal surgery. It is essential that constipation is recognised and actively treated

Contra-indications severe cardiac disorders (e.g. myocarditis; see Cautions); history of neutropenia or agranulocytosis (see Cautions); bone-marrow disorders; paralytic ileus (see Cautions); alcoholic and toxic psychoses; history of circulatory collapse; drug intoxication; coma or severe CNS depression; uncontrolled epilepsy

Hepatic impairment monitor hepatic function regularly; avoid in symptomatic or progressive liver disease or hepatic failure

Renal impairment avoid in severe impairment

Pregnancy see, p. 235; also use with caution

Breast-feeding avoid

Side-effects see notes above; also constipation (see Cautions), hypersalivation, anorexia, speech disorders, malaise, urinary incontinence; *less commonly* agranulocytosis (**important**: see Cautions); *rarely* dysphagia, hepatitis, pancreatitis, circulatory collapse, myocarditis (**important**: see Cautions), pericarditis, pulmonary aspiration, pneumonia; *very rarely* parotid gland enlargement, intestinal obstruction (including fatal cases, see Cautions), cardiomyopathy (**important**: see Cautions), myocardial infarction, respiratory depression, obsessive compulsive disorder, interstitial nephritis, hypertriglyceridaemia, hypercholesterolaemia; *also reported* hepatic disorders and failure, renal failure, muscle disorders

Dose

- Schizophrenia, ADULT over 18 years, 12.5 mg once or twice (ADULT over 60 years, 12.5 mg once) on first day then 25–50 mg (ADULT over 60 years, 25–37.5 mg) on second day then increased gradually (if well tolerated) in steps of 25–50 mg daily (ADULT over 60 years, max. increment 25 mg daily) over 14–21 days up to 300 mg daily in divided doses (larger dose at night, up to 200 mg daily may be taken as a single dose at bedtime); if necessary may be further increased in steps of 50–100 mg once (preferably) or twice weekly; usual dose 200–450 mg daily (max. 900 mg daily); CHILD 12–18 years see *BNF for Children*

  Note *Restarting* after *interval of more than 48 hours*, 12.5 mg once or twice on first day (but may be feasible to increase more quickly than on initiation)—extreme caution if previous respiratory or cardiac arrest with initial dosing

- Psychosis in Parkinson's disease, ADULT over 16 years, 12.5 mg at bedtime then increased according to response in steps of 12.5 mg up to twice weekly; usual dose range 25–37.5 mg at bedtime, usual max. 50 mg daily; exceptionally, dose may be increased further in steps of 12.5 mg weekly to max. 100 mg daily in 1–2 divided doses

Clozaril® (Novartis) PoM
Tablets, yellow, clozapine 25 mg (scored), net price 28-tab pack = £3.78, 84-tab pack (hosp. only) = £11.33, 100-tab pack (hosp. only) = £13.48; 100 mg, 28-tab pack = £15.09, 84-tab pack (hosp. only) = £45.28, 100-tab pack (hosp. only) = £53.90. Label: 2, 10, patient information leaflet
Note Patient, prescriber, and supplying pharmacist must be registered with the Clozaril Patient Monitoring Service—takes several days to do this

Denzapine® (Genus) PoM
Tablets, yellow, scored, clozapine 25 mg, net price 84-tab pack = £16.64, 100-tab pack = £19.80; 50 mg, 50-tab pack = £19.80; 100 mg, 84-tab pack = £66.53, 100-tab pack = £79.20; 200 mg, 50-tab pack = £79.20. Label: 2, 10, patient information leaflet
Suspension, clozapine 50 mg/mL, net price 100 mL = £39.60. Label: 2, 10, patient information leaflet, counselling, administration
Counselling Shake well for 90 seconds when dispensing or if visibly settled and stand for 24 hours before use; otherwise shake well for 10 seconds before use
Note May be diluted with water
Note Patient, prescriber, and supplying pharmacist must be registered with the Denzapine Patient Monitoring Service—takes several days to do this

Zaponex® (TEVA UK) PoM
Tablets, yellow, scored, clozapine 25 mg, net price 84-tab pack = £8.28; 100 mg, 84-tab pack = £33.88. Label: 2, 10, patient information leaflet
Note Patient, prescriber, and supplying pharmacist must be registered with the Zaponex Treatment Access System—takes several days to do this

LURASIDONE HYDROCHLORIDE

Indications schizophrenia

Cautions see notes above; also susceptibility to QT-interval prolongation (including concomitant use of drugs that prolong the QT interval); high doses in elderly

Contra-indications concomitant use of potent CYP3A4 inhibitors or inducers

4 Central nervous system

Central nervous system

4

Hepatic impairment initially 18.5 mg once daily, up to max. 74 mg once daily in moderate impairment; use with caution in severe impairment—initially 18.5 mg once daily, up to max. 37 mg once daily

Renal impairment initially 18.5 mg once daily, up to max. 74 mg once daily if eGFR less than 50 mL/minute/1.73m^2; manufacturer advises use only if potential benefit outweighs risk if eGFR less than 15 mL/minute/1.73m^2

Pregnancy use only if potential benefit outweighs risk—limited information available

Breast-feeding see p. 236

Side-effects see notes above; also anxiety, musculoskeletal stiffness; *less commonly* decreased appetite, hot flush, nightmares, catatonia, dysarthria, dysuria, myalgia; *also reported* dysphagia, angina, bradycardia, AV block, suicidal behaviour, panic attacks, vertigo, pruritus

Dose
• ADULT over 18 years, initially 37 mg once daily, increased if necessary to max. 148 mg once daily
Note Initially 18.5 mg once daily, up to max. 74 mg once daily with concomitant moderate CYP3A4 inhibitors (e.g. diltiazem, erythromycin, fluconazole, and verapamil)
Note Patients on doses higher than 111 mg once daily whose treatment is interrupted for longer than 3 days should restart on 111 mg once daily and titrate to usual dose; for all other doses, restart on usual dose

Latuda® (Sunovion) ▼ [PoM]
Tablets, f/c, lurasidone hydrochloride 18.5 mg, net price 28-tab pack = £90.72; 37 mg, 28-tab pack = £90.72; 74 mg, 28-tab pack = £90.72. Label: 2, 21, 25

◀ OLANZAPINE

Indications see under Dose

Cautions see notes above; also paralytic ileus, diabetes mellitus (risk of exacerbation or ketoacidosis), low leucocyte or neutrophil count, bone-marrow depression, hypereosinophilic disorders, myeloproliferative disease; dose adjustment may be necessary if smoking started or stopped during treatment
CNS and respiratory depression Blood pressure, pulse and respiratory rate should be monitored for at least 4 hours after intramuscular injection, particularly in those also receiving a benzodiazepine or another antipsychotic (leave at least one hour between administration of olanzapine intramuscular injection and parenteral benzodiazepines)

Contra-indications *for injection*, acute myocardial infarction, unstable angina, severe hypotension or bradycardia, sick sinus syndrome, recent heart surgery

Hepatic impairment consider initial dose of 5 mg daily

Renal impairment consider initial dose of 5 mg daily

Pregnancy see, p. 235; also use only if potential benefit outweighs risk; neonatal lethargy, tremor, and hypertonia reported when used in third trimester

Breast-feeding avoid—present in milk

Side-effects see notes above; also increased appetite, hypertriglyceridaemia, hypercholesterolaemia, bradycardia, arthralgia, oedema, malaise; *less commonly* epistaxis, amnesia, alopecia; *rarely* hepatitis, pancreatitis, rhabdomyolysis; *with injection*, sinus pause, hypoventilation

Dose
• Schizophrenia, combination therapy for mania, preventing recurrence in bipolar disorder, by mouth, ADULT over 18 years, 10 mg daily adjusted to usual range of 5–20 mg daily; doses greater than 10 mg daily only after reassessment; max. 20 mg daily; CHILD 12–18 years see *BNF for Children*

• Monotherapy for mania, by mouth, ADULT over 18 years, 15 mg daily adjusted to usual range of 5–20 mg daily; doses greater than 15 mg only after reassessment; max. 20 mg daily; CHILD 12–18 years see *BNF for Children*

• Control of agitation and disturbed behaviour in schizophrenia or mania, by intramuscular injection, ADULT over 18 years, initially 5–10 mg (usual dose 10 mg) as a single dose followed by 5–10 mg after 2 hours if necessary; ELDERLY initially 2.5–5 mg as a single dose followed by 2.5–5 mg after 2 hours if necessary; max. 3 injections daily for 3 days; max. daily combined oral and parenteral dose 20 mg
Important When prescribing, dispensing, or administering, check that this injection is the correct preparation—this preparation is usually used in hospital for the rapid control of an *acute episode* and should **not** be confused with depot preparations which are usually used in the community or clinics for *maintenance* treatment
Note When one or more factors present that might result in slower metabolism (e.g. female gender, elderly, non-smoker) consider lower initial dose and more gradual dose increase

Olanzapine (Non-proprietary) [PoM]
Tablets, olanzapine 2.5 mg, net price 28-tab pack = £1.04; 5 mg, 28-tab pack = £1.23; 7.5 mg, 56-tab pack = £2.70; 10 mg, 28-tab pack = £1.56; 15 mg, 28-tab pack = £1.97; 20 mg, 28-tab pack = £2.23. Label: 2
Brands include *Zalasta*®
Orodispersible tablets, olanzapine 5 mg, net price 28-tab pack = £2.73; 10 mg, 28-tab pack =£3.43; 15 mg, 28-tab pack = £4.04; 20 mg, 28-tab pack = £5.36. Label: 2, counselling, administration
Counselling Olanzapine orodispersible tablet may be placed on the tongue and allowed to dissolve, or dispersed in water, orange juice, apple juice, milk, or coffee

Zyprexa® (Lilly) [PoM]
Tablets, f/c, olanzapine 2.5 mg, net price 28-tab pack = £21.85; 5 mg, 28-tab pack = £43.70; 7.5 mg, 56-tab pack = £131.10; 10 mg, 28-tab pack = £87.40, 15 mg (blue), 28-tab pack = £119.18; 20 mg (pink), 28-tab pack = £158.90. Label: 2
Orodispersible tablet (*Velotab*®), yellow, olanzapine 5 mg, net price 28-tab pack = £48.07; 10 mg, 28-tab pack = £87.40; 15 mg, 28-tab pack = £131.10; 20 mg, 28-tab pack = £174.79. Label: 2, counselling, administration
Excipients include aspartame (section 9.4.1)
Counselling *Velotab*® may be placed on the tongue and allowed to dissolve, or dispersed in water, orange juice, apple juice, milk, or coffee

Injection, olanzapine, available from 'special-order' manufacturers or specialist importing companies
Important When prescribing, dispensing, or administering, check that this injection is the correct preparation—this preparation is usually used in hospital for the rapid control of an *acute episode* and should **not** be confused with depot preparations which are usually used in the community or clinics for *maintenance* treatment

◀ **Depot preparation**
Section 4.2.2

◀ PALIPERIDONE

Note Paliperidone is a metabolite of risperidone

Indications schizophrenia; psychotic or manic symptoms of schizoaffective disorder

Cautions see notes above; predisposition to gastro-intestinal obstruction; elderly patients with dementia and risk factors for stroke; prolactin-dependent tumours; cataract surgery (risk of intraoperative floppy iris syndrome)

Hepatic impairment caution in severe impairment—no information available

Renal impairment initially 3 mg once daily if eGFR 50–80 mL/minute/1.73 m² (max. 6 mg once daily); initially 1.5 mg once daily if eGFR 10–50 mL/minute/1.73 m² (max. 3 mg once daily); avoid if eGFR less than 10 mL/minute/1.73 m²

Pregnancy see, p. 235; also use only if potential benefit outweighs risk—toxicity in animal studies; if discontinuation during pregnancy is necessary, withdraw gradually

Breast-feeding avoid—present in milk

Side-effects see notes above; also hypertension, respiratory disorders (including infection), epistaxis, appetite changes, sleep disorders, anxiety, depression, malaise, urinary disorders, arthralgia, myalgia, toothache, oedema; *less commonly* hypoaesthesia, paraesthesia, taste disturbances, elevated plasma-triglyceride and -cholesterol concentrations, visual disorders, tinnitus, alopecia; *rarely* intestinal obstruction, pancreatitis, pulmonary embolism, inappropriate antidiuretic hormone secretion, rhabdomyolysis, intra-operative floppy iris syndrome

Dose
- ADULT over 18 years, 6 mg once daily in the morning, adjusted if necessary in increments of 3 mg over at least 5 days; usual range 3–12 mg daily

Counselling Always take with breakfast or always take on an empty stomach

Invega® (Janssen) PoM
Tablets, m/r, paliperidone 3 mg (white), net price 28-tab pack = £97.28; 6 mg (beige), 28-tab pack = £97.28; 9 mg (pink), 28-tab pack = £145.92. Label: 2, 25, counselling, administration

◢**Depot preparation**
Section 4.2.2

▌ **QUETIAPINE**

Indications schizophrenia; mania, either alone or with mood stabilisers; depression in bipolar disorder; adjunctive treatment in major depressive disorder

Cautions see notes above; also cerebrovascular disease; patients at risk of aspiration pneumonia; treatment of depression in patients under 25 years (increased risk of suicide); elderly, see Prescribing for the Elderly, p. 235

Hepatic impairment for *immediate-release tablets*, initially 25 mg daily, increased daily in steps of 25–50 mg; for *modified-release tablets*, initially 50 mg daily, increased daily in steps of 50 mg

Pregnancy see, p. 235; also use only if potential benefit outweighs risk

Breast-feeding manufacturer advises avoid

Side-effects see notes above; also dyspnoea, elevated plasma-triglyceride and -cholesterol concentrations, peripheral oedema, increased appetite, sleep disorders, irritability, dysarthria, asthenia; *less commonly* rhinitis, restless legs syndrome, hyponatraemia, hypothyroidism; *rarely* pancreatitis, hepatitis; *very*

rarely inappropriate secretion of antidiuretic hormone, rhabdomyolysis, angioedema, Stevens-Johnson syndrome; *also reported* suicidal behaviour (particularly on initiation), toxic epidermal necrolysis

Dose
- Schizophrenia, ADULT over 18 years, 25 mg twice daily on day 1, 50 mg twice daily on day 2, 100 mg twice daily on day 3, 150 mg twice daily on day 4, then adjusted according to response, usual range 300–450 mg daily in 2 divided doses; max. 750 mg daily; CHILD 12–18 years see *BNF for Children*
- Treatment of mania in bipolar disorder, ADULT over 18 years, 50 mg twice daily on day 1, 100 mg twice daily on day 2, 150 mg twice daily on day 3, 200 mg twice daily on day 4, then adjusted according to response in steps of up to 200 mg daily to max. 800 mg daily; usual range 400–800 mg daily in 2 divided doses; CHILD 12–18 years see *BNF for Children*
- Treatment of depression in bipolar disorder, ADULT over 18 years, 50 mg once daily (at bedtime) on day 1, 100 mg once daily on day 2, 200 mg once daily on day 3, 300 mg once daily on day 4; adjust according to response, usual dose 300 mg once daily, max. 600 mg daily
- Prevention of mania and depression in bipolar disorder, ADULT over 18 years, continue at the dose effective for treatment of bipolar disorder and adjust to lowest effective dose; usual range 300–800 mg in 2 divided doses

Note The rate of dose titration may need to be slower and the daily dose lower in elderly patients, see Prescribing for the Elderly, p. 235

Quetiapine (Non-proprietary) PoM
Tablets, quetiapine (as fumarate) 25 mg, net price 60-tab pack = £1.53; 100 mg, 60-tab pack = £2.49; 150 mg, 60-tab pack = £2.69; 200 mg 60-tab pack = £3.19; 300 mg, 60-tab pack = £4.40. Label: 2

Seroquel® (AstraZeneca) PoM
Tablets, f/c, quetiapine (as fumarate) 25 mg (peach), net price 60-tab pack = £40.50; 100 mg (yellow), 60-tab pack = £113.10; 150 mg (pale yellow), 60-tab pack = £113.10; 200 mg (white), 60-tab pack = £113.10; 300 mg (white), 60-tab pack = £170.00. Label: 2

◢**Modified release**

Quetiapine m/r preparations PoM
Tablets, m/r, quetiapine (as fumarate) 50 mg, net price 60-tab pack = £67.66; 150 mg 60-tab pack = £113.10; 200 mg, 60-tab pack = £113.10; 300 mg, 60-tab pack = £170.00; 400 mg, 60-tab pack = £226.20. Label: 2, 23, 25
Brands include *Seroquel® XL, Tenprolide® XL*
Dose schizophrenia, ADULT over 18 years, 300 mg once daily on day 1, then 600 mg once daily on day 2; adjust according to response, usual dose 600 mg once daily; max. 800 mg once daily under specialist supervision; ELDERLY initially 50 mg once daily adjusted according to response in steps of 50 mg daily

Treatment of mania in bipolar disorder, ADULT over 18 years, 300 mg once daily on day 1, then 600 mg once daily on day 2, then adjusted according to response; dose range 400–800 mg once daily; ELDERLY initially 50 mg once daily adjusted according to response in steps of 50 mg daily

Treatment of depression in bipolar disorder, ADULT over 18 years, 50 mg once daily (at bedtime) on day 1, 100 mg once daily on day 2, 200 mg once daily on day 3, 300 mg once daily on day 4; adjust according to response, usual dose 300 mg once daily, max. 600 mg once daily

Prevention of mania and depression in bipolar disorder, ADULT over 18 years, continue at the dose effective for

4

Central nervous system

Central nervous system 4

treatment of bipolar disorder and adjust to lowest effective dose; usual range 300–800 mg once daily

Adjunctive treatment of major depression, ADULT over 18 years, 50 mg once daily at bedtime for 2 days, then 150 mg once daily for 2 days, then adjusted according to response, usual range 150–300 mg once daily; ELDERLY, initially 50 mg once daily for 3 days, then increase if necessary to 100 mg once daily for 4 days; thereafter adjusted in steps of 50 mg according to response, usual range 50–300 mg once daily (dose of 300 mg should not be reached before day 22 of treatment)

▌ RISPERIDONE

Indications acute and chronic psychoses, mania; short-term treatment (up to 6 weeks) of persistent aggression in patients with moderate to severe Alzheimer's dementia unresponsive to non-pharmacological interventions and when there is a risk of harm to self or others; short-term treatment (up to 6 weeks) of persistent aggression in conduct disorder (under specialist supervision)

Cautions see notes above; dementia with Lewy bodies; prolactin-dependent tumours, dehydration; cataract surgery (risk of intra-operative floppy iris syndrome); avoid in acute porphyria (section 9.8.2)

Hepatic impairment initial and subsequent oral doses should be halved

Renal impairment initial and subsequent oral doses should be halved

Pregnancy see Pregnancy notes, p. 235; also use only if potential benefit outweighs risk

Breast-feeding use only if potential benefit outweighs risk—small amount present in milk

Side-effects see notes above; also hypertension, respiratory disorders (including infection), epistaxis, appetite changes, sleep disorders, anxiety, depression, malaise, urinary disorders, arthralgia, myalgia, toothache, oedema; *less commonly* hypoaesthesia, paraesthesia, taste disturbances, elevated plasma-triglyceride and -cholesterol concentrations, visual disorders, tinnitus, alopecia; *rarely* intestinal obstruction, pancreatitis, pulmonary embolism, inappropriate antidiuretic hormone secretion, rhabdomyolysis, intra-operative floppy iris syndrome

Dose

• Psychosis, 2 mg in 1–2 divided doses on first day *then* 4 mg in 1–2 divided doses on second day (slower titration appropriate in some patients); usual dose range 4–6 mg daily; doses above 10 mg daily only if benefit considered to outweigh risk (max. 16 mg daily); ELDERLY initially 500 micrograms twice daily increased in steps of 500 micrograms twice daily to 1–2 mg twice daily; CHILD 12–18 years see *BNF for Children*

• Mania, initially 2 mg once daily, increased if necessary in steps of 1 mg daily; usual dose range 1–6 mg daily; ELDERLY initially 500 micrograms twice daily increased in steps of 500 micrograms twice daily to 1–2 mg twice daily; CHILD 12–18 years see *BNF for Children*

• Persistent aggression in Alzheimer's dementia, initially 250 micrograms twice daily, increased according to response in steps of 250 micrograms twice daily on alternate days; usual dose 500 micrograms twice daily (up to 1 mg twice daily has been required)

• Persistent aggression in conduct disorder, CHILD 5–18 years see *BNF for Children*

Risperidone (Non-proprietary) PoM
Tablets, risperidone 500 micrograms, net price 20-tab pack = £1.09; 1 mg, 20-tab pack = £1.01, 60-tab pack = £1.66; 2 mg, 60-tab pack = £1.78; 3 mg, 60-tab pack = £2.11; 4 mg, 60-tab pack = £2.40; 6 mg, 28-tab pack = £5.19. Label: 2

Orodispersible tablets, risperidone 500 micrograms, net price 28-tab pack = £23.68; 1 mg, 28-tab pack = £20.92; 2 mg, 28-tab pack = £38.39; 3 mg, 28-tab pack = £33.50; 4 mg, 28-tab pack = £37.94. Label: 2, counselling, administration
Counselling Tablets should be placed on the tongue, allowed to dissolve and swallowed

Liquid, risperidone 1 mg/mL, net price 100-mL pack = £37.48. Label: 2, counselling, use of dose syringe
Note Liquid may be diluted with any non-alcoholic drink, except tea

Risperdal® (Janssen) PoM
Tablets, f/c, scored, risperidone 500 micrograms (brown-red), net price 20-tab pack = £5.08; 1 mg (white), 20-tab pack = £8.36, 60-tab pack = £17.56; 2 mg (orange), 60-tab pack = £34.62; 3 mg (yellow), 60-tab pack = £50.91; 4 mg (green), 60-tab pack = £67.20; 6 mg (yellow), 28-tab pack = £67.88. Label: 2

Orodispersible tablets (*Quicklet®*), pink, risperidone 500 micrograms, net price 28-tab pack = £8.23, 1 mg, 28-tab pack = £13.86; 2 mg, 28-tab pack = £26.12; 3 mg, 28-tab pack = £28.99; 4 mg, 28-tab pack = £37.34. Label: 2, counselling, administration
Excipients include aspartame (section 9.4.1)
Counselling Tablets should be placed on the tongue, allowed to dissolve and swallowed

Liquid, risperidone 1 mg/mL, net price 100 mL = £37.01. Label: 2, counselling, use of dose syringe
Note Liquid may be diluted with any non-alcoholic drink, except tea

◀**Depot preparation**
Section 4.2.2

▌ 4.2.2 Antipsychotic depot injections

Long-acting depot injections are used for maintenance therapy especially when compliance with oral treatment is unreliable. However, depot injections of conventional antipsychotics may give rise to a higher incidence of extrapyramidal reactions than oral preparations; extrapyramidal reactions occur less frequently with second-generation antipsychotic depot preparations, such as risperidone and olanzapine embonate.

Administration Depot antipsychotics are administered by deep intramuscular injection at intervals of 1 to 4 weeks. When initiating therapy with sustained-release preparations of conventional antipsychotics, patients should first be given a small test-dose as undesirable side-effects are prolonged. In general not more than 2–3 mL of oily injection should be administered at any one site; correct injection technique (including the use of z-track technique) and rotation of injection sites are essential. If the dose needs to be reduced to alleviate side-effects, it is important to recognise that the plasma-drug concentration may not fall for some time after reducing the dose, therefore it may be a month or longer before side-effects subside.

Dosage

Individual responses to neuroleptic drugs are very variable and to achieve optimum effect, dosage and dosage interval must be titrated according to the patient's response. For the advice of The Royal College of Psychiatrists on doses above the BNF upper limit, see p. 234.

Equivalent doses of depot antipsychotics

These equivalences are intended **only** as an approximate guide; individual dosage instructions should **also** be checked; patients should be carefully monitored after **any** change in medication

Antipsychotic drug	Dose (mg)	Interval
Flupentixol decanoate	40	2 weeks
Fluphenazine decanoate	25	2 weeks
Haloperidol (as decanoate)	100	4 weeks
Pipotiazine palmitate	50	4 weeks
Zuclopenthixol decanoate	200	2 weeks

Important These equivalences must **not** be extrapolated beyond the maximum dose for the drug

Choice There is no clear-cut division in the use of the conventional antipsychotics, but **zuclopenthixol** may be suitable for the treatment of agitated or aggressive patients whereas **flupentixol** can cause over-excitement in such patients. Zuclopenthixol decanoate may be more effective in preventing relapses than other conventional antipsychotic depot preparations. The incidence of extrapyramidal reactions is similar for the conventional antipsychotics.

Cautions See section 4.2.1. Treatment requires careful monitoring for optimum effect. When transferring from oral to depot therapy, the dose by mouth should be reduced gradually.

Contra-indications See section 4.2.1. Do not use in children.

Side-effects See section 4.2.1. Pain may occur at injection site and occasionally erythema, swelling, and nodules. For side-effects of specific antipsychotics see under the relevant drug.

ARIPIPRAZOLE

Indications maintenance in schizophrenia in patients stabilised with oral aripiprazole

Cautions see section 4.2.1; cerebrovascular disease; elderly

Contra-indications see section 4.2.1

Hepatic impairment oral treatment preferred in severe impairment; see Aripiprazole (section 4.2.1)

Pregnancy see Aripiprazole (section 4.2.1)

Breast-feeding see Aripiprazole (section 4.2.1)

Side-effects see Aripiprazole (section 4.2.1) and notes above

Dose

• By intramuscular injection into the gluteal muscle, 400 mg repeated at monthly intervals (minimum 26 days between injections); for dose adjustment due to side-effects or concomitant use of interacting drugs,

consult product literature; CHILD under 18 years not recommended

Note Treatment with 10–20 mg of oral aripiprazole should be continued for 14 consecutive days after the first injection; for missed depot doses see product literature

Abilify Maintena® (Otsuka) PoM
Injection, powder for reconstitution, aripiprazole 400-mg vial (with solvent), net price = £220.41
Important When prescribing, dispensing or administering, check that this is the correct preparation—this preparation is used for *maintenance* treatment and should not be used for the rapid control of an *acute episode*

■ FLUPENTIXOL DECANOATE
(Flupenthixol Decanoate)

Indications maintenance in schizophrenia and other psychoses

Cautions see Flupentixol (section 4.2.1) and notes above; an alternative antipsychotic may be necessary if symptoms such as aggression or agitation appear

Contra-indications see Flupentixol (section 4.2.1) and notes above

Hepatic impairment see section 4.2.1

Renal impairment see section 4.2.1

Pregnancy see section 4.2.1

Breast-feeding see section 4.2.1

Side-effects see Flupentixol (section 4.2.1) and notes above, but may have a mood elevating effect

Dose

• By deep intramuscular injection into the upper outer buttock or lateral thigh, test dose 20 mg, then after at least 7 days 20–40 mg repeated at intervals of 2–4 weeks, adjusted according to response; max. 400 mg weekly; usual maintenance dose 50 mg every 4 weeks to 300 mg every 2 weeks; ELDERLY initially quarter to half adult dose; CHILD not recommended

Depixol® (Lundbeck) PoM
Injection (oily), flupentixol decanoate 20 mg/mL, net price 1-mL amp = £1.52; 2-mL amp = £2.54

Depixol Conc.® (Lundbeck) PoM
Injection (oily), flupentixol decanoate 100 mg/mL, net price 1-mL amp = £6.25

Depixol Low Volume® (Lundbeck) PoM
Injection (oily), flupentixol decanoate 200 mg/mL, net price 1-mL amp = £19.52

■ FLUPHENAZINE DECANOATE

Indications maintenance in schizophrenia and other psychoses

Cautions see section 4.2.1 and notes above; dose adjustment may be necessary if smoking started or stopped during treatment; QT-interval prolongation (avoid concomitant drugs that prolong QT interval)

Contra-indications see section 4.2.1 and notes above; also marked cerebral atherosclerosis

Hepatic impairment see section 4.2.1; avoid in hepatic failure

Renal impairment see section 4.2.1; manufacturer advises caution; avoid in renal failure

Pregnancy see section 4.2.1

Breast-feeding see section 4.2.1

Side-effects see section 4.2.1 and notes above; less sedating and fewer antimuscarinic or hypotensive symptoms, but extrapyramidal symptoms, particularly dystonic reactions and akathisia, more frequent;

4 Central nervous system

systemic lupus erythematosus, inappropriate anti-diuretic hormone secretion, and oedema also reported; extrapyramidal symptoms usually appear a few hours after injection and continue for about 2 days but may be delayed

Dose

- By deep intramuscular injection into the gluteal muscle, test dose 12.5 mg (6.25 mg in elderly), then after 4–7 days 12.5–100 mg repeated at intervals of 14–35 days, adjusted according to response; CHILD not recommended

Fluphenazine decanoate (Non-proprietary) [PoM]
Injection (oily), fluphenazine decanoate 25 mg/mL, net price 1-mL amp = £2.26; 100 mg/mL, 0.5-mL amp = £4.50, 1-mL amp = £8.75
Excipients include sesame oil

Modecate® (Sanofi-Aventis) [PoM]
Injection (oily), fluphenazine decanoate 25 mg/mL, net price 0.5-mL amp = £1.30, 1-mL amp = £2.26, 2-mL amp = £4.44
Excipients include sesame oil

Modecate Concentrate® (Sanofi-Aventis) [PoM]
Injection (oily), fluphenazine decanoate 100 mg/mL, net price 0.5-mL amp = £4.47, 1-mL amp = £8.75
Excipients include sesame oil

HALOPERIDOL

Indications maintenance in schizophrenia and other psychoses

Cautions see Haloperidol (section 4.2.1) and notes above

Contra-indications see Haloperidol (section 4.2.1) and notes above

Hepatic impairment see section 4.2.1

Renal impairment see section 4.2.1

Pregnancy avoid unless benefits outweigh risks; see also section 4.2.1

Breast-feeding see section 4.2.1

Side-effects see Haloperidol (section 4.2.1) and notes above

Dose

- By deep intramuscular injection into the gluteal muscle, initially 50 mg every 4 weeks, if necessary increasing by 50-mg increments to 300 mg every 4 weeks; higher doses may be needed in some patients; ELDERLY, initially 12.5–25 mg every 4 weeks; CHILD not recommended
  Note If 2-weekly administration preferred, doses should be halved

Haldol Decanoate® (Janssen) [PoM]
Injection (oily), haloperidol (as decanoate) 50 mg/mL, net price 1-mL amp = £3.81; 100 mg/mL, 1-mL amp = £5.05
Excipients include sesame oil and benzyl alcohol (see Excipients)
Important When prescribing, dispensing or administering, check that this is the correct preparation—this preparation is used for *maintenance* treatment and should **not** be used for the rapid control of an *acute episode*

OLANZAPINE EMBONATE
(Olanzapine Pamoate)

Indications maintenance in schizophrenia in patients tolerant to olanzapine by mouth

Cautions see under Olanzapine (section 4.2.1) and notes above; observe patient for at least 3 hours after injection

Contra-indications see under Olanzapine (section 4.2.1) and notes above

Hepatic impairment initially 150 mg every 4 weeks; increase with caution in moderate impairment

Renal impairment initially 150 mg every 4 weeks

Pregnancy see under Olanzapine (section 4.2.1)

Breast-feeding see under Olanzapine (section 4.2.1)

Side-effects see under Olanzapine (section 4.2.1) and notes above; post-injection reactions have been reported leading to signs and symptoms of overdose

Dose

- By deep intramuscular injection into the gluteal muscle, ADULT 18–75 years, *patients taking oral olanzapine 10 mg daily*, initially 210 mg every 2 weeks *or* 405 mg every 4 weeks, then maintenance dose after 2 months treatment, 150 mg every 2 weeks *or* 300 mg every 4 weeks; *patients taking oral olanzapine 15 mg daily*, initially 300 mg every 2 weeks, then maintenance dose after 2 months treatment, 210 mg every 2 weeks *or* 405 mg every 4 weeks; *patients taking oral olanzapine 20 mg daily*, initially 300 mg every 2 weeks, then maintenance dose after 2 months treatment 300 mg every 2 weeks; dose adjusted according to response; max. 300 mg every 2 weeks
  Note If supplementation with oral olanzapine required, consult product literature

ZypAdhera® (Lilly) ▼ [PoM]
Injection, powder for reconstitution, olanzapine embonate 210-mg vial, net price = £142.76, 300-mg vial = £222.64, 405-mg vial = £285.52 (all with diluent)
Important When prescribing, dispensing or administering, check that this is the correct preparation—this preparation is used for *maintenance* treatment and should **not** be used for the rapid control of an *acute episode*

PALIPERIDONE

Indications maintenance in schizophrenia in patients previously responsive to paliperidone or risperidone

Cautions see Paliperidone (section 4.2.1) and notes above

Hepatic impairment see Paliperidone (section 4.2.1)

Renal impairment initial dose 100 mg on day 1 and then 75 mg on day 8 if eGFR 50–80 mL/minute/1.73 m^2; recommended maintenance dose 50 mg (range 25–100 mg) monthly if eGFR 50–80 mL/minute/1.73 m^2; avoid if eGFR less than 50 mL/minute/1.73 m^2

Pregnancy see Paliperidone (section 4.2.1)

Breast-feeding see Paliperidone (section 4.2.1)

Side-effects see Paliperidone (section 4.2.1) and notes above

Dose

- By deep intramuscular injection into the deltoid muscle, 150 mg on day 1, then 100 mg on day 8, adjusted at monthly intervals according to response; recommended maintenance dose 75 mg (range 25–150 mg) monthly
  Note Following the second dose, monthly maintenance doses can be administered into either the deltoid or gluteal muscle; for missed doses see product literature; 25 mg prefilled syringe not available in the UK

Xeplion® (Janssen) ▼ PoM

Injection, paliperidone (as palmitate), net price 50 mg prefilled syringe = £183.92; 75 mg prefilled syringe = £244.90; 100 mg prefilled syringe = £314.07; 150 mg prefilled syringe = £392.59

▐ PIPOTIAZINE PALMITATE
(Pipothiazine Palmitate)

Indications   maintenance in schizophrenia and other psychoses

Cautions   see section 4.2.1 and notes above; also thyrotoxicosis; hypothyroidism

Contra-indications   see section 4.2.1 and notes above

Hepatic impairment   see section 4.2.1

Renal impairment   see section 4.2.1

Pregnancy   see section 4.2.1

Breast-feeding   avoid unless essential

Side-effects   see section 4.2.1 and notes above

Dose

- By deep intramuscular injection into the gluteal muscle, test dose 25 mg, then a further 25–50 mg after 4–7 days, then adjusted according to response at intervals of 4 weeks; usual maintenance range 50–100 mg (max. 200 mg) every 4 weeks; ELDERLY initially 5–10 mg; CHILD not recommended

Piportil Depot® (Sanofi-Aventis) PoM

Injection (oily), pipotiazine palmitate 50 mg/mL, net price 1-mL amp = £16.29; 2-mL amp = £26.65
Excipients   include sesame oil

▐ RISPERIDONE

Indications   schizophrenia and other psychoses in patients tolerant to risperidone by mouth

Cautions   see Risperidone (section 4.2.1) and notes above

Hepatic impairment   if an oral dose of at least 2 mg daily tolerated, 25 mg as a depot injection can be given every 2 weeks

Renal impairment   see Risperidone (section 4.2.1)

Pregnancy   see Risperidone (section 4.2.1)

Breast-feeding   see Risperidone (section 4.2.1)

Side-effects   see Risperidone (section 4.2.1) and notes above

Dose

- By deep intramuscular injection into the deltoid or gluteal muscle, patients taking oral risperidone up to 4 mg daily, initially 25 mg every 2 weeks; patients taking oral risperidone over 4 mg daily, initially 37.5 mg every 2 weeks; dose adjusted at intervals of at least 4 weeks in steps of 12.5 mg to max. 50 mg every 2 weeks; CHILD under 18 years not recommended

Note   During initiation risperidone by mouth may need to be continued for 4–6 weeks; risperidone by mouth may also be used during dose adjustment of depot injection

Risperdal Consta® (Janssen) PoM

Injection, powder for reconstitution, risperidone 25-mg vial, net price = £79.69; 37.5-mg vial = £111.32; 50-mg vial = £142.76 (all with diluent)

▐ ZUCLOPENTHIXOL DECANOATE

Indications   maintenance in schizophrenia and paranoid psychoses

Cautions   see section 4.2.1 and notes above; QT-interval prolongation (avoid concomitant use of drugs that prolong QT interval); avoid in acute porphyria (section 9.8.2)

Contra-indications   see section 4.2.1

Hepatic impairment   see section 4.2.1

Renal impairment   see section 4.2.1

Pregnancy   see section 4.2.1

Breast-feeding   see section 4.2.1

Side-effects   see section 4.2.1 and notes above

Dose

- By deep intramuscular injection into the upper outer buttock or lateral thigh, test dose 100 mg, followed after at least 7 days by 200–500 mg or more, repeated at intervals of 1–4 weeks, adjusted according to response; max. 600 mg weekly; ELDERLY quarter to half usual starting dose; CHILD not recommended

Clopixol® (Lundbeck) PoM

Injection (oily), zuclopenthixol decanoate 200 mg/mL, net price 1-mL amp = £3.15
Important   When prescribing, dispensing, or administering, check that this is the correct preparation—this preparation is used for *maintenance* treatment and should **not** be used for the short-term management of an *acute episode*

Clopixol Conc.® (Lundbeck) PoM

Injection (oily), zuclopenthixol decanoate 500 mg/mL, net price 1-mL amp = £7.44
Important   When prescribing, dispensing, or administering, check that this is the correct preparation—this preparation is used for *maintenance* treatment and should **not** be used for the short-term management of an *acute episode*

▐ 4.2.3   Drugs used for mania and hypomania

Antimanic drugs are used to control acute attacks and to prevent recurrence of episodes of mania or hypomania. Long-term treatment of bipolar disorder should continue for at least two years from the last manic episode and up to five years if the patient has risk factors for relapse.

An antidepressant drug (section 4.3) may also be required for the treatment of co-existing depression, but should be avoided in patients with rapid-cycling bipolar disorder, a recent history of hypomania, or with rapid mood fluctuations.

Benzodiazepines

Use of benzodiazepines (such as lorazepam) (section 4.1) may be helpful in the initial stages of treatment for behavioural disturbance or agitation; they should not be used for long periods because of the risk of dependence.

Antipsychotic drugs

Antipsychotic drugs (normally **olanzapine**, **quetiapine**, or **risperidone**) (section 4.2.1) are useful in acute episodes of mania and hypomania; if the response to antipsychotic drugs is inadequate, lithium or valproate may be added. An antipsychotic drug may be used concomitantly with lithium or valproate in the initial treatment of severe acute mania.

Olanzapine can be used for the long-term management of bipolar disorder in patients whose manic episode responded to olanzapine therapy. It can be given either as monotherapy, or in combination with lithium or valproate if the patient has frequent relapses or continuing functional impairment.

4 Central nervous system

Asenapine, a second-generation antipsychotic, is licensed for the treatment of moderate to severe manic episodes associated with bipolar disorder.

When discontinuing antipsychotics, the dose should be reduced gradually over at least 4 weeks if the patient is continuing with other antimanic drugs; if the patient is not continuing with other antimanic drugs or if there is a history of manic relapse, a withdrawal period of up to 3 months should be considered.

High doses of haloperidol or flupentixol may be hazardous when used with lithium; irreversible toxic encephalopathy has been reported.

■ ASENAPINE

Indications treatment of moderate to severe manic episodes associated with bipolar disorder

Cautions see section 4.2.1; also dementia with Lewy Bodies

Hepatic impairment use with caution in moderate impairment; avoid in severe impairment

Renal impairment use with caution if eGFR less than 15 mL/minute/1.73 m^2—no information available

Pregnancy use only if potential benefit outweighs risk—toxicity in *animal* studies; see also section 4.2.1

Breast-feeding avoid—no information available

Side-effects see section 4.2.1; also hypersalivation, taste disturbance, tongue swelling, glossodynia, anxiety, speech disturbance, dysphagia, transient oral hypoaesthesia and paraesthesia, rhabdomyolysis

Dose

- Monotherapy, ADULT over 18 years initially 10 mg twice daily, reduced to 5 mg twice daily according to response

- Combination therapy, ADULT over 18 years initially 5 mg twice daily, increased if necessary to 10 mg twice daily according to response

Sycrest® (Lundbeck) ▼ PoM
Tablets (sublingual), asenapine (as maleate) 5 mg, net price 60-tab pack = £102.60; 10 mg, 60-tab pack = £102.60. Label: 2, 26, counselling, administration

Carbamazepine

Carbamazepine (section 4.8.1) may be used under specialist supervision for the prophylaxis of bipolar disorder (manic-depressive disorder) in patients unresponsive to a combination of other prophylactic drugs; it is used in patients with rapid-cycling manic-depressive illness (4 or more affective episodes per year). The dose of carbamazepine should not normally be increased if an acute episode of mania occurs.

When stopping treatment with carbamazepine, reduce the dose gradually over a period of at least 4 weeks.

Valproate

Valproic acid (as the semisodium salt) and sodium valproate (section 4.8.1) are used for the treatment of manic episodes associated with bipolar disorder.

Valproate (valproic acid and sodium valproate) is also used for the prophylaxis of bipolar disorder; however, it should **not** normally be prescribed for women of child-bearing potential. In patients with frequent relapse or continuing functional impairment, consider switching therapy to lithium or olanzapine, or adding lithium or

olanzapine to valproate. If a patient taking valproate experiences an acute episode of mania that is not ameliorated by increasing the valproate dose, consider concomitant therapy with olanzapine, quetiapine, or risperidone.

If treatment with valproate is stopped, reduce the dose gradually over at least 4 weeks.

■ VALPROIC ACID

Indications treatment of manic episodes associated with bipolar disorder; migraine prophylaxis (section 4.7.4.2)

Cautions see Sodium Valproate, section 4.8.1; monitor closely if dose greater than 45 mg/kg daily

Contra-indications see Sodium Valproate, section 4.8.1

Hepatic impairment see Sodium Valproate, section 4.8.1

Renal impairment see Sodium Valproate, section 4.8.1

Pregnancy see Sodium Valproate, section 4.8.1

Breast-feeding see Sodium Valproate, section 4.8.1

Side-effects see Sodium Valproate, section 4.8.1

Dose

- Mania, initially 750 mg daily in 2–3 divided doses, increased according to response, usual dose 1–2 g daily; doses greater than 45 mg/kg daily require careful monitoring; CHILD under 18 years not recommended

- Migraine prophylaxis [unlicensed], initially 250 mg twice daily, increased if necessary to 1 g daily in divided doses

Depakote® (Sanofi-Aventis) PoM
Tablets, e/c, valproic acid (as semisodium valproate) 250 mg, net price 90-tab pack = £14.60; 500 mg, 90-tab pack = £29.15. Label: 21, 25, counselling, pancreatitis, blood, or hepatic disorder symptoms, pregnancy, see Cautions above
Note Semisodium valproate comprises equimolar amounts of sodium valproate and valproic acid

Convulex® (Pharmacia) PoM
Section 4.8.1 (epilepsy)

Lithium

Lithium salts are used in the prophylaxis and treatment of mania, hypomania and depression in bipolar disorder (manic-depressive disorder), and in the prophylaxis and treatment of recurrent unipolar depression. Lithium is also used as concomitant therapy with antidepressant medication in patients who have had an incomplete response to treatment for acute bipolar depression and to augment other antidepressants in patients with treatment-resistant depression [unlicensed indication] (section 4.3). It is also licensed for the treatment of aggressive or self-harming behaviour.

The decision to give prophylactic lithium requires specialist advice, and must be based on careful consideration of the likelihood of recurrence in the individual patient, and the benefit of treatment weighed against the risks. The full prophylactic effect of lithium may not occur for six to twelve months after the initiation of therapy. Olanzapine or valproate (given alone or as adjunctive therapy with lithium) are alternative prophylactic treatments in patients who experience frequent relapses or continued functional impairment.

Long-term use of lithium has been associated with thyroid disorders and mild cognitive and memory impairment. Long-term treatment should therefore be undertaken only with careful assessment of risk and benefit, and with monitoring of thyroid function every 6 months (more often if there is evidence of deterioration). Renal function should be monitored at baseline and every 6 months thereafter (more often if there is evidence of deterioration or if the patient has other risk factors, such as starting ACE inhibitors, NSAIDs, or diuretics). The need for continued therapy should be assessed regularly and patients should be maintained on lithium after 3–5 years only if benefit persists.

Serum concentrations Lithium salts have a narrow therapeutic/toxic ratio and should therefore not be prescribed unless facilities for monitoring serum-lithium concentrations are available. Samples should be taken 12 hours after the dose to achieve a serum-lithium concentration of 0.4–1 mmol/litre (lower end of the range for maintenance therapy and elderly patients). A target serum-lithium concentration of 0.8–1 mmol/litre is recommended for acute episodes of mania, and for patients who have previously relapsed or have subsyndromal symptoms. It is important to determine the optimum range for each individual patient. Routine serum-lithium monitoring should be performed weekly after initiation and after each dose change until concentrations are stable, then every 3 months thereafter. Additional serum-lithium measurements should be made if a patient develops significant intercurrent disease or if there is a significant change in a patient's sodium or fluid intake.

Overdosage, usually with serum-lithium concentration of over 1.5 mmol/litre, may be fatal and toxic effects include tremor, ataxia, dysarthria, nystagmus, renal impairment, and convulsions. If these potentially hazardous signs occur, treatment should be stopped, serum-lithium concentrations redetermined, and steps taken to reverse lithium toxicity. In mild cases withdraw lithium and ensure adequate hydration and correction of electrolyte imbalance. Use of IV sodium chloride 0.9% should be considered to maintain urine output. A serum-lithium concentration in excess of 2 mmol/litre requires urgent treatment as described under Emergency Treatment of Poisoning, p. 40.

Interactions Lithium toxicity is made worse by sodium depletion, therefore concurrent use of diuretics (particularly thiazides) is hazardous and should be avoided. For other **interactions** with lithium, see Appendix 1 (lithium).

Withdrawal While there is no clear evidence of withdrawal or rebound psychosis, abrupt discontinuation of lithium increases the risk of relapse. If lithium is to be discontinued, the dose should be reduced gradually over a period of at least 4 weeks (preferably over a period of up to 3 months). Patients should be warned of the risk of relapse if lithium is discontinued abruptly. If lithium is stopped or is to be discontinued abruptly, consider changing therapy to an atypical antipsychotic or valproate.

Lithium treatment packs
A lithium treatment pack should be given to patients on initiation of treatment with lithium. The pack consists of a patient information booklet, lithium alert card, and a record book for tracking serum-lithium concentration.   Packs may be purchased from 3M.   Tel: 0845 610 1112 nhsforms@mmm.uk.com

LITHIUM CARBONATE

Indications treatment and prophylaxis of mania, bipolar disorder, and recurrent depression (see also notes above); aggressive or self-harming behaviour

Cautions see notes above; assess cardiac, renal, and thyroid function before initiating, and thereafter every 6 months on stabilised regimens; cardiac disease; QT-interval prolongation (caution with concomitant use of drugs that prolong the QT interval); review dose as necessary in diarrhoea, vomiting, and intercurrent infection (especially if sweating profusely); may lower seizure threshold (caution with epilepsy, concurrent ECT, concomitant use of drugs and any therapy that may lower seizure threshold); psoriasis (risk of exacerbation); elderly (reduce dose); diuretic treatment (risk of toxicity); myasthenia gravis; surgery (section 15.1); avoid abrupt withdrawal (see notes above); **interactions:** Appendix 1 (lithium)

Counselling Patients should be advised to report signs and symptoms of lithium toxicity (see above), hypothyroidism, renal dysfunction (including polyuria and polydipsia), and benign intracranial hypertension (persistent headache and visual disturbance); maintain adequate fluid intake and avoid dietary changes which reduce or increase sodium intake; may impair performance of skilled tasks (e.g. driving, operating machinery); lithium treatment packs are available (see above)

Contra-indications dehydration, low sodium diets, Addison's disease, untreated hypothyroidism, personal or family history of Brugada syndrome, cardiac insufficiency or rhythm disorder

Renal impairment caution in mild to moderate impairment—monitor serum-lithium concentration closely and adjust dose accordingly; avoid in severe impairment

Pregnancy avoid if possible, particularly in the first trimester (risk of teratogenicity, including cardiac abnormalities); dose requirements increased during the second and third trimesters (but on delivery return abruptly to normal); close monitoring of serum-lithium concentration advised (risk of toxicity in neonate); manufacturer advises effective contraception during treatment for women of child bearing potential

Breast-feeding present in milk and risk of toxicity in infant—avoid

Side-effects gastro-intestinal disturbances, gastritis, weight changes, anorexia, oedema, benign intracranial hypertension, Raynaud's phenomena, ECG changes (including arrhythmia, bradycardia, sinus node dysfunction, QT interval prolongation, AV block), cardiomyopathy, hypersalivation, dry mouth, cognitive impairment, hallucinations, extrapyramidal side-effects, fine tremor, speech disorder, vertigo, memory loss, encephalopathy, dysgeusia, malaise, myasthenia gravis, peripheral neuropathy, kidney changes, renal impairment, polydipsia, nephrotic syndrome, nephrogenic diabetes insipidus; electrolyte imbalance, sexual dysfunction; thyroid changes

4 Central nervous system

Central nervous system 4

(including hyperthyroidism, hypothyroidism, euthyroid goitre); hyperparathyroidism, parathyroid adenoma, leucocytosis, arthralgia, myalgia, nystagmus, alopecia, psoriasis exacerbation, acneiform eruptions and other skin disorders; signs of intoxication require withdrawal of treatment and include increasing gastro-intestinal disturbances (vomiting, diarrhoea), visual disturbances, polyuria, muscle weakness, fine tremor increasing to coarse tremor, CNS disturbances (confusion and drowsiness increasing to lack of coordination, restlessness, stupor); abnormal reflexes, myoclonus, incontinence, hypernatraemia; with severe **overdosage** (serum-lithium concentration above 2 mmol/litre) seizures, cardiac arrhythmias (including sino-atrial block, bradycardia and first-degree heart block), blood pressure changes, circulatory failure, renal failure, coma and sudden death reported; see also Emergency Treatment of Poisoning, p. 40

Dose
* See under preparations below, adjusted to achieve a serum-lithium concentration of 0.4–1 mmol/litre 12 hours after a dose on days 4–7 of treatment, then every week until dosage has remained constant for 4 weeks and every 3 months thereafter; doses are initially divided throughout the day, but once daily administration is preferred when serum-lithium concentration stabilised

Note Preparations vary widely in bioavailability; changing the preparation requires the same precautions as initiation of treatment

Camcolit® (Essential) [PoM]
Camcolit 250® tablets, f/c, scored, lithium carbonate 250 mg (Li⁺ 6.8 mmol), net price 100-tab pack = £3.22. Label: 10, lithium card, counselling, driving, fluid and salt intake, toxicity symptoms, see above

Camcolit 400® tablets, m/r, f/c, scored, lithium carbonate 400 mg (Li⁺ 10.8 mmol), net price 100-tab pack = £4.30. Label: 10, lithium card, 25, counselling, driving, fluid and salt intake, toxicity symptoms, see above

Dose (see Dose above for advice on bioavailability and serum monitoring):
Treatment, ADULT over 18 years, initially 1–1.5 g daily, ELDERLY reduce initial dose; prophylaxis, ADULT over 18 years, initially 300–400 mg daily; CHILD under 18 years see BNF for Children

Note Camcolit 400® also available as Lithonate® (TEVA UK)

Liskonum® (GSK) [PoM]
Tablets, m/r, f/c, scored, lithium carbonate 450 mg (Li⁺ 12.2 mmol), net price 60-tab pack = £2.88. Label: 10, lithium card, 25, counselling, driving, fluid and salt intake, toxicity symptoms, see above

Dose (see Dose above for advice on bioavailability and serum monitoring):
Treatment, ADULT over 18 years, initially 450–675 mg twice daily; ELDERLY initially 225 mg twice daily; prophylaxis, ADULT over 18 years, initially 450 mg twice daily; ELDERLY 225 mg twice daily; CHILD under 18 years see BNF for Children

Priadel® (Sanofi-Aventis) [PoM]
Tablets, m/r, both scored, lithium carbonate 200 mg (Li⁺ 5.4 mmol), net price 100-tab pack= £2.30; 400 mg (Li⁺ 10.8 mmol), 100-tab pack = £3.35. Label: 10, lithium card, 25, counselling, driving, fluid and salt intake, toxicity symptoms, see above

Dose (see Dose above for advice on bioavailability and serum monitoring):
Treatment and prophylaxis, ADULT over 18 years, initially 0.4–1.2 g daily as a single dose or in 2 divided doses,

ELDERLY or patients less than 50 kg, initially 200–400 mg daily; CHILD not recommended
Liquid, see under Lithium Citrate below

▌ LITHIUM CITRATE

Indications see Lithium Carbonate
Cautions see Lithium Carbonate
Counselling Patients should be advised to report signs and symptoms of lithium toxicity (see above), hypothyroidism, renal dysfunction (including polyuria and polydipsia), and benign intracranial hypertension (persistent headache and visual disturbance); maintain adequate fluid intake and avoid dietary changes which reduce or increase sodium intake; may impair performance of skilled tasks (e.g. driving, operating machinery); lithium treatment cards are available (see above)

Contra-indications see Lithium Carbonate
Renal impairment see Lithium Carbonate
Pregnancy see Lithium Carbonate
Breast-feeding see Lithium Carbonate
Side-effects see Lithium Carbonate

Dose
* See under preparations below, adjusted to achieve serum-lithium concentration of 0.4–1 mmol/litre as described under Lithium Carbonate

Note Preparations vary widely in bioavailability; changing the preparation requires the same precautions as initiation of treatment

Li-Liquid® (Rosemont) [PoM]
Oral solution, lithium citrate tetrahydrate 509 mg/ 5 mL (Li⁺ 5.4 mmol/5 mL), yellow, net price 150-mL pack = £5.79; 1.018 g/5 mL (Li⁺ 10.8 mmol/5 mL), orange, 150-mL pack = £11.58. Label: 10, lithium card, counselling, driving, fluid and salt intake, toxicity symptoms, see above

Dose (see Dose above for advice on bioavailability and serum monitoring):
Treatment and prophylaxis, ADULT over 18 years, initially 1.018–2.036 g daily in 2 divided doses; ELDERLY or patients less than 50 kg, initially 509 mg twice daily; CHILD under 18 years see BNF for Children

Note Lithium citrate tetrahydrate 509 mg is equivalent to lithium carbonate 200 mg

Priadel® (Sanofi-Aventis) [PoM]
Tablets, see under Lithium Carbonate

Liquid, sugar-free, lithium citrate tetrahydrate 520 mg/5 mL (approx. Li⁺ 5.5 mmol/5 mL), net price 150-mL pack = £5.61. Label: 10, lithium card, counselling, driving, fluid and salt intake, toxicity symptoms, see above

Dose (see Dose above for advice on bioavailability and serum monitoring):
Treatment and prophylaxis, ADULT over 18 years, initially 1.04–3.12 g daily in 2 divided doses; ELDERLY or patients less than 50 kg, 520 mg twice daily; CHILD under 18 years see BNF for Children

Note Lithium citrate tetrahydrate 520 mg is equivalent to lithium carbonate 204 mg

4.3 Antidepressant drugs

4.3.1	**Tricyclic and related antidepressant drugs**
4.3.2	**Monoamine-oxidase inhibitors**
4.3.3	**Selective serotonin re-uptake inhibitors**
4.3.4	**Other antidepressant drugs**

Antidepressant drugs are effective for treating moderate to severe depression associated with psychomotor and physiological changes such as loss of appetite and sleep disturbance; improvement in sleep is usually the first benefit of therapy. Ideally, patients with moderate to severe depression should be treated with psychological therapy in addition to drug therapy. Antidepressant drugs are also effective for dysthymia (lower grade chronic depression (typically of at least 2 years duration)).

Antidepressant drugs should not be used routinely in mild depression, and psychological therapy should be considered initially; however, a trial of antidepressant therapy may be considered in cases refractory to psychological treatments or in those associated with psychosocial or medical problems. Drug treatment of mild depression may also be considered in patients with a history of moderate or severe depression.

Choice   The major classes of antidepressant drugs include the tricyclic and related antidepressants (section 4.3.1), the selective serotonin re-uptake inhibitors (SSRIs) (section 4.3.3), and the monoamine oxidase inhibitors (MAOIs) (section 4.3.2). A number of antidepressant drugs cannot be accommodated easily into this classification; these are included in section 4.3.4.

There is little to choose between the different classes of antidepressant drugs in terms of efficacy, so choice should be based on the individual patient's requirements, including the presence of concomitant disease, existing therapy, suicide risk, and previous response to antidepressant therapy. Since there may be an interval of 2 weeks before the antidepressant action takes place, electroconvulsive treatment may be required in severe depression when delay is hazardous or intolerable. During the first few weeks of treatment, there is an increased potential for agitation, anxiety, and suicidal ideation (see below).

SSRIs are better tolerated and are safer in overdose than other classes of antidepressants and should be considered first-line for treating depression. In patients with unstable angina or who have had a recent myocardial infarction, sertraline has been shown to be safe.

Tricyclic antidepressants have similar efficacy to SSRIs but are more likely to be discontinued because of side-effects; toxicity in overdosage is also a problem. See section 4.3.1 for more details.

MAOIs have dangerous interactions with some foods and drugs, and should be reserved for use by specialists.

Although anxiety is often present in depressive illness (and may be the presenting symptom), the use of an antipsychotic or an anxiolytic may mask the true diagnosis. Anxiolytics (section 4.1.2) or antipsychotic drugs (section 4.2.1) should therefore be used with caution in depression but they are useful adjuncts in agitated patients. Augmenting antidepressants with antipsychotics under specialist supervision may also be necessary in patients who have depression with psychotic symptoms.

See section 4.2.3 for notes on the management of bipolar disorder.

St John's wort (*Hypericum perforatum*) is a popular herbal remedy on sale to the public for treating mild depression. It should not be prescribed or recommended for depression because St John's wort can induce drug metabolising enzymes and a number of important interactions with conventional drugs, including conventional antidepressants, have been identified (see Appendix 1, St John's wort). Furthermore, the amount of active ingredient varies between different preparations of St John's wort and switching from one to another can change the degree of enzyme induction. If a patient stops taking St John's wort, the concentration of interacting drugs may increase, leading to toxicity.

Hyponatraemia and antidepressant therapy

Hyponatraemia (usually in the elderly and possibly due to inappropriate secretion of antidiuretic hormone) has been associated with all types of antidepressants; however, it has been reported more frequently with SSRIs than with other antidepressants. Hyponatraemia should be considered in all patients who develop drowsiness, confusion, or convulsions while taking an antidepressant.

Suicidal behaviour and antidepressant therapy

The use of antidepressants has been linked with suicidal thoughts and behaviour; children, young adults, and patients with a history of suicidal behaviour are particularly at risk. Where necessary patients should be monitored for suicidal behaviour, self-harm, or hostility, particularly at the beginning of treatment or if the dose is changed.

Management   Patients should be reviewed every 1–2 weeks at the start of antidepressant treatment. Treatment should be continued for at least 4 weeks (6 weeks in the elderly) before considering whether to switch antidepressant due to lack of efficacy. In cases of partial response, continue for a further 2–4 weeks (elderly patients may take longer to respond).

Following remission, antidepressant treatment should be continued at the same dose for at least 6 months (about 12 months in the elderly), or for at least 12 months in patients receiving treatment for generalised anxiety disorder (as the likelihood of relapse is high). Patients with a history of recurrent depression should receive maintenance treatment for at least 2 years.

Failure to respond   Failure to respond to initial treatment with an SSRI may require an increase in the dose, or switching to a different SSRI or mirtazapine. Other second-line choices include lofepramine, moclobemide, and reboxetine. Other tricyclic antidepressants and venlafaxine should be considered for more severe forms of depression; irreversible MAOIs should only be prescribed by specialists. Failure to respond to a second antidepressant may require the addition of another antidepressant of a different class, or use of an augmenting agent (such as lithium (section 4.2.3), aripiprazole [unlicensed], olanzapine [unlicensed], quetiapine, or risperidone [unlicensed] (section 4.2.1)), but such adjunctive treatment should be initiated only by doctors with special experience of these combinations. Electroconvulsive therapy may be initiated in severe refractory depression.

Withdrawal   Withdrawal effects may occur within 5 days of stopping treatment with antidepressant drugs; they are usually mild and self-limiting, but in some cases may be severe. Drugs with a shorter half-life, such as paroxetine (p. 262) and venlafaxine (p. 265), are associated with a higher risk of withdrawal symptoms. The risk of withdrawal symptoms is also increased if the antidepressant is stopped suddenly after regular administration for 8 weeks or more. The dose should preferably be reduced gradually over about 4 weeks, or longer if withdrawal symptoms emerge (6 months in patients who have been on long-term maintenance treatment). See also section 4.3.1, section 4.3.2, and section 4.3.3.

Anxiety disorders and obsessive-compulsive disorder Management of acute anxiety generally involves the use of a benzodiazepine or buspirone (section 4.1.2). For chronic anxiety (of longer than 4 weeks' duration) it may be appropriate to use an antidepressant. Combined therapy with a benzodiazepine may be required until the antidepressant takes effect. Patients with *generalised anxiety disorder*, a form of chronic anxiety, should be offered psychological treatment before initiating an antidepressant. If drug treatment is needed, an SSRI such as escitalopram, paroxetine, or sertraline [unlicensed], can be used. Duloxetine and venlafaxine (serotonin and noradrenaline reuptake inhibitors) are also recommended for the treatment of generalised anxiety disorder; if the patient cannot tolerate SSRIs or serotonin and noradrenaline reuptake inhibitors (or if treatment has failed to control symptoms), pregabalin can be considered.

Panic disorder, obsessive-compulsive disorder, post-traumatic stress disorder, and phobic states such as *social anxiety disorder* are treated with SSRIs. Clomipramine or imipramine can be used second-line in panic disorder [unlicensed]; clomipramine can also be used second-line for obsessive-compulsive disorder. Moclobemide is licensed for the treatment of social anxiety disorder.

4.3.1 Tricyclic and related antidepressant drugs

This section covers tricyclic antidepressants and also 1-, 2-, and 4-ring structured drugs with broadly similar properties.

Some tricyclic antidepressants are used in the management of *panic* and other *anxiety disorders* (section 4.3). For reference to the role of some tricyclic antidepressants in some forms of *neuralgia*, see section 4.7.3, and in *nocturnal enuresis* in children, see section 7.4.2.

Cautions Tricyclic and related antidepressant drugs should be used with caution in patients with cardiovascular disease (see also Contra-indications, below); because of the risk of arrhythmias, patients with concomitant conditions such as hyperthyroidism and phaeochromocytoma should be treated with care. Care is also needed in patients with epilepsy and diabetes.

Tricyclic antidepressant drugs have antimuscarinic activity, and therefore caution is needed in patients with prostatic hypertrophy, chronic constipation, increased intra-ocular pressure, urinary retention, or those with a susceptibility to angle-closure glaucoma. Tricyclic and related antidepressant drugs should be used with caution in patients with a significant risk of suicide, or a history of psychosis or bipolar disorder, because antidepressant therapy may aggravate these conditions; treatment should be stopped if the patient enters a manic phase.

Elderly patients are particularly susceptible to many of the side-effects of tricyclic antidepressants; low initial doses should be used, with close monitoring, particularly for psychiatric and cardiac side-effects.

Overdosage Limited quantities of tricyclic antidepressants should be prescribed at any one time because their cardiovascular and epileptogenic effects are dangerous in overdosage. In particular, overdosage with dosulepin and amitriptyline is associated with a relatively high rate of fatality. Lofepramine is associated with the lowest risk of fatality in overdosage, in comparison with other tricyclic antidepressant drugs. For advice on **overdosage** see Emergency Treatment of Poisoning, p. 38.

Withdrawal Withdrawal symptoms include influenza-like symptoms (chills, myalgia, sweating, headache, nausea), insomnia, vivid dreams, and may occasionally include movement disorders and mania. If possible tricyclic and related antidepressants should be withdrawn slowly (see also section 4.3).

Interactions A tricyclic or related antidepressant (or an SSRI or related antidepressant) should not be started until 2 weeks after stopping an MAOI (3 weeks if starting clomipramine or imipramine). Conversely, an MAOI should not be started until at least 7–14 days after a tricyclic or related antidepressant (3 weeks in the case of clomipramine or imipramine) has been stopped. For guidance relating to the reversible monoamine oxidase inhibitor, moclobemide, see p. 259. For other tricyclic antidepressant **interactions**, see Appendix 1 (antidepressants, tricyclic and antidepressants, tricyclic (related)).

Driving Drowsiness may affect the performance of skilled tasks (e.g. driving); effects of alcohol enhanced.

Contra-indications Tricyclic and related antidepressants are contra-indicated in the immediate recovery period after myocardial infarction, in arrhythmias (particularly heart block), and in the manic phase of bipolar disorder. Avoid treatment with tricyclic antidepressant drugs in acute porphyria (section 9.8.2).

Hepatic impairment Tricyclic antidepressants are preferable to MAOIs in hepatic impairment but sedative effects are increased. They should be avoided in severe liver disease.

Breast-feeding The amount of tricyclic antidepressants (including related drugs such as mianserin and trazodone) secreted into breast milk is too small to be harmful (but see Doxepin, p. 256).

Side-effects Arrhythmias and heart block occasionally follow the use of tricyclic antidepressants, particularly amitriptyline, and may be a factor in the sudden death of patients with cardiac disease; other cardiovascular side-effects include postural hypotension, tachycardia, and ECG changes. The tricyclic-related antidepressant drugs may be associated with a lower risk of cardiotoxicity in overdosage.

Central nervous system side-effects are common, particularly in the elderly, and include anxiety, dizziness, agitation, confusion, sleep disturbances, irritability, and paraesthesia; drowsiness is associated with some of the tricyclic antidepressants (see under Choice, below). Convulsions, hallucinations, delusions, mania, and hypomania may occur (see also under Cautions, above), and, *rarely*, extrapyramidal symptoms including tremor and dysarthria.

Antimuscarinic side-effects include dry mouth, blurred vision (*very rarely* precipitation of angle-closure glaucoma), constipation (*rarely* leading to paralytic ileus, particularly in the elderly), and urinary retention. Tricyclic-related antidepressant drugs have a lower incidence of antimuscarinic side-effects than older tricyclics.

Endocrine effects include breast enlargement, galactorrhoea, and gynaecomastia. Sexual dysfunction may occur. Changes in blood sugar, increased appetite, and weight gain can accompany treatment with tricyclic antidepressant drugs, but anorexia and weight loss are also seen. Hepatic and haematological reactions may occur and have been particularly associated with mianserin. Another side-effect to which the elderly are particularly susceptible is hyponatraemia (see Hyponatraemia and Antidepressant Therapy, p. 253). Other class side-effects include nausea, vomiting, taste disturbance, tinnitus, rash, urticaria, pruritus, photosensitivity, alopecia, and sweating.

The patient should be encouraged to persist with treatment as some tolerance to these side-effects seems to develop. They are reduced if low doses are given initially and then gradually increased, but this must be balanced against the need to obtain a full therapeutic effect as soon as possible.

Neuroleptic malignant syndrome (section 4.2.1) may, very rarely, occur in the course of antidepressant drug treatment.

Suicidal behaviour has been linked with antidepressants (see p. 253).

Dosage About 10 to 20% of patients fail to respond to tricyclic and related antidepressant drugs and inadequate dosage may account for some of these failures. It is important to use doses that are sufficiently high for effective treatment but not so high as to cause toxic effects. Low doses should be used for initial treatment in the **elderly** (see under Side-effects, below).

In most patients the long half-life of tricyclic antidepressant drugs allows **once-daily** administration, usually at night; the use of modified-release preparations is therefore unnecessary.

Choice Tricyclic and related antidepressants block the re-uptake of both serotonin and noradrenaline, although to different extents. For example, clomipramine is more selective for serotonergic transmission, and imipramine is more selective for noradrenergic transmission. Tricyclic and related antidepressant drugs can be roughly divided into those with additional sedative properties and those that are less sedating. Agitated and anxious patients tend to respond best to the sedative compounds, whereas withdrawn and apathetic patients will often obtain most benefit from the less sedating ones. Those with **sedative** properties include amitriptyline, clomipramine, dosulepin, doxepin, mianserin, trazodone, and trimipramine. Those with **less sedative** properties include imipramine, lofepramine, and nortriptyline.

Tricyclic and related antidepressants also have varying degrees of antimuscarinic side-effects and cardiotoxicity in overdosage, which may be important in individual patients. **Lofepramine** has a lower incidence of side-effects and is less dangerous in overdosage but is infrequently associated with hepatic toxicity. **Imipramine** is also well established, but has more marked antimuscarinic side-effects than other tricyclic and related antidepressants. **Amitriptyline** and **dosulepin** are effective but they are particularly dangerous in overdosage (see Overdosage, above) and are not

recommended for the treatment of depression; dosulepin should be initiated by a specialist.

Children and adolescents Studies have shown that tricyclic antidepressants are not effective for treating depression in children; see also Depressive Illness in Children and Adolescents, p. 260.

Tricyclic antidepressants

▌ AMITRIPTYLINE HYDROCHLORIDE

Indications depressive illness (but not recommended, see notes above); neuropathic pain [unlicensed] (section 4.7.3); migraine prophylaxis [unlicensed] (section 4.7.4.2)

Cautions see notes above

Contra-indications see notes above

Hepatic impairment see notes above

Pregnancy use only if potential benefit outweighs risk

Breast-feeding see notes above

Side-effects see notes above; also abdominal pain, stomatitis, palpitation, oedema, hypertension, restlessness, fatigue, mydriasis, and increased intra-ocular pressure; high rate of fatality in overdose—see notes above

Dose

- Depression (but not recommended, see notes above), ADULT and CHILD over 16 years, initially 75 mg (ELDERLY and ADOLESCENTS 30–75 mg) daily in divided doses *or* as a single dose at bedtime increased gradually as necessary to 150–200 mg
- Neuropathic pain [unlicensed indication], initially 10 mg daily at night, gradually increased if necessary to 75 mg daily; higher doses under specialist supervision
- Migraine prophylaxis [unlicensed indication], initially 10 mg at night, increased if necessary to maintenance of 50–75 mg at night; max. 150 mg at night

Amitriptyline (Non-proprietary) ⓅⓄⓂ

Tablets, coated, amitriptyline hydrochloride 10 mg, net price 28-tab pack = £1.02; 25 mg, 28-tab pack = £1.02; 50 mg, 28-tab pack = £1.09. Label: 2

Oral solution, amitriptyline hydrochloride 25 mg/ 5 mL, net price 150 mL = £17.92; 50 mg/5 mL, 150 mL = £19.04. Label: 2

◢**Compound preparations**

Triptafen® (AMCo) ⓅⓄⓂ

Tablets, pink, s/c, amitriptyline hydrochloride 25 mg, perphenazine 2 mg, net price 100-tab pack = £33.13. Label: 2

Dose depression with anxiety, ADULT over 18 years, 1 tablet 3 times daily; an additional tablet may be taken at bedtime when required

▌ CLOMIPRAMINE HYDROCHLORIDE

Indications depressive illness, phobic and obsessional states; adjunctive treatment of cataplexy associated with narcolepsy

Cautions see notes above

Contra-indications see notes above

Hepatic impairment see notes above

Pregnancy neonatal withdrawal symptoms reported if used during third trimester

Breast-feeding see notes above

Side-effects see notes above; also abdominal pain, diarrhoea, hypertension, flushing, restlessness, fatigue, aggression, impaired memory, muscle weakness, muscle hypertonia, myoclonus, mydriasis, and yawning; *very rarely* allergic alveolitis

Dose

- Depressive illness, ADULT over 18 years, initially 10 mg daily, increased gradually as necessary to 30–150 mg daily in divided doses *or* as a single dose at bedtime; max. 250 mg daily; ELDERLY initially 10 mg daily increased carefully over approx. 10 days to 30–75 mg daily
- Phobic and obsessional states, ADULT over 18 years, initially 25 mg daily (ELDERLY 10 mg daily) increased over 2 weeks to 100–150 mg daily; max. 250 mg daily
- Adjunctive treatment of cataplexy associated with narcolepsy, ADULT over 18 years, initially 10 mg daily, gradually increased until satisfactory response (range 10–75 mg daily)

Clomipramine (Non-proprietary) ▱oM▱

Capsules, clomipramine hydrochloride 10 mg, net price 28-cap pack = £1.53; 25 mg, 28-cap pack = £1.92; 50 mg, 28-cap pack = £2.31. Label: 2

◢**Modified release**

Anafranil SR® (Novartis) ▱oM▱ ◢

Tablets, m/r, grey-red, f/c, clomipramine hydrochloride 75 mg, net price 28-tab pack = £8.83. Label: 2, 25

Dose see above; to be taken once daily

DOSULEPIN HYDROCHLORIDE ◢

(Dothiepin hydrochloride)

Indications depressive illness, particularly where sedation is required (initiated by a specialist)

Cautions see notes above

Contra-indications see notes above

Hepatic impairment see notes above

Pregnancy use only if potential benefit outweighs risk

Breast-feeding see notes above

Side-effects see notes above; also increased intra-ocular pressure; high rate of fatality in overdose—see notes above

Dose

- Initially 75 mg (ELDERLY 50–75 mg) daily in divided doses *or* as a single dose at bedtime, increased gradually as necessary to 150 mg daily (ELDERLY 75 mg may be sufficient); up to 225 mg daily in some circumstances (e.g. hospital use); CHILD not recommended

Note A maximum prescription equivalent to 2 weeks' supply of 75 mg daily should be considered in patients with increased risk factors for suicide at initiation of treatment, during any dose adjustment, and until improvement occurs

Dosulepin (Non-proprietary) ▱oM▱ ◢

Capsules, dosulepin hydrochloride 25 mg, net price 28-cap pack = £1.70. Label: 2

Tablets, dosulepin hydrochloride 75 mg, net price 28-tab pack = £1.85. Label: 2

Prothiaden® (Teofarma) ▱oM▱ ◢

Capsules, red/red-brown, dosulepin hydrochloride 25 mg, net price 28-cap pack = £1.70. Label: 2

Tablets, red, s/c, dosulepin hydrochloride 75 mg, net price 28-tab pack = £2.97. Label: 2

DOXEPIN

Indications depressive illness, particularly where sedation is required; pruritus in eczema (section 13.3)

Cautions see notes above

Contra-indications see notes above

Hepatic impairment see notes above

Renal impairment use with caution

Pregnancy use with caution—limited information available

Breast-feeding see notes above; accumulation of metabolite may cause sedation and respiratory depression in neonate

Side-effects see notes above; also abdominal pain, stomatitis, diarrhoea, flushing, and oedema

Dose

- ADULT and CHILD over 12 years, initially 75 mg daily in divided doses *or* as a single dose at bedtime, adjusted according to response; usual maintenance 25–300 mg daily (doses above 100 mg given in 3 divided doses); ELDERLY start with lower doses and adjust according to response

Sinepin® (Marlborough) ▱oM▱

Capsules, doxepin (as hydrochloride) 25 mg (blue/red), net price 28-cap pack = £3.77; 50 mg (blue), 28-cap pack = £5.71. Label: 2

IMIPRAMINE HYDROCHLORIDE

Indications depressive illness; nocturnal enuresis in children (section 7.4.2)

Cautions see notes above

Contra-indications see notes above

Hepatic impairment see notes above

Renal impairment use with caution in severe impairment

Pregnancy colic, tachycardia, dyspnoea, irritability, muscle spasms, respiratory depression, and withdrawal symptoms reported in neonates when used in the third trimester

Breast-feeding see notes above

Side-effects see notes above; also palpitation, flushing, restlessness, headache, fatigue; *very rarely* abdominal pain, stomatitis, hypertension, oedema, cardiac decompensation, allergic alveolitis, aggression, myoclonus, peripheral vasospasm, and mydriasis

Dose

- Depression, initially up to 75 mg daily in divided doses increased gradually to 150–200 mg (up to 300 mg in hospital patients); up to 150 mg may be given as a single dose at bedtime; ELDERLY initially 10 mg daily, increased gradually to 30–50 mg daily; CHILD not recommended for depression
- Nocturnal enuresis, CHILD 6–8 years 25 mg, 8–11 years 25–50 mg, over 11 years 50–75 mg at bedtime; initial period of treatment (including gradual withdrawal) 3 months—full physical examination before further course

Imipramine (Non-proprietary) ▱oM▱

Tablets, coated, imipramine hydrochloride 10 mg, net price 28-tab pack = £1.35; 25 mg, 28-tab pack = £1.37. Label: 2

Oral solution, imipramine hydrochloride 25 mg/5 mL, net price 150-mL = £31.25. Label: 2

LOFEPRAMINE

Indications depressive illness

Cautions see notes above

Contra-indications see notes above

Hepatic impairment see notes above

Renal impairment avoid in severe impairment

Pregnancy neonatal withdrawal symptoms and respiratory depression reported if used during third trimester

Breast-feeding see notes above

Side-effects see notes above; also diarrhoea, headache, and oedema reported

Dose

- 140–210 mg daily in divided doses; ELDERLY may respond to lower doses; CHILD under 18 years not recommended

Lofepramine (Non-proprietary) PoM
Tablets, lofepramine 70 mg (as hydrochloride), net price 56-tab pack = £5.93. Label: 2
Brands include *Feprapax*®

Oral suspension, lofepramine 70 mg/5 mL (as hydrochloride), net price 150 mL = £22.22. Label: 2
Brands include *Lomont*® (sugar-free)

NORTRIPTYLINE

Indications depressive illness; neuropathic pain [unlicensed] (section 4.7.3)

Cautions see notes above; manufacturer advises plasma-nortriptyline concentration monitoring if dose above 100 mg daily, but evidence of practical value uncertain

Contra-indications see notes above

Hepatic impairment see notes above

Pregnancy use only if potential benefit outweighs risk

Breast-feeding see notes above

Side-effects see notes above; also abdominal pain, stomatitis, diarrhoea, hypertension, oedema, flushing, restlessness, fatigue, and mydriasis

Dose

- Depression, low dose initially increased as necessary to 75–100 mg daily in divided doses or as a single dose (max. 150 mg daily); ADOLESCENT and ELDERLY 30–50 mg daily in divided doses; CHILD not recommended for depression

- Neuropathic pain [unlicensed], initially 10 mg daily at night, gradually increased if necessary to 75 mg daily; higher doses under specialist supervision

Allegron® (King) PoM
Tablets, nortriptyline (as hydrochloride) 10 mg, net price 100-tab pack = £12.06; 25 mg (orange, scored), 100-tab pack = £24.02. Label: 2

TRIMIPRAMINE

Indications depressive illness, particularly where sedation is required

Cautions see notes above

Contra-indications see notes above

Hepatic impairment see notes above

Pregnancy use only if potential benefit outweighs risk

Breast-feeding see notes above

Side-effects see notes above

Dose

- Initially 50–75 mg daily in divided doses or as a single dose at bedtime, increased as necessary to 150–300 mg daily; ELDERLY initially 10–25 mg 3 times daily, maintenance half adult dose may be sufficient; CHILD not recommended

Surmontil® (Sanofi-Aventis) PoM
Capsules, green/white, trimipramine 50 mg (as maleate), net price 28-cap pack = £8.36. Label: 2
Tablets, trimipramine (as maleate) 10 mg, net price 28-tab pack = £3.77, 84-tab pack = £11.30; 25 mg, 28-tab pack = £4.98, 84-tab pack = £14.91. Label: 2

Tricyclic-related antidepressants

MIANSERIN HYDROCHLORIDE

Indications depressive illness, particularly where sedation is required

Cautions see notes above
Blood counts A full **blood count** is recommended every 4 weeks during the first 3 months of treatment; clinical monitoring should continue subsequently and treatment should be stopped and a full blood count obtained if *fever, sore throat, stomatitis,* or other signs of infection develop

Contra-indications see notes above

Hepatic impairment see notes above

Renal impairment caution in renal impairment

Pregnancy avoid

Breast-feeding see notes above

Side-effects see notes above; also jaundice, oedema, blood dyscrasias, arthritis, and arthralgia

Dose

- ADULT over 18 years, initially 30–40 mg (elderly 30 mg) daily in divided doses or as a single dose at bedtime, increased gradually as necessary; usual dose range 30–90 mg

Mianserin (Non-proprietary) PoM
Tablets, mianserin hydrochloride 10 mg, net price 28-tab pack = £8.14; 30 mg, 28-tab pack = £18.34. Label: 2, 25

TRAZODONE HYDROCHLORIDE

Indications depressive illness, particularly where sedation is required; anxiety

Cautions see notes above

Contra-indications see notes above

Hepatic impairment see notes above

Renal impairment use with caution in severe impairment

Pregnancy avoid during first trimester—limited information available; monitor infant for signs of withdrawal if used until delivery

Breast-feeding see notes above

Side-effects see notes above; also dyspepsia, hypersalivation, hypertension, palpitation, dyspnoea, priapism (discontinue immediately), myalgia, arthralgia

Dose

- Depression, initially 150 mg (elderly 100 mg) daily in divided doses after food or as a single dose at bedtime; may be increased to 300 mg daily; hospital patients up to max. 600 mg daily in divided doses; CHILD not recommended

- Anxiety, 75 mg daily, increasing if necessary to 300 mg daily; CHILD not recommended

4

Central nervous system

Trazodone (Non-proprietary) PoM

Capsules, trazodone hydrochloride 50 mg, net price 84-cap pack = £27.14; 100 mg, 56-cap pack = £27.26. Label: 2, 21

Tablets, trazodone hydrochloride 150 mg, net price 28-tab pack = £21.23. Label: 2, 21

Liquid, sugar-free, trazodone hydrochloride 50 mg/ 5 mL, net price 120 mL = £27.22. Label: 2, 21

Molipaxin® (Sanofi-Aventis) PoM

Capsules, trazodone hydrochloride 50 mg (violet/ green), net price 84-cap pack = £23.92; 100 mg (vio-let/fawn), 56-cap pack = £28.14. Label: 2, 21

Tablets, pink, f/c, trazodone hydrochloride 150 mg, net price 28-tab pack = £16.08. Label: 2, 21

4.3.2 Monoamine-oxidase inhibitors
(MAOIs)

Monoamine-oxidase inhibitors are used much less frequently than tricyclic and related antidepressants, or SSRIs and related antidepressants because of the dangers of dietary and drug interactions and the fact that it is easier to prescribe MAOIs when tricyclic antidepressants have been unsuccessful than vice versa. Tranyl-cypromine has a greater stimulant action than phenel-zine or isocarboxazid and is more likely to cause a hypertensive crisis. Isocarboxazid and phenelzine are more likely to cause hepatotoxicity than tranylcypromine.

Phobic patients and depressed patients with atypical, hypochondriacal, or hysterical features are said to respond best to MAOIs. However, MAOIs should be tried in any patients who are refractory to treatment with other antidepressants as there is occasionally a dramatic response. Response to treatment may be delayed for 3 weeks or more and may take an additional 1 or 2 weeks to become maximal.

Withdrawal MAOIs are associated with withdrawal symptoms on cessation of therapy. Symptoms include agitation, irritability, ataxia, movement disorders, insomnia, drowsiness, vivid dreams, cognitive impairment, and slowed speech. Withdrawal symptoms occasionally experienced when discontinuing MAOIs include hallucinations and paranoid delusions. If possible MAOIs should be withdrawn slowly (see also section 4.3).

Hepatic impairment MAOIs may cause idiosyncratic hepatotoxicity if used in patients with hepatic impairment. See also individual monographs.

Pregnancy There is an increased risk of neonatal malformations when phenelzine, isocarboxazid, or tranylcypromine is used during pregnancy. The safety of moclobemide in pregnancy has not been established. Manufacturers advise avoid use unless there are compelling reasons.

Interactions MAOIs inhibit monoamine oxidase, thereby causing an accumulation of amine neurotransmitters. The metabolism of some amine drugs such as *indirect-acting sympathomimetics* (present in many cough and decongestant preparations, section 3.10) is also inhibited and their pressor action may be potentiated; the pressor effect of tyramine (in some foods, such as mature cheese, pickled herring, broad bean pods, and *Bovril®*, *Oxo®*, *Marmite®* or any similar meat or yeast extract or fermented soya bean extract) may also be

dangerously potentiated. These interactions may cause a dangerous rise in blood pressure. An early warning symptom may be a throbbing headache. Patients should be advised to eat only fresh foods and avoid food that is suspected of being stale or 'going off'. This is especially important with meat, fish, poultry or offal; game should be avoided. The danger of interaction persists for up to 2 weeks after treatment with MAOIs is discontinued. Patients should also avoid alcoholic drinks or de-alco-holised (low alcohol) drinks.

Other antidepressants should **not** be started for 2 weeks after treatment with MAOIs has been stopped (3 weeks if starting clomipramine or imipramine). Some psychiatrists use selected tricyclics in conjunction with MAOIs but this is hazardous, indeed potentially lethal, except in experienced hands and there is no evidence that the combination is more effective than when either constituent is used alone. The combination of tranyl-cypromine with clomipramine is particularly **dangerous**.

Conversely, an MAOI should not be started until at least 7–14 days after a tricyclic or related antidepressant (3 weeks in the case of clomipramine or imipramine) has been stopped.

In addition, an MAOI should not be started for at least 2 weeks after a previous MAOI has been stopped (then started at a reduced dose).

For other interactions with MAOIs including those with opioid analgesics (notably pethidine), see Appendix 1 (MAOIs). For guidance on interactions relating to the reversible monoamine oxidase inhibitor, moclobemide, see p. 259; for guidance on interactions relating to SSRIs, see p. 260.

PHENELZINE

Indications depressive illness

Cautions diabetes mellitus, cardiovascular disease, epilepsy, blood disorders, concurrent electroconvulsive therapy; elderly (great caution); monitor blood pressure (risk of postural hypotension and hypertensive responses—discontinue if palpitations or frequent headaches); if possible avoid abrupt withdrawal; severe hypertensive reactions to certain drugs and foods—see notes above; avoid in agitated patients; acute porphyria (section 9.8.2); surgery (section 15.1); **interactions:** see notes above and Appendix 1 (MAOIs)

Driving Drowsiness may affect performance of skilled tasks (e.g. driving)

Contra-indications cerebrovascular disease, phaeochromocytoma; not indicated in manic phase

Hepatic impairment avoid in hepatic impairment or if abnormal liver function tests; see also notes above

Pregnancy see notes above

Breast-feeding avoid—no information available

Side-effects commonly postural hypotension (especially in elderly) and dizziness; less common side-effects include drowsiness, insomnia, headache, weakness and fatigue, dry mouth, constipation and other gastro-intestinal disturbances, oedema, myoclonic movement, hyperreflexia, elevated liver enzymes; agitation and tremors, nervousness, euphoria, arrhythmias, blurred vision, nystagmus, difficulty in micturition, sweating, convulsions, rashes, purpura, leucopenia, sexual disturbances, and weight gain with inappropriate appetite may also occur; psychotic episodes with hypomanic behaviour, confusion, and hallucinations may be induced in susceptible persons; suicidal behaviour (see p. 253); jaundice has been reported and, on rare occasions, fatal progressive hepatocellular necrosis; paraesthesia, peripheral neuritis, peripheral neuropathy may be due to pyridoxine deficiency; hyponatraemia (see Hyponatraemia and Antidepressant Therapy, p. 253)

Dose

• 15 mg 3 times daily, increased if necessary to 4 times daily after 2 weeks (hospital patients, max. 30 mg 3 times daily), then reduced gradually to lowest possible maintenance dose (15 mg on alternate days may be adequate); CHILD not recommended

Nardil® (Archimedes) (PoM)

Tablets, orange, f/c, phenelzine (as sulfate) 15 mg, net price 100-tab pack = £22.50. Label: 3, 10, patient information leaflet

◼ ISOCARBOXAZID

Indications depressive illness

Cautions see under Phenelzine

Contra-indications see under Phenelzine

Hepatic impairment avoid in hepatic impairment; see also notes above

Renal impairment use with caution

Pregnancy see notes above

Breast-feeding avoid

Side-effects see under Phenelzine

Dose

• Initially 30 mg daily in single or divided doses until improvement occurs (increased after 4 weeks if necessary to max. 60 mg daily for 4–6 weeks under close supervision), then reduced to usual maintenance dose 10–20 mg daily (but up to 40 mg daily may be required); ELDERLY 5–10 mg daily; CHILD not recommended

Isocarboxazid (Non-proprietary) (PoM)

Tablets, pink, scored, isocarboxazid 10 mg, net price 56-tab pack = £110.33. Label: 3, 10, patient information leaflet

◼ TRANYLCYPROMINE

Indications depressive illness

Cautions see under Phenelzine

Contra-indications see under Phenelzine; hyperthyroidism; congestive heart failure; history of hepatic disease (see below)

Hepatic impairment avoid if history of hepatic disease or if abnormal liver function tests, see also notes above

Pregnancy see notes above

Breast-feeding present in milk in *animal* studies

Side-effects see under Phenelzine; also insomnia; *less commonly* speech disturbances, hypernatraemia, lupus erythematosus-like syndrome; *very rarely* angle-closure glaucoma; hypertensive crises with throbbing headache requiring discontinuation of treatment more frequent than with other MAOIs; liver damage less frequent than with phenelzine; blood dyscrasias also reported

Dose

• Initially 10 mg twice daily not later than 3 p.m., increasing the second daily dose to 20 mg after 1 week if necessary; doses above 30 mg daily under

close supervision only; usual maintenance dose 10 mg daily; CHILD not recommended

Tranylcypromine (Non-proprietary) (PoM)

Tablets, tranylcypromine (as sulfate) 10 mg, net price 28-tab pack = £243.98. Label: 3, 10, patient information leaflet

Reversible MAOIs

Moclobemide is indicated for major depression and social anxiety disorder; it is reported to act by reversible inhibition of monoamine oxidase type A (it is therefore termed a RIMA). It should be reserved as a second-line treatment.

Interactions Moclobemide is claimed to cause less potentiation of the pressor effect of tyramine than the traditional (irreversible) MAOIs, but patients should avoid consuming large amounts of tyramine-rich food (such as mature cheese, yeast extracts and fermented soya bean products).

The risk of drug interactions is also claimed to be less but patients still need to avoid sympathomimetics such as ephedrine and pseudoephedrine. In addition, moclobemide should not be given with another antidepressant. Owing to its short duration of action no treatment-free period is required after it has been stopped but it should not be started until at least a week after a tricyclic or related antidepressant or an SSRI or related antidepressant has been stopped (at least 5 weeks in the case of fluoxetine), or for at least a week after an MAOI has been stopped. For other interactions, see Appendix 1 (moclobemide).

◼ MOCLOBEMIDE

Indications depressive illness; social anxiety disorder

Cautions avoid in agitated or excited patients (or give with sedative for up to 2–3 weeks), thyrotoxicosis, may provoke manic episodes in bipolar disorders; **interactions:** see notes above and Appendix 1 (moclobemide)

Contra-indications acute confusional states, phaeochromocytoma

Hepatic impairment reduce dose in severe disease

Pregnancy see notes above, p. 258

Breast-feeding amount too small to be harmful, but patient information leaflet advises avoid

Side-effects sleep disturbances, dizziness, gastrointestinal disorders, headache, restlessness, agitation; paraesthesia, dry mouth, visual disturbances, oedema, skin reactions, confusional states reported; *rarely* raised liver enzymes, galactorrhoea; hyponatraemia (see Hyponatraemia and Antidepressant Therapy, p. 253)

Dose

• Depression, initially 300 mg daily usually in divided doses after food, adjusted according to response; usual range 150–600 mg daily; CHILD not recommended

• Social anxiety disorder, initially 300 mg daily increased on fourth day to 600 mg daily in 2 divided doses, continued for 8–12 weeks to assess efficacy; CHILD not recommended

Moclobemide (Non-proprietary) (PoM)

Tablets, moclobemide 150 mg, net price 30-tab pack = £20.47; 300 mg, 30-tab pack = £13.99. Label: 10, patient information leaflet, 21

4

Central nervous system

4 Central nervous system

Manerix® (Meda)
Tablets, yellow, f/c, scored, moclobemide 150 mg, net price 30-tab pack = £9.33; 300 mg, 30-tab pack = £13.99. Label: 10, patient information leaflet, 21

4.3.3 Selective serotonin re-uptake inhibitors

Citalopram, escitalopram, fluoxetine, fluvoxamine, paroxetine, and **sertraline** selectively inhibit the re-uptake of serotonin (5-hydroxytryptamine, 5-HT); they are termed selective serotonin re-uptake inhibitors (SSRIs). For a general comment on the management of depression and on the comparison between *tricyclic and related antidepressants* and the *SSRIs and related antidepressants*, see section 4.3.

> **Depressive illness in children and adolescents**
>
> The balance of risks and benefits for the treatment of depressive illness in individuals under 18 years is considered unfavourable for the SSRIs citalopram, escitalopram, paroxetine, and sertraline, and for mirtazapine and venlafaxine. Clinical trials have failed to show efficacy and have shown an increase in harmful outcomes. However, it is recognised that specialists may sometimes decide to use these drugs in response to individual clinical need; children and adolescents should be monitored carefully for suicidal behaviour, self-harm or hostility, particularly at the beginning of treatment.
>
> Only fluoxetine has been shown in clinical trials to be effective for treating depressive illness in children and adolescents. However, it is possible that, in common with the other SSRIs, it is associated with a small risk of self-harm and suicidal thoughts. Overall, the balance of risks and benefits for fluoxetine in the treatment of depressive illness in individuals under 18 years is considered favourable, but children and adolescents must be carefully monitored as above.

Cautions   SSRIs should be used with caution in patients with epilepsy (avoid if poorly controlled, discontinue if convulsions develop), cardiac disease, diabetes mellitus, susceptibility to angle-closure glaucoma, a history of mania or bleeding disorders (especially gastro-intestinal bleeding), and if used with other drugs that increase the risk of bleeding. They should also be used with caution in those receiving concurrent electroconvulsive therapy (prolonged seizures reported with fluoxetine). SSRIs may also impair performance of skilled tasks (e.g. driving, operating machinery). **Interactions:** see below and Appendix 1 (antidepressants, SSRI).

Withdrawal   The risk of withdrawal reactions is higher with paroxetine (see also Withdrawal, section 4.3). Gastro-intestinal disturbances, headache, anxiety, dizziness, paraesthesia, electric shock sensation in the head, neck, and spine, tinnitus, sleep disturbances, fatigue, influenza-like symptoms, and sweating are the most common features of abrupt withdrawal of an SSRI or marked reduction of the dose; palpitation and visual disturbances can occur less commonly. The dose should be tapered over at least a few weeks to avoid these effects. For some patients, it may be necessary to withdraw treatment over a longer period; consider obtaining specialist advice if symptoms persist.

Interactions   An SSRI or related antidepressant should not be started until 2 weeks after stopping an MAOI. Conversely, an MAOI should not be started until at least a week after an SSRI or related antidepressant has been stopped (2 weeks in the case of sertraline, at least 5 weeks in the case of fluoxetine). For guidance relating to the reversible monoamine oxidase inhibitor, moclobemide, see above. For other SSRI antidepressant interactions, see Appendix 1 (antidepressants, SSRI).

Serotonin syndrome   Serotonin syndrome or serotonin toxicity is a relatively uncommon adverse drug reaction caused by excessive central and peripheral serotonergic activity. Onset of symptoms, which range from mild to life-threatening, can occur within hours or days following the initiation, dose escalation, or overdose of a serotonergic drug, the addition of a new serotonergic drug, or the replacement of one serotonergic drug by another without allowing a long enough washout period in-between, particularly when the first drug is an irreversible MAOI or a drug with a long half-life. Severe toxicity, which is a medical emergency, usually occurs with a combination of serotonergic drugs, one of which is generally an MAOI.

The characteristic symptoms of serotonin syndrome fall into 3 main areas, although features from each group may not be seen in all patients—neuromuscular hyperactivity (such as tremor, hyperreflexia, clonus, myoclonus, rigidity), autonomic dysfunction (tachycardia, blood pressure changes, hyperthermia, diaphoresis, shivering, diarrhoea), and altered mental state (agitation, confusion, mania).

Treatment consists of withdrawal of the serotonergic medication and supportive care; specialist advice should be sought; see also Emergency Treatment of Poisoning, p. 39.

Contra-indications   SSRIs should not be used if the patient enters a manic phase.

Pregnancy   Manufacturers advise that SSRIs should not be used during pregnancy unless the potential benefit outweighs the risk. There is a small increased risk of congenital heart defects when SSRIs are taken during early pregnancy. If SSRIs are used during the third trimester there is a risk of neonatal withdrawal symptoms, and persistent pulmonary hypertension in the newborn has been reported; see also individual monographs.

Side-effects   SSRIs are less sedating and have fewer antimuscarinic and cardiotoxic effects than tricyclic antidepressants (section 4.3.1). Side-effects of the SSRIs include gastro-intestinal effects (dose-related and fairly common—include nausea, vomiting, dyspepsia, abdominal pain, diarrhoea, constipation), anorexia with weight loss (increased appetite and weight gain also reported) and hypersensitivity reactions including rash (consider discontinuation—may be sign of impending serious systemic reaction, possibly associated with vasculitis); urticaria, angioedema, anaphylaxis, arthralgia, myalgia and photosensitivity; other side-effects include dry mouth, nervousness, anxiety, headache, insomnia, tremor, dizziness, asthenia, hallucinations, drowsiness, convulsions (see Cautions above), galactorrhoea, sexual dysfunction, urinary retention, sweating, hypomania or mania (see Cautions above), movement disorders and dyskinesias, visual disturbances, hyponatraemia (see Hyponatraemia and Antidepressant Therapy, p. 253), and bleeding disorders including ecchymoses and purpura. Suicidal behaviour has been linked with antidepressants (see p. 253). Angle-closure glaucoma may very rarely be precipitated by treatment with SSRIs.

Overdosage: for advice on overdosage with SSRIs see Emergency Treatment of Poisoning, p. 38

CITALOPRAM

Indications depressive illness, panic disorder

Cautions see notes above; susceptibility to QT-interval prolongation

Contra-indications see notes above; QT-interval prolongation (avoid concomitant administration of drugs that prolong QT interval)

Hepatic impairment use doses at lower end of range; for *tablets* up to max. 20 mg; for *oral solution* up to max. 16 mg

Renal impairment no information available for eGFR less than 20 mL/minute/1.73 m^2

Pregnancy see notes above

Breast-feeding present in milk—use with caution

Side-effects see notes above; also hepatitis, palpitation, tachycardia, oedema, bradycardia, postural hypotension, haemorrhage, QT-interval prolongation, coughing, yawning, confusion, impaired concentration, aggression, malaise, amnesia, migraine, paraesthesia, abnormal dreams, euphoria, mydriasis, taste disturbance, increased salivation, rhinitis, tinnitus, polyuria, micturition disorders, hypokalaemia, pruritus; paradoxical increased anxiety during initial treatment of panic disorder (reduce dose)

Dose

- By mouth as tablets, depressive illness, 20 mg once daily increased if necessary in steps of 20 mg daily at intervals of 3–4 weeks; max. 40 mg daily (ELDERLY over 65 years, max. 20 mg daily); CHILD under 18 years see *BNF for Children* and Depressive Illness in Children and Adolescents, p. 260

  Panic disorder, ADULT over 18 years, initially 10 mg daily increased gradually if necessary in steps of 10 mg daily, usual dose 20–30 mg daily; max. 40 mg daily (ELDERLY over 65 years, max. 20 mg daily)

- By mouth as oral drops, depressive illness, 16 mg daily as a single dose increased if necessary in steps of 16 mg daily at intervals of 3–4 weeks; max. 32 mg daily (ELDERLY over 65 years, max. 16 mg daily); CHILD under 18 years see *BNF for Children* and Depressive Illness in Children and Adolescents, p. 260

  Panic disorder, ADULT over 18 years, initially 8 mg daily as a single dose increased gradually if necessary in steps of 8 mg, usual dose 16–24 mg daily; max. 32 mg daily (ELDERLY over 65 years, max. 16 mg daily)

Citalopram (Non-proprietary) ꟼⓄⓂ

Tablets, citalopram (as hydrobromide) 10 mg, net price 28-tab pack = £1.04; 20 mg, 28-tab pack = £1.10; 40 mg, 28-tab pack = £1.28. Counselling, driving

Oral drops, citalopram (as hydrochloride) 40 mg/mL, net price 15 mL = £7.20. Counselling, driving, administration

Note 4 drops (8 mg) is equivalent in therapeutic effect to 10-mg tablet

Cipramil® (Lundbeck) ꟼⓄⓂ

Tablets, f/c, citalopram (as hydrobromide), 20 mg (scored), net price 28-tab pack = £8.95. Counselling, driving

Oral drops, sugar-free, citalopram (as hydrochloride) 40 mg/mL, net price 15 mL = £10.08. Counselling, driving, administration

Excipients include alcohol

Note 4 drops (8 mg) is equivalent in therapeutic effect to 10-mg tablet

Mix with water, orange juice, or apple juice before taking

ESCITALOPRAM

Note Escitalopram is the active enantiomer of citalopram

Indications see under Dose

Cautions see notes above; susceptibility to QT-interval prolongation

Contra-indications see notes above; QT-interval prolongation (avoid concomitant administration of drugs that prolong QT interval)

Hepatic impairment initial dose 5 mg daily for 2 weeks, thereafter increased to max. 10 mg daily according to response; particular caution in severe impairment

Renal impairment caution if eGFR less than 30 mL/minute/1.73 m^2

Pregnancy see notes above

Breast-feeding present in milk; avoid

Side-effects see notes above; also sinusitis, yawning; fatigue, restlessness, abnormal dreams, paraesthesia; pyrexia; *less commonly* taste disturbance, bruxism, syncope, tachycardia, oedema, confusion, menstrual disturbances, epistaxis, mydriasis, tinnitus, pruritus, and alopecia; *rarely* bradycardia, aggression, and depersonalisation; hepatitis, postural hypotension, QT interval prolongation, and thrombocytopenia also reported; paradoxical increased anxiety during initial treatment of panic disorder (reduce dose)

Dose

- ADULT over 18 years, depressive illness, generalised anxiety disorder, and obsessive-compulsive disorder, 10 mg once daily increased if necessary to max. 20 mg daily; ELDERLY over 65 years, initially half adult dose; max. 10 mg daily; CHILD not recommended (see Depressive Illness in Children and Adolescents, p. 260)

- ADULT over 18 years, panic disorder, initially 5 mg once daily increased to 10 mg daily after 7 days; max. 20 mg daily; ELDERLY over 65 years, initially half adult dose; max. 10 mg daily

- ADULT over 18 years, social anxiety disorder, initially 10 mg once daily adjusted after 2–4 weeks; usual dose 5–20 mg daily; ELDERLY over 65 years, not recommended

Cipralex® (Lundbeck) ꟼⓄⓂ

Tablets, f/c, escitalopram (as oxalate) 5 mg, net price 28-tab pack = £8.97; 10 mg (scored), 28-tab pack = £14.91; 20 mg (scored), 28-tab pack = £25.20. Counselling, driving

Oral drops, sugar-free, escitalopram (as oxalate) 20 mg/mL (1 mg/drop), net price 15 mL = £20.16. Counselling, driving, administration

Note Can be mixed with water, orange juice, or apple juice before taking

Central nervous system   4

FLUOXETINE

Indications see under Dose

Cautions see notes above

Contra-indications see notes above

Hepatic impairment reduce dose or increase dose interval

Pregnancy see notes above

Breast-feeding present in milk—avoid

Side-effects see notes above; also diarrhoea, dysphagia, vasodilatation, hypotension, flushing, palpitation, pharyngitis, dyspnoea, chills, taste disturbance, sleep disturbances, malaise, euphoria, confusion, yawning, impaired concentration, changes in blood sugar, alopecia, urinary frequency; haemorrhage, pulmonary inflammation and fibrosis, hepatitis, toxic epidermal necrolysis, priapism, and neuroleptic malignant syndrome-like event also reported

Dose

- Major depression, 20 mg daily increased after 3–4 weeks if necessary, and at appropriate intervals thereafter; max. 60 mg daily (ELDERLY usual max. 40 mg daily but 60 mg can be used); CHILD 8–18 years, 10 mg daily increased after 1–2 weeks if necessary, max. 20 mg daily (but see also Depressive Illness in Children and Adolescents, p. 260)
- Bulimia nervosa, ADULT over 18 years, 60 mg daily as a single or divided dose (ELDERLY usual max. 40 mg daily but 60 mg can be used)
- Obsessive-compulsive disorder, ADULT over 18 years, 20 mg daily; increased gradually if necessary to max. 60 mg daily (ELDERLY usual max. 40 mg daily but 60 mg can be used); review treatment if inadequate response after 10 weeks

Note Daily dose may be administered as a single or divided dose

Long duration of action Consider the long half-life of fluoxetine when adjusting dosage (or in overdosage)

Fluoxetine (Non-proprietary) ℞

Capsules, fluoxetine (as hydrochloride) 20 mg, net price 30-cap pack = £1.09; 60 mg, 30-cap pack = £27.97. Counselling, driving
Brands include *Oxactin*®

Liquid, fluoxetine (as hydrochloride) 20 mg/5 mL, net price 70 mL = £3.55. Counselling, driving
Brands include *Prozep*®

Olena® (AMCo) ℞

Dispersible tablets, scored, fluoxetine (as hydrochloride) 20 mg, net price 28-tab pack = £3.44.
Label: 10, counselling, administration, see below, driving
Counselling Tablets can be dispersed in water for administration or swallowed whole with plenty of water

Prozac® (Lilly) ℞

Capsules, fluoxetine (as hydrochloride) 20 mg (green/yellow), net price 30-cap pack = £1.50 Counselling, driving

Liquid, fluoxetine (as hydrochloride) 20 mg/5 mL, net price 70 mL = £11.12. Counselling, driving

FLUVOXAMINE MALEATE

Indications depressive illness, obsessive-compulsive disorder

Cautions see notes above

Contra-indications see notes above

Hepatic impairment start with low dose

Renal impairment start with low dose

Pregnancy see notes above

Breast-feeding present in milk—avoid

Side-effects see notes above; palpitation, tachycardia, malaise; *less commonly* postural hypotension, confusion, ataxia; *rarely* abnormal liver function, usually symptomatic (discontinue treatment); *also reported* paraesthesia, taste disturbance, neuroleptic malignant syndrome-like event

Dose

- Depression, ADULT over 18 years, initially 50–100 mg daily in the evening, increased gradually if necessary to max. 300 mg daily (over 150 mg in divided doses); usual maintenance dose 100 mg daily
- Obsessive-compulsive disorder, initially 50 mg in the evening increased gradually if necessary after some weeks to max. 300 mg daily (over 150 mg in divided doses); usual maintenance dose 100–300 mg daily; CHILD over 8 years initially 25 mg daily increased if necessary in steps of 25 mg every 4–7 days to max. 200 mg daily (over 50 mg in 2 divided doses)

Note If no improvement in obsessive-compulsive disorder within 10 weeks, treatment should be reconsidered

Fluvoxamine (Non-proprietary) ℞

Tablets, fluvoxamine maleate 50 mg, net price 60-tab pack = £16.93; 100 mg, 30-tab pack = £16.93. Counselling, driving

Faverin® (Abbott Healthcare) ℞

Tablets, f/c, scored, fluvoxamine maleate 50 mg, net price 60-tab pack = £17.10; 100 mg, 30-tab pack = £17.10. Counselling, driving

PAROXETINE

Indications major depression, obsessive-compulsive disorder, panic disorder; social anxiety disorder; post-traumatic stress disorder; generalised anxiety disorder

Cautions see notes above; also achlorhydria or high gastric pH (reduced absorption of oral suspension)

Contra-indications see notes above

Hepatic impairment reduce dose

Renal impairment reduce dose if eGFR less than 30 mL/minute/1.73 m^2

Pregnancy increased risk of congenital malformations, especially if used in the first trimester; see also notes above

Breast-feeding present in milk but amount too small to be harmful

Side-effects see notes above; also yawning; abnormal dreams; raised cholesterol; *less commonly* arrhythmias, confusion, urinary incontinence; *rarely* panic attacks and paradoxical increased anxiety during initial treatment of panic disorder (reduce dose), depersonalisation, and neuroleptic malignant syndrome-like event; *rarely* restless legs syndrome; *very rarely* peripheral oedema, acute glaucoma, hepatic disorders (e.g. hepatitis), and priapism; *also reported* tinnitus, extrapyramidal reactions (including orofacial dystonias) and withdrawal reactions (see notes above)

Dose

- Major depression, social anxiety disorder, post-traumatic stress disorder, generalised anxiety disorder, ADULT over 18 years, recommended dose 20 mg each morning (no evidence of greater efficacy at higher doses); max. 50 mg daily (ELDERLY 40 mg daily); CHILD under 18 years not recommended (see Depressive Illness in Children and Adolescents, p. 260)

- Obsessive-compulsive disorder, ADULT over 18 years, initially 20 mg each morning, increased gradually in steps of 10 mg to recommended dose of 40 mg daily (no evidence of greater efficacy at higher doses); max. 60 mg daily (ELDERLY 40 mg daily)
- Panic disorder, ADULT over 18 years, initially 10 mg each morning, increased gradually in steps of 10 mg to recommended dose of 40 mg daily (no evidence of greater efficacy at higher doses); max. 60 mg daily (ELDERLY 40 mg daily)

Paroxetine (Non-proprietary) [PoM]
Tablets, paroxetine (as hydrochloride) 20 mg, net price 30-tab pack = £1.89; 30 mg, 30-tab pack = £1.87. Label: 21, counselling, driving

Seroxat® (GSK) [PoM]
Tablets, f/c, scored, paroxetine (as hydrochloride) 10 mg, net price 28-tab pack = £14.21; 20 mg, 30-tab pack = £15.23; 30 mg (blue), 30-tab pack = £26.74. Label: 21, counselling, driving
Oral suspension, orange, sugar-free, paroxetine (as hydrochloride) 10 mg/5 mL, net price 150-mL pack = £9.12. Label: 5, 21, counselling, driving

SERTRALINE

Indications   see under Dose
Cautions   see notes above
Contra-indications   see notes above
Hepatic impairment   reduce dose or increase dose interval in mild or moderate impairment; avoid in severe impairment
Renal impairment   use with caution
Pregnancy   see notes above
Breast-feeding   not known to be harmful but consider discontinuing breast-feeding
Side-effects   see notes above; pancreatitis, hepatitis, jaundice, liver failure, stomatitis, palpitation, hypertension, hypercholesterolaemia, tachycardia, postural hypotension, bronchospasm, amnesia, paraesthesia, aggression, hypoglycaemia, hypothyroidism, hyperprolactinaemia, urinary incontinence, menstrual irregularities, leucopenia, and tinnitus also reported

Dose

- Depressive illness, initially 50 mg daily, increased if necessary by increments of 50 mg at intervals of at least 1 week to max. 200 mg daily; usual maintenance dose 50 mg daily; CHILD under 18 years see *BNF for Children* and Depressive Illness in Children and Adolescents, p. 260
- Obsessive-compulsive disorder, ADULT and CHILD over 12 years initially 50 mg daily, increased if necessary in steps of 50 mg at intervals of at least 1 week; max. 200 mg daily; CHILD 6–12 years initially 25 mg daily, increased to 50 mg daily after 1 week, further increased if necessary in steps of 50 mg at intervals of at least 1 week; max. 200 mg daily
- Panic disorder, post-traumatic stress disorder, or social anxiety disorder, ADULT over 18 years, initially 25 mg daily, increased after 1 week to 50 mg daily; if response is partial and if drug tolerated, dose increased in steps of 50 mg at intervals of at least 1 week to max. 200 mg daily

Sertraline (Non-proprietary) [PoM]
Tablets, sertraline (as hydrochloride) 50 mg, net price 28-tab pack = £1.75; 100 mg, 28-tab pack = £2.15. Counselling, driving

Lustral® (Pfizer) [PoM]
Tablets, f/c, sertraline (as hydrochloride) 50 mg (scored), net price 28-tab pack = £17.82; 100 mg, 28-tab pack = £29.16. Counselling, driving

4.3.4   Other antidepressant drugs

Agomelatine is a melatonin receptor agonist and a selective serotonin-receptor antagonist; it does not affect the uptake of serotonin, noradrenaline, or dopamine.

Duloxetine inhibits the re-uptake of both serotonin and noradrenaline and is licensed to treat major depressive disorder.

The thioxanthene **flupentixol** (*Fluanxol*®) has antidepressant properties when given by mouth in low doses. Flupentixol is also used for the treatment of psychoses (section 4.2.1 and section 4.2.2)

Mirtazapine, a presynaptic alpha$_2$-adrenoreceptor antagonist, increases central noradrenergic and serotonergic neurotransmission. It has few antimuscarinic effects, but causes sedation during initial treatment.

Reboxetine, a selective inhibitor of noradrenaline re-uptake, has been introduced for the treatment of depressive illness.

Venlafaxine is a serotonin and noradrenaline re-uptake inhibitor; it lacks the sedative and antimuscarinic effects of the tricyclic antidepressants. Treatment with venlafaxine is associated with a higher risk of withdrawal effects compared with other antidepressants.

AGOMELATINE

Indications   major depression
Cautions   bipolar disorder, mania or hypomania; concomitant use of drugs associated with hepatic injury; excessive alcohol consumption; obesity; diabetes; non-alcoholic fatty liver disease; dose adjustment may be necessary if smoking started or stopped during treatment; **interactions**: Appendix 1 (agomelatine)
Hepatotoxicity Hepatic injury, including hepatitis and hepatic failure reported rarely; test liver function before treatment (do not start if serum transaminases exceed 3 times the upper limit of reference range), and after 3, 6, 12 and 24 weeks of treatment, and then regularly thereafter when clinically indicated (restart monitoring schedule if dose increased); discontinue if serum transaminases exceed 3 times the upper limit of reference range or symptoms of liver disorder (counselling, see below)
Counselling Patients should be given a booklet with more information on the risk of hepatic side-effects, told how to recognise signs of liver disorder, and advised to seek immediate medical attention if symptoms such as dark urine, light coloured stools, jaundice, bruising, fatigue, abdominal pain, or pruritus develop
Contra-indications   dementia; patients over 75 years of age; see also Hepatotoxicity above
Hepatic impairment   avoid
Renal impairment   caution in moderate to severe impairment
Pregnancy   manufacturer advises avoid
Breast-feeding   avoid—present in milk in *animal* studies

4

Central nervous system

Side-effects nausea, vomiting, diarrhoea, constipation, abdominal pain, increased serum transaminases (see Hepatoxicity above), headache, dizziness, drowsiness, agitation, sleep disturbances, fatigue, anxiety, back pain, sweating; *less commonly* paraesthesia, restless legs syndrome, blurred vision, tinnitus, eczema; *rarely* hepatitis, hepatic failure (see Hepatotoxicity above), weight changes, rash; suicidal behaviour (see Suicidal Behaviour and Antidepressant Therapy, p. 253) and pruritus also reported

Dose

- ADULT over 18 years, 25 mg at bedtime, increased if necessary after 2 weeks to 50 mg at bedtime

Valdoxan® (Servier) [PoM]

Tablets, orange-yellow, f/c, agomelatine 25 mg, net price 28-tab pack = £30.00

▌ DULOXETINE

Indications major depressive disorder; generalised anxiety disorder; diabetic neuropathy (section 6.1.5); stress urinary incontinence (section 7.4.2)

Cautions section 7.4.2

Contra-indications section 7.4.2

Hepatic impairment section 7.4.2

Renal impairment section 7.4.2

Pregnancy toxicity in *animal* studies—use only if potential benefit outweighs risk; risk of neonatal withdrawal symptoms if used near term

Breast-feeding section 7.4.2

Side-effects section 7.4.2

Dose

- Major depression, ADULT over 18 years, 60 mg once daily
- Generalised anxiety disorder, ADULT over 18 years, initially 30 mg daily, increased if necessary to 60 mg once daily; max. 120 mg daily
- Diabetic neuropathy, ADULT over 18 years, 60 mg once daily; max. 120 mg daily in divided doses

Note In diabetic neuropathy, discontinue if inadequate response after 2 months; review treatment at least every 3 months

Cymbalta® (Lilly) [PoM]

Capsules, duloxetine (as hydrochloride) 30 mg (white/blue), net price 28-cap pack = £22.40; 60 mg (green/blue), 28-cap pack = £27.72. Label: 2

Note The *Scottish Medicines Consortium* has advised (September 2006) that duloxetine (*Cymbalta*®) should be restricted for use by specialists when other treatments for diabetic peripheral neuropathic pain are unsuitable or inadequate

Yentreve® (Lilly) [PoM]

Section 7.4.2 (stress urinary incontinence)

▌ FLUPENTIXOL

(Flupenthixol)

Indications depressive illness; psychoses (section 4.2.1)

Cautions cardiovascular disease (including cardiac disorders and cerebral arteriosclerosis), QT-interval prolongation (avoid concomitant administration of drugs that prolong QT interval); diabetes; senile confusional states, parkinsonism; elderly; acute porphyria (section 9.8.2); see also section 4.2.1; **interactions**: Appendix 1 (antipsychotics)

Contra-indications excitable and overactive patients; impaired consciousness; circulatory collapse; coma

Hepatic impairment can precipitate coma; consider serum-flupentixol concentration monitoring

Renal impairment increased cerebral sensitivity in severe impairment; manufacturer advises caution in renal failure

Pregnancy avoid unless potential benefit outweighs risk

Breast-feeding present in milk—avoid

Side-effects section 4.2.1; also hypersalivation, dyspnoea, asthenia, hyperglycaemia, myalgia; torsade de pointes and sudden death also reported

Dose

- ADULT over 18 years, initially 1 mg (ELDERLY 500 micrograms) in the morning, increased after 1 week to 2 mg (ELDERLY 1 mg) if necessary; max. 3 mg (ELDERLY 1.5 mg) daily, doses above 2 mg (ELDERLY 1 mg) in divided doses, last dose before 4 pm; discontinue if no response after 1 week at max. dosage

Counselling Although drowsiness may occur, can also have an alerting effect so should not be taken in the evening

Fluanxol® (Lundbeck) [PoM]

Tablets, yellow, s/c, flupentixol (as dihydrochloride) 500 micrograms, net price 60-tab pack = £2.88; 1 mg, 60-tab pack = £4.86. Label: 2, counselling, administration

Depixol® (Lundbeck) [PoM]

Section 4.2.1 (psychoses)

▌ MIRTAZAPINE

Indications major depression

Cautions elderly, cardiac disorders, hypotension, history of urinary retention, susceptibility to angle-closure glaucoma, diabetes mellitus, psychoses (may aggravate psychotic symptoms), history of seizures or bipolar depression; **interactions**: Appendix 1 (mirtazapine)

Blood disorders Patients should be advised to report any fever, sore throat, stomatitis or other signs of infection during treatment. Blood count should be performed and the drug stopped immediately if blood dyscrasia suspected

Withdrawal Nausea, vomiting, dizziness, agitation, anxiety, and headache are most common features of withdrawal if treatment stopped abruptly or if dose reduced markedly; dose should be reduced over several weeks

Hepatic impairment use with caution; discontinue if jaundice occurs

Renal impairment clearance reduced by 30% if eGFR less than 40 mL/minute/1.73 m^2; clearance reduced by 50% if eGFR less than 10 mL/minute/1.73 m^2

Pregnancy use with caution—limited experience; monitor neonate for withdrawal effects

Breast-feeding present in milk; use only if potential benefit outweighs risk

Side-effects increased appetite, weight gain, dry mouth, postural hypotension, oedema, drowsiness, fatigue, tremor, dizziness, abnormal dreams, confusion, anxiety, insomnia, arthralgia, myalgia *less commonly* syncope, mania, hallucinations, movement disorders; *rarely* pancreatitis, aggression, myoclonus; *also reported* hypersalivation, dysarthria, convulsions, suicidal behaviour (see Suicidal Behaviour and Antidepressant Therapy, p. 253), blood disorders (see Cautions), hyponatraemia (see Hyponatraemia and Antidepressant Therapy, p. 253), inappropriate secretion of antidiuretic hormone, angle-closure glaucoma, Stevens-Johnson syndrome, toxic epidermal necrolysis

Dose

- Initially 15–30 mg daily at bedtime increased within 2–4 weeks according to response; max. 45 mg daily as a single dose at bedtime or in 2 divided doses; CHILD under 18 years not recommended (see Depressive Illness in Children and Adolescents, p. 260)

Mirtazapine (Non-proprietary) [PoM]

Tablets, mirtazapine 15 mg, net price 28-tab pack = £1.94; 30 mg, 28-tab pack = £1.67; 45 mg, 28-tab pack = £2.24. Label: 2, 25

Orodispersible tablets, mirtazapine 15 mg, net price 30-tab pack = £1.67; 30 mg, 30-tab pack = £1.79; 45 mg, 30-tab pack = £2.36. Label: 2, counselling, administration

Oral solution, mirtazapine 15 mg/mL, net price 66 mL = £47.19. Label: 2

Zispin SolTab® (MSD) [PoM]

Orodispersible tablets, mirtazapine 15 mg, net price 6-tab pack = £3.84, 30-tab pack = £15.06; 30 mg, 30-tab pack = £15.06; 45 mg, 30-tab pack = £15.06. Label: 2, counselling, administration

Excipients include aspartame (section 9.4.1)

Counselling *Zispin SolTab®* should be placed on the tongue, allowed to disperse and swallowed

REBOXETINE

Indications major depression

Cautions history of cardiovascular disease and epilepsy; bipolar disorder; urinary retention; prostatic hypertrophy; susceptibility to angle-closure glaucoma; avoid abrupt withdrawal; **interactions:** Appendix 1 (reboxetine)

Hepatic impairment initial dose 2 mg twice daily, increased according to tolerance

Renal impairment initial dose 2 mg twice daily, increased according to tolerance

Pregnancy use only if potential benefit outweighs risk—limited information available

Breast-feeding small amount present in milk—use only if potential benefit outweighs risk

Side-effects nausea, dry mouth, constipation, anorexia; tachycardia, palpitation, vasodilation, postural hypotension; headache, insomnia, dizziness; chills; impotence; urinary retention; impaired visual accommodation; sweating; lowering of plasma-potassium concentration on prolonged administration in the elderly; *very rarely* angle-closure glaucoma; *also reported* vomiting, hypertension, paraesthesia, agitation, anxiety, irritability, hallucinations, aggression, Raynaud's syndrome, hyponatraemia, testicular pain, cold extremities, and rash; suicidal behaviour (see p. 253)

Dose

- 4 mg twice daily increased if necessary after 3–4 weeks to 10 mg daily in divided doses, max. 12 mg daily; CHILD under 18 years and ELDERLY not recommended

Edronax® (Pharmacia) [PoM]

Tablets, scored, reboxetine (as mesilate) 4 mg, net price 60-tab pack = £18.91. Counselling, driving

VENLAFAXINE

Indications major depression, generalised anxiety disorder

Cautions heart disease (monitor blood pressure); diabetes; history of epilepsy; history or family history of mania; susceptibility to angle-closure glaucoma; concomitant use of drugs that increase risk of bleeding, history of bleeding disorders; **interactions:** Appendix 1 (venlafaxine)

Driving May affect performance of skilled tasks (e.g. driving)

Withdrawal Gastro-intestinal disturbances, headache, anxiety, dizziness, paraesthesia, tremor, sleep disturbances, and sweating are most common features of withdrawal if treatment stopped abruptly or if dose reduced markedly; dose should be reduced over several weeks

Contra-indications conditions associated with high risk of cardiac arrhythmia, uncontrolled hypertension

Hepatic impairment consider reducing dose by 50% in mild or moderate impairment; use with caution and reduce dose by at least 50% in severe impairment

Renal impairment use with caution; use half normal dose (immediate-release tablets may be given once daily) if eGFR less than 30 mL/minute/1.73 m^2

Pregnancy avoid unless potential benefit outweighs risk—toxicity in *animal* studies; risk of withdrawal effects in neonate

Breast-feeding present in milk—avoid

Side-effects constipation, nausea, anorexia, weight changes, vomiting; hypertension, palpitation, vasodilatation, changes in serum cholesterol; chills, yawning; dizziness, dry mouth, insomnia, nervousness, drowsiness, asthenia, headache, abnormal dreams, anxiety, confusion, hypertonia, sensory disturbances, tremor, difficulty with micturition, sexual dysfunction, menstrual disturbances; visual disturbances, mydriasis (*very rarely* angle-closure glaucoma); sweating; *less commonly* bruxism, diarrhoea, taste disturbance, postural hypotension, arrhythmias, agitation, apathy, incoordination, hallucinations, myoclonus, angioedema, urinary retention, bleeding disorders (including ecchymosis and gastro-intestinal haemorrhage), tinnitus, alopecia, photosensitivity, and rash; *rarely* mania, hypomania, seizures, extrapyramidal symptoms including akathisia, urinary incontinence; *also reported* hepatitis, pancreatitis, hypotension, QT-interval prolongation, aggression, neuroleptic malignant syndrome, delirium, vertigo, syndrome of inappropriate anti-diuretic hormone secretion (see Hyponatraemia and Antidepressant Therapy, p. 253), hyperprolactinaemia, blood dyscrasias, rhabdomyolysis, pruritus, urticaria, Stevens-Johnson syndrome; suicidal behaviour (see p. 253)

Dose

- Depression, ADULT over 18 years, initially 75 mg daily in 2 divided doses increased if necessary at intervals of at least 2 weeks; max. 375 mg daily; CHILD under 18 years not recommended (see Depressive Illness in Children and Adolescents, p. 260)

Note Faster dose titration may be necessary in some patients

- Generalised anxiety disorder and social anxiety disorder, see under preparations below

Venlafaxine (Non-proprietary) [PoM]

Tablets, venlafaxine (as hydrochloride) 37.5 mg, net price 56-tab pack = £2.32; 75 mg, 56-tab pack = £2.59. Label: 3, counselling, driving

◢**Modified release**

Venlafaxine m/r preparations PoM

Capsules, m/r, venlafaxine (as hydrochloride) 75 mg; 150 mg. Label: 3, 21, 25, counselling, driving
Brands include *Alventa XL®, Bonilux XL®, Depefex® XL, Foraven XL®, Politid XL®, Ranfaxine XL®, Tifaxin XL®, Venaxx XL®, Vensir XL®, Winfex® XL*
Dose depression, ADULT over 18 years, 75 mg once daily, increased if necessary at intervals of at least 2 weeks; max. 375 mg once daily; CHILD under 18 years not recommended (see Depressive Illness in Children and Adolescents, p. 260)
Note Faster dose titration may be necessary in some patients

Generalised anxiety disorder, ADULT over 18 years, 75 mg once daily, increased if necessary at intervals of at least 2 weeks; max. 225 mg once daily

Social anxiety disorder, ADULT over 18 years, recommended dose 75 mg once daily (no evidence of greater efficacy at higher doses); dose may be increased at intervals of at least 2 weeks; max. 225 mg once daily

Tablets, m/r, venlafaxine (as hydrochloride) 37.5 mg; 75 mg; 150 mg; 225 mg. Label: 3, 21, 25, counselling, driving
Brands include *Venlalic® XL*
Dose depression, ADULT over 18 years, 75 mg once daily, increased if necessary at intervals of at least 2 weeks; max. 375 mg once daily; CHILD under 18 years not recommended (see Depressive Illness in Children and Adolescents, p. 260)
Note Faster dose titration may be necessary in some patients

Efexor® XL (Pfizer) PoM

Capsules, m/r, venlafaxine (as hydrochloride) 75 mg (peach), net price 28-cap pack = £22.08; 150 mg (orange), 28-cap pack = £36.81. Label: 3, 21, 25, counselling, driving
Dose depression, ADULT over 18 years, 75 mg once daily, increased if necessary at intervals of at least 2 weeks; max. 375 mg once daily; CHILD under 18 years not recommended (see Depressive Illness in Children and Adolescents, p. 260)
Note Faster dose titration may be necessary in some patients

Generalised anxiety disorder, ADULT over 18 years, 75 mg once daily, increased if necessary at intervals of at least 2 weeks; max. 225 mg once daily

Social anxiety disorder, ADULT over 18 years, recommended dose 75 mg once daily (no evidence of greater efficacy at higher doses); dose may be increased at intervals of at least 2 weeks; max. 225 mg once daily

4.4 CNS stimulants and drugs used for attention deficit hyperactivity disorder

Central nervous system stimulants include the **amfetamines** (dexamfetamine and lisdexamfetamine) **and related drugs** (e.g. methylphenidate). They have very few indications and in particular, should **not** be used to treat depression, obesity, senility, debility, or for relief of fatigue.

CNS stimulants should be prescribed for children with severe and persistent symptoms of *attention deficit hyperactivity disorder* (ADHD), when the diagnosis has been confirmed by a specialist; children with moderate symptoms of ADHD can be treated with CNS stimulants when psychological interventions have been unsuccessful or are unavailable. Prescribing of CNS stimulants may be continued by general practitioners, under a shared-care arrangement. Treatment of ADHD often needs to be continued into adolescence, and may need to be continued into adulthood.

Drug treatment of ADHD should be part of a comprehensive treatment programme. The choice of medication should take into consideration co-morbid conditions (such as tic disorders, Tourette syndrome, and epilepsy), the adverse effect profile, potential for drug misuse, tolerance and dependance; and preferences of the patient and carers. **Methylphenidate** and **atomoxetine** are used for the management of ADHD; **dexamfetamine** and **lisdexamfetamine** are an alternative in children who do not respond to these drugs. Pulse, blood pressure, psychiatric symptoms, appetite, weight and height should be recorded at initiation of therapy, following each dose adjustment, and at least every 6 months thereafter.

The need to continue drug treatment for ADHD should be reviewed at least annually. This may involve suspending treatment.

Modafinil is used for the treatment of excessive sleepiness associated with narcolepsy with or without cataplexy; dependence with long-term use cannot be excluded and it should therefore be used with caution.

Dexamfetamine and methylphenidate [unlicensed indication] are also used to treat narcolepsy.

▶ ATOMOXETINE

Indications attention deficit hyperactivity disorder (initiated by a specialist physician experienced in managing the condition)

Cautions see notes above; also cardiovascular disease including hypertension and tachycardia (avoid in severe cardiovascular disease); structural cardiac abnormalities; QT-interval prolongation (avoid concomitant use of drugs that prolong QT interval); cerebrovascular disease (avoid in severe cerebrovascular disease); psychosis or mania; monitor for appearance or worsening of anxiety, depression or tics; history of seizures; aggressive behaviour, hostility, or emotional lability; susceptibility to angle-closure glaucoma; **interactions**: Appendix 1 (atomoxetine)
Hepatic disorders Following rare reports of hepatic disorders, patients and carers should be advised of the risk and be told how to recognise symptoms; prompt medical attention should be sought in case of abdominal pain, unexplained nausea, malaise, darkening of the urine, or jaundice
Suicidal ideation Following reports of suicidal thoughts and behaviour, patients and their carers should be informed about the risk and told to report clinical worsening, suicidal thoughts or behaviour, irritability, agitation, or depression

Contra-indications phaeochromocytoma

Hepatic impairment halve dose in moderate impairment; quarter dose in severe impairment; see also Hepatic Disorders above

Pregnancy manufacturer advises avoid unless potential benefit outweighs risk

Breast-feeding avoid—present in milk in *animal* studies

Side-effects anorexia, dry mouth, nausea, vomiting, abdominal pain, constipation, dyspepsia, flatulence, palpitation, tachycardia, increased blood pressure, flushing, sleep disturbances, dizziness, headache, malaise, lethargy, drowsiness, anxiety, depression, irritability, taste disturbances, paraesthesia, tremor, chills, urinary dysfunction, prostatitis, sexual dysfunction, mydriasis, dermatitis, rash, sweating; *less commonly* QT-interval prolongation, syncope, suicidal ideation (see Suicidal Ideation, above), aggression, hostility, emotional lability, tics, psychosis, hypoaesthesia, cold extremities, menstrual disturbances, muscle spasms, pruritus; *rarely* seizures, Raynaud's phenomenon; *very rarely* hepatic disorders (see Hepatic Disorders, above), angle-closure glaucoma

Dose

- ADULT over 18 years, body-weight over 70 kg, initially 40 mg daily for 7 days, increased according to response; usual maintenance 80–100 mg daily, but may be increased to max. 120 mg daily [unlicensed] under the direction of a specialist; CHILD 6–18 years, body-weight over 70 kg, initially 40 mg daily for 7 days, increased according to response; usual maintenance 80 mg daily, but may be increased to max. 120 mg daily [unlicensed] under the direction of a specialist; ADULT and CHILD over 6 years, body-weight under 70 kg, initially 500 micrograms/kg daily for 7 days, increased according to response; usual maintenance 1.2 mg/kg daily, but may be increased to 1.8 mg/kg daily (max. 120 mg daily) [unlicensed] under the direction of a specialist

Note Total daily dose may be given *either* as a single dose in the morning *or* in 2 divided doses with last dose no later than early evening

Note Atomoxetine doses in BNF may differ from those in product literature

Strattera® (Lilly) PoM

Capsules, atomoxetine (as hydrochloride) 10 mg (white), net price 7-cap pack = £15.62, 28-cap pack = £62.46; 18 mg (gold/white), 7-cap pack = £15.62, 28-cap pack = £62.46; 25 mg (blue/white), 7-cap pack = £15.62, 28-cap pack = £62.46; 40 mg (blue), 7-cap pack = £15.62, 28-cap pack = £62.46; 60 mg (blue/gold), 28-cap pack = £62.46; 80 mg (brown/white), 28-cap pack = £83.28; 100 mg (brown), 28-cap pack = £83.28. Label: 3

DEXAMFETAMINE SULFATE
(Dexamphetamine sulfate)

Indications narcolepsy; refractory attention deficit hyperactivity disorder (under specialist supervision)

Cautions see notes above; also anorexia; mild hypertension (contra-indicated if moderate or severe); psychosis or bipolar disorder; monitor for aggressive behaviour or hostility during initial treatment; history of epilepsy (discontinue if seizures occur); tics and Tourette syndrome (use with caution)—discontinue if tics occur; monitor growth in children (see also below); susceptibility to angle-closure glaucoma; avoid abrupt withdrawal; data on safety and efficacy of long-term use not complete; acute porphyria (section 9.8.2); **interactions:** Appendix 1 (sympathomimetics)

Special cautions in children Monitor height and weight as growth restriction may occur during prolonged therapy (drug-free periods may allow catch-up in growth but withdraw slowly to avoid inducing depression or renewed hyperactivity)

Driving May affect performance of skilled tasks (e.g. driving); effects of alcohol unpredictable; see also Drugs and Driving, p. 3

Contra-indications cardiovascular disease including moderate to severe hypertension, structural cardiac abnormalities, advanced arteriosclerosis, hyperexcitability or agitated states, hyperthyroidism, history of drug or alcohol abuse

Renal impairment use with caution

Pregnancy avoid (retrospective evidence of uncertain significance suggesting possible embryotoxicity)

Breast-feeding significant amount in milk—avoid

Side-effects nausea, diarrhoea, dry mouth, abdominal cramps, anorexia (increased appetite also reported), weight loss, taste disturbance, ischaemic colitis, palpitations, tachycardia, chest pain, hypertension, hypotension, cardiomyopathy, myocardial infarction, cardiovascular collapse, cerebral vasculitis, stroke, headache, restlessness, depression, hyperreflexia, hyperactivity, impaired concentration, ataxia, anxiety, aggression, dizziness, confusion, sleep disturbances, dysphoria, euphoria, irritability, nervousness, malaise, obsessive-compulsive behaviour, paranoia, psychosis, panic attack, tremor, seizures (see also Cautions), neuroleptic malignant syndrome, anhedonia, growth restriction in children (see also under Cautions and notes above), pyrexia, renal impairment, sexual dysfunction, acidosis, rhabdomyolysis, mydriasis, visual disturbances, alopecia, rash, sweating, urticaria; central stimulants have provoked choreoathetoid movements and dyskinesia, tics and Tourette syndrome in predisposed individuals (see also Cautions); *very rarely* angle-closure glaucoma; **overdosage:** see Emergency Treatment of Poisoning, p. 40

Dose

- Narcolepsy, initially 10 mg (ELDERLY 5 mg) daily in divided doses increased at weekly intervals by 10 mg (ELDERLY 5 mg) daily to a max. of 60 mg daily
- Refractory attention deficit hyperactivity disorder, ADULT over 18 years [unlicensed use], initially 5 mg twice daily, increased at weekly intervals according to response; max. 60 mg daily; CHILD 6–18 years, initially 2.5 mg 2–3 times daily, increased if necessary at weekly intervals by 5 mg daily, usual max. 1 mg/kg (up to 20 mg) daily (40 mg daily has been required in some children)

Note Maintenance dose given in 2–4 divided doses

Dexamfetamine (Non-proprietary) ▼ CD2

Tablets, scored, dexamfetamine sulfate 5 mg, net price 28-tab pack = £24.28. Counselling, driving

LISDEXAMFETAMINE MESILATE

Note Lisdexamfetamine is a prodrug of dexamfetamine

Indications attention deficit hyperactivity disorder refractory to methylphenidate (under specialist supervision)

Cautions see notes above; also anorexia; history of cardiovascular disease or abnormalities; psychosis or bipolar disorder; monitor for aggressive behaviour or hostility during initial treatment; history of drug or alcohol abuse; may lower seizure threshold (discontinue if seizures occur); tics and Tourette syndrome (use with caution)—discontinue if tics occur; monitor growth in children (see also below); susceptibility to angle-closure glaucoma; avoid abrupt withdrawal; acute porphyria (section 9.8.2); **interactions:** Appendix 1 (sympathomimetics)

Special cautions in children Monitor height and weight as growth restriction may occur during prolonged therapy (drug-free periods may allow catch-up in growth but withdraw slowly to avoid inducing depression or renewed hyperactivity)

Driving See Drugs and Driving, p. 3

Contra-indications symptomatic cardiovascular disease including moderate to severe hypertension and advanced arteriosclerosis, hyperexcitability or agitated states, hyperthyroidism

Renal impairment use with caution

Pregnancy manufacturer advises use only if potential benefit outweighs risk

Breast-feeding manufacturer advises avoid—present in human milk

Side-effects nausea, decreased appetite, vomiting, diarrhoea, dry mouth, abdominal cramps, dyspnoea, sleep disturbances, tics, aggression, headache, dizziness, drowsiness, mydriasis, labile mood, weight loss, pyrexia, malaise, growth restriction in children (see also under Cautions and notes above); *less commonly* anorexia, tachycardia, palpitation, hypertension, logorrhoea, anxiety, paranoia, restlessness, depression, dysphoria, dermatillomania, mania, hallucination, sweating, tremor, visual disturbances, sexual dysfunction, rash; *very rarely* angle-closure glaucoma; *also reported* cardiomyopathy, euphoria, seizures (see also Cautions), central stimulants have provoked choreoathetoid movements and dyskinesia, and Tourette syndrome in predisposed individuals (see also Cautions); **overdosage**: see Emergency Treatment of Poisoning, p. 40

Dose

- ADULT over 18 years [unlicensed use] and CHILD 6–18 years, initially 30 mg once daily in the morning, increased if necessary at weekly intervals by 20 mg; max. 70 mg daily (discontinue if response insufficient after 1 month)

Elvanse® (Shire) ▼ CD2

Capsule, lisdexamfetamine mesilate 30 mg (white/pink), net price 28-cap pack = £58.24; 50 mg (white/blue), 28-cap pack = £68.60; 70 mg (blue/pink), 28-cap pack = £83.16. Label: 3, 25, counselling, administration, driving

Counselling Swallow whole or dissolve contents of capsule in a glass of water

METHYLPHENIDATE HYDROCHLORIDE

Indications attention deficit hyperactivity disorder (under specialist supervision); narcolepsy [unlicensed indication]

Cautions see notes above; also monitor for psychiatric disorders; anxiety or agitation; tics or a family history of Tourette syndrome; drug or alcohol dependence; epilepsy (discontinue if increased seizure frequency); susceptibility to angle-closure glaucoma; avoid abrupt withdrawal; **interactions**: Appendix 1 (sympathomimetics)

Driving See Drugs and Driving, p. 3

Contra-indications severe depression, suicidal ideation; anorexia nervosa; psychosis; uncontrolled bipolar disorder; hyperthyroidism; cardiovascular disease (including heart failure, cardiomyopathy, severe hypertension, and arrhythmias), structural cardiac abnormalities; phaeochromocytoma; vasculitis; cerebrovascular disorders

Pregnancy limited experience—avoid unless potential benefit outweighs risk

Breast-feeding limited information available—avoid

Side-effects abdominal pain, nausea, vomiting, diarrhoea, dyspepsia, dry mouth, anorexia, reduced weight gain; tachycardia, palpitation, arrhythmias, changes in blood pressure; cough, nasopharyngitis; tics (*very rarely* Tourette syndrome), insomnia, nervousness, asthenia, depression, irritability, aggression, head-

ache, drowsiness, dizziness, movement disorders; fever; arthralgia; rash, pruritus, alopecia; growth restriction; *less commonly* constipation, dyspnoea, abnormal dreams, confusion, suicidal ideation, urinary frequency, haematuria, muscle cramps, epistaxis; *rarely* angina, sweating, and visual disturbances; *very rarely* hepatic dysfunction, myocardial infarction, cerebral arteritis, psychosis, seizures, neuroleptic malignant syndrome, tolerance and dependence, blood disorders including leucopenia and thrombocytopenia, angle-closure glaucoma, exfoliative dermatitis, and erythema multiforme; supraventricular tachycardia, bradycardia, and convulsions *also reported*

Dose

- Attention deficit hyperactivity disorder, ADULT over 18 years [unlicensed use], 5 mg 2–3 times daily increased if necessary at weekly intervals according to response, max. 100 mg daily in 2–3 divided doses; CHILD 6–18 years, initially 5 mg 1–2 times daily, increased if necessary at weekly intervals by 5–10 mg daily; usual max. 60 mg daily in 2–3 divided doses; may be increased to 2.1 mg/kg daily in 2–3 divided doses (max. 90 mg daily) [unlicensed] under the direction of a specialist; discontinue if no response after 1 month; CHILD 4–6 years see *BNF for Children*
  Evening dose If effect wears off in evening (with rebound hyperactivity) a dose at bedtime may be appropriate (establish need with trial bedtime dose)
  Note Treatment may be started using a modified-release preparation

- Narcolepsy [unlicensed indication], 10–60 mg (usually 20–30 mg) daily in divided doses before meals

Methylphenidate Hydrochloride (Non-proprietary) CD2

Tablets, methylphenidate hydrochloride 5 mg, net price 30-tab pack = £3.03; 10 mg, 30-tab pack = £5.49; 20 mg, 30-tab pack = £10.92. Counselling, driving

Brands include *Medikinet®*

Ritalin® (Novartis) CD2

Tablets, scored, methylphenidate hydrochloride 10 mg, net price 30-tab pack = £5.57. Counselling, driving

◢ Modified release

Note Different versions of modified-release preparations may not have the same clinical effect. To avoid confusion between these different formulations of methylphenidate, prescribers should specify the brand to be dispensed.

Concerta® XL (Janssen) CD2

Tablets, m/r, methylphenidate hydrochloride 18 mg (yellow), net price 30-tab pack = £31.19; 27 mg (grey), 30-tab pack = £36.81; 36 mg (white), 30-tab pack = £42.45. Label: 25, counselling, driving

Note *Concerta® XL* tablets consist of an immediate-release component (22% of the dose) and a modified-release component (78% of the dose)

Counselling Tablet membrane may pass through gastro-intestinal tract unchanged

Cautions dose form not appropriate for use in dysphagia or if gastro-intestinal lumen restricted

Dose attention deficit hyperactivity disorder, ADULT over 18 years [initiation unlicensed], initially 18 mg once daily in the morning, adjusted at weekly intervals according to response, max. 108 mg daily; CHILD 6–18 years, initially 18 mg once daily (in the morning), increased if necessary at weekly intervals by 18 mg according to response, usual max. 54 mg once daily, but may be increased to 2.1 mg/kg daily (max. 108 mg daily) [unlicensed] under the direction of a specialist; discontinue if no response after 1 month

Note Total daily dose of 15 mg of standard-release formulation is equivalent to *Concerta® XL* 18 mg once daily

Equasym XL® (Shire) CD2

Capsules, m/r, methylphenidate hydrochloride 10 mg (white/green), net price 30-cap pack = £25.00; 20 mg (white/blue), 30-cap pack = £30.00; 30 mg (white/brown), 30-cap pack = £35.00. Label: 25, counselling, driving

Note *Equasym XL*® capsules consist of an immediate-release component (30% of the dose) and a modified-release component (70% of the dose)

Dose attention deficit hyperactivity disorder, ADULT over 18 years [unlicensed use], initially 10 mg once daily in the morning before breakfast, increased gradually at weekly intervals if necessary, max. 100 mg daily; CHILD 6–18 years, initially 10 mg once daily in the morning before breakfast, increased gradually at weekly intervals if necessary, usual max. 60 mg daily but may be increased to 2.1 mg/kg daily (max. 90 mg daily) [unlicensed] under the direction of a specialist; discontinue if no response after 1 month

Note Contents of capsule can be sprinkled on a tablespoon of apple sauce (then swallowed immediately without chewing)

Medikinet XL® (Flynn) CD2

Capsules, m/r, methylphenidate hydrochloride 5 mg (white), net price 30-cap pack = £24.04; 10 mg (lilac/white), 30-cap pack = £24.04; 20 mg (lilac), 30-cap pack = £28.86; 30 mg (purple/light grey), 30-cap pack = £33.66; 40 mg (purple/grey), 30-cap pack = £57.72. Label: 25, counselling, driving

Note *Medikinet XL*® capsules consist of an immediate-release component (50% of the dose) and a modified-release component (50% of the dose)

Dose attention deficit hyperactivity disorder, ADULT over 18 years [unlicensed use], initially 10 mg once daily in the morning with breakfast, adjusted at weekly intervals according to response, max. 100 mg daily; CHILD 6–18 years, initially 10 mg once daily in the morning with breakfast, adjusted at weekly intervals according to response, usual max. 60 mg daily but may be increased to 2.1 mg/kg daily (max. 90 mg daily) [unlicensed] under the direction of a specialist; discontinue if no response after 1 month

Note Contents of capsule can be sprinkled on a tablespoon of apple sauce or yoghurt (then swallowed immediately without chewing)

▲ MODAFINIL

Indications excessive sleepiness associated with narcolepsy with or without cataplexy

Cautions monitor blood pressure and heart rate in hypertensive patients (but see Contra-indications); ECG required before initiation; history of psychosis, depression, mania, alcohol or drug abuse; discontinue treatment if psychiatric symptoms develop; possibility of dependence; discontinue treatment if rash develops; **interactions**: Appendix 1 (modafinil)

Contra-indications moderate to severe uncontrolled hypertension, arrhythmia; history of left ventricular hypertrophy, cor pulmonale, or of clinically significant signs of CNS stimulant-induced mitral valve prolapse (including ischaemic ECG changes, chest pain and arrhythmias)

Hepatic impairment halve dose in severe impairment

Renal impairment use with caution—limited information available

Pregnancy avoid

Breast-feeding avoid—present in milk in *animal* studies

Side-effects dry mouth, appetite changes, gastro-intestinal disturbances (including nausea, diarrhoea,

constipation, and dyspepsia), abdominal pain; tachycardia, vasodilatation, chest pain, palpitation; headache (uncommonly migraine), anxiety, sleep disturbances, dizziness, drowsiness, depression, confusion, paraesthesia, asthenia; visual disturbances; *less commonly* flatulence, reflux, vomiting, mouth ulcers, glossitis, dysphagia, taste disturbance, weight changes, hypertension, hypotension, bradycardia, arrhythmia, peripheral oedema, hypercholesterolaemia, rhinitis, dyspnoea, epistaxis, dyskinesia, amnesia, emotional lability, abnormal dreams, suicidal ideation, tremor, decreased libido, agitation, aggression, hyperglycaemia, thirst, urinary frequency, menstrual disturbances, eosinophilia, leucopenia, myasthenia, muscle cramps, hypertonia, myalgia, arthralgia, dry eye, sinusitis, acne, sweating, rash, and pruritus; *rarely* hallucinations, mania, psychosis; multi-organ hypersensitivity reaction, Stevens-Johnson syndrome, and toxic epidermal necrolysis also reported

Dose

• Narcolepsy ADULT over 18 years, initially 200 mg daily, *either* in 2 divided doses morning and at noon *or* as a single dose in the morning, dose adjusted according to response to 200–400 mg daily in 2 divided doses or as a single dose; ELDERLY initiate at 100 mg daily

Provigil® (TEVA UK) PoM

Tablets, modafinil 100 mg, net price 30-tab pack = £52.60; 200 mg (scored), 30-tab pack = £105.21

4.5 Drugs used in the treatment of obesity

4.5.1 Anti-obesity drugs acting on the gastro-intestinal tract

4.5.2 Centrally acting appetite suppressants

Obesity is associated with many health problems including cardiovascular disease, diabetes mellitus, gallstones and osteoarthritis. Factors that aggravate obesity may include depression, other psychosocial problems, and some drugs.

The main treatment of the obese individual is a suitable diet, carefully explained to the individual, with appropriate support and encouragement; the individual should also be advised to increase physical activity. Smoking cessation (while maintaining body weight) may be worthwhile before attempting supervised weight loss since cigarette smoking may be more harmful than obesity. Attendance at weight loss groups helps some individuals.

Obesity should be managed in an appropriate setting by staff who have been trained in the management of obesity; the individual should receive advice on diet and lifestyle modification and be monitored for changes in weight as well as in blood pressure, blood lipids and other associated conditions.

An anti-obesity drug should be considered only for those with a body mass index (BMI, individual's bodyweight divided by the square of the individual's height) of 30 kg/m^2 or greater in whom at least 3 months of managed care involving supervised diet, exercise and behaviour modification fails to achieve a realistic reduction in weight. In the presence of associated risk factors, it may be appropriate to prescribe an anti-obesity drug to individuals with a BMI of 28 kg/m² or greater (see below). Drugs should **never** be used as the sole element of treatment. The individual should be monitored on a regular basis; drug treatment should be discontinued if the individual regains weight at any time whilst receiving drug treatment.

Combination therapy involving more than one anti-obesity drug is **contra-indicated** by the manufacturers; there is no evidence-base to support such treatment.

Thyroid hormones have **no** place in the treatment of obesity except in biochemically proven hypothyroid patients. The use of diuretics, chorionic gonadotrophin, or amfetamines is **not** appropriate for weight reduction.

Central nervous system

4

4.5.1 Anti-obesity drugs acting on the gastro-intestinal tract

Orlistat, a lipase inhibitor, reduces the absorption of dietary fat. It is used in conjunction with a mildly hypocaloric diet in individuals with a body mass index (BMI) of 30 kg/m² or more *or* in individuals with a BMI of 28 kg/m² or more in the presence of other risk factors such as type 2 diabetes, hypertension, or hyper-cholesterolaemia.

Orlistat should be used in conjunction with other life-style measures to manage obesity (section 4.5); treatment should only be continued beyond 12 months after discussing potential benefits and risks with the patient. On stopping orlistat, there may be a gradual reversal of weight loss.

Some of the weight loss in those taking orlistat probably results from individuals reducing their fat intake to avoid severe gastro-intestinal effects including steatorrhoea. Vitamin supplementation (especially of vitamin D) may be considered if there is concern about deficiency of fat-soluble vitamins.

Methylcellulose is claimed to reduce food intake by producing a feeling of satiety, but there is little evidence to support its use in the management of obesity.

▌ ORLISTAT

Indications   adjunct in obesity (see notes above)

Cautions   may impair absorption of fat-soluble vita-mins; chronic kidney disease or volume depletion; **interactions:** Appendix 1 (orlistat)

> **Multivitamins**   If a multivitamin supplement is required, it should be taken at least 2 hours after orlistat dose or at bedtime

Contra-indications   chronic malabsorption syndrome; cholestasis

Pregnancy   use with caution

Breast-feeding   avoid—no information available

Side-effects   oily leakage from rectum, flatulence, faecal urgency, liquid or oily stools, faecal incontinence, abdominal distension and pain (gastro-intestinal effects minimised by reduced fat intake), tooth and gingival disorders, respiratory infections, malaise, anxiety, headache, menstrual disturbances, urinary-tract infection, hypoglycaemia; *also reported* rectal

bleeding, diverticulitis, cholelithiasis, hepatitis, hypo-thyroidism, oxalate nephropathy, bullous eruptions

Dose

- ADULT over 18 years, 120 mg taken immediately before, during, or up to 1 hour after each main meal (max. 120 mg 3 times daily); continue treatment beyond 12 weeks only if weight loss since start of treatment exceeds 5% (target for initial weight loss may be lower in patients with type 2 diabetes); CHILD over 12 years see *BNF for Children*

> **Note**   If a meal is missed or contains no fat, the dose of orlistat should be omitted

Xenical® (Roche)
Capsules, turquoise, orlistat 120 mg, net price 84-cap pack = £31.63

4.5.2 Centrally acting appetite suppressants

Phentermine and **diethylpropion** are central stimulants; they are not recommended for the treatment of obesity. Phentermine has been associated with a risk of pulmonary hypertension.

Sibutramine, dexfenfluramine, and fenfluramine have been withdrawn because the benefit of treatment does not outweigh the risk of serious adverse effects.

4.6 Drugs used in nausea and vertigo

Antiemetics should be prescribed only when the cause of vomiting is known because otherwise they may delay diagnosis, particularly in children. Antiemetics are unnecessary and sometimes harmful when the cause can be treated, such as in diabetic ketoacidosis, or in digoxin or antiepileptic overdose.

If antiemetic drug treatment is indicated, the drug is chosen according to the aetiology of vomiting.

Antihistamines are effective against nausea and vomiting resulting from many underlying conditions. There is no evidence that any one antihistamine is superior to another but their duration of action and incidence of adverse effects (drowsiness and antimuscarinic effects) differ.

The **phenothiazines** are dopamine antagonists and act centrally by blocking the chemoreceptor trigger zone. They are of considerable value for the prophylaxis and treatment of nausea and vomiting associated with diffuse neoplastic disease, radiation sickness, and the emesis caused by drugs such as opioids, general anaesthetics, and cytotoxics. **Prochlorperazine**, **perphenazine**, and **trifluoperazine** are less sedating than **chlorpromazine**; severe dystonic reactions sometimes occur with phenothiazines, especially in children. Some phenothiazines are available as rectal suppositories, which can be useful in patients with persistent vomiting or with severe nausea; prochlorperazine can also be administered as a buccal tablet which is placed between the upper lip and the gum.

Droperidol is a butyrophenone, structurally related to haloperidol, which blocks dopamine receptors in the chemoreceptor trigger zone.

Other antipsychotic drugs including **haloperidol** and **levomepromazine** are used for the relief of nausea and vomiting in terminal illness, see Palliative Care, (p. 22).

Metoclopramide is an effective antiemetic and its activity closely resembles that of the phenothiazines. Metoclopramide also acts directly on the gastro-intestinal tract and it may be superior to the phenothiazines for emesis associated with gastroduodenal, hepatic, and biliary disease. As with the phenothiazines, metoclopramide can induce acute dystonic reactions involving facial and skeletal muscle spasms and oculogyric crises. These dystonic effects are more common in the young (especially girls and young women) and the very old; they usually occur shortly after starting treatment with metoclopramide and subside within 24 hours of stopping it. Injection of an antiparkinsonian drug such as procyclidine (section 4.9.2) will abort dystonic attacks, see also MHRA advice below.

> **MHRA/CHM advice**
> **Metoclopramide: risk of neurological adverse effects—restricted dose and duration of use (August 2013)**
> The benefits and risks of metoclopramide have been reviewed by the European Medicines Agency's Committee on Medicinal Products for Human Use, which concluded that the risk of neurological effects such as extrapyramidal disorders and tardive dyskinesia outweigh the benefits in long-term or high-dose treatment. To help minimise the risk of potentially serious neurological adverse effects, the following restrictions to indications, dose, and duration of use have been made:
> - In adults over 18 years, metoclopramide should only be used for prevention of postoperative nausea and vomiting, radiotherapy-induced nausea and vomiting, delayed (but not acute) chemotherapy-induced nausea and vomiting, and symptomatic treatment of nausea and vomiting, including that associated with acute migraine (where it may also be used to improve absorption of oral analgesics);
> - Metoclopramide should only be prescribed for short-term use (up to 5 days);
> - Usual dose is 10 mg, repeated up to 3 times daily; max. daily dose is 500 micrograms/kg;
> - Intravenous doses should be administered as a slow bolus over at least 3 minutes;
> - Oral liquid formulations should be given via an appropriately designed, graduated oral syringe to ensure dose accuracy.
> **Note** This advice does not apply to unlicensed uses of metoclopramide (e.g. palliative care, p. 20)

Domperidone acts at the chemoreceptor trigger zone; it is licensed only for the relief of nausea and vomiting. It has the advantage over metoclopramide and the phenothiazines of being less likely to cause central effects such as sedation and dystonic reactions because it does not readily cross the blood-brain barrier. In Parkinson's disease, it can be used to treat nausea caused by dopaminergic drugs (section 4.9.1). See also MHRA advice below.

> **MHRA/CHM advice**
> **Domperidone: risk of cardiac side-effects—restricted indication, new contra-indications, reduced dose and duration of use**
> The benefits and risks of domperidone have been reviewed. As domperidone is associated with a small increased risk of serious cardiac side-effects, the following restrictions to indication, dose and duration of treatment have been made, and new contra-indications added:
> - Domperidone should only be used for the relief of the symptoms of nausea and vomiting;
> - Domperidone should be used at the lowest effective dose for the shortest possible duration (max. treatment duration should not normally exceed 1 week);
> - Domperidone is contra-indicated for use in conditions where cardiac conduction is, or could be impaired, or where there is underlying cardiac disease, when administered concomitantly with drugs that prolong the QT interval or potent CYP3A4 inhibitors, and in severe hepatic impairment;
> - The recommended dose in adults and adolescents over 12 years and over 35 kg is 10 mg up to 3 times daily;
> - The recommended dose in children under 35 kg is 250 micrograms/kg up to 3 times daily;
> - Oral liquid formulations should be given via an appropriately designed, graduated oral syringe to ensure dose accuracy.
> **Note** This advice does not apply to unlicensed uses of domperidone (e.g palliative care, p. 20)

Granisetron, **ondansetron**, and **palonosetron** are specific $5HT_3$-receptor antagonists which block $5HT_3$ receptors in the gastro-intestinal tract and in the CNS. Granisetron and ondansetron are of value in the management of nausea and vomiting in patients receiving cytotoxics and in postoperative nausea and vomiting. Palonosetron is licensed for prevention of nausea and vomiting associated with moderately or highly emetogenic cytotoxic chemotherapy.

Dexamethasone (section 6.3.2) has antiemetic effects and it is used in vomiting associated with cancer chemotherapy. It can be used alone or with metoclopramide, prochlorperazine, lorazepam, or a $5HT_3$-receptor antagonist (section 8.1).

Aprepitant and **fosaprepitant** are neurokinin 1-receptor antagonists licensed for the prevention of acute and delayed nausea and vomiting associated with cisplatin-based cytotoxic chemotherapy; they are given with dexamethasone and a $5HT_3$-receptor antagonist.

Nabilone is a synthetic cannabinoid with antiemetic properties. It may be used for nausea and vomiting caused by cytotoxic chemotherapy that is unresponsive to conventional antiemetics. Side-effects such as drowsiness and dizziness occur frequently with standard doses.

Vomiting during pregnancy   Nausea in the first trimester of pregnancy is generally mild and does not require drug therapy. On rare occasions if vomiting is severe, short-term treatment with an antihistamine, such as **promethazine**, may be required. **Prochlorperazine** or **metoclopramide** are alternatives, see also MHRA advice above. If symptoms do not settle in 24 to 48 hours then specialist opinion should be sought. Hyperemesis gravidarum is a more serious condition, which requires regular antiemetic therapy, intravenous fluid and electrolyte replacement, and sometimes nutri-

Central nervous system 4

tional support. Supplementation with thiamine must be considered in order to reduce the risk of Wernicke's encephalopathy.

Postoperative nausea and vomiting The incidence of postoperative nausea and vomiting depends on many factors including the anaesthetic used, and the type and duration of surgery. Other risk factors include female sex, non-smokers, a history of postoperative nausea and vomiting or motion sickness, and intra-operative and postoperative use of opioids. Therapy to prevent postoperative nausea and vomiting should be based on the assessed risk of postoperative nausea and vomiting in each patient. Drugs used include **5HT₃-receptor antagonists**, **droperidol**, **dexamethasone** (section 6.3.2), some **phenothiazines** (e.g. prochlorperazine), and **antihistamines** (e.g. cyclizine). A combination of two or more antiemetic drugs that have different mechanisms of action is often indicated in those at high risk of postoperative nausea and vomiting or where postoperative vomiting presents a particular danger (e.g. in some types of surgery). When a prophylactic antiemetic drug has failed, postoperative nausea and vomiting should be treated with one or more drugs from a different class.

Motion sickness Antiemetics should be given to prevent motion sickness rather than after nausea or vomiting develop. The most effective drug for the prevention of motion sickness is **hyoscine hydrobromide**. For children over 10 years old, a transdermal hyoscine patch provides prolonged activity but it needs to be applied several hours before travelling. The sedating antihistamines are slightly less effective against motion sickness, but are generally better tolerated than hyoscine. If a sedative effect is desired **promethazine** is useful, but generally a slightly less sedating antihistamine such as **cyclizine** or **cinnarizine** is preferred. Domperidone, metoclopramide, 5HT₃-receptor antagonists, and the phenothiazines (except the antihistamine phenothiazine promethazine) are **ineffective** in motion sickness.

Other vestibular disorders Management of vestibular diseases is aimed at treating the underlying cause as well as treating symptoms of the balance disturbance and associated nausea and vomiting. Vertigo and nausea associated with Ménière's disease and middle-ear surgery can be difficult to treat.

Betahistine is an analogue of histamine and is claimed to reduce endolymphatic pressure by improving the microcirculation. Betahistine is licensed for vertigo, tinnitus, and hearing loss associated with Ménière's disease.

A **diuretic** alone or combined with salt restriction may provide some benefit in vertigo associated with Ménière's disease; **antihistamines** (such as cinnarizine), and **phenothiazines** (such as prochlorperazine) are also used. Where possible, prochlorperazine should be reserved for the treatment of acute symptoms.

For advice to avoid the inappropriate prescribing of drugs (notably phenothiazines) for dizziness in the elderly, see Prescribing for the Elderly, (p. 25).

Cytotoxic chemotherapy For the management of nausea and vomiting induced by cytotoxic chemotherapy, see section 8.1.

Palliative care For the management of nausea and vomiting in palliative care, see Palliative Care (Nausea and Vomiting), (p. 22) and Syringe Drivers (Nausea and Vomiting), (p. 23).

Migraine For the management of nausea and vomiting associated with migraine, see section 4.7.4.1, (p. 301)

Antihistamines

▌ CINNARIZINE

Indications vestibular disorders, such as vertigo, tinnitus, nausea, and vomiting in Ménière's disease; motion sickness

Cautions section 3.4.1; also Parkinson's disease

Contra-indications section 3.4.1

Hepatic impairment section 3.4.1

Renal impairment use with caution—no information available

Pregnancy section 3.4.1

Breast-feeding section 3.4.1

Side-effects section 3.4.1; also *rarely* weight gain, sweating, lichen planus, and lupus-like skin reactions

Dose
- Vestibular disorders, 30 mg 3 times daily; CHILD 5–12 years 15 mg 3 times daily
- Motion sickness, 30 mg 2 hours before travel then 15 mg every 8 hours during journey if necessary; CHILD 5–12 years, 15 mg 2 hours before travel then 7.5 mg every 8 hours during journey if necessary

Cinnarizine (Non-proprietary)
Tablets, cinnarizine 15 mg, net price 84-tab pack = £4.26. Label: 2

Stugeron® (Janssen)
Tablets, scored, cinnarizine 15 mg, net price 15-tab pack = £1.77, 100-tab pack = £4.18. Label: 2

◢**With dimenhydrinate**

Arlevert® (Hennig Arzneimittel) [PoM]
Tablets, cinnarizine 20 mg, dimenhydrinate 40 mg, net price 100-tab pack = £24.00. Label: 2, 21
Dose vertigo, ADULT over 18 years, 1 tablet 3 times daily

▌ CYCLIZINE

Indications nausea, vomiting, vertigo, motion sickness, labyrinthine disorders

Cautions section 3.4.1; severe heart failure—may cause fall in cardiac output and associated increase in heart rate, mean arterial pressure and pulmonary wedge pressure; may counteract haemodynamic benefits of opioids; neuromuscular disorders—increased risk of transient paralysis with intravenous use; interactions: Appendix 1 (antihistamines)

Contra-indications section 3.4.1

Hepatic impairment section 3.4.1

Pregnancy section 3.4.1

Breast-feeding no information available

Side-effects section 3.4.1; also tachycardia, hypertension, hypotension (with *injection*), transient speech disorders, movement disorders, paraesthesia, hallucinations, twitching, oculogyric crisis; *rarely* transient paralysis (with intravenous use)

Dose

- By mouth, cyclizine hydrochloride 50 mg up to 3 times daily; CHILD 6–12 years 25 mg up to 3 times daily
  Note For motion sickness, take 1–2 hours before departure
- By intramuscular *or* intravenous injection, cyclizine lactate 50 mg 3 times daily; CHILD under 18 years see *BNF for Children*

Cyclizine (Non-proprietary)
Tablets, cyclizine hydrochloride 50 mg, net price 100-tab pack = £11.26.Label: 2

Valoid® (AMCo) PoM
Injection, cyclizine lactate 50 mg/mL, net price 1-mL amp = 65p

PROMETHAZINE HYDROCHLORIDE

Indications nausea, vomiting, vertigo, labyrinthine disorders, motion sickness; allergy and urticaria (section 3.4.1); sedation (section 4.1.1)

Cautions see Promethazine Hydrochloride, section 3.4.1

Contra-indications see notes in section 3.4.1

Hepatic impairment see notes in section 3.4.1

Renal impairment see Promethazine Hydrochloride, section 3.4.1

Pregnancy see notes in section 3.4.1

Breast-feeding see notes in section 3.4.1

Side-effects see Promethazine Hydrochloride, section 3.4.1

Dose

- By mouth, 20–25 mg at bedtime on night before travel, repeat following morning if necessary; CHILD 2–5 years 5 mg at night, and following morning if necessary, 5–10 years 10 mg at night, and following morning if necessary

◢Preparations
Section 3.4.1

PROMETHAZINE TEOCLATE

Indications nausea, vertigo, labyrinthine disorders, motion sickness (acts longer than the hydrochloride)

Cautions section 3.4.1; severe coronary artery disease; asthma, bronchitis, bronchiectasis; Reye's syndrome

Contra-indications section 3.4.1

Hepatic impairment section 3.4.1

Renal impairment use with caution

Pregnancy section 3.4.1

Breast-feeding section 3.4.1

Side-effects section 3.4.1

Dose

- 25–75 mg, max. 100 mg, daily; CHILD 5–10 years, 12.5–37.5 mg daily
- Motion sickness prevention, ADULT and CHILD over 10 years, 25 mg at bedtime on night before travel *or* 25 mg 1–2 hours before travel; CHILD 5–10 years, 12.5 mg at bedtime on night before travel *or* 12.5 mg 1–2 hours before travel
- Motion sickness treatment, ADULT and CHILD over 10 years, 25 mg at onset, then 25 mg at bedtime for 2 days; CHILD 5–10 years, 12.5 mg at onset, then 12.5 mg at bedtime for 2 days

Avomine® (Manx)
Tablets, scored, promethazine teoclate 25 mg, net price 10-tab pack = £1.13; 28-tab pack = £3.13. Label: 2

Phenothiazines and related drugs

CHLORPROMAZINE HYDROCHLORIDE

Indications nausea and vomiting of terminal illness (where other drugs have failed or are not available); other indications (section 4.2.1)

Cautions see Chlorpromazine Hydrochloride, section 4.2.1

Contra-indications see notes in section 4.2.1

Hepatic impairment see notes in section 4.2.1

Renal impairment see notes in section 4.2.1

Pregnancy see notes in section 4.2.1

Breast-feeding see notes in section 4.2.1

Side-effects see Chlorpromazine Hydrochloride, section 4.2.1

Dose

- By mouth, 10–25 mg every 4–6 hours; CHILD 500 micrograms/kg every 4–6 hours (1–5 years max. 40 mg daily, 6–12 years max. 75 mg daily)
- By deep intramuscular injection initially 25 mg then 25–50 mg every 3–4 hours until vomiting stops; CHILD 500 micrograms/kg every 6–8 hours (1–5 years max. 40 mg daily, 6–12 years max. 75 mg daily)
- By rectum in suppositories, chlorpromazine 100 mg every 6–8 hours [unlicensed]

◢Preparations
Section 4.2.1

DROPERIDOL

Indications prevention and treatment of postoperative nausea and vomiting

Cautions section 4.2.1; also chronic obstructive pulmonary disease or respiratory failure; electrolyte disturbances; history of alcohol abuse; continuous pulse oximetry required if risk of ventricular arrhythmia—continue for 30 minutes following administration; **interactions**: Appendix 1 (droperidol)

Contra-indications section 4.2.1; QT-interval prolongation (avoid concomitant administration of drugs that prolong QT interval); hypokalaemia; hypomagnesaemia; bradycardia

Hepatic impairment in postoperative nausea and vomiting, max. 625 micrograms repeated every 6 hours as required; for nausea and vomiting caused by opioid analgesics in postoperative patient-controlled analgesia, reduce dose

Renal impairment in postoperative nausea and vomiting, max. 625 micrograms repeated every 6 hours as required; for nausea and vomiting caused by opioid analgesics in postoperative patient-controlled analgesia, reduce dose

Pregnancy section 4.2.1

Breast-feeding limited information available—avoid repeated administration

Side-effects section 4.2.1; also anxiety, cardiac arrest, hallucinations, and inappropriate antidiuretic hormone secretion

4

Central nervous system

Central nervous system · **4**

Dose

- Prevention and treatment of postoperative nausea and vomiting, ADULT over 18 years, by intravenous injection, 0.625–1.25 mg (ELDERLY 625 micrograms) 30 minutes before end of surgery, repeated every 6 hours as required; CHILD over 2 years (second-line use only) 20–50 micrograms/kg (max. 1.25 mg)

- Prevention of nausea and vomiting caused by opioid analgesics in postoperative patient-controlled analgesia (PCA), ADULT over 18 years, by intravenous injection, 15–50 micrograms of droperidol for every 1 mg of morphine in PCA (max. 5 mg droperidol daily); ELDERLY reduce dose

Xomolix® (ProStrakan) [PoM]

Injection, droperidol 2.5 mg/mL, net price 1–mL amp = £3.94

▮ PERPHENAZINE

Indications   severe nausea, vomiting (see notes above); other indications (section 4.2.1)

Cautions   see notes in section 4.2.1

Contra-indications   see Perphenazine, section 4.2.1

Hepatic impairment   see notes in section 4.2.1

Renal impairment   see notes in section 4.2.1

Pregnancy   see notes in section 4.2.1

Breast-feeding   see notes in section 4.2.1

Side-effects   see Perphenazine, section 4.2.1

Dose

- 4 mg 3 times daily, adjusted according to response; max. 24 mg daily (chemotherapy-induced); ELDERLY quarter to half adult dose; CHILD under 14 years not recommended

▮ Preparations

Section 4.2.1

▮ PROCHLORPERAZINE

Indications   severe nausea, vomiting, vertigo, labyrinthine disorders (see notes above); other indications section 4.2.1

Cautions   see Prochlorperazine, section 4.2.1; elderly (see notes above)

Contra-indications   see Prochlorperazine, section 4.2.1; avoid oral route in child under 10 kg

Hepatic impairment   see notes in section 4.2.1

Renal impairment   see notes in section 4.2.1

Pregnancy   see notes in section 4.2.1

Breast-feeding   see notes in section 4.2.1

Side-effects   see Prochlorperazine, section 4.2.1

Dose

Note Doses are expressed as prochlorperazine maleate or mesilate; 1 mg prochlorperazine maleate ≡ 1 mg prochlorperazine mesilate

- By mouth, nausea and vomiting, acute attack, 20 mg initially then 10 mg after 2 hours; prevention 5–10 mg 2–3 times daily; CHILD (over 10 kg only) 250 micrograms/kg 2–3 times daily

  Labyrinthine disorders, 5 mg 3 times daily, gradually increased if necessary to 30 mg daily in divided doses, then reduced after several weeks to 5–10 mg daily; CHILD not recommended

- By deep intramuscular injection, nausea and vomiting, 12.5 mg when required followed if necessary after 6 hours by an oral dose, as above; CHILD and ADOLESCENT under 18 years see BNF for Children

Prochlorperazine (Non-proprietary) [PoM]

Tablets, prochlorperazine maleate 5 mg, net price 28-tab pack = £1.03, 84-tab pack = £1.37. Label: 2

Injection, prochlorperazine mesilate 12.5 mg/mL, net price 1-mL amp = 52p

Stemetil® (Sanofi-Aventis) [PoM]

Tablets, prochlorperazine maleate 5 mg (off-white), net price 28-tab pack = £1.98, 84-tab pack = £5.94. Label: 2

Syrup, straw-coloured, prochlorperazine mesilate 5 mg/5 mL, net price 100-mL pack = £3.34. Label: 2

Injection, prochlorperazine mesilate 12.5 mg/mL, net price 1-mL amp = 52p

▮ Buccal preparation

Buccastem® (Alliance) [PoM]

Tablets (buccal), pale yellow, prochlorperazine maleate 3 mg, net price 5 × 10-tab pack = £6.49. Label: 2, counselling, administration, see under Dose below

Dose ADULT and CHILD over 12 years, 1–2 tablets twice daily; tablets are placed high between upper lip and gum and left to dissolve

▮ TRIFLUOPERAZINE

Indications   severe nausea and vomiting (see notes above); other indications (section 4.2.1)

Cautions   see notes in section 4.2.1

Contra-indications   see notes in section 4.2.1

Hepatic impairment   see notes in section 4.2.1

Renal impairment   see notes in section 4.2.1

Pregnancy   see notes in section 4.2.1

Breast-feeding   see notes in section 4.2.1

Side-effects   see Trifluoperazine, section 4.2.1

Dose

- 2–4 mg daily in divided doses; max. 6 mg daily; CHILD 3–5 years up to 1 mg daily, 6–12 years up to 4 mg daily

▮ Preparations

Section 4.2.1

Domperidone and metoclopramide

▮ DOMPERIDONE

Indications   relief of nausea and vomiting

Cautions   children; patients over 60 years—increased risk of ventricular arrhythmia; **interactions:** Appendix 1 (domperidone)

Counselling Patients should be told how to recognise signs of arrhythmia and advised to seek medical attention if symptoms such as palpitation or syncope develop

Contra-indications   prolactinoma; if increased gastrointestinal motility harmful; conditions where cardiac conduction is, or could be, impaired; concomitant use of drugs that prolong the QT interval, or of potent CYP3A4 inhibitors; cardiac disease

Hepatic impairment   avoid in moderate or severe impairment

Renal impairment   reduce frequency

Pregnancy   use only if potential benefit outweighs risk

Breast-feeding   amount too small to be harmful

Side-effects   dry mouth; *less commonly* diarrhoea, drowsiness, malaise, headache, anxiety, decreased libido, galactorrhoea, breast pain, rash, pruritus; *also reported* QT-interval prolongation, ventricular arrhythmias, sudden cardiac death, agitation, nervousness, convulsions, extrapyramidal disorders, gynaecomastia, amenorrhoea, urinary retention, oculogyric crisis

Dose

- By mouth, ADULT and CHILD over 12 years and body-weight over 35 kg, 10 mg up to 3 times daily; max. 30 mg daily; CHILD body-weight up to 35 kg, 250 micrograms/kg up to 3 times daily; max. 750 micrograms/kg daily
  Note See also MHRA advice above

Domperidone (Non-proprietary) ▼ PoM

Tablets, 10 mg (as maleate), net price 30-tab pack = £2.06; 100-tab pack = £6.87. Label: 22, counselling, arrhythmias

Suspension, domperidone 5 mg/5 mL, net price 200-mL pack = £13.21. Label: 22, counselling, arrhythmias

Motilium® (Zentiva) ▼ PoM

Tablets, f/c, domperidone 10 mg (as maleate), net price 30-tab pack = £2.71; 100-tab pack = £9.04. Label: 22, counselling, arrhythmias

METOCLOPRAMIDE HYDROCHLORIDE

Indications symptomatic treatment of nausea and vomiting, including that associated with acute migraine (section 4.7.4.1), delayed (but not acute) chemotherapy-induced nausea and vomiting, radiotherapy-induced nausea and vomiting, prevention of postoperative nausea and vomiting

Cautions elderly, young adults (15–19 years old), and children; atopic allergy (including asthma); cardiac conduction disturbances (and concomitant use of other drugs affecting cardiac conduction); uncorrected electrolyte imbalance; bradycardia; may mask underlying disorders such as cerebral irritation; epilepsy; Parkinson's disease; **interactions:** Appendix 1 (metoclopramide)

Contra-indications gastro-intestinal obstruction, perforation or haemorrhage; 3–4 days after gastrointestinal surgery; phaeochromocytoma

Hepatic impairment reduce dose

Renal impairment avoid or use small dose in severe impairment; increased risk of extrapyramidal reactions

Pregnancy not known to be harmful

Breast-feeding small amount present in milk; avoid

Side-effects extrapyramidal effects (especially in children and young adults (15–19 years old)—see p. 271), hyperprolactinaemia, galactorrhoea, gynaecomastia, menstrual changes; *very rarely* cardiac conduction abnormalities following intravenous administration, depression, neuroleptic malignant syndrome, methaemoglobinaemia (more severe in G6PD deficiency); *also reported* diarrhoea, hypotension, dyspnoea, anxiety, confusion, restlessness, drowsiness, dizziness, tremor, tardive dyskinesia on prolonged administration, visual disturbances, rash, urticaria, pruritus, oedema

Dose

- By mouth *or* by intramuscular injection *or* by slow intravenous injection (over at least 3 minutes), ADULT over 18 years, body-weight over 60 kg, 10 mg up to 3 times daily; body-weight under 60 kg, max. daily dose 500 micrograms/kg in 3 divided doses; CHILD under 18 years see *BNF for Children*
  Note See also MHRA advice above

Metoclopramide (Non-proprietary) PoM

Tablets, metoclopramide hydrochloride 10 mg, net price 28-tab pack = 97p

Oral solution, metoclopramide hydrochloride 5 mg/5 mL, net price 150-mL pack = £19.42. Counselling, use of pipette

Injection, metoclopramide hydrochloride 5 mg/mL, net price 2-mL amp = 32p

Maxolon® (AMCo) PoM

Tablets, scored, metoclopramide hydrochloride 10 mg, net price 84-tab pack = £5.24

Injection, metoclopramide hydrochloride 5 mg/mL, net price 2-mL amp = 27p

◢**Compound preparations (for migraine)**
Section 4.7.1

5HT₃-receptor antagonists

GRANISETRON

Indications see under Dose

Cautions susceptibility to QT-interval prolongation (including concomitant use of drugs that prolong QT interval, and electrolyte disturbances); subacute intestinal obstruction; **interactions:** Appendix 1 (5HT₃-receptor Antagonists)

Hepatic impairment manufacturer advises use with caution

Pregnancy manufacturer advises avoid

Breast-feeding avoid—no information available

Side-effects constipation, diarrhoea, headache, insomnia; *less commonly* QT-interval prolongation, extrapyramidal reactions, rash; also application-site reactions with transdermal patch

Dose

- Nausea and vomiting induced by cytotoxic chemotherapy or radiotherapy, by mouth, 1–2 mg within 1 hour before start of treatment, then 2 mg daily in 1–2 divided doses for up to 1 week following treatment; when intravenous infusion also used, max. combined total 9 mg in 24 hours; CHILD under 18 years see *BNF for Children*

  By intravenous injection (each 1 mg granisetron diluted to 5 mL and given over not less than 30 seconds) *or* by intravenous infusion (over 5 minutes), prevention, 10–40 micrograms/kg (max. 3 mg) 5 minutes before start of chemotherapy or radiotherapy; treatment, dose as for prevention (further maintenance doses must not be given less than 10 minutes apart); max. 9 mg in 24 hours; CHILD under 18 years see *BNF for Children*

- Nausea and vomiting induced by cytotoxic chemotherapy for planned duration of 3–5 days where oral antiemetics cannot be used, by transdermal route, apply one 3.1 mg/24 hours patch to clean, dry, non-irritated, non-hairy skin on upper arm (or abdomen if upper arm cannot be used) 24–48 hours before treatment; remove at least 24 hours after completing chemotherapy (patch may be worn for up to 7 days); CHILD not recommended

- Postoperative nausea and vomiting, by intravenous injection (diluted to 5 mL and given over 30 seconds), prevention, 1 mg before induction of anaesthesia; treatment, 1 mg, given as for prevention; max. 3 mg in 24 hours; CHILD not recommended

Granisetron (Non-proprietary) [PoM]

Tablets, granisetron (as hydrochloride) 1 mg, net price 10-tab pack = £50.38

Injection, granisetron (as hydrochloride) 1 mg/mL, for dilution before use, net price 1-mL amp = £1.60, 3-mL amp = £2.40

Kytril® (Roche) [PoM]

Tablets, f/c, granisetron (as hydrochloride) 1 mg, net price 10-tab pack = £52.39; 2 mg, 5-tab pack = £52.39

Sancuso® (ProStrakan) [PoM]

Patches, self-adhesive, granisetron 3.1 mg/24 hours, net price 1 patch = £56.00. Counselling, administration

Note Patients should be advised not to expose the site of the patch to sunlight during use and for 10 days after removal

ONDANSETRON

Indications see under Dose

Cautions susceptibility to QT-interval prolongation (including concomitant use of drugs that prolong QT interval, and electrolyte disturbances); subacute intestinal obstruction; adenotonsillar surgery; **interactions**: Appendix 1 (5HT$_3$-receptor Antagonists)

Contra-indications congenital long QT syndrome

Hepatic impairment max. 8 mg daily in moderate or severe impairment

Pregnancy no information available; avoid unless potential benefit outweighs risk

Breast-feeding present in milk in *animal* studies—avoid

Side-effects constipation; headache; flushing; injection site-reactions; *less commonly* hiccups, hypotension, bradycardia, chest pain, arrhythmias, movement disorders, seizures; *on intravenous administration, rarely* dizziness, transient visual disturbances (*very rarely* transient blindness); suppositories may cause rectal irritation

Dose
- Moderately emetogenic chemotherapy or radiotherapy, ADULT 18–65 years, by mouth, 8 mg 1–2 hours before treatment *or* by rectum, 16 mg 1–2 hours before treatment *or* by intramuscular injection *or* slow intravenous injection, 8 mg immediately before treatment; ELDERLY over 65 years, by mouth, 8 mg 1–2 hours before treatment *or* by rectum, 16 mg 1–2 hours before treatment *or* by intramuscular injection *or* intravenous infusion (over at least 15 minutes), 8 mg immediately before treatment

  then by mouth, 8 mg every 12 hours for up to 5 days *or* by rectum, 16 mg daily for up to 5 days; CHILD under 18 years see *BNF for Children*
- Severely emetogenic chemotherapy (consult product literature for dose of concomitant corticosteroid), ADULT 18–65 years, by mouth, 24 mg 1–2 hours before treatment *or* by rectum, 16 mg 1–2 hours before treatment *or* by intramuscular injection *or* slow intravenous injection, 8 mg immediately before treatment, where necessary followed by 2 further doses of 8 mg at 4 hourly intervals (*or* followed by 1 mg/hour by continuous intravenous infusion for up to 24 hours); ELDERLY 65–75 years, by mouth, 24 mg 1–2 hours before treatment *or* by rectum, 16 mg 1–2 hours before treatment *or* by intramuscular injection *or* intravenous infusion (over at least 15 minutes), 8 mg immediately before treatment, where necessary followed by 2 further doses of 8 mg at 4 hourly intervals (*or* followed by 1 mg/hour by continuous

intravenous infusion for up to 24 hours); ELDERLY over 75 years, by mouth, 24 mg 1–2 hours before treatment *or* by rectum, 16 mg 1–2 hours before treatment *or* by intravenous infusion (over at least 15 minutes), 8 mg immediately before treatment, where necessary followed by 2 further doses of 8 mg at 4 hourly intervals *alternatively* ADULT 18–65 years, by intravenous infusion (over at least 15 minutes), 16 mg immediately before treatment, where necessary followed by 2 further doses of 8 mg by intramuscular injection *or* slow intravenous injection at 4 hourly intervals; ELDERLY 65–75 years, by intravenous infusion (over at least 15 minutes), 16 mg immediately before treatment, where necessary followed by 2 further doses of 8 mg by intramuscular injection *or* intravenous infusion (over at least 15 minutes) at 4 hourly intervals

then by mouth, 8 mg every 12 hours for up to 5 days *or* by rectum, 16 mg daily for up to 5 days; CHILD under 18 years see *BNF for Children*
- Prevention of postoperative nausea and vomiting, ADULT over 18 years by mouth, 16 mg 1 hour before anaesthesia

  alternatively, by intramuscular injection *or* slow intravenous injection, 4 mg at induction of anaesthesia; CHILD under 18 years see *BNF for Children*
- Treatment of postoperative nausea and vomiting, ADULT over 18 years by intramuscular injection *or* slow intravenous injection, 4 mg; CHILD under 18 years see *BNF for Children*

Ondansetron (Non-proprietary) [PoM]

Tablets, ondansetron (as hydrochloride) 4 mg, net price 30-tab pack = £5.37; 8 mg, 10-tab pack = £45.05

Brands include *Ondemet®*

Oral solution, ondansetron (as hydrochloride) 4 mg/5 mL, net price 50-mL pack = £36.64

Brands include *Demorem®*

Orodispersible film, ondansetron 4 mg, net price 10-film pack = £28.50; 8 mg, 10-film pack = £57.00. Counselling, administration

Counselling Films should be placed on the tongue, allowed to disperse and swallowed

Brands include *Setofilm®*

Injection, ondansetron (as hydrochloride) 2 mg/mL, net price 2-mL amp = £1.00, 4-mL amp = £11.39

Zofran® (GSK) [PoM]

Tablets, yellow, f/c, ondansetron (as hydrochloride) 4 mg, net price 30-tab pack = £107.91; 8 mg, 10-tab pack = £71.94

Oral lyophilisates (*Zofran Melt®*), ondansetron 4 mg, net price 10-tab pack = £35.97; 8 mg, 10-tab pack = £71.94. Counselling, administration

Excipients include aspartame (section 9.4.1)

Counselling Tablets should be placed on the tongue, allowed to disperse and swallowed

Oral solution, sugar-free, strawberry-flavoured, ondansetron (as hydrochloride) 4 mg/5 mL, net price 50-mL pack = £35.97

Injection, ondansetron (as hydrochloride) 2 mg/mL, net price 2-mL amp = £5.99, 4-mL amp = £11.99

Suppositories, ondansetron 16 mg, net price 1 = £14.39

PALONOSETRON

Indications see under Dose

Cautions history of constipation; intestinal obstruction; susceptibility to QT-interval prolongation

(including concomitant use of drugs that prolong QT interval, and electrolyte disturbances)

Driving Dizziness or drowsiness may affect performance of skilled tasks (e.g. driving)

Pregnancy avoid—no information available

Breast-feeding avoid—no information available

Side-effects diarrhoea, constipation, headache, dizziness; *less commonly* dyspepsia, abdominal pain, dry mouth, flatulence, changes in blood pressure, tachycardia, bradycardia, arrhythmia, myocardial ischaemia, atrioventricular block, extrasystoles, hiccups, dyspnoea, asthenia, insomnia, anxiety, euphoria, peripheral neuropathy, anorexia, motion sickness, influenza-like symptoms, urinary retention, glycosuria, hyperglycaemia, electrolyte disturbance, myalgia, arthralgia, eye irritation, eye swelling, amblyopia, tinnitus, rash

Dose

- Moderately emetogenic chemotherapy, ADULT over 18 years, by mouth, 500 micrograms 1 hour before treatment *or* by intravenous injection (over 30 seconds), 250 micrograms as a single dose 30 minutes before treatment
- Severely emetogenic chemotherapy, ADULT over 18 years, by intravenous injection (over 30 seconds), 250 micrograms as a single dose 30 minutes before treatment

Aloxi® (Sinclair IS) PoM

Capsules, palonosetron (as hydrochloride) 500 micrograms, net price 1-cap pack = £55.89
Injection, palonosetron (as hydrochloride) 50 micrograms/mL, net price 5-mL amp = £55.89

Neurokinin-receptor antagonists

◼ APREPITANT

Indications adjunct to dexamethasone and a 5HT$_3$-receptor antagonist in preventing nausea and vomiting associated with moderately and highly emetogenic chemotherapy

Cautions interactions: Appendix 1 (aprepitant)

Contra-indications acute porphyria (section 9.8.2)

Hepatic impairment caution in moderate to severe impairment

Pregnancy avoid unless potential benefit outweighs risk—no information available; effectiveness of hormonal contraceptives reduced—effective non-hormonal methods of contraception necessary during treatment and for 2 months after stopping aprepitant

Breast-feeding avoid—present in milk in *animal* studies

Side-effects hiccups, dyspepsia, diarrhoea, constipation, anorexia; asthenia, headache, dizziness; *less commonly* weight changes, dry mouth, colitis, flatulence, stomatitis, abdominal pain, duodenal ulcer, taste disturbance, oedema, bradycardia, palpitations, cough, euphoria, anxiety, confusion, drowsiness, thirst, abnormal dreams, chills, hyperglycaemia, polyuria, anaemia, dysuria, haematuria, hyponatraemia, neutropenia, myalgia, conjunctivitis, pharyngitis, sneezing, tinnitus, sweating, pruritus, rash, acne, photosensitivity, and flushing; dyspnoea, insomnia, visual disturbances, dysarthria, urticaria, and Stevens-Johnson syndrome also reported

Dose

- ADULT over 18 years 125 mg 1 hour before chemotherapy, then 80 mg daily as a single dose for the next

2 days; consult product literature for dose of concomitant corticosteroid and 5HT$_3$-receptor antagonist

Emend® (MSD) PoM

Capsules, aprepitant 80 mg (white), net price 2-cap pack = £31.61; 125 mg (white/pink), 5-cap pack = £79.03; 3-day pack of one 125-mg capsule and two 80-mg capsules = £47.42

◼ FOSAPREPITANT

Note Fosaprepitant is a prodrug of aprepitant

Indications adjunct to dexamethasone and a 5HT$_3$-receptor antagonist in preventing nausea and vomiting associated with moderately and highly emetogenic chemotherapy

Cautions interactions: Appendix 1 (aprepitant)

Contra-indications acute porphyria (section 9.8.2)

Hepatic impairment see Aprepitant

Pregnancy see Aprepitant

Breast-feeding see Aprepitant

Side-effects see Aprepitant

Dose

- By intravenous infusion, over 20–30 minutes, ADULT over 18 years, 150 mg 30 minutes before chemotherapy on day 1 of cycle only; consult product literature for dose of concomitant corticosteroid and 5HT$_3$-receptor antagonist

Ivemend® (MSD) PoM

Injection, powder for reconstitution, fosaprepitant (as dimeglumine), net price 150-mg vial = £47.42
The *Scottish Medicines Consortium* (p. 4) has advised (January 2011) that fosaprepitant (*Ivemend®*) is accepted for restricted use within NHS Scotland for the prevention of acute and delayed nausea and vomiting associated with highly emetogenic cisplatin-based chemotherapy

Cannabinoid

◼ NABILONE

Indications nausea and vomiting caused by cytotoxic chemotherapy, unresponsive to conventional antiemetics (under close observation, preferably in hospital setting)

Cautions history of psychiatric disorder; elderly; hypertension; heart disease; adverse effects on mental state can persist for 48–72 hours after stopping

Driving Drowsiness may affect performance of skilled tasks (e.g. driving); effects of alcohol enhanced

Hepatic impairment avoid in severe impairment

Pregnancy avoid unless essential

Breast-feeding avoid—no information available

Side-effects drowsiness, vertigo, euphoria, dry mouth, ataxia, visual disturbance, concentration difficulties, sleep disturbance, dysphoria, hypotension, headache and nausea; also confusion, disorientation, hallucinations, psychosis, depression, decreased coordination, tremors, tachycardia, decreased appetite, and abdominal pain

Behavioural effects Patients should be made aware of possible changes of mood and other adverse behavioural effects

Dose

- Initially 1 mg twice daily, increased if necessary to 2 mg twice daily, throughout each cycle of cytotoxic therapy and, if necessary, for 48 hours after the last dose of each cycle; max. 6 mg daily given in 3 divided doses. The first dose should be taken the night before

4 Central nervous system

Central nervous system 4

initiation of cytotoxic treatment and the second dose 1–3 hours before the first dose of cytotoxic drug; ADOLESCENT and CHILD under 18 years consult local treatment protocol [unlicensed use]

Nabilone (Meda) CD2
Capsules, blue/white, nabilone 1 mg, net price 20-cap pack = £125.84. Label: 2, counselling, behavioural effects

Hyoscine

■ **HYOSCINE HYDROBROMIDE**
(Scopolamine Hydrobromide)

Indications motion sickness; hypersalivation associated with clozapine therapy; premedication (section 15.1.3); excessive respiratory secretions (see Prescribing in Palliative Care, p. 21)

Cautions section 1.2; also epilepsy

Contra-indications section 1.2

Hepatic impairment section 15.1.3

Renal impairment section 15.1.3

Pregnancy section 15.1.3

Breast-feeding section 15.1.3

Side-effects section 1.2

Dose
• Motion sickness, by mouth, ADULT and CHILD over 10 years, 150–300 micrograms up to 30 minutes before start of journey repeated every 6 hours if required; max. 900 micrograms daily; CHILD 3–4 years 75 micrograms up to 30 minutes before start of journey repeated after 6 hours if required, max. 150 micrograms daily; 4–10 years 75–150 micrograms up to 30 minutes before start of journey repeated every 6 hours if required; max. 450 micrograms daily
• Hypersalivation associated with clozapine therapy [unlicensed indication], by mouth, 300 micrograms up to 3 times daily; max. 900 micrograms daily; CHILD under 18 years see BNF for Children

Joy Rides® (Forest)
Tablets, chewable, raspberry-flavoured, hyoscine hydrobromide 150 micrograms, net price 12-tab pack = £1.55. Label: 2, 24

Kwells® (Bayer Consumer Care)
Tablets, chewable, scored, hyoscine hydrobromide 150 micrograms (Kwells® Kids) (white), net price 12-tab pack = £1.67; 300 micrograms (pink), 12-tab pack = £1.67. Label: 2

■Patches
Scopoderm TTS® (Novartis Consumer Health) PoM
Patch, self-adhesive, pink, releasing hyoscine approx. 1 mg/72 hours when in contact with skin, net price 5 = £8.64. Label: 19, counselling, see below
Dose motion sickness prevention, apply 1 patch to hairless area of skin behind ear 5–6 hours before journey; replace if necessary after 72 hours, siting replacement patch behind other ear; CHILD under 10 years not recommended
Counselling Explain accompanying instructions to patient and in particular emphasise advice to wash hands after handling and to wash application site after removing, and to use one patch at a time

■Parenteral preparations
Section 15.1.3

Other drugs for Ménière's disease

Betahistine has been promoted as a specific treatment for Ménière's disease.

■ **BETAHISTINE DIHYDROCHLORIDE**

Indications vertigo, tinnitus and hearing loss associated with Ménière's disease

Cautions asthma, history of peptic ulcer; **interactions:** Appendix 1 (betahistine)

Contra-indications phaeochromocytoma

Pregnancy avoid unless clearly necessary—no information available

Breast-feeding use only if potential benefit outweighs risk—no information available

Side-effects gastro-intestinal disturbances; headache, rashes and pruritus reported

Dose
• Initially 16 mg 3 times daily, preferably with food; maintenance 24–48 mg daily; CHILD not recommended

Betahistine Dihydrochloride (Non-proprietary) PoM
Tablets, betahistine dihydrochloride 8 mg, net price 84-tab pack = £2.05, 120-tab pack = £1.55; 16 mg, 84-tab pack = £2.89. Label: 21

Serc® (Abbott Healthcare) PoM
Tablets, betahistine dihydrochloride 8 mg (Serc®-8), net price 120-tab pack = £9.04; 16 mg (Serc®-16) (scored), 84-tab pack = £12.65. Label: 21

4.7 Analgesics

4.7.1	Non-opioid analgesics and compound analgesic preparations
4.7.2	Opioid analgesics
4.7.3	Neuropathic pain
4.7.4	Antimigraine drugs

The non-opioid drugs (section 4.7.1), paracetamol and aspirin (and other NSAIDs), are particularly suitable for pain in musculoskeletal conditions, whereas the opioid analgesics (section 4.7.2) are more suitable for moderate to severe pain, particularly of visceral origin.

Pain in palliative care For advice on pain relief in palliative care, see p. 20.

Pain in sickle-cell disease The pain of mild sickle-cell crises is managed with paracetamol, a NSAID (section 10.1.1), codeine, or dihydrocodeine. Severe crises may require the use of morphine or diamorphine; concomitant use of a NSAID may potentiate analgesia and allow lower doses of the opioid to be used. Pethidine should be avoided if possible because accumulation of a neurotoxic metabolite can precipitate seizures; the relatively short half-life of pethidine necessitates frequent injections.

Dental and orofacial pain Analgesics should be used judiciously in dental care as a **temporary** measure until the cause of the pain has been dealt with.

Dental pain of inflammatory origin, such as that associated with pulpitis, apical infection, localised osteitis or pericoronitis is usually best managed by treating the infection, providing drainage, restorative procedures, and other local measures. Analgesics provide temporary relief of pain (usually for about 1 to 7 days) until the causative factors have been brought under control. In the case of pulpitis, intra-osseous infection or abscess, reliance on analgesics alone is usually inappropriate.

Similarly the pain and discomfort associated with acute problems of the oral mucosa (e.g. acute herpetic gingivostomatitis, erythema multiforme) may be relieved by **benzydamine** mouthwash or spray (p. 787) until the cause of the mucosal disorder has been dealt with. However, where a patient is febrile, the antipyretic action of **paracetamol** (p. 281) or **ibuprofen** (p. 722) is often helpful.

The *choice* of an analgesic for dental purposes should be based on its suitability for the patient. Most dental pain is relieved effectively by non-steroidal anti-inflammatory drugs (NSAIDs). NSAIDs that are used for dental pain include **ibuprofen**, **diclofenac**, and **aspirin**; for further details see section 4.7.1 and section 10.1.1. **Paracetamol** has analgesic and antipyretic effects but no anti-inflammatory effect.

Opioid analgesics (section 4.7.2) such as **dihydrocodeine** act on the central nervous system and are traditionally used for *moderate to severe pain*. However, opioid analgesics are relatively ineffective in dental pain and their side-effects can be unpleasant. Paracetamol, ibuprofen, or aspirin are adequate for most cases of dental pain and an opioid is rarely required.

Combining a non-opioid with an opioid analgesic can provide greater relief of pain than either analgesic given alone. However, this applies only when an adequate dose of each analgesic is used. Most combination analgesic preparations have not been shown to provide greater relief of pain than an adequate dose of the non-opioid component given alone. Moreover, combination preparations have the disadvantage of an increased number of side-effects.

Any analgesic given before a dental procedure should have a low risk of increasing postoperative bleeding. In the case of pain after the dental procedure, taking an analgesic before the effect of the local anaesthetic has worn off can improve control. Postoperative analgesia with ibuprofen or aspirin is usually continued for about 24 to 72 hours.

Temporomandibular dysfunction can be related to anxiety in some patients who may clench or grind their teeth (bruxism) during the day or night. The muscle spasm (which appears to be the main source of pain) may be treated empirically with an overlay appliance which provides a free sliding occlusion and may also interfere with grinding. In addition, **diazepam** (section 4.1.2), which has muscle relaxant as well as anxiolytic properties, may be helpful but it should only be prescribed on a short-term basis during the acute phase. Analgesics such as aspirin (section 4.7.1) or ibuprofen (section 10.1.1) may also be required.

For the management of neuropathic pain, persistent idiopathic facial pain, and trigeminal neuralgia, see section 4.7.3.

Dysmenorrhoea   Use of an oral contraceptive prevents the pain of dysmenorrhoea which is generally associated with ovulatory cycles. If treatment is necessary paracetamol or a NSAID (section 10.1.1) will generally provide adequate relief of pain. The vomiting and severe pain associated with dysmenorrhoea in women with endometriosis may call for an antiemetic (in addition to an analgesic). Antispasmodics (such as alverine citrate, section 1.2) have been advocated for dysmenorrhoea but the antispasmodic action does not generally provide significant relief.

4.7.1 Non-opioid analgesics and compound analgesic preparations

Aspirin is indicated for headache, transient musculoskeletal pain, dysmenorrhoea, and pyrexia. In inflammatory conditions, most physicians prefer anti-inflammatory treatment with another NSAID which may be better tolerated and more convenient for the patient. Aspirin is used increasingly for its antiplatelet properties (section 2.9). Aspirin tablets or dispersible aspirin tablets are adequate for most purposes as they act rapidly.

Gastric irritation may be a problem; it is minimised by taking the dose after food. Enteric-coated preparations are available, but have a slow onset of action and are therefore unsuitable for single-dose analgesic use (though their prolonged action may be useful for night pain).

Aspirin interacts significantly with a number of other drugs and its interaction with warfarin is a **special hazard**, see **interactions:** Appendix 1 (aspirin).

Paracetamol is similar in efficacy to aspirin, but has no demonstrable anti-inflammatory activity; it is less irritant to the stomach and for that reason is now generally preferred to aspirin, particularly in the elderly. **Overdosage** with paracetamol is particularly dangerous as it may cause hepatic damage which is sometimes not apparent for 4 to 6 days (see Emergency Treatment of Poisoning, p. 35).

Nefopam may have a place in the relief of persistent pain unresponsive to other non-opioid analgesics. It causes little or no respiratory depression, but sympathomimetic and antimuscarinic side-effects may be troublesome.

Non-steroidal anti-inflammatory analgesics (NSAIDs, section 10.1.1) are particularly useful for the treatment of patients with chronic disease accompanied by pain and inflammation. Some of them are also used in the short-term treatment of mild to moderate pain including transient musculoskeletal pain but paracetamol is now often preferred, particularly in the elderly (see also p. 25). They are also suitable for the relief of pain in *dysmenorrhoea* and to treat pain caused by *secondary bone tumours*, many of which produce lysis of bone and release prostaglandins (see Prescribing in Palliative Care, p. 20). Selective inhibitors of cyclo-oxygenase-2 may be used in preference to non-selective NSAIDs for patients at high risk of developing serious gastro-intestinal side-effects. Several NSAIDs are also used for postoperative analgesia (section 15.1.4.2).

A non-opioid analgesic administered by intrathecal infusion (**ziconotide** (*Prialt®*), available from Eisai) is licensed for the treatment of chronic severe pain; ziconotide can be used by a hospital specialist as an adjunct to opioid analgesics.

Dental and orofacial pain   Most dental pain is relieved effectively by NSAIDs (section 10.1.1). **Aspirin** (p. 280) is effective against mild to moderate dental pain; dispersible tablets provide a rapidly absorbed form of aspirin suitable for most purposes.

The analgesic effect of **paracetamol** in mild to moderate dental pain is probably less than that of aspirin, but it does not affect bleeding time or interact significantly with warfarin. Moreover, it is less irritant to the stomach. Paracetamol is a suitable analgesic for children; sugar-free versions can be requested by specifying 'sugar-free' on the prescription.

For further information on the management of dental and orofacial pain, see p. 278.

Compound analgesic preparations

Compound analgesic preparations that contain a simple analgesic (such as aspirin or paracetamol) with an opioid component reduce the scope for effective titration of the individual components in the management of pain of varying intensity.

Compound analgesic preparations containing paracetamol or aspirin with a *low dose* of an opioid analgesic (e.g. 8 mg of codeine phosphate per compound tablet) are commonly used, but the advantages have not been substantiated. The low dose of the opioid may be enough to cause opioid side-effects (in particular, constipation) and can complicate the treatment of **overdosage** (see p. 38) yet may not provide significant additional relief of pain.

A *full dose* of the opioid component (e.g. 60 mg codeine phosphate) in compound analgesic preparations effectively augments the analgesic activity but is associated with the full range of opioid side-effects (including nausea, vomiting, severe constipation, drowsiness, respiratory depression, and risk of dependence on long-term administration). For details of the **side-effects** of opioid analgesics, see p. 284 (**important:** the elderly are particularly susceptible to opioid side-effects and should receive lower doses).

In general, when assessing pain, it is necessary to weigh up carefully whether there is a need for a non-opioid and an opioid analgesic to be taken simultaneously.

For information on the use of combination analgesic preparations in dental and orofacial pain, see p. 279.

Caffeine is a weak stimulant that is often included, in small doses, in analgesic preparations. It is claimed that the addition of caffeine may enhance the analgesic effect, but the alerting effect, mild habit-forming effect and possible provocation of headache may not always be desirable. Moreover, in excessive dosage or on withdrawal caffeine may itself induce headache.

Co-proxamol tablets (dextropropoxyphene in combination with paracetamol) are no longer licensed because of safety concerns, particularly toxicity in overdose. Co-proxamol tablets [unlicensed] may still be prescribed for patients who find it difficult to change, because alternatives are not effective or suitable.

ASPIRIN
(Acetylsalicylic Acid)

Indications   mild to moderate pain, pyrexia; antiplatelet (section 2.9)

Cautions   asthma, allergic disease, dehydration; preferably avoid during fever or viral infection in children (risk of Reye's syndrome, see below); elderly; G6PD-deficiency (section 9.1.5); concomitant use of drugs that increase risk of bleeding; anaemia; thyrotoxicosis; **interactions:** Appendix 1 (aspirin)

Contra-indications   children under 16 years (Reye's syndrome, see below); previous or active peptic ulceration, haemophilia; severe cardiac failure; not for treatment of gout

Hypersensitivity Aspirin and other NSAIDs are **contra-**

indicated in patients with a history of hypersensitivity to aspirin or any other NSAID—*which includes those* in whom attacks of *asthma, angioedema, urticaria or rhinitis* have been precipitated by aspirin or any other NSAID

Reye's syndrome Owing to an association with Reye's syndrome, aspirin-containing preparations should not be given to children under 16 years, unless specifically indicated, e.g. for Kawasaki disease

Hepatic impairment   avoid in severe impairment—increased risk of gastro-intestinal bleeding

Renal impairment   use with caution; avoid in severe impairment; sodium and water retention; deterioration in renal function; increased risk of gastro-intestinal bleeding

Pregnancy   high doses may be related to intrauterine growth restriction and teratogenic effects; impaired platelet function with risk of haemorrhage, and delayed onset and increased duration of labour with increased blood loss, can occur if used during delivery; avoid analgesic doses if possible in last few weeks (low doses probably not harmful); with high doses, closure of fetal ductus arteriosus in utero and possibly persistent pulmonary hypertension of newborn; kernicterus in jaundiced neonates

Breast-feeding   avoid—possible risk of Reye's syndrome; regular use of high doses could impair platelet function and produce hypoprothrombinaemia in infant if neonatal vitamin K stores low

Side-effects   generally mild and infrequent but high incidence of gastro-intestinal irritation with slight asymptomatic blood loss, blood disorders have occurred (including increased bleeding time), confusion, tinnitus, bronchospasm and skin reactions in hypersensitive patients. Prolonged administration, see section 10.1.1. **Overdosage:** see Emergency Treatment of Poisoning, p. 35

Dose
- By mouth, 300–900 mg every 4–6 hours when necessary; max. 4 g daily; CHILD under 16 years not recommended (see Reye's Syndrome, above)
- By rectum, 450–900 mg every 4 hours (max. 3.6 g daily); CHILD under 16 years not recommended (see Reye's Syndrome, above)

Aspirin (Non-proprietary)
Tablets [PoM]¹, aspirin 300 mg, net price 32-tab pack = £3.35. Label: 21, 32

Tablets [PoM]¹, e/c, aspirin 300 mg, net price 100-tab pack = £14.00; 75 mg, see section 2.9. Label: 5, 25, 32

Dispersible tablets [PoM]¹, aspirin 300 mg, net price 100-tab pack = £3.19; 75 mg, see section 2.9. Label: 13, 21, 32

Note BP directs that when no strength is stated the 300-mg strength should be dispensed, and that when soluble aspirin tablets are prescribed, dispersible aspirin tablets shall be dispensed.

Dental prescribing on NHS Aspirin Dispersible Tablets 300 mg may be prescribed

Suppositories [PoM], aspirin 150 mg, net price 10 = £16.05; 300 mg, 12 = £13.89. Label: 32
Brands include Resprin®

Nu-Seals® Aspirin (Alliance)
Tablets [PoM]¹, e/c, aspirin 300 mg, net price 100-tab pack = £4.15; 75 mg, see section 2.9. Label: 5, 25, 32

1. Can be sold to the public provided packs contain no more than 32 capsules or tablets; pharmacists can sell multiple packs up to a total quantity of 100 capsules or tablets in justifiable circumstances.

◢**With codeine phosphate 8 mg**

For prescribing information on codeine, see section 4.7.2

[1]**Co-codaprin** (Non-proprietary) PoM ◢

Dispersible tablets, co-codaprin 8/400 (codeine phosphate 8 mg, aspirin 400 mg), net price 100-tab pack = £89.83. Label: 13, 21, 32

Dose ADULT and CHILD over 16 years, 1–2 tablets in water every 4–6 hours when necessary; max. 8 tablets daily

Note When co-codaprin tablets or dispersible tablets are prescribed and no strength is stated, tablets or dispersible tablets, respectively, containing codeine phosphate 8 mg and aspirin 400 mg should be dispensed

◢**With metoclopramide**

For prescribing information on metoclopramide, see section 4.6

MigraMax® (Zentiva) PoM

Oral powder, lemon flavour, aspirin (as lysine acetylsalicylate) 900 mg, metoclopramide hydrochloride 10 mg/sachet, net price 6-sachet pack = £6.61. Label: 13, 21, 32

Excipients include aspartame (section 9.4.1)

Dose acute migraine, ADULT over 18 years, 1 sachet in water at onset of attack, repeated after 2 hours if necessary (max. 3 sachets in 24 hours); CHILD under 18 years, not recommended

Important Metoclopramide can cause **severe extrapyramidal effects**, particularly in children and young adults (for further details, see p. 271)

Note Treatment should not exceed 3 months due to risk of tardive dyskinesia, but see also MHRA advice on Metoclopramide, section 4.6

PARACETAMOL

(Acetaminophen)

Indications mild to moderate pain, pyrexia (pyrexia with discomfort in children)

Cautions alcohol dependence; hepatocellular insufficiency, chronic alcoholism, chronic malnutrition, or dehydration, max. daily infusion dose 3 g in patients greater than 50 kg body-weight with risk factors for hepatotoxicity; before administering, check when paracetamol last administered and cumulative paracetamol dose over previous 24 hours; **interactions**: Appendix 1 (paracetamol)

Hepatic impairment dose-related toxicity—avoid large doses; see also Cautions

Renal impairment increase infusion dose interval to every 6 hours if eGFR less than 30 mL/minute/ 1.73 m^2; note also sodium content of effervescent tablets (see under relevant preparation entry)

Pregnancy not known to be harmful

Breast-feeding amount too small to be harmful

Side-effects side-effects *rare*, malaise, skin reactions including Stevens-Johnson syndrome, toxic epidermal necrolysis, acute generalised exanthematous pustulosis; blood disorders including thrombocytopenia, leucopenia, neutropenia reported; hypotension, flushing, and tachycardia reported on infusion; **important**: liver damage (and less frequently renal damage) following **overdosage**, see Emergency Treatment of Poisoning, p. 35

Dose

• By mouth, 0.5–1 g every 4–6 hours to a max. of 4 g daily; CHILD 2–3 months 60 mg for post-immunisation pyrexia, repeated once after 4–6 hours if necessary;

otherwise under 3 months see *BNF for Children*; 3–6 months 60 mg, 6 months–2 years 120 mg, 2–4 years 180 mg, 4–6 years 240 mg, 6–8 years 240–250 mg, 8–10 years 360–375 mg, 10–12 years 480–500 mg, 12–16 years 480–750 mg; these doses may be repeated every 4–6 hours when necessary (max. of 4 doses in 24 hours); postoperative pain in children see *BNF for Children*

• By intravenous infusion over 15 minutes, ADULT and CHILD over 50 kg, 1 g every 4–6 hours, max. 4 g daily; ADULT and CHILD 10–50 kg, 15 mg/kg every 4–6 hours, max. 60 mg/kg daily; CHILD less than 10 kg see *BNF for Children*

• By rectum, 0.5–1 g every 4–6 hours to a max. of 4 g daily; CHILD under 3 months see *BNF for Children*, 3 months–1 year 60–125 mg, 1–5 years 125–250 mg, 5–12 years 250–500 mg, 12–18 years 500 mg; these doses may be repeated every 4–6 hours as necessary (max. 4 doses in 24 hours); postoperative pain in children see *BNF for Children*

Note For full Joint Committee on Vaccination and Immunisation recommendation on post-immunisation pyrexia, see section 14.1

Paracetamol (Non-proprietary)

Tablets (and caplets) PoM [1], paracetamol 500 mg, net price 32–tab pack = £1.02, 100-tab pack = £3.19. Label: 29, 30

Dental prescribing on NHS Paracetamol Tablets may be prescribed

Capsules PoM [1], paracetamol 500 mg, net price 32-cap pack = £1.32, 100-cap pack = £4.13. Label: 29, 30

Soluble tablets (= Dispersible tablets) PoM, paracetamol 500 mg, net price 24-tab pack = £2.12, 100-tab pack = £8.83. Label: 13, 29, 30

Dental prescribing on NHS Paracetamol Soluble Tablets 500 mg may be prescribed

Oral suspension 120 mg/5 mL, paracetamol 120 mg/5 mL, net price 100 mL = 66p, 500 mL = £3.10. Label: 30

Note BP directs that when Paediatric Paracetamol Oral Suspension or Paediatric Paracetamol Mixture is prescribed Paracetamol Oral Suspension 120 mg/5 mL should be dispensed; sugar-free versions can be ordered by specifying 'sugar-free' on the prescription

Oral suspension 250 mg/5 mL, paracetamol 250 mg/5 mL, net price 100 mL = £1.38, 200 mL = £1.65. Label: 30

Dental prescribing on NHS Paracetamol Oral Suspension may be prescribed

Oral suspension 500 mg/5 mL PoM, paracetamol 500 mg/5 mL sugar-free, net price 150 mL = £20.00. Label: 30

Suppositories, paracetamol 60 mg, net price 10 = £11.95; 120 mg, 10 = £11.26; 125 mg, 10 = £13.80; 240 mg, 10 = £22.01; 250 mg, 10 = £27.60; 500 mg, 10 = £36.50; 1 g, 12 = £60.00. Label: 30

Note Other strengths available from 'special-order' manufacturers or specialist importing companies, see p. 1124

Intravenous infusion PoM, paracetamol 10 mg/mL, net price 100-mL vial = £1.20

Panadol OA® (GSK) PoM

Tablets, f/c, paracetamol 1 g, net price 100-tab pack = £3.45. Label: 30

Dose ADULT and CHILD over 12 years, 1 tablet up to 4 times daily, not more often than every 4 hours

Perfalgan® (Bristol-Myers Squibb) PoM

Intravenous infusion, paracetamol 10 mg/mL, net price 50-mL vial = £1.13, 100-mL vial = £1.25

---

1. Can be sold to the public provided packs contain no more than 32 capsules or tablets; pharmacists can sell multiple packs up to a total quantity of 100 capsules or tablets in justifiable circumstances.

4 Central nervous system

◢**With codeine phosphate 8 mg**

When co-codamol tablets, dispersible (or effervescent) tablets, or capsules are prescribed and **no strength is stated**, tablets, dispersible (or effervescent) tablets, or capsules, respectively, containing codeine phosphate 8 mg and paracetamol **500 mg** should be dispensed.

See notes on p. 280

For prescribing information on codeine, see p. 286

[1]**Co-codamol 8/500** (Non-proprietary) PoM ◢

Tablets, co-codamol 8/500 (codeine phosphate 8 mg, paracetamol 500 mg), net price 30-tab pack = £1.19, 32-tab pack = 50p, 100-tab pack = £3.97. Label: 29, 30

Dose ADULT over 18 years, 1–2 tablets every 4–6 hours when necessary; max. 8 tablets daily; CHILD under 18 years see *BNF for Children*

Effervescent *or* dispersible tablets, co-codamol 8/500 (codeine phosphate 8 mg, paracetamol 500 mg), net price 32-tab pack = £2.51, 100-tab pack = £7.84. Label: 13, 29, 30

Brands include *Paracodol®*[PHS]

Note The Drug Tariff allows tablets of co-codamol labelled 'dispersible' to be dispensed against an order for 'effervescent' and *vice versa*

Dose ADULT over 18 years, 1–2 tablets in water every 4–6 hours when necessary; max. 8 tablets daily; CHILD under 18 years see *BNF for Children*

Capsules, co-codamol 8/500 (codeine phosphate 8 mg, paracetamol 500 mg), net price 10-cap pack = £1.29, 20-cap pack = £1.71. Label: 29, 30

Brands include *Paracodol®*[PHS]

Dose ADULT over 18 years, 1–2 capsules every 4–6 hours when necessary; max. 8 capsules daily; CHILD under 18 years see *BNF for Children*

◢**With codeine phosphate 15 mg**

When co-codamol tablets, dispersible (or effervescent) tablets, or capsules are prescribed and **no strength is stated**, tablets, dispersible (or effervescent) tablets, or capsules, respectively, containing codeine phosphate **8 mg** and paracetamol **500 mg** should be dispensed (see preparations above).

See warnings and notes on p. 280 (**important:** special care in elderly—reduce dose)

For prescribing information on codeine, see p. 286

Codipar® (AMCo) PoM ◢

Tablets, co-codamol 15/500 (codeine phosphate 15 mg, paracetamol 500 mg), net price 100-tab pack = £8.25. Label: 2, 29, 30

Dose ADULT over 18 years, 1–2 tablets every 4–6 hours when necessary; max. 8 tablets daily; CHILD under 18 years see *BNF for Children*

Capsules, co-codamol 15/500 (codeine phosphate 15 mg, paracetamol 500 mg), net price 100-cap pack = £7.25. Label: 2, 29, 30

Dose ADULT over 18 years, 1–2 capsules every 4–6 hours when necessary; max. 8 capsules daily; CHILD under 18 years see *BNF for Children*

Effervescent tablets, co-codamol 15/500 (codeine phosphate 15 mg, paracetamol 500 mg), net price 100-tab pack = £8.25. Label: 2, 13, 29, 30

Electrolytes Na^+ 16.5 mmol/tablet

Dose ADULT over 18 years, 2 tablets every 4–6 hours when necessary; max. 8 tablets daily; CHILD not recommended

Kapake® (Galen) PoM ◢

Tablets, co-codamol 15/500 (codeine phosphate 15 mg, paracetamol 500 mg), net price 100-tab pack = £7.01. Label: 2, 29, 30

Dose ADULT over 18 years, 2 tablets every 4–6 hours when necessary; max. 8 tablets daily; CHILD under 18 years see *BNF for Children*

---

1. Can be sold to the public in certain circumstances; for exemptions see *Medicines, Ethics and Practice*, London, Pharmaceutical Press (always consult latest edition)

◢**With codeine phosphate 30 mg**

When co-codamol tablets, dispersible (or effervescent) tablets, or capsules are prescribed and **no strength is stated**, tablets, dispersible (or effervescent) tablets, or capsules, respectively, containing codeine phosphate **8 mg** and paracetamol **500 mg** should be dispensed (see preparations above).

See warnings and notes on p. 280 (**important:** special care in elderly—reduce dose)

For prescribing information on codeine, see p. 286

Co-codamol 30/500 (Non-proprietary) PoM ◢

Tablets (and caplets), co-codamol 30/500 (codeine phosphate 30 mg, paracetamol 500 mg), net price 100-tab pack = £4.67. Label: 2, 29, 30

Dose ADULT over 18 years, severe pain, 1–2 tablets every 4–6 hours when necessary; max. 8 tablets daily; CHILD under 18 years see *BNF for Children*

Capsules, co-codamol 30/500 (codeine phosphate 30 mg, paracetamol 500 mg), net price 100-cap pack = £3.95. Label: 2, 29, 30

Brands include *Medocodene®*, *Zapain®*

Dose ADULT over 18 years, severe pain, 1–2 capsules every 4–6 hours when necessary; max. 8 capsules daily; CHILD under 18 years see *BNF for Children*

Effervescent tablets, co-codamol 30/500 (codeine phosphate 30 mg, paracetamol 500 mg), net price 100-tab pack = £8.19. Label: 2, 13, 29, 30

Brands include *Medocodene® Effervescent* (contains Na^+ 13.6 mmol/tablet)

Dose ADULT over 18 years, severe pain, 1–2 tablets in water every 4–6 hours when necessary; max. 8 tablets daily; CHILD under 18 years see *BNF for Children*

Kapake® (Galen) PoM ◢

Tablets, scored, co-codamol 30/500 (codeine phosphate 30 mg, paracetamol 500 mg), net price 30-tab pack = £2.26 (hosp. only), 100-tab pack = £6.04. Label: 2, 29, 30

Dose ADULT over 18 years, severe pain, 1–2 tablets every 4–6 hours when necessary; max. 8 tablets daily; CHILD under 18 years see *BNF for Children*

Capsules, co-codamol 30/500 (codeine phosphate 30 mg, paracetamol 500 mg), net price 100-cap pack = £6.04. Label: 2, 29, 30

Dose ADULT over 18 years, severe pain, 1–2 capsules every 4–6 hours when necessary; max. 8 capsules daily; CHILD under 18 years see *BNF for Children*

Solpadol® (Sanofi-Aventis) PoM ◢

Caplets (= tablets), co-codamol 30/500 (codeine phosphate 30 mg, paracetamol 500 mg), net price 100-tab pack = £6.74. Label: 2, 29, 30

Dose ADULT over 18 years, severe pain, 2 tablets every 4–6 hours when necessary; max. 8 tablets daily; CHILD under 18 years see *BNF for Children*

Capsules, grey/purple, co-codamol 30/500 (codeine phosphate 30 mg, paracetamol 500 mg), net price 100-cap pack = £6.74. Label: 2, 29, 30

Dose ADULT over 18 years, severe pain, 2 capsules every 4–6 hours when necessary; max. 8 capsules daily; CHILD under 18 years see *BNF for Children*

Effervescent tablets, co-codamol 30/500 (codeine phosphate 30 mg, paracetamol 500 mg), net price 32-tab pack = £2.59, 100-tab pack = £8.90. Label: 2, 13, 29, 30

Electrolytes Na^+ 16.9 mmol/tablet

Dose ADULT over 18 years, severe pain, 2 tablets in water every 4–6 hours when necessary; max. 8 tablets daily; CHILD under 18 years see *BNF for Children*

4 Central nervous system

Tylex® (UCB Pharma) PoM ▰

Capsules, co-codamol 30/500 (codeine phosphate 30 mg, paracetamol 500 mg), net price 100-cap pack = £7.93. Label: 2, 29, 30

Excipients include sulphites

Dose ADULT over 18 years, severe pain, 1–2 capsules every 4–6 hours when necessary; max. 8 capsules daily; CHILD under 18 years see *BNF for Children*

Effervescent tablets, co-codamol 30/500 (codeine phosphate 30 mg, paracetamol 500 mg), net price 100-tab pack = £9.06. Label: 2, 13, 29, 30

Electrolytes Na⁺ 14.2 mmol/tablet

Excipients include aspartame 25 mg/tablet (section 9.4.1)

Dose ADULT over 18 years, severe pain, 1–2 tablets in water every 4–6 hours when necessary; max. 8 tablets daily; CHILD under 18 years see *BNF for Children*

◢**With dihydrocodeine tartrate 10 mg**

When co-dydramol tablets are prescribed and **no strength is stated**, tablets containing dihydrocodeine tartrate **10 mg** and paracetamol **500 mg** should be dispensed.

See notes on p. 280

For prescribing information on dihydrocodeine, see p. 287

Co-dydramol (Non-proprietary) PoM ▰

Tablets, scored, co-dydramol 10/500 (dihydrocodeine tartrate 10 mg, paracetamol 500 mg), net price 30-tab pack = £1.15. Label: 29, 30

Dose ADULT over 18 years, 1–2 tablets every 4–6 hours when necessary; max. 8 tablets daily; CHILD under 18 years see *BNF for Children*

◢**With dihydrocodeine tartrate 20 mg**

When co-dydramol tablets are prescribed and **no strength is stated**, tablets containing dihydrocodeine tartrate **10 mg** and paracetamol **500 mg** should be dispensed (see preparation above).

See warnings and notes on p. 280 (important: special care in elderly—reduce dose)

For prescribing information on dihydrocodeine, see p. 287

Remedeine® (Crescent) PoM ▰

Tablets, paracetamol 500 mg, dihydrocodeine tartrate 20 mg, net price 112-tab pack = £10.63. Label: 2, 29, 30

Dose ADULT over 18 years, severe pain, 1–2 tablets every 4–6 hours when necessary; max. 8 tablets daily; CHILD under 18 years see *BNF for Children*

◢**With dihydrocodeine tartrate 30 mg**

When co-dydramol tablets are prescribed and **no strength is stated**, tablets containing dihydrocodeine tartrate **10 mg** and paracetamol **500 mg** should be dispensed (see preparation above).

See warnings and notes on p. 280 (important: special care in elderly—reduce dose)

For prescribing information on dihydrocodeine, see p. 287

Remedeine Forte® (Crescent) PoM ▰

Tablets, paracetamol 500 mg, dihydrocodeine tartrate 30 mg, net price 56-tab pack = £6.57. Label: 2, 29, 30

Dose ADULT over 18 years, severe pain, 1–2 tablets every 4–6 hours when necessary; max. 8 tablets daily; CHILD under 18 years see *BNF for Children*

◢**With isometheptene mucate**

Isometheptene mucate (in combination with paracetamol) is licensed for the treatment of acute attacks of migraine; other more effective treatments are available.

Midrid® (Manx) PoM ▰

Capsules, red, isometheptene mucate 65 mg, paracetamol 325 mg, net price 30-cap pack = £5.50. Label: 30, counselling, dosage

Dose migraine, 2 capsules at onset of attack, followed by 1 capsule every hour if necessary; max. 5 capsules in 12 hours; CHILD not recommended

◢**With tramadol**

For prescribing information on tramadol, see section 4.7.2

Tramacet® (Grünenthal) CD3

Tablets, f/c, yellow, tramadol hydrochloride 37.5 mg, paracetamol 325 mg, net price 60-tab pack = £9.68. Label: 2, 25, 29, 30

Dose 2 tablets not more often than every 6 hours; max. 8 tablets daily; CHILD under 12 years not recommended

Effervescent tablets, pink, tramadol hydrochloride 37.5 mg, paracetamol 325 mg, net price 60-tab pack = £9.68. Label: 2, 13, 29, 30

Electrolytes Na⁺ 7.8 mmol/tablet

Dose 2 tablets not more often than every 6 hours; max. 8 tablets daily; CHILD under 12 years not recommended

◢**With antiemetics**

For prescribing information on codeine, see Codeine Phosphate, section 4.7.2. For prescribing information on buclizine hydrochloride, see Antihistamines, section 3.4.1.

Migraleve® (McNeil) ▰

Tablets, f/c, *pink tablets*, buclizine hydrochloride 6.25 mg, paracetamol 500 mg, codeine phosphate 8 mg; *yellow tablets*, paracetamol 500 mg, codeine phosphate 8 mg, net price 48-tab *Migraleve* PoM (32 pink + 16 yellow) = £3.64; 48 pink (*Migraleve Pink*) = £3.97; 48 yellow (*Migraleve Yellow*) = £4.70. Label: 2, (*Migraleve Pink*), 17, 30

Dose acute migraine, ADULT and CHILD over 15 years, 2 pink tablets at onset of attack, followed by 2 yellow tablets every 4 hours if necessary; max. 2 pink and 6 yellow tablets in 24 hours; CHILD 12–14 years, half adult dose

Paramax® (Zentiva) PoM

Tablets, scored, paracetamol 500 mg, metoclopramide hydrochloride 5 mg, net price 42-tab pack = £9.64. Label: 17, 30

Dose acute migraine, ADULT over 18 years, 2 tablets at the onset of attack then repeat every 4 hours when necessary to max. 6 tablets in 24 hours

Sachets, effervescent powder, sugar-free, paracetamol 500 mg, metoclopramide hydrochloride 5 mg, net price 42-sachet pack = £12.52. Label: 13, 17, 30

Dose acute migraine, ADULT over 18 years, 2 sachets dissolved in a quarter tumblerful of water at onset of attack then repeat every 4 hours when necessary to max. 6 sachets in 24 hours

Important Metoclopramide can cause **severe extrapyramidal effects**, particularly in young adults (for further details, see p. 271)

Note Treatment should not exceed 3 months due to risk of tardive dyskinesia, but see also MHRA advice on Metoclopramide, section 4.6

NEFOPAM HYDROCHLORIDE

Indications moderate pain

Cautions elderly, urinary retention; **interactions:** Appendix 1 (nefopam)

Contra-indications convulsive disorders; not indicated for myocardial infarction

4 Central nervous system

Hepatic impairment   caution

Renal impairment   caution

Pregnancy   no information available—avoid unless no safer treatment

Side-effects   nausea, nervousness, urinary retention, dry mouth, lightheadedness; *less commonly* vomiting, blurred vision, drowsiness, sweating, insomnia, tachycardia, headache; confusion and hallucinations *also reported*; may colour urine (pink)

Dose

- By mouth, initially 60 mg (ELDERLY 30 mg) 3 times daily, adjusted according to response; usual range 30–90 mg 3 times daily; CHILD not recommended

Acupan® (Meda) PoM

Tablets, f/c, nefopam hydrochloride 30 mg, net price 90-tab pack = £10.59. Label: 2, 14

4.7.2 Opioid analgesics

Opioid analgesics are usually used to relieve moderate to severe pain particularly of visceral origin. Repeated administration may cause dependence and tolerance, but this is no deterrent in the control of pain in terminal illness, for guidelines see Prescribing in Palliative Care, p. 20. Regular use of a potent opioid may be appropriate for certain cases of chronic non-malignant pain; treatment should be supervised by a specialist and the patient should be assessed at regular intervals.

Cautions   Opioids should be used with caution in patients with impaired respiratory function (avoid in chronic obstructive pulmonary disease) and asthma (avoid during an acute attack), hypotension, urethral stenosis, shock, myasthenia gravis, prostatic hypertrophy, obstructive or inflammatory bowel disorders, diseases of the biliary tract, and convulsive disorders. A reduced dose is recommended in elderly or debilitated patients, in hypothyroidism, and in adrenocortical insufficiency. Repeated use of opioid analgesics is associated with the development of psychological and physical dependence; although this is rarely a problem with therapeutic use, caution is advised if prescribing for patients with a history of drug dependence. Avoid abrupt withdrawal after long-term treatment. Transdermal preparations (fentanyl or buprenorphine patches) are not suitable for acute pain or in those patients whose analgesic requirements are changing rapidly because the long time to steady state prevents rapid titration of the dose. **Interactions**: Appendix 1 (opioid analgesics; **important**: special hazard with *pethidine and possibly other opioids* and MAOIs).

Palliative care In the control of pain in terminal illness, the cautions listed above should not necessarily be a deterrent to the use of opioid analgesics.

Contra-indications   Opioid analgesics should be avoided in patients with acute respiratory depression and when there is a risk of paralytic ileus. They are also contra-indicated in conditions associated with raised intracranial pressure and in head injury (opioid analgesics interfere with pupillary responses vital for neurological assessment). Comatose patients should not be treated with opioid analgesics.

Hepatic impairment   Opioid analgesics may precipitate coma in patients with hepatic impairment; avoid use or reduce dose.

Renal impairment   The effects of opioid analgesia are increased and prolonged and there is increased cerebral sensitivity when patients with renal impairment are treated with opioid analgesics; avoid use or reduce dose.

Pregnancy   Respiratory depression and withdrawal symptoms can occur in the neonate if opioid analgesics are used during delivery; also gastric stasis and inhalation pneumonia has been reported in the mother if opioid analgesics are used during labour.

Side-effects   Opioid analgesics share many side-effects, although qualitative and quantitative differences exist. The most common side-effects include nausea and vomiting (particularly in initial stages), constipation, dry mouth, and biliary spasm; larger doses produce muscle rigidity, hypotension, and respiratory depression (for reversal of opioid-induced respiratory depression, see section 15.1.7). Other common side-effects of opioid analgesics include bradycardia, tachycardia, palpitation, oedema, postural hypotension, hallucinations, vertigo, euphoria, dysphoria, mood changes, dependence, dizziness, confusion, drowsiness, sleep disturbances, headache, sexual dysfunction, difficulty with micturition, urinary retention, ureteric spasm, miosis, visual disturbances, sweating, flushing, rash, urticaria, and pruritus. **Overdosage**: see Emergency Treatment of Poisoning, p. 38.

Long-term use of opioid analgesics can cause hypogonadism and adrenal insufficiency in both men and women. This is thought to be dose related and can lead to amenorrhoea, reduced libido, infertility, depression, and erectile dysfunction. Long-term use of opioid analgesics has also been associated with a state of abnormal pain sensitivity (hyperalgesia). Pain associated with hyperalgesia is usually distinct from pain associated with disease progression or breakthrough pain, and is often more diffuse and less defined. Treatment of hyperalgesia involves reducing the dose of opioid medication or switching therapy; cases of suspected hyperalgesia should be referred to a specialist pain team.

Driving   Drowsiness may affect performance of skilled tasks (e.g. driving); effects of alcohol enhanced. Driving at the start of therapy with opioid analgesics, and following dose changes, should be avoided; see also Drugs and Driving, p. 3

Strong opioids   Morphine remains the most valuable opioid analgesic for severe pain although it frequently causes nausea and vomiting. It is the standard against which other opioid analgesics are compared. In addition to relief of pain, morphine also confers a state of euphoria and mental detachment.

Morphine is the opioid of choice for the oral treatment of *severe pain in palliative care*. It is given regularly every 4 hours (or every 12 or 24 hours as modified-release preparations). For guidelines on dosage adjustment in palliative care, see p. 20.

A modified-release epidural preparation of morphine is available from Flynn Pharma Ltd (*Depodur®*▼).

Buprenorphine has both opioid agonist and antagonist properties and may precipitate withdrawal symptoms, including pain, in patients dependent on other opioids. It has abuse potential and may itself cause dependence.

It has a much longer duration of action than morphine and sublingually is an effective analgesic for 6 to 8 hours. Unlike most opioid analgesics, the effects of buprenorphine are only partially reversed by naloxone.

Dipipanone used alone is less sedating than morphine but the only preparation available contains an anti-emetic and is therefore not suitable for regular regimens in palliative care.

Diamorphine (heroin) is a powerful opioid analgesic. It may cause less nausea and hypotension than morphine. In *palliative care* the greater solubility of diamorphine allows effective doses to be injected in smaller volumes and this is important in the emaciated patient.

Alfentanil, fentanyl and **remifentanil** are used by injection for intra-operative analgesia (section 15.1.4.3); fentanyl is available in a transdermal drug delivery system as a self-adhesive patch which is changed every 72 hours.

Methadone is less sedating than morphine and acts for longer periods. In prolonged use, methadone should not be administered more often than twice daily to avoid the risk of accumulation and opioid overdosage. Methadone may be used instead of morphine in the occasional patient who experiences excitation (or exacerbation of pain) with morphine.

Oxycodone has an efficacy and side-effect profile similar to that of morphine. It is used primarily for control of *pain in palliative care.*

Papaveretum is rarely used; morphine is easier to prescribe and less prone to error with regard to the strength and dose.

Pentazocine has both agonist and antagonist properties and precipitates withdrawal symptoms, including pain in patients dependent on other opioids. By injection it is more potent than dihydrocodeine or codeine, but hallucinations and thought disturbances may occur. It is not recommended and, in particular, should be avoided after myocardial infarction as it may increase pulmonary and aortic blood pressure as well as cardiac work.

Pethidine produces prompt but short-lasting analgesia; it is less constipating than morphine, but even in high doses is a less potent analgesic. It is not suitable for severe continuing pain. It is used for analgesia in labour; however, other opioids, such as morphine or diamorphine, are often preferred for obstetric pain.

Tapentadol produces analgesia by two mechanisms. It is an opioid-receptor agonist and it also inhibits noradrenaline reuptake. Nausea, vomiting, and constipation are less likely to occur with tapentadol than with other strong opioid analgesics.

Tramadol produces analgesia by two mechanisms: an opioid effect and an enhancement of serotonergic and adrenergic pathways. It has fewer of the typical opioid side-effects (notably, less respiratory depression, less constipation and less addiction potential); psychiatric reactions have been reported.

Weak opioids   **Codeine** can be used for the relief of mild to moderate pain where other painkillers such as paracetamol or ibuprofen have proved ineffective, but see Variation in Metabolism, p. 286

Dihydrocodeine has an analgesic efficacy similar to that of codeine. Higher doses may provide some additional pain relief but this may be at the cost of more nausea and vomiting.

Meptazinol is claimed to have a low incidence of respiratory depression. It has a reported length of action of 2 to 7 hours with onset within 15 minutes.

Dose The dose of opioids in the BNF may need to be adjusted **individually** according to the degree of analgesia and side-effects; patients' response to opioids varies widely.

Postoperative analgesia A combination of opioid and non-opioid analgesics (section 4.7.1 and section 15.1.4.2) is used to treat postoperative pain. The use of intra-operative opioids affects the prescribing of post-operative analgesics. A postoperative opioid analgesic should be given with care since it may potentiate any residual respiratory depression (for the treatment of opioid-induced respiratory depression, see section 15.1.7).

Morphine is used most widely. **Tramadol** is not as effective in severe pain as other opioid analgesics. **Buprenorphine** may antagonise the analgesic effect of previously administered opioids and is generally not recommended. **Pethidine** is generally not recommended for postoperative pain because it is metabolised to norpethidine which may accumulate, particularly in renal impairment; norpethidine stimulates the central nervous system and may cause convulsions.

Opioids are also given epidurally [unlicensed route] in the postoperative period but are associated with side-effects such as pruritus, urinary retention, nausea and vomiting; respiratory depression can be delayed, particularly with morphine.

For details of patient-controlled analgesia (PCA) to relieve postoperative pain, consult hospital protocols.

Dental and orofacial pain Opioid analgesics are **relatively ineffective** in dental pain. Like other opioids, **dihydrocodeine** often causes nausea and vomiting which limits its value in dental pain; if taken for more than a few doses it is also liable to cause constipation. Dihydrocodeine is not very effective in postoperative dental pain.

For the management of dental and orofacial pain, see p. 278.

Pain management and opioid dependence
Although caution is necessary, patients who are dependent on opioids or have a history of drug dependence may be treated with opioid analgesics when there is a clinical need. Treatment with opioid analgesics in this patient group should normally be carried out with the advice of specialists. However, doctors do not require a special licence to prescribe opioid analgesics to patients with opioid dependence for relief of pain due to organic disease or injury.

4 Central nervous system

BUPRENORPHINE

Indications see under Dose and under Patches; opioid dependence (section 4.10.3)

Cautions see notes above; also impaired consciousness; effects only partially reversed by naloxone; monitor liver function

> **Fever or external heat** Monitor patients using patches for increased side-effects if fever present (increased absorption possible); avoid exposing application site to external heat (may also increase absorption)

Contra-indications see notes above

4 Central nervous system

Hepatic impairment   see notes above

Renal impairment   see notes above

Pregnancy   see notes above and section 4.10.3

Breast-feeding   present in low levels in breast milk—monitor neonate for drowsiness, adequate weight gain, and developmental milestones

Side-effects   see notes above; can induce mild withdrawal symptoms in patients dependent on opioids; also diarrhoea, abdominal pain, anorexia, dyspepsia; vasodilatation; dyspnoea; paraesthesia, asthenia, fatigue, agitation, anxiety; *less commonly* flatulence, taste disturbance, angina, hypertension, syncope, hypoxia, wheezing, cough, restlessness, depersonalisation, dysarthria, impaired memory, hypoaesthesia, tremor, influenza-like symptoms, pyrexia, rhinitis, rigors, muscle cramp, myalgia, tinnitus, dry eye, and dry skin; *rarely* paralytic ileus, dysphagia, impaired concentration, and psychosis; *very rarely* retching, hyperventilation, hiccups, and muscle fasciculation; hepatic necrosis and hepatitis also reported

Dose
- Moderate to severe pain, by sublingual administration, 200–400 micrograms every 6–8 hours; CHILD over 6 years, 16–25 kg, 100 micrograms every 6–8 hours; 25–37.5 kg, 100–200 micrograms every 6–8 hours; 37.5–50 kg, 200–300 micrograms every 6–8 hours

  By intramuscular *or* slow intravenous injection, 300–600 micrograms every 6–8 hours; CHILD over 6 months 3–6 micrograms/kg every 6–8 hours (max. 9 micrograms/kg)
- Premedication, by sublingual administration, 400 micrograms

  By intramuscular injection, 300 micrograms
- Intra-operative analgesia, by slow intravenous injection, 300–450 micrograms

Temgesic® (Reckitt Benckiser) [CD3]
Tablets (sublingual), buprenorphine (as hydrochloride), 200 micrograms, net price 50-tab pack = £5.04; 400 micrograms, 50-tab pack = £10.07. Label: 2, 26

Injection, buprenorphine (as hydrochloride) 300 micrograms/mL, net price 1-mL amp = 49p

◢**Patches**

BuTrans® (Napp) [CD3]
Patches, self-adhesive, beige, buprenorphine, '5' patch (releasing 5 micrograms/hour for 7 days), net price 4 = £17.60; '10' patch (releasing 10 micrograms/hour for 7 days), 4 = £31.55; '20' patch (releasing 20 micrograms/hour for 7 days), 4 = £57.46. Label: 2

Dose   moderate, non-malignant pain unresponsive to non-opioid analgesics, ADULT over 18 years, initially one '5 micrograms/hour' patch; apply to dry, non-irritated, non-hairy skin on upper torso, removing after 7 days and siting replacement patch on a different area (avoid same area for at least 3 weeks)

Dose adjustment   When starting, analgesic effect should **not** be evaluated until the system has been worn for **72 hours** (to allow for gradual increase in plasma-buprenorphine concentration)—if necessary, dose should be adjusted at intervals of at least 3 days using a patch of the next strength or a combination of 2 patches applied in different places (applied at *same time* to avoid confusion). Max. 2 patches can be used at any one time

Long duration of action   In view of the long duration of action, other opioids should not be administered within 24 hours of patch removal

Hapoctasin® (Actavis) [CD3]
Patches, self-adhesive, skin-coloured, buprenorphine, '35' patch (releasing 35 micrograms/hour for 72 hours), net price 4 = £9.48; '52.5' patch (releasing 52.5 micrograms/hour for 72 hours), 4 = £14.23; '70' patch (releasing 70 micrograms/hour for 72 hours), 4 = £18.96. Label: 2

Dose   moderate to severe chronic cancer pain and severe pain unresponsive to non-opioid analgesics, ADULT over 18 years, apply to dry, non-irritated, non-hairy skin on upper torso, removing after no longer than 72 hours and siting replacement patch on a different area (avoid same area for at least 7 days). Patients who have not previously received strong opioid analgesic, initially, one '35 micrograms/hour' patch replaced after no longer than 72 hours; patients who have received strong opioid analgesic, initial dose based on previous 24-hour opioid requirement, consult product literature

Dose adjustment   When starting, analgesic effect should **not** be evaluated until the system has been worn for **24 hours** (to allow for gradual increase in plasma-buprenorphine concentration)—if necessary, dose should be adjusted at intervals of no longer than 72 hours using a patch of the next strength *or* using 2 patches of the same strength (applied at *same time* to avoid confusion). Max. 2 patches can be used at any one time. For breakthrough pain, consider 200–400 micrograms buprenorphine sublingually.

Important: it may take approx. 25 hours for the plasma-buprenorphine concentration to decrease by 50% after patch is removed

Long duration of action   In view of the long duration of action, patients who have severe side-effects should be monitored for up to 25 hours after removing patch; other opioids should not be administered within 24 hours of patch removal

Transtec® (Napp) [CD3]
Patches, self-adhesive, skin-coloured, buprenorphine, '35' patch (releasing 35 micrograms/hour for 96 hours), net price 4 = £15.80; '52.5' patch (releasing 52.5 micrograms/hour for 96 hours), 4 = £23.71; '70' patch (releasing 70 micrograms/hour for 96 hours), 4 = £31.60. Label: 2

Dose   moderate to severe chronic cancer pain and severe pain unresponsive to non-opioid analgesics, ADULT over 18 years, apply to dry, non-irritated, non-hairy skin on upper torso, removing after no longer than 96 hours and siting replacement patch on a different area (avoid same area for at least 6 days). Patients who have not previously received strong opioid analgesic, initially, one '35 micrograms/hour' patch replaced after no longer than 96 hours; patients who have received strong opioid analgesic, initial dose based on previous 24-hour opioid requirement, consult product literature

Dose adjustment   When starting, analgesic effect should **not** be evaluated until the system has been worn for **24 hours** (to allow for gradual increase in plasma-buprenorphine concentration)—if necessary, dose should be adjusted at intervals of no longer than 96 hours using a patch of the next strength *or* using 2 patches of the same strength (applied at *same time* to avoid confusion). Max. 2 patches can be used at any one time. For breakthrough pain, consider 200–400 micrograms buprenorphine sublingually.

Important: it may take approx. 30 hours for the plasma-buprenorphine concentration to decrease by 50% after patch is removed

Long duration of action   In view of the long duration of action, patients who have severe side-effects should be monitored for up to 30 hours after removing patch; other opioids should not be administered within 24 hours of patch removal

◢ CODEINE PHOSPHATE

Indications   mild to moderate pain; diarrhoea (section 1.4.2); cough suppression (section 3.9.1)

Cautions   see notes above; also cardiac arrhythmias; acute abdomen; gallstones

Variation in metabolism   The capacity to metabolise codeine to morphine can vary considerably between individuals; there is a marked increase in morphine toxicity in patients who are ultra-rapid codeine metabolisers (CYP2D6 ultra-rapid metabolisers) and a reduced therapeutic effect in poor codeine metabolisers

Contra-indications see notes above; also in children under 18 years who undergo the removal of tonsils or adenoids for the treatment of sleep apnoea; known ultra-rapid codeine metabolisers (see Variation in Metabolism above)

Hepatic impairment see notes above

Renal impairment see notes above

Pregnancy see notes above

Breast-feeding Avoid—although amount usually too small to be harmful, mothers vary considerably in their capacity to metabolise codeine—risk of morphine overdose in infant

Side-effects see notes above; also abdominal pain, anorexia, seizures, malaise, hypothermia, antidiuretic effect, and muscle fasciculation; pancreatitis also reported

Dose

- By mouth, ADULT over 18 years, 30–60 mg every 4 hours when necessary, to a max. of 240 mg daily; CHILD under 18 years see *BNF for Children*
- By intramuscular injection, ADULT over 18 years, 30–60 mg every 4 hours when necessary; CHILD under 18 years see *BNF for Children*

Codeine Phosphate (Non-proprietary)

Tablets (PoM), codeine phosphate 15 mg, net price 28-tab pack = £1.34; 30 mg, 28-tab pack = £1.64; 60 mg, 28-tab pack = £3.28. Label: 2

Syrup (PoM), codeine phosphate 25 mg/5 mL, net price 100 mL = 98p. Label: 2

Injection (CD2), codeine phosphate 60 mg/mL, net price 1-mL amp = £2.37

◀**Linctus**
Section 3.9.1

◀**With paracetamol**
Section 4.7.1

DIAMORPHINE HYDROCHLORIDE
(Heroin Hydrochloride)

Indications see under Dose

Cautions see notes above; also severe diarrhoea; toxic psychosis, CNS depression; severe cor pulmonale

Contra-indications see notes above; also delayed gastric emptying; phaeochromocytoma

Hepatic impairment see notes above

Renal impairment see notes above

Pregnancy see notes above

Breast-feeding therapeutic doses unlikely to affect infant; withdrawal symptoms in infants of dependent mothers; breast-feeding not best method of treating dependence in offspring

Side-effects see notes above; also anorexia, taste disturbance; syncope; asthenia, raised intracranial pressure; myocardial infarction also reported

Dose

- Acute pain, by subcutaneous *or* intramuscular injection, 5 mg repeated every 4 hours if necessary (up to 10 mg for heavier well-muscled patients); by slow intravenous injection, quarter to half corresponding intramuscular dose

- Myocardial infarction, by slow intravenous injection (1–2 mg/minute), 5 mg followed by a further 2.5–5 mg if necessary; ELDERLY or frail patients, reduce dose by half
- Acute pulmonary oedema, by slow intravenous injection (1 mg/minute) 2.5–5 mg
- Chronic pain, by subcutaneous *or* intramuscular injection, ADULT **not currently treated** with a strong opioid analgesic, initially 2.5–5 mg every 4 hours, adjusted according to response; ADULT **currently treated** with a strong opioid analgesic—see Prescribing in Palliative Care, p. 21; by subcutaneous infusion, ADULT **not currently treated** with a strong opioid analgesic, initially 5–10 mg over 24 hours, adjusted according to response; ADULT **currently treated** with a strong opioid analgesic—see Prescribing in Palliative Care, p. 24

Diamorphine (Non-proprietary) (CD2)

Tablets, diamorphine hydrochloride 10 mg, net price 100-tab pack = £24.09. Label: 2

Injection, powder for reconstitution, diamorphine hydrochloride, net price 5-mg amp = £2.27, 10-mg amp = £2.79, 30-mg amp = £2.85, 100-mg amp = £8.48, 500-mg amp = £37.54

DIHYDROCODEINE TARTRATE

Indications moderate to severe pain

Cautions see notes above; also pancreatitis; severe cor pulmonale

Contra-indications see notes above

Hepatic impairment see notes above

Renal impairment see notes above

Pregnancy see notes above

Breast-feeding use only if potential benefit outweighs risk

Side-effects see notes above; also paralytic ileus, abdominal pain, diarrhoea, seizures, and paraesthesia

Dose

- By mouth, 30 mg every 4–6 hours when necessary (see also notes above); CHILD over 4 years 0.5–1 mg/kg every 4–6 hours
- By deep subcutaneous *or* intramuscular injection, up to 50 mg repeated every 4–6 hours if necessary; CHILD over 4 years 0.5–1 mg/kg every 4–6 hours

Dihydrocodeine (Non-proprietary)

Tablets (PoM), dihydrocodeine tartrate 30 mg, net price 28-tab pack = £1.31. Label: 2

Dental prescribing on NHS Dihydrocodeine Tablets 30 mg may be prescribed

Oral solution (PoM), dihydrocodeine tartrate 10 mg/5 mL, net price 150 mL = £6.20. Label: 2

Injection (CD2), dihydrocodeine tartrate 50 mg/mL, net price 1-mL amp = £7.89

DF118 Forte® (Martindale) (PoM)

Tablets, dihydrocodeine tartrate 40 mg, net price 100-tab pack = £11.51. Label: 2

Dose ADULT and CHILD over 12 years, severe pain, 40–80 mg 3 times daily; max. 240 mg daily

4

Central nervous system

◢Modified release

DHC Continus® (Napp) PoM

Tablets, m/r, dihydrocodeine tartrate 60 mg, net price 56-tab pack = £5.20; 90 mg, 56-tab pack = £8.66; 120 mg, 56-tab pack = £10.95. Label: 2, 25

Dose ADULT and CHILD over 12 years, chronic severe pain, 60–120 mg every 12 hours

Note Dihydrocodeine is an ingredient of some compound analgesic preparations, section 4.7.1

◢With paracetamol

section 4.7.1

DIPIPANONE HYDROCHLORIDE

Indications   moderate to severe pain

Cautions   see notes above; also diabetes mellitus; phaeochromocytoma

Contra-indications   see notes above

Hepatic impairment   see notes above

Renal impairment   see notes above

Pregnancy   see notes above

Breast-feeding   no information available

Side-effects   see notes above; also psychosis, restlessness, raised intracranial pressure

Dose

• See preparation below

Dipipanone and cyclizine (Non-proprietary) CD2

Tablets, dipipanone hydrochloride 10 mg, cyclizine hydrochloride 30 mg, net price 50-tab pack = £129.74

Dose *acute pain*, 1 tablet gradually increased to 3 tablets every 6 hours; CHILD not recommended

Caution Not recommended in palliative care, see Nausea and Vomiting, p. 22

FENTANYL

Indications   severe chronic pain, breakthrough pain; parenteral indications (section 15.1.4.3)

Cautions   see notes above; also diabetes mellitus (with *Actiq®* lozenges); impaired consciousness; cerebral tumour; mucositis—absorption from oral preparations may be increased, caution during dose titration; see also Transdermal Fentanyl, p. 290

Contra-indications   see notes above

Hepatic impairment   see notes above

Renal impairment   see notes above

Pregnancy   see notes above

Breast-feeding   monitor infant for opioid-induced side-effects

Side-effects   see notes above; also abdominal pain, dyspepsia, diarrhoea, gastro-oesophageal reflux disease, stomatitis, anorexia, hypertension, vasodilation, dyspnoea, aesthenia, myoclonus, anxiety, tremor, appetite changes, rhinitis, pharyngitis, paraesthesia, application-site reactions; *less commonly* ileus, flatulence, hypoventilation, impaired concentration, impaired coordination, amnesia, speech disorder, malaise, seizures, depressed level of consciousness, loss of consciousness, dysgeusia, parosmia, pyrexia, thirst, blood disorders (including thrombocytopenia), arthralgia, chills; *rarely* hiccups; *very rarely* arrhythmia, apnoea, haemoptysis, ataxia, delusions, bladder pain

Dose

• Chronic intractable pain, by transdermal route, apply to dry, non-irritated, non-irradiated, non-hairy skin on torso or upper arm, removing after 72 hours and siting replacement patch on a different area (avoid using the same area for several days). ADULT over 16 years **not currently treated** with a strong opioid analgesic (but see Transdermal Fentanyl, p. 290), initial dose, one '12' or '25 micrograms/hour' patch replaced after 72 hours; ADULT and CHILD over 2 years **currently treated** with a strong opioid analgesic, initial dose based on previous 24-hour opioid requirement (consult product literature)

Dose adjustment When starting, evaluation of the analgesic effect should **not** be made before the system has been worn for **24 hours** (to allow for the gradual increase in plasma-fentanyl concentration)—previous analgesic therapy should be phased out gradually from time of first patch application; if necessary dose should be adjusted at 48–72-hour intervals in steps of 12–25 micrograms/hour. More than one patch may be used at a time (but applied at the *same time* to avoid confusion)—consider additional or alternative analgesic therapy if dose required exceeds 300 micrograms/hour (**important:** it takes 17 hours or more for the plasma-fentanyl concentration to decrease by 50%— replacement opioid therapy should be initiated at a low dose and increased gradually).

Long duration of action In view of the long duration of action, patients who have had severe side-effects should be monitored for up to 24 hours after patch removal

• Breakthrough pain, see under preparations below

Important Fentanyl preparations for the treatment of breakthrough pain are not interchangeable; if patients are switched from another fentanyl-containing preparation, a new dose titration is required

Conversion (from long-term oral morphine to transdermal fentanyl) see Prescribing in Palliative Care, p. 21

◢Tablets

Abstral® (ProStrakan) CD2

Tablets (sublingual), fentanyl (as citrate) 100 micrograms, net price 10-tab pack = £49.99, 30-tab pack = £149.70; 200 micrograms, 10-tab pack = £49.99, 30-tab pack = £149.70; 300 micrograms, 10-tab pack = £49.99, 30-tab pack = £149.70; 400 micrograms, 10-tab pack = £49.99, 30-tab pack = £149.70; 600 micrograms, 30-tab pack = £149.70; 800 micrograms, 30-tab pack = £149.70. Label: 2, 26, counselling, administration

Dose breakthrough pain in patients receiving opioid therapy for chronic cancer pain, ADULT over 18 years, initially 100 micrograms repeated if necessary after 15–30 minutes; adjust dose according to response—consult product literature; no more than 2 dose units 15–30 minutes apart, for each pain episode; max. 800 micrograms per episode of breakthrough pain; leave at least 2 hours between treatment of episodes of breakthrough pain

Note If more than 4 episodes of breakthrough pain each day, adjust background analgesia

Counselling Patients should be advised not to eat or drink until the tablet is completely dissolved. In patients with a dry mouth, the buccal mucosa may be moistened with water before administration of tablet

The *Scottish Medicines Consortium* (p. 4) has advised (January 2009) that *Abstral®* sublingual tablets should be restricted for the management of breakthrough pain in adult patients using opioid therapy for chronic cancer pain, when other short-acting opioids are unsuitable

Effentora® (TEVA UK) CD2

Tablets (buccal), fentanyl, sugar-free (as citrate) 100 micrograms, net price 4-tab pack = £19.96, 28-tab pack = £139.72; 200 micrograms, 4-tab pack = £19.96, 28-tab pack = £139.72; 400 micrograms, 4-tab pack = £19.96, 28-tab pack = £139.72; 600 micrograms, 4-tab pack = £19.96; 800 micrograms, 4-tab pack = £19.96, 28-tab pack = £139.72. Label: 2, counselling, administration

Electrolytes Na$^+$ 0.35 mmol/100 microgram tablet, Na$^+$ 0.70 mmol/tablet (all other strengths)

Dose breakthrough pain in patients receiving opioid therapy for chronic cancer pain, ADULT over 18 years, initially 100 micrograms repeated if necessary 30 minutes after first dose (no more than 2 dose units for each pain episode); adjust dose according to response—consult product literature; max. 800 micrograms per episode of breakthrough pain; leave at least 4 hours between treatment of episodes of breakthrough pain during titration

Counselling Place tablet between cheek and gum and leave to dissolve; if more than 1 tablet required, place second tablet on the other side of the mouth; tablet may alternatively be placed under the tongue (sublingually). Patients should be advised not to eat or drink until the tablet is completely dissolved; after 30 minutes, if any remnants remain, they may be swallowed with a glass of water. Patients with a dry mouth should be advised to drink water to moisten the buccal mucosa before administration of the tablets; if appropriate effervescence does not occur, a switch of therapy may be advised

The *Scottish Medicines Consortium* (p. 4) has advised that *Effentora*® buccal tablets should be restricted for the management of breakthrough pain in adult patients using opioid therapy for chronic cancer pain, when other short-acting opioids are unsuitable

Recivit® (Grünenthal) CD2

Tablets (sublingual), fentanyl (as citrate) 133 micrograms, net price 30-tab pack = £127.20; 267 micrograms, 30-tab pack = £127.20; 400 micrograms, 30-tab pack = £127.20; 533 micrograms, 30-tab pack = £127.20; 800 micrograms, 30-tab pack = £127.20. Label: 2, 26, counselling, administration

Electrolytes Na$^+$ 0.03 mmol/tablet (all tablet strengths)

Dose breakthrough pain in patients receiving opioid therapy for chronic cancer pain, ADULT over 18 years, initially 133 micrograms repeated if necessary after 15–30 minutes; adjust dose according to response—consult product literature; no more than 2 dose units, 15–30 minutes apart, for each pain episode; max. 800 micrograms per episode of breakthrough pain; max. four doses per day

Note If more than 4 episodes of breakthrough pain each day, adjust background analgesia

Counselling Patients should be advised not to eat or drink until the tablet is completely dissolved; after 30 minutes, if any remnants remain, they may be swallowed. In patients with a dry mouth, the buccal mucosa may be moistened with water before administration of tablet

◀**Lozenges**

Actiq® (TEVA UK) CD2

Lozenge (buccal), with oromucosal applicator, fentanyl (as citrate) 200 micrograms, net price 3 = £21.05, 30 = £210.41; 400 micrograms, 3 = £21.05, 30 = £210.41; 600 micrograms, 3 = £21.05, 30 = £210.41; 800 micrograms, 3 = £21.05, 30 = £210.41; 1.2 mg, 3 = £21.05, 30 = £210.41; 1.6 mg, 3 = £21.05, 30 = £210.41. Label: 2, counselling, administration

Excipients include propylene glycol (see Excipients)

Dose breakthrough pain in patients receiving opioid therapy for chronic cancer pain, ADULT and CHILD over 16 years initially 200 micrograms (over 15 minutes) repeated if necessary 15 minutes after first dose (no more than 2 dose units for each pain episode); if adequate pain relief not achieved with 1 dose unit for consecutive breakthrough pain episodes, increase the strength of the dose unit until adequate pain relief achieved with 4 lozenges or less daily

Note If more than 4 episodes of breakthrough pain each day, adjust background analgesia

Counselling Patients should be advised to place the lozenge in the mouth against the cheek and move it around the mouth using the applicator; each lozenge should be sucked over a 15 minute period. In patients with a dry mouth, water may be used to moisten the buccal mucosa. Patients with diabetes should be advised each lozenge contains approximately 2 g glucose

◀**Films**

Breakyl® (Meda) CD2

Film (buccal), fentanyl (as citrate) 200 micrograms, net price 10 = £49.90; 400 micrograms, 10 = £49.90; 800 micrograms, 28 = £139.72. Label: 2, counselling, administration

Excipients include propylene glycol (see Excipients, p. 2)

Dose breakthrough pain in patients receiving opioid therapy for chronic cancer pain, ADULT over 18 years, initially 200 micrograms; adjust dose according to response—consult product literature; max. 1.2 mg per episode of breakthrough pain; leave at least 4 hours between treatment of episodes of breakthrough pain

Note If more than 4 episodes of breakthrough pain each day occur on more than 4 consecutive days, adjust background analgesia

Counselling Moisten mouth, place film on inner lining of cheek (pink side to cheek), hold for at least 5 seconds until it sticks, and leave to dissolve (15–30 minutes); if more than 1 film required do not overlap, but use another area of the mouth. Avoid liquids for 5 minutes after application; avoid food until the film has dissolved

◀**Nasal spray**

Instanyl® (Takeda) CD2

Nasal spray, fentanyl (as citrate) 50 micrograms/metered spray, net price single-dose pack = £5.95, 10-dose pack = £59.50, 20-dose pack = £119.00; 100 micrograms/metered spray, single-dose pack = £5.95, 10-dose pack = £59.50, 20-dose pack = £119.00; 200 micrograms/metered spray, single-dose pack = £5.95, 10-dose pack = £59.50, 20-dose pack = £119.00. Label: 2, counselling, administration

Dose breakthrough pain in patients receiving opioid therapy for chronic cancer pain, ADULT over 18 years, initially 50 micrograms into one nostril, repeated once if necessary after 10 minutes; adjust dose according to response; max. 2 sprays for each pain episode and minimum 4 hours between treatment of each pain episode

Note If more than 4 breakthrough pain episodes daily, adjust background analgesia

Counselling Patient should sit or stand during administration. Avoid concomitant use of other nasal preparations

The *Scottish Medicines Consortium* (p. 4) has advised that *Instanyl*® nasal spray should be restricted for use within NHS Scotland for the management of breakthrough pain in adult patients using opioid therapy for chronic cancer pain, when other short-acting opioids are unsuitable

PecFent® (Archimedes) CD2

Nasal spray, fentanyl (as citrate) 100 micrograms/metered spray, net price 8-dose pack = £36.48, 32-dose pack = £145.92; 400 micrograms/metered spray, 8-dose pack = £36.48, 32-dose pack = £145.92. Label: 2, counselling, administration

Dose breakthrough pain in patients receiving opioid therapy for chronic cancer pain, ADULT over 18 years, initially 100 micrograms into one nostril; adjust dose according to response; max. 2 sprays for each pain episode and minimum 4 hours between treatment of each pain episode

Note If more than 4 breakthrough pain episodes daily, adjust background analgesia

Counselling Avoid concomitant use of other nasal preparations

The *Scottish Medicines Consortium* (p. 4) has advised (September 2008) that *PecFent*® nasal spray should be restricted for use within NHS Scotland for the management of breakthrough pain in adult patients using opioid therapy for chronic cancer pain, when other short-acting opioids are unsuitable

4 Central nervous system

◢Patches

Transdermal fentanyl

Fever or external heat Monitor patients using patches for increased side-effects if fever present (increased absorption possible); avoid exposing application site to external heat, for example a hot bath or sauna (may also increase absorption)

Respiratory depression Risk of fatal respiratory depression, particularly in patients not previously treated with a strong opioid analgesic; manufacturer recommends use only in opioid tolerant patients

Counselling Patients and carers should be informed about safe use, including correct administration and disposal, strict adherence to dosage instructions, and the symptoms and signs of opioid overdosage. Patches should be removed immediately in case of breathing difficulties, marked drowsiness, confusion, dizziness, or impaired speech, and patients and carers should seek prompt medical attention.

Prescriptions Prescriptions for fentanyl patches can be written to show the strength in terms of the release rate and it is acceptable to write '*Fentanyl 25 patches*' to prescribe patches that release fentanyl 25 micrograms per hour. The dosage should be expressed in terms of the interval between applying a patch and replacing it with a new one, e.g. '*one patch to be applied every 72 hours*'. The total quantity of patches to be supplied should be written in words and figures.

Fentanyl (Non-proprietary) [CD2]
Patches, self-adhesive, fentanyl, '12' patch (releasing approx. 12 micrograms/hour for 72 hours), net price 5 = £12.59; '25' patch (releasing approx. 25 micrograms/hour for 72 hours), 5 = £17.99; '37.5' patch (releasing approx. 37.5 micrograms/hour for 72 hours; *Mezolar*® brand only), 5 = £15.45; '50' patch (releasing approx. 50 micrograms/hour for 72 hours), 5 = £33.66; '75' patch (releasing approx. 75 micrograms/hour for 72 hours), 5 = £46.99; '100' patch (releasing approx. 100 micrograms/hour for 72 hours), 5 = £57.86. Label: 2, counselling, administration
Brands include *Fencino*®, *Fentalis*®, *Matrifen*®, *Mezolar*®, *Opiodur*®, *Osmanil*®, *Tilofyl*®, *Victanyl*®

Durogesic DTrans® (Janssen) [CD2]
Patches, self-adhesive, transparent, fentanyl, '12' patch (releasing approx. 12 micrograms/hour for 72 hours), net price 5 = £12.59; '25' patch (releasing approx. 25 micrograms/hour for 72 hours), 5 = £17.99; '50' patch (releasing approx. 50 micrograms/hour for 72 hours), 5 = £33.66; '75' patch (releasing approx. 75 micrograms/hour for 72 hours), 5 = £46.99; '100' patch (releasing approx. 100 micrograms/hour for 72 hours), 5 = £57.86. Label: 2, counselling, administration

HYDROMORPHONE HYDROCHLORIDE

Indications severe pain in cancer

Cautions see notes above; also pancreatitis; toxic psychosis

Contra-indications see notes above; also acute abdomen

Hepatic impairment see notes above

Renal impairment see notes above

Pregnancy see notes above

Breast-feeding avoid—no information available

Side-effects see notes above; also abdominal pain, anorexia, anxiety; *less commonly* diarrhoea, paralytic ileus, peripheral oedema, dysgeusia, seizures, paraesthesia, dyskinesia, myoclonus, agitation, tremor

Dose
• See under preparations below

Palladone® (Napp) [CD2]
Capsules, hydromorphone hydrochloride 1.3 mg (orange/clear), net price 56-cap pack = £8.82; 2.6 mg (red/clear), 56-cap pack = £17.64. Label: 2, counselling, see below
Dose 1.3 mg every 4 hours, increased if necessary according to severity of pain; CHILD under 12 years not recommended
Counselling Swallow whole or open capsule and sprinkle contents on soft food

◢Modified release
Palladone® **SR** (Napp) [CD2]
Capsules, m/r, hydromorphone hydrochloride 2 mg (yellow/clear), net price 56-cap pack = £20.98; 4 mg (pale blue/clear), 56-cap pack = £28.75; 8 mg (pink/clear), 56-cap pack = £56.08; 16 mg (brown/clear), 56-cap pack = £106.53; 24 mg (dark blue/clear), 56-cap pack = £159.82. Label: 2, counselling, see below
Dose 4 mg every 12 hours, increased if necessary according to severity of pain; CHILD under 12 years not recommended
Counselling Swallow whole or open capsule and sprinkle contents on soft cold food (swallow the pellets within the capsule whole; do not chew or crush)

■ MEPTAZINOL

Indications moderate to severe pain, including postoperative and obstetric pain and renal colic; perioperative analgesia, section 15.1.4.3

Cautions see notes above; effects only partially reversed by naloxone

Contra-indications see notes above; also myocardial infarction; phaeochromocytoma

Hepatic impairment see notes above

Renal impairment see notes above

Pregnancy see notes above

Breast-feeding use only if potential benefit outweighs risk

Side-effects see notes above; can induce withdrawal symptoms in patients dependent on opioids; also diarrhoea, abdominal pain, dyspepsia, and hypothermia

Dose
• By mouth, 200 mg every 3–6 hours as required; CHILD not recommended
• By intramuscular injection, 75–100 mg every 2–4 hours if necessary; obstetric analgesia, 100–150 mg according to patient's weight (2 mg/kg); CHILD not recommended
• By slow intravenous injection, 50–100 mg every 2–4 hours if necessary; CHILD not recommended

Meptid® (Almirall) [PoM]
Tablets, orange, f/c, meptazinol 200 mg, net price 112-tab pack = £22.11. Label: 2
Injection, meptazinol 100 mg (as hydrochloride)/mL, net price 1-mL amp = £1.92

METHADONE HYDROCHLORIDE

Indications severe pain, see notes above; cough in terminal disease (section 3.9.1); adjunct in treatment of opioid dependence (section 4.10.3)

Cautions see notes above; also history of cardiac conduction abnormalities, family history of sudden death (ECG monitoring recommended; see also QT-Interval Prolongation, below)

QT-interval prolongation Patients with the following risk factors for QT-interval prolongation should be carefully monitored while taking methadone: heart or liver disease, electrolyte abnormalities, or concomitant treatment with drugs that can prolong QT interval; patients requiring more than 100 mg daily should also be monitored

Contra-indications see notes above; also phaeochromocytoma

Hepatic impairment see notes above

Renal impairment see notes above

Pregnancy see notes above

Breast-feeding withdrawal symptoms in infant; breast-feeding permissible during maintenance but dose should be as low as possible and infant monitored to avoid sedation

Side-effects see notes above; also QT-interval prolongation, torsade de pointes, hypothermia, restlessness, raised intracranial pressure, dysmenorrhoea, dry eyes, and hyperprolactinaemia

Dose

- By mouth or by subcutaneous or intramuscular injection, 5–10 mg every 6–8 hours, adjusted according to response; on prolonged use not to be given more frequently than every 12 hours; CHILD not recommended

Methadone (Non-proprietary) [CD2]

Tablets, methadone hydrochloride 5 mg, net price 50 = £3.39. Label: 2
Brands include *Physeptone*®

Injection, methadone hydrochloride, 10 mg/mL, net price 1-mL amp = 84p, 2-mL amp = £1.32, 3.5-mL amp = £1.51, 5-mL amp = £1.89
Brands include *Physeptone*®, *Synastone*®

◢Linctus

Section 3.9.1

◢Oral solution and oral concentrate

Section 4.10.3

MORPHINE SALTS

Indications see notes above and under Dose; acute diarrhoea (section 1.4.2); cough in terminal care (section 3.9.1)

Cautions see notes above; also pancreatitis, cardiac arrhythmias, severe cor pulmonale

Contra-indications see notes above; also delayed gastric emptying, acute abdomen; heart failure secondary to chronic lung disease; phaeochromocytoma

Hepatic impairment see notes above

Renal impairment see notes above

Pregnancy see notes above

Breast-feeding therapeutic doses unlikely to affect infant

Side-effects see notes above; also paralytic ileus, abdominal pain, anorexia, dyspepsia, exacerbation of pancreatitis, taste disturbance; hypertension, hypothermia, syncope; bronchospasm, inhibition of cough

reflex; restlessness, seizures, paraesthesia, asthenia, malaise, disorientation, excitation, agitation, delirium, raised intracranial pressure; amenorrhoea; myoclonus, muscle fasciculation, rhabdomyolysis, and nystagmus

Dose

> The patient should be closely monitored for pain relief as well as for side-effects especially respiratory depression. See also notes above.

- Acute pain, by subcutaneous injection (not suitable for oedematous patients) or by intramuscular injection, initially 10 mg (ELDERLY or frail 5 mg) every 4 hours (or more frequently during titration), adjusted according to response; NEONATE initially 100 micrograms/kg every 6 hours, adjusted according to response; CHILD 1–6 months initially 100–200 micrograms/kg every 6 hours, adjusted according to response; CHILD 6 months–2 years initially 100–200 micrograms/kg every 4 hours, adjusted according to response; CHILD 2–12 years initially 200 micrograms/kg every 4 hours, adjusted according to response; CHILD 12–18 years initially 2.5–10 mg every 4 hours, adjusted according to response

  By slow intravenous injection, initially 5 mg (reduce dose in ELDERLY or frail) every 4 hours (or more frequently during titration), adjusted according to response; NEONATE initially 50 micrograms/kg every 6 hours, adjusted according to response; CHILD 1–6 months initially 100 micrograms/kg every 6 hours, adjusted according to response; CHILD 6 months–12 years initially 100 micrograms/kg every 4 hours, adjusted according to response

- Premedication, by subcutaneous or intramuscular injection, up to 10 mg 60–90 minutes before operation; CHILD, by intramuscular injection, 150 micrograms/kg

- Patient controlled analgesia (PCA), consult hospital protocols

- Myocardial infarction, by slow intravenous injection (1–2 mg/minute), 5–10 mg followed by a further 5–10 mg if necessary; ELDERLY or frail patients, reduce dose by half

- Acute pulmonary oedema, by slow intravenous injection (2 mg/minute) 5–10 mg; ELDERLY or frail patients, reduce dose by half

- Chronic pain, by mouth or by subcutaneous injection (not suitable for oedematous patients) or by intramuscular injection, initially 5–10 mg every 4 hours, adjusted according to response; see also Prescribing in Palliative Care, p. 20

  By rectum, initially 15–30 mg every 4 hours, adjusted according to response

  Note The doses stated above refer equally to morphine hydrochloride and sulfate

◢Oral solutions

Note For advice on transfer from oral solutions of morphine to modified-release preparations of morphine, see Prescribing in Palliative Care, p. 20

Morphine Oral Solutions

[PoM] or [CD2]

Oral solutions of morphine can be prescribed by writing the formula:
Morphine hydrochloride 5 mg
Chloroform water to 5 mL

Note The proportion of morphine hydrochloride may be altered when specified by the prescriber; if above 13 mg per 5 mL the solution becomes [CD2]. For sample prescription see Controlled Drugs and Drug Dependence, p. 8. It is usual to adjust the strength so that the dose volume is 5 or 10 mL.

Oramorph® (Boehringer Ingelheim)

Oramorph® oral solution (PoM), morphine sulfate 10 mg/5 mL, net price 100-mL pack = £1.89; 300-mL pack = £5.45; 500-mL pack = £8.50. Label: 2

Oramorph® concentrated oral solution (CD2), sugar-free, morphine sulfate 100 mg/5 mL, net price 30-mL pack = £4.98; 120-mL pack = £19.50 (both with calibrated dropper). Label: 2

◾**Tablets**

Sevredol® (Napp) (CD2)

Tablets, f/c, scored, morphine sulfate 10 mg (blue), net price 56-tab pack = £5.31; 20 mg (pink), 56-tab pack = £10.61; 50 mg (pale green), 56-tab pack = £28.02. Label: 2

◾**Modified-release 12-hourly oral preparations**

Filnarine® SR (TEVA UK) (CD2)

Tablets, m/r, f/c, morphine sulfate 10 mg (pink), net price 60-tab pack = £3.30; 30 mg (blue), 60-tab pack = £7.89; 60 mg (pink), 60-tab pack = £15.39; 100 mg (white), 60-tab pack = £21.79; 200 mg (white), 60-tab pack = £43.59. Label: 2, 25

Dose every 12 hours, dose adjusted according to daily morphine requirements; for further advice on determining dose, see Prescribing in Palliative Care, p. 20; dosage requirements should be reviewed if the brand is altered

Note Prescriptions must also specify 'tablets' (i.e. Filnarine SR tablets)

Morphgesic® SR (AMCo) (CD2)

Tablets, m/r, f/c, morphine sulfate 10 mg (buff), net price 60-tab pack = £3.85; 30 mg (violet), 60-tab pack = £9.24; 60 mg (orange), 60-tab pack = £18.04; 100 mg (grey), 60-tab pack = £28.54. Label: 2, 25

Dose every 12 hours, dose adjusted according to daily morphine requirements; for further advice on determining dose, see Prescribing in Palliative Care, p. 20; dosage requirements should be reviewed if the brand is altered

Note Prescriptions must also specify 'tablets' (i.e. Morphgesic SR tablets)

MST Continus® (Napp) (CD2)

Tablets, m/r, f/c, morphine sulfate 5 mg (white), net price 60-tab pack = £3.29; 10 mg (brown), 60-tab pack = £5.18; 15 mg (green), 60-tab pack = £9.10; 30 mg (purple), 60-tab pack = £12.47; 60 mg (orange), 60-tab pack = £24.32; 100 mg (grey), 60-tab pack = £38.50; 200 mg (green), 60-tab pack = £81.34. Label: 2, 25

Suspension (= sachet of granules to mix with water), m/r, pink, morphine sulfate 20 mg/sachet, net price 30-sachet pack = £24.58; 30 mg/sachet, 30-sachet pack = £25.54; 60 mg/sachet, 30-sachet pack = £51.09; 100 mg/sachet, 30-sachet pack = £85.15; 200 mg/sachet pack, 30-sachet pack = £170.30. Label: 2, 13

Dose every 12 hours, dose adjusted according to daily morphine requirements; for further advice on determining dose, see Prescribing in Palliative Care, p. 20; dosage requirements should be reviewed if the brand is altered

Note Prescriptions must also specify 'tablets' or 'suspension' (i.e. 'MST Continus tablets' or 'MST Continus suspension')

Zomorph® (Archimedes) (CD2)

Capsules, m/r, morphine sulfate 10 mg (yellow/clear enclosing pale yellow pellets), net price 60-cap pack = £3.47; 30 mg (pink/clear enclosing pale yellow pellets), 60-cap pack = £8.30; 60 mg (orange/clear enclosing pale yellow pellets), 60-cap pack = £16.20; 100 mg (white/clear enclosing pale yellow pellets), 60-cap pack = £21.80; 200 mg (clear enclos-

ing pale yellow pellets), 60-cap pack = £43.60. Label: 2, counselling, see below

Dose every 12 hours, dose adjusted according to daily morphine requirements; for further advice on determining doses, see Prescribing in Palliative Care, p. 20; dosage requirements should be reviewed if the brand is altered

Counselling Swallow whole or open capsule and sprinkle contents on soft food

Note Prescriptions must also specify 'capsules' (i.e. 'Zomorph capsules')

◾**Modified-release 24-hourly oral preparations**

MXL® (Napp) (CD2)

Capsules, m/r, morphine sulfate 30 mg (light blue), net price 28-cap pack = £10.91; 60 mg (brown), 28-cap pack = £14.95; 90 mg (pink), 28-cap pack = £22.04; 120 mg (green), 28-cap pack = £29.15; 150 mg (blue), 28-cap pack = £36.43; 200 mg (red-brown), 28-cap pack = £46.15. Label: 2, counselling, see below

Dose every 24 hours, dose adjusted according to daily morphine requirements; for further advice on determining dose, see Prescribing in Palliative Care, p. 20; dosage requirements should be reviewed if the brand is altered

Counselling Swallow whole or open capsule and sprinkle contents on soft food

Note Prescriptions must also specify 'capsules' (i.e. 'MXL capsules')

◾**Suppositories**

Morphine (Non-proprietary) (CD2)

Suppositories, morphine sulfate 10 mg, net price 12 = £11.21; 15 mg, 12 = £16.45; 20 mg, 12 = £33.22; 30 mg, 12 = £18.60. Label: 2

Note Both the strength of the suppositories and the morphine salt contained in them must be specified by the prescriber

◾**Injections**

Morphine Sulfate (Non-proprietary) (CD2)

Injection, morphine sulfate 10, 15, 20, and 30 mg/mL, net price 1- and 2-mL amp (all) = 72p–£4.48

Intravenous infusion, morphine sulfate 1 mg/mL, net price 50-mL vial = £5.25; 2 mg/mL, 50-mL vial = £5.89

Minijet® Morphine Sulphate (UCB Pharma) (CD2)

Injection, morphine sulfate 1 mg/mL, net price 10-mL disposable syringe = £15.00

◾**Injection with antiemetic**

For prescribing information on cyclizine, see section 4.6.

Caution In myocardial infarction cyclizine may aggravate severe heart failure and counteract the haemodynamic benefits of opioids, section 4.6. Not recommended in palliative care, see Nausea and Vomiting, p. 22

Cyclimorph® (AMCo) (CD2)

Cyclimorph-10® Injection, morphine tartrate 10 mg, cyclizine tartrate 50 mg/mL, net price 1-mL amp = £1.75

Dose ADULT and CHILD over 12 years, moderate to severe pain (short-term use only) by subcutaneous, intramuscular, or intravenous injection, 1 mL, repeated not more often than every 4 hours; max. 3 doses in any 24-hour period

Cyclimorph-15® Injection, morphine tartrate 15 mg, cyclizine tartrate 50 mg/mL, net price 1-mL amp = £1.82

Dose ADULT and CHILD over 12 years, moderate to severe pain (short-term use only) by subcutaneous, intramuscular, or intravenous injection, 1 mL, repeated not more often than every 4 hours; max. 3 doses in any 24-hour period

◼ OXYCODONE HYDROCHLORIDE

Indications moderate to severe pain in patients with cancer; postoperative pain; severe pain

Cautions see notes above; also toxic psychosis; pancreatitis

Contra-indications see notes above; also acute abdomen; delayed gastric emptying; chronic constipation; cor pulmonale

Hepatic impairment initially 2.5 mg every 6 hours in patients not currently treated with an opioid with mild impairment; avoid in moderate to severe impairment; see also notes above

Renal impairment initially 2.5 mg every 6 hours in patients not currently treated with an opioid with mild to moderate impairment; avoid if eGFR less than $10 \text{ mL/minute}/1.73\text{m}^2$; see also notes above

Pregnancy see notes above

Breast-feeding present in milk—avoid

Side-effects see notes above; also diarrhoea, abdominal pain, anorexia, dyspepsia; bronchospasm, dyspnoea, impaired cough reflex; asthenia, anxiety; chills; *less commonly* paralytic ileus, cholestasis, gastritis, flatulence, dysphagia, taste disturbance, belching, hiccups, vasodilatation, supraventricular tachycardia, syncope, amnesia, hypoaesthesia, restlessness, seizures, hypotonia, paraesthesia, disorientation, malaise, agitation, speech disorder, tremor, pyrexia, amenorrhoea, thirst, dehydration, muscle fasciculation, and dry skin

Dose

- By mouth, initially 5 mg every 4–6 hours, increased if necessary according to severity of pain, usual max. 400 mg daily, but some patients may require higher doses; CHILD under 18 years see *BNF for Children*
- By slow intravenous injection, 1–10 mg every 4 hours when necessary; CHILD under 18 years not recommended
- By intravenous infusion, initially 2 mg/hour, adjusted according to response; CHILD under 18 years not recommended
- By subcutaneous injection, initially 5 mg every 4 hours when necessary; CHILD under 18 years not recommended
- By subcutaneous infusion, initially 7.5 mg/24 hours adjusted according to response; CHILD under 18 years not recommended
- Patient controlled analgesia (PCA), consult hospital protocols

Note 2 mg oral oxycodone is approximately equivalent to 1 mg parenteral oxycodone

Oxycodone (Non-proprietary) ⓒⒹ2

Capsules, oxycodone hydrochloride 5 mg, net price 56 = £11.43; 10 mg, 56 = £22.86; 20 mg, 56 = £45.71. Label: 2

Oral solution, oxycodone hydrochloride 5 mg/5 mL, net price 250-mL pack = £9.71. Label: 2

Concentrated oral solution, oxycodone hydrochloride 10 mg/mL, net price 120-mL pack = £46.63. Label: 2

Injection, oxycodone hydrochloride 10 mg/mL, net price 1-mL amp = £1.60, 2-mL amp = £3.20

OxyNorm® (Napp) ⓒⒹ2

Capsules, oxycodone hydrochloride 5 mg (orange/beige), net price 56-cap pack = £11.43; 10 mg (white/beige), 56-cap pack = £22.86; 20 mg (pink/beige), 56-cap pack = £45.71. Label: 2

Liquid (= oral solution), sugar-free, oxycodone hydrochloride 5 mg/5 mL, net price 250 mL = £9.71. Label: 2

Concentrate (= concentrated oral solution), sugar-free, oxycodone hydrochloride 10 mg/mL, net price 120 mL = £46.63. Label: 2

Injection, oxycodone hydrochloride 10 mg/mL, net price 1-mL amp = £1.60, 2-mL amp = £3.20; 50 mg/mL, 1-mL amp = £14.02

Note The *Scottish Medicines Consortium* (p. 4) has advised (October 2004 and November 2010) that *OxyNorm®* injection is restricted for use within NHS Scotland for patients with cancer who have difficulty in tolerating morphine or diamorphine

▲Modified release

Dolocodon® PR (Zentiva) ⓒⒹ2

Tablets, f/c, m/r, oxycodone hydrochloride 5 mg (white), net price 28-tab pack = £12.50; 10 mg (pink), 56-tab pack = £24.99; 20 mg (white), 56-tab pack = £49.98; 40mg (pink), 56-tab pack = £99.98. Label: 2, 25

Dose initially 10 mg every 12 hours, increased if necessary according to severity of pain, usual max. 200 mg every 12 hours, but some patients may require higher doses; CHILD 8–18 years see *BNF for Children*

Longtec® (Qdem) ⓒⒹ2

Tablets, m/r, oxycodone hydrochloride 5 mg (blue), net price 28-tab pack = £8.75; 10 mg (white), 56-tab pack = £17.50; 20 mg (pink), 56-tab pack = £35.00; 40 mg (yellow), 56-tab pack = £70.00; 80 mg (green), 56-tab pack = £140.00. Label: 2, 25

Dose initially 10 mg every 12 hours, increased if necessary according to severity of pain, usual max. 200 mg every 12 hours, but some patients may require higher doses; CHILD 8–18 years see *BNF for Children*

OxyContin® (Napp) ⓒⒹ2

Tablets, f/c, m/r, oxycodone hydrochloride 5 mg (blue), net price 28-tab pack = £12.52; 10 mg (white), 56-tab pack = £25.04; 15 mg (grey), 56-tab pack = £38.12; 20 mg (pink), 56-tab pack = £50.08; 30 mg (brown), 56-tab pack = £76.23; 40 mg (yellow), 56-tab pack = £100.19; 60 mg (red), 56-tab pack = £152.49; 80 mg (green), 56-tab pack = £200.39; 120 mg (purple), 56-tab pack = £305.02. Label: 2, 25

Dose initially, 10 mg every 12 hours, increased if necessary according to severity of pain, usual max. 200 mg every 12 hours, but some patients may require higher doses; CHILD under 18 years see *BNF for Children*

▲With naloxone

Targinact® (Napp) ⓒⒹ2

Tablets 5 mg/2.5 mg, f/c, m/r, oxycodone hydrochloride 5 mg, naloxone hydrochloride 2.5 mg (blue), net price 28-tab pack = £21.16. Label: 2, 25

Tablets 10 mg/5 mg, f/c, m/r, oxycodone hydrochloride 10 mg, naloxone hydrochloride 5 mg (white), net price 56-tab pack = £42.32. Label: 2, 25

Tablets 20 mg/10 mg, f/c, m/r, oxycodone hydrochloride 20 mg, naloxone hydrochloride 10 mg (pink), net price 56-tab pack = £84.62. Label: 2, 25

Tablets 40 mg/20 mg, f/c, m/r, oxycodone hydrochloride 40 mg, naloxone hydrochloride 20 mg (yellow), net price 56-tab pack = £169.28. Label: 2, 25

Dose severe pain responsive only to opioid analgesics, ADULT over 18 years not currently treated with opioid

4

Central nervous system

Central nervous system 4

analgesics, initially 10 mg/5 mg every 12 hours, increased according to response; patients already receiving opioid analgesics can start with a higher dose of *Targinact*®; max. *Targinact*® 40 mg/20 mg every 12 hours

Note Supplemental modified-release oxycodone (without naloxone) can be prescribed for patients who need higher doses—consult product literature

◣ PAPAVERETUM ◢

Important Do **not** confuse with papaverine (section 7.4.5) A mixture of 253 parts of morphine hydrochloride, 23 parts of papaverine hydrochloride and 20 parts of codeine hydrochloride

Indications   postoperative analgesia; severe chronic pain

Cautions   see notes above; supraventricular tachycardia

Contra-indications   see notes above; heart failure secondary to chronic lung disease; phaeochromocytoma

Hepatic impairment   see notes above

Renal impairment   see notes above

Pregnancy   see notes above

Breast-feeding   therapeutic doses unlikely to affect infant

Side-effects   see notes above; also hypothermia

Dose

- By subcutaneous, intramuscular, *or* intravenous injection, 7.7–15.4 mg repeated every 4 hours if necessary (ELDERLY initially 7.7 mg); CHILD up to 1 month 115 micrograms/kg, 1–12 months 154 micrograms/kg, 1–5 years 1.93–3.85 mg, 6–12 years, 3.85–7.7 mg

Intravenous dose In general the intravenous dose should be 25–50% of the corresponding subcutaneous or intramuscular dose

Papaveretum (Non-proprietary) CD2 ◢
Injection, papaveretum 15.4 mg/mL (providing the equivalent of 10 mg of anhydrous morphine/mL), net price 1-mL amp = £4.90
Note The name *Omnopon*® was formerly used for papaveretum preparations

◢ With hyoscine

For prescribing information on hyoscine, see section 4.6.

Papaveretum and Hyoscine Injection (Non-proprietary) CD2 ◢
Injection, papaveretum 15.4 mg (providing the equivalent of 10 mg of anhydrous morphine), hyoscine hydrobromide 400 micrograms/mL, net price 1-mL amp = £3.57
Dose premedication, by subcutaneous or intramuscular injection, 0.5–1 mL

◣ PENTAZOCINE ◢

Indications   moderate to severe pain, but see notes above

Cautions   see notes above; also pancreatitis, arterial or pulmonary hypertension, cardiac arrhythmias, myocardial infarction, phaeochromocytoma; effects only partially reversed by naloxone

Contra-indications   see notes above; patients dependent on opioids (can precipitate withdrawal); heart failure secondary to chronic lung disease; acute porphyria (section 9.8.2)

Hepatic impairment   see notes above

Renal impairment   see notes above

Pregnancy   see notes above

Breast-feeding   use with caution—limited information available

Side-effects   see notes above; also abdominal pain, hypertension, syncope, seizures, paraesthesia, tremor, raised intracranial pressure, disorientation, hypothermia, chills, blood disorders, myalgia, and toxic epidermal necrolysis

Dose

- By mouth, pentazocine hydrochloride 50 mg every 3–4 hours preferably after food (range 25–100 mg); max. 600 mg daily; CHILD 6–12 years 25 mg

- By subcutaneous, intramuscular, or intravenous injection, moderate pain, pentazocine 30 mg, severe pain 45–60 mg every 3–4 hours when necessary; max. 360 mg daily; CHILD over 1 year, by subcutaneous *or* intramuscular injection, up to 1 mg/kg, by intravenous injection up to 500 micrograms/kg

Pentazocine (Non-proprietary) CD3 ◢
Capsules, pentazocine hydrochloride 50 mg, net price 28-cap pack = £28.50. Label: 2, 21
Tablets, pentazocine hydrochloride 25 mg, net price 28-tab pack = £19.31. Label: 2, 21
Injection, pentazocine 30 mg (as lactate)/mL, net price 1-mL amp = £1.67; 2-mL amp = £3.21

◣ PETHIDINE HYDROCHLORIDE
(Meperidine)

Indications   moderate to severe pain, obstetric analgesia; peri-operative analgesia

Cautions   see notes above; not suitable for severe continuing pain; accumulation of metabolites may result in neurotoxicity; cardiac arrhythmias, severe cor pulmonale

Contra-indications   see notes above; phaeochromocytoma

Hepatic impairment   see notes above

Renal impairment   see notes above

Pregnancy   see notes above

Breast-feeding   present in milk but not known to be harmful

Side-effects   see notes above; also restlessness, tremor, and hypothermia; convulsions reported in **overdosage**

Dose

- Acute pain, by mouth, 50–150 mg every 4 hours; CHILD under 18 years not recommended

  By subcutaneous *or* intramuscular injection, 25–100 mg (ELDERLY or debilitated, initially 25 mg), repeated after 4 hours; CHILD under 18 years not recommended

  By slow intravenous injection, 25–50 mg (ELDERLY or debilitated, initially 25 mg), repeated after 4 hours; CHILD under 18 years not recommended

- Obstetric analgesia, by subcutaneous *or* intramuscular injection, 50–100 mg, repeated 1–3 hours later if necessary; max. 400 mg in 24 hours; CHILD 12–18 years see *BNF for Children*

- Premedication, by intramuscular injection, 25–100 mg 1 hour before operation (ELDERLY or debilitated, 25 mg); CHILD under 18 years not recommended

- Postoperative pain, by subcutaneous *or* intramuscular injection, 25–100 mg (ELDERLY or debilitated, initially 25 mg), every 2–3 hours if necessary; CHILD under 18 years not recommended

Note In the postoperative period, the patient should be closely monitored for pain relief as well as for side-effects especially respiratory depression

Pethidine (Non-proprietary) [CD2]

Tablets, pethidine hydrochloride 50 mg, net price 50 = £50.82. Label: 2

Injection, pethidine hydrochloride 50 mg/mL, net price 1-mL amp = 50p, 2-mL amp = 47p; 10 mg/mL, 5-mL amp = £3.17, 10-mL amp = £2.18

◢**With promethazine**

For prescribing information on promethazine hydrochloride, see section 3.4.1.

Pamergan P100® (Martindale) [CD2] ◢

Injection, pethidine hydrochloride 50 mg, promethazine hydrochloride 25 mg/mL, net price 2-mL amp = £1.44

Dose by intramuscular injection, premedication, 2 mL 60–90 minutes before operation; CHILD 8–12 years 0.75 mL, 13–16 years 1 mL

Obstetric analgesia, 1–2 mL every 4 hours if necessary

Severe pain, 1–2 mL every 4–6 hours if necessary

Note Although usually given intramuscularly, may be given intravenously after dilution to at least 10 mL with water for injections

TAPENTADOL

Indications moderate to severe acute pain which can be managed only with opioid analgesics

Cautions see notes above

Contra-indications see notes above

Hepatic impairment see notes above; for *immediate-release tablets*, initial max. daily dose 150 mg; for *modified-release tablets*, initial max. daily dose 50 mg

Renal impairment manufacturer advises no dose adjustment needed in mild or moderate impairment, but avoid in severe impairment; see also notes above

Pregnancy see notes above

Breast-feeding avoid—no information available

Side-effects see notes above; also decreased appetite, diarrhoea, dyspepsia, abdominal discomfort, weight loss, anxiety, tremor, ataxia, dysarthria, hypoaesthesia, paraesthesia, seizures, malaise, muscle spasms

Dose

- ADULT over 18 years, by mouth, initially 50 mg every 4–6 hours (max. 700 mg in the first 24 hours), adjusted according to response; max. 600 mg daily

Note During the first 24 hours of treatment, an additional dose of 50 mg may be taken 1 hour after the initial dose, if pain control not achieved

Palexia® (Grünenthal) [CD2]

Tablets, f/c, tapentadol (as hydrochloride) 50 mg (white), net price 28-tab pack = £12.46, 56-tab pack = £24.91; 75 mg (yellow), 28-tab pack = £18.68, 56-tab pack = £37.37. Label: 2

Oral solution, tapentadol (as hydrochloride) 20 mg/mL, net price 100-mL pack = £17.80; 200-mL pack = £35.60. Label: 2

Excipients include propylene glycol (see Excipients, p. 2)

◢**Modified release**

Palexia® SR (Grünenthal) [CD2]

Tablets, f/c, m/r, tapentadol (as hydrochloride) 50 mg (white), net price 28-tab pack = £12.46, 56-tab pack = £24.91; 100 mg (yellow), 56-tab pack = £49.82, 150 mg (pink), 56-tab pack = £74.73; 200 mg (orange), 56-tab pack = £99.64; 250 mg (red), 56-tab pack = £124.55. Label: 2, 25

Dose severe chronic pain, initally 50 mg every 12 hours, adjusted according to response; max. 500 mg daily

The *Scottish Medicines Consortium* p. 4 has advised (May 2011) that tapentadol (*Palexia® SR*) is accepted for restricted use within NHS Scotland for the management of severe chronic pain in adult patients, which can be adequately managed only with opioid analgesics, when morphine sulfate modified-release has failed to provide adequate pain control or is not tolerated

TRAMADOL HYDROCHLORIDE

Indications moderate to severe pain

Cautions see notes above; impaired consciousness; excessive bronchial secretions; not suitable as a substitute in opioid-dependent patients

General anaesthesia Not recommended for analgesia during potentially light planes of general anaesthesia (possibly increased intra-operative recall reported)

Contra-indications see notes above; uncontrolled epilepsy

Hepatic impairment see notes above

Renal impairment see notes above

Pregnancy embryotoxic in animal studies—manufacturers advise avoid; see also notes above

Breast-feeding amount probably too small to be harmful, but manufacturer advises avoid

Side-effects see notes above; also diarrhoea, retching, fatigue, paraesthesia; *less commonly* gastritis, and flatulence; *rarely* anorexia, syncope, hypertension, bronchospasm, dyspnoea, wheezing, seizures, and muscle weakness; blood disorders also reported

Dose

- ADULT and CHILD over 12 years, by mouth, 50–100 mg not more often than every 4 hours; total of more than 400 mg daily not usually required

- ADULT and CHILD over 12 years, by intramuscular injection *or* by intravenous injection (over 2–3 minutes) *or* by intravenous infusion, 50–100 mg every 4–6 hours

Postoperative pain, 100 mg initially then 50 mg every 10–20 minutes if necessary during first hour to total max. 250 mg (including initial dose) in first hour, *then* 50–100 mg every 4–6 hours; max. 600 mg daily

Tramadol Hydrochloride (Non-proprietary) [CD3]

Capsules, tramadol hydrochloride 50 mg, net price 30-cap pack = £1.24, 100-cap pack = £4.13. Label: 2

Brands include *Zamadol®*

Oral drops, tramadol hydrochloride 100 mg/mL (2.5 mg/drop), net price 10 mL = £3.50. Label: 2, 13

Orodispersible tablets, tramadol hydrochloride 50 mg, net price 60-tab pack = £7.12. Label: 2, counselling, administration

Counselling Tramadol hydrochloride orodispersible tablets should be sucked and then swallowed. May also be dispersed in water

Brands include *Zamadol®*

Injection, tramadol hydrochloride 50 mg/mL, net price 2-mL amp = 98p

Brands include *Zamadol®*

4 Central nervous system

Zydol® (Grünenthal) CD3
Capsules, yellow, tramadol hydrochloride 50 mg, net price 30-cap pack = £2.29, 100-cap pack = £7.63. Label: 2
Soluble tablets, tramadol hydrochloride 50 mg, net price 20-tab pack = £2.79, 100-tab pack = £13.33. Label: 2, 13
Injection, tramadol hydrochloride 50 mg/mL, net price 2-mL amp = 80p

◢**Modified-release 12-hourly preparations**

Tramadol m/r preparations (Non-proprietary) CD3
Tablets, m/r, tramadol hydrochloride 100 mg, net price 60 = £17.21; 150 mg, 60 = £27.39; 200 mg, 60 = £36.52. Label: 2, 25
Brands include *Mabron®, Marol®, Zeridame® SR*
Capsules, m/r, tramadol hydrochloride 50 mg, net price 60 = £6.56; 100 mg, 60 = £14.72; 150 mg, 60 = £22.92; 200 mg, 60 = £29.43. Label: 2, 25
Brands include *Maxitram® SR, Tramquel® SR, Zamadol® SR*
Dose ADULT and CHILD over 12 years, 50–100 mg twice daily increased if necessary to 150–200 mg twice daily; total of more than 400 mg daily not usually required
Note Some capsule preparations may be opened and the contents swallowed immediately without chewing—check individual preparations
Important Do not confuse with modified-release 24-hourly preparations

Zydol SR® (Grünenthal) CD3
Tablets, m/r, f/c, tramadol hydrochloride 100 mg (yellow), net price 60-tab pack = £4.60; 100 mg, 60-tab pack = £18.26; 150 mg (light orange), 60-tab pack = £27.39; 200 mg (dark orange), 60-tab pack = £36.52. Label: 2, 25
Dose ADULT and CHILD over 12 years, 50–100 mg twice daily increased if necessary to 150–200 mg twice daily; total of more than 400 mg daily not usually required

◢**Modified-release 24-hourly preparations**

Tramadol m/r preparations (Non-proprietary) CD3
Tablets, m/r, tramadol hydrochloride 100 mg, net price 30 = £14.10; 150 mg, 28 = £10.70; 200 mg, 30 = £14.98; 300 mg, 30 = £22.47; 400 mg, 28 = £28.51. Label: 2, 25
Brands include *Tradorec XL®, Zamadol® 24hr*
Dose ADULT and CHILD over 12 years, initially 100–150 mg once daily, increased if necessary; usual max. 400 mg once daily
Important Do not confuse with modified-release 12-hourly preparations

Zydol XL® (Grünenthal) CD3
Tablets, m/r, f/c, tramadol hydrochloride 150 mg, net price 30-tab pack = £12.18; 200 mg, 30-tab pack = £17.98; 300 mg, 30-tab pack = £24.94; 400 mg, 30-tab pack = £32.47. Label: 2, 25
Dose ADULT and CHILD over 12 years, 150 mg once daily increased if necessary; usual max. 400 mg once daily

◢**With paracetamol**
Section 4.7.1

4.7.3 Neuropathic pain

Neuropathic pain, which occurs as a result of damage to neural tissue, includes *phantom limb pain, compression neuropathies, peripheral neuropathies* (e.g. due to diabetes (section 6.1.5), chronic excessive alcohol intake, HIV infection, chemotherapy, idiopathic neuropathy), *trauma, central pain* (e.g. pain following stroke, spinal cord injury, and syringomyelia), and *postherpetic neuralgia* (peripheral nerve damage following acute herpes zoster infection (shingles)). The pain may occur in an area of sensory deficit and is sometimes accompanied by pain that is evoked by a non-noxious stimulus (allodynia).

Trigeminal neuralgia is also caused by dysfunction of neural tissue, but its management (see below) is distinct from other forms of neuropathic pain.

Neuropathic pain is generally managed with a tricyclic antidepressant or with certain antiepileptic drugs. **Amitriptyline** (p. 255) [unlicensed indication] and **pregabalin** (p. 310) are effective treatments for neuropathic pain. Amitriptyline and pregabalin can be used in combination if the patient has an inadequate response to either drug at the maximum tolerated dose.

Nortriptyline [unlicensed indication] (p. 257) may be better tolerated than amitriptyline.

Gabapentin (p. 309) is also effective for the treatment of neuropathic pain.

Neuropathic pain may respond to opioid analgesics. There is evidence of efficacy for **tramadol** (p. 295), **morphine** (p. 291), and **oxycodone** (p. 293); however, treatment with morphine or oxycodone should be initiated only under specialist supervision. Tramadol can be prescribed when other treatments have been unsuccessful, while the patient is waiting for assessment by a specialist.

Patients with localised pain who are unable to take oral medicines may benefit from topical local anaesthetic preparations, such as lidocaine medicated plasters (section 15.2), while awaiting specialist review.

Capsaicin (p. 753) is licensed for neuropathic pain (but the intense burning sensation during initial treatment may limit use). Capsaicin 0.075% cream is licensed for the symptomatic relief of postherpetic neuralgia. A self-adhesive patch containing capsaicin 8% is licensed for the treatment of peripheral neuropathic pain in non-diabetic patients. It should be used under specialist supervision.

A **corticosteroid** may help to relieve pressure in compression neuropathy and thereby reduce pain.

Neuromodulation by spinal cord stimulation may be of benefit in some patients. Many patients with chronic neuropathic pain require multidisciplinary management, including physiotherapy and psychological support.

The management of trigeminal neuralgia and chronic facial pain are outlined below; for the management of neuropathic pain in *palliative care*, see p. 20; for the management of diabetic neuropathy, see section 6.1.5.

Trigeminal neuralgia

Surgery may be the treatment of choice in many patients; a neurological assessment will identify those who stand to benefit. **Carbamazepine** (p. 306) taken during the acute stages of trigeminal neuralgia, reduces the frequency and severity of attacks. It is very effective for the severe pain associated with trigeminal neuralgia and (less commonly) glossopharyngeal neuralgia. Blood counts and electrolytes should be monitored when high doses are given. Small doses should be used initially to reduce the incidence of side-effects e.g. dizziness. Some cases respond to **phenytoin** (p. 314); the drug may be given by intravenous infusion (possibly as fosphenytoin) in a crisis (specialist use only).

Chronic facial pain

Chronic oral and facial pain including persistent idiopathic facial pain (also termed 'atypical facial pain') and temporomandibular dysfunction (previously termed temporomandibular joint pain dysfunction syndrome) may call for prolonged use of analgesics or for other drugs. Tricyclic antidepressants (section 4.3.1) may be useful for facial pain [unlicensed indication], but are not on the Dental Practitioners' List. Disorders of this type require specialist referral and psychological support to accompany drug treatment. Patients on long-term therapy need to be monitored both for progress and for side-effects.

4.7.4 Antimigraine drugs

4.7.4.1 **Treatment of acute migraine**

4.7.4.2 **Prophylaxis of migraine**

4.7.4.3 **Cluster headache and the trigeminal autonomic cephalalgias**

4.7.4.1 Treatment of acute migraine

Treatment of a migraine attack should be guided by response to previous treatment and the severity of the attacks. A **simple analgesic** such as aspirin, paracetamol (preferably in a soluble or dispersible form) or a NSAID is often effective; concomitant **antiemetic** treatment may be required. If treatment with an analgesic is inadequate, an attack may be treated with a specific antimigraine compound such as a **5HT₁-receptor agonist** ('triptan'). Ergot alkaloids are rarely required now; oral preparations are associated with many side-effects and should be avoided in cerebrovascular or cardiovascular disease.

Excessive use of acute treatments for migraine (opioid and non-opioid analgesics, 5HT₁ receptor agonists, and ergotamine) is associated with medication-overuse headache (analgesic-induced headache); therefore, increasing consumption of these medicines needs careful management.

Analgesics

Most migraine headaches respond to analgesics such as aspirin (p. 280) or paracetamol (p. 281) but because peristalsis is often reduced during migraine attacks the medication may not be sufficiently well absorbed to be effective; dispersible or effervescent preparations are therefore preferred. Compound preparations containing analgesics and antiemetics are available (section 4.7.1).

The NSAID **tolfenamic acid** is licensed specifically for the treatment of an acute attack of migraine; **diclofenac potassium**, **flurbiprofen**, and **ibuprofen** (section 10.1.1) are also licensed for use in migraine.

▌ TOLFENAMIC ACID

Indications treatment of acute migraine

Cautions see NSAIDs, section 10.1.1

Contra-indications see NSAIDs, section 10.1.1

Hepatic impairment section 10.1.1

Renal impairment section 10.1.1

Pregnancy section 10.1.1

Breast-feeding amount too small to be harmful

Side-effects see NSAIDs, section 10.1.1; also dysuria (most commonly in men), confusion, malaise, hallucination, paraesthesia, tremor, euphoria, fatigue, and visual disturbances reported

Dose

● ADULT over 18 years, 200 mg at onset repeated once after 1–2 hours if necessary

Clotam Rapid® (Galen) PoM
Tablets, tolfenamic acid 200 mg, net price 10-tab pack = £12.75. Label: 21

5HT₁-receptor agonists

A 5HT₁-receptor agonist is of considerable value in the treatment of an acute migraine attack. The 5HT₁-receptor agonists ('triptans') act on the 5HT (serotonin) 1B/1D receptors and they are therefore sometimes referred to as 5HT₁ᵦ/₁ᴅ-receptor agonists. A 5HT₁-receptor agonist may be used during the established headache phase of an attack and is the preferred treatment in those who fail to respond to conventional analgesics.

The 5HT₁-receptor agonists available for treating migraine are **almotriptan**, **eletriptan**, **frovatriptan**, **naratriptan**, **rizatriptan**, **sumatriptan**, and **zolmitriptan**. If a patient does not respond to one 5HT₁-receptor agonist, an alternative 5HT₁-receptor agonist should be tried. For patients who have prolonged attacks that frequently recur despite treatment with a 5HT₁-receptor agonist, combination therapy with a NSAID such as naproxen can be considered. Sumatriptan or zolmitriptan are also used to treat cluster headache (section 4.7.4.3).

Cautions 5HT₁-receptor agonists should be used with caution in the elderly [unlicensed], and in conditions which predispose to coronary artery disease (pre-existing cardiac disease, see Contra-indications below); **interactions**: Appendix 1 (5HT₁ agonists).

Contra-indications 5HT₁-receptor agonists are contra-indicated in ischaemic heart disease, previous myocardial infarction, coronary vasospasm (including Prinzmetal's angina), and uncontrolled or severe hypertension. 5HT₁-receptor agonists are **not** indicated for the treatment of hemiplegic, basilar, or opthalmoplegic migraine.

Pregnancy There is limited experience of using 5HT₁-receptor agonists during pregnancy; manufacturers advise that they should be avoided unless the potential benefit outweighs the risk.

Side-effects Side-effects of the 5HT₁-receptor agonists include sensations of tingling, heat, heaviness, pressure, or tightness of any part of the body (including throat and chest—discontinue if intense, may be due to coronary vasoconstriction or to anaphylaxis), flushing, dizziness, feeling of weakness; fatigue; nausea and vomiting also reported.

▌ ALMOTRIPTAN

Indications treatment of acute migraine

Cautions see under 5HT₁-receptor agonists above; sensitivity to sulfonamides; **interactions**: Appendix 1 (5HT₁ agonists)

Contra-indications see under 5HT₁-receptor agonists above; previous cerebrovascular accident or transient ischaemic attack; peripheral vascular disease

4

Central nervous system

Hepatic impairment   caution in mild to moderate impairment; avoid in severe impairment

Renal impairment   max. 12.5 mg in 24 hours if eGFR less than 30 mL/minute/1.73 m^2

Pregnancy   see notes above

Breast-feeding   present in milk in *animal* studies—withhold breast-feeding for 24 hours

Side-effects   see under 5HT$_1$-receptor agonists above; also transient increase in blood pressure, drowsiness; *less commonly* diarrhoea, dyspepsia, dry mouth, chest pain, palpitation, paraesthesia, headache, myalgia, bone pain, tinnitus; *very rarely* myocardial infarction, and tachycardia; seizures also reported

Dose

• 12.5 mg as soon as possible after onset repeated after 2 hours if migraine recurs (patient not responding should not take second dose for same attack); max. 25 mg in 24 hours; CHILD and ADOLESCENT under 18 years not recommended

Almogran® (Almirall) [PoM]
Tablets, f/c, almotriptan (as hydrogen malate) 12.5 mg, net price 3-tab pack = £9.07; 6-tab pack = £18.14; 9-tab pack = £27.20. Label: 3

ELETRIPTAN

Indications   treatment of acute migraine

Cautions   see under 5HT$_1$-receptor agonists above; **interactions**: Appendix 1 (5HT$_1$ agonists)

Contra-indications   see under 5HT$_1$-receptor agonists above; previous cerebrovascular accident or transient ischaemic attack; arrhythmias; heart failure; peripheral vascular disease

Hepatic impairment   avoid in severe impairment

Renal impairment   reduce initial dose to 20 mg; max. 40 mg in 24 hours; avoid if eGFR less than 30 mL/minute/1.73 m^2

Pregnancy   see notes above

Breast-feeding   present in milk—avoid breast-feeding for 24 hours

Side-effects   see under 5HT$_1$-receptor agonists above; also abdominal pain, dry mouth, dyspepsia; tachycardia, palpitation; drowsiness, headache; pharyngitis, rhinitis, chills; myasthenia, myalgia; sweating; *less commonly* diarrhoea, glossitis, thirst, anorexia, taste disturbance; dyspnoea, yawning, oedema, agitation, confusion, euphoria, depression, insomnia, depersonalisation, tremor, dysarthria, stupor, movement disorders, hypertonia, urinary frequency, arthralgia, photophobia, visual disturbances, tinnitus, rash, and pruritus; *rarely* constipation, oesophagitis, bradycardia, asthma, syncope, lymphadenopathy, and menorrhagia; ischaemic colitis and hypertension also reported

Dose

• ADULT over 18 years, 40 mg repeated after 2 hours if migraine recurs (patient not responding to initial dose should not take second dose for same attack); increase to 80 mg for subsequent attacks if 40-mg dose inadequate; max. 80 mg in 24 hours

Relpax® (Pfizer) [PoM]
Tablets, f/c, orange, eletriptan (as hydrobromide) 20 mg, net price 6-tab pack = £22.50; 40 mg, 6-tab pack = £22.50. Label: 3

FROVATRIPTAN

Indications   treatment of acute migraine

Cautions   see under 5HT$_1$-receptor agonists above; **interactions**: Appendix 1 (5HT$_1$ agonists)

Contra-indications   see under 5HT$_1$-receptor agonists above; previous cerebrovascular attack or transient ischaemic attack; peripheral vascular disease

Hepatic impairment   avoid in severe impairment

Pregnancy   see notes above

Breast-feeding   present in milk in *animal* studies—withhold breast-feeding for 24 hours

Side-effects   see under 5HT$_1$-receptor agonists above; also dry mouth, dyspepsia, abdominal pain, paraesthesia, drowsiness, headache, visual disturbances, sweating; *less commonly* diarrhoea, dysphagia, flatulence, tachycardia, palpitation, hypertension, rhinitis, pharyngitis, sinusitis, laryngitis, tremor, anxiety, asthenia, insomnia, confusion, nervousness, impaired concentration, agitation, depression, depersonalisation, taste disturbance, micturition disorders, thirst, dehydration, arthralgia, muscle stiffness, tinnitus, vertigo, pruritus; *rarely* constipation, gastro-oesophageal reflux, irritable bowel syndrome, hiccup, peptic ulcer, stomatitis, bradycardia, hyperventilation, amnesia, abnormal dreams, hypertonia, hypotonia, breast tenderness, hypocalcaemia, hypoglycaemia, bilirubinaemia, epistaxis, urticaria, pyrexia, and purpura

Dose

• 2.5 mg as soon as possible after onset repeated after 2 hours if migraine recurs (patient not responding should not take second dose for same attack); max. 5 mg in 24 hours; CHILD and ADOLESCENT under 18 years not recommended

Migard® (Menarini) [PoM]
Tablets, f/c, frovatriptan (as succinate) 2.5 mg, net price 6-tab pack = £16.67. Label: 3

NARATRIPTAN

Indications   treatment of acute migraine

Cautions   see under 5HT$_1$-receptor agonists above; sensitivity to sulfonamides; **interactions**: Appendix 1 (5HT$_1$ agonists)
Driving Drowsiness may affect performance of skilled tasks (e.g. driving)

Contra-indications   see under 5HT$_1$-receptor agonists above; moderate hypertension; previous cerebrovascular accident or transient ischaemic attack; peripheral vascular disease

Hepatic impairment   max. 2.5 mg in 24 hours in moderate impairment; avoid if severe

Renal impairment   max. 2.5 mg in 24 hours; avoid if eGFR less than 15 mL/minute/1.73 m^2

Pregnancy   see notes above

Breast-feeding   withhold breast-feeding for 24 hours

Side-effects   see under 5HT$_1$-receptor agonists above; also *less commonly* bradycardia, tachycardia, palpitation, and visual disturbance; *rarely* ischaemic colitis, rash, and pruritus

Dose

• 2.5 mg, repeated after at least 4 hours if migraine recurs (patient not responding should not take second dose for same attack); max. 5 mg in 24 hours; CHILD and ADOLESCENT under 18 years not recommended

Naratriptan (Non-proprietary) PoM

Tablets, naratriptan (as hydrochloride) 2.5 mg, net price 6-tab pack = £2.06. Label: 3

Naramig® (GSK) PoM

Tablets, f/c, green, naratriptan (as hydrochloride) 2.5 mg, net price 6-tab pack = £24.55. Label: 3

RIZATRIPTAN

Indications treatment of acute migraine

Cautions see under $5HT_1$-receptor agonists above; interactions: Appendix 1 ($5HT_1$ agonists)

Driving Drowsiness may affect performance of skilled tasks (e.g. driving)

Contra-indications see under $5HT_1$-receptor agonists above; previous cerebrovascular accident or transient ischaemic attack; peripheral vascular disease

Hepatic impairment reduce dose to 5 mg in mild to moderate impairment; avoid in severe impairment

Renal impairment reduce dose to 5 mg in mild to moderate impairment; avoid in severe impairment

Pregnancy see notes above

Breast-feeding present in milk in *animal* studies—withhold breast-feeding for 24 hours

Side-effects see under $5HT_1$-receptor agonists above; also dry mouth, diarrhoea, drowsiness, palpitation, tachycardia, pharyngeal discomfort, dyspnoea, headache, paraesthesia, decreased alertness, tremor, sweating; *less commonly* dyspepsia, thirst, hypertension, arrhythmias, insomnia, ataxia, nervousness, vertigo, confusion, taste disturbances, myalgia, muscle weakness, blurred vision, urticaria, pruritus; *rarely* syncope, bradycardia; *also reported* seizures, toxic epidermal necrolysis

Dose

- 10 mg as soon as possible after onset repeated after 2 hours if migraine recurs (patient not responding should not take second dose for same attack); max. 20 mg in 24 hours; CHILD and ADOLESCENT under 18 years not recommended

Rizatriptan (Non-proprietary) PoM

Tablets, rizatriptan (as benzoate) 5 mg, net price 6-tab pack =£26.74; 10 mg, 3-tab pack = £3.69. Label: 3

Orodispersible tablets,rizatriptan (as benzoate) 10 mg, net price 3-tab pack = £5.06. Label: 3, counselling, administration

Counselling rizatriptan orodispersible tablets should be placed on the tongue, allowed to disperse and swallowed

Excipients may include aspartame (section 9.4.1)

Maxalt® (MSD) PoM

Tablets, pink, rizatriptan (as benzoate) 5 mg, net price 6-tab pack = £26.74; 10 mg, 3-tab pack = £13.37, 6-tab pack = £26.74. Label: 3

Oral lyophilisates (*Maxalt*® Melt Wafers), rizatriptan (as benzoate) 10 mg, net price 3-wafer pack = £13.37, 6-wafer pack = £26.74. Label: 3, counselling, administration

Counselling *Maxalt*® Melt wafers should be placed on the tongue and allowed to dissolve

Excipients include aspartame equivalent to phenylalanine 2.1 mg (section 9.4.1)

SUMATRIPTAN

Indications treatment of acute migraine; cluster headache

Cautions see under $5HT_1$-receptor agonists above; history of seizures; sensitivity to sulfonamides; interactions: Appendix 1 ($5HT_1$ agonists)

Driving Drowsiness may affect performance of skilled tasks (e.g. driving)

Contra-indications see under $5HT_1$-receptor agonists above; previous cerebrovascular accident or transient ischaemic attack; peripheral vascular disease; moderate and severe hypertension

Hepatic impairment reduce oral dose to 25–50 mg; avoid in severe impairment

Renal impairment use with caution

Pregnancy see notes above

Breast-feeding present in milk but amount probably too small to be harmful; withhold breast-feeding for 12 hours

Side-effects see under $5HT_1$-receptor agonists above; also dyspnoea, drowsiness, transient increase in blood pressure, myalgia; *also reported* diarrhoea, ischaemic colitis, hypotension, bradycardia or tachycardia, palpitation, arrhythmias, myocardial infarction, Raynaud's syndrome, anxiety, seizures, tremor, dystonia, nystagmus, arthralgia, visual disturbances, and sweating; epistaxis with nasal spray

Dose

- By mouth, migraine, 50 mg (some patients may require 100 mg); dose may be repeated after at least 2 hours if migraine recurs; max. 300 mg in 24 hours; CHILD under 18 years see *BNF for Children*

- By subcutaneous injection cluster headache or migraine, using auto-injector, 6 mg; dose may be repeated once after at least 1 hour if headache recurs; max. 12 mg in 24 hours; CHILD 10–18 years see *BNF for Children*

  Important Not for intravenous injection which may cause coronary vasospasm and angina

- Intranasally, cluster headache [unlicensed] or migraine, 10–20 mg into one nostril; dose may be repeated once after at least 2 hours if headache recurs; max. 40 mg in 24 hours; CHILD 12–18 years see *BNF for Children*

Note Patient not responding to initial dose should not take second dose for same attack

Sumatriptan (Non-proprietary) PoM

Tablets, sumatriptan (as succinate) 50 mg, net price 6-tab pack = £1.65; 100 mg, 6-tab pack = £1.96. Label: 3, 10, patient information leaflet

Imigran® (GSK) PoM

Tablets, sumatriptan (as succinate) 50 mg, net price 6-tab pack = £31.85; 100 mg, 6-tab pack = £51.48. Label: 3, 10, patient information leaflet

Injection, sumatriptan (as succinate) 12 mg/mL (= 6 mg/0.5-mL syringe), net price, treatment pack (2 × 0.5-mL prefilled syringes and auto-injector) = £42.47; refill pack 2 × 0.5-mL prefilled cartridges = £40.41. Label: 3, 10, patient information leaflet

Nasal spray, sumatriptan 10 mg/0.1-mL actuation, net price 2 unit-dose spray device = £11.80; 20 mg/0.1-mL actuation, 2 unit-dose spray device = £14.16, 6 unit-dose spray device = £35.39. Label: 3, 10, patient information leaflet

Dose

- ADULT over 18 years, 50 micrograms twice daily, increased after 2 weeks to 75 micrograms twice daily if necessary

Clonidine (Non-proprietary) (PoM)

Tablets, clonidine hydrochloride 25 micrograms, net price 112-tab pack = £4.21

Dixarit® (Boehringer Ingelheim) (PoM)

Tablets, blue, s/c, clonidine hydrochloride 25 micrograms, net price 112-tab pack = £6.99

Catapres® (PoM)

Section 2.5.2 (hypertension)

4.7.4.3 Cluster headache and the trigeminal autonomic cephalalgias

Cluster headache rarely responds to standard analgesics. **Sumatriptan** (p. 299) given by subcutaneous injection is the drug of choice for the *treatment* of cluster headache. If an injection is unsuitable, sumatriptan nasal spray or **zolmitriptan** nasal spray [both unlicensed use] may be used. Alternatively, 100% **oxygen** at a rate of 10–15 litres/minute for 10–20 minutes is useful in aborting an attack.

Prophylaxis of cluster headache is considered if the attacks are frequent, last over 3 weeks, or if they cannot be treated effectively. **Verapamil** (p. 138) or **lithium** [both unlicensed use] are used for prophylaxis.

Prednisolone (section 6.3.2) can be used for short-term prophylaxis of episodic cluster headache [unlicensed use] either as monotherapy, or in combination with verapamil during verapamil titration. The dose of prednisolone for monotherapy or adjunctive therapy is 60–100 mg once daily for 2–5 days followed by a dose reduction of 10 mg every 2–3 days until prednisolone is discontinued.

Ergotamine, used on an intermittent basis is an alternative for patients with short bouts, but it should **not** be used for prolonged periods.

The other trigeminal autonomic cephalalgias, paroxysmal hemicrania (sensitive to indometacin), and short-lasting unilateral neuralgiform headache attacks with conjunctival injection and tearing, are seen rarely and are best managed by a specialist.

4.8 Antiepileptic drugs

- 4.8.1 Control of the epilepsies
- 4.8.2 Drugs used in status epilepticus
- 4.8.3 Febrile convulsions

4.8.1 Control of the epilepsies

NICE guidance

For additional information, see NICE clinical guideline 137 (January 2012).

The object of treatment is to prevent the occurrence of seizures by maintaining an effective dose of one or more antiepileptic drugs. Careful adjustment of doses is necessary, starting with low doses and increasing gradually until seizures are controlled or there are significant adverse effects.

When choosing an antiepileptic drug, the presenting epilepsy syndrome should first be considered. If the syndrome is not clear, the seizure type should determine the choice of treatment. Concomitant medication, co-morbidity, age, and sex should also be taken into account. For women of child-bearing age, see Pregnancy, p. 304 and Breast-feeding, p. 305.

The dosage frequency is often determined by the plasma-drug half-life, and should be kept as low as possible to encourage adherence with the prescribed regimen. Most antiepileptics, when used in the usual dosage, can be given twice daily. Lamotrigine, perampanel, phenobarbital, and phenytoin, which have long half-lives, can be given once daily at bedtime. However, with large doses, some antiepileptics may need to be given more frequently to avoid adverse effects associated with high peak plasma-drug concentration. Young children metabolise some antiepileptics more rapidly than adults and therefore may require more frequent doses and a higher dose in proportion to their body-weight.

Management When monotherapy with a first-line antiepileptic drug has failed, monotherapy with a second drug should be tried; the diagnosis should be checked before starting an alternative drug if the first drug showed lack of efficacy. The change from one antiepileptic drug to another should be cautious, slowly withdrawing the first drug only when the new regimen has been established. Combination therapy with two or more antiepileptic drugs may be necessary, but the concurrent use of antiepileptic drugs increases the risk of adverse effects and drug interactions (see below). If combination therapy does not bring about worthwhile benefits, revert to the regimen (monotherapy or combination therapy) that provided the best balance between tolerability and efficacy. A single antiepileptic drug should be prescribed wherever possible.

MHRA/CHM advice
Antiepileptic drugs: new advice on switching between different manufacturers' products for a particular drug (November 2013)

The CHM has reviewed spontaneous adverse reactions received by the MHRA and publications that reported potential harm arising from switching of antiepileptic drugs in patients previously stabilised on a branded product to a generic. The CHM concluded that reports of loss of seizure control and/or worsening of side-effects around the time of switching between products could be explained as chance associations, but that a causal role of switching could not be ruled out in all cases. The following guidance has been issued to help minimise risk:

- Different antiepileptic drugs vary considerably in their characteristics, which influences the risk of whether switching between different manufacturers' products of a particular drug may cause adverse effects or loss of seizure control;
- Antiepileptic drugs have been divided into three risk-based categories to help healthcare professionals decide whether it is necessary to maintain continuity of supply of a specific manufacturer's product. These categories are listed below;
- If it is felt desirable for a patient to be maintained on a specific manufacturer's product this should be prescribed either by specifying a brand name, or by using the generic drug name and name of the manufacturer (otherwise known as the Marketing Authorisation Holder);
- This advice relates only to antiepileptic drug use for treatment of epilepsy; it does not apply to their use in other indications (e.g. mood stabilisation, neuropathic pain);
- Please report on a Yellow Card any suspected adverse reactions to antiepileptic drugs (see Yellow Card Scheme, p. 12);
- Dispensing pharmacists should ensure the continuity of supply of a particular product when the prescription specifies it. If the prescribed product is unavailable, it may be necessary to dispense a product from a different manufacturer to maintain continuity of treatment of that antiepileptic drug. Such cases should be discussed and agreed with both the prescriber and patient (or carer);
- Usual dispensing practice can be followed when a specific product is not stated.

Category 1
Phenytoin, carbamazepine, phenobarbital, primidone. For these drugs, doctors are advised to ensure that their patient is maintained on a specific manufacturer's product

Category 2
Valproate, lamotrigine, perampanel, retigabine, rufinamide, clobazam, clonazepam, oxcarbazepine, eslicarbazepine, zonisamide, topiramate. For these drugs, the need for continued supply of a particular manufacturer's product should be based on clinical judgement and consultation with the patient and/or carer taking into account factors such as seizure frequency and treatment history

Category 3
Levetiracetam, lacosamide, tiagabine, gabapentin, pregabalin, ethosuximide, vigabatrin. For these drugs, it is usually unnecessary to ensure that patients are maintained on a specific manufacturer's product unless there are specific concerns such as patient anxiety, and risk of confusion or dosing errors

---

Interactions Interactions between antiepileptics are complex and may increase toxicity without a corresponding increase in antiepileptic effect. Interactions are usually caused by hepatic enzyme induction or inhibition; displacement from protein binding sites is not usually a problem. These interactions are highly variable and unpredictable.

For interactions of antiepileptic drugs, see **Appendix 1**; for advice on hormonal contraception and enzyme-inducing drugs, see section 7.3.1 and section 7.3.2.

Significant interactions that occur **between antiepileptics** and that may affect dosing requirements are as follows:

> **Note**
> Check under each drug for possible interactions when two or more antiepileptic drugs are used

Carbamazepine
often lowers plasma concentration of clobazam, clonazepam, lamotrigine, perampanel, phenytoin (but may also raise plasma-phenytoin concentration), tiagabine, topiramate, valproate, zonisamide, and an active metabolite of oxcarbazepine

sometimes lowers plasma concentration of eslicarbazepine, ethosuximide, primidone (but tendency for corresponding increase in phenobarbital level), retigabine, and rufinamide

sometimes raises plasma concentration of phenobarbital and primidone-derived phenobarbital

Eslicarbazepine
often raises plasma concentration of phenytoin

Ethosuximide
sometimes raises plasma concentration of phenytoin

Lamotrigine
sometimes raises plasma concentration of an active metabolite of carbamazepine (but evidence is conflicting)

Oxcarbazepine
often lowers plasma concentration of perampanel

sometimes lowers plasma concentration of carbamazepine (but may raise plasma concentration of an active metabolite of carbamazepine)

sometimes raises plasma concentration of phenytoin

often raises plasma concentration of phenobarbital and primidone-derived phenobarbital

Phenobarbital *or* **primidone**
often lowers plasma concentration of clonazepam, lamotrigine, phenytoin (but may also raise plasma-phenytoin concentration), tiagabine, valproate, zonisamide, and an active metabolite of oxcarbazepine

sometimes lowers plasma concentration of ethosuximide, rufinamide, and topiramate

Phenytoin
often lowers plasma concentration of clonazepam, carbamazepine, eslicarbazepine, lamotrigine, perampanel, tiagabine, topiramate, valproate, zonisamide, and an active metabolite of oxcarbazepine

often raises plasma concentration of phenobarbital and primidone-derived phenobarbital

sometimes lowers plasma concentration of ethosuximide, primidone (by increasing conversion to phenobarbital), retigabine, and rufinamide

4

Central nervous system

Rufinamide

sometimes lowers plasma concentration of carbamazepine

sometimes raises plasma concentration of phenytoin

Topiramate

often lowers plasma concentration of perampanel

sometimes raises plasma concentration of phenytoin

Valproate

sometimes lowers plasma concentration of an active metabolite of oxcarbazepine

often raises plasma concentration of lamotrigine, phenobarbital, primidone-derived phenobarbital, phenytoin (but may also lower), and an active metabolite of carbamazepine

sometimes raises plasma concentration of ethosuximide and rufinamide

Vigabatrin

often lowers plasma concentration of phenytoin

Withdrawal Antiepileptic drugs should be withdrawn under specialist supervision. Avoid abrupt withdrawal, particularly of barbiturates and benzodiazepines, because this can precipitate severe rebound seizures. Reduction in dosage should be gradual and, in the case of barbiturates, withdrawal of the drug may take months.

The decision to withdraw antiepileptic drugs from a seizure-free patient, and its timing, is often difficult and depends on individual circumstances. Even in patients who have been seizure-free for several years, there is a significant risk of seizure recurrence on drug withdrawal.

In patients receiving several antiepileptic drugs, only one drug should be withdrawn at a time.

Antiepileptic hypersensitivity syndrome Antiepileptic hypersensitivity syndrome is a rare but potentially fatal syndrome associated with some antiepileptic drugs (**carbamazepine, lacosamide, lamotrigine, oxcarbazepine, phenobarbital, phenytoin, primidone**, and **rufinamide**); rarely cross-sensitivity occurs between some of these antiepileptic drugs. Some other antiepileptics (**eslicarbazepine, stiripentol**, and **zonisamide**) have a theoretical risk. The symptoms usually start between 1 and 8 weeks of exposure; fever, rash, and lymphadenopathy are most commonly seen. Other systemic signs include liver dysfunction, haematological, renal, and pulmonary abnormalities, vasculitis, and multi-organ failure. If signs or symptoms of hypersensitivity syndrome occur, the drug should be withdrawn immediately, the patient must not be re-exposed, and expert advice should be sought.

Driving Patients with epilepsy may drive a motor vehicle (but not a large goods or passenger carrying vehicle) provided that they have been seizure-free for one year or, if subject to attacks only while asleep, have established a 3-year period of asleep attacks without awake attacks. Those affected by drowsiness should not drive or operate machinery.

Guidance issued by the Drivers Medical Unit of the Driver and Vehicle Licensing Agency (DVLA) recommends that patients should be advised not to drive during medication changes or withdrawal of antiepileptic drugs, and for 6 months afterwards (see also Drugs and Driving under General Guidance, p. 3).

Patients who have had a first or single epileptic seizure must not drive for 6 months (5 years in the case of large goods or passenger carrying vehicles) after the event; driving may then be resumed, provided the patient has been assessed by a specialist as fit to drive because no abnormality was detected on investigation.

Pregnancy Women of child-bearing potential should discuss with a specialist the impact of both epilepsy, and its treatment, on the outcome of pregnancy.

There is an increased risk of teratogenicity associated with the use of antiepileptic drugs (especially if used during the first trimester and particularly if the patient takes two or more antiepileptic drugs). Valproate is associated with the highest risk of major and minor congenital malformations (in particular neural tube defects), and long-term neurodevelopmental effects. Valproate should not be used during pregnancy or in women of child-bearing potential unless there is no safer alternative and only after a careful discussion of the risks. If valproate is to be used during pregnancy, the lowest effective dose should be prescribed in divided doses or as modified-release tablets to avoid peaks in plasma-valproate concentrations; doses greater than 1 g daily are associated with an increased risk of teratogenicity. Specialist prenatal monitoring should be instigated when valproate has been taken in pregnancy. There is also an increased risk of teratogenicity with phenytoin, primidone, phenobarbital, lamotrigine, and carbamazepine. Topiramate carries an increased risk of cleft palate if taken in the first trimester of pregnancy. There is not enough evidence to establish the risk of teratogenicity with other antiepileptic drugs.

Prescribers should also consider carefully the choice of antiepileptic therapy in pre-pubescent girls who may later become pregnant.

Women of child-bearing potential who take antiepileptic drugs should be given contraceptive advice. Some antiepileptic drugs can reduce the efficacy of hormonal contraceptives, and the efficacy of some antiepileptics may be affected by hormonal contraceptives (see section 7.3.1 and interactions of antiepileptics, Appendix 1).

Women who want to become pregnant should be referred to a specialist for advice in advance of conception. For some women, the severity of seizure or the seizure type may not pose a serious threat, and drug withdrawal may be considered; therapy may be resumed after the first trimester. If treatment with antiepileptic drugs must continue throughout pregnancy, then monotherapy is preferable at the lowest effective dose.

Once an unplanned pregnancy is discovered it is usually too late for changes to be made to the treatment regimen; the risk of harm to the mother and fetus from convulsive seizures outweighs the risk of continued therapy. The likelihood of a woman who is taking antiepileptic drugs having a baby with no malformations is at least 90%, and it is important that women do not stop taking essential treatment because of concern over harm to the fetus.

To reduce the risk of neural tube defects, folate supplementation (section 9.1.2) is advised before conception and throughout the first trimester.

The concentration of antiepileptic drugs in the plasma can change during pregnancy. Doses of phenytoin (see p. 314), carbamazepine, and lamotrigine should be adjusted on the basis of plasma-drug concentration monitoring; the dose of other antiepileptic drugs should be monitored carefully during pregnancy and after birth, and adjustments made on a clinical basis. Plasma-drug concentration monitoring during pregnancy is also useful to check compliance. Additionally, in patients taking topiramate or levetiracetam, it is recommended that fetal growth should be monitored.

Women who have seizures in the second half of pregnancy should be assessed for eclampsia before any change is made to antiepileptic treatment. Status epilepticus should be treated according to the standard protocol, see section 4.8.2.

Routine injection of vitamin K (section 9.6.6) at birth minimises the risk of neonatal haemorrhage associated with antiepileptics.

Withdrawal effects in the newborn may occur with some antiepileptic drugs, in particular benzodiazepines and phenobarbital.

> ### Epilepsy and Pregnancy Register
> All pregnant women with epilepsy, whether taking medication or not, should be encouraged to notify the UK Epilepsy and Pregnancy Register (Tel: 0800 389 1248).

Breast-feeding   Women taking antiepileptic monotherapy should generally be encouraged to breast-feed; if a woman is on combination therapy or if there are other risk factors, such as premature birth, specialist advice should be sought.

All infants should be monitored for sedation, feeding difficulties, adequate weight gain, and developmental milestones. Infants should also be monitored for adverse effects associated with the antiepileptic drug particularly with newer antiepileptics, if the antiepileptic is readily transferred into breast-milk causing high infant serum-drug concentrations (e.g. ethosuximide, lamotrigine, primidone, and zonisamide), or if slower metabolism in the infant causes drugs to accumulate (e.g. phenobarbital and lamotrigine). Serum-drug concentration monitoring should be undertaken in breast-fed infants if suspected adverse reactions develop; if toxicity develops it may be necessary to introduce formula feeds to limit the infant's drug exposure, or to wean the infant off breast-milk altogether.

Primidone, phenobarbital, and the benzodiazepines are associated with an established risk of drowsiness in breast-fed babies and caution is required.

Withdrawal effects may occur in infants if a mother suddenly stops breast-feeding, particularly if she is taking phenobarbital, primidone, or lamotrigine.

Focal seizures with or without secondary generalisation

Carbamazepine and lamotrigine are first-line options for treating newly diagnosed focal seizures; oxcarbazepine, sodium valproate and levetiracetam may be used if carbamazepine or lamotrigine are unsuitable or not tolerated. If monotherapy is unsuccessful with two of these first-line antiepileptic drugs, adjunctive treatment may be considered. Options for adjunctive treatment include carbamazepine, clobazam, gabapentin, lamotrigine, levetiracetam, oxcarbazepine, sodium valproate, or topiramate. If adjunctive treatment is ineffective or not tolerated, a tertiary epilepsy specialist should be consulted who may consider eslicarbazepine, lacosamide, phenobarbital, phenytoin, pregabalin, tiagabine, vigabatrin and zonisamide.

Generalised seizures

Tonic-clonic seizures   Sodium valproate is the first-line treatment for newly diagnosed generalised tonic-clonic seizures. Lamotrigine is the alternative choice if sodium valproate is not suitable, but may exacerbate myoclonic seizures. In those with established epilepsy with generalised tonic-clonic seizures only, lamotrigine or sodium valproate may be prescribed as the first-line treatment. Carbamazepine and oxcarbazepine may also be considered in newly diagnosed and established tonic-clonic seizures, but may exacerbate myoclonic and absence seizures. Clobazam, lamotrigine, levetiracetam, sodium valproate or topiramate may be used as adjunctive treatment if monotherapy is ineffective or not tolerated.

Absence seizures   Ethosuximide or sodium valproate are the drugs of choice in absence seizures and syndromes; lamotrigine is a suitable alternative when ethosuximide and sodium valproate are unsuitable, ineffective or not tolerated. Sodium valproate should be used as the first choice if there is a high risk of generalised tonic-clonic seizures. A combination of any two of these drugs may be used if monotherapy is ineffective. Clobazam, clonazepam, levetiracetam, topiramate or zonisamide may be considered by a tertiary epilepsy specialist if adjunctive treatment fails. Carbamazepine, gabapentin, oxcarbazepine, phenytoin, pregabalin, tiagabine and vigabatrin are not recommended in absence seizures or syndromes.

Myoclonic seizures   Myoclonic seizures (myoclonic jerks) occur in a variety of syndromes, and response to treatment varies considerably. Sodium valproate is the drug of choice in newly diagnosed myoclonic seizures; topiramate and levetiracetam are alternative options if sodium valproate is unsuitable but consideration should be given to the less favourable side-effect profile of topiramate. A combination of two of these drugs may be used if monotherapy is ineffective or not tolerated. If adjunctive treatment fails, a tertiary epilepsy specialist should be consulted and may consider clobazam, clonazepam, zonisamide or piracetam. For reference to the adjunctive use of piracetam, see section 4.9.3. Carbamazepine, gabapentin, oxcarbazepine, phenytoin, pregabalin, tiagabine and vigabatrin are not recommended for the treatment of myoclonic seizures.

Sodium valproate and levetiracetam are effective in treating the generalised tonic-clonic seizures that co-exist with myoclonic seizures in idiopathic generalised epilepsy.

Atonic and tonic seizures   Atonic and tonic seizures are usually seen in childhood, in specific epilepsy syndromes, or associated with cerebral damage or mental retardation. They may respond poorly to the traditional drugs. Sodium valproate is the drug of choice; lamotrigine can be added as adjunctive treatment. If adjunctive treatment is ineffective or not tolerated, a tertiary epilepsy specialist should be consulted, and may consider rufinamide or topiramate. Carbamazepine, gabapentin, oxcarbazepine, pregabalin, tiagabine or vigabatrin are not recommended in atonic and tonic seizures.

Epilepsy syndromes

Some drugs are licensed for use in particular epilepsy syndromes, such as lamotrigine and rufinamide in Lennox-Gastaut syndrome. The epilepsy syndromes are specific types of epilepsy that are characterised according to a number of features including seizure type, age of onset, and EEG characteristics.

For more information on epilepsy syndromes in children, see *BNF for Children*, section 4.8.1. Prescribing information for stiripentol (*Diacomit* ®) in severe myoclonic epilepsy of infancy (Dravet syndrome) can also be found in *BNF for Children*.

Carbamazepine and related antiepileptics

Carbamazepine is a drug of choice for simple and complex focal seizures and is a first-line treatment option for generalised tonic-clonic seizures. It can be used as adjunctive treatment for focal seizures when monotherapy has been ineffective. It is essential to initiate carbamazepine therapy at a low dose and build this up slowly with increments of 100–200 mg every two weeks. Some side-effects (such as headache, ataxia, drowsiness, nausea, vomiting, blurring of vision, dizziness, unsteadiness, and allergic skin reactions) are dose-related, and may be dose-limiting. These side-effects are more common at the start of treatment and in the elderly. Patients should be offered a modified-release preparation to reduce the risk of side-effects; altering the timing of medication may also be beneficial. Carbamazepine may exacerbate tonic, atonic, myoclonic and absence seizures and is therefore not recommended if these seizures are present.

Oxcarbazepine is licensed as monotherapy or adjunctive therapy for the treatment of focal seizures with or without secondary generalised tonic-clonic seizures. It can also be considered for the treatment of primary generalised tonic-clonic seizures [unlicensed]. Oxcarbazepine is not recommended in tonic, atonic, absence or myoclonic seizures due to the risk of seizure exacerbation.

Eslicarbazepine is licensed for adjunctive treatment in adults with focal seizures with or without secondary generalisation.

The *Scottish Medicines Consortium* (p. 4) has advised (October 2010) that eslicarbazepine (*Zebinix* ®) is accepted for restricted use within NHS Scotland as adjunctive therapy in adults with focal seizures with or without secondary generalisation. It is restricted for use in refractory epilepsy.

◢ CARBAMAZEPINE

Indications focal and secondary generalised tonic-clonic seizures, primary generalised tonic-clonic seizures; trigeminal neuralgia; prophylaxis of bipolar disorder unresponsive to lithium; adjunct in acute alcohol withdrawal [unlicensed] (section 4.10.1); diabetic neuropathy [unlicensed] (section 6.1.5)

Cautions cardiac disease (see also Contra-indications); skin reactions (see also Blood, Hepatic, or Skin Disorders, below and under Side-effects); test for HLA-B*1502 allele in individuals of Han Chinese or Thai origin (avoid unless no alternative—risk of Stevens-Johnson syndrome in presence of HLA-B*1502 allele); history of haematological reactions to other drugs; manufacturer recommends blood counts and hepatic and renal function tests (but evidence of practical value uncertain); may exacerbate absence and myoclonic seizures; consider vitamin D supplementation in patients who are immobilised for long periods or who have inadequate sun exposure or dietary intake of calcium; susceptibility to angle-closure glaucoma; cross-sensitivity reported with oxcarbazepine and with phenytoin (see Antiepileptic Hypersensitivity Syndrome p. 304); avoid abrupt withdrawal; **interactions:** see p. 303 and Appendix 1 (carbamazepine)

Blood, hepatic, or skin disorders Patients or their carers should be told how to recognise signs of blood, liver, or skin disorders, and advised to seek immediate medical attention if symptoms such as fever, rash, mouth ulcers, bruising, or bleeding develop. Carbamazepine should be withdrawn immediately in cases of aggravated liver dysfunction or acute liver disease. Leucopenia that is severe, progressive, or associated with clinical symptoms requires withdrawal (if necessary under cover of a suitable alternative).

Switching between formulations Different formulations of oral preparations may vary in bioavailability. Patients being treated for epilepsy should be maintained on a specific manufacturer's product (see also MHRA/CHM advice, p. 303)

Contra-indications AV conduction abnormalities (unless paced); history of bone-marrow depression; acute porphyria (section 9.8.2)

Hepatic impairment metabolism impaired in advanced liver disease; see also Blood, Hepatic, or Skin Disorders, above

Renal impairment use with caution

Pregnancy see Pregnancy, p. 304; monitor plasma-carbamazepine concentration

Breast-feeding see Breast-feeding, p. 305

Side-effects see notes above; also dry mouth, nausea, vomiting, oedema, ataxia, dizziness, drowsiness, fatigue, headache, hyponatraemia (leading in rare cases to water intoxication), blood disorders (including eosinophilia, leucopenia, thrombocytopenia, haemolytic anaemia, and aplastic anaemia), dermatitis, urticaria; *less commonly* diarrhoea, constipation, involuntary movements (including nystagmus), visual disturbances; *rarely* abdominal pain, anorexia, hepatitis, jaundice, vanishing bile duct syndrome, cardiac conduction disorders, hypertension, hypotension, peripheral neuropathy, dysarthria, aggression, agitation, confusion, depression, hallucinations, restlessness, paraesthesia, lymph node enlargement, muscle weakness, systemic lupus erythematosus, delayed multi-organ hypersensitivity disorder (see also Antiepileptic Hypersensitivity Syndrome p. 304); *very rarely* pancreatitis, stomatitis, hepatic failure, taste disturbance, exacerbation of coronary artery disease, AV block with syncope, circulatory collapse, hypercholesterolaemia, thrombophlebitis, thromboembolism, pulmonary hypersensitivity (with dyspnoea, pneumonitis, or pneumonia), psychosis, neuroleptic malignant syndrome, osteomalacia (see Cautions), osteoporosis, galactorrhoea, gynaecomastia, impaired male fertility, interstitial nephritis, renal failure, sexual dysfunction, urinary frequency, urinary retention, arthralgia, muscle pain, muscle spasm, conjunctivitis, angle-closure glaucoma, hearing disorders, acne, alterations in skin pigmentation, alopecia, hirsutism, sweating, photosensitivity, purpura, Stevens-Johnson syndrome, toxic epidermal necrolysis, aseptic meningitis; suicidal ideation

Dose
- Epilepsy, by mouth, initially 100–200 mg 1–2 times daily, increased slowly (see notes above) to usual

dose of 0.8–1.2 g daily in divided doses; in some cases 1.6–2 g daily in divided doses may be needed; ELDERLY reduce initial dose; CHILD daily in divided doses, up to 1 year 100–200 mg, 1–5 years 200–400 mg, 5–10 years 400–600 mg, 10–15 years 0.6–1 g

By rectum, for short-term use (max. 7 days) when oral therapy temporarily not possible; 125-mg suppository approx. equivalent to 100-mg tablet, but final adjustment should always depend on clinical response (plasma concentration monitoring recommended); max. 1 g daily in 4 divided doses

- Trigeminal neuralgia, by mouth, initially 100 mg 1–2 times daily (but some patients may require higher initial dose), increased gradually according to response; usual dose 200 mg 3–4 times daily, up to 1.6 g daily in some patients
- Prophylaxis of bipolar disorder unresponsive to lithium (see also section 4.2.3), by mouth, initially 400 mg daily in divided doses increased until symptoms controlled; usual range 400–600 mg daily; max. 1.6 g daily
- Treatment of alcohol withdrawal [unlicensed indication], by mouth, initially 800 mg daily in divided doses, reduced gradually over 5 days to 200 mg daily; usual treatment duration 7–10 days
- Diabetic neuropathy [unlicensed indication], by mouth, initially 100 mg 1–2 times daily, increased gradually according to response; usual dose 200 mg 3–4 times daily, up to 1.6 g daily in some patients

Note Plasma concentration for optimum response 4–12 mg/ litre (20–50 micromol/litre)

Carbamazepine (Non-proprietary) PoM

Tablets, carbamazepine 100 mg, net price 28 = £6.72; 200 mg, 28 = £5.41; 400 mg, 28 = £2.51. Label: 3, 8, counselling, blood, hepatic or skin disorder symptoms (see above), driving (see notes above)

Note Patients being treated for epilepsy should be maintained on a specific manufacturer's branded or generic oral carbamazepine product. See also MHRA/CHM advice, p. 303

Dental prescribing on NHS Carbamazepine Tablets may be prescribed

Tegretol® (Novartis) PoM

Tablets, scored, carbamazepine 100 mg, net price 84-tab pack = £2.07; 200 mg, 84-tab pack = £3.83; 400 mg, 56-tab pack = £5.02. Label: 3, 8, counselling, blood, hepatic or skin disorder symptoms (see above), driving (see notes above)

Chewtabs, orange, carbamazepine 100 mg, net price 56-tab pack = £3.16. Label: 3, 8, 21, 24, counselling, blood, hepatic or skin disorder symptoms (see above), driving (see notes above)

Liquid, sugar-free, carbamazepine 100 mg/5 mL. Net price 300-mL pack = £6.12. Label: 3, 8, counselling, blood, hepatic or skin disorder symptoms (see above), driving (see notes above)

Suppositories, carbamazepine 125 mg, net price 5 = £8.03; 250 mg, 5 = £10.71. Label: 3, 8, counselling, blood, hepatic or skin disorder symptoms (see above), driving (see notes above)

Note Patients being treated for epilepsy should be maintained on a specific manufacturer's branded or generic oral carbamazepine product. See also MHRA/CHM advice, p. 303

◢ Modified release

Carbagen® SR (Generics) PoM

Tablets, m/r, f/c, scored, carbamazepine 200 mg, net price 56-tab pack = £4.16; 400 mg, 56-tab pack = £8.20. Label: 3, 8, 25, counselling, blood, hepatic or skin disorder symptoms (see above), driving (see notes above)

Dose epilepsy, ADULT and CHILD over 5 years, as above; trigeminal neuralgia, as above; bipolar disorder, as above; total daily dose given in 1–2 divided doses

Note Patients being treated for epilepsy should be maintained on a specific manufacturer's branded or generic oral carbamazepine product. See also MHRA/CHM advice, p. 303

Tegretol® Prolonged Release (Novartis) PoM

Tablets, m/r, scored, carbamazepine 200 mg (beige-orange), net price 56-tab pack = £5.20; 400 mg (brown-orange), 56-tab pack = £10.24. Label: 3, 8, 25, counselling, blood, hepatic or skin disorder symptoms (see above), driving (see notes above)

Dose epilepsy, ADULT and CHILD over 5 years, as above; trigeminal neuralgia, as above; bipolar disorder, as above; total daily dose given in 2 divided doses

Note Patients being treated for epilepsy should be maintained on a specific manufacturer's branded or generic oral carbamazepine product. See also MHRA/CHM advice, p. 303

ESLICARBAZEPINE ACETATE

Indications see notes above

Cautions avoid abrupt withdrawal; hyponatraemia (monitor plasma-sodium concentration in patients at risk and discontinue treatment if hyponatraemia occurs); PR-interval prolongation (avoid concomitant administration of drugs that prolong PR interval); elderly; test for HLA-B*1502 allele in individuals of Han Chinese or Thai origin (avoid unless no alternative—risk of Stevens-Johnson syndrome in presence of HLA-B*1502 allele); **interactions:** see p. 303 and Appendix 1 (eslicarbazepine)

Switching between formulations Care should be taken when switching between oral formulations. The need for continued supply of a particular manufacturer's product should be based on clinical judgement and consultation with the patient or their carer, taking into account factors such as seizure frequency and treatment history (see also MHRA/ CHM advice, p. 303)

Contra-indications second- or third-degree AV block

Hepatic impairment avoid in severe impairment—no information available

Renal impairment reduce initial dose to 400 mg every other day for 2 weeks then 400 mg once daily if eGFR 30–60 mL/minute/1.73 m^2, adjusted according to response; avoid if eGFR less than 30 mL/minute/ 1.73 m^2

Pregnancy see Pregnancy, p. 304

Breast-feeding see Breast-feeding, p. 305

Side-effects gastro-intestinal disturbances; dizziness, drowsiness, headache, impaired coordination, tremor, visual disturbances, fatigue; rash; *less commonly* dry mouth, dehydration, gingival hyperplasia, stomatitis; palpitation, bradycardia, hypertension, hypotension, chest pain, epistaxis, appetite changes, weight changes, agitation, hyperactivity, confusion, mood changes, psychosis, impaired memory, insomnia, dysaesthesia, dystonia, parosmia, movement disorders, convulsions, peripheral neuropathy, nystagmus,

4 Central nervous system

dysarthria, taste disturbance, urinary tract infection, liver disorders, hypothyroidism, anaemia, hyponatraemia (see Cautions), electrolyte imbalance, tinnitus, alopecia, sweating, nail disorder, myalgia, nocturia, menstruation changes, malaise, chills, peripheral oedema; *very rarely* pancreatitis, thrombocytopenia, and leucopenia; PR-interval prolongation also reported; suicidal ideation

Dose
- ADULT over 18 years, initially 400 mg once daily, increased after 1–2 weeks to 800 mg once daily; max. 1.2 g

Zebinix® (Eisai) ⟨PoM⟩
Tablets, scored, eslicarbazepine acetate 800 mg, net price 30-tab pack = £136.00. Label: 8, counselling, driving (see notes above)
Note Patients may need to be maintained on a specific manufacturer's branded or generic eslicarbazepine product, see MHRA/CHM advice, p. 303

◼ OXCARBAZEPINE

Indications see notes above

Cautions hypersensitivity to carbamazepine (see also Antiepileptic Hypersensitivity Syndrome p. 304); avoid abrupt withdrawal; hyponatraemia (monitor plasma-sodium concentration in patients at risk); heart failure (monitor body-weight); cardiac conduction disorders; test for HLA-B*1502 allele in individuals of Han Chinese or Thai origin (avoid unless no alternative—risk of Stevens-Johnson syndrome in presence of HLA-B*1502 allele); avoid in acute porphyria (section 9.8.2); **interactions:** see p. 303 and Appendix 1 (oxcarbazepine)

Blood, hepatic, or skin disorders Patients or their carers should be told how to recognise signs of blood, liver, or skin disorders, and advised to seek immediate medical attention if symptoms such as lethargy, confusion, muscular twitching, fever, rash, blistering, mouth ulcers, bruising, or bleeding develop

Switching between formulations Care should be taken when switching between oral formulations. The need for continued supply of a particular manufacturer's product should be based on clinical judgement and consultation with the patient or their carer, taking into account factors such as seizure frequency and treatment history (see also MHRA/CHM advice, p. 303)

Hepatic impairment caution in severe impairment—no information available

Renal impairment halve initial dose if eGFR less than 30 mL/minute/1.73 m²; increase according to response at intervals of at least 1 week

Pregnancy see Pregnancy, p. 304

Breast-feeding see Breast-feeding, p. 305

Side-effects nausea, vomiting, constipation, diarrhoea, abdominal pain, dizziness, headache, drowsiness, agitation, amnesia, asthenia, ataxia, confusion, impaired concentration, depression, tremor, hyponatraemia, acne, alopecia, rash, nystagmus, visual disorders including diplopia; *less commonly* leucopenia, urticaria; *very rarely* arrhythmias, atrioventricular block, thrombocytopenia, hepatitis, pancreatitis, multi-organ hypersensitivity disorders (see also Antiepileptic Hypersensitivity Syndrome p. 304), systemic lupus erythematosus, Stevens-Johnson syndrome, toxic epidermal necrolysis; *also reported* hypertension, suicidal ideation, hypothyroidism, bone marrow depression, aplastic anaemia, neutropenia, pancytopenia, osteoporotic bone disorders

Dose
- Initially 300 mg twice daily increased according to response in steps of up to 600 mg daily at weekly intervals; usual dose range 0.6–2.4 g daily in divided doses; CHILD 6–18 years, 8–10 mg/kg daily in 2 divided doses increased according to response in steps of up to 10 mg/kg daily at weekly intervals (in adjunctive therapy, maintenance dose approx. 30 mg/kg daily); max. 46 mg/kg daily in divided doses
Note In adjunctive therapy, the dose of concomitant antiepileptics may need to be reduced when using high doses of oxcarbazepine

Oxcarbazepine (Non-proprietary) ⟨PoM⟩
Tablets, oxcarbazepine 150 mg, net price 50-tab pack = £12.41; 300 mg, 50-tab pack = £21.71; 600 mg, 50-tab pack = £42.97. Label: 3, 8, counselling, blood, hepatic, or skin disorders (see above), driving (see notes above)
Note Patients may need to be maintained on a specific manufacturer's branded or generic oxcarbazepine product, see MHRA/CHM advice, p. 303

Trileptal® (Novartis) ⟨PoM⟩
Tablets, f/c, scored, oxcarbazepine 150 mg (green), net price 50-tab pack = £10.20; 300 mg (yellow), 50-tab pack = £20.40; 600 mg (pink), 50-tab pack = £40.80. Label: 3, 8, counselling, blood, hepatic or skin disorders (see above), driving (see notes above)
Oral suspension, sugar-free, oxcarbazepine 300 mg/5 mL, net price 250 mL (with oral syringe) = £40.80. Label: 3, 8, counselling, blood, hepatic or skin disorders (see above), driving (see notes above)
Excipients include propylene glycol (see Excipients, p. 2)
Note Patients may need to be maintained on a specific manufacturer's branded or generic oxcarbazepine product, see MHRA/CHM advice, p. 303

Ethosuximide

Ethosuximide is a first-line treatment option for absence seizures. It may also be prescribed as adjunctive treatment for absence seizures when monotherapy is ineffective. Ethosuximide is also licensed for myoclonic seizures.

◼ ETHOSUXIMIDE

Indications see notes above

Cautions avoid abrupt withdrawal; avoid in acute porphyria (section 9.8.2); **interactions:** see p. 303 and Appendix 1 (ethosuximide)

Blood disorders Patients or their carers should be told how to recognise signs of blood disorders, and advised to seek immediate medical attention if symptoms such as fever, mouth ulcers, bruising, or bleeding develop

Hepatic impairment use with caution

Renal impairment use with caution

Pregnancy see Pregnancy, p. 304

Breast-feeding see Breast-feeding, p. 305

Side-effects gastro-intestinal disturbances (including nausea, vomiting, diarrhoea, abdominal pain, anorexia, weight loss); *less frequently* headache, fatigue, drowsiness, dizziness, hiccup, ataxia, euphoria, irritability, aggression, impaired concentration; *rarely* tongue swelling, sleep disturbances, depression, psychosis, photophobia, dyskinesia, increased libido, vaginal bleeding, myopia, gingival hypertrophy, rash; *also reported* hyperactivity, increase in seizure frequency, blood disorders (including leucopenia, agranulocytosis, pancytopenia, and aplastic anae-

(sidebar) **4 Central nervous system**

mia—blood counts required if features of infection), systemic lupus erythematosus, Stevens-Johnson syndrome; suicidal ideation

Dose

- ADULT and CHILD over 6 years, initially 500 mg daily in 2 divided doses, increased by 250 mg every 5–7 days to usual dose of 1–1.5 g daily in 2 divided doses; occasionally up to 2 g daily may be needed; CHILD 1 month–6 years, initially 10 mg/kg (max. 250 mg) daily in 2 divided doses, increased every 5–7 days to usual dose of 20–40 mg/kg (max. 1 g) daily in 2 divided doses; total daily dose may be given in 3 divided doses

Ethosuximide (Non-proprietary) ▣PoM

Capsules, ethosuximide 250 mg, net price 56-cap pack = £48.20. Label: 8, counselling, blood disorders (see above), driving (see notes above)

Emeside® (ChemIdex) ▣PoM

Syrup, black currant, ethosuximide 250 mg/5 mL, net price 200-mL pack = £6.60. Label: 8, counselling, blood disorders (see above), driving (see notes above)

Zarontin® (Pfizer) ▣PoM

Syrup, yellow, ethosuximide 250 mg/5 mL, net price 200-mL pack = £4.22. Label: 8, counselling, blood disorders (see above), driving (see notes above)

Gabapentin and pregabalin

Gabapentin and **pregabalin** are used for the treatment of focal seizures with or without secondary generalisation. They are not recommended if tonic, atonic, absence or myoclonic seizures are present. Both are also licensed for the treatment of neuropathic pain (p. 296). Pregabalin is licensed for the treatment of generalised anxiety disorder (p. 254). Gabapentin is an effective treatment for migraine prophylaxis [unlicensed] (p. 301).

The *Scottish Medicines Consortium* (p. 4) has advised (July 2007) that pregabalin (*Lyrica®*) is not recommended for the treatment of central neuropathic pain.

The *Scottish Medicines Consortium* (p. 4) has advised (April 2009) that pregabalin (*Lyrica®*) is accepted for restricted use within NHS Scotland for the treatment of peripheral neuropathic pain in adults who have not achieved adequate pain relief with, or have not tolerated, first- or second-line treatments; discontinue treatment if sufficient benefit is not achieved within 8 weeks of reaching the maximum tolerated dose.

GABAPENTIN

Indications monotherapy and adjunctive treatment of focal seizures with or without secondary generalisation; peripheral neuropathic pain (section 4.7.3); migraine prophylaxis [unlicensed] (section 4.7.4.2)

Cautions avoid abrupt withdrawal; elderly; diabetes mellitus; mixed seizures (including absences); false positive readings with some urinary protein tests; history of psychotic illness; high doses of oral solution in adolescents and adults with low body-weight—see preparations below; **interactions:** Appendix 1 (gabapentin)

Renal impairment reduce dose to 0.6–1.8 g daily in 3 divided doses if eGFR 50–80 mL/minute/1.73 m²; reduce dose to 300–900 mg daily in 3 divided doses if eGFR 30–50 mL/minute/1.73 m²; reduce dose to

300 mg on alternate days (up to max. 600 mg daily) in 3 divided doses if eGFR 15–30 mL/minute/1.73 m²; reduce dose to 300 mg on alternate days (up to max. 300 mg daily) in 3 divided doses if eGFR less than 15 mL/minute/1.73 m²—consult product literature

Pregnancy see Pregnancy, p. 304

Breast-feeding see Breast-feeding, p. 305

Side-effects nausea, vomiting, gingivitis, diarrhoea, abdominal pain, dyspepsia, constipation, dry mouth or throat, flatulence, weight gain, increased appetite, anorexia, hypertension, vasodilatation, oedema, dyspnoea, cough, pharyngitis, hostility, confusion, emotional lability, depression, vertigo, anxiety, nervousness, abnormal thoughts, drowsiness, dizziness, malaise, ataxia, convulsions, movement disorders, speech disorder, amnesia, tremor, insomnia, headache, paraesthesia, nystagmus, abnormal reflexes, fever, flu syndrome, impotence, leucopenia, arthralgia, myalgia, twitching, visual disturbances, rhinitis, rash, pruritus, acne; *less commonly* palpitation; *also reported* pancreatitis, hepatitis, hallucinations, blood glucose fluctuations in patients with diabetes, breast hypertrophy, gynaecomastia, acute renal failure, incontinence, thrombocytopenia, tinnitus, Stevens-Johnson syndrome, alopecia, hypersensitivity syndrome; suicidal ideation

Dose

- Epilepsy, 300 mg once daily on day 1, then 300 mg twice daily on day 2, then 300 mg 3 times daily on day 3 *or* initially 300 mg 3 times daily on day 1; then increased according to response in steps of 300 mg (in 3 divided doses) every 2–3 days; usual dose 0.9–3.6 g daily in 3 divided doses (max. 4.8 g daily in 3 divided doses); CHILD 6–12 years (adjunctive therapy only) initially 10 mg/kg (max. 300 mg) once daily on day 1, then 10 mg/kg (max. 300 mg) twice daily on day 2, then 10 mg/kg (max. 300 mg) 3 times daily on day 3; usual dose 25–35 mg/kg daily in 3 divided doses; max. 70 mg/kg daily in 3 divided doses; CHILD 2–6 years see *BNF for Children*
- Neuropathic pain, ADULT over 18 years, 300 mg once daily on day 1, then 300 mg twice daily on day 2, then 300 mg 3 times daily on day 3 *or* initially 300 mg 3 times daily on day 1, then increased according to response in steps of 300 mg (in 3 divided doses) every 2–3 days up to max. 3.6 g daily
- Migraine prophylaxis [unlicensed], initially 300 mg daily, increased according to response up to 2.4 g daily in divided doses

Gabapentin (Non-proprietary) ▣PoM

Capsules, gabapentin 100 mg, net price 100-cap pack = £3.34; 300 mg, 100-cap pack = £4.58; 400 mg, 100-cap pack = £4.82. Label: 3, 5, 8, counselling, driving (see notes above)

Tablets, gabapentin 600 mg, net price 100-tab pack = £10.27; 800 mg, 100-tab pack = £31.42. Label: 3, 5, 8, counselling, driving (see notes above)

Oral solution, gabapentin 50 mg/mL, net price 150-mL pack = £57.50. Label: 3, 5, 8, counselling, driving (see notes above)

Excipients include propylene glycol (see Excipients, p. 2)

Important The levels of propylene glycol, acesulfame K and saccharin sodium may exceed the recommended WHO daily intake limits if high doses of gabapentin oral solution (Rosemont brand) are given to adolescents or adults with low body-weight (39–50 kg)—consult product literature

Electrolytes Na⁺ 0.031 mmol/mL, K⁺ 0.097 mmol/mL

4 Central nervous system

Neurontin® (Pfizer) [PoM]

Capsules, gabapentin 100 mg (white), net price 100-cap pack = £18.29; 300 mg (yellow), 100-cap pack = £42.40; 400 mg (orange), 100-cap pack = £49.06. Label: 3, 5, 8, counselling, driving (see notes above)

Tablets, f/c, gabapentin 600 mg, net price 100-tab pack = £84.80; 800 mg, 100-tab pack = £98.13. Label: 3, 5, 8, counselling, driving (see notes above)

PREGABALIN

Indications   peripheral and central neuropathic pain (section 4.7.3); adjunctive therapy for focal seizures with or without secondary generalisation; generalised anxiety disorder (section 4.3)

Cautions   avoid abrupt withdrawal (taper over at least 1 week); severe congestive heart failure; conditions that may precipitate encephalopathy; **interactions:** Appendix 1 (pregabalin)

Renal impairment   initially 75 mg daily and max. 300 mg daily if eGFR 30–60 mL/minute/1.73 m^2; initially 25–50 mg daily and max. 150 mg daily in 1–2 divided doses if eGFR 15–30 mL/minute/1.73 m^2; initially 25 mg once daily and max. 75 mg once daily if eGFR less than 15 mL/minute/1.73 m^2

Pregnancy   see Pregnancy, p. 304

Breast-feeding   see Breast-feeding, p. 305

Side-effects   dry mouth, constipation, vomiting, flatulence, oedema, dizziness, drowsiness, irritability, impaired attention, disturbances in muscle control and movement, speech disorder, impaired memory, paraesthesia, euphoria, confusion, malaise, appetite changes, insomnia, weight gain, sexual dysfunction, visual disturbances (including blurred vision, diplopia, visual field defects); *less commonly* abdominal distension, hypersalivation, gastro-oesophageal reflux disease, thirst, taste disturbance, flushing, hypotension, hypertension, tachycardia, syncope, first-degree AV block, dyspnoea, nasal dryness, stupor, depersonalisation, depression, abnormal dreams, hallucinations, agitation, cognitive impairment, panic attacks, chills, hypoglycaemia, thrombocytopenia, urinary incontinence, dysuria, myalgia, arthralgia, dry eye, lacrimation, hyperacusis, nasopharyngitis, sweating, rash; *rarely* ascites, dysphagia, pancreatitis, weight loss, cold extremities, arrhythmia, bradycardia, cough, epistaxis, rhinitis, parosmia, hyperglycaemia, renal failure, oliguria, menstrual disturbances, breast pain, breast discharge, breast hypertrophy, neutropenia, hypokalaemia, leucopenia, rhabdomyolysis, urticaria; *also reported* diarrhoea, nausea, congestive heart failure, QT-interval prolongation, aggression, headache, convulsions, encephalopathy, urinary retention, keratitis, Stevens-Johnson syndrome, pruritus; suicidal ideation

Dose

• Neuropathic pain, ADULT over 18 years, initially 150 mg daily in 2–3 divided doses, increased if necessary after 3–7 days to 300 mg daily in 2–3 divided doses, increased further if necessary after 7 days to max. 600 mg daily in 2–3 divided doses

• Epilepsy, ADULT over 18 years, initially 25 mg twice daily, increased at 7-day intervals in steps of 50 mg daily to 300 mg daily in 2–3 divided doses, increased further if necessary after 7 days to max. 600 mg daily in 2–3 divided doses

• Generalised anxiety disorder, ADULT over 18 years, initially 150 mg daily in 2–3 divided doses, increased if

necessary at 7-day intervals in steps of 150 mg daily; max. 600 mg daily in 2–3 divided doses

Note   Pregabalin doses in BNF may differ from those in product literature

Lyrica® (Pfizer) [PoM]

Capsules, pregabalin 25 mg (white), net price 56-cap pack = £64.40, 84-cap pack = £96.60; 50 mg (white), 84-cap pack = £96.60; 75 mg (white/orange), 56-cap pack = £64.40; 100 mg (orange), 84-cap pack = £96.60; 150 mg (white), 56-cap pack = £64.40; 200 mg (orange), 84-cap pack = £96.60; 225 mg (white/orange), 56-cap pack = £64.40; 300 mg (white/orange), 56-cap pack = £64.40. Label: 3, 8, counselling, driving (see notes above)

Oral solution, strawberry flavour, pregabalin 20 mg/mL, net price 473 mL = £99.48. Label: 3, 8, counselling, driving (see notes above)

Lacosamide

Lacosamide is licensed for adjunctive treatment of focal seizures with or without secondary generalisation.

The *Scottish Medicines Consortium* (p. 4) has advised (January 2009) that lacosamide (*Vimpat®*) is accepted for restricted use within NHS Scotland as adjunctive treatment for focal seizures with or without secondary generalisation in patients from 16 years. It is restricted for specialist use in refractory epilepsy.

LACOSAMIDE

Indications   see notes above

Cautions   risk of PR-interval prolongation (including conduction problems, severe cardiac disease, and concomitant use of drugs that prolong PR interval), elderly; **interactions:** Appendix 1 (lacosamide)

Contra-indications   second- or third-degree AV block

Hepatic impairment   titrate with caution in mild to moderate impairment if co-existing renal impairment; caution in severe impairment—no information available

Renal impairment   loading dose regimen can be considered in mild to moderate impairment—titrate above 200 mg with caution; titrate with caution in severe impairment, max. 250 mg daily; consult product literature for loading dose if eGFR less than 30 mL/minute/1.73 m^2

Pregnancy   see Pregnancy, p. 304

Breast-feeding   manufacturer advises avoid—present in milk in *animal* studies; see also Breast-feeding, p. 305

Side-effects   nausea, vomiting, constipation, flatulence, dizziness, headache, impaired coordination, cognitive disorder, drowsiness, tremor, depression, fatigue, abnormal gait, blurred vision, nystagmus, pruritus; *rarely* multi-organ hypersensitivity reaction (see Antiepileptic Hypersensitivity Syndrome p. 304); *also reported* dyspepsia, dry mouth, AV block, bradycardia, PR-interval prolongation, atrial fibrillation, atrial flutter, aggression, agitation, psychosis, euphoria, confusion, hypoesthesia, dysarthria, irritability, agranulocytosis, muscle spasm, tinnitus, rash; suicidal ideation

Dose

• By mouth *or* by intravenous infusion over 15–60 minutes (for up to 5 days), ADULT and CHILD over 16 years, initially 50 mg twice daily, increased weekly by 50 mg twice daily according to response and tolerability; initial maintenance dose 100 mg twice daily; max. 200 mg twice daily

- Alternative loading dose regimen (can be used under medical supervision when it is necessary to rapidly attain therapeutic plasma concentrations), by mouth *or* by intravenous infusion over 15–60 minutes (for up to 5 days), ADULT and CHILD over 16 years, initially 200 mg, followed 12 hours later by a maintenance dose of 100 mg twice daily; thereafter increased weekly by 50 mg twice daily according to response and tolerability; max 200 mg twice daily

Vimpat® (UCB Pharma) (PoM)

Tablets, f/c, lacosamide 50 mg (pink), net price 14-tab pack = £10.81; 100 mg (yellow), 14-tab pack = £21.62, 56-tab pack = £86.50; 150 mg (pink), 14-tab pack = £32.44, 56-tab pack £129.74; 200 mg (blue), 56-tab pack = £144.16. Label: 8, counselling, driving (see notes above)

Syrup, yellow-brown, sugar-free, strawberry flavoured, lacosamide 10 mg/1 mL, net price 200-mL pack =£25.74. Label: 8, counselling, driving (see notes above)

Excipients aspartame (section 9.4.1), propylene glycol, (see Excipients)

Electrolytes Na⁺ 0.062 mmol/mL

Intravenous infusion, lacosamide 10 mg/mL, net price 200-mg vial = £29.70

Electrolytes Na⁺ 2.6 mmol/vial

Lamotrigine

Lamotrigine is an antiepileptic drug recommended as a first-line treatment for focal seizures and primary and secondary generalised tonic-clonic seizures. It is also licensed for typical absence seizures in children (but efficacy may not be maintained in all children) and is an unlicensed treatment option in adults if first-line treatments have been unsuccessful. Lamotrigine can also be used as adjunctive treatment in atonic or tonic seizures if first-line treatment has failed [unlicensed]. Myoclonic seizures may be exacerbated by lamotrigine and it can cause serious rashes especially in children; dose recommendations should be adhered to closely.

Lamotrigine is used either as sole treatment or as an adjunct to treatment with other antiepileptic drugs. Valproate increases plasma-lamotrigine concentration, whereas the enzyme-inducing antiepileptics reduce it; care is therefore required in choosing the appropriate initial dose and subsequent titration. When the potential for interaction is not known, treatment should be initiated with lower doses, such as those used with valproate.

◼ LAMOTRIGINE

Indications monotherapy and adjunctive treatment of focal seizures and generalised seizures including tonic-clonic seizures; seizures associated with Lennox-Gastaut syndrome; monotherapy of typical absence seizures in children; prevention of depressive episodes associated with bipolar disorder

Cautions closely monitor and consider withdrawal if rash, fever, or other signs of hypersensitivity syndrome develop; avoid abrupt withdrawal (taper off over 2 weeks or longer) unless serious skin reaction occurs; myoclonic seizures (may be exacerbated); Parkinson's disease (may be exacerbated); **interactions:** see p. 303 and Appendix 1 (lamotrigine)

Blood disorders Patients and their carers should be alert

for symptoms and signs suggestive of bone-marrow failure, such as anaemia, bruising, or infection. Aplastic anaemia, bone-marrow depression, and pancytopenia have been associated rarely with lamotrigine

Switching between formulations Care should be taken when switching between oral formulations in the treatment of epilepsy. The need for continued supply of a particular manufacturer's product should be based on clinical judgement and consultation with the patient or their carer, taking into account factors such as seizure frequency and treatment history (see also MHRA/CHM advice, p. 303)

Hepatic impairment halve dose in moderate impairment; quarter dose in severe impairment

Renal impairment caution in renal failure; metabolite may accumulate; consider reducing maintenance dose in significant impairment

Pregnancy see Pregnancy, p. 304

Breast-feeding see Breast-feeding, p. 305

Side-effects nausea, vomiting, diarrhoea, dry mouth, aggression, agitation, headache, drowsiness, dizziness, tremor, insomnia, ataxia, back pain, arthralgia, nystagmus, diplopia, blurred vision, rash (see Skin Reactions, below); *rarely* conjunctivitis; *very rarely* hepatic failure, movement disorders, unsteadiness, increase in seizure frequency, exacerbation of Parkinson's disease, confusion, hallucination, blood disorders (including anaemia, leucopenia, thrombocytopenia, pancytopenia—see Blood Disorders, above), hypersensitivity syndrome (see Antiepileptic Hypersensitivity Syndrome p. 304), lupus erythematosus-like reactions; *also reported* suicidal ideation, aseptic meningitis

Skin reactions Serious skin reactions including Stevens-Johnson syndrome and toxic epidermal necrolysis have developed (especially in children); most rashes occur in the first 8 weeks. Rash is sometimes associated with hypersensitivity syndrome (see Side-effects, above) and is more common in patients with history of allergy or rash from other antiepileptic drugs. Consider withdrawal if rash or signs of hypersensitivity syndrome develop. Factors associated with increased risk of serious skin reactions include concomitant use of valproate, initial lamotrigine dosing higher than recommended, and more rapid dose escalation than recommended.

Counselling Warn patients to see their doctor immediately if rash or signs or symptoms of hypersensitivity syndrome develop (see Antiepileptic Hypersensitivity Syndrome p. 304)

Dose **Important** Do not confuse the different combinations or indications; see also notes above

Note Dose titration should be repeated if restarting after an interval of more than 5 days

- Monotherapy of seizures, ADULT and CHILD over 12 years, initially 25 mg once daily for 14 days, increased to 50 mg once daily for further 14 days, then increased by max. 100 mg every 7–14 days; usual maintenance 100–200 mg daily in 1–2 divided doses (up to 500 mg daily has been required)

- Monotherapy of typical absence seizures, CHILD 2–12 years see *BNF for Children*

- Adjunctive therapy of seizures *with valproate*, ADULT and CHILD over 12 years, initially 25 mg on alternate days for 14 days then 25 mg once daily for further 14 days, thereafter increased by max. 50 mg every 7–14 days; usual maintenance, 100–200 mg daily in 1–2 divided doses; CHILD 2–12 years initially 150 micrograms/kg once daily for 14 days (those weighing under 13 kg may receive 2 mg on alternate days for first 14 days) then 300 micrograms/kg once daily for further 14 days, thereafter increased by max. 300 micrograms/kg every 7–14 days; usual maintenance 1–5 mg/kg daily in 1–2 divided doses; max. 200 mg daily

4

Central nervous system

- Adjunctive therapy of seizures (with enzyme inducing drugs) *without valproate*, ADULT and CHILD over 12 years, initially 50 mg once daily for 14 days then 50 mg twice daily for further 14 days, thereafter increased by max. 100 mg every 7–14 days; usual maintenance 200–400 mg daily in 2 divided doses (up to 700 mg daily has been required); CHILD 2–12 years initially 600 micrograms/kg daily in 2 divided doses for 14 days then 1.2 mg/kg daily in 2 divided doses for further 14 days, thereafter increased by max. 1.2 mg/kg every 7–14 days; usual maintenance 5–15 mg/kg daily in 1–2 divided doses; max. 400 mg daily
- Adjunctive therapy of seizures (without enzyme inducing drugs) *without valproate*, ADULT and CHILD over 12 years, initially 25 mg once daily for 14 days, increased to 50 mg once daily for further 14 days, then increased by max. 100 mg every 7–14 days; usual maintenance 100–200 mg daily in 1–2 divided doses; CHILD 2–12 years initially 300 micrograms/kg daily in 1–2 divided doses for 14 days then 600 micrograms/kg daily in 1–2 divided doses for further 14 days, thereafter increased by max. 600 micrograms/kg every 7–14 days; usual maintenance 1–10 mg/kg daily in 1–2 divided doses; max. 200 mg daily
- Monotherapy *or* adjunctive therapy of bipolar disorder (without enzyme inducing drugs) *without valproate*, ADULT over 18 years, initially 25 mg once daily for 14 days, then 50 mg daily in 1–2 divided doses for further 14 days, then 100 mg daily in 1–2 divided doses for further 7 days; usual maintenance 200 mg daily in 1–2 divided doses; max. 400 mg daily
- Adjunctive therapy of bipolar disorder *with valproate*, ADULT over 18 years, initially 25 mg on alternate days for 14 days, then 25 mg once daily for further 14 days, then 50 mg daily in 1–2 divided doses for further 7 days; usual maintenance 100 mg daily in 1–2 divided doses; max. 200 mg daily
- Adjunctive therapy of bipolar disorder (with enzyme inducing drugs) *without valproate*, ADULT over 18 years, initially 50 mg once daily for 14 days, then 50 mg twice daily for further 14 days, then 100 mg twice daily for further 7 days, then 150 mg twice daily for further 7 days; usual maintenance 200 mg twice daily

Note Patients stabilised on lamotrigine for bipolar disorder may require dose adjustments if other drugs are added to or withdrawn from their treatment regimens—consult product literature

Lamotrigine (Non-proprietary) PoM
Tablets, lamotrigine 25 mg, net price 56-tab pack = £1.55; 50 mg, 56-tab pack = £1.85; 100 mg, 56-tab pack = £2.47; 200 mg, 30-tab pack = £27.53, 56-tab pack = £3.73. Label: 8, counselling, driving (see notes above), skin reactions (see above)

Dispersible tablets, lamotrigine 5 mg, net price 28-tab pack = £1.86; 25 mg, 56-tab pack = £2.67; 100 mg, 56-tab pack = £4.99. Label: 8, 13, counselling, driving (see notes above), skin reactions (see above)

Note Patients being treated for epilepsy may need to be maintained on a specific manufacturer's branded or generic lamotrigine product, see MHRA/CHM advice, p. 303

Lamictal® (GSK) PoM
Tablets, yellow, lamotrigine 25 mg, net price 56-tab pack = £23.53; 50 mg, 56-tab pack = £40.02; 100 mg, 56-tab pack = £69.04; 200 mg, 56-tab pack = £117.35. Label: 8, counselling, driving (see notes above), skin reactions (above)
Dispersible tablets, chewable, lamotrigine 2 mg, net price 30-tab pack = £12.54; 5 mg, 28-tab pack =

£9.38; 25 mg, 56-tab pack = £23.53; 100 mg, 56-tab pack = £69.04. Label: 8, 13, counselling, driving (see notes above), skin reactions (above)

Note Patients being treated for epilepsy may need to be maintained on a specific manufacturer's branded or generic lamotrigine product, see MHRA/CHM advice, p. 303

Levetiracetam

Levetiracetam is licensed for monotherapy and adjunctive treatment of focal seizures with or without secondary generalisation, and for adjunctive therapy of myoclonic seizures in patients with juvenile myoclonic epilepsy and primary generalised tonic-clonic seizures. Levetiracetam may also be prescribed alone or in combination for the treatment of myoclonic seizures, and under specialist supervision for absence seizures [both unlicensed].

▋ LEVETIRACETAM

Indications see notes above

Cautions avoid abrupt withdrawal; **interactions:** Appendix 1 (levetiracetam)

Hepatic impairment halve dose in severe hepatic impairment if eGFR less than 60 mL/minute/1.73 m^2

Renal impairment max. 2 g daily if eGFR 50–80 mL/minute/1.73 m^2; max. 1.5 g daily if eGFR 30–50 mL/minute/1.73 m^2; max. 1 g daily if eGFR less than 30 mL/minute/1.73 m^2

Pregnancy see Pregnancy, p. 304

Breast-feeding see Breast-feeding, p. 305

Side-effects anorexia, abdominal pain, nausea, vomiting, dyspepsia, diarrhoea, cough, nasopharyngitis, vertigo, drowsiness, ataxia, convulsion, dizziness, headache, tremor, malaise, aggression, depression, insomnia, anxiety, irritability, rash; *less commonly* weight changes, paraesthesia, impaired attention, agitation, amnesia, confusion, psychosis, suicidal ideation (completed suicide also reported), leucopenia, thrombocytopenia, myalgia, blurred vision, diplopia, alopecia, eczema, pruritus; *rarely* pancreatitis, hepatic failure, dyskinesia, choreoathetosis, neutropenia, agranulocytosis, pancytopenia, hyponatraemia, drug reaction with eosinophilia and systemic symptoms (DRESS), toxic epidermal necrolysis, Stevens-Johnson syndrome, erythema multiforme

Dose
- Monotherapy of focal seizures, by mouth *or* by intravenous infusion, ADULT and CHILD over 16 years, initially 250 mg once daily increased after 1–2 weeks to 250 mg twice daily; thereafter, increased according to response in steps of 250 mg twice daily every 2 weeks; max. 1.5 g twice daily
- Adjunctive therapy of focal seizures, by mouth, ADULT and CHILD over 12 years, body-weight over 50 kg, initially 250 mg twice daily, increased by 500 mg twice daily every 2–4 weeks; max. 1.5 g twice daily; CHILD over 6 months, body-weight under 50 kg, initially 10 mg/kg once daily, increased by max. 10 mg/kg twice daily every 2 weeks; max. 30 mg/kg twice daily; CHILD 1–6 months, initially 7 mg/kg once daily, increased by max. 7 mg/kg twice daily every 2 weeks; max. 21 mg/kg twice daily

By intravenous infusion, ADULT and CHILD over 12 years, body-weight over 50 kg, initially 250 mg twice daily, increased by 500 mg twice daily every 2–4 weeks; max. 1.5 g twice daily; CHILD over 4 years, body-weight under 50 kg, initially 10 mg/kg once daily, increased by max. 10 mg/kg twice daily every 2 weeks; max. 30 mg/kg twice daily

- Adjunctive therapy of myoclonic seizures and tonic-clonic seizures, by mouth *or* by intravenous infusion, ADULT and CHILD over 12 years, body-weight over 50 kg, initially 250 mg twice daily, increased by 500 mg twice daily every 2–4 weeks; max. 1.5 g twice daily; CHILD 12–18 years, body-weight under 50 kg, initially 10 mg/kg once daily, increased by max. 10 mg/kg twice daily every 2 weeks; max. 30 mg/kg twice daily

- If switching between oral therapy and intravenous therapy (because oral route temporarily unavailable), by intravenous infusion, same as established oral dose

Note Levetiracetam doses in BNF may differ from those in product literature

Levetiracetam (Non-proprietary) PoM

Tablets, levetiracetam 250 mg, net price 60-tab pack = £3.02; 500 mg, 60-tab pack = £4.27; 750 mg 60-tab pack = £6.09; 1 g, 60-tab pack = £7.00. Label: 8

Oral solution, levetiracetam 100 mg/mL, net price 300-mL pack = £18.37. Label: 8

Brands include *Desitrend*®

Granules, levetiracetam 250 mg/sachet, net price 60-sachet pack = £22.41; 500 mg/sachet, net price 60-sachet pack = £39.46; 1 g/sachet, net price 60-sachet pack = £76.27. Label: 8

Brands include *Desitrend*®

Note Granules not suitable for use in children under 6 years, for initial treatment in children with body-weight less than 25 kg, or for the administration of doses below 250 mg

Keppra® (UCB Pharma) PoM

Tablets, f/c, levetiracetam 250 mg (blue), net price 60-tab pack = £28.01; 500 mg (yellow), 60-tab pack = £49.32; 750 mg (orange) 60-tab pack = £84.02; 1 g (white), 60-tab pack = £95.34. Label: 8

Oral solution, sugar-free, levetiracetam 100 mg/mL, net price 150 mL (with 1-mL or 3-mL syringe) = £33.48, 300 mL (with 10-mL syringe) = £66.95. Label: 8

Concentrate for intravenous infusion, levetiracetam 100 mg/mL, net price 5-mL vial = £12.73

Electrolytes Na⁺ 0.83 mmol/vial

Note For dilution before use

Perampanel

Perampanel is licensed for adjunctive treatment of focal seizures with or without secondary generalised seizures.

▌ PERAMPANEL

Indications see notes above

Cautions interactions: Appendix 1 (perampanel)

Switching between formulations Care should be taken when switching between oral formulations. The need for continued supply of a particular manufacturer's product should be based on clinical judgement and consultation with the patient or their carer, taking into account factors such as seizure frequency and treatment history (see also MHRA/CHM advice, p. 303)

Hepatic impairment increase at intervals of at least 2 weeks, up to max. 8 mg daily in mild or moderate impairment; avoid in severe impairment

Renal impairment avoid in moderate or severe impairment

Pregnancy see Pregnancy, p. 304; manufacturer advises avoid

Breast-feeding avoid—present in milk in *animal* studies

Side-effects nausea, changes in appetite, weight increase, aggression, dizziness, drowsiness, dysarthria, gait disturbance, irritability, anxiety, confusion, suicidal ideation and behaviour, malaise, ataxia, back pain, vertigo, blurred vision, diplopia

Dose

- ADULT and CHILD over 12 years, initially 2 mg once daily before bedtime, increased according to response and tolerability in 2-mg steps at intervals of at least 2 weeks; usual maintenance 4–8 mg once daily; max. 12 mg once daily

Note Titrate at intervals of at least 1 week with concomitant carbamazepine, oxcarbazepine, or phenytoin (see also Appendix 1)

Fycompa® (Eisai) ▼ PoM

Tablets, all f/c, perampanel 2 mg (orange), net price 7-tab pack = £35.00; 4 mg (red) 28-tab pack = £140.00; 6 mg (pink) 28-tab pack = £140.00; 8 mg (purple) 28-tab pack = £140.00; 10 mg (green) 28-tab pack = £140.00; 12 mg (blue) 28-tab pack = £140.00. Label: 3, 8, 25, counselling, driving (see notes above)

Note Patients may need to be maintained on a specific manufacturer's branded or generic perampanel product, see MHRA/CHM advice, p. 303

Phenobarbital and primidone

Phenobarbital is effective for tonic-clonic and focal seizures but may be sedative in adults and cause behavioural disturbances and hyperkinesia in children. It may be tried for atypical absence, atonic, and tonic seizures. Rebound seizures may be a problem on withdrawal. Plasma-phenobarbital concentration for optimum response is 15–40 mg/litre (60–180 micromol/litre); however, monitoring the plasma-drug concentration is less useful than with other drugs because tolerance occurs.

Primidone is largely converted to phenobarbital and this is probably responsible for its antiepileptic action. A low initial dose of primidone is essential.

▌ PHENOBARBITAL
(Phenobarbitone)

Indications all forms of epilepsy except typical absence seizures; status epilepticus (section 4.8.2)

Cautions see notes above; elderly; debilitated; children; respiratory depression (avoid if severe); avoid abrupt withdrawal (dependence with prolonged use); history of drug or alcohol abuse; consider vitamin D supplementation in patients who are immobilised for long periods or who have inadequate sun exposure or dietary intake of calcium; avoid in acute porphyria (section 9.8.2); interactions: see p. 303 and Appendix 1 (phenobarbital)

Switching between formulations Different formulations of oral preparations may vary in bioavailability. Patients should be maintained on a specific manufacturer's product (see also MHRA/CHM advice, p. 303)

Hepatic impairment may precipitate coma; avoid in severe impairment

Renal impairment use with caution

Pregnancy see Pregnancy, p. 304

Breast-feeding see Breast-feeding, p. 305

Side-effects hepatitis, cholestasis; hypotension; respiratory depression; behavioural disturbances,

4 Central nervous system

nystagmus, irritability, drowsiness, lethargy, depression, ataxia, paradoxical excitement, hallucinations, impaired memory and cognition, hyperactivity particularly in the elderly and in children; osteomalacia (see Cautions); megaloblastic anaemia (may be treated with folic acid), agranulocytosis, thrombocytopenia; allergic skin reactions; *very rarely* Stevens-Johnson syndrome and toxic epidermal necrolysis; suicidal ideation; Antiepileptic Hypersensitivity Syndrome (see p. 304); **overdosage:** see Emergency Treatment of Poisoning, p. 34

Dose
● By mouth, 60–180 mg at night; CHILD 5–8 mg/kg daily

Phenobarbital (Non-proprietary) [CD3]
Tablets, phenobarbital 15 mg, net price 28-tab pack = £24.00; 30 mg, 28-tab pack = 96p; 60 mg, 28-tab pack = £7.51. Label: 2, 8, counselling, driving (see notes above)

Elixir, phenobarbital 15 mg/5 mL in a suitable flavoured vehicle, containing alcohol 38%, net price 100 mL = £4.67. Label: 2, 8, counselling, driving (see notes above)

Note Patients should be maintained on a specific manufacturer's branded or generic phenobarbital product. See also MHRA/CHM advice, p. 303

Note Some hospitals supply **alcohol-free** formulations of varying phenobarbital strengths

◢**Injection**
Section 4.8.2

▮ PRIMIDONE

Indications all forms of epilepsy except typical absence seizures; essential tremor (section 4.9.3)

Cautions see under Phenobarbital; **interactions:** see p. 303 and Appendix 1 (phenobarbital)
Switching between formulations Different formulations of oral preparations may vary in bioavailability. Patients being treated for epilepsy should be maintained on a specific manufacturer's product (see also MHRA/CHM advice, p. 303)

Hepatic impairment reduce dose; may precipitate coma
Renal impairment see Phenobarbital
Pregnancy see Pregnancy, p. 304
Breast-feeding see Breast-feeding, p. 305
Side-effects see Phenobarbital; also nausea, visual disturbances; *less commonly* vomiting, headache, dizziness; *rarely* psychosis, lupus erythematosus, arthralgia; *also reported* Dupuytren's contracture

Dose
● Epilepsy, ADULT and CHILD over 9 years, initially 125 mg daily at bedtime, increased by 125 mg every 3 days to 500 mg daily in 2 divided doses, then increased according to response by 250 mg every 3 days to usual maintenance 0.75–1.5 g daily in 2 divided doses; CHILD under 9 years, initially 125 mg daily at bedtime, increased by 125 mg every 3 days according to response; usual maintenance, CHILD under 2 years, 250–500 mg daily in 2 divided doses; 2–5 years, 500–750 mg daily in 2 divided doses; 5–9 years 0.75–1 g daily in 2 divided doses
● Essential tremor, initially 50 mg daily, increased gradually over 2–3 weeks according to response; max. 750 mg daily

Note Monitor plasma concentrations of derived phenobarbital; optimum range as for phenobarbital

Primidone (Non-proprietary) [PoM]
Tablets, primidone 50 mg, net price 100-tab pack = £70.43; 250 mg, 100-tab pack = £79.15. Label: 2, 8, counselling, driving (see notes above)
Note Patients being treated for epilepsy should be maintained on a specific manufacturer's branded or generic primidone product. See also MHRA/CHM advice, p.

Phenytoin

Phenytoin is licensed for tonic-clonic and focal seizures but may exacerbate absence or myoclonic seizures and should be avoided if theses seizures are present. It has a narrow therapeutic index and the relationship between dose and plasma-drug concentration is non-linear; small dosage increases in some patients may produce large increases in plasma concentration with acute toxic side-effects. Similarly, a few missed doses or a small change in drug absorption may result in a marked change in plasma-drug concentration. Monitoring of plasma-drug concentration improves dosage adjustment.

Preparations containing phenytoin sodium are **not** bioequivalent to those containing phenytoin base (such as *Epanutin Infatabs*® and *Epanutin*® suspension); 100 mg of phenytoin sodium is approximately equivalent in therapeutic effect to 92 mg phenytoin base. The dose is the same for all phenytoin products when initiating therapy, however if switching between these products the difference in phenytoin content may be clinically significant. Care is needed when making changes between formulations and plasma-phenytoin concentration monitoring is recommended (see also MHRA/CHM advice, p. 303).

The usual total plasma-phenytoin concentration for optimum response is 10–20 mg/litre (or 40–80 micromol/litre). In pregnancy, the elderly, and certain disease states where protein binding may be reduced, careful interpretation of total plasma-phenytoin concentration is necessary; it may be more appropriate to measure free plasma-phenytoin concentration.

Symptoms of phenytoin toxicity include nystagmus, diplopia, slurred speech, ataxia, confusion, and hyperglycaemia.

Phenytoin may cause coarsening of the facial appearance, acne, hirsutism, and gingival hyperplasia and so may be particularly undesirable in adolescent patients.

When only parenteral administration is possible, **fosphenytoin** (section 4.8.2), a pro-drug of phenytoin, may be convenient to give. Unlike phenytoin (which should only be given intravenously), fosphenytoin may also be given by intramuscular injection.

▮ PHENYTOIN

Indications tonic-clonic seizures; focal seizures; prevention and treatment of seizures during or following neurosurgery or severe head injury; status epilepticus (section 4.8.2); trigeminal neuralgia if carbamazepine inappropriate (see also section 4.7.3)

Cautions cross-sensitivity reported with carbamazepine (see also Antiepileptic Hypersensitivity Syndrome p. 304); avoid abrupt withdrawal; HLA-B*1502 allele in individuals of Han Chinese or Thai origin—avoid unless essential (increased risk of Stevens-Johnson syndrome); manufacturer recommends blood counts (but evidence of practical value uncertain); consider vitamin D supplementation in patients who are immobilised for long periods or who have inadequate sun exposure or dietary intake of calcium; enteral feeding (interrupt feeding for 2 hours before and after dose; more frequent monitoring may be necessary; avoid in acute porphyria (section 9.8.2); **interactions:** see p. 303 and Appendix 1 (phenytoin) **Blood or skin disorders** Patients or their carers should be told how to recognise signs of blood or skin disorders, and advised to seek immediate medical attention if symptoms such as fever, rash, mouth ulcers, bruising, or bleeding develop. Leucopenia that is severe, progressive, or associated with clinical symptoms requires withdrawal (if necessary under cover of a suitable alternative)

Switching between formulations Different formulations of oral preparations may vary in bioavailability. Patients being treated for epilepsy should be maintained on a specific manufacturer's product (see also MHRA/CHM advice, p. 303)

Hepatic impairment reduce dose to avoid toxicity

Pregnancy changes in plasma-protein binding make interpretation of plasma-phenytoin concentrations difficult—monitor unbound fraction; see also Pregnancy, p. 304

Breast-feeding see Breast-feeding, p. 305

Side-effects nausea, vomiting, constipation, drowsiness, insomnia, transient nervousness, tremor, paraesthesia, dizziness, headache, anorexia; gingival hypertrophy and tenderness (maintain good oral hygiene); rash (discontinue; if mild re-introduce cautiously but discontinue immediately if recurrence); acne, hirsutism, coarsening of facial appearance; *rarely* hepatotoxicity (discontinue immediately and do not readminister), peripheral neuropathy, dyskinesia, lymphadenopathy, osteomalacia (see Cautions); blood disorders (including megaloblastic anaemia, leucopenia, thrombocytopenia, and aplastic anaemia), polyarteritis nodosa, lupus erythematosus, Stevens-Johnson syndrome, and toxic epidermal necrolysis; *also reported* polyarthropathy, pneumonitis, interstitial nephritis, hypersensitivity syndrome (see Antiepileptic Hypersensitivity Syndrome p. 304); suicidal ideation

Dose

- By mouth, initially 3–4 mg/kg daily *or* 150–300 mg daily (as a single dose *or* in 2 divided doses) increased gradually as necessary (with plasma-phenytoin concentration monitoring); usual dose 200–500 mg daily (exceptionally, higher doses may be used); CHILD initially 5 mg/kg daily in 2 divided doses, usual dose range 4–8 mg/kg daily (max. 300 mg daily)

Counselling Take preferably with or after food

Phenytoin (Non-proprietary) [PoM]

Tablets, coated, phenytoin sodium 100 mg, net price 28-tab pack = £30.00. Label: 8, counselling, administration, blood or skin disorder symptoms (see above), driving (see notes above)

Capsules, phenytoin sodium 25 mg, net price 28-cap pack =£15.74; 50 mg, 28-cap pack =£15.98; 100 mg, 84-cap pack =£54.00; 300 mg, 28-cap pack = £57.38. Label: 8, counselling, administration, blood or skin disorder symptoms (see above), driving (see notes above)

Note Patients being treated for epilepsy should be maintained on a specific manufacturer's branded or generic phenytoin product. See also MHRA/CHM advice, p. 303

Epanutin® (Pfizer) [PoM]

Chewable tablets (*Infatabs®*), yellow, scored, phenytoin 50 mg, net price 200-tab pack = £13.18. Label: 8, 24, counselling, blood or skin disorder symptoms (see above), driving (see notes above)

Suspension, red, phenytoin 30 mg/5 mL, net price 500 mL = £4.27. Label: 8, counselling, administration, blood or skin disorder symptoms (see above), driving (see notes above)

Note Patients being treated for epilepsy should be maintained on a specific manufacturer's branded or generic phenytoin product, see MHRA/CHM advice, p. 303. For additional information regarding differences in bioavailability of preparations containing phenytoin base and phenytoin sodium see notes above, p. 314

Retigabine

Retigabine is licensed for the adjunctive treatment of drug-resistant focal seizures with or without secondary generalisation; it should only be prescribed when other appropriate drug combinations have proved inadequate or have not been tolerated.

> **NICE guidance**
> **Retigabine for the adjunctive treatment of partial onset seizures in epilepsy (July 2011)**
> Retigabine is recommended as an option for the adjunctive treatment of partial onset seizures with or without secondary generalisation in adults aged 18 years and older with epilepsy, only when previous treatment with carbamazepine, clobazam, gabapentin, lamotrigine, levetiracetam, oxcarbazepine, sodium valproate, and topiramate has not provided an adequate response, or has not been tolerated.
> www.nice.org.uk/TA232

The *Scottish Medicines Consortium* (p. 4) has advised (June 2011) that retigabine (*Trobalt®*) is accepted for restricted use within NHS Scotland as adjunctive therapy in adults with focal seizures with or without secondary generalisation. It is restricted for use in refractory epilepsy.

▌ RETIGABINE

Indications see notes above

Cautions avoid abrupt withdrawal; risk of urinary retention; known QT-interval prolongation (see below); monitor for discoloration of ocular tissue and visual impairment (see Ophthalmological Monitoring below); monitor for blue-grey discoloration of nails, lips and skin—continue treatment only if potential benefit outweighs risk; **interactions:** see p. 303 and Appendix 1 (retigabine)

QT-interval prolongation Patients with known QT-interval prolongation, or with the following risk factors for QT-interval prolongation, should be carefully monitored while taking retigabine: cardiac failure, ventricular hypertrophy, electrolyte abnormalities, or concomitant treatment with drugs that can prolong QT interval

Ophthalmological monitoring A comprehensive ophthalmological examination (including visual acuity test, slit-lamp examination, and dilated fundoscopy) should be performed at initiation of treatment and at least every 6 months thereafter during treatment. Changes in vision or retinal pigment should lead to re-assessment of the benefits and risks of continuing treatment—discontinue unless no other treatment options are available. Monitoring should be increased if treatment is continued

Switching between formulations Care should be taken when switching between oral formulations. The need for continued supply of a particular manufacturer's product should be based on clinical judgement and consultation with the patient or their carer, taking into account factors such as seizure frequency and treatment history (see also MHRA/CHM advice, p. 303)

Hepatic impairment reduce dose by 50% in moderate to severe impairment; increase by 50 mg every week according to response up to max. 600 mg daily (450 mg in ELDERLY)

Renal impairment reduce dose by 50% if eGFR less than 50 mL/minute/1.73 m^2; increase by 50 mg every week according to response up to max. 600 mg daily (450 mg in ELDERLY)

Pregnancy see Pregnancy, p. 304

Breast-feeding see Breast-feeding, p. 305

Side-effects increased appetite, weight gain, nausea, constipation, dyspepsia, dry mouth, peripheral oedema, malaise, drowsiness, dizziness, vertigo, amnesia, paraesthesia, tremor, impaired coordination, impaired speech and attention, myoclonus, confusion, psychosis, anxiety, dysuria, haematuria, diplopia, blurred vision, discoloration of ocular tissue, visual impairment, discoloration of nails, lips and skin; *less commonly* dysphagia, hypokinesia, urinary retention, nephrolithiasis, rash, sweating; suicidal ideation

Dose

- ADULT over 18 years, initially up to 300 mg daily in 3 divided doses, increased according to response by up to 150 mg every week up to maintenance dose of 0.6–1.2 g daily; ELDERLY over 65 years, initially 150 mg daily in 3 divided doses, increased according to response by up to 150 mg every week; max. 900 mg daily

Trobalt® (GSK) ▼ PoM
Tablets, f/c, retigabine 50 mg (purple), net price 21-tab pack = £4.87, 84-tab pack = £19.46; 100 mg (green), 21-tab pack = £9.73, 84-tab pack = £38.93; 200 mg (yellow), 84-tab pack = £77.86; 300 mg (green), 84-tab pack = £116.78; 400 mg (purple), 84-tab pack = £127.68; starter pack of 21 x 50-mg tablets and 42 x 100-mg tablets = £24.33. Label: 8, 14, 25, counselling, driving (see notes above)
Note Patients may need to be maintained on a specific manufacturer's branded or generic retigabine product, see MHRA/CHM advice, p. 303

Rufinamide

Rufinamide is licensed for the adjunctive treatment of seizures in Lennox-Gastaut syndrome. It may be considered by a tertiary specialist for the treatment of refractory tonic or atonic seizures [unlicensed].

The *Scottish Medicines Consortium* (p. 4) has advised (October 2008) that rufinamide (*Inovelon®*) is accepted for restricted use within NHS Scotland as adjunctive therapy in the treatment of seizures associated with Lennox-Gastaut syndrome in patients 4 years and above. It is restricted for use when alternative traditional antiepileptic drugs are unsatisfactory.

◢ RUFINAMIDE

Indications see notes above

Cautions closely monitor and consider withdrawal if rash, fever, or other signs of hypersensitivity syndrome develop (see also Antiepileptic Hypersensitivity Syndrome p. 304); avoid abrupt withdrawal; **interactions**: see p. 303 and Appendix 1 (rufinamide)
Switching between formulations Care should be taken when switching between oral formulations. The need for continued supply of a particular manufacturer's product should be based on clinical judgement and consultation with the patient or their carer, taking into account factors such as

seizure frequency and treatment history (see also MHRA/CHM advice, p. 303)

Hepatic impairment caution and careful dose titration in mild to moderate impairment; avoid in severe impairment

Pregnancy see Pregnancy, p. 304

Breast-feeding see Breast-feeding, p. 305

Side-effects nausea, vomiting, constipation, diarrhoea, dyspepsia, abdominal pain, weight loss, anorexia; rhinitis, epistaxis; dizziness, headache, drowsiness, insomnia, anxiety, fatigue, increase in seizure frequency, impaired coordination, hyperactivity, tremor, gait disturbances; influenza-like symptoms; oligomenorrhoea; back pain; nystagmus, diplopia, blurred vision; rash and acne; hypersensitivity syndrome (see Antiepileptic Hypersensitivity Syndrome p. 304) also reported

Dose

- ADULT and CHILD over 4 years body-weight over 30 kg, initially 200 mg twice daily increased according to response in steps of 200 mg twice daily at intervals of not less than 2 days; body-weight 30–50 kg max. 900 mg twice daily; body-weight 50–70 kg max. 1.2 g twice daily; body-weight over 70 kg max. 1.6 g twice daily; CHILD over 4 years body-weight less than 30 kg, initially 100 mg twice daily increased according to response in steps of 100 mg twice daily at intervals of not less than 2 days; max. 500 mg twice daily (max. 300 mg twice daily if adjunctive therapy *with valproate*)

Inovelon® (Eisai) PoM
Tablets, pink, f/c, scored, rufinamide 100 mg, net price 10-tab pack = £5.15; 200 mg, 60-tab pack = £61.77; 400 mg, 60-tab pack = £102.96. Label: 8, 21, counselling, driving (see notes above), hypersensitivity syndrome (see notes above)

Oral suspension, white, sugar-free, rufinamide 40 mg/mL, net price 460-mL pack = £94.71. Label: 8, 21, counselling, driving, (see notes above), hypersensitivity syndrome (see notes above)
Excipients include propylene glycol (see Excipients)
Note Patients may need to be maintained on a specific manufacturer's branded or generic rufinamide product, see MHRA/CHM advice, p. 303

Tiagabine

Tiagabine is used as adjunctive treatment for focal seizures with or without secondary generalisation that are not satisfactorily controlled by other antiepileptics. It should be avoided in absence, myoclonic, tonic and atonic seizures due to risk of seizure exacerbation.

◢ TIAGABINE

Indications see notes above

Cautions avoid in acute porphyria (section 9.8.2); avoid abrupt withdrawal; **interactions**: Appendix 1 (tiagabine)
Driving May impair performance of skilled tasks (e.g. driving)

Hepatic impairment in mild to moderate impairment reduce dose, prolong the dose interval, or both; avoid in severe impairment

Pregnancy see Pregnancy, p. 304

Breast-feeding see Breast-feeding, p. 305

Side-effects diarrhoea; dizziness, tiredness, nervousness, tremor, impaired concentration, emotional lability, speech impairment; *rarely* confusion, depression, drowsiness, psychosis, non-convulsive status epilepticus, bruising, and visual disturbances; suicidal ideation; leucopenia also reported

Dose

- Adjunctive therapy, ADULT and CHILD over 12 years, initially 5–10 mg daily in 1–2 divided doses, increased in steps of 5–10 mg daily at weekly intervals; usual maintenance dose *with enzyme-inducing drugs*, 30–45 mg daily in 2–3 divided doses; initial maintenance dose *without enzyme-inducing drugs*, 15–30 mg daily in 2–3 divided doses

Gabitril® (TEVA UK) PoM

Tablets, f/c, tiagabine (as hydrochloride) 5 mg, net price 100-tab pack = £52.04; 10 mg, 100-tab pack = £104.09; 15 mg, 100-tab pack = £156.13. Label: 21

Topiramate

Topiramate can be given alone or as adjunctive treatment in generalised tonic-clonic seizures or focal seizures with or without secondary generalisation. It can be used as adjunctive treatment for seizures associated with Lennox-Gastaut syndrome and for absence, tonic and atonic seizures under specialist supervision [unlicensed]. It can also be considered as an option in myoclonic seizures [unlicensed]. Topiramate is also licensed for prophylaxis of migraine (section 4.7.4.2).

▌ TOPIRAMATE

Indications see notes above

Cautions avoid abrupt withdrawal; risk of metabolic acidosis; risk of nephrolithiasis—ensure adequate hydration (especially in strenuous activity or warm environment); avoid in acute porphyria (section 9.8.2); **interactions:** see p. 303 and Appendix 1 (topiramate)

Important Topiramate has been associated with acute myopia with secondary angle-closure glaucoma, typically occurring within 1 month of starting treatment. Choroidal effusions resulting in anterior displacement of the lens and iris have also been reported. If raised intra-ocular pressure occurs:

- seek specialist ophthalmological advice;
- use appropriate measures to reduce intra-ocular pressure;
- stop topiramate as rapidly as feasible

Switching between formulations Care should be taken when switching between oral formulations in the treatment of epilepsy. The need for continued supply of a particular manufacturer's product should be based on clinical judgement and consultation with the patient or their carer, taking into account factors such as seizure frequency and treatment history (see also MHRA/CHM advice, p. 303)

Hepatic impairment use with caution in moderate to severe impairment—clearance may be reduced

Renal impairment use with caution; half usual starting and maintenance dose if eGFR less than 70 mL/minute/1.73 m² —reduced clearance and longer time to steady-state plasma concentration

Pregnancy see Pregnancy, p. 304

Breast-feeding manufacturer advises avoid—present in milk; see also Breast-feeding, p. 305

Side-effects nausea, diarrhoea, vomiting, constipation, dyspepsia, abdominal pain, dry mouth, taste disturbance, gastritis, appetite changes, dyspnoea, impaired attention, cognitive impairment, movement disorders, seizures, tremor, malaise, impaired coordination, speech disorder, drowsiness, dizziness, sleep disturbance, anxiety, confusion, paraesthesia, aggression, mood changes, depression, agitation, irritability, nephrolithiasis, urinary disorders, anaemia, arthralgia, muscle spasm, myalgia, muscular weakness, visual disturbances, nystagmus, tinnitus, epistaxis, alopecia, rash, pruritus; *less commonly* pancreatitis, flatulence, abdominal distension, gingival bleeding, salivation, halitosis, thirst, glossodynia, bradycardia, palpitation, hypotension, postural hypotension, flushing, altered sense of smell, peripheral neuropathy, suicidal ideation, psychosis, panic attack, influenza-like symptoms, sexual dysfunction, urinary calculus, haematuria, blood disorders (including leucopenia, neutropenia, and thrombocytopenia), hypokalaemia, metabolic acidosis, dry eye, photophobia, blepharospasm, increased lacrimation, mydriasis, hearing loss, reduced sweating, skin discoloration; *rarely* hepatitis, hepatic failure, Raynaud's syndrome, periorbital oedema, unilateral blindness, Stevens-Johnson syndrome, abnormal skin odour, calcinosis; *very rarely* angle-closure glaucoma; *also reported* encephalopathy, hyperammonaemia, maculopathy, toxic epidermal necrolysis

Dose

- Monotherapy in epilepsy, initially 25 mg at night for 1 week *then* increased in steps of 25–50 mg taken in 2 divided doses at intervals of 1–2 weeks; usual dose 100–200 mg daily in 2 divided doses, adjusted according to response; max. 500 mg daily (doses of 1 g daily have been used in refractory epilepsy); CHILD 6–18 years, initially 0.5–1 mg/kg (max. 25 mg) at night for 1 week *then* increased in steps of 0.5–1 mg/kg (max. 50 mg) taken in 2 divided doses at intervals of 1–2 weeks; initial target dose 100 mg daily in 2 divided doses; max. 15 mg/kg (max. 500 mg) daily

- Adjunctive therapy in epilepsy, initially 25–50 mg at night for 1 week *then* increased in steps of 25–50 mg taken in 2 divided doses at intervals of 1–2 weeks; usual dose 200–400 mg daily in 2 divided doses; max. 400 mg daily; CHILD 2–18 years, initially 1–3 mg/kg (max. 25 mg) at night for 1 week *then* increased in steps of 1–3 mg/kg (max. 50 mg) taken in 2 divided doses at intervals of 1–2 weeks; usual dose 5–9 mg/kg daily in 2 divided doses; max. 15 mg/kg (max. 400 mg) daily

- Migraine prophylaxis, ADULT over 18 years, initially 25 mg at night for 1 week *then* increased in steps of 25 mg at weekly intervals; usual dose 50–100 mg daily in 2 divided doses; max. 200 mg daily; CHILD 16–18 years see *BNF for Children*

Topiramate (Non-proprietary) PoM

Tablets, topiramate 25 mg, net price 60-tab pack = £3.71; 50 mg, 60-tab pack = £3.42; 100 mg, 60-tab pack = £3.88; 200 mg, 60-tab pack = £16.14. Label: 3, 8, counselling, driving (see notes above)

Capsules, topiramate 15 mg, net price 60-cap pack = £22.45; 25 mg, 60-cap pack = £15.40; 50 mg, 60-cap pack = £50.78. Label: 3, 8, counselling, driving (see notes above)

Note Patients being treated for epilepsy may need to be maintained on a specific manufacturer's branded or generic topiramate product, see MHRA/CHM advice, p. 303

Topamax® (Janssen) PoM

Tablets, f/c, topiramate 25 mg, net price 60-tab pack = £19.29; 50 mg (light yellow), 60-tab pack = £31.69; 100 mg (yellow), 60-tab pack = £56.76; 200 mg (salmon), 60-tab pack = £110.23. Label: 3, 8, counselling, driving (see notes above)

4 Central nervous system

Capsules (*Sprinkle®*), topiramate 15 mg, net price 60-cap pack = £14.79; 25 mg, 60-cap pack = £22.18; 50 mg, 60-cap pack = £36.45. Label: 3, 8, counselling, administration, driving (see notes above)

Counselling Swallow whole or sprinkle contents of capsule on soft food and swallow immediately without chewing

Note Patients being treated for epilepsy may need to be maintained on a specific manufacturer's branded or generic topiramate product, see MHRA/CHM advice, p. 303

Valproate

Sodium valproate is effective in controlling tonic-clonic seizures, particularly in primary generalised epilepsy. It is a drug of choice in primary generalised tonic-clonic seizures, focal seizures, generalised absences and myoclonic seizures, and can be tried in atypical absence seizures. It is recommended as a first-line option in atonic and tonic seizures. Sodium valproate has widespread metabolic effects and monitoring of liver function tests and full blood count is essential (see Cautions below). Plasma-valproate concentrations are not a useful index of efficacy, therefore routine monitoring is unhelpful.

Valproic acid (as semisodium valproate) (section 4.2.3) is licensed for acute mania associated with bipolar disorder.

Valproate is associated with teratogenic risks—this should be fully considered and discussed before prescribing for women of child-bearing age (see Pregnancy, p. 304)

▌ SODIUM VALPROATE

Indications all forms of epilepsy; migraine prophylaxis [unlicensed] (section 4.7.4.2); mania (section 4.2.3)

Cautions monitor liver function before therapy and during first 6 months especially in patients most at risk (see also below); measure full blood count and ensure no undue potential for bleeding before starting and before surgery; systemic lupus erythematosus; false-positive urine tests for ketones; avoid abrupt withdrawal; consider vitamin D supplementation in patients that are immobilised for long periods or who have inadequate sun exposure or dietary intake of calcium; **interactions**: see p. 303 and Appendix 1 (valproate)

Liver toxicity Liver dysfunction (including fatal hepatic failure) has occurred in association with valproate (especially in children under 3 years and in those with metabolic or degenerative disorders, organic brain disease or severe seizure disorders associated with mental retardation) usually in first 6 months and usually involving multiple antiepileptic therapy. Raised liver enzymes during valproate treatment are usually transient but patients should be reassessed clinically and liver function (including prothrombin time) monitored until return to normal—discontinue if abnormally prolonged prothrombin time (particularly in association with other relevant abnormalities).

Blood or hepatic disorders Patients or their carers should be told how to recognise signs and symptoms of blood or liver disorders and advised to seek immediate medical attention if symptoms develop

Pancreatitis Patients or their carers should be told how to recognise signs and symptoms of pancreatitis and advised to seek immediate medical attention if symptoms such as abdominal pain, nausea, or vomiting develop; discontinue if pancreatitis is diagnosed

Switching between formulations Care should be taken when switching between oral formulations in the treatment of epilepsy. The need for continued supply of a particular manufacturer's product should be based on clinical judgement and consultation with the patient or their carer,

taking into account factors such as seizure frequency and treatment history (see also MHRA/CHM advice, p. 303)

Contra-indications family history of severe hepatic dysfunction; acute porphyria (section 9.8.2)

Hepatic impairment avoid if possible—hepatotoxicity and hepatic failure may occasionally occur (usually in first 6 months); avoid in active liver disease; see also under Cautions

Renal impairment reduce dose

Pregnancy avoid unless there is no safer alternative and only after a careful discussion of the risks; effective contraception advised in women of child-bearing potential; see also Pregnancy, p. 304; neonatal bleeding (related to hypofibrinaemia) and neonatal hepatotoxicity also reported

Breast-feeding see Breast-feeding, p. 305

Side-effects nausea, gastric irritation, diarrhoea; weight gain; hyperammonaemia, thrombocytopenia; transient hair loss (regrowth may be curly); *less frequently* increased alertness, aggression, hyperactivity, behavioural disturbances, ataxia, tremor, and vasculitis; *rarely* hepatic dysfunction (see under Cautions; withdraw treatment immediately if persistent vomiting and abdominal pain, anorexia, jaundice, oedema, malaise, drowsiness, or loss of seizure control), lethargy, drowsiness, confusion, stupor, hallucinations, blood disorders (including anaemia, leucopenia, pancytopenia), hearing loss, and rash; *very rarely* pancreatitis (see under Cautions), peripheral oedema, increase in bleeding time, extrapyramidal symptoms, dementia, encephalopathy, coma, gynaecomastia, Fanconi's syndrome, hirsutism, acne, enuresis, hyponatraemia, toxic epidermal necrolysis, and Stevens-Johnson syndrome; suicidal ideation; reduced bone mineral density (see Cautions); *also reported* menstrual disturbances, male infertility, syndrome of inappropriate secretion of antidiuretic hormone, drug rash with eosinophilia and systemic symptoms (DRESS) syndrome, hypersensitivity reactions

Dose

* Epilepsy, by mouth, initially 600 mg daily in 1–2 divided doses, increased gradually (in steps of 150–300 mg) every 3 days; usual maintenance dose 1–2 g daily (20–30 mg/kg daily), max. 2.5 g daily; CHILD 1 month–12 years, initially 10–15 mg/kg (max. 600 mg) daily in 1–2 divided doses; usual maintenance dose 25–30 mg/kg daily in 2 divided doses

Initiation of valproate treatment by intravenous administration, ADULT and CHILD over 12 years, initially 10 mg/kg (usually 400–800 mg) by intravenous injection (over 3–5 minutes) followed by intravenous infusion *or* intravenous injection (over 3–5 minutes) in 2–4 divided doses *or* by continuous intravenous infusion up to max. 2.5 g daily; usual range 1–2 g daily (20–30 mg/kg daily); CHILD 1 month–12 years, 10 mg/kg by intravenous injection (over 3–5 minutes) followed by intravenous infusion *or* intravenous injection (over 3–5 minutes) in 2–4 divided doses *or* by continuous intravenous infusion up to usual range 20–40 mg/kg daily (doses above 40 mg/kg daily monitor clinical chemistry and haematological parameters)

Continuation of valproate treatment by intravenous injection (over 3–5 minutes) *or* intravenous infusion in 2–4 divided doses, or by continuous intravenous infusion, same as established oral daily dose

- Migraine prophylaxis [unlicensed], by mouth, initially 200 mg twice daily, increased if necessary to 1.2–1.5 g daily in divided doses
- Mania, see under *Episenta*®

◢Oral

Sodium Valproate (Non-proprietary) PoM

Tablets (crushable), scored, sodium valproate 100 mg, net price 100-tab pack = £5.60. Label: 8, 21, counselling, pancreatitis, blood, or hepatic disorder symptoms, pregnancy (see above), driving (see notes above)

Tablets, e/c, sodium valproate 200 mg, net price 100-tab pack = £4.42; 500 mg, 100-tab pack = £8.37. Label: 5, 8, 25, counselling, pancreatitis, blood, or hepatic disorder symptoms, pregnancy (see above), driving (see notes above)

Oral solution, sodium valproate 200 mg/5 mL, net price 300 mL = £9.33. Label: 8, 21, counselling, pancreatitis, blood, or hepatic disorder symptoms, pregnancy (see above), driving (see notes above)

Note Patients being treated for epilepsy may need to be maintained on a specific manufacturer's branded or generic oral sodium valproate product, see MHRA/CHM advice, p. 303

Epilim® (Sanofi-Aventis) PoM

Tablets (crushable), scored, sodium valproate 100 mg, net price 100-tab pack = £5.60. Label: 8, 21, counselling, pancreatitis, blood, or hepatic disorder symptoms, pregnancy (see above), driving (see notes above)

Tablets, e/c, lilac, sodium valproate 200 mg, net price 100-tab pack = £7.70; 500 mg, 100-tab pack = £19.25. Label: 5, 8, 25, counselling, pancreatitis, blood, or hepatic disorder symptoms, pregnancy (see above), driving (see notes above)

Liquid, red, sugar-free, sodium valproate 200 mg/5 mL, net price 300-mL pack = £7.78. Label: 8, 21, counselling, pancreatitis, blood, or hepatic disorder symptoms, pregnancy (see above), driving (see notes above)

Syrup, red, sodium valproate 200 mg/5 mL, net price 300-mL pack = £9.33. Label: 8, 21, counselling, pancreatitis, blood, or hepatic disorder symptoms, pregnancy (see above), driving (see notes above)

Note May be diluted, preferably in Syrup BP; use within 14 days

Note Patients being treated for epilepsy may need to be maintained on a specific manufacturer's branded or generic oral sodium valproate product, see MHRA/CHM advice, p. 303

◢Modified release

Epilim Chrono® (Sanofi-Aventis) PoM

Tablets, m/r, lilac, sodium valproate 200 mg (as sodium valproate and valproic acid), net price 100-tab pack = £11.65; 300 mg, 100-tab pack = £17.47; 500 mg, 100-tab pack = £29.10. Label: 8, 21, 25, counselling, pancreatitis, blood, or hepatic disorder symptoms, pregnancy (see above), driving (see notes above)

Dose epilepsy, ADULT and CHILD over 20 kg, as above, total daily dose given in 1–2 divided doses

Note Patients being treated for epilepsy may need to be maintained on a specific manufacturer's branded or generic oral sodium valproate product, see MHRA/CHM advice, p. 303

Epilim Chronosphere® (Sanofi-Aventis) PoM

Granules, m/r, sodium valproate 50 mg (as sodium valproate and valproic acid), net price 30-sachet pack = £30.00; 100 mg, 30-sachet pack = £30.00; 250 mg, 30-sachet pack = £30.00; 500 mg, 30-sachet pack = £30.00; 750 mg, 30-sachet pack = £30.00; 1 g, 30-sachet pack = £30.00. Label: 8, 21, 25, counselling, administration, pancreatitis, blood, or hepatic disorder symptoms, pregnancy (see above), driving (see notes above)

Dose epilepsy, ADULT and CHILD, as above to the nearest whole 50-mg sachet; total daily dose given in 1–2 divided doses

Counselling Granules may be mixed with soft food or drink that is cold or at room temperature, and swallowed immediately without chewing

Note Patients being treated for epilepsy may need to be maintained on a specific manufacturer's branded or generic oral sodium valproate product, see MHRA/CHM advice, p. 303

Episenta® (Desitin) PoM

Capsules, enclosing m/r granules, sodium valproate 150 mg, net price 100-cap pack = £7.00; 300 mg, 100-cap pack = £13.00. Label: 8, 21, 25, counselling, administration, pancreatitis, blood, or hepatic disorder symptoms, pregnancy (see above), driving (see notes above)

Dose epilepsy, ADULT and CHILD, as above, total daily dose given in 1–2 divided doses

Mania, ADULT over 18 years, initially 750 mg daily, adjusted according to response, usual dose 1–2 g daily; doses greater than 45 mg/kg daily require careful monitoring; total daily dose given in 1–2 divided doses

Counselling Contents of capsule may be mixed with cold soft food or drink and swallowed immediately without chewing

Granules, m/r, sodium valproate 500 mg, net price 100-sachet pack = £21.00; 1 g, 100-sachet pack = £41.00. Label: 8, 21, 25, counselling, administration, pancreatitis, blood, or hepatic disorder symptoms, pregnancy (see above), driving (see notes above)

Dose epilepsy, ADULT and CHILD, as above, total daily dose given in 1–2 divided doses

Mania, ADULT over 18 years, initially 750 mg daily, adjusted according to response, usual dose 1–2 g daily; doses greater than 45 mg/kg daily require careful monitoring; total daily dose given in 1–2 divided doses

Counselling Granules may be mixed with cold soft food or drink and swallowed immediately without chewing

Note Patients being treated for epilepsy may need to be maintained on a specific manufacturer's branded or generic oral sodium valproate product, see MHRA/CHM advice, p. 303

Epival® (Chanelle Medical) PoM

Tablets, m/r, scored, sodium valproate 300 mg, net price 100-tab pack = £12.13; 500 mg, 100-tab pack = £20.21. Label: 8, 21, 25, counselling, pancreatitis, blood, or hepatic disorder symptoms, pregnancy (see above), driving (see notes above)

Dose epilepsy, ADULT and CHILD body-weight over 20 kg, as above, total daily dose given in 1–2 divided doses

Counselling Tablets may be halved but not crushed or chewed

Note Patients being treated for epilepsy may need to be maintained on a specific manufacturer's branded or generic oral sodium valproate product, see MHRA/CHM advice, p. 303

◢Parenteral

Sodium Valproate (Non-proprietary) PoM

Injection, sodium valproate 100 mg/mL, net price 3-mL amp = £7.00; 4-mL amp = £11.58

Brands include *Episenta*®

4 Central nervous system

Epilim® Intravenous (Sanofi-Aventis) PoM
Injection, powder for reconstitution, sodium valproate, net price 400-mg vial (with 4-mL amp water
for injections) = £13.32

◢**Valproic acid**

Convulex® (Pharmacia) PoM
Capsules, e/c, valproic acid 150 mg, net price 100-
cap pack = £3.68; 300 mg, 100-cap pack = £7.35;
500 mg, 100-cap pack = £12.25. Label: 8, 21, 25,
counselling, pancreatitis, blood, or hepatic disorder
symptoms, pregnancy (see above), driving (see
notes above)
Dose epilepsy, ADULT and CHILD, as above, total daily
dose given in 2–4 divided doses
Equivalence to sodium valproate Convulex® has a 1:1
dose relationship with products containing sodium
valproate, but nevertheless care is needed if switching
Note Patients being treated for epilepsy may need to be
maintained on a specific manufacturer's branded or generic
oral valproic acid product, see MHRA/CHM advice, p. 303

Depakote® (Sanofi-Aventis) PoM
Section 4.2.3 (bipolar disorder)

Vigabatrin

Vigabatrin can be prescribed in combination with other
antiepileptic treatment for focal epilepsy with or without
secondary generalisation. It should not be prescribed
unless all other appropriate drug combinations are
ineffective or have not been tolerated, and it should
be initiated and supervised by an appropriate specialist.
Vigabatrin can be prescribed as monotherapy in the
management of infantile spasms in West's syndrome.
Vigabatrin may worsen absence, myoclonic, tonic and
atonic seizures.

About one-third of patients treated with vigabatrin have
suffered visual field defects; counselling and **careful
monitoring** for this side-effect are required (see also
Visual Field Defects under Cautions below). Vigabatrin
has prominent behavioural side-effects in some patients.

▮ VIGABATRIN

Indications see notes above

Cautions elderly; closely monitor neurological function; avoid sudden withdrawal; history of psychosis,
depression, or behavioural problems; absence seizures (may be exacerbated); **interactions:** see p. 303
and Appendix 1 (vigabatrin)
Visual field defects Vigabatrin is associated with visual
field defects. The onset of symptoms varies from 1 month to
several years after starting. In most cases, visual field defects
have persisted despite discontinuation, and further
deterioration after discontinuation cannot be excluded.
Product literature advises visual field testing before
treatment and at 6-month intervals. Patients should be
warned to report any new visual symptoms that develop and
those with symptoms should be referred for an urgent
ophthalmological opinion. Gradual withdrawal of vigabatrin
should be considered.

Contra-indications visual field defects

Renal impairment consider reduced dose or
increased dose interval if eGFR less than 60 mL/
minute/1.73 m^2

Pregnancy see Pregnancy, p. 304

Breast-feeding present in milk—manufacturer
advises avoid; see also Breast-feeding, p. 305

Side-effects nausea, vomiting, abdominal pain,
oedema, drowsiness (*rarely* encephalopathic symptoms including marked sedation, stupor, and confu-

sion with non-specific slow wave EEG—reduce dose
or withdraw), fatigue, excitation (in children), agitation, dizziness, headache, nervousness, depression,
aggression, irritability, paranoia, impaired concentration, impaired memory, tremor, paraesthesia, speech
disorder, weight gain, visual field defects (see under
Cautions), blurred vision, nystagmus, diplopia; *less
commonly* ataxia, psychosis, mania, rash, occasional
increase in seizure frequency (especially if myoclonic); *rarely* suicidal ideation, retinal disorders
(including peripheral retinal neuropathy); *very rarely*
hepatitis, optic neuritis, optic atrophy; *also reported*
movement disorders in infantile spasms

Dose
- With current antiepileptic therapy, by mouth initially
1 g daily in single or 2 divided doses then increased
according to response in steps of 500 mg at weekly
intervals; usual range 2–3 g daily (max. 3 g daily);
NEONATE initially 15–20 mg/kg twice daily, increased
over 2–3 weeks to usual maintenance dose 30–
40 mg/kg twice daily; max. 75 mg/kg twice daily;
CHILD 1 month–12 years, initially 15–20 mg/kg (max.
250 mg) twice daily increased over 2–3 weeks to usual
maintenance dose 30–40 mg/kg twice daily (1
month–2 years, max. 75 mg/kg twice daily; 2–12
years, max. 1.5 g twice daily); CHILD 12–18 years,
initially 250 mg twice daily increased over 2–3 weeks
to usual maintenance dose 1–1.5 g twice daily
- By rectum, [unlicensed route] CHILD 1 month–18 years,
dose as for oral therapy, see above
Note Dissolve contents of sachet in small amount of water
and administer rectally [unlicensed]
- Infantile spasms (West's syndrome), *monotherapy*,
NEONATE and CHILD, initially 15–25 mg/kg twice daily,
adjusted according to response over 7 days to usual
maintenance dose 40–50 mg/kg twice daily; max.
75 mg/kg twice daily
Note Neonate and child vigabatrin doses in BNF may differ
from those in product literature

Sabril® (Sanofi-Aventis) PoM
Tablets, f/c, scored, vigabatrin 500 mg, net price
100-tab pack = £37.01. Label: 3, 8, counselling, driving (see notes above)
Note Tablets may be crushed and dispersed in liquid
[unlicensed use]
Granules, sugar-free, vigabatrin 500 mg/sachet. Net
price 50-sachet pack = £20.50. Label: 3, 8, 13, counselling, driving (see notes above)
Note The contents of a sachet should be dissolved in water
or a soft drink immediately before swallowing; may also be
dissolved in a small amount of water and administered
rectally [unlicensed use]

Zonisamide

Zonisamide can be used alone for the treatment of focal
seizures with or without secondary generalisation in
adults with newly diagnosed epilepsy, and as adjunctive
treatment for refractory focal seizures with or without
secondary generalisation in adults and children aged 6
years and above. It can also be used under the supervision of a specialist for refractory absence and myoclonic seizures [unlicensed indications].

The *Scottish Medicines Consortium* (p. 4) has advised
(February 2014) that zonisamide (*Zonegran®*) is
accepted for restricted use within NHS Scotland as
adjunctive treatment of focal seizures, with or without
secondary generalisation, in adolescents and children
aged 6 years and above. It is restricted to use on advice
from specialists in paediatric neurology or epilepsy.

ZONISAMIDE

Indications   see notes above

Cautions   elderly; avoid overheating and ensure adequate hydration especially in children, during strenuous activity or if in warm environment (fatal cases of heat stroke reported in children, also see Counselling below); risk factors for renal stone formation (particularly predisposition to nephrolithiasis); concomitant use of drugs that increase risk of hyperthermia, metabolic acidosis, or nephrolithiasis—see Contraindications for use in children; metabolic acidosis—monitor serum bicarbonate concentration in children and those with other risk factors (consider dose reduction or discontinuation if metabolic acidosis develops); avoid abrupt withdrawal (consult product literature for recommended withdrawal regimens in children); low body-weight or poor appetite—monitor weight throughout treatment (fatal cases of weight loss reported in children); **interactions:** see p. 303 and Appendix 1 (zonisamide)

Switching between formulations Care should be taken when switching between oral formulations. The need for continued supply of a particular manufacturer's product should be based on clinical judgement and consultation with the patient or their carer, taking into account factors such as seizure frequency and treatment history (see also MHRA/CHM advice, p. 303)

Contra-indications   hypersensitivity to sulfonamides; concomitant use of drugs that increase risk of hyperthermia or metabolic acidosis in children

Hepatic impairment   initially increase dose at 2-week intervals if mild or moderate impairment; avoid in severe impairment

Renal impairment   initially increase dose at 2-week intervals; discontinue if renal function deteriorates

Pregnancy   manufacturer advises women of child-bearing potential should use adequate contraception during treatment and for 4 weeks after last dose; see also Pregnancy, p. 304

Breast-feeding   manufacturer advises avoid for 4 weeks after last dose; see also Breast-feeding, p. 305

Side-effects   nausea, diarrhoea, abdominal pain, constipation, dyspepsia, anorexia, weight loss, peripheral oedema, drowsiness, dizziness, confusion, agitation, irritability, depression, psychosis, ataxia, speech disorder, impaired memory and attention, fatigue, nystagmus, paraesthesia, tremor, pyrexia, insomnia, diplopia, ecchymosis, alopecia, pruritus, rash (consider withdrawal); *less commonly* vomiting, cholelithiasis, cholecystitis, aggression, suicidal ideation, seizures, pneumonia, urinary tract infection, urinary calculus, hypokalaemia; *very rarely* hepatitis, pancreatitis, aspiration, dyspnoea, hallucinations, amnesia, coma, myasthenic syndrome, neuroleptic malignant syndrome, heat stroke, hydronephrosis, renal failure, metabolic acidosis, renal tubular acidosis, blood disorders, rhabdomyolysis, impaired sweating, Stevens-Johnson syndrome, and toxic epidermal necrolysis

Dose

- Monotherapy, ADULT over 18 years, initially 100 mg once daily for 2 weeks, increased by 100 mg at 2-week intervals to usual maintenance 300 mg once daily; max. 500 mg daily

- Adjunctive therapy, ADULT over 18 years, initially 50 mg daily in 2 divided doses, increased after 7 days to 100 mg daily in 2 divided doses; then increased by 100 mg every 7 days; usual maintenance 300–500 mg

daily in 1–2 divided doses; CHILD 6–18 years, initially 1 mg/kg once daily for 7 days, then increased by 1 mg/kg every 7 days; usual maintenance, body-weight 20–55 kg, 6–8 mg/kg once daily (max. 500 mg once daily), body-weight over 55 kg, 300–500 mg once daily

Note In adjunctive therapy, increase dose at 2-week intervals in patients who are **not** receiving concomitant carbamazepine, phenytoin, phenobarbital or other potent inducers of cytochrome P450 enzyme CYP3A4

Counselling Children and their carers should be made aware of how to prevent and recognise overheating and dehydration

Zonegran® (Eisai) [PoM]

Capsules, zonisamide 25 mg (white), net price 14-cap pack = £8.82; 50 mg (white/grey), 56-cap pack = £47.04; 100 mg (white/red), 56-cap pack = £62.72. Label: 3, 8, 10, counselling, overheating (see above)

Note Patients may need to be maintained on a specific manufacturer's branded or generic zonisamide product, see MHRA/CHM advice, p. 303

Benzodiazepines

Clobazam may be used as adjunctive therapy in the treatment of generalised tonic-clonic and refractory focal seizures. It may be prescribed under the care of a specialist for refractory absence and myoclonic seizures. **Clonazepam** may be prescribed by a specialist for refractory absence and myoclonic seizures, but its sedative side-effects may be prominent.

The effectiveness of clobazam and clonazepam may decrease significantly after weeks or months of continuous therapy.

CLOBAZAM

Indications   adjunct in epilepsy; anxiety (short-term use)

Cautions   see Diazepam, section 4.1.2

Switching between formulations Care should be taken when switching between oral formulations in the treatment of epilepsy. The need for continued supply of a particular manufacturer's product should be based on clinical judgement and consultation with the patient or their carer, taking into account factors such as seizure frequency and treatment history (see also MHRA/CHM advice, p. 303)

Contra-indications   see Diazepam, section 4.1.2

Hepatic impairment   see Benzodiazepines, section 4.1.2

Renal impairment   see Benzodiazepines, section 4.1.2

Pregnancy   see Pregnancy, p. 304; in late pregnancy may cause neonatal hypothermia, hypotonia, respiratory depression, and withdrawal

Breast-feeding   see Benzodiazepines, section 4.1.2

Side-effects   see Diazepam, section 4.1.2

Dose

- Epilepsy, 20–30 mg daily, increased if necessary to max. 60 mg daily; CHILD over 6 years, initially 5 mg daily, increased if necessary every 5 days to usual maintenance dose of 0.3–1 mg/kg daily; max. 60 mg daily; daily doses of up to 30 mg may be given as a single dose at bedtime, higher doses should be divided

- Anxiety, 20–30 mg daily in divided doses or as a single dose at bedtime, increased in severe anxiety (in hospital patients) to a max. of 60 mg daily in divided doses; ELDERLY (or debilitated) 10–20 mg daily

4 Central nervous system

¹Clobazam (Non-proprietary) [CD4-1]
Tablets, clobazam 10 mg. Net price 30-tab pack = £2.99. Label: 2 or 19, 8, counselling, driving (see notes above)
Brands include *Frisium*® [᷄ʜ́ˢ]

Oral suspension, clobazam 5 mg/5 mL, net price 150 mL = £128.61; 10 mg/5 mL, net price 150 mL = £134.25. Label: 2, or 19, 8, counselling, driving (see notes above)
Brands include *Tapclob*®

Note Patients being treated for epilepsy may need to be maintained on a specific manufacturer's branded or generic clobazam product, see MHRA/CHM advice, p. 303

◼ CLONAZEPAM

Indications all forms of epilepsy; myoclonus
Cautions see notes above; elderly and debilitated patients, respiratory disease, airways obstruction, spinal or cerebellar ataxia, brain damage; history of alcohol or drug abuse, depression or suicidal ideation; avoid sudden withdrawal (risk of withdrawal symptoms and rebound seizures); myasthenia gravis (avoid if unstable); acute porphyria (section 9.8.2); **interactions:** Appendix 1 (anxiolytics and hypnotics)
Driving Drowsiness may affect performance of skilled tasks (e.g. driving); effects of alcohol enhanced, see Drugs and Driving, p. 3
Switching between formulations Care should be taken when switching between oral formulations in the treatment of epilepsy. The need for continued supply of a particular manufacturer's product should be based on clinical judgement and consultation with the patient or their carer, taking into account factors such as seizure frequency and treatment history (see also MHRA/CHM advice, p. 303)
Contra-indications respiratory depression; acute pulmonary insufficiency; sleep apnoea syndrome; marked neuromuscular respiratory weakness including unstable myasthenia gravis; coma; current alcohol or drug abuse
Hepatic impairment see Benzodiazepines, section 4.1.2
Renal impairment see Benzodiazepines, section 4.1.2
Pregnancy see Benzodiazepines, section 4.1.2
Breast-feeding see Benzodiazepines, section 4.1.2
Side-effects drowsiness, fatigue, dizziness, muscle hypotonia, co-ordination disturbances; also poor concentration, restlessness, confusion, amnesia, dependence; salivary or bronchial hypersecretion in infants and small children; nystagmus; *rarely* gastro-intestinal symptoms, respiratory depression, headache, paradoxical effects including aggression and anxiety, sexual dysfunction, urinary incontinence, urticaria, pruritus, reversible hair loss, skin pigmentation changes; dysarthria, and visual disturbances on long-term treatment; blood disorders reported; suicidal ideation; *very rarely* increase in seizure frequency; **overdosage:** see Emergency Treatment of Poisoning, p. 39
Dose
- 1 mg (ELDERLY 500 micrograms) initially at night for 4 nights, increased according to response over 2–4 weeks to usual maintenance dose of 4–8 mg usually at night (may be given in 3–4 divided doses if necessary); CHILD up to 1 year, initially 250 micrograms increased as above to usual maintenance dose of 0.5–1 mg, 1–5 years, initially 250 micrograms increased as above to 1–3 mg, 5–12 years, initially 500 micrograms increased as above to 3–6 mg
Note Clonazepam doses in BNF may differ from those in product literature

Clonazepam (Non-proprietary) [CD4-1]
Tablets, clonazepam 500 micrograms, net price 100-tab pack = £5.52; 2 mg, 100-tab pack = £7.27. Label: 2, 8, counselling, driving (see notes above)
Oral solution, clonazepam 500 micrograms/5 mL, net price 150 mL = £69.50; 2 mg/5 mL, net price 150 mL = £106.48. Label: 2, 8, counselling, driving (see notes above)
Note Contains ethanol (Rosemont brand); not suitable for use in children

Note Patients being treated for epilepsy may need to be maintained on a specific manufacturer's branded or generic oral clonazepam product, see MHRA/CHM advice, p. 303

Other drugs

Acetazolamide (section 11.6), a carbonic anhydrase inhibitor, has a specific role in treating epilepsy associated with menstruation.

Piracetam (section 4.9.3) is used as adjunctive treatment for cortical myoclonus.

◼ 4.8.2 Drugs used in status epilepticus

Convulsive status epilepticus Immediate measures to manage status epilepticus include positioning the patient to avoid injury, supporting respiration including the provision of oxygen, maintaining blood pressure, and the correction of any hypoglycaemia. Parenteral **thiamine** should be considered if alcohol abuse is suspected; **pyridoxine** (section 9.6.2) should be given if the status epilepticus is caused by pyridoxine deficiency.

Seizures lasting longer than 5 minutes should be treated urgently with intravenous **lorazepam** (repeated once after 10 minutes if seizures recur or fail to respond). Intravenous diazepam is effective but it carries a high risk of thrombophlebitis (reduced by using an emulsion formulation). Absorption of diazepam from intramuscular injection or from suppositories is too slow for treatment of status epilepticus. Patients should be monitored for respiratory depression and hypotension.

Where facilities for resuscitation are not immediately available, **diazepam** can be administered as a rectal solution or **midazolam** oromucosal solution can be given into the buccal cavity.

> **Important**
> If, after initial treatment with benzodiazepines, seizures recur or fail to respond 25 minutes after onset, phenytoin sodium, fosphenytoin, or phenobarbital sodium should be used; contact intensive care unit if seizures continue.
>
> If these measures fail to control seizures 45 minutes after onset, anaesthesia with thiopental (section 15.1.1), midazolam (section 15.1.4), or in adults, a non-barbiturate anaesthetic such as propofol [unlicensed indication] (section 15.1.1), should be instituted with full intensive care support.

Phenytoin sodium can be given by slow intravenous injection, followed by the maintenance dosage if appropriate; monitor ECG and blood pressure and reduce rate of administration if bradycardia or hypotension occurs. Intramuscular phenytoin should not be used (absorption is slow and erratic).

1. [᷄ʜ́ˢ] except for epilepsy and endorsed 'SLS'

Alternatively, **fosphenytoin** (a pro-drug of phenytoin), can be given more rapidly and when given intravenously causes fewer injection-site reactions than phenytoin. Intravenous administration requires ECG monitoring. Although it can also be given intramuscularly, absorption is too slow by this route for treatment of status epilepticus. Doses of fosphenytoin should be expressed in terms of phenytoin sodium.

For advice on the management of epileptic seizures in dental practice, see p. 28.

Non-convulsive status epilepticus The urgency to treat non-convulsive status epilepticus depends on the severity of the patient's condition. If there is incomplete loss of awareness, usual oral antiepileptic therapy should be continued or restarted. Patients who fail to respond to oral antiepileptic therapy or have complete lack of awareness can be treated in the same way as for convulsive status epilepticus, although anaesthesia is rarely needed.

DIAZEPAM

Indications status epilepticus; febrile convulsions (section 4.8.3); convulsions due to poisoning (see p. 34); other indications (section 4.1.2, section 10.2.2, and section 15.1.4.1)

Cautions see Diazepam, section 4.1.2; when given intravenously facilities for reversing respiratory depression with mechanical ventilation must be immediately available (but see also notes above)

Contra-indications see Diazepam, section 4.1.2

Hepatic impairment see Benzodiazepines, section 4.1.2

Renal impairment see Benzodiazepines, section 4.1.2

Pregnancy see Benzodiazepines, section 4.1.2, and Pregnancy, p. 304

Breast-feeding see Benzodiazepines, section 4.1.2

Side-effects see Diazepam, section 4.1.2; hypotension and apnoea

Dose
- Status epilepticus (but see notes above), febrile convulsions, and convulsions due to poisoning, by intravenous injection, 10 mg at a rate of 1 mL (5 mg) per minute, repeated once after 10 minutes if necessary; CHILD under 12 years, 300–400 micrograms/kg (max. 10 mg) [unlicensed dose], repeated once after 10 minutes if necessary

  By rectum as rectal solution, ADULT and CHILD over 12 years, 10–20 mg, repeated once after 10–15 minutes if necessary; ELDERLY 10 mg; NEONATE [unlicensed] 1.25–2.5 mg; CHILD 1 month–1 year [unlicensed] 5 mg; 1–2 years 5 mg; 2–12 years 5–10 mg

Diazepam (Non-proprietary) CD4-1
Injection (solution), diazepam 5 mg/mL. See Appendix 4. Net price 2-mL amp = 45p
Excipients may include benzyl alcohol (avoid in neonates, see Excipients, p. 2), ethanol, propylene glycol

Injection (emulsion), diazepam 5 mg/mL (0.5%). See Appendix 4. Net price 2-mL amp = 91p
Brands include *Diazemuls®*

Rectal tubes (= rectal solution), diazepam 2 mg/mL, net price 1.25-mL (2.5-mg) tube = £1.13, 2.5-mL (5-mg) tube = £1.17; 4 mg/mL, 2.5-mL (10-mg) tube = £1.47
Brands include *Diazepam Desitin®*, *Diazepam Rectubes®*, *Stesolid®*

FOSPHENYTOIN SODIUM

Note Fosphenytoin is a pro-drug of phenytoin

Indications status epilepticus; seizures associated with neurosurgery or head injury; when phenytoin by mouth not possible

Cautions see Phenytoin Sodium; resuscitation facilities must be available; **interactions**: see p. 303 and Appendix 1 (phenytoin)

Contra-indications see Phenytoin Sodium

Hepatic impairment consider 10–25% reduction in dose or infusion rate (except initial dose for status epilepticus)

Renal impairment consider 10–25% reduction in dose or infusion rate (except initial dose for status epilepticus)

Pregnancy see Phenytoin, section 4.8.1, and Pregnancy, p. 304

Breast-feeding see Breast-feeding, p. 305

Side-effects see Phenytoin Sodium; also dry mouth, taste disturbance, vasodilatation, asthenia, dysarthria, euphoria, incoordination, chills, visual disturbances, tinnitus, pruritus, ecchymosis; *less commonly* hypoaesthesia, increased or decreased reflexes, stupor, muscle weakness, muscle spasm, pain, hypoacusis; *also reported* extrapyramidal disorder, twitching, confusion, hyperglycaemia

Important Intravenous infusion of fosphenytoin has been associated with severe cardiovascular reactions including asystole, ventricular fibrillation, and cardiac arrest. Hypotension, bradycardia, and heart block have also been reported. The following are recommended.
- monitor heart rate, blood pressure, and respiratory function for duration of infusion;
- observe patient for at least 30 minutes after infusion;
- if hypotension occurs, reduce infusion rate or discontinue;
- reduce dose or infusion rate in elderly, and in renal or hepatic impairment.

Dose

> **Note**
> Prescriptions for fosphenytoin sodium should state the dose in terms of phenytoin sodium equivalent (PE); fosphenytoin sodium 1.5 mg $\equiv$ phenytoin sodium 1 mg

- Status epilepticus, by intravenous infusion (at a rate of 100–150 mg(PE)/minute), initially 20 mg(PE)/kg then by intravenous infusion (at a rate of 50–100 mg (PE)/minute), 4–5 mg(PE)/kg daily in 1–2 divided doses, dose adjusted according to response and trough plasma-phenytoin concentration

  CHILD 5 years and over, by intravenous infusion (at a rate of 2–3 mg(PE)/kg/minute), initially 20 mg(PE)/kg then by intravenous infusion (at a rate of 1–2 mg (PE)/kg/minute), 4–5 mg(PE)/kg daily in 1–4 divided doses, dose adjusted according to response and trough plasma-phenytoin concentration

- Prophylaxis or treatment of seizures associated with neurosurgery or head injury, by intramuscular injection *or* by intravenous infusion (at a rate of 50–100 mg (PE)/minute), initially 10–15 mg(PE)/kg then by intramuscular injection *or* by intravenous infusion (at a rate of 50–100 mg(PE)/minute), 4–5 mg(PE)/kg daily (in 1–2 divided doses), dose adjusted according to response and trough plasma-phenytoin concentration

  CHILD 5 years and over, by intravenous infusion (at a rate of 1–2 mg(PE)/kg/minute), initially 10–15 mg (PE)/kg then 4–5 mg(PE)/kg daily in 1–4 divided

4 Central nervous system

doses, dose adjusted according to response and trough plasma-phenytoin concentration

- Temporary substitution for oral phenytoin, by intramuscular injection *or* by intravenous infusion (at a rate of 50–100 mg(PE)/minute), same dose and dosing frequency as oral phenytoin therapy; CHILD 5 years and over, by intravenous infusion (at a rate of 1–2 mg (PE)/kg/minute, max. 100 mg(PE)/minute), same dose and dosing frequency as oral phenytoin therapy

Note ELDERLY consider 10–25% reduction in dose or infusion rate

Note Fosphenytoin sodium doses in BNF may differ from those in product literature

Pro-Epanutin® (Pfizer) PoM
Injection, fosphenytoin sodium 75 mg/mL (equivalent to phenytoin sodium 50 mg/mL), net price 10-mL vial = £40.00

Electrolytes phosphate 3.7 micromol/mg fosphenytoin sodium (phosphate 5.6 micromol/mg phenytoin sodium)

LORAZEPAM

Indications status epilepticus; febrile convulsions (section 4.8.3); convulsions due to poisoning (see p. 34); other indications (section 4.1.2 and section 15.1.4.1)

Cautions see Diazepam, section 4.1.2; when given intravenously facilities for reversing respiratory depression with mechanical ventilation must be immediately available (but see also notes above)

Contra-indications see Diazepam, section 4.1.2

Hepatic impairment see Benzodiazepines, section 4.1.2

Renal impairment see Benzodiazepines, section 4.1.2

Pregnancy see Benzodiazepines, section 4.1.2, and Pregnancy, p. 304

Breast-feeding see Benzodiazepines, section 4.1.2

Side-effects see Diazepam, section 4.1.2

Dose

- By slow intravenous injection (into large vein), 4 mg repeated once after 10 minutes if necessary; CHILD under 12 years 100 micrograms/kg (max. 4 mg) repeated once after 10 minutes if necessary

◢ **Preparations**
Section 4.1.2

MIDAZOLAM

Indications status epilepticus; febrile convulsions [unlicensed] (section 4.8.3); other indications (section 15.1.4.1)

Cautions see Midazolam, section 15.1.4.1

Contra-indications see Midazolam, section 15.1.4.1

Hepatic impairment use with caution in mild to moderate impairment; avoid in severe impairment

Renal impairment use with caution in chronic renal failure

Pregnancy see Midazolam, section 15.1.4.1, and Pregnancy, p. 304

Breast-feeding amount probably too small to be harmful after single doses

Side-effects see Midazolam, section 15.1.4.1; also depression of consciousness

Dose

- By buccal administration, ADULT over 18 years [unlicensed], 10 mg repeated once after 10 minutes if

necessary; CHILD up to 3 months [unlicensed], 300 micrograms/kg (max. 2.5 mg), 3 months–1 year 2.5 mg, 1–5 years 5 mg, 5–10 years 7.5 mg, 10–18 years 10 mg; these doses may be repeated once after 10 minutes if necessary

Buccolam (ViroPharma) ▼ CD3
Oromucosal solution, midazolam (as hydrochloride) 5 mg/mL, net price 0.5-mL (2.5 mg) prefilled syringe = £20.50, 1-mL (5 mg) prefilled syringe = £21.38, 1.5-mL (7.5 mg) prefilled syringe = £22.25, 2-mL (10 mg) prefilled syringe = £22.88. Label: 2, counselling, administration

Note Unlicensed formulations are available and may have different doses—refer to product literature

◢ **Parenteral preparations**
Section 15.1.4

PHENOBARBITAL SODIUM
(Phenobarbitone sodium)

Indications status epilepticus; other forms of epilepsy except absence seizures (section 4.8.1)

Cautions see Phenobarbital, section 4.8.1; interactions: see p. 303 and Appendix 1 (phenobarbital)

Hepatic impairment see Phenobarbital, section 4.8.1

Renal impairment see Phenobarbital, section 4.8.1

Pregnancy see Pregnancy, p. 304

Breast-feeding see Breast-feeding, p. 305

Side-effects see Phenobarbital, section 4.8.1

Dose

- Status epilepticus, by intravenous injection (dilute injection 1 in 10 with water for injections), 10 mg/kg at a rate of not more than 100 mg/minute; max. 1 g

Phenobarbital (Non-proprietary) CD3
Injection, phenobarbital sodium 15 mg/mL, net price 1-mL amp = £1.97; 30 mg/mL, 1-mL amp = £6.66; 60 mg/mL, 1-mL amp = £7.08; 200 mg/mL, 1-mL amp = £5.77

Excipients include propylene glycol 90% (see Excipients, p. 2)

Note Must be diluted before intravenous administration (see under Dose)

PHENYTOIN SODIUM

Indications status epilepticus; acute symptomatic seizures associated with head trauma or neurosurgery

Cautions see notes above; respiratory depression; hypotension and heart failure; resuscitation facilities must be available; injection solutions alkaline (irritant to tissues); see also p. 314; interactions: see p. 303 and Appendix 1 (phenytoin)

Contra-indications sinus bradycardia, sino-atrial block, and second- and third-degree heart block; Stokes-Adams syndrome; acute porphyria (section 9.8.2)

Hepatic impairment see Phenytoin, section 4.8.1

Pregnancy see Phenytoin, section 4.8.1, and Pregnancy, p. 304

Breast-feeding see Breast-feeding, p. 305

Side-effects intravenous injection may cause cardiovascular and CNS depression (particularly if injection too rapid) with arrhythmias, hypotension, and cardiovascular collapse; alterations in respiratory function (including respiratory arrest); *also reported* tonic seizures, purple glove syndrome; see also p. 314

Dose

- By slow intravenous injection *or* infusion (with blood pressure and ECG monitoring), 20 mg/kg (max. 2 g) at a rate not exceeding 1 mg/kg/minute (max. 50 mg per minute), as a loading dose (see also notes above); maintenance doses of about 100 mg, by mouth or by intravenous administration, should be given thereafter every 6–8 hours, adjusted according to plasma-phenytoin concentration; CHILD 1 month–12 years, 20 mg/kg at a rate not exceeding 1 mg/kg/minute (max. 50 mg per minute) as a loading dose; maintenance dose of 5–10 mg/kg daily (max. 300 mg daily) in 2 divided doses; NEONATE 20 mg/kg at a rate not exceeding 1 mg/kg/minute, as a loading dose; maintenance dose of 5–10 mg/kg daily in 2 divided doses

Note To avoid local venous irritation each injection or infusion should be preceded and followed by an injection of sterile physiological saline through the same needle or catheter

Note Phenytoin sodium doses in BNF may differ from those in product literature

Phenytoin (Non-proprietary) [PoM]
Injection, phenytoin sodium 50 mg/mL, net price 5-mL amp = £2.91

Epanutin® Ready-Mixed Parenteral (Pfizer) [PoM]
Injection, phenytoin sodium 50 mg/mL, net price 5-mL amp = £4.88
Electrolytes 1.1 mmol Na+ per 5 mL ampoule

4.8.3 Febrile convulsions

Brief febrile convulsions need no specific treatment; antipyretic medication (e.g. **paracetamol**, section 4.7.1) is commonly used to reduce fever and prevent further convulsions but evidence to support this practice is lacking. *Prolonged febrile convulsions* (those lasting 5 minutes or longer), or *recurrent febrile convulsions* without recovery must be treated actively (as for convulsive status epilepticus, section 4.8.2).

Long-term anticonvulsant prophylaxis for febrile convulsions is rarely indicated.

4.9 Drugs used in parkinsonism and related disorders

4.9.1 Dopaminergic drugs used in Parkinson's disease

4.9.2 Antimuscarinic drugs used in parkinsonism

4.9.3 Drugs used in essential tremor, chorea, tics, and related disorders

Parkinson's disease

In idiopathic Parkinson's disease, the progressive degeneration of pigmented neurones in the substantia nigra leads to a deficiency of the neurotransmitter dopamine. The resulting neurochemical imbalance in the basal ganglia causes the characteristic signs and symptoms of the illness. Drug therapy does not prevent disease progression, but it improves most patients' quality of life.

Patients with suspected Parkinson's disease should be referred to a specialist to confirm the diagnosis; the diagnosis should be reviewed every 6–12 months.

Features resembling those of Parkinson's disease can occur in diseases such as progressive supranuclear palsy and multiple system atrophy, but they do not normally show a sustained response to the drugs used in the treatment of idiopathic Parkinson's disease.

When initiating treatment, patients should be advised about its limitations and possible side-effects. About 5–10% of patients with Parkinson's disease respond poorly to treatment.

Treatment is usually not started until symptoms cause significant disruption of daily activities. **Levodopa** (p. 329), **non-ergot-derived dopamine-receptor agonists** (below), or **monoamine-oxidase-B inhibitors** (p. 332) can be prescribed for initial treatment in early Parkinson's disease. Therapy with two or more antiparkinsonian drugs may be necessary as the disease progresses. Most patients eventually require levodopa and subsequently develop motor complications.

Elderly Antiparkinsonian drugs can cause confusion in the elderly. It is particularly important to initiate treatment with low doses and to increase the dose gradually.

4.9.1 Dopaminergic drugs used in Parkinson's disease

Dopamine-receptor agonists

The dopamine-receptor agonists have a direct action on dopamine receptors. Initial treatment of Parkinson's disease is often with the dopamine-receptor agonists **pramipexole**, **ropinirole**, and **rotigotine**. The ergot-derived dopamine-receptor agonists **bromocriptine**, **cabergoline**, and **pergolide** are rarely used because the risk of fibrotic reactions (see notes below).

When used alone, dopamine-receptor agonists cause fewer motor complications in long-term treatment compared with levodopa treatment but the overall motor performance improves slightly less. The dopamine-receptor agonists are associated with more psychiatric side-effects than levodopa.

Dopamine-receptor agonists are also used with levodopa in more advanced disease. If a dopamine-receptor agonist is added to levodopa therapy, the dose of levodopa needs to be reduced (see individual monographs).

Impulse control disorders

Treatment with dopamine-receptor agonists and levodopa is associated with impulse control disorders, including pathological gambling, binge eating, and hypersexuality. Patients and their carers should be informed about the risk of impulse control disorders. There is no evidence that ergot- and non-ergot-derived dopamine-receptor agonists differ in their propensity to cause impulse control disorders, so switching between dopamine-receptor agonists to control these side-effects is not recommended. If the patient develops an impulse control disorder, the dopamine-receptor agonist or levodopa should be withdrawn or the dose reduced until the symptoms resolve.

Antiparkinsonian drug therapy should never be stopped abruptly as this carries a small risk of neuroleptic malignant syndrome.

4 Central nervous system

Fibrotic reactions

Ergot-derived dopamine-receptor agonists, bromocriptine, cabergoline, and pergolide, have been associated with pulmonary, retroperitoneal, and pericardial fibrotic reactions.

Exclude cardiac valvulopathy with echocardiography before starting treatment with these ergot derivatives for Parkinson's disease or chronic endocrine disorders (excludes suppression of lactation); it may also be appropriate to measure the erythrocyte sedimentation rate and serum creatinine and to obtain a chest X-ray. Patients should be monitored for dyspnoea, persistent cough, chest pain, cardiac failure, and abdominal pain or tenderness. If long-term treatment is expected, then lung-function tests may also be helpful. Patients taking cabergoline or pergolide should be regularly monitored for cardiac fibrosis by echocardiography (within 3–6 months of initiating treatment and subsequently at 6–12 month intervals).

Driving

Sudden onset of sleep Excessive daytime sleepiness and sudden onset of sleep can occur with co-careldopa, co-beneldopa, and dopamine-receptor agonists.

Patients starting treatment with these drugs should be warned of the risk and of the need to exercise caution when driving or operating machinery. Those who have experienced excessive sedation or sudden onset of sleep should refrain from driving or operating machines until these effects have stopped occurring.

Management of excessive daytime sleepiness should focus on the identification of an underlying cause, such as depression or concomitant medication. Patients should be counselled on improving sleep behaviour.

Hypotensive reactions Hypotensive reactions can occur in some patients taking dopamine-receptor agonists; these can be particularly problematic during the first few days of treatment and care should be exercised when driving or operating machinery.

Apomorphine is a potent dopamine-receptor agonist that is sometimes helpful in advanced disease for patients experiencing unpredictable 'off' periods with levodopa treatment. Apomorphine should be initiated in a specialist clinic. After an overnight withdrawal of oral antiparkinsonian medication to induce an 'off' episode, the threshold dose of apomorphine is determined. Oral antiparkinsonian medication is then restarted. The patient must be taught to self-administer apomorphine by subcutaneous injection into the lower abdomen or outer thigh at the first sign of an 'off' episode. Once treatment has been established it may be possible to gradually reduce other antiparkinsonian medications. Treatment with apomorphine should remain under specialist supervision.

APOMORPHINE HYDROCHLORIDE

Indications refractory motor fluctuations in Parkinson's disease ('off' episodes) inadequately controlled by co-beneldopa or co-careldopa or other dopaminergics (for capable and motivated patients under specialist supervision)

Cautions see notes above; pulmonary disease, cardiovascular disease, history of postural hypotension (special care on initiation); susceptibility to QT-interval prolongation; neuropsychiatric conditions; monitor hepatic, haemopoietic, renal, and cardiovascular function; *with concomitant levodopa* test initially and every 6 months for haemolytic anaemia and thrombocytopenia (development calls for specialist haematological care with dose reduction and possible discontinuation); **interactions**: Appendix 1 (apomorphine)

Driving See notes above and Drugs and Driving, p. 3

Contra-indications respiratory depression, dementia, hypersensitivity to opioids, psychosis; avoid if 'on' response to levodopa marred by severe dyskinesia or dystonia

Hepatic impairment avoid

Renal impairment use with caution

Pregnancy avoid unless clearly necessary

Breast-feeding no information available; may suppress lactation

Side-effects see notes above; also nausea, vomiting (see notes above); yawning; drowsiness (including sudden onset of sleep), confusion, hallucinations; *less commonly* postural hypotension, dyspnoea, dyskinesia during 'on' periods (may require discontinuation), haemolytic anaemia and thrombocytopenia with levodopa (see Cautions), and rash; *rarely* eosinophilia; peripheral oedema, compulsive behaviour (see notes above), and dizziness also reported

Dose

- By subcutaneous injection, ADULT over 18 years, to determine threshold dose (see also notes above), initially 1 mg at the first sign of 'off' episode; if inadequate or no response after 30 minutes, then a further 2 mg should be given; thereafter increase dose at minimum 40-minute intervals until satisfactory response obtained; usual range 3–30 mg daily in divided doses; subcutaneous infusion may be preferable in those requiring division of injections into more than 10 doses daily; max. single dose 10 mg

- By continuous subcutaneous infusion, ADULT over 18 years, (those requiring division into more than 10 injections daily) initially 1 mg/hour increased according to response (not more often than every 4 hours) in max. steps of 500 micrograms/hour, to usual rate of 1–4 mg/hour (15–60 micrograms/kg/hour); change infusion site every 12 hours and give during waking hours only (tolerance may occur unless there is a 4-hour treatment-free period at night—24-hour infusions not recommended unless severe night-time symptoms); intermittent bolus doses may be needed

Note Total daily dose by either route (or combined routes) max. 100 mg

Apomorphine (Non-proprietary) ℗oM

Injection, apomorphine hydrochloride 10 mg/mL, net price 2-mL amp = £6.07, 5-mL amp = £11.70. Label: 10, counselling, driving, see Cautions above

APO-go® (Genus) ℗oM

Injection, apomorphine hydrochloride 10 mg/mL, net price 2-mL amp = £7.59, 5-mL amp = £14.62. Label: 10, counselling, driving, see Cautions above
Excipients include sulphites

Injection (APO-go® Pen), apomorphine hydrochloride 10 mg/mL, net price 3-mL pen injector = £24.78. Label: 10, counselling, driving, see Cautions above
Excipients include sulphites

Injection (APO-go® PFS), apomorphine hydrochloride 5 mg/mL, net price 10-mL prefilled syringe = £14.62. Label: 10, counselling, driving, see Cautions above
Excipients include sulphites

BROMOCRIPTINE

Indications Parkinson's disease; endocrine disorders (section 6.7.1)

Cautions see Bromocriptine in section 6.7.1 and notes above

Contra-indications see Bromocriptine, section 6.7.1

Hepatic impairment see Bromocriptine, section 6.7.1

Pregnancy see Bromocriptine, section 6.7.1

Breast-feeding see Bromocriptine, section 6.7.1

Side-effects see notes above and Bromocriptine, section 6.7.1

Dose
- First week 1–1.25 mg at night, second week 2–2.5 mg at night, third week 2.5 mg twice daily, fourth week 2.5 mg 3 times daily then increasing by 2.5 mg every 3–14 days according to response to a usual range of 10–30 mg daily

◢Preparations
Section 6.7.1

CABERGOLINE

Indications alone or as adjunct to co-beneldopa or co-careldopa in Parkinson's disease where dopamine-receptor agonists other than ergot derivative not appropriate; endocrine disorders (section 6.7.1)

Cautions see Cabergoline in section 6.7.1 and notes above

Contra-indications see Cabergoline, section 6.7.1

Hepatic impairment see Cabergoline, section 6.7.1

Pregnancy see Cabergoline, section 6.7.1

Breast-feeding see Cabergoline, section 6.7.1

Side-effects see notes above and Cabergoline, section 6.7.1

Dose
- Initially 1 mg daily, increased by increments of 0.5–1 mg at 7 or 14 day intervals; max. 3 mg daily
  Note Concurrent dose of levodopa may be decreased gradually while dose of cabergoline is increased

Cabergoline (Non-proprietary) (PoM)
Tablets, scored, cabergoline 1 mg, net price 20-tab pack = £63.77; 2 mg, 20-tab pack = £72.57. Label: 10, 21, counselling, driving, see notes above
Note Dispense in original container (contains desiccant)

Cabaser® (Pharmacia) (PoM)
Tablets, scored, cabergoline 1 mg, net price 20-tab pack = £83.00; 2 mg, 20-tab pack = £83.00. Label: 10, 21, counselling, driving, see notes above
Note Dispense in original container (contains desiccant)

PERGOLIDE

Indications alone or as adjunct to co-beneldopa or co-careldopa in Parkinson's disease where dopamine-receptor agonists other than ergot derivative not appropriate

Cautions see notes above; arrhythmias or underlying cardiac disease; history of confusion, psychosis, or hallucinations, dyskinesia (may exacerbate); acute porphyria (section 9.8.2); **interactions:** Appendix 1 (pergolide)

Contra-indications history of fibrotic disorders; cardiac valvulopathy (exclude before treatment, see Fibrotic Reactions, p. 326)

Pregnancy use only if potential benefit outweighs risk

Breast-feeding may suppress lactation

Side-effects see notes above; also nausea, vomiting, dyspepsia, abdominal pain; dyspnoea, rhinitis; hallucinations, dyskinesia, drowsiness (including sudden onset of sleep, see p. 326); diplopia; also reported constipation, diarrhoea, hiccups, tachycardia, atrial premature contractions, palpitation, hypotension, syncope, Raynaud's phenomenon, compulsive behaviour (see notes above), insomnia, confusion, dizziness, fever, erythromelalgia, and rash

Dose
- Monotherapy, 50 micrograms at night on day 1, then 50 micrograms twice daily on days 2–4, then increased by 100–250 micrograms daily every 3–4 days to 1.5 mg daily in 3 divided doses at day 28; after day 30, further increases every 3–4 days of up to 250 micrograms daily; usual maintenance dose 2.1–2.5 mg daily; max. 3 mg daily
- Adjunctive therapy with levodopa, 50 micrograms daily for 2 days, increased gradually by 100–150 micrograms every 3 days over next 12 days, usually given in 3 divided doses; further increases of 250 micrograms every 3 days; max. 3 mg daily
  Note During pergolide titration levodopa dose may be reduced cautiously

Pergolide (Non-proprietary) (PoM)
Tablets, pergolide (as mesilate) 50 micrograms, net price 100-tab pack = £32.54; 250 micrograms, 100-tab pack = £35.77; 1 mg, 100-tab pack = £130.70. Label: 10, counselling, driving, see notes above

PRAMIPEXOLE

Indications Parkinson's disease, used alone or as an adjunct to co-beneldopa or co-careldopa; moderate to severe restless legs syndrome

Cautions see notes above; psychotic disorders; ophthalmological testing recommended (risk of visual disorders); severe cardiovascular disease; risk of postural hypotension (especially on initiation)—monitor blood pressure; **interactions:** Appendix 1 (pramipexole)

Renal impairment
- for *immediate-release* tablets in Parkinson's disease, initially 88 micrograms twice daily (max. 1.57 mg daily in 2 divided doses) if eGFR 20–50 mL/minute/1.73m²; initially 88 micrograms once daily (max. 1.1 mg once daily) if eGFR less than 20 mL/minute/1.73 m²; if renal function declines during treatment, reduce dose by the same percentage as the decline in eGFR
- for *immediate-release* tablets in restless legs syndrome, reduce dose if eGFR less than 20 mL/minute/1.73 m²
- for *modified-release* tablets, initially 260 micrograms on alternate days if eGFR 30–50 mL/minute/1.73m², increased to 260 micrograms once daily after 1 week, further increased if necessary by

260 micrograms daily at weekly intervals to max. 1.57 mg daily; avoid if eGFR less than 30 mL/minute/1.73m^2

Pregnancy use only if potential benefit outweighs risk—no information available

Breast-feeding may suppress lactation; avoid—present in milk in *animal* studies

Side-effects see notes above; also nausea, constipation, vomiting, weight changes, decreased appetite, hypotension (including postural hypotension), peripheral oedema, dizziness, dyskinesia, hyperkinesia, drowsiness (including sudden onset of sleep, see p. 326), headache, sleep disturbances, confusion, hallucinations, restlessness, visual disturbances; *less commonly* hiccups, cardiac failure, syncope, pneumonia, dyspnoea, binge eating, compulsive behaviour (see notes above), amnesia, delusion, paranoia, pruritus, rash; *also reported* paradoxical worsening of restless legs syndrome

Dose Important Doses and strengths are stated in terms of pramipexole (base); equivalent strengths in terms of pramipexole dihydrochloride monohydrate (salt) are as follows:
88 micrograms base ≡ 125 micrograms salt;
180 micrograms base ≡ 250 micrograms salt;
350 micrograms base ≡ 500 micrograms salt;
700 micrograms base ≡ 1 mg salt

- Parkinson's disease, ADULT over 18 years, initially 88 micrograms 3 times daily, dose doubled every 5–7 days if tolerated to 350 micrograms 3 times daily; further increased if necessary by 180 micrograms 3 times daily at weekly intervals; max. 3.3 mg daily in 3 divided doses
  Note During dose titration and maintenance, levodopa dose may be reduced

- Restless legs syndrome, ADULT over 18 years, initially 88 micrograms once daily 2–3 hours before bedtime, dose doubled every 4–7 days if necessary; max. 540 micrograms daily
  Note Repeat dose titration if restarting treatment after an interval of more than a few days

Pramipexole (Non-proprietary) PoM
Tablets, pramipexole 88 micrograms, net price 30-tab pack = £2.19; 180 micrograms, 30-tab pack = £2.44, 100-tab pack = £8.76; 350 micrograms 30-tab pack = £15.72, 100-tab pack = £32.95; 700 micrograms, 30-tab pack = £4.27, 100-tab pack = £14.53. Label: 10, counselling, driving, see notes above

Mirapexin® (Boehringer Ingelheim) PoM
Tablets, pramipexole 88 micrograms, net price 30-tab pack = £11.24; 180 micrograms (scored), 30-tab pack = £22.49, 100-tab pack = £74.95; 350 micrograms (scored), 30-tab pack = £44.97, 100-tab pack = £149.90; 700 micrograms (scored), 30-tab pack = £89.94, 100-tab pack = £299.82. Label: 10, counselling, driving, see notes above

◢ Modified release

Mirapexin® Prolonged Release (Boehringer Ingelheim) PoM
Tablets, m/r, pramipexole 260 micrograms, net price 30-tab pack = £30.08; 520 micrograms, 30-tab pack = £60.17; 1.05 mg, 30-tab pack = £129.96; 1.57 mg, 30-tab pack = £202.36; 2.1 mg, 30-tab pack = £259.91; 2.62 mg, 30-tab pack = £337.27; 3.15 mg, 30-tab pack = £389.87. Label: 10, 25, counselling, driving, see notes above
Important Doses and strengths are stated in terms of pramipexole (base); equivalent strengths in terms of

pramipexole dihydrochloride monohydrate (salt) are as follows:
260 micrograms base ≡ 375 micrograms salt;
520 micrograms base ≡ 750 micrograms salt;
1.05 mg base ≡ 1.5 mg salt;
1.57 mg base ≡ 2.25 mg salt;
2.1 mg base ≡ 3 mg salt;
2.62 mg base ≡ 3.75 mg salt;
3.15 mg base ≡ 4.5 mg salt

Dose Parkinson's disease (with or without co-beneldopa or co-careldopa), ADULT over 18 years, initially 260 micrograms once daily, dose doubled every 5–7 days to 1.05 mg once daily; further increased if necessary by 520 micrograms daily at weekly intervals; max. 3.15 mg once daily
Note During dose titration and maintenance, levodopa dose may be reduced according to response

ROPINIROLE

Indications Parkinson's disease, either used alone or as adjunct to co-beneldopa or co-careldopa; moderate to severe restless legs syndrome

Cautions see notes above; severe cardiovascular disease (risk of hypotension—monitor blood pressure), major psychotic disorders; elderly; avoid abrupt withdrawal; dose adjustment may be necessary if smoking started or stopped during treatment; **interactions**: Appendix 1 (ropinirole)

Hepatic impairment avoid—no information available

Renal impairment avoid if eGFR less than 30 mL/minute/1.73 m^2

Pregnancy avoid unless potential benefit outweighs risk—toxicity in *animal* studies

Breast-feeding may suppress lactation—avoid

Side-effects see notes above; also nausea, vomiting, abdominal pain, dyspepsia, gastro-oesophageal reflux disease, constipation; hypotension; syncope, peripheral oedema; drowsiness (including sudden onset of sleep, see p. 326), dizziness, nervousness, fatigue, dyskinesia, hallucinations, confusion; *less commonly* psychosis, compulsive behaviour (see notes above); *very rarely* hepatic disorders; *also reported* paradoxical worsening of restless legs syndrome

Dose
- Parkinson's disease, initially 750 micrograms daily in 3 divided doses, increased by increments of 750 micrograms daily at weekly intervals to 3 mg daily in 3 divided doses; further increased by increments of 1.5–3 mg daily at weekly intervals according to response; usual range 9–16 mg daily in 3 divided doses (but higher doses may be required if used with levodopa); max. 24 mg daily in 3 divided doses
  Note When administered as adjunct to levodopa, concurrent dose of levodopa may be reduced by approx. 20%; ropinirole doses in the BNF may differ from those in product literature

- Restless legs syndrome, ADULT over 18 years initially 250 micrograms at night for 2 days, increased if tolerated to 500 micrograms at night for 5 days and then to 1 mg at night for 7 days; further increased at weekly intervals in steps of 500 micrograms daily according to response; usual dose 2 mg at night; max. 4 mg daily
  Note Repeat dose titration if restarting after interval of more than a few days

Ropinirole (Non-proprietary) PoM
Tablets, ropinirole (as hydrochloride) 250 micrograms, net price 12-tab pack = £1.66; 500 micrograms, 28-tab pack = £2.24; 1 mg, 84-tab pack = £3.03; 2 mg, 84-tab pack = £7.77; 5 mg, 84-tab pack = £16.41. Label: 10, 21, counselling, driving, see notes above

Adartrel® (GSK) PoM

Tablets, f/c, ropinirole (as hydrochloride) 250 micrograms (white), net price 12-tab pack = £3.94; 500 micrograms (yellow), 28-tab pack = £15.75, 84-tab pack = £47.26; 2 mg (pink), 28-tab pack = £31.51, 84-tab pack = £94.53. Label: 10, 21, counselling, driving, see notes above

Note The *Scottish Medicines Consortium*, p. 4 has advised (June 2006) that *Adartrel*® should be restricted for use in patients with a baseline score of 24 points or more on the International Restless Legs Scale

Requip® (GSK) PoM

Tablets, f/c, ropinirole (as hydrochloride) 1 mg (green), net price 84-tab pack = £56.71; 2 mg (pink), 84-tab pack = £113.44; 5 mg (blue), 84-tab pack = £195.92; 28-day starter pack of 42 × 250-microgram (white) tablets, 42 × 500-microgram (yellow) tablets, and 21 × 1-mg (green) tablets = £40.10; 28-day follow-on pack of 42 × 500-microgram (yellow) tablets, 42 × 1-mg (green) tablets, and 63 × 2-mg (pink) tablets = £74.40. Label: 10, 21, counselling, driving, see notes above

◢ **Modified release**

Ropinirole m/r preparations (Non-proprietary) PoM

Tablets, m/r, ropinirole 2 mg; 4 mg; 8 mg. Label: 10, 25, counselling, driving, see notes above

Brands include *Ralnea XL*®, *Repinex XL*®, *Spiroco XL*®

Dose initial treatment of Parkinson's disease, 2 mg once daily for 1 week, then 4 mg once daily; increased according to response by 2 mg at intervals of at least 1 week up to 8 mg once daily; if still no response, increase by 2–4 mg at intervals of at least 2 weeks as necessary; max. 24 mg once daily

Parkinson's disease in patients transferring from ropinirole immediate-release tablets, initially ropinirole modified release once daily substituted for total daily dose equivalent of ropinirole immediate-release tablets; if control not maintained after switching, titrate dose as above

Note Consider slower titration in patients over 75 years

Note When administered as adjunct to levodopa, concurrent dose of levodopa may gradually be reduced by approx. 30%

Note If treatment interrupted for 1 day or more, consider reinitiation with immediate-release tablets

Requip® XL (GSK) PoM

Tablets, m/r, f/c, ropinirole (as hydrochloride) 2 mg (pink), net price 28-tab pack = £12.54; 4 mg (brown), 28-tab pack = £25.09; 8 mg (red), 28-tab pack = £42.11. Label: 10, 25, counselling, driving, see notes above

Dose initial treatment of Parkinson's disease, 2 mg once daily for 1 week, then 4 mg once daily; increased according to response by 2 mg at intervals of at least 1 week up to 8 mg once daily; if still no response, increase by 2–4 mg at intervals of at least 2 weeks as necessary; max. 24 mg once daily

Parkinson's disease in patients transferring from ropinirole immediate-release tablets, initially *Requip*® XL once daily substituted for total daily dose equivalent of ropinirole immediate-release tablets; if control not maintained after switching, titrate dose as above

Note Consider slower titration in patients over 75 years

Note When administered as adjunct to levodopa, concurrent dose of levodopa may gradually be reduced by approx. 30%

Note If treatment interrupted for 1 day or more, consider reinitiation with immediate-release tablets

▎ **ROTIGOTINE**

Indications Parkinson's disease, either used alone or as adjunct to co-beneldopa or co-careldopa; moderate to severe restless legs syndrome

Cautions see notes above; ophthalmic testing recommended; avoid exposure of patch to heat; withdraw gradually; **interactions**: Appendix 1 (rotigotine)

Hepatic impairment caution in severe impairment—no information available

Pregnancy avoid—no information available

Breast-feeding may suppress lactation; avoid—present in milk in *animal* studies

Side-effects see notes above; also constipation, dry mouth, dyspepsia, nausea, vomiting, weight changes, hypertension, postural hypotension, palpitation, peripheral oedema, hiccup, malaise, dizziness, drowsiness (including sudden onset of sleep, see p. 326), sleep disturbances, dyskinesia, abnormal thinking and behaviour (including hallucinations, paranoia, psychosis, aggression, confusion), headache, syncope, sweating, rash, pruritus, application site reactions; *less commonly* abdominal pain, atrial fibrillation, hypotension, impulse control disorders (see notes above), erectile dysfunction, visual disturbances; *rarely* tachycardia, seizures, irritability, obsessive compulsive disorder

Dose

● Monotherapy in Parkinson's disease, initially apply '2 mg/24 hours' patch, increased in steps of 2 mg/24 hours at weekly intervals if required; max. 8 mg/24 hours

● Adjunctive therapy with levodopa in Parkinson's disease, initially apply '4 mg/24 hours' patch, increased in steps of 2 mg/24 hours at weekly intervals if required; max. 16 mg/24 hours

● Restless legs syndrome, initially apply '1 mg/24 hours' patch, increased in steps of 1 mg/24 hours at weekly intervals if required; max. 3 mg/24 hours

Note Apply patch to dry, non-irritated skin on torso, thigh, or upper arm, removing after 24 hours and siting replacement patch on a different area (avoid using the same area for 14 days)

Neupro® (UCB Pharma) ▼ PoM

Patches, self-adhesive, beige, rotigotine 1 mg/24 hours, net price 28 = £77.24; 2 mg/24 hours, 28 = £81.10; 3 mg/24 hours, 28 = £102.35; 4 mg/24 hours, 28 = £123.60; 6 mg/24 hours, 28 = £149.93; 8 mg/24 hours, 28 = £149.93; 28-day starter pack of 7 × 2 mg/24 hours, 7 × 4 mg/24 hours, 7 × 6 mg/24 hours, and 7 × 8 mg/24 hours patches = £142.79. Label: 10, counselling, driving, see notes above

Note Remove patch (aluminium-containing) before magnetic resonance imaging or cardioversion

Note The *Scottish Medicines Consortium* (p. 4) has advised that *Neupro*® is accepted as monotherapy for the treatment of early-stage idiopathic Parkinson's disease (June 2007) and for restricted use for the treatment of advanced Parkinson's disease in combination with levodopa where the transdermal route would facilitate treatment (July 2007)

Note The *Scottish Medicines Consortium* (p. 4) has advised (April 2009) that rotigotine (*Neupro*®) is accepted for restricted use within NHS Scotland for the symptomatic treatment of moderate to severe idiopathic restless legs syndrome in adults with a baseline score of 15 points or more on the International Restless Legs Scale

Levodopa

Levodopa, the amino-acid precursor of dopamine, acts by replenishing depleted striatal dopamine. It is given with an extracerebral **dopa-decarboxylase inhibitor**, which reduces the peripheral conversion of levodopa to dopamine, thereby limiting side-effects such as nausea,

4 Central nervous system

vomiting, and cardiovascular effects; additionally, effective brain-dopamine concentrations are achieved with lower doses of levodopa. The extracerebral dopa-decarboxylase inhibitors used with levodopa are benserazide (in **co-beneldopa**) and carbidopa (in **co-careldopa**).

Levodopa, in combination with a dopa-decarboxylase inhibitor, is useful in the elderly or frail, in patients with other significant illnesses, and in those with more severe symptoms. It is effective and well tolerated in the majority of patients.

Levodopa therapy should be initiated at a low dose and increased in small steps; the final dose should be as low as possible. Intervals between doses should be chosen to suit the needs of the individual patient.

Nausea and vomiting with co-beneldopa or co-careldopa are rarely dose-limiting and domperidone (section 4.6) can be useful in controlling these effects.

Levodopa treatment is associated with potentially troublesome motor complications including response fluctuations and dyskinesias. Response fluctuations are characterised by large variations in motor performance, with normal function during the 'on' period, and weakness and restricted mobility during the 'off' period. 'End-of-dose' deterioration with progressively shorter duration of benefit also occurs. Modified-release preparations may help with 'end-of-dose' deterioration or nocturnal immobility and rigidity. Motor complications are particularly problematic in young patients treated with levodopa.

Cautions   Levodopa should be used with caution in severe pulmonary or cardiovascular disease (including history of myocardial infarction with residual arrhythmia), psychiatric illness (avoid if severe and discontinue if deterioration), endocrine disorders (including hyperthyroidism, Cushing's syndrome, diabetes mellitus, osteomalacia, and phaeochromocytoma), and in those with a history of convulsions or peptic ulcer. Levodopa should be used with caution in patients susceptible to angle-closure glaucoma, and in hepatic or renal impairment. Patients should be advised to avoid abrupt withdrawal (risk of neuroleptic malignant syndrome and rhabdomyolysis), and to be aware of the potential for excessive drowsiness and sudden onset of sleep (see Driving, p. 326); **interactions:** Appendix 1 (levodopa).

Pregnancy   Levodopa should be used with caution in pregnancy—toxicity has occurred in *animal* studies.

Breast-feeding   Levodopa may suppress lactation. It is present in milk—avoid.

Side-effects   Side-effects of levodopa include nausea, vomiting, taste disturbances, dry mouth, anorexia, arrhythmias, palpitations, postural hypotension, syncope, drowsiness (see Driving, p. 326), fatigue, dementia, psychosis, confusion, euphoria, abnormal dreams, insomnia, depression (*very rarely* with suicidal ideation), anxiety, dizziness, dystonia, dyskinesia, and chorea.

Less commonly weight changes, constipation, diarrhoea, hypersalivation, dysphagia, flatulence, hypertension, chest pain, oedema, hoarseness, ataxia, hand tremor, malaise, weakness, muscle cramps, and reddish discoloration of the urine and other body fluids may occur. *Rare* side-effects include abdominal pain, gastro-intestinal bleeding, duodenal ulcer, dyspepsia, phlebitis, dyspnoea, agitation, paraesthesia, bruxism, trismus, hiccups, neuroleptic malignant syndrome (associated

with abrupt withdrawal), convulsions, reduced mental acuity, disorientation, headache, urinary retention, urinary incontinence, priapism, activation of malignant melanoma, leucopenia, haemolytic and non-haemolytic anaemia, thrombocytopenia, agranulocytosis, blurred vision, blepharospasm, diplopia, activation of Horner's syndrome, pupil dilatation, oculogyric crisis, flushing, alopecia, exanthema, Henoch-Schönlein purpura, and sweating; *very rarely* angle-closure glaucoma may occur; compulsive behaviour (see Impulse Control Disorders, p. 325) and false positive tests for urinary ketones have also been reported.

CO-BENELDOPA

A mixture of benserazide hydrochloride and levodopa in mass proportions corresponding to 1 part of benserazide and 4 parts of levodopa

Indications   Parkinson's disease, see notes above

Cautions   see notes above

Pregnancy   see notes above

Breast-feeding   see notes above

Side-effects   see notes above

Dose

- Expressed as levodopa, initially 50 mg 3–4 times daily (100 mg 3 times daily in advanced disease), increased by 100 mg daily once or twice weekly according to response; usual maintenance dose 400–800 mg daily in divided doses; ELDERLY initially 50 mg once or twice daily, increased by 50 mg daily every 3–4 days according to response

  Note   When transferring patients from another levodopa/dopa-decarboxylase inhibitor preparation, the previous preparation should be discontinued 12 hours before (although interval can be shorter)

  Note   When administered as an adjunct to other antiparkinsonian drugs, once therapeutic effect apparent, the other drugs may be reduced or withdrawn

  Note   When switching from modified-release levodopa to dispersible co-beneldopa, reduce dose by approx. 30%

Co-beneldopa (Non-proprietary) PoM
Capsules, co-beneldopa 12.5/50) (benserazide 12.5 mg (as hydrochloride), levodopa 50 mg), net price 100-cap pack = £4.96. Label: 10, 14, 21, counselling, driving, see notes above

Capsules, co-beneldopa 25/100) (benserazide 25 mg (as hydrochloride), levodopa 100 mg), net price 100-cap pack = £6.91. Label: 10, 14, 21, counselling, driving, see notes above

Capsules, co-beneldopa 50/200) (benserazide 50 mg (as hydrochloride), levodopa 200 mg), net price 100-cap pack = £11.78. Label: 10, 14, 21, counselling, driving, see notes above

Madopar® (Roche) PoM
Capsules (*Madopar®-62.5 mg*), blue/grey, co-beneldopa 12.5/50 (benserazide 12.5 mg (as hydrochloride), levodopa 50 mg), net price 100-cap pack = £4.96. Label: 10, 14, 21, counselling, driving, see notes above

Capsules (*Madopar®-125 mg*), blue/pink, co-beneldopa 25/100 (benserazide 25 mg (as hydrochloride), levodopa 100 mg), net price 100-cap pack = £6.91. Label: 10, 14, 21, counselling, driving, see notes above

Capsules (*Madopar®-250 mg*), blue/caramel, co-beneldopa 50/200 (benserazide 50 mg (as hydrochloride), levodopa 200 mg), net price 100-cap pack = £11.78. Label: 10, 14, 21, counselling, driving, see notes above

Dispersible tablets, scored, co-beneldopa 12.5/50 (benserazide 12.5 mg (as hydrochloride), levodopa 50 mg), net price 100-tab pack = £5.90. Label: 10, 14, 21, counselling, administration, see below, driving, see notes above

Dispersible tablets, scored, co-beneldopa 25/100 (benserazide 25 mg (as hydrochloride) levodopa 100 mg), net price 100-tab pack = £10.45. Label: 10, 14, 21, counselling, administration, see below, driving, see notes above

Counselling The dispersible tablets can be dispersed in water or orange squash (not orange juice) or swallowed whole

◀**Modified release**

Madopar® CR (Roche) [PoM]

Capsules, m/r, dark green/light blue, co-beneldopa 25/100 (benserazide 25 mg (as hydrochloride), levodopa 100 mg), net price 100-cap pack = £12.77. Label: 5, 10, 14, 25, counselling, driving, see notes above

Dose patients not taking levodopa/dopa-decarboxylase inhibitor therapy, initially 1 capsule 3 times daily (max. initial dose 6 capsules daily)

Patients transferring from immediate-release levodopa/dopa-decarboxylase inhibitor preparations, initially 1 capsule substituted for every 100 mg of levodopa and given at same dosage frequency, increased every 2–3 days according to response; average increase of 50% needed over previous levodopa dose and titration may take up to 4 weeks

Supplementary dose of immediate-release *Madopar* may be needed with first morning dose; if response still poor to total daily dose of *Madopar® CR* plus *Madopar®* corresponding to 1.2 g levodopa, consider alternative therapy

---

▮ **CO-CARELDOPA**

A mixture of carbidopa and levodopa; the proportions are expressed in the form *x/y* where *x* and *y* are the strengths in milligrams of carbidopa and levodopa respectively

Indications Parkinson's disease, see notes above

Cautions see notes above

Pregnancy see notes above

Breast-feeding see notes above

Side-effects see notes above

Dose

• Expressed as levodopa, *initially* 100 mg (with carbidopa 25 mg) 3 times daily, increased by 50 mg (with carbidopa 12.5 mg) or 100 mg (with carbidopa 25 mg) daily or on alternate days according to response, until a dose of 800 mg (with carbidopa 200 mg) daily in divided doses is reached; then *maintenance dose* adjusted according to response up to max. 2 g (with carbidopa 200 mg) daily in divided doses

• Alternatively, expressed as levodopa, *initially* 50 mg (with carbidopa 12.5 mg) or 100 mg (with carbidopa 10 mg) 3–4 times daily, increased by 50 mg (with carbidopa 12.5 mg) or 100 mg (with carbidopa 10 mg) daily or on alternate days according to response, until a dose of 800 mg (with carbidopa up to 200 mg) daily in divided doses is reached; then *maintenance dose* adjusted according to response to max. 2 g (with carbidopa 200 mg) daily in divided doses

Note When co-careldopa is used, the total daily dose of carbidopa should be at least 70 mg. A lower dose may not achieve full inhibition of extracerebral dopa-decarboxylase, with a resultant increase in side-effects.

Note When transferring patients from another levodopa/dopa-decarboxylase inhibitor preparation, the previous preparation should be discontinued at least 12 hours before

Co-careldopa (Non-proprietary) [PoM]

Tablets, co-careldopa 10/100 (carbidopa 10 mg (anhydrous), levodopa 100 mg), net price 100-tab pack = £7.32. Label: 10, 14, counselling, driving, see notes above

Tablets, co-careldopa 25/100 (carbidopa 25 mg (anhydrous), levodopa 100 mg), net price 100-tab pack = £16.21. Label: 10, 14, counselling, driving, see notes above

Tablets, co-careldopa 25/250 (carbidopa 25 mg (anhydrous), levodopa 250 mg), net price 100-tab pack = £34.74. Label: 10, 14, counselling, driving, see notes above

Sinemet® (MSD) [PoM]

Sinemet® 12.5 mg/50 mg tablets, yellow, scored, co-careldopa 12.5/50 (carbidopa 12.5 mg (anhydrous), levodopa 50 mg), net price 90-tab pack = £6.28. Label: 10, 14, counselling, driving, see notes above

Note 2 tablets *Sinemet®* 12.5 mg/50 mg ≡ 1 tablet *Sinemet®* Plus 25 mg/100 mg

Sinemet® 10 mg/100 mg tablets, blue, scored, co-careldopa 10/100 (carbidopa 10 mg (anhydrous), levodopa 100 mg), net price 100-tab pack = £7.30. Label: 10, 14, counselling, driving, see notes above

Sinemet® Plus 25 mg/100 mg tablets, yellow, scored, co-careldopa 25/100 (carbidopa 25 mg (anhydrous), levodopa 100 mg), net price 100-tab pack = £12.88. Label: 10, 14, counselling, driving, see notes above

Note Co-careldopa 25/100 provides an adequate dose of carbidopa when low doses of levodopa are needed

Sinemet® 25 mg/250 mg tablets, blue, scored, co-careldopa 25/250 (carbidopa 25 mg (anhydrous), levodopa 250 mg), net price 100-tab pack = £18.29. Label: 10, 14, counselling, driving, see notes above

◀**For use with enteral tube**

Duodopa® (AbbVie) [PoM]

Intestinal gel, co-careldopa 5/20 (carbidopa 5 mg as monohydrate, levodopa 20 mg)/mL, net price 100 mL cassette (for use with *Duodopa®* portable pump) = £77.00. Label: 10, 14, counselling, driving, see notes above

Dose severe Parkinson's disease inadequately controlled by other preparations, consult product literature

◀**Modified release**

Caramet® CR (TEVA UK) [PoM]

Tablets, m/r, orange-brown, co-careldopa 25/100 (carbidopa 25 mg (as monohydrate), levodopa 100 mg), net price 60-tab pack = £11.47; co-careldopa 50/200 (carbidopa 50 mg (as monohydrate), levodopa 200 mg), 60-tab pack = £11.47. Label: 10, 14, 25, counselling, driving, see notes above

Dose patients not receiving levodopa/dopa-decarboxylase inhibitor preparations, expressed as levodopa, initially 100–200 mg twice daily (at least 6 hours between doses); dose adjusted according to response at intervals of at least 2 days

Patients transferring from immediate-release levodopa/dopa-decarboxylase inhibitor preparations, discontinue previous preparation at least 12 hours before first dose of *Caramet® CR*; substitute *Caramet® CR* to provide a similar amount of levodopa daily and extend dosing interval by 30–50%; dose then adjusted according to response at intervals of at least 2 days

Half Sinemet® CR (MSD) PoM

Tablets, m/r, pink, co-careldopa 25/100 (carbidopa 25 mg (anhydrous), levodopa 100 mg), net price 60-tab pack = £11.60. Label: 10, 14, 25, counselling, driving, see notes above

Dose for fine adjustment of *Sinemet® CR* dose (see below)

Sinemet® CR (MSD) PoM

Tablets, m/r, peach, scored, co-careldopa 50/200 (carbidopa 50 mg (anhydrous), levodopa 200 mg), net price 60-tab pack = £11.60. Label: 10, 14, 25, counselling, driving, see notes above

Dose patients not receiving levodopa/dopa-decarboxylase inhibitor therapy, initially, 1 *Sinemet® CR* tablet twice daily; both dose and interval then adjusted according to response at intervals of not less than 3 days

Patients transferring from immediate-release levodopa/dopa-decarboxylase inhibitor preparations, 1 *Sinemet® CR* tablet twice daily can be substituted for a daily dose of levodopa 300–400 mg in immediate-release *Sinemet®* tablets (substitute *Sinemet® CR* to provide approx. 10% more levodopa per day and extend dosing interval by 30–50%); dose and interval then adjusted according to response at intervals of not less than 3 days

◢**With entacapone**

For Parkinson's disease and end-of-dose motor fluctuations not adequately controlled with levodopa and dopa-decarboxylase inhibitor treatment

Stalevo® (Orion) PoM

Tablets, f/c, brown, levodopa 50 mg, carbidopa 12.5 mg, entacapone 200 mg, net price 30-tab pack = £20.79, 100-tab pack = £69.31. Label: 10, 14 (urine reddish-brown), 25, counselling, driving, see notes above

Dose only 1 tablet to be taken for each dose; max. 10 tablets daily

Tablets, f/c, brown, levodopa 75 mg, carbidopa 18.75 mg, entacapone 200 mg, net price 30-tab pack = £20.79, 100-tab pack = £69.31. Label: 10, 14 (urine reddish-brown), 25, counselling, driving, see notes above

Dose only 1 tablet to be taken for each dose; max. 10 tablets daily

Tablets, f/c, brown, levodopa 100 mg, carbidopa 25 mg, entacapone 200 mg, net price 30-tab pack = £20.79, 100-tab pack = £69.31. Label: 10, 14 (urine reddish-brown), 25, counselling, driving, see notes above

Dose only 1 tablet to be taken for each dose; max. 10 tablets daily

Tablets, f/c, brown, levodopa 125 mg, carbidopa 31.25 mg, entacapone 200 mg, net price 30-tab pack = £20.79, 100-tab pack = £69.31. Label: 10, 14 (urine reddish-brown), 25, counselling, driving, see notes above

Dose only 1 tablet to be taken for each dose; max. 10 tablets daily

Tablets, f/c, brown, levodopa 150 mg, carbidopa 37.5 mg, entacapone 200 mg, net price 30-tab pack = £20.79, 100-tab pack = £69.31. Label: 10, 14 (urine reddish-brown), 25, counselling, driving, see notes above

Dose only 1 tablet to be taken for each dose; max. 10 tablets daily

Tablets, f/c, brown, levodopa 175 mg, carbidopa 43.75 mg, entacapone 200 mg, net price 30-tab pack =£20.79, 100-tab pack = £69.31. Label: 10, 14 (urine reddish-brown), 25, counselling, driving, see notes above

Dose only 1 tablet to be taken for each dose; max. 8 tablets daily

Tablets, f/c, brown, levodopa 200 mg, carbidopa 50 mg, entacapone 200 mg, net price 30-tab pack = £20.79, 100-tab pack = £69.31. Label: 10, 14 (urine reddish-brown), 25, counselling, driving, see notes above

Dose only 1 tablet to be taken for each dose; max. 7 tablets daily

Note Patients receiving standard-release co-careldopa or co-beneldopa alone, initiate *Stalevo®* at a dose that provides similar (or slightly lower) amount of levodopa

Patients with dyskinesia or receiving more than 800 mg levodopa daily, introduce entacapone before transferring to *Stalevo®* (levodopa dose may need to be reduced by 10–30% initially)

Patients receiving entacapone and standard-release co-careldopa or co-beneldopa, initiate *Stalevo®* at a dose that provides similar (or slightly higher) amount of levodopa

Monoamine-oxidase-B inhibitors

Rasagiline, a monoamine-oxidase-B inhibitor, is licensed for the management of Parkinson's disease used alone or as an adjunct to levodopa for 'end-of-dose' fluctuations.

Selegiline is a monoamine-oxidase-B inhibitor used in conjunction with levodopa to reduce 'end-of-dose' deterioration in advanced Parkinson's disease. Early treatment with selegiline alone can delay the need for levodopa therapy. When combined with levodopa, selegiline should be avoided or used with great caution in postural hypotension.

◼ RASAGILINE

Indications   Parkinson's disease, used alone or as adjunct to co-beneldopa or co-careldopa

Cautions   avoid abrupt withdrawal; **interactions:** Appendix 1 (rasagiline)

Hepatic impairment   use with caution in mild impairment; avoid in moderate to severe impairment

Pregnancy   use with caution

Breast-feeding   use with caution—may suppress lactation

Side-effects   dry mouth, dyspepsia, constipation, flatulence, angina; headache, depression, anorexia, weight loss, abnormal dreams, vertigo, hallucinations; influenza-like symptoms; urinary urgency; leucopenia; arthralgia; conjunctivitis; rhinitis; rash, skin carcinoma; *less commonly* myocardial infarction, and cerebrovascular accident

Dose

● 1 mg daily

Azilect® (Teva) PoM

Tablets, rasagiline (as mesilate) 1 mg, net price 28-tab pack = £70.72

◼ SELEGILINE HYDROCHLORIDE

Indications   Parkinson's disease, used alone or as adjunct to co-beneldopa or co-careldopa; symptomatic parkinsonism

Cautions   avoid abrupt withdrawal; gastric and duodenal ulceration (avoid in active ulceration), uncontrolled hypertension (and avoid drugs that increase blood pressure), arrhythmias, angina, psychosis (and patients predisposed to confusion and psychosis), side-effects of levodopa may be increased—concurrent levodopa dosage can be reduced by 10–30% in steps of 10% every 3–4 days; history of hepatic dysfunction; avoid in acute porphyria (section 9.8.2); **interactions**: Appendix 1 (selegiline)

Driving See Drugs and Driving, p. 3

Hepatic impairment   use with caution in severe impairment

Renal impairment   use with caution in severe impairment

Pregnancy   avoid—no information available

Breast-feeding   avoid—no information available

Side-effects   nausea, constipation, diarrhoea, dry mouth, stomatitis, mouth ulcers, bradycardia, hypertension, hypotension, depression, dizziness, psychosis, impaired balance, tremor, fatigue, movement disorders, sleeping disorders, headache, confusion, arthralgia, myalgia, muscle cramps, myopathy, nasal congestion, hair loss, sweating; *less commonly* loss of appetite, angina, arrhythmias, palpitation, postural hypotension, supraventricular tachycardia, ankle oedema, dyspnoea, agitation, anxiety, micturition difficulties, leucocytopenia, thrombocytopenia, blurred vision; skin reactions; *also reported* hypersexuality

Dose

- Initially 5 mg in the morning; increasing after 2–4 weeks if tolerated to 10 mg in the morning

  Note 1.25-mg oral lyophilisate is equivalent to 10-mg tablet

Selegiline Hydrochloride (Non-proprietary) [PoM]

Tablets, selegiline hydrochloride 5 mg, net price 60-tab pack = £22.16; 10 mg, 30-tab pack = £19.99. Counselling, driving

Eldepryl® (Orion) [PoM]

Tablets, scored, selegiline hydrochloride 5 mg, net price 100-tab pack = £16.52; 10 mg, 100-tab pack = £32.23. Counselling, driving

◢**Oral lyophilisate**

Zelapar® (TEVA UK) [PoM]

Oral lyophilisates (= freeze-dried tablets), yellow, selegiline hydrochloride 1.25 mg, net price 30-tab pack = £43.16. Counselling, administration, driving

Excipients include aspartame (section 9.4.1)

Dose 1.25 mg daily before breakfast

Counselling Tablets should be placed on the tongue and allowed to dissolve. Advise patient not to drink, rinse, or wash mouth out for 5 minutes after taking the tablet

Note Patients receiving 10 mg conventional selegiline hydrochloride tablets can be switched to *Zelapar*® 1.25 mg

Catechol-*O*-methyltransferase inhibitors

Entacapone and **tolcapone** prevent the peripheral breakdown of levodopa, by inhibiting catechol-*O*-methyltransferase, allowing more levodopa to reach the brain. They are licensed for use as an adjunct to co-beneldopa or co-careldopa for patients with Parkinson's disease who experience 'end-of-dose' deterioration and cannot be stabilised on these combinations. Due to the risk of hepatotoxicity, tolcapone should be prescribed under specialist supervision only, when other catechol-*O*-methyltransferase inhibitors combined with co-beneldopa or co-careldopa are ineffective.

█ ENTACAPONE

Indications   adjunct to co-beneldopa or co-careldopa in Parkinson's disease with 'end-of-dose' motor fluctuations

Cautions   ischaemic heart disease; avoid abrupt withdrawal; concurrent levodopa dose may need to be reduced by about 10–30%; **interactions**: Appendix 1 (entacapone)

Contra-indications   phaeochromocytoma; history of neuroleptic malignant syndrome or non-traumatic rhabdomyolysis

Hepatic impairment   avoid

Pregnancy   avoid—no information available

Breast-feeding   avoid—present in milk in *animal* studies

Side-effects   nausea, vomiting, abdominal pain, constipation, diarrhoea, urine may be coloured reddish-brown, dry mouth; ischaemic heart disease; confusion, dizziness, abnormal dreams, fatigue, insomnia, dystonia, dyskinesia, hallucinations; sweating; *less commonly* myocardial infarction; *rarely* rash; *very rarely* anorexia, weight loss, agitation, and urticaria; *also reported* hepatitis, colitis, neuroleptic malignant syndrome, rhabdomyolysis, and skin, hair, and nail discoloration

Dose

- 200 mg with each dose of levodopa with dopa-decarboxylase inhibitor; max. 2 g daily

Entacapone (Non-proprietary) [PoM]

Tablets, entacapone 200 mg, net price 30-tab pack = £6.31, 100-tab pack = £18.07. Label: 14, (urine reddish-brown), counselling, driving, see notes above, avoid iron-containing products at the same time of day

Comtess® (Orion) [PoM]

Tablets, f/c, brown/orange, entacapone 200 mg, net price 30-tab pack = £17.24, 100-tab pack = £57.45. Label: 14, (urine reddish-brown), counselling, driving, see notes above, avoid iron-containing products at the same time of day

█ TOLCAPONE

Indications   adjunct to co-beneldopa or co-careldopa in Parkinson's disease with 'end-of-dose' motor fluctuations if another inhibitor of peripheral catechol-*O*-methyltransferase inappropriate (under specialist supervision)

Cautions   avoid abrupt withdrawal; most patients receiving more than 600 mg levodopa daily require reduction of levodopa dose by about 30%; **interactions**: Appendix 1 (tolcapone)

Hepatotoxicity Potentially life-threatening hepatotoxicity including fulminant hepatitis reported rarely, usually in women and during the first 6 months, but late-onset liver injury also reported; test liver function before treatment, and monitor every 2 weeks for first year, every 4 weeks for next 6 months and then every 8 weeks thereafter (restart monitoring schedule if dose increased); discontinue if abnormal liver function tests or symptoms of liver disorder (counselling, see below); do not re-introduce tolcapone once discontinued

Counselling Patients should be told how to recognise signs of liver disorder and advised to seek immediate medical attention if symptoms such as anorexia, nausea, vomiting, fatigue, abdominal pain, dark urine, or pruritus develop

Contra-indications   severe dyskinesia, phaeochromocytoma, previous history of neuroleptic malignant syndrome, rhabdomyolysis, or hyperthermia

Hepatic impairment   avoid; see also under Cautions

Renal impairment   caution if eGFR less than 30 mL/minute/1.73 m^2

4 Central nervous system

Pregnancy toxicity in *animal* studies—use only if potential benefit outweighs risk

Breast-feeding avoid—present in milk in *animal* studies

Side-effects diarrhoea, constipation, dyspepsia, abdominal pain, nausea, vomiting, anorexia, xerostomia, hepatotoxicity (see above); chest pain; confusion, dystonia, dyskinesia, drowsiness, headache, dizziness, sleep disturbances, excessive dreaming, hallucinations; syncope; urine discoloration; sweating; neuroleptic malignant syndrome and rhabdomyolysis reported on dose reduction or withdrawal

Dose

- 100 mg 3 times daily, leave 6 hours between each dose; max. 200 mg 3 times daily in exceptional circumstances; first daily dose should be taken at the same time as levodopa with dopa-decarboxylase inhibitor

  Note Continue beyond 3 weeks **only** if substantial improvement

Tasmar® (Meda) PoM

Tablets, f/c, yellow, tolcapone 100 mg, net price 100-tab pack = £95.20. Label: 14, 25

Amantadine

Amantadine is a weak dopamine agonist with modest antiparkinsonian effects. Tolerance to its effects may develop and confusion and hallucinations may occasionally occur.

■ AMANTADINE HYDROCHLORIDE

Indications Parkinson's disease; antiviral (section 5.3.4)

Cautions congestive heart disease (may exacerbate oedema), confused or hallucinatory states, elderly; avoid abrupt withdrawal in Parkinson's disease; **interactions:** Appendix 1 (amantadine)

Driving May affect performance of skilled tasks (e.g. driving)

Contra-indications epilepsy; history of gastric ulceration

Hepatic impairment caution

Renal impairment reduce dose; avoid if eGFR less than 15 mL/minute/1.73 m^2

Pregnancy avoid; toxicity in *animal* studies

Breast-feeding avoid; present in milk; toxicity in infant reported

Side-effects gastro-intestinal disturbances, anorexia, dry mouth; palpitation, peripheral oedema, postural hypotension; anxiety, mood changes, dizziness, headache, lethargy, hallucinations, insomnia, impaired concentration, slurred speech; myalgia; sweating and livedo reticularis; *less commonly* confusion, psychosis, tremor, movement disorders, seizure, neuroleptic malignant syndrome, urinary retention, urinary incontinence, visual disturbances, and rash; heart failure, leucopenia, and photosensitisation also reported

Dose

- Parkinson's disease, 100 mg daily increased after one week to 100 mg twice daily, usually in conjunction with other treatment; some patients may require higher doses, max. 400 mg daily; ELDERLY 65 years and over, 100 mg daily adjusted according to response
- Post-herpetic neuralgia, 100 mg twice daily for 14 days, continued for a further 14 days if necessary

Symmetrel® (Alliance) PoM

Capsules, red-brown, amantadine hydrochloride 100 mg. Net price 56-cap pack = £3.30. Counselling, driving, see Cautions

Syrup, amantadine hydrochloride 50 mg/5 mL. Net price 150-mL pack = £6.66. Counselling, driving, see Cautions

Lysovir® (Alliance) PoM

Section 5.3

4.9.2 Antimuscarinic drugs used in parkinsonism

Antimuscarinic drugs exert their antiparkinsonian action by reducing the effects of the relative central cholinergic excess that occurs as a result of dopamine deficiency. Antimuscarinic drugs can be useful in drug-induced parkinsonism, but they are generally not used in idiopathic Parkinson's disease because they are less effective than dopaminergic drugs and they are associated with cognitive impairment.

The antimuscarinic drugs **orphenadrine**, **procyclidine**, and **trihexyphenidyl** reduce the symptoms of parkinsonism induced by antipsychotic drugs, but there is no justification for giving them routinely in the absence of parkinsonian side-effects. Tardive dyskinesia is not improved by antimuscarinic drugs and may be made worse.

In idiopathic Parkinson's disease, antimuscarinic drugs reduce tremor and rigidity but they have little effect on bradykinesia. They may be useful in reducing sialorrhoea.

There are no important differences between the antimuscarinic drugs, but some patients tolerate one better than another.

Procyclidine can be given parenterally and is effective emergency treatment for acute drug-induced dystonic reactions.

If treatment with an antimuscarinic is ineffective, intravenous **diazepam** (p. 232) can be given for life-threatening acute drug-induced dystonic reactions.

Cautions Antimuscarinics should be used with caution in cardiovascular disease, hypertension, psychotic disorders, prostatic hypertrophy, pyrexia, and in those susceptible to angle-closure glaucoma, and in the elderly. Antimuscarinics should not be withdrawn abruptly in patients taking long-term treatment. Antimuscarinics are liable to abuse. **Interactions:** Appendix 1 (Antimuscarinics)

Driving Antimuscarinics can affect performance of skilled tasks (e.g. driving)

Contra-indications Antimuscarinics should be avoided in gastro-intestinal obstruction and myasthenia gravis.

Hepatic and renal impairment Orphenadrine, procyclidine, and trihexyphenidyl should be used with caution in patients with hepatic or renal impairment.

Side-effects Side-effects of antimuscarinics include constipation, dry mouth, nausea, vomiting, tachycardia, dizziness, confusion, euphoria, hallucinations, impaired memory, anxiety, restlessness, urinary retention, blurred vision, and rash. Angle-closure glaucoma occurs very rarely.

ORPHENADRINE HYDROCHLORIDE

Indications   parkinsonism; drug-induced extrapyramidal symptoms (but not tardive dyskinesia, see notes above)

Cautions   see notes above

Contra-indications   see notes above; also acute porphyria (section 9.8.2)

Hepatic impairment   see notes above

Renal impairment   see notes above

Pregnancy   caution

Breast-feeding   caution

Side-effects   see notes above; *less commonly* seizures, drowsiness, insomnia, and impaired coordination

Dose

- Initially 150 mg daily in divided doses, increased gradually in steps of 50 mg every 2–3 days according to response; usual dose range 150–300 mg daily in divided doses; max. 400 mg daily; ELDERLY preferably lower end of range

Orphenadrine Hydrochloride (Non-proprietary) [PoM]
Tablets, orphenadrine hydrochloride 50 mg, net price 100-tab pack = £80.00. Counselling, driving, see notes above
Oral solution, orphenadrine hydrochloride 50 mg/5 mL, net price 200 mL = £9.47. Counselling, driving, see notes above

Biorphen® (Alliance) [PoM]
Liquid, sugar-free, orphenadrine hydrochloride 25 mg/5 mL, net price 200 mL = £8.48. Counselling, driving, see notes above

Disipal® (Astellas) [PoM]
Tablets, yellow, s/c, orphenadrine hydrochloride 50 mg, net price 250-tab pack = £8.59. Counselling, driving, see notes above
Excipients   include tartrazine

PROCYCLIDINE HYDROCHLORIDE

Indications   parkinsonism; drug-induced extrapyramidal symptoms (but not tardive dyskinesia, see notes above)

Cautions   see notes above

Contra-indications   see notes above

Hepatic impairment   see notes above

Renal impairment   see notes above

Pregnancy   use only if potential benefit outweighs risk

Breast-feeding   no information available

Side-effects   see notes above; also gingivitis

Dose

- By mouth, 2.5 mg 3 times daily, increased gradually in steps of 2.5–5 mg daily every 2–3 days if necessary; usual max. 30 mg daily in 2–4 divided doses (60 mg daily in exceptional circumstances); ELDERLY preferably lower end of range
- By intramuscular *or* intravenous injection, acute dystonia, 5–10 mg (occasionally more than 10 mg), usually effective in 5–10 minutes but may need 30 minutes for relief; ELDERLY preferably lower end of range

Procyclidine (Non-proprietary) [PoM]
Tablets, procyclidine hydrochloride 5 mg, net price 28-tab pack = £1.99. Counselling, driving, see notes above

Arpicolin® (Rosemont) [PoM]
Syrup, sugar-free, procyclidine hydrochloride 2.5 mg/5 mL, net price 150 mL = £4.22; 5 mg/5 mL, 150 mL pack = £7.54. Counselling, driving, see notes above

Kemadrin® (Aspen) [PoM]
Tablets, scored, procyclidine hydrochloride 5 mg, net price 100-tab pack = £4.72. Counselling, driving, see notes above

Kemadrin® (Auden Mckenzie) [PoM]
Injection, procyclidine hydrochloride 5 mg/mL, net price 2-mL amp = £1.49

TRIHEXYPHENIDYL HYDROCHLORIDE
(Benzhexol hydrochloride)

Indications   parkinsonism; drug-induced extrapyramidal symptoms (but not tardive dyskinesia, see notes above)

Cautions   see notes above

Contra-indications   see notes above

Hepatic impairment   see notes above

Renal impairment   see notes above

Pregnancy   use only if potential benefit outweighs risk

Breast-feeding   avoid

Side-effects   see notes above

Dose

- 1 mg daily, increased by 2 mg every 3–5 days according to response; usual maintenance dose 5–15 mg daily in 3–4 divided doses (max. 20 mg daily); ELDERLY preferably lower end of range; CHILD under 18 years see BNF for Children

Note   Not recommended for use in Parkinson's disease because of toxicity in the elderly and the risk of aggravating dementia. However, if using in combination with co-careldopa or co-beneldopa the usual maintenance dose is 2–6 mg daily in divided doses

Trihexyphenidyl (Non-proprietary) [PoM]
Tablets, trihexyphenidyl hydrochloride 2 mg, net price 84-tab pack = £9.04; 5 mg, 84-tab pack = £17.91, 100-tab pack = £17.15. Counselling, with or after food, driving, see notes above
Syrup, trihexyphenidyl hydrochloride 5 mg/5 ml, net price 200 mL = £20.00. Counselling, driving, see notes above
Excipients   may include propylene glycol (see Excipients, p. 2)

4.9.3 Drugs used in essential tremor, chorea, tics, and related disorders

Tetrabenazine is mainly used to control movement disorders in Huntington's chorea and related disorders. Tetrabenazine can also be prescribed for the treatment of tardive dyskinesia if switching or withdrawing the causative antipsychotic drug is not effective. It acts by depleting nerve endings of dopamine. It is effective in only a proportion of patients and its use may be limited by the development of depression.

Haloperidol (p. 239) [unlicensed indication], **olanzapine** (p. 244) [unlicensed indication], **risperidone** (p. 246) [unlicensed indication], and **quetiapine** (p. 245) [unlicensed indication], can also be used to suppress chorea in Huntington's disease.

4 Central nervous system

Haloperidol (p. 239) can also improve motor tics and symptoms of Tourette syndrome and related choreas. Other treatments for Tourette syndrome include **pimozide** (p. 240) [unlicensed indication] (**important**: ECG monitoring required), **clonidine** (p. 301) [unlicensed indication], and **sulpiride** (p. 241) [unlicensed indication]. **Trihexyphenidyl** (p. 335) in high dosage can also improve some movement disorders; it is sometimes necessary to build the dose up over many weeks, to 20 to 30 mg daily or higher. **Chlorpromazine** (p. 238) and haloperidol (p. 239) are used to relieve intractable hiccup.

Propranolol or another beta-adrenoceptor blocking drug (section 2.4) may be useful in treating essential tremor or tremors associated with anxiety or thyrotoxicosis.

Primidone (p. 314) in some cases provides relief from benign essential tremor; the dose is increased slowly to reduce side-effects.

Piracetam (below) is used as an adjunctive treatment for myoclonus of cortical origin. After an acute episode, attempts should be made every 6 months to decrease or discontinue treatment.

Riluzole (below) is used to extend life in patients with motor neurone disease who have amyotrophic lateral sclerosis.

> ### NICE guidance
> ### Riluzole for motor neurone disease (January 2001)
> Riluzole is recommended for treating the amyotrophic lateral sclerosis (ALS) form of motor neurone disease (MND). Treatment should be initiated by a specialist in MND but it can then be supervised under a shared-care arrangement involving the general practitioner.
> www.nice.org.uk/TA20

Tafamidis (below) is used for the treatment of transthyretin familial amyloid polyneuropathy (TTR-FAP) in patients with stage 1 symptomatic polyneuropathy to delay peripheral neurological impairment. It acts by inhibiting amyloid formation, and should be prescribed in addition to standard treatment, but before liver transplantation; it should be discontinued in patients who undergo liver transplantation. Treatment should be initiated and supervised by a specialist in TTR-FAP.

PIRACETAM

Indications adjunctive treatment of cortical myoclonus

Cautions avoid abrupt withdrawal; increased risk of bleeding (gastric ulcer, history of haemorrhagic stroke, concomitant drugs that increase bleeding), underlying disorders of haemostasis, major surgery

Contra-indications cerebral haemorrhage; Huntington's chorea

Hepatic impairment adjust dose if both hepatic and renal impairment (see under Renal impairment, below)

Renal impairment use two-thirds of normal dose if eGFR 50–80 mL/minute/1.73 m²; use one-third of normal dose in 2 divided doses if eGFR 30–50 mL/minute/1.73 m²; use one-sixth normal dose as a single dose if eGFR 20–30 mL/minute/1.73 m²; avoid if eGFR less than 20 mL/minute/1.73 m²

Pregnancy avoid
Breast-feeding avoid
Side-effects weight gain, nervousness, hyperkinesia; *less commonly* drowsiness, depression, asthenia; *also reported* abdominal pain, nausea, vomiting, diarrhoea, headache, anxiety, confusion, hallucination, vertigo, ataxia, insomnia, haemorrhagic disorder, dermatitis, pruritus, urticaria

Dose
* Initially 7.2 g daily in 2–3 divided doses, increased according to response by 4.8 g every 3–4 days to max. 24 g daily (subsequently, attempts should be made to reduce dose of concurrent therapy); CHILD under 16 years not recommended
  Oral solution Follow the oral solution with a glass of water (or soft drink) to reduce bitter taste.

Nootropil® (UCB Pharma) PoM
Tablets, f/c, scored, piracetam 800 mg, net price 90-tab pack = £11.75; 1.2 g, 60-tab pack = £10.97. Label: 3
Oral solution, piracetam, 333.3 mg/mL, net price 300-mL pack = £16.31. Label: 3

RILUZOLE

Indications to extend life in patients with amyotrophic lateral sclerosis, initiated by specialists experienced in the management of motor neurone disease

Cautions history of abnormal hepatic function (consult product literature for details)
   Blood disorders Patients or their carers should be told how to recognise signs of neutropenia and advised to seek immediate medical attention if symptoms such as fever occur; white blood cell counts should be determined in febrile illness; neutropenia requires discontinuation of riluzole
   Interstitial lung disease Perform chest radiography if symptoms such as dry cough or dyspnoea develop; discontinue if interstitial lung disease is diagnosed
   Driving Dizziness or vertigo may affect performance of skilled tasks (e.g. driving)

Contra-indications acute porphyria (section 9.8.2)
Hepatic impairment avoid; see also under Cautions
Renal impairment avoid—no information available
Pregnancy avoid—no information available
Breast-feeding avoid—no information available
Side-effects nausea, vomiting, diarrhoea, abdominal pain; tachycardia; asthenia, headache, dizziness, drowsiness, oral paraesthesia; *less commonly* interstitial lung disease, pancreatitis, angioedema, and anaemia; *rarely* neutropenia; *very rarely* hepatitis

Dose
* 50 mg twice daily; CHILD not recommended

Rilutek® (Sanofi-Aventis) PoM
Tablets, f/c, riluzole 50 mg. Net price 56-tab pack = £320.33. Counselling, blood disorders, driving, see Cautions

TAFAMIDIS

Indications see notes above
Hepatic impairment caution in severe impairment—no information available
Pregnancy avoid (toxicity in *animal* studies); exclude pregnancy before treatment and ensure effective contraception during and for one month after stopping treatment

Breast-feeding avoid—present in milk in *animal* studies

Side-effects diarrhoea, abdominal pain, urinary tract infection, vaginal infection

Dose
- ADULT over 18 years, 20 mg once daily

Vyndaqel® (Pfizer) ▼ PoM
Capsules, pale yellow/white, tafamidis (as meglumine) 20 mg, net price 30-cap pack = £10685.00. Label: 25

TETRABENAZINE

Indications see Dose

Cautions avoid abrupt withdrawal; susceptibility to QT-interval prolongation (including concomitant use of drugs that prolong QT interval); **interactions:** Appendix 1 (tetrabenazine)
Driving May affect performance of skilled tasks (e.g. driving)

Contra-indications depression, parkinsonism, phaeochromocytoma, prolactin-dependent tumours

Hepatic impairment use half initial dose and slower dose titration in mild to moderate impairment; use with caution in severe impairment

Renal impairment use with caution

Pregnancy avoid unless essential—toxicity in *animal* studies

Breast-feeding avoid

Side-effects dysphagia, nausea, vomiting, diarrhoea, constipation, hypotension, depression, anxiety, insomnia, confusion, drowsiness, parkinsonism; *less commonly* altered consciousness level, extrapyramidal disorders, hyperthermia; *rarely* neuroleptic malignant syndrome; *very rarely* rhabdomyolysis; *also reported* dry mouth, dyspepsia, bradycardia, disorientation, agitation, dizziness, amnesia, ataxia

Dose
- Movement disorders due to Huntington's chorea, hemiballismus, senile chorea, and related neurological conditions, initially 25 mg 3 times daily, increased by 25 mg every 3–4 days as tolerated to max. 200 mg daily
  Note Lower initial doses may be necessary in elderly patients
- Moderate to severe tardive dyskinesia, initially 12.5 mg daily, gradually increased according to response

Tetrabenazine (Non-proprietary) PoM
Tablets, tetrabenazine 25 mg, net price 112-tab pack = £100.00. Label: 2
Brands include *Tetmodis®*, *Xenazine®*

Torsion dystonias and other involuntary movements

Botulinum toxin type A should be used under specialist supervision.

Botox® and *Dysport®* are licensed for the treatment of focal spasticity (including arm symptoms in conjunction with physiotherapy, dynamic equinus foot deformity caused by spasticity in ambulant paediatric cerebral palsy patients over 2 years, and hand and wrist disability associated with stroke), blepharospasm, hemifacial spasm, and spasmodic torticollis. *Botox®* is also licensed for severe hyperhidrosis of the axillae, and for the prophylaxis of headaches in adults with chronic

migraine (section 4.7.4.2). The *Scottish Medicines Consortium* (p. 4) has advised (March 2011 and March 2013) that *Botox®* is **not** recommended for use within NHS Scotland for prophylaxis of headaches in adults with chronic migraine.

Azzalure®, *Bocouture®*, *Botox®*, and *Vistabel®* are licensed for the temporary improvement of moderate to severe wrinkles between the eyebrows in adults under 65 years. The *Scottish Medicines Consortium* (p. 4) has advised that *Azzalure®* and *Vistabel®* (December 2010), and that *Bocouture®* (February 2011) are **not** recommended for use within NHS Scotland.

Xeomin® is licensed for the treatment of blepharospasm, spasmodic torticollis, and post-stroke spasticity of the upper limb.

Treatment with botulinum toxin type A can be considered after an acquired non-progressive brain injury if rapid-onset spasticity causes postural or functional difficulties.

BOTULINUM TOXIN TYPE A

Indications see notes above; preparations are **not** interchangeable and should be used under specialist supervision

Cautions history of dysphagia or aspiration; chronic respiratory disorder; neuromuscular or neurological disorders (can lead to increased sensitivity and exaggerated muscle weakness including dysphagia and respiratory compromise); excessive weakness, inflammation or atrophy in target muscle; off-label use (fatal adverse events reported)
Specific cautions for blepharospasm or hemifacial spasm Caution if risk of angle-closure glaucoma; reduced blinking can lead to corneal exposure, persistent epithelial defect and corneal ulceration (especially in those with VIIth nerve disorders)—careful testing of corneal sensation in previously operated eyes, avoidance of injection in lower lid area to avoid ectropion, and vigorous treatment of epithelial defect needed

Contra-indications generalised disorders of muscle activity (e.g. myasthenia gravis); infection at injection site

Pregnancy avoid unless essential—toxicity in *animal* studies; avoid in women of child-bearing age unless using effective contraception

Breast-feeding low risk of systemic absorption but avoid unless essential

Side-effects increased electrophysiologic jitter in some distant muscles; misplaced injections may paralyse nearby muscle groups and excessive doses may paralyse distant muscles; influenza-like symptoms; *rarely* arrhythmias, myocardial infarction, seizures, and antibody formation (substantial deterioration in response); *very rarely* exaggerated muscle weakness, dysphagia, dysphonia, respiratory disorders, aspiration (see Counselling below)
Specific side-effects for blepharospasm or hemifacial spasm ptosis; keratitis, lagophthalmos, dry eye, irritation, photophobia, lacrimation; facial oedema, ecchymosis; *less commonly* dry mouth, facial weakness (including drooping), dizziness, paraesthesia, headache, tiredness, ectropion, entropion, diplopia, visual disturbances, conjunctivitis, dermatitis; *rarely* eyelid bruising and swelling (minimised by applying gentle pressure at injection site immediately after injection); *very rarely* angle-closure glaucoma, corneal ulceration, corneal epithelial defect, corneal perforation
Specific side-effects in paediatric cerebral palsy drowsiness, malaise, abnormal gait, paraesthesia, urinary incontinence, myalgia, pain in extremities
Specific side-effects for temporary improvement of

Central nervous system 4

moderate to severe wrinkles between the eyebrows facial oedema, headache; ptosis; *less commonly* nausea, dry mouth, dizziness, asthenia, anxiety, paraesthesia, muscle cramp, visual disturbances, tinnitus, blepharitis, photosensitivity reactions, and dry skin

Specific side-effects in spasmodic torticollis dysphagia and pooling of saliva (occurs most frequently after injection into sternomastoid muscle), nausea, dry mouth; rhinitis; drowsiness, headache, dizziness, malaise, numbness, stiffness, hypertonia, back pain, weakness; *less commonly* diarrhoea, vomiting, colitis, dyspnoea, voice alteration, tremor, skeletal pain, myalgia, diplopia, eye pain, ptosis, and sweating

Specific side-effects in axillary hyperhidrosis paraesthesia, pain in extremities, non-axillary sweating, hot flushes, abnormal skin odour, pruritus, subcutaneous nodule, alopecia; *less commonly* myalgia and joint pain

Specific side-effects in focal upper-limb spasticity associated with stroke dysphagia; hypertonia, purpura; *less commonly* nausea, dry mouth, cough, haematoma, peripheral oedema, depression, insomnia, vertigo, amnesia, malaise, paraesthesia, dysaesthesia, headache, pain in extremities, arthralgia, and bursitis

Dose
- Consult product literature (**important:** specific to **each individual preparation** and **not interchangeable**)

    Counselling Patients should be warned of the signs and symptoms of toxin spread, such as muscle weakness and breathing difficulties; they should be advised to seek immediate medical attention if swallowing, speech or breathing difficulties occur

Azzalure® (Galderma) [PoM]
Injection, powder for reconstitution, botulinum toxin type A-haemagglutinin complex, net price 125-unit vial = £64.00. Counselling, side-effects, see under Dose above

Bocouture® (Merz) [PoM]
Injection, powder for reconstitution, botulinum toxin type A, net price 50-unit vial = £72.00. Counselling, side-effects, see under Dose above

Botox® (Allergan) [PoM]
Injection, powder for reconstitution, botulinum toxin type A complex, net price 50-unit vial = £77.50, 100-unit vial = £138.20, 200-unit vial = £276.40. Counselling, side-effects, see under Dose above

Dysport® (Ipsen) [PoM]
Injection, powder for reconstitution, botulinum type A toxin-haemagglutinin complex, net price 300-unit vial = £92.40; 500-unit vial = £154.00. Counselling, side-effects, see under Dose above

Vistabel® (Allergan) [PoM]
Injection, powder for reconstitution, botulinum toxin type A, net price 50-unit vial = £77.50. Counselling, side-effects, see under Dose above

Xeomin® (Merz) [PoM]
Injection, powder for reconstitution, botulinum toxin type A, net price 50-unit vial = £72.00; 100-unit vial = £129.90. Counselling, side-effects, see under Dose above

BOTULINUM TOXIN TYPE B

Indications spasmodic torticollis (cervical dystonia)—specialist use only

Cautions history of dysphagia or aspiration; off-label use (risk of toxin spread); tolerance may occur

Contra-indications neuromuscular or neuromuscular junctional disorders

Pregnancy low risk of systemic absorption but avoid unless essential

Breast-feeding low risk of systemic absorption but avoid unless essential

Side-effects increased electrophysiologic jitter in some distant muscles; dry mouth, taste disturbances, dyspepsia, dysphagia, worsening torticollis, neck pain, myasthenia, dysphonia, headache, influenza-like symptoms, visual disturbances; *also reported* vomiting, constipation, respiratory disorders, aspiration pneumonia, exaggerated muscle weakness (see Counselling below), malaise, ptosis

Dose
- By intramuscular injection, ADULT over 18 years, initially 5000–10 000 units divided between 2–4 most affected muscles; adjust dose and frequency according to response; **important: not** interchangeable with other botulinum toxin preparations

    Counselling Patients should be warned of the signs and symptoms of toxin spread, such as muscle weakness and breathing difficulties; they should be advised to seek immediate medical attention if swallowing, speech or breathing difficulties occur

NeuroBloc® (Eisai) [PoM]
Injection, botulinum toxin type B 5000 units/mL, net price 0.5-mL vial = £111.20; 1-mL vial = £148.27; 2-mL vial = £197.69. Counselling, side-effects, see under Dose above
Note May be diluted with sodium chloride 0.9%

4.10 Drugs used in substance dependence

4.10.1	Alcohol dependence
4.10.2	Nicotine dependence
4.10.3	Opioid dependence

This section includes drugs used in alcohol dependence, cigarette smoking, and opioid dependence.

The UK health departments have produced guidance on the treatment of drug misuse in the UK. *Drug Misuse and Dependence: UK Guidelines on Clinical Management* (2007) is available at www.nta.nhs.uk/ uploads/clinical_guidelines_2007.pdf.

4.10.1 Alcohol dependence

Excessive drinking of alcoholic beverages over a prolonged period of time can result in an alcohol withdrawal syndrome on abrupt cessation of, or marked reduction in, drinking. The presence and severity of alcohol dependence can be assessed by *The Severity of Alcohol Dependence Questionnaire (SADQ)*; other assessment questionnaires are also available.

Acute alcohol withdrawal People with moderate dependence can generally be treated in a community setting unless they are under 18 years of age, or are at high-risk of severe reactions or treatment failure. People with severe dependence should undergo withdrawal in an inpatient setting; withdrawal in severely dependent patients without medical support may lead to seizures, delirium tremens, and death. Long-acting benzodiazepines, usually **chlordiazepoxide** (p. 233), are used to attenuate alcohol withdrawal symptoms. In primary care, fixed-dose reducing regimens are usually used, whilst a symptom-triggered flexible regimen is used in hospital or other settings where continued assessment and monitoring is carried out for 24–48 hours, usually followed by a fixed 5-day reducing dose schedule (sometimes it may be necessary to continue treatment for up to 10 days). Patients with decompensated liver disease should be treated under specialist supervision.

Carbamazepine [unlicensed indication] (p. 306) is sometimes used as an alternative treatment in acute alcohol withdrawal when benzodiazepines are contra-indicated or not tolerated. **Clomethiazole** (p. 229) is licensed for use in acute alcohol withdrawal, but benzo-diazepines are preferred. It should only be used in an inpatient setting and should not be prescribed if the patient is liable to continue drinking alcohol.

Patients with marked agitation or hallucinations and those at risk of delirium tremens (characterised by delirium, hallucinations, course tremor, and disorienta-tion) may be prescribed antipsychotic drugs, such as **haloperidol** (p. 239) or **olanzapine** (p. 244) [unlicensed indication], as adjunctive therapy to benzodiazepines; antipsychotics should not be used alone because they do not treat alcohol withdrawal and may lower the seizure threshold. Delirium tremens is a medical emer-gency that requires specialist inpatient care.

If a patient taking a benzodiazepine as part of a with-drawal regimen develops alcohol withdrawal seizures, a fast-acting benzodiazepine (such as intravenous **loraze-pam** [unlicensed indication] (p. 324) or rectal **diazepam** (p. 323)) should be prescribed; thereafter an increase in the dose of oral benzodiazepine should be considered to prevent further seizures from occurring.

Alcohol dependence   Acamprosate and **naltrex-one** are effective treatments for relapse prevention in patients with alcohol dependence; **disulfiram** is an alternative (see below). Disulfiram should only be used in patients in whom acamprosate and naltrexone are not suitable, or if the patient prefers disulfiram. **Nalmefene** is licensed for the reduction of alcohol consumption in patients with alcohol dependence who have a high drinking risk level, without physical withdrawal symp-toms, and who do not require immediate detoxification.

Patients with alcohol dependence are at risk of devel-oping Wernicke's encephalopathy; patients at high-risk are those who are malnourished, at risk of malnourish-ment, or have decompensated liver disease. Parenteral **thiamine** (as *Pabrinex*®, section 9.6.2) should be pre-scribed for treatment of suspected or confirmed Wer-nicke's encephalopathy, and for prophylaxis in alcohol-dependent patients attending hospital for acute treat-ment (including treatment unrelated to alcohol depend-ence); parenteral prophylaxis may also be considered for high-risk patients being treated in primary care. High-dose oral thiamine (p. 702) should be prescribed following parenteral treatment until cognitive function is maximised. In primary care, prophylactic high-dose oral thiamine should be prescribed during acute withdrawal of alcohol, before planned withdrawal, and for patients not undergoing withdrawal but who are at high-risk of developing Wernicke's encephalopathy.

Patients with chronic alcohol-related pancreatitis who have symptoms of steatorrhoea or who have poor nutritional status due to exocrine pancreatic insuffi-ciency should be prescribed **pancreatic enzyme sup-plements** (section 1.9.4); supplements are not indicated when pain is the only symptom.

Corticosteroids (section 6.3.2) are used in patients with severe acute alcohol-related hepatitis.

Acamprosate

Acamprosate, in combination with counselling, may be helpful for maintaining abstinence in alcohol-dependent patients. It is useful for patients who are concerned that strong cravings will result in relapse. It should be initiated as soon as possible *after* abstinence has been achieved and continued for 1 year; treatment should be maintained if the patient has a temporary relapse but stopped if the patient returns to regular or excessive drinking that persists 4–6 weeks after starting treatment. Acamprosate is not effective in all patients, so efficacy should be regularly assessed.

▌ACAMPROSATE CALCIUM

Indications   see notes above

Cautions   continued alcohol abuse (risk of treatment failure)

Hepatic impairment   avoid if severe

Renal impairment   avoid if serum-creatinine greater than 120 micromol/litre

Pregnancy   avoid

Breast-feeding   avoid

Side-effects   diarrhoea, nausea, vomiting, abdominal pain; fluctuation in libido; pruritus, maculopapular rash; *rarely* bullous skin reactions

Dose
- ADULT 18–65 years, body-weight 60 kg and over, 666 mg 3 times daily; body-weight less than 60 kg, 666 mg at breakfast, 333 mg at midday, and 333 mg at night
- CHILD 16–18 years (under specialist supervision) [unlicensed], body-weight 60 kg and over, 666 mg 3 times daily; body-weight less than 60 kg, 666 mg at breakfast, 333 mg at midday, and 333 mg at night

Campral EC® (Merck Serono) [PoM]
Tablet, e/c, acamprosate calcium 333 mg, net price 168-tab pack = £28.80. Label: 21, 25
Electrolytes   Ca²⁺ 0.8 mmol/tablet

Disulfiram

Disulfiram is used as an adjunct in the treatment of alcohol dependence (under specialist supervision). It gives rise to an extremely unpleasant systemic reaction after the ingestion of even a small amount of alcohol because it causes accumulation of acetaldehyde in the body; it is only effective if taken daily. Symptoms can occur within 10 minutes of ingesting alcohol and include flushing of the face, throbbing headache, palpitation, tachycardia, nausea, vomiting, and, with large doses of alcohol, arrhythmias, hypotension, and collapse; these reactions can last several hours. Small amounts of alcohol such as those included in many oral medicines may be sufficient to precipitate a reaction—even toile-tries and mouthwashes that contain alcohol should be avoided. Alcohol should be avoided for at least 1 week after stopping treatment.

Before initiating disulfiram, prescribers should evaluate the patient's suitability for treatment, because some patient factors, for example memory impairment or social circumstances, make compliance to treatment or abstinence from alcohol difficult.

4   Central nervous system

During treatment with disulfiram, patients should be monitored at least every 2 weeks for the first 2 months, then each month for the following 4 months, and at least every 6 months thereafter.

DISULFIRAM

Indications see notes above

Cautions ensure that alcohol not consumed for at least 24 hours before initiating treatment; see also notes above; alcohol challenge **not** recommended on routine basis (if considered essential—specialist units only with resuscitation facilities); respiratory disease, diabetes mellitus, epilepsy; avoid in acute porphyria (section 9.8.2); **interactions:** Appendix 1 (disulfiram)

Contra-indications cardiac failure, coronary artery disease, history of cerebrovascular accident, hypertension, psychosis, severe personality disorder, suicide risk

Hepatic impairment use with caution

Renal impairment use with caution

Pregnancy high concentrations of acetaldehyde which occur in presence of alcohol may be teratogenic; avoid in first trimester

Breast-feeding avoid—no information available

Side-effects initially drowsiness and fatigue; nausea, vomiting, halitosis, reduced libido; *rarely* psychotic reactions (depression, paranoia, schizophrenia, mania), allergic dermatitis, peripheral neuritis, hepatic cell damage

Dose
- 200 mg daily increased if necessary; usual max. 500 mg daily; CHILD not recommended

Note Disulfiram doses in BNF may differ from those in product literature

Antabuse® (Actavis) PoM
Tablets, scored, disulfiram 200 mg. Net price 50-tab pack = £31.00. Label: 2, counselling, alcohol reaction

Nalmefene

Nalmefene is licensed for the reduction of alcohol consumption in patients with alcohol dependence who have a high drinking risk level without physical withdrawal symptoms, and who do not require immediate detoxification. It should only be prescribed in conjunction with continuous psychosocial support focused on treatment adherence and reducing alcohol consumption. Nalmefene is not recommended for patients aiming to achieve immediate abstinence.

Before initiating treatment, prescribers should evaluate the patient's clinical status, alcohol dependence, and level of alcohol consumption. Nalmefene should only be prescribed for patients who continue to have a high drinking risk level two weeks after the initial assessment.

During treatment, patients should be monitored regularly and the need for continued treatment assessed. Caution is advised if treatment is continued for more than 1 year.

NICE guidance
Nalmefene for reducing alcohol consumption in people with alcohol dependence (November 2014)
Nalmefene is recommended within its marketing authorisation, as an option for reducing alcohol consumption, for patients with alcohol dependence:
- who have a high drinking risk level (defined as alcohol consumption of more than 60 g per day for men and more than 40 g per day for women, according to the World Health Organization's drinking risk levels) without physical withdrawal symptoms, **and**
- who do not require immediate detoxification.

The marketing authorisation states that nalmefene should:
- only be prescribed in conjunction with continuous psychosocial support focused on treatment adherence and reducing alcohol consumption, **and**
- be initiated only in patients who continue to have a high drinking risk level 2 weeks after initial assessment.

www.nice.org.uk/TA325

NALMEFENE

Indications see notes above

Cautions notes above; also avoid concomitant use of opioids—discontinue treatment 1 week before anticipated use of opioids; if emergency analgesia is required during treatment, an increased dose of opioid analgesic may be necessary (monitor for opioid intoxication); psychiatric illness; history of seizure disorders (including alcohol withdrawal seizures); **interactions:** Appendix 1 (nalmefene)

Contra-indications recent or current opioid use; recent history of acute alcohol withdrawal syndrome

Hepatic impairment use with caution—avoid in severe impairment

Renal impairment use with caution—avoid in severe impairment

Pregnancy manufacturer advises avoid—toxicity in *animal* studies

Breast-feeding manufacturer advises avoid—present in milk in *animal* studies

Side-effects nausea, vomiting, dry mouth, weight loss, decreased appetite, tachycardia, palpitation, dizziness, headache, somnolence, tremor, disturbance in attention, paraesthesia, hypoaesthesia, malaise, sleep disorders, confusion, restlessness, decreased libido, muscle spasms, hyperhidrosis; *also reported* hallucinations, dissociation

Dose
- ADULT over 18 years, 1 tablet as required on each day there is a risk of drinking alcohol, preferably taken 1–2 hours before the anticipated time of drinking; if a dose has not been taken before drinking alcohol, 1 tablet should be taken as soon as possible; max. 1 tablet daily

Selincro® (Lundbeck) ▼ PoM
Tablets, f/c, nalmefene (as hydrochloride dihydrate) 18 mg, net price 14-tab pack = £42.42; 28-tab pack = £84.84. Label: 25

Naltrexone

Naltrexone is an opioid-receptor antagonist (section 4.10.3), but is useful as an adjunct in the treatment of alcohol dependence after a successful withdrawal. Treatment should be initiated by a specialist and continued under specialist supervision. Treatment should be reviewed monthly for the first 6 months, and then at reduced intervals; naltrexone should be stopped if drinking continues for 4–6 weeks after starting treatment.

4.10.2 Nicotine dependence

Smoking cessation interventions are a cost-effective way of reducing ill health and prolonging life. Smokers should be advised to stop and offered help with follow-up when appropriate. If possible, smokers should have access to smoking cessation services for behavioural support.

Therapy to aid smoking cessation is chosen according to the smoker's likely adherence, availability of counselling and support, previous experience of smoking-cessation aids, contra-indications and adverse effects of the preparations, and the smoker's preferences. **Nicotine replacement therapy**, **bupropion**, and **varenicline** are effective aids to smoking cessation. The use of nicotine replacement therapy in an individual who is already accustomed to nicotine introduces few new risks and it is widely accepted that there are no circumstances in which it is safer to smoke than to use nicotine replacement therapy.

Some patients benefit from having more than one type of nicotine replacement therapy prescribed, such as a combination of transdermal and oral preparations. The combination of nicotine replacement therapy with varenicline or bupropion is not recommended.

Concomitant medication Cigarette smoking increases the metabolism of some medicines by stimulating the hepatic enzyme CYP1A2. When smoking is discontinued, the dose of these drugs, in particular theophylline (p. 195), cinacalcet (p. 695), ropinirole (p. 328), and some antipsychotics (including clozapine (p. 242), olanzapine (p. 244), chlorpromazine (p. 238), and haloperidol (p. 239)), may need to be reduced. Regular monitoring for adverse effects is advised.

Bupropion

Bupropion has been used as an antidepressant. Its mode of action in smoking cessation is not clear and may involve an effect on noradrenaline and dopamine neurotransmission.

BUPROPION HYDROCHLORIDE
(Amfebutamone hydrochloride)

Indications see notes above

Cautions elderly; predisposition to seizures (prescribe only if benefit clearly outweighs risk) including concomitant use of drugs that lower seizure threshold, alcohol abuse, history of head trauma, and diabetes; measure blood pressure before and during treatment; interactions: Appendix 1 (bupropion)
Driving May impair performance of skilled tasks (e.g. driving)

Contra-indications acute alcohol or benzodiazepine withdrawal; severe hepatic cirrhosis; CNS tumour; history of seizures, eating disorders, or bipolar disorder

Hepatic impairment reduce dose to 150 mg daily; avoid in severe hepatic cirrhosis

Renal impairment reduce dose to 150 mg daily
Pregnancy avoid—no information available
Breast-feeding present in milk—avoid
Side-effects dry mouth, gastro-intestinal disturbances, taste disturbance; agitation, anxiety, dizziness, depression, headache, impaired concentration, insomnia (reduced by avoiding dose at bedtime), tremor; fever; pruritus, rash, sweating; *less commonly* chest pain, flushing, hypertension, tachycardia, anorexia, asthenia, confusion, tinnitus, and visual disturbances; *rarely* hepatitis, jaundice, palpitation, postural hypotension, vasodilatation, abnormal dreams, ataxia, dystonia, depersonalisation, hallucinations, hostility, incoordination, irritability, impaired memory, paraesthesia, seizures, twitching, blood-glucose changes, urinary frequency, urinary retention, exacerbation of psoriasis, and Stevens-Johnson syndrome; *very rarely* aggression, delusions, paranoid ideation, and restlessness; *also reported* suicidal ideation

Dose
• ADULT over 18 years, start 1–2 weeks before target stop date, initially 150 mg daily for 6 days then 150 mg twice daily (max. single dose 150 mg, max. daily dose 300 mg; minimum 8 hours between doses); period of treatment 7–9 weeks; discontinue if abstinence not achieved at 7 weeks; consider max. 150 mg daily in patients with risk factors for seizures; ELDERLY max. 150 mg daily

Zyban® (GSK) [PoM]
Tablets, m/r, f/c, bupropion hydrochloride 150 mg, net price 60-tab pack = £41.76. Label: 25, counselling, driving, see Cautions

Nicotine replacement therapy

Nicotine replacement therapy can be used in place of cigarettes after abrupt cessation of smoking, or alternatively to reduce the amount of cigarettes used in advance of making a quit attempt. Nicotine replacement therapy can also be used to minimise passive smoking, and to treat cravings and reduce compensatory smoking after enforced abstinence in smoke-free environments. Smokers who find it difficult to achieve abstinence should consult a healthcare professional for advice.

Choice Nicotine patches are a prolonged-release formulation and are applied for 16 hours (with the patch removed overnight) or for 24 hours. If patients experience strong cravings for cigarettes on waking, a 24-hour patch may be more suitable. Immediate-release nicotine preparations (gum, lozenges, sublingual tablets, inhalator, nasal spray, and oral spray) are used whenever the urge to smoke occurs or to prevent cravings.

The choice of nicotine replacement preparation depends largely on patient preference, and should take into account what preparations, if any, have been tried before. Patients with a high level of nicotine dependence, or who have failed with nicotine replacement therapy previously, may benefit from using a combination of an immediate-release preparation and patches to achieve abstinence.

All preparations are licensed for adults and children over 12 years (with the exception of *Nicotinell* lozenges which are licensed for children under 18 years only when recommended by a doctor).

Cautions Most warnings for nicotine replacement therapy also apply to continued cigarette smoking, but

 4 Central nervous system

the risk of continued smoking outweighs any risks of using nicotine preparations. Nicotine replacement therapy should be used with caution in haemodynamically unstable patients hospitalised with severe arrhythmias, myocardial infarction, or cerebrovascular accident, and in patients with phaeochromocytoma or uncontrolled hyperthyroidism. Care is also needed in patients with diabetes mellitus—blood-glucose concentration should be monitored closely when initiating treatment.

Specific cautions for individual preparations are usually related to the local effect of nicotine. *Oral preparations* should be used with caution in patients with oesophagitis, gastritis, or peptic ulcers because swallowed nicotine can aggravate these conditions. The *gum* may also stick to and damage dentures. Acidic beverages, such as coffee or fruit juice, may decrease the absorption of nicotine through the buccal mucosa and should be avoided for 15 minutes before the use of oral nicotine replacement therapy. Care should be taken with the *inhalation cartridges* in patients with obstructive lung disease, chronic throat disease, or bronchospastic disease. The *nasal spray* can cause worsening of bronchial asthma. *Patches* should not be placed on broken skin and should be used with caution in patients with skin disorders.

Hepatic impairment   Nicotine replacement therapy should be used with caution in moderate to severe hepatic impairment.

Renal impairment   Nicotine replacement therapy should be used with caution in severe renal impairment.

Pregnancy   The use of nicotine replacement therapy in pregnancy is preferable to the continuation of smoking, but should be used only if smoking cessation without nicotine replacement fails. Intermittent therapy is preferable to patches but avoid liquorice-flavoured nicotine products. Patches are useful, however, if the patient is experiencing pregnancy-related nausea and vomiting. If patches are used, they should be removed before bed.

Breast-feeding   Nicotine is present in milk; however, the amount to which the infant is exposed is small and less hazardous than second-hand smoke. Intermittent therapy is preferred.

Side-effects   Some systemic effects occur on initiation of therapy, particularly if the patient is using high-strength preparations; however, the patient may confuse side-effects of the nicotine-replacement preparation with nicotine withdrawal symptoms. Common symptoms of nicotine withdrawal include malaise, headache, dizziness, sleep disturbance, coughing, influenza-like symptoms, depression, irritability, increased appetite, weight gain, restlessness, anxiety, drowsiness, aphthous ulcers, decreased heart rate, and impaired concentration.

Mild local reactions at the beginning of treatment are common because of the irritant effect of nicotine. *Oral preparations* and *inhalation cartridges* can cause irritation of the throat, *gum*, *lozenges*, and *oral spray* can cause increased salivation, and *patches* can cause minor skin irritation. The *nasal spray* commonly causes coughing, nasal irritation, epistaxis, sneezing, and watery eyes; the *oral spray* can cause watery eyes and blurred vision.

Gastro-intestinal disturbances are common and may be caused by swallowed nicotine. Nausea, vomiting, dyspepsia, and hiccup occur most frequently. Ulcerative

stomatitis has also been reported. Dry mouth is a common side-effect of *lozenges*, *patches*, *oral spray*, and *sublingual tablets*. *Lozenges* cause diarrhoea, constipation, dysphagia, oesophagitis, gastritis, mouth ulcers, bloating, flatulence, and less commonly, taste disturbance, thirst, gingival bleeding, and halitosis. The *oral spray* may also cause abdominal pain, flatulence, and taste disturbance.

Palpitations may occur with nicotine replacement therapy and rarely *patches* and *oral spray* can cause arrhythmia. *Patches*, *lozenges*, and *oral spray* can cause chest pain. The *inhalator* can very rarely cause reversible atrial fibrillation.

Paraesthesia is a common side-effect of *oral spray*. Abnormal dreams can occur with *patches*; removal of the patch before bed may help. *Lozenges* and *oral spray* may cause rash and hot flushes. Sweating and myalgia can occur with *patches* and *oral spray*; the *patches* can also cause arthralgia.

Nicotine medicated chewing gum   Individuals who smoke fewer than 20 cigarettes each day should use 1 piece of 2-mg strength gum when the urge to smoke occurs or to prevent cravings; individuals who smoke more than 20 cigarettes each day or who require more than 15 pieces of 2-mg strength gum each day should use the 4-mg strength. Patients should not exceed 15 pieces of 4-mg strength gum daily. If attempting smoking cessation, treatment should continue for 3 months before reducing the dose.

Administration   Chew the gum until the taste becomes strong, then rest it between the cheek and gum; when the taste starts to fade, repeat this process. One piece of gum lasts for approximately 30 minutes.

Nicotine inhalation cartridge   The cartridges can be used when the urge to smoke occurs or to prevent cravings. Patients should not exceed 12 cartridges of the 10 mg strength daily, or 6 cartridges of the 15 mg strength daily.

Administration   Insert the cartridge into the device and draw in air through the mouthpiece; each session can last for approximately 5 minutes. The amount of nicotine from 1 puff of the cartridge is less than that from a cigarette, therefore it is necessary to inhale more often than when smoking a cigarette. A single 10 mg cartridge lasts for approximately 20 minutes of intense use; a single 15 mg cartridge lasts for approximately 40 minutes of intense use.

Nicotine lozenge   One lozenge should be used every 1–2 hours when the urge to smoke occurs. Individuals who smoke less than 20 cigarettes each day should usually use the lower-strength lozenges; individuals who smoke more than 20 cigarettes each day and those who fail to stop smoking with the low-strength lozenges should use the higher-strength lozenges. Patients should not exceed 15 lozenges daily. If attempting smoking cessation, treatment should continue for 6–12 weeks before attempting a reduction in dose.

Administration   Slowly allow each lozenge to dissolve in the mouth; periodically move the lozenge from one side of the mouth to the other. Lozenges last for 10–30 minutes, depending on their size.

Nicotine sublingual tablets   Individuals who smoke fewer than 20 cigarettes each day should initially use 1 tablet each hour, increased to 2 tablets each hour if necessary; individuals who smoke more than 20 cigarettes each day should use 2 tablets each hour. Patients should not exceed 40 tablets daily. If attempting smoking cessation, treatment should continue for up to 3 months before reducing the dose.

Administration Each tablet should be placed under the tongue and allowed to dissolve.

Nicotine oral spray Patients can use 1–2 sprays in the mouth when the urge to smoke occurs or to prevent cravings. Individuals should not exceed 2 sprays per episode (up to 4 sprays every hour), and a maximum of 64 sprays daily.

Administration The oral spray should be released into the mouth, holding the spray as close to the mouth as possible and avoiding the lips. The patient should not inhale while spraying and avoid swallowing for a few seconds after use.

Note If using the oral spray for the first time, or if unit not used for 2 or more days, prime the unit before administration

Nicotine nasal spray Patients can use 1 spray in each nostril when the urge to smoke occurs, up to twice every hour for 16 hours daily (maximum 64 sprays daily). If attempting smoking cessation, treatment should continue for 8 weeks before reducing the dose.

Administration Initially 1 spray should be used in both nostrils but when withdrawing from therapy, the dose can be gradually reduced to 1 spray in 1 nostril.

Nicotine transdermal patches As a general guide for smoking cessation, individuals who smoke more than 10 cigarettes daily should apply a high-strength patch daily for 6–8 weeks, followed by the medium-strength patch for 2 weeks, and then the low-strength patch for the final 2 weeks; individuals who smoke fewer than 10 cigarettes daily can usually start with the medium-strength patch for 6–8 weeks, followed by the low-strength patch for 2–4 weeks. A slower titration schedule can be used in patients who are not ready to quit but want to reduce cigarette consumption before a quit attempt.

If abstinence is not achieved, or if withdrawal symptoms are experienced, the strength of the patch used should be maintained or increased until the patient is stabilised. Patients using the high-strength patch who experience excessive side-effects, that do not resolve within a few days, should change to a medium-strength patch for the remainder of the initial period and then use the low-strength patch for 2–4 weeks.

Administration Patches should be applied on waking to dry, non-hairy skin on the hip, trunk, or upper arm and held in position for 10–20 seconds to ensure adhesion; place next patch on a different area and avoid using the same site for several days.

◢ **NICOTINE**

Indications see notes above

Cautions see notes above; **interactions:** Appendix 1 (nicotine)

Hepatic impairment see notes above

Renal impairment see notes above

Pregnancy see notes above

Breast-feeding see notes above

Side-effects see notes above

Dose

• See notes above

Nicorette® (McNeil)

Tablets (sublingual) (*Nicorette Microtab®*), nicotine (as a cyclodextrin complex) 2 mg, net price starter pack of 2 × 15-tablet discs with dispenser = £4.83; pack of 100 = £13.12. Label: 26, counselling, administration, see notes above

Note Also available as *NicAssist®*

Chewing gum, sugar-free, nicotine (as resin) 2 mg, net price pack of 30 = £3.25, pack of 105 = £9.27, pack of 210 = £14.82; 4 mg, pack of 30 = £3.99, pack of 105 = £11.28, pack of 210 = £18.24. Counselling, administration, see notes above

Note Also available in mint, freshfruit, freshmint, and icy white flavours (icy white flavour not available for pack size of 210 pieces). Also available as *NicAssist®*

Mint lozenge, sugar-free, nicotine (as bitartrate) 2 mg, net price pack of 24 = £2.55, pack of 96 = £8.29. Counselling, administration, see notes above

Patches, self-adhesive, beige, nicotine, '*5 mg' patch* (releasing approx. 5 mg/16 hours), net price 7 = £9.97; '*10 mg' patch* (releasing approx. 10 mg/16 hours), 7 = £9.97; '*15 mg' patch* (releasing approx. 15 mg/16 hours), 2 = £2.85, 7 = £9.97. Counselling, administration, see notes above

Note Also available as *NicAssist®*

Invisi patches, self-adhesive, beige, nicotine, '*10 mg' patch* (releasing approx. 10 mg/16 hours), net price 7 = £9.97; '*15 mg' patch* (releasing approx. 15 mg/16 hours), 7 = £9.97; '*25 mg' patch* (releasing approx. 25 mg/16 hours), 7 = £9.97. Counselling, administration, see notes above

Note Also available as *NicAssist® Translucent* patches

Oral spray (*Nicorette Quickmist® mouthspray*), nicotine 1 mg/metered dose, net price 150-dose pack = £12.12, 2 × 150-dose pack = £19.14. Counselling, administration, see notes above

Note Contains < 100 mg ethanol per dose

Nasal spray, nicotine 500 micrograms/metered spray, net price 200-spray unit = £13.40. Counselling, administration, see notes above

Note Also available as *NicAssist®*

Inhalator (nicotine-impregnated plug for use in inhalator mouthpiece), nicotine 10 mg/cartridge, net price 6-cartridge pack = £4.46, 42-cartridge pack = £14.65; 15 mg/cartridge, 4-cartridge pack = £4.14, 20-cartridge pack = £14.67, 36-cartridge pack = £22.33. Counselling, administration, see notes above

Note Also available as *NicAssist®*

Nicotinell® (Novartis Consumer Health)

Chewing gum, sugar-free, nicotine (as polacrilin complex) 2 mg, net price pack of 12 = £1.71, pack of 24 = £3.01, pack of 72 = £6.69, pack of 96 = £8.26, pack of 204 = £14.23; 4 mg, pack of 12 = £1.70, pack of 24 = £3.30, pack of 72 = £8.29, pack of 96 = £10.26. Counselling, administration, see notes above

Note Also available in fruit, liquorice, icemint, and mint flavours

Mint lozenge, sugar-free, nicotine (as bitartrate) 1 mg, net price pack of 12 = £1.59, pack of 36 = £4.27, pack of 96 = £9.12; 2 mg, pack of 12 = £1.99, pack of 36 = £4.95, pack of 96 = £10.60. Counselling, administration, see notes above

Excipients include aspartame (section 9.4.1)

TTS Patches, self-adhesive, all yellowish-ochre, nicotine, '*10' patch* (releasing approx. 7 mg/24 hours), net price 7 = £9.12; '*20' patch* (releasing approx. 14 mg/24 hours), 2 = £2.57, 7 = £9.40; '*30' patch* (releasing approx. 21 mg/24 hours), 2 = £2.85, 7 = £9.97, 21 = £24.51. Counselling, administration, see notes above

4 Central nervous system

NiQuitin® (GSK Consumer Healthcare)

Chewing gum, sugar-free, mint-flavour, nicotine 2 mg (white), net price pack of 12 = £1.71, pack of 24 = £2.85, pack of 96 = £8.55; 4 mg (yellow), pack of 12 = £1.71, pack of 24 = £2.85, pack of 96 = £8.55. Counselling, administration, see notes above

Lozenges, sugar-free, nicotine (as resinate) 1.5 mg (cherry- and mint-flavoured), net price pack of 20 = £3.18, pack of 60 = £8.93; 2 mg (mint-flavoured), pack of 36 = £5.12, pack of 72 = £9.97; 4 mg (mint-flavoured), pack of 20 = £3.18, pack of 60 = £8.93, pack of 36 = £5.12, pack of 72 = £9.97. Counselling, administration, see notes above

Excipients include aspartame (section 9.4.1); contains 0.65 mmol Na⁺/lozenge

Note Nicotine (as resinate) also available as *NiQuitin® Pre-quit* lozenges and *NiQuitin® Minis* lozenges

Patches, self-adhesive, pink/beige, nicotine *'7 mg' patch* (releasing approx. 7 mg/24 hours), net price 7 = £9.97; *'14 mg' patch* (releasing approx. 14 mg/24 hours), 7 = £9.97; *'21 mg' patch* (releasing approx. 21 mg/24 hours), 7 = £9.97, 14 = £18.79. Counselling, administration, see notes above

Note Also available as a clear patch

Varenicline

Varenicline is a selective nicotine-receptor partial agonist used as an aid for smoking cessation.

> ### NICE guidance
> #### Varenicline for smoking cessation (July 2007)
> Varenicline is recommended, within its licensed indications, as an option for smokers who have expressed a desire to quit smoking; it should normally be prescribed only as part of a programme of behavioural support.
> www.nice.org.uk/TA123

▌ VARENICLINE

Indications see notes above

Cautions risk of relapse, irritability, depression, and insomnia on discontinuation (consider dose tapering on completion of 12-week course); history of psychiatric illness (may exacerbate underlying illness including depression); predisposition to seizures, including conditions that may lower seizure threshold; history of cardiovascular disease

> #### MHRA/CHM advice
> #### Suicidal behaviour and varenicline
> Patients should be advised to discontinue treatment and seek prompt medical advice if they develop agitation, depressed mood, or suicidal thoughts. Patients with a history of psychiatric illness should be monitored closely while taking varenicline.

Renal impairment if eGFR less than 30 mL/minute/1.73 m², initial dose 500 micrograms once daily, increased after 3 days to 1 mg once daily

Pregnancy avoid—toxicity in *animal* studies

Breast-feeding avoid—present in milk in *animal* studies

Side-effects gastro-intestinal disturbances, appetite changes, dry mouth, taste disturbance; headache, drowsiness, dizziness, sleep disorders, abnormal dreams; *less commonly* thirst, weight gain, aphthous stomatitis, gingival pain, chest pain, hypertension, tachycardia, atrial fibrillation, palpitation, depression, anxiety, hallucinations, panic attack, mood swings, dysarthria, asthenia, seizure, tremor, incoordination, hypertonia, restlessness, hypoaesthesia, impaired temperature regulation, menorrhagia, vaginal discharge, sexual dysfunction, dysuria, arthralgia, muscle spasm, visual disturbances, eye pain, lacrimation, tinnitus, acne, sweating, rash, pruritus; *rarely* cerebrovascular accident; *also reported* myocardial infarction, aggression, irrational behaviour, psychosis, suicidal ideation (see MHRA/CHM advice above), sleep-walking, hyperglycaemia, diabetes mellitus, Stevens-Johnson syndrome

Dose

● ADULT over 18 years, starting usually 1–2 weeks before target stop date (up to max. 5 weeks before target stop date), initially 500 micrograms once daily for 3 days, increased to 500 micrograms twice daily for 4 days, then 1 mg twice daily for 11 weeks (reduce to 500 micrograms twice daily if not tolerated); 12-week course can be repeated in abstinent individuals to reduce risk of relapse

Champix® (Pfizer) ▼ PoM

Tablets, f/c, varenicline (as tartrate) 500 micrograms (white), net price 56-tab pack = £54.60; 1 mg (blue) 28-tab pack = £27.30, 56-tab pack = £54.60; starter pack of 11 × 500-microgram tabs with 14 × 1-mg tabs = £27.30. Label: 3

4.10.3 Opioid dependence

The management of opioid dependence requires medical, social, and psychological treatment; access to a multidisciplinary team is recommended. Treatment for opioid dependence should be initiated under the supervision of an appropriately qualified prescriber.

Untreated heroin dependence shows early withdrawal symptoms within 8 hours, with peak symptoms at 36–72 hours; symptoms subside substantially after 5 days. Methadone or buprenorphine withdrawal occurs later, with longer-lasting symptoms.

Opioid substitution therapy

Methadone and **buprenorphine** are used as substitution therapy in opioid dependence. Substitute medication should be commenced with a short period of stabilisation, followed by either a withdrawal regimen or by maintenance treatment. Maintenance treatment enables patients to achieve stability, reduces drug use and crime, and improves health; it should be regularly reviewed to ensure the patient continues to derive benefit. The prescriber should monitor for signs of toxicity, and the patient should be told to be aware of warning signs of toxicity on initiation and during titration.

A withdrawal regimen after stabilisation with methadone or buprenorphine should be attempted only after careful consideration. Enforced withdrawal is ineffective for sustained abstinence, and it increases the risk of patients relapsing and subsequently overdosing because of loss of tolerance. Complete withdrawal from opioids usually takes up to 4 weeks in an inpatient or residential setting, and up to 12 weeks in a community setting. If abstinence is not achieved, illicit drug use is resumed, or the patient cannot tolerate withdrawal, the withdrawal regimen should be stopped and maintenance therapy should be resumed at the optimal dose. Following successful withdrawal treatment, further support and monitoring to maintain abstinence should be provided for a period of at least 6 months.

In younger patients (under 18 years), the harmful effects of drug misuse are more often related to acute intoxication than to dependence, so substitution therapy is usually inappropriate. Maintenance treatment with opioid substitution therapy is therefore controversial in young people; however, it may be useful for the older adolescent who has a history of opioid use to undergo a period of stabilisation with buprenorphine or methadone before starting a withdrawal regimen.

> ### Missed doses
>
> Patients who miss 3 days or more of their regular prescribed dose of opioid maintenance therapy are at risk of overdose because of loss of tolerance. Consider reducing the dose in these patients.
>
> If the patient misses 5 or more days of treatment, an assessment of illicit drug use is also recommended before restarting substitution therapy; this is particularly important for patients taking buprenorphine, because of the risk of precipitated withdrawal.

> ### NICE guidance
> ### Methadone and buprenorphine for the management of opioid dependence (January 2007)
>
> Oral methadone and buprenorphine are recommended for maintenance therapy in the management of opioid dependence. Patients should be committed to a supportive care programme including a flexible dosing regimen administered under supervision for at least 3 months, until compliance is assured. Selection of methadone or buprenorphine should be made on a case-by-case basis, but methadone should be prescribed if both drugs are equally suitable.
> www.nice.org.uk/TA114

Buprenorphine Buprenorphine is an opioid-receptor partial agonist (it has opioid agonist and antagonist properties). Buprenorphine is preferred by some patients because it is less sedating than methadone; for this reason it may be more suitable for employed patients or those undertaking other skilled tasks such as driving. Buprenorphine is safer than methadone when used in conjunction with other sedating drugs, and has fewer drug interactions. Dose reductions may be easier than with methadone because the withdrawal symptoms are milder, and patients generally require fewer adjunctive medications; there is also a lower risk of overdose. Buprenorphine can be given on alternate days in higher doses and it requires a shorter drug-free period than methadone before induction with naltrexone for prevention of relapse (p. 347).

Patients dependent on high doses of opioids may be at increased risk of precipitated withdrawal. Precipitated withdrawal can occur in any patient if buprenorphine is administered when other opioid agonist drugs are in circulation. Precipitated opioid withdrawal, if it occurs, starts within 1–3 hours of the first buprenorphine dose and peaks at around 6 hours. Non-opioid adjunctive therapy, such as lofexidine (p. 347), may be required if symptoms are severe.

To reduce the risk of precipitated withdrawal, the first dose of buprenorphine should be given when the patient is exhibiting signs of withdrawal, or 6–12 hours after the last use of heroin (or other short-acting opioid), or 24–48 hours after the last dose of methadone. It is possible to titrate the dose of buprenorphine within one week—more rapidly than with methadone therapy—but care is still needed to avoid toxicity or precipitated withdrawal; dividing the dose on the first day may be useful.

In patients taking methadone who want to switch to buprenorphine, the dose of methadone should be reduced to a maximum of 30 mg daily before starting buprenorphine treatment. If the dose of methadone is over 10 mg daily, buprenorphine can be started at a dose of 4 mg daily and titrated according to requirements; if the methadone dose is below 10 mg daily, buprenorphine can be started at a dose of 2 mg daily.

Buprenorphine should not normally be used in patients with liver dysfunction. Baseline liver function tests and documentation of viral hepatitis status is recommended before commencing therapy, and regular liver function tests should be performed throughout treatment.

A combination preparation containing buprenorphine with naloxone (*Suboxone®*, p. 346) can be prescribed for patients when there is a risk of dose diversion for parenteral administration; the naloxone component precipitates withdrawal if the preparation is injected, but it has little effect when the preparation is taken sublingually.

Methadone Methadone, a long-acting opioid agonist, is usually administered in a single daily dose as methadone oral solution 1 mg/mL. Patients with a long history of opioid misuse, those who typically abuse a variety of sedative drugs and alcohol, and those who experience increased anxiety during withdrawal of opioids may prefer methadone to buprenorphine because it has a more pronounced sedative effect.

Methadone is initiated at least 8 hours after the last heroin dose, provided that there is objective evidence of withdrawal symptoms. A supplementary dose on the first day may be considered if there is evidence of persistent opioid withdrawal symptoms. Because of the long half-life, plasma concentrations progressively rise during initial treatment even if the patient remains on the same daily dose (it takes 3–10 days for plasma concentrations to reach steady-state in patients on a stable dose); a dose tolerated on the first day of treatment may become a toxic dose on the third day as cumulative toxicity develops. Thus, titration to the optimal dose in methadone maintenance treatment may take several weeks.

Pregnancy Acute withdrawal of opioids should be avoided in pregnancy because it can cause fetal death. Opioid substitution therapy is recommended during pregnancy because it carries a lower risk to the fetus than continued use of illicit drugs. If a woman who is stabilised on methadone or buprenorphine for treatment of opioid dependence becomes pregnant, therapy should be continued [buprenorphine is not licensed for use in pregnancy]. Many pregnant patients choose a withdrawal regimen, but withdrawal during the first trimester should be avoided because it is associated with an increased risk of spontaneous miscarriage. Withdrawal of methadone or buprenorphine should be undertaken gradually during the second trimester; for example, the dose of methadone may be reduced by 2–3 mg every 3–5 days. If illicit drug use occurs, the

4 Central nervous system

4 Central nervous system

patient should be re-stabilised at the optimal mainte-nance dose and consideration should be given to stop-ping the withdrawal regimen.

Further withdrawal of methadone or buprenorphine in the third trimester is not recommended because mater-nal withdrawal, even if mild, is associated with fetal distress, stillbirth, and the risk of neonatal mortality. Drug metabolism can be increased in the third trimester; it may be necessary to either increase the dose of methadone or change to twice-daily consumption (or a combination of both strategies) to prevent withdrawal symptoms from developing.

The neonate should be monitored for respiratory depression and signs of withdrawal if the mother is prescribed high doses of opioid substitute.

Signs of neonatal withdrawal from opioids usually develop 24–72 hours after delivery but symptoms may be delayed for up to 14 days, so monitoring may be required for several weeks. Symptoms include a high-pitched cry, rapid breathing, hungry but ineffective suckling, and excessive wakefulness; severe, but rare symptoms include hypertonicity and convulsions.

Breast-feeding   The dose of methadone should be kept as low as possible in breast-feeding mothers and the infant should be monitored for sedation (high doses of methadone carry an increased risk of sedation and respiratory depression in the neonate).

Buprenorphine is excreted in low concentrations in breast milk and has low oral bioavailability; however, neonates should be monitored for drowsiness, adequate weight gain, and developmental milestones.

Increased sleepiness, breathing difficulties, or limpness in breast-fed babies of mothers taking opioid substitutes should be reported urgently to a healthcare professional.

BUPRENORPHINE

Indications   adjunct in the treatment of opioid dep-endence; premedication, peri-operative analgesia, analgesia in other situations (section 4.7.2)

Cautions   see Buprenorphine in section 4.7.2 and notes above; caution if pre-existing liver enzyme abnormalities, hepatitis B or C infection, or conco-mitant use of hepatotoxic drugs

Contra-indications   see notes in section 4.7.2

Hepatic impairment   see notes in section 4.7.2

Renal impairment   see notes in section 4.7.2

Pregnancy   see notes above

Breast-feeding   see notes above

Side-effects   see Buprenorphine, section 4.7.2

Dose

• By sublingual administration, ADULT and CHILD over 16 years, initially, 0.8–4 mg on day 1, adjusted if neces-sary by 2–4 mg daily to usual dose of 12–24 mg daily (max. 32 mg daily); withdraw gradually

Buprenorphine (Non-proprietary) CD3
Tablets (sublingual), buprenorphine (as hydro-chloride) 400 micrograms, net price 7-tab pack = £1.60; 2 mg, 7-tab pack = £2.12; 8 mg, 7-tab pack = £4.13. Label: 2, 26

Subutex® (Reckitt Benckiser) CD3
Tablets (sublingual), buprenorphine (as hydro-chloride) 400 micrograms, net price 7-tab pack = £1.60; 2 mg, 7-tab pack = £6.35; 8 mg, 7-tab pack = £19.05. Label: 2, 26

◢ With naloxone

Suboxone® (Reckitt Benckiser) ▼ CD3
Suboxone 2 mg/500 micrograms tablets (sublingual), buprenorphine (as hydrochloride) 2 mg, naloxone (as hydrochloride) 500 micrograms, net price 28-tab pack = £25.40. Label: 2, 26
Suboxone 8 mg/2 mg tablets (sublingual), bupren-orphine (as hydrochloride) 8 mg, naloxone (as hydrochloride) 2 mg, net price 28-tab pack = £76.19. Label: 2, 26
Dose expressed as buprenorphine, ADULT and CHILD over 15 years, initially 2-4 mg once daily (an additional dose of 2–4 mg may be administered on day 1 depending on the individual patient's requirement), increased in steps of 2–8 mg according to response; max. 24 mg daily; total weekly dose may be divided and given on alternate days or 3 times weekly (but max. 24 mg daily)
Note The *Scottish Medicines Consortium* (p. 4) has advised (February 2007) that *Suboxone*® should be restricted for use in patients in whom methadone is not suitable

METHADONE HYDROCHLORIDE

Indications   adjunct in treatment of opioid depend-ence, see notes above; analgesia (section 4.7.2); cough in terminal disease (section 3.9.1)

Cautions   see Methadone, section 4.7.2

Contra-indications   see Methadone, section 4.7.2

Hepatic impairment   see notes in section 4.7.2

Renal impairment   see notes in section 4.7.2

Pregnancy   see notes above

Breast-feeding   see notes above

Side-effects   see Methadone, section 4.7.2; overdo-sage: see Emergency Treatment of Poisoning, p. 38
Important Methadone, even in low doses is a **special hazard** for children; non-dependent adults are also at risk of toxicity; dependent adults are at risk if tolerance is incorrectly assessed during induction
Incompatibility Syrup preserved with hydroxybenzoate (parabens) esters may be incompatible with methadone hydrochloride.

Dose

• Initially 10–30 mg daily, (10–20 mg daily if tolerance low or not known, up to 40 mg daily if tolerance high and under supervision of experienced prescriber); increased as necessary during first week by 5–10 mg daily (max. weekly increase 30 mg) until no signs of withdrawal nor evidence of intoxication; then increased every few days as necessary up to usual dose range 60–120 mg daily; CHILD not recommended (see also important note above)

Note Methadone hydrochloride doses in the BNF may differ from those in the product literature

Methadone (Non-proprietary) CD2
Oral solution 1 mg/mL, methadone hydrochloride 1 mg/mL, net price 100 mL = £1.39, 500 mL = £6.95, 2.5 L = £32.10. Label: 2
Sugar free oral solution 1 mg/mL, methadone hydro-chloride 1 mg/mL, net price 30 mL = 62p, 50 mL = £1.04, 100 mL = £2.08, 500 mL = £6.30, 2.5 L = £32.50. Label: 2
Brands include *Metharose*® (sugar-free), *Physeptone* (sugar-free)
Important Methadone oral solution 1 mg/mL is 2½ times the strength of Methadone Linctus (section 3.9.1). Many preparations of Methadone oral solution are licensed for opioid drug addiction only but some are also licensed for analgesia in severe pain
Injection, methadone hydrochloride 25 mg/mL, net price 2-mL amp = £1.77; 50 mg/mL, 1-mL amp = £1.77
Brands include *Synastone*®

Methadose® (Rosemont) CD2

Oral concentrate, methadone hydrochloride 10 mg/mL (blue), net price 150 mL = £12.01; 20 mg/mL (brown), 150 mL = £24.02. Label: 2

Note The final strength of the methadone mixture to be dispensed to the patient must be specified on the prescription

Important Care is required in prescribing and dispensing the **correct strength** since any confusion could lead to an overdose; this preparation should be dispensed only **after dilution** as appropriate with *Methadose® Diluent* (life of diluted solution 3 months) and is for drug dependent persons

---

Adjunctive therapy and symptomatic treatment

Adjunctive therapy may be required for the management of opioid withdrawal symptoms. **Loperamide** (p. 59) may be used for the control of diarrhoea; **mebeverine** (p. 49) for controlling stomach cramps; **paracetamol** (p. 281) and **non-steroidal anti-inflammatory drugs** (p. 716) for muscular pains and headaches; **metoclopramide** (p. 275) or **prochlorperazine** (p. 274) may be useful for nausea or vomiting. Topical **rubefacients** (p. 752) can be helpful for relieving muscle pain associated with methadone withdrawal. If a patient is suffering from insomnia, short-acting **benzodiazepines** (section 4.1) or **zopiclone** (p. 229) may be prescribed, but because of the potential for abuse, prescriptions should be limited to a short course of a few days only. If anxiety or agitation is severe, specialist advice should be sought.

Lofexidine   Lofexidine is an alpha₂-adrenergic agonist. It may alleviate some of the physical symptoms of opioid withdrawal by attenuating the increase in adrenergic neurotransmission that occurs during opioid withdrawal. Lofexidine can be prescribed as an adjuvant to opioid substitution therapy, initiated either at the same time as the opioid substitute or during withdrawal of the opioid substitute. Alternatively, lofexidine may be prescribed instead of an opioid substitute in patients who have mild or uncertain dependence (including young people), and those with a short history of illicit drug use. The patient should take part of the dose at bedtime to offset insomnia associated with opioid withdrawal.

Monitoring of blood pressure and pulse rate is recommended on initiation, for at least 72 hours or until a stable dose is achieved, and on discontinuation; treatment should be discontinued gradually over 2–4 days to reduce the risk of rebound hypertension.

▌LOFEXIDINE HYDROCHLORIDE

Indications   management of symptoms of opioid withdrawal

Cautions   severe coronary insufficiency, recent myocardial infarction, cerebrovascular disease, bradycardia, hypotension (monitor pulse rate and blood pressure); history of QT prolongation, concomitant administration of drugs that prolong QT interval; metabolic disturbances; withdraw gradually over 2–4 days (or longer) to minimise risk of rebound hypertension and associated symptoms; depression; **interactions:** Appendix 1 (lofexidine)

Renal impairment   caution in chronic impairment

Pregnancy   use only if benefit outweighs risk—no information available

Breast-feeding   use only if benefit outweighs risk—no information available

Side-effects   dry mucous membranes; hypotension; bradycardia; dizziness; drowsiness; QT-interval prolongation also reported

Dose

- ADULT and CHILD over 12 years, initially 800 micrograms daily in divided doses, increased as necessary in steps of 400–800 micrograms daily to max. 2.4 mg daily in divided doses; max. single dose 800 micrograms; recommended duration of treatment 7–10 days if no opioid use (but longer may be required)

Note Lofexidine unlicensed for children under 18 years of age

BritLofex® (Genus) PoM

Tablets, peach, f/c, lofexidine hydrochloride 200 micrograms, net price 60-tab pack = £61.79. Label: 2

Opioid-receptor antagonists

Naloxone is an opioid-receptor antagonist used to reverse opioid overdose. Patients dependant on opioids can be given a supply of naloxone to be used in case of accidental overdose; see Emergency Treatment of Poisoning, p. 38.

Naltrexone is an opioid-receptor antagonist that precipitates withdrawal symptoms in opioid-dependent subjects. Because the effects of opioid-receptor agonists are blocked by naltrexone, it is prescribed as an aid to prevent relapse in formerly opioid-dependent patients.

> **NICE guidance**
> **Naltrexone for the management of opioid dependence** (January 2007)
> Naltrexone is recommended for the prevention of relapse in formerly opioid-dependent patients who are motivated to remain in a supportive care abstinence programme. Naltrexone should be administered under supervision and its effectiveness in preventing opioid misuse reviewed regularly.
> www.nice.org.uk/TA115

▌NALTREXONE HYDROCHLORIDE

Indications   adjunct to prevent relapse in formerly opioid-dependent patients (who have remained opioid-free for at least 7–10 days); adjunct to prevent relapse in formerly alcohol-dependent patients (section 4.10.1); treatment should be initiated and supervised by an appropriate specialist

Cautions   liver function tests needed before and during treatment; test for opioid dependence with naloxone before treatment; avoid concomitant use of opioids but increased dose of opioid analgesic may be required for pain (monitor for opioid intoxication)

Note Patients should be warned that an attempt to overcome the blockade of opioid receptors by overdosing could result in acute opioid intoxication

Contra-indications   patients currently dependent on opioids

Hepatic impairment   avoid in acute hepatitis, hepatic failure, or severe impairment

Renal impairment   avoid in severe impairment

Pregnancy   use only if benefit outweighs risk

Breast-feeding   avoid—potential toxicity

4

Central nervous system

Central nervous system 4

Side-effects nausea, vomiting, abdominal pain, diarrhoea, constipation, reduced appetite, increased thirst, chest pain, anxiety, sleep disorders, headache, increased energy, irritability, mood swings, dizziness, chills, urinary retention, delayed ejaculation, decreased potency, joint and muscle pain, increased lacrimation, rash, increased sweating; *rarely* hepatic dysfunction, depression, suicidal ideation, tinnitus, speech disorders; *very rarely* hallucinations, tremor, idiopathic thrombocytopenia, exanthema

Dose

- Relapse prevention in opioid dependence, ADULT over 18 years (initiate in specialist clinics only), 25 mg initially then 50 mg daily; total weekly dose (350 mg) may be divided and given on 3 days of the week for improved compliance (e.g. 100 mg on Monday and Wednesday, and 150 mg on Friday)
- Relapse prevention in alcohol dependence, ADULT and CHILD over 16 years [unlicensed under 18 years], 25 mg [unlicensed dose] on first day, increased to 50 mg daily if tolerated

Naltrexone (Non-proprietary) PoM

Tablets, naltrexone hydrochloride 50 mg, net price 28-tab pack = £22.34

Brands include *Adepend®*, *Opizone®*

Nalorex® (Bristol-Myers Squibb) PoM

Tablets, yellow, f/c, scored, naltrexone hydrochloride 50 mg, net price 28-tab pack = £22.34

4.11 Drugs for dementia

Acetylcholinesterase inhibiting drugs are used in the treatment of Alzheimer's disease, specifically for mild to moderate disease. Rivastigmine is also licensed for mild to moderate dementia associated with Parkinson's disease. The evidence to support the use of these drugs relates to their cognitive enhancement.

Treatment with drugs for dementia should be initiated and supervised only by a specialist experienced in the management of dementia.

Benefit is assessed by repeating the cognitive assessment at around 3 months. Such assessment cannot demonstrate how the disease may have progressed in the absence of treatment but it can give a good guide to response. Up to half the patients given these drugs will show a slower rate of cognitive decline. Drugs for dementia should be discontinued in those thought not to be responding. Many specialists repeat the cognitive assessment 4 to 6 weeks after discontinuation to assess deterioration; if significant deterioration occurs during this short period, consideration should be given to restarting therapy.

Donepezil is a reversible inhibitor of acetylcholinesterase. **Galantamine** is a reversible inhibitor of acetylcholinesterase and it also has nicotinic receptor agonist properties. **Rivastigmine** is a reversible non-competitive inhibitor of acetylcholinesterases; it is also licensed for treating mild to moderate dementia in Parkinson's disease.

Acetylcholinesterase inhibitors can cause unwanted dose-related cholinergic effects and should be started at a low dose and the dose increased according to response and tolerability.

Memantine is a glutamate receptor antagonist; it is licensed for treating moderate to severe Alzheimer's disease.

> **NICE guidance**
> **Donepezil, galantamine, rivastigmine, and memantine for the treatment of Alzheimer's disease (March 2011)**
>
> Donepezil, galantamine, and rivastigmine can be used for the treatment of mild to moderate Alzheimer's disease. Memantine can be used for moderate Alzheimer's disease in patients who are unable to take acetylcholinesterase inhibitors, and for patients with severe disease; combination treatment with memantine and an acetylcholinesterase inhibitor is not recommended. Treatment should only be prescribed under the following conditions:
>
> - Alzheimer's disease must be diagnosed and treatment initiated by a specialist; treatment can be continued by general practitioners under a shared-care protocol;
> - the carers' views of the condition should be sought before and during treatment;
> - treatment should continue only if it is considered to have a worthwhile effect on cognitive, global, functional, or behavioural symptoms.
>
> Healthcare professionals should not rely solely on assessment scales to determine the severity of Alzheimer's disease when the patient has learning or other disabilities, or other communication difficulties.
>
> www.nice.org.uk/TA217

DONEPEZIL HYDROCHLORIDE

Indications mild to moderate dementia in Alzheimer's disease

Cautions sick sinus syndrome or other supraventricular conduction abnormalities; susceptibility to peptic ulcers; asthma, chronic obstructive pulmonary disease; concomitant antipsychotic treatment— increased risk of neuroleptic malignant syndrome; **interactions**: Appendix 1 (parasympathomimetics)

Hepatic impairment caution in mild to moderate impairment, no information available for severe impairment

Side-effects nausea, vomiting, anorexia, diarrhoea; fatigue, insomnia, headache, dizziness, syncope, abnormal dreams, hallucinations, agitation, aggression; muscle cramps; urinary incontinence; rash, pruritus; *less commonly* gastric and duodenal ulcers, gastro-intestinal haemorrhage, bradycardia, seizures; *rarely* sino-atrial block, AV block, hepatitis, extra-pyramidal symptoms; potential for bladder outflow obstruction; *very rarely* neuroleptic malignant syndrome

Dose

- Initially 5 mg once daily at bedtime, increased if necessary after one month to max. 10 mg daily

Donepezil (Non-proprietary) PoM

Tablets, donepezil hydrochloride 5 mg, net price 28-tab pack =£1.33; 10 mg, 28-tab pack = £1.76.

Orodispersible tablets, donepezil hydrochloride 5 mg, net price 28-tab pack = £7.17; 10 mg, 28-tab pack = £9.57. Counselling, administration

Counselling Donepezil orodispersible tablet should be placed on the tongue, allowed to disperse, and swallowed

Aricept® (Eisai) [PoM]

Tablets, f/c, donepezil hydrochloride 5 mg (white), net price 28-tab pack = £59.85; 10 mg (yellow), 28-tab pack = £83.89.

Aricept Evess® (Eisai) [PoM]

Orodispersible tablets, donepezil hydrochloride 5 mg (white), net price 28-tab pack = £59.85; 10 mg (yellow), 28-tab pack = £83.89. Counselling, administration

Counselling *Aricept Evess®* should be placed on the tongue, allowed to disperse, and swallowed

---

GALANTAMINE

Indications mild to moderate dementia in Alzheimer's disease

Cautions cardiac disease (including sick sinus syndrome or other supraventricular conduction abnormalities; unstable angina, congestive heart failure); electrolyte disturbances; susceptibility to peptic ulcers; asthma, chronic obstructive pulmonary disease, pulmonary infection; avoid in urinary retention, gastro-intestinal obstruction, and while recovering from bladder or gastro-intestinal surgery; history of seizures; **interactions**: Appendix 1 (parasympathomimetics)

Hepatic impairment

* for *immediate-release* preparations in moderate impairment, initially 4 mg once daily (preferably in the morning) for at least 7 days, then 4 mg twice daily for at least 4 weeks; max. 8 mg twice daily; avoid in severe impairment

* for *modified-release* preparations in moderate impairment, initially 8 mg on alternate days (preferably in the morning) for 7 days, then 8 mg once daily for 4 weeks; max. 16 mg daily; avoid in severe impairment

Renal impairment avoid if eGFR less than 9 mL/minute/1.73m²

Pregnancy use with caution

Breast-feeding avoid—no information available

Side-effects vomiting, nausea, abdominal pain, diarrhoea, dyspepsia, anorexia, weight loss, bradycardia, hypertension, syncope, hallucination, depression, dizziness, tremor, headache, drowsiness, malaise, muscle spasm, sweating; *less commonly* taste disturbance, palpitation, arrhythmias, first-degree AV block, hypotension, flushing, paraesthesia, dehydration, seizures, muscular weakness, blurred vision, tinnitus; *rarely* hepatitis, exacerbation of Parkinson's disease

Dose

* Initially 4 mg twice daily for 4 weeks increased to 8 mg twice daily for 4 weeks; maintenance 8–12 mg twice daily

Galantamine (Non-proprietary) [PoM]

Tablets, galantamine (as hydrobromide) 8 mg, net price, 56-tab pack = £59.29; 12 mg, 56-tab pack = £74.10. Label: 3, 21

Oral solution, galantamine (as hydrobromide) 4 mg/mL, net price 100 mL =£437.00. Label: 3, 21

Note Sugar-free versions are available and can be ordered by specifying sugar-free on the prescription

Reminyl® (Shire) [PoM]

Tablets, f/c, galantamine (as hydrobromide) 8 mg (pink), net price 56-tab pack = £68.32; 12 mg (orange-brown), 56-tab pack = £84.00 Label: 3, 21

Oral solution, sugar-free, galantamine (as hydrobromide) 4 mg/mL, net price 100 mL with pipette = £120.00. Label: 3, 21

◢ **Modified release**

Galantamine m/r preparations [PoM]

Capsules, m/r, galantamine 8 mg; 16 mg; 24 mg. Label: 3, 21, 25

Brands include *Acumor XL®, Galsya XL®, Gatalin XL®, Lotprosin XL®, Reminyl XL®*

Dose initially 8 mg once daily for 4 weeks increased to 16 mg once daily for 4 weeks; maintenance 16–24 mg daily

---

MEMANTINE HYDROCHLORIDE

Indications moderate to severe dementia in Alzheimer's disease

Cautions history of convulsions; **interactions**: Appendix 1 (memantine)

Hepatic impairment avoid in severe impairment—no information available

Renal impairment reduce dose to 10 mg daily if eGFR 30–49 mL/minute/1.73 m², if well tolerated after at least 7 days dose can be increased in steps to 20 mg daily; reduce dose to 10 mg daily if eGFR 5–29 mL/minute/1.73 m²; avoid if eGFR less than 5 mL/minute/1.73 m²

Side-effects constipation; hypertension; dyspnoea; headache, dizziness, drowsiness; *less commonly* vomiting, thrombosis, heart failure, confusion, fatigue, hallucinations, and abnormal gait; *very rarely* seizures; pancreatitis, psychosis, depression, and suicidal ideation also reported

Dose

* Initially 5 mg once daily, increased in steps of 5 mg at weekly intervals to max. 20 mg daily

Memantine (Non-proprietary) [PoM]

Tablets, memantine 10 mg, net price 28-tab pack = £4.89, 56-tab pack = £15.67; 20 mg, 28-tab pack = £12.71

Brands include *Maruxa®, Nemdatine®*

Ebixa® (Lundbeck) [PoM]

Tablets, f/c, scored, memantine hydrochloride 10 mg (yellow), net price 28-tab pack = £34.50, 56-tab pack = £69.01, 112-tab pack = £138.01; 20 mg (red), 28-tab pack = £69.01; treatment initiation pack, 7 × 5 mg (white), 7 × 10 mg, 7 × 15 mg (orange), and 7 × 20 mg = £43.13

Oral solution, memantine hydrochloride 5 mg/actuation (10 mg/mL), net price 50-mL pump pack = £61.61, 100-mL pump pack = £123.23

Counselling Solution should be dosed onto a spoon or into a glass of water

---

RIVASTIGMINE

Indications see under Dose

Cautions gastric or duodenal ulcers (or susceptibility to ulcers); monitor body-weight; sick sinus syndrome, conduction abnormalities; history of asthma or chronic obstructive pulmonary disease; history of

4 Central nervous system

4 Central nervous system

seizures; bladder outflow obstruction; risk of fatal overdose with patch administration errors (see Counselling below); **interactions:** Appendix 1 (parasympathomimetics)

Hepatic impairment titrate according to individual tolerability in mild to moderate impairment; use with caution in severe impairment—no information available

Renal impairment titrate according to individual tolerability

Side-effects nausea, vomiting, diarrhoea, dyspepsia, anorexia, weight loss, increased salivation, abdominal pain, bradycardia, dizziness, headache, drowsiness, malaise, agitation, anxiety, tremor, confusion, insomnia, extrapyramidal symptoms (and worsening of Parkinson's disease), urinary incontinence, sweating; *less commonly* atrial fibrillation, AV block, depression, syncope; *rarely* gastric and duodenal ulceration, angina, seizures, rash; *very rarely* gastrointestinal haemorrhage, pancreatitis, tachycardia, hypertension, hallucinations; *also reported* dehydration, hepatitis, restlessness, aggression, sick sinus syndrome, skin hypersensitivity reactions

Note Transdermal administration less likely to cause gastrointestinal disturbance

Note Treatment should be interrupted if gastro-intestinal side-effects occur and withheld until their resolution—retitrate dose if necessary

Dose

- Mild to moderate dementia in Alzheimer's disease or in Parkinson's disease, by mouth, initially 1.5 mg twice daily, increased in steps of 1.5 mg twice daily at intervals of at least 2 weeks according to response and tolerance; usual range 3–6 mg twice daily; max. 6 mg twice daily; if treatment interrupted for more than several days, treatment should be retitrated from 1.5 mg twice daily

- Mild to moderate dementia in Alzheimer's disease, by transdermal application, initially apply 4.6 mg/24 hours patch to clean, dry, non-hairy, non-irritated skin on back, upper arm, or chest, removing after 24 hours and siting a replacement patch on a different area (avoid using the same area for 14 days); after at least 4 weeks, and if well tolerated, increase to usual maintenance dose of 9.5 mg/24 hours patch daily; after a further 6 months if well tolerated and cognitive deterioration or functional decline are demonstrated, the dose can be increased to 13.3 mg/24 hours patch daily (caution in patients with body-weight less than 50 kg); if treatment interrupted for more than three days, treatment should be retitrated from 4.6 mg/24 hours patch

Note When switching from oral to transdermal therapy, patients taking 3–6 mg by mouth daily should initially switch to 4.6 mg/24 hours patch, then titrate as above. Patients taking 9 mg by mouth daily should switch to 9.5 mg/24 hours patch if oral dose stable and well tolerated; if oral dose not stable or well tolerated. patients should switch to 4.6 mg/24 hours patch, then titrate as above. Patients taking 12 mg by mouth daily should switch to 9.5 mg/24 hours patch. The first patch should be applied on the day following the last oral dose

Rivastigmine (Non-proprietary) ⒫ℴⓂ

Capsules, rivastigmine (as hydrogen tartrate) 1.5 mg, net price 28-cap pack = £3.14, 56-cap pack = £11.98; 3 mg, 28-cap pack = £3.27, 56-cap pack = £6.54; 4.5 mg, 28-cap pack = £17.95, 56-cap pack = £21.01; 6 mg, 28-cap pack = £16.35, 56-cap pack = £18.76. Label: 21, 25

Brands include *Kerstipon*®

Exelon® (Novartis) ⒫ℴⓂ

Capsules, rivastigmine (as hydrogen tartrate) 1.5 mg (yellow), net price 28-cap pack = £33.25, 56-cap pack = £66.51; 3 mg (orange), 28-cap pack = £33.25, 56-cap pack = £66.51; 4.5 mg (red), 28-cap pack = £33.25, 56-cap pack = £66.51; 6 mg (red/orange), 28-cap pack = £33.25, 56-cap pack = £66.51. Label: 21, 25

Oral solution, rivastigmine (as hydrogen tartrate) 2 mg/mL, net price 120 mL (with oral syringe) = £99.14. Label: 21

Patches, self-adhesive, beige, rivastigmine 4.6 mg/ 24 hours, net price 30 = £77.97; 9.5 mg/24 hours, 30 = £77.97; 13.3 mg/24 hours, 30 = £77.97. Counselling, administration

Counselling Advise patients and carers of patch administration instructions, particularly to remove the previous day's patch before applying the new patch—consult product literature

Note The *Scottish Medicines Consortium* (p. 4) has advised (October 2007) that *Exelon*® patches should be restricted for use in patients with moderately severe Alzheimer's disease under the conditions of the NICE guidance (September 2007) and when a transdermal patch is an appropriate choice of formulation

5 Infections

This chapter also includes advice on the drug management of the following:

anthrax, p. 406

Clostridium difficile infection, p. 353

bacterial infections: table 1, summary of antibacterial treatment, p. 353

bacterial infections: table 2, summary of antibacterial prophylaxis, p. 363

Lyme disease, p. 369

MRSA infections, p. 368

oral infections, p. 352, p. 360, p. 411

Notifiable diseases

Doctors must notify the Proper Officer of the local authority (usually the consultant in communicable disease control) when attending a patient suspected of suffering from any of the diseases listed below; a form is available from the Proper Officer.

Anthrax	Mumps
Botulism	Paratyphoid fever
Brucellosis	Plague
Cholera	Poliomyelitis, acute
Diarrhoea (infectious bloody)	Rabies
Diphtheria	Rubella
Encephalitis, acute	SARS
Food poisoning	Scarlet fever
Haemolytic uraemic syndrome	Smallpox
	Streptococcal disease
Haemorrhagic fever (viral)	(Group A, invasive)
Hepatitis, viral	Tetanus
Legionnaires' disease	Tuberculosis
Leprosy	Typhoid fever
Malaria	Typhus
Measles	Whooping cough
Meningitis	Yellow fever
Meningococcal septicaemia	

Note It is good practice for doctors to also inform the consultant in communicable disease control of

5 Infections

instances of other infections (e.g. psittacosis) where there could be a public health risk.

5.1 Antibacterial drugs

Choice of a suitable drug   Before selecting an antibacterial the clinician must first consider two factors—the patient and the known or likely causative organism. Factors related to the patient which must be considered include history of allergy, renal and hepatic function, susceptibility to infection (i.e. whether immunocompromised), ability to tolerate drugs by mouth, severity of illness, ethnic origin, age, whether taking other medication and, if female, whether pregnant, breast-feeding or taking an oral contraceptive.

The known or likely organism and its antibacterial sensitivity, in association with the above factors, will suggest one or more antibacterials, the final choice depending on the microbiological, pharmacological, and toxicological properties.

An example of a rational approach to the selection of an antibacterial is treatment of a urinary-tract infection in a patient complaining of nausea and symptoms of a urinary-tract infection in early pregnancy. The organism is reported as being resistant to ampicillin but sensitive to nitrofurantoin (can cause nausea), gentamicin (can be given only by injection and best avoided in pregnancy), tetracycline (causes dental discoloration) and trimethoprim (folate antagonist therefore theoretical teratogenic risk), and cefalexin. The safest antibiotics in pregnancy are the penicillins and cephalosporins; therefore, cefalexin would be indicated for this patient.

The principles involved in selection of an antibacterial must allow for a number of variables including changing renal and hepatic function, increasing bacterial resistance, and information on side-effects. Duration of therapy, dosage, and route of administration depend on site, type and severity of infection and response.

Antibacterial policies   Local policies often limit the antibacterials that may be used to achieve reasonable economy consistent with adequate cover, and to reduce the development of resistant organisms. A policy may indicate a range of drugs for general use, and permit other drugs only on the advice of the microbiologist or physician responsible for the control of infectious diseases.

Before starting therapy   The following precepts should be considered before starting:

- Viral infections should not be treated with antibacterials. However, antibacterials may be used to treat secondary bacterial infection (e.g. bacterial pneumonia secondary to influenza);

- Samples should be taken for culture and sensitivity testing; **'blind'** antibacterial prescribing for unexplained pyrexia usually leads to further difficulty in establishing the diagnosis;

- Knowledge of **prevalent organisms** and their current sensitivity is of great help in choosing an antibacterial before bacteriological confirmation is available. Generally, narrow-spectrum antibacterials are preferred to broad-spectrum antibacterials unless there is a clear clinical indication (e.g. life-threatening sepsis);

- The **dose** of an antibacterial varies according to a number of factors including age, weight, hepatic function, renal function, and severity of infection. The prescribing of the so-called 'standard' dose in serious infections may result in failure of treatment or even death of the patient; therefore it is important to prescribe a dose appropriate to the condition. An inadequate dose may also increase the likelihood of antibacterial resistance. On the other hand, for an antibacterial with a narrow margin between the toxic and therapeutic dose (e.g. an aminoglycoside) it is also important to avoid an excessive dose and the concentration of the drug in the plasma may need to be monitored;

- The **route** of administration of an antibacterial often depends on the severity of the infection. Life-threatening infections require intravenous therapy. Antibacterials that are well absorbed may be given by mouth even for some serious infections. Parenteral administration is also appropriate when the oral route cannot be used (e.g. because of vomiting) or if absorption is inadequate. Whenever possible, painful intramuscular injections should be avoided in children;

- **Duration** of therapy depends on the nature of the infection and the response to treatment. Courses should not be unduly prolonged because they encourage resistance, they may lead to side-effects and they are costly. However, in certain infections such as tuberculosis or osteomyelitis it may be necessary to treat for prolonged periods. Conversely a single dose of an antibacterial may cure uncomplicated urinary-tract infections. The prescription for an antibacterial should specify the duration of treatment or the date when treatment is to be reviewed.

Oral bacterial infections   Antibacterial drugs should only be prescribed for the *treatment* of oral infections on the basis of defined need. They may be used in conjunction with (but not as an alternative to) other appropriate measures, such as providing drainage or extracting a tooth.

The 'blind' prescribing of an antibacterial for unexplained pyrexia, cervical lymphadenopathy, or facial swelling can lead to difficulty in establishing the diagnosis. In severe oral infections, a sample should always be taken for bacteriology.

Oral infections which may require antibacterial treatment include acute periapical or periodontal abscess, cellulitis, acutely created oral-antral communication (and acute sinusitis), severe pericoronitis, localised osteitis, acute necrotising ulcerative gingivitis, and destructive forms of chronic periodontal disease. Most of these infections are readily resolved by the early establishment of drainage and removal of the cause (typically an infected necrotic pulp). Antibacterials may be required if treatment has to be delayed, in immunocompromised patients, or in those with conditions such as diabetes or Paget's disease; see also Table 1, section 5.1. Certain rarer infections including bacterial sialadenitis, osteomyelitis, actinomycosis, and infections involving fascial spaces such as Ludwig's angina, require antibiotics and specialist hospital care.

Antibacterial drugs may also be useful after dental surgery in some cases of spreading infection. Infection may spread to involve local lymph nodes, to fascial spaces (where it can cause airway obstruction), or into the bloodstream (where it can lead to cavernous sinus thrombosis and other serious complications). Extension of an infection can also lead to maxillary sinusitis; osteomyelitis is a complication, which usually arises when host resistance is reduced.

If the oral infection fails to respond to antibacterial treatment within 48 hours the antibacterial should be changed, preferably on the basis of bacteriological investigation. Failure to respond may also suggest an incorrect diagnosis, lack of essential additional mea-sures (such as drainage), poor host resistance, or poor patient compliance.

Combination of a penicillin (or a macrolide) with metronidazole may sometimes be helpful for the treatment of severe oral infections or oral infections that have not responded to initial antibacterial treatment.

See also **Penicillins** (section 5.1.1), **Cephalosporins** (section 5.1.2), **Tetracyclines** (section 5.1.3), **Macrolides** (section 5.1.5), **Clindamycin** (section 5.1.6), **Metronidazole** (section 5.1.11), **Fusidic acid** (section 13.10.1.2).

Superinfection   In general, broad-spectrum antibacterial drugs such as the cephalosporins are more likely to be associated with adverse reactions related to the selection of resistant organisms e.g. *fungal infections* or *antibiotic-associated colitis* (pseudomembranous colitis); other problems associated with superinfection include vaginitis and pruritus ani.

Therapy   Suggested treatment is shown in table 1. When the pathogen has been isolated treatment may be changed to a more appropriate antibacterial if necessary. If no bacterium is cultured the antibacterial can be continued or stopped on clinical grounds. Infections for which prophylaxis is useful are listed in table 2.

Table 1. Summary of antibacterial therapy

> If treating a patient suspected of suffering from a notifiable disease, the consultant in communicable disease control should be informed (see p. 351)

Gastro-intestinal system

Gastro-enteritis

Frequently self-limiting and may not be bacterial.

> Antibacterial not usually indicated

Campylobacter enteritis

Frequently self-limiting; treat if immunocompromised or if severe infection.

> Clarithromycin[1]
>
> *Alternative*, ciprofloxacin
>> Strains with decreased sensitivity to ciprofloxacin isolated frequently

Salmonella (non-typhoid)

Treat invasive or severe infection. Do not treat less severe infection unless there is a risk of developing invasive infection (e.g. immunocompromised patients, those with haemoglobinopathy, or children under 6 months of age).

> Ciprofloxacin *or* cefotaxime

Shigellosis

Antibacterial not indicated for mild cases.

> Ciprofloxacin *or* azithromycin
>
> *Alternatives if micro-organism sensitive*, amoxicillin *or* trimethoprim

---

1. Where clarithromycin is suggested azithromycin or erythromycin may be used

Typhoid fever

Infections from Middle-East, South Asia, and South-East Asia may be multiple-antibacterial-resistant and sensitivity should be tested.

Cefotaxime[1]

> Azithromycin may be an alternative in mild or moderate disease caused by multiple-antibacterial-resistant organisms.

Alternative if micro-organism sensitive, ciprofloxacin

Clostridium difficile infection

For first episode of mild to moderate infection, oral metronidazole
> *Suggested duration of treatment* 10–14 days

For second or subsequent episode of infection, for severe infection, for infection not responding to metronidazole, or in patients intolerant of metronidazole, oral vancomycin
> For severe infection in patients with multiple co-morbidities who are receiving treatment with other antibacterials, or for second or subsequent episode of infection, fidaxomicin can replace vancomycin
> *Suggested duration of treatment* 10–14 days

For infection not responding to vancomycin or fidaxomicin, for life-threatening infection, or in patients with ileus, oral vancomycin + i/v metronidazole
> For infection not responding to vancomycin in patients without life-threatening infection or ileus, fidaxomicin can be used instead of vancomycin + metronidazole
> *Suggested duration of treatment* 10–14 days

Biliary-tract infection

Ciprofloxacin *or* gentamicin *or* a cephalosporin

Peritonitis

A cephalosporin + metronidazole *or* gentamicin + metronidazole *or* gentamicin + clindamycin *or* piperacillin with tazobactam alone

Peritonitis: peritoneal dialysis-associated

Vancomycin[2] + ceftazidime added to dialysis fluid *or* vancomycin added to dialysis fluid + ciprofloxacin by mouth
> *Suggested duration of treatment* 14 days or longer

Cardiovascular system

Endocarditis: initial 'blind' therapy

Native valve endocarditis, amoxicillin[3]
> Consider adding low-dose gentamicin
> If penicillin-allergic, or if meticillin-resistant *Staphylococcus aureus* suspected, or if severe sepsis, use vancomycin + low-dose gentamicin
> If severe sepsis with risk factors for Gram-negative infection, use vancomycin + meropenem

If prosthetic valve endocarditis, vancomycin + rifampicin + low-dose gentamicin

Native-valve endocarditis caused by staphylococci

Flucloxacillin
> *Suggested duration of treatment* 4 weeks (at least 6 weeks if secondary lung abscess or osteomyelitis also present)

If penicillin-allergic or if meticillin-resistant Staphylococcus aureus, vancomycin + rifampicin
> *Suggested duration of treatment* 4 weeks (at least 6 weeks if secondary lung abscecess or osteomyelitis also present)

Prosthetic valve endocarditis caused by staphylococci

Flucloxacillin + rifampicin + low-dose gentamicin
> *Suggested duration of treatment* at least 6 weeks; review need to continue gentamicin at 2 weeks—seek specialist advice if gentamicin considered necessary beyond 2 weeks

If penicillin-allergic or if meticillin-resistant Staphylococcus aureus, vancomycin + rifampicin + low-dose gentamicin
> *Suggested duration of treatment* at least 6 weeks; review need to continue gentamicin at 2 weeks—seek specialist advice if gentamicin considered necessary beyond 2 weeks

---

1. Where cefotaxime is suggested ceftriaxone may be used
2. Where vancomycin is suggested teicoplanin may be used
3. Where amoxicillin is suggested ampicillin may be used

Endocarditis caused by fully-sensitive streptococci

Benzylpenicillin

Suggested duration of treatment 4–6 weeks (6 weeks for prosthetic valve endocarditis)

If penicillin-allergic, vancomycin[1] + low-dose gentamicin

Suggested duration of treatment 4–6 weeks (stop gentamicin after 2 weeks)

Endocarditis caused by less-sensitive streptococci

Benzylpenicillin + low-dose gentamicin

Suggested duration of treatment 4–6 weeks (6 weeks for prosthetic valve endocarditis); review need to continue gentamicin at 2 weeks—seek specialist advice if gentamicin considered necessary beyond 2 weeks; stop gentamicin at 2 weeks if micro-organisms moderately sensitive to penicillin

If penicillin-allergic or highly penicillin-resistant, vancomycin[1] + low-dose gentamicin

Suggested duration of treatment 4–6 weeks (6 weeks for prosthetic valve endocarditis); review need to continue gentamicin at 2 weeks—seek specialist advice if gentamicin considered necessary beyond 2 weeks; stop gentamicin at 2 weeks if micro-organisms moderately sensitive to penicillin

Endocarditis caused by enterococci

Amoxicillin[2] + low dose gentamicin *or* benzylpenicillin + low-dose gentamicin

Suggested duration of treatment 4–6 weeks (6 weeks for prosthetic valve endocarditis); review need to continue gentamicin at 2 weeks—seek specialist advice if gentamicin considered necessary beyond 2 weeks

If penicillin-allergic or penicillin-resistant, vancomycin[1] + low-dose gentamicin

Suggested duration of treatment 4–6 weeks (6 weeks for prosthetic valve endocarditis); review need to continue gentamicin at 2 weeks—seek specialist advice if gentamicin considered necessary beyond 2 weeks

If gentamicin resistant, amoxicillin[2]

Add streptomycin (if susceptible) for 2 weeks

Suggested duration of treatment at least 6 weeks

Endocarditis caused by *Haemophilus, Actinobacillus, Cardiobacterium, Eikenella,* and *Kingella* species ('HACEK' micro-organisms)

Amoxicillin[2] + low-dose gentamicin

Suggested duration of treatment 4 weeks (6 weeks for prosthetic valve endocarditis); stop gentamicin after 2 weeks

If amoxicillin-resistant, ceftriaxone[3] + low-dose gentamicin

Suggested duration of treatment 4 weeks (6 weeks for prosthetic valve endocarditis); stop gentamicin after 2 weeks

Respiratory system

Haemophilus influenzae epiglottitis

Cefotaxime[4]

If history of immediate hypersensitivity reaction to penicillin or to cephalosporins, chloramphenicol

Chronic bronchitis: acute exacerbations

Treat if increase in sputum purulence accompanied by an increase in sputum volume or increase in dyspnoea.

Amoxicillin[2] *or* a tetracycline

Some pneumococci and *Haemophilus influenzae* strains tetracycline-resistant; approx. 20% *H. influenzae* strains amoxicillin-resistant.

Suggested duration of treatment 5 days; longer treatment may be necessary in severely ill patients

Alternative, clarithromycin[5]

Suggested duration of treatment 5 days; longer treatment may be necessary in severely ill patients

---

1. Where vancomycin is suggested teicoplanin may be used
2. Where amoxicillin is suggested ampicillin may be used
3. Where ceftriaxone is suggested cefotaxime may be used
4. Where cefotaxime is suggested ceftriaxone may be used
5. Where clarithromycin is suggested azithromycin or erythromycin may be used

Pneumonia: low-severity community-acquired

Amoxicillin[1]

Pneumococci with decreased penicillin sensitivity being isolated, but not yet common in UK.
If atypical pathogens suspected, add clarithromycin[2].
If staphylococci suspected (e. g. in influenza or measles), add flucloxacillin.
Suggested duration of treatment 7 days (14–21 days for infections caused by staphylococci)

Alternatives, doxycycline *or* clarithromycin[2]
Suggested duration of treatment 7 days (14–21 days for infections caused by staphylococci)

Pneumonia: moderate-severity community-acquired

Amoxicillin[1] + clarithromycin[2] *or* doxycycline alone

Pneumococci with decreased penicillin sensitivity being isolated, but not yet common in UK.
If meticillin-resistant *Staphylococcus aureus* suspected, add vancomycin[3].
Suggested duration of treatment 7 days (14–21 days for infections caused by staphylococci)

Pneumonia: high-severity community-acquired

Benzylpenicillin + clarithromycin[2] *or* benzylpenicillin + doxycycline

If meticillin-resistant *Staphylococcus aureus* suspected, add vancomycin[3].
Suggested duration of treatment 7–10 days (may extend treatment to 14–21 days in some cases e.g. if staphylococci suspected)

If life-threatening infection, or if Gram-negative infection suspected, or if co-morbidities present, or if living in long-term residential or nursing home, co-amoxiclav + clarithromycin[2]

If meticillin-resistant *Staphylococcus aureus* suspected, add vancomycin[3]
Suggested duration of treatment 7–10 days (may extend treatment to 14–21 days in some cases e.g. if staphylococci or Gram-negative enteric bacilli suspected)

Alternatives if life-threatening infection, or if Gram-negative infection suspected, or if co-morbidities present, or if living in long-term residential or nursing home, cefuroxime + clarithromycin[2] *or* cefotaxime[4] + clarithromycin[2]

If meticillin-resistant *Staphylococcus aureus* suspected, add vancomycin[3].
Suggested duration of treatment 7–10 days (may extend treatment to 14–21 days in some cases e.g. if staphylococci or Gram-negative enteric bacilli suspected)

Pneumonia possibly caused by atypical pathogens

Clarithromycin[2]

If high-severity Legionella infection, add rifampicin for the first few days.
Suggested duration of treatment 14 days (usually 7–10 days for Legionella)

Alternative if Legionella infection suspected, a quinolone

If high-severity Legionella infection, add clarithromycin[2] or rifampicin for the first few days.
Suggested duration of treatment usually 7–10 days

Alternative for chlamydial or mycoplasma infections, doxycycline
Suggested duration of treatment 14 days

Pneumonia: hospital-acquired

Early-onset infection (less than 5 days after admission to hospital), co-amoxiclav *or* cefuroxime

If life-threatening infection, or if history of antibacterial treatment in the last 3 months, or if resistant microorganisms suspected, treat as for late-onset hospital-acquired pneumonia.
Suggested duration of treatment 7 days

Late-onset infection (more than 5 days after admission to hospital), an antipseudomonal penicillin (e.g. piperacillin with tazobactam) *or* a broad-spectrum cephalosporin (e.g. ceftazidime) *or* another antipseudomonal beta-lactam *or* a quinolone (e.g. ciprofloxacin)

If meticillin-resistant *Staphylococcus aureus* suspected, add vancomycin.
For severe illness caused by *Pseudomonas aeruginosa*, consider adding an aminoglycoside.
Suggested duration of treatment 7 days (longer if *Pseudomonas aeruginosa* confirmed)

---

1. Where amoxicillin is suggested ampicillin may be used
2. Where clarithromycin is suggested azithromycin or erythromycin may be used
3. Where vancomycin is suggested teicoplanin may be used
4. Where cefotaxime is suggested ceftriaxone may be used

██████████ **Central nervous system**

Meningitis: initial empirical therapy

- Transfer patient to hospital urgently
- If *meningococcal disease* (meningitis with non-blanching rash or meningococcal septicaemia) suspected, benzylpenicillin (see p. 367 for dose) should be given before transfer to hospital, so long as this does not delay the transfer. If a patient with suspected bacterial meningitis without non-blanching rash cannot be transferred to hospital urgently, benzylpenicillin (see p. 367 for dose) should be given before the transfer. Cefotaxime (section 5.1.2) may be an alternative in penicillin allergy; chloramphenicol (section 5.1.7) may be used if history of immediate hypersensitivity reaction to penicillin or to cephalosporins.
- In hospital, consider adjunctive treatment with dexamethasone (particularly if pneumococcal meningitis suspected in adults; section 6.3.2), preferably starting before or with first dose of antibacterial, but no later than 12 hours after starting antibacterial; avoid dexamethasone in septic shock, meningococcal septicaemia, or if immunocompromised, or in meningitis following surgery.

In hospital, if aetiology unknown

Adult and child 3 months–50 years, cefotaxime[1]

> Consider adding vancomycin if prolonged or multiple use of other antibacterials in the last 3 months, or if travelled, in the last 3 months, to areas outside the UK with highly penicillin- and cephalosporin-resistant pneumococci.
>
> *Suggested duration of treatment* at least 10 days

Adult over 50 years, cefotaxime[1] + amoxicillin[2]

> Consider adding vancomycin if prolonged or multiple use of other antibacterials in the last 3 months, or if travelled, in the last 3 months, to areas outside the UK with highly penicillin- and cephalosporin-resistant pneumococci.
>
> *Suggested duration of treatment* at least 10 days

Meningitis caused by meningococci

Benzylpenicillin *or* cefotaxime[1]

> *Suggested duration of treatment* 7 days.
>
> To eliminate nasopharyngeal carriage in patients treated with benzylpenicillin or cefotaxime see Table 2, section 5.1

If history of immediate hypersensitivity reaction to penicillin or to cephalosporins, chloramphenicol

> *Suggested duration of treatment* 7 days.
>
> To eliminate nasopharyngeal carriage see Table 2, section 5.1

Meningitis caused by pneumococci

Cefotaxime[1]

> Consider adjunctive treatment with dexamethasone (section 6.3.2), preferably starting before or with first dose of antibacterial, but no later than 12 hours after starting antibacterial (may reduce penetration of vancomycin into cerebrospinal fluid).
>
> If micro-organism penicillin-sensitive, replace cefotaxime with benzylpenicillin.
>
> If micro-organism highly penicillin- and cephalosporin-resistant, add vancomycin and if necessary rifampicin.
>
> *Suggested duration of antibacterial treatment* 14 days

Meningitis caused by *Haemophilus influenzae*

Cefotaxime[1]

> Consider adjunctive treatment with dexamethasone (section 6.3.2), preferably starting before or with first dose of antibacterial, but no later than 12 hours after starting antibacterial.
>
> *Suggested duration of antibacterial treatment* 10 days.
>
> For *H. influenzae* type b give rifampicin for 4 days before hospital discharge to those under 10 years of age or to those in contact with vulnerable household contacts (see Table 2, section 5.1)

If history of immediate hypersensitivity reaction to penicillin or to cephalosporins, or if micro-organism resistant to cefotaxime, chloramphenicol

> Consider adjunctive treatment with dexamethasone (section 6.3.2), preferably starting before or with first dose of antibacterial, but no later than 12 hours after starting antibacterial.
>
> *Suggested duration of antibacterial treatment* 10 days.
>
> For *H. influenzae* type b give rifampicin for 4 days before hospital discharge to those under 10 years of age or to those in contact with vulnerable household contacts (see Table 2, section 5.1)

---

1. Where cefotaxime is suggested ceftriaxone may be used
2. Where amoxicillin is suggested ampicillin may be used

5
Infections

Meningitis caused by Listeria

Amoxicillin[1] + gentamicin

Suggested duration of treatment 21 days.
Consider stopping gentamicin after 7 days

If history of immediate hypersensitivity reaction to penicillin, co-trimoxazole
Suggested duration of treatment 21 days

Urinary tract

Pyelonephritis: acute

A broad-spectrum cephalosporin *or* a quinolone

Suggested duration of treatment 10–14 days (longer treatment may be necessary in complicated pyelonephritis)

Prostatitis: acute

Ciprofloxacin *or* ofloxacin

Suggested duration of treatment 28 days

Alternative, trimethoprim

Suggested duration of treatment 28 days

Urinary-tract infection: 'lower'

Trimethoprim *or* nitrofurantoin

Suggested duration of treatment 7 days, but a short course (e.g. 3 days) is usually adequate for uncomplicated urinary-tract infections in women. See also section 5.1.13

Alternative, amoxicillin[1] *or* oral cephalosporin

Suggested duration of treatment 7 days, but a short course (e.g. 3 days) is usually adequate for uncomplicated urinary-tract infections in women. See also section 5.1.13

Genital system

Bacterial vaginosis

Oral metronidazole

Suggested duration of treatment 5–7 days (or high-dose metronidazole as a single dose)

Alternative, topical metronidazole *or* topical clindamycin

Suggested duration of treatment 5 days with metronidazole or 7 days with clindamycin

Uncomplicated genital chlamydial infection, non-gonococcal urethritis, and non-specific genital infection

Contact tracing recommended.

Azithromycin *or* doxycycline

Suggested duration of treatment azithromycin as a single dose or doxycycline for 7 days

Alternative, erythromycin

Suggested duration of treatment 14 days

Gonorrhoea: uncomplicated

Contact tracing recommended. Consider chlamydia co-infection. Choice of alternative antibacterial regimen depends on locality where infection acquired.

Azithromycin + i/m ceftriaxone

Suggested duration of treatment single-dose of each antibacterial

Alternative when parenteral administration not possible, cefixime + azithromycin

Suggested duration of treatment single-dose of each antibacterial

Alternative if micro-organism sensitive to a quinolone, ciprofloxacin + azithromycin

Suggested duration of treatment single-dose of each antibacterial

Pharyngeal infection, azithromycin + i/m ceftriaxone

Suggested duration of treatment single-dose of each antibacterial

---

1. Where amoxicillin is suggested ampicillin may be used

Pelvic inflammatory disease
Contact tracing recommended.

Doxycycline + metronidazole + i/m ceftriaxone *or* ofloxacin + metronidazole
Suggested duration of treatment 14 days (use i/m ceftriaxone as a single dose).
In severely ill patients initial treatment with doxycycline + i/v ceftriaxone + i/v metronidazole, then switch to oral treatment with doxycycline + metronidazole to complete 14 days' treatment

Early syphilis (infection of less than 2 years)
Contact tracing recommended.

Benzathine benzylpenicillin [unlicensed]
Suggested duration of treatment single-dose (repeat dose after 7 days for women in the third trimester of pregnancy)

Alternatives, doxycycline *or* erythromycin
Suggested duration of treatment 14 days

Late latent syphilis (asymptomatic infection of more than 2 years)
Contact tracing recommended.

Benzathine benzylpenicillin [unlicensed]
Suggested duration of treatment once weekly for 2 weeks

Alternative, doxycycline
Suggested duration of treatment 28 days

Asymptomatic contacts of patients with infectious syphilis

Doxycycline
Suggested duration of treatment 14 days

Blood

Septicaemia: community-acquired
A broad-spectrum antipseudomonal penicillin (e.g. piperacillin with tazobactam, ticarcillin with clavulanic acid) *or* a broad-spectrum cephalosporin (e.g. cefuroxime)
If meticillin-resistant *Staphylococcus aureus* suspected, add vancomycin[1].
If anaerobic infection suspected, add metronidazole to broad-spectrum cephalosporin.
If other resistant micro-organisms suspected, use a more broad-spectrum beta-lactam antibacterial (e.g. meropenem)

Septicaemia: hospital-acquired
A broad-spectrum antipseudomonal beta-lactam antibacterial (e.g. piperacillin with tazobactam, ticarcillin with clavulanic acid, ceftazidime, imipenem with cilastatin, *or* meropenem)
If meticillin-resistant *Staphylococcus aureus* suspected, add vancomycin[1].
If anaerobic infection suspected, add metronidazole to broad-spectrum cephalosporin

Septicaemia related to vascular catheter
Vancomycin[1]
If Gram-negative sepsis suspected, especially in the immunocompromised, add a broad-spectrum anti-pseudomonal beta-lactam.
Consider removing vascular catheter, particularly if infection caused by *Staphylococcus aureus*, pseudomonas, or *Candida* species

Meningococcal septicaemia
If meningococcal disease suspected, a single dose of benzylpenicillin (see p. 367 for dose) should be given before urgent transfer to hospital, so long as this does not delay the transfer; cefotaxime (section 5.1.2) may be an alternative in penicillin allergy; chloramphenicol may be used if history of immediate hypersensitivity reaction to penicillin or to cephalosporins.

Benzylpenicillin or cefotaxime[2]
To eliminate nasopharyngeal carriage in patients treated with benzylpenicillin or cefotaxime see Table 2, section 5.1

If history of immediate hypersensitivity reaction to penicillin or to cephalosporins, chloramphenicol
To eliminate nasopharyngeal carriage see Table 2, section 5.1

1. Where vancomycin is suggested teicoplanin may be used
2. Where cefotaxime is suggested ceftriaxone may be used

Musculoskeletal system

Osteomyelitis

Seek specialist advice if chronic infection or prostheses present.

Flucloxacillin

Consider adding fusidic acid or rifampicin for initial 2 weeks.
Suggested duration of treatment 6 weeks for acute infection

If penicillin-allergic, clindamycin

Consider adding fusidic acid or rifampicin for initial 2 weeks.
Suggested duration of treatment 6 weeks for acute infection

If meticillin-resistant Staphylococcus aureus suspected, vancomycin[1]

Consider adding fusidic acid or rifampicin for initial 2 weeks.
Suggested duration of treatment 6 weeks for acute infection

Septic arthritis

Seek specialist advice if prostheses present.

Flucloxacillin

Suggested duration of treatment 4–6 weeks (longer if infection complicated)

If penicillin-allergic, clindamycin

Suggested duration of treatment 4–6 weeks (longer if infection complicated)

If meticillin-resistant Staphylococcus aureus suspected, vancomycin[1]

Suggested duration of treatment 4–6 weeks (longer if infection complicated)

If gonococcal arthritis or Gram-negative infection suspected, cefotaxime[2]

Suggested duration of treatment 4–6 weeks (longer if infection complicated; treat gonococcal infection for 2 weeks)

Eye

Purulent conjunctivitis

Chloramphenicol eye-drops

See also section 11.3.1

Ear, nose, and oropharynx

Pericoronitis

Antibacterial required only in presence of systemic features of infection, or of trismus, or persistent swelling despite local treatment.

Metronidazole

Suggested duration of treatment 3 days or until symptoms resolve

Alternative, amoxicillin

Suggested duration of treatment 3 days or until symptoms resolve

Gingivitis: acute necrotising ulcerative

Antibacterial required only if systemic features of infection.

Metronidazole

Suggested duration of treatment 3 days or until symptoms resolve

Alternative, amoxicillin

Suggested duration of treatment 3 days or until symptoms resolve

Periapical or periodontal abscess

Antibacterial required only in severe disease with cellulitis or if systemic features of infection.

Amoxicillin

Suggested duration of treatment 5 days

Alternative, metronidazole

Suggested duration of treatment 5 days

1. Where vancomycin is suggested teicoplanin may be used
2. Where cefotaxime is suggested ceftriaxone may be used

Periodontitis

Antibacterial used as an adjunct to debridement in severe disease or disease unresponsive to local treatment alone.

>Metronidazole
>
>*Alternative*, doxycycline

Throat infections

Most throat infections are caused by viruses and many do not require antibacterial therapy. Consider antibacterial, if history of valvular heart disease, if marked systemic upset, if peritonsillar cellulitis or abscess, or if at increased risk from acute infection (e.g. in immunosuppression, cystic fibrosis); prescribe antibacterial for beta-haemolytic streptococcal pharyngitis.

>Phenoxymethylpenicillin
>
>In severe infection, initial parenteral therapy with benzylpenicillin, then oral therapy with phenoxymethyl-penicillin *or* amoxicillin[1]. **Avoid** amoxicillin if possibility of glandular fever, see section 5.1.1.3.
>*Suggested duration of treatment* 10 days
>
>*If penicillin-allergic*, clarithromycin[2]
>*Suggested duration of treatment* 10 days

Sinusitis

Antibacterial should usually be used only for persistent symptoms and purulent discharge lasting at least 7 days or if severe symptoms. Also, consider antibacterial for those at high risk of serious complications (e.g. in immunosuppression, cystic fibrosis).

>Amoxicillin[1] *or* doxycycline *or* clarithromycin[2]
>*Suggested duration of treatment* 7 days.
>Consider oral co-amoxiclav if no improvement after 48 hours.
>In severe infection, initial parenteral therapy with co-amoxiclav or cefuroxime may be required

Otitis externa

Consider systemic antibacterial if spreading cellulitis or patient systemically unwell.

>For topical preparations see section 12.1.1.
>Flucloxacillin
>
>*If penicillin-allergic*, clarithromycin[2]
>
>*If pseudomonas suspected*, ciprofloxacin (*or* an aminoglycoside)

Otitis media

Many infections caused by viruses. Most uncomplicated cases resolve without antibacterial treatment. In children without systemic features, antibacterial treatment may be started after 72 hours if no improvement. Consider earlier treatment if deterioration, if systemically unwell, if at high risk of serious complications (e.g. in immunosuppression, cystic fibrosis), if mastoiditis present, or in children under 2 years of age with bilateral otitis media.

>Amoxicillin[1]
>
>Consider co-amoxiclav if no improvement after 48 hours.
>In severe infection, initial parenteral therapy with co-amoxiclav or cefuroxime.
>*Suggested duration of treatment* 5 days (longer if severely ill)
>
>*If penicillin-allergic*, clarithromycin[2]
>*Suggested duration of treatment* 5 days (longer if severely ill)

1. Where amoxicillin is suggested ampicillin may be used
2. Where clarithromycin is suggested azithromycin or erythromycin may be used

Skin

Impetigo: small areas of skin infected

Seek local microbiology advice before using topical treatment in hospital.

Topical fusidic acid

Suggested duration of treatment 7 days is usually adequate (max. 10 days)

Alternative if meticillin-resistant Staphylococcus aureus, topical mupirocin

Suggested duration of treatment 7 days is usually adequate (max. 10 days)

Impetigo: widespread infection

Oral flucloxacillin

If streptococci suspected in severe infection, add phenoxymethylpenicillin.

Suggested duration of treatment 7 days

If penicillin-allergic, oral clarithromycin[1]

Suggested duration of treatment 7 days

Erysipelas

Phenoxymethylpenicillin *or* benzylpenicillin

If severe infection, replace phenoxymethylpenicillin or benzylpenicillin with high-dose flucloxacillin; if meticillin-resistant *S. aureus* suspected, see section 5.1.1.2.

Suggested duration of treatment at least 7 days

If penicillin-allergic, clindamycin *or* clarithromycin[1]

If meticillin-resistant *S. aureus* suspected in severe infection, see section 5.1.1.2.

Suggested duration of treatment at least 7 days

Cellulitis

Flucloxacillin (high-dose)

If streptococcal infection confirmed, replace flucloxacillin with phenoxymethylpenicillin *or* benzylpenicillin.

If Gram-negative bacteria or anaerobes suspected, use broad-spectrum antibacterials.

If meticillin-resistant *S. aureus* suspected, see section 5.1.1.2

If penicillin-allergic, clindamycin *or* clarithromycin[1] *or* vancomycin[2]

If Gram-negative bacteria suspected, use broad-spectrum antibacterials.

If meticillin-resistant *S. aureus* suspected, see section 5.1.1.2

Animal and human bites

Cleanse wound thoroughly. For tetanus-prone wound, give human tetanus immunoglobulin (with a tetanus-containing vaccine if necessary, according to immunisation history and risk of infection), see under Tetanus Vaccines, section 14.4. Consider rabies prophylaxis (section 14.4) for bites from animals in endemic countries. Assess risk of blood-borne viruses (including HIV, hepatitis B and C) and give appropriate prophylaxis to prevent viral spread.

Co-amoxiclav

If penicillin-allergic, doxycycline + metronidazole

Mastitis during breast-feeding

Treat if severe, if systemically unwell, if nipple fissure present, if symptoms do not improve after 12–24 hours of effective milk removal, or if culture indicates infection.

Flucloxacillin

Continue breast-feeding or expressing milk during treatment.

Suggested duration of treatment 10–14 days

If penicillin-allergic, erythromycin

Continue breast-feeding or expressing milk during treatment.

Suggested duration of treatment 10–14 days

Acne

See section 13.6

---

1. Where clarithromycin is suggested azithromycin or erythromycin may be used
2. Where vancomycin is suggested teicoplanin may be used

Table 2. Summary of antibacterial prophylaxis

Prevention of recurrence of rheumatic fever

Phenoxymethylpenicillin 250 mg twice daily or sulfadiazine 1 g daily (500 mg daily for patients under 30 kg)

Prevention of secondary case of invasive group A streptococcal infection[1]

Phenoxymethylpenicillin 250–500 mg every 6 hours for 10 days; CHILD under 1 year 62.5 mg every 6 hours, 1–5 years 125 mg every 6 hours, 6–12 years 250 mg every 6 hours

Patients who are penicillin allergic,

either erythromycin ADULT and CHILD over 8 years, 250–500 mg every 6 hours for 10 days; CHILD under 2 years 125 mg every 6 hours, 2–8 years 250 mg every 6 hours

or azithromycin [unlicensed indication] 500 mg once daily for 5 days; CHILD over 6 months, 12 mg/kg (max. 500 mg) once daily

Prevention of secondary case of meningococcal meningitis[2]

Ciprofloxacin 500 mg as a single dose; CHILD [unlicensed] under 5 years 30 mg/kg (max. 125 mg) as a single dose; 5–12 years 250 mg as a single dose

or rifampicin 600 mg every 12 hours for 2 days; CHILD under 1 year 5 mg/kg every 12 hours for 2 days; 1–12 years 10 mg/kg every 12 hours for 2 days

or i/m ceftriaxone [unlicensed indication] 250 mg as a single dose; CHILD under 12 years 125 mg

Prevention of secondary case of *Haemophilus influenzae* type b disease[2]

Rifampicin 600 mg once daily for 4 days; CHILD 1–3 months 10 mg/kg once daily for 4 days, over 3 months 20 mg/kg once daily for 4 days (max. 600 mg daily)

or (if rifampicin cannot be used) i/m or i/v ceftriaxone [unlicensed indication] 1 g once daily for 2 days; CHILD 1 month–12 years 50 mg/kg (max. 1 g) once daily for 2 days by i/v infusion only

Within 4 weeks of illness onset in an index case with confirmed or suspected invasive *Haemophilus influenzae* type b disease, give antibacterial prophylaxis to all household contacts if there is a vulnerable individual in the household. Also, give antibacterial prophylaxis to the index case if they are in contact with vulnerable household contacts or if they are under 10 years of age. Vulnerable individuals include the immunocompromised, those with asplenia, or children under 10 years of age. If there are 2 or more cases of invasive *Haemophilus influenzae* type b disease within 120 days in a pre-school or primary school, antibacterial prophylaxis should also be given to all room contacts (including staff). For immunisation against *Haemophilus influenzae* type b disease, see section 14.4

1. For details of those who should receive chemoprophylaxis contact a consultant in communicable disease control (or a consultant in infectious diseases or the local Health Protection Agency Laboratory)
2. For details of those who should receive chemoprophylaxis contact a consultant in communicable disease control (or a consultant in infectious diseases or the local Health Protection Agency laboratory). Unless there has been direct exposure of the mouth or nose to infectious droplets from a patient with meningococcal disease who has received less than 24 hours of antibacterial treatment, healthcare workers do not generally require chemoprophylaxis

Prevention of secondary case of diphtheria in non-immune patient

Erythromycin[3] 500 mg every 6 hours for 7 days; CHILD up to 2 years 125 mg every 6 hours, 2–8 years 250 mg every 6 hours

Treat for further 10 days if nasopharyngeal swabs positive after first 7 days' treatment. For immunisation against diphtheria see section 14.4

Prevention of pertussis

Clarithromycin[4] ADULT and CHILD over 12 years, 500 mg twice daily for 7 days; CHILD body–weight under 8 kg, 7.5 mg/kg twice daily for 7 days; 8–11 kg, 62.5 mg twice daily for 7 days; 12–19 kg, 125 mg twice daily for 7 days; 20–29 kg, 187.5 mg twice daily for 7 days; 30–40 kg, 250 mg twice daily for 7 days

Within 3 weeks of onset of cough in the index case, give antibacterial prophylaxis to all close contacts if amongst them there is at least one unimmunised or partially immunised child under under 1 year of age, *or* if there is at least one individual who has not received a pertussis-containing vaccine more than 1 week and less than 5 years ago (so long as that individual lives or works with children under 4 months of age, is pregnant at over 32 weeks gestation, or is a healthcare worker who works with children under 1 year of age or with pregnant women). For immunisation against pertussis see section 14.4

Prevention of pneumococcal infection in asplenia or in patients with sickle-cell disease

Phenoxymethylpenicillin ADULT and CHILD over 5 years, 250 mg twice daily; CHILD under 1 year 62.5 mg twice daily, 1–5 years 125 mg twice daily—if cover also needed for *H. influenzae* in CHILD give amoxicillin instead (1 month–5 years 125 mg twice daily, 5–12 years 250 mg twice daily, 12–18 years 500 mg twice daily)

If penicillin-allergic, erythromycin ADULT and CHILD over 8 years, 500 mg twice daily; CHILD 1 month–2 years 125 mg twice daily, 2–8 years 250 mg twice daily

Note Antibiotic prophylaxis is not fully reliable; for vaccines in asplenia see p. 845. Antibacterial prophylaxis may be discontinued in those over 5 years of age with sickle-cell disease who have received pneumococcal immunisation and who do not have a history of severe pneumococcal infection

Prevention of tuberculosis in susceptible close contacts or those who have become tuberculin positive[5]

Isoniazid 300 mg daily for 6 months; CHILD 10 mg/kg daily (max. 300 mg daily)

or isoniazid 300 mg daily + rifampicin 600 mg daily (450 mg if less than 50 kg) for 3 months; CHILD isoniazid 10 mg/kg daily (max. 300 mg daily) + rifampicin 15 mg/kg daily (max. 450 mg daily if body-weight less than 50 kg; max. 600 mg daily if body-weight over 50 kg)

or (if isoniazid-resistant tuberculosis in patients under 35 years) rifampicin 600 mg daily (450 mg if less than 50 kg) for 6 months; CHILD 15 mg/kg daily (max. 450 mg daily if body-weight less than 50 kg; max. 600 mg daily if body-weight over 50 kg)

3. Where erythromycin is suggested another macrolide (e.g. azithromycin or clarithromycin) may be used
4. Where clarithromycin is suggested azithromycin or erythromycin may be used
5. For details of those who should receive chemoprophylaxis contact the lead clinician for local tuberculosis services (or a consultant in communicable disease control). See also section 5.1.9, for advice on immunocompromised patients and on prevention of tuberculosis

Prevention of infection from animal and human bites

Co-amoxiclav alone (or doxycycline + metronidazole if penicillin-allergic)

Cleanse wound thoroughly. For tetanus-prone wound, give human tetanus immunoglobulin (with a tetanus-containing vaccine if necessary, according to immunisation history and risk of infection), see under Tetanus vaccines, section 14.4. Consider rabies prophylaxis (section 14.4) for bites from animals in endemic countries. Assess risk of blood-borne viruses (including HIV, hepatitis B and C) and give appropriate prophylaxis to prevent viral spread. Antibacterial prophylaxis recommended for wounds less than 48–72 hours old when the risk of infection is high (e.g. bites from humans or cats; bites to the hand, foot, face, or genital area; bites involving oedema, crush or puncture injury, or other moderate to severe injury; wounds that cannot be debrided adequately; patients with diabetes mellitus, cirrhosis, asplenia, prosthetic joints or valves, or those who are immunocompromised. Give antibacterial prophylaxis for up to 5 days

Prevention of early-onset neonatal infection

i/v benzylpenicillin (or i/v clindamycin if history of allergy to penicillins)

Give intrapartum prophylaxis to women with group B streptococcal colonisation, bacteriuria, or infection in the current pregnancy, or to women who had a previous baby with an invasive group B streptococcal infection. Consider prophylaxis for women in preterm labour if there is prelabour rupture of membranes or if intrapartum rupture of membranes lasting more than 18 hours is suspected.

Prevention of infection in gastro-intestinal procedures

Operations on stomach or oesophagus[1]

Single dose[2] of i/v gentamicin or i/v cefuroxime or i/v co-amoxiclav

Add i/v teicoplanin[3] if high risk of meticillin-resistant *Staphylococcus aureus*

Open biliary surgery[1]

Single dose[2] of i/v cefuroxime + i/v metronidazole[4] or i/v gentamicin + i/v metronidazole[4] or i/v co-amoxiclav alone

Add i/v teicoplanin[3] if high risk of meticillin-resistant *Staphylococcus aureus*

Resections of colon and rectum for carcinoma, and resections in inflammatory bowel disease, and appendicectomy[1]

Single dose[2] of i/v gentamicin + i/v metronidazole[4] or i/v cefuroxime + i/v metronidazole[4] or i/v co-amoxiclav alone

Add i/v teicoplanin[3] if high risk of meticillin-resistant *Staphylococcus aureus*

---

1. Intravenous antibacterial prophylaxis should be given up to 30 minutes before the procedure
2. Additional intra-operative or postoperative doses of antibacterial may be given for prolonged procedures or if there is major blood loss
3. Where teicoplanin is suggested vancomycin may be used
4. Metronidazole may alternatively be given by suppository but to allow adequate absorption, it should be given 2 hours before surgery

Endoscopic retrograde cholangiopancreatography[1]

Single dose of i/v gentamicin or oral or i/v ciprofloxacin

Prophylaxis recommended if pancreatic pseudocyst, immunocompromised, history of liver transplantation, or risk of incomplete biliary drainage. For biliary complications following liver transplantation, add i/v amoxicillin or i/v teicoplanin[3]

Percutaneous endoscopic gastrostomy or jejunostomy[1]

Single dose of i/v co-amoxiclav or i/v cefuroxime

Use single dose of i/v teicoplanin[3] if history of allergy to penicillins or cephalosporins, or if high risk of meticillin-resistant *Staphylococcus aureus*

Prevention of infection in orthopaedic surgery

Joint replacement including hip and knee[1]

Single dose[2] of i/v cefuroxime alone or i/v flucloxacillin + i/v gentamicin

If history of allergy to penicillins or to cephalosporins or if high risk of meticillin-resistant *Staphylococcus aureus*, use single dose[2] of i/v teicoplanin[3] + i/v gentamicin

Closed fractures[1]

Single dose[2] of i/v cefuroxime or i/v flucloxacillin

If history of allergy to penicillins or to cephalosporins or if high risk of meticillin-resistant *Staphylococcus aureus*, use single dose[2] of i/v teicoplanin[3]

Open fractures

i/v co-amoxiclav alone or i/v cefuroxime + i/v metronidazole (or i/v clindamycin alone if history of allergy to penicillins or to cephalosporins)

Add i/v teicoplanin[3] if high risk of meticillin-resistant *Staphylococcus aureus*. Start prophylaxis within 3 hours of injury and continue until soft tissue closure (max. 72 hours). At first debridement also use a single dose of i/v cefuroxime + i/v metronidazole + i/v gentamicin or i/v co-amoxiclav + i/v gentamicin (or i/v clindamycin + i/v gentamicin if history of allergy to penicillins or to cephalosporins). At time of skeletal stabilisation and definitive soft tissue closure[1] use a single dose of i/v gentamicin + i/v teicoplanin[3]

High lower-limb amputation[1]

i/v co-amoxiclav alone or i/v cefuroxime + i/v metronidazole[4]

Continue antibacterial prophylaxis for at least 2 doses after procedure (max. duration of prophylaxis 5 days). If history of allergy to penicillin or to cephalosporins, or if high risk of meticillin-resistant *Staphylococcus aureus*, use i/v teicoplanin[3] + i/v gentamicin + i/v metronidazole[4]

Prevention of infection in urological procedures

Transrectal prostate biopsy[1]

Single dose[2] of oral ciprofloxacin + oral metronidazole or i/v gentamicin + i/v metronidazole[4]

Use single dose[2] of i/v gentamicin + i/v metronidazole[4] if high risk of meticillin-resistant *Staphylococcus aureus*

Transurethral resection of prostate[1]

Single dose[2] of oral ciprofloxacin or i/v gentamicin or i/v cefuroxime

Use single dose[2] of i/v gentamicin if high risk of meticillin-resistant *Staphylococcus aureus*

Prevention of infection in obstetric and gynaecological surgery

Caesarean section[1]

Single dose[2] of i/v cefuroxime

Substitute i/v clindamycin if history of allergy to penicillins or cephalosporins. Add i/v teicoplanin[3] if high risk of meticillin-resistant *Staphylococcus aureus*

Hysterectomy[1]

Single dose[2] of i/v cefuroxime + i/v metronidazole[4] *or* i/v gentamicin + i/v metronidazole[4] *or* i/v co-amoxiclav alone

Use single dose[2] of i/v gentamicin + i/v metronidazole[4] *or* add i/v teicoplanin[3] to other regimens if high risk of meticillin-resistant *Staphylococcus aureus*

Termination of pregnancy

Single dose[2] of oral metronidazole

If genital chlamydial infection cannot be ruled out, give doxycycline (section 5.1.3) postoperatively

Prevention of infection in cardiology procedures

Cardiac pacemaker insertion[1]

Single dose[2] of i/v cefuroxime alone *or* i/v flucloxacillin + i/v gentamicin *or* i/v teicoplanin[3] + i/v gentamicin

Use single dose[2] of i/v teicoplanin[3] + i/v cefuroxime *or* i/v teicoplanin[3] + i/v gentamicin if high risk of meticillin-resistant *Staphylococcus aureus*

Prevention of infection in vascular surgery

Reconstructive arterial surgery of abdomen, pelvis or legs[1]

Single dose[2] of i/v cefuroxime alone *or* i/v flucloxacillin + i/v gentamicin

Add i/v metronidazole for patients at risk from anaerobic infections including those with diabetes, gangrene, or undergoing amputation. Use single dose[2] of i/v teicoplanin[3] + i/v gentamicin if history of allergy to penicillins or cephalosporins, or if high risk of meticillin-resistant *Staphylococcus aureus*

Prevention of endocarditis

> ### NICE guidance
> ### Antimicrobial prophylaxis against infective endocarditis in adults and children undergoing interventional procedures (March 2008)
>
> Antibacterial prophylaxis and chlorhexidine mouthwash are **not** recommended for the prevention of endocarditis in patients undergoing dental procedures.
>
> Antibacterial prophylaxis is **not** recommended for the prevention of endocarditis in patients undergoing procedures of the:
>
> - upper and lower respiratory tract (including ear, nose, and throat procedures and bronchoscopy);
> - genito-urinary tract (including urological, gynaecological, and obstetric procedures);
> - upper and lower gastro-intestinal tract.
>
> Whilst these procedures can cause bacteraemia, there is no clear association with the development of infective endocarditis. Prophylaxis may expose patients to the adverse effects of antimicrobials when the evidence of benefit has not been proven.
>
> Any infection in patients at risk of endocarditis[5] should be investigated promptly and treated appropriately to reduce the risk of endocarditis.
>
> If patients at risk of endocarditis[5] are undergoing a gastro-intestinal or genito-urinary tract procedure at a site where infection is suspected, they should receive appropriate antibacterial therapy that includes cover against organisms that cause endocarditis.
>
> Patients at risk of endocarditis[5] should be:
>
> - advised to maintain good oral hygiene;
> - told how to recognise signs of infective endocarditis, and advised when to seek expert advice.

> ### Dermatological procedures
> Advice of a Working Party of the British Society for Antimicrobial Chemotherapy is that patients who undergo dermatological procedures[6] do not require antibacterial prophylaxis against endocarditis.

---

5. Patients at risk of endocarditis include those with valve replacement, acquired valvular heart disease with stenosis or regurgitation, structural congenital heart disease (including surgically corrected or palliated structural conditions, but excluding isolated atrial septal defect, fully repaired ventricular septal defect, fully repaired patent ductus arteriosus, and closure devices considered to be endothelialised), hypertrophic cardiomyopathy, or a previous episode of infective endocarditis

6. The British Association of Dermatologists Therapy Guidelines and Audit Subcommittee advise that such dermatological procedures include skin biopsies and excision of moles or of malignant lesions

---

1. Intravenous antibacterial prophylaxis should be given up to 30 minutes before the procedure
2. Additional intra-operative or postoperative doses of antibacterial may be given for prolonged procedures or if there is major blood loss
3. Where teicoplanin is suggested vancomycin may be used
4. Metronidazole may alternatively be given by suppository but to allow adequate absorption, it should be given 2 hours before surgery

5 Infections

Joint prostheses and dental treatment

Joint prostheses and dental treatment

Advice of a Working Party of the British Society for Antimicrobial Chemotherapy is that patients with prosthetic joint implants (including total hip replacements) do not require antibiotic prophylaxis for dental treatment. The Working Party considers that it is unacceptable to expose patients to the adverse effects of antibiotics when there is no evidence that such prophylaxis is of any benefit, but that those who develop any intercurrent infection require prompt treatment with antibiotics to which the infecting organisms are sensitive.

The Working Party has commented that joint infections have rarely been shown to follow dental procedures and are even more rarely caused by oral streptococci.

Immunosuppression and indwelling intraperitoneal catheters

Immunosuppression and indwelling intraperitoneal catheters

Advice of a Working Party of the British Society for Antimicrobial Chemotherapy is that patients who are immunosuppressed (including transplant patients) and patients with indwelling intraperitoneal catheters do not require antibiotic prophylaxis for dental treatment provided there is no other indication for prophylaxis.

The Working Party has commented that there is little evidence that dental treatment is followed by infection in immunosuppressed and immunodeficient patients nor is there evidence that dental treatment is followed by infection in patients with indwelling intraperitoneal catheters.

5.1.1   Penicillins

5.1.1.1   Benzylpenicillin and phenoxymethylpenicillin

5.1.1.2   Penicillinase-resistant penicillins

5.1.1.3   Broad-spectrum penicillins

5.1.1.4   Antipseudomonal penicillins

5.1.1.5   Mecillinams

The penicillins are bactericidal and act by interfering with bacterial cell wall synthesis. They diffuse well into body tissues and fluids, but penetration into the cerebrospinal fluid is poor except when the meninges are inflamed. They are excreted in the urine in therapeutic concentrations.

Hypersensitivity reactions The most important side-effect of the penicillins is hypersensitivity which causes rashes and anaphylaxis and can be fatal. Allergic reactions to penicillins occur in 1–10% of exposed individuals; anaphylactic reactions occur in fewer than 0.05% of treated patients. Patients with a history of atopic allergy (e.g. asthma, eczema, hay fever) are at a higher risk of anaphylactic reactions to penicillins. Individuals with a history of anaphylaxis, urticaria, or rash immediately after penicillin administration are at risk of immediate hypersensitivity to a penicillin; these individuals should not receive a penicillin. Patients who are

allergic to one penicillin will be allergic to all because the hypersensitivity is related to the basic penicillin structure. As patients with a history of immediate hypersensitivity to penicillins may also react to the cephalosporins and other beta-lactam antibiotics, they should not receive these antibiotics; aztreonam may be less likely to cause hypersensitivity in penicillin-sensitive patients and can be used with caution. If a penicillin (or another beta-lactam antibiotic) is essential in an individual with immediate hypersensitivity to penicillin then specialist advice should be sought on hypersensitivity testing or using a beta-lactam antibiotic with a different structure to the penicillin that caused the hypersensitivity (see also p. 374).

Individuals with a history of a minor rash (i.e. non-confluent, non-pruritic rash restricted to a small area of the body) or a rash that occurs more than 72 hours after penicillin administration are probably not allergic to penicillin and in these individuals a penicillin should not be withheld unnecessarily for serious infections; the possibility of an allergic reaction should, however, be borne in mind. Other beta-lactam antibiotics (including cephalosporins) can be used in these patients.

Other side-effects A rare but serious toxic effect of the penicillins is encephalopathy due to cerebral irritation. This may result from excessively high doses or in patients with severe renal failure. The penicillins should **not** be given by intrathecal injection because they can cause encephalopathy which may be fatal.

Another problem relating to high doses of penicillin, or normal doses given to patients with renal failure, is the accumulation of electrolyte since most injectable penicillins contain either sodium or potassium.

Diarrhoea frequently occurs during oral penicillin therapy. It is most common with broad-spectrum penicillins, which can also cause antibiotic-associated colitis.

5.1.1.1   Benzylpenicillin and phenoxymethylpenicillin

Benzylpenicillin sodium (Penicillin G) remains an important and useful antibiotic but is inactivated by bacterial beta-lactamases. It is effective for many streptococcal (including pneumococcal), gonococcal, and meningococcal infections and also for anthrax (section 5.1.12), diphtheria, gas-gangrene, leptospirosis, and treatment of Lyme disease (section 5.1.1.3). Pneumococci, meningococci, and gonococci which have decreased sensitivity to penicillin have been isolated; benzylpenicillin is no longer the drug of first choice for pneumococcal meningitis. Although benzylpenicillin is effective in the treatment of tetanus, metronidazole (section 5.1.11) is preferred. Benzylpenicillin is inactivated by gastric acid and absorption from the gut is low; therefore it is best given by injection.

Benzathine benzylpenicillin (available from 'special-order' manufacturers or specialist importing companies, see p. 1124) is used for the treatment of early syphilis and late latent syphilis; it is given by intramuscular injection.

Phenoxymethylpenicillin (Penicillin V) has a similar antibacterial spectrum to benzylpenicillin, but is less active. It is gastric acid-stable, so is suitable for oral administration. It should not be used for serious infections because absorption can be unpredictable and plasma concentrations variable. It is indicated principally for respiratory-tract infections in children, for streptococcal tonsillitis, and for continuing treatment after one or more injections of benzylpenicillin when clinical response has begun. It should not be used for meningococcal or gonococcal infections. Phenoxymethylpenicillin is used for prophylaxis against streptococcal infections following rheumatic fever and against pneumococcal infections following splenectomy or in sickle-cell disease.

Oral infections Phenoxymethylpenicillin is effective for dentoalveolar abscess.

■ BENZYLPENICILLIN SODIUM
(Penicillin G)

Indications throat infections, otitis media, endocarditis, meningococcal disease, pneumonia, cellulitis (Table 1, section 5.1); anthrax; intrapartum prophylaxis against group B streptococcal infection; see also notes above

Cautions history of allergy; false-positive urinary glucose (if tested for reducing substances); **interactions:** Appendix 1 (penicillins)

Contra-indications penicillin hypersensitivity

Renal impairment reduce dose—consult product literature; high doses may cause cerebral irritation, convulsions, or coma

Pregnancy not known to be harmful

Breast-feeding trace amounts in milk, but appropriate to use

Side-effects hypersensitivity reactions including urticaria, fever, joint pains, rashes, angioedema, anaphylaxis, serum sickness-like reaction; *rarely* CNS toxicity including convulsions (especially with high doses or in severe renal impairment), interstitial nephritis, haemolytic anaemia, leucopenia, thrombocytopenia, and coagulation disorders; also reported diarrhoea (including antibiotic-associated colitis)

Dose

- By intramuscular *or* by slow intravenous injection *or* by infusion, 0.6–1.2 g every 6 hours, increased if necessary in more serious infections (single doses over 1.2 g intravenous route only; see also below); CHILD under 18 years see *BNF for Children*
- Endocarditis (in combination with another antibacterial if necessary, see Table 1, section 5.1), by slow intravenous injection *or* by infusion, 1.2 g every 4 hours, increased if necessary (e.g. in enterococcal endocarditis) to 2.4 g every 4 hours; CHILD 1 month–18 years see *BNF for Children*
- Anthrax (in combination with other antibacterials, see also section 5.1.12), by slow intravenous injection *or* by infusion, ADULT over 18 years, 2.4 g every 4 hours
- Intrapartum prophylaxis against group B streptococcal infection, by slow intravenous injection *or* by infusion, initially 3 g then 1.5 g every 4 hours until delivery
- Meningitis, meningococcal disease, by slow intravenous injection *or* by infusion, 2.4 g every 4 hours; NEONATE under 7 days, 50 mg/kg every 12 hours; NEONATE 7–28 days, 50 mg/kg every 8 hours; CHILD 1 month–18 years, 50 mg/kg every 4–6 hours (max. 2.4 g every 4 hours)

Important. If meningococcal disease (meningitis with non-blanching rash or meningococcal septicaemia) is suspected, a single dose of benzylpenicillin should be given before transferring the patient to hospital urgently, so long as this does not delay the transfer. If a patient with suspected bacterial meningitis without non-blanching rash cannot be

transferred to hospital urgently, a single dose of benzylpenicillin should be given before the transfer. Suitable doses of benzylpenicillin by intravenous injection (or by intramuscular injection) are: ADULT 1.2 g; INFANT under 1 year 300 mg; CHILD 1–9 years 600 mg, 10 years and over as for adult. In **penicillin allergy**, cefotaxime (section 5.1.2) may be an alternative; chloramphenicol (section 5.1.7) may be used if there is a history of anaphylaxis to penicillins

- By intrathecal injection, **not** recommended

Note Benzylpenicillin doses in BNF may differ from those in product literature

Crystapen® (Genus) PoM

Injection, powder for reconstitution, benzylpenicillin sodium (unbuffered), net price 600-mg vial = 95p, 2-vial 'GP pack' = £2.64; 1.2-g vial = £1.89

Electrolytes Na^+ 1.68 mmol/600-mg vial; 3.36 mmol/1.2-g vial

■ PHENOXYMETHYLPENICILLIN
(Penicillin V)

Indications oral infections (see notes above); tonsillitis, otitis media, erysipelas, cellulitis; group A streptococcal infection, rheumatic fever and pneumococcal infection prophylaxis (Table 2, section 5.1)

Cautions see under Benzylpenicillin; **interactions:** Appendix 1 (penicillins)

Contra-indications see under Benzylpenicillin

Pregnancy not known to be harmful

Breast-feeding trace amounts in milk, but appropriate to use

Side-effects see under Benzylpenicillin

Dose

- 500 mg every 6 hours, increased up to 1 g every 6 hours if necessary; CHILD up to 1 year 62.5 mg every 6 hours, increased up to 12.5 mg/kg every 6 hours if necessary; 1–6 years, 125 mg every 6 hours, increased up to 12.5 mg/kg every 6 hours if necessary; 6–12 years, 250 mg every 6 hours, increased up to 12.5 mg/kg every 6 hours if necessary

Note Phenoxymethylpenicillin doses in the BNF may differ from those in product literature

Phenoxymethylpenicillin (Non-proprietary) PoM

Tablets, phenoxymethylpenicillin (as potassium salt) 250 mg, net price 28-tab pack = £1.19. Label: 9, 23

Dental prescribing on NHS Phenoxymethylpenicillin Tablets may be prescribed

Oral solution, phenoxymethylpenicillin (as potassium salt) for reconstitution with water, net price 125 mg/5 mL, 100 mL = £14.73; 250 mg/5 mL, 100 mL = £14.66. Label: 9, 23

Note Sugar-free versions are available and can be ordered by specifying 'sugar-free' on the prescription

Dental prescribing on NHS Phenoxymethylpenicillin Oral Solution may be prescribed

5.1.1.2 Penicillinase-resistant penicillins

Most staphylococci are now resistant to benzylpenicillin because they produce penicillinases. **Flucloxacillin**, however, is not inactivated by these enzymes and is thus effective in infections caused by penicillin-resistant staphylococci, which is the sole indication for its use. Flucloxacillin is acid-stable and can, therefore, be given by mouth as well as by injection.

Flucloxacillin is well absorbed from the gut. For a warning on hepatic disorders see under Flucloxacillin.

5 Infections

Temocillin is active against Gram-negative bacteria and is stable against a wide range of beta-lactamases. It should be reserved for the treatment of infections caused by beta-lactamase-producing strains of Gram-negative bacteria, including those resistant to third-generation cephalosporins. Temocillin is not active against *Pseudomonas aeruginosa* or *Acinetobacter* spp.

MRSA Infection from *Staphylococcus aureus* strains resistant to meticillin [now discontinued] (meticillin-resistant *Staph. aureus*, MRSA) and to flucloxacillin can be difficult to manage. Treatment is guided by the sensitivity of the infecting strain.

Rifampicin (section 5.1.9) or **sodium fusidate** (section 5.1.7) should **not** be used alone because resistance may develop rapidly. A **tetracycline** alone or a combination of rifampicin and sodium fusidate can be used for *skin and soft-tissue infections* caused by MRSA; **clindamycin** alone is an alternative. A **glycopeptide** (e.g. vancomycin, section 5.1.7) can be used for severe skin and soft-tissue infections associated with MRSA; if a glycopeptide is unsuitable, **linezolid** (section 5.1.7) can be used on expert advice. As linezolid is **not** active against Gram-negative organisms, it can be used for mixed skin and soft-tissue infections only when other treatments are not available; linezolid must be given with other antibacterials if the infection also involves Gram-negative organisms. A combination of a glycopeptide and sodium fusidate *or* a glycopeptide and rifampicin can be considered for skin and soft-tissue infections that have failed to respond to a single antibacterial.

Tigecycline (section 5.1.3) and **daptomycin** (section 5.1.7) are licensed for the treatment of complicated skin and soft-tissue infections involving MRSA.

A **tetracycline** or **clindamycin** can be used for *bronchiectasis* caused by MRSA. A **glycopeptide** can be used for *pneumonia* associated with MRSA; if a glycopeptide is unsuitable, **linezolid** can be used on expert advice. Linezolid must be given with other antibacterials if the infection also involves Gram-negative organisms.

A **tetracycline** can be used for *urinary-tract infections* caused by MRSA; **trimethoprim** or **nitrofurantoin** are alternatives. A **glycopeptide** can be used for urinary-tract infections that are severe or resistant to other antibacterials.

A **glycopeptide** can be used for *septicaemia* associated with MRSA.

For the management of *endocarditis, osteomyelitis,* or *septic arthritis* associated with MRSA, see Table 1, section 5.1.

Prophylaxis with vancomycin or teicoplanin (alone or in combination with another antibacterial active against other pathogens) is appropriate for patients undergoing surgery if:

- there is a history of MRSA colonisation or infection without documented eradication;
- there is a risk that the patient's MRSA carriage has recurred;
- the patient comes from an area with a high prevalence of MRSA.

For eradication of nasal carriage of MRSA, see section 12.2.3.

FLUCLOXACILLIN

Indications infections due to beta-lactamase-producing staphylococci including otitis externa; adjunct in pneumonia, impetigo, cellulitis, osteomyelitis and in staphylococcal endocarditis (Table 1, section 5.1)

Cautions see under Benzylpenicillin (section 5.1.1.1); risk of kernicterus in jaundiced neonates when high doses given parenterally; **interactions:** Appendix 1 (penicillins)

> ### Hepatic disorders
> Cholestatic jaundice and hepatitis may occur very rarely, up to two months after treatment with flucloxacillin has been stopped. Administration for more than 2 weeks and increasing age are risk factors. Healthcare professionals are reminded that:
> - flucloxacillin should not be used in patients with a history of hepatic dysfunction associated with flucloxacillin;
> - flucloxacillin should be used with caution in patients with hepatic impairment;
> - careful enquiry should be made about hypersensitivity reactions to beta-lactam antibacterials.

Contra-indications see under Benzylpenicillin (section 5.1.1.1)

Hepatic impairment see Cautions and Hepatic Disorders above

Renal impairment reduce dose if eGFR less than $10\,mL/minute/1.73\,m^2$

Pregnancy not known to be harmful

Breast-feeding trace amounts in milk, but appropriate to use

Side-effects see under Benzylpenicillin (section 5.1.1.1); also gastro-intestinal disturbances; *very rarely* hepatitis and cholestatic jaundice (see also Hepatic disorders above)

Dose
- By mouth, 250–500 mg every 6 hours, at least 30 minutes before food; NEONATE see *BNF for Children*; CHILD 1 month–2 years, 62.5–125 mg every 6 hours, at least 30 minutes before food; 2–10 years, 125–250 mg every 6 hours, at least 30 minutes before food
- By intramuscular injection, 250–500 mg every 6 hours; CHILD 1 month–18 years see *BNF for Children*
- By slow intravenous injection *or* by intravenous infusion, 0.25–2 g every 6 hours; CHILD under 18 years see *BNF for Children*

  Endocarditis (in combination with another antibacterial if necessary, see Table 1, section 5.1), body-weight under 85 kg, 8 g daily in 4 divided doses; body-weight over 85 kg, 12 g daily in 6 divided doses; CHILD 1 month–18 years see *BNF for Children*

  Osteomyelitis (see Table 1, section 5.1), up to 8 g daily in 3–4 divided doses; CHILD under 18 years see *BNF for Children*
- Surgical prophylaxis, by slow intravenous injection *or* by intravenous infusion, 1–2 g up to 30 minutes before the procedure; up to 4 further doses of 500 mg may be given every 6 hours by mouth, *or* by intramuscular injection, *or* by slow intravenous injection *or* by intravenous infusion for high risk procedures

Note Flucloxacillin doses in BNF may differ from those in product literature

Flucloxacillin (Non-proprietary) [PoM]
Capsules, flucloxacillin (as sodium salt) 250 mg, net price 28 = £1.58; 500 mg, 28 = £2.63. Label: 9, 23
Brands include *Floxapen®, Fluclomix®, Ladropen®*

Oral solution (= elixir or syrup), flucloxacillin (as sodium salt) for reconstitution with water, 125 mg/ 5 mL, net price 100 mL = £5.19; 250 mg/5 mL, 100 mL = £26.04. Label: 9, 23

Brands include *Ladropen®*

Note Sugar-free versions are available and can be ordered by specifying 'sugar-free' on the prescription

Injection, powder for reconstitution, flucloxacillin (as sodium salt), net price 250-mg vial = £1.23; 500-mg vial = £2.45; 1-g vial = £4.90

▎ TEMOCILLIN

Indications   septicaemia, urinary-tract infections, lower respiratory-tract infections caused by susceptible Gram-negative bacteria

Cautions   see under Benzylpenicillin (section 5.1.1.1); **interactions:** Appendix 1 (penicillins)

Contra-indications   see under Benzylpenicillin (section 5.1.1.1)

Renal impairment   1 g every 12 hours if eGFR 30–60 mL/minute/1.73 m^2; 1 g every 24 hours if eGFR 10–30 mL/minute/1.73 m^2; 1 g every 48 hours *or* 500 mg every 24 hours if eGFR less than 10 mL/minute/1.73 m^2

Pregnancy   not known to be harmful

Breast-feeding   trace amounts in milk

Side-effects   see under Benzylpenicillin (section 5.1.1.1)

Dose
- ADULT over 18 years, by intramuscular injection *or* by intravenous injection over 3–4 minutes, *or* by intravenous infusion, 1–2 g every 12 hours

Negaban® (Eumedica) ▢PoM▢
Injection, powder for reconstitution, temocillin (as sodium salt), net price 1-g vial = £25.45
Electrolytes Na$^+$ 5 mmol/g

� 5.1.1.3   Broad-spectrum penicillins

Ampicillin is active against certain Gram-positive and Gram-negative organisms but is inactivated by penicillinases including those produced by *Staphylococcus aureus* and by common Gram-negative bacilli such as *Escherichia coli*. Almost all staphylococci, approx. 60% of *E. coli* strains and approx. 20% of *Haemophilus influenzae* strains are now resistant. The likelihood of resistance should therefore be considered before using ampicillin for the 'blind' treatment of infections; in particular, it should not be used for hospital patients without checking sensitivity.

Ampicillin is well excreted in the bile and urine. It is principally indicated for the treatment of exacerbations of chronic bronchitis and middle ear infections, both of which may be due to *Streptococcus pneumoniae* and *H. influenzae*, and for urinary-tract infections (section 5.1.13).

Ampicillin can be given by mouth but less than half the dose is absorbed, and absorption is further decreased by the presence of food in the gut.

Maculopapular rashes commonly occur with ampicillin (and amoxicillin) but are not usually related to true penicillin allergy. They almost always occur in patients with glandular fever; broad-spectrum penicillins should not therefore be used for 'blind' treatment of a sore throat. The risk of rash is also increased in patients with

acute or chronic lymphocytic leukaemia or in cytomegalovirus infection.

Amoxicillin is a derivative of ampicillin and has a similar antibacterial spectrum. It is better absorbed than ampicillin when given by mouth, producing higher plasma and tissue concentrations; unlike ampicillin, absorption is not affected by the presence of food in the stomach. Amoxicillin may also be used for the treatment of Lyme disease [not licensed], see below.

Co-amoxiclav consists of amoxicillin with the beta-lactamase inhibitor clavulanic acid. Clavulanic acid itself has no significant antibacterial activity but, by inactivating beta-lactamases, it makes the combination active against beta-lactamase-producing bacteria that are resistant to amoxicillin. These include resistant strains of *Staph. aureus*, *E. coli*, and *H. influenzae*, as well as many *Bacteroides* and *Klebsiella* spp. Co-amoxiclav should be reserved for infections likely, or known, to be caused by amoxicillin-resistant beta-lactamase-producing strains.

A combination of ampicillin with flucloxacillin (as co-fluampicil) is available to treat infections involving either streptococci or staphylococci (e.g. cellulitis).

Lyme disease   Lyme disease should generally be treated by those experienced in its management. **Doxycycline** (p. 381), **amoxicillin** [unlicensed indication] or **cefuroxime axetil** are the antibacterials of choice for *early Lyme disease* or *Lyme arthritis*. If these antibacterials are contra-indicated, a **macrolide** (e.g. clarithromycin) can be used for early Lyme disease. Intravenous administration of **ceftriaxone**, **cefotaxime** (p. 374), or **benzylpenicillin** (p. 367) is recommended for Lyme disease associated with cardiac or neurological complications. The duration of treatment is usually 2–4 weeks; Lyme arthritis may require further treatment.

Oral infections   Amoxicillin is as effective as phenoxymethylpenicillin (section 5.1.1.1) but is better absorbed; however, it may encourage emergence of resistant organisms. Like phenoxymethylpenicillin, amoxicillin is ineffective against bacteria that produce beta-lactamases. Amoxicillin may be useful for short-course oral regimens. Co-amoxiclav is active against beta-lactamase-producing bacteria that are resistant to amoxicillin. Co-amoxiclav may be used for severe dental infection with spreading cellulitis or dental infection not responding to first-line antibacterial treatment.

▎ AMOXICILLIN
(Amoxycillin)

Indications   see under Ampicillin; also oral infections, Lyme disease (see notes above); endocarditis treatment (Table 1, section 5.1); anthrax (section 5.1.12); adjunct in listerial meningitis (Table 1, section 5.1); pneumococcal infection prophylaxis (Table 2, section 5.1); *Helicobacter pylori* eradication (section 1.3)

Cautions   see under Ampicillin; maintain adequate hydration with high doses (particularly during parenteral therapy); **interactions:** Appendix 1 (penicillins)

Contra-indications   see under Ampicillin

Renal impairment   risk of crystalluria with high doses (particularly during parenteral therapy). Reduce dose in severe impairment; rashes more common

Pregnancy   not known to be harmful

5 Infections

Breast-feeding trace amounts in milk, but appropriate to use

Side-effects see under Ampicillin

Dose

- By mouth, 500 mg every 8 hours, dose doubled in severe infection; CHILD 1 month–1 year, 125 mg every 8 hours, increased if necessary up to 30 mg/kg every 8 hours; 1–5 years, 250 mg every 8 hours, increased if necessary up to 30 mg/kg every 8 hours; 5–12 years, 500 mg every 8 hours, increased if necessary up to 30 mg/kg (max. 1 g) every 8 hours; 12–18 years, 500 mg every 8 hours, in severe infection 1 g every 8 hours

  Lyme disease (see also notes above), ADULT and CHILD over 5 years, 500 mg every 8 hours for 14–21 days (for 28 days in Lyme arthritis) [unlicensed indication]; CHILD 1 month–5 years see *BNF for Children*

  Anthrax (treatment and post-exposure prophylaxis— see also section 5.1.12), 500 mg every 8 hours; CHILD body-weight under 20 kg, 80 mg/kg daily in 3 divided doses, body-weight over 20 kg, adult dose

- *Short-course oral therapy*

  Dental abscess, ADULT over 18 years, 3 g repeated after 8 hours

  Urinary-tract infections, ADULT over 18 years, 3 g repeated after 10–12 hours

- By intramuscular injection, ADULT over 18 years, 500 mg every 8 hours

- By intravenous injection *or* infusion, ADULT over 18 years, 500 mg every 8 hours increased to 1 g every 6 hours in severe infection; CHILD 1 month–18 years, 20–30 mg/kg (max. 500 mg) every 8 hours; dose doubled in severe infection

- Listerial meningitis (in combination with another antibiotic, see Table 1, section 5.1), by intravenous infusion, ADULT over 18 years, 2 g every 4 hours; CHILD under 18 years see *BNF for Children*

- Endocarditis (in combination with another antibiotic if necessary, see Table 1, section 5.1), by intravenous infusion, ADULT over 18 years, 2 g every 4 hours; CHILD under 18 years see *BNF for Children*

Note Amoxicillin doses in BNF may differ from those in product literature

Amoxicillin (Non-proprietary) [PoM]

Capsules, amoxicillin (as trihydrate) 250 mg, net price 21 = £1.46; 500 mg, 21 = £1.68. Label: 9
Brands include *Amix®, Amoram®, Amoxident®, Galenamox®, Rimoxallin®*
Dental prescribing on NHS Amoxicillin Capsules may be prescribed

Oral suspension, amoxicillin (as trihydrate) for reconstitution with water, 125 mg/5 mL, net price 100 mL = £1.22; 250 mg/5 mL, 100 mL = £1.38. Label: 9
Note Sugar-free versions are available and can be ordered by specifying 'sugar-free' on the prescription
Brands include *Amoram®, Galenamox®, Rimoxallin®*
Dental prescribing on NHS Amoxicillin Oral Suspension may be prescribed

Sachets, sugar-free, amoxicillin (as trihydrate) 3 g/sachet, net price 2-sachet pack = £9.92, 14-sachet pack = £31.94. Label: 9, 13
Dental prescribing on NHS Amoxicillin Sachets may be prescribed as Amoxicillin Oral Powder

Injection, powder for reconstitution, amoxicillin (as sodium salt), net price 250-mg vial = 32p; 500-mg vial = 55p; 1-g vial = £1.10

Amoxil® (GSK) [PoM]

Capsules, both maroon/gold, amoxicillin (as trihydrate), 250 mg, net price 21-cap pack = £3.38; 500 mg, 21-cap pack = £6.77. Label: 9
Paediatric suspension, amoxicillin 125 mg (as trihydrate)/1.25 mL when reconstituted with water, net price 20 mL (peach- strawberry- and lemon-flavoured) = £3.18. Label: 9, counselling, use of pipette
Excipients include sucrose 600 mg/1.25 mL

Sachets, sugar-free, amoxicillin (as trihydrate) 3 g/sachet, net price 2-sachet pack (peach- strawberry- and lemon-flavoured) = £2.99. Label: 9, 13

Injection, powder for reconstitution, amoxicillin (as sodium salt), net price 500-mg vial = 55p; 1-g vial = £1.10
Electrolytes Na$^+$ 3.3 mmol/g

AMPICILLIN

Indications urinary-tract infections, otitis media, sinusitis, bronchitis, low or moderate-severity community-acquired pneumonia (Table 1, section 5.1), invasive salmonellosis; endocarditis treatment (Table 1, section 5.1); listerial meningitis (Table 1, section 5.1)

Cautions history of allergy; erythematous rashes common in glandular fever (see notes above); increased risk of erythematous rashes in cytomegalovirus infection, and acute or chronic lymphocytic leukaemia (see notes above); **interactions:** Appendix 1 (penicillins)

Contra-indications penicillin hypersensitivity

Renal impairment reduce dose if eGFR less than 10 mL/minute/1.73 m^2; rashes more common

Pregnancy not known to be harmful

Breast-feeding trace amounts in milk, but appropriate to use

Side-effects nausea, vomiting, diarrhoea; rashes (discontinue treatment); rarely, antibiotic-associated colitis; see also under Benzylpenicillin (section 5.1.1.1)

Dose

- By mouth, 0.5–1 g every 6 hours; CHILD 1 month–1 year, 125 mg every 6 hours, increased if necessary up to 30 mg/kg every 6 hours; 1–5 years, 250 mg every 6 hours, increased if necessary up to 30 mg/kg every 6 hours; 5–12 years, 500 mg every 6 hours, increased if necessary up to 30 mg/kg (max. 1 g) every 6 hours; 12–18 years, 500 mg every 6 hours, in severe infection 1 g every 6 hours

- By intramuscular injection *or* intravenous injection *or* infusion, 500 mg every 4–6 hours; CHILD under 18 years see *BNF for Children*

- Endocarditis (in combination with another antibiotic if necessary, see Table 1, section 5.1), by intravenous infusion, ADULT over 18 years, 2 g every 4 hours; CHILD under 18 years see *BNF for Children*

- Listerial meningitis (in combination with another antibiotic, see Table 1, section 5.1), by intravenous infusion, ADULT over 18 years, 2 g every 4 hours; CHILD under 18 years see *BNF for Children*

Note Ampicillin doses in BNF may differ from those in product literature

Ampicillin (Non-proprietary) [PoM]

Capsules, ampicillin 250 mg, net price 28 = £4.75; 500 mg, 28 = £21.37. Label: 9, 23
Brands include *Rimacillin®*

Oral suspension, ampicillin 125 mg/5 mL when reconstituted with water, net price 100 mL = £29.86; 250 mg/5 mL, 100 mL = £7.39. Label: 9, 23
Brands include *Rimacillin*®

Injection, powder for reconstitution, ampicillin (as sodium salt), net price 500-mg vial = £7.83

Penbritin® (Chemidex) PoM

Capsules, grey/red, ampicillin (as trihydrate) 250 mg, net price 28-cap pack = £2.10; 500 mg, 28-cap pack = £5.28. Label: 9, 23

Syrup, apricot- caramel- and peppermint-flavoured, ampicillin (as trihydrate) for reconstitution with water, 250 mg/5 mL, net price 100 mL = £11.84. Label: 9, 23
Excipients include sucrose 3.6 g/5 mL

◢**With flucloxacillin**
See Co-fluampicil

▌ CO-AMOXICLAV

A mixture of amoxicillin (as the trihydrate or as the sodium salt) and clavulanic acid (as potassium clavulanate). The proportions are expressed in the form *x/y* where *x* and *y* are the strengths in milligrams of amoxicillin and clavulanic acid respectively

Indications infections due to beta-lactamase-producing strains (where amoxicillin alone not appropriate) including respiratory-tract infections, bone and joint infections, genito-urinary and abdominal infections, cellulitis, animal bites, severe dental infection with spreading cellulitis or dental infection not responding to first-line antibacterial

Cautions see under Ampicillin and notes above; maintain adequate hydration with high doses (particularly during parenteral therapy); **interactions:** Appendix 1 (penicillins)
Cholestatic jaundice Cholestatic jaundice can occur either during or shortly after the use of co-amoxiclav. An epidemiological study has shown that the risk of acute liver toxicity was about 6 times greater with co-amoxiclav than with amoxicillin. Cholestatic jaundice is more common in patients above the age of 65 years and in men; these reactions have only rarely been reported in children. Jaundice is usually self-limiting and very rarely fatal. The duration of treatment should be appropriate to the indication and should not usually exceed 14 days

Contra-indications penicillin hypersensitivity, history of co-amoxiclav-associated or penicillin-associated jaundice or hepatic dysfunction

Hepatic impairment monitor liver function in liver disease; see also Cholestatic Jaundice above

Renal impairment risk of crystalluria with high doses (particularly during parenteral therapy).
Co-amoxiclav 250/125 tablets or 500/125 tablets: if eGFR 10–30 mL/minute/1.73 m², one *250/125* strength tablet every 12 hours *or* one *500/125* strength tablet every 12 hours; if eGFR less than 10 mL/minute/1.73 m², one *250/125* strength tablet every 24 hours *or* one *500/125* strength tablet every 24 hours.
Co-amoxiclav 400/57 suspension: avoid if eGFR less than 30 mL/minute/1.73 m².
Co-amoxiclav injection (expressed as co-amoxiclav): if eGFR 10–30 mL/minute/1.73 m², 1.2 g initially, then 600 mg every 12 hours; if eGFR less than 10 mL/minute/1.73 m², 1.2 g initially, then 600 mg every 24 hours

Pregnancy not known to be harmful

Breast-feeding trace amounts in milk, but appropriate to use

Side-effects see under Ampicillin; hepatitis, cholestatic jaundice (see above); Stevens-Johnson syndrome, toxic epidermal necrolysis, exfoliative dermatitis, vasculitis reported; rarely prolongation of bleeding time, dizziness, headache, convulsions (particularly with high doses or in renal impairment); superficial staining of teeth with suspension, phlebitis at injection site

Dose

- By mouth, expressed as co-amoxiclav, one *250/125* strength tablet every 8 hours; increased in severe infection to one *500/125* strength tablet every 8 hours; NEONATE 0.25 mL/kg of *125/31* suspension every 8 hours; CHILD 1 month–1 year, 0.25 mL/kg of *125/31* suspension every 8 hours, dose doubled in severe infection; 1–6 years, 5 mL of *125/31* suspension every 8 hours *or* 0.25 mL/kg of *125/31* suspension every 8 hours, dose doubled in severe infection; 6–12 years, 5 mL of *250/62* suspension every 8 hours *or* 0.15 mL/kg of *250/62* suspension every 8 hours, dose doubled in severe infection

  Severe dental infections (but not generally first-line, see notes above), expressed as co-amoxiclav, ADULT and CHILD over 12 years, one *250/125* strength tablet every 8 hours for 5 days

- By intravenous injection over 3–4 minutes *or* by intravenous infusion, expressed as co-amoxiclav, 1.2 g every 8 hours; NEONATE 30 mg/kg every 12 hours; CHILD 1–3 months 30 mg/kg every 12 hours; CHILD 3 months–18 years, 30 mg/kg (max. 1.2 g) every 8 hours

  Surgical prophylaxis, expressed as co-amoxiclav, 1.2 g up to 30 minutes before the procedure; for high risk procedures up to 2–3 further doses of 1.2 g may be given every 8 hours

Co-amoxiclav (Non-proprietary) PoM

Tablets, co-amoxiclav 250/125 (amoxicillin 250 mg as trihydrate, clavulanic acid 125 mg as potassium salt), net price 21-tab pack = £6.47. Label: 9
Dental prescribing on NHS Co-amoxiclav 250/125 Tablets may be prescribed

Tablets, co-amoxiclav 500/125 (amoxicillin 500 mg as trihydrate, clavulanic acid 125 mg as potassium salt), net price 21-tab pack = £6.14. Label: 9

Oral suspension, co-amoxiclav 125/31 (amoxicillin 125 mg as trihydrate, clavulanic acid 31.25 mg as potassium salt)/5 mL when reconstituted with water, net price 100 mL = £1.63. Label: 9
Note Sugar-free versions are available and can be ordered by specifying 'sugar-free' on the prescription
Dental prescribing on NHS Co-amoxiclav 125/31 Suspension may be prescribed

Oral suspension, co-amoxiclav 250/62 (amoxicillin 250 mg as trihydrate, clavulanic acid 62.5 mg as potassium salt)/5 mL when reconstituted with water, net price 100 mL = £1.72. Label: 9
Note Sugar-free versions are available and can be ordered by specifying 'sugar-free' on the prescription
Dental prescribing on NHS Co-amoxiclav 250/62 Suspension may be prescribed

Injection 500/100, powder for reconstitution, co-amoxiclav 500/100 (amoxicillin 500 mg as sodium salt, clavulanic acid 100 mg as potassium salt), net price per vial = £1.21

Injection 1000/200, powder for reconstitution, co-amoxiclav 1000/200 (amoxicillin 1 g as sodium salt, clavulanic acid 200 mg as potassium salt), net price per vial = £2.62

Augmentin® (GSK) [PoM]

Tablets 375 mg, f/c, co-amoxiclav 250/125 (amoxicillin 250 mg as trihydrate, clavulanic acid 125 mg as potassium salt), net price 21-tab pack = £5.03. Label: 9

Tablets 625 mg, f/c, co-amoxiclav 500/125 (amoxicillin 500 mg as trihydrate, clavulanic acid 125 mg as potassium salt), net price 21-tab pack = £9.60. Label: 9

Suspension '125/31 SF', sugar-free, co-amoxiclav 125/31 (amoxicillin 125 mg as trihydrate, clavulanic acid 31.25 mg as potassium salt)/5 mL when reconstituted with water, net price 100 mL (raspberry-and orange-flavoured) = £3.54. Label: 9

Excipients include aspartame 12.5 mg/5 mL (section 9.4.1)

Suspension '250/62 SF', sugar-free, co-amoxiclav 250/62 (amoxicillin 250 mg as trihydrate, clavulanic acid 62.5 mg as potassium salt)/5 mL when reconstituted with water, net price 100 mL (raspberry-and orange-flavoured) = £3.60. Label: 9

Excipients include aspartame 12.5 mg/5 mL (section 9.4.1)

Injection 600 mg, powder for reconstitution, co-amoxiclav 500/100 (amoxicillin 500 mg as sodium salt, clavulanic acid 100 mg as potassium salt), net price per vial = £1.06

Electrolytes Na⁺ 1.35 mmol, K⁺ 0.5 mmol/600-mg vial

Injection 1.2 g, powder for reconstitution, co-amoxiclav 1000/200 (amoxicillin 1 g as sodium salt, clavulanic acid 200 mg as potassium salt), net price per vial = £1.06

Electrolytes Na⁺ 2.7 mmol, K⁺ 1 mmol/1.2-g vial

◀**Other oral preparations**

Co-amoxiclav (Non-proprietary) [PoM]

Suspension '400/57', co-amoxiclav 400/57 (amoxicillin 400 mg as trihydrate, clavulanic acid 57 mg as potassium salt)/5 mL when reconstituted with water, net price 35 mL = £4.13, 70 mL = £5.79. Label: 9

Excipients may include aspartame (section 9.4.1)

Note Sugar-free versions are available and can be ordered by specifying 'sugar-free' on the prescription

Brands include Augmentin-Duo®

Dose ADULT and CHILD over 40 kg 10 mL twice daily, increased to 10 mL three times daily in severe infection; CHILD 2 months–2 years 0.15 mL/kg twice daily, 2–6 years (13–21 kg) 2.5 mL twice daily, 7–12 years (22–40 kg) 5 mL twice daily, doubled in severe infection

---

CO-FLUAMPICIL

A mixture of equal parts by mass of flucloxacillin and ampicillin

Indications mixed infections involving beta-lactamase-producing staphylococci

Cautions see under Ampicillin and Flucloxacillin; interactions: Appendix 1 (penicillins)

Contra-indications see under Ampicillin and Flucloxacillin

Hepatic impairment see under Flucloxacillin

Renal impairment see under Ampicillin and Flucloxacillin

Pregnancy not known to be harmful

Breast-feeding trace amounts in milk, but appropriate to use

Side-effects see under Ampicillin and Flucloxacillin

Dose

- By mouth, co-fluampicil, 250/250 every 6 hours, dose doubled in severe infections; CHILD under 10 years half adult dose, dose doubled in severe infections

- By intramuscular *or* slow intravenous injection *or* by intravenous infusion, co-fluampicil 250/250 every 6 hours, dose doubled in severe infections; CHILD under 2 years quarter adult dose, 2–10 years half adult dose, dose doubled in severe infections

Co-fluampicil (Non-proprietary) [PoM]

Capsules, co-fluampicil 250/250 (flucloxacillin 250 mg as sodium salt, ampicillin 250 mg as trihydrate), net price 28-cap pack = £4.18. Label: 9, 22

Brands include *Flu-Amp®*

Syrup, co-fluampicil 125/125 (flucloxacillin 125 mg as magnesium salt, ampicillin 125 mg as trihydrate)/5 mL when reconstituted with water, net price 100 mL = £23.93. Label: 9, 22

Magnapen® (Wockhardt) [PoM]

Injection 500 mg, powder for reconstitution, co-fluampicil 250/250 (flucloxacillin 250 mg as sodium salt, ampicillin 250 mg as sodium salt), net price per vial = £1.33

Electrolytes Na⁺ 1.3 mmol/vial

5.1.1.4 Antipseudomonal penicillins

Piperacillin, a ureidopenicillin, is only available in combination with the beta-lactamase inhibitor tazobactam. **Ticarcillin**, a carboxypenicillin, is only available in combination with the beta-lactamase inhibitor clavulanic acid (section 5.1.1.3). Both preparations have a broad spectrum of activity against a range of Gram-positive and Gram-negative bacteria, and anaerobes. Piperacillin with tazobactam has activity against a wider range of Gram-negative organisms than ticarcillin with clavulanic acid and it is more active against *Pseudomonas aeruginosa*. These antibacterials are not active against MRSA. They are used in the treatment of septicaemia, hospital-acquired pneumonia, and complicated infections involving the urinary tract, skin and soft tissues, or intra-abdomen.

For severe pseudomonas infections these antipseudomonal penicillins can be given with an aminoglycoside (e.g. gentamicin section 5.1.4) since they have a synergistic effect.

Owing to the sodium content of many of these antibiotics, high doses may lead to hypernatraemia.

PIPERACILLIN WITH TAZOBACTAM

Indications see under Dose

Cautions see under Benzylpenicillin (section 5.1.1.1); interactions: Appendix 1 (penicillins)

Contra-indications see under Benzylpenicillin (section 5.1.1.1)

Renal impairment max. 4.5 g every 8 hours if eGFR 20–40 mL/minute/1.73 m²; max. 4.5 g every 12 hours if eGFR less than 20 mL/minute/1.73 m²

Pregnancy manufacturers advise use only if potential benefit outweighs risk

Breast-feeding trace amounts in milk, but appropriate to use

Side-effects see under Benzylpenicillin (section 5.1.1.1); also nausea, vomiting, diarrhoea; *less commonly* stomatitis, dyspepsia, constipation, jaundice, hypotension, headache, insomnia, injection-site reactions; *rarely* abdominal pain, hepatitis, eosinophilia; *very rarely* hypoglycaemia, hypokalaemia, pancytopenia, Stevens-Johnson syndrome, toxic epidermal necrolysis

Dose

Note Expressed as a combination of piperacillin and tazobactam (both as sodium salts) in a ratio of 8:1

- Hospital-acquired pneumonia, septicaemia, complicated intra-abdominal infections, complicated infections involving the urinary tract or skin and soft tissues, ADULT and CHILD over 12 years, **by intravenous infusion**, 4.5 g every 8 hours, increased to 4.5 g every 6 hours in severe infections
- Complicated intra-abdominal infections, **by intravenous infusion**, CHILD 2–12 years, 112.5 mg/kg (max. 4.5 g) every 8 hours
- Infections in neutropenic patients, **by intravenous infusion**, ADULT and CHILD over 12 years, 4.5 g every 6 hours; CHILD 2–12 years, 90 mg/kg (max. 4.5 g) every 6 hours

Piperacillin with tazobactam (Non-proprietary) [PoM]
Injection 2.25 g, powder for reconstitution, piperacillin 2 g (as sodium salt), tazobactam 250 mg (as sodium salt), net price 2.25-g vial = £6.08
Injection 4.5 g, powder for reconstitution, piperacillin 4 g (as sodium salt), tazobactam 500 mg (as sodium salt), net price 4.5-g vial = £12.90

Tazocin® (Pfizer) [PoM]
Injection 2.25 g, powder for reconstitution, piperacillin 2 g (as sodium salt), tazobactam 250 mg (as sodium salt), net price 2.25-g vial = £7.65
Electrolytes Na+ 5.58 mmol/2.25-g vial
Injection 4.5 g, powder for reconstitution, piperacillin 4 g (as sodium salt), tazobactam 500 mg (as sodium salt), net price 4.5-g vial = £15.17
Electrolytes Na+ 11.16 mmol/4.5-g vial

TICARCILLIN WITH CLAVULANIC ACID

Indications infections due to *Pseudomonas* and *Proteus* spp, see notes above

Cautions see under Benzylpenicillin (section 5.1.1.1); **interactions:** Appendix 1 (penicillins)
Cholestatic jaundice For a warning on cholestatic jaundice possibly associated with clavulanic acid, see under Co-amoxiclav, p. 371.

Contra-indications see under Benzylpenicillin (section 5.1.1.1)

Hepatic impairment manufacturer advises caution in severe impairment; also cholestatic jaundice, see under Co-amoxiclav, p. 371

Renal impairment reduce dose to 3.2 g every eight hours if eGFR 30–60 mL/minute/1.73 m^2; 1.6 g every eight hours if eGFR 10–30 mL/minute/1.73 m^2; 1.6 g every twelve hours if eGFR less than 10 mL/minute/1.73 m^2

Pregnancy not known to be harmful

Breast-feeding trace amounts in milk, but appropriate to use

Side-effects see under Benzylpenicillin (section 5.1.1.1); also nausea, vomiting, coagulation disorders, haemorrhagic cystitis (more frequent in children), injection-site reactions, Stevens-Johnson syndrome, toxic epidermal necrolysis, hypokalaemia, eosinophilia

Dose

Note Expressed as a combination of ticarcillin (as sodium salt) and clavulanic acid (as potassium salt) in a ratio of 15:1

- **By intravenous infusion**, 3.2 g every 6–8 hours increased to every 4 hours in more severe infections; CHILD 1 month–18 years, body-weight under 40 kg, 80 mg/kg every 8 hours, increased to every 6 hours in more severe infections; body-weight over 40 kg, adult dose

Timentin (GSK) [PoM]
Injection 3.2 g, powder for reconstitution, ticarcillin 3 g (as sodium salt), clavulanic acid 200 mg (as potassium salt). Net price per vial = £5.33
Electrolytes Na+ 16 mmol, K+ 1 mmol /3.2-g vial

5.1.1.5 Mecillinams

Pivmecillinam has significant activity against many Gram-negative bacteria including *Escherichia coli*, klebsiella, enterobacter, and salmonellae. It is not active against *Pseudomonas aeruginosa* or enterococci. Pivmecillinam is hydrolysed to mecillinam, which is the active drug.

PIVMECILLINAM HYDROCHLORIDE

Indications see under Dose below

Cautions see under Benzylpenicillin (section 5.1.1.1); also liver and renal function tests required in long-term use; avoid in acute porphyria (section 9.8.2); **interactions:** Appendix 1 (penicillins)

Contra-indications see under Benzylpenicillin (section 5.1.1.1); also carnitine deficiency, oesophageal strictures, gastro-intestinal obstruction, infants under 3 months

Pregnancy not known to be harmful, but manufacturer advises avoid

Breast-feeding trace amounts in milk, but appropriate to use

Side-effects see under Benzylpenicillin (section 5.1.1.1); nausea, vomiting, abdominal pain, headache, dizziness; also reported mouth ulcers, oesophagitis, reduced serum and total body carnitine (especially with long-term or repeated use)

Dose

- Acute uncomplicated cystitis, ADULT and CHILD over 40 kg, initially 400 mg then 200 mg every 8 hours for 3 days
- Chronic or recurrent bacteriuria, ADULT and CHILD over 40 kg, 400 mg every 6–8 hours
- Urinary-tract infections, CHILD under 40 kg, 20–40 mg/kg daily in 3–4 divided doses
- Salmonellosis, not recommended therefore no dose stated
Counselling Tablets should be swallowed whole with plenty of fluid during meals while sitting or standing

Selexid® (LEO) [PoM]
Tablets, f/c, pivmecillinam hydrochloride 200 mg, net price 10-tab pack = £4.50. Label 9, 21, 27, counselling, posture (see Dose above)

5.1.2 Cephalosporins, carbapenems, and other beta-lactams

5.1.2.1 Cephalosporins
5.1.2.2 Carbapenems
5.1.2.3 Other beta-lactam antibiotics

Antibiotics in this section include the **cephalosporins**, such as cefotaxime, ceftazidime, cefuroxime, cefalexin and cefradine, the **monobactam**, aztreonam, and the **carbapenems**, imipenem (a thienamycin derivative), meropenem, and ertapenem.

5.1.2.1 Cephalosporins

The cephalosporins are broad-spectrum antibiotics which are used for the treatment of septicaemia, pneumonia, meningitis, biliary-tract infections, peritonitis, and urinary-tract infections. The pharmacology of the cephalosporins is similar to that of the penicillins, excretion being principally renal. Cephalosporins penetrate the cerebrospinal fluid poorly unless the meninges are inflamed; cefotaxime is a suitable cephalosporin for infections of the CNS (e.g meningitis).

The principal side-effect of the cephalosporins is hypersensitivity and about 0.5–6.5% of penicillin-sensitive patients will also be allergic to the cephalosporins. Patients with a history of immediate hypersensitivity to penicillin should not receive a cephalosporin. If a cephalosporin is essential in these patients because a suitable alternative antibacterial is not available, then cefixime, cefotaxime, ceftazidime, ceftriaxone, or cefuroxime can be used with caution; cefaclor, cefadroxil, cefalexin, cefradine, and ceftaroline fosamil should be avoided.

Antibiotic-associated colitis may occur with the use of broad-spectrum cephalosporins, particularly second- and third-generation cephalosporins.

Cefuroxime is a 'second generation' cephalosporin that is less susceptible than the earlier cephalosporins to inactivation by beta-lactamases. It is, therefore, active against certain bacteria which are resistant to the other drugs and has greater activity against *Haemophilus influenzae*.

Cefotaxime, **ceftazidime** and **ceftriaxone** are 'third generation' cephalosporins with greater activity than the 'second generation' cephalosporins against certain Gram-negative bacteria. However, they are less active than cefuroxime against Gram-positive bacteria, most notably *Staphylococcus aureus*. Their broad antibacterial spectrum may encourage superinfection with resistant bacteria or fungi.

Ceftazidime has good activity against pseudomonas. It is also active against other Gram-negative bacteria.

Ceftriaxone has a longer half-life and therefore needs to be given only once daily. Indications include serious infections such as septicaemia, pneumonia, and meningitis. The calcium salt of ceftriaxone forms a precipitate in the gall bladder which may rarely cause symptoms but these usually resolve when the antibiotic is stopped.

Ceftaroline fosamil is a 'fifth generation' cephalosporin with bactericidal activity similar to cefotaxime; however, ceftaroline fosamil has an extended spectrum of activity against Gram-positive bacteria that includes meticillin-resistant *Staphylococcus aureus* and multi-drug resistant *Streptococcus pneumoniae*. Ceftaroline fosamil is licensed for the treatment of community-acquired pneumonia and complicated skin and soft-tissue infections, but there is no experience of its use in pneumonia caused by meticillin-resistant *S. aureus*.

The *Scottish Medicines Consortium*, p. 4 has advised (Dec 2012) that ceftaroline fosamil (*Zinforo®*) is accepted for restricted use within NHS Scotland when meticillin-resistant *S. aureus* is suspected in complicated skin and soft-tissue infection and vancomycin cannot be used.

Orally active cephalosporins The orally active 'first generation' cephalosporins, **cefalexin**, **cefradine**, and **cefadroxil** and the 'second generation' cephalosporin, **cefaclor**, have a similar antimicrobial spectrum. They are useful for urinary-tract infections which do not respond to other drugs or which occur in pregnancy, respiratory-tract infections, otitis media, sinusitis, and skin and soft-tissue infections. Cefaclor has good activity against *H. influenzae*, but it is associated with protracted skin reactions especially in children. Cefadroxil has a long duration of action and can be given twice daily; it has poor activity against *H. influenzae*. **Cefuroxime axetil**, an ester of the 'second generation' cephalosporin cefuroxime, has the same antibacterial spectrum as the parent compound; it is poorly absorbed.

Cefixime is an orally active 'third generation' cephalosporin. It has a longer duration of action than the other cephalosporins that are active by mouth. It is only licensed for acute infections.

For treatment of Lyme disease, see section 5.1.1.3.

Oral infections The cephalosporins offer little advantage over the penicillins in dental infections, often being less active against anaerobes. Infections due to oral streptococci (often termed viridans streptococci) which become resistant to penicillin are usually also resistant to cephalosporins. This is of importance in the case of patients who have had rheumatic fever and are on long-term penicillin therapy. Cefalexin and cefradine have been used in the treatment of oral infections.

CEFACLOR

Indications infections due to sensitive Gram-positive and Gram-negative bacteria, but see notes above

Cautions sensitivity to beta-lactam antibacterials (avoid if history of immediate hypersensitivity reaction, see also notes above and p. 366); false positive urinary glucose (if tested for reducing substances) and false positive Coombs' test; **interactions:** Appendix 1 (cephalosporins)

Contra-indications cephalosporin hypersensitivity

Renal impairment no dose adjustment required—manufacturer advises caution

Pregnancy not known to be harmful

Breast-feeding present in milk in low concentration, but appropriate to use

Side-effects diarrhoea (rarely antibiotic-associated colitis), nausea and vomiting, abdominal discomfort, headache; allergic reactions including rashes, pruritus, urticaria, serum sickness-like reactions with rashes, fever and arthralgia, and anaphylaxis; Stevens-Johnson syndrome, toxic epidermal necrolysis reported; disturbances in liver enzymes, transient hepatitis and cholestatic jaundice; other side-effects reported include eosinophilia and blood disorders (including thrombocytopenia, leucopenia, agranulocytosis, aplastic anaemia and haemolytic anaemia); reversible interstitial nephritis, hyperactivity, nervousness, sleep disturbances, hallucinations, confusion, hypertonia, and dizziness

Dose

- 250 mg every 8 hours, doubled for severe infections; max. 4 g daily; CHILD over 1 month, 20 mg/kg daily in 3 divided doses, doubled for severe infections, max. 1 g daily; *or* 1 month–1 year, 62.5 mg every 8 hours; 1–5 years, 125 mg; over 5 years, 250 mg; doses doubled for severe infections

Cefaclor (Non-proprietary) ▒PoM▒

Capsules, cefaclor (as monohydrate) 250 mg, net price 21-cap pack = £6.80; 500 mg, 50-cap pack = £24.00. Label: 9
Brands include *Keftid®*

Suspension, cefaclor (as monohydrate) for reconstitution with water, 125 mg/5 mL, net price 100 mL = £5.16; 250 mg/5 mL, 100 mL = £10.32. Label: 9
Note Sugar-free versions are available and can be ordered by specifying 'sugar-free' on the prescription
Brands include *Keftid®*

Distaclor® (Flynn) ▒PoM▒

Capsules, cefaclor (as monohydrate) 500 mg (violet/grey), net price 21-cap pack = £7.50. Label: 9

Suspension, both pink, cefaclor (as monohydrate) for reconstitution with water, 125 mg/5 mL, net price 100 mL = £4.13; 250 mg/5 mL, 100 mL = £8.26. Label: 9

◢Modified release

Distaclor MR® (Flynn) ▒PoM▒

Tablets, m/r, both blue, cefaclor (as monohydrate) 375 mg. Net price 14-tab pack = £9.10. Label: 9, 21, 25

Dose 375 mg every 12 hours with food, dose doubled for pneumonia

Lower urinary-tract infections, 375 mg every 12 hours with food

◢ CEFADROXIL

Indications   see under Cefaclor; see also notes above

Cautions   see under Cefaclor; **interactions:** Appendix 1 (cephalosporins)

Contra-indications   see under Cefaclor

Renal impairment   1 g initially, then 500 mg every 12 hours if eGFR 26–50 mL/minute/1.73 m^2; 1 g initially, then 500 mg every 24 hours if eGFR 11–26 mL/minute/1.73 m^2; 1 g initially, then 500 mg every 36 hours if eGFR less than 11 mL/minute/1.73 m^2

Pregnancy   see under Cefaclor

Breast-feeding   see under Cefaclor

Side-effects   see under Cefaclor

Dose

- 0.5–1 g twice daily; skin, soft-tissue, and uncomplicated urinary-tract infections, 1 g daily; CHILD 6–18 years, body-weight under 40 kg, 500 mg twice daily; body-weight over 40 kg, adult dose

Cefadroxil (Non-proprietary) ▒PoM▒

Capsules, cefadroxil (as monohydrate) 500 mg, net price 20-cap pack = £21.82. Label: 9

◢ CEFALEXIN
(Cephalexin)

Indications   see under Cefaclor

Cautions   see under Cefaclor; **interactions:** Appendix 1 (cephalosporins)

Contra-indications   see under Cefaclor

Renal impairment   max. 3 g daily if eGFR 40–50 mL/minute/1.73 m^2; max. 1.5 g daily if eGFR 10–40 mL/minute/1.73 m^2; max. 750 mg daily if eGFR less than 10 mL/minute/1.73 m^2

Pregnancy   see under Cefaclor

Breast-feeding   see under Cefaclor

Side-effects   see under Cefaclor

Dose

- 250 mg every 6 hours *or* 500 mg every 8–12 hours increased to 1–1.5 g every 6–8 hours for severe infections; CHILD 25 mg/kg daily in divided doses, doubled for severe infections, max. 100 mg/kg daily; *or* under 1 year 125 mg every 12 hours, 1–5 years 125 mg every 8 hours, 5–12 years 250 mg every 8 hours

- Prophylaxis of recurrent urinary-tract infection, ADULT 125 mg at night

Cefalexin (Non-proprietary) ▒PoM▒

Capsules, cefalexin 250 mg, net price 28-cap pack = £1.71; 500 mg, 21-cap pack = £1.89. Label: 9
Dental prescribing on NHS Cefalexin Capsules may be prescribed

Tablets, cefalexin 250 mg, net price 28-tab pack = £2.18; 500 mg, 21-tab pack = £2.65. Label: 9
Dental prescribing on NHS Cefalexin Tablets may be prescribed

Oral suspension, cefalexin for reconstitution with water, 125 mg/5 mL, net price 100 mL = £1.40; 250 mg/5 mL, 100 mL = £1.87. Label: 9
Dental prescribing on NHS Cefalexin Oral Suspension may be prescribed

Ceporex® (Co-Pharma) ▒PoM▒

Capsules, both caramel/grey, cefalexin 250 mg, net price 28-cap pack = £4.02; 500 mg, 28-cap pack = £7.85. Label: 9

Tablets, all pink, f/c, cefalexin 250 mg, net price 28-tab pack = £4.02; 500 mg, 28-tab pack = £7.85. Label: 9

Syrup, all orange, cefalexin for reconstitution with water, 125 mg/5 mL, net price 100 mL = £1.43; 250 mg/5 mL, 100 mL = £2.87; 500 mg/5 mL, 100 mL = £5.57. Label: 9

Keflex® (Flynn) ▒PoM▒

Capsules, cefalexin 250 mg (green/white), net price 28-cap pack = £1.46; 500 mg (pale green/dark green), 21-cap pack = £1.98. Label: 9

Tablets, both peach, cefalexin 250 mg, net price 28-tab pack = £1.60; 500 mg (scored), 21-tab pack = £2.08. Label: 9

Suspension, cefalexin for reconstitution with water, 125 mg/5 mL, net price 100 mL = 84p; 250 mg/5 mL, 100 mL = £1.40. Label: 9

◢ CEFIXIME

Indications   see under Cefaclor (acute infections only); gonorrhoea [unlicensed indication] (see also Table 1, section 5.1)

Cautions   see under Cefaclor; **interactions:** Appendix 1 (cephalosporins)

Contra-indications see under Cefaclor

Renal impairment reduce dose if eGFR less than 20 mL/minute/1.73 m^2 (max. 200 mg once daily)

Pregnancy see under Cefaclor

Breast-feeding manufacturer advises avoid unless essential—no information available

Side-effects see under Cefaclor

Dose

- ADULT and CHILD over 10 years, 200–400 mg daily in 1–2 divided doses; CHILD over 6 months 8 mg/kg daily in 1–2 divided doses or 6 months–1 year 75 mg daily; 1–4 years 100 mg daily; 5–10 years 200 mg daily

- Uncomplicated gonorrhoea [unlicensed indication] (see also Table 1, section 5.1), 400 mg as a single dose

Suprax® (Sanofi-Aventis) [PoM]

Tablets, f/c, scored, cefixime 200 mg. Net price 7-tab pack = £13.23. Label: 9

Paediatric oral suspension, cefixime 100 mg/5 mL when reconstituted with water, net price 100 mL (with spoon for measuring 3.75 mL or 5 mL) = £18.91. Label: 9

CEFOTAXIME

Indications see under Cefaclor; gonorrhoea; surgical prophylaxis; Haemophilus epiglottitis and meningitis (Table 1, section 5.1); see also notes above

Cautions see under Cefaclor; **interactions:** Appendix 1 (cephalosporins)

Contra-indications see under Cefaclor

Renal impairment if eGFR less than 5 mL/minute/1.73 m^2, initial dose of 1 g then use half normal dose

Pregnancy see under Cefaclor

Breast-feeding see under Cefaclor

Side-effects see under Cefaclor; rarely arrhythmias following rapid injection reported

Dose

- By intramuscular or intravenous injection or by intravenous infusion, 1 g every 12 hours increased in severe infections (e.g. meningitis) to 8 g daily in 4 divided doses; higher doses (up to 12 g daily in 3–4 divided doses) may be required; intramuscular doses over 1 g divided between more than one site; NEONATE 50 mg/kg daily in 2–4 divided doses increased to 150–200 mg/kg daily in severe infections; CHILD 100–150 mg/kg daily in 2–4 divided doses increased up to 200 mg/kg daily in very severe infections

- Uncomplicated gonorrhoea, by intramuscular injection, 500 mg as a single dose

  Important. If meningococcal disease (meningitis with non-blanching rash or meningococcal septicaemia) is suspected, and the patient cannot be given benzylpenicillin (e.g. because of an allergy), a single dose of cefotaxime can be given (if available) before urgent transfer to hospital, so long as this does not delay the transfer. If a patient with suspected bacterial meningitis without non-blanching rash cannot be transferred to hospital urgently and cannot be given benzylpenicillin, a single dose of cefotaxime can be given before transfer. Suitable doses of cefotaxime by intravenous injection (or by intramuscular injection) are ADULT and CHILD over 12 years 1 g; CHILD under 12 years 50 mg/kg; chloramphenicol (section 5.1.7) may be used if there is a history of anaphylaxis to penicillins or cephalosporins

Cefotaxime (Non-proprietary) [PoM]

Injection, powder for reconstitution, cefotaxime (as sodium salt), net price 500-mg vial = £2.25; 1-g vial = £4.20; 2-g vial = £8.57

CEFRADINE
(Cephradine)

Indications see under Cefaclor; surgical prophylaxis

Cautions see under Cefaclor; **interactions:** Appendix 1 (cephalosporins)

Contra-indications see under Cefaclor

Renal impairment use half normal dose if eGFR 5–20 mL/minute/1.73 m^2; use one-quarter normal dose if eGFR less than 5 mL/minute/1.73 m^2

Pregnancy see under Cefaclor

Breast-feeding see under Cefaclor

Side-effects see under Cefaclor

Dose

- 250–500 mg every 6 hours or 0.5–1 g every 12 hours; up to 1 g every 6 hours in severe infections; CHILD 7–12 years, 25–50 mg/kg daily in 2–4 divided doses

Cefradine (Non-proprietary) [PoM]

Capsules, cefradine 250 mg, net price 20-cap pack = £2.24; 500 mg, 20-cap pack = £3.35. Label: 9
Brands include Nicef®
Dental prescribing on NHS Cefradine Capsules may be prescribed

---

CEFTAROLINE FOSAMIL

Indications community-acquired pneumonia; complicated skin and soft-tissue infections; see also notes above

Cautions see under Cefaclor; also seizure disorders; **interactions:** Appendix 1 (cephalosporins)

Contra-indications see under Cefaclor

Renal impairment 400 mg every 12 hours if eGFR 30–50 mL/minute/1.73 m^2; manufacturer advises avoid if eGFR less than 30 mL/minute/1.73 m^2

Pregnancy manufacturer advises avoid unless essential—no information available

Breast-feeding manufacturer advises avoid—no information available

Side-effects see under Cefaclor

Dose

- By intravenous infusion, ADULT over 18 years 600 mg every 12 hours for 5–7 days in community-acquired pneumonia or 5–14 days in complicated skin and soft-tissue infections

Zinforo® (AstraZeneca) ▼ [PoM]

Intravenous infusion, powder for reconstitution, ceftaroline fosamil (as acetate), net price 600-mg vial = £37.50

CEFTAZIDIME

Indications see under Cefaclor; see also notes above

Cautions see under Cefaclor; **interactions:** Appendix 1 (cephalosporins)

Contra-indications see under Cefaclor

Hepatic impairment manufacturer advises caution in severe impairment

Renal impairment reduce dose if eGFR less than 50 mL/minute/1.73 m^2—consult product literature

Pregnancy see under Cefaclor

Breast-feeding see under Cefaclor

Side-effects see under Cefaclor; also taste disturbances, paraesthesia

Dose

- By intravenous injection *or* infusion (*or by deep intramuscular injection if intravenous administration not possible*) 1–2 g every 8 hours; in meningitis, septicaemia, hospital-acquired pneumonia, or in febrile patients with neutropenia, 2 g every 8 hours; single doses over 1 g intravenous route only; ELDERLY over 80 years usual max. 3 g daily

  Complicated urinary-tract infection, 1–2 g every 8–12 hours; single doses over 1 g intravenous route only; ELDERLY over 80 years usual max. 3 g daily

  Pseudomonal lung infection in cystic fibrosis, ADULT 100–150 mg/kg daily (max. 9 g daily) in 3 divided doses; single doses over 1 g intravenous route only

  Prophylaxis for transurethral resection of prostate, 1 g up to 30 minutes before the procedure, repeated if necessary when catheter removed

- CHILD under 18 years see *BNF for Children*

Ceftazidime (Non-proprietary) PoM

Injection, powder for reconstitution, ceftazidime (as pentahydrate), with sodium carbonate, net price 1-g vial = £1.40; 2-g vial = £17.90

Fortum® (GSK) PoM

Injection, powder for reconstitution, ceftazidime (as pentahydrate), with sodium carbonate, net price 500-mg vial = £4.40, 1-g vial = £8.79, 2-g vial = £17.59, 3-g vial = £25.76

Electrolytes Na⁺ 2.3 mmol/g

Kefadim® (Flynn) PoM

Injection, powder for reconstitution, ceftazidime (as pentahydrate), with sodium carbonate, net price 1-g vial = £7.92; 2-g vial = £15.84

Electrolytes Na⁺ 2.3 mmol/g

CEFTRIAXONE

Indications see under Cefaclor and notes above; surgical prophylaxis; prophylaxis of meningococcal meningitis and *Haemophilus influenzae* type b disease [unlicensed indications] (Table 2, section 5.1)

Cautions see under Cefaclor; may displace bilirubin from serum albumin, administer over 60 minutes in neonates (see also Contra-indications); treatment longer than 14 days, renal failure, dehydration—risk of ceftriaxone precipitation in gall bladder; **interactions:** Appendix 1 (cephalosporins)

Contra-indications see under Cefaclor; neonates less than 41 weeks corrected gestational age; neonates over 41 weeks corrected gestational age with jaundice, hypoalbuminaemia, or acidosis; concomitant treatment with intravenous calcium (including total parenteral nutrition containing calcium) in neonates over 41 weeks corrected gestational age—risk of precipitation in urine and lungs

Hepatic impairment reduce dose and monitor plasma concentration if both hepatic and severe renal impairment

Renal impairment reduce dose if eGFR less than 10 mL/minute/1.73 m² (max. 2 g daily); monitor plasma concentration if both hepatic and severe renal impairment

Pregnancy see under Cefaclor

Breast-feeding see under Cefaclor

Side-effects see under Cefaclor; calcium ceftriaxone precipitates in urine (particularly in very young, dehydrated or those who are immobilised) or in gall

bladder—consider discontinuation if symptomatic; rarely prolongation of prothrombin time, pancreatitis

Dose

- By deep intramuscular injection, *or* by intravenous injection over at least 2–4 minutes, *or* by intravenous infusion, 1 g daily; 2–4 g daily in severe infections; intramuscular doses over 1 g divided between more than one site; single intravenous doses above 1 g by intravenous infusion only

  NEONATE, by intravenous infusion over 60 minutes, 20–50 mg/kg daily (max. 50 mg/kg daily); INFANT and CHILD under 50 kg, by deep intramuscular injection, *or* by intravenous injection over 2–4 minutes, *or* by intravenous infusion, 20–50 mg/kg daily; up to 80 mg/kg daily in severe infections; doses of 50 mg/kg and over by intravenous infusion only; 50 kg and over, adult dose

- Endocarditis caused by haemophilus, actinobacillus, cardiobacterium, eikenella, and kingella species ('HACEK organisms') (in combination with another antibacterial, see Table 1, section 5.1; [unlicensed indication]), by intravenous infusion, 2–4 g daily

- Early syphilis [unlicensed indication], by deep intramuscular injection, 500 mg daily for 10 days

- Uncomplicated gonorrhoea, pelvic inflammatory disease (see also Table 1, section 5.1), by deep intramuscular injection, 500 mg as a single dose [unlicensed dose]

- Surgical prophylaxis, by deep intramuscular injection *or* by intravenous injection over at least 2–4 minutes, 1 g up to 30 minutes before the procedure; colorectal surgery, by deep intramuscular injection *or* by intravenous infusion, 2 g up to 30 minutes before the procedure; intramuscular doses over 1 g divided between more than one site

Ceftriaxone (Non-proprietary) PoM

Injection, powder for reconstitution, ceftriaxone (as sodium salt), net price 1-g vial = £9.58; 2-g vial = £19.18

Rocephin® (Roche) PoM

Injection, powder for reconstitution, ceftriaxone (as sodium salt), net price 250-mg vial = £2.40; 1-g vial = £9.58; 2-g vial = £19.18

Electrolytes Na⁺ 3.6 mmol/g

CEFUROXIME

Indications see under Cefaclor; surgical prophylaxis; more active against *Haemophilus influenzae*; Lyme disease

Cautions see under Cefaclor; **interactions:** Appendix 1 (cephalosporins)

Contra-indications see under Cefaclor

Renal impairment use parenteral dose of 750 mg twice daily if eGFR 10–20 mL/minute/1.73 m²; use parenteral dose of 750 mg once daily if eGFR less than 10 mL/minute/1.73 m²

Pregnancy see under Cefaclor

Breast-feeding see under Cefaclor

Side-effects see under Cefaclor

Dose

- By mouth (as cefuroxime axetil), 250 mg twice daily in most infections including mild to moderate lower respiratory-tract infections (e.g. bronchitis); doubled for more severe lower respiratory-tract infections or if pneumonia suspected

Urinary-tract infection, 125 mg twice daily, doubled in pyelonephritis

CHILD over 3 months, 125 mg twice daily, if necessary doubled in child over 2 years with otitis media

Lyme disease (see also section 5.1.1.3), ADULT and CHILD over 12 years, 500 mg twice daily for 14–21 days (for 28 days in Lyme arthritis) [unlicensed duration]

- By intramuscular injection *or* intravenous injection *or* infusion, 750 mg every 6–8 hours; 1.5 g every 6–8 hours in severe infections; single doses over 750 mg intravenous route only

CHILD usual dose 60 mg/kg daily (range 30–100 mg/kg daily) in 3–4 divided doses (2–3 divided doses in neonates)

- Surgical prophylaxis, 1.5 g by intravenous injection up to 30 minutes before the procedure; up to 3 further doses of 750 mg may be given by intramuscular *or* intravenous injection every 8 hours for high-risk procedures

- Open fractures, prophylaxis (see also Table 2, section 5.1), by intravenous injection *or* infusion, 1.5 g every 8 hours until soft-tissue closure (max. duration 72 hours)

Cefuroxime (Non-proprietary) ▣PoM

Tablets, cefuroxime (as axetil) 250 mg, net price 14-tab pack = £17.00. Label: 9, 21, 25

Injection, powder for reconstitution, cefuroxime (as sodium salt), net price 750-mg vial =£2.52; 1.5-g vial = £5.05

Zinacef® (GSK) ▣PoM

Injection, powder for reconstitution, cefuroxime (as sodium salt). Net price 250-mg vial = 94p; 750-mg vial = £2.34; 1.5-g vial = £4.70

Electrolytes Na⁺ 1.8 mmol/750-mg vial

Zinnat® (GSK) ▣PoM

Tablets, both f/c, cefuroxime (as axetil) 125 mg, net price 14-tab pack = £4.56; 250 mg, 14-tab pack = £9.11. Label: 9, 21, 25

Suspension, cefuroxime (as axetil) 125 mg/5 mL when reconstituted with water, net price 70 mL (tutti-frutti-flavoured) = £5.20. Label: 9, 21

Excipients include aspartame (section 9.4.1), sucrose 3.1 g/5 mL

5.1.2.2 Carbapenems

The carbapenems are beta-lactam antibacterials with a broad-spectrum of activity which includes many Gram-positive and Gram-negative bacteria, and anaerobes; **imipenem** and **meropenem** have good activity against *Pseudomonas aeruginosa*. The carbapenems are not active against meticillin-resistant *Staphylococcus aureus* and *Enterococcus faecium*.

Imipenem and meropenem are used for the treatment of severe hospital-acquired infections and polymicrobial infections including septicaemia, hospital-acquired pneumonia, intra-abdominal infections, skin and soft-tissue infections, and complicated urinary-tract infections.

Ertapenem is licensed for treating abdominal and gynaecological infections and for community-acquired pneumonia, but it is not active against atypical respiratory pathogens and it has limited activity against penicillin-resistant pneumococci. It is also licensed for treating foot infections of the skin and soft tissue in patients with diabetes. Unlike the other carbapenems, ertape-

nem is not active against *Pseudomonas* or against *Acinetobacter* spp.

Imipenem is partially inactivated in the kidney by enzymatic activity and is therefore administered in combination with **cilastatin**, a specific enzyme inhibitor, which blocks its renal metabolism. Meropenem and ertapenem are stable to the renal enzyme which inactivates imipenem and therefore can be given without cilastatin.

Side-effects of imipenem with cilastatin are similar to those of other beta-lactam antibiotics; neurotoxicity has been observed at very high dosage, in renal failure, or in patients with CNS disease. Ertapenem has been associated with seizures uncommonly. Meropenem has less seizure-inducing potential and can be used to treat central nervous system infection.

▮ ERTAPENEM

Indications abdominal infections; acute gynaecological infections; community-acquired pneumonia; diabetic foot infections of the skin and soft-tissue; prophylaxis for colorectal surgery

Cautions sensitivity to beta-lactam antibacterials (avoid if history of immediate hypersensitivity reaction, see also p. 366); elderly, CNS disorders—risk of seizures; **interactions**: Appendix 1 (ertapenem)

Renal impairment risk of seizures; max. 500 mg daily if eGFR less than 30 mL/minute/1.73 m²

Pregnancy manufacturer advises avoid unless potential benefit outweighs risk

Breast-feeding present in milk—manufacturer advises avoid

Side-effects diarrhoea, nausea, vomiting, headache, injection-site reactions, rash (also reported with eosinophilia and systemic symptoms), pruritus, raised platelet count; *less commonly* dry mouth, taste disturbances, dyspepsia, abdominal pain, anorexia, constipation, melaena, antibiotic-associated colitis, bradycardia, hypotension, chest pain, oedema, pharyngeal discomfort, dyspnoea, dizziness, sleep disturbances, confusion, asthenia, seizures, raised glucose, petechiae; *rarely* dysphagia, cholecystitis, liver disorder (including jaundice), arrhythmia, increase in blood pressure, syncope, nasal congestion, cough, wheezing, anxiety, depression, agitation, tremor, pelvic peritonitis, renal impairment, muscle cramp, scleral disorder, blood disorders (including neutropenia, thrombocytopenia, haemorrhage), hypoglycaemia, electrolyte disturbances; also reported hallucinations, dyskinesia

Dose

- By intravenous infusion, ADULT and ADOLESCENT over 13 years, 1 g once daily; CHILD 3 months–13 years, 15 mg/kg every 12 hours (max. 1 g daily)

Surgical prophylaxis, colorectal surgery, ADULT over 18 years, 1 g completed within 1 hour before surgery

Invanz® (MSD) ▣PoM

Intravenous infusion, powder for reconstitution, ertapenem (as sodium salt), net price 1-g vial = £31.65

Electrolytes Na⁺ 6 mmol/1-g vial

▮ IMIPENEM WITH CILASTATIN

Indications aerobic and anaerobic Gram-positive and Gram-negative infections; hospital-acquired septicaemia (Table 1, section 5.1); not indicated for CNS infections

Cautions sensitivity to beta-lactam antibacterials (avoid if history of immediate hypersensitivity reaction, see also p. 366); CNS disorders (e.g. epilepsy); **interactions:** Appendix 1 (imipenem with cilastatin)

Renal impairment risk of CNS side-effects; reduce dose if eGFR less than 70 mL/minute/1.73 m²—consult product literature

Pregnancy manufacturer advises avoid unless potential benefit outweighs risk (toxicity in *animal* studies)

Breast-feeding present in milk but unlikely to be absorbed

Side-effects nausea (may reduce rate of infusion), vomiting, diarrhoea (rarely antibiotic-associated colitis), eosinophilia, rash (rarely toxic epidermal necrolysis and Stevens-Johnson syndrome); *less commonly* hypotension, seizures, myoclonic activity, dizziness, drowsiness, hallucinations, confusion, leucopenia, thrombocytopenia, thrombocytosis, positive Coombs' test; *rarely* taste disturbances, hepatitis, encephalopathy, anaphylactic reactions, paraesthesia, tremor, acute renal failure, polyuria, tooth, tongue or urine discoloration, hearing loss; *very rarely*, abdominal pain, heartburn, glossitis, tachycardia, palpitation, flushing, cyanosis, dyspnoea, hyperventilation, headache, asthenia, haemolytic anaemia, aggravation of myasthenia gravis, polyarthralgia, tinnitus, hypersalivation, hyperhidrosis

Dose

- By intravenous infusion, in terms of imipenem, 500 mg every 6 hours *or* 1 g every 8 hours; infection caused by *Pseudomonas* or other less sensitive organisms, life-threatening infection, or empirical treatment of infection in febrile patients with neutropenia, 1 g every 6 hours; CHILD under 1 year see *BNF for Children*; 1 year and older, 15 mg/kg (max. 500 mg) every 6 hours; infection caused by *Pseudomonas* or other less sensitive organisms, life-threatening infection, or empirical treatment of infection in febrile patients with neutropenia, 25 mg/kg (max. 1 g) every 6 hours

Imipenem with cilastatin (Non-proprietary) PoM

Intravenous infusion, powder for reconstitution, imipenem (as monohydrate) 500 mg with cilastatin (as sodium salt) 500 mg, net price per vial = £12.00

Primaxin® (MSD) PoM

Intravenous infusion, powder for reconstitution, imipenem (as monohydrate) 500 mg with cilastatin (as sodium salt) 500 mg, net price per vial = £12.00
Electrolytes Na⁺ 1.6 mmol/vial

MEROPENEM

Indications aerobic and anaerobic Gram-positive and Gram-negative infections (see notes above); hospital-acquired septicaemia (Table 1, section 5.1)

Cautions sensitivity to beta-lactam antibacterials (avoid if history of immediate hypersensitivity reaction, see also p. 366); **interactions:** Appendix 1 (meropenem)

Hepatic impairment monitor liver function

Renal impairment use normal dose every 12 hours if eGFR 26–50 mL/minute/1.73 m²; use half normal dose every 12 hours if eGFR 10–25 mL/minute/1.73 m²; use half normal dose every 24 hours if eGFR less than 10 mL/minute/1.73 m²

Pregnancy use only if potential benefit outweighs risk—no information available

Breast-feeding unlikely to be absorbed (however, manufacturer advises avoid)

Side-effects nausea, vomiting, diarrhoea (antibiotic-associated colitis reported), abdominal pain, disturbances in liver function tests, headache, thrombocythaemia, rash, pruritus; *less commonly* paraesthesia, eosinophilia, thrombocytopenia, leucopenia; *rarely* convulsions; also reported haemolytic anaemia, positive Coombs' test, Stevens-Johnson syndrome, toxic epidermal necrolysis

Dose

- By intravenous injection over 5 minutes *or* by intravenous infusion, 0.5–1 g every 8 hours; CHILD 3 months–12 years 10–20 mg/kg every 8 hours, bodyweight over 50 kg, adult dose
  Exacerbations of chronic lower respiratory-tract infection in cystic fibrosis, meningitis, 2 g every 8 hours; CHILD 3 months–12 years 40 mg/kg every 8 hours, body-weight over 50 kg, adult dose
  Endocarditis (in combination with another antibacterial [unlicensed], see Table 1, section 5.1), ADULT over 18 years, 2 g every 8 hours

Meropenem (Non-proprietary) PoM

Injection, powder for reconstitution, meropenem (as trihydrate), net price 500-mg vial = £8.00; 1-g vial = £16.00

Meronem® (AstraZeneca) PoM

Injection, powder for reconstitution, meropenem (as trihydrate), net price 500-mg vial = £10.31; 1-g vial = £20.63
Electrolytes Na⁺ 3.9 mmol/g

5.1.2.3 Other beta-lactam antibiotics

Aztreonam is a monocyclic beta-lactam ('monobactam') antibiotic with an antibacterial spectrum limited to Gram-negative aerobic bacteria including *Pseudomonas aeruginosa*, *Neisseria meningitidis*, and *Haemophilus influenzae*; it should not be used alone for 'blind' treatment since it is not active against Gram-positive organisms. Aztreonam is also effective against *Neisseria gonorrhoeae* (but not against concurrent chlamydial infection). Side-effects are similar to those of the other beta-lactams although aztreonam may be less likely to cause hypersensitivity in penicillin-sensitive patients.

Aztreonam may be administered by nebuliser for the treatment of chronic *Ps. aeruginosa* infection in cystic fibrosis. The *Scottish Medicines Consortium* (p. 4) has advised (January 2012) that aztreonam powder for nebuliser solution (*Cayston®*) is **not** recommended for use within NHS Scotland.

AZTREONAM

Indications Gram-negative infections including *Pseudomonas aeruginosa*, *Haemophilus influenzae*, and *Neisseria meningitidis*

Cautions hypersensitivity to beta-lactam antibiotics; **interactions:** Appendix 1 (aztreonam)
Specific cautions for inhaled treatment Other inhaled drugs should be administered before aztreonam; a bronchodilator should be administered before each dose. Measure lung function before and after initial dose of aztreonam and monitor for bronchospasm. Haemoptysis—risk of further haemorrhage

Contra-indications aztreonam hypersensitivity

Hepatic impairment use injection with caution and monitor liver function

Renal impairment if eGFR 10–30 mL/minute/ 1.73 m², usual initial dose of injection, then half normal dose; if eGFR less than 10 mL/minute/1.73 m², usual initial dose of injection, then one-quarter normal dose

Pregnancy no information available; manufacturer of injection advises avoid; manufacturer of powder for nebuliser solution advises avoid unless essential

Breast-feeding amount in milk probably too small to be harmful

Side-effects

Specific side-effects for parenteral treatment *Rarely* gastro-intestinal bleeding, antibiotic-associated colitis, jaundice, hepatitis, hypotension, chest pain, dyspnoea, seizures, paraesthesia, confusion, dizziness, asthenia, headache, insomnia, breast tenderness, blood disorders (including thrombocytopenia and neutropenia), myalgia, diplopia, tinnitus, halitosis; also reported nausea, vomiting, abdominal pain, diarrhoea, mouth ulcers, taste disturbances, flushing, bronchospasm, rash (including toxic epidermal necrolysis and erythema multiforme)

Specific side-effects for inhaled treatment Wheezing, bronchospasm, cough, haemoptysis, pyrexia, arthralgia, rash, rhinorrhoea, pharyngolaryngeal pain

Dose

• By deep intramuscular injection *or* by intravenous injection over 3–5 minutes *or* by intravenous infusion, 1 g every 8 hours *or* 2 g every 12 hours; 2 g every 6–8 hours for severe infections (including systemic *Pseudomonas aeruginosa* and lung infections in cystic fibrosis); single doses over 1 g intravenous route only Urinary-tract infections, 0.5–1 g every 8–12 hours

• CHILD over 1 week, by intravenous injection *or* infusion, 30 mg/kg every 6–8 hours increased in severe infections for child of 2 years or older to 50 mg/kg every 6–8 hours; max. 8 g daily

• Gonorrhoea, cystitis, by intramuscular injection, 1 g as a single dose

• Chronic pulmonary *Pseudomonas aeruginosa* infection in patients with cystic fibrosis, by inhalation of nebulised solution, ADULT and CHILD over 6 years, 75 mg 3 times daily (at least 4 hours apart) for 28 days, subsequent courses repeated after 28-day interval without aztreonam nebuliser solution

◢ **Parenteral**

Azactam® (Squibb) [PoM]
Injection, powder for reconstitution, aztreonam, net price 1-g vial = £9.40; 2-g vial = £18.82

◢ **Inhalation**

Cayston® (Gilead) [PoM]
Powder for nebuliser solution, aztreonam (as lysine), net price 84 × 75 mg vials (with solvent and nebuliser handset) = £2181.53

5.1.3 Tetracyclines

The tetracyclines are broad-spectrum antibiotics whose value has decreased owing to increasing bacterial resistance. They remain, however, the treatment of choice for infections caused by chlamydia (trachoma, psittacosis, salpingitis, urethritis, and lymphogranuloma venereum), rickettsia (including Q-fever), brucella (doxycycline with either streptomycin or rifampicin), and the spirochaete, *Borrelia burgdorferi* (Lyme disease—see section 5.1.1.3). They are also used in respiratory and genital mycoplasma infections, in acne, in destructive (refractory) periodontal disease, in exacerbations of chronic bronchitis (because of their activity against

Haemophilus influenzae), and for leptospirosis in penicillin hypersensitivity (as an alternative to erythromycin).

For the role of tetracyclines in the management of meticillin-resistant *Staphylococcus aureus* (MRSA) infection, see p. 368.

Microbiologically, there is little to choose between the various tetracyclines, the only exception being **minocycline** which has a broader spectrum; it is active against *Neisseria meningitidis* and has been used for meningococcal prophylaxis but is no longer recommended because of side-effects including dizziness and vertigo (see section 5.1, table 2 for current recommendations). Compared to other tetracyclines, minocycline is associated with a greater risk of lupus-erythematosus-like syndrome. Minocycline sometimes causes irreversible pigmentation.

Oral infections In adults, tetracyclines can be effective against oral anaerobes but the development of resistance (especially by oral streptococci) has reduced their usefulness for the treatment of acute oral infections; they may still have a role in the treatment of destructive (refractory) forms of periodontal disease. Doxycycline has a longer duration of action than tetracycline or oxytetracycline and need only be given once daily; it is reported to be more active against anaerobes than some other tetracyclines.

For the use of doxycycline in the treatment of recurrent aphthous ulceration, or as an adjunct to gingival scaling and root planing for periodontitis, see section 12.3.1.

Cautions Tetracyclines may increase muscle weakness in patients with myasthenia gravis, and exacerbate systemic lupus erythematosus. Antacids, and aluminium, calcium, iron, magnesium and zinc salts decrease the absorption of tetracyclines; milk also reduces the absorption of demeclocycline, oxytetracycline, and tetracycline. Other **interactions:** Appendix 1 (tetracyclines).

Contra-indications Deposition of tetracyclines in growing bone and teeth (by binding to calcium) causes staining and occasionally dental hypoplasia, and they should **not** be given to children under 12 years, or to pregnant or breast-feeding women. However, doxycycline may be used in children for treatment and post-exposure prophylaxis of anthrax when an alternative antibacterial cannot be given [unlicensed indication].

Hepatic impairment Tetracyclines should be avoided or used with caution in patients with hepatic impairment. Tetracyclines should also be used with caution in those receiving potentially hepatotoxic drugs.

Renal impairment With the exception of **doxycycline** and **minocycline**, the tetracyclines may exacerbate renal failure and should **not** be given to patients with renal impairment.

Pregnancy Tetracyclines should **not** be given to pregnant women. Effects on skeletal development have been documented when tetracyclines have been used in the first trimester in *animal* studies. Administration during the second or third trimester may cause discoloration of the child's teeth, and maternal hepatotoxicity has been reported with large parenteral doses. However, when travel to malarious areas is unavoidable during pregnancy, doxycycline can be used for malaria prophylaxis if other regimens are unsuitable (section

5.4.1), and if the entire course of doxycycline can be completed before 15 weeks' gestation [unlicensed].

Breast-feeding Tetracyclines should **not** be given to women who are breast-feeding (although absorption and therefore discoloration of teeth in the infant is probably usually prevented by chelation with calcium in milk)..

Side-effects Side-effects of the tetracyclines include nausea, vomiting, diarrhoea (antibiotic-associated colitis reported occasionally), dysphagia, and oesophageal irritation. Other rare side-effects include hepatotoxicity, pancreatitis, blood disorders, photosensitivity (particularly with demeclocycline), and hypersensitivity reactions (including rash, exfoliative dermatitis, Stevens-Johnson syndrome, urticaria, angioedema, anaphylaxis, pericarditis). Headache and visual disturbances may indicate benign intracranial hypertension (discontinue treatment); bulging fontanelles have been reported in infants.

TETRACYCLINE

Indications see notes above; acne vulgaris, rosacea (section 13.6)

Cautions see notes above

Contra-indications see notes above

Hepatic impairment see notes above; max. 1 g daily in divided doses

Renal impairment see notes above

Pregnancy see notes above

Breast-feeding see notes above

Side-effects see notes above; also acute renal failure, skin discoloration

Dose
- 250 mg every 6 hours, increased in severe infections to 500 mg every 6–8 hours
- Acne, see section 13.6.2
- Non-gonococcal urethritis, 500 mg every 6 hours for 7–14 days (21 days if failure or relapse after first course)

Counselling Tablets should be swallowed whole with plenty of fluid while sitting or standing

Tetracycline (Non-proprietary) [PoM]
Tablets, coated, tetracycline hydrochloride 250 mg, net price 28-tab pack = £2.61. Label: 7, 9, 23, counselling, posture

Dental prescribing on NHS Tetracycline Tablets may be prescribed

DEMECLOCYCLINE HYDROCHLORIDE

Indications see notes above; also inappropriate secretion of antidiuretic hormone, section 6.5.2

Cautions see notes above, but photosensitivity more common (avoid exposure to sunlight or sun lamps)

Contra-indications see notes above

Hepatic impairment see notes above; max. 1 g daily in divided doses

Renal impairment see notes above

Pregnancy see notes above

Breast-feeding see notes above

Side-effects see notes above; also reversible nephrogenic diabetes insipidus, acute renal failure

Dose
- 150 mg every 6 hours or 300 mg every 12 hours

Demeclocycline hydrochloride (Non-proprietary) [PoM]
Capsules, demeclocycline hydrochloride 150 mg, net price 28-cap pack = £81.49. Label: 7, 9, 11, 23

DOXYCYCLINE

Indications see notes above; chronic prostatitis; sinusitis, syphilis, pelvic inflammatory disease (Table 1, section 5.1); treatment and prophylaxis of anthrax [unlicensed indication]; malaria treatment and prophylaxis (section 5.4.1); recurrent aphthous ulceration, adjunct to gingival scaling and root planing for periodontitis (section 12.3.1); rosacea, acne vulgaris (section 13.6)

Cautions see notes above; alcohol dependence; photosensitivity reported (avoid exposure to sunlight or sun lamps)

Contra-indications see notes above

Hepatic impairment see notes above

Renal impairment use with caution (avoid excessive doses)

Pregnancy see notes above

Breast-feeding see notes above

Side-effects see notes above; also anorexia, dry mouth, flushing, anxiety, and tinnitus

Dose
- 200 mg on first day, then 100 mg daily; severe infections (including refractory urinary-tract infections), 200 mg daily
- Early syphilis, 100 mg twice daily for 14 days; late latent syphilis, 100 mg twice daily for 28 days; neurosyphilis, 200 mg twice daily for 28 days
- Uncomplicated genital chlamydia, non-gonococcal urethritis, 100 mg twice daily for 7 days (14 days in pelvic inflammatory disease, see also Table 1, section 5.1)
- Lyme disease (see also section 5.1.1.3), 100 mg twice daily for 10–14 days (28 days in Lyme arthritis)
- Anthrax (treatment or post-exposure prophylaxis; see also section 5.1.12), 100 mg twice daily; CHILD (only if alternative antibacterial cannot be given) [unlicensed dose] 5 mg/kg daily in 2 divided doses (max. 200 mg daily)

Counselling Capsules should be swallowed whole with plenty of fluid during meals while sitting or standing
Note Doxycycline doses in BNF may differ from those in product literature

Doxycycline (Non-proprietary) [PoM]
Capsules, doxycycline (as hyclate) 50 mg, net price 28-cap pack = £1.70; 100 mg, 8-cap pack = £1.14. Label: 6, 9, 11, 27, counselling, posture
Brands include *Doxylar®*
Dental prescribing on NHS Doxycycline Capsules 100 mg may be prescribed

Vibramycin-D® (Pfizer) [PoM]
Dispersible tablets, yellow, scored, doxycycline 100 mg, net price 8-tab pack = £4.91. Label: 6, 9, 11, 13
Dental prescribing on NHS May be prescribed as Dispersible Doxycycline Tablets

◢Modified-release
Efracea® (Galderma) [PoM]
Capsules, m/r, beige, doxycycline (as monohydrate) 40 mg, net price 56-cap pack = £21.71. Label: 6, 11, 27, counselling, posture
Dose papulopustular, facial rosacea (without ocular involvement), 40 mg daily in the morning for 16 weeks; consider discontinuing treatment if no response after 6 weeks

5

Infections

Infections (side tab) 5

▌LYMECYCLINE

Indications see notes above
Cautions see notes above
Contra-indications see notes above
Hepatic impairment see notes above
Renal impairment see notes above
Pregnancy see notes above
Breast-feeding see notes above
Side-effects see notes above
Dose
• 408 mg every 12 hours, increased to 1.224–1.632 g daily in severe infections
• Acne, 408 mg daily for at least 8 weeks

Lymecycline (Non-proprietary) PoM
Capsules, lymecycline 408 mg (= tetracycline 300 mg), net price 28-cap pack = £7.49. Label: 6, 9

Tetralysal 300® (Galderma) PoM
Capsules, red/yellow, lymecycline 408 mg (= tetracycline 300 mg), net price 28-cap pack = £5.95, 56-cap pack = £11.53. Label: 6, 9

▌MINOCYCLINE

Indications see notes above; meningococcal carrier state; acne vulgaris (section 13.6.2)
Cautions see notes above; if treatment continued for longer than 6 months, monitor every 3 months for hepatotoxicity, pigmentation and for systemic lupus erythematosus—discontinue if these develop or if pre-existing systemic lupus erythematosus worsens
Contra-indications see notes above
Hepatic impairment see notes above
Renal impairment use with caution (avoid excessive doses)
Pregnancy see notes above
Breast-feeding see notes above
Side-effects see notes above; also dizziness and vertigo (more common in women); *rarely* anorexia, tinnitus, impaired hearing, hyperaesthesia, paraesthesia, acute renal failure, pigmentation (sometimes irreversible), and alopecia; *very rarely* systemic lupus erythematosus, discoloration of conjunctiva, tears, and sweat
Dose
• 100 mg twice daily
• Acne, see section 13.6.2 and under preparations, below
• Prophylaxis of asymptomatic meningococcal carrier state (but no longer recommended, see notes above), 100 mg twice daily for 5 days usually followed by rifampicin
Counselling Tablets or capsules should be swallowed whole with plenty of fluid while sitting or standing

Minocycline (Non-proprietary) PoM ◢
Capsules, minocycline (as hydrochloride) 50 mg, net price 56-cap pack = £15.27; 100 mg, 28-cap pack = £13.09. Label: 6, 9, counselling, posture
Brands include *Aknemin®*

Tablets, minocycline (as hydrochloride) 50 mg, net price 28-tab pack = £5.63, 100 mg, 28-tab pack = £11.62. Label: 6, 9, counselling, posture

◢Modified release
Minocycline m/r preparations PoM ◢
Capsules, m/r, minocycline (as hydrochloride) 100 mg, net price 56-cap pack = £20.08. Label: 6, 25
Brands include *Acnamino®* MR, *Minocin MR®*, *Sebomin MR®*
Dose acne, 100 mg daily

▌OXYTETRACYCLINE

Indications see notes above; acne vulgaris, rosacea (section 13.6)
Cautions see notes above
Contra-indications see notes above
Hepatic impairment see notes above
Renal impairment see notes above
Pregnancy see notes above
Breast-feeding see notes above
Side-effects see notes above
Dose
• 250–500 mg every 6 hours
• Acne, see section 13.6.2

Oxytetracycline (Non-proprietary) PoM
Tablets, coated, oxytetracycline dihydrate 250 mg, net price 28-tab pack = £1.22. Label: 7, 9, 23
Brands include *Oxymycin®*
Dental prescribing on NHS Oxtetracycline Tablets may be prescribed

Tigecycline

Tigecycline is a glycylcycline antibacterial structurally related to the tetracyclines; side-effects similar to those of the tetracyclines can potentially occur. Tigecycline is active against Gram-positive and Gram-negative bacteria, including tetracycline-resistant organisms, and some anaerobes. It is also active against meticillin-resistant *Staphylococcus aureus* and vancomycin-resistant enterococci, but *Pseudomonas aeruginosa* and many strains of *Proteus spp* are resistant to tigecycline. Tigecycline should be reserved for the treatment of complicated skin and soft-tissue infections and complicated abdominal infections caused by multiple-antibacterial resistant organisms when other antibacterials cannot be used; it is not recommended for the treatment of foot infections in patients with diabetes.

▌TIGECYCLINE

Indications see notes above
Cautions cholestasis; **interactions:** Appendix 1 (tigecycline)
Contra-indications hypersensitivity to tetracyclines
Hepatic impairment initially 100 mg then 25 mg every 12 hours in severe impairment
Pregnancy see under Tetracyclines, p. 380
Breast-feeding manufacturer advises caution—present in milk in *animal* studies
Side-effects see notes above; also nausea, vomiting, abdominal pain, dyspepsia, diarrhoea, anorexia, bilirubinaemia, dizziness, headache, hypoglycaemia, prolonged prothrombin time, prolonged activated partial thromboplastin time, rash, pruritus, and injec-

tion-site reactions; *less commonly* pancreatitis, chole-static jaundice, and hypoproteinaemia; also reported, antibiotic-associated colitis, hepatic failure, thrombocytopenia, Stevens-Johnson syndrome

Dose
• By intravenous infusion, ADULT over 18 years, initially 100 mg, then 50 mg every 12 hours for 5–14 days

Tygacil® (Pfizer) ▼ PoM
Intravenous infusion, powder for reconstitution, tigecycline, net price 50-mg vial = £32.31

5.1.4 Aminoglycosides

These include amikacin, gentamicin, neomycin, streptomycin, and tobramycin. All are bactericidal and active against some Gram-positive and many Gram-negative organisms. Amikacin, gentamicin, and tobramycin are also active against *Pseudomonas aeruginosa*; streptomycin is active against *Mycobacterium tuberculosis* and is now almost entirely reserved for tuberculosis (section 5.1.9).

The aminoglycosides are not absorbed from the gut (although there is a risk of absorption in inflammatory bowel disease and liver failure) and must therefore be given by injection for systemic infections.

The important side-effects of aminoglycosides are ototoxicity and nephrotoxicity; they occur most commonly in the elderly and in patients with renal failure.

Gentamicin is the aminoglycoside of choice in the UK and is used widely for the treatment of serious infections. It has a broad spectrum but is inactive against anaerobes and has poor activity against haemolytic streptococci and pneumococci. When used for the 'blind' therapy of undiagnosed serious infections it is usually given in conjunction with a penicillin or metronidazole (or both). Gentamicin is used together with another antibiotic for the treatment of endocarditis (see below and Table 1, section 5.1).

Loading and maintenance doses of gentamicin may be calculated on the basis of the patient's weight and renal function (e.g. using a nomogram); adjustments are then made according to serum-gentamicin concentrations. High doses are occasionally indicated for serious infections, especially in the neonate, in the patient with cystic fibrosis, or in the immunocompromised patient. Whenever possible treatment should not exceed 7 days.

Amikacin is more stable than gentamicin to enzyme inactivation. Amikacin is used in the treatment of serious infections caused by gentamicin-resistant Gram-negative bacilli.

Tobramycin has similar activity to gentamicin. It is slightly more active against *Ps. aeruginosa* but shows less activity against certain other Gram-negative bacteria. Tobramycin can be administered by nebuliser or by inhalation of powder on a cyclical basis (28 days of tobramycin followed by a 28–day tobramycin-free interval) for the treatment of chronic pulmonary *Ps. aeruginosa* infection in cystic fibrosis; however, resistance may develop and some patients do not respond to treatment.

Neomycin is too toxic for parenteral administration and can only be used for infections of the skin or mucous membranes or to reduce the bacterial population of the colon prior to bowel surgery or in hepatic failure. Oral administration may lead to malabsorption. Small amounts of neomycin may be absorbed from the gut in patients with hepatic failure and, as these patients may also be uraemic, cumulation may occur with resultant ototoxicity.

Endocarditis **Gentamicin** is used in combination with other antibiotics for the treatment of bacterial endocarditis (Table 1, section 5.1). Serum-gentamicin concentration should be measured after 3 or 4 doses, then at least every 3 days and after a dose change (more frequently in renal impairment). **Streptomycin** may be used as an alternative in gentamicin-resistant enterococcal endocarditis.

Once daily dosage *Once daily administration* of aminoglycosides is more convenient, provides adequate serum concentrations, and in many cases has largely superseded *multiple daily dose regimens* (given in 2–3 divided doses during the 24 hours). Local guidelines on dosage and serum concentrations should be consulted. A once-daily, high-dose regimen of an aminoglycoside should be avoided in patients with endocarditis due to Gram-positive bacteria, HACEK endocarditis, burns of more than 20% of the total body surface area, or creatinine clearance less than 20 mL/minute. There is insufficient evidence to recommend a once daily, high-dose regimen of an aminoglycoside in pregnancy.

Serum concentrations Serum concentration monitoring avoids both excessive and subtherapeutic concentrations thus preventing toxicity and ensuring efficacy. Serum-aminoglycoside concentrations should be measured in all patients receiving parenteral aminoglycosides, and **must** be determined in the elderly, in obesity, and in cystic fibrosis, *or* if high doses are being given, *or* if there is renal impairment.

In patients with normal renal function, aminoglycoside concentrations should be measured after 3 or 4 doses of a multiple daily dose regimen and after a dose change; patients with renal impairment may require earlier and more frequent measurement of aminoglycoside concentration.

For multiple daily dose regimens, blood samples should be taken approximately 1 hour after intramuscular or

5

Infections

intravenous administration ('peak' concentration) and also just before the next dose ('trough' concentration). If the pre-dose ('trough') concentration is high, the interval between doses must be increased. If the post-dose ('peak') concentration is high, the dose must be decreased. For once daily dose regimens, consult local guidelines on serum concentration monitoring.

Cautions The main side-effects of the aminoglycosides are dose-related, therefore, care must be taken with dosage, and, whenever possible, parenteral treatment should not exceed 7 days. Renal function should be assessed before starting an aminoglycoside and during treatment. If possible, dehydration should be corrected before starting an aminoglycoside. Auditory and vestibular function should also be monitored during treatment. In order to optimise the dose and avoid toxicity, serum-aminoglycoside concentrations should be monitored in patients receiving parenteral aminoglycosides (see also Serum Concentrations). Ototoxicity and nephrotoxicity occur most commonly in the elderly; therefore, monitoring is particularly important in these patients, who may require reduced doses.

Aminoglycosides should be used with caution in those with conditions characterised by muscular weakness (avoid in myasthenia gravis). If possible, aminoglycosides should not be given with potentially ototoxic drugs (e.g. cisplatin). Administration of an aminoglycoside and of an ototoxic diuretic (e.g. furosemide) should be separated by as long a period as practicable. **Interactions**: Appendix 1 (aminoglycosides)

Contra-indications Aminoglycosides may impair neuromuscular transmission and should not be given to patients with myasthenia gravis

Renal impairment Excretion of aminoglycosides is principally via the kidney and accumulation occurs in renal impairment. Ototoxicity and nephrotoxicity occur commonly in patients with renal failure. If there is impairment of renal function, the interval between doses must be increased; if the renal impairment is severe, the dose itself should be reduced as well. Serum-aminoglycoside concentrations **must** be monitored in patients with renal impairment, see Serum Concentrations above; renal, auditory, and vestibular function should also be monitored. A once-daily, high-dose regimen of an aminoglycoside should be avoided in patients with a creatinine clearance less than 20 mL/minute.

Pregnancy There is a risk of auditory or vestibular nerve damage in the infant when aminoglycosides are used in the second and third trimesters of pregnancy. The risk is greatest with streptomycin (section 5.1.9). The risk is probably very small with gentamicin and tobramycin, but their use should be avoided unless essential (if given, serum-aminoglycoside concentration monitoring is essential).

Side-effects The important side-effects of the aminoglycosides are nephrotoxicity and irreversible ototoxicity (including vestibular and auditory damage). Rash occurs commonly with streptomycin, but less frequently with the other aminoglycosides. Rare side-effects include nausea, vomiting, antibiotic-associated colitis, peripheral neuropathy, electrolyte disturbances (notably hypomagnesaemia on prolonged therapy, but also hypocalcaemia and hypokalaemia), and stomatitis. Side-effects reported very rarely include blood disorders and CNS effects (including headache, encephalopathy,

and convulsions). Aminoglycosides may impair neuromuscular transmission; large doses given during surgery have been responsible for a transient myasthenic syndrome in patients with normal neuromuscular function.

GENTAMICIN

Indications septicaemia and neonatal sepsis; meningitis and other CNS infections; biliary-tract infection, acute pyelonephritis or prostatitis, endocarditis (see notes above); pneumonia in hospital patients, adjunct in listerial meningitis (Table 1, section 5.1); eye (section 11.3.1); ear (section 12.1.1)

Cautions see above; **interactions**: Appendix 1 (aminoglycosides)

Contra-indications see notes above

Renal impairment see notes above

Pregnancy see notes above

Side-effects see notes above

Dose

> To avoid excessive dosage in obese patients, use ideal weight for height to calculate dose and monitor serum-gentamicin concentration closely

- Multiple daily dose regimen, by intramuscular *or* by slow intravenous injection over at least 3 minutes *or* by intravenous infusion, 3–5 mg/kg daily (in divided doses every 8 hours), see also notes above; CHILD under 18 years see *BNF for Children*
  Gram-positive bacterial endocarditis or HACEK endocarditis (in combination with other antibacterials, see Table 1, section 5.1), ADULT 1 mg/kg every 12 hours; CHILD under 18 years see *BNF for Children*
- Once daily dose regimen (see notes above and also consult local guidelines), by intravenous infusion, initially 5–7 mg/kg, then adjust according to serum-gentamicin concentration; CHILD under 18 years see *BNF for Children*
- Surgical prophylaxis, ADULT over 18 years, by slow intravenous injection over at least 3 minutes, 1.5 mg/kg up to 30 minutes before the procedure (up to 3 further doses of 1.5 mg/kg may be given every 8 hours for high-risk procedures) *or* (for joint replacement surgery) by intravenous infusion, 5 mg/kg as a single dose up to 30 minutes before the procedure
- By intrathecal injection, seek specialist advice, 1 mg daily (increased if necessary to 5 mg daily); only preservative-free, intrathecal preparation should be used; CHILD under 18 years see *BNF for Children*

Note For multiple daily dose regimen, one-hour ('peak') serum concentration should be 5–10 mg/litre (3–5 mg/litre for endocarditis); pre-dose ('trough') concentration should be less than 2 mg/litre (less than 1 mg/litre for endocarditis). For once-daily dose regimen, consult local guidelines on monitoring serum-gentamicin concentration

Gentamicin (Non-proprietary) ⓅoⓂ
  Injection, gentamicin (as sulfate), net price 40 mg/mL, 1-mL amp = £1.40, 2-mL amp = £1.00, 2-mL vial = £4.00

  Paediatric injection, gentamicin (as sulfate) 10 mg/mL, net price 2-mL vial = £2.25

  Intrathecal injection, gentamicin (as sulfate) 5 mg/mL, net price 1-mL amp = 74p

  Intravenous infusion, gentamicin (as sulfate) 1 mg/mL in sodium chloride intravenous infusion 0.9%, net price 80-mL (80 mg) bottle = £1.95; 3 mg/mL, 80-mL (240 mg) bottle = £5.95, 120-mL (360 mg) bottle = £8.45

Cidomycin® (Sanofi-Aventis) [PoM]

Injection, gentamicin (as sulfate) 40 mg/mL. Net price 2-mL amp or vial = £1.38

Genticin® (AMCo) [PoM]

Injection, gentamicin (as sulfate) 40 mg/mL. Net price 2-mL amp = £1.00

Isotonic Gentamicin Injection (Baxter) [PoM]

Intravenous infusion, gentamicin (as sulfate) 800 micrograms/mL in sodium chloride intravenous infusion 0.9%. Net price 100-mL (80-mg) *Viaflex®* bag = £1.61

Electrolytes Na⁺ 15.4 mmol/100-mL bag

◼ AMIKACIN

Indications serious Gram-negative infections resistant to gentamicin

Cautions see notes above; **interactions:** Appendix 1 (aminoglycosides)

Contra-indications see notes above

Renal impairment see notes above

Pregnancy see notes above

Side-effects see notes above

Dose

> To avoid excessive dosage in obese patients, use ideal weight for height to calculate dose and monitor serum-amikacin concentration closely

- Multiple daily dose regimen, by intramuscular *or* by slow intravenous injection *or* by infusion, 15 mg/kg daily in 2 divided doses, increased to 22.5 mg/kg daily in 3 divided doses in severe infections; max. 1.5 g daily for up to 10 days (max. cumulative dose 15 g); CHILD under 18 years see *BNF for Children*
- Once daily dose regimen (not for endocarditis, febrile neutropenia, or meningitis; see notes above and also consult local guidelines), by intravenous infusion, initially 15 mg/kg (max. 1.5 g), then adjust according to serum-amikacin concentration; max. cumulative dose 15 g; CHILD under 18 years see *BNF for Children*

Note For multiple daily dose regimen, one-hour ('peak') serum concentration should not exceed 30 mg/litre; pre-dose ('trough') concentration should be less than 10 mg/litre. For once daily dose regimen, pre-dose ('trough') concentration should be less than 5 mg/litre

Amikacin (Non-proprietary) [PoM]

Injection, amikacin (as sulfate) 250 mg/mL. Net price 2-mL vial = £9.64

Electrolytes Na⁺ 0.56 mmol/500-mg vial

Amikin® (Bristol-Myers Squibb) [PoM]

Injection, amikacin (as sulfate) 50 mg/mL. Net price 2-mL vial = £2.07

Electrolytes Na⁺ < 0.5 mmol/vial

◼ NEOMYCIN SULFATE

Indications bowel sterilisation before surgery; see also notes above

Cautions see notes above, but too toxic for systemic use; **interactions:** Appendix 1 (aminoglycosides)

Contra-indications see notes above; also intestinal obstruction

Hepatic impairment absorbed from gastro-intestinal tract in liver disease—increased risk of ototoxicity

Renal impairment avoid; ototoxic; nephrotoxic

Pregnancy see notes above

Side-effects see notes above, but poorly absorbed on oral administration; increased salivation, impaired intestinal absorption with steatorrhoea and diarrhoea

Dose

- By mouth, pre-operative bowel sterilisation, 1 g every hour for 4 hours, then 1 g every 4 hours for 2–3 days

Hepatic coma, up to 4 g daily in divided doses usually for 5–7 days

Neomycin (Non-proprietary) [PoM]

Tablets, neomycin sulfate 500 mg. Net price 100= £24.78

Brands include *Nivemycin®*

◼ TOBRAMYCIN

Indications see under Gentamicin and notes above

Cautions see notes above; **interactions:** Appendix 1 (aminoglycosides)

Specific cautions for inhaled treatment Other inhaled drugs should be administered before tobramycin. Measure lung function before and after initial dose of tobramycin and monitor for bronchospasm; if bronchospasm occurs in a patient not using a bronchodilator, repeat test using bronchodilator. Monitor renal function before treatment and then annually. Severe haemoptysis—risk of further haemorrhage.

Contra-indications see notes above

Renal impairment see notes above

Pregnancy see notes above

Side-effects see notes above; *on inhalation,* cough (more frequent by inhalation of powder), bronchospasm (see Cautions), dysphonia, taste disturbances, pharyngitis, mouth ulcers, salivary hypersecretion, laryngitis, haemoptysis, epistaxis

Dose

> To avoid excessive dosage in obese patients, use ideal weight for height to calculate parenteral dose and monitor serum-tobramycin concentration closely

- By intramuscular injection *or* by slow intravenous injection *or* by intravenous infusion, 3 mg/kg daily in divided doses every 8 hours, see also notes above; in severe infections up to 5 mg/kg daily in divided doses every 6–8 hours (reduced to 3 mg/kg as soon as clinically indicated); CHILD under 18 years see *BNF for Children*
- Urinary-tract infection, by intramuscular injection, 2–3 mg/kg daily as a single dose

Note One-hour ('peak') serum concentration should not exceed 10 mg/litre; pre-dose ('trough') concentration should be less than 2 mg/litre

- Chronic pulmonary *Pseudomonas aeruginosa* infection in patients with cystic fibrosis, by inhalation of nebulised solution, ADULT and CHILD over 6 years, 300 mg every 12 hours for 28 days, subsequent courses repeated after 28-day interval without tobramycin nebuliser solution

By inhalation of powder, ADULT and CHILD over 6 years, 112 mg every 12 hours for 28 days, subsequent courses repeated after 28-day interval without tobramycin inhalation powder

◢ **Parenteral**

Tobramycin (Non-proprietary) [PoM]

Injection, tobramycin (as sulfate) 40 mg/mL, net price 1-mL (40-mg) vial = £3.70, 2-mL (80-mg) vial = £3.77, 6-mL (240-mg) vial = £45.00

◢ **Inhalation**

Bramitob® (Chiesi) [PoM]

Nebuliser solution, tobramycin 75 mg/mL, net price 56 × 4-mL (300-mg) unit = £1187.00

Tobi® (Novartis) [PoM]

Nebuliser solution, tobramycin 60 mg/mL, net price 56 × 5-mL (300-mg) unit = £1187.20

Podhaler (dry powder for inhalation), tobramycin 28 mg/capsule, net price 56-cap pack (with *Tobi® Podhaler* device) = £447.50, 224-cap pack (with 5 *Tobi® Podhaler* devices) = £1790.00. Counselling, administration

5.1.5 Macrolides

The macrolides have an antibacterial spectrum that is similar but not identical to that of penicillin; they are thus an alternative in penicillin-allergic patients. They are active against many-penicillin-resistant staphylococci, but some are now also resistant to the macrolides.

Indications for the macrolides include campylobacter enteritis, respiratory infections (including pneumonia, whooping cough, Legionella, chlamydia, and mycoplasma infection), and skin infections.

Erythromycin is also used in the treatment of early syphilis, uncomplicated genital chlamydial infection, and non-gonococcal urethritis. Erythromycin has poor activity against *Haemophilus influenzae*. Erythromycin causes nausea, vomiting, and diarrhoea in some patients; in mild to moderate infections this can be avoided by giving a lower dose (250 mg 4 times daily), but if a more serious infection, such as Legionella pneumonia, is suspected higher doses are needed.

Azithromycin is a macrolide with slightly less activity than erythromycin against Gram-positive bacteria, but enhanced activity against some Gram-negative organisms including *H. influenzae*. Plasma concentrations are very low, but tissue concentrations are much higher. It has a long tissue half-life and once daily dosage is recommended. Azithromycin is also used in the treatment of uncomplicated genital chlamydial infection, non-gonococcal urethritis, uncomplicated gonorrhoea, typhoid [unlicensed indication], and trachoma [unlicensed indication] (section 11.3.1).

Clarithromycin is an erythromycin derivative with slightly greater activity than the parent compound. Tissue concentrations are higher than with erythromycin. It is given twice daily. Clarithromycin is also used in regimens for *Helicobacter pylori* eradication (section 1.3).

For the role of erythromycin, azithromycin, and clarithromycin in the treatment of Lyme disease, see section 5.1.1.3

Spiramycin is also a macrolide (section 5.4.7).

Oral infections The macrolides are an alternative for oral infections in penicillin-allergic patients or where a beta-lactamase producing organism is involved. However, many organisms are now resistant to macrolides or rapidly develop resistance; their use should therefore be limited to short courses. Metronidazole (section 5.1.11) may be preferred as an alternative to a penicillin.

Cautions Macrolides should be used with caution in patients with a predisposition to QT interval prolongation (including electrolyte disturbances and concomitant use of drugs that prolong the QT interval). Macrolides may aggravate myasthenia gravis. **Interactions:** Appendix 1 (macrolides).

Side-effects Nausea, vomiting, abdominal discomfort, and diarrhoea are the most common side-effects of the macrolides, but they are mild and less frequent with azithromycin and clarithromycin than with erythromycin. Hepatotoxicity (including cholestatic jaundice) and rash occur less frequently. Other side-effects reported rarely or very rarely include pancreatitis, antibiotic-associated colitis, QT interval prolongation, arrhythmias, Stevens-Johnson syndrome, and toxic epidermal necrolysis. Generally reversible hearing loss (sometimes with tinnitus) can occur after large doses of a macrolide; it occurs commonly after long-term therapy with azithromycin. Intravenous infusion may cause local tenderness and phlebitis.

▌ AZITHROMYCIN

Indications see under Dose; prophylaxis of group A streptococcal infection (Table 2, section 5.1); antibacterial prophylaxis for insertion of intra-uterine device (section 7.3.5); eye (section 11.3.1)

Cautions see notes above; **interactions:** Appendix 1 (macrolides)

Hepatic impairment use with caution in severe liver disease; may cause hepatotoxicity

Renal impairment use with caution if eGFR less than 10 mL/minute/1.73 m²

Pregnancy manufacturers advise use only if adequate alternatives not available

Breast-feeding present in milk; use only if no suitable alternatives

Side-effects see notes above; also anorexia, dyspepsia, flatulence, dizziness, headache, malaise, paraesthesia, arthralgia, disturbances in taste and vision; *less commonly* constipation, gastritis, chest pain, oedema, anxiety, sleep disturbances, hypoaesthesia, leucopenia, photosensitivity; *rarely* agitation; also reported syncope, convulsions, smell disturbances, interstitial nephritis, acute renal failure, thrombocytopenia, haemolytic anaemia, tongue discoloration

Dose

- Respiratory-tract infections (but see also below for community acquired pneumonia), otitis media, skin and soft-tissue infections, by mouth, 500 mg once daily for 3 days *or* 500 mg on first day then 250 mg once daily for 4 days; CHILD over 6 months 10 mg/kg once daily (max. 500 mg once daily) for 3 days; *or* body-weight 15–25 kg, 200 mg once daily for 3 days; body-weight 26–35 kg, 300 mg once daily for 3 days; body-weight 36–45 kg, 400 mg once daily for 3 days

- Community-acquired pneumonia, low to moderate severity, ADULT over 18 years, by mouth, 500 mg once daily for 3 days *or* 500 mg on first day then 250 mg once daily for 4 days

- Community-acquired pneumonia, high severity, ADULT over 18 years, by intravenous infusion, 500 mg once daily for at least 2 days, then by mouth, 500 mg once daily; total duration 7–10 days [unlicensed when used by mouth for over 3 days]

- Uncomplicated gonorrhoea [unlicensed indication] (see also Table 1, section 5.1), ADULT over 18 years, by mouth, 1 g as a single dose

- Uncomplicated genital chlamydial infections and non-gonococcal urethritis (see also Table 1, section 5.1), ADULT and CHILD over 12 years, by mouth, 1 g as a single dose

- Lyme disease (see also section 5.1.1.3), mild to moderate typhoid due to multiple-antibacterial-resistant organisms [unlicensed indications], ADULT over 18 years, by mouth, 500 mg once daily for 7–10 days (7 days in typhoid); CHILD 6 months–18 years, see *BNF for Children*

Azithromycin (Non-proprietary) PoM

Capsules, azithromycin (as dihydrate) 250 mg, net price 4-cap pack = £10.00, 6-cap pack = £15.02. Label: 5, 9, 23

Dental prescribing on NHS Azithromycin Capsules may be prescribed

Tablets, azithromycin (as monohydrate hemi-ethanolate) 250 mg, net price 4-tab pack = £1.97; 500 mg, 3-tab pack = £1.78. Label: 5, 9

Dental prescribing on NHS Azithromycin Tablets may be prescribed

Note Azithromycin tablets can be sold to the public for the treatment of confirmed, asymptomatic *Chlamydia trachomatis* genital infection in those over 16 years of age, and for the epidemiological treatment of their sexual partners, subject to max. single dose of 1 g, max. daily dose 1 g, and a pack size of 1 g

Oral suspension, azithromycin (as monohydrate) 200 mg/5 mL when reconstituted with water, net price 15-mL pack = £4.06, 30-mL pack = £11.04. Label: 5, 9

Dental prescribing on NHS Azithromycin Oral Suspension 200 mg/5 mL may be prescribed

Zithromax® (Pfizer) PoM

Capsules, azithromycin (as dihydrate) 250 mg, net price 4-cap pack = £7.16, 6-cap pack = £10.74. Label: 5, 9, 23

Oral suspension, cherry/banana-flavoured, azithromycin (as dihydrate) 200 mg/5 mL when reconstituted with water. Net price 15-mL pack = £4.06, 22.5-mL pack = £6.10, 30-mL pack = £11.04. Label: 5, 9

Zedbac® (Aspire) PoM

Intravenous infusion, powder for reconstitution, azithromycin (as dihydrate), net price 500-mg vial = £9.50.

Electrolytes Na+ 7.3 mmol/vial

CLARITHROMYCIN

Indications respiratory-tract infections, mild to moderate skin and soft-tissue infections, otitis media; Lyme disease (see also section 5.1.1.3); prevention of pertussis (Table 2, section 5.1); *Helicobacter pylori* eradication (section 1.3)

Cautions see notes above; **interactions:** Appendix 1 (macrolides)

Hepatic impairment hepatic dysfunction including jaundice reported; avoid in severe impairment if renal impairment also present

Renal impairment use half normal dose if eGFR less than 30 mL/minute/1.73 m², max. duration 14 days; avoid *Klaricid XL*® or clarithromycin m/r preparations if eGFR less than 30 mL/minute/1.73 m²

Pregnancy manufacturer advises avoid, particularly in the first trimester, unless potential benefit outweighs risk

Breast-feeding manufacturer advises avoid unless potential benefit outweighs risk—present in milk

Side-effects see notes above; also dyspepsia, taste disturbances, headache, insomnia, hyperhidrosis; *less commonly* gastritis, flatulence, constipation, dry mouth, stomatitis, glossitis, anorexia, chest pain, anxiety, dizziness, tremor, malaise, blood disorders (including leucopenia), myalgia, tinnitus; *also reported* confusion, psychotic disorders, depression, abnormal dreams, convulsions, paraesthesia, hypoglycaemia, renal failure, interstitial nephritis, myopathy, tooth and tongue discoloration, smell disturbances

Dose

* By mouth, ADULT and CHILD over 12 years, 250 mg every 12 hours, increased in pneumonia or severe infections to 500 mg every 12 hours; usual duration 7–14 days (see also Table 1, section 5.1); CHILD body-weight under 8 kg, 7.5 mg/kg twice daily; 8–11 kg, 62.5 mg twice daily; 12–19 kg, 125 mg twice daily; 20–29 kg, 187.5 mg twice daily; 30–40 kg, 250 mg twice daily

Lyme disease (see also section 5.1.1.3), ADULT and CHILD over 12 years, 500 mg every 12 hours for 14–21 days; CHILD 1 month–12 years see *BNF for Children*

* By intravenous infusion into larger proximal vein, ADULT and CHILD over 12 years, 500 mg twice daily; max. duration 5 days (switch to oral route when appropriate); CHILD 1 month–12 years see *BNF for Children*

Clarithromycin (Non-proprietary) PoM

Tablets, clarithromycin 250 mg, net price 14-tab pack = £1.63; 500 mg, 14-tab pack = £2.87. Label: 9

Dental prescribing on NHS Clarithromycin Tablets may be prescribed

Oral suspension, clarithromycin for reconstitution with water 125 mg/5 mL, net price 70 mL = £4.09; 250 mg/5 mL, 70 mL = £6.22. Label: 9

Dental prescribing on NHS Clarithromycin Oral Suspension may be prescribed

Intravenous infusion, powder for reconstitution, clarithromycin, net price 500-mg vial = £9.45

Klaricid® (Abbott Healthcare) PoM

Tablets, both yellow, f/c, clarithromycin 250 mg, net price 14-tab pack = £7.00; 500 mg, 14-tab pack = £11.30, 20-tab pack = £16.15. Label: 9

Paediatric suspension, clarithromycin for reconstitution with water 125 mg/5 mL, net price 70 mL = £5.26, 100 mL = £9.04; 250 mg/5 mL, 70 mL = £10.51. Label: 9

Granules, clarithromycin 250 mg/sachet, net price 14-sachet pack = £11.68. Label: 9, 13

Intravenous infusion, powder for reconstitution, clarithromycin. Net price 500-mg vial = £9.45

Electrolytes Na+ < 0.5 mmol/500-mg vial

◢Modified release

Clarithromycin m/r preparations PoM

Tablets, m/r, clarithromycin 500 mg, net price 7 = £6.72, 14 = £13.23. Label: 9, 21, 25

Brands include *Mycifor XL*®

Dose ADULT and CHILD over 12 years, 500 mg once daily (doubled in severe infections) for 7–14 days

Klaricid XL® (Abbott Healthcare) PoM

Tablets, m/r, yellow, clarithromycin 500 mg, net price 7-tab pack = £6.72, 14-tab pack = £13.23. Label: 9, 21, 25

Dose ADULT and CHILD over 12 years, 500 mg once daily (doubled in severe infections) for 7–14 days

ERYTHROMYCIN

Indications susceptible infections in patients with penicillin hypersensitivity; oral infections (see notes above); campylobacter enteritis, syphilis, non-gonococcal urethritis, respiratory-tract infections (including Legionella infection), skin infections (Table 1, section 5.1); chronic prostatitis; prophylaxis of diphtheria, group A streptococcal infection, and pneumococcal infection (Table 2, section 5.1), and pertussis; acne vulgaris and rosacea (section 13.6)

5 Infections

Cautions   see notes above; neonate under 2 weeks (risk of hypertrophic pyloric stenosis); avoid in acute porphyria (section 9.8.2); **interactions:** Appendix 1 (macrolides)

Hepatic impairment   may cause idiosyncratic hepatotoxicity

Renal impairment   max. 1.5 g daily in severe renal impairment (ototoxicity)

Pregnancy   not known to be harmful

Breast-feeding   only small amounts in milk—not known to be harmful

Side-effects   see notes above

Dose

● By mouth, ADULT and CHILD over 8 years, 250–500 mg every 6 hours *or* 0.5–1 g every 12 hours (see notes above); up to 4 g daily in divided doses in severe infections; NEONATE 12.5 mg/kg every 6 hours; CHILD 1 month–2 years 125 mg every 6 hours *or* 250 mg every 12 hours, 2–8 years 250 mg every 6 hours *or* 500 mg every 12 hours, doses doubled for severe infections

   Early syphilis, 500 mg 4 times daily for 14 days; CHILD 12–18 years see *BNF for Children*

   Uncomplicated genital chlamydia, non-gonococcal urethritis, 500 mg twice daily for 14 days; CHILD under 18 years see *BNF for Children*

   Lyme disease (see also section 5.1.1.3), 500 mg 4 times daily for 14–21 days; CHILD under 18 years see *BNF for Children*

● By intravenous infusion, ADULT and CHILD severe infections, 12.5 mg/kg every 6 hours; mild infections (when oral treatment not possible), 6.25 mg/kg every 6 hours; NEONATE see *BNF for Children*

Erythromycin (Non-proprietary) [PoM]

Capsules, enclosing e/c microgranules, erythromycin 250 mg, net price 28-cap pack = £5.61. Label: 5, 9, 25

Brands include *Tiloryth®*

Tablets, e/c, erythromycin 250 mg, net price 28 = £1.89. Label: 5, 9, 25

Dental prescribing on NHS Erythromycin Tablets e/c may be prescribed

Erythromycin Ethyl Succinate (Non-proprietary) [PoM]

Oral suspension, erythromycin (as ethyl succinate) for reconstitution with water 125 mg/5 mL, net price 100 mL = £2.94; 250 mg/5 mL, 100 mL = £4.43; 500 mg/5 mL, 100 mL = £7.65. Label: 9

Note Sugar-free versions are available and can be ordered by specifying 'sugar-free' on the prescription

Brands include *Primacine®*

Dental prescribing on NHS Erythromycin Ethyl Succinate Oral Suspension may be prescribed

Erythromycin Lactobionate (Non-proprietary) [PoM]

Intravenous infusion, powder for reconstitution, erythromycin (as lactobionate), net price 1-g vial = £10.98

Erymax® (TEVA UK) [PoM]

Capsules, opaque orange/clear orange, enclosing orange and white e/c pellets, erythromycin 250 mg, net price 28-cap pack = £5.61, 112-cap pack = £22.44. Label: 5, 9, 25

Dose 1 capsule every 6 hours *or* 2 capsules every 12 hours; acne, 1 capsule twice daily for 1 month then 1 capsule daily

Erythrocin® (AMCo) [PoM]

Tablets, both f/c, erythromycin (as stearate), 250 mg, net price 100 = £18.20; 500 mg, 100 = £36.40. Label: 9

Dental prescribing on NHS May be prescribed as Erythromycin Stearate Tablets

Erythroped® (AMCo) [PoM]

Suspension SF, sugar-free, banana-flavoured, erythromycin (as ethyl succinate) for reconstitution with water, 125 mg/5 mL (*Suspension PI SF*), net price 140 mL = £3.06; 250 mg/5 mL, 140 mL = £5.95; 500 mg/5 mL (*Suspension SF Forte*), 140 mL = £10.56. Label: 9

Erythroped A® (AMCo) [PoM]

Tablets, yellow, f/c, erythromycin 500 mg (as ethyl succinate). Net price 28-tab pack = £10.78. Label: 9

Dental prescribing on NHS May be prescribed as Erythromycin Ethyl Succinate Tablets

Telithromycin

The ketolide **telithromycin** is a derivative of erythromycin. The antibacterial spectrum of telithromycin is similar to that of macrolides and it is also active against penicillin- and erythromycin-resistant *Streptococcus pneumoniae*. Telithromycin should only be used to treat beta-haemolytic streptococcal pharyngitis and tonsillitis, sinusitis, community-acquired pneumonia, and exacerbations of chronic bronchitis if caused by organisms resistant to beta-lactam antibacterials and other macrolides, or if conventional treatment is contra-indicated.

■ TELITHROMYCIN

Indications   see notes above

Cautions   coronary heart disease, ventricular arrhythmias, bradycardia, hypokalaemia, hypomagnesaemia—risk of QT interval prolongation; concomitant administration of drugs that prolong QT-interval; avoid in acute porphyria (section 9.8.2); **interactions:** Appendix 1 (telithromycin)

Hepatic disorders Patients should be told how to recognise signs of liver disorder, and advised to discontinue treatment and seek prompt medical attention if symptoms such as anorexia, nausea, vomiting, abdominal pain, jaundice, or dark urine develop

Driving Visual disturbances or transient loss of consciousness may affect performance of skilled tasks (e.g. driving); effects may occur after the first dose. Administration at bedtime may reduce these side-effects. Patients should be advised not to drive or operate machinery if affected

Contra-indications   myasthenia gravis; history of telithromycin-associated hepatitis or jaundice; prolongation of QT interval; congenital or family history of QT interval prolongation (if not excluded by ECG)

Hepatic impairment   manufacturer advises caution; see also Hepatic Disorders above

Renal impairment   manufacturer advises avoid if possible if eGFR less than 30 mL/minute/1.73 m² —if no alternative, use alternating daily doses of 800 mg and 400 mg, starting with 800 mg dose

Pregnancy   toxicity in *animal* studies—manufacturer advises use only if potential benefit outweighs risk

Breast-feeding   manufacturer advises avoid—present in milk in *animal* studies

Side-effects   diarrhoea, nausea, vomiting, flatulence, abdominal pain, taste disturbances; dizziness, headache; *less commonly* constipation, stomatitis, anorexia, hepatitis, flushing, palpitations, drowsiness, insomnia, nervousness, eosinophilia, blurred vision, rash, urticaria, and pruritus; *rarely* cholestatic jaundice, arrhythmias, hypotension, transient loss of consciousness, paraesthesia, and diplopia; *very rarely* antibiotic-associated colitis, altered sense of smell, muscle cramp, erythema multiforme; also reported pancreatitis, confusion, hallucinations and arthralgia

Dose

- 800 mg once daily for 5 days for sinusitis or exacerbation of chronic bronchitis *or* for 7–10 days in community-acquired pneumonia; CHILD under 18 years safety and efficacy not established
- Tonsillitis or pharyngitis caused by *Streptococcus pyogenes*, ADULT and CHILD over 12 years, 800 mg once daily for 5 days

Ketek® (Sanofi-Aventis) [PoM]

Tablets, orange, f/c, telithromycin 400 mg, net price 10-tab pack = £18.56. Label: 9, counselling, driving, hepatic disorders

5.1.6 Clindamycin

Clindamycin is active against Gram-positive cocci, including streptococci and penicillin-resistant staphylococci, and also against many anaerobes, especially *Bacteroides fragilis*. It is well concentrated in bone and excreted in bile and urine.

Clindamycin is recommended for staphylococcal joint and bone infections such as osteomyelitis, and intra-abdominal sepsis; it is an alternative to macrolides for erysipelas or cellulitis in penicillin-allergic patients. Clindamycin can also be used for infections associated with meticillin-resistant *Staphylococcus aureus* (MRSA) in bronchiectasis, bone and joint infections, and skin and soft-tissue infections.

Clindamycin has been associated with antibiotic-associated colitis (section 1.5), which may be fatal; it is most common in middle-aged and elderly women, especially following an operation. Although antibiotic-associated colitis can occur with most antibacterials, it occurs more frequently with clindamycin. Patients should therefore discontinue treatment immediately if diarrhoea develops.

Oral infections   Clindamycin should not be used routinely for the treatment of oral infections because it may be no more effective than penicillins against anaerobes and there may be cross-resistance with erythromycin-resistant bacteria. Clindamycin can be used for the treatment of dentoalveolar abscess that has not responded to penicillin or to metronidazole.

CLINDAMYCIN

Indications   see notes above; staphylococcal bone and joint infections, peritonitis; falciparum malaria (section 5.4.1)

Cautions   discontinue immediately if diarrhoea or colitis develops; monitor liver and renal function if treatment exceeds 10 days, and in neonates and infants; avoid rapid intravenous administration; avoid in acute porphyria (section 9.8.2); **interactions:** Appendix 1 (clindamycin)

Contra-indications   diarrhoeal states; avoid injections containing benzyl alcohol in neonates (see under preparations below)

Pregnancy   not known to be harmful

Breast-feeding   amount probably too small to be harmful but bloody diarrhoea reported in 1 infant

Side-effects   diarrhoea (discontinue treatment), abdominal discomfort, oesophagitis, oesophageal ulcers, taste disturbances, nausea, vomiting, antibio-

tic-associated colitis; jaundice; leucopenia, eosinophilia, and thrombocytopenia reported; polyarthritis reported; rash, pruritus, urticaria, anaphylactoid reactions, Stevens-Johnson syndrome, toxic epidermal necrolysis, exfoliative and vesiculobullous dermatitis reported; pain, induration, and abscess after intramuscular injection; thrombophlebitis after intravenous injection

Dose

- By mouth, 150–300 mg every 6 hours; up to 450 mg every 6 hours in severe infections; NEONATE see *BNF for Children*; CHILD 1 month–18 years, 3–6 mg/kg (max. 450 mg) every 6 hours
  Counselling Patients should discontinue treatment immediately and contact doctor if diarrhoea develops; capsules should be swallowed with a glass of water.
- By deep intramuscular injection *or* by intravenous infusion, 0.6–2.7 g daily (in 2–4 divided doses); life-threatening infection, up to 4.8 g daily; single doses above 600 mg by intravenous infusion only; single doses by intravenous infusion not to exceed 1.2 g; CHILD over 1 month, see *BNF for Children*

Clindamycin (Non-proprietary) [PoM]

Capsules, clindamycin (as hydrochloride) 150 mg, net price 24-cap pack = £4.53. Label: 9, 27, counselling, see above (diarrhoea)
Dental prescribing on NHS Clindamycin Capsules may be prescribed

Injection, clindamycin (as phosphate) 150 mg/mL, net price 2-mL amp = £5.90, 4-mL amp = £11.80

Dalacin C® (Pharmacia) [PoM]

Capsules, clindamycin (as hydrochloride) 75 mg (green/white), net price 24-cap pack = £7.45; 150 mg, (white), 24-cap pack = £13.72. Label: 9, 27, counselling, see above (diarrhoea)
Dental prescribing on NHS May be prescribed as Clindamycin Capsules

Injection, clindamycin (as phosphate) 150 mg/mL, net price 2-mL amp = £6.20, 4-mL amp = £12.35
Excipients include benzyl alcohol (avoid in neonates, see Excipients, p. 2)

5.1.7 Some other antibacterials

Antibacterials discussed in this section include chloramphenicol, fusidic acid, glycopeptide antibiotics (vancomycin and teicoplanin), daptomycin, linezolid, fidaxomicin, the polymyxin, colistimethate sodium, and the rifamycin, rifaximin.

Chloramphenicol

Chloramphenicol is a potent broad-spectrum antibiotic; however, it is associated with serious haematological side-effects when given systemically and should therefore be reserved for the treatment of life-threatening infections, particularly those caused by *Haemophilus influenzae*, and also for typhoid fever.

Chloramphenicol eye drops (section 11.3.1) and chloramphenicol ear drops (section 12.1.1) are also available.

CHLORAMPHENICOL

Indications   see notes above

Cautions   avoid repeated courses and prolonged treatment; blood counts required before and periodically during treatment; monitor plasma-chloramphenicol concentration in neonates (see below); **interactions:** Appendix 1 (chloramphenicol)

Contra-indications acute porphyria (section 9.8.2)

Hepatic impairment avoid if possible—increased risk of bone-marrow depression; reduce dose and monitor plasma-chloramphenicol concentration

Renal impairment avoid in severe renal impairment unless no alternative; dose-related depression of haematopoiesis

Pregnancy manufacturer advises avoid; neonatal 'grey syndrome' if used in third trimester

Breast-feeding manufacturer advises avoid; use another antibiotic; may cause bone-marrow toxicity in infant; concentration in milk usually insufficient to cause 'grey syndrome'

Side-effects blood disorders including reversible and irreversible aplastic anaemia (with reports of resulting leukaemia), peripheral neuritis, optic neuritis, headache, depression, urticaria, erythema multiforme, nausea, vomiting, diarrhoea, stomatitis, glossitis, dry mouth; nocturnal haemoglobinuria reported; grey syndrome (abdominal distension, pallid cyanosis, circulatory collapse) may follow excessive doses in neonates with immature hepatic metabolism

Dose

- By mouth *or* by intravenous injection *or* infusion, 12.5 mg/kg every 6 hours (exceptionally, can be doubled for severe infections such as septicaemia and meningitis, providing high doses reduced as soon as clinically indicated); CHILD over 1 month, haemophilus epiglottitis and pyogenic meningitis, 12.5–25 mg/kg every 6 hours (high dosages decreased as soon as clinically indicated); NEONATE under 2 weeks, 12.5 mg/kg twice daily; 2 weeks–1 month, 12.5 mg/kg 2–4 times daily

  Note Plasma concentration monitoring required in neonates and preferred in those under 4 years of age, in the elderly, and in hepatic impairment; recommended peak plasma concentration (approx. 2 hours after administration by mouth, intravenous injection or infusion) 10–25 mg/litre; pre-dose ('trough') concentration should not exceed 15 mg/litre

Chloramphenicol (Non-proprietary) [PoM]

Capsules, chloramphenicol 250 mg. Net price 60 = £377.00

Kemicetine® (Pharmacia) [PoM]

Injection, powder for reconstitution, chloramphenicol (as sodium succinate). Net price 1-g vial = £1.39

Electrolytes Na⁺ 3.14 mmol/g

Fosfomycin

Fosfomycin, a phosphonic acid antibacterial, is active against a range of Gram-positive and Gram-negative bacteria including *Staphylococcus aureus* and Enterobacteriaceae. It is licensed intravenously for the treatment of acute osteomyelitis, complicated urinary-tract infections, hospital-acquired lower respiratory-tract infections, and bacterial meningitis only when first-line treatments are inappropriate or ineffective. Although oral preparations containing fosfomycin are not marketed in the UK, they can be used, on the advice of a microbiologist, for the treatment of uncomplicated lower urinary-tract infections caused by multiple-antibacterial resistant organisms when other antibacterials cannot be used.

▌ FOSFOMYCIN

Indications see Dose below

Cautions interactions: Appendix 1 (fosfomycin)
Specific cautions for intravenous treatment Monitor electrolytes and fluid balance; cardiac insufficiency;

hypertension; hyperaldosteronism; hypernatraemia; pulmonary oedema; elderly (high doses)

Renal impairment avoid *oral* treatment if eGFR less than 10 mL/minute/1.73m²; use *intravenous* treatment with caution if eGFR 40–80 mL/minute/1.73m² and consult product literature for dose if eGFR less than 40 mL/minute/1.73m²

Pregnancy manufacturer advises use only if potential benefit outweighs risk

Breast-feeding manufacturer advises use only if potential benefit outweighs risk—present in milk

Side-effects gastro-intestinal disturbances (including nausea, vomiting, heartburn, abdominal pain, diarrhoea), rash

Specific side-effects for intravenous treatment Decreased appetite, taste disturbances, dyspnoea, headache, fatigue, vertigo, hypernatraemia, hypokalaemia; *rarely* blood disorders (including aplastic anaemia, eosinophilia); *very rarely* visual impairment, fatty liver; *also reported* antibiotic-associated colitis, hepatitis, jaundice, tachycardia, bronchospasm, confusion

Dose

Note Doses expressed as fosfomycin base

- By mouth [unlicensed], uncomplicated lower urinary-tract infections caused by multiple-antibacterial resistant organisms (when other antibacterials cannot be used), ADULT over 18 years 3 g as a single dose (in men, repeat dose after 3 days)

- By intravenous infusion, osteomyelitis or hospital-acquired lower respiratory tract infections when first-line treatment ineffective or inappropriate, 12–24 g daily in 2–3 divided doses; use the high-dose regimen in severe infection suspected or known to be caused by less sensitive organisms; max. single dose 8 g; CHILD under 18 years see *BNF for Children*
  Complicated urinary-tract infections when first-line treatment ineffective or inappropriate, 12–16 g daily in 2–3 divided doses; max. single dose 8 g; CHILD under 18 years see *BNF for Children*
  Bacterial meningitis when first-line treatment ineffective or inappropriate, 16–24 g daily in 3–4 divided doses; use the high-dose regimen in severe infection suspected or known to be caused by less sensitive organisms; max. single dose 8 g; CHILD under 18 years see *BNF for Children*

Fosfomycin [PoM]

Granules, fosfomycin (as trometamol) 3 g/sachet. Label: 9, 13, 23
Available from 'special order' manufacturers or specialist importing companies, see p. 1124

Fomicyt® (Nordic) [PoM]

Intravenous infusion, powder for reconstitution, fosfomycin (as sodium), net price 2-g vial = £15.00
Electrolytes Na⁺ 28 mmol/2-g vial

Fusidic acid

Fusidic acid and its salts are narrow-spectrum antibiotics. The only indication for their use is in infections caused by penicillin-resistant staphylococci, especially osteomyelitis, as they are well concentrated in bone; they are also used for staphylococcal endocarditis. A second antistaphylococcal antibiotic is usually required to prevent emergence of resistance.

▌ SODIUM FUSIDATE

Indications penicillin-resistant staphylococcal infection including osteomyelitis; staphylococcal endocarditis in combination with other antibacterials (Table 1, section 5.1)

Cautions monitor liver function with high doses or on prolonged therapy; elimination may be reduced in biliary disease or biliary obstruction; **interactions:** Appendix 1 (fusidic acid)

Hepatic impairment impaired biliary excretion; possibly increased risk of hepatotoxicity; avoid or reduce dose; monitor liver function

Pregnancy not known to be harmful; manufacturer advises use only if potential benefit outweighs risk

Breast-feeding present in milk—manufacturer advises caution

Side-effects nausea, vomiting, abdominal pain, dyspepsia, diarrhoea, drowsiness, dizziness; *less commonly* anorexia, headache, malaise, rash, pruritus; also reported reversible jaundice especially after high dosage (withdraw therapy if persistent), acute renal failure (usually with jaundice), blood disorders

Dose

- See under Preparations, below

Fucidin® (LEO) PoM
Tablets, f/c, sodium fusidate 250 mg, net price 10-tab pack = £6.02. Label: 9
Dose as sodium fusidate, 500 mg every 8 hours, doubled for severe infections
Skin infection, as sodium fusidate, 250 mg every 12 hours for 5–10 days
Suspension, off-white, banana- and orange-flavoured, fusidic acid 250 mg/5 mL, net price 50 mL = £6.73. Label: 9, 21
Dose as fusidic acid, ADULT 750 mg every 8 hours; CHILD up to 1 year 50 mg/kg daily (in 3 divided doses), 1–5 years 250 mg every 8 hours, 5–12 years 500 mg every 8 hours
Note Fusidic acid is incompletely absorbed and doses recommended for suspension are proportionately higher than those for sodium fusidate tablets

Glycopeptides

The glycopeptide antibiotics **vancomycin**, **teicoplanin**, and **telavancin** have bactericidal activity against aerobic and anaerobic Gram-positive bacteria including multi-resistant staphylococci. However, there are reports of *Staphylococcus aureus* with reduced susceptibility to glycopeptides. There are increasing reports of glycopeptide-resistant enterococci.

Vancomycin and teicoplanin are used *parenterally* in the treatment of endocarditis and other serious infections caused by Gram-positive cocci. Vancomycin has a long duration of action and can therefore be given every 12 hours. Teicoplanin is similar to vancomycin, but has a significantly longer duration of action, allowing once daily administration after the loading dose. Teicoplanin is associated with a lower incidence of nephrotoxicity than vancomycin. Telavancin is licensed only for the treatment of adults with hospital-acquired pneumonia, including ventilator-associated pneumonia, known or suspected to be caused by meticillin-resistant *Staphylococcus aureus* (MRSA), and should only be used when other antibacterials are not suitable. Telavancin may be associated with a higher incidence of nephrotoxicity than vancomycin.

Either vancomycin or teicoplanin (added to dialysis fluid) is used in the treatment of peritonitis associated with peritoneal dialysis (Table 1, section 5.1); this is an [unlicensed route] for vancomycin.

Vancomycin and teicoplanin are also used for surgical prophylaxis when there is a high risk of MRSA (Table 2, section 5.1).

Vancomycin given *by mouth* for 10–14 days is effective in the treatment of *Clostridium difficile* infection (see also section 1.5); low doses are considered adequate (higher dose may be considered if the infection fails to respond or it is life threatening). Teicoplanin given *by mouth* is licensed for the treatment of *Clostridium difficile* infection. Vancomycin and teicoplanin should **not** be given by mouth for systemic infections because they are not absorbed significantly.

◢ VANCOMYCIN

Indications see notes above

Cautions avoid rapid infusion (risk of anaphylactoid reactions, see Side-effects); rotate infusion sites; elderly; avoid if history of deafness; all patients require plasma-vancomycin measurement (after 3 or 4 doses if renal function normal, earlier if renal impairment), blood counts, urinalysis, and renal function tests; monitor auditory function in elderly or if renal impairment; teicoplanin sensitivity; systemic absorption may follow oral administration especially in inflammatory bowel disorders or following multiple doses; **interactions:** Appendix 1 (vancomycin)

Renal impairment reduce dose—monitor plasma-vancomycin concentration and renal function regularly; see also Cautions above

Pregnancy manufacturer advises use only if potential benefit outweighs risk—plasma-vancomycin concentration monitoring essential to reduce risk of fetal toxicity

Breast-feeding present in milk—significant absorption following oral administration unlikely

Side-effects after parenteral administration: nephrotoxicity including renal failure and interstitial nephritis; ototoxicity (discontinue if tinnitus occurs); blood disorders including neutropenia (usually after 1 week or cumulative dose of 25 g), rarely agranulocytosis and thrombocytopenia; nausea; chills; fever; eosinophilia, anaphylaxis, rashes (including exfoliative dermatitis, Stevens-Johnson syndrome, toxic epidermal necrolysis, and vasculitis); phlebitis (irritant to tissue); on rapid infusion, severe hypotension (including shock and cardiac arrest), wheezing, dyspnoea, urticaria, pruritus, flushing of the upper body ('red man' syndrome), pain and muscle spasm of back and chest

Dose

- By mouth, *Clostridium difficile* infection, (see also notes above), 125 mg every 6 hours for 10–14 days (increased up to 500 mg every 6 hours if infection fails to respond or is life-threatening)
- By intravenous infusion, 1–1.5 g every 12 hours; ELDERLY over 65 years, 500 mg every 12 hours *or* 1 g once daily
  Note Plasma concentration monitoring required (see Cautions above); pre-dose ('trough') concentration should be 10–15 mg/litre (15–20 mg/litre for endocarditis or less sensitive strains of meticillin-resistant *Staphylococcus aureus* or for complicated infections caused by *S. aureus*). An initial loading dose, by intravenous infusion, may be considered—consult local guidelines
- Surgical prophylaxis, by intravenous infusion, 1 g
- CHILD under 18 years see *BNF for Children*
Note Vancomycin doses in BNF may differ from those in product literature

Vancomycin (Non-proprietary) PoM
Capsules, vancomycin (as hydrochloride) 125 mg, net price 28-cap pack = £132.47; 250 mg, 28-cap pack = £140.08. Label: 9

5 Infections

Injection, powder for reconstitution, vancomycin (as hydrochloride), for use as an infusion, net price 500-mg vial = £6.25; 1-g vial = £12.99

Note Can be used to prepare solution for oral administration

Vancocin® (Flynn) PoM

Matrigel capsules, vancomycin (as hydrochloride) 125 mg, net price 28-cap pack = £88.31. Label: 9

Injection, powder for reconstitution, vancomycin (as hydrochloride), for use as an infusion, net price 500-mg vial = £6.25; 1-g vial = £12.50

Note Can be used to prepare solution for oral administration

TEICOPLANIN

Indications see notes above and under Dose

Cautions vancomycin sensitivity; blood counts and liver and kidney function tests required; monitor renal and auditory function during prolonged treatment in renal impairment or if other nephrotoxic or neurotoxic drugs given; monitor plasma-teicoplanin concentration during parenteral maintenance treatment if severe sepsis or burns, deep-seated staphylococcal infection (including bone and joint infection), endocarditis, renal impairment, in elderly, and in intravenous drug abusers; **interactions:** Appendix 1 (teicoplanin)

Renal impairment use normal dose regimen on days 1–4, then use normal maintenance dose every 48 hours if eGFR 30–80 mL/minute/1.73 m² and use normal maintenance dose every 72 hours if eGFR less than 30 mL/minute/1.73 m²; see also Cautions above

Pregnancy manufacturer advises use only if potential benefit outweighs risk

Breast-feeding no information available

Side-effects rash, pruritus; *less commonly* nausea, vomiting, diarrhoea, bronchospasm, dizziness, headache, fever, leucopenia, thrombocytopenia, eosinophilia, tinnitus, mild hearing loss, vestibular disorders, thrombophlebitis; *also reported* renal failure, exfoliative dermatitis, Stevens-Johnson syndrome, toxic epidermal necrolysis

Dose

- By mouth, *Clostridium difficile* infection, ADULT, 100–200 mg twice daily for 10–14 days
- By intravenous injection *or* infusion *or* by intramuscular injection, ADULT body-weight under 70 kg, initially 400 mg every 12 hours for 3 doses, subsequently 400 mg once daily; body-weight over 70 kg, initially 6 mg/kg every 12 hours for 3 doses, then 6 mg/kg once daily
- Streptococcal or enterococcal endocarditis (in combination with another antibacterial, see Table 1, section 5.1), by intravenous injection *or* infusion, ADULT initially 10 mg/kg every 12 hours for 3–5 doses, subsequently 10 mg/kg once daily (subsequent doses can be given by intramuscular injection)
- Bone and joint infections, by intravenous injection *or* by intravenous infusion, ADULT, initially 12 mg/kg every 12 hours for 3–5 doses, subsequently 12 mg/kg once daily (subsequent doses can be given by intramuscular injection); increased risk of fever and rash with doses of 12 mg/kg
- Surgical prophylaxis [unlicensed indication], ADULT, by intravenous injection, 400 mg up to 30 minutes before the procedure; open fractures, by intravenous infusion, 800 mg up to 30 minutes before skeletal stabilisation and definitive soft-tissue closure

- CHILD under 18 years see *BNF for Children*

Note Plasma-teicoplanin concentration is not measured routinely because a relationship between plasma concentration and toxicity has not been established. However, the plasma-teicoplanin concentration can be used to optimise parenteral treatment in some patients (see Cautions). Pre-dose ('trough') concentrations should be greater than 15 mg/litre (greater than 20 mg/litre in endocarditis or deep-seated infection such as bone and joint infection), but less than 60 mg/litre. Teicoplanin doses in BNF may differ from those in product literature

Targocid® (Sanofi-Aventis) ▼ PoM

Injection, powder for reconstitution, teicoplanin, net price 200-mg vial (with diluent) = £3.93; 400-mg vial (with diluent) = £7.32

Electrolytes Na⁺< 0.5 mmol/200- and 400-mg vial

Note Can be used to prepare solution for oral administration

TELAVANCIN

Indications hospital-acquired pneumonia, known or suspected to be caused by meticillin-resistant *Staphylococcus aureus* when other antibacterials cannot be used

Cautions avoid rapid infusion ('red man' syndrome); vancomycin or teicoplanin sensitivity; monitor renal function daily for at least the first 3–5 days, then every 2–3 days thereafter; concomitant use with nephrotoxic drugs; conditions that predispose to renal impairment; predisposition to QT interval prolongation (including electrolyte disturbances, congenital long QT syndrome, concomitant use of drugs that prolong the QT interval, uncompensated heart failure, severe left ventricular hypertrophy); concomitant use with potentially ototoxic drugs; **interactions:** Appendix 1 (telavancin)

Hepatic impairment manufacturer advises caution in severe impairment—no information available

Renal impairment avoid in acute renal failure—risk of mortality increased; in chronic renal failure, use 7.5 mg/kg once daily if eGFR 30–50 mL/minute/1.73m² and avoid if eGFR less than 30 mL/minute/1.73m²

Pregnancy avoid (teratogenic in *animal* studies); effective contraception required during treatment

Breast-feeding manufacturer advises avoid unless potential benefit outweighs risk—no information available

Side-effects diarrhoea, nausea, vomiting, constipation, taste disturbances, insomnia, headache, dizziness, malaise, chills, fungal infection, acute renal failure, pruritus, rash; *less commonly* abdominal pain, dry mouth, dyspepsia, decreased appetite, flatulence, oral hypoaesthesia, hepatitis, angina, atrial fibrillation, bradycardia, congestive cardiac failure, QT interval prolongation, palpitation, sinus tachycardia, supraventricular extrasystoles, ventricular extrasystoles, oedema, flushing, hypertension, hypotension, dyspnoea, hiccup, nasal congestion, pharyngolaryngeal pain, paraesthesia, altered sense of smell, somnolence, tremor, agitation, anxiety, confusion, depression, antibiotic-associated colitis, urinary tract infection, pyrexia, dysuria, haematuria, microalbuminuria, oliguria, pollakiuria, electrolyte disturbances, increased INR, blood disorders, arthralgia, back pain, myalgia, eye irritation, blurred vision, tinnitus, erythema, hyperhidrosis, urticaria, phlebitis, non-cardiac chest pain, flushing of the upper body ('red man' syndrome); *rarely* deafness

Dose

• By intravenous infusion, ADULT over 18 years, 10 mg/kg once daily for 7–21 days

Vibativ® (Clinigen) ▼ PoM
Concentrate for intravenous infusion, powder for reconstitution, telavancin (as hydrochloride), net price 750-mg vial = £645.00

Daptomycin

Daptomycin is a lipopeptide antibacterial with a spectrum of activity similar to vancomycin but its efficacy against enterococci has not been established. Daptomycin should be reserved for complicated skin and soft-tissue infections caused by resistant Gram-positive bacteria including meticillin-resistant *Staphylococcus aureus* (MRSA). It needs to be given with other antibacterials for mixed infections involving Gram-negative bacteria and some anaerobes. Daptomycin is used (in combination with other antibacterials) for staphylococcal endocarditis caused by organisms resistant to vancomycin or in patients intolerant of vancomycin.

The *Scottish Medicines Consortium* (p. 4) has advised (February 2008) that daptomycin (*Cubicin®*) is accepted for restricted use within NHS Scotland for the treatment of MRSA bacteraemia associated with right-sided endocarditis or with complicated skin and soft-tissue infections.

◢ DAPTOMYCIN

Indications see under Dose

Cautions interference with assay for prothrombin time and INR—take blood sample immediately before daptomycin dose; **interactions:** Appendix 1 (daptomycin)

Muscle effects Myalgia, muscle weakness, and myositis may occur uncommonly; rhabdomyolysis is very rare. Monitor creatine kinase before treatment and then weekly during treatment (more frequently if creatine kinase elevated more than 5 times upper limit of normal before treatment, or if receiving another drug known to cause myopathy (preferably avoid concomitant use), or if eGFR less than 80 mL/minute/1.73 m²). If unexplained muscle pain, tenderness, weakness, or cramps develop during treatment, measure creatine kinase every 2 days; discontinue if unexplained muscular symptoms and creatine kinase elevated markedly

Hepatic impairment manufacturer advises caution in severe hepatic impairment—no information available

Renal impairment see Muscle Effects above; also monitor renal function if eGFR less than 80 mL/minute/1.73 m²; use normal dose every 48 hours if eGFR less than 30 mL/minute/1.73 m²

Pregnancy manufacturer advises use only if potential benefit outweighs risk—no information available

Breast-feeding present in milk in small amounts, but absorption from gastro-intestinal tract negligible

Side-effects nausea, vomiting, abdominal pain, flatulence, diarrhoea (antibiotic-associated colitis reported), constipation, hypertension, hypotension, headache, anxiety, insomnia, dizziness, asthenia, anaemia, arthralgia, rash, pruritus, injection-site reactions; *less commonly* dyspepsia, anorexia, taste disturbance, glossitis, flushing, arrhythmias, tremor, paraesthesia, hyperglycaemia, renal failure, eosinophilia, thrombocytopenia, electrolyte disturbances, muscle effects (see Cautions); *rarely* jaundice; also reported syncope, wheezing, eosinophilic pneumonia, peripheral neuropathy

Dose

• By slow intravenous injection over 2 minutes *or* by intravenous infusion, complicated skin and soft-tissue infections caused by Gram-positive bacteria, ADULT over 18 years, 4 mg/kg once daily; increased to 6 mg/kg once daily if associated with *Staphylococcus aureus* bacteraemia

Staphylococcal endocarditis, ADULT over 18 years, 6 mg/kg once daily

Note not licensed for use in left-sided endocarditis

Cubicin® (Novartis) PoM
Intravenous infusion, powder for reconstitution, daptomycin, net price 350-mg vial = £62.00; 500-mg vial = £88.57

Linezolid

Linezolid, an oxazolidinone antibacterial, is active against Gram-positive bacteria including meticillin-resistant *Staphylococcus aureus* (MRSA), and vancomycin-resistant enterococci. Resistance to linezolid can develop with prolonged treatment or if the dose is less than that recommended. Linezolid is an option if a glycopeptide, such as vancomycin, cannot be used to treat pneumonia or severe skin and soft-tissue infections caused by MRSA. Linezolid is **not** active against Gram-negative organisms and must be given with other antibacterials if the infection also involves Gram-negative organisms (the combination should be used for mixed skin and soft tissue infections only when other treatments are not available). A higher incidence of blood disorders and optic neuropathy have been reported in patients receiving linezolid for more than the maximum recommended duration of 28 days.

◢ LINEZOLID

Indications pneumonia, complicated skin and soft-tissue infections caused by Gram-positive bacteria (initiated under expert supervision)

Cautions monitor full blood count (including platelet count) weekly (see also Blood disorders below); history of seizures; unless close observation and blood-pressure monitoring possible, avoid in uncontrolled hypertension, phaeochromocytoma, carcinoid tumour, thyrotoxicosis, bipolar depression, schizophrenia, or acute confusional states; **interactions:** Appendix 1 (MAOIs)

> **Blood disorders**
>
> Haematopoietic disorders (including thrombocytopenia, anaemia, leucopenia, and pancytopenia) have been reported in patients receiving linezolid, particularly the elderly. It is recommended that full blood counts are monitored weekly. Close monitoring is recommended in patients who:
>
> • receive treatment for more than 10–14 days;
> • have pre-existing myelosuppression;
> • are receiving drugs that may have adverse effects on haemoglobin, blood counts, or platelet function;
> • have severe renal impairment.
>
> If significant myelosuppression occurs, treatment should be stopped unless it is considered essential, in which case intensive monitoring of blood counts and appropriate management should be implemented.

5

Infections

CHM advice (optic neuropathy)

Severe optic neuropathy may occur rarely, particularly if linezolid is used for longer than 28 days. The CHM recommends that:

- patients should be warned to report symptoms of visual impairment (including blurred vision, visual field defect, changes in visual acuity and colour vision) immediately;
- patients experiencing new visual symptoms (regardless of treatment duration) should be evaluated promptly, and referred to an ophthalmologist if necessary;
- visual function should be monitored regularly if treatment is required for longer than 28 days.

Monoamine oxidase inhibition Linezolid is a reversible, non-selective monoamine oxidase inhibitor (MAOI). Patients should avoid consuming large amounts of tyramine-rich foods (such as mature cheese, yeast extracts, undistilled alcoholic beverages, and fermented soya bean products). In addition, linezolid should not be given with another MAOI or within 2 weeks of stopping another MAOI. Unless close observation and blood-pressure monitoring is possible, avoid in those receiving SSRIs, 5HT$_1$ agonists ('triptans'), tricyclic antidepressants, sympathomimetics, dopaminergics, buspirone, pethidine and possibly other opioid analgesics. For other interactions see Appendix 1 (MAOIs)

Contra-indications see Monoamine Oxidase Inhibition above

Hepatic impairment in severe hepatic impairment manufacturer advises use only if potential benefit outweighs risk

Renal impairment manufacturer advises metabolites may accumulate if eGFR less than 30 mL/minute/1.73 m^2; see also Blood Disorders, above

Pregnancy manufacturer advises use only if potential benefit outweighs risk—no information available

Breast-feeding manufacturer advises avoid—present in milk in *animal* studies

Side-effects diarrhoea (antibiotic-associated colitis reported), nausea, vomiting, taste disturbances, headache; *less commonly* thirst, dry mouth, glossitis, stomatitis, tongue discoloration, abdominal pain, dyspepsia, gastritis, constipation, pancreatitis, hypertension, fever, fatigue, dizziness, insomnia, hypoaesthesia, paraesthesia, tinnitus, polyuria, leucopenia, thrombocytopenia, eosinophilia, electrolyte disturbances, blurred vision, rash, pruritus, diaphoresis, injection-site reactions; *rarely* tachycardia, transient ischaemic attacks, renal failure; also reported tooth discoloration, convulsions, lactic acidosis, hyponatraemia, pancytopenia, anaemia, Stevens-Johnson syndrome, toxic epidermal necrolysis; peripheral and optic neuropathy reported on prolonged therapy (see also CHM advice above)

Dose

- By mouth, 600 mg every 12 hours usually for 10–14 days (max. duration of treatment 28 days); CHILD [unlicensed] 1 week–12 years, 10 mg/kg every 8 hours; 12–18 years, adult dose
- By intravenous infusion over 30–120 minutes, 600 mg every 12 hours, CHILD [unlicensed] 1 week–12 years, 10 mg/kg every 8 hours; 12–18 years, adult dose

Zyvox® (Pharmacia) [PoM]

Tablets, f/c, linezolid 600 mg, net price 10-tab pack = £445.00. Label: 9, 10, patient information leaflet

Suspension, yellow, linezolid 100 mg/5 mL when reconstituted with water, net price 150 mL (orange-flavoured) = £222.50. Label: 9, 10 patient information leaflet

Excipients include aspartame 20 mg/5 mL (section 9.4.1)

Intravenous infusion, linezolid 2 mg/mL, net price 300-mL *Excel®* bag = £44.50

Excipients include Na$^+$ 5 mmol/300-mL bag, glucose 13.71 g/300-mL bag

Polymyxins

The polymyxin antibiotic, **colistimethate sodium** (colistin sulfomethate sodium), is active against Gram-negative organisms including *Pseudomonas aeruginosa*, *Acinetobacter baumanii*, and *Klebsiella pneumoniae*. It is not absorbed by mouth and thus needs to be given by injection for a systemic effect. Intravenous administration of colistimethate sodium should be reserved for Gram-negative infections resistant to other antibacterials; its major adverse effects are dose-related neurotoxicity and nephrotoxicity.

Colistimethate sodium is also given by inhalation as an adjunct to standard antibacterial therapy in patients with cystic fibrosis.

NICE guidance

Colistimethate sodium by dry powder inhalation for pseudomonal lung infection in cystic fibrosis (March 2013)

Colistimethate sodium dry powder for inhalation is recommended for chronic pulmonary infection caused by *Pseudomonas aeruginosa* in patients with cystic fibrosis who would benefit from continued treatment, but do not tolerate the drug in its nebulised form. The manufacturer must provide colistimethate sodium dry powder for inhalation at the discount agreed as part of the patient access scheme to primary, secondary and tertiary care in the NHS. Patients currently receiving colistimethate sodium dry powder for inhalation can continue treatment until they and their clinician consider it appropriate to stop.

www.nice.org.uk/TA276

Both colistimethate sodium and polymyxin B are included in some preparations for topical application.

COLISTIMETHATE SODIUM
(Colistin sulfomethate sodium)

Indications see notes above

Cautions acute porphyria (section 9.8.2); **interactions:** Appendix 1 (polymyxins)

Specific cautions for parenteral treatment Monitor renal function

Specific cautions for inhaled treatment Other inhaled drugs should be administered before colistimethate sodium. Measure lung function before and after initial dose of colistimethate sodium and monitor for bronchospasm; if bronchospasm occurs in a patient not using a bronchodilator, repeat test using a bronchodilator before the dose of colistimethate sodium. Severe haemoptysis—risk of further haemorrhage

Contra-indications myasthenia gravis

Renal impairment reduce dose and monitor plasma-colistimethate sodium concentration during parenteral treatment—consult product literature

Pregnancy clinical use suggests probably safe when used by inhalation; use parenteral treatment only if potential benefit outweighs risk

Breast-feeding present in milk but poorly absorbed from gut; manufacturers advise avoid (or use only if potential benefit outweighs risk)

Side-effects

Specific side-effects for parenteral treatment Neurotoxicity reported especially with excessive doses (including apnoea, perioral and peripheral paraesthesia, vertigo, headache, muscle weakness; rarely vasomotor instability, slurred speech, confusion, psychosis, visual disturbances), nephrotoxicity, rash **Specific side-effects for inhaled treatment** Sore throat, sore mouth, taste disturbances, nausea, vomiting, cough, bronchospasm, dysphonia; *less commonly* thirst, hypersalivation

Dose

- By slow intravenous injection into a totally implantable venous access device, *or* by intravenous infusion (but see notes above), ADULT and CHILD body-weight under 60 kg, 50 000–75 000 units/kg daily in 3 divided doses; body-weight over 60 kg, 1–2 million units every 8 hours

  Note Plasma concentration monitoring recommended in renal impairment; recommended 'peak' plasma-colistimethate sodium concentration (approx. 1 hour after intravenous injection or infusion) 5–15 mg/litre, pre-dose ('trough') concentration 2–6 mg/litre

- By inhalation of nebulised solution, ADULT and CHILD over 2 years, 1–2 million units twice daily; increased to 2 million units 3 times daily for subsequent respiratory isolates of *Ps. aeruginosa*; CHILD 1 month–2 years, 0.5–1 million units twice daily; increased to 1 million units 3 times daily for subsequent respiratory isolates of *Ps. aeruginosa*

- By inhalation of powder, ADULT and CHILD over 6 years, 1.66 million units twice daily

Colistimethate sodium (Non-proprietary) ℗ℴ𝓜

Injection, powder for reconstitution, colistimethate sodium, net price 1 million-unit vial = £1.68

Colomycin® (Forest) ℗ℴ𝓜

Injection, powder for reconstitution, colistimethate sodium, net price 1 million-unit vial = £1.80; 2 million-unit vial = £3.24

Electrolytes (before reconstitution) Na⁺< 0.5 mmol/1 million-unit and 2 million-unit vial

Note *Colomycin*® Injection may be used for nebulisation; administer required dose in 2–4 mL of sodium chloride 0.9%, (*or* water for injections) *or* a 1:1 mixture of sodium chloride 0.9% and water for injection

Promixin® (Profile) ℗ℴ𝓜

Powder for nebuliser solution, colistimethate sodium, net price 1 million-unit vial = £4.60

Injection, powder for reconstitution, colistimethate sodium, net price 1 million unit-vial = £2.30

Electrolytes (before reconstitution) Na⁺< 0.5 mmol/1 million-unit vial

Colobreathe® (Forest) ℗ℴ𝓜

Dry powder for inhalation, hard capsule, colistimethate sodium 1.66 million units/capsule, net price 56-cap pack (with *Turbospin*® inhaler device) = £968.80. Counselling, administration

Counselling Rinse mouth with water after each dose

Rifaximin

Rifaximin is a rifamycin that is poorly absorbed from the gastro-intestinal tract, and, therefore, should not be used to treat systemic infections. It is licensed for the treatment of travellers' diarrhoea that is not complicated by fever and blood in the stools, but see section 1.4. It is not recommended for diarrhoea associated with invasive organisms such as *Campylobacter* and *Shigella*. Rifaximin is also licensed to reduce the risk of recurrence of hepatic encephalopathy.

▌ RIFAXIMIN

Indications see under Dose

Contra-indications rifamycin hypersensitivity; intestinal obstruction

Hepatic impairment manufacturer advises caution when used for hepatic encephalopathy in patients with severe hepatic impairment

Pregnancy manufacturer advises avoid—toxicity in *animal* studies

Breast-feeding unlikely to be present in milk in significant amounts, but manufacturer advises avoid

Side-effects nausea, vomiting, abdominal pain, flatulence, diarrhoea, dyspnoea, headache, depression, dizziness, muscle spasm, rash, pruritus; *less commonly* anorexia, taste disturbances, dry mouth, peripheral oedema, sleep disturbances, anxiety, memory impairment, convulsions, hypoaesthesia, paraesthesia, antibiotic-associated colitis, influenza-like symptoms, dysuria, polyuria, glycosuria, polymenorrhoea, blood disorders, hyperkalaemia; *rarely* blood pressure changes, constipation; also reported syncope

Dose

- Travellers' diarrhoea that is not associated with fever, bloody diarrhoea, blood or leucocytes in the stool, or 8 or more unformed stools in the previous 24 hours, ADULT over 18 years, 200 mg every 8 hours for 3 days

- Reduction in recurrence of hepatic encephalopathy, ADULT over 18 years, 550 mg twice daily

Targaxan® (Norgine) ℗ℴ𝓜

Tablets, pink, f/c, rifaximin 550 mg, net price 56-tab pack = £259.23. Label: 14

Xifaxanta® (Norgine) ℗ℴ𝓜

Tablets, pink, f/c, rifaximin 200 mg, net price 9-tab pack = £15.15. Label: 9

Fidaxomicin

Fidaxomicin is a macrocyclic antibacterial that is poorly absorbed from the gastro-intestinal tract, and, therefore, it should not be used to treat systemic infections. It is licensed for the treatment of *Clostridium difficile* infection (see also section 1.5), but limited clinical data is available on the use of fidaxomicin in severe or life-threatening *C. difficile* infection.

The *Scottish Medicines Consortium* (p. 4) has advised (June 2012) that fidaxomicin (*Dificlir*®) is accepted for restricted use within NHS Scotland to treat the first recurrence of *C. difficile* infection, on the advice of a microbiologist or specialist in infectious diseases.

▌ FIDAXOMICIN

Indications *Clostridium difficile* infection

Cautions macrolide hypersensitivity; severe or life-threatening *C. difficile* infection; inflammatory bowel disease; **interactions**: Appendix 1 (fidaxomicin)

Hepatic impairment manufacturer advises caution in moderate to severe impairment—no information available

Renal impairment manufacturer advises caution in severe impairment—no information available

Pregnancy manufacturer advises avoid—no information available

Breast-feeding manufacturer advises avoid—no information available

Side-effects nausea, vomiting, constipation; *less commonly* taste disturbance, abdominal distension, flatulence, headache, dizziness, decreased appetite, dry mouth

Dose
- ADULT over 18 years, 200 mg every 12 hours for 10 days

Dificlir® (Astellas) ▼ PoM
Tablets, f/c, fidaxomicin 200 mg, net price 20-tab pack = £1350.00. Label: 9

5.1.8 Sulfonamides and trimethoprim

The importance of the sulfonamides has decreased as a result of increasing bacterial resistance and their replacement by antibacterials which are generally more active and less toxic.

Sulfamethoxazole and trimethoprim are used in combination (as **co-trimoxazole**) because of their synergistic activity. However, co-trimoxazole is associated with rare but serious side-effects (e.g. Stevens-Johnson syndrome and blood dyscrasias, notably bone marrow depression and agranulocytosis) especially in the elderly (see Restrictions on the use of Co-trimoxazole below)

Restrictions on the use of co-trimoxazole
Co-trimoxazole is the drug of choice in the prophylaxis and treatment of *Pneumocystis jirovecii* (*Pneumocystis carinii*) pneumonia; it is also indicated for nocardiasis, *Stenotrophomonas maltophilia* infection [unlicensed indication], and toxoplasmosis. It should only be considered for use in *acute exacerbations of chronic bronchitis* and *infections of the urinary tract* when there is bacteriological evidence of sensitivity to co-trimoxazole and good reason to prefer this combination to a single antibacterial; similarly it should only be used in *acute otitis media in children* when there is good reason to prefer it. Co-trimoxazole is also used for the treatment of infections caused by *Burkholderia cepacia* in cystic fibrosis [unlicensed indication].

Trimethoprim can be used alone for urinary- and respiratory-tract infections and for prostatitis, shigellosis, and invasive salmonella infections. Trimethoprim has side-effects similar to co-trimoxazole but they are less severe and occur less frequently.

For *topical preparations* of sulfonamides used in the treatment of burns see section 13.10.1.1.

CO-TRIMOXAZOLE

A mixture of trimethoprim and sulfamethoxazole (sulphamethoxazole) in the proportions of 1 part to 5 parts

Indications see restrictions above

Cautions maintain adequate fluid intake; avoid in blood disorders (unless under specialist supervision); monitor blood counts on prolonged treatment; discontinue immediately if blood disorders or rash develop; predisposition to folate deficiency or hyperkalaemia; elderly (see Restrictions on the use of Co-trimoxazole above); asthma; G6PD deficiency (section 9.1.5); avoid in infants under 6 weeks (except for treatment or prophylaxis of pneumocystis pneu-

monia); **interactions:** Appendix 1 (trimethoprim, sulfamethoxazole)

Contra-indications acute porphyria (section 9.8.2)

Hepatic impairment manufacturer advises avoid in severe liver disease

Renal impairment use half normal dose if eGFR 15–30 mL/minute/1.73 m²; avoid if eGFR less than 15 mL/minute/1.73 m² and if plasma-sulfamethoxazole concentration cannot be monitored

Pregnancy teratogenic risk in first trimester (trimethoprim a folate antagonist). Neonatal haemolysis and methaemoglobinaemia in third trimester; fear of increased risk of kernicterus in neonates appears to be unfounded

Breast-feeding small risk of kernicterus in jaundiced infants and of haemolysis in G6PD-deficient infants (due to sulfamethoxazole)

Side-effects nausea, diarrhoea; headache; hyperkalaemia; rash (very rarely including Stevens-Johnson syndrome, toxic epidermal necrolysis, photosensitivity)—discontinue immediately; *less commonly* vomiting; *very rarely* glossitis, stomatitis, anorexia, liver damage (including jaundice and hepatic necrosis), pancreatitis, antibiotic-associated colitis, myocarditis, cough and shortness of breath, pulmonary infiltrates, aseptic meningitis, depression, convulsions, peripheral neuropathy, ataxia, tinnitus, vertigo, hallucinations, hypoglycaemia, blood disorders (including leucopenia, thrombocytopenia, megaloblastic anaemia, eosinophilia), hyponatraemia, renal disorders including interstitial nephritis, arthralgia, myalgia, vasculitis, systemic lupus erythematosus and uveitis; rhabdomyolysis reported in HIV-infected patients

Dose
- By mouth, 960 mg every 12 hours; CHILD, every 12 hours, 6 weeks–5 months, 120 mg; 6 months–5 years, 240 mg; 6–12 years, 480 mg
- By intravenous infusion, 960 mg every 12 hours increased to 1.44 g every 12 hours in severe infections; CHILD 36 mg/kg daily in 2 divided doses increased to 54 mg/kg daily in severe infections
- Treatment of *Pneumocystis jirovecii* (*Pneumocystis carinii*) infections (undertaken where facilities for appropriate monitoring available—consult microbiologist and product literature), by mouth *or* by intravenous infusion, ADULT and CHILD over 4 weeks, 120 mg/kg daily in 2–4 divided doses for 14–21 days
- Prophylaxis of *Pneumocystis jirovecii* (*Pneumocystis carinii*) infections, by mouth, 960 mg once daily (may be reduced to 480 mg once daily to improve tolerance) *or* 960 mg on alternate days (3 times a week) *or* 960 mg twice daily on alternate days (3 times a week); CHILD 6 weeks–5 months, 120 mg twice daily on 3 consecutive or alternate days per week *or* on 7 days per week; 6 months–5 years, 240 mg; 6–12 years, 480 mg

Note 480 mg of co-trimoxazole consists of sulfamethoxazole 400 mg and trimethoprim 80 mg

Co-trimoxazole (Non-proprietary) PoM
Tablets, co-trimoxazole 480 mg, net price 28-tab pack = £3.46, 960 mg, 100 = £23.46. Label: 9
Brands include *Fectrim®, Fectrim® Forte*
Paediatric oral suspension, co-trimoxazole 240 mg/5 mL, net price 100 mL = £1.12. Label: 9
Oral suspension, co-trimoxazole 480 mg/5 mL. Net price 100 mL = £4.41. Label: 9

5 Infections

Septrin® (Aspen) [PoM]

Tablets, co-trimoxazole 480 mg, net price 100-tab pack= £15.52. Label: 9

Forte tablets, scored, co-trimoxazole 960 mg, net price 100-tab pack = £23.46. Label: 9

Adult suspension, co-trimoxazole 480 mg/5 mL, net price 100 mL (vanilla-flavoured) = £4.41. Label: 9

Paediatric suspension, sugar-free, co-trimoxazole 240 mg/5 mL, net price 100 mL (banana- and vanilla-flavoured) = £2.45. Label: 9

Intravenous infusion, co-trimoxazole 96 mg/mL. To be diluted before use. Net price 5-mL amp = £1.78
Electrolytes Na$^+$ 1.7 mmol/5 mL
Excipients include alcohol 13.2%, propylene glycol, sulfites

SULFADIAZINE
(Sulphadiazine)

Indications prevention of rheumatic fever recurrence, toxoplasmosis [unlicensed]—see section 5.4.7

Cautions see under Co-trimoxazole; **interactions:** Appendix 1 (sulfonamides)

Contra-indications see under Co-trimoxazole

Hepatic impairment use with caution in mild to moderate impairment; avoid in severe impairment

Renal impairment use with caution in mild to moderate impairment; avoid in severe impairment; high risk of crystalluria

Pregnancy neonatal haemolysis and methaemoglobinaemia in third trimester; fear of increased risk of kernicterus in neonates appears to be unfounded

Breast-feeding small risk of kernicterus in jaundiced infants and of haemolysis in G6PD-deficient infants

Side-effects see under Co-trimoxazole; also hypothyroidism, benign intracranial hypertension, optic neuropathy

Dose
- Prevention of rheumatic fever, *by mouth*, 1 g daily (500 mg daily for patients less than 30 kg)

Sulfadiazine (Non-proprietary) [PoM]

Tablets, sulfadiazine 500 mg, net price 56-tab pack = £69.00. Label: 9, 27

TRIMETHOPRIM

Indications urinary-tract infections, acute and chronic bronchitis; pneumocystis pneumonia (section 5.4.8)

Cautions predisposition to folate deficiency; elderly; manufacturer recommends blood counts on long-term therapy (but evidence of practical value unsatisfactory); neonates (specialist supervision required); acute porphyria (section 9.8.2); **interactions:** Appendix 1 (trimethoprim)
Blood disorders On long-term treatment, patients and their carers should be told how to recognise signs of blood disorders and advised to seek immediate medical attention if symptoms such as fever, sore throat, rash, mouth ulcers, purpura, bruising or bleeding develop

Contra-indications blood dyscrasias

Renal impairment use half normal dose after 3 days if eGFR 15–30 mL/minute/1.73 m^2; use half normal dose if eGFR less than 15 mL/minute/1.73 m^2 (monitor plasma-trimethoprim concentration if eGFR less than 10 mL/minute/1.73 m^2)

Pregnancy teratogenic risk in first trimester (folate antagonist); manufacturers advise avoid

Breast-feeding present in milk—short-term use not known to be harmful

Side-effects gastro-intestinal disturbances including nausea and vomiting, pruritus, rashes, hyperkalaemia, depression of haematopoiesis; rarely erythema multiforme, toxic epidermal necrolysis, photosensitivity and other allergic reactions including angioedema and anaphylaxis; aseptic meningitis and uveitis reported

Dose
- Acute infections, 200 mg every 12 hours; CHILD 1 month–12 years, 4 mg/kg (max. 200 mg) every 12 hours; *or* 6 weeks–6 months 25 mg every 12 hours, 6 months–6 years 50 mg every 12 hours, 6–12 years 100 mg every 12 hours
- Prophylaxis, 100 mg at night; CHILD under 12 years, 2 mg/kg (max.100 mg) at night; *or* [unlicensed dose] 6 weeks–6 months 12.5 mg at night, 6 months–6 years 25 mg at night, 6–12 years 50 mg at night

Trimethoprim (Non-proprietary) [PoM]

Tablets, trimethoprim 100 mg, net price 28 = £1.08; 200 mg, 14-tab pack = £1.01. Label: 9
Brands include *Trimopan®*

Suspension, trimethoprim 50 mg/5 mL, net price 100 mL = £1.59. Label: 9

5.1.9　Antituberculosis drugs

Tuberculosis is treated in two phases—an *initial phase* using 4 drugs and a *continuation phase* using 2 drugs in fully sensitive cases. Treatment requires specialised knowledge, particularly where the disease involves resistant organisms or non-respiratory organs.

The regimens given below are recommended for the treatment of tuberculosis in the UK; variations occur in other countries. Either the unsupervised regimen or the supervised regimen described below should be used; the two regimens should **not** be used concurrently.

Initial phase The concurrent use of 4 drugs during the initial phase is designed to reduce the bacterial population as rapidly as possible and to prevent the emergence of drug-resistant bacteria. The drugs are best given as combination preparations unless one of the components cannot be given because of resistance or intolerance. The treatment of choice for the initial phase is the daily use of isoniazid, rifampicin, pyrazinamide and ethambutol. Treatment should be started without waiting for culture results if clinical features or histology results are consistent with tuberculosis; treatment should be continued even if initial culture results are negative. The initial phase drugs should be continued for 2 months. Where a positive culture for *M. tuberculosis* has been obtained, but susceptibility results are not available after 2 months, treatment with rifampicin, isoniazid, pyrazinamide and ethambutol should be continued until full susceptibility is confirmed, even if this is for longer than 2 months.

Streptomycin is rarely used in the UK but it may be used in the initial phase of treatment if resistance to isoniazid has been established before therapy is commenced.

Continuation phase After the initial phase, treatment is continued for a further 4 months with isoniazid and rifampicin (preferably given as a combination preparation). Longer treatment is necessary for meningitis, direct spinal cord involvement, and for resistant organisms which may also require modification of the regimen.

5 Infections

Unsupervised treatment The following regimen should be used for patients who are likely to take antituberculous drugs reliably **without supervision**. Patients who are unlikely to comply with daily administration of antituberculous drugs should be treated with the regimen described under Supervised Treatment.

ment regimen. These patients are given isoniazid, rifampicin, pyrazinamide and ethambutol (or streptomycin) 3 times a week under supervision for the first 2 months followed by isoniazid and rifampicin 3 times a week for a further 4 months.

Recommended dosage for standard unsupervised 6-month treatment

2-month initial phase

Rifater® [rifampicin, isoniazid, and pyrazinamide]	ADULT body-weight under 40 kg 3 tablets daily; body-weight 40–49 kg 4 tablets daily; body-weight 50–64 kg 5 tablets daily; body-weight over 65 kg 6 tablets daily
Ethambutol	ADULT 15 mg/kg daily

4-month continuation phase following initial treatment with Rifater® and ethambutol

Rifinah® [rifampicin and isoniazid]	ADULT body-weight under 50 kg 3 tablets daily of *Rifinah® 150/100*; body-weight 50 kg and over 2 tablets daily of *Rifinah® 300/150*

or (if combination preparations not appropriate):

Isoniazid (for 6 months)	ADULT 300 mg daily; CHILD 10 mg/kg (max. 300 mg) daily
Rifampicin (for 6 months)	ADULT body-weight under 50 kg 450 mg daily; body-weight 50 kg and over 600 mg daily; CHILD 15 mg/kg daily (max. 450 mg daily if body-weight under 50 kg; max. 600 mg daily if body-weight 50 kg and over)
Pyrazinamide (for 2-month initial phase only)	ADULT body-weight under 50 kg 1.5 g daily; body-weight 50 kg and over 2 g daily; CHILD 35 mg/kg daily (max. 1.5 g daily if body-weight under 50 kg; max. 2 g daily if body-weight 50 kg and over)
Ethambutol (for 2-month initial phase only)	ADULT 15 mg/kg daily; CHILD 20 mg/kg daily

Pregnancy The standard regimen (above) may be used during pregnancy. Streptomycin should not be given in pregnancy.

Breast-feeding The standard regimen (above) may be used during breast-feeding

Children Children are given isoniazid, rifampicin, pyrazinamide, and ethambutol for the first 2 months followed by isoniazid and rifampicin during the next 4 months. However, care is needed in young children receiving ethambutol because of the difficulty in testing eyesight and in obtaining reports of visual symptoms (see below).

Supervised treatment Drug administration needs to be **fully supervised** (directly observed therapy, DOT) in patients who cannot comply reliably with the treat-

Recommended dosage for intermittent supervised 6-month treatment

Isoniazid (for 6 months)	ADULT and CHILD 15 mg/kg (max. 900 mg) 3 times a week
Rifampicin (for 6 months)	ADULT 600–900 mg 3 times a week; CHILD 15 mg/kg (max. 900 mg) 3 times a week
Pyrazinamide (for 2-month initial phase only)	ADULT body-weight under 50 kg 2 g 3 times a week; body-weight 50 kg and over 2.5 g 3 times a week; CHILD 50 mg/kg 3 times a week (max. 2 g 3 times a week if body-weight under 50 kg; max. 2.5 g 3 times a week if body-weight 50 kg and over)
Ethambutol (for 2-month initial phase only)	ADULT and CHILD 30 mg/kg 3 times a week

Immunocompromised patients Multi-resistant *Mycobacterium tuberculosis* may be present in immunocompromised patients. The organism should always be cultured to confirm its type and drug sensitivity. Confirmed *M. tuberculosis* infection sensitive to first-line drugs should be treated with a standard 6-month regimen; after completing treatment, patients should be closely monitored. The regimen may need to be modified if infection is caused by resistant organisms, and specialist advice is needed.

Specialist advice should be sought about tuberculosis treatment or chemoprophylaxis in a HIV-positive individual; care is required in choosing the regimen and in avoiding potentially serious interactions. Starting antiretroviral treatment in the first 2 months of antituberculosis treatment increases the risk of immune reconstitution syndrome.

Infection may also be caused by other mycobacteria e.g. *M. avium* complex in which case specialist advice on management is needed.

Corticosteroids In meningeal or pericardial tuberculosis, a corticosteroid should be started at the same time as antituberculosis therapy.

Prevention of tuberculosis Some individuals may develop tuberculosis owing to reactivation of previously latent disease. Chemoprophylaxis may be required in those who have evidence of latent tuberculosis and are receiving treatment with immunosuppressants (including cytotoxics and possibly long-term treatment with systemic corticosteroids). In these cases, chemoprophylaxis involves use of either isoniazid alone for 6 months or of isoniazid and rifampicin for 3 months, see Table 2, section 5.1; longer chemoprophylaxis is not recommended.

For prevention of tuberculosis in susceptible close contacts or those who have become tuberculin-positive, see Table 2, section 5.1. For advice on immunisation against tuberculosis, see section 14.4

Monitoring Since isoniazid, rifampicin and pyrazinamide are associated with liver toxicity, *hepatic function* should be checked before treatment with these drugs. Those with pre-existing liver disease or alcohol dependence should have frequent checks particularly in the first 2 months. If there is no evidence of liver disease (and pre-treatment liver function is normal), further checks are only necessary if the patient develops fever, malaise, vomiting, jaundice or unexplained deterioration during treatment. In view of the need to comply fully with antituberculous treatment on the one hand and to guard against serious liver damage on the other, patients and their carers should be informed carefully how to recognise signs of liver disorders and advised to discontinue treatment and seek **immediate** medical attention should symptoms of liver disease occur.

Renal function should be checked before treatment with antituberculous drugs and appropriate dosage adjustments made. Streptomycin or ethambutol should preferably be avoided in patients with renal impairment, but if used, the dose should be reduced and the plasma-drug concentration monitored.

Visual acuity should be tested before ethambutol is used (see below).

> Major causes of treatment failure are incorrect prescribing by the physician and inadequate compliance by the patient. Monthly tablet counts and urine examination (rifampicin imparts an orange-red coloration) may be useful indicators of compliance with treatment. Avoid both excessive and inadequate dosage. Treatment should be supervised by a specialist physician.

Isoniazid is cheap and highly effective. Like rifampicin it should always be included in any antituberculous regimen unless there is a specific contra-indication. Its only common side-effect is peripheral neuropathy which is more likely to occur where there are pre-existing risk factors such as diabetes, alcohol dependence, chronic renal failure, pregnancy, malnutrition and HIV infection. In these circumstances pyridoxine 10 mg daily (or 20 mg daily if suitable product not available) (section 9.6.2) should be given prophylactically from the start of treatment. The risk of peripheral neuropathy may also be increased by high doses of isoniazid; pyridoxine should, therefore, be considered for those receiving *Voractiv*®(p. 403) 5 tablets daily. Other side-effects such as hepatitis (important: see Monitoring above) and psychosis are rare.

Rifampicin, a rifamycin, is a key component of any antituberculous regimen. Like isoniazid it should always be included unless there is a specific contra-indication.

During the first two months ('initial phase') of rifampicin administration transient disturbance of liver function with elevated serum transaminases is common but generally does not require interruption of treatment. Occasionally more serious liver toxicity requires a change of treatment particularly in those with pre-existing liver disease (important: see Monitoring above).

On intermittent treatment six toxicity syndromes have been recognised—influenza-like, abdominal, and respiratory symptoms, shock, renal failure, and thrombocytopenic purpura—and can occur in 20 to 30% of patients.

Rifampicin induces hepatic enzymes which accelerate the metabolism of several drugs including oestrogens,

corticosteroids, phenytoin, sulfonylureas, and anticoagulants; **interactions**: Appendix 1 (rifamycins). **Important**: the effectiveness of hormonal contraceptives is reduced and alternative family planning advice should be offered (section 7.3.1).

Rifabutin, another rifamycin, is indicated for *prophylaxis* against *M. avium* complex infections in patients with a low CD4 count; it is also licensed for the *treatment* of non-tuberculous mycobacterial disease and pulmonary tuberculosis. **Important**: as with rifampicin it induces hepatic enzymes and the effectiveness of hormonal contraceptives is reduced requiring alternative family planning methods.

Pyrazinamide is a bactericidal drug only active against intracellular dividing forms of *Mycobacterium tuberculosis*; it exerts its main effect only in the first two or three months. It is particularly useful in tuberculous meningitis because of good meningeal penetration. It is not active against *M. bovis*. Serious liver toxicity may occasionally occur (important: see Monitoring above).

Ethambutol is included in a treatment regimen if isoniazid resistance is suspected; it can be omitted if the risk of resistance is low.

Side-effects of ethambutol are largely confined to visual disturbances in the form of loss of acuity, colour blindness, and restriction of visual fields. These toxic effects are more common where excessive dosage is used or if the patient's renal function is impaired. The earliest features of ocular toxicity are subjective and patients should be advised to discontinue therapy immediately if they develop deterioration in vision and promptly seek further advice. Early discontinuation of the drug is almost always followed by recovery of eyesight. Patients who cannot understand warnings about visual side-effects should, if possible, be given an alternative drug. In particular, ethambutol should be used with caution in children until they are at least 5 years old and capable of reporting symptomatic visual changes accurately.

Visual acuity should be tested by Snellen chart before treatment with ethambutol.

Streptomycin [unlicensed] is now rarely used in the UK except for resistant organisms. Plasma-drug concentration should be measured in patients with impaired renal function in whom streptomycin must be used with great care.

Drug-resistant tuberculosis should be treated by a specialist physician with experience in such cases, and where appropriate facilities for infection-control exist. Second-line drugs available for infections caused by resistant organisms, or when first-line drugs cause unacceptable side-effects, include **aminosalicylic acid**, **amikacin**, **capreomycin**, **cycloserine**, newer macrolides (e.g. **azithromycin** and **clarithromycin**), **moxifloxacin** and **protionamide** (prothionamide; no longer on UK market). **Bedaquiline** and **delamanid** are licensed for the treatment of multiple-drug resistant pulmonary tuberculosis. Bedaquiline has a long half-life.

AMINOSALICYLIC ACID

Indications in combination with other drugs, multiple-drug resistant tuberculosis

Cautions monitor liver function - discontinue immediately if signs or symptoms of hepatic toxicity (including rash, fever and gastrointestinal disturbance); monitor for hypersensitivity reaction during the first 3 months of treatment—for desensitisation dosing regimen consult product literature; peptic ulcer

Hepatic impairment   use with caution

Renal impairment   use with caution in mild to moderate impairment; avoid in severe impairment due to accumulation of inactive metabolites

Pregnancy   manufacturer advises avoid unless essential—toxicity in *animal* studies (highest risk during first trimester)

Breast-feeding   present in milk—manufacturer advises avoid

Side-effects   abdominal pain, vomiting, nausea, bloating, diarrhoea, vestibular syndrome, rash; *less commonly* anorexia; *rarely* malabsorption syndrome, peptic ulcer, gastrointestinal bleeding, jaundice, metallic taste, hypothyroidism, urticaria; *very rarely* weight loss, headache, peripheral neuropathy, dizziness, hypoglycaemia, thrombocytopenia, purpura, leucopenia, anaemia, methemoglobinaemia, agranulocytosis, crystalluria, tendon pain, visual abnormalities; *also reported* hepatitis, hypersensitivity

Dose

- By mouth, ADULT over 18 years, 4 g every 8 hours (max. 12 g daily), usual treatment duration 24 months
- Desensitisation regimen, consult product literature

Granupas® (Lucane) [PoM]

Granules, e/c, sugar-free, aminosalicyclic acid 4 g/sachet, net price 30-sachet pack = £331.00. Label: 9, 25, counselling, administration

Counselling Disperse granules in orange or tomato juice and take immediately (granules will not dissolve, ensure all granules are swallowed). Granules can be sprinkled on apple sauce or yoghurt for administration.

Patients should be advised that the skeletons of the granules may be seen in the stools.

▌BEDAQUILINE

Indications   in combination with other drugs, multiple-drug resistant pulmonary tuberculosis

Cautions   determine serum potassium, calcium, and magnesium before starting treatment (correct if abnormal)—remeasure if QT prolongation occurs during treatment; obtain ECG before starting treatment, and then at least monthly during treatment or more frequently if concomitant use with other drugs known to prolong the QT interval; also obtain ECG if syncope occurs; QTc interval (derived using Fridericia's formula) 450–500 milliseconds—discontinue if QTc interval more than 500 milliseconds; risk factors for QT interval prolongation (e.g. electrolyte disturbances, heart failure with reduced left ventricular ejection fraction, history of symptomatic arrhythmias (avoid if ventricular arrhythmia present), bradycardia, congenital long QT syndrome); hypothyroidism; monitor liver function before starting treatment and then at least monthly during treatment—discontinue treatment if severe abnormalities in liver function tests; concomitant use of hepatotoxic drugs; **interactions**: Appendix 1 (bedaquiline)

Driving Dizziness may affect performance of skilled tasks (e.g. driving)

Contra-indications   ventricular arrhythmia; QTc interval more than 500 milliseconds (derived using Fridericia's formula)

Hepatic impairment   avoid concomitant use of hepatotoxic drugs unless essential; manufacturer advises caution in moderate impairment; avoid in severe impairment—no information available

Renal impairment   manufacturer advises caution if eGFR less than 30 mL/minute/1.73 m²

Pregnancy   manufacturer advises avoid unless potential benefit outweighs risk

Breast-feeding   manufacturer advises avoid—present in milk in *animal* studies

Side-effects   nausea, vomiting, diarrhoea, QT interval prolongation, headache, dizziness, arthralgia, myalgia

Dose

- ADULT over 18 years, initially 400 mg once daily for 2 weeks, then 200 mg three times a week (with at least 48 hours between each dose) for 22 weeks; continue appropriate combination therapy after bedaquiline
  Missed dose If a dose is missed during the first two weeks of treatment, the missed dose should not be taken and the next dose should be taken at the usual time; if a dose is missed during weeks 3–24 of treatment, the missed dose should be taken as soon as possible and then the usual regimen resumed

Sirturo® (Janssen) ▼ [PoM]

Tablets, bedaquiline (as fumarate) 100 mg, net price 188-tab pack = £18700.00. Label: 4, 8, 21, counselling, driving

▌CAPREOMYCIN

Indications   in combination with other drugs, tuberculosis resistant to first-line drugs

Cautions   auditory impairment; monitor renal, hepatic, auditory, and vestibular function and electrolytes; **interactions**: Appendix 1 (capreomycin)

Hepatic impairment   use with caution

Renal impairment   reduce dose—consult product literature; nephrotoxic; ototoxic

Pregnancy   manufacturer advises use only if potential benefit outweighs risk—teratogenic in *animal* studies

Breast-feeding   manufacturer advises caution—no information available

Side-effects   hypersensitivity reactions including urticaria and rashes; leucocytosis or leucopenia, rarely thrombocytopenia; changes in liver function tests; nephrotoxicity, electrolyte disturbances; hearing loss with tinnitus and vertigo; neuromuscular block after large doses, pain and induration at injection site

Dose

- By deep intramuscular injection, 1 g daily (not more than 20 mg/kg) for 2–4 months, then 1 g 2–3 times each week

Capreomycin (King) [PoM]

Injection, powder for reconstitution, capreomycin sulfate 1 million units (= capreomycin approx. 1 g). Net price per vial = £16.01

▌CYCLOSERINE

Indications   in combination with other drugs, tuberculosis resistant to first-line drugs

Cautions   monitor haematological, renal, and hepatic function; **interactions**: Appendix 1 (cycloserine)

Contra-indications   epilepsy, depression, severe anxiety, psychotic states, alcohol dependence

Renal impairment   increase interval between doses if creatinine clearance less than 50 mL/minute and monitor blood-cycloserine concentration

Pregnancy   manufacturer advises use only if potential benefit outweighs risk—crosses the placenta

Breast-feeding amount too small to be harmful

Side-effects mainly neurological, including headache, dizziness, vertigo, drowsiness, tremor, convulsions, confusion, psychosis, depression (discontinue or reduce dose if symptoms of CNS toxicity); rashes, allergic dermatitis (discontinue or reduce dose); megaloblastic anaemia; changes in liver function tests; heart failure at high doses reported

Dose

- Initially 250 mg every 12 hours for 2 weeks increased according to blood concentration and response to max. 500 mg every 12 hours; CHILD 2–18 years see *BNF for Children*

   Note Blood concentration monitoring required especially in renal impairment or if dose exceeds 500 mg daily or if signs of toxicity; blood concentration should not exceed 30 mg/litre

Cycloserine (King) [PoM]

Capsules, red/grey cycloserine 250 mg, net price 100-cap pack = £402.63. Label: 2, 8

◼ DELAMANID

Indications in combination with other drugs, multiple-drug resistant pulmonary tuberculosis

Cautions monitor serum albumin and electrolytes before starting treatment and then during treatment—discontinue treatment if serum albumin less than 28 g/litre; obtain ECG before starting treatment and then monthly during treatment (more frequently if serum albumin 28–34 g/litre, or if concomitant use of potent CYP3A4 inhibitors, or if risk factors for QT interval prolongation, or if QTc interval 450–500 milliseconds in men or 470–500 milliseconds in women)—discontinue treatment if QTc interval more than 500 milliseconds (derived using Fridericia's formula); risk factors for QT interval prolongation (e.g. electrolyte disturbances, acute myocardial infarction, heart failure with reduced left ventricular ejection fraction, severe hypertension, left ventricular hypertrophy, bradycardia, congenital long QT syndrome, concomitant use with other drugs known to prolong the QT interval, history of symptomatic arrhythmias); **interactions**: Appendix 1 (delamanid)

Contra-indications serum albumin less than 28 g/litre; QTc interval more than 500 milliseconds (derived using Fridericia's formula); concomitant use of potent CYP3A4 inducers

Hepatic impairment manufacturer advises avoid in moderate to severe impairment

Renal impairment manufacturer advises avoid in severe impairment—no information available

Pregnancy manufacturer advises avoid—toxicity in *animal* studies; effective contraception required during treatment

Breast-feeding manufacturer advises avoid—present in milk in *animal* studies

Side-effects nausea, vomiting, abdominal pain, dyspepsia, decreased appetite, palpitation, QT interval prolongation, chest pain, hypertension, hypotension, hyperlipidaemia, haemoptysis, dyspnoea, cough, malaise, headache, peripheral neuropathy, tremor, insomnia, anxiety, depression, agitation, psychiatric disorder, hypokalaemia, reticulocytosis, osteochondrosis, photophobia, tinnitus, earache, oropharyngeal pain, dermatitis, acne, hyperhidrosis; *less commonly* dysphagia, arrhythmias, balance disorder, herpes zoster, nocturia, urinary retention, hypocalcaemia, dehydration, leucopenia, thrombocytopenia, rash

Dose

- ADULT over 18 years, 100 mg twice daily for 24 weeks; continue appropriate combination therapy after delamanid

Deltyba® (Otsuka Novel) ▼ [PoM]

Tablets, yellow, f/c, delamanid 50 mg, net price 40-tab pack = £1045.83. Label: 8, 21

   Note Dispense in orginal container (contains desiccant)

◼ ETHAMBUTOL HYDROCHLORIDE

Indications tuberculosis, in combination with other drugs

Cautions elderly; test visual acuity before treatment and warn patients to report visual changes—see Monitoring in notes above; young children (see notes above)—routine ophthalmological monitoring recommended; **interactions**: Appendix 1 (ethambutol)

Contra-indications optic neuritis, poor vision

Renal impairment if creatinine clearance less than 30 mL/minute, use 15–25 mg/kg (max. 2.5 g) 3 times a week and monitor plasma-ethambutol concentration; optic nerve damage

Pregnancy not known to be harmful; see also p. 398

Breast-feeding amount too small to be harmful; see also p. 398

Side-effects optic neuritis, red/green colour blindness, peripheral neuritis, rarely rash, pruritus, urticaria, thrombocytopenia

Dose

- See notes above

   Note 'Peak' concentration (2–2.5 hours after dose) should be 2–6 mg/litre (7–22 micromol/litre); 'trough' (pre-dose) concentration should be less than 1 mg/litre (4 micromol/litre); see Renal Impairment above

Ethambutol (Non-proprietary) [PoM]

Tablets, ethambutol hydrochloride 100 mg, net price 56-tab pack = £11.52; 400 mg, 56-tab pack = £42.74. Label: 8

◼ ISONIAZID

Indications tuberculosis, in combination with other drugs; prophylaxis—Table 2, section 5.1

Cautions see Monitoring in notes above; also slow acetylator status (increased risk of side-effects); epilepsy; history of psychosis; alcohol dependence, malnutrition, diabetes mellitus, HIV infection (risk of peripheral neuritis); acute porphyria (section 9.8.2); **interactions**: Appendix 1 (isoniazid)

   Hepatic disorders Patients or their carers should be told how to recognise signs of liver disorder, and advised to discontinue treatment and seek immediate medical attention if symptoms such as persistent nausea, vomiting, malaise or jaundice develop

Contra-indications drug-induced liver disease

Hepatic impairment use with caution; monitor liver function regularly and particularly frequently in first 2 months; see also Hepatic Disorders above

Renal impairment risk of ototoxicity and peripheral neuropathy; prophylactic pyridoxine recommended, see notes above

Pregnancy not known to be harmful; prophylactic pyridoxine recommended; see also p. 398

Breast-feeding monitor infant for possible toxicity; theoretical risk of convulsions and neuropathy; prophylactic pyridoxine advisable in mother; see also p. 398

5
Infections

Side-effects nausea, vomiting, constipation, dry mouth; peripheral neuritis with high doses (pyridoxine prophylaxis, see notes above), optic neuritis, convulsions, psychotic episodes, vertigo; hypersensitivity reactions including fever, Stevens-Johnson syndrome, purpura; blood disorders including agranulocytosis, haemolytic anaemia, aplastic anaemia; hepatitis (especially over age of 35 years); pancreatitis; interstitial pneumonitis; systemic lupus erythematosus-like syndrome, pellagra, hyperreflexia, difficulty with micturition, hyperglycaemia, and gynaecomastia reported; hearing loss and tinnitus (in patients with end-stage renal impairment); when used with tyramine or histamine rich foods, tachycardia, palpitation, hypotension, flushing, headache, dizziness, and sweating also reported

Dose

- By mouth *or* by intramuscular *or* intravenous injection, see notes above

Isoniazid (Non-proprietary) PoM
Tablets, isoniazid 50 mg, net price 56-tab pack = £14.40; 100 mg, 28-tab pack = £14.40. Label: 8, 22
Injection, isoniazid 25 mg/mL, net price 2-mL amp = £24.11

◣ PYRAZINAMIDE

Indications tuberculosis in combination with other drugs

Cautions see Monitoring in notes above; also diabetes; gout (avoid in acute attack); **interactions:** Appendix 1 (pyrazinamide)
Hepatic disorders Patients or their carers should be told how to recognise signs of liver disorder, and advised to discontinue treatment and seek immediate medical attention if symptoms such as persistent nausea, vomiting, malaise or jaundice develop

Hepatic impairment monitor hepatic function—idiosyncratic hepatotoxicity more common; avoid in severe hepatic impairment; see also Hepatic Disorders above

Renal impairment monitor for gout; 25–30 mg/kg 3 times a week if eGFR less than 30 mL/minute/1.73 m^2

Pregnancy manufacturer advises use only if potential benefit outweighs risk; see also p. 398

Breast-feeding amount too small to be harmful; see also p. 398

Side-effects hepatotoxicity including fever, anorexia, hepatomegaly, splenomegaly, jaundice, liver failure; nausea, vomiting, flushing, dysuria, arthralgia, sideroblastic anaemia, thrombocytopenia, rash and occasionally photosensitivity

Dose

- See notes above

Zinamide® (Genus) PoM
Tablets, scored, pyrazinamide 500 mg, net price 30-tab pack = £31.35. Label: 8

◣ RIFABUTIN

Indications see under Dose

Cautions see under Rifampicin; acute porphyria (section 9.8.2)

Contra-indications rifamycin hypersensitivity

Hepatic impairment reduce dose in severe impairment

Renal impairment use half normal dose if eGFR less than 30 mL/minute/1.73 m^2

Pregnancy manufacturer advises avoid—no information available

Breast-feeding manufacturer advises avoid—no information available

Side-effects nausea, pyrexia, blood disorders (including leucopenia, anaemia, thrombocytopenia, and rarely haemolysis), myalgia, rash; *less commonly* vomiting, raised liver enzymes, jaundice, arthralgia, corneal deposits, uveitis especially following high doses or concomitant use with drugs that increase plasma concentration—see also **interactions**: Appendix 1 (rifamycins), hypersensitivity reactions (including eosinophilia, bronchospasm); skin, urine, saliva and other body secretions coloured orange-red; *also reported* hepatitis, influenza-like symptoms, chest pain, dyspnoea

Dose

- Prophylaxis of *Mycobacterium avium* complex infections in immunosuppressed patients with low CD4 count (see product literature), 300 mg daily as a single dose
- Treatment of non-tuberculous mycobacterial disease, in combination with other drugs, 450–600 mg daily as a single dose for up to 6 months after cultures negative
- Treatment of pulmonary tuberculosis, in combination with other drugs, 150–450 mg daily as a single dose for at least 6 months
- CHILD not recommended

Mycobutin® (Pharmacia) PoM
Capsules, red-brown, rifabutin 150 mg. Net price 30-cap pack = £90.38. Label: 8, 14, counselling, lenses, see under Rifampicin

---

◣ RIFAMPICIN

Indications see under Dose

Cautions see Monitoring in notes above; also liver function tests and blood counts in hepatic disorders, alcohol dependence, and on prolonged therapy, see also below; **important:** effectiveness of hormonal contraceptives is reduced and alternative family planning advice should be offered (see also section 7.3.1); discolours soft contact lenses; see also notes above; **interactions:** Appendix 1 (rifamycins)
Note If treatment interrupted re-introduce with low dosage and increase gradually; discontinue permanently if serious side-effects develop
Hepatic disorders Patients or their carers should be told how to recognise signs of liver disorder, and advised to discontinue treatment and seek immediate medical attention if symptoms such as persistent nausea, vomiting, malaise or jaundice develop

Contra-indications jaundice; rifamycin hypersensitivity; acute porphyria (section 9.8.2)

Hepatic impairment impaired elimination; monitor liver function; avoid or do not exceed 8 mg/kg daily; see also Cautions above

Renal impairment use with caution if dose above 600 mg daily

Pregnancy manufacturers advise very high doses teratogenic in *animal* studies in first trimester; risk of neonatal bleeding may be increased in third trimester; see also p. 398

Breast-feeding amount too small to be harmful; see also p. 398

Side-effects gastro-intestinal symptoms including anorexia, nausea, vomiting, diarrhoea (antibiotic-associated colitis reported); headache, drowsiness; those occurring mainly on intermittent therapy include influenza-like symptoms (with chills, fever, dizziness, bone pain), respiratory symptoms (including shortness of breath), collapse and shock, haemolytic anaemia, thrombocytopenic purpura, disseminated intravascular coagulation, and acute renal failure; alterations of liver function, jaundice; flushing, urticaria, and rashes; other side-effects reported include oedema, psychoses, adrenal insufficiency, muscular weakness and myopathy, exfoliative dermatitis, toxic epidermal necrolysis, Stevens-Johnson syndrome, pemphigoid reactions, leucopenia, eosinophilia, menstrual disturbances; urine, saliva, and other body secretions coloured orange-red; thrombophlebitis reported if infusion used for prolonged period

Dose

- Brucellosis, legionnaires' disease, endocarditis and serious staphylococcal infections, in combination with other drugs, by mouth *or* by intravenous infusion, 0.6–1.2 g daily (in 2–4 divided doses)
- Tuberculosis, in combination with other drugs, see notes above
- Leprosy, section 5.1.10
- Prophylaxis of meningococcal meningitis and *Haemophilus influenzae* (type b) infection, Table 2, section 5.1

Rifampicin (Non-proprietary) ᴘᴏᴹ
Capsules, rifampicin 150 mg, net price 100 = £14.76; 300 mg, 100 = £47.20. Label: 8, 14, 22, counselling, see lenses above

Rifadin® (Sanofi-Aventis) ᴘᴏᴹ
Capsules, rifampicin 150 mg (blue/red), net price 100-cap pack= £18.32; 300 mg (red), 100-cap pack= £36.63. Label: 8, 14, 22, counselling, see lenses above
Syrup, red, rifampicin 100 mg/5 mL (raspberry-flavoured), net price 120 mL = £3.56. Label: 8, 14, 22, counselling, see lenses above
Intravenous infusion, powder for reconstitution, rifampicin, net price 600-mg vial (with solvent) = £7.67
Electrolytes Na⁺< 0.5 mmol/vial

Rimactane® (Sandoz) ᴘᴏᴹ
Capsules, rifampicin 150 mg (red), net price 60-cap pack = £15.83; 300 mg (red/brown), 60-cap pack = £25.92. Label: 8, 14, 22, counselling, see lenses above

◀**Combined preparations**

Rifater® (Sanofi-Aventis) ᴘᴏᴹ
Tablets, pink, s/c, rifampicin 120 mg, isoniazid 50 mg, pyrazinamide 300 mg, net price 100-tab pack= £21.95. Label: 8, 14, 22, counselling, see lenses above
Dose initial treatment of pulmonary tuberculosis, patients up to 40 kg 3 tablets daily preferably before breakfast, 40–49 kg 4 tablets daily, 50–64 kg 5 tablets daily, 65 kg or more, 6 tablets daily; not suitable for use in children

Rifinah® 150/100 (Sanofi-Aventis) ᴘᴏᴹ
Tablets, pink, s/c, rifampicin 150 mg, isoniazid 100 mg, net price 84-tab pack = £15.91. Label: 8, 14, 22, counselling, see lenses above
Dose ADULT under 50 kg, 3 tablets daily, preferably before breakfast

Rifinah® 300/150 (Sanofi-Aventis) ᴘᴏᴹ
Tablets, orange, s/c, rifampicin 300 mg, isoniazid 150 mg, net price 56-tab pack = £26.24. Label: 8, 14, 22, counselling, see lenses above
Dose ADULT 50 kg and over, 2 tablets daily, preferably before breakfast
Note Some stock packaged as *Rifinah 150/300*

Voractiv® (Sandoz) ᴘᴏᴹ
Tablets, brown, f/c, rifampicin 150 mg, isoniazid 75 mg, pyrazinamide 400 mg, ethambutol hydrochloride 275 mg, net price 60-tab pack = £39.50. Label: 8, 14, 22, counselling, see lenses above
Dose initial treatment of tuberculosis ADULT 30–39 kg 2 tablets daily, 40–54 kg 3 tablets daily, 55–70 kg 4 tablets daily, over 70 kg 5 tablets daily
Note Risk of peripheral neuropathy may be increased by high doses of isoniazid—consider prescribing pyridoxine for those receiving *Voractiv®* 5 tablets daily (see also Isoniazid prescribing notes, p. 399)

▌ STREPTOMYCIN

Indications tuberculosis, in combination with other drugs; adjunct to doxycycline in brucellosis; enterococcal endocarditis (Table 1, section 5.1)

Cautions see under Aminoglycosides, section 5.1.4; interactions: Appendix 1 (aminoglycosides)

Contra-indications see under Aminoglycosides, section 5.1.4

Renal impairment see under Aminoglycosides, section 5.1.4

Pregnancy see under Aminoglycosides, section 5.1.4

Side-effects see under Aminoglycosides, section 5.1.4; also hypersensitivity reactions, paraesthesia of mouth

Dose

- By deep intramuscular injection, tuberculosis [unlicensed], 15 mg/kg (max. 1 g) daily (reduced in those under 50 kg, those over 40 years, or those with renal impairment)

Brucellosis, expert advice essential

Important Side-effects increase after a cumulative dose of 100 g, which should only be exceeded in exceptional circumstances

Note One-hour ('peak') concentration should be 15–40 mg/litre; pre-dose ('trough') concentration should be less than 5 mg/litre (less than 1 mg/litre in renal impairment or in those over 50 years)

Streptomycin Sulfate (Non-proprietary) ᴘᴏᴹ
Injection, powder for reconstitution, streptomycin (as sulfate), net price 1-g vial = £15.00
Available from 'special-order' manufacturers or specialist importing companies, see p. 1124

▌5.1.10 Antileprotic drugs

Advice from a member of the Panel of Leprosy Opinion is essential for the treatment of leprosy (Hansen's disease). Details can be obtained from the Hospital for Tropical Diseases, London (telephone (020) 3456 7890).

The World Health Organization has made recommendations to overcome the problem of dapsone resistance and to prevent the emergence of resistance to other antileprotic drugs. Drugs recommended are **dapsone**, **rifampicin** (section 5.1.9), and **clofazimine**. Other drugs with significant activity against *Mycobacterium leprae* include ofloxacin, minocycline and clarithromycin, but none of these are as active as rifampicin;

5 Infections

at present they should be reserved as second-line drugs for leprosy.

A three-drug regimen is recommended for *multibacillary leprosy* (lepromatous, borderline-lepromatous, and borderline leprosy) and a two-drug regimen for *paucibacillary leprosy* (borderline-tuberculoid, tuberculoid, and indeterminate). The following regimens are widely used throughout the world (with minor local variations):

Multibacillary leprosy (3-drug regimen)

Rifampicin	600 mg once-monthly, supervised (450 mg for adults weighing less than 35 kg)
Dapsone	100 mg daily, self-administered (50 mg daily or 1–2 mg/kg daily for adults weighing less than 35 kg)
Clofazimine	300 mg once-monthly, supervised, *and* 50 mg daily (or 100 mg on alternate days), self-administered

Multibacillary leprosy should be treated for at least 2 years. Treatment should be continued unchanged during both type I (reversal) or type II (erythema nodosum leprosum) reactions. During reversal reactions neuritic pain or weakness can herald the rapid onset of permanent nerve damage. Treatment with prednisolone (initially 40–60 mg daily) should be instituted at once. Mild type II reactions may respond to aspirin. Severe type II reactions may require corticosteroids; thalidomide [unlicensed] is also useful in patients who have become corticosteroid dependent, but it should be used only under **specialist supervision**. Thalidomide is teratogenic and, therefore, contra-indicated in pregnancy; it must **not** be given to women of child-bearing potential unless they comply with a pregnancy prevention programme (see section 8.2.4). Increased doses of clofazimine 100 mg 3 times daily for the first month with subsequent reductions, are also useful but may take 4–6 weeks to attain full effect.

Paucibacillary leprosy (2-drug regimen)

| Rifampicin | 600 mg once-monthly, supervised (450 mg for those weighing less than 35 kg) |
| Dapsone | 100 mg daily, self-administered (50 mg daily or 1–2 mg/kg daily for adults weighing less than 35 kg) |

Paucibacillary leprosy should be treated for 6 months. If treatment is interrupted the regimen should be recommenced where it was left off to complete the full course.

Neither the multibacillary nor the paucibacillary antileprosy regimen is sufficient to treat tuberculosis.

◼ DAPSONE

Indications leprosy, dermatitis herpetiformis; *Pneumocystis jirovecii* (*Pneumocystis carinii*) pneumonia (section 5.4.8)

Cautions cardiac or pulmonary disease; anaemia (treat severe anaemia before starting); susceptibility to haemolysis including G6PD deficiency (section 9.1.5); avoid in acute porphyria (section 9.8.2); **interactions:** Appendix 1 (dapsone)

Blood disorders On long-term treatment, patients and their carers should be told how to recognise signs of blood disorders and advised to seek immediate medical attention if symptoms such as fever, sore throat, rash, mouth ulcers, purpura, bruising or bleeding develop

Pregnancy folic acid 5 mg daily should be given to mother throughout pregnancy; neonatal haemolysis and methaemoglobinaemia reported in third trimester

Breast-feeding haemolytic anaemia; although significant amount in milk, risk to infant very small unless infant is G6PD deficient

Side-effects (dose-related and uncommon at doses used for leprosy), haemolysis, methaemoglobinaemia, neuropathy, allergic dermatitis (rarely including toxic epidermal necrolysis and Stevens-Johnson syndrome), anorexia, nausea, vomiting, tachycardia, headache, insomnia, psychosis, hepatitis, agranulocytosis; dapsone syndrome (rash with fever and eosinophilia)—discontinue immediately (may progress to exfoliative dermatitis, hepatitis, hypoalbuminaemia, psychosis and death)

Dose
- Leprosy, 1–2 mg/kg daily, see notes above
- Dermatitis herpetiformis, see specialist literature

Dapsone (Non-proprietary) ℗ₒₘ [PoM]
Tablets, dapsone 50 mg, net price 28-tab pack = £49.29; 100 mg, 28-tab pack = £92.69 Label: 8

◼ CLOFAZIMINE

Indications leprosy

Cautions may discolour soft contact lenses; avoid if persistent abdominal pain and diarrhoea; **interactions:** Appendix 1 (clofazimine)

Hepatic impairment use with caution

Renal impairment use with caution

Pregnancy use with caution

Breast-feeding may alter colour of milk; skin discoloration of infant

Side-effects nausea, vomiting (hospitalise if persistent), abdominal pain; headache, tiredness; brownish-black discoloration of lesions and skin including areas exposed to light; reversible hair discoloration; dry skin; red discoloration of faeces, urine and other body fluids; also rash, pruritus, photosensitivity, acne-like eruptions, anorexia, eosinophilic enteropathy, bowel obstruction, dry eyes, dimmed vision, macular and subepithelial corneal pigmentation; elevation of blood sugar, weight loss, splenic infarction, lymphadenopathy

Dose
- Leprosy, see notes above
- Lepromatous lepra reactions, dosage increased to 300 mg daily for max. of 3 months

Clofazimine (Non-proprietary) [PoM]
Capsules, clofazimine 100 mg. Label: 8, 14, 21
Available on named-patient basis

5.1.11 Metronidazole and tinidazole

Metronidazole is an antimicrobial drug with high activity against anaerobic bacteria and protozoa; indications include trichomonal vaginitis (section 5.4.3), bacterial vaginosis (notably *Gardnerella vaginalis* infections), and *Entamoeba histolytica* and *Giardia lamblia* infections (section 5.4.2). It is also used for surgical and gynaecological sepsis in which its activity against colonic anaerobes, especially *Bacteroides fragilis*, is important. Metronidazole by the rectal route is an effective alternative to the intravenous route when oral administration is not possible. Intravenous metronidazole is used for the treatment of established cases of tetanus; diazepam (section 10.2.2) and tetanus immunoglobulin (section 14.5.2) are also used.

Metronidazole by mouth is effective for the treatment of *Clostridium difficile* infection , see also section 1.5; it can be given by intravenous infusion if oral treatment is inappropriate.

Topical metronidazole (section 13.10.1.2) reduces the odour produced by anaerobic bacteria in fungating tumours; it is also used in the management of rosacea (section 13.6).

Tinidazole is similar to metronidazole but has a longer duration of action.

Oral infections   Metronidazole is an alternative to a penicillin for the treatment of many oral infections where the patient is allergic to penicillin or the infection is due to beta-lactamase-producing anaerobes (Table 1, section 5.1). It is the drug of first choice for the treatment of acute necrotising ulcerative gingivitis (Vincent's infection) and pericoronitis; amoxicillin is a suitable alternative (section 5.1.1.3). For these purposes metronidazole in a dose of 200 mg 3 times daily for 3 days is sufficient, but the duration of treatment may need to be longer in pericoronitis. Tinidazole is licensed for the treatment of acute ulcerative gingivitis.

METRONIDAZOLE

Indications   anaerobic infections (including dental), see under Dose below; protozoal infections (section 5.4.2); *Helicobacter pylori* eradication (section 1.3); fistulating Crohn's disease (section 1.5); skin (section 13.10.1.2)

Cautions   disulfiram-like reaction with alcohol; clinical and laboratory monitoring advised if treatment exceeds 10 days; **interactions:** Appendix 1 (metronidazole)

Hepatic impairment   in severe liver disease reduce total daily dose to one-third, and give once daily; use with caution in hepatic encephalopathy

Pregnancy   manufacturer advises avoidance of high-dose regimens

Breast-feeding   significant amount in milk; manufacturer advises avoid large single doses

Side-effects   gastro-intestinal disturbances (including nausea and vomiting), taste disturbances, furred tongue, oral mucositis, anorexia; *very rarely* hepatitis, jaundice, pancreatitis, drowsiness, dizziness, headache, ataxia, psychotic disorders, darkening of urine, thrombocytopenia, pancytopenia, myalgia, arthralgia, visual disturbances, rash, pruritus, and erythema multiforme; on prolonged or intensive therapy peripheral neuropathy, transient epileptiform seizures, and leucopenia; also reported aseptic meningitis, optic neuropathy

Dose

- Anaerobic infections (usually treated for 7 days and for 10–14 days in *Clostridium difficile* infection), by mouth, *either* 400 mg every 8 hours *or* 500 mg every 8 hours, CHILD 1–2 months 7.5 mg/kg every 12 hours, 2 months–12 years 7.5 mg/kg (max. 400 mg) every 8 hours; by rectum, 1 g every 8 hours for 3 days, then 1 g

every 12 hours, CHILD every 8 hours for 3 days, then every 12 hours, 1 month–1 year 125 mg, 1–5 years 250 mg, 5–10 years 500 mg, over 10 years, adult dose; by intravenous infusion over 20 minutes, 500 mg every 8 hours; CHILD under 18 years see *BNF for Children*
- Leg ulcers and pressure sores, by mouth, 400 mg every 8 hours for 7 days
- Bacterial vaginosis, by mouth, 400–500 mg twice daily for 5–7 days *or* 2 g as a single dose
- Pelvic inflammatory disease (see also Table 1, section 5.1), by mouth, 400 mg twice daily for 14 days; CHILD 12–18 years see *BNF for Children*
- Acute ulcerative gingivitis, by mouth, 200–250 mg every 8 hours for 3 days; CHILD 1–3 years 50 mg every 8 hours for 3 days; 3–7 years 100 mg every 12 hours; 7–10 years 100 mg every 8 hours
- Acute oral infections, by mouth, 200 mg every 8 hours for 3–7 days (see also notes above); CHILD 1–3 years 50 mg every 8 hours for 3–7 days; 3–7 years 100 mg every 12 hours; 7–10 years 100 mg every 8 hours
- Surgical prophylaxis, by mouth, 400–500 mg 2 hours before surgery; up to 3 further doses of 400–500 mg may be given every 8 hours for high-risk procedures; CHILD 1 month–18 years see *BNF for Children*
  By rectum, 1 g 2 hours before surgery; up to 3 further doses of 1 g may be given every 8 hours for high-risk procedures; CHILD 5–18 years see *BNF for Children*
  By intravenous infusion (if rectal administration inappropriate), 500 mg up to 30 minutes before the procedure; up to 3 further doses of 500 mg may be given every 8 hours for high-risk procedures; CHILD under 18 years see *BNF for Children*

Note Metronidazole doses in BNF may differ from those in product literature

Metronidazole (Non-proprietary) ᴾᵒᴹ
Tablets, metronidazole 200 mg, net price 21-tab pack = £9.17; 400 mg, 21-tab pack = £1.34. Label: 4, 9, 21, 25, 27
Brands include *Vaginyl®*
Dental prescribing on NHS Metronidazole Tablets may be prescribed

Tablets, metronidazole 500 mg, net price 21-tab pack = £37.82. Label: 4, 9, 21, 25, 27
Dental prescribing on NHS Metronidazole Tablets may be prescribed

Suspension, metronidazole (as benzoate) 200 mg/5 mL. Net price 100 mL = £32.35. Label: 4, 9
Brands include *Norzol®*
Dental prescribing on NHS Metronidazole Oral Suspension may be prescribed

Intravenous infusion, metronidazole 5 mg/mL. Net price 20-mL amp = £1.56, 100-mL container = £3.10

Flagyl® (Zentiva) ᴾᵒᴹ
Tablets, both f/c, ivory, metronidazole 200 mg, net price 21-tab pack = £4.49; 400 mg, 14-tab pack = £6.34. Label: 4, 9, 21, 25, 27
Suppositories, metronidazole 500 mg, net price 10 = £15.18; 1 g, 10 = £23.06. Label: 4, 9

Metrolyl® (Sandoz) ᴾᵒᴹ
Intravenous infusion, metronidazole 5 mg/mL, net price 100-mL Steriflex® bag = £1.22
Electrolytes Na⁺ 14.53 mmol/100-mL bag
Suppositories, metronidazole 500 mg, net price 10 = £12.34; 1 g, 10 = £18.34. Label: 4, 9

5

Infections

TINIDAZOLE

Indications anaerobic infections, see under Dose below; protozoal infections (section 5.4.2); *Helicobacter pylori* eradication (section 1.3)

Cautions see under Metronidazole; avoid in acute porphyria (section 9.8.2); **interactions:** Appendix 1 (tinidazole)

Pregnancy manufacturer advises avoid in first trimester

Breast-feeding present in milk—manufacturer advises avoid breast-feeding during and for 3 days after stopping treatment

Side-effects see under Metronidazole

Dose
- Anaerobic infections, 2 g initially, followed by 1 g daily *or* 500 mg twice daily, usually for 5–6 days
- Bacterial vaginosis and acute ulcerative gingivitis, a single 2-g dose
- Abdominal surgery prophylaxis, a single 2-g dose approximately 12 hours before surgery

Fasigyn® (Pfizer) PoM
Tablets, f/c, tinidazole 500 mg. Net price 16-tab pack = £11.04. Label: 4, 9, 21, 25

5.1.12 Quinolones

Nalidixic acid and **norfloxacin** are effective in uncomplicated urinary-tract infections (section 5.1.13).

Ciprofloxacin is active against both Gram-positive and Gram-negative bacteria. It is particularly active against Gram-negative bacteria, including salmonella, shigella, campylobacter, neisseria, and pseudomonas. Ciprofloxacin has only moderate activity against Gram-positive bacteria such as *Streptococcus pneumoniae* and *Enterococcus faecalis*; it should not be used for pneumococcal pneumonia. It is active against chlamydia and some mycobacteria. Most anaerobic organisms are not susceptible. Ciprofloxacin can be used for respiratory tract infections (but not for pneumococcal pneumonia), urinary-tract infections (section 5.1.13), infections of the gastro-intestinal system (including typhoid fever), bone and joint infections, gonorrhoea and septicaemia caused by sensitive organisms.

Ofloxacin is used for urinary-tract infections (section 5.1.13), lower respiratory-tract infections, gonorrhoea, and non-gonococcal urethritis and cervicitis.

Levofloxacin is active against Gram-positive and Gram-negative organisms. It has greater activity against pneumococci than ciprofloxacin. Levofloxacin is licensed for the treatment of acute sinusitis, acute exacerbations of chronic bronchitis, and community-acquired pneumonia, but it should only be considered for these infections when first-line treatment cannot be used or is ineffective. Levofloxacin is also licensed for the treatment of urinary-tract infections (section 5.1.13).

Although ciprofloxacin, levofloxacin, moxifloxacin, and ofloxacin are licensed for skin and soft-tissue infections, many staphylococci are resistant to the quinolones and their use should be avoided in MRSA infections.

Moxifloxacin should be reserved for the treatment of sinusitis, community-acquired pneumonia, exacerbations of chronic bronchitis, mild to moderate pelvic inflammatory disease, or complicated skin and soft-tissue infections which have failed to respond to other antibacterials or for patients who cannot be treated with other antibacterials. It has been associated with QT interval prolongation and life-threatening hepatotoxicity. Moxifloxacin is active against Gram-positive and Gram-negative organisms. It has greater activity against Gram-positive organisms, including pneumococci, than ciprofloxacin. Moxifloxacin is not active against *Pseudomonas aeruginosa* or meticillin-resistant *Staphylococcus aureus* (MRSA).

Anthrax *Inhalation* or *gastro-intestinal anthrax* should be treated initially with either **ciprofloxacin** [not licensed for gastro-intestinal anthrax] or **doxycycline** [unlicensed indication] (section 5.1.3) combined with one or two other antibacterials (such as amoxicillin, benzylpenicillin, chloramphenicol, clarithromycin, clindamycin, imipenem with cilastatin, rifampicin [unlicensed indication], and vancomycin). When the condition improves and the sensitivity of the *Bacillus anthracis* strain is known, treatment may be switched to a single antibacterial. Treatment should continue for 60 days because germination may be delayed.

Cutaneous anthrax should be treated with either ciprofloxacin [unlicensed indication] or doxycycline [unlicensed indication] (section 5.1.3) for 7 days. Treatment may be switched to amoxicillin (section 5.1.1.3) if the infecting strain is susceptible. Treatment may need to be extended to 60 days if exposure is due to aerosol. A combination of antibacterials for 14 days is recommended for cutaneous anthrax with systemic features, extensive oedema, or lesions of the head or neck.

Ciprofloxacin or doxycycline may be given for *post-exposure prophylaxis*. If exposure is confirmed, antibacterial prophylaxis should continue for 60 days. Antibacterial prophylaxis may be switched to amoxicillin after 10–14 days if the strain of *B. anthracis* is susceptible. Vaccination against anthrax (section 14.4) may allow the duration of antibacterial prophylaxis to be shortened.

Cautions Quinolones should be used with caution in patients with a history of epilepsy or conditions that predispose to seizures, in G6PD deficiency (section 9.1.5), myasthenia gravis (risk of exacerbation), and in children or adolescents (arthropathy has developed in weight-bearing joints in young *animals*—see below). Exposure to excessive sunlight should be avoided (discontinue if photosensitivity occurs). Quinolones can prolong the QT interval. Moxifloxacin is contra-indicated in patients with risk factors for QT interval prolongation (e.g. electrolyte disturbances, acute myocardial infarction, heart failure with reduced left ventricular ejection fraction, bradycardia, congenital long QT syndrome, concomitant use with other drugs known to prolong the QT interval, history of symptomatic arrhythmias) and the other quinolones should be used with caution in these patients. The CSM has warned that quinolones may induce **convulsions** in patients with or without a history of convulsions; taking NSAIDs at the same time may also induce them. Other **interactions:** Appendix 1 (quinolones).

Use in children Quinolones cause arthropathy in the weight-bearing joints of immature *animals* and are therefore generally not recommended in children and growing adolescents. However, the significance of this effect in humans is uncertain and in some specific circumstances short-term use of either ciprofloxacin or nalidixic acid may be justified in children. For further details see *BNF for Children*.

> ### Tendon damage
>
> Tendon damage (including rupture) has been reported rarely in patients receiving quinolones. Tendon rupture may occur within 48 hours of starting treatment; cases have also been reported several months after stopping a quinolone. Healthcare professionals are reminded that:
>
> - quinolones are contra-indicated in patients with a history of tendon disorders related to quinolone use;
> - patients over 60 years of age are more prone to tendon damage;
> - the risk of tendon damage is increased by the concomitant use of corticosteroids;
> - if tendinitis is suspected, the quinolone should be discontinued immediately.

Contra-indications   quinolone hypersensitivity. See also Cautions above.

Pregnancy   Quinolones should be avoided in pregnancy because they have been shown to cause arthropathy in *animal* studies; safer alternatives are available; however, a single dose of ciprofloxacin may be used for the prevention of a secondary case of meningococcal meningitis

Side-effects   Side-effects of the quinolones include nausea, vomiting, diarrhoea (rarely antibiotic-associated colitis), headache, and dizziness. Less frequent side-effects include dyspepsia, abdominal pain, anorexia, sleep disturbances, asthenia, confusion, anxiety, depression, hallucinations, tremor, blood disorders (including eosinophilia, leucopenia, thrombocytopenia), arthralgia, myalgia, rash (very rarely Stevens-Johnson syndrome and toxic epidermal necrolysis), disturbances in vision and taste. Other side-effects reported rarely or very rarely include hepatic dysfunction (including jaundice and hepatitis), hypotension, vasculitis, dyspnoea (more frequent with levofloxacin and moxifloxacin), convulsions, psychoses, symptoms of peripheral neuropathy (sometimes irreversible), renal failure, interstitial nephritis, tendon inflammation and damage (see also Tendon Damage above), photosensitivity, disturbances in hearing and smell. The drug should be **discontinued** if psychiatric, neurological or hypersensitivity reactions (including severe rash) occur.

▐ CIPROFLOXACIN

Indications   see notes above and under Dose; fistulating Crohn's disease (section 1.5); eye infections (section 11.3.1)

Cautions   see notes above; avoid excessive alkalinity of urine and ensure adequate fluid intake (risk of crystalluria); **interactions:** Appendix 1 (quinolones)
Driving May impair performance of skilled tasks (e.g. driving); effects enhanced by alcohol

Contra-indications   see notes above

Renal impairment   by mouth, 250–500 mg every 12 hours if eGFR 30–60 mL/minute/1.73 m^2 (every 24 hours if eGFR less than 30 mL/minute/1.73 m^2); by intravenous infusion (200 mg over 30 minutes), 200–400 mg every 12 hours if eGFR 30–60 mL/minute/1.73 m^2 (every 24 hours if eGFR less than 30 mL/minute/1.73 m^2)

Pregnancy   see notes above

Breast-feeding   amount too small to be harmful but manufacturer advises avoid

Side-effects   see notes above; also flatulence, pain and phlebitis at injection site; *rarely* dysphagia, pancreatitis, chest pain, tachycardia, syncope, oedema, hot flushes, abnormal dreams, sweating, hyperglycaemia, hypoglycaemia, and erythema nodosum; *very rarely* movement disorders, tinnitus, intracranial hypertension, and tenosynovitis; *also reported* peripheral neuropathy and polyneuropathy

Dose

- By mouth, respiratory-tract infections, 500–750 mg twice daily (750 mg twice daily in pseudomonal lower respiratory-tract infection in cystic fibrosis)

  Urinary-tract infections, 250–750 mg twice daily (250 mg twice daily for 3 days usually adequate for acute uncomplicated cystitis in women)

  Acute or chronic prostatitis, 500 mg twice daily for 28 days

  Gonorrhoea (see also Table 1, section 5.1), 500 mg as a single dose

  Most other infections, 500 mg twice daily (increased to 750 mg twice daily in severe or deep-seated infection)

  Surgical prophylaxis [unlicensed], 750 mg 60 minutes before procedure

  Prophylaxis of meningococcal meningitis, Table 2, section 5.1

- By intravenous infusion over 60 minutes, 400 mg every 8–12 hours

- Anthrax (treatment and post-exposure prophylaxis, see notes above), by mouth, 500 mg twice daily

  By intravenous infusion over 60 minutes, 400 mg every 12 hours

- CHILD under 18 years see *BNF for Children*

Ciprofloxacin (Non-proprietary) PoM
Tablets, ciprofloxacin (as hydrochloride) 100 mg, net price 6-tab pack = £1.41; 250 mg, 10-tab pack = 92p, 20-tab pack = £1.48; 500 mg, 10-tab pack = £1.10, 20-tab pack = £1.47; 750 mg, 10-tab pack = £8.00. Label: 7, 9, 25, counselling, driving

Intravenous infusion, ciprofloxacin (as lactate) 2 mg/mL, net price 50-mL bottle = £7.57, 100-mL bottle = £14.49, 200-mL bottle = £19.79

Ciproxin® (Bayer) PoM
Tablets, all f/c, ciprofloxacin (as hydrochloride) 250 mg (scored), net price 10-tab pack = £6.59; 500 mg (scored), 10-tab pack = £12.49; 750 mg, 10-tab pack = £17.78. Label: 7, 9, 25, counselling, driving

Suspension, strawberry-flavoured, ciprofloxacin for reconstitution with diluent provided, 250 mg/5 mL, net price 100 mL = £19.80. Label: 7, 9, 25, counselling, driving

Intravenous infusion, ciprofloxacin (as lactate) 2 mg/mL, in sodium chloride 0.9%, net price 50-mL bottle = £7.61, 100-mL bottle = £15.01, 200-mL bottle = £22.85
Electrolytes Na$^+$ 15.4 mmol/100-mL bottle

▐ LEVOFLOXACIN

Indications   see notes above and under Dose

Cautions   see notes above; history of psychiatric illness; **interactions:** Appendix 1 (quinolones)
Driving May impair performance of skilled tasks (e.g. driving)

Contra-indications   see notes above

Renal impairment   usual initial dose then use half normal dose if eGFR 20–50 mL/minute/1.73 m^2;

5 Infections

consult product literature if eGFR less than 20 mL/minute/1.73 m^2

Pregnancy see notes above

Breast-feeding manufacturer advises avoid

Side-effects see notes above; also flatulence, constipation, hyperhidrosis; *rarely* tachycardia, palpitation, abnormal dreams, tinnitus, hypoglycaemia; also reported potentially life-threatening hepatic failure, syncope, benign intracranial hypertension, pneumonitis, peripheral neuropathy, extrapyramidal symptoms, hyperglycaemia, rhabdomyolysis, stomatitis; local reactions and transient hypotension reported with infusion

Dose

- By mouth, acute sinusitis, 500 mg once daily for 10–14 days

  Acute exacerbation of chronic bronchitis, 500 mg once daily for 7–10 days

  Community-acquired pneumonia, 500 mg once or twice daily for 7–14 days

  Urinary-tract infections, 500 mg once daily for 7–14 days (250 mg once daily for 3 days in uncomplicated infection)

  Chronic prostatitis, 500 mg once daily for 28 days

  Complicated skin and soft tissue infections, 500 mg once or twice daily for 7–14 days

  Inhalation anthrax (treatment and post-exposure prophylaxis), 500 mg once daily for 8 weeks

- By intravenous infusion (over at least 60 minutes for 500 mg), community-acquired pneumonia, 500 mg once or twice daily

  Complicated urinary-tract infections, chronic prostatitis, 500 mg once daily

  Complicated skin and soft tissue infections, 500 mg once or twice daily

  Inhalation anthrax (treatment and post-exposure prophylaxis), 500 mg once daily

Levofloxacin (Non-proprietary) ℗ₒ𝖬

Tablets, levofloxacin 250 mg, net price 5-tab pack = £5.00, 10-tab pack = £10.68; 500 mg, 5-tab pack = £7.80, 10-tab pack = £16.22. Label: 6, 9, 25, counselling, driving

Brands include *Evoxil*®

Intravenous infusion, levofloxacin 5 mg/mL, net price 100-mL bottle = £25.00, 100-mL infusion bag = £23.75

Tavanic® (Sanofi-Aventis) ℗ₒ𝖬

Tablets, yellow-red, f/c, scored, levofloxacin 250 mg, net price 5-tab pack = £7.23, 10-tab pack = £14.45; 500 mg, 5-tab pack = £12.93, 10-tab pack = £25.85. Label: 6, 9, 25, counselling, driving

Intravenous infusion, levofloxacin 5 mg/mL, net price 100-mL bottle = £26.40

Electrolytes Na$^+$ 15.8 mmol/100-mL bottle

▌ MOXIFLOXACIN

Indications sinusitis, community-acquired pneumonia, exacerbations of chronic bronchitis, mild to moderate pelvic inflammatory disease, or complicated skin and soft-tissue infections which have failed to respond to other antibacterials or for patients who cannot be treated with other antibacterials

Cautions see notes above; **interactions**: Appendix 1 (quinolones)

Driving May impair performance of skilled tasks (e.g. driving)

Contra-indications see notes above

Hepatic impairment manufacturer advises avoid in severe impairment

Pregnancy see notes above

Breast-feeding manufacturer advises avoid—present in milk in *animal* studies

Side-effects see notes above; also gastritis, flatulence, constipation, arrhythmias, palpitation, angina, vasodilatation, hyperlipidaemia, sweating; *rarely* oedema, hypertension, syncope, dysphagia, abnormal dreams, incoordination, amnesia, peripheral neuropathy, hyperglycaemia, hyperuricaemia, myopathy, stomatitis; *very rarely* rhabdomyolysis, potentially life-threatening hepatic failure; *on intravenous infusion*, pain and phlebitis at injection site

Dose

- By mouth, 400 mg once daily
- By intravenous infusion over 60 minutes, community-acquired pneumonia, complicated skin and soft-tissue infections, 400 mg once daily

Note Recommended duration of treatment is 7–14 days for community-acquired pneumonia, 5–10 days in exacerbations of chronic bronchitis, 7 days in sinusitis, 14 days in pelvic inflammatory disease, 7–21 days for complicated skin and soft-tissue infections

Avelox® (Bayer) ℗ₒ𝖬

Tablets, red, f/c, moxifloxacin (as hydrochloride) 400 mg, net price 5-tab pack = £12.43. Label: 6, 9, counselling, driving

Intravenous infusion, moxifloxacin (as hydrochloride) 1.6 mg/mL, net price 250-mL bottle (400 mg) = £39.95

Electrolytes Na$^+$ 34 mmol/250-mL bottle

▌ NALIDIXIC ACID

Indications urinary-tract infections

Cautions see notes above; avoid in acute porphyria (section 9.8.2); false positive urinary glucose (if tested for reducing substances); monitor blood counts, renal and liver function if treatment exceeds 2 weeks; **interactions**: Appendix 1 (quinolones)

Contra-indications see notes above

Hepatic impairment manufacturer advises caution in liver disease

Renal impairment use with caution; avoid if eGFR less than 20 mL/minute/1.73 m^2

Pregnancy see notes above

Breast-feeding risk to infant very small but one case of haemolytic anaemia reported

Side-effects see notes above; also reported toxic psychosis, increased intracranial pressure, cranial nerve palsy, peripheral neuropathy, and metabolic acidosis

Dose

- 900 mg every 6 hours for 7 days, reduced in chronic infections to 600 mg every 6 hours; CHILD 3 months–18 years see *BNF for Children*

Nalidixic Acid (Rosemont) ℗ₒ𝖬

Suspension, pink, nalidixic acid 300 mg/5 mL, net price 150 mL (raspberry- and strawberry-flavoured) = £17.00. Label: 9, 11

Excipients include sucrose 450 mg/5 mL

▌ NORFLOXACIN

Indications see under Dose

Cautions see notes above; **interactions**: Appendix 1 (quinolones)

Driving May impair performance of skilled tasks (e.g. driving)

Contra-indications see notes above

Renal impairment use 400 mg once daily if eGFR less than 30 mL/minute/1.73 m^2

Pregnancy see notes above

Breast-feeding no information available—manufacturer advises avoid

Side-effects see notes above; also tinnitus, epiphora; *rarely* pancreatitis; *very rarely* arrhythmias; also reported, polyneuropathy and exfoliative dermatitis

Dose

- 'Lower' urinary-tract infections, 400 mg twice daily for 7–10 days (for 3 days for uncomplicated infections in women)
- Chronic relapsing 'lower' urinary-tract infections, 400 mg twice daily for up to 12 weeks; may be reduced to 400 mg once daily if adequate suppression within first 4 weeks
- Chronic prostatitis, 400 mg twice daily for 28 days

Norfloxacin (Non-proprietary) PoM

Tablets, norfloxacin 400 mg, net price 6-tab pack = £5.40, 14-tab pack = £12.00. Label: 7, 9, 23, counselling, driving

---

■ OFLOXACIN

Indications see under Dose

Cautions see notes above; history of psychiatric illness; **interactions**: Appendix 1 (quinolones)

Driving May affect performance of skilled tasks (e.g. driving); effects enhanced by alcohol

Contra-indications see notes above

Hepatic impairment use with caution; elimination may be reduced in severe impairment

Renal impairment usual initial dose, then use half normal dose if eGFR 20–50 mL/minute/1.73 m^2; 100 mg every 24 hours if eGFR less than 20 mL/minute/1.73 m^2

Pregnancy see notes above

Breast-feeding amount probably too small to be harmful but manufacturer advises avoid

Side-effects see notes above; also cough, nasopharyngitis, eye irritation; *rarely* arrhythmias, bronchospasm, abnormal dreams, hot flushes, hyperhidrosis; *very rarely* neuropathy, extrapyramidal symptoms, tinnitus; also reported pneumonitis, changes in blood sugar, myopathy, rhabdomyolysis; on intravenous infusion, hypotension and local reactions (including thrombophlebitis)

Dose

- By mouth, urinary-tract infections, 200–400 mg daily preferably in the morning, increased if necessary in upper urinary-tract infections to 400 mg twice daily

  Acute or chronic prostatitis, 200 mg twice daily for 28 days

  Lower respiratory-tract infections, 400 mg daily preferably in the morning, increased if necessary to 400 mg twice daily

  Skin and soft-tissue infections, 400 mg twice daily

  Uncomplicated gonorrhoea, 400 mg as a single dose

  Uncomplicated genital chlamydial infection, nongonococcal urethritis, 400 mg daily in single or divided doses for 7 days

  Pelvic inflammatory disease (see also section 5.1, table 1), 400 mg twice daily for 14 days

- By intravenous infusion (over at least 30 minutes for each 200 mg), complicated urinary-tract infection, 200 mg daily

Lower respiratory-tract infection, 200 mg twice daily

Septicaemia, 200 mg twice daily

Skin and soft-tissue infections, 400 mg twice daily

Severe or complicated infections, dose may be increased to 400 mg twice daily

Ofloxacin (Non-proprietary) PoM

Tablets, ofloxacin 200 mg, net price 10-tab pack = £4.75; 400 mg, 5-tab pack = £10.82, 10-tab pack = £4.59. Label: 6, 9, 11, counselling, driving

Tarivid® (Sanofi-Aventis) PoM

Tablets, f/c, scored, ofloxacin 200 mg, net price 10-tab pack = £7.53, 20-tab pack = £15.05; 400 mg (yellow), 10-tab pack = £7.52, 10-tab pack = £14.99. Label: 6, 9, 11, counselling, driving

Intravenous infusion, ofloxacin (as hydrochloride) 2 mg/mL, net price 100-mL bottle = £16.16 (hosp. only)

5.1.13 Urinary-tract infections

Urinary-tract infection is more common in women than in men; when it occurs in men there is frequently an underlying abnormality of the renal tract. Recurrent episodes of infection are an indication for radiological investigation especially in children in whom untreated pyelonephritis may lead to permanent kidney damage.

Escherichia coli is the most common cause of urinary-tract infection; *Staphylococcus saprophyticus* is also common in sexually active young women. Less common causes include Proteus and Klebsiella spp. *Pseudomonas aeruginosa* infections usually occur in the hospital setting and may be associated with functional or anatomical abnormalities of the renal tract. *Staphylococcus epidermidis* and *Enterococcus faecalis* infection may complicate catheterisation or instrumentation.

A specimen of urine should be collected for culture and sensitivity testing before starting antibacterial therapy;

- in men;
- in pregnant women;
- in children under 3 years of age;
- in patients with suspected upper urinary-tract infection, complicated infection, or recurrent infection;
- if resistant organisms are suspected;
- if urine dipstick testing gives a single positive result for leucocyte esterase or nitrite;
- if clinical symptoms are not consistent with results of dipstick testing.

Treatment should not be delayed while waiting for results. The antibacterial chosen should reflect current local bacterial sensitivity to antibacterials.

Uncomplicated lower urinary-tract infections often respond to trimethoprim, nitrofurantoin, or amoxicillin given for 7 days (3 days may be adequate for infections in women; see also Table 1, section 5.1); those caused by fully sensitive bacteria respond to two 3-g doses of amoxicillin (section 5.1.1.3). Widespread bacterial resistance to ampicillin, amoxicillin, and trimethoprim has been reported. Alternatives for resistant organisms include co-amoxiclav (amoxicillin with clavulanic acid), an oral cephalosporin, nitrofurantoin, pivmecillinam, or a quinolone.

Fosfomycin [unlicensed] (section 5.1.7) can be used, on the advice of a microbiologist, for the treatment of uncomplicated lower urinary-tract infections caused

5 Infections

by multiple-antibacterial resistant organisms when other antibacterials cannot be used.

Long-term low dose therapy may be required in selected patients to prevent *recurrence of infection*; indications include frequent relapses and significant kidney damage. Trimethoprim, nitrofurantoin and cefalexin have been recommended for long-term therapy.

Methenamine (hexamine) should **not** generally be used because it requires an acidic urine for its antimicrobial activity and it is ineffective for upper urinary-tract infections; it may, however, have a role in the prophylaxis and treatment of chronic or recurrent uncomplicated lower urinary-tract infections.

Acute pyelonephritis can lead to septicaemia and is treated initially by injection of a broad-spectrum antibacterial such as cefuroxime or a quinolone if the patient is severely ill; gentamicin can also be used.

Prostatitis can be difficult to cure and requires treatment for several weeks with an antibacterial which penetrates prostatic tissue such as trimethoprim, or some quinolones.

Where infection is localised and associated with an indwelling *catheter* a bladder instillation is often effective (section 7.4.4).

Pregnancy   Urinary-tract infection in pregnancy may be asymptomatic and requires prompt treatment to prevent progression to acute pyelonephritis. Penicillins and cephalosporins are suitable for treating urinary-tract infection during pregnancy. Nitrofurantoin may also be used but it should be avoided at term. Sulfonamides and quinolones should be avoided during pregnancy; trimethoprim should also preferably be avoided particularly in the first trimester.

Renal impairment   In renal failure antibacterials normally excreted by the kidney accumulate with resultant toxicity unless the dose is reduced. This applies especially to the aminoglycosides which should be used with great caution; tetracyclines, methenamine, and nitrofurantoin should be avoided altogether.

Children   Urinary-tract infections in children require prompt antibacterial treatment to minimise the risk of renal scarring. Uncomplicated 'lower' urinary-tract infections in *children over 3 months of age* can be treated with trimethoprim, nitrofurantoin, a first generation cephalosporin (e.g. cefalexin), or amoxicillin for 3 days; children should be reassessed if they continue to be unwell 24–48 hours after the initial assessment. Amoxicillin should only be used if the organism causing the infection is sensitive to it.

Acute pyelonephritis in children over 3 months of age can be treated with a first generation cephalosporin or co-amoxiclav for 7–10 days. If the patient is severely ill, then the infection is best treated initially by injection of a broad-spectrum antibacterial such as cefotaxime or co-amoxiclav; gentamicin is an alternative.

Children under 3 months of age should be transferred to hospital and treated initially with intravenous antibacterial drugs such as ampicillin with gentamicin, or cefotaxime alone, until the infection responds; full doses of oral antibacterials are then given for a further period.

Recurrent episodes of infection are an indication for imaging tests. *Antibacterial prophylaxis* with low doses of trimethoprim or nitrofurantoin may be considered for children with recurrent infection, significant urinary-tract anomalies, or significant kidney damage.

NITROFURANTOIN

Indications   urinary-tract infections

Cautions   anaemia; diabetes mellitus; electrolyte imbalance; vitamin B and folate deficiency; pulmonary disease; on long-term therapy, monitor liver function and monitor for pulmonary symptoms, especially in the elderly (discontinue if deterioration in lung function); susceptibility to peripheral neuropathy; false positive urinary glucose (if tested for reducing substances); urine may be coloured yellow or brown; **interactions**: Appendix 1 (nitrofurantoin)

Contra-indications   infants less than 3 months old, G6PD deficiency (section 9.1.5); acute porphyria (section 9.8.2)

Hepatic impairment   use with caution; cholestatic jaundice and chronic active hepatitis reported

Renal impairment   avoid if eGFR less than 45 mL/minute/1.73 m^2; may be used with caution if eGFR 30–44 mL/minute/1.73 m^2 as a short-course only (3 to 7 days), to treat uncomplicated lower urinary-tract infection caused by suspected or proven multidrug resistant bacteria and only if potential benefit outweighs risk; risk of peripheral neuropathy; antibacterial efficacy depends on renal secretion of the drug into the urinary tract

Pregnancy   avoid at term—may produce neonatal haemolysis

Breast-feeding   avoid; only small amounts in milk but could be enough to produce haemolysis in G6PD-deficient infants (section 9.1.5)

Side-effects   anorexia, nausea, vomiting, and diarrhoea; acute and chronic pulmonary reactions (pulmonary fibrosis reported; possible association with lupus erythematosus-like syndrome); peripheral neuropathy; also reported, hypersensitivity reactions (including angioedema, anaphylaxis, sialadenitis, urticaria, rash and pruritus); rarely, cholestatic jaundice, hepatitis, exfoliative dermatitis, erythema multiforme, pancreatitis, arthralgia, blood disorders (including agranulocytosis, thrombocytopenia, and aplastic anaemia), benign intracranial hypertension, and transient alopecia

Dose

- Acute uncomplicated infection, 50 mg every 6 hours with food for 7 days (3 days usually adequate in women); CHILD over 3 months, 750 micrograms/kg every 6 hours

- Severe chronic recurrent infection, 100 mg every 6 hours with food for 7 days (dose reduced or discontinued if severe nausea)

- Prophylaxis (but see Cautions), 50–100 mg at night; CHILD over 3 months, 1 mg/kg at night

Nitrofurantoin (Non-proprietary) PoM
Tablets, nitrofurantoin 50 mg, net price 28-tab pack = £20.63; 100 mg, 28-tab pack = £11.03. Label: 9, 14, 21
Oral suspension, nitrofurantoin 25 mg/5 mL, net price 300 mL = £195.83. Label: 9, 14, 21
Note Sugar-free versions are available and can be ordered by specifying 'sugar-free' on the prescription

◢**Modified release**

Macrobid® (AMCo) PoM
Capsules, m/r, blue/yellow, nitrofurantoin 100 mg (as nitrofurantoin macrocrystals and nitrofurantoin monohydrate), net price 14-cap pack = £9.50. Label: 9, 14, 21, 25
Dose uncomplicated urinary-tract infection, 1 capsule twice daily with food
Genito-urinary surgical prophylaxis, 1 capsule twice daily on day of procedure and for 3 days after

5 Infections

METHENAMINE HIPPURATE ◢
(Hexamine hippurate)

Indications   prophylaxis and long-term treatment of chronic or recurrent lower urinary-tract infections

Cautions   avoid concurrent administration with sulfonamides (risk of crystalluria) or urinary alkalinising agents; **interactions:** Appendix 1 (methenamine)

Contra-indications   severe dehydration, gout, metabolic acidosis

Hepatic impairment   avoid

Renal impairment   avoid if eGFR less than 10 mL/minute/1.73 m^2—risk of hippurate crystalluria

Pregnancy   use with caution

Breast-feeding   amount too small to be harmful

Side-effects   gastro-intestinal disturbances, bladder irritation, rash

Dose
- 1 g every 12 hours (may be increased in patients with catheters to 1 g every 8 hours); CHILD 6–12 years 500 mg every 12 hours

Hiprex® (Meda)
Tablets, scored, methenamine hippurate 1 g, net price 60-tab pack = £19.74. Label: 9

5.2 Antifungal drugs

5.2.1   Triazole antifungals

5.2.2   Imidazole antifungals

5.2.3   Polyene antifungals

5.2.4   Echinocandin antifungals

5.2.5   Other antifungals

Treatment of fungal infections

The systemic treatment of common fungal infections is outlined below; specialist treatment is required in most forms of systemic or disseminated fungal infections. For local treatment of fungal infections, see section 7.2.2 (genital), section 7.4.4 (bladder), section 11.3.2 (eye), section 12.1.1 (ear), section 12.3.2 (oropharynx), and section 13.10.2 (skin).

Aspergillosis   Aspergillosis most commonly affects the respiratory tract but in severely immunocompromised patients, invasive forms can affect the heart, brain, and skin. **Voriconazole** (section 5.2.1) is the treatment of choice for aspergillosis; **liposomal amphotericin** (section 5.2.3) is an alternative first-line treatment when voriconazole cannot be used. **Caspofungin** (section 5.2.4), **itraconazole** (section 5.2.1), or **posaconazole** (section 5.2.1) can be used in patients who are refractory to, or intolerant of voriconazole and liposomal amphotericin. Itraconazole is also used for the treatment of chronic pulmonary aspergillosis or as an adjunct in the treatment of allergic bronchopulmonary aspergillosis [unlicensed indication].

Candidiasis   Many superficial candidal infections including infections of the skin (section 13.10.2) are treated locally; widespread or intractable infection requires systemic antifungal treatment. Vaginal candidiasis (section 7.2.2) may be treated with locally acting antifungals or with **fluconazole** (section 5.2.1) given by mouth; for resistant organisms, **itraconazole** (section 5.2.1) can be given by mouth.

Oropharyngeal candidiasis generally responds to topical therapy (section 12.3.2); fluconazole is given by mouth for unresponsive infections; it is effective and is reliably absorbed. Itraconazole may be used for infections that do not respond to fluconazole. Topical therapy may not be adequate in immunocompromised patients and an oral triazole antifungal is preferred.

For *invasive or disseminated candidiasis*, an **echinocandin** (section 5.2.4) can be used. **Fluconazole** (section 5.2.1) is an alternative for *Candida albicans* infection in clinically stable patients who have not received an azole antifungal recently. **Amphotericin** (section 5.2.3) is an alternative when an echinocandin or fluconazole cannot be used, however, amphotericin should be considered for the initial treatment of CNS candidiasis. **Voriconazole** (section 5.2.1) can be used for infections caused by fluconazole-resistant *Candida* spp. when oral therapy is required, or in patients intolerant of amphotericin or an echinocandin. In refractory cases, **flucytosine** (section 5.2.5) can be used with intravenous amphotericin.

Cryptococcosis   Cryptococcosis is uncommon but infection in the immunocompromised, especially in HIV-positive patients, can be life-threatening; cryptococcal meningitis is the most common form of fungal meningitis. The treatment of choice in cryptococcal meningitis is **amphotericin** (section 5.2.3) by intravenous infusion and **flucytosine** (section 5.2.5) by intravenous infusion for 2 weeks, followed by **fluconazole** (section 5.2.1) by mouth for 8 weeks or until cultures are negative. In cryptococcosis, **fluconazole** is sometimes given alone as an alternative in HIV-positive patients with mild, localised infections or in those who cannot tolerate amphotericin. Following successful treatment, fluconazole can be used for prophylaxis against relapse until immunity recovers.

Histoplasmosis   Histoplasmosis is rare in temperate climates; it can be life-threatening, particularly in HIV-infected persons. **Itraconazole** (section 5.2.1) can be used for the treatment of immunocompetent patients with indolent non-meningeal infection, including chronic pulmonary histoplasmosis. **Amphotericin** (section 5.2.3) by intravenous infusion is used for the initial treatment of fulminant or severe infections, followed by a course of itraconazole by mouth. Following successful treatment, itraconazole can be used for prophylaxis against relapse until immunity recovers.

Skin and nail infections   Mild localised fungal infections of the skin (including tinea corporis, tinea cruris, and tinea pedis) respond to topical therapy (section 13.10.2). Systemic therapy is appropriate if topical therapy fails, if many areas are affected, or if the site of infection is difficult to treat such as in infections of the nails (onychomycosis) and of the scalp (tinea capitis). Oral imidazole or triazole antifungals (particularly **itraconazole**) and **terbinafine** are used more frequently than griseofulvin because they have a broader spectrum of activity and require a shorter duration of treatment.

Tinea capitis is treated systemically; additional topical application of an antifungal (section 13.10.2) may reduce transmission. **Griseofulvin** (section 5.2.5) is used for tinea capitis in adults and children; it is effective against infections caused by *Trichophyton tonsurans* and *Microsporum* spp. **Terbinafine** (section 5.2.5) is used for tinea capitis caused by *T. tonsurans* [unlicensed indication]. The role of terbinafine in the management of *Microsporum* infections is uncertain.

Pityriasis versicolor (section 13.10.2) may be treated with **itraconazole** (section 5.2.1) by mouth if topical therapy is ineffective; **fluconazole** (section 5.2.1) by mouth is an alternative. Oral **terbinafine** is **not** effective for pityriasis versicolor.

Antifungal treatment may not be necessary in asymptomatic patients with tinea infection of the nails. If treatment is necessary, a systemic antifungal is more effective than topical therapy. **Terbinafine** (section 5.2.5) and **itraconazole** (section 5.2.1) have largely replaced griseofulvin for the systemic treatment of *onychomycosis*, particularly of the toenail; terbinafine is considered to be the drug of choice. Itraconazole can be administered as intermittent 'pulse' therapy. For the role of topical antifungals in the treatment of onychomycosis, see section 13.10.2.

Immunocompromised patients Immunocompromised patients are at particular risk of fungal infections and may receive antifungal drugs prophylactically; oral triazole antifungals are the drugs of choice for prophylaxis. **Fluconazole** (section 5.2.1) is more reliably absorbed than **itraconazole** (section 5.2.1), but fluconazole is not effective against *Aspergillus* spp. Itraconazole is preferred in patients at risk of invasive aspergillosis. **Posaconazole** (section 5.2.1) can be used for prophylaxis in patients who are undergoing haematopoietic stem cell transplantation or receiving chemotherapy for acute myeloid leukaemia and myelodysplastic syndrome, if they are intolerant of fluconazole or itraconazole. **Micafungin** (section 5.2.4) can be used for prophylaxis of candidiasis in patients undergoing haematopoietic stem cell transplantation when fluconazole, itraconazole or posaconazole cannot be used.

Amphotericin (section 5.2.3) by intravenous infusion or **caspofungin** (section 5.2.4) is used for the empirical *treatment* of serious fungal infections; caspofungin is not effective against fungal infections of the CNS.

5.2.1 Triazole antifungals

For the role of triazole antifungal drugs in the prevention and systemic treatment of fungal infections, see p. 411.

Fluconazole is very well absorbed after oral administration. It also achieves good penetration into the cerebrospinal fluid to treat fungal meningitis. Fluconazole is excreted largely unchanged in the urine and can be used to treat candiduria.

Itraconazole is active against a wide range of dermatophytes. Itraconazole capsules require an acid environment in the stomach for optimal absorption.

Itraconazole has been associated with liver damage and should be avoided or used with caution in patients with liver disease; fluconazole is less frequently associated with hepatotoxicity.

Posaconazole is licensed for the treatment of invasive fungal infections unresponsive to conventional treatment.

Voriconazole is a broad-spectrum antifungal drug which is licensed for use in life-threatening infections.

▌ FLUCONAZOLE

Indications see under Dose
Cautions concomitant use with hepatotoxic drugs, monitor liver function with high doses or extended courses—discontinue if signs or symptoms of hepatic disease (risk of hepatic necrosis); susceptibility to QT interval prolongation; **interactions:** Appendix 1 (antifungals, triazole)

Contra-indications acute porphyria (section 9.8.2)

Hepatic impairment toxicity with related drugs

Renal impairment usual initial dose then halve subsequent doses if eGFR less than 50 mL/minute/ 1.73 m^2

Pregnancy manufacturer advises avoid—multiple congenital abnormalities reported with long-term high doses

Breast-feeding present in milk but amount probably too small to be harmful

Side-effects nausea, abdominal discomfort, diarrhoea, flatulence, headache, rash (discontinue treatment or monitor closely if infection invasive or systemic); less frequently dyspepsia, vomiting, taste disturbance, hepatic disorders, hypersensitivity reactions, anaphylaxis, dizziness, seizures, alopecia, pruritus, toxic epidermal necrolysis, Stevens-Johnson syndrome (severe cutaneous reactions more likely in HIV-positive patients), hyperlipidaemia, leucopenia, thrombocytopenia, and hypokalaemia reported

Dose
- Vaginal candidiasis (see also Recurrent Vulvovaginal Candidiasis, section 7.2.2) and candidal balanitis, ADULT and CHILD over 16 years, by mouth, a single dose of 150 mg
- Mucosal candidiasis (except genital), by mouth, 50 mg daily (100 mg daily in unusually difficult infections) given for 7–14 days in oropharyngeal candidiasis (max. 14 days except in severely immunocompromised patients); for 14 days in atrophic oral candidiasis associated with dentures; for 14–30 days in other mucosal infections (e.g. oesophagitis, candiduria, non-invasive bronchopulmonary infections); CHILD by mouth *or* by intravenous infusion, 3–6 mg/ kg on first day then 3 mg/kg daily (every 72 hours in NEONATE up to 2 weeks old, every 48 hours in neonate 2–4 weeks old)
- Tinea pedis, corporis, cruris, pityriasis versicolor, and dermal candidiasis, by mouth, 50 mg daily for 2–4 weeks (for up to 6 weeks in tinea pedis); max. duration of treatment 6 weeks
- Invasive candidal infections (including candidaemia and disseminated candidiasis) and cryptococcal infections (including meningitis), by mouth *or* intravenous infusion, 400 mg on first day then 200–400 mg daily; max. 800 mg daily in severe infections [unlicensed dose]; treatment continued according to response (at least 8 weeks for cryptococcal meningitis); CHILD 6–12 mg/kg daily (every 72 hours in NEONATE up to 2 weeks old, every 48 hours in NEONATE 2–4 weeks old); max. 800 mg daily [unlicensed dose]
- Prevention of relapse of cryptococcal meningitis in HIV-infected patients after completion of primary therapy, by mouth *or* by intravenous infusion, 200 mg daily
- Prevention of fungal infections in immunocompromised patients, by mouth *or* by intravenous infusion, 50–400 mg daily adjusted according to risk; 400 mg daily if high risk of systemic infections e.g. following bone-marrow transplantation; commence treatment before anticipated onset of neutropenia and continue for 7 days after neutrophil count in desirable range; CHILD according to extent and duration of neutropenia, 3–12 mg/kg daily (every 72 hours in NEONATE up to 2 weeks old, every 48 hours in NEONATE 2–4 weeks old); max. 400 mg daily

Fluconazole (Non-proprietary) [PoM]

[1]Capsules, fluconazole 50 mg, net price 7-cap pack = £1.06; 150 mg, single-capsule pack = £1.02; 200 mg, 7-cap pack = £6.86. Label: 9, (50 and 200 mg)

Dental prescribing on NHS Fluconazole Capsules 50 mg may be prescribed

Intravenous infusion, fluconazole 2 mg/mL, net price 25-mL bottle = £7.31; 100-mL bottle = £27.45; 50-mL infusion bag = £2.70; 100-mL infusion bag = £27.82

Diflucan® (Pfizer) [PoM]

[1]Capsules, fluconazole 50 mg (blue/white), net price 7-cap pack = £16.61; 150 mg (blue), single-capsule pack = £7.12; 200 mg (purple/white), 7-cap pack = £66.42. Label: 9, (50 and 200 mg)

Oral suspension, orange-flavoured, fluconazole for reconstitution with water, 50 mg/5 mL, net price 35 mL = £16.61; 200 mg/5 mL, 35 mL = £66.42. Label: 9

Dental prescribing on NHS May be prescribed as Fluconazole Oral Suspension 50 mg/5 mL

Intravenous infusion, fluconazole 2 mg/mL in sodium chloride intravenous infusion 0.9%, net price 100-mL bottle = £29.28

Electrolytes Na$^+$ 15 mmol/100-mL bottle

ITRACONAZOLE

Indications see under Dose

Cautions absorption reduced in HIV-infection and neutropenia (monitor plasma-itraconazole concentration and increase dose if necessary); susceptibility to congestive heart failure (see also Heart Failure, below); **interactions**: Appendix 1 (antifungals, triazole)

Hepatotoxicity Potentially life-threatening hepatotoxicity reported very rarely—discontinue if signs of hepatitis develop. Avoid or use with caution if history of hepatotoxicity with other drugs or in active liver disease. Monitor liver function if treatment continues for longer than one month, if receiving other hepatotoxic drugs, if history of hepatotoxicity with other drugs, or in hepatic impairment

Counselling Patients should be told how to recognise signs of liver disorder and advised to seek prompt medical attention if symptoms such as anorexia, nausea, vomiting, fatigue, abdominal pain or dark urine develop

Heart failure

Following reports of heart failure, caution is advised when prescribing itraconazole to patients at high risk of heart failure. Those at risk include:

- patients receiving high doses and longer treatment courses;
- older patients and those with cardiac disease;
- patients with chronic lung disease (including chronic obstructive pulmonary disease) associated with pulmonary hypertension;
- patients receiving treatment with negative inotropic drugs, e.g. calcium channel blockers.

Itraconazole should be avoided in patients with ventricular dysfunction or a history of heart failure unless the infection is serious.

Contra-indications acute porphyria (section 9.8.2)

Hepatic impairment use only if potential benefit outweighs risk of hepatotoxicity (see Hepatotoxicity above); dose reduction may be necessary

Renal impairment risk of congestive heart failure; bioavailability of oral formulations possibly reduced; use intravenous infusion with caution if eGFR 30–80 mL/minute/1.73 m^2; avoid intravenous infusion if eGFR less than 30 mL/minute/1.73 m^2

Pregnancy manufacturer advises use only in life-threatening situations (toxicity at high doses in *animal* studies); ensure effective contraception during treatment and until the next menstrual period following end of treatment

Breast-feeding small amounts present in milk—may accumulate; manufacturer advises avoid

Side-effects nausea, vomiting, taste disturbances, abdominal pain, diarrhoea, hepatitis (see Hepatotoxicity above), dyspnoea, headache, hypokalaemia, rash; *less commonly* dyspepsia, flatulence, constipation, oedema, dizziness, peripheral neuropathy (discontinue treatment), menstrual disorder, myalgia; *rarely* pancreatitis, heart failure (see Cautions above), hypertriglyceridaemia, erectile dysfunction, urinary frequency, leucopenia, visual disturbances, tinnitus, deafness, alopecia, photosensitivity, toxic epidermal necrolysis, Stevens-Johnson syndrome; also reported, blood pressure changes, confusion, drowsiness, tremor, thrombocytopenia, renal impairment, arthralgia; *with intravenous injection* hyperglycaemia

Dose

- By mouth, oropharyngeal candidiasis, see under *Sporanox*® oral liquid below

Vulvovaginal candidiasis (see also Recurrent Vulvovaginal Candidiasis, section 7.2.2), 200 mg twice daily for 1 day

Pityriasis versicolor, 200 mg once daily for 7 days

Tinea corporis and tinea cruris, *either* 100 mg once daily for 15 days *or* 200 mg once daily for 7 days

Tinea pedis and tinea manuum, *either* 100 mg once daily for 30 days *or* 200 mg twice daily for 7 days

Onychomycosis, *either* 200 mg once daily for 3 months *or* course ('pulse') of 200 mg twice daily for 7 days, subsequent courses repeated after 21-day interval; fingernails 2 courses, toenails 3 courses

Aspergillosis, 200 mg twice daily

Histoplasmosis, 200 mg 3 times daily for 3 days, then 200 mg once or twice daily

Systemic candidiasis and cryptococcosis including cryptococcal meningitis where other antifungal drugs inappropriate or ineffective, 200 mg once daily (candidiasis 100–200 mg once daily) increased in invasive or disseminated disease and in cryptococcal meningitis to 200 mg twice daily

Maintenance in HIV-infected patients to prevent relapse of underlying fungal infection and prophylaxis in neutropenia when standard therapy inappropriate, 200 mg once daily, increased to 200 mg twice daily if low plasma-itraconazole concentration (see Cautions)

Prophylaxis in patients with haematological malignancy or undergoing bone-marrow transplant, see under *Sporanox*® oral liquid below

- By intravenous infusion, systemic aspergillosis, candidiasis and cryptococcosis including cryptococcal meningitis where other antifungal drugs inappropriate or ineffective, histoplasmosis, 200 mg every 12 hours for 2 days, then 200 mg once daily for max. 12 days

- CHILD under 18 years see *BNF for Children*

Note Itraconazole doses in BNF may differ from those in product literature

---

1. Capsules can be sold to the public for vaginal candidiasis and associated candidal balanitis in those aged 16–60 years, in a container or packaging containing not more than 150 mg and labelled to show a max. dose of 150 mg

Itraconazole (Non-proprietary) PoM

Capsules, enclosing coated beads, itraconazole 100 mg, net price 15-cap pack = £4.58. Label: 5, 9, 21, 25, counselling, hepatotoxicity

Sporanox® (Janssen) PoM

Capsules, blue/pink, enclosing coated beads, itraconazole 100 mg, net price 4-cap pack = £3.67; 15-cap pack = £13.77; 28-cap pack (*Sporanox®-Pulse*) = £25.72; 60-cap pack = £55.10. Label: 5, 9, 21, 25, counselling, hepatotoxicity

Oral liquid, sugar-free, cherry-flavoured, itraconazole 10 mg/mL, net price 150 mL (with 10-mL measuring cup) = £58.34. Label: 9, 23, counselling, administration, hepatotoxicity

Dose oral or oesophageal candidiasis in HIV-positive or other immunocompromised patients, 20 mL (2 measuring cups) daily in 1–2 divided doses for 1 week (continue for another week if no response)

Oral or oesophageal candidiasis that has not responded to fluconazole, 10–20 mL (1–2 measuring cups) twice daily for 2 weeks (continue for another 2 weeks if no response; the higher dose should not be used for longer than 2 weeks if no signs of improvement)

Prophylaxis of deep fungal infections (when standard therapy is inappropriate) in patients with haematological malignancy or undergoing bone-marrow transplantation who are expected to become neutropenic, 5 mg/kg daily in 2 divided doses; starting before transplantation or before chemotherapy (taking care to avoid interaction with cytotoxic drugs) and continued until neutrophil count recovers; CHILD and ELDERLY safety and efficacy not established

Counselling Do not take with food; swish around mouth and swallow, do not rinse afterwards

Concentrate for intravenous infusion, itraconazole 10 mg/mL. For dilution before use. Net price 25-mL amp (with infusion bag and filter) = £79.71

Excipients include propylene glycol

POSACONAZOLE

Indications invasive aspergillosis (see notes above); fusariosis either unresponsive to, or in patients intolerant of, amphotericin; chromoblastomycosis and mycetoma either unresponsive to, or in patients intolerant of, itraconazole; coccidioidomycosis either unresponsive to, or in patients intolerant of, amphotericin, itraconazole, or fluconazole; see also under preparations below

Cautions cardiomyopathy, bradycardia, symptomatic arrhythmias, history of QT interval prolongation, concomitant use with other drugs known to cause QT-interval prolongation; monitor electrolytes (including potassium, magnesium, and calcium) before and during therapy, monitor liver function before and during therapy; body-weight under 60 kg—risk of side-effects increased; body-weight over 120 kg—risk of treatment failure possibly increased; **interactions:** Appendix 1 (antifungals, triazole)

Contra-indications acute porphyria (section 9.8.2)

Hepatic impairment monitor liver function; manufacturer advises caution

Pregnancy manufacturer advises avoid unless potential benefit outweighs risk and recommends effective contraception during treatment; toxicity in *animal* studies

Breast-feeding manufacturer advises avoid—present in milk in *animal* studies

Side-effects gastro-intestinal disturbances (including nausea, vomiting, abdominal pain, diarrhoea, constipation, dyspepsia, and flatulence); dizziness, headache, paraesthesia, drowsiness, fatigue, fever, anorexia; blood disorders (including anaemia, neutropenia, and thrombocytopenia), electrolyte disturbances; dry mouth; rash, pruritus; *less commonly* pancreatitis, hepatic disorders, gastro-oesophageal reflux, arrhythmias, bradycardia, tachycardia, palpitation, changes in blood pressure, oedema, vasculitis, cough, hiccups, convulsions, neuropathy, tremor, aphasia, insomnia, hyperglycaemia, menstrual disorders, renal failure, musculoskeletal pain, visual disturbances, mouth ulcers, and alopecia; *rarely* ileus, cardiac failure, myocardial infarction, stroke, thrombosis, syncope, pneumonitis, psychosis, depression, encephalopathy, adrenal insufficiency, breast pain, hearing impairment, and Stevens-Johnson syndrome

Dose
• See under preparations below

Noxafil® (MSD) PoM

Tablets, yellow, e/c, posaconazole 100 mg, net price 24-tab pack = £596.96, 96-tab pack = £2387.85. Label: 3, 9, 25

Note Tablets not licensed for oropharyngeal candidiasis

Dose ADULT over 18 years, 300 mg twice daily on first day, then 300 mg once daily

Prophylaxis of invasive fungal infections in patients undergoing bone-marrow transplantation or receiving chemotherapy for acute myeloid leukaemia and myelodysplastic syndrome who are expected to become neutropenic, and who are intolerant of fluconazole or itraconazole, ADULT over 18 years, 300 mg twice daily on first day, then 300 mg once daily, starting before transplantation or before chemotherapy and continued until neutrophil count recovers

Suspension, posaconazole 200 mg/5 mL, net price 105 mL (cherry-flavoured) = £491.20. Label: 3, 9, 21

Dose ADULT over 18 years, 400 mg twice daily with food *or* if food not tolerated, 200 mg 4 times daily

Oropharyngeal candidiasis (severe infection or in immunocompromised patients only), ADULT over 18 years, 200 mg with food on first day, then 100 mg once daily with food for 13 days

Prophylaxis of invasive fungal infections in patients undergoing bone-marrow transplantation or receiving chemotherapy for acute myeloid leukaemia and myelodysplastic syndrome who are expected to become neutropenic, and who are intolerant of fluconazole or itraconazole, ADULT over 18 years, 200 mg 3 times daily with food, starting before transplantation or before chemotherapy and continued until neutrophil count recovers

Note Where possible, *Noxafil®* tablets should be used in preference to the suspension because the tablets have a higher bioavailability; the suspension is not interchangeable with the tablets on a milligram-for-milligram basis

VORICONAZOLE

Indications invasive aspergillosis; serious infections caused by *Scedosporium* spp., *Fusarium* spp., or invasive fluconazole-resistant *Candida* spp. (including *C. krusei*)

Cautions electrolyte disturbances, cardiomyopathy, bradycardia, symptomatic arrhythmias, history of QT interval prolongation, concomitant use with other drugs that prolong QT interval; patients at risk of pancreatitis; monitor renal function; **interactions:** Appendix 1 (antifungals, triazole)

Hepatotoxicity Hepatitis, cholestasis, and fulminant hepatic failure reported uncommonly; risk increased in patients with haematological malignancy. Monitor liver function before starting treatment, then at least weekly for 1 month, and then monthly during treatment. Consider

5 Infections

treatment discontinuation if severe abnormalities in liver function tests. Patients should be told how to recognise signs of liver disorder, and advised to seek immediate medical attention if symptoms such as persistent nausea, vomiting, malaise or jaundice develop

Phototoxicity Phototoxicity occurs commonly. Patients should be advised to avoid intense or prolonged exposure to direct sunlight, and to avoid use of sunbeds. In sunlight, patients should cover sun-exposed areas of skin and use a sunscreen with a high sun protection factor. Patients should seek medical attention if they experience sunburn or a severe skin reaction following exposure to light or sun. If phototoxicity occurs, consider treatment discontinuation; if treatment is continued, monitor for pre-malignant skin lesions and squamous cell carcinoma, and discontinue treatment if they occur. Patients should be advised to keep the Alert Card with them at all times

Contra-indications acute porphyria (section 9.8.2)

Hepatic impairment in mild to moderate hepatic cirrhosis use usual loading dose then halve maintenance dose; no information available for severe hepatic cirrhosis—manufacturer advises use only if potential benefit outweighs risk. See also Hepatotoxicity above

Renal impairment intravenous vehicle may accumulate if eGFR less than $50\,mL/minute/1.73\,m^2$—use intravenous infusion only if potential benefit outweighs risk, and monitor renal function; alternatively, use tablets or oral suspension (no dose adjustment required)

Pregnancy toxicity in *animal* studies—manufacturer advises avoid unless potential benefit outweighs risk; effective contraception required during treatment

Breast-feeding manufacturer advises avoid—no information available

Side-effects nausea, vomiting, abdominal pain, diarrhoea, jaundice (see Hepatotoxicity above), oedema, hypotension, chest pain, respiratory distress syndrome, sinusitis, headache, dizziness, asthenia, anxiety, depression, confusion, agitation, hallucinations, paraesthesia, tremor, influenza-like symptoms, hypoglycaemia, haematuria, blood disorders (including anaemia, thrombocytopenia, leucopenia, pancytopenia), acute renal failure, hypokalaemia, visual disturbances (including altered perception, blurred vision, and photophobia), rash, pruritus, photosensitivity, alopecia, cheilitis, injection-site reactions; *less commonly* dyspepsia, duodenitis, cholecystitis, pancreatitis, hepatitis (see Hepatotoxicity above), constipation, arrhythmias (including QT interval prolongation), syncope, hyponatraemia, raised serum cholesterol, hypersensitivity reactions (including flushing), ataxia, nystagmus, hypoaesthesia, adrenocortical insufficiency, arthritis, blepharitis, optic neuritis, scleritis, glossitis, gingivitis, psoriasis, Stevens-Johnson syndrome; *rarely* pseudomembranous colitis, taste disturbances (more common with oral suspension), convulsions, extrapyramidal effects, insomnia, tinnitus, hearing disturbances, hypertonia, hypothyroidism, hyperthyroidism, discoid lupus erythematosus, toxic epidermal necrolysis, pseudoporphyria, retinal haemorrhage, optic atrophy; also reported on long-term treatment squamous cell carcinoma of skin (particularly in presence of phototoxicity) and periostitis (particularly in transplant patients)

Dose

- By mouth, ADULT over 18 years, body-weight over 40 kg, 400 mg every 12 hours for 2 doses then 200 mg every 12 hours, increased if necessary to 300 mg every 12 hours; body-weight under 40 kg, 200 mg every 12 hours for 2 doses then 100 mg every 12

hours, increased if necessary to 150 mg every 12 hours; CHILD 2–18 years see *BNF for Children*

- By intravenous infusion, 6 mg/kg every 12 hours for 2 doses, then 4 mg/kg every 12 hours (reduced to 3 mg/kg every 12 hours if not tolerated) for max. 6 months; CHILD 2–18 years see *BNF for Children*

Vfend® (Pfizer) (PoM)

Tablets, f/c, voriconazole 50 mg, net price 28-tablet pack = £275.68; 200 mg, 28-tab pack = £1102.74. Label: 9, 11, 23, counselling, hepatotoxicity, phototoxicity

Oral suspension, voriconazole 200 mg/5 mL when reconstituted with water, net price 75 mL (orange-flavoured) = £551.37. Label: 9, 11, 23, counselling, hepatotoxicity, phototoxicity

Intravenous infusion, powder for reconstitution, voriconazole, net price 200-mg vial = £77.14; 200-mg vial (with solvent) = £77.14

Excipients include sulfobutylether beta cyclodextrin sodium (risk of accumulation in renal impairment)

Electrolytes Na^+ 9.47 mmol/vial

5.2.2 Imidazole antifungals

The imidazole antifungals include clotrimazole, econazole, ketoconazole, and tioconazole. They are used for the local treatment of vaginal candidiasis (section 7.2.2) and for dermatophyte infections (section 13.10.2).

> ### CHMP advice
> ### Ketoconazole (July 2013)
>
> The CHMP has recommended that the marketing authorisation for oral ketoconazole should be suspended. The CHMP concluded that the risk of hepatotoxicity associated with oral ketoconazole is greater than the benefit in treating fungal infections. Doctors should review patients who are being treated with oral ketoconazole for fungal infections, with a view to stopping treatment or choosing an alternative treatment. Patients with a prescription of oral ketoconazole for fungal infections should be referred back to their doctors.
>
> Topical products containing ketoconazole are not affected by this advice.

Miconazole (section 12.3.2) can be used locally for oral infections; it is also effective in intestinal infections. Systemic absorption may follow use of miconazole oral gel and may result in significant drug interactions.

5.2.3 Polyene antifungals

The polyene antifungals include amphotericin and nystatin; neither drug is absorbed when given by mouth. Nystatin is used for oral, oropharyngeal, and perioral infections by local application in the mouth (section 12.3.2). Nystatin is also used for *Candida albicans* infection of the skin (section 13.10.2).

Amphotericin by intravenous infusion is used for the treatment of systemic fungal infections and is active against most fungi and yeasts. It is highly protein bound and penetrates poorly into body fluids and tissues. When given parenterally amphotericin is toxic and side-effects are common. Lipid formulations of amphotericin (*Abelcet®* and *AmBisome®*) are significantly less toxic and are recommended when the conventional formulation of amphotericin is contra-indicated because of toxicity, especially nephrotoxicity or when response to conventional amphotericin is inadequate; lipid formulations are more expensive. For the role of amphotericin in the systemic treatment of fungal infections, see p. 411.

AMPHOTERICIN
(Amphotericin B)

Indications See under Dose

Cautions when given parenterally, toxicity common (close supervision necessary and test dose required; see Anaphylaxis below); hepatic and renal function tests, blood counts, and plasma electrolyte (including plasma-potassium and magnesium concentration) monitoring required; corticosteroids (avoid except to control reactions); avoid rapid infusion (risk of arrhythmias); **interactions**: Appendix 1 (amphotericin)

Anaphylaxis Anaphylaxis can occur with any intravenous amphotericin product and a test dose is advisable before the first infusion; the patient should be carefully observed for at least 30 minutes after the test dose. Prophylactic antipyretics or hydrocortisone should only be used in patients who have previously experienced acute adverse reactions (in whom continued treatment with amphotericin is essential)

Renal impairment use only if no alternative; nephrotoxicity may be reduced with use of lipid formulation

Pregnancy not known to be harmful but manufacturers advise avoid unless potential benefit outweighs risk

Breast-feeding no information available

Side-effects nausea, vomiting, abdominal pain, diarrhoea, cardiovascular effects (including arrhythmias, blood pressure changes, chest pain), dyspnoea, headache, febrile reactions, electrolyte disturbances (including hypokalaemia and hypomagnesaemia), disturbances in renal function (including renal tubular acidosis), abnormal liver function (discontinue treatment), blood disorders (including anaemia, thrombocytopenia), rash; *less commonly* anaphylactoid reactions (see Anaphylaxis, above), bronchospasm, neurological disorders (including convulsions, peripheral neuropathy, tremor, encephalopathy, hearing loss, diplopia); also reported anorexia, myalgia, arthralgia, toxic epidermal necrolysis, Stevens-Johnson syndrome

Dose
- By intravenous infusion, see preparations

Note Different preparations of intravenous amphotericin vary in their pharmacodynamics, pharmacokinetics, dosage, and administration; these preparations should **not** be considered interchangeable. To avoid confusion, prescribers should specify the brand to be dispensed.

Fungizone® (Squibb) PoM
Intravenous infusion, powder for reconstitution, amphotericin (as sodium deoxycholate complex), net price 50-mg vial = £3.88
Electrolytes Na⁺ < 0.5 mmol/vial
Dose by intravenous infusion, systemic fungal infections, initial test dose of 1 mg over 20–30 minutes then 250 micrograms/kg daily, gradually increased over 2–4 days, if tolerated, to 1 mg/kg daily; max. (severe infection) 1.5 mg/kg daily or on alternate days; CHILD under 18 years see BNF for Children
Note Prolonged treatment usually necessary; if interrupted for longer than 7 days recommence at 250 micrograms/kg daily and increase gradually

◀ **Lipid formulations**

Abelcet® (TEVA UK) PoM
Intravenous infusion, amphotericin 5 mg/mL as lipid complex with L-α-dimyristoylphosphatidylcholine and L-α-dimyristoylphosphatidylglycerol, net price 20-mL vial = £77.50 (hosp. only)
Electrolytes Na⁺ 3.12 mmol/vial
Dose by intravenous infusion, severe invasive candidiasis; severe systemic fungal infections in patients not responding to conventional amphotericin or to other antifungal drugs or where toxicity or renal impairment precludes conventional amphotericin, including invasive aspergillosis, cryptococcal meningitis and disseminated cryptococcosis in HIV patients, initial test dose 1 mg over 15 minutes then 5 mg/kg once daily for at least 14 days; CHILD under 18 years see BNF for Children

AmBisome® (Gilead) PoM
Intravenous infusion, powder for reconstitution, amphotericin 50 mg encapsulated in liposomes, net price 50-mg vial = £82.19
Electrolytes Na⁺ < 0.5 mmol/vial
Excipients include sucrose 900 mg/vial
Dose by intravenous infusion, severe systemic or deep mycoses where toxicity (particularly nephrotoxicity) precludes use of conventional amphotericin; suspected or proven infection in febrile neutropenic patients unresponsive to broad-spectrum antibacterials; aspergillosis, initial test dose 1 mg over 10 minutes then 3 mg/kg once daily; max. 5 mg/kg once daily [unlicensed dose]; CHILD under 18 years see BNF for Children
Visceral leishmaniasis, see section 5.4.5 and product literature

5.2.4 Echinocandin antifungals

The echinocandin antifungals include **anidulafungin**, **caspofungin** and **micafungin**. They are only active against *Aspergillus* spp. and *Candida* spp.; however, anidulafungin and micafungin are not used for the treatment of aspergillosis. Echinocandins are not effective against fungal infections of the CNS. For the role of echinocandin antifungals in the prevention and systemic treatment of fungal infections, see p. 411.

ANIDULAFUNGIN

Indications invasive candidiasis (see notes above)

Pregnancy manufacturer advises avoid—no information available

Breast-feeding manufacturer advises avoid unless potential benefit outweighs risk—present in milk in *animal* studies

Side-effects diarrhoea, nausea, vomiting, flushing, convulsion, headache, coagulopathy, hypokalaemia, raised serum creatinine, rash, pruritus; *less commonly* abdominal pain, cholestasis, hypertension, hyperglycaemia, urticaria, injection-site pain; also reported, hypotension, dyspnoea, bronchospasm, hepatitis

Dose
- By intravenous infusion, ADULT over 18 years, 200 mg on first day then 100 mg once daily

Ecalta® (Pfizer) PoM
Intravenous infusion, powder for reconstitution, anidulafungin, net price 100-mg vial = £299.99

CASPOFUNGIN

Indications invasive aspergillosis (see notes above); invasive candidiasis (see notes above); empirical treatment of systemic fungal infections in patients with neutropenia

Cautions interactions: Appendix 1 (caspofungin)

Hepatic impairment 70 mg on first day then 35 mg once daily in moderate impairment; no information available for severe impairment

Pregnancy manufacturer advises avoid unless essential—toxicity in *animal* studies

Breast-feeding present in milk in *animal* studies—manufacturer advises avoid

Side-effects nausea, diarrhoea, vomiting; dyspnoea; headache; hypokalaemia; arthralgia; rash, pruritus, sweating, injection-site reactions; *less commonly* abdominal pain, dyspepsia, dry mouth, dysphagia, taste disturbances, anorexia, constipation, flatulence, cholestasis, hepatic dysfunction, ascites, palpitation, arrhythmia, chest pain, heart failure, thrombophlebitis, flushing, hypotension, hypertension, bronchospasm, cough, dizziness, fatigue, paraesthesia, hypoaesthesia, sleep disturbances, tremor, anxiety, disorientation, hyperglycaemia, renal failure, hypomagnesaemia, hypocalcaemia, metabolic acidosis, anaemia, thrombocytopenia, leucopenia, myalgia, muscular weakness, blurred vision, and erythema multiforme; also reported, adult respiratory distress syndrome and anaphylaxis

Dose
- By intravenous infusion, 70 mg on first day then 50 mg once daily (70 mg once daily if body-weight over 80 kg); CHILD under 18 years see *BNF for Children*

Cancidas® (MSD) (PoM)
Intravenous infusion, powder for reconstitution, caspofungin (as acetate), net price 50-mg vial = £327.67; 70-mg vial = £416.78

MICAFUNGIN

Indications see under Dose

Cautions monitor renal function; **interactions:** Appendix 1 (micafungin)

Hepatotoxicity Potentially life-threatening hepatotoxicity reported. Monitor liver function—discontinue if significant and persistent abnormalities in liver function tests develop. Use with caution in hepatic impairment (avoid if severe) or if receiving other hepatotoxic drugs. Risk of hepatic side-effects greater in children under 1 year of age

Hepatic impairment use with caution in mild to moderate impairment; avoid in severe impairment; see also Hepatotoxicity above

Renal impairment use with caution; renal function may deteriorate

Pregnancy manufacturer advises avoid unless essential—toxicity in *animal* studies

Breast-feeding manufacturer advises use only if potential benefit outweighs risk—present in milk in *animal* studies

Side-effects nausea, vomiting, diarrhoea, abdominal pain; headache, fever; hypokalaemia, hypomagnesaemia, hypocalcaemia, leucopenia, anaemia; rash, phlebitis; *less commonly* dyspepsia, constipation, hepatomegaly, hepatitis and cholestasis (see also Hepatotoxicity above), taste disturbances, anorexia, tachycardia, palpitation, bradycardia, blood pressure changes, flushing, dyspnoea, sleep disturbances, anxiety, confusion, dizziness, tremor, pancytopenia, thrombocytopenia, eosinophilia, hyponatraemia, hypophosphataemia, hyperkalaemia, hyperhidrosis, and pruritus; *rarely* haemolytic anaemia; also reported disseminated intravascualr coagulation, renal failure (more frequent in children), Stevens-Johnson syndrome, toxic epidermal necrolysis

Dose
- By intravenous infusion, invasive candidiasis, ADULT body-weight over 40 kg, 100 mg once daily (increased to 200 mg daily if inadequate response) for at least 14 days; body-weight under 40 kg, 2 mg/kg once daily (increased to 4 mg/kg daily if inadequate response) for at least 14 days; CHILD under 18 years see *BNF for Children*

  Oesophageal candidiasis, ADULT body-weight over 40 kg, 150 mg once daily; body-weight under 40 kg, 3 mg/kg once daily; CHILD 16–18 years see *BNF for Children*

  Prophylaxis of candidiasis in patients undergoing bone-marrow transplantation or who are expected to become neutropenic for over 10 days, ADULT body-weight over 40 kg, 50 mg once daily; body-weight under 40 kg, 1 mg/kg once daily; continue for at least 7 days after neutrophil count in desirable range; CHILD under 18 years see *BNF for Children*

Mycamine® (Astellas) (PoM)
Intravenous infusion, powder for reconstitution, micafungin (as sodium), net price 50-mg vial = £196.08; 100-mg vial = £341.00

5.2.5 Other antifungals

Flucytosine is used with amphotericin in a synergistic combination. Bone marrow depression can occur which limits its use, particularly in HIV-positive patients; weekly blood counts are necessary during prolonged therapy. Resistance to flucytosine can develop during therapy and sensitivity testing is essential before and during treatment. For the role of flucytosine in the treatment of systemic candidiasis and cryptococcal meningitis, see p. 411.

Griseofulvin is effective for widespread or intractable dermatophyte infections but has been superseded by newer antifungals, particularly for nail infections. It is the drug of choice for trichophyton infections in children. Duration of therapy is dependent on the site of the infection and may extend to a number of months. For the role of griseofulvin in the treatment of tinea capitis, see p. 411.

Terbinafine is the drug of choice for fungal nail infections and is also used for ringworm infections where oral treatment is considered appropriate (see p. 411).

FLUCYTOSINE

Indications systemic yeast and fungal infections; adjunct to amphotericin in cryptococcal meningitis (see Cryptococcosis, p. 411), adjunct to amphotericin in severe systemic candidiasis and in other severe or long-standing infections

Cautions elderly; blood disorders; liver- and kidney-function tests and blood counts required (weekly in blood disorders); **interactions:** Appendix 1 (flucytosine)

Renal impairment liver- and kidney-function tests and blood counts required weekly; use 50 mg/kg every 12 hours if creatinine clearance 20–40 mL/minute; use 50 mg/kg every 24 hours if creatinine clearance 10–20 mL/minute; use initial dose of 50 mg/kg if creatinine clearance less than 10 mL/minute and then adjust dose according to plasma-flucytosine concentration

Pregnancy teratogenic in *animal* studies; manufacturer advises use only if potential benefit outweighs risk

5 Infections

Breast-feeding   manufacturer advises avoid

Side-effects   nausea, vomiting, diarrhoea, rashes; less frequently cardiotoxicity, confusion, hallucinations, convulsions, headache, sedation, vertigo, alterations in liver function tests (hepatitis and hepatic necrosis reported), and toxic epidermal necrolysis; blood disorders including thrombocytopenia, leucopenia, and aplastic anaemia reported

Dose

- By intravenous infusion over 20–40 minutes, 200 mg/ kg daily in 4 divided doses usually for not more than 7 days; extremely sensitive organisms, 100–150 mg/kg daily may be sufficient; CHILD under 18 years see *BNF for Children*

    Cryptococcal meningitis (adjunct to amphotericin, see Cryptococcosis, p. 411) 100 mg/kg daily in 4 divided doses for 2 weeks [unlicensed duration]; CHILD under 18 years see *BNF for Children*

    Note For plasma concentration monitoring, blood should be taken shortly before starting the next infusion; plasma concentration for optimum response 25–50 mg/litre (200–400 micromol/litre)—should not be allowed to exceed 80 mg/litre (620 micromol/litre)

Ancotil® (Meda) ⒫ℴⓜ

Intravenous infusion, flucytosine 10 mg/mL, net price 250-mL infusion bottle = £30.33 (hosp. only)

Electrolytes Na⁺ 34.5 mmol/250-mL bottle

Note Flucytosine tablets [unlicensed] may be available from 'special-order' manufacturers or specialist-importing companies, see p. 1124

GRISEOFULVIN

Indications   dermatophyte infections of the skin, scalp, hair and nails where topical therapy has failed or is inappropriate

Cautions   interactions: Appendix 1 (griseofulvin)

Driving May impair performance of skilled tasks (e.g. driving); effects of alcohol enhanced

Contra-indications   severe liver disease; systemic lupus erythematosus (risk of exacerbation); acute porphyria (section 9.8.2)

Hepatic impairment   avoid in severe liver disease

Pregnancy   avoid (fetotoxicity and teratogenicity in *animals*); effective contraception required during and for at least 1 month after administration to women (**important:** effectiveness of oral contraceptives may be reduced, additional contraceptive precautions e.g. barrier method, required); also men should avoid fathering a child during and for at least 6 months after administration

Breast-feeding   avoid—no information available

Side-effects   nausea, vomiting, diarrhoea; headache; also reported, abdominal pain, dyspepsia, hepatotoxicity, glossitis, taste disturbances, sleep disturbances, dizziness, fatigue, confusion, agitation, depression, impaired coordination and hearing, peripheral neuropathy, menstrual disturbances, renal failure, leucopenia, systemic lupus erythematosus, rash (including rarely erythema multiforme, toxic epidermal necrolysis), and photosensitivity

Dose

- Dermatophyte infections, 500 mg once daily or in divided doses; in severe infection dose may be doubled, reducing when response occurs; CHILD under 50 kg, 10 mg/kg once daily or in divided doses
- Tinea capitis caused by *Trichophyton tonsurans*, 1 g once daily or in divided doses; CHILD under 50 kg, 15–20 mg/kg once daily or in divided doses

Note Griseofulvin doses in BNF may differ from those in product literature

Griseofulvin (Non-proprietary) ⒫ℴⓜ

Tablets, griseofulvin 125 mg, net price 100 = £81.67; 500 mg, 100= £92.74. Label: 9, 21, counselling, driving

TERBINAFINE

Indications   dermatophyte infections of the nails, ringworm infections (including tinea pedis, cruris, and corporis) where oral therapy appropriate (due to site, severity or extent)

Cautions   psoriasis (risk of exacerbation); autoimmune disease (risk of lupus-erythematosus-like effect); monitor hepatic function before treatment and then every 4–6 weeks during treatment — discontinue if abnormalities in liver function tests; **interactions:** Appendix 1 (terbinafine)

Hepatic impairment   manufacturer advises avoid— elimination reduced

Renal impairment   use half normal dose if eGFR less than 50 mL/minute/1.73 m² and no suitable alternative available

Pregnancy   manufacturer advises use only if potential benefit outweighs risk—no information available

Breast-feeding   avoid—present in milk

Side-effects   abdominal discomfort, anorexia, nausea, diarrhoea, dyspepsia, headache, arthralgia, myalgia, rash, urticaria; *less commonly* taste disturbance; *rarely* liver toxicity (including jaundice, cholestasis, and hepatitis)—discontinue treatment, dizziness, malaise, paraesthesia, hypoaesthesia; *very rarely* blood disorders (including neutropenia and thrombocytopenia), lupus erythematosus-like effect, photosensitivity, alopecia, serious skin reactions (including Stevens-Johnson syndrome and toxic epidermal necrolysis)— discontinue treatment if progressive skin rash; also reported, pancreatitis, vasculitis, influenza-like symptoms, rhabdomyolysis, disturbances in smell, hearing disturbances, exacerbation of psoriasis

Dose

- By mouth, 250 mg daily usually for 2–6 weeks in tinea pedis, 2–4 weeks in tinea cruris, 4 weeks in tinea corporis, 6 weeks–3 months in nail infections (occasionally longer in toenail infections); CHILD [unlicensed] usually for 4 weeks, tinea capitis, over 1 year, body-weight 10–20 kg, 62.5 mg once daily; body-weight 20–40 kg, 125 mg once daily; body-weight over 40 kg, 250 mg once daily

Terbinafine (Non-proprietary) ⒫ℴⓜ

Tablets, terbinafine (as hydrochloride) 250 mg, net price 14-tab pack = £1.62, 28-tab pack = £2.63. Label: 9

Lamisil® (Novartis) ⒫ℴⓜ

Tablets, off-white, scored, terbinafine (as hydrochloride) 250 mg, net price 14-tab pack = £21.30, 28-tab pack = £41.09. Label: 9

5.3 Antiviral drugs

5.3.1	**HIV infection**
5.3.2	**Herpesvirus infections**
5.3.3	**Viral hepatitis**
5.3.4	**Influenza**
5.3.5	**Respiratory syncytial virus**

The majority of virus infections resolve spontaneously in immunocompetent subjects. A number of specific treatments for viral infections are available, particularly for the immunocompromised. This section includes notes on herpes simplex and varicella-zoster, human immunodeficiency virus, cytomegalovirus, respiratory syncytial virus, viral hepatitis and influenza.

5.3.1 HIV infection

There is no cure for infection caused by the human immunodeficiency virus (HIV) but a number of drugs slow or halt disease progression. Drugs for HIV infection (antiretrovirals) may be associated with serious side-effects. Although antiretrovirals increase life expectancy considerably and decrease the risk of complications associated with premature ageing, mortality and morbidity remain slightly higher than in uninfected individuals. Treatment should be undertaken only by those experienced in their use.

Principles of treatment Treatment aims to prevent the mortality and morbidity associated with chronic HIV infection whilst minimising drug toxicity. Although it should be started before the immune system is irreversibly damaged, the need for early drug treatment should be balanced against the risk of toxicity. Commitment to treatment and strict adherence over many years are required; the regimen chosen should take into account convenience and patient tolerance. The development of drug resistance is reduced by using a combination of drugs; such combinations should have synergistic or additive activity while ensuring that their toxicity is not additive. It is recommended that viral sensitivity to antiretroviral drugs is established before starting treatment or before switching drugs if the infection is not responding.

Treatment also reduces the risk of HIV transmission to sexual partners, but the risk is not eliminated completely; this risk and strategies to reduce HIV transmission should be discussed with patients and their sexual partners.

Initiation of treatment The optimum time for initiating antiretroviral treatment depends primarily on the CD4 cell count. The timing and choice of treatment should also take account of clinical symptoms, co-morbidities, and the possible effect of antiretroviral drugs on factors such as the risk of cardiovascular events. Treatment includes a combination of drugs known as 'highly active antiretroviral therapy'. Treatment of HIV-1 infection is initiated with 2 nucleoside reverse transcriptase inhibitors and *either* a non-nucleoside reverse transcriptase inhibitor, *or* a boosted protease inhibitor, *or* an integrase inhibitor; the regimens of choice contain tenofovir and emtricitabine with *either* efavirenz *or* ritonavir-boosted atazanavir, *or* ritonavir-boosted darunavir, *or* raltegravir. Alternative regimens contain abacavir and lamivudine with *either* ritonavir-boosted lopinavir, *or* ritonavir-boosted fosamprenavir, *or* nevirapine, *or* rilpivirine. Patients who require treatment for both HIV and chronic hepatitis B should be treated with antivirals active against both diseases (section 5.3.3.1).

Switching therapy Deterioration of the condition (including clinical and virological changes) may require a change in therapy. The choice of an alternative regimen depends on factors such as the response to previous treatment, tolerance and the possibility of cross-resistance.

Pregnancy Treatment of HIV infection in pregnancy aims to reduce the risk of toxicity to the fetus (although information on the teratogenic potential of most antiretroviral drugs is limited), to minimise the viral load and disease progression in the mother, and to prevent transmission of infection to the neonate. **All treatment options require careful assessment by a specialist.** Combination antiretroviral therapy maximises the chance of preventing transmission and represents optimal therapy for the mother. However, it may be associated with a greater risk of preterm delivery. Pregnancies in HIV-positive women and babies born to them should be reported prospectively to the National Study of HIV in Pregnancy and Childhood at www.nshpc.ucl.ac.uk **and** to the Antiretroviral Pregnancy Registry at www.apregistry.com.

Mitochondrial dysfunction has been reported in infants exposed to nucleoside reverse transcriptase inhibitors in utero; the main effects include haematological, metabolic, and neurological disorders; all infants whose mothers received nucleoside reverse transcriptase inhibitors during pregnancy should be monitored for relevant signs or symptoms.

Breast-feeding Breast-feeding by HIV-positive mothers may cause HIV infection in the infant and should be avoided.

Children HIV disease in children has a different natural progression to adults. Children infected with HIV should be managed within a formal paediatric HIV clinical network by specialists with access to guidelines and information on antiretroviral drugs for children.

Post-exposure prophylaxis Prophylaxis with antiretroviral drugs [unlicensed indication] may be appropriate following exposure to HIV-contaminated material. Immediate expert advice should be sought in such cases; national guidelines on post-exposure prophylaxis for healthcare workers have been developed (by the Chief Medical Officer's Expert Advisory Group on AIDS, www.gov.uk/dh) and local ones may also be available. Antiretrovirals for prophylaxis are chosen on the basis of efficacy and potential for toxicity. Prompt prophylaxis with antiretroviral drugs [unlicensed indication] is also appropriate following potential sexual exposure to HIV; recommendations have been developed by the British Association for Sexual Health and HIV, www.bashh.org

Drugs for HIV infection Zidovudine, a nucleoside reverse transcriptase inhibitor (or 'nucleoside analogue'), was the first anti-HIV drug to be introduced. Other nucleoside reverse transcriptase inhibitors include **abacavir, didanosine, emtricitabine, lamivudine, stavudine,** and **tenofovir.**

The protease inhibitors include **atazanavir, darunavir, fosamprenavir** (a pro-drug of amprenavir), **indinavir, lopinavir, ritonavir, saquinavir,** and **tipranavir.** Indinavir is rarely used in the treatment of HIV-infection because it is associated with nephrolithiasis. Ritonavir in low doses boosts the activity of atazanavir, darunavir, fosamprenavir, indinavir, lopinavir, saquinavir, and tipranavir increasing the persistence of plasma concentrations of these drugs; at such a low dose, ritonavir has no intrinsic antiviral activity. A combination of lopinavir with low-dose ritonavir is available. The protease inhibitors are metabolised by cytochrome P450 enzyme systems and therefore have a significant potential for drug interactions. Protease inhibitors are associated with lipodystrophy and metabolic effects (see below).

5 Infections

The non-nucleoside reverse transcriptase inhibitors **efavirenz**, **etravirine**, **nevirapine**, and **rilpivirine** are used in the treatment of HIV-1 infection, but not against the subtype HIV-2, a subtype that is rare in the UK. Nevirapine is associated with a high incidence of rash (including Stevens-Johnson syndrome) and occasionally fatal hepatitis. Rash is also associated with efavirenz and etravirine but it is usually milder. Psychiatric or CNS disturbances are common with efavirenz; CNS disturbances are often self-limiting and can be reduced by taking the dose at bedtime (especially in the first 2–4 weeks of treatment). Efavirenz has also been associated with an increased plasma-cholesterol concentration. Etravirine is used in regimens containing a boosted protease inhibitor for HIV infection resistant to other non-nucleoside reverse transcriptase inhibitors and protease inhibitors.

Enfuvirtide, which inhibits the fusion of HIV to the host cell, is licensed for managing infection that has failed to respond to a regimen of other antiretroviral drugs; enfuvirtide should be combined with other potentially active antiretroviral drugs.

Maraviroc is an antagonist of the CCR5 chemokine receptor. It is licensed for patients exclusively infected with CCR5-tropic HIV. The *Scottish Medicines Consortium* (p. 4) has advised (March 2008) that maraviroc (*Celsentri*®) is **not** recommended for use within NHS Scotland.

Dolutegravir and **raltegravir** are inhibitors of HIV integrase. They are licensed for the treatment of HIV infection in combination with other antiretroviral drugs. The *Scottish Medicines Consortium* (p. 4) has advised (April 2010) that raltegravir (*Isentress*®) is accepted for restricted use within NHS Scotland for the treatment of HIV infection when non-nucleoside reverse transcriptase inhibitors or protease inhibitors cannot be used because of intolerance, drug interactions, or resistance.

Elvitegravir is also an inhibitor of HIV integrase that is only available as a component of a fixed-dose combination product containing **cobicistat**, emtricitabine, and tenofovir disoproxil.

Cobicistat is a pharmacokinetic enhancer that boosts the concentrations of other antiretrovirals, but it has no antiretroviral activity itself.

Immune reconstitution syndrome Improvement in immune function as a result of antiretroviral treatment may provoke a marked inflammatory reaction against residual opportunistic organisms; these reactions may occur within the first few weeks or months of initiating treatment. Autoimmune disorders (such as Graves' disease) have also been reported many months after initiation of treatment.

Lipodystrophy syndrome Metabolic effects associated with antiretroviral treatment include *fat redistribution*, *insulin resistance*, and *dyslipidaemia*; collectively these have been termed *lipodystrophy syndrome*. The usual risk factors for cardiovascular disease should be taken into account before starting antiretroviral therapy and patients should be advised about lifestyle changes to reduce their cardiovascular risk. Plasma lipids and blood glucose should be measured before starting antiretroviral therapy, after 3–6 months of treatment, and then annually.

Fat redistribution (with loss of subcutaneous fat, increased abdominal fat, 'buffalo hump' and breast enlargement) is associated with regimens containing protease inhibitors and nucleoside reverse transcriptase inhibitors. Stavudine (especially in combination with didanosine), and to a lesser extent zidovudine, are associated with a higher risk of lipoatrophy and should be used only if alternative regimens are not suitable.

Dyslipidaemia is associated with antiretroviral treatment, particularly with protease inhibitors. Protease inhibitors and some nucleoside reverse transcriptase inhibitors are associated with insulin resistance and hyperglycaemia. Of the protease inhibitors, atazanavir and darunavir may be less likely to cause dyslipidaemia, while saquinavir and atazanavir may be less likely to impair glucose tolerance.

Osteonecrosis Osteonecrosis has been reported in patients with advanced HIV disease or following long-term exposure to combination antiretroviral therapy.

Nucleoside reverse transcriptase inhibitors

Cautions

Lactic acidosis Life-threatening lactic acidosis associated with hepatomegaly and hepatic steatosis has been reported with nucleoside reverse transcriptase inhibitors. They should be used with caution in patients (particularly obese women) with hepatomegaly, hepatitis (especially hepatitis C treated with interferon alfa and ribavirin), liver-enzyme abnormalities and with other risk factors for liver disease and hepatic steatosis (including alcohol abuse). Treatment with the nucleoside reverse transcriptase inhibitor should be **discontinued** in case of symptomatic hyperlactataemia, lactic acidosis, progressive hepatomegaly or rapid deterioration of liver function. Stavudine, especially with didanosine, is associated with a higher risk of lactic acidosis and should be used only if alternative regimens are not suitable.

Hepatic impairment Nucleoside reverse transcriptase inhibitors should be used with caution in patients with chronic hepatitis B or C (greater risk of hepatic side-effects); see also Lactic acidosis above.

Pregnancy see p. 419

Breast-feeding see p. 419

Side-effects Side-effects of the nucleoside reverse transcriptase inhibitors include gastro-intestinal disturbances (such as nausea, vomiting, abdominal pain, flatulence and diarrhoea), anorexia, pancreatitis, liver damage (see also Lactic Acidosis, above), dyspnoea, cough, headache, insomnia, dizziness, fatigue, blood disorders (including anaemia, neutropenia, and thrombocytopenia), myalgia, arthralgia, rash, urticaria, and fever. See notes above for metabolic effects and lipodystrophy (Lipodystrophy Syndrome), and Osteonecrosis.

◢ ABACAVIR

Indications HIV infection in combination with other antiretroviral drugs

Cautions see notes above; also test for HLA-B*5701 allele before treatment or if restarting treatment and HLA-B*5701 status not known—increased risk of hypersensitivity reaction in presence of HLA-B*5701 allele; HIV load greater than 100 000 copies/mL; patients at high risk of cardiovascular disease (espe-

5 Infections *(vertical side tab)*

cially if 10-year cardiovascular risk greater than 20%);
interactions: Appendix 1 (abacavir)

Hypersensitivity reactions Life-threatening hypersensitivity reactions reported—characterised by fever or rash and possibly nausea, vomiting, diarrhoea, abdominal pain, dyspnoea, cough, lethargy, malaise, headache, and myalgia; less frequently mouth ulceration, oedema, hypotension, sore throat, acute respiratory distress syndrome, anaphylaxIs, paraesthesia, arthralgia, conjunctivitis, lymphadenopathy, lymphocytopenia and renal failure; rarely myolysis; laboratory abnormalities may include raised liver function tests (see Lactic Acidosis p. 420) and creatine kinase; symptoms usually appear in the first 6 weeks, but may occur at any time; monitor for symptoms every 2 weeks for 2 months; discontinue immediately if any symptom of hypersensitivity develops and do not rechallenge (risk of more severe hypersensitivity reaction); discontinue if hypersensitivity cannot be ruled out, even when other diagnoses possible—if rechallenge necessary it must be carried out in hospital setting; if abacavir is stopped for any reason other than hypersensitivity, exclude hypersensitivity reaction as the cause and rechallenge only if medical assistance is readily available; care needed with concomitant use of drugs which cause skin toxicity

Counselling Patients should be told the importance of regular dosing (intermittent therapy may increase the risk of sensitisation), how to recognise signs of hypersensitivity, and advised to seek immediate medical attention if symptoms develop or before re-starting treatment; patients should be advised to keep Alert Card with them at all times

Hepatic impairment see notes above; monitor closely in mild impairment (combination preparations not recommended as reduced abacavir dose may be required); avoid in moderate impairment unless essential—close monitoring recommended; avoid in severe impairment

Renal impairment manufacturer advises avoid in end-stage renal disease; avoid *Kivexa*®, *Triumeq*® or *Trizivir*® if eGFR less than 50 mL/minute/1.73 m² (consult product literature)

Pregnancy see p. 419

Breast-feeding see p. 419

Side-effects see notes above; also hypersensitivity reactions (see above); *very rarely* Stevens-Johnson syndrome and toxic epidermal necrolysis; rash and gastro-intestinal disturbances more common in children

Dose
- 600 mg daily in 1–2 divided doses; CHILD 3 months–18 years see *BNF for Children*

Ziagen® (ViiV) [PoM]
Tablets, yellow, f/c, scored, abacavir (as sulfate) 300 mg, net price 60-tab pack = £177.60. Counselling, hypersensitivity reactions
Oral solution, sugar-free, banana and strawberry flavoured, abacavir (as sulfate) 20 mg/mL, net price 240-mL = £47.36. Counselling, hypersensitivity reactions

◢**With lamivudine**
For **cautions, contra-indications, side-effects**, and other prescribing information see under individual drugs

Kivexa® (ViiV) [PoM]
Tablets, orange, f/c, abacavir (as sulfate) 600 mg, lamivudine 300 mg, net price 30-tab pack = £299.41. Counselling, hypersensitivity reactions
Dose ADULT body-weight over 40 kg, 1 tablet once daily; CHILD 12–18 years see *BNF for Children*

◢**With lamivudine and zidovudine**
Note For patients stabilised (for 6–8 weeks) on the individual components in the same proportions. For **cautions, contra-indications, side-effects**, and other prescribing information see under individual drugs

Trizivir® (ViiV) [PoM]
Tablets, blue-green, f/c, abacavir (as sulfate) 300 mg, lamivudine 150 mg, zidovudine 300 mg, net price 60-tab pack = £432.70. Counselling, hypersensitivity reactions
Dose 1 tablet twice daily; CHILD under 18 years, body-weight over 30 kg see *BNF for Children*

◢**With lamivudine and dolutegravir**
For **cautions, contra-indications, side-effects**, and other prescribing information see under individual drugs

Triumeq® (ViiV) ▼ [PoM]
Tablet, purple, f/c, abacavir (as sulfate) 600 mg, dolutegravir (as sodium) 50 mg, lamivudine 300 mg, net price 30-tab pack = £798.16. Counselling, hypersensitivity reactions
Dose HIV infection, ADULT over 18 years and body-weight over 40 kg, 1 tablet once daily; CHILD 12–18 years and body-weight over 40 kg see *BNF for Children*
Missed dose If a dose is more than 20 hours late, the missed dose should not be taken and the next dose should be taken at the normal time

DIDANOSINE
(ddI, DDI)

Indications HIV infection in combination with other antiretroviral drugs

Cautions see notes above; also history of pancreatitis (preferably avoid, otherwise extreme caution, see also below); peripheral neuropathy or hyperuricaemia (see under Side-effects); ophthalmological examination (including visual acuity, colour vision, and dilated fundus examination) recommended annually or if visual changes occur; **interactions:** Appendix 1 (didanosine)

Pancreatitis Suspend treatment if serum lipase raised (even if asymptomatic) or if symptoms of pancreatitis develop; discontinue if pancreatitis confirmed. Whenever possible avoid concomitant treatment with other drugs known to cause pancreatic toxicity (e.g. intravenous pentamidine isetionate); monitor closely if concomitant therapy unavoidable. Since significant elevations of triglycerides cause pancreatitis monitor closely if elevated

Hepatic impairment see notes above; also insufficient information but monitor for toxicity

Renal impairment reduce dose if eGFR less than 60 mL/minute/1.73 m²; consult product literature

Pregnancy manufacturer advises use only if potential benefit outweighs risk

Breast-feeding see p. 419

Side-effects see notes above; also pancreatitis (see also under Cautions), liver failure, non-cirrhotic portal hypertension, anaphylactic reactions, peripheral neuropathy (switch to another antiretroviral if peripheral neuropathy develops), diabetes mellitus, hypoglycaemia, acute renal failure, rhabdomyolysis, dry eyes, retinal and optic nerve changes, dry mouth, parotid gland enlargement, sialadenitis, alopecia, hyperuricaemia (suspend if raised significantly)

Dose
- ADULT under 60 kg, 250 mg daily in 1–2 divided doses; 60 kg and over, 400 mg daily in 1–2 divided doses; CHILD under 18 years see *BNF for Children*

Videx® (Bristol-Myers Squibb) [PoM]
Tablets, with calcium and magnesium antacids, didanosine 25 mg, net price 60-tab pack = £25.06. Label: 23, counselling, administration, see below
Excipients include aspartame equivalent to phenylalanine 36.5 mg per tablet (section 9.4.1)
Note Antacids in formulation may affect absorption of other drugs—see **interactions:** Appendix 1 (antacids)

Counselling To ensure sufficient antacid, each dose to be taken as at least 2 tablets chewed thoroughly, crushed or dispersed in water; clear apple juice may be added for flavouring; tablets to be taken 2 hours after lopinavir with ritonavir capsules and oral solution or atazanavir with ritonavir

Videx® EC capsules, enclosing e/c granules, didanosine 125 mg, net price 30-cap pack = £48.18; 200 mg, 30-cap pack = £77.09; 250 mg, 30-cap pack = £96.37; 400 mg, 30-cap pack = £154.19. Label: 25, counselling, administration, see below

Counselling Capsules to be taken at least 2 hours before or 2 hours after food

EMTRICITABINE
(FTC)

Indications HIV infection in combination with other antiretroviral drugs

Cautions see notes above; also on discontinuation, monitor patients with hepatitis B (risk of exacerbation of hepatitis); **interactions:** Appendix 1 (emtricitabine)

Hepatic impairment see notes above and Cautions above

Renal impairment reduce dose if eGFR less than 50 mL/minute/1.73 m^2; consult product literature

Pregnancy see p. 419

Breast-feeding see p. 419

Side-effects see notes above; also abnormal dreams, pruritus, and hyperpigmentation

Dose
• See preparations

Emtriva® (Gilead) PoM

Capsules, white/blue, emtricitabine 200 mg, net price 30-cap pack = £138.98

Dose 200 mg once daily; CHILD body-weight over 33 kg see BNF for Children

Oral solution, orange, emtricitabine 10 mg/mL, net price 170-mL pack (candy-flavoured) = £39.53

Electrolytes Na⁺ 460 micromol/mL

Dose 240 mg once daily; CHILD 4 months–18 years see BNF for Children

Note 240 mg oral solution ≡ 200 mg capsule; where appropriate the capsule may be used instead of the oral solution

Missed dose If a dose is more than 12 hours late, the missed dose should not be taken and the next dose should be taken at the normal time

◢ With tenofovir
See under Tenofovir

◢ With efavirenz and tenofovir
See under Tenofovir

◢ With rilpivirine and tenofovir
See under Tenofovir

◢ With cobicistat, elvitegravir, and tenofovir
See under Tenofovir

LAMIVUDINE
(3TC)

Indications see preparations below

Cautions see notes above; **interactions:** Appendix 1 (lamivudine)

Chronic hepatitis B Recurrent hepatitis in patients with chronic hepatitis B may occur on discontinuation of lamivudine. When treating chronic hepatitis B with lamivudine, monitor liver function tests every 3 months, and viral markers of hepatitis B every 3–6 months, more frequently in patients with advanced liver disease or following transplantation (monitoring to continue for at least 1 year after discontinuation)

Hepatic impairment see notes above and Cautions above

Renal impairment reduce dose if eGFR less than 50 mL/minute/1.73 m^2; consult product literature

Pregnancy see p. 419

Breast-feeding can be used with caution in women infected with chronic hepatitis B alone, providing that adequate measures are taken to prevent hepatitis B infection in infants; for women infected with HIV, see p. 419

Side-effects see notes above; also peripheral neuropathy, muscle disorders including rhabdomyolysis, nasal symptoms, alopecia

Dose
• See preparations below

Epivir® (ViiV) PoM

Tablets, f/c, lamivudine 150 mg (scored, white), net price 60-tab pack = £121.82; 300 mg (grey), 30-tab pack = £133.89

Oral solution, banana- and strawberry-flavoured, lamivudine 50 mg/5 mL, net price 240-mL pack = £33.16

Excipients include sucrose 1 g/5 mL

Dose HIV infection in combination with other antiretroviral drugs, 150 mg every 12 hours or 300 mg once daily; CHILD 1 month–18 years see BNF for Children

Zeffix® (ViiV) PoM

Tablets, brown, f/c, lamivudine 100 mg, net price 28-tab pack = £78.09

Dose chronic hepatitis B infection either with compensated liver disease (with evidence of viral replication and histology of active liver inflammation or fibrosis) when first-line treatments cannot be used, or (in combination with another antiviral drug without cross-resistance to lamivudine) with decompensated liver disease, 100 mg daily; CHILD [unlicensed indication] 2–11 years, 3 mg/kg once daily (max. 100 mg daily); 12–17 years, adult dose

Note Patients receiving lamivudine for concomitant HIV infection should continue to receive lamivudine in a dose appropriate for HIV infection

◢ With abacavir
See under Abacavir

◢ With zidovudine
See under Zidovudine

◢ With abacavir and zidovudine
See under Abacavir

◢ With abacavir and dolutegravir
See under Abacavir

STAVUDINE
(d4T)

Indications HIV infection in combination with other antiretroviral drugs when no suitable alternative available and when prescribed for shortest period possible

Cautions see notes above; also history of peripheral neuropathy, excessive alcohol intake, concomitant use of isoniazid—risk of peripheral neuropathy (see under Side-effects); history of pancreatitis or concomitant use with other drugs associated with pancreatitis; **interactions:** Appendix 1 (stavudine)

Hepatic impairment see notes above

Renal impairment risk of peripheral neuropathy; use half normal dose every 12 hours if eGFR 25–50 mL/minute/1.73 m^2; use half normal dose every 24 hours if eGFR less than 25 mL/minute/1.73 m^2

Pregnancy manufacturer advises use only if potential benefit outweighs risk

Breast-feeding see p. 419

Side-effects see notes above; also peripheral neuropathy (switch to another antiretroviral if peripheral neuropathy develops), abnormal dreams, cognitive dysfunction, drowsiness, depression, pruritus; *less commonly* anxiety, gynaecomastia

Dose

- ADULT under 60 kg, 30 mg every 12 hours preferably at least 1 hour before food; 60 kg and over, 40 mg every 12 hours; CHILD 1 month–18 years see *BNF for Children*

Zerit® (Bristol-Myers Squibb) [PoM] ▰

Capsules, stavudine 20 mg (brown), net price 56-cap pack = £139.46; 30 mg (light orange/dark orange), 56-cap pack = £146.25; 40 mg (dark orange), 56-cap pack = £150.66 (all hosp. only)

Oral solution, cherry-flavoured, stavudine for reconstitution with water, 1 mg/mL, net price 200 mL = £22.94

◼ TENOFOVIR DISOPROXIL

Indications HIV infection in combination with other antiretroviral drugs; chronic hepatitis B infection with *either* compensated liver disease (with evidence of viral replication, and histologically documented active liver inflammation or fibrosis) *or* decompensated liver disease

Cautions see notes above; also test renal function and serum phosphate before treatment, then every 4 weeks (more frequently if at increased risk of renal impairment) for 1 year and then every 3 months, interrupt treatment if renal function deteriorates or serum phosphate decreases; concomitant or recent use of nephrotoxic drugs; **interactions**: Appendix 1 (tenofovir)

Chronic hepatitis B When treating chronic hepatitis B with tenofovir, monitor liver function tests every 3 months and viral markers for hepatitis B every 3–6 months during treatment (continue monitoring for at least 1 year after discontinuation—recurrent hepatitis may occur on discontinuation)

Hepatic impairment see notes above and Cautions above; manufacturer of *Atripla*® advises caution in mild impairment; avoid *Atripla*® in moderate to severe impairment; manufacturer of *Eviplera*® advises caution in moderate impairment; avoid *Eviplera*® or *Stribild*® in severe impairment

Renal impairment monitor renal function—interrupt treatment if further deterioration.

Granules: 132 mg once daily if eGFR 30–50 mL/minute/1.73 m^2; 66 mg once daily if eGFR 20–30 mL/minute/1.73 m^2; 33 mg once daily if eGFR 10–20 mL/minute/1.73 m^2.

Tablets: 245 mg every 2 days if eGFR 30–50 mL/minute/1.73 m^2; 245 mg every 3–4 days if eGFR 10–30 mL/minute/1.73 m^2.

Avoid *Atripla*® if eGFR less than 50 mL/minute/1.73 m^2; avoid *Eviplera*® if eGFR less than 50 mL/minute/1.73m^2; use normal dose of *Truvada*® every 2 days if eGFR 30–50 mL/minute/1.73 m^2; avoid *Truvada*® if eGFR less than 30 mL/minute/1.73 m^2; if eGFR less than 90 mL/minute/1.73 m^2, only *initiate Stribild*® if other treatments cannot be used (avoid *initiating Stribild*® if eGFR less than 70 mL/minute/1.73 m^2); if eGFR less than 70 mL/minute/1.73 m^2, only *continue Stribild*® if potential benefit outweighs risk (discontinue *Stribild*® if eGFR less than 50 mL/minute/1.73 m^2)

Pregnancy see p. 419

Breast-feeding see p. 419

Side-effects see notes above; also hypophosphataemia; *rarely* renal failure, proximal renal tubulopathy, nephrogenic diabetes insipidus; also reported reduced bone density

Dose

- ADULT over 18 years, 245 mg once daily; CHILD 2–18 years see *BNF for Children*

Missed dose If a dose is more than 12 hours late, the missed dose should not be taken and the next dose should be taken at the normal time

Viread® (Gilead) [PoM]

Tablets, f/c, blue, tenofovir disoproxil (as fumarate) 245 mg, net price 30-tab pack = £204.39. Label: 21

Granules, sugar-free, tenofovir disoproxil (as fumarate) 33 mg/g, net price 60 g (with 1-g scoop) = £54.50. Label: 21, counselling, administration

Note 7.5 scoops of granules contains approx. 245 mg tenofovir disoproxil (as fumarate)

Counselling Mix 1 scoop of granules with 1 tablespoon of soft food (e.g. yoghurt, apple sauce) and take immediately without chewing. Do **not** mix granules with liquids

◢With emtricitabine

For **cautions**, **contra-indications**, **side-effects**, and other prescribing information see under individual drugs

Truvada® (Gilead) [PoM]

Tablets, blue, f/c, tenofovir disoproxil (as fumarate) 245 mg, emtricitabine 200 mg, net price 30-tab pack = £355.73. Label: 21, counselling, administration

Counselling Patients with swallowing difficulties may disperse tablet in half a glass of water, orange juice, or grape juice (but bitter taste)

Dose HIV infection in combination with other antiretroviral drugs, ADULT over 18 years, 1 tablet once daily

Missed dose If a dose is more than 12 hours late, the missed dose should not be taken and the next dose should be taken at the normal time

◢With efavirenz and emtricitabine

For **cautions**, **contra-indications**, **side-effects**, and other prescribing information see under individual drugs

Atripla® (Gilead) [PoM]

Tablets, pink, f/c, efavirenz 600 mg, emtricitabine 200 mg, tenofovir disoproxil (as fumarate) 245 mg, net price 30-tab pack = £532.87. Label: 23, 25

Dose HIV infection stabilised on antiretroviral therapy for more than 3 months, ADULT over 18 years, 1 tablet once daily

Missed dose If a dose is more than 12 hours late, the missed dose should not be taken and the next dose should be taken at the normal time

◢With emtricitabine and rilpivirine

For **cautions**, **contra-indications**, **side-effects**, and other prescribing information see under individual drugs

Eviplera® (Gilead) ▼ [PoM]

Tablets, purple-pink, f/c, emtricitabine 200 mg, rilpivirine (as hydrochloride) 25 mg, tenofovir disoproxil (as fumarate) 245 mg, net price 30-tab pack = £525.95. Label: 21, 25, counselling, antacids

Counselling avoid antacids 2 hours before or 4 hours after taking *Eviplera*®

Dose HIV infection in patients with plasma HIV-1 RNA concentration less than 100 000 copies/mL, ADULT over 18 years, 1 tablet once daily

Missed dose If a dose is more than 12 hours late, the missed dose should not be taken and the next dose should be taken at the normal time

◢With cobicistat, elvitegravir, and emtricitabine

Stribild® (Gilead) ▼ PoM

Tablets, green, f/c, cobicistat 150 mg, elvitegravir 150 mg, emtricitabine 200 mg, tenofovir disoproxil (as fumarate) 245 mg, net price 30-tab pack = £1034.72. Label: 21, counselling, antacids

Counselling Avoid antacids 4 hours before or 4 hours after taking *Stribild®*

Cautions see notes above and also Cautions under Emtricitabine and Tenofovir Disoproxil; also test urine glucose before treatment, then every 4 weeks for 1 year and then every 3 months; women of child-bearing potential should use effective contraception during treatment (if using a hormonal contraceptive, it must contain norgestimate as the progestogen and at least 30 micrograms ethinylestradiol); **interactions**: Appendix 1 (cobicistat, elvitegravir, emtricitabine, and tenofovir)

Hepatic impairment see notes above and also Cautions under Tenofovir Disoproxil

Renal impairment see Tenofovir Disoproxil

Pregnancy see also Cautions; manufacturer advises use only if potential benefit outweighs risk

Breast-feeding see p. 419

Side-effects see notes above and also Side-effects under Emtricitabine and Tenofovir Disoproxil; also *less commonly* depression and suicidal ideation (in patients with history of psychiatric illness)

Dose HIV infection, ADULT over 18 years, 1 tablet once daily

Missed dose If a dose is more than 18 hours late, the missed dose should not be taken and the next dose should be taken at the normal time

Note Dispense in original container (contains desiccant)

ZIDOVUDINE

(Azidothymidine, AZT)

Note The abbreviation AZT which is sometimes used for zidovudine has also been used for another drug

Indications HIV infection in combination with other antiretroviral drugs; prevention of maternal-fetal HIV transmission (see notes above under Pregnancy and Breast-feeding)

Cautions see notes above; also haematological toxicity particularly with high dose and advanced disease—monitor full blood count after 4 weeks of treatment, then every 3 months; vitamin B_{12} deficiency (increased risk of neutropenia); if anaemia or myelosuppression occur, reduce dose or interrupt treatment according to product literature, or consider other treatment; elderly; **interactions**: Appendix 1 (zidovudine)

Contra-indications abnormally low neutrophil counts or haemoglobin concentration (consult product literature); neonates with hyperbilirubinaemia requiring treatment other than phototherapy, or with raised transaminase (consult product literature); acute porphyria (section 9.8.2)

Hepatic impairment see notes above; also accumulation may occur

Renal impairment reduce oral dose to 300–400 mg daily in divided doses or intravenous dose to 1 mg/kg 3–4 times daily if eGFR is less than 10 mL/minute/ 1.73 m²; avoid *Combivir®* (or non-proprietary equivalents) if eGFR less than 50 mL/minute/1.73m² (consult product literature)

Pregnancy see p. 419

Breast-feeding see p. 419

Side-effects see notes above; also anaemia (may require transfusion), taste disturbance, chest pain, influenza-like symptoms, paraesthesia, neuropathy, convulsions, dizziness, drowsiness, anxiety, depression, loss of mental acuity, myopathy, gynaecomastia,

urinary frequency, sweating, pruritus, pigmentation of nails, skin and oral mucosa

Dose

● By mouth, 250–300 mg twice daily; CHILD 1 month–18 years see *BNF for Children*

● Prevention of maternal-fetal HIV transmission, seek specialist advice (combination therapy preferred)

● Patients temporarily unable to take zidovudine by mouth, by intravenous infusion over 1 hour, 0.8– 1 mg/kg every 4 hours (approximating to 1.2–1.5 mg/ kg every 4 hours by mouth) usually for not more than 2 weeks; CHILD 3 months–18 years see *BNF for Children*

Zidovudine (Non-proprietary) PoM

Capsules, zidovudine 100 mg, net price 60-cap pack = £50.17; 250 mg, 60-cap pack = £125.44

Retrovir® (ViiV) PoM

Capsules, zidovudine 100 mg (white), net price 100-cap pack = £88.86; 250 mg (blue/white), 40-cap pack = £88.86

Oral solution, sugar-free, strawberry-flavoured, zidovudine 50 mg/5 mL, net price 200-mL pack with 10-mL oral syringe = £17.78

Injection, zidovudine 10 mg/mL. For dilution and use as an intravenous infusion. Net price 20-mL vial = £8.92

◢With lamivudine

For **cautions**, **contra-indications**, **side-effects**, and other prescribing information see under individual drugs

Zidovudine and lamivudine (Non-proprietary) PoM

Tablets, f/c, scored, zidovudine 300 mg, lamivudine 150 mg, net price 60-tab pack = £70.61

Dose 1 tablet twice daily; CHILD body-weight over 14 kg see *BNF for Children*

Combivir® (ViiV) PoM

Tablets, f/c, scored, zidovudine 300 mg, lamivudine 150 mg, net price 60-tab pack = £255.10

Dose 1 tablet twice daily; CHILD body-weight over 14 kg see *BNF for Children*

Note Tablets may be crushed and mixed with semi-solid food or liquid just before administration

◢With abacavir and lamivudine

See under Abacavir

Protease inhibitors

Cautions Protease inhibitors are associated with hyperglycaemia and should be used with caution in diabetes (see Lipodystrophy Syndrome, p. 420). Caution is also needed in patients with haemophilia who may be at increased risk of bleeding.

Contra-indications Protease inhibitors should not be given to patients with acute porphyria (but see section 9.8.2).

Hepatic impairment Protease inhibitors should be used with caution in patients with chronic hepatitis B or C (increased risk of hepatic side-effects)

Pregnancy See p. 419

Breast-feeding See p. 419

Side-effects Side-effects of the protease inhibitors include gastro-intestinal disturbances (including diarrhoea, nausea, vomiting, abdominal pain, flatulence), anorexia, hepatic dysfunction, pancreatitis; blood disorders including anaemia, neutropenia, and thrombocytopenia; sleep disturbances, fatigue, headache, dizziness, paraesthesia, myalgia, myositis, rhabdomyolysis; taste disturbances; rash, pruritus, Stevens-Johnson syndrome, hypersensitivity reactions including anaphylaxis; see also notes above for lipodystrophy and metabolic effects (Lipodystrophy Syndrome), and Osteonecrosis.

ATAZANAVIR

Indications HIV infection in combination with other antiretroviral drugs

Cautions see notes above; also concomitant use with drugs that prolong PR interval; cardiac conduction disorders; predisposition to QT interval prolongation (including electrolyte disturbances, concomitant use of drugs that prolong QT interval); **interactions:** Appendix 1 (atazanavir)

> **Rash** Mild to moderate rash occurs commonly, usually within the first 3 weeks of therapy. Severe rash occurs less frequently and may be accompanied by systemic symptoms. Discontinue if severe rash develops

Contra-indications see notes above

Hepatic impairment see notes above; also manufacturer advises caution in mild impairment; avoid in moderate to severe impairment

Pregnancy see p. 419; monitor viral load and plasma-atazanavir concentration during third trimester; theoretical risk of hyperbilirubinaemia in neonate if used at term

Breast-feeding see p. 419

Side-effects see notes above; also AV block (in children); *less commonly* mouth ulcers, dry mouth, cholelithiasis, hypertension, syncope, chest pain, torsade de pointes, dyspnoea, peripheral neuropathy, abnormal dreams, amnesia, disorientation, depression, anxiety, weight changes, increased appetite, gynaecomastia, nephrolithiasis, urinary frequency, haematuria, proteinuria, arthralgia, and alopecia; *rarely* cholecystitis, hepatosplenomegaly, oedema, palpitation, abnormal gait

Dose

- With cobicistat *or* low-dose ritonavir, 300 mg once daily; CHILD 6–18 years see *BNF for Children*

Reyataz® (Bristol-Myers Squibb) ▼ PoM

> Capsules, atazanavir (as sulfate) 150 mg (dark blue/light blue), net price 60-cap pack = £303.38; 200 mg (dark blue), 60-cap pack = £303.38; 300 mg (red/blue), 30-cap pack = £303.38. Label: 5, 21

DARUNAVIR

Indications HIV infection in combination with other antiretroviral drugs

Cautions see notes above; also sulfonamide sensitivity; monitor liver function before and during treatment; **interactions:** Appendix 1 (darunavir)

> **Rash** Mild to moderate rash occurs commonly, usually within the first 4 weeks of therapy and resolves without stopping treatment. Severe skin rash (including Stevens-Johnson syndrome and toxic epidermal necrolysis) occurs less frequently and may be accompanied by fever, malaise, arthralgia, myalgia, oral lesions, conjunctivitis, hepatitis, or eosinophilia; treatment should be stopped if severe rash develops

Contra-indications see notes above

Hepatic impairment see notes above; also manufacturer advises caution in mild to moderate impairment; avoid in severe impairment—no information available

Pregnancy manufacturer advises use only if potential benefit outweighs risk; if required, use the twice daily dose regimen; see also p. 419

Breast-feeding see p. 419

Side-effects see notes above; also peripheral neuropathy; *less commonly* myocardial infarction, angina, QT interval prolongation, tachycardia, hypertension, flushing, peripheral oedema, dyspnoea, cough, anxiety, memory impairment, depression, abnormal dreams, increased appetite, weight changes, pyrexia, hypothyroidism, osteoporosis, gynaecomastia, erectile dysfunction, reduced libido, dysuria, polyuria, nephrolithiasis, renal failure, arthralgia, dry eyes, conjunctival hyperaemia, throat irritation, dry mouth, stomatitis, nail discoloration, acne, eczema, increased sweating, alopecia; *rarely* haematemesis, syncope, bradycardia, palpitation, confusion, convulsions, visual disturbances, rhinorrhoea, seborrhoeic dermatitis

Dose

- ADULT over 18 years previously treated with antiretroviral therapy, 600 mg twice daily with low-dose ritonavir *or* (if no resistance to darunavir, if plasma HIV-RNA concentration less than 100 000 copies/mL, and if CD4 cell count greater than 100 cells × 10^6/litre) 800 mg once daily with cobicistat or with low-dose ritonavir; CHILD 3–18 years see *BNF for Children*

- ADULT over 18 years not previously treated with antiretroviral therapy, 800 mg once daily with cobicistat or with low-dose ritonavir; CHILD 12–18 years see *BNF for Children*

Missed dose If a dose is more than 6 hours late on the twice daily regimen (or more than 12 hours late on the once daily regimen), the missed dose should not be taken and the next dose should be taken at the normal time

Prezista® (Janssen) PoM

> Tablets, f/c, darunavir (as ethanolate) 75 mg (white), net price 480-tab pack = £446.70; 150 mg (white), 240-tab pack = £446.70; 400 mg (light orange), 60-tab pack = £297.80; 600 mg (orange), 60-tab pack = £446.70; 800 mg (red), 30-tab pack = £297.80. Label: 21

> Oral suspension, sugar-free, strawberry-flavoured, darunavir (as ethanolate) 100 mg/mL, net price 200-mL = £248.17. Label: 21

FOSAMPRENAVIR

Note Fosamprenavir is a pro-drug of amprenavir

Indications HIV infection in combination with other antiretroviral drugs

Cautions see notes above; **interactions:** Appendix 1 (fosamprenavir)

> **Rash** Rash may occur, usually in the second week of therapy; discontinue permanently if severe rash with systemic or allergic symptoms or, mucosal involvement; if rash mild or moderate, may continue without interruption—usually resolves within 2 weeks and may respond to antihistamines

Contra-indications see notes above

Hepatic impairment see notes above; also manufacturer advises caution in mild impairment; reduce dose to 450 mg twice daily in moderate impairment; reduce dose to 300 mg twice daily in severe impairment

Pregnancy toxicity in *animal* studies; manufacturer advises use only if potential benefit outweighs risk

Breast-feeding see p. 419

Side-effects see notes above; also reported, rash including rarely Stevens-Johnson syndrome (see also Rash above)

5 Infections

Dose

- With low-dose ritonavir, 700 mg twice daily; CHILD 6–18 years see *BNF for Children*

  Note 700 mg fosamprenavir is equivalent to approx. 600 mg amprenavir

Telzir® (ViiV) [PoM]

Tablets, f/c, pink, fosamprenavir (as calcium) 700 mg, net price 60-tab pack = £220.13

Oral suspension, fosamprenavir (as calcium) 50 mg/mL, net price 225-mL pack (grape-bubblegum-and peppermint-flavoured) (with 10-mL oral syringe) = £58.70. Counselling, administration

Counselling In adults, oral suspension should be taken on an empty stomach

---

◣ INDINAVIR ◢

Indications HIV infection in combination with nucleoside reverse transcriptase inhibitors

Cautions see notes above; also ensure adequate hydration (risk of nephrolithiasis); patients at risk of nephrolithiasis (monitor for nephrolithiasis); patients at high risk of cardiovascular disease (especially if 10-year cardiovascular risk greater than 20%); **interactions**: Appendix 1 (indinavir)

Contra-indications see notes above

Hepatic impairment see notes above; also increased risk of nephrolithiasis; reduce dose in mild to moderate impairment; not studied in severe impairment

Renal impairment use with caution; monitor for nephrolithiasis

Pregnancy toxicity in *animal* studies; manufacturer advises use only if potential benefit outweighs risk; theoretical risk of hyperbilirubinaemia and renal stones in neonate if used at term

Breast-feeding see p. 419

Side-effects see notes above; also reported, dry mouth, hypoaesthesia, dry skin, hyperpigmentation, alopecia, paronychia, interstitial nephritis (with medullary calcification and cortical atrophy in asymptomatic severe leucocyturia), nephrolithiasis (may require interruption or discontinuation), dysuria, haematuria, crystalluria, proteinuria, pyelonephritis; haemolytic anaemia

Dose

- ADULT over 18 years, seek specialist advice

Crixivan® (MSD) [PoM] ◢

Capsules, indinavir (as sulfate), 200 mg, net price 360-cap pack = £181.02; 400 mg, 180-cap pack = £181.02. Label: 27, counselling, administration

Counselling Administer 1 hour before or 2 hours after a meal; may be administered with a low-fat light meal; in combination with didanosine tablets, allow 1 hour between each drug (antacids in didanosine tablets reduce absorption of indinavir); in combination with low-dose ritonavir, give with food

Note Dispense in original container (contains desiccant)

◣ LOPINAVIR WITH RITONAVIR

Indications HIV infection in combination with other antiretroviral drugs

Cautions see notes above; concomitant use with drugs that prolong QT or PR interval; cardiac conduction disorders, structural heart disease; patients at high risk of cardiovascular disease (especially if 10-year cardiovascular risk greater than 20%); pancreatitis

(see below); monitor liver function before and during treatment; **interactions**: Appendix 1 (lopinavir, ritonavir)

Pancreatitis Signs and symptoms suggestive of pancreatitis (including raised serum lipase) should be evaluated—discontinue if pancreatitis diagnosed

Contra-indications see notes above

Hepatic impairment see notes above; also avoid oral solution due to propylene glycol content; manufacturer advises avoid capsules and tablets in severe impairment

Renal impairment avoid oral solution due to propylene glycol content; use tablets with caution in severe impairment

Pregnancy avoid oral solution due to high propylene glycol content; use tablets only if potential benefit outweighs risk (toxicity in *animal* studies); for tablets see also p. 419

Breast-feeding see p. 419

Side-effects see notes above; also colitis, weight changes, hypertension, anxiety, neuropathy, sexual dysfunction, amenorrhoea, menorrhagia, arthralgia, night sweats; *less commonly* gastro-intestinal ulcer, rectal bleeding, dry mouth, stomatitis, myocardial infarction, AV block, cerebrovascular accident, deep vein thrombosis, abnormal dreams, convulsions, tremor, nephritis, haematuria, visual disturbances, tinnitus, alopecia

Dose

- See preparations below

Kaletra® (AbbVie) [PoM]

Tablets, pale yellow, f/c, lopinavir 100 mg, ritonavir 25 mg, net price 60-tab pack = £76.85. Label: 25

Dose CHILD 2–18 years see *BNF for Children*

Tablets, yellow, f/c, lopinavir 200 mg, ritonavir 50 mg, net price 120-tab pack = £285.41. Label: 25

Dose 2 tablets twice daily; alternatively, in adults with a HIV strain that has less than 3 mutations to protease inhibitors, 4 tablets may be taken once daily; CHILD 2–18 years see *BNF for Children*

Oral solution, lopinavir 400 mg, ritonavir 100 mg/5 mL, net price 5 × 60-mL packs = £307.39. Label: 21

Excipients include propylene glycol 153 mg/mL (see Excipients, p. 2), alcohol 42%

Dose 5 mL twice daily with food; CHILD 2–18 years see *BNF for Children*

◣ RITONAVIR

Indications HIV infection in combination with other antiretroviral drugs; low doses used to increase effect of some protease inhibitors

Cautions see notes above; concomitant use with drugs that prolong PR interval; cardiac conduction disorders, structural heart disease; pancreatitis (see below); **interactions**: Appendix 1 (ritonavir)

Pancreatitis Signs and symptoms suggestive of pancreatitis (including raised serum lipase) should be evaluated—discontinue if pancreatitis diagnosed

Contra-indications see notes above

Hepatic impairment see notes above; also avoid in decompensated liver disease; in severe impairment without decompensation, use 'booster' doses with caution (avoid treatment doses)

Pregnancy only use low-dose booster to increase the effect of other protease inhibitors; see also p. 419

Breast-feeding see p. 419

Side-effects see notes and Cautions above; also gastro-intestinal haemorrhage, blood pressure changes, oedema, syncope, flushing, cough, pharyngitis, anxiety, confusion, seizures, peripheral neuropathy, fever, decreased blood thyroxine concentration, menorrhagia, renal impairment, arthralgia, blurred vision, mouth ulcers, acne; *less commonly* myocardial infarction, electrolyte disturbances; *rarely* toxic epidermal necrolysis

Dose
- Initially 300 mg every 12 hours for 3 days, increased in steps of 100 mg every 12 hours over not longer than 14 days to 600 mg every 12 hours; CHILD 2–18 years see *BNF for Children*
- Low-dose booster to increase effect of other protease inhibitors, 100–200 mg once or twice daily; CHILD 2–18 years see *BNF for Children*

Norvir® (AbbVie) PoM
Tablets, f/c, ritonavir 100 mg, net price 30-tab pack = £19.44. Label: 21, 25

Oral solution, sugar-free, ritonavir 400 mg/5 mL, net price 5 × 90-mL packs (with measuring cup) = £403.20. Label: 21, counselling, administration
Excipients include propylene glycol 26% (see Excipients, p. 2), alcohol 43%
Counselling Bitter taste of oral solution can be masked by mixing with chocolate milk; do not mix with water, measuring cup must be dry

◢ **With lopinavir**
See under Lopinavir with Ritonavir

SAQUINAVIR

Indications HIV infection in combination with other antiretroviral drugs

Cautions see notes above; monitor ECG before starting treatment (do not initiate treatment if QT interval over 450 milliseconds); if baseline QT interval less than 450 milliseconds, monitor ECG during treatment (particularly 10 days after starting treatment in patients not previously treated with antiretroviral therapy)—discontinue if QT interval increases over 480 milliseconds, if QT interval more than 20 milliseconds above baseline, if prolongation of PR interval, or if arrhythmias occur; concomitant use of garlic (avoid garlic capsules—reduces plasma-saquinavir concentration); **interactions**: Appendix 1 (saquinavir)
Counselling Patients should be told how to recognise signs of arrhythmia and advised to seek medical attention if symptoms such as palpitation or syncope develop

Contra-indications see notes above; predisposition to cardiac arrhythmias (including congenital QT prolongation, bradycardia, history of symptomatic arrhythmias, heart failure with reduced left ventricular ejection fraction, electrolyte disturbances, concomitant use of drugs that prolong QT or PR interval); concomitant use of drugs that increase plasma-saquinavir concentration (avoid unless no alternative treatment available)

Hepatic impairment see notes above; also manufacturer advises caution in moderate impairment; avoid in decompensated liver disease

Renal impairment use with caution if eGFR less than 30 mL/minute/1.73 m²

Pregnancy see p. 419

Breast-feeding see p. 419

Side-effects see notes above; also dyspnoea, increased appetite, peripheral neuropathy, changes in libido, dry mouth, alopecia; *less commonly* mucosal ulceration, convulsions, renal impairment, visual impairment

Dose
- With low-dose ritonavir, ADULT over 18 years previously treated with antiretroviral therapy, 1 g every 12 hours
- With low-dose ritonavir, ADULT over 18 years not previously treated with antiretroviral therapy, 500 mg every 12 hours for 7 days then 1 g every 12 hours

Invirase® (Roche) PoM
Tablets, orange, f/c, saquinavir (as mesilate) 500 mg, net price 120-tab pack = £251.26. Label: 21, counselling, arrhythmias

TIPRANAVIR

Indications HIV infection resistant to other protease inhibitors, in combination with other antiretroviral drugs in patients previously treated with anti-retrovirals

Cautions see notes above; also patients at risk of increased bleeding from trauma, surgery or other pathological conditions; concomitant use of drugs that increase risk of bleeding; **interactions**: Appendix 1 (tipranavir)
Hepatotoxicity Potentially life-threatening hepatotoxicity reported; monitor liver function before treatment then every 2 weeks for 1 month, then every 3 months. Discontinue if signs or symptoms of hepatitis develop or if liver-function abnormality develops (consult product literature)

Contra-indications see notes above

Hepatic impairment see notes above; also manufacturer advises caution in mild impairment; avoid in moderate or severe impairment—no information available

Pregnancy manufacturer advises use only if potential benefit outweighs risk—toxicity in *animal* studies

Breast-feeding see p. 419

Side-effects see notes above; also dyspnoea, anorexia, peripheral neuropathy, influenza-like symptoms, renal impairment and photosensitivity; *rarely* dehydration

Dose
- See preparations

Aptivus® (Boehringer Ingelheim) PoM
Capsules, pink, tipranavir 250 mg, net price 120–cap pack = £441.00. Label: 5, 21
Excipients include ethanol 100 mg per capsule
Dose with low-dose ritonavir, 500 mg twice daily; CHILD 12–18 years see *BNF for Children*

Oral Solution, toffee-and mint-flavoured, tipranavir 100 mg/mL, net price 95–mL pack = £129.65.
Label: 5, 21, counselling, crystallisation
Excipients include vitamin E 78 mg/mL
Dose with low-dose ritonavir, CHILD 2–12 years see *BNF for Children*

Note The bioavailability of *Aptivus*® oral solution is higher than that of the capsules; the oral solution is **not** interchangeable with the capsules on a milligram-for-milligram basis
Counselling Patients should be told to observe the oral solution for crystallisation; the bottle should be replaced if more than a thin layer of crystals form (doses should continue to be taken at the normal time until the bottle is replaced)

5 **Infections**

Non-nucleoside reverse transcriptase inhibitors

EFAVIRENZ

Indications   HIV infection in combination with other antiretroviral drugs

Cautions   elderly; history of mental illness or seizures; monitor liver function if receiving other hepatotoxic drugs; **interactions**: Appendix 1 (efavirenz)
Rash   Rash, usually in the first 2 weeks, is the most common side-effect; discontinue if severe rash with blistering, desquamation, mucosal involvement or fever; if rash mild or moderate, may continue without interruption—usually resolves within 1 month
Psychiatric disorders   Patients or their carers should be advised to seek immediate medical attention if symptoms such as severe depression, psychosis or suicidal ideation occur

Contra-indications   acute porphyria (but see section 9.8.2)

Hepatic impairment   in mild liver disease, monitor for dose related side-effects (e.g. CNS effects) and monitor liver function; avoid in moderate to severe impairment; greater risk of hepatic side-effects in chronic hepatitis B or C

Renal impairment   manufacturer advises caution in severe renal failure—no information available

Pregnancy   see p. 419; reports of neural tube defects when used in first trimester

Breast-feeding   see p. 419

Side-effects   rash including Stevens-Johnson syndrome (see Rash above); abdominal pain, diarrhoea, nausea, vomiting; anxiety, depression, sleep disturbances, abnormal dreams, dizziness, headache, fatigue, impaired concentration (administration at bedtime especially in first 2–4 weeks reduces CNS effects); pruritus; *less commonly* pancreatitis, hepatitis, flushing, psychosis, mania, suicidal ideation, amnesia, ataxia, tremor, convulsions, gynaecomastia, blurred vision, tinnitus; *rarely* hepatic failure, suicide, photosensitivity; also reported raised serum cholesterol (see Lipodystrophy Syndrome, p. 420); see also Osteonecrosis, p. 420

Dose
● See preparations below

Sustiva® (Bristol-Myers Squibb) [PoM]
Capsules, efavirenz 50 mg (yellow/white), net price 30-cap pack = £16.73; 100 mg (white), 30-cap pack = £33.41; 200 mg (yellow), 90-cap pack = £200.27. Label: 23
Dose   600 mg once daily; CHILD 3–18 years see *BNF for Children*

Tablets, f/c, yellow, efavirenz 600 mg, net price 30-tab pack = £200.27. Label: 23
Dose   600 mg once daily; CHILD body-weight over 40 kg see *BNF for Children*

Oral solution, sugar-free, strawberry and mint flavour, efavirenz 30 mg/mL, net price 180-mL pack = £53.84
Dose   720 mg once daily; CHILD 3–18 years see *BNF for Children*
Note The bioavailability of *Sustiva®* oral solution is lower than that of the capsules and tablets; the oral solution is **not** interchangeable with either capsules or tablets on a milligram-for-milligram basis

◢**With emtricitabine and tenofovir**
See under Tenofovir

ETRAVIRINE

Indications   in combination with other antiretroviral drugs (including a boosted protease inhibitor) for HIV infection resistant to other non-nucleoside reverse transcriptase inhibitors and protease inhibitors

Cautions   **interactions**: Appendix 1 (etravirine)
Hypersensitivity reactions   Rash, usually in the second week, is the most common side-effect and appears more frequently in women. Life-threatening hypersensitivity reactions reported usually during week 3–6 of treatment and characterised by rash, eosinophilia, and systemic symptoms (including fever, general malaise, myalgia, arthralgia, blistering, oral lesions, conjunctivitis, and hepatitis). Discontinue permanently if hypersensitivity reaction or severe rash develop. If rash mild or moderate (without signs of hypersensitivity reaction), may continue without interruption—usually resolves within 2 weeks
Counselling   Patients should be told how to recognise hypersensitivity reactions and advised to seek immediate medical attention if hypersensitivity reaction or severe rash develop

Contra-indications   acute porphyria (but see section 9.8.2)

Hepatic impairment   manufacturer advises caution in moderate impairment; avoid in severe impairment—no information available; greater risk of hepatic side-effects in chronic hepatitis B or C

Pregnancy   see p. 419

Breast-feeding   see p. 419

Side-effects   rash (including Stevens-Johnson syndrome rarely and toxic epidermal necrolysis very rarely; see also Hypersensitivity Reactions above); gastro-oesophageal reflux, nausea, abdominal pain, flatulence, gastritis; myocardial infarction, hypertension; peripheral neuropathy; diabetes, hyperlipidaemia (see also Lipodystrophy Syndrome, p. 420); renal failure; anaemia; *less commonly* pancreatitis, haematemesis, hepatitis, angina, bronchospasm, drowsiness, malaise, gynaecomastia, blurred vision, dry mouth, and sweating; also reported, haemorrhagic stroke and hypersensitivity reactions; see also Osteonecrosis, p. 420

Dose
● 200 mg twice daily after food; CHILD 6–18 years see *BNF for Children*
Missed dose   If a dose is more than 6 hours late, the missed dose should not be taken and the next dose should be taken at the normal time

Intelence® (Janssen) ▼ [PoM]
Tablets, etravirine 100 mg, net price 120-tab pack = £301.27; 200 mg, 60-tab pack = £301.27. Label: 21, counselling, rash and hypersensitivity reactions
Note Dispense in original container (contains desiccant). Patients with swallowing difficulties may disperse tablets in a glass of water just before administration

NEVIRAPINE

Indications   HIV infection in combination with other antiretroviral drugs

Cautions   chronic hepatitis B or C, high CD4 cell count, and women (all at greater risk of hepatic side-effects—if plasma HIV-1 RNA detectable, manufacturer advises avoid in women with CD4 cell count greater than 250 cells/mm^3 or in men with CD4 cell count greater than 400 cells/mm^3 unless potential benefit outweighs risk); **interactions**: Appendix 1 (nevirapine)
Hepatic disease   Potentially life-threatening hepatotoxicity including fatal fulminant hepatitis reported usually in first 6 weeks; close monitoring required during first 18 weeks; monitor liver function before treatment then every 2 weeks

for 2 months then after 1 month and then regularly; discontinue permanently if abnormalities in liver function tests accompanied by hypersensitivity reaction (rash, fever, arthralgia, myalgia, lymphadenopathy, hepatitis, renal impairment, eosinophilia, granulocytopenia); suspend if severe abnormalities in liver function tests but no hypersensitivity reaction—discontinue permanently if significant liver function abnormalities recur; monitor patient closely if mild to moderate abnormalities in liver function tests with no hypersensitivity reaction

Rash Rash, usually in first 6 weeks, is most common side-effect; incidence reduced if introduced at low dose and dose increased after 14 days; monitor closely for skin reactions during first 18 weeks; discontinue permanently if severe rash or if rash accompanied by blistering, oral lesions, conjunctivitis, facial oedema, general malaise or hypersensitivity reactions; if rash mild or moderate may continue without interruption but dose should not be increased until rash resolves

Counselling Patients should be told how to recognise hypersensitivity reactions and advised to discontinue treatment and seek immediate medical attention if severe skin reaction, hypersensitivity reactions, or symptoms of hepatitis develop

Contra-indications acute porphyria (but see section 9.8.2); post-exposure prophylaxis

Hepatic impairment manufacturer advises avoid modified-release preparation—no information available; use 'immediate-release' preparation with caution in moderate impairment and avoid in severe impairment; see also Hepatic Disease, above

Renal impairment manufacturer advises avoid modified-release preparation—no information available

Pregnancy see p. 419

Breast-feeding see p. 419

Side-effects rash including Stevens-Johnson syndrome and toxic epidermal necrolysis (see also Cautions above), nausea, vomiting, abdominal pain, diarrhoea, hepatitis (see also Hepatic Disease above), hypersensitivity reactions (may involve hepatic reactions and rash, see also Hepatic Disease above), headache, fatigue, fever, granulocytopenia; *less commonly* anaemia, myalgia, arthralgia; see also Osteonecrosis, p. 420

Dose

● 200 mg once daily of 'immediate-release' preparation for first 14 days then (if no rash present) 200 mg twice daily of 'immediate-release' preparation or 400 mg once daily of modified-release preparation; CHILD under 18 years see *BNF for children*

Note Duration of once daily dose regimen of 'immediate-release' preparation should not exceed 28 days; if rash not resolved within 28 days, alternative treatment should be sought. If treatment interrupted for more than 7 days, restart using the once daily dose regimen of the 'immediate-release' preparation for the first 14 days as for new treatment

Missed dose If a dose is more than 8 hours late with the 'immediate-release' preparation (or more than 12 hours late with the modified-release preparation), the missed dose should not be taken and the next dose should be taken at the usual time

Nevirapine (Non-proprietary) (PoM)
Tablets, nevirapine 200 mg, net price 60 = £122.00. Counselling, hypersensitivity reactions

Viramune® (Boehringer Ingelheim) (PoM)
Tablets, nevirapine 200 mg, net price 14-tab pack = £39.67, 60-tab pack = £170.00. Counselling, hypersensitivity reactions

Suspension, nevirapine 50 mg/5 mL, net price 240-mL pack = £50.40. Counselling, hypersensitivity reactions

Prolonged-release tablets, m/r, yellow, nevirapine 400 mg, net price 30-tab pack = £170.00. Label: 25, counselling, hypersensitivity reactions

RILPIVIRINE

Indications see preparations below

Cautions concomitant use with drugs that prolong QT interval; **interactions**: Appendix 1 (rilpivirine)

Hepatic impairment manufacturer advises caution in moderate impairment; avoid in severe impairment—no information available; greater risk of hepatic side-effects in chronic hepatitis B or C

Renal impairment manufacturer advises caution in severe impairment

Pregnancy manufacturer advises avoid unless essential—no information available

Breast-feeding see p. 419

Side-effects nausea, vomiting, abdominal pain, anorexia, dry mouth, raised serum amylase and lipase, hyperlipidaemia (see also Lipodystrophy Syndrome, p. 420), depression, abnormal dreams, sleep disturbances, headache, dizziness, malaise, rash; see also Osteonecrosis, p. 420

Dose

● See preparations below

Edurant® (Janssen) ▼ (PoM)
Tablets, f/c, rilpivirine (as hydrochloride) 25 mg, net price 30-tab pack = £200.27. Label: 21, 25, counselling, antacids

Counselling Avoid antacids 2 hours before or 4 hours after taking rilpivirine

Dose HIV infection in combination with other antiretroviral drugs in patients not previously treated with antiretroviral therapy and if plasma HIV-1 RNA concentration less than 100 000 copies/mL, ADULT over 18 years, 25 mg once daily

Missed dose If a dose is more than 12 hours late, the missed dose should not be taken and the next dose should be taken at the normal time

With emtricitabine and tenofovir
See under Tenofovir

Other antiretrovirals

DOLUTEGRAVIR

Indications HIV infection in combination with other antiretroviral drugs

Cautions avoid concomitant use with etravirine, unless used in combination with atazanavir, darunavir, or lopinavir; **interactions**: Appendix 1 (dolutegravir)

Hypersensitivity reactions Hypersensitivity reactions (including severe rash, or rash accompanied by fever, malaise, arthralgia, myalgia, blistering, oral lesions, conjunctivitis, angioedema, eosinophilia, or raised liver enzymes) reported uncommonly. Discontinue immediately if any sign or symptoms of hypersensitivity reactions develop

Hepatic impairment manufacturer advises caution in severe impairment—no information available

Pregnancy manufacturer advises use only if potential benefit outweighs risk

Breast-feeding see p. 419

Side-effects diarrhoea, nausea, vomiting, abdominal pain, flatulence, headache, dizziness, insomnia, abnormal dreams, fatigue, rash, pruritus, raised creatine kinase; *less commonly* hepatitis, hypersensitivity reactions (see Cautions); see also Osteonecrosis, p. 420

Dose

- 50 mg once daily; if resistance to other inhibitors of HIV integrase suspected, 50 mg twice daily with food; CHILD 12–18 years see *BNF for Children*

Note 50 mg twice daily with concomitant efavirenz, nevirapine, tipranavir, or rifampicin, however, avoid concomitant use with these drugs if resistance to other inhibitors of HIV integrase suspected

Missed dose If a dose is more than 20 hours late on the once daily regimen (or more than 8 hours late on the twice daily regimen), the missed dose should not be taken and the next dose should be taken at the normal time

Tivicay® (GSK) ▼ [PoM]

Tablets, yellow, f/c, dolutegravir (as sodium salt) 50 mg, net price 30-tab pack = £498.75. Counselling, antacids

Counselling Avoid antacids 6 hours before or 2 hours after taking dolutegravir

◢**With abacavir and lamivudine**

See under Abacavir

◼ ENFUVIRTIDE

Indications HIV infection in combination with other antiretroviral drugs for resistant infection or for patients intolerant to other antiretroviral regimens

Cautions interactions: Appendix 1 (enfuvirtide)
Hypersensitivity reactions Hypersensitivity reactions including rash, fever, nausea, vomiting, chills, rigors, low blood pressure, respiratory distress, glomerulonephritis, and raised liver enzymes reported; discontinue immediately if any signs or symptoms of systemic hypersensitivity develop and do not rechallenge
Counselling Patients should be told how to recognise signs of hypersensitivity, and advised to discontinue treatment and seek immediate medical attention if symptoms develop

Hepatic impairment manufacturer advises caution— no information available; chronic hepatitis B or C (possibly greater risk of hepatic side-effects)

Pregnancy manufacturer advises use only if potential benefit outweighs risk

Breast-feeding see p. 419

Side-effects injection-site reactions; pancreatitis, gastro-oesophageal reflux disease, anorexia, weight loss; hypertriglyceridaemia; peripheral neuropathy, asthenia, tremor, anxiety, nightmares, irritability, impaired concentration, vertigo; pneumonia, sinusitis, influenza-like illness; diabetes mellitus; haematuria; renal calculi, lymphadenopathy; myalgia; conjunctivitis; dry skin, acne, erythema, skin papilloma; *less commonly* hypersensitivity reactions (see Cautions); see also Osteonecrosis, p. 420

Dose

- By subcutaneous injection, 90 mg twice daily; CHILD 6–18 years see *BNF for Children*

Fuzeon® (Roche) [PoM]

Injection, powder for reconstitution, enfuvirtide 108 mg (= enfuvirtide 90 mg/mL when reconstituted with 1.1 mL Water for Injections), net price 108-mg vial = £18.03 (with solvent, syringe, and alcohol swabs). Counselling, hypersensitivity reactions
Electrolytes Na⁺ < 1 mmol/mL

◼ MARAVIROC

Indications CCR5-tropic HIV infection in combination with other antiretroviral drugs in patients previously treated with antiretrovirals

Cautions cardiovascular disease; chronic hepatitis B or C; **interactions**: Appendix 1 (maraviroc)

Hepatic impairment manufacturer advises caution
Renal impairment if eGFR less than 80 mL/minute/ 1.73 m², consult product literature

Pregnancy manufacturer advises use only if potential benefit outweighs risk—toxicity in *animal* studies

Breast-feeding see p. 419

Side-effects nausea, diarrhoea, abdominal pain, flatulence, anorexia, depression, insomnia, malaise, headache, anaemia, rash; *less commonly* seizures, renal failure, proteinuria, myositis; *rarely* hepatitis, angina, pancytopenia, granulocytopenia, Stevens-Johnson syndrome, toxic epidermal necrolysis; also reported hypersensitivity reactions (including rash, fever, eosinophilia, and hepatic reactions); see also Osteonecrosis, p. 420

Dose

- ADULT over 18 years, 300 mg twice daily

Celsentri® (ViiV) [PoM]

Tablets, blue, f/c, maraviroc, 150 mg, net price 60-tab pack = £441.27; 300 mg, 60-tab pack = £441.27

◼ RALTEGRAVIR

Indications HIV infection in combination with other antiretroviral drugs

Cautions risk factors for myopathy or rhabdomyolysis; chronic hepatitis B or C (greater risk of hepatic side-effects); psychiatric illness (may exacerbate underlying illness including depression); **interactions**: Appendix 1 (raltegravir)
Rash Rash occurs commonly. Discontinue if severe rash or rash accompanied by fever, malaise, arthralgia, myalgia, blistering, mouth ulceration, conjunctivitis, angioedema, hepatitis, or eosinophilia

Hepatic impairment manufacturer advises caution in severe impairment—no information available

Pregnancy manufacturer advises avoid—toxicity in *animal* studies

Breast-feeding see p. 419

Side-effects diarrhoea, nausea, vomiting, dyspepsia, abdominal pain, flatulence, hypertriglyceridaemia, dizziness, headache, depression, insomnia, abnormal dreams, hyperactivity, asthenia, rash (including less commonly Stevens-Johnson syndrome, rash with eosinophilia and systemic symptoms; see also Rash above); *less commonly* gastritis, hepatitis, pancreatitis, dry mouth, taste disturbances, pain on swallowing, peptic ulcer, constipation, rectal bleeding, lipodystrophy (see Lipodystrophy Syndrome, p. 420), palpitation, ventricular extrasystoles, bradycardia, hypertension, flushing, chest pain, oedema, dysphonia, epistaxis, nasal congestion, drowsiness, anxiety, appetite changes, confusion, impaired memory and attention, suicidal ideation, pyrexia, chills, carpal tunnel syndrome, tremor, peripheral neuropathy, erectile dysfunction, gynaecomastia, menopausal symptoms, osteopenia, renal failure, nocturia, polydipsia, anaemia, thrombocytopenia, neutropenia, arthralgia, myalgia, rhabdomyolysis, visual disturbances, tinnitus, gingivitis, glossitis, acne, pruritus, hyperhidrosis, dry skin, skin papilloma, alopecia; see also Osteonecrosis, p. 420

Dose

- 400 mg twice daily; CHILD 2–18 years see *BNF for Children*

Isentress® (MSD) [PoM]

Tablets, pink, f/c, raltegravir (as potassium salt) 400 mg, net price 60-tab pack = £471.41. Label: 25

Pharmacokinetic enhancers of antiretrovirals

▰ COBICISTAT

Indications pharmacokinetic enhancer used to increase the effect of atazanavir or darunavir

Cautions interactions: Appendix 1(cobicistat)

Hepatic impairment manufacturer advises avoid in severe impairment—no information available

Renal impairment no dose adjustment required; inhibits tubular secretion of creatinine; when any co-administered drug requires dose adjustment based on renal function, avoid initiating cobicistat if eGFR less than $70 \, mL/minute/1.73m^2$

Pregnancy manufacturer advises avoid unless essential

Breast-feeding see p. 419

Dose

• With atazanavir or darunavir, ADULT over 18 years, 150 mg once daily

  Missed dose If a dose is more than 12 hours late, the missed dose should not be taken and the next dose should be taken at the normal time

Tybost® (Gilead) ▼ PoM

Tablets, orange, f/c, cobicistat 150 mg, net price 30-tab pack = £21.38 Label: 21

Note dispense in original container (contains desiccant)

◢**With elvitegravir, emtricitabine, and tenofovir**

See under Tenofovir

5.3.2 Herpesvirus infections

5.3.2.1	Herpes simplex and varicella–zoster infection
5.3.2.2	Cytomegalovirus infection

5.3.2.1 Herpes simplex and varicella–zoster infection

The two most important herpesvirus pathogens are herpes simplex virus (herpesvirus hominis) and varicella–zoster virus.

Herpes simplex infections Herpes infection of the mouth and lips and in the eye is generally associated with herpes simplex virus serotype 1 (HSV-1); other areas of the skin may also be infected, especially in immunodeficiency. Genital infection is most often associated with HSV-2 and also HSV-1. Treatment of herpes simplex infection should start as early as possible and usually within 5 days of the appearance of the infection.

In individuals with good immune function, mild infection of the eye (ocular herpes, section 11.3.3) and of the lips (herpes labialis or cold sores, section 13.10.3) is treated with a topical antiviral drug. Primary herpetic gingivostomatitis is managed by changes to diet and with analgesics (section 12.3.2). Severe infection, neonatal herpes infection or infection in immunocompromised individuals requires treatment with a systemic antiviral drug. Primary or recurrent genital herpes simplex infection is treated with an antiviral drug given by mouth. Persistence of a lesion or recurrence in an immunocompromised patient may signal the development of resistance.

Specialist advice should be sought for systemic treatment of herpes simplex infection in pregnancy.

Varicella-zoster infections Regardless of immune function and the use of any immunoglobulins, neonates with *chickenpox* should be treated with a parenteral antiviral to reduce the risk of severe disease. Chickenpox in otherwise healthy children between 1 month and 12 years is usually mild and antiviral treatment is not usually required.

Chickenpox is more severe in adolescents and adults than in children; antiviral treatment started within 24 hours of the onset of rash may reduce the duration and severity of symptoms in otherwise healthy adults and adolescents. Antiviral treatment is generally recommended in immunocompromised patients and those at special risk (e.g. because of severe cardiovascular or respiratory disease or chronic skin disorder); in such cases, an antiviral is given for 10 days with at least 7 days of parenteral treatment.

Pregnant women who develop severe chickenpox may be at risk of complications, especially varicella pneumonia. Specialist advice should be sought for the treatment of chickenpox during pregnancy.

Those who have been exposed to chickenpox and are at special risk of complications may require prophylaxis with varicella-zoster immunoglobulin (see under Disease Specific Immunoglobulins, section 14.5.2).

In *herpes zoster* (shingles) systemic antiviral treatment can reduce the severity and duration of pain, reduce complications, and reduce viral shedding. Treatment with the antiviral should be started within 72 hours of the onset of rash and is usually continued for 7–10 days. Immunocompromised patients at high risk of disseminated or severe infection should be treated with a parenteral antiviral drug.

Chronic pain which persists after the rash has healed (postherpetic neuralgia) requires specific management (section 4.7.3).

Choice Aciclovir is active against herpesviruses but does not eradicate them. Uses of aciclovir include systemic treatment of varicella–zoster and the systemic and topical treatment of herpes simplex infections of the skin (section 13.10.3) and mucous membranes (section 7.2.2). It is used by mouth for severe herpetic stomatitis (see also p. 790). Aciclovir eye ointment (section 11.3.3) is used for herpes simplex infections of the eye; it is combined with systemic treatment for ophthalmic zoster.

Famciclovir, a pro-drug of penciclovir, is similar to aciclovir and is licensed for use in herpes zoster and genital herpes.

Valaciclovir is an ester of aciclovir, licensed for herpes zoster and herpes simplex infections of the skin and mucous membranes (including genital herpes); it is also licensed for preventing cytomegalovirus disease following solid organ transplantation. Famciclovir or valaciclovir are suitable alternatives to aciclovir for oral lesions associated with herpes zoster. Valaciclovir once daily may reduce the risk of transmitting genital herpes to heterosexual partners—specialist advice should be sought.

Foscarnet (section 5.3.2.2) is used for mucocutaneous herpes simplex virus infection unresponsive to aciclovir in immunocompromised patients; it is toxic and can cause renal impairment.

Inosine pranobex has been used by mouth for herpes simplex infections; its effectiveness remains unproven.

5 Infections

ACICLOVIR
(Acyclovir)

Indications herpes simplex and varicella–zoster (see also under Dose)

Cautions maintain adequate hydration (especially with infusion or high doses, or during renal impairment); elderly (risk of neurological reactions); **interactions**: Appendix 1 (aciclovir)

Renal impairment see Cautions above; also risk of neurological reactions increased; use normal intravenous dose every 12 hours if eGFR 25–50 mL/minute/1.73 m² (every 24 hours if eGFR 10–25 mL/minute/1.73 m²); consult product literature for intravenous dose if eGFR less than 10 mL/minute/1.73 m²; for *herpes zoster*, use normal oral dose every 8 hours if eGFR 10–25 mL/minute/1.73 m² (every 12 hours if eGFR less than 10 mL/minute/1.73 m²); for *herpes simplex*, use normal oral dose every 12 hours if eGFR less than 10 mL/minute/1.73 m²

Pregnancy not known to be harmful—manufacturers advise use only when potential benefit outweighs risk

Breast-feeding significant amount in milk after systemic administration—not known to be harmful but manufacturer advises caution

Side-effects nausea, vomiting, abdominal pain, diarrhoea, headache, fatigue, rash, urticaria, pruritus, photosensitivity; *very rarely* hepatitis, jaundice, dyspnoea, neurological reactions (including dizziness, confusion, hallucinations, convulsions, ataxia, dysarthria, and drowsiness), acute renal failure, anaemia, thrombocytopenia and leucopenia; on *intravenous infusion*, severe local inflammation (sometimes leading to ulceration), and *very rarely* agitation, tremors, psychosis and fever

Dose

- By mouth, non-genital herpes simplex, treatment, 200 mg (400 mg in the immunocompromised or if absorption impaired) 5 times daily, usually for 5 days (longer if new lesions appear during treatment or if healing incomplete); CHILD 1 month–2 years, half adult dose, over 2 years, adult dose

  Genital herpes simplex, treatment of *first episode*, 200 mg 5 times daily *or* 400 mg 3 times daily usually for 5 days, longer if new lesions appear during treatment or if healing is incomplete (400 mg 5 times daily for 7–10 days in immunocompromised or HIV-positive patients); treatment of *recurrent infection*, 800 mg 3 times daily for 2 days *or* 200 mg 5 times daily for 5 days *or* 400 mg 3 times daily for 3–5 days (400 mg 3 times daily for 5–10 days in immunocompromised or HIV-positive patients)

  Herpes simplex, suppression, 400 mg twice daily *or* 200 mg 4 times daily; increased to 400 mg 3 times daily if recurrences occur on standard suppressive therapy or for suppression of genital herpes during late pregnancy (from 36 weeks gestation); therapy interrupted every 6–12 months to reassess recurrence frequency—consider restarting after two or more recurrences

  Herpes simplex, prophylaxis in the immunocompromised, 200–400 mg 4 times daily; CHILD 1 month–2 years, half adult dose, over 2 years, adult dose

  Varicella and herpes zoster, treatment, 800 mg 5 times daily for 7 days (for herpes zoster in immunocompromised continue for 2 days after crusting of lesions); CHILD 1 month–2 years 200 mg 4 times daily for 5 days (for herpes zoster in immunocompromised continue for 2 days after crusting of lesions); 2–6

  years 400 mg 4 times daily for 5 days (for herpes zoster in immunocompromised continue for 2 days after crusting of lesions); 6–12 years 800 mg 4 times daily for 5 days (for herpes zoster in immunocompromised continue for 2 days after crusting of lesions)

  Attenuation of chickenpox (if varicella–zoster immunoglobulin not indicated) [unlicensed use], ADULT and CHILD 40 mg/kg daily in 4 divided doses for 7 days starting 1 week after exposure

- By intravenous infusion, treatment of herpes simplex in the immunocompromised, severe initial genital herpes, 5 mg/kg every 8 hours usually for 5 days, doubled to 10 mg/kg every 8 hours if resistant organisms suspected or in simplex encephalitis (given for at least 14 days in encephalitis (at least 21 days if also immunocompromised)—confirm cerebrospinal fluid negative for herpes simplex virus before stopping treatment)

  Treatment of varicella-zoster 5 mg/kg every 8 hours usually for 5 days, doubled to 10 mg/kg every 8 hours in the immunocompromised or in encephalitis (given for 10–14 days in encephalitis, possibly longer if also immunocompromised or if severe infection)

  Prophylaxis of herpes simplex in the immunocompromised, 5 mg/kg every 8 hours

  Note To avoid excessive dosage in obese patients, parenteral dose should be calculated on the basis of ideal weight for height

  CHILD under 18 years, see *BNF for Children*

- By topical application, see section 13.10.3 (skin) and section 11.3.3 (eye)

Note Aciclovir doses in BNF may differ from those in product literature

Aciclovir (Non-proprietary) ᴾᵒᴹ

Tablets, aciclovir 200 mg, net price 25-tab pack = £1.76; 400 mg, 56-tab pack = £4.41; 800 mg, 35-tab pack = £4.47. Label: 9

Dental prescribing on NHS Aciclovir Tablets 200 mg or 800 mg may be prescribed

Dispersible tablets, aciclovir 200 mg, net price 25-tab pack = £2.44; 400 mg, 56-tab pack = £11.15; 800 mg, 35-tab pack = £10.30. Label: 9

Suspension, aciclovir 200 mg/5 mL, net price 125 mL = £35.76; 400 mg/5 mL, 100 mL = £39.47. Label: 9

Note Sugar-free versions are available and can be ordered by specifying 'sugar-free' on the prescription

Dental prescribing on NHS Aciclovir Oral Suspension 200 mg/5 mL may be prescribed

Intravenous infusion, powder for reconstitution, aciclovir (as sodium salt), net price 250-mg vial = £9.13; 500-mg vial = £20.22

Electrolytes Na⁺ 1.1 mmol/250-mg vial

Intravenous infusion, aciclovir (as sodium salt), 25 mg/mL, net price 10-mL (250-mg) vial = £10.18; 20-mL (500-mg) vial = £19.61; 40-mL (1-g) vial = £40.44

Electrolytes Na⁺ 1.16 mmol/250-mg vial

Zovirax® (GSK) ᴾᵒᴹ

Tablets, all dispersible, f/c, aciclovir 200 mg, net price 25-tab pack = £2.85; 800 mg (scored, *Shingles Treatment Pack*), 35-tab pack = £10.50. Label: 9

Suspension, both off-white, sugar-free, aciclovir 200 mg/5 mL (banana-flavoured), net price 125 mL = £29.56; 400 mg/5 mL (*Double Strength Suspension*, orange-flavoured) 100 mL = £33.02. Label: 9

Intravenous infusion, powder for reconstitution, aciclovir (as sodium salt), net price 250-mg vial = £3.34; 500-mg vial = £3.40

Electrolytes Na⁺ 1.1 mmol/250-mg vial

■ FAMCICLOVIR

Note Famciclovir is a pro-drug of penciclovir

Indications see under Dose

Cautions interactions: Appendix 1 (famciclovir)

Hepatic impairment usual dose in well compensated liver disease (information not available on decompensated)

Renal impairment reduce dose; consult product literature

Pregnancy manufacturers advise avoid unless potential benefit outweighs risk

Breast-feeding no information available—present in milk in *animal* studies

Side-effects nausea, vomiting, abdominal pain, diarrhoea; headache, fatigue; sweating, pruritus; *rarely* confusion; *very rarely* jaundice, dizziness, drowsiness, hallucinations, thrombocytopenia, rash (including Stevens-Johnson syndrome); also reported, constipation and fever

Dose

- Herpes zoster, treatment, 500 mg 3 times daily for 7 days *or* 750 mg 1–2 times daily for 7 days (in immunocompromised, 500 mg 3 times daily for 10 days, continue for 2 days after crusting of lesions)
- Genital herpes, treatment of *first episode*, 250 mg 3 times daily for 5 days, longer if new lesions appear during treatment or if healing incomplete (500 mg twice daily for 10 days in immunocompromised or HIV-positive patients); treatment of *recurrent infection*, 125 mg twice daily for 5 days *or* 1 g twice daily for 1 day (500 mg twice daily for 5–10 days in immunocompromised or HIV-positive patients)
- Genital herpes, suppression, 250 mg twice daily (500 mg twice daily in immunocompromised or HIV-positive patients); therapy interrupted every 6–12 months to reassess recurrence frequency—consider restarting after two or more recurrences
- Non-genital herpes simplex, treatment in the immunocompromised, 500 mg twice daily for 7 days
- CHILD not recommended

Note Famciclovir doses in BNF may differ from those in product literature

Famciclovir (Non-proprietary) [PoM]
Tablets, famciclovir 125 mg, net price 10-tab pack = £30.50; 250 mg, 15-tab pack = £103.03, 21-tab pack = £144.24, 56-tab pack = £384.64; 500 mg, 14-tab pack = £178.37, 30-tab pack = £399.34, 56-tab pack = £831.46; 750 mg, 7-tab pack = £134.88. Label: 9

Famvir® (Novartis) [PoM]
Tablets, all f/c, famciclovir 125 mg, net price 10-tab pack = £44.54; 250 mg, 15-tab pack = £133.62, 21-tab pack = £187.04; 56-tab pack = £498.80; 500 mg, 14-tab pack = £249.43, 30-tab pack = £534.34, 56-tab pack = £997.75. Label: 9

■ INOSINE PRANOBEX ▱

(Inosine acedoben dimepranol)

Indications see under Dose

Cautions history of gout or hyperuricaemia

Renal impairment manufacturer advises caution; metabolised to uric acid

Pregnancy manufacturer advises avoid

Side-effects reversible increase in serum and urinary uric acid; *less commonly* nausea, vomiting, epigastric discomfort, headache, vertigo, fatigue, arthralgia,

rashes and itching; *rarely* diarrhoea, constipation, anxiety, sleep disturbances, and polyuria

Dose

- Mucocutaneous herpes simplex, 1 g 4 times daily for 7–14 days
- Adjunctive treatment of genital warts, 1 g 3 times daily for 14–28 days
- Subacute sclerosing panencephalitis, 50–100 mg/kg daily in 6 divided doses

Imunovir® (KoRa) [PoM] ▱
Tablets, scored, inosine pranobex 500 mg, net price 100-tab pack = £39.50. Label: 9

■ VALACICLOVIR

Note Valaciclovir is a pro-drug of aciclovir

Indications treatment of herpes zoster; treatment of initial and suppression of recurrent herpes simplex infections of skin and mucous membranes including initial and recurrent genital herpes; reduction of transmission of genital herpes; prevention of cytomegalovirus disease following solid organ transplantation when valganciclovir or ganciclovir cannot be used

Cautions see under Aciclovir

Hepatic impairment manufacturer advises caution with high doses used for herpes labialis and prevention of cytomegalovirus disease—no information available

Renal impairment maintain adequate hydration; for *herpes zoster*, 1 g every 12 hours if eGFR 30–50 mL/minute/1.73 m^2 (1 g every 24 hours if eGFR 10–30 mL/minute/1.73 m^2; 500 mg every 24 hours if eGFR less than 10 mL/minute/1.73 m^2); for *treatment of herpes simplex*, 500 mg (1 g in immunocompromised or HIV-positive patients) every 24 hours if eGFR less than 30 mL/minute/1.73 m^2; for *treatment of herpes labialis*, if eGFR 30–50 mL/minute/1.73 m^2, initially 1 g, then 1 g 12 hours after initial dose (if eGFR 10–30 mL/minute/1.73 m^2, initally 500 mg, then 500 mg 12 hours after initial dose; if eGFR less than 10 mL/minute/1.73 m^2, 500 mg as a single dose); for *suppression of herpes simplex*, 250 mg (500 mg in immunocompromised or HIV-positive patients) every 24 hours if eGFR less than 30 mL/minute/1.73 m^2; for *reduction of genital herpes transmission*, 250 mg every 24 hours if eGFR less than 15 mL/minute/1.73 m^2; reduce dose according to eGFR for *cytomegalovirus prophylaxis* following solid organ transplantation (consult product literature)

Pregnancy see under Aciclovir

Breast-feeding see under Aciclovir

Side-effects see under Aciclovir but neurological reactions more frequent with high doses

Dose

- Herpes zoster, 1 g 3 times daily for 7 days (in immunocompromised continue for 2 days after crusting of lesions); CHILD 12–18 years see *BNF for Children*
- Herpes simplex, treatment of *first episode*, 500 mg twice daily for 5 days, longer if new lesions appear during treatment or if healing incomplete (1 g twice daily for 10 days in immunocompromised or HIV-positive patients); treatment of *recurrent infection*, 500 mg twice daily for 3–5 days (1 g twice daily for 5–10 days in immunocompromised or HIV-positive patients); CHILD 12–18 years see *BNF for Children*
- Herpes labialis, treatment, ADULT and CHILD over 12 years, initially 2 g, then 2 g 12 hours after initial dose

- Herpes simplex, suppression, 500 mg daily in 1–2 divided doses (in immunocompromised or HIV positive patients, 500 mg twice daily); therapy interrupted every 6–12 months to reassess recurrence frequency—consider restarting after two or more recurrences; CHILD 12–18 years see *BNF for Children*
- Reduction of transmission of genital herpes, seek specialist advice, 500 mg once daily to be taken by the infected partner
- Prevention of cytomegalovirus disease following solid organ transplantation (preferably starting within 72 hours of transplantation), 2 g 4 times daily usually for 90 days; CHILD 12–18 years see *BNF for Children*

Valaciclovir (Non-proprietary) PoM
Tablets, valaciclovir 500 mg, net price 10-tab pack = £3.80, 42 tab-pack = £8.50. Label: 9

Valtrex® (GSK) PoM
Tablets, f/c, valaciclovir (as hydrochloride) 250 mg, net price 60-tab pack = £123.28; 500 mg, 10-tab pack = £20.59, 42-tab pack = £86.30. Label: 9

5.3.2.2 Cytomegalovirus infection

Ganciclovir is related to aciclovir but it is more active against cytomegalovirus (CMV); it is also much more toxic than aciclovir and should therefore be prescribed only when the potential benefit outweighs the risks. Ganciclovir is administered by intravenous infusion for the *initial treatment* of CMV infection. Ganciclovir causes profound myelosuppression when given with zidovudine; the two should not normally be given together particularly during initial ganciclovir therapy. The likelihood of ganciclovir resistance increases in patients with a high viral load or in those who receive the drug over a long duration.

Valaciclovir (see p. 433) is licensed for prevention of cytomegalovirus disease following renal transplantation.

Valganciclovir is an ester of ganciclovir which is licensed for the *initial treatment* and *maintenance treatment* of CMV retinitis in AIDS patients. Valganciclovir is also licensed for preventing CMV disease following solid organ transplantation from a cytomegalovirus-positive donor.

Foscarnet is also active against cytomegalovirus; it is toxic and can cause renal impairment.

For local treatment of CMV retinitis, see section 11.3.3.

GANCICLOVIR

Indications life-threatening or sight-threatening cytomegalovirus infections in immunocompromised patients only; prevention of cytomegalovirus disease during immunosuppressive therapy following organ transplantation; local treatment of CMV retinitis (section 11.3.3)

Cautions close monitoring of full blood count (severe deterioration may require correction and possibly treatment interruption); history of cytopenia; potential carcinogen and teratogen; radiotherapy; ensure adequate hydration during intravenous administration; vesicant—infuse into vein with adequate flow preferably using plastic cannula; children (possible risk of long-term carcinogenic or reproductive toxicity); **interactions:** Appendix 1 (ganciclovir)

Contra-indications hypersensitivity to valganciclovir, ganciclovir, aciclovir, or valaciclovir; abnormally low

haemoglobin, neutrophil, or platelet counts (consult product literature)

Renal impairment reduce dose if eGFR less than 70 mL/minute/1.73 m^2; consult product literature

Pregnancy avoid—teratogenic risk; ensure effective contraception during treatment and barrier contraception for men during and for at least 90 days after treatment

Breast-feeding avoid—no information available

Side-effects diarrhoea, nausea, vomiting, dyspepsia, abdominal pain, constipation, flatulence, dysphagia, taste disturbance, hepatic dysfunction; dyspnoea, chest pain, cough; headache, insomnia, convulsions, dizziness, peripheral neuropathy, depression, anxiety, confusion, abnormal thinking, fatigue, weight loss, anorexia; infection, pyrexia, night sweats; anaemia, leucopenia, thrombocytopenia, pancytopenia, renal impairment; myalgia, arthralgia; macular oedema, retinal detachment, vitreous floaters, eye pain; ear pain; dermatitis, pruritus; injection-site reactions; *less commonly* mouth ulcers, pancreatitis, arrhythmias, hypotension, anaphylactic reactions, psychosis, tremor, male infertility, haematuria, disturbances in hearing and vision, and alopecia

Dose
- By intravenous infusion, initially (induction) 5 mg/kg every 12 hours for 14–21 days for treatment or for 7–14 days for prevention; maintenance (for patients at risk of relapse of retinitis) 6 mg/kg daily on 5 days per week *or* 5 mg/kg daily until adequate recovery of immunity; if retinitis progresses initial induction treatment may be repeated; CHILD under 18 years, see *BNF for Children*

Cymevene® (Roche) PoM
Intravenous infusion, powder for reconstitution, ganciclovir (as sodium salt). Net price 500-mg vial = £29.77
Electrolytes Na$^+$ 2 mmol/500-mg vial
Caution in handling Ganciclovir is toxic and personnel should be adequately protected during handling and administration; if solution comes into contact with skin or mucosa, wash off immediately with soap and water

FOSCARNET SODIUM

Indications cytomegalovirus disease [licensed for cytomegalovirus retinitis in AIDS patients only]; mucocutaneous herpes simplex virus infections unresponsive to aciclovir in immunocompromised patients

Cautions monitor electrolytes, particularly calcium and magnesium; monitor serum creatinine every second day during induction and every week during maintenance; ensure adequate hydration; avoid rapid infusion; men should avoid fathering a child during and for 6 months after treatment; **interactions:** Appendix 1 (foscarnet)

Renal impairment reduce dose; consult product literature

Pregnancy manufacturer advises avoid

Breast-feeding avoid—present in milk in *animal* studies

Side-effects nausea (reduce infusion rate), vomiting, diarrhoea, abdominal pain, constipation, dyspepsia, anorexia, hepatic dysfunction, pancreatitis, changes in blood pressure and ECG, palpitation, oedema, dizziness, headache, malaise, aggression, agitation, anxiety, confusion, depression, paraesthesia (reduce infusion rate), convulsions, tremor, and other neurological disorders, anaemia, granulocytopenia, leucopenia, thrombocytopenia, dysuria, polyuria, renal impairment (including acute renal failure), electrolyte disturbances (including hypokalaemia, hypomagnesaemia, and hypocalcaemia), myalgia, rash, pruritus, thrombophlebitis if given undiluted by peripheral vein, genital irritation and ulceration (due to high concentrations excreted in urine); *less commonly* acidosis; also reported oesophageal ulceration, ventricular arrhythmias, diabetes insipidus, myasthenia, myositis, rhabdomyolysis

Dose

- CMV disease [licensed for CMV retinitis only], by intravenous infusion, initially (induction) 60 mg/kg every 8 hours *or* 90 mg/kg every 12 hours, for 2–3 weeks; maintenance 60 mg/kg daily, increased to 90–120 mg/kg if tolerated; if disease progresses on maintenance dose, repeat induction regimen
- Mucocutaneous herpes simplex infection, by intravenous infusion, 40 mg/kg every 8 hours for 2–3 weeks or until lesions heal
  Note Foscarnet doses in BNF may differ from those in product literature

Foscavir® (Clinigen) ⓅⓄⓂ
Intravenous infusion, foscarnet sodium hexahydrate 24 mg/mL, net price 250-mL bottle = £119.85
Electrolytes Na⁺ 0.24 mmol/mL

VALGANCICLOVIR

Note Valganciclovir is a pro-drug of ganciclovir

Indications induction and maintenance treatment of cytomegalovirus retinitis in AIDS patients; prevention of cytomegalovirus disease following solid organ transplantation from a cytomegalovirus-positive donor.

Cautions see under Ganciclovir

Contra-indications see under Ganciclovir

Renal impairment reduce dose; consult product literature

Pregnancy see under Ganciclovir

Breast-feeding see under Ganciclovir

Side-effects see under Ganciclovir

Dose

- CMV retinitis, induction, ADULT over 18 years, 900 mg twice daily for 21 days then 900 mg once daily; induction regimen may be repeated if retinitis progresses
- Prevention of cytomegalovirus disease following solid organ transplantation (starting within 10 days of transplantation), ADULT over 18 years, 900 mg once daily for 100 days (for 100–200 days following kidney transplantation)
  Note Oral valganciclovir 900 mg twice daily is equivalent to intravenous ganciclovir 5 mg/kg twice daily

Valcyte® (Roche) ⓅⓄⓂ
Tablets, pink, f/c, valganciclovir (as hydrochloride) 450 mg, net price 60-tab pack = £1081.46. Label: 21
Oral solution, tutti-frutti flavoured, valganciclovir (as hydrochloride) 250 mg/5 mL when reconstituted with water, net price 100 mL = £230.32. Label: 21
Caution in handling Valganciclovir is a potential teratogen and carcinogen and caution is advised when handling the powder, reconstituted solution, or broken tablets; if these come into contact with skin or mucosa, wash off immediately with water; avoid inhalation of powder

---

5.3.3 Viral hepatitis

5.3.3.1 Chronic hepatitis B
5.3.3.2 Chronic hepatitis C

Treatment for viral hepatitis should be initiated by a specialist. The management of uncomplicated acute viral hepatitis is largely symptomatic. Early treatment of acute hepatitis C with interferon alfa [unlicensed indication] may reduce the risk of chronic infection. Hepatitis B and hepatitis C viruses are major causes of chronic hepatitis. For details on immunisation against hepatitis A and B infections, see section 14.4 (active immunisation), section 14.5.1 (passive immunisation against hepatitis A), and section 14.5.2 (passive immunisation against hepatitis B).

5.3.3.1 Chronic hepatitis B

Peginterferon alfa (section 8.2.4) is an option for the initial treatment of chronic hepatitis B and may be preferable to **interferon alfa**. The use of peginterferon alfa and interferon alfa is limited by a response rate of 30–40% and relapse is frequent. Treatment should be discontinued if no improvement occurs after 4 months. The manufacturers of peginterferon alfa-2a and interferon alfa contraindicate use in decompensated liver disease, but low doses can be used with great caution in these patients. Although interferon alfa is contra-indicated in patients receiving immunosuppressant treatment (or who have received it recently), cautious use of peginterferon alfa-2a may be justified in some cases.

Entecavir or tenofovir disoproxil (see p. 423) are options for the initial treatment of chronic hepatitis B. If the response is inadequate after 6–9 months of treatment, a change in treatment should be considered. Other drugs that are licensed for the treatment of chronic hepatitis B include **adefovir dipivoxil, lamivudine** (see p. 422), or **telbivudine** (but see NICE guidance below).

Entecavir alone, tenofovir disoproxil alone, or a combination of lamivudine with either adefovir dipivoxil or tenofovir disoproxil can be used in patients with decompensated liver disease.

If drug-resistant hepatitis B virus emerges during treatment, another antiviral drug to which the virus is sensitive should be added. Hepatitis B viruses with reduced susceptibility to lamivudine have emerged following extended therapy. Adefovir or tenofovir can be given with lamivudine in lamivudine-resistant chronic hepatitis B; telbivudine or entecavir should not be used because cross-resistance can occur.

If there is no toxicity or loss in efficacy, treatment with adefovir, entecavir, lamivudine, telbivudine, or tenofovir is usually continued until 6 months after adequate seroconversion has occurred. Treatment is usually continued long-term in patients with decompensated liver disease.

Tenofovir, or a combination of tenofovir with either emtricitabine or lamivudine may be used with other antiretrovirals, as part of 'highly active antiretroviral therapy' (section 5.3.1) in patients who require treatment for both HIV and chronic hepatitis B. If patients infected with both HIV and chronic hepatitis B only require treatment for chronic hepatitis B, they should receive antivirals that are not active against HIV, such

5 Infections

as peginterferon alfa or adefovir. Treatment may be continued long-term, even if adequate seroconversion occurs. Management of these patients should be coordinated between HIV and hepatology specialists.

> **NICE guidance**
> **Entecavir for chronic hepatitis B (August 2008)**
> Entecavir is an option for the treatment of chronic hepatitis B.
> www.nice.org.uk/TA153

> **NICE guidance**
> **Telbivudine for chronic hepatitis B (August 2008)**
> Telbivudine is not recommended for the treatment of chronic hepatitis B. Patients currently receiving telbivudine can continue treatment until they and their clinician consider it appropriate to stop.
> www.nice.org.uk/TA154

> **NICE guidance**
> **Tenofovir disoproxil for the treatment of chronic hepatitis B (July 2009)**
> Tenofovir is an option for the treatment of chronic hepatitis B.
> www.nice.org.uk/TA173

ADEFOVIR DIPIVOXIL

Indications chronic hepatitis B infection with *either* compensated liver disease with evidence of viral replication, and histologically documented active liver inflammation and fibrosis, when other treatment not appropriate *or* decompensated liver disease in combination with another antiviral for chronic hepatitis B that has no cross-resistance to adefovir

Cautions monitor liver function tests every 3 months, and viral markers for hepatitis B every 3–6 months during treatment (continue monitoring for at least 1 year after discontinuation—recurrent hepatitis may occur on discontinuation); monitor renal function before treatment then every 3 months, more frequently in renal impairment or in patients receiving nephrotoxic drugs; elderly; discontinue if deterioration in liver function, hepatic steatosis, progressive hepatomegaly or unexplained lactic acidosis

Renal impairment 10 mg every 48 hours if eGFR 30–50 mL/minute/1.73 m^2; 10 mg every 72 hours if eGFR 10–30 mL/minute/1.73 m^2; no information available if eGFR less than 10 mL/minute/1.73 m^2; see also Cautions above

Pregnancy toxicity in *animal* studies—manufacturer advises use only if potential benefit outweighs risk; effective contraception required during treatment

Breast-feeding manufacturer advises avoid—no information available

Side-effects nausea, vomiting, dyspepsia, abdominal pain, flatulence, diarrhoea; asthenia, headache; renal failure; hypophosphataemia; rash and pruritus; also reported pancreatitis

Dose
- ADULT over 18 years, 10 mg once daily

Hepsera® (Gilead) [PoM]
Tablets, adefovir dipivoxil 10 mg, net price 30-tab pack = £252.22

ENTECAVIR

Indications chronic hepatitis B infection *either* with compensated liver disease (with evidence of viral replication, and histologically documented active liver inflammation or fibrosis) *or* decompensated liver disease

Cautions monitor liver function tests every 3 months, and viral markers for hepatitis B every 3–6 months during treatment (continue monitoring for at least 1 year after discontinuation—recurrent hepatitis may occur on discontinuation); HIV infection—risk of HIV resistance in patients not receiving 'highly active antiretroviral therapy'; lamivudine-resistant chronic hepatitis B—risk of entecavir resistance; discontinue if deterioration in liver function, hepatic steatosis, progressive hepatomegaly or unexplained lactic acidosis

Renal impairment reduce dose if eGFR less than 50 mL/minute/1.73 m^2; consult product literature

Pregnancy toxicity in *animal* studies—manufacturer advises use only if potential benefit outweighs risk; effective contraception required during treatment

Breast-feeding manufacturer advises avoid—present in milk in *animal* studies

Side-effects nausea, vomiting, dyspepsia, diarrhoea, raised serum amylase and lipase, headache, fatigue, dizziness, sleep disturbances; *less commonly* thrombocytopenia, rash, alopecia

Dose
- Compensated liver disease not previously treated with nucleoside analogues, ADULT over 18 years, 500 micrograms once daily
- Compensated liver disease with lamivudine-resistant chronic hepatitis B (but see notes above), ADULT over 18 years, 1 mg once daily; consider other treatment if inadequate response after 6 months
  Counselling To be taken at least 2 hours before or 2 hours after food
- Decompensated liver disease, ADULT over 18 years, 1 mg once daily
  Counselling To be taken at least 2 hours before or 2 hours after food

Baraclude® (Bristol-Myers Squibb) [PoM]
Tablets, f/c, entecavir (as monohydrate) 500 micrograms (white), net price 30-tab pack = £363.26; 1 mg (pink), 30-tab pack = £363.26. Counselling, administration
Oral solution, entecavir (as monohydrate) 50 micrograms/mL, net price 210-mL pack (orange-flavoured) = £423.80. Counselling, administration

TELBIVUDINE

Indications chronic hepatitis B infection with compensated liver disease, evidence of viral replication, and histologically documented active liver inflammation or fibrosis, when other treatment is not appropriate

Cautions monitor liver function tests every 3 months, and viral markers of hepatitis B every 3–6 months during treatment (continue monitoring for at least 1 year after discontinuation—recurrent hepatitis may occur on discontinuation); lamivudine-resistant chronic hepatitis B—risk of telbivudine resistance; discontinue if deterioration in liver function, hepatic steatosis, progressive hepatomegaly or unexplained lactic acidosis; **interactions:** Appendix 1 (telbivudine)
Counselling Patients should be advised to promptly report unexplained muscle pain, tenderness, or weakness, or numbness, tingling or burning sensations

Renal impairment   600 mg every 48 hours if eGFR 30–
49 mL/minute/1.73 m^2; 600 mg every 72 hours if
eGFR less than 30 mL/minute/1.73 m^2

Pregnancy   manufacturer advises use only if potential
benefit outweighs risk

Breast-feeding   manufacturer advises avoid—present
in milk in *animal* studies

Side-effects   nausea, diarrhoea, abdominal pain,
raised serum amylase and lipase; cough; dizziness,
headache, fatigue; rash; *less commonly* taste disturbance, arthralgia, myalgia, myopathy (discontinue
treatment), and peripheral neuropathy; *rarely* lactic
acidosis, rhabdomyolysis

Dose

● ADULT over 18 years, 600 mg once daily

Sebivo® (Novartis) [PoM]
Tablets, f/c, telbivudine 600 mg, net price 28-tab
pack = £290.33. Counselling, muscle effects, peripheral neuropathy

5.3.3.2   Chronic hepatitis C

Before starting treatment, the genotype of the infecting
hepatitis C virus should be determined and the viral load
measured as this may affect the choice and duration of
treatment. A combination of **ribavirin** (see p. 442) and
peginterferon alfa (section 8.2.4) is used for the treatment of chronic hepatitis C (see NICE guidance, below).
The combination of ribavirin and interferon alfa is less
effective than the combination of peginterferon alfa and
ribavirin. Peginterferon alfa alone should be used if
ribavirin is contra-indicated or not tolerated. Ribavirin
monotherapy is ineffective.

> **NICE guidance**
> **Peginterferon alfa and ribavirin for mild
> chronic hepatitis C (August 2006 and
> September 2010)**
> The combination of peginterferon alfa and ribavirin
> can be used for treating mild chronic hepatitis C in
> patients over 18 years. Alternatively, treatment can be
> delayed until the disease has reached a moderate stage
> ('watchful waiting'). Peginterferon alfa alone can be
> used if ribavirin is contra-indicated or not tolerated.
> www.nice.org.uk/TA200

> **NICE guidance**
> **Peginterferon alfa, interferon alfa, and
> ribavirin for moderate to severe chronic
> hepatitis C (January 2004 and September
> 2010)**
> The combination of peginterferon alfa and ribavirin
> should be used for treating moderate to severe
> chronic hepatitis C in patients aged over 18 years:
> ● not previously treated with interferon alfa or peginter-
>   feron alfa;
> ● treated previously with interferon alfa alone or in
>   combination with ribavirin;
> ● whose condition did not respond to peginterferon alfa
>   alone or to a combination of peginterferon alfa and
>   ribavirin, or responded but subsequently relapsed;
> ● co-infected with HIV.
> Peginterferon alfa alone should be used if ribavirin is
> contra-indicated or not tolerated. Interferon alfa for
> either monotherapy or combined therapy should be
> used only if neutropenia and thrombocytopenia are a
> particular risk. Patients receiving interferon alfa may
> be switched to peginterferon alfa.
> www.nice.org.uk/TA200

Boceprevir and **telaprevir** are protease inhibitors that
inhibit the replication of hepatitis C virus genotype 1,
but they are less effective against other genotypes of the
virus. Monotherapy is not recommended because there
is a high likelihood of resistance developing. Either
boceprevir or telaprevir is licensed for use in combination with ribavirin and peginterferon alfa for the treatment of chronic hepatitis C infection of genotype 1 in
patients with compensated liver disease; these combinations are more effective than dual therapy with ribavirin and peginterferon alfa. However, triple therapy is
associated with a higher incidence and greater severity
of anaemia than dual therapy. Neutropenia seems to be
more frequent during treatment with regimens containing boceprevir than with those containing telaprevir.
Rash is a particular concern with telaprevir, and to a
lesser extent with boceprevir.

> **NICE guidance**
> **Boceprevir for chronic hepatitis C infection
> of genotype 1 (April 2012)**
> Boceprevir in combination with ribavirin and pegin-
> terferon alfa is an option for the treatment of chronic
> hepatitis C infection of genotype 1 in adults with
> compensated liver disease:
> ● who have not been treated previously;
> ● in whom previous treatment (e.g. with peginterferon
>   alfa in combination with ribavirin) has failed.
> www.nice.org.uk/TA253

> **NICE guidance**
> **Telaprevir for chronic hepatitis C infection of
> genotype 1 (April 2012)**
> Telaprevir in combination with ribavirin and pegin-
> terferon alfa is an option for the treatment of chronic
> hepatitis C infection of genotype 1 in adults with
> compensated liver disease:
> ● who have not been treated previously;
> ● in whom previous treatment (e.g. with peginterferon
>   alfa in combination with ribavirin) has failed.
> www.nice.org.uk/TA252

Daclatasvir is an inhibitor of the multifunctional protein
NS5A, which is an essential component of the hepatitis
C virus replication process. It is licensed for use in
combination with sofosbuvir (see below) for the treatment of chronic hepatitis C infection of genotypes 1 or
4, with or without compensated cirrhosis; the addition of
ribavirin should be considered for patients with
advanced liver disease or with other negative prognostic factors, such as prior treatment experience. It is also
licensed in combination with sofosbuvir and ribavirin for
the treatment of chronic hepatitis C infection of genotype 3 in patients who are treatment experienced, with
or without compensated cirrhosis, and in combination
with peginterferon alfa and ribavirin for the treatment of
chronic hepatitis C infection of genotype 4. Daclatasvir
must not be given as monotherapy.

Sofosbuvir is a pro-drug of a nucleoside inhibitor that is
effective against hepatitis C virus polymerase NS5B. It is
licensed for use in combination with ribavirin, with or
without peginterferon alfa, for the treatment of chronic
hepatitis C infection of genotypes 1, 2, 3, 4, 5, or 6 in
patients with compensated liver disease. Sofosbuvir
monotherapy is not recommended because it is less
effective than combination therapy. For the use of
sofosbuvir in combination with daclatasvir and ribavirin,
see notes above.

5 Infections

The *Scottish Medicines Consortium* (p. 4) has advised (June 2014) that sofosbuvir (*Sovaldi®*) is accepted for use within NHS Scotland for the treatment of chronic hepatitis C infection of genotypes 1 to 6; its use in combination with ribavirin as dual therapy for chronic hepatitis C infection of either genotype 2 (in treatment naive patients) or genotype 3 is restricted to those who cannot use peginterferon alfa because of intolerance or contra-indications.

Simeprevir is a protease inhibitor that is licensed for use in combination with ribavirin and peginterferon alfa for the treatment of chronic hepatitis C infection of genotype 1 or 4; regimens containing peginterferon alfa-2b are less effective than those containing peginterferon alfa-2a. Simeprevir may also be used in combination with sofosbuvir, with or without ribavirin, for the urgent treatment of chronic hepatitis C infection of genotypes 1 or 4 only when peginterferon alfa cannot be used because of intolerance or contra-indications. Simeprevir monotherapy is not recommended.

BOCEPREVIR

Indications in combination with ribavirin and peginterferon alfa for chronic hepatitis C infection of genotype 1 in patients with compensated liver disease

Cautions monitor full blood count before starting treatment and then on weeks 2, 4, 8, and 12 of treatment, then as indicated clinically; not recommended in patients with low platelets, hypoalbuminaemia or coagulopathy—if initiated in these patients monitor closely for signs of infection, worsening liver impairment and anaemia (increased risk of severe morbidity and mortality); predisposition to QT interval prolongation (including concomitant use with other drugs known to prolong QT interval); **interactions:** Appendix 1 (boceprevir)

Contra-indications autoimmune hepatitis

Pregnancy manufacturer advises avoid; see also under Ribavirin

Breast-feeding manufacturer advises avoid; present in milk in *animal* studies

Side-effects in combination with ribavirin and peginterferon alfa, anaemia, nausea, vomiting, abdominal pain, gastro-oesophageal reflux, flatulence, diarrhoea, constipation, haemorrhoids, dry mouth, disturbances in taste and smell, mouth ulcers, stomatitis, tooth disorder, palpitation, blood pressure changes, syncope, peripheral oedema, hypertriglyceridaemia, cough, dyspnoea, dizziness, headache, decreased appetite, weight loss, anxiety, depression, insomnia, agitation, amnesia, asthenia, hypoaesthesia, paraesthesia, tremor, influenza-like symptoms, hyperglycaemia, hypothyroidism, changes in libido, erectile dysfunction, polyuria, leucopenia, thrombocytopenia, pancytopenia, arthralgia, myalgia, muscle spasms, hyperuricaemia, visual disturbances, dry eyes, tinnitus, alopecia, rash (also reported Stevens-Johnson syndrome, rash with eosinophilia and systemic symptoms), pruritus, hyperhidrosis, psoriasis; *less commonly* gingivitis, tongue discoloration, hypersalivation, dysphagia, pancreatitis, colitis, hyperbilirubinaemia, arrhythmias, venous thromboembolism, flushing, pallor, dysphonia, hyperaesthesia, homicidal and suicidal ideation, hyperthyroidism, amenorrhoea, menorrhagia, dysuria, hypokalaemia, hypercalcaemia, gout, retinal ischaemia, retinopathy, conjunctival haemorrhage, eye pain, increased lacrima-

tion, photophobia, hearing impairment, photosensitivity, skin ulceration; *rarely* cholecystitis, acute myocardial infarction, coronary artery disease, pericarditis, pleural fibrosis, respiratory failure, bipolar disorder, hallucinations, encephalopathy, thyroid neoplasms, aspermia, sarcoidosis

Dose
● In combination with ribavirin and peginterferon alfa, ADULT over 18 years, 800 mg 3 times daily (for duration of treatment consult product literature)

　Missed dose If a dose is more than 6 hours late, the missed dose should not be taken and the next dose should be taken at the normal time

Victrelis® (MSD) ▼ PoM
Capsules, brown-yellow/white, boceprevir 200 mg, net price 336-cap pack = £2800.00. Label: 21

DACLATASVIR

Indications in combination with sofosbuvir for the treatment of chronic hepatitis C infection of genotypes 1 or 4, with or without compensated cirrhosis; in combination with sofosbuvir and ribavirin for the treatment of chronic hepatitis C infection of genotype 3 in patients who are treatment experienced, with or without compensated cirrhosis; in combination with peginterferon alfa and ribavirin for the treatment of chronic hepatitis C infection of genotype 4

Cautions decompensated liver disease; organ transplant patients; human immunodeficiency virus co-infection; hepatitis B virus co-infection; retreatment—efficacy not established in patients with prior exposure to a NS5A inhibitor; **interactions:** Appendix 1 (daclatasvir)

　Driving May affect performance of skilled tasks (e.g. driving)

Pregnancy manufacturer advises avoid (toxicity in *animal* studies); highly effective contraception required during and for 5 weeks after treatment; see also under Ribavirin and Sofosbuvir

Breast-feeding manufacturer advises avoid—present in milk in *animal* studies

Side-effects *in combination with sofosbuvir with or without ribavirin*, nausea, abdominal pain, constipation, diarrhoea, dry mouth, flatulence, gastro-oesophageal reflux, vomitting, hot flush, cough, dyspnoea, nasal congestion, anxiety, depression, dizziness, migraine, insomnia, headache, irritability, malaise, decreased appetite, anaemia, arthralgia, myalgia, alopecia, dry skin, pruritus, rash; *in combination with ribavirin and peginterferon alfa*, also decreased appetite, dizziness, disturbance in attention, pyrexia, neutropenia, anaemia, lymphopenia, arthralgia, myalgia, blurred vision, reduced visual acuity, dry skin, rash, alopecia

Dose
● In combination with sofosbuvir with or without ribavirin, *or* in combination with ribavirin and peginterferon alfa, ADULT over 18 years, 60 mg once daily (for duration of treatment consult product literature)

　Note Reduce dose to 30 mg once daily with concomitant use of potent CYP3A4 inhibitors (e.g. atazanavir boosted with ritonavir, boceprevir, clarithromycin, cobicistat, itraconazole, posaconazole, telaprevir, telithromycin, and voriconazole). Increase dose to 90 mg once daily with concomitant use of moderate CYP3A4 inducers (e.g. efavirenz)

　Missed dose If a dose is more than 20 hours late, the missed dose should not be taken and the next dose should be taken at the normal time

Daklinza® (Bristol-Myers Squibb) ▼ PoM
Tablets, f/c, daclatasvir (as dihydrochloride) 30 mg
(green), net price 28-tab pack = £8172.61; 60 mg
(light green), 28-tab pack = £8172.61. Label: 25,
counselling, driving

SIMEPREVIR

Indications in combination with ribavirin and peginterferon alfa for chronic hepatitis C infection of genotype 1 or 4; in combination with sofosbuvir (with or
without ribavirin) for urgent treatment of chronic
hepatitis C infection of genotype 1 or 4 when peginterferon alfa cannot be used because of intolerance or
contra-indications

Cautions test for NS3 Q80K polymorphism before
combination treatment with ribavirin and peginterferon alfa in patients with chronic hepatitis C infection
of genotype 1a—in presence of NS3 Q80K polymorphism, consider alternative treatment because
efficacy of simeprevir is reduced; consider testing for
NS3 Q80K polymorphism before combination treatment with sofosbuvir (with or without ribavirin) in
patients with chronic hepatitis C infection of genotype
1a; patients of East Asian origin; **interactions**:
Appendix 1 (simeprevir)

Hepatic impairment manufacturer advises caution in
moderate to severe impairment or in decompensated
cirrhosis—elimination reduced in severe impairment

Renal impairment manufacturer advises caution if
eGFR less than 30 mL/minute/1.73m²—elimination
may be reduced

Pregnancy manufacturer advises use only if potential
benefit outweighs risk—toxicity in *animal* studies;
effective contraception required during treatment; see
also under Ribavirin and Sofosbuvir

Breast-feeding manufacturer advises avoid—present
in plasma of breast-fed *animals*

Side-effects nausea, constipation, raised bilirubin
concentration, dyspnoea, rash (monitor for deterioration if mild or moderate; discontinue if severe),
pruritus, photosensitivity; *in combination with sofosbuvir,* also fatigue, insomnia, headache

Dose
• ADULT over 18 years, 150 mg once daily (for duration
of treatment consult product literature)
  Missed dose If a dose is more than 12 hours late, the
  missed dose should not be taken and the next dose should be
  taken at the normal time

Olysio® (Janssen) ▼ PoM
Capsules, simeprevir (as sodium) 150 mg, net price
7-cap pack = £1866.50. Label: 11, 21

SOFOSBUVIR

Indications in combination with ribavirin, with or
without peginterferon alfa, for chronic hepatitis C
infection of genotypes 1, 3, 4, 5, or 6 in patients with
compensated liver disease; in combination with ribavirin for chronic hepatitis C infection of genotype 2 in
patients with compensated liver disease; in combination with daclatasvir for chronic hepatitis C infection of genotype 1, 3, or 4, see Daclatasvir

Cautions in chronic hepatitis C of genotype 1, 4, 5, or
6, only use sofosbuvir with ribavirin in those with
intolerance or contra-indications to peginterferon alfa
who require urgent treatment; **interactions**: Appendix 1 (sofosbuvir)

Renal impairment safety and efficacy not established
if eGFR less than 30 mL/minute/1.73m²—accumulation may occur

Pregnancy manufacturer advises avoid; see also
under Ribavirin, Simeprevir, and Daclatasvir

Breast-feeding manufacturer advises avoid—metabolites present in milk in *antmal* studies

Side-effects *in combination with ribavirin (with or
without peginterferon alfa),* anaemia, nausea, constipation, abdominal discomfort, gastro-oesophageal
reflux, dyspnoea, cough, insomnia, depression,
headache, disturbance in attention, irritability, asthenia, influenza-like symptoms, myalgia, arthralgia,
alopecia, rash; *in combination with ribavirin and
peginterferon alfa,* also vomiting, diarrhoea, dry mouth,
chest pain, decreased appetite, weight loss, anxiety,
agitation, dizziness, migraine, memory impairment,
neutropenia, blurred vision

Dose
• In combination with *Copegus*®, with or without
peginterferon alfa, *or* in combination with daclatasvir,
ADULT over 18 years, 400 mg once daily (for duration
of treatment consult product literature)
  Missed dose If a dose is more than 18 hours late, the
  missed dose should not be taken and the next dose should be
  taken at the normal time

Sovaldi® (Gilead) ▼ PoM
Tablets, yellow, f/c, sofosbuvir 400 mg, net price 28-
tab pack = £11660.98 Label: 21, 25
Note Dispense in original container (contains desiccant)

TELAPREVIR

Indications in combination with ribavirin and peginterferon alfa for chronic hepatitis C infection of genotype 1 in patients with compensated liver disease

Cautions monitor full blood count, platelets, electrolytes, serum creatinine, uric acid, and liver and thyroid function tests before starting treatment and then
on weeks 2, 4, 8, and 12 of treatment, then as
indicated clinically; not recommended in patients
with low platelets or hypoalbuminaemia—if initiated
in these patients monitor closely for signs of infection,
worsening liver impairment and anaemia (increased
risk of severe morbidity and mortality); electrolyte
disturbances; prolongation of QT interval, bradycardia, heart failure with reduced left ventricular
ejection fraction, concomitant use with other drugs
known to prolong QT interval; congenital or family
history of QT interval prolongation, family history of
sudden death; effectiveness of hormonal contraceptives reduced during treatment and for 2 months
after stopping telaprevir—effective non-hormonal
methods of contraception necessary during this time
(see also Cautions under Ribavirin); **interactions**:
Appendix 1 (telaprevir)
Rash Rash occurs very commonly. If rash mild or moderate,
may continue without interruption, but monitor for
deterioration. If moderate rash deteriorates, consider
permanent discontinuation of telaprevir; if rash does not
improve within 7 days of discontinuation, suspend ribavirin.
If severe rash or if rash accompanied by blistering or
mucosal ulceration, discontinue telaprevir permanently; if
rash does not improve within 7 days of discontinuation,
consider discontinuation of ribavirin and peginterferon alfa.
If serious rash, or if severe rash deteriorates, or if rash
accompanied by systemic symptoms, discontinue telaprevir,
ribavirin, and peginterferon alfa permanently
Counselling Patients should be told to seek immediate
medical attention if a rash develops or if an existing rash
worsens

Hepatic impairment manufacturer advises avoid in
moderate to severe impairment

Pregnancy manufacturer advises avoid; see Cautions above and also see under Ribavirin

Breast-feeding manufacturer advises avoid—present in milk in *animal* studies

Side-effects in combination with ribavirin and peginterferon alfa, rash (including eczema and rarely Stevens-Johnson syndrome and toxic epidermal necrolysis; see also Rash above), pruritus, anaemia, nausea, vomiting, diarrhoea, haemorrhoids, anal fissure, hyperbilirubinaemia, taste disturbances, syncope, peripheral oedema, hypothyroidism, hypokalaemia, thrombocytopenia, lymphopenia, hyperuricaemia; *less commonly* proctitis, gout, retinopathy, urticaria

Dose

- In combination with ribavirin and peginterferon alfa, ADULT over 18 years, 1.125 g every 12 hours *or* 750 mg every 8 hours (for duration of treatment consult product literature)

  Missed dose If a dose is more than 6 hours late with the 12 hourly regimen (or more than 4 hours late with the 8 hourly regimen), the missed dose should not be taken and the next dose should be taken at the normal time

Incivo® (Janssen) ▼ PoM

Tablets, yellow, f/c, telaprevir 375 mg, net price 42-tab pack = £1866.50. Label: 21, counselling, rash
Note Dispense in original container (contains desiccant)

5.3.4 Influenza

For advice on immunisation against influenza, see section 14.4.

Oseltamivir and **zanamivir** reduce replication of influenza A and B viruses by inhibiting viral neuraminidase. They are most effective for the treatment of influenza if started within a few hours of the onset of symptoms; they are licensed for use within 48 hours (within 36 hours for zanamivir in children) of the first symptoms. In otherwise healthy individuals they reduce the duration of symptoms by about 1–1.5 days. Oseltamivir or zanamivir can reduce the risk of complications from influenza in the elderly and in patients with chronic disease (see also NICE guidance, below).

Oseltamivir and zanamivir are licensed for post-exposure prophylaxis of influenza when influenza is circulating in the community. Oseltamivir should be given within 48 hours of exposure to influenza while zanamivir should be given within 36 hours of exposure to influenza (see also NICE guidance, below). However, in patients with severe influenza or in those who are immunocompromised, antivirals may still be effective after this time if viral shedding continues [unlicensed use]. Oseltamivir and zanamivir are also licensed for use in exceptional circumstances (e.g. when vaccination does not cover the infecting strain) to prevent influenza in an epidemic.

There is evidence that some strains of influenza A virus have reduced susceptibility to oseltamivir, but may retain susceptibility to zanamivir. Resistance to oseltamivir may be greater in severely immunocompromised patients.

Zanamivir should be reserved for patients who are severely immunocompromised, or when oseltamivir cannot be used, or when resistance to oseltamivir is suspected. For those unable to use the dry powder for inhalation, zanamivir is available as a solution that can be administered by nebuliser or intravenously [unlicensed].

Amantadine is licensed for prophylaxis and treatment of influenza A but it is no longer recommended (see NICE guidance).

Information on pandemic influenza, avian influenza, and swine influenza may be found at www.hpa.org.uk

Oseltamivir in children under 1 year of age
Data on the use of oseltamivir in children under 1 year of age is limited. Furthermore, oseltamivir may be ineffective in neonates because they may not be able to metabolise oseltamivir to its active form. However, oseltamivir can be used (under specialist supervision) for the treatment or post-exposure prophylaxis of influenza in children under 1 year of age. The Department of Health has advised (May 2009) that during a pandemic, treatment with oseltamivir can be overseen by healthcare professionals experienced in assessing children.

Pregnancy and breast-feeding Although safety data are limited, either oseltamivir or zanamivir can be used in women who are pregnant or breast-feeding when the potential benefit outweighs the risk (e.g. during a pandemic). Oseltamivir is the preferred drug in women who are breast-feeding.

NICE guidance
Oseltamivir, zanamivir, and amantadine for prophylaxis of influenza (September 2008)
The drugs described here are not a substitute for vaccination, which remains the most effective way of preventing illness from influenza.

- Amantadine is **not** recommended for prophylaxis of influenza.
- Oseltamivir *or* zanamivir are **not** recommended for seasonal prophylaxis against influenza.
- When influenza is circulating in the community[1], either oseltamivir or zanamivir is recommended (in accordance with UK licensing) for post-exposure prophylaxis in at-risk patients who are not effectively protected by influenza vaccine, and who have been in close contact with someone suffering from influenza-like illness in the same household or residential setting. Oseltamivir should be given within 48 hours of exposure to influenza while zanamivir should be given within 36 hours of exposure to influenza.
- During local outbreaks of influenza-like illness, when there is a high level of certainty that influenza is present, either oseltamivir or zanamivir may be used for post-exposure prophylaxis in at-risk patients (regardless of influenza vaccination) living in long-term residential or nursing homes.

At risk[2] patients include those aged over 65 years *or* those who have one or more of the following conditions:

- chronic respiratory disease (including asthma and chronic obstructive pulmonary disease);
- chronic heart disease;
- chronic renal disease;
- chronic liver disease;
- chronic neurological disease;
- immunosuppression;
- diabetes mellitus.

This guidance does not cover the circumstances of a pandemic, an impending pandemic, or a widespread epidemic of a new strain of influenza to which there is little or no immunity in the community.
www.nice.org.uk/TA158

---

1. National surveillance schemes, including those run by Public Health England, should be used to indicate when influenza is circulating in the community.
2. The Department of Health in England has advised (November 2010 and April 2011) that 'at risk patients' also includes patients under 65 years of age who are at risk of developing medical complications from influenza (treatment only) or women who are pregnant.

NICE guidance
Oseltamivir, zanamivir, and amantadine for treatment of influenza (February 2009)
The drugs described here are not a substitute for vaccination, which remains the most effective way of preventing illness from influenza.

- Amantadine is **not** recommended for treatment of influenza.
- When influenza is circulating in the community[1], either oseltamivir or zanamivir is recommended (in accordance with UK licensing) for the treatment of influenza in at-risk patients who can start treatment within 48 hours (within 36 hours for zanamivir in children) of the onset of symptoms.
- During local outbreaks of influenza-like illness, when there is a high level of certainty that influenza is present, either oseltamivir or zanamivir may be used for treatment in at-risk patients living in long-term residential or nursing homes.

At risk[2] patients include those aged over 65 years *or* those who have one or more of the following conditions:

- chronic respiratory disease (including asthma and chronic obstructive pulmonary disease);
- chronic heart disease;
- chronic renal disease;
- chronic liver disease;
- chronic neurological disease;
- immunosuppression;
- diabetes mellitus.

This guidance does not cover the circumstances of a pandemic, an impending pandemic, or a widespread epidemic of a new strain of influenza to which there is little or no immunity in the community.
www.nice.org.uk/TA168

AMANTADINE HYDROCHLORIDE

Indications see under Dose; parkinsonism (section 4.9.1)
Cautions section 4.9.1
Contra-indications section 4.9.1
Renal impairment section 4.9.1
Pregnancy section 4.9.1
Breast-feeding section 4.9.1
Side-effects section 4.9.1
Dose

- Influenza A (see also notes above), ADULT and CHILD over 10 years, treatment, 100 mg daily for 4–5 days; prophylaxis, 100 mg daily usually for 6 weeks *or* with influenza vaccination for 2–3 weeks after vaccination

Lysovir® (Alliance) PoM
Capsules, red-brown, amantadine hydrochloride 100 mg, net price 5-cap pack = £2.40, 14-cap pack = £3.00. Counselling, driving

Symmetrel® (Alliance) PoM
Section 4.9.1

OSELTAMIVIR

Indications see notes above
Renal impairment for *treatment*, use 30 mg twice daily if eGFR 30–60 mL/minute/1.73 m^2 (30 mg once daily

---

1. National surveillance schemes, including those run by Public Health England, should be used to indicate when influenza is circulating in the community.
2. The Department of Health in England has advised (November 2010 and April 2011) that 'at risk patients' also includes patients under 65 years of age who are at risk of developing medical complications from influenza (treatment only) or women who are pregnant.

---

if eGFR 10–30 mL/minute/1.73 m^2); for *prevention*, use 30 mg once daily if eGFR 30–60 mL/minute/1.73 m^2 (30 mg every 48 hours if eGFR 10–30 mL/minute/1.73 m^2); avoid for *treatment* and *prevention* if eGFR less than 10 mL/minute/1.73 m^2

Pregnancy use only if potential benefit outweighs risk (e.g. during a pandemic); see also p. 440
Breast-feeding amount probably too small to be harmful; use only if potential benefit outweighs risk (e.g. during a pandemic); see also p. 440
Side-effects nausea, vomiting, abdominal pain, dyspepsia, headache; *less commonly* arrhythmias, convulsions and altered consciousness (usually in children and adolescents), eczema, rash; *rarely* hepatitis, gastro-intestinal bleeding, neuropsychiatric disorders (usually in children and adolescents), thrombocytopenia, visual disturbances, Stevens-Johnson syndrome, toxic epidermal necrolysis

Dose

- Prevention of influenza, ADULT and CHILD over 13 years, 75 mg once daily for 10 days for post-exposure prophylaxis; for up to 6 weeks during an epidemic; NEONATE (see notes above), 2 mg/kg once daily for 10 days for post-exposure prophylaxis; CHILD 1–3 months (see notes above), 2.5 mg/kg once daily for 10 days for post–exposure prophylaxis; 3 months–1 year (see notes above), 3 mg/kg once daily for 10 days for post-exposure prophylaxis; 1–13 years, body-weight 10–15 kg, 30 mg once daily for 10 days for post-exposure prophylaxis (for up to 6 weeks during an epidemic); body-weight 15–23 kg, 45 mg once daily for 10 days for post-exposure prophylaxis (for up to 6 weeks during an epidemic); body-weight 23–40 kg, 60 mg once daily for 10 days for post-exposure prophylaxis (for up to 6 weeks during an epidemic); body-weight over 40 kg, adult dose

- Treatment of influenza, ADULT and CHILD over 13 years, 75 mg every 12 hours for 5 days; NEONATE (see notes above), 2 mg/kg every 12 hours for 5 days; CHILD 1–3 months (see notes above), 2.5 mg/kg every 12 hours for 5 days; 3 months–1 year (see notes above), 3 mg/kg every 12 hours for 5 days; 1–13 years, body-weight 10–15 kg, 30 mg every 12 hours for 5 days, body-weight 15–23 kg, 45 mg every 12 hours for 5 days, body-weight 23–40 kg, 60 mg every 12 hours for 5 days, body-weight over 40 kg, adult dose

Note Not licensed for use in children under 1 year of age unless there is a pandemic

[3]**Tamiflu®** (Roche) PoM
Capsules, oseltamivir (as phosphate) 30 mg (yellow), net price 10-cap pack = £7.71; 45 mg (grey), 10-cap pack = £15.41; 75 mg (grey-yellow), 10-cap pack = £15.41. Label: 9
Note If suspension not available, capsules can be opened and the contents mixed with a small amount of sweetened food, such as sugar water or chocolate syrup, just before administration

Oral suspension, sugar-free, tutti-frutti-flavoured, oseltamivir (as phosphate) for reconstitution with water, 30 mg/5 mL, net price 65 mL = £10.27.
Label: 9
Excipients include sorbitol 900 mg/5 mL
Note Solutions prepared by 'special order' manufacturers may be a different concentration

---

3. NHS except for the treatment and prophylaxis of influenza as indicated in the notes above and NICE guidance; endorse prescription 'SLS'

5 Infections

ZANAMIVIR

Indications see notes above

Cautions asthma and chronic pulmonary disease (risk of bronchospasm—short-acting bronchodilator should be available; avoid in severe asthma unless close monitoring possible and appropriate facilities available to treat bronchospasm); uncontrolled chronic illness; other inhaled drugs should be administered before zanamivir

Pregnancy use only if potential benefit outweighs risk (e.g. during a pandemic); see also p. 440

Breast-feeding amount probably too small to be harmful; use only if potential benefit outweighs risk (e.g. during a pandemic); see also p. 440

Side-effects rash; *less commonly* bronchospasm, dyspnoea, angioedema, urticaria; *rarely* Stevens-Johnson syndrome, toxic epidermal necrolysis; also reported neuropsychiatric disorders (especially in children and adolescents)

Dose

● By inhalation of powder, post-exposure prophylaxis of influenza, ADULT and CHILD over 5 years, 10 mg once daily for 10 days

Prevention of influenza during an epidemic, ADULT and CHILD over 5 years, 10 mg once daily for up to 28 days

Treatment of influenza, ADULT and CHILD over 5 years, 10 mg twice daily for 5 days (for up to 10 days if resistance to oseltamivir suspected [unlicensed duration])

¹Relenza® (GSK) [PoM]
Dry powder for inhalation disks containing 4 blisters of zanamivir 5 mg/blister, net price 5 disks with *Diskhaler*® device = £16.36

5.3.5 Respiratory syncytial virus

Ribavirin inhibits a wide range of DNA and RNA viruses. It is licensed for administration by inhalation for the treatment of severe bronchiolitis caused by the respiratory syncytial virus (RSV) in infants, especially when they have other serious diseases. However, there is no evidence that ribavirin produces clinically relevant benefit in RSV bronchiolitis. Ribavirin is given by mouth with peginterferon alfa or interferon alfa for the treatment of chronic hepatitis C infection (see section 5.3.3.2, p. 437). Ribavirin is also effective in Lassa fever [unlicensed indication].

Palivizumab is a monoclonal antibody licensed for preventing serious lower respiratory-tract disease caused by respiratory syncytial virus in children at high risk of the disease; it should be prescribed under specialist supervision and on the basis of the likelihood of hospitalisation.

Palivizumab is recommended for:

● children under 9 months of age with chronic lung disease (defined as requiring oxygen for at least 28 days from birth) and who were born preterm²;

1. [NHS] except for the treatment and prophylaxis of influenza as indicated in the notes above and NICE guidance; endorse prescription 'SLS'
2. For details of the preterm age groups included in the recommendations, see *Immunisation against Infectious Disease* (2006), available at www.gov.uk/dh

● children under 6 months of age with haemodynamically significant, acyanotic congenital heart disease who were born preterm².

Palivizumab should be considered for:

● children under 2 years of age with severe combined immunodeficiency syndrome;

● children under 1 year of age who require long-term ventilation;

● children 1–2 years of age who require long-term ventilation and have an additional co-morbidity (including cardiac disease or pulmonary hypertension).

PALIVIZUMAB

Indications see notes above

Cautions moderate to severe acute infection or febrile illness; thrombocytopenia; serum-palivizumab concentration may be reduced after cardiac surgery; hypersensitivity to humanised monoclonal antibodies

Side-effects fever, injection-site reactions, nervousness; *less commonly* diarrhoea, vomiting, constipation, haemorrhage, rhinitis, cough, wheeze, pain, drowsiness, asthenia, hyperkinesia, leucopenia, and rash; also reported, apnoea, hypersensitivity reactions (including anaphylaxis), convulsions and thombocytopenia

Dose

● By intramuscular injection (preferably in anterolateral thigh), 15 mg/kg once a month during season of RSV risk (child undergoing cardiac bypass surgery, 15 mg/kg as soon as stable after surgery, then once a month during season of risk); injection volume over 1 mL should be divided between more than one site

Synagis® (AbbVie) [PoM]
Injection, powder for reconstitution, palivizumab, net price 50-mg vial = £306.34; 100-mg vial = £563.64

RIBAVIRIN
(Tribavirin)

Indications severe respiratory syncytial virus bronchiolitis in infants and children; in combination with peginterferon alfa or interferon alfa for chronic hepatitis C in patients without liver decompensation (see also section 5.3.3.2)

Cautions

Specific cautions for inhaled treatment Maintain standard supportive respiratory and fluid management therapy; monitor electrolytes closely; monitor equipment for precipitation; pregnant women (and those planning pregnancy) should avoid exposure to aerosol

Specific cautions for oral treatment Exclude pregnancy before treatment; effective contraception essential during treatment and for 4 months after treatment in women and for 7 months after treatment in men; routine monthly pregnancy tests recommended; condoms must be used if partner of male patient is pregnant (ribavirin excreted in semen); cardiac disease (assessment including ECG recommended before and during treatment—discontinue if deterioration); gout; determine full blood count, platelets, electrolytes, serum creatinine, liver function tests and uric acid before starting treatment and then on weeks 2 and 4 of treatment, then as indicated clinically—adjust dose if adverse reactions or laboratory abnormalities develop (consult product literature); eye examination recommended before treatment; eye examination also recommended during treatment if pre-existing ophthalmological disorder or if decrease in vision reported—discontinue treatment if ophthalmological disorder deteriorates or if new ophthalmological disorder develops; patients with a transplant—risk of rejection; test thyroid function before treatment and then every 3 months in children; risk of growth retardation in children, the reversibility of which is uncertain—if possible, consider starting treatment after pubertal growth spurt

Interactions: Appendix 1 (ribavirin)

Contra-indications

Specific contra-indications for oral treatment Severe cardiac disease, including unstable or uncontrolled cardiac disease in previous 6 months; haemoglobinopathies; severe debilitating medical conditions; autoimmune disease (including autoimmune hepatitis); uncontrolled severe psychiatric condition; history of severe psychiatric condition in children

Hepatic impairment   no dosage adjustment required; use oral ribavirin with caution in severe hepatic dysfunction or decompensated cirrhosis

Renal impairment   plasma-ribavirin concentration increased; avoid oral ribavirin unless essential if eGFR less than 50 mL/minute/1.73 m^2—monitor haemoglobin concentration closely

Pregnancy   avoid; teratogenicity in *animal* studies; see also Cautions above

Breast-feeding   avoid—no information available

Side-effects

Specific side-effects for inhaled treatment Worsening respiration, bacterial pneumonia, and pneumothorax reported; rarely non-specific anaemia and haemolysis
Specific side-effects for oral treatment Haemolytic anaemia (anaemia may be improved by epoetin); also (in combination with peginterferon alfa or interferon alfa) nausea, vomiting, dyspepsia, abdominal pain, flatulence, constipation, diarrhoea, colitis, chest pain, palpitation, tachycardia, peripheral oedema, changes in blood pressure, syncope, flushing, cough, dyspnoea, headache, dizziness, asthenia, impaired concentration and memory, sleep disturbances, abnormal dreams, anxiety, depression, suicidal ideation (more frequent in children), psychoses, dysphagia, weight loss, dysphonia, paraesthesia, hypoaesthesia, ataxia, hypertonia, influenza-like symptoms, thyroid disorders, hyperglycaemia, menstrual disturbances, breast pain, prostatitis, sexual dysfunction, micturition disorders, leucopenia, thrombocytopenia, lymphadenopathy, dehydration, hypocalcaemia, myalgia, arthralgia, hyperuricaemia, visual disturbances, eye pain, dry eyes, hearing impairment, tinnitus, earache, dry mouth, taste disturbances, mouth ulcers, stomatitis, glossitis, tooth disorder, gingivitis, alopecia, pruritus, dry skin, rash (including very rarely Stevens-Johnson syndrome and toxic epidermal necrolysis), increased sweating, psoriasis, photosensitivity, and acne; *less commonly* pancreatitis, gastro-intestinal bleeding, and hypertriglyceridaemia; *rarely* peptic ulcer, arrhythmias, cardiomyopathy, myocardial infarction, pericarditis, stroke, interstitial pneumonitis, pulmonary embolism, seizures, renal failure, vasculitis, rheumatoid arthritis, systemic lupus erythematosus, sarcoidosis, optic neuropathy, and retinal haemorrhage; *very rarely* aplastic anaemia and peripheral ischaemia; *in children* also growth retardation (including decrease in height and weight), pallor, tachypnoea, hyperkinesia, virilism, and skin discoloration

Dose

• See preparations below

Copegus® (Roche) [PoM]
Tablets, f/c, ribavirin 200 mg (pink), net price 42-tab pack = £92.50, 112-tab pack = £246.65, 168-tab pack = £369.98; 400 mg (red-brown), 56-tab pack = £246.65. Label: 21
Dose chronic hepatitis C (in combination with interferon alfa or peginterferon alfa), ADULT over 18 years, body-weight under 75 kg, 400 mg in the morning and 600 mg in the evening; body-weight 75 kg and over, 600 mg twice daily
Note Patients with chronic hepatitis C genotype 2 or 3 (not previously treated), or patients infected with HIV and hepatitis C require a lower dose of *Copegus*® (in combination with peginterferon alfa), usual dose 400 mg twice daily

Rebetol® (MSD) [PoM]
Capsules, ribavirin 200 mg, net price 84-cap pack = £160.69, 140-cap pack = £267.81, 168-cap pack = £321.38. Label: 21
Oral solution, ribavirin 200 mg/5 mL, net price 100 mL (bubble-gum-flavoured) = £67.08. Label: 21
Dose chronic hepatitis C (in combination with interferon alfa or peginterferon alfa), ADULT over 18 years, body-weight under 65 kg, 400 mg twice daily; body-weight 65–81 kg, 400 mg in the morning and 600 mg in the evening; body-weight 81–105 kg, 600 mg twice daily; body-weight over 105 kg, 600 mg in the morning and 800 mg in the evening; CHILD 3–18 years see *BNF for Children*

Virazole® (Meda) [PoM]
Inhalation, ribavirin 6 g for reconstitution with 300 mL water for injections. Net price 3 × 6-g vials = £349.00
Dose bronchiolitis, by aerosol inhalation *or* nebulisation (via small particle aerosol generator) of solution containing 20 mg/mL for 12–18 hours for at least 3 days; max. 7 days

5.4 Antiprotozoal drugs

5.4.1	**Antimalarials**
5.4.2	**Amoebicides**
5.4.3	**Trichomonacides**
5.4.4	**Antigiardial drugs**
5.4.5	**Leishmaniacides**
5.4.6	**Trypanocides**
5.4.7	**Drugs for toxoplasmosis**
5.4.8	**Drugs for pneumocystis pneumonia**

Advice on specific problems available from:

Advice for healthcare professionals

PHE (Public Health England) Malaria Reference Laboratory	(020) 7637 0248 (fax) (prophylaxis only)
www.malaria-reference.co.uk	
National Travel Health Network and Centre	0845 602 6712
Travel Medicine Team, Health Protection Scotland (registered users of Travax only) www.travax.nhs.uk (for registered users of the NHS Travax website only)	(0141) 300 1100 (weekdays 2–4 p.m. only)
Birmingham	(0121) 424 2358
Liverpool	(0151) 705 3100
London	0845 155 5000 (treatment)
Oxford	(01865) 225 430

Advice for travellers

Hospital for Tropical Diseases Travel Healthline	(020) 7950 7799
www.fitfortravel.nhs.uk	
WHO advice on international travel and health www.who.int/ith	

National Travel Health Network and Centre (NaTHNaC)
www.nathnac.org/travel/index.htm

5.4.1 Antimalarials

Recommendations on the prophylaxis and treatment of malaria reflect guidelines agreed by UK malaria specialists.

5 Infections

The centres listed above should be consulted for advice on special problems.

Treatment of malaria

If the infective species is **not known**, or if the infection is **mixed**, initial treatment should be as for *falciparum malaria* with quinine, *Malarone*® (proguanil with atovaquone), or *Riamet*® (artemether with lumefantrine). Falciparum malaria can progress rapidly in unprotected individuals and antimalarial treatment should be considered in those with features of severe malaria and possible exposure, even if the initial blood tests for the organism are negative.

Falciparum malaria (treatment)

Falciparum malaria (malignant malaria) is caused by *Plasmodium falciparum*. In most parts of the world *P. falciparum* is now resistant to chloroquine which should not therefore be given for treatment.

Quinine, *Malarone*® (proguanil with atovaquone), or *Riamet*® (artemether with lumefantrine) can be given *by mouth* if the patient can swallow and retain tablets and there are no serious manifestations (e.g. impaired consciousness); quinine should be given by *intravenous infusion* (see below) if the patient is seriously ill or unable to take tablets. Mefloquine is now rarely used for treatment because of concerns about resistance.

Oral. The adult dosage regimen for **quinine** *by mouth* is:
600 mg (of quinine salt[1]) every 8 hours for 5–7 days *together with or followed by*
either **doxycycline** 200 mg once daily for 7 days
or **clindamycin** 450 mg every 8 hours for 7 days [unlicensed indication].
If the parasite is likely to be sensitive, **pyrimethamine** 75 mg with **sulfadoxine** 1.5 g as a single dose [unlicensed] may be given (instead of either clindamycin or doxycycline) together with, or after, a course of quinine.

Alternatively, *Malarone*® or *Riamet*® may be given instead of quinine. It is not necessary to give doxycycline, clindamycin or pyrimethamine with sulfadoxine after *Malarone*® or *Riamet*® treatment.

The adult dose of *Malarone*® *by mouth* is:
4 ('standard') tablets once daily for 3 days.

The dose of *Riamet*® *by mouth* for adult with body-weight over 35 kg is:
4 tablets initially, followed by 5 further doses of 4 tablets each given at 8, 24, 36, 48, and 60 hours (total 24 tablets over 60 hours).

Parenteral. If the patient is seriously ill or unable to take tablets, or if more than 2% of red blood cell are parasitized, **quinine** should be given *by intravenous infusion* [unlicensed]. The adult dosage regimen for quinine *by infusion* is:
loading dose[2] of 20 mg/kg[3] (up to maximum 1.4 g)

of quinine salt[1] infused over 4 hours *then 8 hours after the start of the loading dose*, maintenance dose of 10 mg/kg[4] (up to maximum 700 mg) of quinine salt[1] infused over 4 hours every 8 hours (until patient can swallow tablets to complete the 7-day course *together with or followed by either* doxycycline or clindamycin as above).

Specialist advice should be sought in difficult cases (e.g. very high parasite count, deterioration on optimal doses of quinine, infection acquired in quinine-resistant areas of south east Asia) because intravenous **artesunate** may be available for 'named-patient' use.

Children

Oral. **Quinine** is well tolerated by children although the salts are bitter. The dosage regimen for quinine *by mouth* for children is:
10 mg/kg (of quinine salt[1]; max. 600 mg) every 8 hours for 7 days *together with or followed by*
Clindamycin 7–13 mg/kg (max. 450 mg) every 8 hours for 7 days [unlicensed indication]
or in children over 12 years, **doxycycline** 200 mg once daily for 7 days
or if the parasite is likely to be sensitive, **pyrimethamine** with **sulfadoxine** as a single dose [unlicensed]: up to 4 years and body-weight over 5 kg, pyrimethamine 12.5 mg with sulfadoxine 250 mg; 5–6 years, pyrimethamine 25 mg with sulfadoxine 500 mg; 7–9 years, pyrimethamine 37.5 mg with sulfadoxine 750 mg; 10–14 years, pyrimethamine 50 mg with sulfadoxine 1 g; 14–18 years, pyrimethamine 75 mg with sulfadoxine 1.5 g

Alternatively, *Malarone*® or *Riamet*® may be given instead of quinine; it is not necessary to give clindamycin, doxycycline, or pyrimethamine with sulfadoxine after *Malarone*® or *Riamet*® treatment. The dose regimen for *Malarone*® *by mouth* for children over 40 kg is the same as for adults (see above); the dose regimen for *Malarone*® for smaller children is reduced as follows:
body-weight 5–9 kg, 2 'paediatric' tablets once daily for 3 days; body-weight 9–11 kg, 3 'paediatric' tablets once daily for 3 days; body-weight 11–21 kg, 1 'standard' tablet once daily for 3 days; body-weight 21–31 kg, 2 'standard' tablets once daily for 3 days; body-weight 31–40 kg, 3 'standard' tablets once daily for 3 days.

The dose regimen of *Riamet*® *by mouth* for children over 12 years and body-weight over 35 kg is the same as for adults (see above). The dose regimen for *Riamet*® for children under 12 years is as follows:
body-weight 5–15 kg 1 tablet initially, followed by 5 further doses of 1 tablet each given at 8, 24, 36, 48, and 60 hours (total 6 tablets over 60 hours); body-weight 15–25 kg 2 tablets initially, followed by 5 further doses of 2 tablets each given at 8, 24, 36, 48, and 60 hours (total 12 tablets over 60 hours); body-weight 25–35 kg 3 tablets initially, followed by 5 further doses of 3 tablets each given at 8, 24, 36, 48, and 60 hours (total 18 tablets over 60 hours)

Parenteral. The dose regimen for quinine *by intravenous infusion* for children is calculated on a mg/kg basis as for adults (see above).

---

1. Valid for quinine hydrochloride, dihydrochloride, and sulfate; not valid for quinine bisulfate which contains a correspondingly smaller amount of quinine.
2. In intensive care units the loading dose can alternatively be given as quinine salt[1] 7 mg/kg infused over 30 minutes followed immediately by 10 mg/kg over 4 hours then (after 8 hours) maintenance dose as described.
3. **Important:** the loading dose of 20 mg/kg should **not** be used if the patient has received quinine or mefloquine during the previous 12 hours.
4. Maintenance dose should be reduced to 5–7 mg/kg of quinine salt[1] in patients with severe renal impairment, severe hepatic impairment, or if parenteral treatment is required for more than 48 hours.

Pregnancy Falciparum malaria is particularly dangerous in pregnancy, especially in the last trimester. The adult treatment doses of oral and intravenous quinine given above (including the loading dose) can safely be given to pregnant women. Clindamycin 450 mg every 8 hours for 7 days [unlicensed indication] should be given with or after quinine. Doxycycline should be avoided in pregnancy (affects teeth and skeletal development); pyrimethamine with sulfadoxine, *Malarone*®, and *Riamet*® are also best avoided until more information is available. Specialist advice should be sought in difficult cases (e.g. very high parasite count, deterioration on optimal doses of quinine, infection acquired in quinine-resistant areas of south east Asia) because intravenous artesunate may be available for 'named patient' use.

Non-falciparum malaria (treatment)

Non-falciparum malaria is usually caused by *Plasmodium vivax* and less commonly by *P. ovale* and *P. malariae*. *P. knowlesi* is also present in the Asia-Pacific region. **Chloroquine**[1] is the drug of choice for the treatment of non-falciparum malaria (but chloroquine-resistant *P. vivax* has been reported in the Indonesian archipelago, the Malay Peninsula, including Myanmar, and eastward to Southern Vietnam).

The adult dosage regimen for **chloroquine** *by mouth* is:

initial dose of 620 mg of base *then*

a single dose of 310 mg of base after 6 to 8 hours *then*

a single dose of 310 mg of base daily for 2 days

(approximate total cumulative dose of 25 mg/kg of base)

Chloroquine alone is adequate for *P. malariae* and *P. knowlesi* infections but in the case of *P. vivax* and *P. ovale*, a *radical cure* (to destroy parasites in the liver and thus prevent relapses) is required. This is achieved with **primaquine**[2] [unlicensed] given after chloroquine; in *P. vivax* infection primaquine is given in an adult dosage of 30 mg daily for 14 days and for *P. ovale* infection it is given in an adult dosage of 15 mg daily for 14 days.

Children The dosage regimen of chloroquine for non-falciparum malaria in children is:

initial dose of 10 mg/kg of base (max. 620 mg) *then*

a single dose of 5 mg/kg of base (max. 310 mg) after 6–8 hours *then*

a single dose of 5 mg/kg of base (max. 310 mg) daily for 2 days

For a *radical cure*, primaquine[2] [unlicensed] is then given to children over 6 months of age; specialist advice should be sought for children under 6 months of age. In *P. vivax* infection primaquine is given in a dose of 500 micrograms/kg (max. 30 mg) daily for 14 days, and

for *P. ovale* infection it is given in a dose of 250 micrograms/kg (max. 15 mg) daily for 14 days.

Parenteral If the patient is unable to take oral therapy, **quinine** can be given by *intravenous infusion* [unlicensed]. The dose (for adults and children) is 10 mg/kg[3] (max. 700 mg) of quinine salt[4] infused over 4 hours every 8 hours, changed to oral chloroquine as soon as the patient's condition permits.

Pregnancy The adult treatment doses of chloroquine can be given for non-falciparum malaria. In the case of *P. vivax* or *P. ovale*, however, the radical cure with primaquine should be **postponed** until the pregnancy is over; instead chloroquine should be continued at a dose of 310 mg each week during the pregnancy.

Prophylaxis against malaria

The recommendations on prophylaxis reflect guidelines agreed by UK malaria specialists; the advice is aimed at residents of the UK who travel to endemic areas. The choice of drug for a particular individual should take into account:

risk of exposure to malaria;

extent of drug resistance;

efficacy of the recommended drugs;

side-effects of the drugs;

patient-related factors (e.g. age, pregnancy, renal or hepatic impairment, compliance with prophylactic regimen).

Protection against bites Prophylaxis is not absolute, and breakthrough infection can occur with any of the drugs recommended. Personal protection against being bitten is very important. Mosquito nets impregnated with permethrin provide the most effective barrier protection against insects; mats and vaporised insecticides are also useful. Diethyltoluamide (DEET) 20–50% in lotions, sprays, or roll-on formulations is safe and effective when applied to the skin of adults and children over 2 months of age. It can also be used during pregnancy and breast-feeding. The duration of protection varies according to the concentration of DEET and is longest for DEET 50%. When sunscreen is also required, DEET should be applied after the sunscreen. Long sleeves and trousers worn after dusk also provide protection against bites.

Length of prophylaxis In order to determine tolerance and to establish habit, prophylaxis should generally be started one week (2–3 weeks in the case of mefloquine) before travel into an endemic area; *Malarone*® or doxycycline prophylaxis should be started 1–2 days before travel. Prophylaxis should be continued for **4 weeks after leaving** (except for *Malarone*® prophylaxis which should be stopped 1 week after leaving).

In those requiring long-term prophylaxis, chloroquine and proguanil may be used for periods of over 5 years. Mefloquine is licensed for up to 1 year (although, if it is tolerated in the short term, there is no evidence of harm when it is used for up to 3 years). Doxycycline can be used for up to 2 years. *Malarone*® can be used for up to

---

1. For the treatment of chloroquine-resistant non-falciparum malaria, *Malarone*® [unlicensed indication], quinine, or *Riamet*® [unlicensed indication] can be used; as with chloroquine, primaquine should be given for radical cure.
2. Before starting primaquine, blood should be tested for glucose-6-phosphate dehydrogenase (G6PD) activity since the drug can cause haemolysis in G6PD-deficient patients. Specialist advice should be obtained in G6PD deficiency; in mild G6PD deficiency primaquine in a dose for adults of 45 mg once a week (children 750 micrograms/kg once a week; max. 45 mg once a week) for 8 weeks, has been found useful and without undue harmful effects.

---

3. Maintenance dose should be reduced to 5–7 mg/kg of quinine salt[4] in patients with severe renal impairment, severe hepatic impairment, or if parenteral treatment is required for more than 48 hours.
4. Valid for quinine hydrochloride, dihydrochloride, and sulfate; not valid for quinine bisulfate which contains a correspondingly smaller amount of quinine.

1 year. Prophylaxis with mefloquine, doxycycline, or *Malarone*® may be considered for longer durations if it is justified by the risk of exposure to malaria. Specialist advice should be sought for long-term prophylaxis.

Return from malarial region   It is important to be aware that **any illness** that occurs within 1 year and **especially within 3 months of return might be malaria** even if all recommended precautions against malaria were taken. Travellers should be **warned** of this and told that if they develop any illness **particularly within 3 months** of their return they should go **immediately** to a doctor and specifically mention their exposure to malaria.

Children   Prophylactic doses are based on guidelines agreed by UK malaria experts and may differ from advice in product literature. Weight is a better guide than age. If in doubt telephone centres listed on p. 443.

Epilepsy   Both chloroquine and mefloquine are unsuitable for malaria prophylaxis in individuals with a history of epilepsy. In areas *without chloroquine resistance* proguanil 200 mg daily alone is recommended; in areas *with chloroquine resistance*, doxycycline or *Malarone*® may be considered; the metabolism of doxycycline may be influenced by antiepileptics (see **interactions**: Appendix 1 (tetracyclines)).

Asplenia   Asplenic individuals (or those with severe splenic dysfunction) are at particular risk of severe malaria. If travel to malarious areas is unavoidable, rigorous precautions are required against contracting the disease.

Renal impairment   Avoidance (or dosage reduction) of proguanil is recommended since it is excreted by the kidneys. *Malarone*® should not be used for prophylaxis in patients with estimated glomerular filtration rate less than 30 mL/minute/1.73 m². Chloroquine is only partially excreted by the kidneys and reduction of the dose for prophylaxis is not required except in severe impairment. Mefloquine is considered to be appropriate to use in renal impairment and does not require dosage reduction. Doxycycline is also considered to be appropriate.

Pregnancy   Travel to malarious areas should be avoided during pregnancy; if travel is unavoidable, effective prophylaxis must be used. Chloroquine and proguanil can be given in the usual doses during pregnancy, but these drugs are not appropriate for most areas because their effectiveness has declined, particularly in Sub-Saharan Africa; in the case of proguanil, folic acid 5 mg daily should be given for at least the first trimester. The centres listed on p. 443 should be consulted for advice on prophylaxis in chloroquine-resistant areas. Although the manufacturer advises that mefloquine should not be used during pregnancy, particularly in the first trimester, unless the potential benefit outweighs the risk, studies of mefloquine in pregnancy (including use in the first trimester) indicate that it can be considered for travel to chloroquine-resistant areas. Doxycycline is contra-indicated during pregnancy (see section 5.1.3); however, it can be used for malaria prophylaxis if other regimens are unsuitable, and if the entire course of doxycycline can be completed before 15 weeks' gestation [unlicensed]. *Malarone*® should be avoided during pregnancy, however, it can be considered during the second and third trimesters if there is no suitable alternative.

Breast-feeding   Prophylaxis is required in **breast-fed infants**; although antimalarials are present in milk, the amounts are too variable to give reliable protection.

Anticoagulants   Travellers taking warfarin should begin chemoprophylaxis 2–3 weeks before departure. The INR should be stable before departure. It should be measured before starting chemoprophylaxis, 7 days after starting, and after completing the course. For prolonged stays, the INR should be checked at regular intervals.

Specific recommendations

Where a journey requires two regimens, the regimen for the higher risk area should be used for the whole journey. Those travelling to remote or little-visited areas may require expert advice.

> **Important**
>
> Settled immigrants (or long-term visitors) to the UK may be unaware that **any immunity they may have acquired while living in malarious areas is lost rapidly** after migration to the UK, or that any non-malarious areas where they lived previously **may now be malarious**

Key to recommended regimens for prophylaxis against malaria

Codes for regimens	Details of regimens for prophylaxis against malaria
1	Chemoprophylaxis not recommended, but avoid mosquito bites and consider malaria if fever presents
2	Chloroquine only
3	Chloroquine + proguanil hydrochloride
4	*Malarone®* or doxycycline *or* mefloquine
5	*Malarone®* or doxycycline

Specific recommendations: Afghanistan–Burundi

Country	Comments on risk of malaria and regional or seasonal variation	Codes for regimens
Afghanistan	Risk below 2000 m from May–November	3
	Low risk below 2000 m from December–April	1
Algeria	Very low risk in Illizi department only	1
Andaman and Nicobar Islands (India)	Risk present	1
Angola	High risk	4
Argentina	Low risk in low altitude areas of Salta provinces bordering Bolivia and in Chaco, Corrientes, and Misiones provinces close to border with Paraguay and Brazil	2
	No risk in Iguaçu Falls and areas other than those above	1
Armenia	No risk	1
Azerbaijan	Low to no risk	1
Bangladesh	High risk in Chittagong Hill Tract districts (but not Chittagong city)	4
	Low to no risk in Chittagong city and other areas, except Chittagong Hill Tract districts	1
Belize	Low risk in rural areas	2
	No risk in Belize district (including Belize city and islands)	1
Benin	High risk	4
Bhutan	Risk in southern belt districts, along border with India: Chukha, Geyleg-phug, Samchi, Samdrup Jonkhar, and Shemgang	3
	Low to no risk in areas other than those above	1
Bolivia	High risk in Amazon basin	4
	Risk in rural areas below 2500 m (other than above)	2
	No risk above 2500 m	1
Botswana	High risk from November–June in northern half, including Okavango Delta area	4
	Low risk from July–October in northern half; low to no risk all year in southern half	1
Brazil	Risk in Amazon basin, including city of Manaus	4
	Very low risk in areas other than those above, and no risk in Iguaçu Falls	1
Brunei Darussalam	Very low risk	1
Burkina Faso	High risk	4
Burundi	High risk	4

5

Infections

Key to recommended regimens for prophylaxis against malaria

Codes for regimens	Details of regimens for prophylaxis against malaria
1	Chemoprophylaxis not recommended, but avoid mosquito bites and consider malaria if fever presents
2	Chloroquine only
3	Chloroquine + proguanil hydrochloride
4	*Malarone®* or doxycycline *or* mefloquine
5	*Malarone®* or doxycycline

Specific recommendations: Cambodia–Ethiopia

Country	Comments on risk of malaria and regional or seasonal variation	Codes for regimens
Cambodia	High risk, with widespread chloroquine and mefloquine resistance, in western provinces bordering Thailand	5
	High risk in areas other than those above and below	4
	Very low risk in Angkor Wat and Lake Tonle Sap, including Siem Reap; no risk in Phnom Penh	1
Cameroon	High risk	4
Cape Verde	Very low risk on island of Santiago (Sao Tiago) and Boa Vista	1
Central African Republic	High risk	4
Chad	High risk	4
China	High risk in Yunnan and Hainan provinces	4
	Very low risk in areas other than those above and below	1
	No risk in Hong Kong	–
Colombia	High risk in rural areas below 1600 m	4
	Low to no risk above 1600 m and in Cartagena	1
Comoros	High risk	4
Congo	High risk	4
Costa Rica	Risk in Limon province (but not city of Limon)	2
	Very low risk in areas other than those above	1
Cote d'Ivoire (Ivory Coast)	High risk	4
Democratic Republic of the Congo	High risk	4
Djibouti	High risk	4
Dominican Republic	Risk in all areas except cities of Santiago and Santo Domingo	2
	Cities of Santiago and Santo Domingo	1
East Timor (Timor-Leste)	High risk	4
Ecuador	Risk in areas below 1500 m including coastal provinces and Amazon basin (no risk in Galapagos islands or city of Guayaquil)	4
Egypt	No risk	1
El Salvador	Low risk in rural areas of Santa Ana, Ahuachapán, and La Unión provinces in western part of country; low to no risk in other areas	1
Equatorial Guinea	High risk	4
Eritrea	High risk below 2200 m	4
Ethiopia	High risk below 2000 m	4

Specific recommendations: French Guiana–Iraq

Country	Comments on risk of malaria and regional or seasonal variation	Codes for regimens
French Guiana	High risk (particularly in border areas) except city of Cayenne or Devil's Island (Ile du Diable)	4
	No risk In clty of Cayenne or Devil's Island (Ile du Diable)	1
Gabon	High risk	4
Gambia	HIgh risk	4
Georgia	Very low risk in rural south east from June–October	1
Ghana	High risk	4
Guatemala	Low risk below 1500 m	2
	No risk in Guatemala City, Antigua, or Lake Atitlan	–
Guinea	High risk	4
Guinea-Bissau	High risk	4
Guyana	High risk in all interior regions	4
	Very low risk in Georgetown and coastal region	1
Haiti	Risk present	2
Honduras	Risk below 1000 m and in Roatán and other Bay Islands (no risk in San Pedro Sula or Tegucigalpa)	2
India	High risk in states of Assam and Orissa, districts of East Godavari, Srikakulam, Vishakhapatnam, and Vizianagaram in the state of Andhra Pradesh, and districts of Balaghat, Dindori, Mandla, and Seoni in the state of Madhya Pradesh	4
	Risk in areas other than those above or below (including Goa, Andaman and Nicobar islands)	1
	No risk in Lakshadweep islands	–
Indonesia	High risk in Lombok and Irian Jaya (Papua)	4
	Risk in areas other than those above or below	3
	Very low risk in Bali, and cities on islands of Java and Sumatra	1
	No rIsk In clty of Jakarta	–
Indonesia (Borneo)	High risk	4
Iran	Risk from March–November in rural south eastern provinces and in north, along Azerbaijan border in Ardabil, and near Turkmenistan border In North Khorasan	3
	Low to no risk in areas other than those above	1
Iraq	Very low risk from May–November in rural northern area below 1500 m	1

Specific recommendations: Kenya–Myanmar

Country	Comments on risk of malaria and regional or seasonal variation	Codes for regimens
Kenya	High risk below 2500 m (except city of Nairobi)	4
	Very low risk in the highlands above 2500 m and in city of Nairobi	1
Kyrgyzstan	Very low risk from June–October in southwest areas bordering Tajikistan and Uzbekistan	1
Laos	High risk along the border with Myanmar in the provinces of Bokeo and Louang Namtha, and along the border with Thailand in the province of Champasak and Saravan	5
	High risk in areas other than those above or below	4
	Low to no risk in cIty of Vientiane	1
Liberia	High risk	4
Libya	No risk	1
Madagascar	High risk	4
Malawi	High risk	4

Key to recommended regimens for prophylaxis against malaria

Codes for regimens	Details of regimens for prophylaxis against malaria
1	Chemoprophylaxis not recommended, but avoid mosquito bites and consider malaria if fever presents
2	Chloroquine only
3	Chloroquine + proguanil hydrochloride
4	*Malarone*® or doxycycline *or* mefloquine
5	*Malarone*® or doxycycline

Specific recommendations: Kenya–Myanmar (*continued*)

Country	Comments on risk of malaria and regional or seasonal variation	Codes for regimens
Malaysia	Risk in inland forested areas of peninsular Malaysia	4
	Very low risk in rest of peninsular Malaysia, including Cameron Highlands and city of Kuala Lumpur	1
Malaysia (Borneo)	High risk in inland areas of eastern Sabah and in inland, forested areas of Sarawak	4
	Very low risk in areas other than those above, including coastal areas of Sabah and Sarawak	1
Mali	High risk	4
Mauritania	High risk all year in southern provinces, and from July–October in the north	4
	Low risk from November–June in north	1
Mauritius	No risk	1
Mayotte	Risk present	4
Mexico	Low risk in Oaxaca and Chiapas	2
	Very low risk in areas other than those above	1
Mozambique	High risk	4
Myanmar	High risk (but not in cities of Mandalay and Yangon)	5
	No risk in cities of Mandalay and Yangon	1

Specific recommendations: Namibia–Rwanda

Country	Comments on risk of malaria and regional or seasonal variation	Codes for regimens
Namibia	High risk all year in regions of Caprivi Strip, Kavango, and Kunene river, and from November–June in northern third of country	4
	Low to no risk in areas other than those above; low risk from July–October in northern third of country	1
Nepal	Risk below 1500 m, particularly in Terai district	3
	No risk in city of Kathmandu and on typical Himalayan treks	1
Nicaragua	Low risk (except Managua)	2
	Very low risk in Managua	1
Niger	High risk	4
Nigeria	High risk	4
North Korea	Very low risk in some southern areas	1
Pakistan	Risk below 2000 m	3
	Low to no risk above 2000 m	1

Specific recommendations: Namibia–Rwanda (*continued*)

Country	Comments on risk of malaria and regional or seasonal variation	Codes for regimens
Panama	Risk east of Canal Zone	3
	Low risk west of Canal Zone	2
	No risk in Panama City or Canal Zone itself	1
Papua New Guinea	High risk below 1800 m	4
	Low to no risk above 1800 m	1
Paraguay	Low risk in departments of Alto Paraná and Caaguazú	2
	Very low risk in areas other than those above	1
Peru	High risk in Amazon basin along border with Brazil, particularly in Loreto province	4
	Risk in rural areas below 2000 m (other than those above and below) and in part of the Amazon basin that borders Bolivia	2
	No risk in city of Lima and coastal region south of Chiclayo	1
Philippines	Risk in rural areas below 600 m and on islands of Luzon, Mindanao, Mindoro, and Palawan	3
	No risk in cities or on islands of Boracay, Bohol, Catanduanes, Cebu, or Leyte	1
Rwanda	High risk	4

Specific recommendations: São Tomé and Principe–Syria

Country	Comments on risk of malaria and regional or seasonal variation	Codes for regimens
São Tomé and Principe	High risk	4
Saudi Arabia	Risk in south-western provinces along border with Yemen, including below 2000 m in Asir province	3
	No risk in cities of Jeddah, Makkah (Mecca), Medina, Riyadh, or Ta'if, or above 2000 m in Asir province	1
Senegal	High risk	4
Sierra Leone	High risk	4
Solomon Islands	High risk	4
Somalia	High risk	4
South Africa	Moderate risk from September–May in low altitude areas of Mpumalanga and Limpopo, which border Mozambique and Zimbabwe (including Kruger National Park)	4
	Low risk in north-east KwaZulu-Natal	1
	Low risk in areas bordering those above	1
South Korea	Very low risk in northern areas, in Gangwon-do and Gyeonggi-do provinces, and Incheon city (towards Demilitarized Zone)	1
South Sudan	High risk	4
Sri Lanka	Low risk north of Vavuniya	1
	Very low risk in areas other than those above and below	1
	No risk in Colombo or Kandy	–
Sudan	High risk in central and southern areas; risk also present in rest of country (except Khartoum)	4
	Very low risk in Khartoum	1
Suriname	High risk (except coastal districts or city of Paramaribo)	4
	Very low risk in coastal districts; no risk in city of Paramaribo	1
Swaziland	High risk in northern and eastern regions bordering Mozambique and South Africa, including all of Lubombo district and Big Bend, Mhlume, Simunye, and Tshaneni regions	4
	Very low risk in the areas other than those above	1
Syria	Very low risk in small, remote foci of El Hasakah	1

Key to recommended regimens for prophylaxis against malaria

Codes for regimens	Details of regimens for prophylaxis against malaria
1	Chemoprophylaxis not recommended, but avoid mosquito bites and consider malaria if fever presents
2	Chloroquine only
3	Chloroquine + proguanil hydrochloride
4	*Malarone®* or doxycycline *or* mefloquine
5	*Malarone®* or doxycycline

Specific recommendations: Tajikistan–Zimbabwe

Country	Comments on risk of malaria and regional or seasonal variation	Codes for regimens
Tajikistan	Risk below 2000 m from June–October	3
	Low risk below 2000 m from November–May	1
Tanzania	High risk below 1800 m; risk also in Zanzibar	4
Thailand	High risk, with chloroquine and mefloquine resistance, in rural forested borders with Cambodia, Laos, and Myanmar	5
	Very low risk in areas other than those above, including Kanchanaburi (Kwai Bridge); no risk in cities of Bangkok, Chiang Mai, Chiang Rai, Koh Phangan, Koh Samui, and Pattaya	1
Togo	High risk	4
Turkey	Low risk from May–October along the border plain with Syria, around Adana and east of Adana	2
	Very low risk from November–April along the border plain with Syria, around Adana and east of Adana; very low risk all year in rest of country	1
Uganda	High risk	4
Uzbekistan	Very low risk in extreme south-east	1
Vanuatu	Risk present	4
Venezuela	High risk in all areas south of, and including, the Orinoco river and Angel Falls	4
	Risk in rural areas of Apure, Monagas, Sucre, and Zulia states	3
	No risk in city of Caracas or on Margarita Island	1
Vietnam	Risk in rural areas, and in southern provinces of Tay Ninh, Lam Dong, Dac Lac, Gia Lai, and Kon Tum	5
	Very low risk in Mekong river delta until border area with Cambodia; no risk in large cities (including Ho Chi Minh (Saigon) and Hanoi), Red river delta, and coastal areas north of Nha Trang	1
Western Sahara	No risk	1
Yemen	Risk below 2000 m	3
	Very low risk on Socrota Island; no risk above 2000 m, including Sana'a city	1
Zambia	High risk	4
Zimbabwe	High risk all year in Zambezi valley, and from November–June in areas below 1200 m	4
	Low risk from July–October in areas below 1200 m; very low risk all year in Harare and Bulawayo	1

Standby treatment

> Travellers visiting remote, malarious areas for pro-
> longed periods should carry standby treatment if
> they are likely to be more than 24 hours away
> from medical care. Self-medication should be
> **avoided** if medical help is accessible.
>
> In order to avoid excessive self-medication, the
> traveller should be provided with **written instruc-
> tions** that urgent medical attention should be sought
> if fever (38°C or more) develops 7 days (or more)
> after arriving in a malarious area and that self-treat-
> ment is indicated if medical help is not available
> within 24 hours of fever onset.
>
> In view of the continuing emergence of resistant
> strains and of the different regimens required for
> different areas expert advice should be sought on
> the best treatment course for an individual traveller.
> A drug used for chemoprophylaxis should not be
> considered for standby treatment for the same tra-
> veller.

Artemether with lumefantrine

Artemether with lumefantrine is licensed for the *treatment of acute uncomplicated falciparum malaria.*

■ ARTEMETHER WITH LUMEFANTRINE

Indications treatment of acute uncomplicated falciparum malaria; treatment of non-falciparum malaria
[unlicensed indication]

Cautions electrolyte disturbances, concomitant use
with other drugs known to cause QT-interval prolongation; monitor patients unable to take food
(greater risk of recrudescence); avoid in acute porphyria (section 9.8.2); **interactions:** Appendix 1
(artemether with lumefantrine)

Driving Dizziness may affect performance of skilled tasks
(e.g. driving)

Contra-indications history of arrhythmias, of clinically relevant bradycardia, and of congestive heart
failure accompanied by reduced left ventricular ejection fraction; family history of sudden death or of
congenital QT interval prolongation

Hepatic impairment manufacturer advises caution in
severe impairment

Renal impairment manufacturer advises caution in
severe impairment—monitor ECG and plasma
potassium concentration

Pregnancy toxicity in *animal* studies with artemether;
manufacturer advises use only if potential benefit
outweighs risk

Breast-feeding manufacturer advises avoid breast-
feeding for at least 1 week after last dose; present in
milk in *animal* studies

Side-effects abdominal pain, anorexia, diarrhoea,
vomiting, nausea; palpitation, prolonged QT interval;
cough; headache, dizziness, sleep disturbances, asthenia, paraesthesia; arthralgia, myalgia; pruritus, rash;
less commonly ataxia, hypoaesthesia, and clonus

Dose
● Treatment of malaria, see p. 444

Riamet® (Novartis) [PoM]
Tablets, yellow, artemether 20 mg, lumefantrine
120 mg, net price 24-tab pack = £22.50. Label: 21,
counselling, driving
Note Tablets may be crushed just before administration

Chloroquine

Chloroquine is used for the *prophylaxis of malaria* in
areas of the world where the *risk of chloroquine-resistant
falciparum malaria is still low.* It is also used with proguanil when chloroquine-resistant falciparum malaria is
present but this regimen may not give optimal protection (see specific recommendations by country, p. 446).

Chloroquine is **no longer recommended** for the *treatment of falciparum malaria* owing to widespread resistance, nor is it recommended if the infective species is
not known or if the infection is *mixed*; in these cases
treatment should be with quinine, *Malarone®*, or *Ria-
met®* (for details, see p. 444). It is still recommended for
the *treatment of non-falciparum malaria* (for details, see
p. 445).

■ CHLOROQUINE

Indications chemoprophylaxis and treatment of malaria; rheumatoid arthritis and lupus erythematosus
(section 10.1.3)

Cautions may exacerbate psoriasis; neurological disorders (avoid for prophylaxis if history of epilepsy, see
notes above); may aggravate myasthenia gravis;
severe gastro-intestinal disorders; G6PD deficiency
(see section 9.1.5); ophthalmic examination and long-
term therapy, see under Chloroquine, section 10.1.3;
avoid concurrent therapy with hepatotoxic drugs—
other **interactions:** Appendix 1 (chloroquine and
hydroxychloroquine)

Hepatic impairment use with caution in moderate to
severe impairment

Renal impairment manufacturers advise caution; see
also Prophylaxis Against Malaria, p. 446

Pregnancy benefit of prophylaxis and treatment in
malaria outweighs risk; see also Non-falciparum
Malaria (treatment), p. 445 and Prophylaxis Against
Malaria, p. 446

Breast-feeding amount in milk probably too small to
be harmful; see also Prophylaxis Against Malaria,
p. 446

Side-effects gastro-intestinal disturbances, headache,
skin reactions (rashes, pruritus); also hypotension,
convulsions, extrapyramidal symptoms, visual disturbances, depigmentation or loss of hair; rarely bone-
marrow suppression, hypersensitivity reactions such
as urticaria and angioedema; other side-effects (not
usually associated with malaria prophylaxis or treatment), see under Chloroquine, section 10.1.3; very
toxic in **overdosage**—immediate advice from poisons
centres essential (see also p. 39)

Dose
Note Doses expressed as chloroquine base
● Prophylaxis of malaria, started 1 week before entering
endemic area and continued for 4 weeks after leaving
(see notes above), 310 mg once weekly; CHILD up to 6
weeks body-weight under 4.5 kg, 25 mg once weekly;
6 weeks–6 months body-weight 4.5–8 kg, 50 mg once
weekly; 6 months–1 year body-weight 8–11 kg, 75 mg
once weekly; 1–3 years body-weight 11–15 kg,
100 mg once weekly; 3–4 years body-weight 15–

5

Infections

5 Infections

16.5 kg, 125 mg once weekly; 4–8 years body-weight 16.5–25 kg, 150 mg once weekly (or 155 mg once weekly if tablets used); 8–13 years body-weight 25–45 kg, 225 mg once weekly (or 232.5 mg once weekly if tablets used); over 13 years body-weight over 45 kg, adult dose

Counselling Warn travellers about **importance** of avoiding mosquito bites, **importance** of taking prophylaxis regularly, and **importance** of immediate visit to doctor if ill within 1 year and **especially** within 3 months of return. For details, see notes above

• Treatment of non-falciparum malaria, see p. 445

Note Chloroquine doses in BNF may differ from those in product literature

¹Avloclor® (Alliance) PoM
Tablets, scored, chloroquine phosphate 250 mg (≡ chloroquine base 155 mg). Net price 20-tab pack = £4.90. Label: 5, counselling, prophylaxis, see above

¹Malarivon® (Wallace Mfg) PoM
Syrup, chloroquine phosphate 80 mg/5 mL (≡ chloroquine base 50 mg/5 mL), net price 75 mL = £10.85. Label: 5, counselling, prophylaxis, see above

¹Nivaquine® (Sanofi-Aventis) PoM
Syrup, golden, chloroquine sulfate 68 mg/5 mL (≡ chloroquine base 50 mg/5 mL), net price 100 mL = £4.60. Label: 5, counselling, prophylaxis, see above

◀With proguanil
For cautions and side-effects of proguanil see Proguanil; for dose see Chloroquine and Proguanil

¹Paludrine/Avloclor® (Alliance)
Tablets, travel pack of 14 tablets of chloroquine phosphate 250 mg (≡ chloroquine base 155 mg) and 98 tablets of proguanil hydrochloride 100 mg, net price 112-tab pack = £11.75. Label: 5, 21, counselling, prophylaxis, see above

---

Mefloquine

Mefloquine is used for the *prophylaxis of malaria* in areas of the world where there is a *high risk of chloroquine-resistant falciparum malaria* (for details, see specific recommendations by country, p. 446).

Mefloquine is now rarely used for the *treatment of falciparum malaria* because of increased resistance. It is rarely used for the *treatment of non-falciparum malaria* because better tolerated alternatives are available. Mefloquine should not be used for treatment if it has been used for prophylaxis.

▌ MEFLOQUINE

Indications chemoprophylaxis of malaria, treatment of malaria, see notes above

Cautions cardiac conduction disorders; epilepsy (avoid for prophylaxis); traumatic brain injury; not recommended in infants under 3 months (5 kg); interactions: Appendix 1 (mefloquine)
Neuropsychiatric reactions Mefloquine is associated with potentially serious neuropsychiatric reactions. Abnormal dreams, insomnia, anxiety, and depression occur commonly. Psychosis, suicidal ideation, and suicide have also been

reported. Psychiatric symptoms such as nightmares, acute anxiety, depression, restlessness, or confusion should be regarded as potentially prodromal for a more serious event. If neuropsychiatric symptoms occur, patients should be advised to discontinue mefloquine and to seek immediate medical attention so that mefloquine can be replaced with an alternative antimalarial. Adverse reactions may occur and persist up to several months after discontinuation because mefloquine has a long half-life. Mefloquine is contra-indicated for malaria prophylaxis in those with a history of psychiatric disorders or convulsions
Driving Dizziness or a disturbed sense of balance may affect performance of skilled tasks (e.g. driving); effects may occur and persist up to several months after stopping mefloquine

Contra-indications hypersensitivity to quinine; history of blackwater fever; avoid for standby treatment if history of convulsions; avoid for prophylaxis if history of psychiatric disorders (including depression) or convulsions

Hepatic impairment elimination may be prolonged; avoid in severe impairment

Renal impairment manufacturer advises caution

Pregnancy manufacturer advises adequate contraception during prophylaxis and for 3 months after stopping (teratogenicity in *animal* studies), but see also p. 446

Breast-feeding present in milk but risk to infant minimal; see also p. 446

Side-effects nausea, vomiting, abdominal pain, diarrhoea, headache, dizziness, visual disturbances, pruritus; see also Neuropsychiatric Reactions above; *also reported* anorexia, dyspepsia, hepatic failure, hypotension, hypertension, flushing, chest pain, bradycardia, tachycardia, palpitation, arrhythmias, syncope, oedema, dyspnoea, pneumonitis, drowsiness, sensory and motor neuropathies, tremor, ataxia, panic attacks, confusion, amnesia, seizures, encephalopathy, speech disturbances, malaise, fever, blood disorders (including leucopenia, leucocytosis, thrombocytopenia), muscle weakness, myalgia, arthralgia, cataract, optic neuropathy, vestibular disorders, rash (including Stevens-Johnson syndrome), alopecia, hyperhidrosis

Dose

• Prophylaxis of malaria, started 2–3 weeks before entering endemic area and continued for 4 weeks after leaving (see notes above), ADULT and CHILD body-weight over 45 kg, 250 mg once weekly; body-weight 5–16 kg, 62.5 mg once weekly; body-weight 16–25 kg, 125 mg once weekly; body-weight 25–45 kg, 187.5 mg once weekly

• Treatment of malaria, see notes above

Counselling Inform travellers about adverse reactions of mefloquine and, if they occur, to seek medical advice on alternative antimalarials before the next dose is due (see also Neuropsychiatric Reactions and Driving above). Also warn travellers about **importance** of avoiding mosquito bites, **importance** of taking prophylaxis regularly, and **importance** of immediate visit to doctor if ill within 1 year and **especially** within 3 months of return. For details, see notes above

Note Mefloquine doses in BNF may differ from those in product literature

²Lariam® (Roche) PoM
Tablets, scored, mefloquine (as hydrochloride) 250 mg. Net price 8-tab pack = £14.53. Label: 21, 27, counselling, driving, prophylaxis, see above
Note Tablet may be crushed and mixed with food such as jam or honey just before administration

---

1. Can be sold to the public provided it is licensed and labelled for the prophylaxis of malaria. Drugs for malaria prophylaxis not prescribable on the NHS; health authorities may investigate circumstances under which antimalarials are prescribed

2. Drugs for malaria prophylaxis not prescribable on the NHS; health authorities may investigate circumstances under which antimalarials prescribed

Piperaquine with artenimol

Piperaquine with artenimol is not recommended for the first-line treatment of acute uncomplicated falciparum malaria because there is limited experience of its use in travellers who usually reside in areas where malaria is not endemic. Piperaquine has a long half-life.

▌ PIPERAQUINE PHOSPHATE WITH ARTENIMOL

(Piperaquine tetraphosphate with dihydroartemisinin)

Indications see notes above

Cautions obtain ECG as soon as possible after starting treatment then continue monitoring in those taking medicines that increase plasma-piperaquine concentration, in children who are vomiting, in females, or in the elderly; consider obtaining ECG in all patients before third dose and 4–6 hours after third dose; if QT_C interval more than 500 milliseconds, discontinue treatment and monitor ECG for a further 24–48 hours; **interactions**: Appendix 1 (piperaquine with artenimol)

Contra-indications risk factors for QT interval prolongation (e.g. electrolyte disturbances, acute myocardial infarction, severe hypertension, left ventricular hypertrophy, heart failure with reduced left ventricular ejection fraction, bradycardia, congenital long QT syndrome, family history of sudden death, concomitant use with other drugs known to prolong the QT interval, history of symptomatic arrhythmias)

Hepatic impairment no information available in moderate to severe impairment—manufacturer advises monitor ECG and plasma-potassium concentration

Renal impairment no information available in moderate to severe impairment—manufacturer advises monitor ECG and plasma-potassium concentration

Pregnancy teratogenic in *animal* studies—manufacturer advises use only if other antimalarials cannot be used

Breast-feeding manufacturer advises avoid—present in milk in *animal* studies

Side-effects QT interval prolonged, tachycardia, headache, malaise, anaemia; *less commonly* nausea, vomiting, abdominal pain, diarrhoea, anorexia, hepatitis, hepatomegaly, arrhythmias, bradycardia, cough, dizziness, convulsions, influenza-like symptoms, arthralgia, myalgia, pruritus; also reported in children stomatitis, jaundice, heart murmur, blood disorders (including leucopenia and thrombocytopenia), conjunctivitis, rash, acanthosis

Dose
• See preparations

Eurartesim® (Sigma-Tau) ▼ PoM
Tablets, f/c, scored, piperaquine phosphate 320 mg, artenimol 40 mg, net price 12-tab pack = £40.00. Counselling, administration
Counselling Tablets to be taken at least 3 hours before and at least 3 hours after food. Tablets may be crushed and mixed with water immediately before administration
Dose Treatment of uncomplicated falciparum malaria, ADULT and CHILD over 6 months, body-weight 7–13 kg, ½ tablet once daily for 3 days; body-weight 13–24 kg, 1 tablet once daily for 3 days; body-weight 24–36 kg, 2 tablets once daily for 3 days; body-weight 36–75 kg,

3 tablets once daily for 3 days; body-weight 75–100 kg, 4 tablets once daily for 3 days
Note Max. 2 courses in 12 months; second course given at least 2 months after first course

Primaquine

Primaquine is used to eliminate the liver stages of *P. vivax or P. ovale following chloroquine treatment* (for details, see p. 445).

▌ PRIMAQUINE

Indications adjunct in the treatment of *Plasmodium vivax* and *P. ovale* malaria (eradication of liver stages)

Cautions G6PD deficiency (test blood, see under Non-falciparum Malaria (treatment), p. 445); systemic diseases associated with granulocytopenia (e.g. rheumatoid arthritis, lupus erythematosus); **interactions**: Appendix 1 (primaquine)

Pregnancy risk of neonatal haemolysis and methaemoglobinaemia in third trimester; see also p. 445

Breast-feeding no information available; theoretical risk of haemolysis in G6PD-deficient infants

Side-effects nausea, vomiting, anorexia, abdominal pain; less commonly methaemoglobinaemia, haemolytic anaemia especially in G6PD deficiency, leucopenia

Dose
• Treatment of non-falciparum malaria, see p. 445

Primaquine (Non-proprietary)
Tablets, primaquine (as phosphate) 7.5 mg or 15 mg
Available from 'special-order' manufacturers or specialist-importing companies, see p. 1124

Proguanil

Proguanil is used (usually *with chloroquine*, but occasionally *alone*) for the *prophylaxis of malaria*, (for details, see specific recommendations by country, p. 446).

Proguanil used alone is not suitable for the *treatment of malaria*; however, *Malarone®* (a combination of atovaquone with proguanil) is licensed for the treatment of acute uncomplicated falciparum malaria. *Malarone®* is also used for the *prophylaxis of falciparum malaria* in areas of *widespread mefloquine or chloroquine resistance*. *Malarone®* is also used as an alternative to mefloquine or doxycycline. *Malarone®* is particularly suitable for short trips to highly chloroquine-resistant areas because it needs to be taken only for 7 days after leaving an endemic area.

▌ PROGUANIL HYDROCHLORIDE

Indications chemoprophylaxis of malaria

Cautions interactions: Appendix 1 (proguanil)

Renal impairment 100 mg once daily if eGFR 20–60 mL/minute/1.73 m²; 50 mg on alternate days if eGFR 10–20 mL/minute/1.73 m²; 50 mg once weekly if eGFR less than 10 mL/minute/1.73 m² (increased risk of haematological toxicity)

Pregnancy benefit of prophylaxis in malaria outweighs risk; adequate folate supplements should be given to mother; see also p. 446

Breast-feeding amount in milk probably too small to be harmful when used for malaria prophylaxis; see also p. 446

5 Infections

Side-effects mild gastric intolerance, diarrhoea, and constipation; occasionally mouth ulcers and stomatitis; *very rarely* cholestasis, vasculitis, skin reactions, and hair loss

Dose

- Prophylaxis of malaria, started 1 week before entering endemic area and continued for 4 weeks after leaving (see notes above), 200 mg once daily; INFANT up to 12 weeks body-weight under 6 kg, 25 mg once daily; 12 weeks–1 year body-weight 6–10 kg, 50 mg once daily; CHILD 1–4 years body-weight 10–16 kg, 75 mg once daily; 4–8 years body-weight 16–25 kg, 100 mg once daily; 8–13 years, body-weight 25–45 kg, 150 mg once daily; over 13 years body-weight over 45 kg, adult dose

  Counselling Warn travellers about **importance** of avoiding mosquito bites, **importance** of taking prophylaxis regularly, and **importance** of immediate visit to doctor if ill within 1 year and **especially** within 3 months of return. For details, see notes above

  Note Proguanil doses in BNF may differ from those in product literature.

[1]Paludrine® (Alliance)

Tablets, scored, proguanil hydrochloride 100 mg. Net price 98-tab pack = £10.45. Label: 21, counselling, prophylaxis, see above

Note Tablet may be crushed and mixed with food such as milk, jam, or honey just before administration

◢**With chloroquine**

See under Chloroquine

PROGUANIL HYDROCHLORIDE WITH ATOVAQUONE

Indications treatment of acute uncomplicated falciparum malaria and prophylaxis of falciparum malaria, particularly where resistance to other antimalarial drugs suspected; treatment of non-falciparum malaria [unlicensed indication]

Cautions diarrhoea or vomiting (reduced absorption of atovaquone); efficacy not evaluated in cerebral or complicated malaria (including hyperparasitaemia, pulmonary oedema or renal failure); **interactions:** see Appendix 1 (proguanil, atovaquone)

Renal impairment avoid for malaria prophylaxis (and if possible for malaria treatment) if eGFR less than 30 mL/minute/1.73 m^2

Pregnancy manufacturer advises avoid unless essential; see also p. 446

Breast-feeding use only if no suitable alternative available; see also p. 446

Side-effects abdominal pain, nausea, vomiting, diarrhoea; cough; headache, dizziness, insomnia, abnormal dreams, depression, anorexia, fever; rash, pruritus; *less frequently* stomatitis, palpitation, anxiety, blood disorders, hyponatraemia, and hair loss; also reported, hepatitis, cholestasis, tachycardia, hallucinations, seizures, vasculitis, mouth ulcers, photosensitivity, and Stevens-Johnson syndrome

Dose

- See preparations

  Counselling Warn travellers about **importance** of avoiding mosquito bites, **importance** of taking prophylaxis regularly, and **importance** of immediate visit to doctor if ill within 1

year and **especially** within 3 months of return. For details, see notes above

[2]Malarone® (GSK) [PoM]

Tablets ('standard'), pink, f/c, proguanil hydrochloride 100 mg, atovaquone 250 mg. Net price 12-tab pack = £25.21. Label: 21, counselling, prophylaxis, see above

Dose prophylaxis of malaria, started 1–2 days before entering endemic area and continued for 1 week after leaving, ADULT and CHILD over 40 kg, 1 tablet daily

Treatment of malaria, ADULT and CHILD body-weight over 40 kg, 4 tablets once daily for 3 days; CHILD body-weight 11–21 kg 1 tablet daily for 3 days; body-weight 21–31 kg 2 tablets once daily for 3 days; body-weight 31–40 kg 3 tablets once daily for 3 days

[2]Malarone® Paediatric (GSK) [PoM]

Paediatric tablets, pink, f/c proguanil hydrochloride 25 mg, atovaquone 62.5 mg, net price 12-tab pack = £6.26. Label: 21, counselling, prophylaxis, see above

Dose prophylaxis of malaria, started 1–2 days before entering endemic area and continued for 1 week after leaving, CHILD body-weight 5–10 kg, see *BNF for Children*; body-weight 10–20 kg, 1 tablet once daily; body-weight 20–30 kg, 2 tablets once daily; body-weight 30–40 kg, 3 tablets once daily; body-weight over 40 kg use *Malarone®* ('standard') tablets

Treatment of malaria, CHILD body-weight 5–9 kg, 2 tablets once daily for 3 days; body-weight 9–11 kg, 3 tablets once daily for 3 days; body-weight 11 kg and over use *Malarone®* ('standard') tablets

Note *Malarone® Paediatric* doses in BNF may differ from those in product literature. Tablets may be crushed and mixed with food or milky drink just before administration

Pyrimethamine

Pyrimethamine should not be used alone, but is used with sulfadoxine.

Pyrimethamine with sulfadoxine is not recommended for the *prophylaxis of malaria*, but it can be used in the treatment of *falciparum malaria with (or following) quinine*.

PYRIMETHAMINE

Indications malaria (but used only in combined preparations incorporating sulfadoxine); toxoplasmosis—section 5.4.7

Cautions blood counts required with prolonged treatment; predisposition to folate deficiency; history of seizures—avoid large loading doses; **interactions:** Appendix 1 (pyrimethamine)

Hepatic impairment manufacturer advises caution

Renal impairment manufacturer advises caution

Pregnancy theoretical teratogenic risk in *first trimester* (folate antagonist); adequate folate supplements should be given to mother

Breast-feeding significant amount in milk—avoid administration of other folate antagonists to infant; avoid breast-feeding during toxoplasmosis treatment

Side-effects nausea, vomiting, diarrhoea, headache, dizziness, blood disorders with high doses (including anaemia, leucopenia, thrombocytopenia), rash; *less commonly* fever, abnormal skin pigmentation; *very rarely* colic, buccal ulceration, convulsions

---

1. Can be sold to the public provided it is licensed and labelled for the prophylaxis of malaria. Drugs for malaria prophylaxis not prescribable on the NHS; health authorities may investigate circumstances under which antimalarials are prescribed

2. Drugs for malaria prophylaxis not prescribable on the NHS; health authorities may investigate circumstances under which antimalarials prescribed

5 Infections

Dose

- Malaria, no dose stated because not recommended alone, see Pyrimethamine with Sulfadoxine below
- Toxoplasmosis, section 5.4.7

Daraprim® (GSK) PoM ▨

Tablets, scored, pyrimethamine 25 mg. Net price 30-tab pack = £13.00

PYRIMETHAMINE WITH SULFADOXINE

Indications adjunct to quinine in treatment of *Plasmodium falciparum* malaria; **not** recommended for prophylaxis

Cautions see under Pyrimethamine and under Co-trimoxazole (section 5.1.8); not recommended for prophylaxis (severe side-effects on long-term use); **interactions:** Appendix 1 (pyrimethamine, sulfonamides)

Contra-indications see under Pyrimethamine and under Co-trimoxazole (section 5.1.8); sulfonamide allergy

Pregnancy possible teratogenic risk in *first trimester* (pyrimethamine a folate antagonist); in *third trimester*—risk of neonatal haemolysis and methaemoglobinaemia; fear of increased risk of kernicterus in neonates appears to be unfounded; see also p. 445

Breast-feeding small risk of kernicterus in jaundiced infants and of haemolysis in G6PD-deficient infants (due to sulfadoxine)

Side-effects see under Pyrimethamine and under Co-trimoxazole (section 5.1.8); pulmonary infiltrates (e.g. eosinophilic or allergic alveolitis) reported—discontinue if cough or shortness of breath

Dose

- Treatment of falciparum malaria, see p. 444
- Prophylaxis, not recommended by UK malaria experts

Pyrimethamine with sulfadoxine (Non-proprietary) PoM

Tablets, scored, pyrimethamine 25 mg, sulfadoxine 500 mg, net price 3-tab pack = 74p

Note Also known as *Fansidar®*

Available from 'special-order' manufacturers or specialist importing companies, see p. 1124

Quinine

Quinine is not suitable for the *prophylaxis of malaria*.

Quinine is used for the *treatment of falciparum malaria* or if the infective species is *not known* or if the infection is *mixed* (for details see p. 444).

QUININE

Indications falciparum malaria; nocturnal leg cramps, see section 10.2.2

Cautions cardiac disease (including atrial fibrillation, conduction defects, heart block), elderly—monitor ECG during parenteral treatment; monitor blood glucose and electrolyte concentration during parenteral treatment; G6PD deficiency (see section 9.1.5); **interactions:** Appendix 1 (quinine)

Contra-indications haemoglobinuria, myasthenia gravis, optic neuritis, tinnitus

Hepatic impairment for treatment of malaria in severe impairment, reduce parenteral maintenance dose to 5–7 mg/kg of quinine salt

Renal impairment for treatment of malaria in severe impairment, reduce parenteral maintenance dose to 5–7 mg/kg of quinine salt

Pregnancy high doses are teratogenic in *first trimester*, but in malaria benefit of treatment outweighs risk; see also p. 445

Breast-feeding present in milk but not known to be harmful

Side-effects cinchonism, including tinnitus, hearing impairment, vertigo, headache, nausea, vomiting, abdominal pain, diarrhoea, visual disturbances (including temporary blindness); agitation, confusion; cardiovascular effects (see Cautions); dyspnoea; hypersensitivity reactions including angioedema, rashes, hot and flushed skin; hypoglycaemia (especially after parenteral administration); blood disorders (including thrombocytopenia and intravascular coagulation); acute renal failure; muscle weakness; photosensitivity; very toxic in **overdosage**—immediate advice from poisons centres essential (see also p. 39)

Dose

- Treatment of malaria, see p. 444

Note Quinine (anhydrous base) 100 mg ≡ quinine bisulfate 169 mg ≡ quinine dihydrochloride 122 mg ≡ quinine hydrochloride 122 mg ≡ quinine sulfate 121 mg. Quinine bisulfate 300-mg tablets are available but provide less quinine than 300 mg of the dihydrochloride, hydrochloride, or sulfate

Quinine Sulfate (Non-proprietary) PoM

Tablets, coated, quinine sulfate 200 mg, net price 28-tab pack = £2.07; 300 mg, 28-tab pack = £2.24

Quinine Dihydrochloride (Non-proprietary) PoM

Injection, quinine dihydrochloride 300 mg/mL. For dilution and use as an infusion. 1- and 2-mL amps

Available from 'special-order' manufacturers or specialist importing companies, see p. 1124

Note Intravenous injection of quinine is so hazardous that it has been superseded by infusion

Tetracyclines

Doxycycline (section 5.1.3) is used for the *prophylaxis of malaria* in areas of *widespread mefloquine or chloroquine resistance*. Doxycycline is also used as an alternative to mefloquine or *Malarone®* (for details, see specific recommendations by country, p. 446).

Doxycycline is also used as an *adjunct to quinine in the treatment of falciparum malaria* (for details see p. 444).

DOXYCYCLINE

Indications prophylaxis of malaria; adjunct to quinine in treatment of *Plasmodium falciparum* malaria; see also section 5.1.3

Cautions section 5.1.3

Contra-indications section 5.1.3

Hepatic impairment section 5.1.3

Renal impairment section 5.1.3

Pregnancy section 5.1.3

Breast-feeding section 5.1.3

Side-effects section 5.1.3

Dose

- Prophylaxis of malaria, started 1–2 days before entering endemic area and continued for 4 weeks after leaving (see notes above), ADULT and CHILD over 12 years, 100 mg once daily
- Treatment of falciparum malaria, see p. 444

◢**Preparations**

Section 5.1.3

5.4.2   Amoebicides

Metronidazole is the drug of choice for *acute invasive amoebic dysentery* since it is very effective against vegetative forms of *Entamoeba histolytica* in ulcers; it is given in an adult dose of 800 mg three times daily for 5 days. **Tinidazole** is also effective. Metronidazole and tinidazole are also active against amoebae which may have migrated to the liver. Treatment with metronidazole (or tinidazole) is followed by a 10-day course of diloxanide furoate.

Diloxanide furoate is the drug of choice for asymptomatic patients with *E. histolytica* cysts in the faeces; metronidazole and tinidazole are relatively ineffective. Diloxanide furoate is relatively free from toxic effects and the usual course is of 10 days, given alone for chronic infections or following metronidazole or tinidazole treatment.

For *amoebic abscesses* of the liver **metronidazole** is effective; tinidazole is an alternative. Aspiration of the abscess is indicated where it is suspected that it may rupture or where there is no improvement after 72 hours of metronidazole; the aspiration may need to be repeated. Aspiration aids penetration of metronidazole and, for abscesses with more than 100 mL of pus, if carried out in conjunction with drug therapy, may reduce the period of disability.

Diloxanide furoate is not effective against hepatic amoebiasis, but a 10-day course should be given at the completion of metronidazole or tinidazole treatment to destroy any amoebae in the gut.

▮ DILOXANIDE FUROATE

Indications   see notes above; chronic amoebiasis and as adjunct to metronidazole or tinidazole in acute amoebiasis

Pregnancy   manufacturer advises avoid—no information available

Breast-feeding   manufacturer advises avoid

Side-effects   flatulence, vomiting, urticaria, pruritus

Dose

- 500 mg every 8 hours for 10 days; CHILD body-weight over 25 kg, 20 mg/kg daily in 3 divided doses for 10 days; body-weight under 25 kg, see *BNF for Children* See also notes above

Diloxanide (Non-proprietary) PoM

Tablets, diloxanide furoate 500 mg, net price 30-tab pack = £93.50. Label: 9

▮ METRONIDAZOLE

Indications   see under Dose below; anaerobic infections, section 5.1.11

Cautions   section 5.1.11

Hepatic impairment   section 5.1.11

Pregnancy   section 5.1.11

Breast-feeding   section 5.1.11

Side-effects   section 5.1.11

Dose

- By mouth, invasive intestinal amoebiasis, extra-intestinal amoebiasis (including liver abscess), 800 mg every 8 hours for 5 days in intestinal infection (for 5–10 days in extra-intestinal infection); CHILD 1–3 years 200 mg every 8 hours; 3–7 years 200 mg every 6 hours; 7–10 years 400 mg every 8 hours

  Urogenital trichomoniasis, 200 mg every 8 hours for 7 days *or* 400–500 mg every 12 hours for 5–7 days, *or* 2 g as a single dose; CHILD 1–3 years 50 mg every 8 hours for 7 days; 3–7 years 100 mg every 12 hours; 7–10 years 100 mg every 8 hours

  Giardiasis, 2 g daily for 3 days *or* 400 mg 3 times daily for 5 days *or* 500 mg twice daily for 7–10 days; CHILD 1–3 years 500 mg daily for 3 days; 3–7 years 600–800 mg daily; 7–10 years 1 g daily

◢**Preparations**

Section 5.1.11

▮ TINIDAZOLE

Indications   see under Dose below; anaerobic infections, section 5.1.11

Cautions   section 5.1.11

Pregnancy   section 5.1.11

Breast-feeding   section 5.1.11

Side-effects   section 5.1.11

Dose

- Intestinal amoebiasis, 2 g daily for 2–3 days; CHILD 50–60 mg/kg daily for 3 days
- Amoebic involvement of liver, 1.5–2 g daily for 3–6 days; CHILD 50–60 mg/kg daily for 5 days
- Urogenital trichomoniasis and giardiasis, single 2 g dose; CHILD single dose of 50–75 mg/kg (repeated once if necessary)

◢**Preparations**

Section 5.1.11

5.4.3   Trichomonacides

Metronidazole (section 5.4.2) is the treatment of choice for *Trichomonas vaginalis* infection. Contact tracing is recommended and sexual contacts should be treated simultaneously. If metronidazole is ineffective, **tinidazole** (section 5.4.2) may be tried.

5.4.4   Antigiardial drugs

Metronidazole (section 5.4.2) is the treatment of choice for *Giardia lamblia* infections. Alternative treatments are **tinidazole** (section 5.4.2) or **mepacrine hydrochloride**.

▮ MEPACRINE HYDROCHLORIDE

Indications   giardiasis; discoid lupus erythematosus (Antimalarials, section 10.1.3)

Cautions   hepatic impairment, elderly, history of psychosis; avoid in psoriasis; **interactions:** Appendix 1 (mepacrine)

Side-effects   gastro-intestinal disturbances; dizziness, headache; with large doses nausea, vomiting and occasionally transient acute toxic psychosis and CNS stimulation; on prolonged treatment yellow discoloration of skin and urine, chronic dermatoses (including severe exfoliative dermatitis), hepatitis, aplastic anaemia; also reported blue/black discoloration of palate and nails and corneal deposits with visual disturbances

Dose
- Giardiasis [unlicensed], 100 mg every 8 hours for 5–7 days

Mepacrine Hydrochloride

Tablets, mepacrine hydrochloride 100 mg. Label: 4, 9, 14, 21

Available from 'special-order' manufacturers or specialist importing companies, see p. 1124

5.4.5 Leishmaniacides

Cutaneous leishmaniasis frequently heals spontaneously but if skin lesions are extensive or unsightly, treatment is indicated, as it is in visceral leishmaniasis (kala-azar). Leishmaniasis should be treated under specialist supervision.

Sodium stibogluconate, an organic pentavalent antimony compound, is used for visceral leishmaniasis. The dose is 20 mg/kg daily by intramuscular or intravenous injection for 28 days in visceral leishmaniasis and for 20 days in cutaneous infection; the dosage varies with different geographical regions and expert advice should be obtained. Some early non-inflamed lesions of cutaneous leishmaniasis can be treated with intralesional injections of sodium stibogluconate under specialist supervision.

Amphotericin is used with or after an antimony compound for visceral leishmaniasis unresponsive to the antimonial alone; side-effects may be reduced by using liposomal amphotericin (*AmBisome®*—section 5.2.3) at a dose of 1–3 mg/kg daily for 10–21 days to a cumulative dose of 21–30 mg/kg *or* at a dose of 3 mg/kg for 5 consecutive days followed by a single dose of 3 mg/kg 6 days later. *Abelcet®*, a lipid formulation of amphotericin is also likely to be effective but less information is available.

Pentamidine isetionate (pentamidine isethionate) (section 5.4.8) has been used in antimony-resistant visceral leishmaniasis, but although the initial response is often good, the relapse rate is high; it is associated with serious side-effects. Other treatments include paromomycin [unlicensed] (available from 'special-order' manufacturers or specialist importing companies, see p. 1124).

SODIUM STIBOGLUCONATE

Indications leishmaniasis

Cautions intravenous injections must be given slowly over 5 minutes (to reduce risk of local thrombosis) and stopped if coughing or substernal pain; mucocutaneous disease (see below); treat intercurrent infection (e.g. pneumonia); monitor ECG before and during treatment; heart disease (withdraw if conduction disturbances occur); predisposition to QT interval prolongation (including concomitant use with drugs that prolong QT interval); **interactions:** Appendix 1 (sodium stibogluconate)

Mucocutaneous disease Successful treatment of mucocutaneous leishmaniasis may induce severe inflammation around the lesions (may be life-threatening if

pharyngeal or tracheal involvement)—may require corticosteroid

Hepatic impairment use with caution

Renal impairment avoid in significant impairment

Pregnancy manufacturer advises use only if potential benefit outweighs risk

Breast-feeding amount probably too small to be harmful

Side-effects anorexia, nausea, vomiting, abdominal pain, diarrhoea; ECG changes; coughing (see Cautions); headache, lethargy; arthralgia, myalgia; *rarely* jaundice, flushing, bleeding from nose or gum, substernal pain (see Cautions), vertigo, fever, sweating, and rash; also reported pancreatitis and anaphylaxis; pain and thrombosis on intravenous administration, intramuscular injection also painful

Dose
- See notes above

Pentostam® (GSK) (PoM)

Injection, sodium stibogluconate equivalent to pentavalent antimony 100 mg/mL. Net price 100-mL bottle = £66.43

Note Injection should be filtered immediately before administration using a filter of 5 microns or less

5.4.6 Trypanocides

The prophylaxis and treatment of trypanosomiasis is difficult and differs according to the strain of organism. Expert advice should therefore be obtained.

5.4.7 Drugs for toxoplasmosis

Most infections caused by *Toxoplasma gondii* are self-limiting, and treatment is not necessary. Exceptions are patients with eye involvement (toxoplasma choroidoretinitis), and those who are immunosuppressed. Toxoplasmic encephalitis is a common complication of AIDS. The treatment of choice is a combination of pyrimethamine and sulfadiazine, given for several weeks (expert advice **essential**). Pyrimethamine is a folate antagonist, and adverse reactions to this combination are relatively common (folinic acid supplements and weekly blood counts needed). Alternative regimens use combinations of pyrimethamine with clindamycin or clarithromycin or azithromycin. Long-term secondary prophylaxis is required after treatment of toxoplasmosis in immunocompromised patients; prophylaxis should continue until immunity recovers.

If toxoplasmosis is acquired in pregnancy, transplacental infection may lead to severe disease in the fetus. Spiramycin [unlicensed] (available from 'special-order' manufacturers or specialist importing companies, see p. 1124) may reduce the risk of transmission of maternal infection to the fetus.

5.4.8 Drugs for pneumocystis pneumonia

Pneumonia caused by *Pneumocystis jirovecii (Pneumocystis carinii)* occurs in immunosuppressed patients; it is a common cause of pneumonia in AIDS. Pneumocystis pneumonia should generally be treated by those experienced in its management. Blood gas measurement is used to assess disease severity.

5   Infections

5 Infections

Treatment

Mild to moderate disease Co-trimoxazole (section 5.1.8) in high dosage is the drug of choice for the treatment of mild to moderate pneumocystis pneumonia.

Atovaquone is licensed for the treatment of mild to moderate pneumocystis infection in patients who cannot tolerate co-trimoxazole. A combination of **dapsone** 100 mg daily (section 5.1.10) with **trimethoprim** 5 mg/kg every 6–8 hours (section 5.1.8) is given by mouth for the treatment of mild to moderate disease [unlicensed indication].

A combination of **clindamycin** 600 mg by mouth every 8 hours (section 5.1.6) and **primaquine** 30 mg daily by mouth (section 5.4.1) is used in the treatment of mild to moderate disease [unlicensed indication]; this combination is associated with considerable toxicity.

Severe disease Co-trimoxazole (section 5.1.8) in high dosage, given by mouth or by intravenous infusion, is the drug of choice for the treatment of severe pneumocystis pneumonia. **Pentamidine isetionate** given by intravenous infusion is an alternative for patients who cannot tolerate co-trimoxazole, or who have not responded to it. Pentamidine isetionate is a potentially toxic drug that can cause severe hypotension during or immediately after infusion.

Corticosteroid treatment can be lifesaving in those with severe pneumocystis pneumonia (see Adjunctive Therapy below).

Adjunctive therapy In moderate to severe infections associated with HIV infection, prednisolone 50–80 mg daily is given by mouth for 5 days (alternatively, hydrocortisone may be given parenterally); the dose is then reduced to complete 21 days of treatment. Corticosteroid treatment should ideally be started at the same time as the anti-pneumocystis therapy and certainly no later than 24–72 hours afterwards. The corticosteroid should be withdrawn before anti-pneumocystis treatment is complete.

Prophylaxis

Prophylaxis against pneumocystis pneumonia should be given to all patients with a history of the infection. Prophylaxis against pneumocystis pneumonia should also be considered for severely immunocompromised patients. Prophylaxis should continue until immunity recovers sufficiently. It should not be discontinued if the patient has oral candidiasis, continues to lose weight, or is receiving cytotoxic therapy or long-term immunosuppressant therapy.

Co-trimoxazole by mouth is the drug of choice for prophylaxis against pneumocystis pneumonia. It is given in a dose of 960 mg daily or 960 mg on alternate days (3 times a week); the dose may be reduced to co-trimoxazole 480 mg daily to improve tolerance.

Inhaled **pentamidine isetionate** is better tolerated than parenteral pentamidine. Intermittent inhalation of pentamidine isetionate is used for prophylaxis against pneumocystis pneumonia in patients unable to tolerate co-trimoxazole. It is effective but patients may be prone to extrapulmonary infection. Alternatively, **dapsone** 100 mg daily (section 5.1.10) can be used. **Atovaquone**

750 mg twice daily has also been used for prophylaxis [unlicensed indication].

▌ ATOVAQUONE

Indications treatment of mild to moderate *Pneumocystis jirovecii (Pneumocystis carinii)* pneumonia in patients intolerant of co-trimoxazole

Cautions initial diarrhoea and difficulty in taking with food may reduce absorption (and require alternative therapy); other causes of pulmonary disease should be sought and treated; elderly; **interactions:** Appendix 1 (atovaquone)

Hepatic impairment manufacturer advises caution—monitor more closely

Renal impairment manufacturer advises caution—monitor more closely

Pregnancy manufacturer advises avoid unless potential benefit outweighs risk—no information available

Breast-feeding manufacturer advises avoid

Side-effects nausea, diarrhoea, vomiting; headache, insomnia; fever; anaemia, neutropenia, hyponatraemia; rash, pruritus; also reported, Stevens-Johnson syndrome

Dose
* 750 mg twice daily with food (particularly high fat) for 21 days; CHILD not recommended

Wellvone® (GSK) PoM
Suspension, sugar-free, atovaquone 750 mg/5 mL, net price 226 mL (tutti-frutti-flavoured) = £486.37. Label: 21

◢ **With proguanil hydrochloride**
See section 5.4.1

▌ PENTAMIDINE ISETIONATE

Indications see under Dose (should only be given by specialists)

Cautions risk of severe hypotension following administration (monitor blood pressure before starting treatment, during administration, and at regular intervals, until treatment concluded; patient should be lying down when receiving drug parenterally); hypokalaemia, hypomagnesaemia, coronary heart disease, bradycardia, history of ventricular arrhythmias, concomitant use with other drugs which prolong QT-interval; hypertension or hypotension; hyperglycaemia or hypoglycaemia; leucopenia, thrombocytopenia, or anaemia; carry out laboratory monitoring according to product literature; care required to protect personnel during handling and administration; **interactions:** Appendix 1 (pentamidine isetionate)

Hepatic impairment manufacturer advises caution

Renal impairment reduce intravenous dose for pneumocystis pneumonia if creatinine clearance less than 10 mL/minute: in *life-threatening infection*, use 4 mg/kg once daily for 7–10 days, then 4 mg/kg on alternate days to complete course of at least 14 doses; in *less severe infection*, use 4 mg/kg on alternate days for at least 14 doses

Pregnancy manufacturer advises avoid unless essential

Breast-feeding manufacturer advises avoid unless essential—no information available

Side-effects severe reactions, sometimes fatal, due to hypotension, hypoglycaemia, pancreatitis, and arrhythmias; also leucopenia, thrombocytopenia, acute renal failure, hypocalcaemia; also reported: azotaemia, abnormal liver-function tests, anaemia, hyperkalaemia, nausea and vomiting, dizziness, syncope, flushing, hyperglycaemia, rash, and taste disturbances; Stevens-Johnson syndrome reported; on inhalation, bronchoconstriction (may be prevented by prior use of bronchodilators), cough, and shortness of breath; discomfort, pain, induration, abscess formation, and muscle necrosis at injection site

Dose

- Treatment of *Pneumocystis jirovecii (Pneumocystis carinii)* pneumonia, by intravenous infusion, 4 mg/kg once daily for at least 14 days
- Prophylaxis of *Pneumocystis jirovecii (Pneumocystis carinii)* pneumonia, by inhalation of nebulised solution (using suitable equipment—consult product literature), 300 mg every 4 weeks *or* 150 mg every 2 weeks [unlicensed for primary prevention]
- Visceral leishmaniasis (kala-azar, section 5.4.5), by deep intramuscular injection, 3–4 mg/kg on alternate days to max. total of 10 injections; course may be repeated if necessary
- Cutaneous leishmaniasis, by deep intramuscular injection, 3–4 mg/kg once or twice weekly until condition resolves (but see also section 5.4.5)
- Trypanosomiasis, by deep intramuscular injection *or* intravenous infusion, 4 mg/kg daily or on alternate days to total of 7–10 injections

  Note Direct intravenous injection should be avoided whenever possible and **never** given rapidly; intramuscular injections should be deep and preferably given into the buttock

Pentacarinat® (Sanofi-Aventis) [PoM]

Injection, powder for reconstitution, pentamidine isetionate, net price 300-mg vial = £31.77

Caution in handling Pentamidine isetionate is toxic and personnel should be adequately protected during handling and administration—consult product literature

Note *Pentacarinat*® Injection (dissolved in water for injection) may be used for nebulisation

5.5 Anthelmintics

Advice on prophylaxis and treatment of helminth infections is available from:

Birmingham	(0121) 424 0357
Scottish Centre for Infection and Environmental Health (registered users of Travax only)	(0141) 300 1100 (weekdays 12–5 p.m. only)
Liverpool	(0151) 705 3100
London	0845 155 5000 (treatment)

5.5.1 Drugs for threadworms
(pinworms, Enterobius vermicularis)

Anthelmintics are effective in threadworm infections, but their use needs to be combined with hygienic measures to break the cycle of auto-infection. All members of the family require treatment.

Adult threadworms do not live for longer than 6 weeks and for development of fresh worms, ova must be swallowed and exposed to the action of digestive juices in the upper intestinal tract. Direct multiplication of worms does not take place in the large bowel. Adult female worms lay ova on the perianal skin which causes pruritus; scratching the area then leads to ova being transmitted on fingers to the mouth, often via food eaten with unwashed hands. Washing hands and scrubbing nails before each meal and after each visit to the toilet is essential. A bath taken immediately after rising will remove ova laid during the night.

Mebendazole is the drug of choice for treating threadworm infection in patients of all ages over 2 years. It is given as a single dose; as reinfection is very common, a second dose may be given after 2 weeks.

█ MEBENDAZOLE

Indications threadworm, roundworm, whipworm, and hookworm infections

Cautions interactions: Appendix 1 (mebendazole)

Note The package insert in the *Vermox*® pack includes the statement that it is not suitable for women known to be pregnant or children under 2 years

Pregnancy manufacturer advises toxicity in *animal* studies

Breast-feeding amount too small to be harmful but manufacturer advises avoid

Side-effects abdominal pain; *less commonly* diarrhoea, flatulence; *rarely* hepatitis, convulsions, dizziness, neutropenia, urticaria, alopecia, rash (including Stevens-Johnson syndrome and toxic epidermal necrolysis)

Dose

- Threadworms, ADULT and CHILD over 2 years, 100 mg as a single dose; if reinfection occurs second dose may be needed after 2 weeks; CHILD under 2 years, see *BNF for Children*
- Whipworms, ADULT and CHILD over 2 years, 100 mg twice daily for 3 days; CHILD under 2 years, see *BNF for Children*
- Roundworms—section 5.5.2
- Hookworms—section 5.5.4

[1]**Mebendazole** (Non-proprietary) [PoM]

Tablets, chewable, mebendazole 100 mg

Vermox® (Janssen) [PoM]

Tablets, orange, scored, chewable, mebendazole 100 mg. Net price 6-tab pack = £1.36

Oral suspension, mebendazole 100 mg/5 mL (banana-flavoured). Net price 30 mL = £1.59

1. Mebendazole tablets can be sold to the public if supplied for oral use in the treatment of enterobiasis in adults and children over 2 years provided its container or package is labelled to show a max. single dose of 100 mg and it is supplied in a container or package containing not more than 800 mg

5

Infections

5.5.2 Ascaricides
(common roundworm infections)

Mebendazole (section 5.5.1) is effective against *Ascaris lumbricoides* and is generally considered to be the drug of choice; the usual dose is 100 mg twice daily for 3 days or 500 mg as a single dose [unlicensed single dose].

Levamisole [unlicensed] (available from 'special-order' manufacturers or specialist importing companies, see p. 1124) is an alternative when mebendazole cannot be used. It is very well tolerated; mild nausea or vomiting has been reported in about 1% of treated patients; it is given as a single dose of 120–150 mg in adults.

5.5.3 Drugs for tapeworm infections

Taenicides

Niclosamide [unlicensed] (available from 'special-order' manufacturers or specialist importing companies, see p. 1124) is the most widely used drug for tapeworm infections and side-effects are limited to occasional gastro-intestinal upset, lightheadedness, and pruritus; it is not effective against larval worms. Fears of developing cysticercosis in *Taenia solium* infections have proved unfounded. All the same, an antiemetic can be given before treatment and a laxative can be given 2 hours after niclosamide.

Praziquantel [unlicensed] (available from 'special-order' manufacturers or specialist importing companies, see p. 1124) is as effective as niclosamide and is given as a single dose of 5–10 mg/kg after a light breakfast (a single dose of 25 mg/kg for *Hymenolepis nana*).

Hydatid disease

Cysts caused by *Echinococcus granulosus* grow slowly and asymptomatic patients do not always require treatment. Surgical treatment remains the method of choice in many situations. **Albendazole** [unlicensed] (available from 'special-order' manufacturers or specialist importing companies, see p. 1124) is used in conjunction with surgery to reduce the risk of recurrence or as primary treatment in inoperable cases. Alveolar echinococcosis due to *E. multilocularis* is usually fatal if untreated. Surgical removal with albendazole cover is the treatment of choice, but where effective surgery is impossible, repeated cycles of albendazole (for a year or more) may help. Careful monitoring of liver function is particularly important during drug treatment.

5.5.4 Drugs for hookworms
(ancylostomiasis, necatoriasis)

Hookworms live in the upper small intestine and draw blood from the point of their attachment to their host. An iron-deficiency anaemia may occur and, if present, effective treatment of the infection requires not only expulsion of the worms but treatment of the anaemia.

Mebendazole (section 5.5.1) has a useful broad-spectrum activity, and is effective against hookworms; the usual dose is 100 mg twice daily for 3 days. **Albendazole** [unlicensed] (available from 'special-order' manufacturers or specialist importing companies, see p. 1124) given as a single dose of 400 mg, is an alternative.

5.5.5 Schistosomicides
(bilharziasis)

Adult *Schistosoma haematobium* worms live in the genito-urinary veins and adult *S. mansoni* in those of the colon and mesentery. *S. japonicum* is more widely distributed in veins of the alimentary tract and portal system.

Praziquantel [unlicensed] is available from Merck Serono (*Cysticide*®) and is effective against all human schistosomes. The dose is 20 mg/kg followed after 4–6 hours by one further dose of 20 mg/kg (20 mg/kg given 3 times on one day for *S. japonicum* infections). No serious adverse effects have been reported. Of all the available schistosomicides, it has the most attractive combination of effectiveness, broad-spectrum activity, and low toxicity.

Hycanthone, lucanthone, niridazole, oxamniquine, and sodium stibocaptate have now been superseded.

5.5.6 Filaricides

Diethylcarbamazine [unlicensed] (available from 'special-order' manufacturers or specialist importing companies, see p. 1124) is effective against microfilariae and adults of *Loa loa*, *Wuchereria bancrofti*, and *Brugia malayi*. To minimise reactions treatment is commenced with a dose of diethylcarbamazine citrate 1 mg/kg on the first day and increased gradually over 3 days to 6 mg/kg daily in divided doses (up to 9 mg/kg daily in divided doses for *Loa loa*); this dosage is maintained for a further period. Close medical supervision is necessary particularly in the early phase of treatment.

In heavy infections there may be a febrile reaction, and in heavy *Loa loa* infection there is a small risk of encephalopathy. In such cases specialist advice should be sought, and treatment must be given under careful in-patient supervision and stopped at the first sign of cerebral involvement.

Ivermectin [unlicensed] (available from 'special-order' manufacturers or specialist importing companies, see p. 1124) is very effective in onchocerciasis and it is now the drug of choice. A single dose of 150 micrograms/kg by mouth produces a prolonged reduction in microfilarial levels. Retreatment at intervals of 6 to 12 months depending on symptoms must be given until the adult worms die out. Reactions are usually slight and most commonly take the form of temporary aggravation of itching and rash. Diethylcarbamazine or suramin should no longer be used for onchocerciasis because of their toxicity.

5.5.7 Drugs for cutaneous larva migrans
(creeping eruption)

Dog and cat hookworm larvae may enter human skin where they produce slowly extending itching tracks usually on the foot. Single tracks can be treated with topical tiabendazole (no commercial preparation available). Multiple infections respond to **ivermectin**, **albendazole** or **tiabendazole** (thiabendazole) by mouth [all unlicensed] and available from 'special-order' manufacturers or specialist importing companies, see p. 1124).

5.5.8   Drugs for strongyloidiasis

Adult *Strongyloides stercoralis* live in the gut and produce larvae which penetrate the gut wall and invade the tissues, setting up a cycle of auto-infection. **Ivermectin** [unlicensed] (available from 'special-order' manufacturers or specialist importing companies, see p. 1124) in a dose of 200 micrograms/kg daily for 2 days is the treatment of choice for chronic *Strongyloides* infection. **Albendazole** [unlicensed] (available from 'special-order' manufacturers or specialist importing companies, see p. 1124) is an alternative given in a dose of 400 mg twice daily for 3 days, repeated after 3 weeks if necessary.

6 Endocrine system

This chapter also includes advice on the drug management of the following:

Adrenal suppression during illness, trauma or surgery, p. 495

Serious infections in patients taking corticosteroids, p. 496

Osteoporosis, p. 521

Breast pain (mastalgia), p. 536

For hormonal contraception, see section 7.3.

6.1 Drugs used in diabetes

6.1.1 Insulins

6.1.2 Antidiabetic drugs

6.1.3 Diabetic ketoacidosis

6.1.4 Treatment of hypoglycaemia

6.1.5 Treatment of diabetic nephropathy and neuropathy

6.1.6 Diagnostic and monitoring devices for diabetes mellitus

Diabetes mellitus occurs because of a lack of insulin or resistance to its action. It is diagnosed by measuring fasting or random blood-glucose concentration (and occasionally by oral glucose tolerance test). Although there are many subtypes, the two principal classes of diabetes are type 1 diabetes and type 2 diabetes.

Type 1 diabetes, (formerly referred to as insulin-dependent diabetes mellitus (IDDM)), occurs as a result of a deficiency of insulin following autoimmune destruction of pancreatic beta cells. Patients with type 1 diabetes require administration of insulin.

Type 2 diabetes, (formerly referred to as non-insulin-dependent diabetes (NIDDM)), is due to reduced secretion of insulin or to peripheral resistance to the action of insulin or to a combination of both. Although patients may be controlled on diet alone, many also require oral antidiabetic drugs or insulin (or both) to maintain satisfactory control. In overweight individuals, type 2 diabetes may be prevented by losing weight and increasing physical activity; use of the anti-obesity drug orlistat (section 4.5.1) may be considered in obese patients.

Treatment of diabetes Treatment of all forms of diabetes should be aimed at alleviating symptoms and minimising the risk of long-term complications (see below); tight control of diabetes is essential.

Diabetes is a strong risk factor for cardiovascular disease (section 2.12). Other risk factors for cardiovascular disease such as smoking (section 4.10.2), hypertension (section 2.5), obesity (section 4.5), and hyperlipidaemia (section 2.12) should be addressed. Cardiovascular risk in patients with diabetes can be further reduced by the use of an ACE inhibitor (section 2.5.5.1), low-dose aspirin (section 2.9) and a lipid-regulating drug (section 2.12).

Prevention of diabetic complications Optimal glycaemic control in both type 1 diabetes and type 2 diabetes reduces, in the long term, the risk of microvascular complications including retinopathy, development of proteinuria and to some extent neuropathy. However, a temporary deterioration in established diabetic retinopathy may occur when normalising blood-glucose concentration. For reference to the use of an ACE inhibitor or an angiotensin-II receptor antagonist in the management of diabetic nephropathy, see section 6.1.5.

A measure of the total glycosylated (or glycated) haemoglobin (HbA_1) or a specific fraction (HbA_{1c}) provides a good indication of glycaemic control over the previous 2–3 months. Overall it is ideal to aim for an HbA_{1c} (glycosylated haemoglobin) concentration of 48–59 mmol/mol or less (reference range 20–42 mmol/mol) but this cannot always be achieved and for those using insulin there is a significantly increased risk of disabling hypoglycaemia; in those at risk of arterial disease, the aim should be to maintain the HbA_{1c} concentration at 48 mmol/mol or less. HbA_{1c} should be measured every 3–6 months.

> **Measurement of HbA_{1c}**
>
> HbA_{1c} values are expressed in *mmol of glycosylated haemoglobin per mol of haemoglobin (mmol/mol)*, a standardised unit specific for HbA_{1c} created by the International Federation of Clinical Chemistry and Laboratory Medicine (IFCC). HbA_{1c} values were previously aligned to the assay used in the Diabetes Control and Complications Trial (DCCT) and expressed as a percentage.
>
> **Equivalent values**
>
> | IFCC-HbA_{1c} (mmol/mol) | DCCT-HbA_{1c} (%) |
> | --- | --- |
> | 42 | 6.0 |
> | 48 | 6.5 |
> | 53 | 7.0 |
> | 59 | 7.5 |
> | 64 | 8.0 |
> | 75 | 9.0 |

Laboratory measurement of serum-fructosamine concentration is technically simpler and cheaper than the measurement of HbA_{1c} and can be used to assess control over short periods of time, particularly when HbA_{1c} monitoring is invalid (e.g. disturbed erythrocyte turnover or abnormal haemoglobin type).

Tight control of blood pressure in hypertensive patients with type 2 diabetes reduces mortality and protects visual acuity (by reducing considerably the risks of maculopathy and retinal photocoagulation) (see also section 2.5).

Driving Drivers with diabetes may be required to notify the Driver and Vehicle Licensing Agency (DVLA) of their condition depending on their treatment, the type of licence, and whether they have diabetic complications. Detailed guidance on eligibility to drive, and precautions required, is available from the DVLA (www.gov.uk/government/publications/at-a-glance).

Drivers need to be particularly careful to avoid hypoglycaemia and should be warned of the problems. Drivers treated with insulin should normally check their blood-glucose concentration before driving and, on long journeys, at 2-hour intervals as specified by DVLA guidance; depending on the type of licence, monitoring may also be necessary for drivers taking oral antidiabetic drugs which carry a risk of hypoglycaemia (e.g. sulfonylureas, nateglinide, repaglinide). Drivers treated with insulin should ensure that a supply of sugar is always available in the vehicle and they should avoid driving if their meal is delayed. If hypoglycaemia occurs, or warning signs develop, the driver should:

- stop the vehicle in a safe place;

- switch off the ignition and move from the driver's seat;

- eat or drink a suitable source of sugar;

- wait until 45 minutes after blood glucose has returned to normal, before continuing journey.

6.1.1 Insulins

6.1.1.1	**Short-acting insulins**
6.1.1.2	**Intermediate- and long-acting insulins**
6.1.1.3	**Hypodermic equipment**

Insulin plays a key role in the regulation of carbohydrate, fat, and protein metabolism. It is a polypeptide hormone of complex structure. There are differences in the amino-acid sequence of animal insulins, human insulins and the human insulin analogues. Insulin may be extracted from pork pancreas and purified by crystallisation; it may also be extracted from beef pancreas, but beef insulins are now rarely used. Human sequence insulin may be produced semisynthetically by enzymatic modification of porcine insulin (emp) or biosynthetically by recombinant DNA technology using bacteria (crb, prb) or yeast (pyr).

All insulin preparations are to a greater or lesser extent immunogenic in man but immunological resistance to insulin action is uncommon. Preparations of human sequence insulin should theoretically be less immunogenic, but no real advantage has been shown in trials.

Insulin is inactivated by gastro-intestinal enzymes, and must therefore be given by injection; the subcutaneous route is ideal in most circumstances. Insulin is usually injected into the upper arms, thighs, buttocks, or abdomen; absorption from a limb site may be increased if the limb is used in strenuous exercise after the injection. Generally subcutaneous insulin injections cause few problems; lipodystrophy may occur but can be minimised by using different injection sites in rotation. Local allergic reactions are rare.

6   Endocrine system

Insulin is needed by all patients with ketoacidosis, and it is likely to be needed by most patients with:

- rapid onset of symptoms;
- substantial loss of weight;
- weakness;
- ketonuria;
- a first-degree relative who has type 1 diabetes.

Insulin is required by almost all children with diabetes. It is also needed for type 2 diabetes when other methods have failed to achieve good control, and temporarily in the presence of intercurrent illness or peri-operatively. Pregnant women with type 2 diabetes may be treated with insulin when diet alone fails. For advice on use of oral antidiabetic drugs in the management of diabetes in pregnancy, see section 6.1.2.

> **NHS Diabetes guidance**
> **Safe and Effective Use of Insulin in Hospitalised Patients (March 2010)**
> Available at www.diabetes.nhs.uk

Management of diabetes with insulin The aim of treatment is to achieve the best possible control of blood-glucose concentration without making the patient obsessional and to avoid disabling hypoglycaemia; close co-operation is needed between the patient and the medical team because good control reduces the risk of complications.

Insulin preparations can be divided into 3 types:

- those of **short** duration which have a relatively rapid onset of action, namely soluble insulin and the rapid-acting insulin analogues, insulin aspart, insulin glulisine, and insulin lispro (section 6.1.1.1);
- those with an **intermediate** action, e.g. isophane insulin (section 6.1.1.2); and
- those whose action is slower in onset and lasts for **long** periods, e.g. protamine zinc insulin, insulin detemir, and insulin glargine (section 6.1.1.2).

The duration of action of a particular type of insulin varies considerably from one patient to another, and needs to be assessed individually.

Mixtures of insulin preparations may be required and appropriate combinations have to be determined for the individual patient. Treatment should be started with a short-acting insulin (e.g. soluble insulin) or a rapid-acting insulin analogue (e.g. insulin aspart) given before meals with intermediate-acting or long-acting insulin once or twice daily. Alternatively, for those who have difficulty with, or prefer not to use, multiple injection regimens, a mixture of premixed short-acting insulin or rapid acting insulin analogue with an intermediate-acting or long-acting insulin (most commonly in a proportion of 30% soluble insulin and 70% isophane insulin) can be given once or twice daily. The dose of short-acting or rapid-acting insulin (or the proportion of the short-acting soluble insulin component in premixed insulin) can be increased in those with excessive post-prandial hyperglycaemia. The dose of insulin is increased gradually according to the patient's individual requirements, taking care to avoid troublesome hypoglycaemic reactions.

Insulin requirements may be increased by infection, stress, accidental or surgical trauma, and during puberty. Requirements may be decreased in those with certain endocrine disorders (e.g. Addison's disease, hypopituitarism), or in coeliac disease.

Examples of recommended insulin regimens

- Multiple injection regimen: short-acting insulin or rapid-acting insulin analogue, before meals With intermediate-acting or long-acting insulin, once or twice daily;
- Short-acting insulin or rapid-acting insulin analogue mixed with intermediate-acting or long-acting insulin, once or twice daily (before meals);
- Intermediate-acting or long-acting insulin, once or twice daily With or without short-acting insulin or rapid-acting insulin before meals;
- Continuous subcutaneous insulin infusion (see below).

Hepatic impairment Insulin requirements may be decreased in patients with hepatic impairment.

Renal impairment Insulin requirements may decrease in patients with renal impairment and therefore dose reduction may be necessary. The compensatory response to hypoglycaemia is impaired in renal impairment.

Pregnancy and breast-feeding During pregnancy and breast-feeding, insulin requirements may alter and doses should be assessed frequently by an experienced diabetes physician. The dose of insulin generally needs to be increased in the second and third trimesters of pregnancy. The short-acting insulin analogues, insulin aspart and insulin lispro, are not known to be harmful, and may be used during pregnancy and lactation. Evidence of the safety of long-acting insulin analogues in pregnancy is limited, therefore isophane insulin is recommended where longer-acting insulins are needed; insulin detemir may also be considered.

Insulin administration Insulin is generally given by *subcutaneous injection*; the injection site should be rotated to prevent lipodystrophy. Injection devices ('pens') (section 6.1.1.3), which hold the insulin in a cartridge and meter the required dose, are convenient to use. Insulin syringes (for use with needles) are required for insulins not available in cartridge form.

For intensive insulin regimens multiple subcutaneous injections (3 or more times daily) are usually recommended.

Short-acting injectable insulins (soluble insulin, insulin aspart, insulin glulisine, and insulin lispro) can also be given by *continuous subcutaneous infusion* using a portable infusion pump. This device delivers a continuous basal insulin infusion and patient-activated bolus doses at meal times. This technique can be useful for patients who suffer recurrent hypoglycaemia or marked morning rise in blood-glucose concentration despite optimised multiple-injection regimens (see also NICE guidance, below). Patients on subcutaneous insulin infusion must be highly motivated, able to monitor their blood-glucose concentration, and have expert training, advice and supervision from an experienced healthcare team.

Soluble insulin by the *intravenous route* is reserved for urgent treatment, e.g. in diabetic ketoacidosis, and for fine control in serious illness and in the peri-operative period (see under Diabetes and Surgery, below).

Units   The word 'unit' should **not** be abbreviated.

Monitoring   Many patients now monitor their own blood-glucose concentrations (section 6.1.6). Since blood-glucose concentration varies substantially throughout the day, 'normoglycaemia' cannot always be achieved throughout a 24-hour period without causing damaging hypoglycaemia. It is therefore best to recommend that patients should maintain a blood-glucose concentration of between 4 and 9 mmol/litre for most of the time (4–7 mmol/litre before meals and less than 9 mmol/litre after meals), while accepting that on occasions, for brief periods, it will be above these values; strenuous efforts should be made to prevent the blood-glucose concentration from falling below 4 mmol/litre. Patients using multiple injection regimens should understand how to adjust their insulin dose according to their carbohydrate intake. With fixed-dose insulin regimens, the carbohydrate intake needs to be regulated, and should be distributed throughout the day to match the insulin regimen. The intake of energy and of simple and complex carbohydrates should be adequate to allow normal growth and development but obesity must be avoided.

Hypoglycaemia   Hypoglycaemia is a potential problem with insulin therapy. All patients must be carefully instructed on how to avoid it.

Loss of warning of hypoglycaemia among insulin-treated patients can be a serious hazard, especially for drivers and those in dangerous occupations. Very tight control of diabetes lowers the blood-glucose concentration needed to trigger hypoglycaemic symptoms; an increase in the frequency of hypoglycaemic episodes may reduce the warning symptoms experienced by the patient. Beta-blockers can also blunt hypoglycaemic awareness (and also delay recovery).

To restore the warning signs, episodes of hypoglycaemia must be minimised; this involves appropriate adjustment of insulin type, dose and frequency together with suitable timing and quantity of meals and snacks.

Some patients have reported loss of hypoglycaemia warning after transfer to human insulin. Clinical studies do not confirm that human insulin decreases hypoglycaemia awareness. If a patient believes that human insulin is responsible for the loss of warning it is reasonable to revert to animal insulin and essential to educate the patient about avoiding hypoglycaemia. Great care should be taken to specify whether a human or an animal preparation is required.

Few patients are now treated with beef insulins; when undertaking conversion from beef to human insulin, the total dose should be reduced by about 10% with careful monitoring for the first few days. When changing between pork and human-sequence insulins, a dose change is not usually needed, but careful monitoring is still advised.

Diabetes and surgery   Perioperative control of blood-glucose concentrations in patients with type 1 diabetes is achieved via an adjustable, continuous, intravenous infusion of insulin. Detailed local protocols should be available to all healthcare professionals involved in the treatment of these patients; in general, the following steps should be followed:

- Give an injection of the patient's usual insulin on the night before the operation;

- Early on the day of the operation, start an intravenous infusion of glucose containing potassium chloride (provided that the patient is not hyperkalaemic) and infuse at a constant rate appropriate to the patient's fluid requirements (usually 125 mL per hour); make up a solution of soluble insulin in sodium chloride 0.9% and infuse intravenously using a syringe pump piggy-backed to the intravenous infusion. Glucose and potassium infusions, and insulin infusions should be made up according to locally agreed protocols;

- The rate of the insulin infusion should be adjusted according to blood-glucose concentration (frequent monitoring necessary) in line with locally agreed protocols. Other factors affecting the rate of infusion include the patient's volume depletion, cardiac function, and age.

Protocols should include specific instructions on how to manage resistant cases (such as patients who are in shock or severely ill or those receiving corticosteroids or sympathomimetics) and those with hypoglycaemia.

If a syringe pump is not available, soluble insulin should be added to the intravenous infusion of glucose and potassium chloride (provided the patient is not hyperkalaemic), and the infusion run at the rate appropriate to the patient's fluid requirements (usually 125 mL per hour) with the insulin dose adjusted according to blood-glucose concentration in line with locally agreed protocols.

Once the patient starts to eat and drink, give subcutaneous insulin before breakfast and stop intravenous insulin 30 minutes later; the dose may need to be 10–20% more than usual if the patient is still in bed or unwell. If the patient was not previously receiving insulin, an appropriate initial dose is 30–40 units daily in four divided doses using soluble insulin before meals and intermediate-acting insulin at bedtime and the dose adjusted from day to day. Patients with hyperglycaemia often relapse after conversion back to subcutaneous insulin calling for one of the following approaches:

- additional doses of soluble insulin at any of the four injection times (before meals or bedtime) *or*

- temporary addition of intravenous insulin infusion (while continuing the subcutaneous regimen) until blood-glucose concentration is satisfactory *or*

- complete reversion to the intravenous regimen (especially if the patient is unwell).

Insulin Passport   Insulin Passports and patient information booklets should be offered to patients receiving insulin. The Insulin Passport provides a record of the patient's current insulin preparations and contains a section for emergency information. The patient information booklet provides advice on the safe use of insulin. They are available for purchase from:

3M Security Print and Systems Limited
Gorse Street, Chadderton
Oldham
OL9 9QH
Tel: 0845 610 1112

GP practices can obtain supplies through their Local Area Team stores.

NHS Trusts can order supplies from www.nhsforms.co. uk or by emailing nhsforms@mmm.com.

Further information is available at www.npsa.nhs.uk.

6.1.1.1 Short-acting insulins

Soluble insulin is a short-acting form of insulin. For maintenance regimens it is usual to inject it 15 to 30 minutes before meals.

Soluble insulin is the most appropriate form of insulin for use in diabetic emergencies e.g. diabetic ketoacidosis (section 6.1.3) and at the time of surgery. It can be given intravenously and intramuscularly, as well as subcutaneously.

When injected subcutaneously, soluble insulin has a rapid onset of action (30 to 60 minutes), a peak action between 2 and 4 hours, and a duration of action of up to 8 hours.

When injected intravenously, soluble insulin has a very short half-life of only about 5 minutes and its effect disappears within 30 minutes.

The rapid-acting human insulin analogues, **insulin aspart**, **insulin glulisine**, and **insulin lispro** have a faster onset and shorter duration of action than soluble insulin; as a result, compared to soluble insulin, fasting and preprandial blood-glucose concentrations are a little higher, postprandial blood-glucose concentration is a little lower, and hypoglycaemia occurs slightly less frequently. Subcutaneous injection of insulin analogues may be convenient for those who wish to inject shortly before or, when necessary, shortly after a meal. They can also help those susceptible to hypoglycaemia before lunch and those who eat late in the evening and are prone to nocturnal hypoglycaemia. They can also be administered by subcutaneous infusion (see Insulin Administration, above). Insulin aspart and insulin lispro can be administered intravenously and can be used as alternatives to soluble insulin for diabetic emergencies and at the time of surgery.

INSULIN

(Insulin Injection; Neutral Insulin; Soluble Insulin)

A sterile solution of insulin (i.e. bovine or porcine) or of human insulin; pH 6.6–8.0

Indications   diabetes mellitus; diabetic ketoacidosis (section 6.1.3)

Cautions   section 6.1.1; **interactions:** Appendix 1 (antidiabetics)

Hepatic impairment   section 6.1.1

Renal impairment   section 6.1.1

Pregnancy   section 6.1.1

Breast-feeding   section 6.1.1

Side-effects   see notes above; transient oedema; local reactions and fat hypertrophy at injection site; *rarely* hypersensitivity reactions including urticaria, rash; overdose causes hypoglycaemia

Dose

- By subcutaneous, intramuscular *or* intravenous injection *or* intravenous infusion, according to requirements

◢**Highly purified animal**
Counselling Show container to patient and confirm that patient is expecting the version dispensed

Hypurin® Bovine Neutral (Wockhardt) [PoM]
Injection, soluble insulin (bovine, highly purified) 100 units/mL. Net price 10-mL vial = £27.72; cartridges (for *Autopen® Classic*) 5 × 3 mL = £41.58

Hypurin® Porcine Neutral (Wockhardt) [PoM]
Injection, soluble insulin (porcine, highly purified) 100 units/mL. Net price 10-mL vial = £25.20; cartridges (for *Autopen® Classic*) 5 × 3 mL = £37.80

◢**Human sequence**
Counselling Show container to patient and confirm that patient is expecting the version dispensed

Actrapid® (Novo Nordisk) [PoM]
Injection, soluble insulin (human, pyr) 100 units/mL. Net price 10-mL vial = £7.48
Note Not recommended for use in subcutaneous insulin infusion pumps—may precipitate in catheter or needle

Humulin S® (Lilly) [PoM]
Injection, soluble insulin (human, prb) 100 units/mL. Net price 10-mL vial = £15.68; 5 × 3-mL cartridge (for most *Autopen® Classic* or *HumaPen®*) = £19.08

Insuman® Rapid (Sanofi-Aventis) [PoM]
Injection, soluble insulin (human, crb) 100 units/mL, net price 5 × 3-mL cartridge (for *ClikSTAR®* and *Autopen® 24*) = £17.50
Note Not recommended for use in subcutaneous insulin infusion pumps

◢**Mixed preparations**
See Biphasic Isophane Insulin (section 6.1.1.2)

INSULIN ASPART

(Recombinant human insulin analogue)

Indications   diabetes mellitus

Cautions   section 6.1.1; **interactions:** Appendix 1 (antidiabetics)

Hepatic impairment   section 6.1.1

Renal impairment   section 6.1.1

Pregnancy   section 6.1.1

Breast-feeding   section 6.1.1

Side-effects see under Insulin

Dose

- By subcutaneous injection, ADULT and CHILD over 2 years, immediately before meals or when necessary shortly after meals, according to requirements
- By subcutaneous infusion, *or* intravenous injection, *or* intravenous infusion, ADULT and CHILD over 2 years, according to requirements

NovoRapid® (Novo Nordisk) ᴾᵒᴹ

Injection, insulin aspart (recombinant human insulin analogue) 100 units/mL, net price 10-mL vial = £14.08; *Penfill®* cartridge (for *NovoPen®* devices) 5 × 3-mL = £28.31; 5 × 3-mL *FlexPen®* prefilled disposable injection devices (range 1–60 units, allowing 1-unit dosage adjustment) = £30.60; 5 × 3-mL *Flex-Touch®* prefilled disposable injection devices (range 1–80 units, allowing 1-unit dosage adjustment) = £32.13

Counselling Show container to patient and confirm that patient is expecting the version dispensed

▌INSULIN GLULISINE

(Recombinant human insulin analogue)

Indications diabetes mellitus

Cautions section 6.1.1; **interactions:** Appendix 1 (antidiabetics)

Hepatic impairment section 6.1.1

Renal impairment section 6.1.1

Pregnancy section 6.1.1

Breast-feeding section 6.1.1

Side-effects see under Insulin

Dose

- By subcutaneous injection, ADULT and CHILD over 6 years, immediately before meals or when necessary shortly after meals, according to requirements
- By subcutaneous infusion *or* intravenous infusion ADULT and CHILD over 6 years, according to requirements

Apidra® (Sanofi-Aventis) ᴾᵒᴹ

Injection, insulin glulisine (recombinant human insulin analogue) 100 units/mL, net price 10-mL vial = £16.00; 5 × 3-mL cartridge (for *ClikSTAR®* and *Autopen® 24*) = £28.30; 5 × 3-mL *Apidra® SoloStar®* prefilled disposable injection devices (range 1–80 units, allowing 1-unit dosage adjustment) = £28.30

Counselling Show container to patient and confirm that patient is expecting the version dispensed

Note The *Scottish Medicines Consortium* (p. 4) has advised (October 2008) that *Apidra®* is accepted for restricted use within NHS Scotland for the treatment of adults and children over 6 years with diabetes mellitus in whom the use of a short-acting insulin analogue is appropriate

▌INSULIN LISPRO

(Recombinant human insulin analogue)

Indications diabetes mellitus

Cautions section 6.1.1; children (use only if benefit likely compared to soluble insulin); **interactions:** Appendix 1 (antidiabetics)

Hepatic impairment section 6.1.1

Renal impairment section 6.1.1

Pregnancy section 6.1.1

Breast-feeding section 6.1.1

Side-effects see under Insulin

Dose

- By subcutaneous injection shortly before meals or when necessary shortly after meals, according to requirements
- By subcutaneous infusion, *or* intravenous injection, *or* intravenous infusion, according to requirements

Humalog® (Lilly) ᴾᵒᴹ

Injection, insulin lispro (recombinant human insulin analogue) 100 units/mL, net price 10-mL vial = £16.61; 5 × 3-mL cartridge (for *Autopen® Classic* or *HumaPen®*) = £28.31; 5 × 3-mL *Humalog® KwikPen* prefilled disposable injection devices (range 1–60 units, allowing 1-unit dosage adjustment) = £29.46

Counselling Show container to patient and confirm that patient is expecting the version dispensed

6.1.1.2 Intermediate- and long-acting insulins

When given by subcutaneous injection, intermediate- and long-acting insulins have an onset of action of approximately 1–2 hours, a maximal effect at 4–12 hours, and a duration of 16–42 hours. Some are given twice daily in conjunction with short-acting (soluble) insulin, and others are given once daily, particularly in elderly patients. Soluble insulin can be mixed with intermediate and long-acting insulins (except insulin detemir, insulin glargine, and insulin degludec) in the syringe, essentially retaining the properties of the two components, although there may be some blunting of the initial effect of the soluble insulin component (especially on mixing with protamine zinc insulin, see below).

Isophane insulin is a suspension of insulin with protamine; it is of particular value for initiation of twice-daily insulin regimens. Patients usually mix isophane with soluble insulin but ready-mixed preparations may be appropriate (**biphasic isophane insulin**, **biphasic insulin aspart**, or **biphasic insulin lispro**).

Insulin zinc suspension (30% amorphous, 70% crystalline) has a more prolonged duration of action.

Protamine zinc insulin is usually given once daily with short-acting (soluble) insulin. It has the drawback of binding with the soluble insulin when mixed in the same syringe and is now rarely used.

Insulin glargine and **insulin detemir** are both long-acting human insulin analogues with a prolonged duration of action; insulin glargine is given once daily and insulin detemir is given once or twice daily. NICE (December 2002) has recommended that insulin glargine should be available as an option for patients with type 1 diabetes.

NICE (May 2009) has recommended that, if insulin is required in patients with type 2 diabetes, insulin detemir or insulin glargine may be considered for those:

- who require assistance with injecting insulin *or*
- whose lifestyle is significantly restricted by recurrent symptomatic hypoglycaemia *or*
- who would otherwise need twice-daily basal insulin injections in combination with oral antidiabetic drugs *or*
- who cannot use the device needed to inject isophane insulin.

6 Endocrine system

Insulin detemir is also licensed as add-on therapy in patients receiving treatment with liraglutide.

Insulin degludec is a long-acting human insulin analogue for once daily subcutaneous administration.

INSULIN DEGLUDEC
(Recombinant human insulin analogue—long acting)

Indications diabetes mellitus

Cautions section 6.1.1; **interactions:** Appendix 1 (antidiabetics)

Hepatic impairment section 6.1.1

Renal impairment section 6.1.1

Pregnancy section 6.1.1

Breast-feeding section 6.1.1

Side-effects see under Insulin (section 6.1.1.1)

Dose

> **Important**
> Insulin degludec (*Tresiba*®) is available in strengths of 100 units/mL (allows 1-unit dose adjustment) and 200 units/mL (allows 2-unit dose adjustment)—ensure correct strength prescribed

- By subcutaneous injection, ADULT over 18 years, according to requirements

Tresiba® (Novo Nordisk) ▼ PoM
Injection, insulin degludec (recombinant human insulin analogue) 100 units/mL, net price 5 × 3-mL *Penfill*® cartridges (for *Novo Nordisk*® devices) = £72.00; 100 units/mL, 5 × 3-mL *FlexTouch*® prefilled disposable injection devices (range 1– 80 units, allowing 1-unit dosage adjustment) = £72.00; 200 units/mL, 3 × 3-mL *FlexTouch*® prefilled disposable injection devices (range 2–160 units, allowing 2-unit dosage adjustment) = £86.52
Counselling Show container to patient and confirm that patient is expecting the version dispensed

◢**With liraglutide**
Section 6.1.2.3

INSULIN DETEMIR
(Recombinant human insulin analogue—long acting)

Indications diabetes mellitus

Cautions section 6.1.1.1; **interactions:** Appendix 1 (antidiabetics)

Hepatic impairment section 6.1.1

Renal impairment section 6.1.1

Pregnancy section 6.1.1

Breast-feeding section 6.1.1

Side-effects see under Insulin (section 6.1.1.1)

Dose

- By subcutaneous injection, ADULT and CHILD over 2 years, according to requirements

Levemir® (Novo Nordisk) PoM
Injection, insulin detemir (recombinant human insulin analogue) 100 units/mL, net price 5 × 3-mL cartridge (for *NovoPen*® devices) = £42.00; 5 × 3-mL *FlexPen*® prefilled disposable injection device (range 1–60 units, allowing 1-unit dosage adjustment) = £42.00; 5 × 3-mL *Levemir InnoLet*® prefilled disposable injection devices (range 1–50 units, allowing 1-unit dosage adjustment) = £44.85
Counselling Show container to patient and confirm that patient is expecting the version dispensed

INSULIN GLARGINE
(Recombinant human insulin analogue—long acting)

Indications diabetes mellitus

Cautions section 6.1.1.1; **interactions:** Appendix 1 (antidiabetics)

Hepatic impairment section 6.1.1

Renal impairment section 6.1.1

Pregnancy section 6.1.1

Breast-feeding section 6.1.1

Side-effects see under Insulin (section 6.1.1.1)

Dose

- By subcutaneous injection, ADULT and CHILD over 2 years, according to requirements

Lantus® (Sanofi-Aventis) PoM
Injection, insulin glargine (recombinant human insulin analogue) 100 units/mL, net price 10-mL vial = £30.68; 5 × 3-mL cartridge (for *ClikSTAR*® and *Autopen*® 24) = £41.50; 5 × 3-mL *Lantus*® *SoloStar*® prefilled disposable injection devices (range 1– 80 units, allowing 1-unit dosage adjustment) = £41.50
Note The *Scottish Medicines Consortium* (p. 4) has advised (March 2013) that insulin glargine is accepted for restricted use within NHS Scotland for the treatment of type 1 diabetes:

- in those who are at risk of or experience unacceptable frequency or severity of nocturnal hypoglycaemia on attempting to achieve better hypoglycaemic control during treatment with other insulins

- as a once daily insulin therapy for patients who require a carer to administer their insulin.

It is **not** recommended for routine use in patients with type 2 diabetes unless they suffer from recurrent episodes of hypoglycaemia or require assistance with their insulin injections.
Counselling Show container to patient and confirm that patient is expecting the version dispensed

INSULIN ZINC SUSPENSION
(Insulin Zinc Suspension (Mixed)—long acting)
A sterile neutral suspension of bovine and/or porcine insulin or of human insulin in the form of a complex obtained by the addition of a suitable zinc salt; consists of rhombohedral crystals (10–40 microns) and of particles of no uniform shape (not exceeding 2 microns)

Indications diabetes mellitus

Cautions section 6.1.1.1; **interactions:** Appendix 1 (antidiabetics)

Hepatic impairment section 6.1.1

Renal impairment section 6.1.1

Pregnancy section 6.1.1

Breast-feeding section 6.1.1

Side-effects see under Insulin (section 6.1.1.1)

Dose

- By subcutaneous injection, according to requirements

◢**Highly purified animal**

Hypurin® **Bovine Lente** (Wockhardt) PoM
Injection, insulin zinc suspension (bovine, highly purified) 100 units/mL. Net price 10-mL vial = £27.72
Counselling Show container to patient and confirm that patient is expecting the version dispensed

ISOPHANE INSULIN

(Isophane Insulin Injection; Isophane
Protamine Insulin Injection; Isophane Insulin
(NPH)—intermediate acting)

A sterile suspension of bovine or porcine insulin or of human
insulin in the form of a complex obtained by the addition of
protamine sulfate or another suitable protamine

Indications   diabetes mellitus

Cautions   section 6.1.1.1; **interactions:** Appendix 1
(antidiabetics)

Hepatic impairment   section 6.1.1

Renal impairment   section 6.1.1

Pregnancy   section 6.1.1

Breast-feeding   section 6.1.1

Side-effects   see under Insulin (section 6.1.1.1); protamine may cause allergic reactions

Dose

● By subcutaneous injection, according to requirements

◢ **Highly purified animal**

Counselling Show container to patient and confirm that
patient is expecting the version dispensed

Hypurin® **Bovine Isophane** (Wockhardt)   PoM

Injection, isophane insulin (bovine, highly purified)
100 units/mL. Net price 10-mL vial = £27.72; cartridges (for *Autopen® Classic*) 5 × 3 mL = £41.58

Hypurin® **Porcine Isophane** (Wockhardt)   PoM

Injection, isophane insulin (porcine, highly purified)
100 units/mL. Net price 10-mL vial = £25.20; cartridges (for *Autopen® Classic*) 5 × 3 mL = £37.80

◢ **Human sequence**

Counselling Show container to patient and confirm that
patient is expecting the version dispensed

Insulatard® (Novo Nordisk)   PoM

Injection, isophane insulin (human, pyr) 100 units/
mL. Net price 10-mL vial = £7.48; *Insulatard Penfill®*
cartridge (for *Novopen®* devices) 5 × 3 mL =
£22.90; 5 × 3-mL *Insulatard InnoLet®* prefilled disposable injection devices (range 1–50 units, allowing
1-unit dosage adjustment) = £20.40

Humulin I® (Lilly)   PoM

Injection, isophane insulin (human, prb) 100 units/
mL, net price 10-mL vial = £15.68; 5 × 3-mL cartridge (for *Autopen® Classic* or *HumaPen®*) = £19.08;
5 × 3-mL *Humulin I KwikPen®* prefilled disposable
injection devices (range 1–60 units, allowing 1-unit
dosage adjustment) = £21.70

Insuman® **Basal** (Sanofi-Aventis)   PoM

Injection, isophane insulin (human, crb) 100 units/
mL, net price 5-mL vial = £5.61; 5 × 3-mL cartridge (for *ClikSTAR®* and *Autopen® 24*) = £17.50; 5
× 3-mL *Insuman® Basal Solostar®* prefilled disposable injection devices (range 1–80 units, allowing 1-
unit dosage adjustment) = £19.80

◢ **Mixed preparations**

See Biphasic Isophane Insulin (p. 472)

PROTAMINE ZINC INSULIN

(Protamine Zinc Insulin Injection—long acting)

A sterile suspension of insulin in the form of a complex
obtained by the addition of a suitable protamine and zinc
chloride; this preparation was included in BP 1980 but is not
included in BP 1988

Indications   diabetes mellitus

Cautions   section 6.1.1.1; see also notes above; **interactions:** Appendix 1 (antidiabetics)

Hepatic impairment   section 6.1.1

Renal impairment   section 6.1.1

Pregnancy   section 6.1.1

Breast-feeding   section 6.1.1

Side-effects   see under Insulin (section 6.1.1.1); protamine may cause allergic reactions

Dose

● By subcutaneous injection, according to requirements

Hypurin® **Bovine Protamine Zinc** (Wockhardt)   PoM

Injection, protamine zinc insulin (bovine, highly purified) 100 units/mL. Net price 10-mL vial = £27.72

Counselling Show container to patient and confirm that
patient is expecting the version dispensed

Biphasic insulins

BIPHASIC INSULIN ASPART

(Intermediate-acting insulin)

Indications   diabetes mellitus

Cautions   see section 6.1.1.1; **interactions:** Appendix
1 (antidiabetics)

Hepatic impairment   section 6.1.1

Renal impairment   section 6.1.1

Pregnancy   section 6.1.1

Breast-feeding   section 6.1.1

Side-effects   see under Insulin (section 6.1.1.1); protamine may cause allergic reactions

Dose

● By subcutaneous injection, up to 10 minutes before
or soon after a meal, according to requirements

NovoMix® **30** (Novo Nordisk)   PoM

Injection, biphasic insulin aspart (recombinant
human insulin analogue), 30% insulin aspart, 70%
insulin aspart protamine, 100 units/mL, net price 5
× 3-mL *Penfill®* cartridges (for *NovoPen®* devices)
= £28.79; 5 × 3-mL *FlexPen®* prefilled disposable
injection devices (range 1–60 units, allowing 1-unit
dosage adjustment) = £29.89

Counselling Show container to patient and confirm that
patient is expecting the version dispensed; the proportions of
the two components should be checked **carefully** (the order
in which the proportions are stated may not be the same in
other countries)

BIPHASIC INSULIN LISPRO

(Intermediate-acting insulin)

Indications   diabetes mellitus

Cautions   see section 6.1.1.1 and Insulin Lispro;
interactions: Appendix 1 (antidiabetics)

Hepatic impairment   section 6.1.1

Renal impairment   section 6.1.1

Pregnancy   section 6.1.1

Breast-feeding   section 6.1.1

Side-effects   see under Insulin (section 6.1.1.1); protamine may cause allergic reactions

6 Endocrine system

Dose

- By subcutaneous injection, up to 15 minutes before or soon after a meal, according to requirements

Humalog® Mix25 (Lilly) [PoM]

Injection, biphasic insulin lispro (recombinant human insulin analogue), 25% insulin lispro, 75% insulin lispro protamine, 100 units/mL, net price 10-mL vial = £16.61; 5 × 3-mL cartridge (for *Autopen® Classic* or *HumaPen®*) = £29.46; 5 × 3-mL *Humalog® Mix25 KwikPen* prefilled disposable injection devices (range 1–60 units, allowing 1-unit dosage adjustment) = £30.98

Counselling Show container to patient and confirm that patient is expecting the version dispensed; the proportions of the two components should be checked **carefully** (the order in which the proportions are stated may not be the same in other countries)

Humalog® Mix50 (Lilly) [PoM]

Injection, biphasic insulin lispro (recombinant human insulin analogue), 50% insulin lispro, 50% insulin lispro protamine, 100 units/mL, net price 5 × 3-mL cartridge (for *Autopen® Classic* or *HumaPen®*) = £29.46; 5 × 3-mL *Humalog® Mix50 KwikPen* prefilled disposable injection devices (range 1–60 units, allowing 1-unit dosage adjustment) = £30.98

Counselling Show container to patient and confirm that patient is expecting the version dispensed; the proportions of the two components should be checked **carefully** (the order in which the proportions are stated may not be the same in other countries)

BIPHASIC ISOPHANE INSULIN

(Biphasic Isophane Insulin Injection— intermediate acting)

A sterile buffered suspension of either porcine or human insulin complexed with protamine sulfate (or another suitable protamine) in a solution of insulin of the same species

Indications diabetes mellitus

Cautions section 6.1.1.1; **interactions**: Appendix 1 (antidiabetics)

Hepatic impairment section 6.1.1

Renal impairment section 6.1.1

Pregnancy section 6.1.1

Breast-feeding section 6.1.1

Side-effects see under Insulin (section 6.1.1.1); protamine may cause allergic reactions

Dose

- By subcutaneous injection, according to requirements

◢**Highly purified animal**

Counselling Show container to patient and confirm that patient is expecting the version dispensed; the proportions of the two components should be checked **carefully** (the order in which the proportions are stated may not be the same in other countries)

Hypurin® Porcine 30/70 Mix (Wockhardt) [PoM]

Injection, biphasic isophane insulin (porcine, highly purified), 30% soluble, 70% isophane, 100 units/mL, net price 10-mL vial = £25.20; cartridges (for *Autopen® Classic*) 5 × 3 mL = £37.80

◢**Human sequence**

Counselling Show container to patient and confirm that patient is expecting the version dispensed; the proportions of the two components should be checked **carefully** (the order in which the proportions are stated may not be the same in other countries)

Humulin M3® (Lilly) [PoM]

Injection, biphasic isophane insulin (human, prb), 30% soluble, 70% isophane, 100 units/mL, net price 10-mL vial = £15.68; 5 × 3-mL cartridge (for most *Autopen® Classic* or *HumaPen®*) = £19.08; 5 × 3-mL *Humulin M3 KwikPen®* prefilled disposable injection devices (range 1–60 units, allowing 1-unit dosage adjustment) = £21.70

Insuman® Comb 15 (Sanofi-Aventis) [PoM]

Injection, biphasic isophane insulin (human, crb), 15% soluble, 85% isophane, 100 units/mL, net price 5 × 3-mL cartridge (for *ClikSTAR®* and *Autopen® 24*) = £17.50

Insuman® Comb 25 (Sanofi-Aventis) [PoM]

Injection, biphasic isophane insulin (human, crb), 25% soluble, 75% isophane, 100 units/mL, net price 5-mL vial = £5.61; 5 × 3-mL cartridge (for *ClikSTAR®* and *Autopen® 24*) = £17.50; 5 × 3-mL *Insuman® Comb 25 SoloStar®* prefilled disposable injection devices (range 1–80 units, allowing 1-unit dosage adjustment) = £19.80

Insuman® Comb 50 (Sanofi-Aventis) [PoM]

Injection, biphasic isophane insulin (human, crb), 50% soluble, 50% isophane, 100 units/mL, net price 5 × 3-mL cartridge (for *ClikSTAR®* and *Autopen® 24*) = £17.50

6.1.1.3 Hypodermic equipment

Patients should be advised on the safe disposal of lancets, single-use syringes, and needles. Suitable arrangements for the safe disposal of contaminated waste must be made before these products are prescribed for patients who are carriers of infectious diseases.

◢**Injection devices**

Autopen® (Owen Mumford)

Injection device, *Autopen® 24* (for use with Sanofi-Aventis 3-mL insulin cartridges), allowing 1-unit dosage adjustment, max. 21 units (single-unit version) *or* 2-unit dosage adjustment, max. 42 units (2-unit version), net price (both) = £16.47; *Autopen® Classic* (for use with Lilly and Wockhardt 3-mL insulin cartridges), allowing 1-unit dosage adjustment, max. 21 units (single-unit version) *or* 2-unit dosage adjustment, max. 42 units (2-unit version), net price (all) = £16.72

ClikSTAR® (Sanofi-Aventis)

Injection device, for use with *Lantus®*, *Apidra®*, and *Insuman®* 3-mL insulin cartridges; allowing 1-unit dose adjustment, max. 80 units, net price = £25.00

HumaPen® Luxura (Lilly)

Injection device, for use with *Humulin®* and *Humalog®* 3-mL cartridges; allowing 1-unit dosage adjustment, max. 60 units, net price = £26.82

HumaPen® Luxura HD (Lilly)

Injection device, for use with *Humulin®* and *Humalog®* 3-mL cartridges; allowing 0.5-unit dosage adjustment, max. 30 units, net price = £26.82

Endocrine system

6

HumaPen® Memoir (Lilly)

Injection device, for use with *Humalog®* 3-mL cartridges; allowing 1-unit dosage adjustment, max. 60 units, net price = £26.82

Injex (Injex UK)

Needle-free insulin delivery device, for use with any 10-mL vial of insulin, allowing 1-unit dosage adjustment, max. 30 units, net price *starter set* (*Injex®* device, reset box, transporter, 9 × 10-mL vial adaptors, 165 ampoules) = £149.36; *4-month refill pack* (6 × 10-mL vial adaptors, 100 ampoules) = £24.47; *ampoule pack* (50 ampoules) = £12.28; *vial adaptor pack* (20 × 10-mL vial adaptors) = £12.23

InsuJet (European Pharma)

Needle-free insulin delivery device, for use with any 10-mL vial or 3-mL cartridge of insulin, allowing 1-unit dosage adjustment, max 40 units, net price *starter set* (*InsuJet®* device, nozzle cap, nozzle and piston, 1 × 10-mL adaptor, 1 × 3-mL adaptor, 1 cartridge cap removal key) = £143.60; *nozzle pack* (15 nozzles) = £28.40, *cartridge adaptor pack* (15 adaptors) = £21.70, *vial adaptor pack* (15 adaptors) = £21.70

NovoPen® 4 (Novo Nordisk)

Injection device, for use with *Penfill®* 3-mL insulin cartridges; allowing 1-unit dosage adjustment, max. 60 units, net price = £26.86

◢**Lancets, needles, syringes, and accessories**

Lancets, **needles**, **syringes**, and **accessories** are listed under Hypodermic Equipment in Part IXA of the Drug Tariff (Part III of the Northern Ireland Drug Tariff, Part 3 of the Scottish Drug Tariff).

> The Drug Tariffs can be accessed online at:
> National Health Service Drug Tariff for England and Wales: www.ppa.org.uk/ppa/edt_intro.htm
> Health and Personal Social Services for Northern Ireland Drug Tariff: www.dhsspsni.gov.uk/pas-tariff
> Scottish Drug Tariff: www.isdscotland.org/Health-Topics/Prescribing-and-Medicines/Scottish-Drug-Tariff/

6.1.2   Antidiabetic drugs

6.1.2.1   Sulfonylureas

6.1.2.2   Biguanides

6.1.2.3   Other antidiabetic drugs

Oral antidiabetic drugs are used for the treatment of type 2 diabetes mellitus. They should be prescribed only if the patient fails to respond adequately to at least 3 months' restriction of energy and carbohydrate intake and an increase in physical activity. They should be used to augment the effect of diet and exercise, and not to replace them.

For patients not adequately controlled by diet and oral hypoglycaemic drugs, insulin may be added to the treatment regimen or substituted for oral therapy. When insulin is added to oral therapy, it is generally given at bedtime as isophane or long-acting insulin, and when insulin replaces an oral regimen it may be given as twice-daily injections of a biphasic insulin (or isophane insulin mixed with soluble insulin), or a multiple injection regimen. Weight gain and hypoglycaemia may be

complications of insulin therapy but weight gain may be reduced if the insulin is given in combination with metformin.

Exenatide, liraglutide, and lixisenatide, given by subcutaneous injection, are also available for the treatment of type 2 diabetes, see section 6.1.2.3.

Pregnancy and breast-feeding   During pregnancy, women with *pre-existing diabetes* can be treated with metformin [unlicensed use], either alone or in combination with insulin (section 6.1.1). Metformin can be continued, or glibenclamide resumed, during breast-feeding for those with pre-existing diabetes. Women with *gestational diabetes* may be treated, with or without concomitant insulin (section 6.1.1), with glibenclamide from 11 weeks gestation (after organogenesis) [unlicensed use] or with metformin [unlicensed use]. Women with gestational diabetes should discontinue hypoglycaemic treatment after giving birth.

Other oral hypoglycaemic drugs, exenatide, liraglutide, and lixisenatide are contra-indicated in pregnancy.

6.1.2.1   Sulfonylureas

The sulfonylureas act mainly by augmenting insulin secretion and consequently are effective only when some residual pancreatic beta-cell activity is present; during long-term administration they also have an extrapancreatic action. All may cause hypoglycaemia but this is uncommon and usually indicates excessive dosage. Sulfonylurea-induced hypoglycaemia may persist for many hours and must always be treated in hospital.

Sulfonylureas are considered for patients who are not overweight, or in whom metformin is contra-indicated or not tolerated. Several sulfonylureas are available and choice is determined by side-effects and the duration of action as well as the patient's age and renal function. **Glibenclamide**, a long-acting sulfonylurea, is associated with a greater risk of hypoglycaemia; for this reason it should be avoided in the elderly, and shorter-acting alternatives, such as **gliclazide** or **tolbutamide**, should be used instead.

When the combination of strict diet and sulfonylurea treatment fails, other options include:

- combining with metformin (section 6.1.2.2);
- combining with pioglitazone, but see section 6.1.2.3;
- combining with alogliptin, linagliptin, saxagliptin, sitagliptin, or vildagliptin (section 6.1.2.3);
- combining with canagliflozin, dapagliflozin, or empagliflozin (section 6.1.2.3);
- combining with exenatide, liraglutide, or lixisenatide (section 6.1.2.3);
- combining with acarbose (section 6.1.2.3), which may have a small beneficial effect, but flatulence can be a problem;
- combining with bedtime isophane insulin (section 6.1.1) but weight gain and hypoglycaemia can occur.

The risk of hypoglycaemia associated with sulfonylureas (see notes above) should be discussed with the patient, especially when concomitant glucose-lowering drugs are prescribed.

6 Endocrine system

Insulin therapy should be instituted temporarily during intercurrent illness (such as myocardial infarction, coma, infection, and trauma). Sulfonylureas should be omitted on the morning of surgery; insulin is required because of the ensuing hyperglycaemia in these circumstances.

Cautions Sulfonylureas can encourage weight gain and should be prescribed only if poor control and symptoms persist despite adequate attempts at dieting; metformin (section 6.1.2.2) is considered the drug of choice in obese patients. Caution is needed in the elderly and in patients with G6PD deficiency (section 9.1.5).

Contra-indications Sulfonylureas should be avoided where possible in acute porphyria (section 9.8.2) but glipizide and glimepiride are thought to be safe. Sulfonylureas are contra-indicated in the presence of ketoacidosis.

Hepatic impairment Sulfonylureas should be avoided or a reduced dose should be used in severe hepatic impairment, because there is an increased risk of hypoglycaemia. Jaundice may occur.

Renal impairment Sulfonylureas should be used with care in those with mild to moderate renal impairment, because of the hazard of hypoglycaemia; they should be avoided where possible in severe renal impairment. Glipizide should also be avoided if the patient has both renal and hepatic impairment. If necessary, the short-acting drug tolbutamide can be used in renal impairment, as can gliclazide which is principally metabolised in the liver, but careful monitoring of blood-glucose concentration is essential; care is required to use the lowest dose that adequately controls blood glucose.

Pregnancy The use of sulfonylureas in pregnancy should generally be avoided because of the risk of neonatal hypoglycaemia; however, glibenclamide can be used during the second and third trimesters of pregnancy in women with gestational diabetes, see section 6.1.2.

Breast-feeding The use of sulfonylureas (except glibenclamide [unlicensed use], see section 6.1.2) in breast-feeding should be avoided because there is a theoretical possibility of hypoglycaemia in the infant.

Side-effects Side-effects of sulfonylureas are generally mild and infrequent and include gastro-intestinal disturbances such as nausea, vomiting, diarrhoea, and constipation. Hyponatraemia has been reported with glimepiride and glipizide.

Sulfonylureas can occasionally cause a disturbance in liver function, which may rarely lead to cholestatic jaundice, hepatitis, and hepatic failure. Hypersensitivity reactions can occur, usually in the first 6–8 weeks of therapy. They consist mainly of allergic skin reactions which progress rarely to erythema multiforme and exfoliative dermatitis, fever, and jaundice; photosensitivity has rarely been reported with glipizide. Blood disorders are also rare but may include leucopenia, thrombocytopenia, agranulocytosis, pancytopenia, haemolytic anaemia, and aplastic anaemia.

GLIBENCLAMIDE

Indications type 2 diabetes mellitus

Cautions see notes above; **interactions**: Appendix 1 (antidiabetics)

Contra-indications see notes above

Hepatic impairment see notes above

Renal impairment see notes above

Pregnancy see notes above

Breast-feeding see notes above

Side-effects see notes above

Dose
- Initially 5 mg daily with or immediately after breakfast, dose adjusted according to response (ELDERLY avoid, see notes above); max. 15 mg daily

Glibenclamide (Non-proprietary) ⓅⓄⓂ
Tablets, glibenclamide 2.5 mg, net price 28-tab pack = £14.07; 5 mg, 28-tab pack = £1.10

GLICLAZIDE

Indications type 2 diabetes mellitus

Cautions see notes above; **interactions**: Appendix 1 (antidiabetics)

Contra-indications see notes above

Hepatic impairment see notes above

Renal impairment see notes above

Pregnancy see notes above

Breast-feeding see notes above

Side-effects see notes above

Dose
- Initially, 40–80 mg daily, adjusted according to response; up to 160 mg as a single dose, with breakfast; higher doses divided; max. 320 mg daily

Gliclazide (Non-proprietary) ⓅⓄⓂ
Tablets, gliclazide 40 mg, net price 28-tab pack = £3.36; 80 mg, 28-tab pack = £1.31, 60-tab pack = £2.12
Brands include *Zicron*®

Diamicron® (Servier) ⓅⓄⓂ
Tablets, scored, gliclazide 80 mg, net price 60-tab pack = £4.38

◢**Modified release**

Gliclazide (Non-proprietary) ⓅⓄⓂ
Tablets, m/r, gliclazide 30 mg, net price 28-tab pack = £2.06, 56-tab pack = £4.10. Label: 25
Brands include *Dacadis*® MR, *Vitile*® XL
Dose ADULT over 18 years, initially 30 mg daily with breakfast, adjusted according to response every 4 weeks (after 2 weeks if no decrease in blood glucose); max. 120 mg daily
Note Gliclazide modified release 30 mg may be considered to be approximately equivalent in therapeutic effect to standard formulation gliclazide 80 mg

Diamicron® MR (Servier) ⓅⓄⓂ
Tablets, m/r, gliclazide 30 mg, net price 28-tab pack = £2.81, 56-tab pack = £5.62. Label: 25
Dose ADULT initially 30 mg daily with breakfast, adjusted according to response every 4 weeks (after 2 weeks if no decrease in blood glucose); max. 120 mg daily
Note *Diamicron*® MR 30 mg may be considered to be approximately equivalent in therapeutic effect to standard formulation *Diamicron*® 80 mg

GLIMEPIRIDE

Indications   type 2 diabetes mellitus

Cautions   see notes above; manufacturer recommends regular hepatic and haematological monitoring but limited evidence of clinical value; **interactions**: Appendix 1 (antidiabetics)

Contra-indications   see notes above

Hepatic impairment   see notes above

Renal impairment   see notes above

Pregnancy   see notes above

Breast-feeding   see notes above

Side-effects   see notes above

Dose

- Initially 1 mg daily, adjusted according to response in 1-mg steps at 1–2 week intervals; usual max. 4 mg daily (exceptionally, up to 6 mg daily may be used); taken shortly before or with first main meal

Glimepiride (Non-proprietary) PoM
Tablets, glimepiride 1 mg, net price 30-tab pack = £1.21; 2 mg, 30-tab pack = £1.18; 3 mg, 30-tab pack = £8.56; 4 mg, 30-tab pack = £1.48

Amaryl® (Sanofi-Aventis) PoM
Tablets, all scored, glimepiride 1 mg (pink), net price 30-tab pack = £4.33; 2 mg (green), 30-tab pack = £7.13; 3 mg (yellow), 30-tab pack = £10.75; 4 mg (blue), 30-tab pack = £14.24

GLIPIZIDE

Indications   type 2 diabetes mellitus

Cautions   see notes above; **interactions**: Appendix 1 (antidiabetics)

Contra-indications   see notes above

Hepatic impairment   see notes above

Renal impairment   see notes above

Pregnancy   see notes above

Breast-feeding   see notes above

Side-effects   see notes above; also dizziness, drowsiness

Dose

- Initially 2.5–5 mg daily shortly before breakfast or lunch, adjusted according to response; max. 20 mg daily; up to 15 mg may be given as a single dose; higher doses divided

Glipizide (Non-proprietary) PoM
Tablets, glipizide 5 mg, net price 56-tab pack = £5.36

Minodiab® (Pharmacia) PoM
Tablets, scored, glipizide 5 mg, net price 28-tab pack = £1.26

TOLBUTAMIDE

Indications   type 2 diabetes mellitus

Cautions   see notes above; **interactions**: Appendix 1 (antidiabetics)

Contra-indications   see notes above

Hepatic impairment   see notes above

Renal impairment   see notes above

Pregnancy   see notes above

Breast-feeding   see notes above

Side-effects   see notes above; also headache, tinnitus

Dose

- 0.5–1.5 g (max. 2 g) daily in divided doses with or immediately after meals *or* as a single dose with or immediately after breakfast

Tolbutamide (Non-proprietary) PoM
Tablets, tolbutamide 500 mg, net price 28-tab pack = £22.18

6.1.2.2   Biguanides

Metformin, the only available biguanide, has a different mode of action from the sulfonylureas, and is not interchangeable with them. It exerts its effect mainly by decreasing gluconeogenesis and by increasing peripheral utilisation of glucose; since it acts only in the presence of endogenous insulin it is effective only if there are some residual functioning pancreatic islet cells.

Metformin is the drug of first choice in overweight patients in whom strict dieting has failed to control diabetes, if appropriate it may also be considered as an option in patients who are not overweight. It is also used when diabetes is inadequately controlled with sulfonylurea treatment. When the combination of strict diet and metformin treatment fails, other options include:

- combining with a sulfonylurea (section 6.1.2.1);
- combining with pioglitazone (section 6.1.2.3);
- combining with repaglinide or nateglinide (section 6.1.2.3);
- combining with alogliptin, linagliptin, saxagliptin, sitagliptin, or vildagliptin (section 6.1.2.3);
- combining with canagliflozin, dapagliflozin, or empagliflozin (section 6.1.2.3);
- combining with exenatide, liraglutide, or lixisenatide (section 6.1.2.3);
- combining with acarbose (section 6.1.2.3), which may have a small beneficial effect, but flatulence can be a problem;
- combining with insulin (section 6.1.1) but weight gain and hypoglycaemia can be problems (weight gain minimised if insulin given at night).

Insulin treatment is almost always required in medical and surgical emergencies; insulin should also be substituted before elective surgery (omit metformin on the morning of surgery and give insulin if required).

Hypoglycaemia does not usually occur with metformin; other advantages are the lower incidence of weight gain and lower plasma-insulin concentration. It does not exert a hypoglycaemic action in non-diabetic subjects unless given in overdose.

Gastro-intestinal side-effects are initially common with metformin, and may persist in some patients, particularly when very high doses such as 3 g daily are given.

Very rarely, metformin can provoke lactic acidosis. It is most likely to occur in patients with renal impairment, see Lactic Acidosis below.

Metformin is used for the symptomatic management of polycystic ovary syndrome [unlicensed indication]; however, treatment should be initiated by a specialist.

6 Endocrine system

Metformin improves insulin sensitivity, may aid weight reduction, helps to normalise menstrual cycle (increasing the rate of spontaneous ovulation), and may improve hirsutism.

■ METFORMIN HYDROCHLORIDE

Indications diabetes mellitus (see notes above); polycystic ovary syndrome [unlicensed indication]

Cautions see notes above; determine renal function before treatment and at least annually (at least twice a year in patients with additional risk factors for renal impairment, or if deterioration suspected); **interactions:** Appendix 1 (antidiabetics)

Lactic acidosis Use with caution in renal impairment—increased risk of lactic acidosis; avoid in significant renal impairment. NICE[1] recommends that the dose should be reviewed if eGFR less than 45 mL/minute/1.73 m² and to avoid if eGFR less than 30 mL/minute/1.73 m². Withdraw or interrupt treatment in those at risk of tissue hypoxia or sudden deterioration in renal function, such as those with dehydration, severe infection, shock, sepsis, acute heart failure, respiratory failure or hepatic impairment, or those who have recently had a myocardial infarction

Contra-indications ketoacidosis, see also Lactic Acidosis above; use of general anaesthesia (suspend metformin on the morning of surgery and restart when renal function returns to baseline)

Iodine-containing X-ray contrast media Intravascular administration of iodinated contrast agents can cause renal failure, which can increase the risk of lactic acidosis with metformin—see Lactic Acidosis above. Suspend metformin prior to the test; restart no earlier than 48 hours after the test if renal function has returned to baseline

Hepatic impairment withdraw if tissue hypoxia likely

Renal impairment see under Cautions

Pregnancy used in pregnancy for both pre-existing and gestational diabetes—see also p. 473

Breast-feeding may be used during breast-feeding—see p. 473

Side-effects anorexia, nausea, vomiting, diarrhoea (usually transient), abdominal pain, taste disturbance, *rarely* lactic acidosis (withdraw treatment), decreased vitamin-B₁₂ absorption, erythema, pruritus and urticaria; hepatitis also reported

Dose
* Diabetes mellitus, ADULT and CHILD over 10 years initially 500 mg with breakfast for at least 1 week then 500 mg with breakfast and evening meal for at least 1 week then 500 mg with breakfast, lunch and evening meal; usual max. 2 g daily in divided doses
* Polycystic ovary syndrome [unlicensed], initially 500 mg with breakfast for 1 week, then 500 mg with breakfast and evening meal for 1 week, then 1.5–1.7 g daily in 2–3 divided doses

Note Metformin doses in the BNF may differ from those in the product literature

Metformin (Non-proprietary) [PoM]
Tablets, coated, metformin hydrochloride 500 mg, net price 28-tab pack = £1.32, 84-tab pack = £1.00; 850 mg, 56-tab pack = £1.91. Label: 21

Oral solution, sugar-free, metformin hydrochloride 500 mg/5 mL, net price 100 mL = £40.00. Label: 21

Glucophage® (Merck Serono) [PoM]
Tablets, f/c, metformin hydrochloride 500 mg, net price 84-tab pack = £2.88; 850 mg, 56-tab pack = £3.20. Label: 21

1. NICE clinical guideline 87 (May 2009): Type 2 diabetes: The management of type 2 diabetes

◢ Modified release

Metformin (Non-proprietary) [PoM]
Tablets, m/r, metformin hydrochloride 500 mg, net price 28 tab-pack = £2.66, 56 tab-pack = £5.32. Label: 21, 25
Brands include *Bolamyn*® *SR*, *Glucient*® *SR*, *Metabet*® *SR*
Dose initially 500 mg once daily, increased every 10–15 days, max. 2 g once daily with evening meal; if control not achieved, use 1 g twice daily with meals, and if control still not achieved change to standard-release tablets
Note Patients taking up to 2 g daily of the standard-release metformin may start with the same daily dose of metformin modified release; not suitable if dose of standard-release tablets more than 2 g daily

Glucophage® **SR** (Merck Serono) [PoM]
Tablets, m/r, metformin hydrochloride 500 mg, net price 28-tab pack = £2.66, 56-tab pack = £5.32; 750 mg, 28-tab pack = £3.20, 56-tab pack = £6.40; 1 g, 28-tab pack = £4.26, 56-tab pack = £8.52. Label: 21, 25

Dose initially 500 mg once daily, increased every 10–15 days, max. 2 g once daily with evening meal; if control not achieved, use 1 g twice daily with meals, and if control still not achieved change to standard-release tablets
Note Patients taking up to 2 g daily of the standard-release metformin may start with the same daily dose of *Glucophage*® *SR*; not suitable if dose of standard-release tablets more than 2 g daily

The *Scottish Medicines Consortium* (p. 4) has advised (September 2009) that *Glucophage*® *SR* is accepted for restricted use within NHS Scotland for the treatment of type 2 diabetes mellitus in adult patients who are intolerant of standard-release metformin, and in whom the prolonged-release tablet allows the use of a dose of metformin not previously tolerated, or in patients for whom a once daily preparation offers a clinically significant benefit.

◢ With alogliptin
Section 6.1.2.3

◢ With canagliflozin
Section 6.1.2.3

◢ With dapagliflozin
Section 6.1.2.3

◢ With linagliptin
Section 6.1.2.3

◢ With pioglitazone
Section 6.1.2.3

◢ With saxagliptin
Section 6.1.2.3

◢ With sitagliptin
Section 6.1.2.3

◢ With vildagliptin
Section 6.1.2.3

6.1.2.3 Other antidiabetic drugs

Acarbose, an inhibitor of intestinal alpha glucosidases, delays the digestion and absorption of starch and sucrose; it has a small but significant effect in lowering blood glucose. Use of acarbose is usually reserved for when other oral hypoglycaemics are not tolerated or are contra-indicated. Postprandial hyperglycaemia in type 1 diabetes can be reduced by acarbose, but it has been little used for this purpose. Flatulence deters some from using acarbose although this side-effect tends to decrease with time.

Nateglinide and **repaglinide** stimulate insulin secretion. Both drugs have a rapid onset of action and short duration of activity, and should be administered shortly before each main meal. Repaglinide may be given as monotherapy for patients who are not overweight or for those in whom metformin is contra-indicated or not tolerated, or it may be given in combination with metformin. Nateglinide is licensed only for use with metformin.

The thiazolidinedione, **pioglitazone**, reduces peripheral insulin resistance, leading to a reduction of blood-glucose concentration. Pioglitazone can be used alone or in combination with metformin or with a sulfonylurea (if metformin inappropriate), or with both; the combination of pioglitazone plus metformin is preferred to pioglitazone plus sulfonylurea, particularly for obese patients. Inadequate response to a combination of metformin and sulfonylurea may indicate failing insulin release; the introduction of pioglitazone has a limited role in these circumstances and the initiation of insulin is often more appropriate. Pioglitazone is also licensed in combination with insulin, in patients who have not achieved adequate glycaemic control with insulin alone, when metformin is inappropriate. Blood-glucose control may deteriorate temporarily when pioglitazone is substituted for an oral antidiabetic drug that is being used in combination with another. Long-term benefits of pioglitazone have not yet been demonstrated. NICE (May 2009) has recommended that, when glycaemic control is inadequate with existing treatment, pioglitazone can be added to:

- a sulfonylurea, if metformin is contra-indicated or not tolerated;

- metformin, if risks of hypoglycaemia with sulfonylurea are unacceptable or a sulfonylurea is contra-indicated or not tolerated;

- a combination of metformin and a sulfonylurea, if insulin is unacceptable because of lifestyle or other personal issues, or because the patient is obese.

NICE has recommended that treatment with pioglitazone is continued only if HbA_{1c} concentration is reduced by at least 0.5 percentage points within 6 months of starting treatment.

The *Scottish Medicines Consortium* (p. 4) accepts use of pioglitazone (February 2007) with metformin and a sulfonylurea, for patients (especially if overweight) whose glycaemic control is inadequate despite the use of 2 oral hypoglycaemic drugs and who are unable or unwilling to take insulin; treatment should be initiated and monitored by an experienced diabetes physician.

MHRA/CHM advice
Pioglitazone cardiovascular safety
(December 2007 and January 2011)

Incidence of heart failure is increased when pioglitazone is combined with insulin especially in patients with predisposing factors e.g. previous myocardial infarction. Patients who take pioglitazone should be closely monitored for signs of heart failure; treatment should be discontinued if any deterioration in cardiac status occurs.

Pioglitazone should not be used in patients with heart failure or a history of heart failure.

Pioglitazone: risk of bladder cancer (July 2011)

The European Medicines Agency has advised that there is a small increased risk of bladder cancer associated with pioglitazone use. However, in patients who respond adequately to treatment, the benefits of pioglitazone continue to outweigh the risks.

Pioglitazone should not be used in patients with active bladder cancer or a past history of bladder cancer, or in those who have uninvestigated macroscopic haematuria. Pioglitazone should be used with caution in elderly patients as the risk of bladder cancer increases with age.

Before initiating treatment with pioglitazone, patients should be assessed for risk factors of bladder cancer (including age, smoking status, exposure to certain occupational or chemotherapy agents, or previous radiation therapy to the pelvic region) and any macroscopic haematuria should be investigated. The safety and efficacy of pioglitazone should be reviewed after 3–6 months and pioglitazone should be stopped in patients who do not respond adequately to treatment.

Patients already receiving treatment with pioglitazone should be assessed for risk factors of bladder cancer and treatment should be reviewed after 3–6 months, as above.

Patients should be advised to report promptly any haematuria, dysuria, or urinary urgency during treatment.

Alogliptin, **linagliptin**, **saxagliptin**, **sitagliptin**, and **vildagliptin** inhibit dipeptidylpeptidase-4 to increase insulin secretion and lower glucagon secretion. Linagliptin is licensed for use in type 2 diabetes as monotherapy (if metformin inappropriate), or in combination with metformin (when treatment with metformin alone fails to achieve adequate glycaemic control), or both metformin and a sulfonylurea (when dual therapy with these drugs fails to achieve adequate glycaemic control). Linagliptin may also be used in combination with insulin (with or without metformin) when a stable dose of insulin has not provided adequate glycaemic control. Saxagliptin and vildagliptin are licensed for use in type 2 diabetes as monotherapy (if metformin inappropriate), or in combination with metformin or a sulfonylurea (if metformin inappropriate), or pioglitazone (when treatment with either metformin or a sulfonylurea or pioglitazone fails to achieve adequate glycaemic control), and also in combination with both metformin and a sulfonylurea (when dual therapy with these drugs fails to achieve adequate glycaemic control). The combination of either saxagliptin or vildagliptin, and insulin (with or without metformin) is also licensed for use when a stable dose of insulin has not provided adequate glycaemic control. Sitagliptin is licensed for use in type 2 diabetes as monotherapy (if metformin inappropriate), or in combination with metformin or a sulfonylurea (if metformin inappropriate), or pioglitazone (when treatment with either metformin or a sulfonylurea or pioglitazone fails to achieve adequate glycaemic control), and also in combination with both metformin and a sulfonylurea (when dual therapy with these drugs fails to achieve adequate glycaemic control). Sitagliptin is also licensed for use in combination with both metformin and pioglitazone when dual therapy with these drugs

6

Endocrine system

fails to achieve adequate glycaemic control, and may also be used in combination with insulin (with or without metformin) when a stable dose of insulin has not provided adequate glycaemic control. Alogliptin is licensed for use in type 2 diabetes as dual therapy in combination with either metformin, pioglitazone, a sulfonylurea, or insulin (when treatment with these drugs alone fails to achieve adequate glycaemic control); it is also licensed for use as triple therapy in combination with metformin and either pioglitazone or insulin.

NICE (May 2009) has recommended that, when glycaemic control is inadequate with existing treatment:

- sitagliptin or vildagliptin (instead of a sulfonylurea) can be added to metformin, if there is a significant risk of hypoglycaemia or if a sulfonylurea is contraindicated or not tolerated;

- sitagliptin or vildagliptin can be added to a sulfonylurea, if metformin is contra-indicated or not tolerated;

- sitagliptin can be added to both metformin and a sulfonylurea, if insulin is unacceptable because of lifestyle or other personal issues, or because the patient is obese.

NICE has recommended that treatment with sitagliptin or vildagliptin is continued only if HbA$_{1c}$ concentration is reduced by at least 0.5 percentage points within 6 months of starting treatment.

The Scottish Medicines Consortium (p. 4) has advised that vildagliptin (Galvus®) is accepted for restricted use within NHS Scotland for the treatment of type 2 diabetes mellitus as monotherapy when treatment with metformin or a sulfonylurea is inappropriate (December 2012), and in combination with metformin when addition of a sulfonylurea is inappropriate (March 2008), and in combination with a sulfonylurea if metformin is inappropriate (September 2009), and also as triple therapy in combination with metformin and a sulfonylurea, as an alternative to existing dipeptidyl peptidase-4 inhibitors, when treatment with metformin and a sulfonylurea is inadequate (November 2013).

The Scottish Medicines Consortium (p. 4) has advised that linagliptin (Trajenta®) is accepted for restricted use within NHS Scotland for the treatment of type 2 diabetes mellitus as monotherapy when both metformin and a sulfonylurea are inappropriate (January 2013), and in combination with metformin when addition of a sulfonylurea is inappropriate (December 2011), and also in combination with both a sulfonylurea and metformin when dual therapy is ineffective (January 2013).

The Scottish Medicines Consortium (p. 4) has advised that saxagliptin (Onglyza®) is accepted for restricted use within NHS Scotland for the treatment of type 2 diabetes mellitus as triple therapy in combination with metformin and a sulfonylurea, as an alternative to existing dipeptidyl peptidase-4 inhibitors, when treatment with metformin and a sulfonylurea is inadequate (November 2013).

Exenatide, liraglutide, and **lixisenatide** bind to, and activate, the GLP-1 (glucagon-like peptide-1) receptor to increase insulin secretion, suppress glucagon secretion, and slow gastric emptying. Treatment with exenatide, liraglutide, and lixisenatide is associated with the prevention of weight gain and possible promotion of weight loss which can be beneficial in overweight patients. They are given by subcutaneous injection for the treatment of type 2 diabetes mellitus.

Exenatide is licensed in combination with metformin or a sulfonylurea, or both, or with pioglitazone, or with both metformin and pioglitazone, in patients who have not achieved adequate glycaemic control with these drugs alone or in combination; standard-release exenatide is also licensed in combination with basal insulin alone or with metformin or pioglitazone (or both).

NICE (May 2009) has recommended that, when glycaemic control is inadequate with metformin and sulfonylurea treatment, the addition of standard-release exenatide may be considered if the patient has:

- a body mass index of 35 kg/m^2 or over and is of European descent (with appropriate adjustment for other ethnic groups) and weight-related psychological or medical problems or

- a body mass index less than 35 kg/m^2, and insulin would be unacceptable for occupational reasons or weight loss would benefit other significant obesity-related comorbidities.

NICE has recommended that treatment with standard-release exenatide is continued only if HbA$_{1c}$ concentration is reduced by at least 1 percentage point and a weight loss of at least 3% is achieved within 6 months of starting treatment.

The Scottish Medicines Consortium (p. 4) has advised (June 2007) that standard-release exenatide (Byetta®) is accepted for restricted use within NHS Scotland for the treatment of type 2 diabetes in combination with metformin or sulfonylurea (or both), as an alternative to treatment with insulin in patients where treatment with metformin or sulfonylurea (or both) at maximally tolerated doses has been inadequate, and treatment with insulin would be the next option.

The Scottish Medicines Consortium (p. 4) has also advised (February 2011) that standard-release exenatide (Bye-tta®) is accepted for restricted use within NHS Scotland for the treatment of type 2 diabetes in combination with metformin and pioglitazone as a third-line pre-insulin treatment option.

The *Scottish Medicines Consortium* (p. 4) has advised (December 2011) that modified-release exenatide (*Bydureon*®) is accepted for restricted use within NHS Scotland for the treatment of type 2 diabetes as a third-line treatment option.

Liraglutide is licensed for the treatment of type 2 diabetes mellitus in combination with metformin or a sulfonylurea, or both, in patients who have not achieved adequate glycaemic control with these drugs alone or in combination. Liraglutide is also licensed for use in combination with basal insulin or both metformin and pioglitazone when dual therapy with these drugs fails to achieve adequate glycaemic control.

Lixisenatide is licensed for the treatment of type 2 diabetes mellitus in combination with oral antidiabetic drugs (e.g. metformin, pioglitazone, or a sulfonylurea) or basal insulin, or both, when adequate glycaemic control has not been achieved with these drugs; lixisenatide should not be used in combination with both basal insulin and a sulfonylurea because of an increased risk of hypoglycaemia.

The *Scottish Medicines Consortium* (p. 4) has advised (August 2013) that lixisenatide (*Lyxumia*®) is accepted for restricted use within NHS Scotland for the treatment of type 2 diabetes in combination with oral antidiabetic drugs or basal insulin (or both), when adequate glycaemic control has not been achieved with these drugs; use is restricted to patients in whom a GLP-1 agonist is appropriate, as an alternative to an existing GLP-1 agonist (exenatide or liraglutide).

Canagliflozin, dapagliflozin, and **empagliflozin** reversibly inhibit sodium-glucose co-transporter 2 (SGLT2) in the renal proximal convoluted tubule to reduce glucose reabsorption and increase urinary glucose excretion. Canagliflozin, dapagliflozin, and empagliflozin are licensed for use in type 2 diabetes as monotherapy (if metformin inappropriate), or in combination with insulin or other antidiabetic drugs (if existing treatment fails to achieve adequate glycaemic control). Dapagliflozin is not recommended in combination with pioglitazone.

6 Endocrine system

NICE guidance
Dapagliflozin in combination therapy for treating type 2 diabetes (June 2013)

Dapagliflozin in a dual therapy regimen in combination with metformin is recommended for the treatment of type 2 diabetes, only if glycaemic control is inadequate, and the patient has a significant risk of hypoglycaemia *or* if a sulfonylurea is contra-indicated or not tolerated.

Dapagliflozin in combination with insulin (alone or with other antidiabetic drugs) is an option for the treatment of type 2 diabetes.

Dapagliflozin in combination with metformin and a sulfonylurea as triple therapy is not recommended for the treatment of type 2 diabetes except as part of a clinical trial.

Patients currently receiving dapagliflozin in a dual or triple therapy regimen that is not recommended according to the above criteria should have the option to continue treatment until they and their clinician consider it appropriate to stop.

www.nice.org.uk/TA288

The *Scottish Medicines Consortium* (p. 4) has advised that dapagliflozin (*Forxiga*®) is accepted for restricted use within NHS Scotland for the treatment of type 2 diabetes in combination with metformin, when treatment with metformin alone is inadequate and a sulfonylurea is inappropriate (December 2012), or in combination with insulin when treatment with insulin alone is inadequate (February 2014).

NICE guidance
Canagliflozin in combination therapy for treating type 2 diabetes (June 2014)

Canagliflozin in a dual therapy regimen in combination with metformin is recommended for the treatment of type 2 diabetes, only if a sulfonylurea is contra-indicated or not tolerated *or* the patient has a significant risk of hypoglycaemia.

Canagliflozin in a triple therapy regimen is an option for the treatment of type 2 diabetes in combination with metformin and a sulfonylurea *or* metformin and a thiazolidinedione.

Canagliflozin in combination with insulin (alone or with other antidiabetic drugs) is an option for the treatment of type 2 diabetes.

Patients currently receiving canagliflozin in a dual or triple therapy regimen that is not recommended according to the above criteria should have the option to continue treatment until they and their clinician consider it appropriate to stop.

www.nice.org.uk/TA315

The *Scottish Medicines Consortium* (p. 4) has advised (May 2014) that canagliflozin (*Invokana*®) is accepted for restricted use within NHS Scotland for the treatment of type 2 diabetes in combination with metformin as dual therapy, or in combination with metformin and standard of care as triple therapy, or in combination with insulin and standard of care.

ACARBOSE

Indications   diabetes mellitus inadequately controlled by diet or by diet with oral antidiabetic drugs

Cautions   monitor liver function; may enhance hypoglycaemic effects of insulin and sulfonylureas (hypo-glycaemic episodes may be treated with oral glucose but not with sucrose); **interactions:** Appendix 1 (antidiabetics)

Contra-indications   inflammatory bowel disease, predisposition to partial intestinal obstruction; hernia, previous abdominal surgery

Hepatic impairment   avoid

Renal impairment   avoid if eGFR less than 25 mL/minute/1.73 m^2

Pregnancy   avoid

Breast-feeding   avoid

Side-effects   flatulence, soft stools, diarrhoea (may need to reduce dose or withdraw), abdominal distention and pain; *rarely*, nausea, abnormal liver function tests and skin reactions; *very rarely* ileus, oedema, jaundice, and hepatitis
Note Antacids unlikely to be beneficial for treating side-effects

Dose
- ADULT over 18 years, initially 50 mg daily increased to 50 mg 3 times daily, then increased if necessary after 6–8 weeks to 100 mg 3 times daily; max. 200 mg 3 times daily
  Counselling Tablets should be chewed with first mouthful of food or swallowed whole with a little liquid immediately before food. To counteract possible hypoglycaemia, patients receiving insulin or a sulfonylurea as well as acarbose need to carry glucose (not sucrose—acarbose interferes with sucrose absorption)

Glucobay® (Bayer) [PoM]
Tablets, acarbose 50 mg, net price 90-tab pack = £7.35; 100 mg (scored), 90-tab pack = £13.50. Counselling, administration

ALOGLIPTIN

Indications   see notes above

Cautions   determine renal function before treatment and periodically thereafter; history of pancreatitis; discontinue if symptoms of acute pancreatitis (persistent, severe abdominal pain); not recommended in moderate to severe heart failure (limited experience); **interactions:** Appendix 1 (antidiabetics)

Contra-indications   history of serious hypersensitivity to dipeptidylpeptidase-4 inhibitors; ketoacidosis

Hepatic impairment   manufacturer advises avoid in severe impairment—no information available

Renal impairment   reduce dose to 12.5 mg once daily if eGFR 30–50 mL/minute/1.73 m^2; reduce dose to 6.25 mg once daily if eGFR less than 30 mL/minute/1.73 m^2 and use with caution

Pregnancy   manufacturer advises avoid—no information available

Breast-feeding   avoid—present in milk in *animal* studies

Side-effects   abdominal pain, gastro-oesophageal reflux, nasopharyngitis, upper respiratory-tract infection, headache, pruritus, rash; *also reported* pancreatitis, hepatic impairment, angioedema, urticaria, Stevens-Johnson syndrome

Dose
- ADULT over 18 years, 25 mg once daily
Note Dose of concomitant sulfonylurea or insulin may need to be reduced; caution with use in combination with both metformin and pioglitazone—risk of hypoglycaemia (dose of metformin or pioglitazone may need to be reduced)

Vipidia® (Takeda) ▼ PoM

Tablets, f/c, alogliptin (as benzoate) 6.25 mg (pink), net price 28-tab pack = £26.60; 12.5 mg (yellow), 28-tab pack = £26.60; 25 mg (red), 28-tab pack = £26.60

◢With metformin

For prescribing information on metformin, see section 6.1.2.2

Vipdomet® (Takeda) ▼ PoM

Tablets, f/c, yellow, alogliptin (as benzoate) 12.5 mg, metformin hydrochloride 1 g, net price 56-tab pack = £26.60. Label: 21

Dose type 2 diabetes mellitus not controlled by metformin alone *or* by metformin in combination with either pioglitazone or insulin, ADULT over 18 years, 1 tablet twice daily (based on patient's current metformin dose)

Note Dose of concomitant insulin may need to be reduced; caution with use in combination with pioglitazone—risk of hypoglycaemia (dose of pioglitazone may need to be reduced)

▌ CANAGLIFLOZIN

Indications see notes above

Cautions determine renal function before treatment and at least annually thereafter, and before initiation of concomitant drugs that reduce renal function and periodically thereafter; elderly or cardiovascular disease (risk of hypotension); history of hypotension; elevated haematocrit; **interactions**: Appendix 1 (antidiabetics)

Volume depletion Correct hypovolaemia before starting treatment. Patients should be advised to report symptoms of volume depletion including postural hypotension and dizziness—consider interrupting treatment if volume depletion occurs

Contra-indications ketoacidosis

Hepatic impairment manufacturer advises avoid in severe impairment—no information available

Renal impairment monitor renal function at least twice a year in moderate impairment; avoid initiation if eGFR less than 60 mL/minute/1.73 m²; avoid in combination with metformin (*Vokanamet*®) if eGFR less than 60 mL/minute/1.73 m²; reduce dose to 100 mg once daily if eGFR falls persistently below 60 mL/minute/1.73m² and existing canagliflozin treatment tolerated; avoid if eGFR less than 45 mL/minute/1.73m²

Pregnancy avoid—toxicity in *animal* studies

Breast-feeding avoid—present in milk in *animal* studies

Side-effects constipation, thirst, nausea, dyslipidaemia, urinary-tract infection, hypoglycaemia (in combination with insulin or sulfonylurea), genital infection, polyuria, urinary frequency, raised haematocrit; *less commonly* postural hypotension, dizziness, syncope, dehydration, hypovolaemia, rash, raised serum creatinine and urea

Dose

- ADULT over 18 years, 100 mg once daily preferably before breakfast; if necessary and if tolerated, increase to 300 mg once daily

Note Dose of concomitant insulin or drugs that stimulate insulin secretion may need to be reduced

Invokana® (Janssen) ▼ PoM

Tablets, f/c, canagliflozin 100 mg (yellow), net price 30-tab pack = £39.20; 300 mg (white), 30-tab pack = £49.99. Counselling, volume depletion, see above

◢With metformin

For prescribing information on metformin, see section 6.1.2.2

Vokanamet® (Janssen) ▼ PoM

Vokanamet® 50 mg/850 mg tablets, f/c, pink, canagliflozin 50 mg, metformin hydrochloride 850 mg, net price 60-tab pack = £39.20. Label: 21, counselling, volume depletion, see above

Vokanamet® 50 mg/1 g tablets, f/c, beige, canagliflozin 50 mg, metformin hydrochloride 1 g, net price 60-tab pack = £39.20 Label: 21, counselling, volume depletion, see above

Dose type 2 diabetes mellitus not controlled by metformin alone *or* by metformin in combination with insulin or other antidiabetic drugs, ADULT over 18 years, 1 tablet twice daily (based on patient's current metformin dose); daily dose of metformin should not exceed 2 g

Note Dose of concomitant insulin or drugs that stimulate insulin secretion may need to be reduced

---

▌ DAPAGLIFLOZIN

Indications see notes above

Cautions determine renal function before treatment and at least annually thereafter; hypotension; electrolyte disturbances; cardiovascular disease or elderly (risk of hypotension); raised haematocrit; **interactions**: Appendix 1 (antidiabetics)

Volume depletion Correct hypovolaemia before starting treatment. Consider interrupting treatment if volume depletion occurs

Contra-indications ketoacidosis

Hepatic impairment initial dose 5 mg daily in severe impairment, increased according to response; in combination with metformin (*Xigduo*®), avoid

Renal impairment avoid if eGFR less than 60 mL/minute/1.73 m² (ineffective)

Pregnancy avoid—toxicity in *animal* studies

Breast-feeding avoid—present in milk in *animal* studies

Side-effects hypoglycaemia (in combination with insulin or sulphonylurea), constipation, dyslipidaemia, back pain, genital infection, urinary-tract infection, dysuria, polyuria, thirst, sweating; *less commonly* nausea, hypotension, dizziness, rash, nocturia, dehydration, hypovolaemia, raised serum creatinine and urea

Dose

- ADULT over 18 years, 10 mg once daily; ELDERLY over 75 years, initiation not recommended

Note Dose of concomitant insulin or drugs that stimulate insulin secretion may need to be reduced

Forxiga® (AstraZeneca) ▼ PoM

Tablets, yellow, f/c, dapagliflozin (as propanediol monohydrate) 5 mg, net price 28-tab pack = £36.59; 10 mg, 28-tab pack = £36.59

◢With metformin

For prescribing information on metformin, see section 6.1.2.2

Xigduo® (AstraZeneca) ▼ PoM

Xigduo® 5 mg/850 mg tablets, f/c, brown, dapagliflozin (as propanediol monohydrate) 5 mg, metformin hydrochloride 850 mg, net price 56 tab-pack = £36.59. Label: 21

5

Endocrine system

Xigduo® 5 mg/1 g tablets, f/c, yellow, dapagliflozin (as propanediol monohydrate) 5 mg, metformin hydrochloride 1 g, net price 56 tab-pack = £36.59. Label: 21

Dose type 2 diabetes mellitus not controlled by metformin alone *or* by metformin in combination with insulin or other antidiabetic drugs, ADULT over 18 years, 1 tablet twice daily (based on patient's current metformin dose); ELDERLY over 75 years, initiation not recommended

Note Dose of concomitant insulin or drugs that stimulate insulin secretion may need to be reduced

The *Scottish Medicines Consortium* (p.) has advised (July 2014) that dapagliflozin plus metformin (*Xigduo®*) is accepted for restricted use within NHS Scotland in patients for whom a combination of dapagliflozin and metformin is an appropriate choice of therapy i.e. when metformin alone does not provide adequate glycaemic control and a sulfonylurea is inappropriate, *or* in combination with insulin, when insulin and metformin does not provide adequate control, *or* in combination with a sulfonylurea, when a sulfonylurea and metformin does not provide adequate control

EMPAGLIFLOZIN

Indications see notes above

Cautions determine renal function before treatment and before initiation of concomitant drugs that may reduce renal function, then at least annually thereafter; patients at increased risk of volume depletion (risk factors include elderly patients aged over 75 years, cardiovascular disease, concomitant antihypertensive therapy, history of hypotension, predisposition to fluid disturbances e.g. gastro-intestinal illness, concomitant use of diuretics) see below; heart failure; complicated urinary tract infections—consider temporarily interrupting treatment; **interactions**: Appendix 1 (antidiabetics)

Volume depletion Correct hypovolaemia before starting treatment. Consider interrupting treatment if volume depletion occurs

Contra-indications diabetic ketoacidosis

Hepatic impairment manufacturer advises avoid in severe impairment—no information available

Renal impairment avoid initiation if eGFR below 60 mL/minute/1.73 m²; reduce dose to 10 mg once daily if eGFR falls persistently below 60 mL/minute/1.73 m²; avoid if eGFR is persistently below 45 mL/minute/1.73 m²

Pregnancy manufacturer advises avoid—toxicity in *animal* studies

Breast-feeding manufacturer advises avoid—present in milk in *animal* studies

Side-effects Hypoglycaemia (in combination with insulin or sulfonylurea), urinary tract infection, genital infection, polyuria, pruritus; *less commonly* dysuria, volume depletion

Dose

● ADULT over 18 years, 10 mg once daily, if necessary and if tolerated, increase to max. 25 mg once daily; ELDERLY over 85 years, initiation not recommended

Note Dose of concomitant insulin or drugs that stimulate insulin secretion may need to be reduced

Jardiance® (Boehringer Ingelheim) ▼ PoM
Tablets, pale yellow, f/c, empagliflozin 10mg, net price 28-tab pack = £36.59; 25 mg, 28-tab pack = £36.59.

EXENATIDE

Indications see notes above

Cautions elderly; pancreatitis (see below); may cause weight loss greater than 1.5 kg weekly; **interactions**: Appendix 1 (antidiabetics)

Pancreatitis Severe pancreatitis (sometimes fatal), including haemorrhagic or necrotising pancreatitis, has been reported rarely. Patients or their carers should be told how to recognise signs and symptoms of pancreatitis and advised to seek prompt medical attention if symptoms such as abdominal pain, nausea, and vomiting develop; discontinue permanently if pancreatitis is diagnosed

Contra-indications ketoacidosis; severe gastro-intestinal disease

Renal impairment

● for *standard-release* injection, use with caution if eGFR 30–50 mL/minute/1.73 m²; avoid if eGFR less than 30 mL/minute/1.73m²

● for *modified-release* injection, avoid if eGFR less than 50 mL/minute/1.73 m²

Pregnancy avoid—toxicity in *animal* studies. Women of child-bearing age should use effective contraception during treatment with modified-release exenatide and for 12 weeks after discontinuation

Breast-feeding avoid—no information available

Side-effects gastro-intestinal disturbances including nausea, vomiting, diarrhoea, dyspepsia, abdominal pain and distension, gastro-oesophageal reflux disease, decreased appetite, weight loss, headache, dizziness, agitation, asthenia, hypoglycaemia, increased sweating, injection-site reactions, antibody formation; *less commonly* pancreatitis (see Cautions above); *rarely* alopecia; *very rarely* anaphylactic reactions; also reported constipation, flatulence, eructation, dehydration, taste disturbance, renal impairment, drowsiness, rash, pruritus, urticaria, and angioedema

Dose

● By subcutaneous injection, ADULT over 18 years, initially 5 micrograms twice daily within 1 hour before 2 main meals (at least 6 hours apart), increased if necessary after at least 1 month to max. 10 micrograms twice daily

Counselling If a dose is missed, continue with the next scheduled dose—do not administer after a meal. Some oral medications should be taken at least 1 hour before or 4 hours after exenatide injection—consult product literature for details

Note Dose of concomitant sulfonylurea may need to be reduced

Byetta® (AstraZeneca) ▼ PoM
Injection, exenatide 250 micrograms/mL, net price 5 microgram/dose prefilled pen (60 doses) = £68.24, 10 microgram/dose prefilled pen (60 doses) = £68.24. Label: 10, counselling, administration

◢Modified release

Bydureon® (AstraZeneca) ▼ PoM
Injection, m/r, powder for reconstitution, exenatide, net price 2-mg vial (with solvent) = £18.34. Label: 10, counselling, administration

Dose by subcutaneous injection, ADULT over 18 years, 2 mg once weekly

Counselling Patients changing from standard-release exenatide formulation may experience initial transient increase in blood glucose. Some oral medications should be taken at least 1 hour before or 4 hours after exenatide injection—consult product literature for details

Note Dose of concomitant sulfonylurea may need to be reduced

Important Effect of *Bydureon®* may persist for 10 weeks after discontinuation

Endocrine system

6

■ LINAGLIPTIN

Indications see notes above

Cautions discontinue if symptoms of acute pancreatitis (persistent, severe abdominal pain); **interactions:** Appendix 1 (antidiabetics)

Pregnancy avoid—no information available

Breast-feeding avoid—present in milk in *animal* studies

Side-effects *less commonly* cough, nasopharyngitis; *also reported* pancreatitis

Dose

● ADULT over 18 years, 5 mg once daily
Note Dose of concomitant sulfonylurea or insulin may need to be reduced

Trajenta® (Boehringer Ingelheim) ▼ PoM
Tablets, light red, f/c, linagliptin 5 mg, net price 28-tab pack = £33.26

◢With metformin

For prescribing information on metformin, see section 6.1.2.2

Jentadueto® (Boehringer Ingelheim) ▼ PoM
Jentadueto® 2.5 mg/850 mg tablets, f/c, light orange, linagliptin 2.5 mg, metformin hydrochloride 850 mg, net price 56-tab pack = £33.26. Label: 21
Jentadueto® 2.5 mg/1 g tablets, f/c, light pink, linagliptin 2.5 mg, metformin hydrochloride 1 g, net price 56-tab pack = £33.26. Label: 21
Dose type 2 diabetes mellitus not controlled by metformin alone *or* by metformin in combination with either a sulfonylurea *or* insulin, ADULT over 18 years, 1 *Jentadueto*® tablet twice daily (based on patient's current metformin dose)
Note Dose of concomitant sulfonyurea or insulin may need to be reduced

■ LIRAGLUTIDE

Indications see notes above

Cautions discontinue if symptoms of acute pancreatitis (persistent, severe abdominal pain); thyroid disease; **interactions:** Appendix 1 (antidiabetics)

Contra-indications ketoacidosis; inflammatory bowel disease; diabetic gastroparesis

Hepatic impairment avoid—limited experience

Renal impairment avoid if eGFR less than 60 mL/minute/1.73 m^2—limited experience

Pregnancy avoid—toxicity in *animal* studies

Breast-feeding avoid—no information available

Side-effects gastro-intestinal disturbances including nausea, vomiting, constipation, diarrhoea, dyspepsia, abdominal pain and distension, flatulence, gastritis, gastro-oesophageal reflux disease, decreased appetite; headache, dizziness, fatigue; fever, bronchitis, nasopharyngitis; hypoglycaemia; injection site reactions; *less commonly* dehydration; *also reported* acute pancreatitis, thyroid neoplasm, goitre, increased blood calcitonin, angioedema

Dose

● By subcutaneous injection, ADULT over 18 years, initially 0.6 mg once daily, increased after at least 1 week to 1.2 mg once daily, further increased if necessary after an interval of at least 1 week to max. 1.8 mg once daily
Note Dose of concomitant insulin or sulfonylurea may need to be reduced

Victoza® (Novo Nordisk) PoM
Injection, liraglutide 6 mg/mL, net price 2 × 3-mL prefilled pens = £78.48, 3 × 3-mL prefilled pens = £117.72. Counselling, administration

◢With insulin degludec

For prescribing information on insulin degludec, see section 6.1.1.2

Xultophy® (Novo Nordisk) ▼ PoM
Injection, insulin degludec (recombinant human insulin analogue) 1 unit/dose-step, liraglutide 36 micrograms/dose-step), net price 5 × 3-mL (300 dose-step) prefilled pens = £159.22. Counselling, administration
Dose type 2 diabetes mellitus not controlled by oral antidiabetics alone *or* by oral antidiabetics in combination with basal insulin, by subcutaneous injection, ADULT over 18 years, *as add-on to oral antidiabetics*, initially 10 dose-steps once daily (adjusted according to response); *when transferring from basal insulin*, initially 16 dose-steps once daily (adjusted according to response); max. 50 dose-steps once daily
Note Dose of concomitant sulfonylurea may need to be reduced
Counselling Show container to patient and confirm that patient is expecting the version dispensed

■ LIXISENATIDE

Indications see notes above

Cautions discontinue if symptoms of acute pancreatitis (persistent, severe abdominal pain); **interactions:** Appendix 1 (antidiabetics)

Contra-indications ketoacidosis; severe gastro-intestinal disease

Renal impairment use with caution if eGFR 30–50 mL/minute/1.73 m^2; avoid if eGFR less than 30 mL/minute/1.73 m^2—no information available

Pregnancy avoid—toxicity in *animal* studies; women of child-bearing age should use effective contraception

Breast-feeding avoid—no information available

Side-effects nausea, vomiting, diarrhoea, dyspepsia, palpitation, headache, dizziness, drowsiness, hypoglycaemia, injection-site reactions; *less commonly* tachycardia, urticaria

Dose

● By subcutaneous injection, ADULT over 18 years, initially 10 micrograms once daily within 1 hour before the first meal of the day or the evening meal for 14 days, increased to 20 micrograms once daily thereafter
Counselling If a dose is missed, inject within 1 hour before the next meal—do not administer **after** a meal. Some oral medications should be taken at least 1 hour before or 4 hours after lixisenatide injection—consult product literature for details
Note Dose of concomitant sulfonylurea or insulin may need to be reduced

Lyxumia® (Sanofi-Aventis) ▼ PoM
Injection, 50 micrograms/mL, net price 10 micrograms/dose prefilled pen (14 doses) = £27.07; 100 micrograms/mL, 20 micrograms/dose prefilled pen (14 doses) × 2 = £54.14; treatment initiation pack, 10 micrograms/dose prefilled pen and 20 micrograms/dose prefilled pen = £54.14. Label: 10, counselling, administration

Endocrine system

▌ NATEGLINIDE

Indications type 2 diabetes mellitus in combination with metformin (section 6.1.2.2) when metformin alone inadequate

Cautions substitute insulin during intercurrent illness (such as myocardial infarction, coma, infection, and trauma) and during surgery (omit nateglinide on morning of surgery and recommence when eating and drinking normally); elderly, debilitated and malnourished patients; **interactions:** Appendix 1 (antidiabetics)

Contra-indications ketoacidosis

Hepatic impairment caution in moderate hepatic impairment; avoid in severe impairment—no information available

Pregnancy avoid—toxicity in *animal* studies

Breast-feeding avoid—present in milk in *animal* studies

Side-effects hypoglycaemia; hypersensitivity reactions including pruritus, rashes and urticaria

Dose
- ADULT over 18 years, initially 60 mg 3 times daily within 30 minutes before main meals, adjusted according to response up to max. 180 mg 3 times daily

Starlix® (Novartis) (PoM)
Tablets, f/c, nateglinide 60 mg (pink), net price 84-tab pack = £22.71; 120 mg (yellow), 84-tab pack = £25.88; 180 mg (red), 84-tab pack = £25.88

▌ PIOGLITAZONE

Indications type 2 diabetes mellitus (alone or combined with metformin or a sulfonylurea, or with both, or with insulin—see also notes above)

Cautions monitor liver function (see below); cardiovascular disease or in combination with insulin (risk of heart failure—see MHRA/CHM advice p. 477); substitute insulin during peri-operative period (omit pioglitazone on morning of surgery and recommence when eating and drinking normally); increased risk of bone fractures, particularly in women; avoid in acute porphyria (but see section 9.8.2); risk factors for bladder cancer (see Risk of Bladder Cancer, p. 477); elderly (increased risk of heart failure, fractures, and bladder cancer); **interactions:** Appendix 1 (antidiabetics)

Liver toxicity Rare reports of liver dysfunction; monitor liver function before treatment, and periodically thereafter; advise patients to seek immediate medical attention if symptoms such as nausea, vomiting, abdominal pain, fatigue and dark urine develop; discontinue if jaundice occurs

Contra-indications history of heart failure; uninvestigated macroscopic haematuria, previous or active bladder cancer

Hepatic impairment avoid; see also Cautions above

Pregnancy avoid—toxicity in *animal* studies

Breast-feeding avoid—present in milk in *animal* studies

Side-effects gastro-intestinal disturbances, weight gain, oedema, anaemia, headache, visual disturbances, dizziness, arthralgia, hypoaesthesia, haematuria, impotence; *less commonly* hypoglycaemia, fatigue, insomnia, vertigo, sweating, altered blood lipids, proteinuria, bladder cancer; see also Liver Toxicity above

Dose
- ADULT over 18 years, initially 15–30 mg once daily increased to 45 mg once daily according to response, (ELDERLY, initiate with lowest possible dose and increase gradually); review treatment after 3–6 months and regularly thereafter

Note Dose of concomitant sulfonylurea or insulin may need to be reduced

Pioglitazone (Non-proprietary) (PoM)
Tablets, pioglitazone (as hydrochloride) 15 mg, net price 28-tab pack = £1.32; 30 mg, 28-tab pack = £1.57; 45 mg, 28-tab pack = £1.86

Actos® (Takeda) (PoM)
Tablets, pioglitazone (as hydrochloride) 15 mg, net price 28-tab pack = £25.83; 30 mg, 28-tab pack = £35.89; 45 mg, 28-tab pack = £39.55

◢With metformin
For prescribing information on metformin, see section 6.1.2.2

Competact® (Takeda) (PoM)
Tablets, f/c, pioglitazone (as hydrochloride) 15 mg, metformin hydrochloride 850 mg, net price 56-tab pack = £35.89. Label: 21

Dose ADULT over 18 years, type 2 diabetes not controlled by metformin alone, 1 tablet twice daily

Note Titration with the individual components (pioglitazone and metformin) desirable before initiating *Competact®*

▌ REPAGLINIDE

Indications type 2 diabetes mellitus (as monotherapy or in combination with metformin when metformin alone inadequate)

Cautions substitute insulin during intercurrent illness (such as myocardial infarction, coma, infection, and trauma) and during surgery (omit repaglinide on morning of surgery and recommence when eating and drinking normally); debilitated and malnourished patients; **interactions:** Appendix 1 (antidiabetics)

Contra-indications ketoacidosis

Hepatic impairment avoid in severe liver disease

Renal impairment use with caution

Pregnancy avoid

Breast-feeding avoid—present in milk in *animal* studies

Side-effects abdominal pain, diarrhoea, constipation, nausea, vomiting; *rarely* hypoglycaemia, hypersensitivity reactions including pruritus, rashes, vasculitis, urticaria, and visual disturbances

Dose
- ADULT over 18 years, initially 500 micrograms within 30 minutes before main meals (1 mg if transferring from another oral hypoglycaemic), adjusted according to response at intervals of 1–2 weeks; up to 4 mg may be given as a single dose, max. 16 mg daily; ELDERLY over 75 years, not recommended

Repaglinide (Non-proprietary) (PoM)
Tablets, repaglinide 500 micrograms, net price 30-tab pack = £2.90, 90-tab pack = £9.38; 1 mg, 30-tab pack = £3.03, 90-tab pack = £10.14; 2 mg, 90-tab pack = £5.84

Prandin® (Daiichi Sankyo) (PoM)
Tablets, repaglinide 500 micrograms, net price 30-tab pack = £3.92, 90-tab pack = £11.76; 1 mg (yellow), 30-tab pack = £3.92, 90-tab pack = £11.76; 2 mg (peach), 90-tab pack = £11.76
Formerly marketed as *NovoNorm®*

6 Endocrine system

▮ SAXAGLIPTIN

Indications see notes above

Cautions elderly; determine renal function before treatment and periodically thereafter; discontinue if symptoms of acute pancreatitis (persistent, severe abdominal pain); **interactions:** Appendix 1 (antidiabetics)

Contra-indications history of serious hypersensitivity to dipeptidylpeptidase-4 inhibitors

Hepatic impairment use with caution in moderate impairment; avoid in severe impairment

Renal impairment reduce dose to 2.5 mg once daily in moderate to severe impairment; use with caution in severe impairment

Pregnancy avoid unless essential—toxicity in *animal* studies

Breast-feeding avoid—present in milk in *animal* studies

Side-effects vomiting, dyspepsia, gastritis; peripheral oedema; headache, dizziness, fatigue; upper respiratory tract infection, urinary tract infection, gastroenteritis, sinusitis, nasopharyngitis; hypoglycaemia, myalgia; *less commonly* dyslipidaemia, hypertriglyceridaemia, pancreatitis, erectile dysfunction, arthralgia, hypersensitivity reactions (including anaphylaxis); *also reported* rash

Dose
• ADULT over 18 years, 5 mg once daily

Note Dose of concomitant sulfonylurea or insulin may need to be reduced

Onglyza® (AstraZeneca) [PoM]
Tablets, f/c, saxagliptin (as hydrochloride) 2.5 mg (yellow), net price 28-tab pack = £31.60; 5 mg (pink), net price 28-tab pack = £31.60

◢With metformin

For prescribing information on metformin, see section 6.1.2.2

Komboglyze® (AstraZeneca) [PoM]
Komboglyze® 2.5 mg/850 mg tablets, f/c, brown, saxagliptin (as hydrochloride) 2.5 mg, metformin hydrochloride 850 mg, net price 56-tab pack = £31.60. Label: 21
Komboglyze® 2.5 mg/1 g tablets, f/c, yellow, saxagliptin (as hydrochloride) 2.5 mg, metformin hydrochloride 1 g, net price 56-tab pack = £31.60. Label: 21
Dose type 2 diabetes mellitus not controlled by metformin alone *or* by metformin in combination with either a sulfonylurea *or* insulin, ADULT over 18 years, 1 tablet twice daily (based on patient's current metformin dose)
Note Dose of concomitant sulfonylurea or insulin may need to be reduced
The *Scottish Medicines Consortium* (p. 4) has advised (May 2013) that *Komboglyze*® is accepted for restricted use within NHS Scotland for the treatment of type 2 diabetes mellitus in patients unable to achieve adequate glycaemic control with metformin alone and when the addition of a sulfonylurea is inappropriate

▮ SITAGLIPTIN

Indications see notes above

Cautions discontinue if symptoms of acute pancreatitis (persistent, severe abdominal pain); **interactions:** Appendix 1 (antidiabetics)

Contra-indications ketoacidosis

Renal impairment reduce dose to 50 mg once daily if eGFR 30–50 mL/minute/1.73 m²; reduce dose to 25 mg once daily if eGFR less than 30 mL/minute/1.73 m²

Pregnancy avoid—toxicity in *animal* studies

Breast-feeding avoid—present in milk in *animal* studies

Side-effects gastro-intestinal disturbances; peripheral oedema; upper respiratory tract infection, nasopharyngitis; pain; *less commonly* dry mouth, anorexia, headache, drowsiness, dizziness, hypoglycaemia, osteoarthritis; *also reported* pancreatitis, rash, cutaneous vasculitis, and Stevens-Johnson syndrome

Dose
• ADULT over 18 years, 100 mg once daily

Note Dose of concomitant sulfonylurea or insulin may need to be reduced

Januvia® (MSD) [PoM]
Tablets, f/c, sitagliptin (as phosphate monohydrate) 25 mg (pink), net price 28-tab pack =£33.26; 50 mg (light beige), 28-tab pack =£33.26; 100 mg (beige), 28-tab pack = £33.26
The *Scottish Medicines Consortium* (p. 4) has advised (June 2010) that *Januvia*® is accepted for restricted use within NHS Scotland as monotherapy, to improve glycaemic control in patients with type 2 diabetes mellitus, for whom both metformin and sulfonylureas are not appropriate

◢With metformin

For prescribing information on metformin, see section 6.1.2.2

Janumet® (MSD) [PoM]
Tablets, f/c, red, sitagliptin 50 mg, metformin hydrochloride 1 g, net price 56-tab pack = £33.26. Label: 21
Dose type 2 diabetes mellitus not controlled by metformin alone *or* by metformin in combination with either a sulfonylurea *or* pioglitazone *or* insulin, ADULT over 18 years, 1 tablet twice daily
Note Dose of concomitant sulfonylurea or insulin may need to be reduced
The *Scottish Medicines Consortium* (p. 4) has advised (July 2008) that *Janumet*® is accepted for restricted use within NHS Scotland for the treatment of type 2 diabetes mellitus when the addition of a sulfonylurea to metformin is not appropriate; it is also accepted for use in NHS Scotland in combination with a sulfonylurea in patients inadequately controlled on maximum tolerated doses of metformin and a sulfonylurea.

▮ VILDAGLIPTIN

Indications see notes above

Cautions monitor liver function (see below); manufacturer advises avoid in severe heart failure—no information available; discontinue if symptoms of acute pancreatitis (persistent, severe abdominal pain); **interactions:** Appendix 1 (antidiabetics)
Liver toxicity Rare reports of liver dysfunction; monitor liver function before treatment and every 3 months for first year and periodically thereafter; advise patients to seek prompt medical attention if symptoms such as nausea, vomiting, abdominal pain, fatigue, and dark urine develop; discontinue if jaundice or other signs of liver dysfunction occur

Contra-indications ketoacidosis

Hepatic impairment avoid; see also Cautions above

Renal impairment reduce dose to 50 mg once daily if eGFR less than 50 mL/minute/1.73 m²

Pregnancy avoid—toxicity in *animal* studies

Breast-feeding avoid—present in milk in *animal* studies

Endocrine system

Side-effects nausea, peripheral oedema, headache, tremor, asthenia, dizziness; *less commonly* constipation, hypoglycaemia, arthralgia; *rarely* hepatic dysfunction (see also Liver Toxicity above); *very rarely* nasopharyngitis, upper respiratory tract infection; *also reported* pancreatitis, exfoliative and bullous skin reactions

Dose
- ADULT over 18 years, monotherapy, 50 mg twice daily
- ADULT over 18 years, dual therapy in combination with metformin or pioglitazone, 50 mg twice daily; dual therapy in combination with a sulfonylurea, 50 mg daily in the morning
- ADULT over 18 years, triple therapy in combination with metformin and a sulfonylurea, 50 mg twice daily
- ADULT over 18 years, in combination with insulin (with or without metformin), 50 mg twice daily

Note Dose of concomitant sulfonylurea or insulin may need to be reduced

Galvus® (Novartis) [PoM]
Tablets, pale yellow, vildagliptin 50 mg, net price 56-tab pack = £31.76

◢**With metformin**
For prescribing information on metformin, see section 6.1.2.2

Eucreas® (Novartis) [PoM]
Eucreas® 50 mg/850 mg tablets, f/c, yellow, vildagliptin 50 mg, metformin hydrochloride 850 mg, net price 60-tab pack = £33.98. Label: 21
Eucreas® 50 mg/1 g tablets, f/c, dark yellow, vildagliptin 50 mg, metformin hydrochloride 1 g, net price 60-tab pack = £33.98. Label: 21
Dose type 2 diabetes mellitus not controlled by metformin alone *or* by metformin in combination with either a sulfonylurea *or* insulin, ADULT over 18 years, 1 *Eucreas®* tablet twice daily (based on patient's current metformin dose)
Note Dose of concomitant sulfonylurea or insulin may need to be reduced
The *Scottish Medicines Consortium* (p. 4) has advised (June 2008) that *Eucreas®* is accepted for restricted use within NHS Scotland for the treatment of type 2 diabetes mellitus in patients unable to achieve adequate glycaemic control with metformin alone or those already treated with vildagliptin and metformin as separate tablets

6.1.3 Diabetic ketoacidosis

The management of diabetic ketoacidosis involves the replacement of fluid and electrolytes and the administration of insulin. Guidelines for the Management of Diabetic Ketoacidosis in Adults, published by the Joint British Diabetes Societies Inpatient Care Group[1], should be followed.

- To restore circulating volume if systolic blood pressure is below 90 mmHg (adjusted for age, sex, and medication as appropriate), give 500 mL **sodium chloride 0.9%** by intravenous infusion over 10–15 minutes; repeat if blood pressure remains below 90 mmHg and seek senior medical advice.

- When blood pressure is over 90 mmHg, **sodium chloride 0.9%** should be given by intravenous infusion at a rate that replaces deficit and provides maintenance; see guideline for suggested regimen.

- Include **potassium chloride** in the fluids unless anuria is suspected; adjust according to plasma-potassium concentration (measure at 60 minutes, 2 hours, and 2 hourly thereafter; measure hourly if outside the normal range).

- Start an intravenous insulin infusion: **soluble insulin** should be diluted (and **mixed thoroughly**) with **sodium chloride 0.9%** intravenous infusion to a concentration of 1 unit/mL; infuse at a fixed rate of 0.1 units/kg/hour.

- Established subcutaneous therapy with long-acting insulin analogues (insulin detemir or insulin glargine) should be continued during treatment of diabetic ketoacidosis.

- Monitor blood-ketone and blood-glucose concentrations hourly and adjust the insulin infusion rate accordingly. Blood-ketone concentration should fall by at least 0.5 mmol/litre/hour and blood-glucose concentration should fall by at least 3 mmol/litre/hour.

- Once blood-glucose concentration falls below 14 mmol/litre, **glucose 10%** should be given by intravenous infusion (into a large vein through a large-gauge needle) at a rate of 125 mL/hour, in addition to the **sodium chloride 0.9%** infusion.

- Continue insulin infusion until blood-ketone concentration is below 0.3 mmol/litre, blood pH is above 7.3 *and* the patient is able to eat and drink; ideally give subcutaneous fast-acting insulin and a meal, and stop the insulin infusion 1 hour later.

For the management of diabetic ketoacidosis in children under 18 years, see *BNF for Children*.

The management of hyperosmolar hyperglycaemic state or hyperosmolar hyperglycaemic nonketotic coma is similar to that of diabetic ketoacidosis, although lower rates of insulin infusion are usually necessary and slower rehydration may be required.

6.1.4 Treatment of hypoglycaemia

Initially glucose 10–20 g is given by mouth either in liquid form or as granulated sugar or sugar lumps. Approximately 10 g of glucose is available from non-diet versions of *Lucozade® Energy Original* 55 mL, *Coca-Cola®* 100 mL, *Ribena® Blackcurrant* 19 mL (to be diluted), 2 teaspoons of sugar, and also from 3 sugar lumps[2]. If necessary this may be repeated in 10–15 minutes. After initial treatment, a snack providing sustained availability of carbohydrate (e.g. a sandwich, fruit, milk, or biscuits) or the next meal, if it is due, can prevent blood-glucose concentration from falling again.

Hypoglycaemia which causes unconsciousness is an emergency. **Glucagon**, a polypeptide hormone produced by the alpha cells of the islets of Langerhans, increases plasma-glucose concentration by mobilising glycogen stored in the liver. In hypoglycaemia, if sugar cannot be given by mouth, glucagon can be given by injection. Carbohydrates should be given as soon as possible to restore liver glycogen; glucagon is not appropriate for chronic hypoglycaemia. Glucagon may

---

1. Available at www.diabetes.org.uk/About_us/What-we-say/Improving-diabetes-healthcare/The-Management-of-Diabetic-Ketoacidosis-in-Adults

2. Proprietary products of quick-acting carbohydrate (e.g. GlucoGel®, Dextrogel®, GSF-Syrup®, Rapilose® gel) are available on prescription for the patient to keep to hand in case of hypoglycaemia.

be issued to close relatives of insulin-treated patients for emergency use in hypoglycaemic attacks. It is often advisable to prescribe on an 'if necessary' basis to hospitalised insulin-treated patients, so that it may be given rapidly by the nurses during an hypoglycaemic emergency. If not effective in 10 minutes intravenous glucose should be given.

Alternatively, 50 mL of **glucose intravenous infusion 20%** (section 9.2.2) may be given intravenously into a large vein through a large-gauge needle; care is required since this concentration is irritant especially if extravasation occurs. Glucose intravenous infusion 10% may also be used but larger volumes are needed. Glucose intravenous infusion 50% is not recommended because of the higher risk of extravasation injury and because administration is difficult. Close monitoring is necessary in the case of an overdose with a long-acting insulin because further administration of glucose may be required. Patients whose hypoglycaemia is caused by an oral antidiabetic drug should be transferred to hospital because the hypoglycaemic effects of these drugs may persist for many hours.

For advice on the emergency management of hypoglycaemia in dental practice, see p. 29.

GLUCAGON

Indications see notes above and under Dose

Cautions see notes above, insulinoma, glucagonoma; ineffective in chronic hypoglycaemia, starvation, and adrenal insufficiency

Contra-indications phaeochromocytoma

Side-effects nausea, vomiting, abdominal pain, hypokalaemia, hypotension, rarely hypersensitivity reactions

Dose
- Insulin-induced hypoglycaemia, by subcutaneous *or* intramuscular injection, ADULT and CHILD over 8 years (or body-weight over 25 kg), 1 mg; CHILD under 8 years (or body-weight under 25 kg), 500 micrograms; if no response within 10 minutes intravenous glucose must be given
- Diagnostic aid, consult product literature
- Beta-blocker poisoning, see p. 39

Note 1 unit of glucagon = 1 mg of glucagon

¹GlucaGen® HypoKit (Novo Nordisk) `PoM`
Injection, powder for reconstitution, glucagon (rys) as hydrochloride with lactose, net price 1-mg vial with prefilled syringe containing water for injection = £11.52

Chronic hypoglycaemia

Diazoxide, administered by mouth, is useful in the management of patients with chronic hypoglycaemia from excess endogenous insulin secretion, either from an islet cell tumour or islet cell hyperplasia. It has no place in the management of acute hypoglycaemia.

DIAZOXIDE

Indications chronic intractable hypoglycaemia

Cautions impaired cardiac or cerebral circulation; heart failure; aortic coarctation; aortic stenosis; arteriovenous shunt; monitor blood pressure; hyper-

uricaemia; during prolonged use monitor white cell and platelet count; **interactions:** Appendix 1 (diazoxide)

Renal impairment dose reduction may be required

Pregnancy use only if essential; alopecia and hypertrichosis reported in neonates with prolonged use; may inhibit uterine activity during labour

Breast-feeding manufacturer advises avoid—no information available

Side-effects nausea, vomiting, abdominal pain, diarrhoea, constipation, ileus, pancreatitis, anorexia (prolonged use), taste disturbance, bleeding, heart failure, hypotension, pulmonary hypertension, dyspnoea, extrapyramidal effects, headache, dizziness, galactorrhoea, hyperglycaemia, decreased libido, leucopenia, thrombocytopenia, anaemia, eosinophilia, hyperosmolar non-ketotic coma, raised serum creatinine and urea, reversible nephritic syndrome, sodium and fluid retention, hyperuricaemia (prolonged use), musculoskeletal pain, visual disturbances, transient cataracts, lacrimation, tinnitus, hypertrichosis, pruritus, dermatitis, lichenoid eruption

Dose
- By mouth, ADULT, initially 5 mg/kg daily in 2–3 divided doses, then adjusted according to response; usual maintenance dose 3–8 mg/kg daily in 2–3 divided doses; CHILD 1 month–18 years see *BNF for Children*

Eudemine® (PharSafer) `PoM`
Tablets, diazoxide 50 mg. Net price 100 = £46.45

6.1.5 Treatment of diabetic nephropathy and neuropathy

Diabetic nephropathy

Regular review of diabetic patients should include an annual test for urinary protein (using *Albustix®*) and serum creatinine measurement. If the urinary protein test is negative, the urine should be tested for microalbuminuria (the earliest sign of nephropathy). If reagent strip tests (*Micral-Test II®* `JHS` or *Microbumintest®* `JHS`) are used and prove positive, the result should be confirmed by laboratory analysis of a urine sample. Provided there are no contra-indications, all diabetic patients with nephropathy causing proteinuria or with established microalbuminuria (at least 3 positive tests) should be treated with an ACE inhibitor (section 2.5.5.1) or an angiotensin-II receptor antagonist (section 2.5.5.2) even if the blood pressure is normal; in any case, to minimise the risk of renal deterioration, blood pressure should be carefully controlled (section 2.5). Patients with diabetic nephropathy are particularly susceptible to developing hyperkalaemia and should not be given an ACE inhibitor together with an angiotensin-II receptor antagonist.

ACE inhibitors can potentiate the hypoglycaemic effect of insulin and oral antidiabetic drugs; this effect is more likely during the first weeks of combined treatment and in patients with renal impairment.

For the treatment of hypertension in diabetes, see section 2.5.

---

1. `PoM` restriction does not apply where administration is for saving life in emergency

6 Endocrine system

Meter (all NHS)	Type of monitoring	Compatible test strips	Test strip net price	Sensitivity range (mmol/litre)	Manufacturer
Mendor Discreet®	Blood glucose	Mendor Discreet®	50-strip pack = £14.75	1.1–33.3	Merck Serono
Microdot®+[1]	Blood glucose	Microdot®+	50-strip pack = £9.99	1.1–29.2	Cambridge Sensors
MyGlucoHealth®	Blood glucose	MyGlucoHealth®	50-strip pack = £15.50	0.6–33.3	Entra Health
Omnitest® 3	Blood glucose	Omnitest® 3	50-strip pack = £9.89	0.6–33.3	B. Braun
One Touch Ultra®[2]	Blood glucose	One Touch Ultra®	50-strip pack = £11.99	1.1–33.3	LifeScan
One Touch Ultra 2®[1]	Blood glucose	One Touch Ultra®	50-strip pack = £11.99	1.1–33.3	LifeScan
One Touch UltraEasy®[1]	Blood glucose	One Touch Ultra®	50-strip pack = £11.99	1.1–33.3	LifeScan
One Touch UltraSmart®[1]	Blood glucose	One Touch Ultra®	50-strip pack = £11.99	1.1–33.3	LifeScan
One Touch® VerioPro[1]	Blood glucose	One Touch® Verio	50-strip pack = £15.12	1.1–33.3	LifeScan
One Touch® Vita[1]	Blood glucose	One Touch® Vita	50-strip pack = £15.07	1.1–33.3	LifeScan
SD CodeFree®	Blood glucose	SD CodeFree®	50-strip pack = £6.99	0.6–33.3	SD Biosensor
Sensocard Plus®[2]	Blood glucose	Sensocard®	50-strip pack= £16.30	1.1–33.3	BBI Healthcare
SuperCheck2®[1]	Blood glucose	SuperCheck2®	50-strip pack = £8.49	1.1–33.3	Apollo Medical
TRUEone®	Blood glucose	All-in-one test strips and meter	50-strip pack with meter = £14.99	1.1–33.3	Nipro Diagnostics
TRUEresult®[1]	Blood glucose	TRUEresult®	50-strip pack = £14.99	1.1–33.3	Nipro Diagnostics
TRUEresult twist®[1]	Blood glucose	TRUEresult®	50-strip pack = £14.99	1.1–33.3	Nipro Diagnostics
TRUEtrack®	Blood glucose	TRUEtrack®	50-strip pack = £14.99	1.1–33.3	Nipro Diagnostics
TRUEyou mini®	Blood glucose	TRUEyou®	50-strip pack = £9.92	1.1–33.3	Nipro Diagnostics
WaveSense JAZZ®[1]	Blood glucose	WaveSense JAZZ®	50-strip pack = £9.87	1.1–33.3	AgaMatrix

1. Free of charge from diabetes healthcare professionals
2. Meter no longer available

Patients using multiple injection regimens should understand how to adjust their insulin dose according to their carbohydrate intake. With fixed-dose insulin regimens, the carbohydrate intake needs to be regulated, and should be distributed throughout the day to match the insulin regimen.

Self-monitoring of blood-glucose concentration is appropriate for patients with type 2 diabetes:

- who are treated with insulin;
- who are treated with oral hypoglycaemic drugs e.g. sulfonylureas, to provide information on hypoglycaemia;
- to monitor changes in blood-glucose concentration resulting from changes in lifestyle or medication, and during intercurrent illness;
- to ensure safe blood-glucose concentration during activities, including driving.

Note In the UK blood-glucose concentration is expressed in mmol/litre and Diabetes UK advises that these units should be used for self-monitoring of blood glucose. In other European countries units of mg/100 mL (or mg/dL) are commonly used.
It is advisable to check that the meter is pre-set in the correct units.

If the patient is unwell and diabetic ketoacidosis is suspected, blood **ketones** should be measured according to local guidelines (section 6.1.3). Patients and their carers should be trained in the use of blood ketone monitoring systems and to take appropriate action on the results obtained, including when to seek medical attention.

Urinalysis

Reagent strips are available for measuring for glucose in the urine. Tests for ketones by patients are rarely required unless they become unwell—see also Blood Monitoring, p. 488.

Microalbuminuria can be detected with *Micral-Test II*® JHS but this should be followed by confirmation in the laboratory, since false positive results are common.

◢**Glucose**

Diabur-Test 5000® (Roche Diagnostics)
Reagent strips, for detection of glucose in urine. Net price 50-strip pack = £2.87

Diastix® (Bayer Diabetes Care)
Reagent strips, for detection of glucose in urine. Net price 50-strip pack = £2.78

Medi-Test® **Glucose** (BHR)
Reagent strips, for detection of glucose in urine. Net price 50-strip pack = £2.33

Mission® **Glucose** (Spirit)
Reagent strips, for detection of glucose in urine. Net price 50-strip pack = £2.29

◢**Ketones**

Ketostix® (Bayer Diabetes Care)
Reagent strips, for detection of ketones in urine. Net price 50-strip pack = £3.03

Mission® **Ketone** (Spirit)
Reagent strips, for detection of ketones in urine. Net price 50-strip pack = £2.50

◢**Protein**

Albustix® (Siemens)
Reagent strips, for detection of protein in urine. Net price 50-strip pack = £4.10

Medi-Test® **Protein 2** (BHR)
Reagent strips, for detection of protein in urine. Net price 50-strip pack = £3.27

◢**Other reagent strips available for urinalysis include:**

Combur-3 Test® JHS (glucose and protein—Roche Diagnostics)

Clinitek Microalbumin® JHS (albumin and creatinine—Siemens)

Ketodiastix® JHS (glucose and ketones—Bayer Diagnostics)

Medi-Test Combi 2® JHS (glucose and protein—BHR)

Micral-Test II® JHS (albumin—Roche Diagnostics)

Microalbustix® JHS (albumin and creatinine—Siemens)

Uristix® JHS (glucose and protein—Siemens)

Oral glucose tolerance test

The oral glucose tolerance test is used mainly for diagnosis of impaired glucose tolerance; it is not recommended or necessary for routine diagnostic use when severe symptoms of hyperglycaemia are present. In patients who have less severe symptoms and blood glucose levels that do not establish or exclude diabetes (e.g. impaired fasting glycaemia), an oral glucose tolerance test may be required. It is also used to establish the presence of gestational diabetes. The oral glucose tolerance test generally involves giving anhydrous glucose 75 g (equivalent to Glucose BP 82.5 g) by mouth to the fasting patient, and measuring blood-glucose concentrations at intervals.

The appropriate amount of glucose should be given with 200–300 mL fluid. Anhydrous glucose 75 g may alternatively be given as 113 mL *Polycal*® with extra fluid to administer a total volume of 200–300 mL, or as *Rapilose*® OGTT oral solution.

6.2 Thyroid and antithyroid drugs

6.2.1 Thyroid hormones
6.2.2 Antithyroid drugs

6.2.1 Thyroid hormones

Thyroid hormones are used in hypothyroidism (myxoedema), and also in diffuse non-toxic goitre, Hashimoto's thyroiditis (lymphadenoid goitre), and thyroid carcinoma. Neonatal hypothyroidism requires prompt treatment for normal development. **Levothyroxine sodium** (thyroxine sodium) is the treatment of choice for *maintenance* therapy.

In infants and children with congenital hypothyroidism and juvenile myxoedema, the dose of levothyroxine should be titrated according to clinical response, growth assessment, and measurements of plasma thyroxine and thyroid-stimulating hormone. See *BNF for Children* (section 6.2.1) for suitable dosage regimens.

Liothyronine sodium has a similar action to levothyroxine but is more rapidly metabolised and has a more rapid effect; 20–25 micrograms is equivalent to 100 micrograms of levothyroxine. Its effects develop after a few hours and disappear within 24 to 48 hours of discontinuing treatment. It may be used in *severe hypothyroid states* when a rapid response is desired.

Liothyronine by intravenous injection is the treatment of choice in *hypothyroid coma*. Adjunctive therapy includes intravenous fluids, hydrocortisone, and treatment of infection; assisted ventilation is often required.

LEVOTHYROXINE SODIUM
(Thyroxine sodium)

Indications hypothyroidism; see also notes above

Cautions panhypopituitarism or predisposition to adrenal insufficiency (initiate corticosteroid therapy before starting levothyroxine), elderly, cardiovascular disorders (including hypertension, myocardial insufficiency or myocardial infarction, see Initial Dosage below), long-standing hypothyroidism, diabetes insipidus, diabetes mellitus (dose of antidiabetic drugs including insulin may need to be increased); **interactions:** Appendix 1 (thyroid hormones)
Initial dosage Baseline ECG is valuable because changes induced by hypothyroidism can be confused with ischaemia. If metabolism increases too rapidly (causing diarrhoea, nervousness, rapid pulse, insomnia, tremors and sometimes anginal pain where there is latent myocardial ischaemia), reduce dose or withhold for 1–2 days and start again at a lower dose

Contra-indications thyrotoxicosis

Pregnancy levothyroxine may cross the placenta; excessive or insufficient maternal thyroid hormones can be detrimental to fetus; levothyroxine requirement may increase during pregnancy; assess maternal thyroid function before conception (if possible), at diagnosis of pregnancy, at antenatal booking, during

Endocrine system

both the second and third trimesters, and after delivery (more frequent monitoring required on initiation or adjustment of levothyroxine)

Breast-feeding   amount too small to affect tests for neonatal hypothyroidism

Side-effects   usually at excessive dosage (see Initial Dosage above) include diarrhoea, vomiting, anginal pain, arrhythmias, palpitation, tachycardia, tremor, restlessness, excitability, insomnia; headache, flushing, sweating, fever, heat intolerance, weight-loss, muscle cramp, and muscular weakness; transient hair loss in children; hypersensitivity reactions including rash, pruritus and oedema also reported

Dose

- ADULT over 18 years, initially 50–100 micrograms once daily, preferably taken at least 30 minutes before breakfast, caffeine-containing liquids (e.g. coffee, tea), or other medication, adjusted in steps of 25–50 micrograms every 3–4 weeks according to response (usual maintenance dose 100–200 micrograms once daily); in cardiac disease, severe hypothyroidism, and patients over 50 years, initially 25 micrograms once daily, adjusted in steps of 25 micrograms every 4 weeks according to response (usual maintenance dose 50–200 micrograms once daily); CHILD under 18 years see *BNF for Children* (section 6.2.1)
- Congenital hypothyroidism and juvenile myxoedema, see *BNF for Children* (section 6.2.1)

Levothyroxine (Non-proprietary) PoM

Tablets, levothyroxine sodium 25 micrograms, net price 28-tab pack = £2.82; 50 micrograms, 28-tab pack = £1.97; 100 micrograms, 28-tab pack = £1.98
Brands include *Eltroxin*®

Oral solution, levothyroxine sodium 25 micrograms/5 mL, net price 100 mL = £69.25; 50 micrograms/5 mL, 100 mL = £77.22; 100 micrograms/5 mL, 100 mL = £110.14

LIOTHYRONINE SODIUM
(L-Tri-iodothyronine sodium)

Indications   see notes above

Cautions   see under Levothyroxine Sodium; **interactions:** Appendix 1 (thyroid hormones)

Contra-indications   see under Levothyroxine Sodium

Pregnancy   does not cross the placenta in significant amounts; excessive or insufficient maternal thyroid hormones can be detrimental to fetus; liothyronine requirement may increase during pregnancy; assess maternal thyroid function before conception (if possible), at diagnosis of pregnancy, at antenatal booking, during both the second and third trimesters, and after delivery (more frequent monitoring required on initiation or adjustment of liothyronine)

Breast-feeding   amount too small to affect tests for neonatal hypothyroidism

Side-effects   see under Levothyroxine Sodium

Dose

- By mouth, initially 10–20 micrograms daily gradually increased to 60 micrograms daily in 2–3 divided doses; ELDERLY smaller initial doses; CHILD, adult dose reduced in proportion to body-weight
- By slow intravenous injection, hypothyroid coma, 5–20 micrograms repeated every 12 hours or as often as every 4 hours if necessary; *alternatively* initially 50 micrograms then 25 micrograms every 8 hours reducing to 25 micrograms twice daily

Liothyronine sodium (Non-proprietary) PoM

Tablets, scored, liothyronine sodium 20 micrograms, net price 28-tab pack = £102.30

Important Patients switched to a different brand should be monitored (particularly if pregnant or if heart disease present) as brands without a UK licence may not be bioequivalent and dose adjustment may be necessary; pregnant women or those with heart disease should undergo an early review of thyroid status, and other patients should have thyroid function assessed if experiencing a significant change in symptoms. If liothyronine is continued long-term, thyroid function tests should be repeated 1–2 months after any change in brand.

Injection, powder for reconstitution, liothyronine sodium, net price 20-microgram vial = £22.50

6.2.2 Antithyroid drugs

Antithyroid drugs are used for hyperthyroidism either to prepare patients for thyroidectomy or for long-term management. In the UK **carbimazole** is the most commonly used drug. **Propylthiouracil** should be reserved for patients who are intolerant of carbimazole or for those who experience sensitivity reactions to carbimazole (sensitivity is not necessarily displayed to both drugs), and for whom other treatments are inappropriate. Both drugs act primarily by interfering with the synthesis of thyroid hormones.

> **Neutropenia and agranulocytosis**
> Doctors are reminded of the importance of recognising bone marrow suppression induced by carbimazole and the need to stop treatment promptly.
> 1. Patient should be asked to report symptoms and signs suggestive of infection, especially sore throat.
> 2. A white blood cell count should be performed if there is any clinical evidence of infection.
> 3. Carbimazole should be stopped promptly if there is clinical or laboratory evidence of neutropenia.

Carbimazole is given in a dose of 15 to 40 mg daily; higher doses should be prescribed under specialist supervision only. This dose is continued until the patient becomes euthyroid, usually after 4 to 8 weeks and the dose is then gradually reduced to a maintenance dose of 5 to 15 mg. Therapy is usually given for 12 to 18 months. Treatment in children should be undertaken by a specialist, see *BNF for Children*. Rashes and pruritus are common but they can be treated with antihistamines without discontinuing therapy; alternatively propylthiouracil can be substituted. All patients should be advised to report any sore throat immediately because of the rare complication of agranulocytosis (see Neutropenia and Agranulocytosis, above).

Propylthiouracil is given in a dose of 200 to 400 mg daily in divided doses in adults and this dose is maintained until the patient becomes euthyroid; the dose may then be gradually reduced to a maintenance dose of 50 to 150 mg daily in divided doses.

Over-treatment with antithyroid drugs can result in the rapid development of hypothyroidism and should be avoided particularly during pregnancy because it can cause fetal goitre.

A combination of carbimazole, 40 to 60 mg daily with levothyroxine, 50 to 150 micrograms daily, may be used in a *blocking-replacement regimen*; therapy is usually

Endocrine system

6

given for 18 months. The blocking-replacement regimen is **not** suitable during pregnancy.

Iodine has been used as an adjunct to antithyroid drugs for 10 to 14 days before partial thyroidectomy; however, there is little evidence of a beneficial effect. Iodine should not be used for long-term treatment because its antithyroid action tends to diminish.

Radioactive sodium iodide (^{131}I) solution is used increasingly for the treatment of thyrotoxicosis at all ages, particularly where medical therapy or compliance is a problem, in patients with cardiac disease, and in patients who relapse after thyroidectomy.

Propranolol is useful for rapid relief of thyrotoxic symptoms and may be used in conjunction with anti-thyroid drugs or as an adjunct to radioactive iodine. Beta-blockers are also useful in neonatal thyrotoxicosis and in supraventricular arrhythmias due to hyper-thyroidism. Propranolol has been used in conjunction with iodine to prepare mildly thyrotoxic patients for surgery but it is preferable to make the patient euthyroid with carbimazole. Laboratory tests of thyroid function are not altered by beta-blockers. Most experience in treating thyrotoxicosis has been gained with propranolol but **nadolol** is also used. For doses and preparations of beta-blockers see section 2.4.

Thyrotoxic crisis ('thyroid storm') requires emergency treatment with intravenous administration of fluids, propranolol (5 mg) and hydrocortisone (100 mg every 6 hours, as sodium succinate), as well as oral iodine solution and carbimazole or propylthiouracil which may need to be administered by nasogastric tube.

Pregnancy Radioactive iodine therapy is contra-indicated during pregnancy. Propylthiouracil and carbimazole can be given but the blocking-replacement regimen (see above) is **not** suitable. Rarely, carbimazole has been associated with congenital defects, including aplasia cutis of the neonate, therefore propylthiouracil remains the drug of choice during the first trimester of pregnancy. In the second trimester, consider switching to carbimazole because of the potential risk of hepatotoxicity with propylthiouracil. Both propylthiouracil and carbimazole cross the placenta and in high doses may cause fetal goitre and hypothyroidism—the lowest dose that will control the hyperthyroid state should be used (requirements in Graves' disease tend to fall during pregnancy).

Breast-feeding Carbimazole and propylthiouracil are present in breast milk but this does not preclude breast-feeding as long as neonatal development is closely monitored and the lowest effective dose is used.

CARBIMAZOLE

Indications hyperthyroidism

Contra-indications severe blood disorders

Hepatic impairment use with caution in mild to moderate impairment; avoid in severe impairment

Pregnancy neonatal goitre and hypothyroidism; has been associated with congenital defects including aplasia cutis of the neonate; see also notes above

Breast-feeding amount in milk may be sufficient to affect neonatal thyroid function therefore lowest effective dose should be used; see also notes above

Side-effects nausea, mild gastro-intestinal disturbances, taste disturbance, headache, fever, malaise, rash, pruritus, arthralgia; *rarely* myopathy, alopecia,

bone marrow suppression (including pancytopenia and agranulocytosis, see Neutropenia and Agranulocytosis above), and jaundice

Counselling Warn patient to tell doctor **immediately** if sore throat, mouth ulcers, bruising, fever, malaise, or non-specific illness develops

Dose
- See notes above

Carbimazole (Non-proprietary) [PoM]

Tablets, carbimazole 5 mg, net price 100-tab pack = £64.79; 20 mg, 100-tab pack = £160.09. Counselling, blood disorder symptoms

IODINE AND IODIDE

Indications thyrotoxicosis (pre-operative)

Cautions children; not for long-term treatment

Pregnancy neonatal goitre and hypothyroidism; see also notes above

Breast-feeding stop breast-feeding; danger of neonatal hypothyroidism or goitre; appears to be concentrated in milk; see also notes above

Side-effects hypersensitivity reactions including coryza-like symptoms, headache, lacrimation, conjunctivitis, pain in salivary glands, laryngitis, bronchitis, rashes; on prolonged treatment depression, insomnia, impotence; goitre in infants of mothers taking iodides

Dose
- See under preparation

Aqueous Iodine Oral Solution

Oral solution, iodine 5%, potassium iodide 10% in purified water, freshly boiled and cooled, total iodine 130 mg/mL, net price 500 mL = £9.57. Label: 27

Dose 0.1–0.3 mL 3 times daily well diluted with milk or water

PROPYLTHIOURACIL

Indications hyperthyroidism

Cautions monitor for hepatotoxicity

Hepatotoxicity Severe hepatic reactions have been reported, including fatal cases and cases requiring liver transplant—discontinue if significant liver-enzyme abnormalities develop

Counselling Patients should be told how to recognise signs of liver disorder and advised to seek prompt medical attention if symptoms such as anorexia, nausea, vomiting, fatigue, abdominal pain, jaundice, dark urine, or pruritus develop

Hepatic impairment reduce dose (see also Hepatotoxicity above)

Renal impairment use three-quarters normal dose if eGFR 10–50 mL/minute/1.73 m^2; use half normal dose if eGFR less than 10 mL/minute/1.73 m^2

Pregnancy neonatal goitre and hypothyroidism; see also notes above

Breast-feeding monitor infant's thyroid status but amount in milk probably too small to affect infant; high doses may affect neonatal thyroid function; see also notes above

Side-effects see under Carbimazole; leucopenia; rarely cutaneous vasculitis, thrombocytopenia, aplastic anaemia, hypoprothrombinaemia, hepatic disorders (including hepatitis, hepatic failure, encephalopathy, hepatic necrosis; see also Hepatotoxicity above), nephritis, lupus erythematous-like syndromes

6

Endocrine system

Dose
- See notes above

Propylthiouracil (Non-proprietary) [PoM]
  Tablets, propylthiouracil 50 mg, net price 56-tab pack = £60.00, 100-tab pack = £87.52

6.3 Corticosteroids

6.3.1 Replacement therapy
6.3.2 Glucocorticoid therapy

6.3.1 Replacement therapy

The adrenal cortex normally secretes hydrocortisone (cortisol) which has glucocorticoid activity and weak mineralocorticoid activity. It also secretes the mineralocorticoid aldosterone.

In deficiency states, physiological replacement is best achieved with a combination of **hydrocortisone** (section 6.3.2) and the mineralocorticoid **fludrocortisone**; hydrocortisone alone does not usually provide sufficient mineralocorticoid activity for complete replacement.

In *Addison's disease* or following adrenalectomy, **hydrocortisone** 20 to 30 mg daily by mouth is usually required. This is given in 2 doses, the larger in the morning and the smaller in the evening, mimicking the normal diurnal rhythm of cortisol secretion. The optimum daily dose is determined on the basis of clinical response. Glucocorticoid therapy is supplemented by fludrocortisone 50 to 300 micrograms daily.

In *acute adrenocortical insufficiency*, **hydrocortisone** is given intravenously (preferably as sodium succinate) in doses of 100 mg every 6 to 8 hours in sodium chloride intravenous infusion 0.9%.

In *hypopituitarism* glucocorticoids should be given as in adrenocortical insufficiency, but since production of aldosterone is also regulated by the renin-angiotensin system a mineralocorticoid is not usually required. Additional replacement therapy with levothyroxine (section 6.2.1) and sex hormones (section 6.4) should be given as indicated by the pattern of hormone deficiency.

FLUDROCORTISONE ACETATE

Indications mineralocorticoid replacement in adrenocortical insufficiency
Cautions section 6.3.2; **interactions:** Appendix 1 (corticosteroids)
Contra-indications section 6.3.2
Hepatic impairment section 6.3.2
Renal impairment section 6.3.2
Pregnancy section 6.3.2
Breast-feeding section 6.3.2
Side-effects section 6.3.2
Dose
- 50–300 micrograms daily; CHILD 1 month–18 years see *BNF for Children*

Florinef® (Squibb) [PoM]
  Tablets, scored, fludrocortisone acetate 100 micrograms. Net price 100-tab pack = £5.05. Label: 10, steroid card

6.3.2 Glucocorticoid therapy

In comparing the relative potencies of corticosteroids in terms of their anti-inflammatory (glucocorticoid) effects it should be borne in mind that high glucocorticoid activity in itself is of no advantage unless it is accompanied by relatively low mineralocorticoid activity (see Disadvantages of Corticosteroids below). The mineralocorticoid activity of **fludrocortisone** (section 6.3.1) is so high that its anti-inflammatory activity is of no clinical relevance. The table below shows equivalent anti-inflammatory doses.

Equivalent anti-inflammatory doses of corticosteroids

This table takes no account of mineralocorticoid effects, nor does it take account of variations in duration of action

Prednisolone 5 mg	
≡	Betamethasone 750 micrograms
≡	Deflazacort 6 mg
≡	Dexamethasone 750 micrograms
≡	Hydrocortisone 20 mg
≡	Methylprednisolone 4 mg
≡	Prednisone 5 mg
≡	Triamcinolone 4 mg

The relatively high mineralocorticoid activity of **hydrocortisone**, and the resulting fluid retention, makes it unsuitable for disease suppression on a long-term basis. However, hydrocortisone can be used for adrenal replacement therapy (section 6.3.1). Hydrocortisone is used on a short-term basis by intravenous injection for the emergency management of some conditions. The relatively moderate anti-inflammatory potency of hydrocortisone also makes it a useful topical corticosteroid for the management of inflammatory skin conditions because side-effects (both topical and systemic) are less marked (section 13.4).

Prednisolone and **prednisone** have predominantly glucocorticoid activity. Prednisolone is the corticosteroid most commonly used by mouth for long-term disease suppression.

Betamethasone and **dexamethasone** have very high glucocorticoid activity in conjunction with insignificant mineralocorticoid activity. This makes them particularly suitable for high-dose therapy in conditions where fluid retention would be a disadvantage.

Betamethasone and dexamethasone also have a long duration of action and this, coupled with their lack of mineralocorticoid action makes them particularly suitable for conditions which require suppression of corticotropin (corticotrophin) secretion (e.g. congenital adrenal hyperplasia). Some esters of betamethasone and of **beclometasone** (beclomethasone) exert a considerably more marked topical effect (e.g. on the skin or the lungs) than when given by mouth; use is made of this to obtain topical effects whilst minimising systemic side-effects (e.g. for skin applications and asthma inhalations).

Deflazacort has a high glucocorticoid activity; it is derived from prednisolone.

Use of corticosteroids

Dosages of corticosteroids vary widely in different diseases and in different patients. If the use of a corticosteroid can save or prolong life, as in exfoliative dermatitis, pemphigus, acute leukaemia or acute transplant rejection, high doses may need to be given, because the complications of therapy are likely to be less serious than the effects of the disease itself.

When long-term corticosteroid therapy is used in some chronic diseases, the adverse effects of treatment may become greater than the disabilities caused by the disease. To minimise side-effects the maintenance dose should be kept as low as possible.

When potentially less harmful measures are ineffective corticosteroids are used topically for the treatment of inflammatory conditions of the skin (section 13.4). Corticosteroids should be avoided or used only under specialist supervision in psoriasis (section 13.5).

Corticosteroids are used both topically (by rectum) and systemically (by mouth or intravenously) in the management of ulcerative colitis and Crohn's disease (section 1.5). They are also included in locally applied creams for haemorrhoids (section 1.7.2).

Use can be made of the mineralocorticoid activity of fludrocortisone to treat postural hypotension in autonomic neuropathy (section 6.1.5).

High-dose corticosteroids should be avoided for the management of septic shock. However, there is evidence that administration of lower doses of hydrocortisone (50 mg intravenously every 6 hours) and fludrocortisone (50 micrograms daily by mouth) is of benefit in adrenocortical insufficiency resulting from septic shock.

Dexamethasone and betamethasone have little if any mineralocorticoid action and their long duration of action makes them particularly suitable for suppressing corticotropin secretion in congenital adrenal hyperplasia where the dose should be tailored to clinical response and by measurement of adrenal androgens and 17-hydroxyprogesterone. In common with all glucocorticoids their suppressive action on the hypothalamic-pituitary-adrenal axis is greatest and most prolonged when they are given at night. In most individuals a single dose of 1 mg of dexamethasone at night, is sufficient to inhibit corticotropin secretion for 24 hours. This is the basis of the 'overnight dexamethasone suppression test' for diagnosing Cushing's syndrome.

Betamethasone and dexamethasone are also appropriate for conditions where water retention would be a disadvantage.

A corticosteroid may be used in the management of raised intracranial pressure or cerebral oedema that occurs as a result of malignancy (see also Prescribing in Palliative Care p.); high doses of betamethasone or dexamethasone are generally used. However, a corticosteroid should **not** be used for the management of head injury or stroke because it is unlikely to be of benefit and may even be harmful.

In acute hypersensitivity reactions such as angioedema of the upper respiratory tract and anaphylaxis, corticosteroids are indicated as an adjunct to emergency treatment with adrenaline (epinephrine) (section 3.4.3). In such cases hydrocortisone (as sodium succinate) by intravenous injection in a dose of 100 to 300 mg may be required.

Corticosteroids are preferably used by inhalation in the management of asthma (section 3.2) but systemic therapy in association with bronchodilators is required for the emergency treatment of severe acute asthma (section 3.1.1).

Corticosteroids may also be useful in conditions such as autoimmune hepatitis, rheumatoid arthritis and sarcoidosis; they may also lead to remissions of acquired haemolytic anaemia (section 9.1.3), and some cases of the nephrotic syndrome (particularly in children) and thrombocytopenic purpura (section 9.1.4).

Corticosteroids can improve the prognosis of serious conditions such as systemic lupus erythematosus, temporal arteritis, and polyarteritis nodosa; the effects of the disease process may be suppressed and symptoms relieved, but the underlying condition is not cured, although it may ultimately remit. It is usual to begin therapy in these conditions at fairly high dose, such as 40 to 60 mg prednisolone daily, and then to reduce the dose to the lowest commensurate with disease control.

For other references to the use of corticosteroids see Prescribing in Palliative Care, section 8.2.2 (immunosuppression), section 10.1.2 (rheumatic diseases), section 11.4 (eye), section 12.1.1 (otitis externa), section 12.2.1 (allergic rhinitis), and section 12.3.1 (aphthous ulcers).

Administration

Whenever possible *local treatment* with creams, intra-articular injections, inhalations, eye-drops, or enemas should be used in preference to *systemic treatment*. The suppressive action of a corticosteroid on cortisol secretion is least when it is given as a single dose in the morning. In an attempt to reduce pituitary-adrenal suppression further, the total dose for two days can sometimes be taken as a single dose on alternate days; alternate-day administration has not been very successful in the management of asthma (section 3.2). Pituitary-adrenal suppression can also be reduced by means of intermittent therapy with short courses. In some conditions it may be possible to reduce the dose of corticosteroid by adding a small dose of an immunosuppressive drug (section 8.2.1).

Cautions and contra-indications of corticosteroids

Adrenal suppression

During prolonged therapy with corticosteroids, adrenal atrophy develops and can persist for years after stopping. Abrupt withdrawal after a prolonged period can lead to acute adrenal insufficiency, hypotension or death (see Withdrawal of Corticosteroids, below). Withdrawal can also be associated with fever, myalgia, arthralgia, rhinitis, conjunctivitis, painful itchy skin nodules and weight loss.

To compensate for a diminished adrenocortical response caused by prolonged corticosteroid treatment, any significant intercurrent illness, trauma, or surgical procedure requires a temporary increase in corticosteroid dose, or if already stopped, a temporary reintroduction of corticosteroid treatment. To avoid a precipitous fall in blood pressure during anaesthesia or in the immediate postoperative period, anaesthetists **must** know whether a patient is taking or has been taking a corticosteroid. A suitable regimen for corticosteroid replacement, in patients who have taken more than 10 mg prednisolone daily (or equivalent) within 3 months of surgery, is:

- *Minor surgery under general anaesthesia*—usual oral corticosteroid dose on the morning of surgery or hydrocortisone 25–50 mg (usually the sodium succinate) intravenously at induction; the usual oral corticosteroid dose is recommenced after surgery

- *Moderate or major surgery*—usual oral corticosteroid dose on the morning of surgery and hydrocortisone 25–50 mg intravenously at induction, followed by hydrocortisone 25–50 mg 3 times a day by intravenous injection for 24 hours after moderate surgery or for 48–72 hours after major surgery; the usual pre-operative oral corticosteroid dose is recommenced on stopping hydrocortisone injections

Patients on long-term corticosteroid treatment should carry a Steroid Treatment Card (see p. 498) which gives guidance on minimising risk and provides details of prescriber, drug, dosage and duration of treatment.

Infections

Prolonged courses of corticosteroids increase susceptibility to infections and severity of infections; clinical presentation of infections may also be atypical. Serious infections e.g. *septicaemia* and *tuberculosis* may reach an advanced stage before being recognised, and *amoebiasis* or *strongyloidiasis* may be activated or exacerbated (exclude before initiating a corticosteroid in those at risk or with suggestive symptoms). Fungal or viral *ocular infections* may also be exacerbated (see also section 11.4.1).

Chickenpox   Unless they have had chickenpox, patients receiving oral or parenteral corticosteroids for purposes other than replacement should be regarded as being *at risk of severe chickenpox* (see Steroid Treatment Card). Manifestations of fulminant illness include pneumonia, hepatitis and disseminated intravascular coagulation; rash is not necessarily a prominent feature.

Passive immunisation with varicella–zoster immunoglobulin (section 14.5.2) is needed for exposed non-immune patients receiving systemic corticosteroids or for those who have used them within the previous 3 months. Confirmed chickenpox warrants specialist care and urgent treatment (section 5.3.2.1). Corticosteroids should not be stopped and dosage may need to be increased.

Topical, inhaled or rectal corticosteroids are less likely to be associated with an increased risk of severe chickenpox.

Measles   Patients taking corticosteroids should be advised to take particular care to avoid exposure to measles and to seek immediate medical advice if exposure occurs. Prophylaxis with intramuscular normal immunoglobulin (section 14.5.1) may be needed.

Withdrawal of corticosteroids

The magnitude and speed of dose reduction in corticosteroid withdrawal should be determined on a case-by-case basis, taking into consideration the underlying condition that is being treated, and individual patient factors such as the likelihood of relapse and the duration of corticosteroid treatment. *Gradual* withdrawal of systemic corticosteroids should be considered in those whose disease is unlikely to relapse and have:

- received more than 40 mg prednisolone (or equivalent) daily for more than 1 week;

- been given repeat doses in the evening;

- received more than 3 weeks' treatment;

- recently received repeated courses (particularly if taken for longer than 3 weeks);

- taken a short course within 1 year of stopping long-term therapy;

- other possible causes of adrenal suppression.

Systemic corticosteroids may be stopped abruptly in those whose disease is unlikely to relapse *and* who have received treatment for 3 weeks or less *and* who are not included in the patient groups described above.

During corticosteroid withdrawal the dose may be reduced rapidly down to physiological doses (equivalent to prednisolone 7.5 mg daily) and then reduced more slowly. Assessment of the disease may be needed during withdrawal to ensure that relapse does not occur.

STEROID TREATMENT CARD

I am a patient on STEROID treatment which must not be stopped suddenly

- If you have been taking this medicine for more than three weeks, the dose should be reduced gradually when you stop taking steroids unless your doctor says otherwise.

- Read the patient information leaflet given with the medicine.

- Always carry this card with you and show it to anyone who treats you (for example a doctor, nurse, pharmacist or dentist). For one year after you stop the treatment, you must mention that you have taken steroids.

- If you become ill, or if you come into contact with anyone who has an infectious disease, consult your doctor promptly. If you have never had chickenpox, you should avoid close contact with people who have chickenpox or shingles. If you do come into contact with chickenpox, see your doctor urgently.

- Make sure that the information on the card is kept up to date.

Psychiatric reactions

Systemic corticosteroids, particularly in high doses, are linked to psychiatric reactions including euphoria, nightmares, insomnia, irritability, mood lability, suicidal thoughts, psychotic reactions, and behavioural disturbances. A serious paranoid state or depression with risk of suicide can be induced, particularly in patients with a history of mental disorder. These reactions frequently subside on reducing the dose or discontinuing the corticosteroid but they may also require specific management. Patients should be advised to seek medical advice if psychiatric symptoms (especially depression and suicidal thoughts) occur and they should also be alert to the rare possibility of such reactions during withdrawal of corticosteroid treatment.

Systemic corticosteroids should be prescribed with care in those predisposed to psychiatric reactions, including those who have previously suffered corticosteroid-induced psychosis, or who have a personal or family history of psychiatric disorders.

Advice to patients
A patient information leaflet should be supplied to every patient when a systemic corticosteroid is prescribed. Patients should especially be advised of the following (for details, see Infections, Adrenal Suppression, Psychiatric Reactions, and Withdrawal of Corticosteroids above):

- **Immunosuppression** Prolonged courses of corticosteroids can increase susceptibility to infection and serious infections can go unrecognised. Unless already immune, patients are at risk of severe **chickenpox** and should avoid close contact with people who have chickenpox or shingles. Similarly, precautions should also be taken against contracting **measles**;

- **Adrenal suppression** If the corticosteroid is given for longer than 3 weeks, treatment must not be stopped abruptly. Adrenal suppression can last for a year or more after stopping treatment and the patient must mention the course of corticosteroid when receiving treatment for any illness or injury;

- **Mood and behaviour changes** Corticosteroid treatment, especially with high doses, can alter mood and behaviour early in treatment—the patient can become confused, irritable and suffer from delusion and suicidal thoughts. These effects can also occur when corticosteroid treatment is being withdrawn. Medical advice should be sought if worrying psychological changes occur;

- **Other serious effects** Serious gastro-intestinal, musculoskeletal, and ophthalmic effects which require medical help can also occur; for details see Side-effects of Corticosteroids, p. 498.

Steroid treatment cards
Steroid treatment cards (see p. 498) should be issued where appropriate, and are available for purchase from:

3M Security Print and Systems Limited
Gorse Street, Chadderton
Oldham, OL9 9QH
Tel: 0845 610 1112

GP practices can obtain supplies through their Local Area Team Stores.

NHS Trusts can order supplies from www.nhsforms. co.uk or by emailing nhsforms@mmm.com.

In **Scotland**, steroid treatment cards can be obtained from APS Group Scotland by emailing stockorders. dppas@theapsgroup.com or by fax on 0131 629 9967.

Other cautions and contra-indications

Other cautions include: children and adolescents (growth restriction possibly irreversible), elderly (close supervision required particularly on long-term treatment); frequent monitoring required if history of tuberculosis (or X-ray changes), hypertension, recent myocardial infarction (rupture reported), congestive heart failure, diabetes mellitus including family history, osteoporosis (post-menopausal women at special risk), glaucoma (including family history), ocular herpes simplex—risk of corneal perforation, severe affective disorders (particularly if history of steroid-induced psychosis—see also Psychiatric Reactions, above), epilepsy, peptic ulcer, hypothyroidism, history of steroid myopathy, ulcerative colitis, diverticulitis, recent intestinal anastomoses, thromboembolic disorders; myasthenia gravis; **interactions:** Appendix 1 (corticosteroids).

Other contra-indications include: systemic infection (unless specific therapy given); avoid live virus vaccines in those receiving immunosuppressive doses (serum antibody response diminished).

Hepatic impairment

When corticosteroids are administered orally or parenterally, the plasma-drug concentration may be increased in patients with hepatic impairment. Corticosteroids should be used with caution in hepatic impairment and the patient should be monitored closely.

Renal impairment

Oral and parenteral preparations of corticosteroids should be used with caution in patients with renal impairment.

Pregnancy and breast-feeding

The benefit of treatment with corticosteroids during pregnancy and breast-feeding outweighs the risk; pregnant women with fluid retention should be monitored closely. Corticosteroid cover is required during labour.

Following a review of the data on the safety of systemic corticosteroids used in pregnancy and breast-feeding the CSM (May 1998) has concluded:

- corticosteroids vary in their ability to cross the placenta; betamethasone and dexamethasone cross the placenta readily while 88% of prednisolone is inactivated as it crosses the placenta;

- there is no convincing evidence that systemic corticosteroids increase the incidence of congenital abnormalities such as cleft palate or lip;

- when administration is prolonged or repeated during pregnancy, systemic corticosteroids increase the risk of intra-uterine growth restriction; there is no evidence of intra-uterine growth restriction following short-term treatment (e.g. prophylactic treatment for neonatal respiratory distress syndrome);

- any adrenal suppression in the neonate following prenatal exposure usually resolves spontaneously after birth and is rarely clinically important;

- prednisolone appears in small amounts in breast milk but maternal doses of up to 40 mg daily are unlikely to cause systemic effects in the infant; infants should be monitored for adrenal suppression if the mothers are taking a higher dose.

6 Endocrine system

Side-effects of corticosteroids

Overdosage or prolonged use can exaggerate some of the normal physiological actions of corticosteroids leading to mineralocorticoid and glucocorticoid side-effects.

Mineralocorticoid side-effects include hypertension, sodium and water retention, and potassium and calcium loss. They are most marked with fludrocortisone, but are significant with hydrocortisone, corticotropin, and tetracosactide. Mineralocorticoid actions are negligible with the high potency glucocorticoids, betamethasone and dexamethasone, and occur only slightly with methylprednisolone, prednisolone, and triamcinolone.

Glucocorticoid side-effects include diabetes and osteoporosis (section 6.6), which is a danger, particularly in the elderly, as it can result in osteoporotic fractures for example of the hip or vertebrae; in addition high doses are associated with avascular necrosis of the femoral head. Muscle wasting (proximal myopathy) can also occur. Corticosteroid therapy is also weakly linked with peptic ulceration and perforation; there is no conclusive evidence that the use of enteric-coated preparations of prednisolone reduces the risk of peptic ulceration. See also Psychiatric Reactions, p. 497.

High doses of corticosteroids can cause Cushing's syndrome, with moon face, striae, and acne; it is usually reversible on withdrawal of treatment, but this must always be gradually tapered to avoid symptoms of acute adrenal insufficiency (**important**: see also Adrenal Suppression, p. 495).

In children, administration of corticosteroids may result in suppression of growth. For the effect of corticosteroids given in pregnancy, see Pregnancy and Breast-feeding, p. 497.

Side-effects can be minimised by using lowest effective dose for minimum period possible.

Other side-effects include: *gastro-intestinal effects*: dyspepsia, abdominal distension, acute pancreatitis, oesophageal ulceration and candidiasis; *musculoskeletal effects*: muscle weakness, vertebral and long bone fractures, tendon rupture; *endocrine effects*: menstrual irregularities and amenorrhoea, hirsutism, weight gain, hypercholesterolaemia, hyperlipidaemia, negative nitrogen and calcium balance, increased appetite; increased susceptibility to and severity of infection, reactivation of dormant tuberculosis; *neuropsychiatric effects*: psychological dependence, insomnia, increased intracranial pressure with papilloedema in children (usually after withdrawal), aggravation of schizophrenia, aggravation of epilepsy; *ophthalmic effects*: glaucoma, papilloedema, posterior subcapsular cataracts, corneal or scleral thinning and exacerbation of ophthalmic viral or fungal disease, increased intra-ocular pressure, exophthalmos; *also* impaired healing, petechiae, ecchymoses, facial erythema, suppression of skin test reactions, urticaria, hyperhidrosis, skin atrophy, bruising, telangiectasia, myocardial rupture following recent myocardial infarction, congestive heart failure, leucocytosis, hyperglycaemia, thromboembolism, nausea, malaise, hiccups, headache, vertigo.

For other references to the side-effects of corticosteroids see section 3.2 (asthma), section 11.4 (eye) and section 13.4 (skin).

Endocrine system

6

▌ BETAMETHASONE

Indications suppression of inflammatory and allergic disorders; congenital adrenal hyperplasia; see also notes above; ear (section 12.1.1); eye (section 11.4.1); nose (section 12.2.1); oral ulceration (section 12.3.1)

Cautions see notes above

Contra-indications see notes above

Hepatic impairment see notes above

Renal impairment see notes above

Pregnancy see notes above; transient effect on fetal movements and heart rate

Breast-feeding see notes above

Side-effects see notes above

Dose

● By mouth, usual range 0.5–5 mg daily; see also Administration (above)

● By intramuscular injection *or* slow intravenous injection *or* infusion, 4–20 mg, repeated up to 4 times in 24 hours; CHILD, by slow intravenous injection, up to 1 year 1 mg, 1–5 years 2 mg, 6–12 years 4 mg, repeated up to 4 times in 24 hours according to response

Betamethasone (Non-proprietary) ⒫ⓄⓂ
   Soluble tablets, betamethasone (as sodium phosphate) 500 micrograms, net price 100-tab pack = £22.34. Label: 10, steroid card, 13, 21

Betnesol® (RPH) ⒫ⓄⓂ
   Injection, betamethasone (as sodium phosphate) 4 mg/mL, net price 1-mL amp = £1.22. Label: 10, steroid card

▌ DEFLAZACORT

Indications suppression of inflammatory and allergic disorders

Cautions see notes above

Contra-indications see notes above

Hepatic impairment see notes above

Renal impairment see notes above

Pregnancy see notes above

Breast-feeding see notes above

Side-effects see notes above

Dose

● Usual maintenance 3–18 mg daily (acute disorders, initially up to 120 mg daily); see also Administration (above)

   CHILD 0.25–1.5 mg/kg daily (or on alternate days); see also Administration (above)

Calcort® (Sanofi-Aventis) ⒫ⓄⓂ
   Tablets, deflazacort 6 mg, net price 60-tab pack = £15.82. Label: 5, 10, steroid card

▌ DEXAMETHASONE

Indications suppression of inflammatory and allergic disorders; diagnosis of Cushing's disease, congenital adrenal hyperplasia; cerebral oedema associated with malignancy; croup (section 3.1); nausea and vomiting with chemotherapy (section 8.1); rheumatic disease (section 10.1.2); eye (section 11.4.1); see also notes above

Cautions see notes above

Contra-indications see notes above

Hepatic impairment see notes above

Renal impairment see notes above

Pregnancy see notes above

Breast-feeding see notes above

Side-effects see notes above; also perineal irritation may follow intravenous administration of the phosphate ester

Dose

- By mouth, usual range 0.5–10 mg daily; CHILD 10–100 micrograms/kg daily; see also Administration (above)
- By intramuscular injection *or* slow intravenous injection *or* infusion, see under preparations

Dexamethasone (Non-proprietary) [PoM]

Tablets, dexamethasone 500 micrograms, net price 28-tab pack = £59.52; 2 mg, 50-tab pack = £46.39, 100-tab pack = £78.00. Label: 10, steroid card, 21

Oral solution, sugar-free, dexamethasone (as sodium phosphate) 2 mg/5 mL, net price 75-mL = £32.50, 150-mL = £42.30. Label: 10, steroid card, 21

Brands include *Dexsol®*, *Martapan®*

Injection, dexamethasone (as sodium phosphate) 3.8 mg/mL, net price 1-mL vial = £1.99. Label: 10, steroid card

Note Dexamethasone 3.8 mg/mL Injection has replaced Dexamethasone 4 mg/mL Injection

Dose By intramuscular injection *or* slow intravenous injection *or* infusion, 0.4–20 mg; CHILD 200–400 micrograms/kg daily

Cerebral oedema, by intravenous injection 8–16 mg initially, then 5 mg by intramuscular injection *or* intravenous injection every 6 hours until adequate response achieved then taper-off gradually

Adjunctive treatment of bacterial meningitis, (starting before or with first dose of antibacterial treatment), [unlicensed indication], by intravenous injection 8.3 mg every 6 hours for 4 days; CHILD 3 months–18 years see *BNF for Children*

Injection, dexamethasone (as sodium phosphate) 3.3 mg/mL, net price 1-mL amp = £1.20, 2-mL vial = £4.80. Label: 10, steroid card

Dose by intramuscular injection *or* slow intravenous injection *or* infusion, 0.4–20 mg; CHILD 167–333 micrograms/kg daily

Cerebral oedema associated with malignancy, by intravenous injection 8.3 mg initially, then 3.3 mg by intramuscular injection every 6 hours as required for 2–4 days then gradually reduced and stopped over 5–7 days

Adjunctive treatment of bacterial meningitis, (starting before or with first dose of antibacterial treatment), [unlicensed indication], by intravenous injection 8.3 mg every 6 hours for 4 days; CHILD 3 months–18 years see *BNF for Children*

HYDROCORTISONE

Indications adrenocortical insufficiency (section 6.3.1); shock; see also notes above; hypersensitivity reactions e.g. anaphylaxis and angioedema (section 3.4.3); asthma (section 3.1); severe inflammatory bowel disease (section 1.5); haemorrhoids (section 1.7.2); rheumatic disease (section 10.1.2); skin (section 13.4)

Cautions see notes above

Contra-indications see notes above

Hepatic impairment see notes above

Renal impairment see notes above

Pregnancy see notes above

Breast-feeding see notes above

Side-effects see notes above; also phosphate ester associated with paraesthesia and pain (particularly in the perineal region)

Dose

- By mouth, replacement therapy, 20–30 mg daily in divided doses—see section 6.3.1; CHILD 1 month–18 years see *BNF for Children*
- By intramuscular injection *or* slow intravenous injection *or* infusion, 100–500 mg, 3–4 times in 24 hours or as required; CHILD by slow intravenous injection up to 1 year 25 mg, 1–5 years 50 mg, 6–12 years 100 mg

Hydrocortisone (Non-proprietary) [PoM]

Tablets, scored, hydrocortisone 10 mg, net price 30-tab pack = £64.79; 20 mg, 30-tab pack = £78.62. Label: 10, steroid card, 21

¹Efcortesol® (AMCo) [PoM] ◢

Injection, hydrocortisone 100 mg (as sodium phosphate)/mL, net price 1-mL amp = £1.08, 5-mL amp = £4.89. Label: 10, steroid card

Note Paraesthesia and pain (particularly in the perineal region) may follow intravenous injection of the phosphate ester

¹Solu-Cortef® (Pharmacia) [PoM]

Injection, powder for reconstitution, hydrocortisone (as sodium succinate). Net price 100-mg vial = 92p, 100-mg vial with 2-mL amp water for injections = £1.16. Label: 10, steroid card

◢ **Modified release**

Plenadren® (ViroPharma) ▼ [PoM]

Tablets, m/r, hydrocortisone 5 mg (pink), net price 50-tab pack = £242.50; 20 mg (white), 50-tab pack = £400.00. Label: 10, steroid card, 22, 25

Dose replacement in adrenocortical insufficiency, ADULT over 18 years, usual dose 20–30 mg once daily in the morning, adjusted according to response

Note When switching from immediate-release hydrocortisone tablets to *Plenadren®* use same total daily dose. Bioavailability of *Plenadren®* lower than immediate-release tablets—monitor clinical response

METHYLPREDNISOLONE

Indications suppression of inflammatory and allergic disorders; severe inflammatory bowel disease (section 1.5); cerebral oedema associated with malignancy; see also notes above; rheumatic disease (section 10.1.2); skin (section 13.4)

Cautions see notes above; also rapid intravenous administration of large doses associated with cardiovascular collapse

Contra-indications see notes above

Hepatic impairment see notes above

Renal impairment see notes above

Pregnancy see notes above

Breast-feeding see notes above

Side-effects see notes above

Dose

- By mouth, usual range 2–40 mg daily; see also Administration (above)
- By intramuscular injection *or* slow intravenous injection *or* infusion, initially 10–500 mg; graft rejection, up to 1 g daily by intravenous infusion for up to 3 days

Medrone® (Pfizer) [PoM]

Tablets, scored, methylprednisolone 2 mg (pink), net price 30-tab pack = £3.88; 4 mg, 30-tab pack = £6.19; 16 mg, 30-tab pack = £17.17; 100 mg (blue), 20-tab pack = £48.32. Label: 10, steroid card, 21

---

1. [PoM] restriction does not apply where administration is for saving life in emergency

6   Endocrine system

Solu-Medrone® (Pharmacia) [PoM]

Injection, powder for reconstitution, methylprednisolone (as sodium succinate) (all with solvent). Net price 40-mg vial = £1.58; 125-mg vial = £4.75; 500-mg vial = £9.60; 1-g vial = £17.30; 2-g vial = £32.86. Label: 10, steroid card

◢ **Intramuscular depot**

Depo-Medrone® (Pharmacia) [PoM]

Injection (aqueous suspension), methylprednisolone acetate 40 mg/mL. Net price 1-mL vial = £3.44; 2-mL vial = £6.18; 3-mL vial = £8.96. Label: 10, steroid card

> Dose by deep intramuscular injection into gluteal muscle, 40–120 mg, a second injection may be given after 2–3 weeks if required

▮ PREDNISOLONE

Indications suppression of inflammatory and allergic disorders; see also notes above; inflammatory bowel disease (section 1.5); asthma (section 3.1 and section 3.2); croup (section 3.1); immunosuppression (section 8.2.2); rheumatic disease (section 10.1.2); eye (section 11.4.1); ear (section 12.1.1)

Cautions see notes above; also Duchenne's muscular dystrophy (possible transient rhabdomyolysis and myoglobinuria following strenuous physical activity)

Contra-indications see notes above

Hepatic impairment see notes above

Renal impairment see notes above

Pregnancy see notes above

Breast-feeding see notes above

Side-effects see notes above

Dose

- By mouth, initially, up to 10–20 mg daily (severe disease, up to 60 mg daily), preferably taken in the morning after breakfast; can often be reduced within a few days but may need to be continued for several weeks or months
  Maintenance, usual range, 2.5–15 mg daily, but higher doses may be needed; cushingoid side-effects increasingly likely with doses above 7.5 mg daily
- By intramuscular injection, prednisolone acetate (section 10.1.2.2), 25–100 mg once or twice weekly

Prednisolone (Non-proprietary) [PoM]

Tablets, prednisolone 1 mg, net price 28-tab pack = £1.18; 5 mg, 28-tab pack = £1.33; 25 mg, 56-tab pack = £50.00. Label: 10, steroid card, 21

Tablets, e/c, prednisolone 2.5 mg (brown), net price 28-tab pack = £1.74, 100-tab pack = £13.43; 5 mg (red), 28-tab pack = £1.82, 100-tab pack = £13.54. Label: 5, 10, steroid card, 25
Brands include *Deltacortril®*

Soluble tablets, prednisolone 5 mg (as sodium phosphate), net price 30-tab pack = £42.78. Label: 10, steroid card, 13, 21

Injection, see section 10.1.2.2

▮ PREDNISONE

Indications moderate to severe rheumatoid arthritis (section 10.1.2.1)

Cautions see notes above

Contra-indications see notes above

Hepatic impairment see notes above

Renal impairment see notes above

Pregnancy see notes above

Breast-feeding see notes above

Side-effects see notes above

Dose

- ADULT over 18 years, initially 10–20 mg at bedtime, adjusted according to response

Lodotra® (Napp) [PoM]

Tablets, m/r, yellow, prednisone 1 mg, net price 30-tab pack = £26.70; 2 mg, 30-tab pack = £26.70, 100-tab pack = £89.00; 5 mg, 30-tab pack = £26.70, 100-tab pack = £89.00. Label: 10, steroid card, 21, 25

▮ TRIAMCINOLONE

Indications suppression of inflammatory and allergic disorders; see also notes above; rheumatic disease (section 10.1.2); skin (section 13.4)

Cautions see notes above; also high dosage may cause proximal myopathy, avoid in chronic therapy

Contra-indications see notes above

Hepatic impairment see notes above

Renal impairment see notes above

Pregnancy see notes above

Breast-feeding see notes above

Side-effects see notes above

Dose

- By deep intramuscular injection, into gluteal muscle, 40 mg of acetonide for depot effect, repeated at intervals according to the patient's response; max. single dose 100 mg

Kenalog® Intra-articular/Intramuscular (Squibb) [PoM]

Injection (aqueous suspension), triamcinolone acetonide 40 mg/mL, net price 1-mL vial = £1.49. Label: 10, steroid card

6.4 Sex hormones

6.4.1 Female sex hormones and their modulators

6.4.2 Male sex hormones and antagonists

6.4.3 Anabolic steroids

6.4.1 Female sex hormones and their modulators

6.4.1.1 Oestrogens and HRT

6.4.1.2 Progestogens and progesterone receptor modulators

6.4.1.1 Oestrogens and HRT

Oestrogens are necessary for the development of female secondary sexual characteristics; they also stimulate myometrial hypertrophy with endometrial hyperplasia.

In terms of oestrogenic activity *natural oestrogens* (estradiol (oestradiol), estrone (oestrone), and estriol (oestriol)) have a more appropriate profile for hormone replacement therapy (HRT) than *synthetic oestrogens* (ethinylestradiol (ethinyloestradiol) and mestranol). Tibolone has oestrogenic, progestogenic and weak androgenic activity.

Oestrogen therapy is given cyclically or continuously for a number of gynaecological conditions. If long-term therapy is required in women with a uterus, a progestogen should normally be added to reduce the risk of cystic hyperplasia of the endometrium (or of endometriotic foci in women who have had a hysterectomy) and possible transformation to cancer.

Oestrogens are no longer used to suppress lactation because of their association with thromboembolism.

Hormone replacement therapy

Hormone replacement therapy (HRT) with small doses of an oestrogen (together with a progestogen in women with a uterus) is appropriate for alleviating menopausal symptoms such as vaginal atrophy or vasomotor instability. Oestrogen given systemically in the perimenopausal and postmenopausal period or tibolone given in the postmenopausal period also diminish postmenopausal osteoporosis (section 6.6.1) but other drugs (section 6.6) are preferred. Menopausal atrophic vaginitis may respond to a short course of a topical vaginal oestrogen preparation (section 7.2.1) used for a few weeks and repeated if necessary.

Systemic therapy with an oestrogen or drugs with oestrogenic properties alleviates the symptoms of oestrogen deficiency such as vasomotor symptoms. Tibolone combines oestrogenic and progestogenic activity with weak androgenic activity; it is given continuously, without cyclical progestogen.

HRT may be used in women with early natural or surgical menopause (before age 45 years), since they are at high risk of osteoporosis. For early menopause, HRT can be given until the approximate age of natural menopause (i.e. until age 50 years). Alternatives to HRT should be considered if osteoporosis is the main concern (section 6.6).

Clonidine (section 2.5.2 and section 4.7.4.2) may be used to reduce vasomotor symptoms in women who cannot take an oestrogen, but clonidine may cause unacceptable side-effects.

HRT increases the risk of venous thromboembolism, stroke, endometrial cancer (reduced by a progestogen), breast cancer, and ovarian cancer; there is an increased risk of coronary heart disease in women who start combined HRT more than 10 years after menopause. For details of these risks see HRT Risk table, below.

HRT Risk

Risk	Age range (years)	Background incidence per 1000 women in Europe not using HRT		Additional cases per 1000 women using oestrogen only HRT (estimated)		Additional cases per 1000 women using combined (oestrogen-progestogen) HRT (estimated)	
		Over 5 years	Over 10 years	For 5 years' use	For 10 years' use	For 5 years' use	For 10 years' use
Breast cancer[1]	50–59	10	20	2	6	6	24
	60–69	15	30	3	9	9	36
Endometrial cancer[2,3]	50–59	2	4	4	32	NS	NS
	60–69	3	6	6	48	NS	NS
Ovarian cancer	50–59	2	4	<1	1	<1	1
	60–69	3	6	<1	2	<1	2
Venous thromboembolism[4,5]	50–59	5	–	2	–	7	–
	60–69	8	–	2	–	10	–
Stroke[6]	50–59	4	–	1	–	1	–
	60–69	9	–	3	–	3	–
Coronary heart disease[7,8]	70–79	29–44	–	NS	–	15	–

Note Where background incidence or additional cases have not been included in the table, this indicates a lack of available data. NS indicates a non-significant difference
Taken from MHRA/CHM (*Drug Safety Update* 2007; **1** (2): 2–6) available at www.mhra.gov.uk/drugsafetyupdate

1. Tibolone increases the risk of breast cancer but to a lesser extent than with combined HRT.
2. Evidence suggests an increased risk of endometrial cancer with tibolone. After 2.7 years of use (in women of average age 68 years), 1 extra case of endometrial hyperplasia and 4 extra cases of endometrial cancer were diagnosed compared with placebo users.
3. The risk of endometrial cancer cannot be reliably estimated in those using combined HRT because the addition of progestogen for at least 10 days per 28-day cycle greatly reduces the additional risk, and addition of a daily progestogen eliminates the additional risk. The risk of endometrial cancer in women who have not used HRT increases with body mass index (BMI); the increased risk of endometrial cancer in users of oestrogen-only HRT or tibolone is more apparent in women who are not overweight.
4. Limited data does not suggest an increased risk of thromboembolism with tibolone compared with combined HRT or women not taking HRT.
5. Although the level of risk of thromboembolism associated with non-oral routes of administration of HRT has not been established, it may be lower for the transdermal route.
6. Tibolone increases the risk of stroke about 2.2 times from the first year of treatment; risk of stroke is age-dependent and therefore the absolute risk of stroke with tibolone increases with age.
7. Increased risk of coronary heart disease in women who start combined HRT more than 10 years after menopause.
8. There is insufficient data to draw a conclusion on the risk of coronary heart disease with tibolone.

6 Endocrine system

The minimum effective dose of HRT should be used for the shortest duration. Treatment should be reviewed at least annually and for osteoporosis alternative treatments considered (section 6.6). HRT does not prevent coronary heart disease or protect against a decline in cognitive function and it should **not** be prescribed for these purposes. Experience of treating women over 65 years with HRT is limited.

For the treatment of menopausal symptoms the benefits of short-term HRT outweigh the risks in the majority of women, especially in those aged under 60 years.

Risk of breast cancer   It is estimated that using *all* types of HRT, including tibolone, increases the risk of breast cancer within 1–2 years of initiating treatment, see HRT Risk table, p. 501 for details. The increased risk is related to the duration of HRT use (but not to the age at which it is started) and this excess risk disappears within 5 years of stopping.

Radiological detection of breast cancer can be made more difficult as mammographic density can increase with HRT use; tibolone has only a limited effect on mammographic density.

Risk of endometrial cancer   The increased risk of endometrial cancer depends on the dose and duration of oestrogen-only HRT, see HRT Risk table, p. 501 for details.

In women with a uterus, the addition of a progestogen cyclically (for at least 10 days per 28-day cycle) reduces the additional risk of endometrial cancer; this additional risk is eliminated if a progestogen is given continuously. However, this should be weighed against the increased risk of breast cancer.

Risk of ovarian cancer   Long-term use of combined HRT or oestrogen-only HRT is associated with a small increased risk of ovarian cancer, see HRT Risk table, p. 501 for details; this excess risk disappears within a few years of stopping.

Risk of venous thromboembolism   Women using combined or oestrogen-only HRT are at an increased risk of deep vein thrombosis and of pulmonary embolism especially in the first year of use, see HRT Risk table, p. 501 for details.

In *women who have predisposing factors* (such as a personal or family history of deep vein thrombosis or pulmonary embolism, severe varicose veins, obesity, trauma, or prolonged bed-rest) it is prudent to review the need for HRT, as in some cases the risks of HRT may exceed the benefits. See below for advice on surgery.

Travel involving prolonged immobility further increases the risk of deep vein thrombosis, see under Travel in section 7.3.1.

Risk of stroke   Risk of stroke increases with age, therefore older women have a greater absolute risk of stroke. Combined HRT or oestrogen-only HRT slightly increases the risk of stroke. Tibolone increases the risk of stroke about 2.2 times from the first year of treatment, see HRT Risk table, p. 501 for details.

Risk of coronary heart disease   HRT does not prevent coronary heart disease and should not be prescribed for this purpose. There is an increased risk of coronary heart disease in women who start combined HRT more than 10 years after menopause, see HRT Risk table, p. 501 for details. Although very little infor-

mation is available on the risk of coronary heart disease in younger women who start HRT close to the menopause, studies suggest a lower relative risk compared with older women.

Choice   The choice of HRT for an individual depends on an overall balance of indication, risk, and convenience. A woman with a uterus normally requires oestrogen with cyclical progestogen for the last 12 to 14 days of the cycle *or* a preparation which involves continuous administration of an oestrogen and a progestogen (*or* one which provides both oestrogenic and progestogenic activity in a single preparation). Continuous combined preparations or tibolone are **not suitable** for use in the perimenopause or within 12 months of the last menstrual period; women who use such preparations may bleed irregularly in the early stages of treatment—if bleeding continues endometrial abnormality should be ruled out and consideration given to changing to cyclical HRT.

An oestrogen alone is suitable for continuous use in women without a uterus. However, in endometriosis, endometrial foci may remain despite hysterectomy and the addition of a progestogen should be considered in these circumstances.

An oestrogen may be given by mouth or by transdermal administration, which avoids first-pass metabolism. For the use of topical HRT preparations see section 7.2.1.

Contraception   HRT does **not** provide contraception and a woman is considered potentially fertile for 2 years after her last menstrual period if she is under 50 years, and for 1 year if she is over 50 years. A woman who is under 50 years and free of all risk factors for venous and arterial disease can use a low-oestrogen combined oral contraceptive pill (section 7.3.1) to provide both relief of menopausal symptoms and contraception; it is recommended that the oral contraceptive be stopped at 50 years of age since there are more suitable alternatives. If any potentially fertile woman needs HRT, non-hormonal contraceptive measures (such as condoms) are necessary.

Measurement of follicle-stimulating hormone can help to determine fertility, but high measurements alone (particularly in women aged under 50 years) do not necessarily preclude the possibility of becoming pregnant.

Surgery   Major surgery under general anaesthesia, including orthopaedic and vascular leg surgery, is a predisposing factor for venous thromboembolism and it may be prudent to stop HRT 4–6 weeks before surgery (see Risk of Venous Thromboembolism, above); it should be restarted only after full mobilisation. If HRT is continued or if discontinuation is not possible (e.g. in non-elective surgery), prophylaxis with unfractionated or low molecular weight heparin and graduated compression hosiery is advised.

Reasons to stop HRT   For circumstances in which HRT should be stopped, see p. 549.

▌ OESTROGENS FOR HRT

Note   Relates only to small amounts of oestrogens given for hormone replacement therapy

Indications   see notes above and under preparations

Cautions   prolonged exposure to unopposed oestrogens may increase risk of developing endometrial

cancer (see notes above); migraine (or migraine-like headaches); diabetes (increased risk of heart disease); history of breast nodules or fibrocystic disease—closely monitor breast status (risk of breast cancer, see notes above); risk factors for oestrogen-dependent tumours (e.g. breast cancer in first-degree relative); uterine fibroids may increase in size, symptoms of endometriosis may be exacerbated; history of endometrial hyperplasia; factors predisposing to thromboembolism (see notes above); presence of antiphospholipid antibodies (increased risk of thrombotic events); increased risk of gall-bladder disease reported; hypophyseal tumours; acute porphyria (see section 9.8.2); **interactions:** Appendix 1 (oestrogens)
Other conditions The product literature advises caution in other conditions including hypertension, renal disease, asthma, epilepsy, sickle-cell disease, melanoma, otosclerosis, multiple sclerosis, and systemic lupus erythematosus (but care required if antiphospholipid antibodies present, see above). Evidence for caution in these conditions is unsatisfactory and many women with these conditions may stand to benefit from HRT.

Contra-indications oestrogen-dependent cancer, history of breast cancer, active thrombophlebitis, active or recent arterial thromboembolic disease (e.g. angina or myocardial infarction), venous thromboembolism, or history of recurrent venous thromboembolism (unless already on anticoagulant treatment), thrombophilic disorder, liver disease (where liver function tests have failed to return to normal), Dubin-Johnson and Rotor syndromes (or monitor closely), untreated endometrial hyperplasia, undiagnosed vaginal bleeding

Hepatic impairment see Combined Hormonal Contraceptives, section 7.3.1

Renal impairment see Other Conditions, above

Pregnancy see Combined Hormonal Contraceptives, section 7.3.1

Breast-feeding see Combined Hormonal Contraceptives, section 7.3.1

Side-effects see notes above for risks of long-term use; nausea and vomiting, abdominal cramps and bloating, weight changes, breast enlargement and tenderness, premenstrual-like syndrome, sodium and fluid retention, cholestatic jaundice, glucose intolerance, altered blood lipids—may lead to pancreatitis, rashes and chloasma, changes in libido, depression, mood changes, headache, migraine, dizziness, leg cramps (rule out venous thrombosis), vaginal candidiasis, contact lenses may irritate; transdermal delivery systems may cause contact sensitisation (possible severe hypersensitivity reaction on continued exposure), and headache has been reported on vigorous exercise

Withdrawal bleeding Cyclical HRT (where a progestogen is taken for 12–14 days of each 28-day oestrogen treatment cycle) usually results in *regular withdrawal bleeding* towards the end of the progestogen. The aim of continuous combined HRT (where a combination of oestrogen and progestogen is taken, usually in a single tablet, throughout each 28-day treatment cycle) is to avoid bleeding, but *irregular bleeding* may occur during the early treatment stages (if it continues endometrial abnormality should be excluded and consideration given to cyclical HRT instead)

Dose
- See under preparations

  Counselling on patches Patch should be removed after 3–4 days (or once a week in case of 7-day patch) and replaced with fresh patch on slightly different site; recommended sites: clean, dry, unbroken areas of skin on trunk below waistline; not to be applied on or near breasts or under waistband. If patch falls off in bath allow skin to cool before applying new patch

◄ **Conjugated oestrogens with progestogen**
For prescribing information on progestogens, see section 6.4.1.2

Premique® (Pfizer) [PoM]
Premique® Low Dose tablets, m/r, ivory, s/c, conjugated oestrogen (equine) 300 micrograms and medroxyprogesterone acetate 1.5 mg, net price 3 × 28-tab pack = £6.52
Dose menopausal symptoms in women with a uterus, 1 tablet daily continuously
Premique® tablets, s/c, blue, conjugated oestrogen (equine) 625 micrograms and medroxyprogesterone acetate 5 mg, net price 3 × 28-tab pack = £10.61
Dose menopausal symptoms and osteoporosis prophylaxis (see section 6.6), in women with a uterus, 1 tablet daily continuously

Prempak-C® (Pfizer) [PoM]
Prempak C® 0.625 Calendar pack, s/c, 28 maroon tablets, conjugated oestrogens (equine) 625 micrograms; 12 light brown tablets, norgestrel 150 micrograms (≡ levonorgestrel 75 micrograms), net price 3 × 40-tab pack = £6.25
Dose menopausal symptoms and osteoporosis prophylaxis (see section 6.6), in women with a uterus, 1 maroon tablet daily continuously, starting on day 1 of menstruation (or at any time if cycles have ceased or are infrequent), and 1 brown tablet daily on days 17–28 of each 28-day treatment cycle; subsequent courses are repeated without interval
Prempak C® 1.25 Calendar pack, s/c, 28 yellow tablets, conjugated oestrogens (equine) 1.25 mg; 12 light brown tablets, norgestrel 150 micrograms (≡ levonorgestrel 75 micrograms), net price 3 × 40-tab pack = £7.40
Dose see under 0.625 Calendar pack, but taking 1 yellow tablet daily continuously (instead of 1 maroon tablet) if symptoms not fully controlled with lower strength

◄ **Estradiol with progestogen**
For prescribing information on progestogens, see section 6.4.1.2

Angeliq® (Bayer) [PoM]
Tablets, f/c, red, estradiol 1 mg, drospirenone 2 mg, net price 3 × 28-tab pack = £29.00
Dose menopausal symptoms and osteoporosis prophylaxis (see section 6.6) in women with a uterus whose last menstrual period occurred over 12 months previously, 1 tablet daily continuously (if changing from cyclical HRT begin treatment the day after finishing oestrogen plus progestogen phase)
Cautions use with care if an increased concentration of potassium might be hazardous
Renal impairment avoid if eGFR less than 30 mL/minute/1.73 m²

Climagest® (Novartis) [PoM]
Climagest® 1-mg tablets, 16 grey-blue, estradiol valerate 1 mg; 12 white, estradiol valerate 1 mg and norethisterone 1 mg, net price 28-tab pack = £5.51; 3 × 28-tab pack = £16.02
Dose menopausal symptoms, 1 grey-blue tablet daily for 16 days, starting on day 1 of menstruation (or at any time if cycles have ceased or are infrequent) then 1 white tablet for 12 days; subsequent courses are repeated without interval
Climagest® 2-mg tablets, 16 blue, estradiol valerate 2 mg; 12 yellow, estradiol valerate 2 mg and norethisterone 1 mg, net price 28-tab pack = £5.51; 3 × 28-tab pack = £16.02
Dose see *Climagest® 1-mg*, but starting with 1 blue tablet daily (instead of 1 grey-blue tablet) if symptoms not controlled with lower strength

6

Endocrine system

Endocrine system · **6** (side tab)

Climesse® (Novartis) [PoM]

Tablets, pink, estradiol valerate 2 mg, norethisterone 700 micrograms, net price 1 × 28-tab pack = £9.92; 3 × 28-tab pack = £29.78

Dose menopausal symptoms and osteoporosis prophylaxis (see section 6.6) in women with a uterus whose last menstrual period occurred over 12 months previously, 1 tablet daily continuously

Clinorette® (ReSource Medical) [PoM]

Tablets, f/c, 16 white, estradiol 2 mg; 12 pink, estradiol 2 mg and norethisterone 1 mg, net price 3 × 28-tab pack = £9.23

Dose menopausal symptoms and osteoporosis prophylaxis (see section 6.6), in women with a uterus, 1 white tablet daily for 16 days starting on day 5 of menstruation (or at any time if cycles have ceased or are infrequent), then 1 pink tablet daily for 12 days; subsequent courses repeated without interval

Cyclo-Progynova® (Meda) [PoM]

Cyclo-Progynova® 2-mg tablets, s/c, 11 white, estradiol valerate 2 mg; 10 brown, estradiol valerate 2 mg and norgestrel 500 micrograms (≡ levonorgestrel 250 micrograms), net price per pack = £3.11

Dose menopausal symptoms and osteoporosis prophylaxis (see section 6.6) in women with a uterus, 1 white tablet daily for 11 days, starting on day 5 of menstruation (or at any time if cycles have ceased or are infrequent), then 1 brown tablet daily for 10 days, followed by a 7-day tablet-free interval

Elleste-Duet® (Meda) [PoM]

Elleste-Duet® 1-mg tablets, 16 white, estradiol 1 mg; 12 green, estradiol 1 mg and norethisterone acetate 1 mg, net price 3 × 28-tab pack = £9.20

Dose menopausal symptoms, 1 white tablet daily for 16 days starting on day 1 of menstruation (or at any time if cycles have ceased or are infrequent), then 1 green tablet daily for 12 days; subsequent courses are repeated without interval

Elleste-Duet® 2-mg tablets, 16 orange, estradiol 2 mg; 12 grey, estradiol 2 mg, norethisterone acetate 1 mg, net price 3 × 28-tab pack = £9.20

Dose menopausal symptoms and osteoporosis prophylaxis (see section 6.6), 1 orange tablet daily for 16 days, starting on day 1 of menstruation (or at any time if cycles have ceased or are infrequent) then 1 grey tablet daily for 12 days; subsequent courses are repeated without interval

Elleste-Duet Conti® tablets, f/c, grey, estradiol 2 mg, norethisterone acetate 1 mg, net price 3 × 28-tab pack = £17.02

Dose menopausal symptoms and osteoporosis prophylaxis (see section 6.6) in women with a uterus whose last menstrual period occurred over 12 months previously, 1 tablet daily on a continuous basis (if changing from cyclical HRT begin treatment at the end of scheduled bleed)

Evorel® (Janssen) [PoM]

Evorel® Conti patches, self-adhesive, (releasing estradiol approx. 50 micrograms/24 hours and norethisterone acetate approx. 170 micrograms/24 hours), net price 8-patch pack = £13.00, 24-patch pack = £37.22. Counselling, administration

Dose menopausal symptoms and osteoporosis prophylaxis (see section 6.6), in women with a uterus, 1 patch to be applied twice weekly continuously

Evorel® Sequi combination pack, 4 self-adhesive patches of Evorel® 50 (releasing estradiol approx. 50 micrograms/24 hours) and 4 self-adhesive patches of Evorel® Conti (releasing estradiol approx. 50 micrograms/24 hours and norethisterone acetate approx. 170 micrograms/24 hours), net price 8-patch pack = £11.09. Counselling, administration

Dose menopausal symptoms and osteoporosis prophylaxis (see section 6.6), in women with a uterus, 1 Evorel® 50 patch to be applied twice weekly for 2 weeks, starting within 5 days of onset of menstruation (or at any time if cycles have ceased or are infrequent), followed by 1 Evorel® Conti patch twice weekly for 2 weeks; subsequent courses are repeated without interval

Femoston® (Abbott Healthcare) [PoM]

Femoston® 1 mg/10 mg tablets, f/c, 14 white, estradiol 1 mg; 14 grey, estradiol 1 mg, dydrogesterone 10 mg, net price 3 × 28-tab pack = £16.16

Dose menopausal symptoms and osteoporosis prophylaxis (see section 6.6), in women with a uterus, 1 white tablet daily for 14 days, starting within 5 days of onset of menstruation (or any time if cycles have ceased or are infrequent) then 1 grey tablet daily for 14 days; subsequent courses repeated without interval

Femoston® 2 mg/10 mg tablets, f/c, 14 red, estradiol 2 mg; 14 yellow, estradiol 2 mg, dydrogesterone 10 mg, net price 3 × 28-tab pack = £16.16

Dose menopausal symptoms and osteoporosis prophylaxis (see section 6.6), in women with a uterus, 1 red tablet daily for 14 days, starting within 5 days of onset of menstruation (or any time if cycles have ceased or are infrequent) then 1 yellow tablet daily for 14 days; subsequent courses repeated without interval; where therapy required for menopausal symptoms alone, Femoston® 1 mg/10 mg given initially and Femoston® 2 mg/10 mg substituted if symptoms not controlled

Femoston®-conti 0.5 mg/2.5 mg tablets, f/c, yellow, estradiol 0.5 mg, dydrogesterone 2.5 mg, net price 3 × 28-tab pack = £20.36

Dose menopausal symptoms in women with a uterus whose last menstrual period occurred over 12 months previously, 1 tablet daily continuously (if changing from cyclical HRT begin treatment the day after finishing oestrogen plus progestogen phase)

Femoston®-conti 1 mg/5 mg tablets, f/c, salmon, estradiol 1 mg, dydrogesterone 5 mg, net price 3 × 28-tab pack = £24.43

Dose menopausal symptoms and osteoporosis prophylaxis (see section 6.6) in women with a uterus whose last menstrual period occurred over 12 months previously, 1 tablet daily continuously (if changing from cyclical HRT begin treatment the day after finishing oestrogen plus progestogen phase)

FemSeven® Conti (TEVA UK) [PoM]

Patches, self-adhesive (releasing estradiol approx. 50 micrograms/24 hours and levonorgestrel approx. 7 micrograms/24 hours); net price 4-patch pack = £15.48, 12-patch pack = £ 44.12. Counselling, administration

Dose menopausal symptoms in women with a uterus whose last menstrual period occurred over 12 months previously, 1 patch to be applied once a week continuously

FemSeven® Sequi (TEVA UK) [PoM]

Combination pack, self-adhesive patches of FemSeven® Sequi Phase 1 (releasing estradiol approx. 50 micrograms/24 hours) and of FemSeven® Sequi Phase 2 (releasing estradiol approx. 50 micrograms/24 hours and levonorgestrel approx. 10 micrograms/24 hours); net price 1-month pack (2 of each) = £13.18, 3-month pack (6 of each) = £37.54. Counselling, administration

Dose menopausal symptoms in women with a uterus, 1 Phase 1 patch applied once a week for 2 weeks followed by 1 Phase 2 patch applied once a week for 2 weeks; subsequent courses are repeated without interval

Indivina® (Orion) [PoM]

Indivina® 1 mg/2.5 mg tablets, estradiol valerate 1 mg, medroxyprogesterone acetate 2.5 mg, net price 3 × 28-tab pack = £20.58

Indivina® 1 mg/5 mg tablets, estradiol valerate 1 mg, medroxyprogesterone acetate 5 mg, net price 3 × 28-tab pack = £20.58

Indivina® 2 mg/5 mg tablets, estradiol valerate 2 mg, medroxyprogesterone acetate 5 mg, net price 3 × 28-tab pack = £20.58

Dose menopausal symptoms and osteoporosis prophylaxis (see section 6.6) in women with a uterus whose last menstrual period occurred over 3 years previously, 1 tablet daily continuously; initiate therapy with *Indivina® 1 mg/ 2.5 mg* tablets and adjust according to response; start at end of scheduled bleed if changing from cyclical HRT

Kliofem® (Novo Nordisk) PoM
Tablets, f/c yellow, estradiol 2 mg, norethisterone acetate 1 mg, net price 3 × 28-tab pack = £11.43

Dose menopausal symptoms and osteoporosis prophylaxis (see section 6.6) in women with a uterus whose last menstrual period occurred over 12 months previously, 1 tablet daily continuously; start at end of scheduled bleed if changing from cyclical HRT

Kliovance® (Novo Nordisk) PoM
Tablets, f/c, estradiol 1 mg, norethisterone acetate 500 micrograms, net price 3 × 28-tab pack = £13.20

Dose menopausal symptoms and osteoporosis prophylaxis (see section 6.6) in women with a uterus whose last menstrual period occurred over 12 months previously, 1 tablet daily continuously; start at end of scheduled bleed if changing from cyclical HRT

Novofem® (Novo Nordisk) PoM
Tablets, f/c, 16 red, estradiol 1 mg; 12 white, estradiol 1 mg, norethisterone acetate 1 mg, net price 3 × 28-tab pack = £11.43

Dose menopausal symptoms and osteoporosis prophylaxis (see section 6.6), in women with a uterus, 1 red tablet daily for 16 days then 1 white tablet daily for 12 days; subsequent courses are repeated without interval; start treatment with red tablet at any time or if changing from cyclical HRT, start treatment the day after finishing oestrogen plus progestogen phase

Nuvelle® Continuous (Bayer) PoM
Tablets, f/c, pink, estradiol 2 mg, norethisterone acetate 1 mg, net price 3 × 28-tab pack = £19.00

Dose menopausal symptoms and osteoporosis prophylaxis (see section 6.6) in women with a uterus whose last menstrual period occurred over 12 months previously, 1 tablet daily continuously; if changing from cyclical HRT, start treatment the day after finishing oestrogen plus progestogen phase

Tridestra® (Orion) PoM
Tablets, 70 white, estradiol valerate 2 mg; 14 blue, estradiol valerate 2 mg and medroxyprogesterone acetate 20 mg; 7 yellow, inactive, net price 91-tab pack = £20.49

Dose menopausal symptoms and osteoporosis prophylaxis (see section 6.6), in women with a uterus, 1 white tablet daily for 70 days, then 1 blue tablet daily for 14 days, then 1 yellow tablet daily for 7 days; subsequent courses are repeated without interval

Trisequens® (Novo Nordisk) PoM
Tablets, 12 blue, estradiol 2 mg; 10 white, estradiol 2 mg, norethisterone acetate 1 mg; 6 red, estradiol 1 mg, net price 3 × 28-tab pack = £11.10

Dose menopausal symptoms and osteoporosis prophylaxis (see section 6.6), in women with a uterus, 1 blue tablet daily for 12 days followed by 1 white tablet for 10 days, then 1 red tablet daily for 6 days; subsequent courses are repeated without interval

◢ **Conjugated oestrogens only**

Premarin® (Pfizer) PoM
Tablets, all s/c, conjugated oestrogens (equine) 300 micrograms (green) net price 3 × 28-tab pack = £6.07; 625 micrograms (maroon), 3 × 28-tab pack = £4.02; 1.25 mg (yellow), 3 × 28-tab pack = £3.58

Dose menopausal symptoms, 0.3–1.25 mg daily continuously; osteoporosis prophylaxis (see section 6.6), 0.625–1.25 mg daily continuously; with cyclical progestogen for 12–14 days of each cycle in women with a uterus

◢ **Estradiol only**

Bedol® (ReSource Medical) PoM
Tablets, f/c, estradiol 2 mg, net price 3 × 28-tab pack = £5.07

Dose menopausal symptoms and osteoporosis prophylaxis (see section 6.6), with cyclical progestogen for 12–14 days of each cycle in women with a uterus, 2 mg daily starting on day 1–5 of menstruation (or at any time if cycles have ceased or are infrequent)

Climaval® (Novartis) PoM
Tablets, estradiol valerate 1 mg (grey-blue), net price 1 × 28-tab pack = £2.94, 3 × 28-tab pack = £8.82; 2 mg (blue), 1 × 28-tab pack = £2.94, 3 × 28-tab pack = £8.82

Dose menopausal symptoms (if patient has had a hysterectomy), 1–2 mg daily

Elleste-Solo® (Meda) PoM
Elleste-Solo® 1-mg tablets, estradiol 1 mg, net price 3 × 28-tab pack = £5.06

Dose menopausal symptoms, with cyclical progestogen for 12–14 days of each cycle in women with a uterus, 1 mg daily starting on day 1 of menstruation (or at any time if cycles have ceased or are infrequent)

Elleste-Solo® 2-mg tablets, orange, estradiol 2 mg, net price 3 × 28-tab pack = £5.06

Dose menopausal symptoms not controlled with lower strength and osteoporosis prophylaxis (see section 6.6), with cyclical progestogen for 12–14 days of each cycle in women with a uterus, 2 mg daily starting on day 1 of menstruation (or at any time if cycles have ceased or are infrequent)

Elleste Solo® MX (Meda) PoM
Patches, self-adhesive, estradiol, *MX 40 patch* (releasing approx. 40 micrograms/24 hours), net price 8-patch pack = £5.19; *MX 80 patch* (releasing approx. 80 micrograms/24 hours), 8-patch pack = £5.99. Counselling, administration

Dose menopausal symptoms and osteoporosis prophylaxis (see section 6.6), 1 patch to be applied twice weekly continuously starting within 5 days of onset of menstruation (or at any time if cycles have ceased or are infrequent); with cyclical progestogen for 12–14 days of each cycle in women with a uterus; for menopausal symptoms initiate therapy with *MX 40*, subsequently adjust according to response; for osteoporosis prophylaxis, initiate therapy with *MX 80*

Estraderm MX® (Novartis) PoM
Patches, self-adhesive, estradiol, *MX 25 patch* (releasing approx. 25 micrograms/24 hours), net price 8-patch pack = £5.50, 24-patch pack = £16.46; *MX 50 patch* (releasing approx. 50 micrograms/24 hours), 8-patch pack = £5.51, 24-patch pack = £16.46, 20-patch pack (hosp. only) = £13.04; *MX 75 patch* (releasing approx. 75 micrograms/24 hours), 8-patch pack = £6.42, 24-patch pack = £19.27; *MX 100 patch* (releasing approx. 100 micrograms/24 hours), 8-patch pack = £6.66, 24-patch pack = £19.99. Counselling, administration

Dose menopausal symptoms and osteoporosis prophylaxis (see section 6.6), 1 patch to be applied twice weekly continuously starting within 5 days of onset of menstruation (or at any time if cycles have ceased or are infrequent), with cyclical progestogen for at least 12 days of each cycle in women with a uterus; for menopausal symptoms, initiate therapy with *MX25* for first 3 months; for osteoporosis prophylaxis, initiate therapy with *MX50*; subsequently adjust according to response

Estradot® (Novartis) PoM
Patches, self-adhesive, estradiol, *'25' patch* (releasing approx. 25 micrograms/24 hours), net price 8-patch pack = £4.99; *'37.5' patch* (releasing approx. 37.5 micrograms/24 hours), 8-patch pack = £5.00;

6
Endocrine system

'50' patch (releasing approx. 50 micrograms/24 hours), 8-patch pack = £5.02; *'75' patch* (releasing approx. 75 micrograms/24 hours), 8-patch pack = £5.83; *'100' patch* (releasing approx. 100 micrograms/24 hours), 8-patch pack = £6.06. Counselling, administration

Dose menopausal symptoms and osteoporosis prophylaxis (see section 6.6), 1 patch to be applied twice weekly continuously, with cyclical progestogen for 12–14 days of each cycle in women with a uterus; for menopausal symptoms, initiate therapy with *25 patch* for 3 months; for osteoporosis prophylaxis initiate therapy with *50 patch*; subsequently adjust according to response

Evorel® (Janssen) PoM

Patches, self-adhesive, estradiol, *'25' patch* (releasing approx. 25 micrograms/24 hours), net price 8-patch pack = £3.42; *'50' patch* (releasing approx. 50 micrograms/24 hours), 8-patch pack = £3.88, 24-patch pack = £11.66; *'75' patch* (releasing approx. 75 micrograms/24 hours), 8-patch pack = £4.12; *'100' patch* (releasing approx. 100 micrograms/24 hours), 8-patch pack = £4.28. Counselling, administration

Dose menopausal symptoms and osteoporosis prophylaxis (see section 6.6), 1 patch to be applied twice weekly continuously starting within 5 days of onset of menstruation (or at any time if cycles have ceased or are infrequent), with cyclical progestogen for 12–14 days of each cycle in women with a uterus; therapy should be initiated with *Evorel 50* patch; subsequently adjust according to response; dose may be reduced to *Evorel 25* patch after first month if necessary for menopausal symptoms **only**

FemSeven® (TEVA UK) PoM

Patches, self-adhesive, estradiol, *'50' patch* (releasing approx. 50 micrograms/24 hours), net price 4-patch pack = £6.04, 12-patch pack = £18.02; *'75' patch* (releasing approx. 75 micrograms/24 hours), net price 4-patch pack = £6.98; *'100' patch* (releasing approx. 100 micrograms/24 hours), net price 4-patch pack = £7.28. Counselling, administration

Dose menopausal symptoms and osteoporosis prophylaxis (see section 6.6), 1 patch to be applied once a week continuously, with cyclical progestogen for 12–14 days of each cycle in women with a uterus; initiate therapy with *FemSeven 50* patches for the first few months, subsequently adjust according to response

Oestrogel® (Besins) PoM

Gel, estradiol 0.06%, net price 64-dose pump pack = £4.80. Counselling, administration

Dose menopausal symptoms and osteoporosis prophylaxis (see section 6.6), 2 measures (estradiol 1.5 mg) to be applied over an area twice that of the template provided once daily continuously, starting within 5 days of menstruation (or anytime if cycles have ceased or are infrequent), with cyclical progestogen for at least 12 days of each cycle in women with a uterus; for menopausal symptoms may be increased if necessary after 1 month to max. 4 measures daily

Counselling Apply gel to clean, dry, intact skin such as arms, shoulders or inner thighs and allow to dry for 5 minutes before covering with clothing. Not to be applied on or near breasts or on vulval region. Avoid skin contact with another person (particularly male) and avoid other skin products or washing the area for at least 1 hour after application

Progynova® (Bayer) PoM

Tablets, s/c, estradiol valerate 1 mg (beige), net price 3 × 28-tab pack = £7.30; 2 mg (blue), 3 × 28-tab pack = £7.30

Dose menopausal symptoms, 1–2 mg daily continuously starting on day 1 of menstruation (or at any time if cycles have ceased or are infrequent); osteoporosis prophylaxis (see section 6.6), 2 mg daily continuously; with cyclical progestogen for 12–14 days of each cycle in women with a uterus

Progynova® TS (Bayer) PoM

Patches, self-adhesive, *Progynova® TS 50* (releasing estradiol approx. 50 micrograms/24 hours), net price 12-patch pack = £18.90; *Progynova® TS 100* (releasing estradiol approx. 100 micrograms/24 hours), 12-patch pack = £20.70. Counselling, administration

Dose menopausal symptoms and osteoporosis prophylaxis (see section 6.6), 1 patch to be applied once a week continuously *or* 1 patch per week for 3 weeks followed by a 7-day patch-free interval (cyclical); with cyclical progestogen for 12–14 days of each cycle in women with a uterus; initiate therapy with *Progynova TS 50*, subsequently adjust according to response

Note Women receiving *Progynova TS 100* patches for menopausal symptoms may continue with this strength for osteoporosis prophylaxis (see section 6.6)

Sandrena® (Orion) PoM

Gel, estradiol (0.1%), 500 microgram/500 mg sachet, net price 28-sachet pack = £5.08, 1 mg/1 g sachet, 28-sachet pack = £5.85. Counselling, administration

Excipients include propylene glycol (see section 13.1.3)

Dose menopausal symptoms, estradiol 1 mg (1 g gel) to be applied once daily over area 1–2 times size of hand; with cyclical progestogen for 12–14 days of each cycle in women with a uterus; dose may be adjusted after 2–3 cycles to lowest effective dose (usual dose of estradiol 0.5–1.5 mg (0.5–1.5 g gel) daily)

Counselling Apply gel to intact areas of skin such as lower trunk or thighs, using right and left sides on alternate days. Wash hands after application. Not to be applied on the breasts or face and avoid contact with eyes. Allow area of application to dry for 5 minutes and do not wash area for at least 1 hour

Zumenon® (Abbott Healthcare) PoM

Tablets, f/c, estradiol 1 mg, net price 84-tab pack = £6.89; 2 mg (red), 84-tab pack = £6.89

Dose menopausal symptoms, initially 1 mg daily starting within 5 days of onset of menstruation (or any time if cycles have ceased or are infrequent) increased to 2 mg daily if required; osteoporosis prophylaxis (see section 6.6), 2 mg daily; with cyclical progestogen for 12–14 days of each cycle in women with a uterus

◢ Estradiol, estriol and estrone

Hormonin® (AMCo) PoM

Tablets, pink, estradiol 600 micrograms, estriol 270 micrograms, estrone 1.4 mg, net price 84-tab pack = £7.93

Dose menopausal symptoms and osteoporosis prophylaxis (see section 6.6), 1–2 tablets daily starting within 5 days of onset of menstruation (or at any time if cycles have ceased or are infrequent), with cyclical progestogen for 12–14 days of each cycle in women with a uterus

Note *Hormonin®* tablets can be given continuously or cyclically (21 days out of 28)

◢ TIBOLONE

Indications short-term treatment of symptoms of oestrogen deficiency (including women being treated with gonadotrophin releasing hormone analogues); osteoporosis prophylaxis in women at high risk of fractures when other prophylaxis contra-indicated or not tolerated

Cautions see Hormone Replacement Therapy, p. 501 and under Oestrogens for HRT; vaginal bleeding (investigate for endometrial cancer if bleeding continues beyond 6 months or after stopping treatment); history of liver disease, epilepsy, migraine, diabetes mellitus, hypertriglyceridaemia; withdraw if signs of thromboembolic disease, abnormal liver function tests or cholestatic jaundice; see also Note below; **interactions:** Appendix 1 (tibolone)

Contra-indications　see notes above and under Oestrogens for HRT; history of cardiovascular or cerebrovascular disease (e.g. thrombophlebitis, thromboembolism), uninvestigated vaginal bleeding; acute porphyria (section 9.8.2)

Hepatic impairment　avoid in acute liver disease or if history of liver disease and liver function tests not returned to normal

Renal impairment　risk of fluid retention—patients with renal impairment should be closely monitored

Pregnancy　avoid; toxicity in *animal* studies

Breast-feeding　avoid

Side-effects　see notes above; also abdominal pain, weight changes, vaginal bleeding, leucorrhoea, facial hair, and *rarely* amnesia; gastro-intestinal disturbances, oedema, dizziness, headache, migraine, depression, breast cancer (see notes above and section 6.4.1.1), arthralgia, myalgia, visual disturbances, seborrhoeic dermatitis, rash and pruritus also reported

Dose

● 2.5 mg daily

　Note Unsuitable for use in the premenopause (unless being treated with gonadotrophin-releasing hormone analogue) and as (or with) an oral contraceptive; also unsuitable for use within 12 months of last menstrual period (may cause irregular bleeding). If transferring from cyclical HRT, start at end of regimen; if transferring from continuous-combined HRT, start at any time

Livial® (MSD) PoM
　Tablets, tibolone 2.5 mg, net price 28-tab pack = £10.36; 3 × 28-tab pack = £31.08

Ethinylestradiol

Ethinylestradiol (ethinyloestradiol) is licensed for short-term treatment of symptoms of oestrogen deficiency, for osteoporosis prophylaxis if other drugs (section 6.6) cannot be used and for the treatment of female hypogonadism and menstrual disorders.

Ethinylestradiol is occasionally used under **specialist supervision** for the management of *hereditary haemorrhagic telangiectasia* (but evidence of benefit is limited). Side-effects include nausea, fluid retention, and thrombosis. Impotence and gynaecomastia have been reported in men.

For use in prostate cancer, see section 8.3.1.

ETHINYLESTRADIOL
(Ethinyloestradiol)

Indications　see notes above

Cautions　cardiovascular disease (sodium retention with oedema, thromboembolism); see also under Combined Hormonal Contraceptives (section 7.3.1) and under Oestrogens for HRT (p. 502)

Contra-indications　see under Combined Hormonal Contraceptives (section 7.3.1) and under Oestrogens for HRT (p. 502)

Hepatic impairment　avoid; see also Combined Hormonal Contraceptives, section 7.3.1

Pregnancy　see Combined Hormonal Contraceptives, section 7.3.1

Breast-feeding　see Combined Hormonal Contraceptives, section 7.3.1

Side-effects　feminising effects in men; see also under Combined Hormonal Contraceptives (section 7.3.1) and under Oestrogens for HRT (p. 503)

Dose

● Menopausal symptoms and osteoporosis prophylaxis, (with progestogen for 12–14 days per cycle in women with intact uterus), 10–50 micrograms daily for 21 days, repeated after 7-day tablet-free period

● Female hypogonadism, 10–50 micrograms daily, usually on cyclical basis; initial oestrogen therapy should be followed by combined oestrogen and progestogen therapy

● Menstrual disorders, 20–50 micrograms daily from day 5 to 25 of each cycle, with progestogen added either throughout the cycle or from day 15 to 25

Ethinylestradiol (Non-proprietary) PoM
　Tablets, ethinylestradiol 10 micrograms, net price 21-tab pack = £200.00; 50 micrograms, 21-tab pack = £200.00; 1 mg, 28-tab pack = £200.00

Raloxifene

Raloxifene is licensed for the treatment and prevention of *postmenopausal osteoporosis*; unlike hormone replacement therapy, raloxifene does not reduce menopausal vasomotor symptoms.

Raloxifene may reduce the incidence of oestrogen-receptor-positive breast cancer but its role in established breast cancer is not yet clear. The manufacturer advises avoiding its use during treatment for breast cancer.

RALOXIFENE HYDROCHLORIDE

Indications　treatment and prevention of postmenopausal osteoporosis

Cautions　risk factors for venous thromboembolism (discontinue if prolonged immobilisation); risk factors for stroke; breast cancer (see notes above); history of oestrogen-induced hypertriglyceridaemia (monitor serum triglycerides); avoid in acute porphyria (section 9.8.2); **interactions:** Appendix 1 (raloxifene)

Contra-indications　history of venous thromboembolism, undiagnosed uterine bleeding, endometrial cancer, cholestasis

Hepatic impairment　avoid

Renal impairment　caution in mild to moderate impairment; avoid in severe impairment

Side-effects　hot flushes, leg cramps, peripheral oedema, influenza-like symptoms; *less commonly* venous thromboembolism, thrombophlebitis; *rarely* rashes, gastro-intestinal disturbances, hypertension, arterial thromboembolism, headache (including migraine), breast discomfort, thrombocytopenia

Dose

● 60 mg once daily

Evista® (Daiichi Sankyo) PoM
　Tablets, f/c, raloxifene hydrochloride 60 mg, net price 28-tab pack = £17.06; 84-tab pack = £59.59

6.4.1.2　Progestogens and progesterone receptor modulators

There are two main groups of progestogen, progesterone and its analogues (dydrogesterone and medroxyprogesterone) and testosterone analogues (norethisterone and norgestrel). The newer progestogens (desogestrel, norgestimate, and gestodene) are all derivatives of norgestrel; levonorgestrel is the active isomer of norgestrel and has twice its potency. Progesterone and its analogues are less androgenic than the testosterone derivatives and neither progesterone nor dydrogesterone causes virilisation.

Where endometriosis requires drug treatment, it may respond to a progestogen, e.g. norethisterone, administered on a continuous basis. Danazol and gonadorelin analogues are also available (section 6.7.2).

Although oral progestogens have been used widely for menorrhagia they are relatively ineffective compared with tranexamic acid (section 2.11) or, particularly where dysmenorrhoea is also a factor, mefenamic acid (section 10.1.1); the levonorgestrel-releasing intra-uterine system (section 7.3.2.3) may be particularly useful for women also requiring contraception. Oral progestogens have also been used for severe dysmenorrhoea, but where contraception is also required in younger women the best choice is a combined oral contraceptive (section 7.3.1).

Progestogens have also been advocated for the alleviation of premenstrual symptoms, but no convincing physiological basis for such treatment has been shown.

Progestogens have been used for the prevention of miscarriage in women with a history of recurrent miscarriage but there is no evidence of benefit and they are **not** recommended for this purpose. In pregnant women with antiphospholipid antibody syndrome who have suffered recurrent miscarriage, administration of low-dose aspirin (section 2.9) and a prophylactic dose of a low molecular weight heparin (section 2.8.1) may decrease the risk of fetal loss (use under specialist supervision only).

Hormone replacement therapy In women with a uterus a progestogen needs to be added to long-term oestrogen therapy for hormone replacement, to prevent cystic hyperplasia of the endometrium and possible transformation to cancer; it can be added on a cyclical or a continuous basis (see section 6.4.1.1). Combined packs incorporating suitable progestogen tablets are available, see p. 503.

Oral contraception Desogestrel, gestodene, levonorgestrel, norethisterone, and norgestimate are used in combined oral contraceptives and in progestogen-only contraceptives (section 7.3.1 and section 7.3.2).

Cancer Progestogens also have a role in neoplastic disease (section 8.3.2).

Cautions Progestogens should be used with caution in conditions that may worsen with fluid retention e.g. epilepsy, hypertension, migraine, asthma, or cardiac dysfunction, and in those susceptible to thromboembolism (particular caution with high dose). Care is also required in those with a history of depression. Progestogens can decrease glucose tolerance and patients with diabetes should be monitored closely. For **interactions** see Appendix 1 (progestogens).

Contra-indications Progestogens should be avoided in patients with a history of liver tumours. They are also contra-indicated in those with genital or breast cancer (unless progestogens are being used in the management of these conditions), severe arterial disease, undiagnosed vaginal bleeding and acute porphyria (section 9.8.2). Progestogens should not be used if there is a history during pregnancy of idiopathic jaundice, severe pruritus, or pemphigoid gestationis.

Side-effects Side-effects of progestogens include menstrual disturbances, premenstrual-like syndrome (including bloating, fluid retention, breast tenderness), weight change, nausea, headache, dizziness, insomnia, drowsiness, depression, change in libido; also skin reactions (including urticaria, pruritus, rash, and acne), hirsutism and alopecia. Jaundice and anaphylactoid reactions have also been reported.

DYDROGESTERONE

Indications HRT (section 6.4.1.1)

Cautions see notes above

Contra-indications see notes above

Hepatic impairment avoid; see also Combined Hormonal Contraceptives, section 7.3.1

Renal impairment use with caution

Pregnancy not known to be harmful

Breast-feeding present in milk—no adverse effects reported

Side-effects see notes above

Dose
- See under combined preparations (section 6.4.1.1)

MEDROXYPROGESTERONE ACETATE

Indications see under Dose; contraception (section 7.3.2.2); malignant disease (section 8.3.2)

Cautions see notes above

Contra-indications see notes above

Hepatic impairment section 8.3.2

Renal impairment use with caution

Pregnancy section 8.3.2

Breast-feeding section 8.3.2

Side-effects see notes above; indigestion

Dose
- By mouth, 2.5–10 mg daily for 5–10 days beginning on day 16 to 21 of cycle, repeated for 2 cycles in dysfunctional uterine bleeding and 3 cycles in secondary amenorrhoea
- Mild to moderate endometriosis, 10 mg 3 times daily for 90 consecutive days, beginning on day 1 of cycle
- Progestogenic opposition of oestrogen HRT, 10 mg daily for the last 14 days of each 28-day oestrogen HRT cycle

Provera® (Pharmacia) PoM
Tablets, all scored, medroxyprogesterone acetate 2.5 mg (orange), net price 30-tab pack = £1.84; 5 mg (blue), 10-tab pack = £1.23; 10 mg (white), 10-tab pack = £2.47, 90-tab pack = £22.16

Climanor® (ReSource Medical) PoM
Tablets, f/c, medroxyprogesterone acetate 5 mg, net price 28-tab pack = £3.27

◢**Combined preparations**
Section 6.4.1.1

NORETHISTERONE

Indications see under Dose; HRT (section 6.4.1.1); contraception (section 7.3.1 and section 7.3.2); malignant disease (section 8.3.2)

Cautions see notes above

Contra-indications see notes above

Hepatic impairment section 8.3.2

Renal impairment use with caution

Pregnancy section 8.3.2

Breast-feeding section 8.3.2

Side-effects see notes above

Dose

- Endometriosis, by mouth, 10–15 mg daily for 4–6 months or longer, starting on day 5 of cycle (if spotting occurs increase dose to 20–25 mg daily, reduced once bleeding has stopped)

- Dysfunctional uterine bleeding, menorrhagia (but see notes above), by mouth, 5 mg 3 times daily for 10 days to arrest bleeding; to prevent bleeding 5 mg twice daily from day 19 to 26

- Dysmenorrhoea (but see notes above), by mouth, 5 mg 3 times daily from day 5 to 24 for 3–4 cycles

- Premenstrual syndrome (but not recommended, see notes above), by mouth, 5 mg 2–3 times daily from day 19 to 26 for several cycles

- Postponement of menstruation, by mouth, 5 mg 3 times daily starting 3 days before expected onset (menstruation occurs 2–3 days after stopping)

Norethisterone (Non-proprietary) [PoM]

Tablets, norethisterone 5 mg, net price 30-tab pack = £2.23

Primolut N® (Bayer) [PoM]

Tablets, norethisterone 5 mg, net price 30-tab pack = £2.26

Utovlan® (Pharmacia) [PoM]

Tablets, norethisterone 5 mg, net price 30-tab pack = £1.40, 90-tab pack = £4.21

◄**Combined preparations**

Section 6.4.1.1

PROGESTERONE

Indications see under preparations

Cautions see notes above

Contra-indications see notes above; missed or incomplete miscarriage

Hepatic impairment avoid; see also Combined Hormonal Contraceptives, section 7.3.1

Renal impairment use with caution

Pregnancy not known to be harmful

Breast-feeding avoid—present in milk

Side-effects see notes above; injection-site reactions; *with rectal administration*, pain, diarrhoea and flatulence; *with vaginal administration*, local irritation

Dose

- See under preparations

Crinone® (Merck Serono) [PoM]

Vaginal gel, progesterone 90 mg/application (8%), net price 15 = £30.83

Dose by vagina, infertility due to inadequate luteal phase, insert 1 applicatorful daily starting either after documented ovulation or on day 18–21 of cycle. *In vitro* fertilisation, daily application continued for 30 days after laboratory evidence of pregnancy

Cyclogest® (Actavis) [PoM] ◢

Pessaries, progesterone 200 mg, net price 15 = £8.95; 400 mg, 15 = £12.96

Dose by vagina or rectum, premenstrual syndrome and post-natal depression, 200 mg daily to 400 mg twice daily; for premenstrual syndrome start on day 12–14 and continue until onset of menstruation (but not recommended, see notes above); rectally if barrier methods of contraception are used, in patients who have recently given birth or in those who suffer from vaginal infection or recurrent cystitis

Gestone® (Nordic) [PoM]

Injection, progesterone 50 mg/mL, net price 1-mL amp = £4.50, 2-mL amp = £4.50

Dose by deep intramuscular injection into buttock, dysfunctional uterine bleeding, 5–10 mg daily for 5–10 days until 2 days before expected onset of menstruation

Recurrent miscarriage due to inadequate luteal phase (but not recommended, see notes above) or following *in vitro* fertilisation *or* gamete intra-fallopian transfer, 25–100 mg 2–7 times a week from day 15, or day of embryo *or* gamete transfer, until 8–16 weeks of pregnancy; max. 200 mg daily

Lubion® (Pharmasure) [PoM]

Injection, progesterone, net price 25-mg vial = £8.00

Dose by subcutaneous *or* intramuscular injection, supplementation of luteal phase during assisted reproductive technology (ART) treatment in women for whom vaginal preparations are inappropriate, 25 mg once daily from day of oocyte retrieval up to week 12 of pregnancy

Utrogestan® (Besins) [PoM]

Capsules, progesterone (micronised) 100 mg, net price 30-cap pack = £5.13. Counselling, administration

Excipients include arachis (peanut) oil

Counselling Capsules should be taken at bedtime on an empty stomach

Dose by mouth, progestogenic opposition of oestrogen HRT 200 mg once daily on days 15–26, *or* 100 mg once daily on days 1–25, of each 28-day oestrogen HRT cycle

Vaginal capsule, progesterone (micronised) 200 mg, net price 21 vaginal capsules = £21.00

Excipients include arachis (peanut) oil

Dose by vagina, supplementation of luteal phase during assisted reproductive technology (ART) cycles, insert 1 vaginal capsule 3 times daily from day of embryo transfer until at least week 7 of pregnancy up to week 12 of pregnancy

---

Progesterone receptor modulators

Ulipristal acetate is a progesterone receptor modulator with a partial progesterone antagonist effect. Ulipristal is used in the pre-operative treatment of moderate to severe symptoms of uterine fibroids; it is also used as an hormonal emergency contraceptive (see section 7.3.5).

ULIPRISTAL ACETATE

Indications pre-operative treatment of moderate to severe symptoms of uterine fibroids

Cautions uncontrolled severe asthma; non-hormonal contraceptive methods (barrier methods or intra-uterine device) should be used during treatment and for 12 days after stopping, if required; **interactions:** see Appendix 1 (ulipristal)

Contra-indications undiagnosed vaginal bleeding, vaginal bleeding not caused by uterine fibroids; uterine, ovarian, cervical, or breast cancer

Hepatic impairment caution in moderate to severe impairment—no information available

Renal impairment caution in severe impairment—no information available

Pregnancy manufacturer advises avoid—no information available

Breast-feeding manufacturer advises avoid—no information available

Side-effects nausea, abdominal pain, oedema, hot flushes, headache, dizziness, malaise, menstrual disturbances, uterine haemorrhage, endometrial thickening, ovarian cyst (including rupture), breast pain, pelvic pain, myalgia, acne, hyperhidrosis; *less commonly* dyspepsia, dry mouth, flatulence, constipation, epistaxis, anxiety, urinary incontinence

Dose

● ADULT over 18 years, 5 mg daily for up to 3 months starting during the first week of menstruation; if necessary, repeat course once, starting during the second menstruation after first course completed; max. 2 courses of 3 months

Esmya® (Gedeon Richter) ▼ PoM
Tablets, ulipristal acetate 5 mg, net price 28-tab pack = £114.13

6.4.2 Male sex hormones and antagonists

Androgens cause masculinisation; they may be used as replacement therapy in castrated adults and in those who are hypogonadal due to either pituitary or testicular disease. In the normal male they inhibit pituitary gonadotrophin secretion and depress spermatogenesis. Androgens also have an anabolic action which led to the development of anabolic steroids (section 6.4.3).

Androgens are useless as a treatment of impotence and impaired spermatogenesis unless there is associated hypogonadism; they should not be given until the hypogonadism has been properly investigated. Treatment should be under expert supervision.

When given to patients with hypopituitarism they can lead to normal sexual development and potency but not to fertility. If fertility is desired, the usual treatment is with gonadotrophins or pulsatile gonadotrophin-releasing hormone (section 6.5.1) which will stimulate spermatogenesis as well as androgen production.

Caution should be used when androgens or chorionic gonadotrophin are used in treating boys with delayed puberty since the fusion of epiphyses is hastened and may result in short stature; skeletal maturation should be monitored.

Intramuscular depot preparations of **testosterone esters** are preferred for replacement therapy. Testosterone enantate, propionate or undecanoate, or alternatively *Sustanon®*, which consists of a mixture of testosterone esters and has a longer duration of action, may be used. Satisfactory replacement therapy can sometimes be obtained with 1 mL of *Sustanon 250®*, given by intramuscular injection once a month, although more frequent dose intervals are often necessary.

▉ TESTOSTERONE AND ESTERS

Indications see under preparations
Cautions cardiac impairment, elderly, ischaemic heart disease, hypertension, epilepsy, migraine, diabetes mellitus, skeletal metastases (risk of hypercalcaemia), undertake regular examination of the prostate and breast during treatment; monitor full blood count, lipid profile and liver function; pre-pubertal boys (see notes above and under Side-effects); **interactions**: Appendix 1 (testosterone)
Women Regularly assess for androgenic side-effects; women should be advised to report any signs of virilisation e.g. deepening of the voice or hirsutism

Contra-indications breast cancer in men, prostate cancer, history of primary liver tumours, hypercalcaemia, nephrotic syndrome
Hepatic impairment avoid if possible—fluid retention and dose-related toxicity
Renal impairment caution—potential for fluid retention
Pregnancy avoid; causes masculinisation of female fetus
Breast-feeding avoid; may cause masculinisation in the female infant or precocious development in the male infant; high doses suppress lactation
Side-effects prostate abnormalities and prostate cancer, headache, depression, gastro-intestinal bleeding, nausea, vomiting, cholestatic jaundice, changes in libido, gynaecomastia, polycythaemia, anxiety, irritability, nervousness, asthenia, paraesthesia, hypertension, electrolyte disturbances including sodium retention with oedema and hypercalcaemia, weight gain; increased bone growth; muscle cramps, arthralgia; androgenic effects such as hirsutism, male-pattern baldness, seborrhoea, acne, pruritus, excessive frequency and duration of penile erection, precocious sexual development and premature closure of epiphyses in pre-pubertal males, suppression of spermatogenesis in men and virilism in women; *rarely* liver tumours; sleep apnoea also reported; *with buccal tablets and gel*, local irritation and allergic reactions, and taste disturbances
Dose
● See under preparations

▉ Oral

Restandol® Testocaps (MSD) CD4-2
Capsules, orange, testosterone undecanoate 40 mg in oily solution, net price 30-cap pack = £8.55; 60-cap pack = £17.10. Label: 21, 25
Dose androgen deficiency, 120–160 mg daily for 2–3 weeks; maintenance 40–120 mg daily

▉ Buccal

Striant® SR (The Urology Co.) CD4-2
Mucoadhesive buccal tablets, m/r, testosterone 30 mg, net price 60-tab pack = £28.00. Counselling, see under Dose below
Dose hypogonadism, 30 mg every 12 hours; CHILD and ADOLESCENT under 18 years not recommended
Counselling Place rounded side of tablet on gum above front teeth and hold lip firmly over the gum for 30 seconds. If tablet detaches within 4 hours of next dose, replace with new tablet which is considered the second dose for the day.

▉ Intramuscular

Testosterone Enantate (Non-proprietary) CD4-2
Injection (oily), testosterone enantate 250 mg/mL, net price 1-mL amp = £19.62
Dose by slow intramuscular injection, hypogonadism, initially 250 mg every 2–3 weeks; maintenance 250 mg every 3–6 weeks
Breast cancer, 250 mg every 2–3 weeks

Nebido® (Bayer) CD4-2
Injection (oily), testosterone undecanoate 250 mg/mL, net price 4-mL amp = £80.00; 4-mL vial = £80.00
Dose by deep intramuscular injection over 2 minutes, hypogonadism in men over 18 years, 1 g every 10–14 weeks; if necessary, second dose may be given after 6 weeks to achieve rapid steady state plasma testosterone levels and then every 10–14 weeks

Sustanon 250® (Aspen) CD4-2

Injection (oily), testosterone propionate 30 mg, testosterone phenylpropionate 60 mg, testosterone isocaproate 60 mg, and testosterone decanoate 100 mg/mL, net price 1-mL amp = £2.45

Excipients include arachis (peanut) oil, benzyl alcohol (see Excipients p. 2)

Dose by deep intramuscular injection, androgen deficiency, 1 mL usually every 3 weeks

Virormone® (Nordic) CD4-2

Injection, testosterone propionate 50 mg/mL, net price 2-mL amp = £4.50

Dose by intramuscular injection, androgen deficiency, 50 mg 2–3 times weekly

Delayed puberty, 50 mg weekly

Breast cancer in women, 100 mg 2–3 times weekly

◢**Transdermal preparations**

Testim® (Ferring) CD4-2

Gel, testosterone 50 mg/5 g tube, net price 30-tube pack = £32.00. Counselling, administration

Excipients include propylene glycol (see section 13.1.3)

Dose hypogonadism due to testosterone deficiency in men (over 18 years), 50 mg testosterone (5 g gel) applied once daily; subsequent application adjusted according to response; max. 100 mg (10 g gel) daily

Counselling Squeeze entire content of tube on to one palm and apply as a thin layer on clean, dry, healthy skin of shoulder or upper arm, preferably in the morning after washing or bathing (if 2 tubes required use 1 per shoulder or upper arm); rub in and allow to dry before putting on clothing to cover site; wash hands with soap after application; avoid washing application site for at least 6 hours

Avoid skin contact with application sites to prevent testosterone transfer to other people, especially pregnant women and children—consult product literature

Testogel® (Besins) CD4-2

Gel, testosterone 50 mg/5 g sachet, net price 30-sachet pack = £31.11. Counselling, administration

Dose hypogonadism due to androgen deficiency in men (over 18 years), 50 mg testosterone (5 g gel) to be applied once daily; subsequent application adjusted according to response in 25-mg (2.5 g gel) increments to max. 100 mg (10 g gel) daily

Counselling Apply thin layer of gel on clean, dry, healthy skin such as shoulders, arms or abdomen, immediately after sachet is opened. Not to be applied on genital area as high alcohol content may cause local irritation. Allow to dry for 3–5 minutes before dressing. Wash hands with soap and water after applying gel, avoid shower or bath for at least 6 hours

Avoid skin contact with gel application sites to prevent testosterone transfer to other people, especially pregnant women and children—consult product literature

Tostran® (ProStrakan) CD4-2

Gel, testosterone 2% (10 mg/metered application), net price 60-g multidose dispenser = £28.67. Counselling, administration

Excipients include butylhydroxytoluene, propylene glycol (see section 13.1.3)

Dose hypogonadism due to testosterone deficiency in men (over 18 years), initially 60 mg testosterone (3 g gel) applied once daily; subsequent applications adjusted according to response; max. 80 mg (4 g gel) daily

Counselling Apply gel on clean, dry, intact skin of abdomen or both inner thighs, preferably in the morning. Gently rub in with a finger until dry before dressing. Wash hands with soap and water after applying gel; avoid washing application site for at least 2 hours. Not to be applied on genital area.

Avoid skin contact with gel application sites to prevent testosterone transfer to other people, especially pregnant women and children—consult product literature

MESTEROLONE

Indications see under Dose

Cautions see under Testosterone and Esters

Contra-indications see under Testosterone and Esters

Hepatic impairment see under Testosterone and Esters

Renal impairment see under Testosterone and Esters

Pregnancy see under Testosterone and Esters

Breast-feeding see under Testosterone and Esters

Side-effects see under Testosterone and Esters but spermatogenesis unimpaired

Dose

• Androgen deficiency and male infertility associated with hypogonadism, 25 mg 3–4 times daily for several months, reduced to 50–75 mg daily in divided doses for maintenance; CHILD not recommended

Pro-Viron® (Bayer) CD4-2

Tablets, scored, mesterolone 25 mg. Net price 30-tab pack = £4.19

Anti-androgens

Cyproterone acetate

Cyproterone acetate is an anti-androgen used in the treatment of severe hypersexuality and sexual deviation in the male. It inhibits spermatogenesis and produces reversible infertility (but is not a male contraceptive); abnormal sperm forms are produced. Fully informed consent is recommended and an initial spermatogram. As hepatic tumours have been produced in *animal* studies, careful consideration should be given to the risk/benefit ratio before treatment. Cyproterone acetate is also used as an adjunct in prostatic cancer (section 8.3.4.2) and in the treatment of acne and hirsutism in women (section 13.6.2).

CYPROTERONE ACETATE

Indications see notes above; prostate cancer (section 8.3.4.2)

Cautions ineffective for male hypersexuality in chronic alcoholism (relevance to prostate cancer not known); blood counts initially and throughout treatment; monitor hepatic function regularly (liver function tests should be performed before treatment, see also under Side-effects below); monitor adrenocortical function regularly; diabetes mellitus (see also Contra-indications)

Driving Fatigue and lassitude may impair performance of skilled tasks (e.g. driving)

Contra-indications (do not apply in prostate cancer), severe diabetes (with vascular changes), sickle-cell anaemia, liver-disease including Dubin-Johnson and Rotor syndromes, previous or existing liver tumours, malignant or wasting diseases, meningioma or history of meningioma, severe depression, history of thromboembolic disorders; youths under 18 years (may arrest bone maturation and testicular development)

Hepatic impairment avoid—dose-related toxicity; see also side-effects, p. 657

Side-effects fatigue and lassitude, breathlessness, weight changes, reduced sebum production (may clear acne), changes in hair pattern, gynaecomastia (rarely leading to galactorrhoea and benign breast nodules); rarely hypersensitivity reactions, rash and

6

Endocrine system

osteoporosis; inhibition of spermatogenesis (see notes above); hepatotoxicity reported (including jaundice, hepatitis and hepatic failure (fatalities reported at dosages of 100 mg and above, usually in men treated for advanced prostate cancer), see section 8.3.4.2 for details and warnings)

Dose

- ADULT over 18 years, male hypersexuality, 50 mg twice daily after food

Cyproterone Acetate (Non-proprietary) (PoM)

Tablets, cyproterone acetate 50 mg, net price 56-tab pack = £29.00. Label: 21, counselling, driving

Androcur® (Bayer) (PoM)

Tablets, scored, cyproterone acetate 50 mg, net price 56-tab pack = £29.25. Label: 21, counselling, driving

Dutasteride and finasteride

Dutasteride and **finasteride** are specific inhibitors of the enzyme 5α-reductase, which metabolises testosterone into the more potent androgen, dihydrotestosterone. This inhibition of testosterone metabolism leads to reduction in prostate size, with improvement in urinary flow rate and in obstructive symptoms. Dutasteride and finasteride are alternatives to alpha-blockers (section 7.4.1) particularly in men with a significantly enlarged prostate. Finasteride is also licensed for use with doxazosin in the management of benign prostatic hyperplasia.

A low strength of finasteride is licensed for treating male-pattern baldness in men (section 13.9).

Cautions Dutasteride and finasteride decrease serum concentration of prostate cancer markers such as prostate-specific antigen; reference values may need adjustment. Both dutasteride and finasteride are excreted in semen and use of a condom is recommended if sexual partner is pregnant or likely to become pregnant. Women of childbearing potential should avoid handling crushed or broken tablets of finasteride and leaking capsules of dutasteride.

Side-effects The side-effects of dutasteride and finasteride include impotence, decreased libido, ejaculation disorders, and breast tenderness and enlargement.

◢ DUTASTERIDE

Indications benign prostatic hyperplasia

Cautions see notes above; **interactions:** Appendix 1 (dutasteride)

Male breast cancer Cases of male breast cancer have been reported. Patients or their carers should be told to promptly report to their doctor any changes in breast tissue such as lumps, pain, or nipple discharge

Hepatic impairment avoid in severe impairment—no information available

Side-effects see notes above

Dose

- 500 micrograms daily, review treatment at 3–6 months and then every 6–12 months (may require several months treatment before benefit is obtained)

Avodart® (GSK) (PoM)

Capsules, yellow, dutasteride 500 micrograms, net price 30-cap pack = £16.80. Label: 25

◢ **With tamsulosin**

Section 7.4.1

◢ FINASTERIDE

Indications benign prostatic hyperplasia; male-pattern baldness in men (section 13.9)

Cautions see notes above; also obstructive uropathy

Male breast cancer Cases of male breast cancer have been reported. Patients or their carers should be told to promptly report to their doctor any changes in breast tissue such as lumps, pain, or nipple discharge

Side-effects see notes above; also testicular pain, hypersensitivity reactions (including lip and face swelling, pruritus and rash); male breast cancer also reported (see Cautions above)

Dose

- 5 mg daily, review treatment at 3–6 months and then every 6–12 months (may require several months' treatment before benefit is obtained)

Finasteride (Non-proprietary) (PoM)

Tablets, finasteride 5 mg, net price 28-tab pack = £1.73

Proscar® (MSD) (PoM)

Tablets, blue, f/c, finasteride 5 mg, net price 28-tab pack = £13.94

6.4.3 Anabolic steroids

Anabolic steroids have some androgenic activity but they cause less virilisation than androgens in women. They are used in the treatment of some *aplastic anaemias* (section 9.1.3). Anabolic steroids have been given for osteoporosis in women but they are no longer advocated for this purpose.

The protein-building properties of anabolic steroids have not proved beneficial in the clinical setting. Their use as body builders or tonics is unjustified; some athletes abuse them.

◢ NANDROLONE

Indications osteoporosis in postmenopausal women (but not recommended, see notes above); aplastic anaemia (section 9.1.3)

Cautions cardiac impairment, hypertension, diabetes mellitus, epilepsy, migraine; monitor skeletal maturation in young patients; skeletal metastases (risk of hypercalcaemia); **interactions:** Appendix 1 (anabolic steroids)

Contra-indications prostate cancer, male breast cancer, acute porphyria (section 9.8.2)

Hepatic impairment use in severe hepatic impairment only if benefit outweighs risk

Renal impairment use with caution—may cause sodium and water retention

Side-effects acne, sodium retention with oedema, virilisation with high doses including voice changes (sometimes irreversible), amenorrhoea, inhibition of spermatogenesis, premature epiphyseal closure; abnormal liver-function tests reported with high doses; liver tumours reported occasionally on prolonged treatment with anabolic steroids

Dose

- See below

Deca-Durabolin® (Aspen) [CD4-2]
Injection (oily), nandrolone decanoate 50 mg/mL, net price 1-mL amp = £3.17
Excipients include arachis (peanut) oil, benzyl alcohol (see Excipients, p. 2)
Dose by deep intramuscular injection, 50 mg every 3 weeks

6.5 Hypothalamic and pituitary hormones and anti-oestrogens

6.5.1 Hypothalamic and anterior pituitary hormones and anti-oestrogens

6.5.2 Posterior pituitary hormones and antagonists

> Use of preparations in these sections requires detailed prior investigation of the patient and *should be reserved for specialist centres*.

6.5.1 Hypothalamic and anterior pituitary hormones and anti-oestrogens

Anti-oestrogens

The anti-oestrogens **clomifene** (clomiphene) and **tamoxifen** (section 8.3.4.1) are used in the treatment of female infertility due to oligomenorrhoea or secondary amenorrhoea (e.g. associated with polycystic ovarian disease). They induce gonadotrophin release by occupying oestrogen receptors in the hypothalamus, thereby interfering with feedback mechanisms; chorionic gonadotrophin is sometimes used as an adjunct. Patients should be warned that there is a risk of multiple pregnancy (*rarely* more than twins).

CLOMIFENE CITRATE
(Clomiphene Citrate)

Indications anovulatory infertility—see notes above
Cautions see notes above; polycystic ovary syndrome (cysts may enlarge during treatment, also risk of exaggerated response to usual doses), ovarian hyperstimulation syndrome, uterine fibroids, ectopic pregnancy, incidence of multiple births increased (consider ultrasound monitoring), visual symptoms (discontinue and initiate ophthalmological examination)
CSM Advice The CSM has recommended that clomifene should not normally be used for longer than 6 cycles (possibly increased risk of ovarian cancer)
Contra-indications ovarian cysts, hormone-dependent tumours or abnormal uterine bleeding of undetermined cause
Hepatic impairment avoid in severe liver disease
Pregnancy exclude pregnancy before treatment; possible effects on fetal development
Breast-feeding may inhibit lactation
Side-effects visual disturbances (withdraw), ovarian hyperstimulation (withdraw), hot flushes, abdominal discomfort, occasionally nausea, vomiting, depression, insomnia, breast tenderness, headache, inter-

menstrual spotting, menorrhagia, endometriosis, convulsions, weight gain, rashes, dizziness, hair loss
Dose
● 50 mg daily for 5 days, starting within about 5 days of onset of menstruation (preferably on 2nd day) or at any time (normally preceded by a progestogen-induced withdrawal bleed) if cycles have ceased; second course of 100 mg daily for 5 days may be given in absence of ovulation; most patients who are going to respond will do so to first course; 3 courses should constitute adequate therapeutic trial; long-term cyclical therapy not recommended—see CSM advice, above

Clomifene (Non-proprietary) [PoM]
Tablets, clomifene citrate 50 mg, net price 30-tab pack = £21.74

Clomid® (Sanofi-Aventis) [PoM]
Tablets, yellow, scored, clomifene citrate 50 mg. Net price 30-tab pack = £8.46

Anterior pituitary hormones

Corticotrophins

Tetracosactide (tetracosactrin), an analogue of corticotropin (ACTH), is used to test adrenocortical function; failure of the plasma cortisol concentration to rise after administration of tetracosactide indicates adrenocortical insufficiency.

Both corticotropin and tetracosactide were formerly used as alternatives to corticosteroids in conditions such as Crohn's disease or rheumatoid arthritis; their value was limited by the variable and unpredictable therapeutic response and by the waning of their effect with time.

TETRACOSACTIDE
(Tetracosactrin)

Indications see notes above
Cautions as for corticosteroids, section 6.3.2; **important**: risk of anaphylaxis (medical supervision; consult product literature); history of atopic allergy (e.g. asthma, eczema, hayfever); history of hypersensitivity; **interactions**: Appendix 1 (corticosteroids)
Contra-indications as for corticosteroids, section 6.3.2; avoid injections containing benzyl alcohol in neonates (see under preparations); history of hypersensitivity to corticotrophins
Hepatic impairment see section 6.3.2
Renal impairment see section 6.3.2
Pregnancy avoid (but may be used diagnostically if essential)
Breast-feeding avoid (but may be used diagnostically if essential)
Side-effects as for corticosteroids, section 6.3.2
Dose
● See under preparations below

Synacthen® (Alliance) [PoM]
Injection, tetracosactide 250 micrograms (as acetate)/mL. Net price 1-mL amp = £2.93
Dose diagnostic (30-minute test), by intramuscular *or* intravenous injection, 250 micrograms as a single dose

Synacthen Depot® (Alliance) [PoM]
Injection (aqueous suspension), tetracosactide
acetate 1 mg/mL, with zinc phosphate complex. Net
price 1-mL amp = £4.18

Excipients include benzyl alcohol (avoid in neonates, see
Excipients p. 2)

Dose diagnostic (5-hour test), by intramuscular injection,
1 mg as a single dose

Note Formerly used therapeutically by intramuscular
injection, in an initial dose of 1 mg daily (or every 12 hours in
acute cases); reduced to 1 mg every 2–3 days, then 1 mg
weekly (or 500 micrograms every 2–3 days) but value was
limited (see notes above)

Gonadotrophins

Follicle-stimulating hormone (FSH) and luteinising
hormone (LH) together (as in **human menopausal
gonadotrophin**), follicle-stimulating hormone alone
(as in **follitropin**), or chorionic gonadotrophin, are
used in the treatment of infertility in women with proven
hypopituitarism or who have not responded to clomifene, or in superovulation treatment for assisted conception (such as *in vitro* fertilisation).

The gonadotrophins are also occasionally used in the
treatment of hypogonadotrophic hypogonadism and
associated oligospermia. There is no justification for
their use in primary gonadal failure.

Chorionic gonadotrophin has also been used in delayed
puberty in the male to stimulate endogenous testosterone production, but has little advantage over testosterone (section 6.4.2).

■ CHORIONIC GONADOTROPHIN
(Human Chorionic Gonadotrophin; HCG)

A preparation of a glycoprotein fraction secreted by the
placenta and obtained from the urine of pregnant women
having the action of the pituitary luteinising hormone

Indications see notes above

Cautions cardiac impairment, asthma, epilepsy,
migraine; prepubertal boys (risk of premature epiphyseal closure or precocious puberty)

Contra-indications androgen-dependent tumours

Renal impairment use with caution

Side-effects oedema (particularly in males—reduce
dose), headache, tiredness, mood changes, gynaecomastia, local reactions; may aggravate ovarian
hyperstimulation, multiple pregnancy

Dose
• By subcutaneous *or* intramuscular injection, according to patient's response

Choragon® (Ferring) [CD4-2]
Injection, powder for reconstitution, chorionic
gonadotrophin. Net price 5000-unit amp (with solvent) = £3.26. For intramuscular injection

Pregnyl® (MSD) [CD4-2]
Injection, powder for reconstitution, chorionic
gonadotrophin. Net price 1500-unit amp = £2.12;
5000-unit amp = £3.15 (both with solvent). For subcutaneous or intramuscular injection

■ CHORIOGONADOTROPIN ALFA
(Human chorionic gonadotropin)

Indications see notes above

Cautions acute porphyria (section 9.8.2)

Contra-indications ovarian enlargement or cyst
(unless caused by polycystic ovarian disease); ectopic
pregnancy in previous 3 months; active thromboembolic disorders; hypothalamus, pituitary, ovarian,
uterine or mammary malignancy

Side-effects nausea, vomiting, abdominal pain;
headache, tiredness; injection-site reactions; ovarian
hyperstimulation syndrome; rarely diarrhoea,
depression, irritability, breast pain; ectopic pregnancy
and ovarian torsion reported

Dose
• By subcutaneous injection, according to patient's
response

Ovitrelle® (Merck Serono) [CD4-2]
Injection, choriogonadotropin alfa, net price 6500-
unit/0.5 mL (250-micrograms/0.5 mL) prefilled
syringe or prefilled pen = £31.38

■ CORIFOLLITROPIN ALFA

Indications controlled ovarian stimulation in combination with a gonadotrophin-releasing hormone
antagonist

Cautions risk factors for thromboembolism; risk of
ovarian hyperstimulation syndrome; acute porphyria
(section 9.8.2)

Contra-indications ovarian enlargement or cyst;
polycystic ovarian syndrome; tumours of hypothalamus, pituitary, ovaries, uterus, or breast; vaginal
bleeding of unknown cause; history of ovarian
hyperstimulation syndrome

Renal impairment avoid

Breast-feeding avoid

Side-effects nausea; headache, fatigue; ovarian
hyperstimulation, pelvic pain, breast pain; *less commonly* vomiting, abdominal distension and pain,
diarrhoea, constipation, dizziness, ovarian torsion;
also reported ectopic pregnancy, miscarriage, and
multiple pregnancies

Dose
• By subcutaneous injection, body-weight under 60 kg,
100 micrograms; body-weight over 60 kg, 150 micrograms

Elonva® (MSD) ▼ [PoM]
Injection, prefilled syringe, corifollitropin alfa, net
price 100 micrograms/0.5 mL = £638.00; 150 micr-
ograms/0.5 mL = £638.00

■ FOLLITROPIN ALFA and BETA
(Recombinant human follicle stimulating hormone)

Indications see notes above

Cautions acute porphyria (section 9.8.2)

Contra-indications see under Human Menopausal
Gonadotrophins

Pregnancy avoid

Breast-feeding avoid

Side-effects see under Human Menopausal Gonadotrophins

Dose
• By subcutaneous *or* intramuscular injection, according to patient's response

◢ **Follitropin alfa**

Gonal-F® (Merck Serono) PoM
Injection, powder for reconstitution, follitropin alfa. Net price 75-unit amp = £21.02; 450 units/0.75 mL, multidose vial = £126.10; 1050 units/1.75 mL, multi-dose vial = £294.22 (all with solvent). For subcutaneous injection

Injection, prefilled pen, follitropin alfa 600 units/mL, net price 0.5 mL (300 units) = £94.00, 0.75 mL (450 units) = £141.00, 1.5 mL (900 units) = £282.00. For subcutaneous injection

◢ **Follitropin alfa with lutropin alfa**

Pergoveris® (Merck Serono) PoM
Injection, powder for reconstitution, follitropin alfa 150 units (11 micrograms), lutropin alfa 75 units (3 micrograms), net price per vial (with solvent) = £60.29. For subcutaneous injection
Electrolytes Na⁺<1 mmol/vial

◢ **Follitropin beta**

Puregon® (MSD) PoM
Injection, follitropin beta 100 units/mL, net price 0.5-mL (50-unit) vial = £18.03; 200 units/mL, 0.5-mL (100-unit) vial = £36.06; 0.36-mL (300-unit) cartridge = £97.41, 0.72-mL (600-unit) cartridge = £194.82, 1.08-mL (900-unit) cartridge = £292.23, (cartridges for use with *Puregon®* pen). For subcutaneous (cartridges and vials) or intramuscular injection (vials)
Excipients may include neomycin and streptomycin

■ **HUMAN MENOPAUSAL GONADOTROPHINS**

Indications see notes above
Cautions acute porphyria (section 9.8.2)
Contra-indications ovarian cysts (not caused by polycystic ovarian syndrome); tumours of pituitary, hypothalamus, breast, uterus, ovaries, testes or prostate; vaginal bleeding of unknown cause
Pregnancy avoid
Breast-feeding avoid
Side-effects ovarian hyperstimulation, increased risk of multiple pregnancy and miscarriage, hypersensitivity reactions, gastro-intestinal disturbances, headache, joint pain, fever, injection site reactions, *very rarely* thromboembolism; gynaecomastia, acne, and weight gain reported in men
Dose
● By deep intramuscular *or* subcutaneous injection, according to patient's response

◢ **Menotrophin**

Purified extract of human post-menopausal urine containing follicle-stimulating hormone (FSH) and luteinising hormone (LH) in a ratio of 1:1

Merional® (Pharmasure) PoM
Injection, powder for reconstitution, menotrophin as follicle-stimulating hormone 75 units and luteinising hormone 75 units, net price per vial (with solvent) = £27.90; follicle-stimulating hormone 150 units, luteinising hormone 150 units, net price per vial (with solvent) = £55.80. For intramuscular or subcutaneous injection

Menopur® (Ferring) PoM
Injection, powder for reconstitution, menotrophin as follicle-stimulating hormone 75 units and luteinising hormone 75 units, net price per vial (with solvent) = £16.38; follicle-stimulating hormone 150 units and luteinising hormone 150 units, net price per vial (with solvent) = £32.76; follicle-stimulating hormone 600 units and luteinising hormone 600 units, net price per multidose vial (with solvent) = £131.04; follicle-stimulating hormone 1200 units and luteinising hormone 1200 units, net price per multidose vial (with solvent) = £262.08. For intramuscular or subcutaneous injection

◢ **Urofollitropin**

Purified extract of human post-menopausal urine containing follicle-stimulating hormone (FSH)

Fostimon® (Pharmasure) PoM
Injection, powder for reconstitution, urofollitropin as follicle-stimulating hormone 75 units, net price per vial (with solvent) = £27.90; follicle-stimulating hormone 150 units, net price per vial (with solvent) = £55.80. For intramuscular or subcutaneous injection

■ **LUTROPIN ALFA**
(Recombinant human luteinising hormone)

Indications see notes above
Cautions acute porphyria (section 9.8.2)
Contra-indications ovarian enlargement or cyst (unless caused by polycystic ovarian disease); undiagnosed vaginal bleeding; tumours of hypothalamus and pituitary; ovarian, uterine or mammary carcinoma
Side-effects nausea, vomiting, abdominal and pelvic pain; headache, somnolence; injection-site reactions; ovarian hyperstimulation syndrome, ovarian cyst, breast pain, ectopic pregnancy; thromboembolism; adnexal torsion, and haemoperitoneum
Dose
● By subcutaneous injection, in conjunction with follicle-stimulating hormone, according to response

Luveris® (Merck Serono) PoM
Injection, powder for reconstitution, lutropin alfa, net price 75-unit vial = £31.38 (with solvent)

Growth hormone

Growth hormone is used to treat deficiency of the hormone in children and in adults (see NICE guidance below). In children it is used in Prader-Willi syndrome, Turner syndrome, chronic renal insufficiency, short children considered small for gestational age at birth, and short stature homeobox-containing gene (SHOX) deficiency.

Growth hormone of human origin (HGH; somatotrophin) has been replaced by a growth hormone of human sequence, **somatropin**, produced using recombinant DNA technology.

6
Endocrine system

Endocrine system

6

NICE guidance
Somatropin for the treatment of growth failure in children (May 2010)

Somatropin is recommended for children with growth failure who:

- have growth-hormone deficiency;
- have Turner syndrome;
- have Prader-Willi syndrome;
- have chronic renal insufficiency;
- are born small for gestational age with subsequent growth failure at 4 years of age or later;
- have short stature homeobox-containing gene (SHOX) deficiency.

Treatment should be discontinued if growth velocity increases by less than 50% from baseline in the first year of treatment.

www.nice.org.uk/TA188

NICE guidance
Somatropin for adults with growth hormone deficiency (August 2003)

Somatropin is recommended in adults **only** if the following 3 criteria are fulfilled:

- Severe growth hormone deficiency, established by an appropriate method,
- Impaired quality of life, measured by means of a specific questionnaire,
- Already receiving treatment for another pituitary hormone deficiency.

Somatropin treatment should be discontinued if the quality of life has not improved sufficiently by 9 months.

Severe growth hormone deficiency developing after linear growth is complete but before the age of 25 years should be treated with growth hormone; treatment should continue until adult peak bone mass has been achieved. Treatment for adult-onset growth hormone deficiency should be stopped only when the patient and the patient's physician consider it appropriate.

Treatment with somatropin should be initiated and managed by a physician with expertise in growth hormone disorders; maintenance treatment can be prescribed in the community under a shared-care protocol.

www.nice.org.uk/TA64

Mecasermin, a human insulin-like growth factor-I (rhIGF-I), is licensed to treat growth failure in children and adolescents with severe primary insulin-like growth factor-I deficiency (section 6.7.4).

▌ SOMATROPIN
(Recombinant Human Growth Hormone)

Indications see under Dose

Cautions diabetes mellitus (adjustment of antidiabetic therapy may be necessary), papilloedema (see under Side-effects), relative deficiencies of other pituitary hormones (notably hypothyroidism—manufacturers recommend periodic thyroid function tests but limited evidence of clinical value), history of malignant disease, disorders of the epiphysis of the hip (monitor for limping), resolved intracranial hypertension (monitor closely), initiation of treatment close to puberty not

recommended in child born small for gestational age; Silver-Russell syndrome; rotate subcutaneous injection sites to prevent lipoatrophy; **interactions:** Appendix 1 (somatropin)

Contra-indications evidence of tumour activity (complete antitumour therapy and ensure intracranial lesions inactive before starting); not to be used after renal transplantation or for growth promotion in children with closed epiphyses (or near closure in Prader-Willi syndrome); severe obesity or severe respiratory impairment in Prader-Willi syndrome

Pregnancy discontinue if pregnancy occurs—no information available

Breast-feeding no information available

Side-effects headache, funduscopy for papilloedema recommended if severe or recurrent headache, visual problems, nausea and vomiting occur—if papilloedema confirmed consider benign intracranial hypertension (rare cases reported); fluid retention (peripheral oedema), arthralgia, myalgia, carpal tunnel syndrome, paraesthesia, antibody formation, hypothyroidism, insulin resistance, hyperglycaemia, hypoglycaemia, reactions at injection site; leukaemia in children with growth hormone deficiency also reported

Dose

- Gonadal dysgenesis (Turner syndrome), by subcutaneous injection, 45–50 micrograms/kg daily *or* 1.4 mg/m^2 daily
- Deficiency of growth hormone in children, by subcutaneous *or* intramuscular injection, 23–39 micrograms/kg daily *or* 0.7–1 mg/m^2 daily
- Growth disturbance in short children born small for gestational age whose growth has not caught up by 4 years or later, by subcutaneous injection, 35 micrograms/kg daily *or* 1 mg/m^2 daily
- Prader-Willi syndrome, by subcutaneous injection in children with growth velocity greater than 1 cm/year, in combination with energy-restricted diet, 35 micrograms/kg daily *or* 1 mg/m^2 daily; max. 2.7 mg daily
- Chronic renal insufficiency in children (renal function decreased to less than 50%), by subcutaneous injection, 45–50 micrograms/kg daily *or* 1.4 mg/m^2 daily (higher doses may be needed) adjusted if necessary after 6 months
- Adult growth hormone deficiency, by subcutaneous injection, initially 150–300 micrograms daily, gradually increased if required to max. 1 mg daily; use minimum effective dose (requirements may decrease with age)
- SHOX deficiency in children, by subcutaneous injection, 45–50 micrograms/kg daily

Note Dose formerly expressed in units; somatropin 1 mg ≡ 3 units

Genotropin® (Pharmacia) CD4-2

Injection, two-compartment cartridge containing powder for reconstitution, somatropin (rbe) and diluent, net price 5.3-mg (16-unit) cartridge = £92.15, 12-mg (36-unit) cartridge = £208.65. For use with *Genotropin® Pen* NHS device (available free of charge from clinics). For subcutaneous injection

GoQuick® injection, two-compartment, multi-dose disposable, prefilled pen containing powder for reconstitution, somatropin (rbe) and diluent, net price 5.3-mg (16-unit) prefilled pen = £92.15; 12-mg (36-unit) prefilled pen = £208.65. For subcutaneous injection

MiniQuick® injection, two-compartment single-dose syringe containing powder for reconstitution, somatropin (rbe) and diluent, net price 0.2-mg (0.6-unit) syringe = £3.48; 0.4-mg (1.2-unit) syringe = £6.95; 0.6-mg (1.8-unit) syringe = £10.43; 0.8-mg (2.4-unit) syringe = £13.91; 1-mg (3-unit) syringe = £17.39; 1.2-mg (3.6-unit) syringe = £20.87; 1.4-mg (4.2-unit) syringe = £24.34; 1.6-mg (4.8-unit) syringe = £27.82; 1.8-mg (5.4-unit) syringe = £31.30; 2-mg (6-unit) syringe = £34.77. For subcutaneous injection

Humatrope® (Lilly) CD4-2

Injection, powder for reconstitution, somatropin (rbe), net price 6-mg (18-unit) cartridge = £108.00; 12-mg (36-unit) cartridge = £216.00; 24-mg (72-unit) cartridge = £432.00; all supplied with diluent. For subcutaneous or intramuscular injection; cartridges for subcutaneous injection

Norditropin® (Novo Nordisk) CD4-2

SimpleXx® injection, somatropin (epr) 3.3 mg (10 units)/mL, net price 1.5-mL (5-mg, 15-unit) cartridge = £106.35; 6.7 mg (20 units)/mL, 1.5-mL (10-mg, 30-unit) cartridge = £212.70; 10 mg (30 units)/mL, 1.5-mL (15-mg, 45-unit) cartridge = £319.05. For use with appropriate *NordiPen* JHS device (available free of charge from clinics). For subcutaneous injection

NordiFlex® injection, multidose disposable prefilled pen, somatropin (rbe) 10 mg (30 units)/mL, net price 1.5 mL (15-mg, 45-unit) prefilled pen = £347.70. For use with *NovoFine®* or *NovoTwist®* needles. For subcutaneous injection

NutropinAq® (Ipsen) CD4-2

Injection, somatropin (rbe), net price 10 mg (30 units) 2-ml cartridge = £203.00. For use with *NutropinAq® Pen* JHS device (available free of charge from clinics). For subcutaneous injection

Omnitrope® (Sandoz) CD4-2

Injection, somatropin (rbe) 3.3 mg (10 units)/mL, net price 1.5 mL (5-mg, 15-unit) cartridge = £73.75; 6.7 mg (20 units)/mL, 1.5 mL (10-mg, 30-unit) cartridge = £147.50. For use with *Omnitrope Pen 5®* JHS and *Omnitrope Pen 10®* JHS devices respectively (available free of charge from clinics). For subcutaneous injection

Excipients include benzyl alcohol (in 5-mg cartridge) (avoid in neonates, see Excipients, p. 2)

Note Biosimilar medicine, see p. 1

Saizen® (Merck Serono) CD4-2

Injection, somatropin (rmc), 5.83 mg (17.5 units)/ mL, net price 1.03-mL (6-mg, 18-unit) cartridge = £139.08; 8 mg (24 units)/mL, 1.5-mL (12-mg, 36-unit) cartridge = £278.16, 2.5-mL (20-mg, 60-unit) cartridge = £463.60. For use with *cool.click®* JHS needle-free autoinjector device or *easypod®* JHS autoinjector device (available free of charge from clinics). For subcutaneous injection

Click.easy®, powder for reconstitution, somatropin (rmc), net price 8-mg (24-unit) vial (in *click.easy®* device with diluent) = £185.44. For use with *one. click®* JHS autoinjector device or *cool.click®* JHS needle-free autoinjector device or *easypod®* JHS autoinjector device (available free of charge from clinics). For subcutaneous injection

Zomacton® (Ferring) CD4-2

Injection, powder for reconstitution, somatropin (rbe), net price 4-mg (12-unit) vial (with diluent) = £79.69, for use with *ZomaJet 2® Vision* JHS needle-free device (available free of charge from clinics) or with needles and syringes; 10 mg (30-unit) vial (with diluent) = £199.23, for use with *ZomaJet Vision X®* JHS needle-free device (available free of charge from clinics) or with needles and syringes. For subcutaneous injection

Excipients include benzyl alcohol (in 4-mg vial) (avoid in neonates, see Excipients p. 2)

Growth hormone receptor antagonists

Pegvisomant is a genetically modified analogue of human growth hormone and is a highly selective growth hormone receptor antagonist. Pegvisomant is licensed for the treatment of acromegaly in patients with inadequate response to surgery, radiation, or both, and to treatment with somatostatin analogues. Pegvisomant should be initiated only by physicians experienced in the treatment of acromegaly.

█ PEGVISOMANT

Indications see notes above

Cautions liver disease (monitor liver enzymes every 4–6 weeks for 6 months or if symptoms of hepatitis develop); diabetes mellitus (adjustment of antidiabetic therapy may be necessary); possible increase in female fertility

Pregnancy avoid

Breast-feeding avoid

Side-effects diarrhoea, constipation, nausea, vomiting, abdominal distension, dyspepsia, flatulence, elevated liver enzymes; hypertension; headache, asthenia, dizziness, drowsiness, tremor, sleep disturbances; influenza-like syndrome, weight gain, hyperglycaemia, hypoglycaemia; arthralgia; myalgia; injection-site reactions (rotate injection sites to avoid lipohypertrophy), sweating, pruritus, rash; fatigue; hypercholesterolaemia; less commonly thrombocytopenia, leucopenia, leucocytosis, bleeding tendency

Dose

- By subcutaneous injection, initially 80 mg, then 10 mg daily, increased in steps of 5 mg daily according to response; max. 30 mg daily; CHILD not recommended

Somavert® (Pfizer) PoM

Injection, powder for reconstitution, pegvisomant, net price 10-mg vial = £50.00; 15-mg vial = £75.00; 20-mg vial = £100.00 (all with solvent)

Thyrotrophin

Thyrotropin alfa is a recombinant form of thyrotrophin (thyroid stimulating hormone). It is licensed for use with or without radioiodine imaging, together with serum thyroglobulin testing, for the detection of thyroid remnants and thyroid cancer in post-thyroidectomy patients. It is also licensed to increase radio-iodine uptake for the ablation of thyroid remnant tissue in suitable post-thyroidectomy patients.

█ THYROTROPIN ALFA

(Recombinant human thyroid stimulating hormone, rhTSH)

Indications see notes above and product literature

Cautions presence of thyroglobulin autoantibodies may give false negative results

 6 **Endocrine system**

Contra-indications hypersensitivity to bovine or human thyrotropin

Pregnancy avoid

Breast-feeding avoid

Side-effects nausea, vomiting; headache, dizziness, fatigue; *less commonly* asthenia, paraesthesia, back pain, influenza-like symptoms, rash, urticaria; *rarely* diarrhoea; *very rarely* palpitation, flushing, dyspnoea, pain at site of metastases, tremor, arthralgia, myalgia, hyperhidrosis, and injection-site reactions including pain, pruritus, and rash

Dose

• By intramuscular injection into the gluteal muscle, 900 micrograms every 24 hours for 2 doses, consult product literature

Thyrogen® (Genzyme) [PoM]
Injection, powder for reconstitution, thyrotropin alfa 900 micrograms/vial, net price = £291.52

Hypothalamic hormones

Gonadorelin when injected intravenously in normal subjects leads to a rapid rise in plasma concentrations of both luteinising hormone (LH) and follicle-stimulating hormone (FSH). It has not proved to be very helpful, however, in distinguishing hypothalamic from pituitary lesions. **Gonadorelin analogues** are indicated in endometriosis and infertility (section 6.7.2) and in breast and prostate cancer (section 8.3.4).

■ GONADORELIN

(Gonadotrophin-releasing hormone; GnRH; LH–RH)

Indications see preparations below

Cautions pituitary adenoma

Pregnancy avoid

Breast-feeding avoid

Side-effects rarely, nausea, headache, abdominal pain, increased menstrual bleeding; rarely, hypersensitivity reaction on repeated administration of large doses; irritation at injection site

Dose

• See under preparations

Gonadorelin (Intrapharm) [PoM]
Injection, powder for reconstitution, gonadorelin. Net price 100-microgram vial (with diluent) = £67.00 (hosp. only)
Excipients include benzyl alcohol (avoid in neonates, see Excipients p. 2)
Dose for assessment of pituitary function (adults), by subcutaneous *or* intravenous injection, 100 micrograms

6.5.2 Posterior pituitary hormones and antagonists

Posterior pituitary hormones

Diabetes insipidus Vasopressin (antidiuretic hormone, ADH) is used in the treatment of *pituitary* ('cranial') *diabetes insipidus* as is its analogue **desmopressin**. Dosage is tailored to produce a slight diuresis every 24 hours to avoid water intoxication. Treatment may be required for a limited period only in diabetes insipidus following trauma or pituitary surgery.

Desmopressin is more potent and has a longer duration of action than vasopressin; unlike vasopressin it has no vasoconstrictor effect. It is given by mouth or intranasally for maintenance therapy, and by injection in the postoperative period or in unconscious patients. Desmopressin is also used in the differential diagnosis of diabetes insipidus. Following a dose of 2 micrograms intramuscularly or 20 micrograms intranasally, restoration of the ability to concentrate urine after water deprivation confirms a diagnosis of cranial diabetes insipidus. Failure to respond occurs in nephrogenic diabetes insipidus.

In *nephrogenic* and *partial pituitary diabetes insipidus* benefit may be gained from the paradoxical antidiuretic effect of thiazides (section 2.2.1) e.g. chlortalidone 100 mg twice daily reduced to maintenance dose of 50 mg daily.

Carbamazepine (section 4.8.1) is sometimes useful in partial pituitary diabetes insipidus (in a dose of 200 mg once or twice daily) [unlicensed]; it may act by sensitising the renal tubules to the action of remaining endogenous vasopressin.

Other uses Desmopressin is also used to boost factor VIII concentration in mild to moderate haemophilia and in von Willebrand's disease; it is also used to test fibrinolytic response. For a comment on use of desmopressin in nocturnal enuresis see section 7.4.2.

Vasopressin infusion is used to control variceal bleeding in portal hypertension, prior to more definitive treatment and with variable results. **Terlipressin**, a derivative of vasopressin with reportedly less pressor and antidiuretic activity, is used similarly.

Oxytocin, another posterior pituitary hormone, is indicated in obstetrics (section 7.1.1).

■ DESMOPRESSIN

Indications see under Dose

Cautions see under Vasopressin; less pressor activity, but still considerable caution in cardiovascular disease and in hypertension (not indicated for nocturnal enuresis or nocturia in these circumstances); elderly (avoid for nocturnal enuresis and nocturia in those over 65 years); also considerable caution in cystic fibrosis; in nocturia and nocturnal enuresis limit fluid intake to minimum from 1 hour before dose until 8 hours afterwards; in nocturia periodic blood pressure and weight checks needed to monitor for fluid overload; **interactions:** Appendix 1 (desmopressin)
Hyponatraemic convulsions Patients being treated for primary nocturnal enuresis should be warned to avoid fluid overload (including during swimming) and to stop taking desmopressin during an episode of vomiting or diarrhoea (until fluid balance normal). The risk of hyponatraemic convulsions can also be minimised by keeping to the recommended starting doses and by avoiding concomitant use of drugs which increase secretion of vasopressin (e.g. tricyclic antidepressants)

Contra-indications cardiac insufficiency and other conditions treated with diuretics; psychogenic polydipsia and polydipsia in alcohol dependence

Renal impairment use with caution; antidiuretic effect may be reduced

Pregnancy small oxytocic effect in third trimester; increased risk of pre-eclampsia

Breast-feeding not known to be harmful

Side-effects fluid retention, and hyponatraemia (in more serious cases with convulsions) on administration without restricting fluid intake; stomach pain, headache, nausea, vomiting, allergic reactions, and emotional disturbance in children also reported; epistaxis, nasal congestion, rhinitis with nasal spray

Dose

- By mouth (as desmopressin acetate)

  Diabetes insipidus, treatment, ADULT and CHILD initially 300 micrograms daily (in 3 divided doses); maintenance, 300–600 micrograms daily in 3 divided doses; range 0.2–1.2 mg daily

  Primary nocturnal enuresis, ADULT (under 65 years) and CHILD over 5 years 200 micrograms at bedtime, only increased to 400 micrograms if lower dose not effective (**important:** see also Cautions); withdraw for at least 1 week for reassessment after 3 months

  Postoperative polyuria or polydipsia, adjust dose according to urine osmolality

- Sublingually (as desmopressin base)

  Diabetes insipidus, treatment, ADULT and CHILD initially 180 micrograms daily in 3 divided doses; range 120–720 micrograms daily

  Primary nocturnal enuresis, ADULT (under 65 years) and CHILD over 5 years 120 micrograms at bedtime, only increased to 240 micrograms if lower dose not effective (**important:** see also Cautions); withdraw for at least 1 week for reassessment after 3 months

  Polyuria or polydipsia after hypophysectomy, adjust dose according to urine osmolality

- Intranasally (as desmopressin acetate)

  Diabetes insipidus, diagnosis, ADULT and CHILD 20 micrograms (limit fluid intake to 500 mL from 1 hour before to 8 hours after administration)

  Diabetes insipidus, treatment, ADULT 10–40 micrograms daily (in 1–2 divided doses); CHILD 5–20 micrograms daily; infants may require lower doses

  Nocturia associated with multiple sclerosis (when other treatments have failed), ADULT (under 65 years) 10–20 micrograms at bedtime (**important:** see also Cautions), dose not to be repeated within 24 hours

  Renal function testing (empty bladder at time of administration and limit fluid intake to 500 mL from 1 hour before until 8 hours after administration), ADULT 40 micrograms; INFANT under 1 year 10 micrograms (restrict fluid intake to 50% at next 2 feeds to avoid fluid overload), CHILD 1–15 years 20 micrograms

  Mild to moderate haemophilia and von Willebrand's disease, ADULT 300 micrograms (one 150-microgram spray into each nostril) 30 minutes before surgery or when bleeding; may be repeated at intervals of 12 hours (or at intervals of at least 3 days if self-administered)

  Fibrinolytic response testing, ADULT 300 micrograms (one 150-microgram spray into each nostril); blood sampled after 1 hour for fibrinolytic activity

- By injection (as desmopressin acetate)

  Diabetes insipidus, diagnosis (subcutaneous or intramuscular), ADULT and CHILD 2 micrograms (limit fluid intake to 500 mL from 1 hour before to 8 hours after administration)

  Diabetes insipidus, treatment (subcutaneous, intramuscular or intravenous), ADULT 1–4 micrograms daily; INFANT and CHILD 400 nanograms

  Renal function testing (empty bladder at time of administration and limit fluid intake to 500 mL from 1 hour before until 8 hours after administration) (subcutaneous or intramuscular), ADULT and CHILD

2 micrograms; INFANT 400 nanograms (restrict fluid intake to 50% at next 2 feeds)

Mild to moderate haemophilia and von Willebrand's disease, (subcutaneous or intravenous), ADULT and CHILD over 1 month 300 nanograms/kg as a single dose immediately before surgery or after trauma; may be repeated at intervals of 12 hours

Fibrinolytic response testing, (subcutaneous or intravenous), ADULT and CHILD 300 nanograms/kg; blood sampled after 20 minutes for fibrinolytic activity

Lumbar-puncture-associated headache, consult product literature

Desmopressin acetate (Non-proprietary) [PoM]

Tablets, desmopressin acetate 100 micrograms, net price 90-tab pack = £60.98; 200 micrograms, 30-tab pack = £9.86, 90-tab pack = £39.20. Counselling, fluid intake, see above

Nasal spray, desmopressin acetate 10 micrograms/ metered spray, net price 6-mL unit (60 metered sprays) = £9.88. Counselling, fluid intake, see above
Brands include Presinex®

Note Children requiring dose of less than 10 micrograms should be given *DDAVP*® intranasal solution

DDAVP® (Ferring) [PoM]

Tablets, both scored, desmopressin acetate 100 micrograms, net price 90-tab pack = £44.12; 200 micrograms, 90-tab pack = £88.23. Counselling, fluid intake, see above

Oral lyophilisates (DDAVP® Melt), desmopressin (as acetate) 60 micrograms, net price 100-tab pack = £50.53; 120 micrograms, 100-tab pack = £101.07; 240 micrograms, 100-tab pack = £202.14. Label: 26, counselling, fluid intake, see above. For sublingual administration

Intranasal solution, desmopressin acetate 100 micrograms/mL. Net price 2.5-mL dropper bottle and catheter = £9.72. Counselling, fluid intake, see above

Injection, desmopressin acetate 4 micrograms/mL. Net price 1-mL amp = £1.32

DesmoMelt® (Ferring) [PoM]

Oral lyophilisates, desmopressin (as acetate) 120 micrograms, net price 30-tab pack = £30.34; 240 micrograms, 30-tab pack = £60.68. Label: 26, counselling, fluid intake, see above. For sublingual administration

Desmotabs® (Ferring) [PoM]

Tablets, scored, desmopressin acetate 200 micrograms, net price 30-tab pack = £29.43. Counselling, fluid intake, see above

Desmospray® (Ferring) [PoM]

Nasal spray, desmopressin acetate 10 micrograms/ metered spray. Net price 6-mL unit (60 metered sprays) = £25.02. Counselling, fluid intake, see above

Note Children requiring dose of less than 10 micrograms should be given *DDAVP*® intranasal solution

Octim® (Ferring) [PoM]

Nasal spray, desmopressin acetate 150 micrograms/ metered spray, net price 2.5-mL unit (25 metered sprays) = £576.60. Counselling, fluid intake, see above

Injection, desmopressin acetate 15 micrograms/mL, net price 1-mL amp = £19.22

◢ TERLIPRESSIN ACETATE

Indications bleeding from oesophageal varices

Cautions elderly; uncontrolled hypertension; vascular disease; heart disease; history of QT-interval prolongation; concomitant use of drugs that prolong the QT-interval; arrhythmia; respiratory disease; septic shock; electrolyte and fluid disturbances

Renal impairment use with caution in chronic renal failure

Pregnancy avoid unless benefits outweigh risk—uterine contractions and increased intra-uterine pressure in early pregnancy, and decreased uterine blood flow reported

Breast-feeding avoid unless benefits outweigh risk—no information available

Side-effects abdominal cramps, diarrhoea, hypertension, hypotension, peripheral ischaemia, pallor, arrhythmia, bradycardia, headache; *less commonly* nausea, vomiting, hot flushes, angina, myocardial infarction, tachycardia, intestinal ischaemia, bronchospasm, respiratory failure, pulmonary oedema, convulsions, hyponatraemia; *rarely* dyspnoea; *very rarely* stroke, hyperglycaemia; *also reported* heart failure, skin necrosis

Dose
* See under preparations

Glypressin® (Ferring) ℗ℴℳ
Injection, powder for reconstitution, terlipressin acetate, net price 1-mg vial with 5 mL diluent = £18.47

Injection, solution for injection, terlipressin acetate, 0.12 mg/mL, net price 1-mg (8.5 mL) amp = £19.39
Dose by intravenous injection, 2 mg every 4 hours until bleeding controlled (after initial dose, may reduce to 1 mg every 4 hours if not tolerated or body-weight under 50 kg); max. duration 48 hours; CHILD under 18 years see *BNF for Children*

Variquel® (Sinclair IS) ℗ℴℳ
Injection, powder for reconstitution, terlipressin acetate, net price 1-mg vial with 5 mL diluent = £17.90
Dose by intravenous injection over 1 minute, initially 1 mg if body-weight under 50 kg (initial dose 1.5 mg if body-weight 50–70 kg, or 2 mg if body-weight over 70 kg), then 1 mg every 4–6 hours for up to 72 hours; CHILD under 18 years see *BNF for Children*

◢ VASOPRESSIN

Indications pituitary diabetes insipidus; bleeding from oesophageal varices

Cautions heart failure, hypertension, asthma, epilepsy, migraine or other conditions which might be aggravated by water retention; avoid fluid overload

Contra-indications vascular disease (especially disease of coronary arteries) unless extreme caution, chronic nephritis (until reasonable blood nitrogen concentrations attained)

Renal impairment see Contra-indications

Pregnancy oxytocic effect in third trimester

Breast-feeding not known to be harmful

Side-effects fluid retention, pallor, tremor, sweating, vertigo, headache, nausea, vomiting, belching, abdominal cramps, desire to defaecate, hypersensitivity reactions (including anaphylaxis), constriction of coronary arteries (may cause anginal attacks and

myocardial ischaemia), peripheral ischaemia and rarely gangrene

Dose
* By subcutaneous *or* intramuscular injection, diabetes insipidus, 5–20 units every four hours
* By intravenous infusion, initial control of variceal bleeding, 20 units over 15 minutes

◢ Synthetic vasopressin

Argipressin (Non-proprietary) ℗ℴℳ
Injection, argipressin (synthetic vasopressin) 20 units/mL, net price 1-mL amp = £22.50 (hosp. only)

Antidiuretic hormone antagonists

Demeclocycline (section 5.1.3) can be used in the treatment of hyponatraemia resulting from inappropriate secretion of antidiuretic hormone, if fluid restriction alone does not restore sodium concentration or is not tolerable. Demeclocycline is thought to act by directly blocking the renal tubular effect of antidiuretic hormone. Initially 0.9–1.2 g is given daily in divided doses, reduced to 600–900 mg daily for maintenance.

Tolvaptan

Tolvaptan is a vasopressin V_2-receptor antagonist licensed for the treatment of hyponatraemia secondary to syndrome of inappropriate antidiuretic hormone secretion; treatment duration with tolvaptan is determined by the underlying disease and its treatment.

Rapid correction of hyponatraemia during tolvaptan therapy can cause osmotic demyelination, leading to serious neurological events; close monitoring of serum-sodium concentration and fluid balance is essential

◢ TOLVAPTAN

Indications see notes above

Cautions ensure adequate fluid intake (monitor for dehydration in patients who are fluid-restricted); monitor serum-sodium concentration and fluid balance no later than 6 hours after initiating treatment and every 6 hours during the first 1–2 days of treatment and until dose stabilised; discontinue if rapid rise in serum-sodium concentration (greater than 12 mmol/litre in 24 hours or 18 mmol/litre in 48 hours); diabetes mellitus; pseudohyponatraemia associated with diabetes mellitus (exclude before treatment); increased risk of demyelination syndrome in alcoholism, hypoxia, or malnutrition if rapid correction of hyponatraemia; avoid concomitant drugs that increase serum-sodium concentration; discontinue and perform liver-function tests promptly if symptoms of hepatic impairment (anorexia, nausea, vomiting, fatigue, abdominal pain, jaundice, dark urine, pruritus); **interactions:** Appendix 1 (tolvaptan)

Contra-indications anuria; volume depletion; hypovolaemic hyponatraemia; hypernatraemia; impaired perception of thirst

Hepatic impairment use with caution in severe impairment—no information available; see also Cautions above

Renal impairment no information available in severe impairment

Pregnancy avoid—toxicity in *animal* studies

Breast-feeding avoid—present in milk in *animal* studies

Side-effects nausea, constipation, dry mouth, postural hypotension, thirst, decreased appetite, fever, malaise, hyperglycaemia, urinary frequency, hyperkalaemia, dehydration, ecchymosis, increased blood creatinine, pruritus, neurological disturbance (following rapid correction of hyponatraemia); *less commonly* taste disturbance, renal impairment; *also reported* hepatic impairment (discontinue), hypernatraemia, hyperuricaemia, hypoglycaemia, syncope, dizziness

Dose

- ADULT over 18 years, 15 mg once daily, increased as required to max. 60 mg daily

Samsca® (Otsuka) PoM

Tablets, blue, tolvaptan 15 mg, net price 10-tab pack = £746.80; 30 mg, 10-tab pack = £746.80

6.6 Drugs affecting bone metabolism

6.6.1   Calcitonin and parathyroid hormone
6.6.2   Bisphosphonates and other drugs affecting bone metabolism

See also calcium (section 9.5.1.1), phosphorus (section 9.5.2), vitamin D (section 9.6.4), and oestrogens in postmenopausal osteoporosis (section 6.4.1.1).

Osteoporosis

Osteoporosis occurs most commonly in postmenopausal women and in those taking long-term oral corticosteroids (glucocorticosteroids). Other risk factors for osteoporosis include low body weight, cigarette smoking, excess alcohol intake, lack of physical activity, family history of osteoporosis, and early menopause.

> Those at risk of osteoporosis should maintain an adequate intake of **calcium and vitamin D** and any deficiency should be corrected by increasing dietary intake or taking supplements.

Elderly patients, especially those who are housebound or live in residential or nursing homes, are at increased risk of calcium and vitamin D deficiency and may benefit from supplements (section 9.5.1.1 and section 9.6.4). Reversible secondary causes of osteoporosis such as hyperthyroidism, hyperparathyroidism, osteomalacia or hypogonadism should be excluded, in both men and women, before treatment for osteoporosis is initiated.

Postmenopausal osteoporosis The bisphosphonates (alendronic acid and risedronate, section 6.6.2) are effective for preventing postmenopausal osteoporosis. **Hormone replacement therapy** (HRT section 6.4.1.1) is an option where other therapies are contra-indicated, cannot be tolerated, or if there is a lack of response. The CSM has advised that HRT should **not** be considered first-line therapy for long-term prevention of osteoporosis in women over 50 years of age. HRT is of most benefit for the prophylaxis of postmenopausal osteoporosis if started early in menopause and continued for up to 5 years, but bone loss resumes (possibly at an accelerated rate) on stopping HRT. Women of Afro-Caribbean origin appear to be less susceptible to osteoporosis than those who are white or of Asian origin.

Postmenopausal osteoporosis may be *treated* with a **bisphosphonate** (section 6.6.2). The bisphosphonates (such as alendronate and risedronate) decrease the risk of vertebral fracture; alendronate and risedronate have also been shown to reduce non-vertebral fractures. If bisphosphonates are unsuitable **calcitriol** (section 9.6.4) or **strontium ranelate** (but see section 6.6.2) may be considered. **Calcitonin** is no longer recommended for the treatment of postmenopausal osteoporosis as the benefits are outweighed by the risk of malignancy associated with long-term use. Calcitonin [unlicensed indication] has been used for pain relief for up to 3 months after a vertebral fracture when other analgesics were ineffective, but the benefits of treatment should be balanced against the risks. **Parathyroid hormone**, and **teriparatide** (section 6.6.1) have been introduced for the treatment of postmenopausal osteoporosis.

Raloxifene (section 6.4.1.1) is licensed for the *prophylaxis* and *treatment* of vertebral fractures in postmenopausal women.

> **NICE guidance**
> **Alendronate, etidronate, risedronate, raloxifene and strontium ranelate for the primary prevention of osteoporotic fragility fractures in postmenopausal women (October 2008)**
>
> **Alendronate** is recommended as a treatment option for the primary prevention of osteoporotic fractures in the following susceptible postmenopausal women:
>
> - Women over 70 years who have an independent risk factor for fracture (parental history of hip fracture, alcohol intake of 4 or more units per day, or rheumatoid arthritis) *or* an indicator of low bone mineral density (body mass index under 22 kg/m², ankylosing spondylitis, Crohn's disease, prolonged immobility, untreated premature menopause, or rheumatoid arthritis) **and** confirmed osteoporosis
> - Women aged 65–69 years who have an independent risk factor for fracture **and** confirmed osteoporosis
> - Women under 65 years who have an independent risk factor for fracture **and** at least one additional indicator of low bone mineral density **and** confirmed osteoporosis
>
> **Risedronate** or **etidronate** [now discontinued] are recommended as alternatives for women:
>
> - in whom alendronate is contra-indicated or not tolerated **and**
> - who comply with particular combinations of bone mineral density measurement, age, and independent risk factors for fracture, as indicated in the full NICE guidance[1]
>
> **Strontium ranelate** [but see also Strontium Ranelate, p. 530] is recommended as an alternative for women:
>
> - in whom alendronate and either risedronate or editronate are contra-indicated or not tolerated **and**
> - who comply with particular combinations of bone mineral density measurement, age, and independent risk factors for fracture, as indicated in the full NICE guidance[1]
>
> **Raloxifene** is **not** recommended as a treatment option in postmenopausal women for primary prevention of osteoporotic fractures.
>
> www.nice.org.uk/TA160

6

Endocrine system

NICE guidance
Alendronate, etidronate, risedronate, raloxifene, strontium ranelate, and teriparatide for the secondary prevention of osteoporotic fragility fractures in postmenopausal women (October 2008)

This guideline recommends treatment options for the secondary prevention of osteoporotic fractures in postmenopausal women with confirmed osteoporosis who have also sustained a clinically apparent osteoporotic fracture.

Alendronate is recommended as a treatment option for the secondary prevention of osteoporotic fractures in susceptible postmenupausal women.

Risedronate or **etidronate** [now discontinued] are recommended as alternatives for women:

- in whom alendronate is contra-indicated or not tolerated **and**
- who comply with particular combinations of bone mineral density measurement, age, and independent risk factors for fracture (parental history of hip fracture, alcohol intake of 4 or more units per day, or rheumatoid arthritis, as indicated in the full NICE guidance[1]

Strontium ranelate [but see also Strontium Ranelate, p. 530] or **raloxifene** are recommended as alternatives for women:

- in whom alendronate and either risedronate or editronate are contra-indicated or not tolerated **and**
- who comply with particular combinations of bone mineral density measurement, age, and independent risk factors for fracture, as indicated in the full NICE guidance[1]

Teriparatide is recommended as an alternative for women:

- in whom alendronate and either risedronate or editronate, *or* strontium ranelate are contra-indicated or not tolerated, **or** where treatment with alendronate, risedronate or editronate has been unsatisfactory (indicated by another fragility fracture and a decline in bone mineral density despite treatment for 1 year) **and**
- who comply with particular combinations of bone mineral density measurement, age, and number of fractures, as indicated in the full NICE guidance[1]

www.nice.org.uk/TA161

Corticosteroid-induced osteoporosis To reduce the risk of osteoporosis doses of oral corticosteroids should be as low as possible and courses of treatment as short as possible. The risk of osteoporosis may be related to cumulative dose of corticosteroids; even intermittent courses can therefore increase the risk. The greatest rate of bone loss occurs during the first 6–12 months of corticosteroid use and so early steps to prevent the development of osteoporosis are important. Long-term use of high-dose inhaled corticosteroids may also contribute to corticosteroid-induced osteoporosis (section 3.2).

Patients taking (or who are likely to take) an oral corticosteroid for 3 months or longer should be assessed and where necessary given prophylactic treatment; those aged over 65 years are at greater risk. Patients taking oral corticosteroids who have sustained a low-trauma fracture should receive treatment for osteoporosis. The therapeutic options for *prophylaxis* and *treatment* of corticosteroid-induced osteoporosis are the same:

- a bisphosphonate (section 6.6.2);
- calcitriol [unlicensed indication] (section 9.6.4);
- hormone replacement (HRT in women (section 6.4.1), testosterone in men [unlicensed indication] (section 6.4.2)).

6.6.1 Calcitonin and parathyroid hormone

Calcitonin is involved with parathyroid hormone in the regulation of bone turnover and hence in the maintenance of calcium balance and homoeostasis. **Calcitonin (salmon)** (**salcatonin**, synthetic or recombinant salmon calcitonin) is used to lower the plasma-calcium concentration in patients with hypercalcaemia associated with malignancy, see also section 9.5.1.2. Calcitonin is also licensed for treatment of Paget's disease of bone when other treatments are ineffective or inappropriate; it is also licensed for the prevention of acute bone loss due to sudden immobility. Calcitonin is no longer recommended for the prevention or treatment of postmenopausal osteoporosis because the benefits are outweighed by the risk of malignancy associated with long-term use.

Recombinant **parathyroid hormone** is used for the treatment of postmenopausal osteoporosis. **Teriparatide** (a recombinant fragment of parathyroid hormone) is used for the treatment of postmenopausal osteoporosis, osteoporosis in men at increased risk of fracture, and corticosteroid-induced osteoporosis. *The Scottish Medicines Consortium*, p. 4 has advised (February 2007) that parathyroid hormone (*Preotact*®) should be initiated by specialists experienced in the treatment of osteoporosis; also that the use of teriparatide (*Forsteo*®) (December 2003) in postmenopausal women should be restricted to the treatment of established (severe) osteoporosis and should be initiated by specialists experienced in the treatment of osteoporosis.

Cinacalcet (section 9.5.1.2) is licensed for the treatment of hypercalcaemia in parathyroid carcinoma.

▌ **CALCITONIN (SALMON)/ SALCATONIN**

Indications see notes above

Cautions history of allergy (skin test advised); heart failure; avoid prolonged use—risk of malignancy (use lowest effective dose for shortest possible time)

Contra-indications hypocalcaemia

Renal impairment use with caution

Pregnancy avoid unless potential benefit outweighs risk (toxicity in *animal* studies)

Breast-feeding avoid; inhibits lactation in *animals*

Side-effects nausea, vomiting, diarrhoea, abdominal pain, taste disturbances, flushing, dizziness, headache, fatigue, malignancy (with long-term use), musculo-skeletal pain; *less commonly* hypertension, oedema, cough, polyuria, visual disturbances, injection-site reactions, rash, hypersensitivity reactions including pruritus; *also reported* tremor

Dose

- Hypercalcaemia of malignancy (see also section 9.5.1.2), ADULT over 18 years, *by subcutaneous or intramuscular injection*, 100 units every 6–8 hours adjusted according to response; max. 400 units every 6–8 hours; in severe or emergency cases, *by intravenous infusion*, up to 10 units/kg over at least 6 hours

- Paget's disease of bone, ADULT over 18 years, *by subcutaneous or intramuscular injection*, 50 units 3 times weekly to 100 units daily adjusted according to response; max. duration of treatment 3 months (6 months in exceptional circumstances)

- Prevention of acute bone loss due to sudden immobility, ADULT over 18 years, *by subcutaneous or intramuscular injection*, 100 units daily in 1–2 divided doses, reduced to 50 units daily at start of mobilisation; duration of treatment 2 weeks, max. 4 weeks

Miacalcic® (Novartis) PoM

Injection, calcitonin (salmon) 50 units/mL, net price 1-mL amp = £3.42; 100 units/mL, 1-mL amp = £6.84; 200 units/mL, 2-mL vial = £24.60
For subcutaneous or intramuscular injection and for dilution and use as an intravenous infusion

---

■ PARATHYROID HORMONE
(Human recombinant parathyroid hormone)

Indications treatment of osteoporosis in postmenopausal women at high risk of fractures (to reduce the risk of vertebral fractures) (see also notes above)

Cautions monitor serum or urinary calcium concentration at 1, 3 and 6 months after initiation of treatment (consult product literature for guidance if serum-calcium concentration raised); active or previous urolithiasis; concomitant cardiac glycosides

Contra-indications previous radiation therapy to skeleton, pre-existing hypercalcaemia, metabolic bone disease (including hyperparathyroidism and Paget's disease), unexplained raised levels of alkaline phosphatase

Hepatic impairment avoid

Renal impairment avoid if eGFR less than 30 mL/minute/1.73m²

Pregnancy avoid

Breast-feeding avoid

Side-effects nausea, vomiting, dyspepsia, constipation, diarrhoea; palpitation; headache, dizziness, fatigue, asthenia; transient hypercalcaemia, hypercalciuria; muscle cramp, pain in extremities, back pain; injection-site reactions; *less commonly* abdominal pain, altered sense of smell, taste disturbance, anorexia, influenza, hyperuricaemia

Dose

- *By subcutaneous injection*, 100 micrograms daily, max. duration of treatment 24 months

Preotact® (Nycomed) PoM

Injection, dual-chamber cartridge containing powder for reconstitution, parathyroid hormone (rdna) and diluent, net price 1.61-mg (14-dose) cartridge = £156.24. For use with *Preotact*® pen device.

■ TERIPARATIDE

Indications treatment of osteoporosis in postmenopausal women and in men at increased risk of fractures; treatment of corticosteroid-induced osteoporosis; see also notes above

Contra-indications pre-existing hypercalcaemia, skeletal malignancies or bone metastases, metabolic bone diseases, including Paget's disease and hyperparathyroidism, unexplained raised alkaline phosphatase, previous radiation therapy to the skeleton

Renal impairment caution in moderate impairment; avoid if severe

Pregnancy avoid

Breast-feeding avoid

Side-effects gastro-intestinal disorders (including nausea, reflux and haemorrhoids); palpitation; dyspnoea; headache, fatigue, asthenia, depression, dizziness, vertigo; anaemia, increased sweating, muscle cramps, sciatica, myalgia, arthralgia; *less commonly* urinary disorders, hypercalcaemia; injection-site reactions; *rarely* hypersensitivity reactions

Dose

- *By subcutaneous injection*, 20 micrograms daily; max. duration of treatment 24 months (course not to be repeated)

Forsteo® (Lilly) PoM

Injection, teriparatide 250 micrograms/mL, net price 2.4-mL prefilled pen = £271.88

6.6.2   Bisphosphonates and other drugs affecting bone metabolism

Bisphosphonates

Bisphosphonates are adsorbed onto hydroxyapatite crystals in bone, slowing both their rate of growth and dissolution, and therefore reducing the rate of bone turnover. Bisphosphonates have an important role in the prophylaxis and treatment of osteoporosis and corticosteroid-induced osteoporosis; **alendronic acid** or **risedronate sodium** are considered the drugs of choice for these conditions (see also section 6.6).

Bisphosphonates are also used in the treatment of *Paget's disease*, hypercalcaemia of malignancy (section 9.5.1.2), and in bone metastases in breast cancer (section 8.3.4.1). Etidronate disodium can impair bone mineralisation when used continuously or in high doses.

Bisphosphonates: osteonecrosis of the jaw

The risk of osteonecrosis of the jaw is substantially greater for patients receiving intravenous bisphosphonates in the treatment of cancer than for patients receiving oral bisphosphonates for osteoporosis or Paget's disease.

Risk factors for developing osteonecrosis of the jaw that should be considered are: potency of bisphosphonate (highest for zoledronate), route of administration, cumulative dose, duration and type of malignant disease, concomitant treatment, smoking, comorbid conditions, and history of dental disease. All patients should have a dental check-up (and any necessary remedial work should be performed) before bisphosphonate treatment, or as soon as possible after starting treatment.

During bisphosphonate treatment patients should maintain good oral hygiene, receive routine dental check-ups, and report any oral symptoms.

Guidance for dentists in primary care is included in *Oral Health Management of Patients Prescribed Bisphosphonates: Dental Clinical Guidance*, Scottish Dental Clinical Effectiveness Programme, April 2011 (available at www.sdcep.org.uk).

MHRA/CHM advice
Bisphosphonates: atypical femoral fractures (June 2011)

Atypical femoral fractures have been reported rarely with bisphosphonate treatment, mainly in patients receiving long-term treatment for osteoporosis.

The need to continue bisphosphonate treatment for osteoporosis should be re-evaluated periodically based on an assessment of the benefits and risks of treatment for individual patients, particularly after 5 or more years of use.

Patients should be advised to report any thigh, hip, or groin pain during treatment with a bisphosphonate.

Discontinuation of bisphosphonate treatment in patients suspected to have an atypical femoral fracture should be considered after an assessment of the benefits and risks of continued treatment.

ALENDRONIC ACID

Indications see under Dose

Cautions upper gastro-intestinal disorders (dysphagia, symptomatic oesophageal disease, gastritis, duodenitis, or ulcers—see also under Contra-indications and Side-effects); history (within 1 year) of ulcers, active gastro-intestinal bleeding, or surgery of the upper gastro-intestinal tract; correct disturbances of calcium and mineral metabolism (e.g. vitamin-D deficiency, hypocalcaemia) before starting and monitor serum-calcium concentration during treatment; consider dental check-up before initiating bisphosphonate (risk of osteonecrosis of the jaw, see Bisphosphonates: Osteonecrosis of the Jaw, above); exclude other causes of osteoporosis; atypical femoral fractures, see MHRA/CHM advice, above; **interactions:** Appendix 1 (bisphosphonates)

Contra-indications abnormalities of oesophagus and other factors which delay emptying (e.g. stricture or achalasia), hypocalcaemia

Renal impairment avoid if eGFR less than 35 mL/minute/1.73 m^2

Pregnancy avoid

Breast-feeding no information available

Side-effects oesophageal reactions (see below), abdominal pain and distension, dyspepsia, regurgitation, melaena, diarrhoea or constipation, flatulence, musculoskeletal pain, headache; *rarely* rash, pruritus, erythema, photosensitivity, uveitis, scleritis, transient decrease in serum calcium and phosphate; nausea, vomiting, gastritis, peptic ulceration, hypersensitivity reactions (including urticaria and angioedema), atypical femoral fractures with long-term use (see MHRA/CHM advice, above); myalgia, malaise, and fever at initiation of treatment; *very rarely* severe skin reactions (including Stevens-Johnson syndrome), osteonecrosis of the jaw (see Bisphosphonates: Osteonecrosis of the Jaw, above)

Oesophageal reactions Severe oesophageal reactions (oesophagitis, oesophageal ulcers, oesophageal stricture and oesophageal erosions) have been reported; patients should be advised to stop taking the tablets and to seek medical attention if they develop symptoms of oesophageal irritation such as dysphagia, new or worsening heartburn, pain on swallowing or retrosternal pain

Dose
* Treatment of postmenopausal osteoporosis, 10 mg daily *or* 70 mg once weekly
* Treatment of osteoporosis in men, 10 mg daily
* Prevention and treatment of corticosteroid-induced osteoporosis in postmenopausal women not receiving hormone replacement therapy, 10 mg daily

Counselling Tablets should be swallowed whole with plenty of water while sitting or standing; to be taken on an empty stomach at least 30 minutes before breakfast (or another oral medicine); patient should stand or sit upright for at least 30 minutes after taking tablet

Alendronic acid (Non-proprietary) PoM

Tablets, alendronic acid (as sodium alendronate) 10 mg, net price 28-tab pack = £1.66; 70 mg, 4-tab pack = £1.17. Counselling, administration

Oral solution, sugar-free, alendronic acid (as sodium alendronate) 70 mg/100 mL, net price 4 × 100-mL = £22.80. Counselling, administration

Counselling Oral solution should be swallowed as a single 100 mL dose with plenty of water while sitting or standing; to be taken on an empty stomach at least 30 minutes before breakfast (or another oral medicine); patients should stand or sit upright for at least 30 minutes after taking the solution.

Fosamax® (MSD) PoM

Tablets, alendronic acid (as sodium alendronate) 10 mg, net price 28-tab pack = £23.12. Counselling, administration

Fosamax® Once Weekly (MSD) PoM

Tablets, alendronic acid (as sodium alendronate) 70 mg, net price 4-tab pack = £22.80. Counselling, administration

◀ **With colecalciferol**

For prescribing information on colecalciferol, see section 9.6.4

Fosavance® (MSD) PoM

Tablets, alendronic acid (as sodium alendronate) 70 mg, colecalciferol 70 micrograms (2 800 units), net price 4-tab pack = £22.80. Counselling, administration

Dose treatment of postmenopausal osteoporosis in women at risk of vitamin D deficiency, 1 tablet once weekly

Counselling Tablets should be swallowed whole with plenty of water while sitting or standing; to be taken on an empty stomach at least 30 minutes before breakfast (or another oral medicine); patient should stand or sit upright for at least 30 minutes after taking tablet

ETIDRONATE DISODIUM

Indications Paget's disease of bone

Cautions consider dental check-up before initiating bisphosphonate (risk of osteonecrosis of the jaw, see Bisphosphonates: Osteonecrosis of the Jaw, p. 524); atypical femoral fractures, see MHRA/CHM advice, p. 524; **interactions:** Appendix 1 (bisphosphonates)

Contra-indications osteomalacia

Renal impairment reduce dose in mild impairment; avoid in moderate to severe renal impairment

Pregnancy avoid

Breast-feeding no information available

Side-effects nausea, diarrhoea or constipation, abdominal pain, increased bone pain, also increased risk of fractures with high doses (discontinue if fractures occur); *rarely* exacerbation of asthma, skin reactions (including angioedema, rash, urticaria and pruritus), transient hyperphosphataemia, headache, paraesthesia, peripheral neuropathy, atypical femoral fractures (see MHRA/CHM advice, p. 524); *very rarely* osteonecrosis of the jaw (see Bisphosphonates: Osteonecrosis of the Jaw, p. 524); blood disorders (including leucopenia, agranulocytosis and pancytopenia) also reported

Dose

* Paget's disease of bone, 5 mg/kg as a single daily dose for up to 6 months; doses above 10 mg/kg daily for up to 3 months may be used with caution but doses above 20 mg/kg daily are not recommended; after interval of not less than 3 months may be repeated where evidence of reactivation—including biochemical indices (avoid premature retreatment)

Monitoring Serum phosphate, serum alkaline phosphatase, and (if possible) urinary hydroxyproline should be measured before starting and at intervals of 3 months—consult product literature for further details

Counselling Avoid food for at least 2 hours before and after treatment, particularly calcium-containing products e.g. milk; also avoid iron and mineral supplements and antacids

Didronel® (Warner Chilcott) [PoM]
Tablets, etidronate disodium 200 mg. Net price 60-tab pack = £19.48. Counselling, food and calcium (see above)

IBANDRONIC ACID

Indications see under Dose

Cautions consider dental check-up before initiating bisphosphonate (risk of osteonecrosis of the jaw, see Bisphosphonates: Osteonecrosis of the Jaw, p. 524; atypical femoral fractures, see MHRA/CHM advice, p. 524; monitor renal function and serum calcium, phosphate and magnesium; cardiac disease (avoid fluid overload); **interactions:** Appendix 1 (bisphosphonates)

Contra-indications hypocalcaemia; *oral route* abnormalities of the oesophagus and other factors which delay emptying (e.g. stricture or achalasia)

Renal impairment for treatment of osteoporosis, avoid if eGFR less than 30 mL/minute/1.73 m²; for reduction of bone damage in bone metastases, if eGFR 30–50 mL/minute/1.73 m² reduce *intravenous dose* to 4 mg and infuse over 1 hour, reduce *oral dose* to 50 mg on alternative days, if eGFR less than 30 mL/minute/1.73 m² reduce *intravenous dose* to

2 mg and infuse over 1 hour, reduce *oral dose* to 50 mg once weekly

Pregnancy avoid

Breast-feeding avoid—present in milk in *animal* studies

Side-effects hypocalcaemia, hypophosphataemia, influenza-like symptoms (including fever, chills, and muscle pain), bone pain; oesophageal reactions (see below), diarrhoea, nausea, vomiting, gastritis, abdominal pain, dyspepsia, pharyngitis; headache, asthenia, rash; *rarely* anaemia, atypical femoral fractures (see MHRA/CHM advice, p. 524); hypersensitivity reactions (pruritus, bronchospasm and angioedema reported); urticaria; injection-site reactions; *very rarely* osteonecrosis of the jaw (see Bisphosphonates: Osteonecrosis of the Jaw, p. 524)

Oesophageal reactions Severe oesophageal reactions reported with all **oral** bisphosphonates; patients should be advised to stop tablets and seek medical attention for symptoms of oesophageal irritation such as dysphagia, pain on swallowing, retrosternal pain, or heartburn

Dose

* Reduction of bone damage in bone metastases in breast cancer, by mouth, 50 mg daily, *or* by intravenous infusion, 6 mg every 3–4 weeks
* Hypercalcaemia of malignancy by intravenous infusion, according to serum calcium concentration, 2–4 mg in single infusion
* Treatment of postmenopausal osteoporosis, by mouth, 150 mg once a month *or* by intravenous injection over 15–30 seconds, 3 mg every 3 months
* CHILD not recommended

Counselling Tablets should be swallowed whole with plenty of water while sitting or standing; to be taken on an empty stomach at least 30 minutes (ibandronic acid tablets, 50 mg) or 1 hour (*Bonviva*® tablets, 150 mg) before first food or drink (other than water) of the day, or another oral medicine; patient should stand or sit upright for at least 1 hour after taking tablet

Ibandronic acid (Non-proprietary) [PoM]
Tablets, ibandronic acid 50 mg, net price 28-tab pack = £12.29. Counselling, administration
Brands include *Iasibon*®

Bondronat® (Roche) [PoM]
Tablets, f/c, ibandronic acid 50 mg, net price 28-tab pack = £183.69. Counselling, administration
Concentrate for intravenous infusion, ibandronic acid 1 mg/mL, net price 2-mL vial = £89.36, 6-mL vial = £183.69

Bonviva® (Roche) [PoM]
Tablets, f/c, ibandronic acid 150 mg, net price 1-tab pack = £18.40, 3-tab pack = £55.21. Counselling, administration
Injection, ibandronic acid 1 mg/mL, net price 3-mL prefilled syringe = £68.64

PAMIDRONATE DISODIUM

Pamidronate disodium was formerly called aminohydroxypropylidenediphosphonate disodium (APD)

Indications see under Dose

Cautions assess renal function before each dose; ensure adequate hydration; cardiac disease (especially in elderly); previous thyroid surgery (risk of hypocalcaemia); monitor serum electrolytes, calcium and phosphate—possibility of convulsions due to electrolyte changes; avoid concurrent use with other bisphosphonates; consider dental check-up before initiating bisphosphonate (risk of osteonecrosis of the

6 **Endocrine system**

jaw, see Bisphosphonates: Osteonecrosis of the Jaw, p. 524); atypical femoral fractures, see MHRA/CHM advice, p. 524; **interactions:** Appendix 1 (bisphosphonates)

Driving Patients should be warned against driving or operating machinery immediately after treatment (somnolence or dizziness can occur)

Hepatic impairment caution in severe hepatic impairment—no information available

Renal impairment max. infusion rate 20 mg/hour; avoid if eGFR less than 30 mL/minute/1.73 m², except in life-threatening hypercalcaemia if benefit outweighs risk; if renal function deteriorates in patients with bone metastases, withhold dose until serum creatinine returns to within 10% of baseline value

Pregnancy avoid

Breast-feeding avoid

Side-effects hypophosphataemia, fever and influenza-like symptoms (sometimes accompanied by malaise, rigors, fatigue and flushes); nausea, vomiting, anorexia, abdominal pain, diarrhoea, constipation; symptomatic hypocalcaemia (paraesthesia, tetany), hypomagnesaemia, headache, insomnia, drowsiness; hypertension; anaemia, thrombocytopenia, lymphocytopenia; rash; arthralgia, myalgia, bone pain; *rarely* muscle cramps, atypical femoral fractures (see MHRA/CHM advice, p. 524); dyspepsia, agitation, confusion, dizziness, lethargy; leucopenia, hypotension, pruritus, hyperkalaemia or hypokalaemia, and hypernatraemia; osteonecrosis of the jaw (see Bisphosphonates: Osteonecrosis of the Jaw, p. 524), isolated cases of seizures, hallucinations, haematuria, acute renal failure, deterioration of renal disease, conjunctivitis, and other ocular symptoms; atrial fibrillation, and reactivation of herpes simplex and zoster also reported; also injection-site reactions

Dose

- By slow intravenous infusion (via cannula in a relatively large vein), see also Appendix 4

  Hypercalcaemia of malignancy, according to serum calcium concentration 15–60 mg in single infusion or in divided doses over 2–4 days; max. 90 mg per treatment course

  Osteolytic lesions and bone pain in bone metastases associated with breast cancer or multiple myeloma, 90 mg every 4 weeks (or every 3 weeks to coincide with chemotherapy in breast cancer)

  Paget's disease of bone, 30 mg once a week for 6 weeks (total dose 180 mg) *or* 30 mg in first week then 60 mg every other week (total dose 210 mg); max. total 360 mg (in divided doses of 60 mg) per treatment course; may be repeated every 6 months

- CHILD not recommended

Calcium and vitamin D supplements Oral supplements are advised to minimise potential risk of hypocalcaemia for those with mainly lytic bone metastases or multiple myeloma at risk of calcium or vitamin D deficiency (e.g. through malabsorption or lack of exposure to sunlight) and in those with Paget's disease

Pamidronate disodium (Non-proprietary) ▣PoM▣

Concentrate for intravenous infusion, pamidronate disodium 3 mg/mL, net price 5-mL vial = £13.33, 10-mL vial = £26.66; 6 mg/mL, 10-mL vial = £53.33; 9 mg/mL, 10-mL vial = £80.00; 15 mg/mL, 1-mL vial = £29.83, 2-mL vial = £59.66, 4-mL vial = £119.32, 6-mL vial £170.46

Aredia Dry Powder® (Novartis) ▣PoM▣

Intravenous infusion, powder for reconstitution, pamidronate disodium, net price 15-mg vial = £29.83; 30-mg vial = £59.66; 90-mg vial = £170.45 (all with diluent)

▌ **RISEDRONATE SODIUM**

Indications see under Dose

Cautions oesophageal abnormalities and other factors which delay transit or emptying (e.g. stricture or achalasia—see also under Side-effects); correct hypocalcaemia before starting, correct other disturbances of bone and mineral metabolism (e.g. vitamin-D deficiency) at onset of treatment; consider dental check-up before initiating bisphosphonate (risk of osteonecrosis of the jaw, see Bisphosphonates: Osteonecrosis of the Jaw, p. 524); atypical femoral fractures, see MHRA/CHM advice, p. 524; **interactions:** Appendix 1 (bisphosphonates)

Contra-indications hypocalcaemia (see Cautions above)

Renal impairment avoid if eGFR less than 30 mL/minute/1.73 m²

Pregnancy avoid

Breast-feeding avoid

Side-effects abdominal pain, dyspepsia, nausea, diarrhoea, constipation, headache, musculoskeletal pain; *less commonly* oesophagitis, oesophageal ulcer, dysphagia, gastritis, duodenitis, uveitis; *rarely* glossitis, oesophageal stricture, atypical femoral fractures (see MHRA/CHM advice, p. 524); *also reported* gastroduodenal ulceration, hepatic disorders, Stevens-Johnson syndrome, toxic epidermal necrolysis, hair loss, cutaneous vasculitis, osteonecrosis of the jaw (see Bisphosphonates: Osteonecrosis of the Jaw, p. 524)

Oesophageal reactions Patients should be advised to stop taking the tablets and seek medical attention if they develop symptoms of oesophageal irritation such as dysphagia, pain on swallowing, retrosternal pain, or heartburn

Dose

- Paget's disease of bone, 30 mg daily for 2 months; may be repeated if necessary after at least 2 months
- Treatment of postmenopausal osteoporosis to reduce risk of vertebral or hip fractures, 5 mg daily *or* 35 mg once weekly
- Prevention of osteoporosis (including corticosteroid-induced osteoporosis) in postmenopausal women, 5 mg daily
- Treatment of osteoporosis in men at high risk of fractures, 35 mg once weekly
- CHILD see *BNF for Children*

  Counselling Swallow tablets whole with full glass of water; on rising, take on an empty stomach at least 30 minutes before first food or drink of the day **or**, if taking at any other time of the day, avoid food and drink for at least 2 hours before or after risedronate (particularly avoid calcium-containing products e.g. milk; also avoid iron and mineral supplements and antacids); stand or sit upright for at least 30 minutes; do not take tablets at bedtime or before rising

Risedronate Sodium (Non-proprietary) ▣PoM▣

Tablets, risedronate sodium 5 mg, net price 28-tab pack = £13.24; 30 mg, 28-tab pack = £109.10; 35 mg, 4-tab pack = £1.25. Counselling, administration, food, and calcium (see above)

Actonel® (Warner Chilcott) [PoM]

Tablets, f/c, risedronate sodium 5 mg (yellow), net price 28-tab pack = £17.99; 30 mg (white), 28-tab pack = £143.95. Counselling, administration, food and calcium (see above)

Actonel Once a Week® (Warner Chilcott) [PoM]

Tablets, f/c, orange, risedronate sodium 35 mg, net price 4-tab pack = £19.12. Counselling, administration, food and calcium (see above)

◢**With calcium carbonate and colecalciferol**

For cautions, contra-indications, and side-effects of calcium carbonate, see section 9.5.1.1 and of colecalciferol, see section 9.6.4

Actonel® Combi (Warner Chilcott) [PoM]

Tablets, f/c, orange, risedronate sodium 35 mg (*Actonel Once a Week®*);

Granules, effervescent, lemon flavour, calcium carbonate 2.5 g (calcium 1 g or Ca^{2+} 25 mmol) and colecalciferol 22 micrograms (880 units)/sachet, net price 24-sachet plus 4-tab pack = £19.12. Counselling, administration, food and calcium (see above)

Dose treatment of postmenopausal osteoporosis to reduce risk of vertebral or hip fractures, given in weekly cycles, 1 *Actonel Once a Week®* tablet on the first day followed by 1 calcium and colecalciferol sachet daily for 6 days

Counselling Tablets should be swallowed whole with plenty of water while sitting or standing; to be taken on an empty stomach at least 30 minutes before breakfast (or another oral medicine); patient should stand or sit upright for at least 30 minutes after taking tablet. Granules should be stirred into a glass of water and after dissolution complete taken immediately

---

▮ SODIUM CLODRONATE

Indications see under Dose

Cautions monitor renal function, serum calcium and serum phosphate before and during treatment; renal dysfunction reported in patients receiving concomitant NSAIDs; maintain adequate fluid intake during treatment; consider dental check-up before initiating bisphosphonate (risk of osteonecrosis of the jaw, see Bisphosphonates: Osteonecrosis of the Jaw, p. 524); atypical femoral fractures, see MHRA/CHM advice, p. 524; **interactions**: Appendix 1 (bisphosphonates)

Contra-indications acute gastro-intestinal inflammatory conditions

Renal impairment max. initial dose 1200 mg daily if eGFR 30–50 mL/minute/1.73 m²; use half normal dose if eGFR 10–30 mL/minute/1.73 m²; avoid if eGFR less than 10 mL/minute/1.73 m²

Pregnancy avoid

Breast-feeding manufacturer advises avoid—no information available

Side-effects nausea, vomiting, diarrhoea, skin reactions, bronchospasm; *rarely* atypical femoral fractures (see MHRA/CHM advice, p. 524); *very rarely* osteonecrosis of the jaw (see Bisphosphonates: Osteonecrosis of the Jaw, p. 524); *also reported* renal impairment and uveitis

Dose

• Osteolytic lesions, hypercalcaemia and bone pain associated with skeletal metastases in patients with breast cancer or multiple myeloma, by mouth, 1.6 g daily in single or 2 divided doses increased if necessary to a max. of 3.2 g daily in 2 divided doses

Counselling Avoid food for 2 hours before and 1 hour after

treatment, particularly calcium-containing products e.g. milk; also avoid iron and mineral supplements and antacids; maintain adequate fluid intake

Bonefos® (Bayer) [PoM]

Capsules, yellow, sodium clodronate 400 mg, net price 120-cap pack = £139.83. Counselling, food and calcium

Tablets, f/c, scored, sodium clodronate 800 mg, net price 60-tab pack = £146.43. Counselling, food and calcium

Clasteon® (Beacon) [PoM]

Capsules, blue/white, sodium clodronate 400 mg, net price 30-cap pack = £34.96, 120-cap pack = £139.83. Counselling, food and calcium

Tablets, f/c, sodium clodronate 800 mg, net price 60-tab pack = £146.43. Counselling, food and calcium

Loron 520® (Intrapharm) [PoM]

Tablets, f/c, scored, sodium clodronate 520 mg, net price 60-tab pack = £152.59. Label: 10, patient information leaflet, counselling, food and calcium

Dose 2 tablets daily in single or two divided doses; may be increased to max. 4 tablets daily

---

▮ ZOLEDRONIC ACID

Indications see under preparations

Cautions correct disturbances of calcium metabolism (e.g. vitamin D deficiency, hypocalcaemia) before starting; monitor serum electrolytes, calcium, phosphate and magnesium; cardiac disease (avoid fluid overload); consider dental check-up before initiating bisphosphonate (risk of osteonecrosis of the jaw, see Bisphosphonates: Osteonecrosis of the Jaw, p. 524); atypical femoral fractures, see MHRA/CHM advice, p. 524; **interactions**: Appendix 1 (bisphosphonates)

Renal function Renal impairment and renal failure have been reported. Before each dose ensure patient is hydrated and assess renal function. Continue to monitor renal function in patients at risk, such as those with pre-existing renal impairment, those of advanced age, those taking concomitant nephrotoxic drugs or diuretics, or those who are dehydrated. Use with caution with concomitant medicines that affect renal function

Contra-indications women of child-bearing potential

Hepatic impairment caution in severe hepatic impairment—limited information available

Renal impairment avoid if serum creatinine above 400 micromol/litre in tumour-induced hypercalcaemia; in advanced malignancies involving bone, if eGFR 50–60 mL/minute/1.73 m² reduce dose to 3.5 mg every 3–4 weeks, if eGFR 40–50 mL/minute/1.73 m² reduce dose to 3.3 mg every 3–4 weeks, if eGFR 30–40 mL/minute/1.73 m² reduce dose to 3 mg every 3–4 weeks, avoid if eGFR less than 30 mL/minute/1.73 m² (or if serum creatinine greater than 265 micromol/litre); if renal function deteriorates in patients with bone metastases, withhold dose until serum creatinine returns to within 10% of baseline value; avoid in Paget's disease, treatment of postmenopausal osteoporosis and osteoporosis in men if eGFR less than 35 mL/minute/1.73 m²; see also Cautions above

Pregnancy avoid—toxicity in *animal* studies

Breast-feeding avoid—no information available

Side-effects hypophosphataemia, anaemia, influenza-like symptoms including bone pain, myalgia, arthralgia, fever and rigors; gastro-intestinal disturbances; atrial fibrillation; headache, dizziness, conjunctivitis, renal impairment (rarely acute renal failure); *less commonly* anorexia, taste disturbance, dry mouth, stomatitis, chest pain, hypertension, hypotension, dyspnoea, cough, paraesthesia, tremor, anxiety, lethargy, sleep disturbance, blurred vision, weight gain, pruritus, rash, sweating, muscle cramps, haematuria, proteinuria, urinary frequency, hypersensitivity reactions (including angioedema), asthenia, peripheral oedema, thrombocytopenia, leucopenia, hypomagnesaemia, hypokalaemia, also injection-site reactions; *rarely* bradycardia, confusion, hyperkalaemia, hypernatraemia, pancytopenia, osteonecrosis of the jaw (see Bisphosphonates: Osteonecrosis of the Jaw, p. 524), atypical femoral fractures (see MHRA/CHM advice, p. 524); *very rarely* uveitis and episcleritis

Dose
● See under preparations

Aclasta® (Novartis) [PoM]
Intravenous infusion, zoledronic acid 50 micrograms/mL, net price 100-mL bottle = £253.38
Dose treatment of Paget's disease of bone, by intravenous infusion, 5 mg as a single dose over at least 15 minutes
Note At least 500 mg elemental calcium twice daily (with vitamin D, section 9.6.4) for at least 10 days is recommended following infusion
Treatment of postmenopausal osteoporosis and osteoporosis in men (including corticosteroid-induced osteoporosis), by intravenous infusion, 5 mg over at least 15 minutes once a year
Note In patients with a recent low-trauma hip fracture, the dose should be given 2 or more weeks following hip fracture repair; before first infusion give 50 000–125 000 units of vitamin D (section 9.6.4)
Note The *Scottish Medicines Consortium* (p. 4) has advised (February 2008) that in postmenopausal women *Aclasta®* is accepted for restricted use within the NHS Scotland for the treatment of osteoporosis in those for whom oral treatment options for osteoporosis are inappropriate and when initiated by a specialist

Zometa® (Novartis) [PoM]
Concentrate for intravenous infusion, zoledronic acid, 800 micrograms/mL, net price 5-mL (4-mg) vial = £174.17
Solution for intravenous infusion, zoledronic acid, 40 micrograms/mL, net price 100-mL (4-mg) bottle = £174.14
Dose reduction of bone damage in advanced malignancies involving bone, by intravenous infusion, 4 mg over at least 15 minutes every 3–4 weeks; CHILD not recommended
Note Calcium 500 mg daily and vitamin D 400 units daily should also be taken
Hypercalcaemia of malignancy, by intravenous infusion, 4 mg as a single dose over at least 15 minutes; CHILD not recommended
Note The *Scottish Medicines Consortium* (p. 4) has advised (May 2003) that for the prevention of skeletal related events *Zometa®* is accepted for restricted use within NHS Scotland for the treatment of patients with breast cancer and multiple myeloma if prescribed by an oncologist

Denosumab

Denosumab is a human monoclonal antibody that inhibits osteoclast formation, function, and survival, thereby decreasing bone resorption.

> **NICE guidance**
> **Denosumab for the prevention of osteoporotic fractures in postmenopausal women (October 2010)**
> Denosumab is recommended as a treatment option for the *primary prevention* of osteoporotic fragility fractures in postmenopausal women at increased risk of fractures:
> ● who are unable to comply with the special instructions for administering alendronate and either risedronate or etidronate, or have an intolerance of, or a contra-indication to, those treatments **and**
> ● who comply with particular combinations of bone mineral density measurement, age, and independent risk factors for fracture, as indicated in the full NICE guidance (available at www.nice.org.uk/TA204).
> Denosumab is recommended as a treatment option for the *secondary prevention* of osteoporotic fragility fractures only in postmenopausal women at increased risk of fractures who are unable to comply with the special instructions for administering alendronate and either risedronate or etidronate, or have an intolerance of, or a contra-indication to, those treatments.
> www.nice.org.uk/TA204

The *Scottish Medicines Consortium* (p. 4) has advised (November 2010) that denosumab (*Prolia®*) is accepted for restricted use within NHS Scotland for the treatment of osteoporosis in postmenopausal women at increased risk of fractures who have a bone mineral density T-score <−2.5 and ≥−4.0 and for whom bisphosphonates are unsuitable.

NICE guidance
Denosumab for the prevention of skeletal-related events in adults with bone metastases from solid tumours (October 2012)

Denosumab is recommended for the prevention of skeletal-related events in adults with bone metastases from breast cancer and from solid tumours other than prostate cancer if:

- bisphosphonates would otherwise be prescribed, **and**
- the manufacturer provides denosumab with the discount agreed in the patient access scheme.

Denosumab is **not** recommended for preventing skeletal-related events in adults with bone metastases from prostate cancer.

Patients with bone metastases from solid tumours currently receiving denosumab whose disease does not meet the above criteria can continue treatment until they and their clinician consider it appropriate to stop.

www.nice.org.uk/TA265

MHRA/CHM advice
Denosumab: atypical femoral fractures (February 2013)

Atypical femoral fractures have been reported rarely in patients receiving denosumab for the long-term treatment (2.5 or more years) of postmenopausal osteoporosis.

Patients should be advised to report any new or unusual thigh, hip, or groin pain during treatment with denosumab.

Discontinuation of denosumab in patients suspected to have an atypical femoral fracture should be considered after an assessment of the benefits and risks of continued treatment.

MHRA/CHM advice
Denosumab: minimising the risk of osteonecrosis of the jaw; monitoring for hypocalcaemia—updated recommendations (September 2014)

Denosumab is associated with a risk of osteonecrosis of the jaw (ONJ) and with a risk of hypocalcaemia.

Osteonecrosis of the jaw

Osteonecrosis of the jaw is a well-known and common side-effect in patients receiving denosumab 120 mg for cancer. Risk factors include smoking, old age, poor oral hygiene, invasive dental procedures (including tooth extractions, dental implants, oral surgery), comorbidity (including dental disease, anaemia, coagulopathy, infection), advanced cancer, previous treatment with bisphosphonates, and concomitant treatments (including chemotherapy, anti-angiogenic biologics, corticosteroids, and radiotherapy to head and neck). The following precautions are now recommended to reduce the risk of ONJ:

Denosumab 120 mg (cancer indication)

- A dental examination and appropriate preventative dentistry before starting treatment are now recommended for all patients
- Do not start denosumab in patients with a dental or jaw condition requiring surgery, or in patients who have not recovered following oral surgery

Denosumab 60 mg (osteoporosis indication)

- Check for ONJ risk factors before starting treatment. A dental examination and appropriate preventative dentistry are now recommended for patients with risk factors

All patients should be informed to maintain good oral hygiene, receive routine dental check-ups, and immediately report any oral symptoms such as dental mobility, pain, or swelling to a doctor and dentist.

Hypocalcaemia

Denosumab is associated with a risk of hypocalcaemia. This risk increases with the degree of renal impairment. Hypocalcaemia usually occurs in the first weeks of denosumab treatment, but it can also occur later in treatment.

Plasma-calcium concentration monitoring is recommended for denosumab 120 mg (cancer indication):

- before the first dose
- within two weeks after the initial dose
- if suspected symptoms of hypocalcaemia occur
- consider monitoring more frequently in patients with risk factors for hypocalcaemia (e.g. severe renal impairment, creatinine clearance less than 30 mL/minute)

Plasma-calcium concentration monitoring is recommended for denosumab 60 mg (osteoporosis indication):

- before each dose
- within two weeks after the initial dose in patients with risk factors for hypocalcaemia (e.g. severe renal impairment, creatinine clearance less than 30 mL/minute)
- if suspected symptoms of hypocalcaemia occur

All patients should be advised to report symptoms of hypocalcaemia to their doctor (e.g. muscle spasms, twitches, cramps, numbness or tingling in the fingers, toes, or around the mouth)

6 Endocrine system

DENOSUMAB

Indications   see under preparations

Cautions   atypical femoral fractures (see MHRA/CHM advice, p. 529); osteonecrosis of the jaw—consider temporary interruption of treatment if occurs (see MHRA/CHM advice, p. 529); hypocalcaemia (see MHRA/CHM advice, p. 529)

Contra-indications   hypocalcaemia

Renal impairment   increased risk of hypocalcaemia if eGFR less than 30 mL/minute/1.73 m²—monitor plasma-calcium concentration; see also Cautions

Pregnancy   avoid during, and for at least 5 months after stopping treatment (toxicity in *animal* studies); ensure effective contraception in women of child-bearing potential; risk of toxicity increases with each trimester—advise women who become pregnant during treatment to enrol in the manufacturer's Pregnancy Surveillance Programme (consult product literature)

Breast-feeding   avoid (if women do decide to breast-feed during treatment, they should enrol in the manufacturer's Lactation Surveillance Programme—consult product literature)

Side-effects   diarrhoea, constipation, abdominal discomfort, dyspnoea, urinary tract infection, upper respiratory tract infection, pain in extremity, sciatica, hypocalcaemia (fatal cases reported, see also Cautions), hypophosphataemia, musculoskeletal pain, osteonecrosis of the jaw (see also Cautions), cataracts, rash, eczema, sweating; *less commonly* diverticulitis, skin infections including cellulitis (seek prompt medical attention), ear infection; *rarely* atypical femoral fractures (see MHRA/CHM advice, p. 529)

Dose
- See under preparations

Prolia® (Amgen) ▼ [PoM]
Injection, denosumab 60 mg/mL, net price 1-mL prefilled syringe = £183.00. Counselling, symptoms of hypocalcaemia, osteonecrosis of the jaw
Dose treatment of osteoporosis in postmenopausal women and in men at increased risk of fractures; treatment of bone loss associated with hormone ablation in men with prostate cancer at increased risk of fractures, by subcutaneous injection, 60 mg every 6 months
Note Supplement with calcium and vitamin D

XGEVA® (Amgen) ▼ [PoM]
Injection, denosumab 70 mg/mL, net price 1.7-mL (120-mg) vial = £309.86. Counselling, symptoms of hypocalcaemia, osteonecrosis of the jaw
Dose prevention of skeletal related events in patients with bone metastases from solid tumours, ADULT over 18 years, by subcutaneous injection, 120 mg every 4 weeks
Treatment of giant cell tumour of bone that is unresectable or where surgical resection is likely to result in severe morbidity, ADULT over 18 years and skeletally mature adolescent, by subcutaneous injection, 120 mg every 4 weeks, with an additional dose on days 8 and 15 of the first month of treatment only
Note Supplementation of at least Calcium 500 mg and vitamin D 400 units daily should also be taken unless hypercalcaemia is present

Strontium ranelate

Strontium ranelate stimulates bone formation and reduces bone resorption. Strontium ranelate treatment has been associated with an increased risk of serious cardiovascular disease, including myocardial infarction, and the risk should be assessed before treatment and regularly during treatment. Strontium ranelate should be initiated only by specialists for the treatment of severe osteoporosis in postmenopausal women or men at high risk of fracture for whom other treatments are contra-indicated or not tolerated.

STRONTIUM RANELATE

Indications   see notes above

Cautions   predisposition to cardiovascular disease—assess risk before and every 6–12 months during treatment; interferes with colorimetric measurements of calcium in blood and urine; **interactions**: Appendix 1 (strontium ranelate)

Contra-indications   current or previous venous thromboembolic event, ischaemic heart disease, peripheral arterial disease, cerebrovascular disease, or uncontrolled hypertension; temporary or prolonged immobilisation

Renal impairment   avoid if eGFR less than 30 mL/minute/1.73 m²

Side-effects   nausea, diarrhoea, venous thromboembolism, myocardial infarction, headache, dermatitis, eczema; *very rarely* hypersensitivity reactions, including rash, pruritus, urticaria, and angioedema—see Severe Allergic Reactions; *also reported* gastro-oesophageal reflux, dyspepsia, abdominal pain, vomiting, constipation, flatulence, stomatitis, peripheral oedema, bone marrow suppression, alopecia

Severe allergic reactions

Severe allergic reactions, including drug rash with eosinophilia and systemic symptoms (DRESS), have been reported in patients taking strontium ranelate. DRESS starts with rash, fever, swollen glands, and increased white cell count, and it can affect the liver, kidneys and lungs; DRESS can also be fatal.

Patients should be advised to stop taking strontium ranelate and consult their doctor immediately if skin rash develops. Treatment with strontium ranelate should not be restarted.

Dose
- 2 g once daily in water, preferably at bedtime
Counselling Avoid food for 2 hours before and after taking granules, particularly calcium-containing products e.g. milk; also preferably avoid concomitant antacids containing aluminium and magnesium hydroxides for 2 hours after taking granules

Protelos® (Servier) ▼ [PoM]
Granules, yellow, strontium ranelate, 2 g/sachet, net price 28-sachets = £27.08. Label: 5, 13, counselling, food and calcium
Excipients include aspartame (section 9.4.1)

6.7   Other endocrine drugs

6.7.1   Bromocriptine and other dopaminergic drugs

Bromocriptine is a stimulant of dopamine receptors in the brain; it also inhibits release of prolactin by the pituitary. Bromocriptine is used for the treatment of galactorrhoea, and for the treatment of prolactinomas (when it reduces both plasma prolactin concentration and tumour size). Bromocriptine also inhibits the release of growth hormone and is sometimes used in the treatment of acromegaly, but somatostatin analogues (such as octreotide, section 8.3.4.3) are more effective.

Cabergoline has actions and uses similar to those of bromocriptine, but its duration of action is longer. It has similar side-effects to bromocriptine, however patients intolerant of bromocriptine may be able to tolerate cabergoline (and *vice versa*).

Quinagolide is a non-ergot dopamine D_2 agonist; it has actions and uses similar to those of ergot-derived dopamine agonists, but its side-effects differ slightly.

Cautions   see notes below; also bromocriptine and cabergoline should be used with caution in patients with a history of peptic ulcer, particularly in acromegalic patients. Treatment should be withdrawn if gastro-intestinal bleeding occurs. In hyperprolactinaemic patients, the source of the hyperprolactinaemia should be established (i.e. exclude pituitary tumour before treatment). Bromocriptine and cabergoline should be used with caution in patients with Raynaud's syndrome and cardiovascular disease (see also Contra-indications under Bromocriptine, below). Monitor for fibrotic disease (see Fibrotic Reactions, below). Caution is also advised in patients with a history of serious mental disorders (especially psychotic disorders) and in those with acute porphyria (see section 9.8.2). Tolerance may be reduced by alcohol.

Contra-indications   Bromocriptine and cabergoline should not be used in patients with hypersensitivity to ergot alkaloids. They are contra-indicated in those with cardiac valvulopathy (exclude before treatment, see Fibrotic Reactions, below). They should also be avoided in pre-eclampsia (see also Contra-indications under Bromocriptine, below).

Side-effects   Nausea, constipation, and headache are common side-effects of bromocriptine and cabergoline. Paraesthesia has been reported rarely. Other reported side-effects include hypotension (see also Hypotensive Reactions, below), drowsiness (see also Driving, below), dyskinesia, pathological gambling, increased libido, hypersexuality, leg cramps, allergic skin reactions, alopecia, and peripheral oedema. Bromocriptine and cabergoline have been associated with pleuritis, pleural effusion, cardiac valvulopathy, pericardial effusion, constrictive pericarditis, and retroperitoneal, pleural, and pulmonary fibrosis (see Fibrotic Reactions).

Suppression of lactation   Although bromocriptine and cabergoline are licensed to suppress lactation, they are **not** recommended for routine suppression (or for the relief of symptoms of postpartum pain and engorgement) that can be adequately treated with simple analgesics and breast support. If a dopamine-receptor agonist is required, cabergoline is preferred. Quinagolide is not licensed for the suppression of lactation.

BROMOCRIPTINE

Indications   see notes above and under Dose; Parkinson's disease (section 4.9.1)

Cautions   see notes above; also specialist evaluation—monitor for pituitary enlargement, particularly during pregnancy; monitor visual field to detect secondary field loss in macroprolactinoma; contraceptive advice if appropriate (oral contraceptives may increase prolactin concentration); **interactions:** Appendix 1 (bromocriptine)

Contra-indications   see notes above; also hypertension in postpartum women or in puerperium (see also below)

Postpartum or puerperium Should not be used postpartum or in puerperium in women with high blood pressure, coronary artery disease, or symptoms (or history) of serious mental disorder; monitor blood pressure carefully (especially during first few days) in postpartum women. Very rarely hypertension, myocardial infarction, seizures or stroke (both sometimes preceded by severe headache or visual disturbances), and mental disorders have been reported in postpartum women given bromocriptine for lactation suppression—caution with antihypertensive therapy and avoid other ergot alkaloids. Discontinue immediately if hypertension, unremitting headache, or signs of CNS toxicity develop

Hepatic impairment dose reduction may be necessary

Pregnancy see Cautions above

Breast-feeding suppresses lactation; avoid breast feeding for about 5 days if lactation prevention fails

Side-effects see notes above; also nasal congestion; *less commonly* vomiting, postural hypotension, fatigue, dizziness, dry mouth; also, particularly with *high doses*, confusion, psychomotor excitation, hallucinations; *rarely* diarrhoea, gastro-intestinal bleeding, gastric ulcer, abdominal pain, tachycardia, bradycardia, arrhythmia, insomnia, psychosis, visual disturbances, tinnitus; *very rarely* vasospasm of fingers and toes particularly in patients with Raynaud's syndrome, and effects like neuroleptic malignant syndrome on withdrawal; urinary incontinence, leucopenia, thrombocytopenia, hyponatraemia, reversible hearing loss, increased libido, and hypersexuality also reported

Dose

- Prevention or suppression of lactation (but see notes above and under Cautions), 2.5 mg on day 1 (prevention) or daily for 2–3 days (suppression); then 2.5 mg twice daily for 14 days

- Hypogonadism, galactorrhoea, infertility, initially 1–1.25 mg at bedtime, increased gradually; usual dose 7.5 mg daily in divided doses, increased if necessary to max. 30 mg daily, usual dose in infertility without hyperprolactinaemia, 2.5 mg twice daily

- Acromegaly, initially 1–1.25 mg at bedtime, increase gradually to 5 mg every 6 hours

- Prolactinoma, initially 1–1.25 mg at bedtime; increased gradually to 5 mg every 6 hours (occasional patients may require up to 30 mg daily)

- CHILD under 15 years, not recommended

Bromocriptine (Non-proprietary) PoM
Tablets, bromocriptine (as mesilate) 1 mg, net price 100-tab pack = £60.10; 2.5 mg, 30-tab pack = £71.36. Label: 10, 21, counselling, driving, see notes above

Parlodel® (Meda) PoM
Capsules, bromocriptine (as mesilate) 5 mg (blue/white), net price 100-cap pack = £37.57; 10 mg (white), 100-cap pack = £69.50. Label: 10, 21, counselling, driving, see notes above

CABERGOLINE

Indications see notes above and under Dose

Cautions see notes above; also monthly pregnancy tests during the amenorrhoeic period; advise non-hormonal contraception if pregnancy not desired (see also Pregnancy, below); **interactions:** Appendix 1 (cabergoline)

Contra-indications see notes above; history of puerperal psychosis; history of pulmonary, pericardial, or retroperitoneal fibrotic disorders (see Fibrotic Reactions in notes above); cardiac valvulopathy

Hepatic impairment reduce dose in severe hepatic impairment

Pregnancy exclude pregnancy before starting and discontinue 1 month before intended conception

(ovulatory cycles persist for 6 months)—discontinue if pregnancy occurs during treatment (specialist advice needed)

Breast-feeding suppresses lactation; avoid breast-feeding if lactation prevention fails

Side-effects see notes above; also cardiac valvulopathy, dyspepsia, gastritis, epigastric and abdominal pain, angina, syncope, depression, confusion, hallucinations, breast pain; *rarely* vomiting, palpitation, epistaxis, digital vasospasm, hot flushes, transient hemianopia, muscle weakness; *also reported* erythromelalgia

Dose

- Prevention of lactation (but see notes above and under Contra-indications), during first day postpartum, 1 mg as a single dose; suppression of established lactation (but see notes above) 250 micrograms every 12 hours for 2 days; CHILD under 16 years, not recommended

- Hyperprolactinaemic disorders, 500 micrograms weekly (as a single dose *or* as 2 divided doses on separate days) increased at monthly intervals in steps of 500 micrograms until optimal therapeutic response (usually 1 mg weekly, range 0.25–2 mg weekly) with monthly monitoring of serum prolactin levels; reduce initial dose and increase more gradually if patient intolerant; over 1 mg weekly give as divided doses; up to 4.5 mg weekly have been used in hyperprolactinaemic patients; CHILD under 16 years, not recommended

- Parkinson's disease, section 4.9.1

Cabergoline (Non-proprietary) PoM
Tablet, scored, cabergoline 500 micrograms, net price 8-tab pack = £34.72. Label: 10, 21, counselling, driving, see notes above
Note Dispense in original container (contains desiccant)

Dostinex® (Pharmacia) PoM
Tablets, scored, cabergoline 500 micrograms. Net price 8-tab pack = £30.04. Label: 10, 21, counselling, driving, see notes above
Note Dispense in original container (contains desiccant)

QUINAGOLIDE

Indications see notes above and under Dose

Cautions see notes above; history of psychotic illness; advise non-hormonal contraception if pregnancy not desired; **interactions:** Appendix 1 (quinagolide)

Contra-indications hypersensitivity to quinagolide (but not ergot alkaloids)

Hepatic impairment avoid—no information available

Renal impairment avoid—no information available

Pregnancy discontinue when pregnancy confirmed unless medical reason for continuing (specialist advice needed)

Breast-feeding suppresses lactation

Side-effects nausea, vomiting, anorexia, abdominal pain, constipation or diarrhoea; syncope, hypotension (see also notes above), oedema, flushing; nasal congestion; headache, dizziness, fatigue, insomnia; *very rarely* psychosis

Dose

- Hyperprolactinaemia, 25 micrograms at bedtime for 3 days; increased at intervals of 3 days in steps of 25 micrograms to usual maintenance dose of 75–150 micrograms daily; for doses higher than 300 micrograms daily increase in steps of 75–150 micrograms at intervals of not less than 4 weeks; CHILD not recommended

Norprolac® (Ferring) ▱PoM▱
Tablets, quinagolide (as hydrochloride) 75 micrograms (white), net price 30-tab pack = £27.00; starter pack of 3 × 25-microgram tabs (pink) with 3 × 50-microgram tabs (blue) = £4.50. Label: 10, 21, counselling, driving, see notes above

6.7.2 Drugs affecting gonadotrophins

Danazol inhibits pituitary gonadotrophins; it combines androgenic activity with antioestrogenic and anti-progestogenic activity. It is licensed for the treatment of *endometriosis* and for the relief of severe pain and tenderness in *benign fibrocystic breast disease* where other measures have proved unsatisfactory. It may also be effective in the long-term management of *hereditary angioedema* [unlicensed indication].

Cetrorelix and **ganirelix** are luteinising hormone releasing hormone antagonists, which inhibit the release of gonadotrophins (luteinising hormone and follicle-stimulating hormone). They are used in the treatment of infertility by assisted reproductive techniques.

CETRORELIX

Indications adjunct in the treatment of female infertility (under specialist supervision)
Hepatic impairment avoid in moderate or severe liver impairment
Renal impairment avoid in moderate or severe renal impairment
Pregnancy avoid in confirmed pregnancy
Breast-feeding avoid
Side-effects nausea, headache, injection site reactions; rarely hypersensitivity reactions
Dose
● By subcutaneous injection into the lower abdominal wall, 250 micrograms in the morning, starting on day 5 or 6 of ovarian stimulation with gonadotrophins (*or* each evening starting on day 5 of ovarian stimulation); continue throughout administration of gonadotrophin including day of ovulation induction (*or* evening before ovulation induction)

Cetrotide® (Merck Serono) ▱PoM▱
Injection, powder for reconstitution, cetrorelix (as acetate), net price 250-micrograms vial (with solvent) = £22.61

DANAZOL

Indications see notes above and under Dose
Cautions cardiac impairment (avoid if severe), elderly, polycythaemia, epilepsy, diabetes mellitus, hypertension, migraine, lipoprotein disorder, history of thrombosis or thromboembolic disease; withdraw if virilisation (may be irreversible on continued use); non-hormonal contraceptive methods should be used, if appropriate; **interactions:** Appendix 1 (danazol)
Contra-indications ensure that patients with amenorrhoea are not pregnant; thromboembolic disease; undiagnosed genital bleeding; androgen-dependent tumours; acute porphyria (section 9.8.2)
Hepatic impairment caution in hepatic impairment (avoid if severe)
Renal impairment caution in renal impairment (avoid if severe)

Pregnancy avoid; has weak androgenic effects and virilisation of female fetus reported
Breast-feeding no data available but avoid because of possible androgenic effects in infant
Side-effects nausea, dizziness, skin reactions including rashes, photosensitivity and exfoliative dermatitis, fever, backache, nervousness, mood changes, anxiety, changes in libido, vertigo, fatigue, epigastric and pleuritic pain, headache, weight gain; menstrual disturbances, vaginal dryness and irritation, flushing and reduction in breast size; musculo-skeletal spasm, joint pain and swelling, hair loss; androgenic effects including acne, oily skin, oedema, hirsutism, voice changes and rarely clitoral hypertrophy (see also Cautions); temporary alteration in lipoproteins and other metabolic changes, insulin resistance; thrombotic events; leucopenia, thrombocytopenia, eosinophilia, reversible erythrocytosis or polycythaemia reported; headache and visual disturbances may indicate benign intracranial hypertension; rarely cholestatic jaundice, pancreatitis, peliosis hepatis and benign hepatic adenomata
Dose Note In women of child-bearing potential, treatment should start during menstruation, preferably on day 1
● Endometriosis, 200–800 mg daily in up to 4 divided doses, adjusted to achieve amenorrhoea, usually for 3–6 months
● Severe pain and tenderness in benign fibrocystic breast disease not responding to other treatment, 300 mg daily in divided doses usually for 3–6 months
● Hereditary angioedema [unlicensed indication], initially 100–200 mg daily, reduced according to response

Danazol (Non-proprietary) ▱CD4-2▱
Capsules, danazol 100 mg, net price 28-cap pack = £7.64, 60-cap pack = £16.38; 200 mg, 56-cap pack = £54.60

Danol® (Sanofi-Aventis) ▱CD4-2▱
Capsules, danazol 100 mg (grey/white), net price 60-cap pack = £16.38; 200 mg (pink/white), 60-cap pack = £32.43

GANIRELIX

Indications adjunct in the treatment of female infertility (under specialist supervision)
Hepatic impairment avoid in moderate or severe hepatic impairment
Renal impairment avoid in moderate to severe renal impairment
Pregnancy avoid in confirmed pregnancy—toxicity in *animal* studies
Breast-feeding avoid—no information available
Side-effects nausea, headache, malaise, injection-site reactions; *very rarely* hypersensitivity reactions including rash, facial oedema, and dyspnoea also reported
Dose
● By subcutaneous injection preferably into the upper leg (rotate injection sites to prevent lipoatrophy), 250 micrograms in the morning (or each afternoon) starting on day 5 or day 6 of ovarian stimulation with gonadotrophins; continue throughout administration of gonadotrophins including day of ovulation induction (if administering in afternoon, give last dose in afternoon *before* ovulation induction)

Orgalutran® (MSD) ▱PoM▱
Injection, ganirelix, 500 micrograms/mL, net price 0.5-mL prefilled syringe = £21.48

 6 Endocrine system

Gonadorelin analogues

Administration of **gonadorelin analogues** produces an initial phase of stimulation; continued administration is followed by down-regulation of gonadotrophin-releasing hormone receptors, thereby reducing the release of gonadotrophins (follicle stimulating hormone and luteinising hormone) which in turn leads to inhibition of androgen and oestrogen production.

Gonadorelin analogues are used in the treatment of endometriosis, precocious puberty, infertility, male hypersexuality with severe sexual deviation, anaemia due to uterine fibroids (together with iron supplementation), breast cancer (section 8.3.4.1), prostate cancer (section 8.3.4.2) and before intra-uterine surgery. Use of leuprorelin and triptorelin for 3 to 4 months before surgery reduces the uterine volume, fibroid size and associated bleeding. For women undergoing hysterectomy or myomectomy, a vaginal procedure is made more feasible following the use of a gonadorelin analogue.

Cautions Non-hormonal, barrier methods of contraception should be used during entire treatment period with gonadorelin analogues; also use with caution in patients with metabolic bone disease because decrease in bone mineral density can occur.

Contra-indications Gonadorelin analogues are contra-indicated for use longer than 6 months in the treatment of endometriosis (do not repeat) and when there is unexplained vaginal bleeding.

Pregnancy The use of gonadorelin analogues in pregnancy is contra-indicated. Pregnancy should be excluded before treatment; the first injection should be given during menstruation or shortly afterwards *or* use barrier contraception for 1 month beforehand.

Breast-feeding Gonadorelin analogues are contra-indicated in breast-feeding.

Side-effects Side-effects of the gonadorelin analogues related to the inhibition of oestrogen production include menopausal-like symptoms (e.g. hot flushes, increased sweating, vaginal dryness, dyspareunia and loss of libido) and a decrease in trabecular bone density; these effects can be reduced by hormone replacement (e.g. with an oestrogen and a progestogen or with tibolone). Side-effects of gonadorelin analogues also include headache (rarely migraine) and hypersensitivity reactions including urticaria, pruritus, rash, asthma and anaphylaxis; when treating uterine fibroids, bleeding associated with fibroid degeneration can occur; spray formulations can cause irritation of the nasal mucosa including nose bleeds; local reactions at injection site can occur; other side-effects also reported with some gonadorelin analogues include palpitation, hypertension, ovarian cysts (may require withdrawal), changes in breast size, musculoskeletal pain or weakness, visual disturbances, paraesthesia, changes in scalp and body hair, oedema of the face and extremities, weight changes, and mood changes including depression.

▌ BUSERELIN

Indications see under Dose; prostate cancer (section 8.3.4.2)

Cautions see notes above; polycystic ovarian disease, depression, hypertension, diabetes

Contra-indications see notes above; hormone-dependent tumours

Pregnancy see notes above

Breast-feeding see notes above

Side-effects see notes above; initially withdrawal bleeding and subsequently breakthrough bleeding, leucorrhoea; nausea, vomiting, constipation, diarrhoea; anxiety, memory and concentration disturbances, sleep disturbances, nervousness, dizziness, drowsiness; breast tenderness, lactation; abdominal pain; fatigue; increased thirst, changes in appetite; acne, dry skin, splitting nails, dry eyes; altered blood lipids, leucopenia, thrombocytopenia; hearing disturbances; reduced glucose tolerance

Dose
- Endometriosis, intranasally, 300 micrograms (one 150-microgram spray in each nostril) 3 times daily (starting on days 1 or 2 of menstruation); max. duration of treatment 6 months (do not repeat)
- Pituitary desensitisation before induction of ovulation by gonadotrophins for *in vitro* fertilisation (under specialist supervision), by subcutaneous injection, 200–500 micrograms daily given as a single injection (occasionally up to 500 micrograms twice daily may be needed) starting in early follicular phase (day 1) *or*, after exclusion of pregnancy, in midluteal phase (day 21) and continued until down-regulation achieved (usually about 1–3 weeks) then maintained during gonadotrophin administration (stopping gonadotrophin and buserelin on administration of chorionic gonadotrophin at appropriate stage of follicular development)

  Intranasally, 150 micrograms (one spray in one nostril) 4 times daily during waking hours (occasionally up to 300 micrograms 4 times daily may be needed) starting in early follicular phase (day 1) *or*, after exclusion of pregnancy, in midluteal phase (day 21) and continued until down-regulation achieved (usually about 2–3 weeks) then maintained during gonadotrophin administration (stopping gonadotrophin and buserelin on administration of chorionic gonadotrophin at appropriate stage of follicular development)

Counselling Avoid use of nasal decongestants before and for at least 30 minutes after treatment

Suprecur® (Sanofi-Aventis) PoM
Nasal spray, buserelin (as acetate) 150 micrograms/metered spray. Net price 2 × 100-dose pack (with metered dose pumps) = £87.63. Counselling, nasal decongestants

Injection, buserelin (as acetate) 1 mg/mL. Net price 5.5-mL vial = £13.76

▌ GOSERELIN

Indications see under Dose; prostate cancer (section 8.3.4.2); early and advanced breast cancer (section 8.3.4.1)

Cautions see notes above; polycystic ovarian disease; diabetes

Contra-indications see notes above

Pregnancy use non-hormonal contraceptives during treatment; see also notes above

Breast-feeding see notes above

Side-effects see notes above; withdrawal bleeding

Dose

- By subcutaneous injection into anterior abdominal wall (as *Zoladex®*)

  Endometriosis, 3.6 mg every 28 days; max. duration of treatment 6 months (do not repeat)

  Endometrial thinning before intra-uterine surgery, 3.6 mg (may be repeated after 28 days if uterus is large or to allow flexible surgical timing)

  Before surgery in women who have anaemia due to uterine fibroids, 3.6 mg every 28 days (with supplementary iron); max. duration of treatment 3 months

  Pituitary desensitisation before induction of ovulation by gonadotrophins for *in vitro* fertilisation (under specialist supervision), after exclusion of pregnancy, 3.6 mg to achieve pituitary down-regulation (usually 1–3 weeks) then gonadotrophin is administered (stopping gonadotrophin on administration of chorionic gonadotrophin at appropriate stage of follicular development)

◢**Preparation**

Section 8.3.4.2

▆ LEUPRORELIN ACETATE

Indications   see under Dose; prostate cancer (section 8.3.4.2)

Cautions   see notes above; monitor liver function; family history of osteoporosis; chronic use of other drugs which reduce bone density including alcohol and tobacco; diabetes

Contra-indications   see notes above

Pregnancy   teratogenic in *animal* studies; see also notes above

Breast-feeding   see notes above

Side-effects   see notes above; breast tenderness; nausea, vomiting, diarrhoea, anorexia; fever, chills; sleep disturbances, dizziness, fatigue, leucopenia, thrombocytopenia, altered blood lipids, pulmonary embolism; spinal fracture, paralysis, hypotension and worsening of depression also reported

Dose

- By subcutaneous injection (as *Prostap® SR DCS*)

  Endometriosis, 3.75 mg as a single dose in first 5 days of menstrual cycle then every month for max. 6 months (course not to be repeated)

  Endometrial thinning before intra-uterine surgery, 3.75 mg as a single dose (given between days 3 and 5 of menstrual cycle) 5–6 weeks before surgery

  Reduction of size of uterine fibroids and of associated bleeding before surgery, 3.75 mg as a single dose every month usually for 3–4 months (max. 6 months)

- By intramuscular injection (as *Prostap® 3 DCS*)

  Endometriosis, 11.25 mg as a single dose in first 5 days of menstrual cycle then every 3 months for max. 6 months (course not to be repeated)

◢**Preparations**

Section 8.3.4.2

▆ NAFARELIN

Indications   see under Dose

Cautions   see notes above

Contra-indications   see notes above

Pregnancy   see notes above

Breast-feeding   see notes above

Side-effects   see notes above; acne

Dose

- Endometriosis, women over 18 years, 200 micrograms twice daily as one spray in one nostril in the morning and one spray in the other nostril in the evening (starting on days 2–4 of menstruation), max. duration of treatment 6 months (do not repeat)

- Pituitary desensitisation before induction of ovulation by gonadotrophins for *in vitro* fertilisation (under specialist supervision), 400 micrograms (one spray in each nostril) twice daily starting in early follicular phase (day 2) or, after exclusion of pregnancy, in midluteal phase (day 21) and continued until down-regulation achieved (usually within 4 weeks) then maintained (usually for 8–12 days) during gonadotrophin administration (stopping gonadotrophin and nafarelin on administration of chorionic gonadotrophin at follicular maturity); discontinue if down-regulation not achieved within 12 weeks

  Counselling Avoid use of nasal decongestants before and for at least 30 minutes after treatment; repeat dose if sneezing occurs during or immediately after administration

Synarel® (Pharmacia) [PoM]
Nasal spray, nafarelin (as acetate) 200 micrograms/metered spray. Net price 30-dose unit = £30.41; 60-dose unit = £52.43. Label: 10, patient information leaflet, counselling, see above

▆ TRIPTORELIN

Indications   endometriosis; precocious puberty; reduction in size of uterine fibroids; male hypersexuality with severe sexual deviation; advanced prostate cancer (section 8.3.4.2)

Cautions   see notes above

Contra-indications   see notes above

Pregnancy   see notes above

Breast-feeding   see notes above

Side-effects   see notes above; also gastro-intestinal disturbances; in precocious puberty, withdrawal bleeding in females may occur in the first month of treatment; asthenia

Dose

- See under preparations below

Decapeptyl® SR (Ipsen) [PoM]
Injection, (powder for suspension), m/r, triptorelin (as acetate), net price 3-mg vial (with diluent) = £69.00

Dose by intramuscular injection, endometriosis and reduction in size of uterine fibroids, 3 mg every 4 weeks starting during first 5 days of menstrual cycle; for uterine fibroids continue treatment for at least 3 months; max. duration of treatment 6 months (not to be repeated)

Note Each vial includes an overage to allow accurate administration of 3-mg dose

Injection, (powder for suspension), m/r, triptorelin (as acetate), net price 11.25-mg vial (with diluent) = £207.00

Dose by intramuscular injection, endometriosis, 11.25 mg every 3 months starting during first 5 days of menstrual cycle; max. duration of treatment 6 months (not to be repeated)

Precocious puberty, 11.25 mg every 3 months; discontinue when bone maturation consistent with age of 12 years in girls or 13–14 years in boys

Note Each vial includes an overage to allow accurate administration of 11.25-mg dose

6 Endocrine system

Gonapeptyl Depot® (Ferring) [PoM]

Injection, (powder for suspension), triptorelin (as acetate), net price 3.75-mg prefilled syringe (with prefilled syringe of vehicle) = £81.69

Dose by subcutaneous *or* deep intramuscular injection, endometriosis and reduction in size of uterine fibroids, 3.75 mg every 4 weeks starting during first 5 days of menstrual cycle; max. duration of treatment 6 months (not to be repeated)

Precocious puberty, body-weight over 30 kg, initially 3.75 mg every 2 weeks for 3 doses, then every 3–4 weeks; body-weight 20–30 kg, initially 2.5 mg every 2 weeks for 3 doses, then every 3–4 weeks; body-weight under 20 kg, initially 1.875 mg every 2 weeks for 3 doses, then every 3–4 weeks; discontinue when bone maturation consistent with age over 12 years in girls or over 13 years in boys

Salvacyl® (Ipsen) [PoM]

Injection, (powder for suspension), triptorelin (as embonate), net price 11.25-mg vial (with diluent) = £248.00

Cautions transient increase in serum testosterone occurs on initiation—consider administration of an anti-androgen; increased risk of sensitivity to restored testosterone if treatment interrupted—consider administration of an anti-androgen before stopping treatment

Contra-indications severe osteoporosis

Dose by intramuscular injection, male hypersexuality with severe sexual deviation, 11.25 mg every 12 weeks

Breast pain (mastalgia)

Once any serious underlying cause for breast pain has been ruled out, most women will respond to reassurance and reduction in dietary fat; withdrawal of an oral contraceptive or of hormone replacement therapy may help to resolve the pain.

Mild, non-cyclical breast pain is treated with simple analgesics (section 4.7.1); moderate to severe pain, cyclical pain or symptoms that persist for longer than 6 months may require specific drug treatment.

Danazol (section 6.7.2) is licensed for the relief of severe pain and tenderness in benign fibrocystic breast disease which has not responded to other treatment.

Tamoxifen (section 8.3.4.1) may be a useful adjunct in the treatment of mastalgia [unlicensed indication] especially when symptoms can definitely be related to cyclic oestrogen production; it may be given on the days of the cycle when symptoms are predicted.

Treatment for breast pain should be reviewed after 6 months and continued if necessary. Symptoms recur in about 50% of women within 2 years of withdrawal of therapy but may be less severe.

6.7.3 Metyrapone

Metyrapone is a competitive inhibitor of 11β-hydroxylation in the adrenal cortex; the resulting inhibition of cortisol (and to a lesser extent aldosterone) production leads to an increase in ACTH production which, in turn, leads to increased synthesis and release of cortisol precursors. It may be used as a test of anterior pituitary function.

Although most types of *Cushing's syndrome* are treated surgically, that which occasionally accompanies carcinoma of the bronchus is not usually amenable to surgery. Metyrapone has been found helpful in controlling the symptoms of the disease; it is also used in other forms of Cushing's syndrome to prepare the patient for surgery. The dosages used are either low, and tailored to

cortisol production, or high, in which case corticosteroid replacement therapy is also needed.

■ METYRAPONE

Indications see notes above and under Dose (specialist supervision in hospital)

Cautions gross hypopituitarism (risk of precipitating acute adrenal failure); hypertension on long-term administration; hypothyroidism (delayed response); many drugs interfere with diagnostic estimation of steroids; avoid in acute porphyria (section 9.8.2)

Driving Drowsiness may affect the performance of skilled tasks (e.g. driving)

Contra-indications adrenocortical insufficiency (see Cautions)

Hepatic impairment use with caution in hepatic impairment (delayed response)

Pregnancy avoid (may impair biosynthesis of fetal-placental steroids)

Breast-feeding avoid—no information available

Side-effects occasional nausea, vomiting, dizziness, headache, hypotension, sedation; rarely abdominal pain, allergic skin reactions, hypoadrenalism, hirsutism

Dose

- Differential diagnosis of ACTH-dependent Cushing's syndrome, 750 mg every 4 hours for 6 doses; CHILD 15 mg/kg (minimum 250 mg) every 4 hours for 6 doses
- Management of Cushing's syndrome, range 0.25–6 g daily, tailored to cortisol production; see notes above
- Resistant oedema due to increased aldosterone secretion in cirrhosis, nephrotic syndrome, and congestive heart failure (with glucocorticoid replacement therapy) 3 g daily in divided doses

Metopirone® (HRA Pharma) [PoM]

Capsules, ivory, metyrapone 250 mg, net price 100-cap pack = £363.66. Label: 21, counselling, driving

6.7.4 Somatomedins

Somatomedins are a group of polypeptide hormones structurally related to insulin and commonly known as insulin-like growth factors (IGFs). **Mecasermin**, a human insulin-like growth factor-I (rhIGF-I), is the principal mediator of the somatotropic effects of human growth hormone and is used to treat growth failure in children and adolescents with severe primary insulin-like growth factor-I deficiency.

■ MECASERMIN

(Recombinant human insulin-like growth factor-I; rhIGF-I)

Indications see notes above

Cautions correct hypothyroidism before initiating treatment; diabetes mellitus (adjustment of antidiabetic therapy may be necessary); monitor ECG before and on termination of treatment (and during treatment if ECG abnormal), papilloedema (see under Side-effects), monitor for disorders of the epiphysis of the hip (monitor for limping), monitor for signs of tonsillar hypertrophy (snoring, sleep apnoea, and chronic middle ear effusions)

Contra-indications evidence of tumour activity (discontinue treatment)

Pregnancy avoid unless essential; contraception advised in women of child-bearing potential

Breast-feeding avoid

Side-effects headache, funduscopy for papilloedema recommended if severe or recurrent headache, visual problems, nausea and vomiting occur—if papilloedema confirmed consider benign intracranial hypertension (rare cases reported); cardiomegaly, ventricular hypertrophy, tachycardia; convulsions, sleep apnoea, night terrors, dizziness, nervousness; tonsillar hypertrophy (see Cautions above); hypoglycaemia (especially in first month, and in younger children), hyperglycaemia, gynaecomastia; arthralgia, myalgia; visual disturbance, impaired hearing; antibody formation; injection-site reactions (rotate site)

Dose

- By subcutaneous injection, ADOLESCENT and CHILD over 2 years, initially 40 micrograms/kg twice daily for 1 week, if tolerated increase dose in steps of 40 micrograms/kg to max. 120 micrograms/kg twice daily; discontinue if no response within 1 year
  Counselling Dose should be administered just before or after food; do not increase dose if a dose is missed
  Note Reduce dose if hypoglycaemia occurs despite adequate food intake; withhold injection if patient unable to eat

Increlex® (Ipsen) ▼ PoM

Injection, mecasermin 10 mg/mL, net price 4-mL vial = £605.00. Counselling, administration
Excipients include benzyl alcohol (avoid in neonates, see Excipients, p. 2)

7 Obstetrics, gynaecology, and urinary-tract disorders

This chapter also includes advice on the drug management of the following:

For hormonal therapy of gynaecological disorders see section 6.4.1 (including HRT), section 6.5.1 and section 6.7.2.

7.1 Drugs used in obstetrics

7.1.1 Prostaglandins and oxytocics
7.1.2 Mifepristone
7.1.3 Myometrial relaxants

Because of the complexity of dosage regimens in obstetrics, in all cases **detailed specialist literature** should be consulted.

7.1.1 Prostaglandins and oxytocics

7.1.1.1 Drugs affecting the ductus arteriosus

Prostaglandins and oxytocics are used to induce abortion or induce or augment labour and to minimise blood loss from the placental site. They include oxytocin, carbetocin, ergometrine, and the prostaglandins. All induce uterine contractions with varying degrees of pain according to the strength of contractions induced.

Induction of abortion Gemeprost, a prostaglandin administered vaginally as pessaries, is suitable for the medical induction of late therapeutic abortion; gemeprost is also used to ripen the cervix before surgical abortion, particularly in primigravidas. The prostaglandin misoprostol (section 7.1.2) is given by mouth, buccally, sublingually, or vaginally, to induce medical abortion [unlicensed indication]; intravaginal use ripens the cervix before surgical abortion [unlicensed indication]. Extra-amniotic dinoprostone is rarely used nowadays.

Pre-treatment with mifepristone (section 7.1.2) can facilitate the process of medical abortion. It sensitises the uterus to subsequent administration of a prostaglandin and, therefore, abortion occurs in a shorter time and with a lower dose of prostaglandin.

Induction and augmentation of labour Dinoprostone is available as vaginal tablets, pessaries and vaginal gels for the induction of labour. The intravenous solution is rarely used; it is associated with more side-effects.

Oxytocin (*Syntocinon®*) is administered by slow intravenous infusion, using an infusion pump, to induce or augment labour, usually in conjunction with amniotomy. Uterine activity must be monitored carefully and hyperstimulation avoided. Large doses of oxytocin may result in excessive fluid retention.

Misoprostol is given orally or vaginally for the induction of labour [unlicensed indication].

> **NICE guidance**
> **Induction of labour (updated July 2008)**
> Available at guidance.nice.org.uk/CG70

Prevention and treatment of haemorrhage
Bleeding due to incomplete miscarriage or abortion can be controlled with **ergometrine** and **oxytocin** (*Syntometrine®*) given intramuscularly, the dose is adjusted according to the patient's condition and blood loss. This is commonly used before surgical evacuation of the uterus, particularly when surgery is delayed. Oxytocin and ergometrine combined are more effective in early pregnancy than either drug alone.

Active management of the third stage of labour reduces the risk of postpartum haemorrhage; oxytocin is given by intramuscular injection [unlicensed] on delivery of the anterior shoulder or, at the latest, immediately after the baby is delivered. Alternatively, ergometrine 500 micrograms with oxytocin 5 units (*Syntometrine®* 1 mL) can be given by intramuscular injection in the absence of hypertension; oxytocin alone causes less nausea, vomiting, and hypertension than when given with ergometrine.

In excessive uterine bleeding, any placental products remaining in the uterus should be removed. Oxytocic drugs are used to treat postpartum haemorrhage caused by uterine atony; treatment options are as follows:

- oxytocin 5 units by slow intravenous injection (dose may be repeated), followed in severe cases by intravenous infusion of oxytocin 40 units in 500 mL infusion fluid (prolonged administration—see Appendix 4) at a rate that controls uterine atony *or*

- ergometrine 250–500 micrograms by intramuscular injection *or*

- ergometrine 250–500 micrograms by slow intravenous injection (use with caution—risk of hypertension) *or*

- ergometrine 500 micrograms with oxytocin 5 units (*Syntometrine®* 1 mL) by intramuscular injection

Carboprost has an important role in severe postpartum haemorrhage unresponsive to ergometrine and oxytocin.

Misoprostol [unlicensed] can be used in postpartum haemorrhage when oxytocin, ergometrine, and carboprost are not available or are inappropriate.

◢ CARBETOCIN

Indications prevention of uterine atony after caesarean section
Cautions hyponatraemia; cardiovascular disease (avoid if severe); migraine; asthma
Contra-indications pre-eclampsia and eclampsia; epilepsy
Hepatic impairment manufacturer advises avoid
Renal impairment manufacturer advises avoid
Side-effects nausea, vomiting, abdominal pain, metallic taste; flushing, hypotension, chest pain; dyspnoea; headache, tremor, dizziness; anaemia; back

pain; pruritus; feeling of warmth, chills; tachycardia and sweating also reported
Dose
- By slow intravenous injection over 1 minute, a single dose of 100 micrograms, as soon as possible after delivery, preferably before removal of placenta

Pabal® (Ferring) (PoM)
Injection, carbetocin 100 micrograms/mL, net price 1-mL amp = £17.64

◢ CARBOPROST

Indications postpartum haemorrhage due to uterine atony in patients unresponsive to ergometrine and oxytocin
Cautions history of glaucoma or raised intra-ocular pressure, asthma, hypertension, hypotension, anaemia, jaundice, diabetes, epilepsy; uterine scars; excessive dosage may cause uterine rupture; **interactions**: Appendix 1 (prostaglandins)
Contra-indications untreated pelvic infection; cardiac or pulmonary disease
Hepatic impairment manufacturer advises avoid
Renal impairment manufacturer advises avoid
Side-effects nausea, vomiting and diarrhoea, hyperthermia and flushing, bronchospasm; less frequent effects include raised blood pressure, dyspnoea, and pulmonary oedema; chills, headache, diaphoresis, dizziness; cardiovascular collapse also reported; erythema and pain at injection site reported
Dose
- By deep intramuscular injection, 250 micrograms repeated if necessary at intervals of not less than 15 minutes; total dose should not exceed 2 mg (8 doses)

Hemabate® (Pharmacia) (PoM)
Injection, carboprost as trometamol salt (tromethamine salt) 250 micrograms/mL, net price 1-mL amp = £18.20 (hosp. only)

◢ DINOPROSTONE

Indications see notes above and under preparations below
Cautions history of asthma, glaucoma and raised intra-ocular pressure; hypertension; history of epilepsy; uterine scarring; monitor uterine activity and fetal status (particular care if history of uterine hypertony); uterine rupture; see also notes above; monitor for disseminated intravascular coagulation after parturition; risk factors for disseminated intravascular coagulation; effect of oxytocin enhanced (care needed in monitoring uterine activity when used in sequence); **interactions**: Appendix 1 (prostaglandins)
Contra-indications active cardiac, or pulmonary disease; placenta praevia or unexplained vaginal bleeding during pregnancy, ruptured membranes, major cephalopelvic disproportion or fetal malpresentation, history of caesarean section or major uterine surgery, untreated pelvic infection, fetal distress, grand multiparas and multiple pregnancy, history of difficult or traumatic delivery; avoid extra-amniotic route in cervicitis or vaginitis
Hepatic impairment manufacturers advise avoid
Renal impairment manufacturers advise avoid
Side-effects nausea, vomiting, diarrhoea; other side-effects include uterine hypertonus, severe uterine

contractions, pulmonary or amniotic fluid embolism, abruptio placenta, fetal distress, maternal hypertension, bronchospasm, rapid cervical dilation, fever, backache; uterine hypercontractility with or without fetal bradycardia, low Apgar scores; cardiac arrest, uterine rupture, stillbirth or neonatal death also reported; vaginal symptoms (warmth, irritation, pain); after intravenous administration—flushing, shivering, headache, dizziness, temporary pyrexia and raised white blood cell count; disseminated intravascular coagulation reported; also local tissue reaction and erythema after intravenous administration and possibility of infection after extra-amniotic administration

Dose
- See under preparations, below

  Important Do not confuse dose of *Prostin E2*® vaginal **gel** with that of *Prostin E2*® vaginal **tablets**—not bioequivalent.

Propess® (Ferring) [PoM]

Pessaries (within retrieval device), releasing dinoprostone approx. 10 mg over 24 hours; net price 1-pessary pack = £30.00

Dose by vagina, cervical ripening and induction of labour at term, 1 pessary (in retrieval device) inserted high into posterior fornix and removed when cervical ripening adequate; if oxytocin necessary, remove 30 minutes before oxytocin infusion; remove if cervical ripening inadequate after 24 hours (dose not to be repeated)

Prostin E2® (Pharmacia) [PoM]

Intravenous solution ◢, for dilution and use as an infusion, dinoprostone 1 mg/mL, net price 0.75-mL amp = £8.52; 10 mg/mL, 0.5-mL amp = £18.40 (both hosp. only; rarely used, consult product literature for dose and indications)

Extra-amniotic solution ◢, dinoprostone 10 mg/mL, net price 0.5-mL amp (with diluent) = £18.40 (hosp. only; less commonly used nowadays, consult product literature for dose and indications)

Vaginal gel, dinoprostone 400 micrograms/mL, net price 2.5 mL (1 mg) = £13.28; 800 micrograms/mL, 2.5 mL (2 mg) = £13.28

Dose by vagina, induction of labour, inserted high into posterior fornix (avoid administration into cervical canal), 1 mg (unfavourable primigravida 2 mg), followed after 6 hours by 1–2 mg if required; max. [gel] 3 mg (unfavourable primigravida 4 mg)

Vaginal tablets, dinoprostone 3 mg, net price 8-vaginal tab pack = £106.23

Dose by vagina, induction of labour, inserted high into posterior fornix, 3 mg, followed after 6–8 hours by 3 mg if labour is not established; max. 6 mg [vaginal tablets]

Note *Prostin E2 Vaginal Gel* and *Vaginal Tablets* are **not** bioequivalent

ERGOMETRINE MALEATE

Indications see notes above

Cautions cardiac disease; hypertension; multiple pregnancy; acute porphyria (section 9.8.2); **interactions:** Appendix 1 (ergot alkaloids)

Contra-indications induction of labour, first and second stages of labour, vascular disease, severe cardiac disease, sepsis, severe hypertension, eclampsia

Hepatic impairment manufacturer advises caution in mild or moderate impairment and avoid in severe impairment

Renal impairment manufacturer advises caution in mild or moderate impairment and avoid in severe impairment

Side-effects nausea, vomiting, abdominal pain; chest pain, arrhythmias (including bradycardia), palpitation, hypertension, vasoconstriction; dyspnoea, pulmonary oedema; headache, dizziness; tinnitus; rash; *very rarely* myocardial infarction

Dose
- See notes above

Ergometrine (Non-proprietary) [PoM]

Injection, ergometrine maleate 500 micrograms/mL, net price 1-mL amp = 93p

◢**With oxytocin**

Syntometrine® (Alliance) [PoM]

Injection, ergometrine maleate 500 micrograms, oxytocin 5 units/mL, net price 1-mL amp = £1.57

Dose by intramuscular injection, 1 mL; by intravenous injection, no longer recommended

GEMEPROST

Indications see under Dose

Cautions obstructive airways disease, cardiovascular insufficiency, raised intra-ocular pressure, cervicitis or vaginitis; **interactions:** Appendix 1 (prostaglandins)

Important For warnings relating to use of gemeprost in a patient undergoing induction of abortion with mifepristone, see under Mifepristone and Note below

Contra-indications unexplained vaginal bleeding, uterine scarring, placenta praevia

Renal impairment manufacturer advises avoid

Side-effects vaginal bleeding and uterine pain; nausea, vomiting, or diarrhoea; headache, muscle weakness, dizziness, flushing, chills, backache, dyspnoea, chest pain, palpitation and mild pyrexia; uterine rupture reported (most commonly in multiparas or if history of uterine surgery or if given with intravenous oxytocics); also reported severe hypotension, coronary artery spasm and myocardial infarction

Dose
- By vagina, cervical ripening prior to first trimester surgical abortion, 1 mg inserted into posterior fornix 3 hours before surgery
- Second trimester abortion, 1 mg inserted into posterior fornix every 3 hours for max. of 5 administrations; second course may begin 24 hours after start of treatment (if treatment fails pregnancy should be terminated by another method)
- Second trimester intra-uterine death, 1 mg inserted into posterior fornix every 3 hours for max. of 5 administrations only; monitor for coagulopathy

Note If used in combination with mifepristone, carefully monitor blood pressure and pulse for 3 hours

Gemeprost (Sanofi-Aventis) [PoM]

Pessaries, gemeprost 1 mg, net price 5-pessary pack = £215.00

OXYTOCIN

Indications see under Dose and notes above

Cautions induction or enhancement of labour—presence of borderline cephalopelvic disproportion (avoid if significant), secondary uterine inertia, mild or moderate pregnancy-induced hypertension or cardiac disease, women over 35 years or with history of lower-uterine segment caesarean section (see also under Contra-indications below); risk factors for disseminated intravascular coagulation; monitor for disseminated intravascular coagulation after parturition; avoid large infusion volumes and restrict fluid intake by mouth (risk of hyponatraemia and water-intoxication—see also Appendix 4); effects enhanced by concomitant prostaglandins (very careful monitoring of uterine activity); caudal block anaesthesia (may enhance hypertensive effects of sympathomimetic vasopressors); see also **interactions**: Appendix 1 (oxytocin)

Contra-indications hypertonic uterine contractions, fetal distress; any condition where spontaneous labour or vaginal delivery inadvisable; avoid prolonged administration in oxytocin-resistant uterine inertia, severe pre-eclamptic toxaemia, or severe cardiovascular disease

Side-effects nausea, vomiting; arrhythmia; headache; *rarely* disseminated intravascular coagulation, rash, and anaphylactoid reactions (with dyspnoea, hypotension, or shock); uterine spasm (may occur at low doses); uterine hyperstimulation (usually with excessive doses—may cause fetal distress, asphyxia, and death, or may lead to hypertonicity, tetanic contractions, soft-tissue damage or uterine rupture); water intoxication and hyponatraemia associated with high doses with large infusion volumes of electrolyte-free fluid (see also under Dose below); placental abruption and amniotic fluid embolism also reported on overdose

Dose

● Induction of labour for medical reasons or stimulation of labour in hypotonic uterine inertia, by intravenous infusion (not to be started for at least 6 hours after administration of vaginal prostaglandin), initially 0.001–0.004 units/minute, increased at intervals of at least 30 minutes until a maximum of 3–4 contractions occur every 10 minutes (0.01 units/minute is often adequate) up to max. 0.02 units/minute; if regular contractions not established after total of 5 units stop induction attempt (may be repeated next day starting again at 0.001–0.004 units/minute)

  Important Careful monitoring of fetal heart rate and uterine motility essential for dose titration (**avoid** intravenous injection during labour); discontinue immediately in uterine hyperactivity or fetal distress

● Caesarean section, by slow intravenous injection immediately after delivery, 5 units

● Prevention of postpartum haemorrhage, after delivery of placenta, by slow intravenous injection, 5 units (if infusion used for induction or enhancement of labour, increase rate during third stage and for next few hours).

  Important Avoid rapid intravenous injection (may transiently reduce blood pressure)

  Note Can be given in a dose of 10 units by intramuscular injection [unlicensed route] instead of oxytocin with ergometrine (*Syntometrine®*), see notes above

● Treatment of postpartum haemorrhage, by slow intravenous injection, 5 units (dose may be repeated), followed in severe cases by intravenous infusion of 40 units in 500 mL infusion fluid at a rate sufficient to control uterine atony

  Important Avoid rapid intravenous injection (may transiently reduce blood pressure); prolonged administration, see warning below

● Incomplete, inevitable, or missed miscarriage, by slow intravenous injection, 5 units followed if necessary by intravenous infusion, 0.02–0.04 units/minute or faster

  Important Prolonged intravenous administration at high doses with large volume of fluid (which is possible in inevitable or missed miscarriage or postpartum haemorrhage) may cause water intoxication with hyponatraemia. To avoid:

use electrolyte-containing diluent (i.e. not glucose), increase oxytocin concentration to reduce fluid, restrict fluid intake by mouth; monitor fluid and electrolytes.

Note Oxytocin doses in the BNF may differ from those in the product literature

Syntocinon® (Novartis) [PoM]

  Injection, oxytocin, net price 5 units/mL, 1-mL amp = 80p; 10 units/mL, 1-mL amp = 91p

◢**With ergometrine**

See *Syntometrine®*, p. 540

7.1.1.1 Drugs affecting the ductus arteriosus

This section is not included in the BNF. For the management of ductus arteriosus, see *BNF for Children* section 2.14.

7.1.2 Mifepristone

Mifepristone, an antiprogestogenic steroid, sensitises the myometrium to prostaglandin-induced contractions and ripens the cervix. For termination of pregnancy, a single dose of mifepristone is followed by administration of a prostaglandin (gemeprost or misoprostol [unlicensed]). Guidelines of the Royal College of Obstetricians and Gynaecologists (November 2011) include the following [unlicensed] regimens for inducing medical abortion:

● For gestation up to 49 days, mifepristone 200 mg by mouth followed 24–48 hours later by misoprostol 400 micrograms by mouth

● For gestation at 50–63 days, mifepristone 200 mg by mouth followed 24–48 hours later by misoprostol 800 micrograms vaginally, buccally, or sublingually; if abortion has not occurred 4 hours after misoprostol dose, a further dose of misoprostol 400 micrograms may be given vaginally or by mouth

● For gestation between 9 and 13 weeks, mifepristone 200 mg by mouth followed 36–48 hours later by misoprostol 800 micrograms vaginally, followed if necessary by a maximum of 4 further doses at 3-hourly intervals of misoprostol 400 micrograms vaginally or by mouth

● For gestation between 13 and 24 weeks, mifepristone 200 mg by mouth followed 36–48 hours later by misoprostol 800 micrograms vaginally, followed if necessary by a maximum of 4 further doses at 3-hourly intervals of misoprostol 400 micrograms vaginally or by mouth; if abortion has not occurred 3 hours after the last dose of misoprostol, a further dose of mifepristone may be given, and misoprostol may be recommenced 12 hours later

MIFEPRISTONE

Indications see under dose

Cautions asthma (avoid if severe and uncontrolled); haemorrhagic disorders and anticoagulant therapy; prosthetic heart valve or history of endocarditis (see section 5.1 table 2); risk factors for or existing cardiovascular disease; adrenal suppression (may require corticosteroid); **interactions**: Appendix 1 (mifepristone)

  Important For warnings relating to use of gemeprost in a patient undergoing induction of abortion with mifepristone, see under Gemeprost

Contra-indications uncontrolled severe asthma; suspected ectopic pregnancy (use other specific means of termination); chronic adrenal failure; acute porphyria (section 9.8.2)

Hepatic impairment manufacturer advises avoid

Renal impairment   manufacturer advises avoid

Side-effects   gastro-intestinal cramps; uterine contractions, vaginal bleeding (sometimes severe) may occur between administration of mifepristone and surgery (and rarely abortion may occur before surgery); *less commonly* hypersensitivity reactions including rash and urticaria; *rarely* hypotension, malaise, headache, fever, hot flushes, dizziness, and chills; infections (including toxic shock syndrome) also reported

Dose

- Medical termination of intra-uterine pregnancy of up to 49 days gestation, by mouth, mifepristone 600 mg as a single dose under medical supervision followed 36–48 hours later (unless abortion already complete) by gemeprost 1 mg by vagina *or* misoprostol 400 micrograms by mouth [unlicensed]; alternative regimen, mifepristone 200 mg by mouth as a single dose followed 36–48 hours later (unless abortion already complete) by gemeprost 1 mg by vagina; observe for at least 3 hours (or until bleeding or pain at acceptable level); follow-up visit within 2 weeks to verify complete expulsion and to assess vaginal bleeding

- Medical termination of intra-uterine pregnancy of 50–63 days gestation, by mouth, mifepristone 600 mg (200 mg also effective) as a single dose under medical supervision, followed 36–48 hours later (unless abortion already complete) by gemeprost 1 mg by vagina; observe for at least 3 hours (or until bleeding or pain at acceptable level); follow-up visit within 2 weeks to verify complete expulsion and to assess vaginal bleeding

- Cervical ripening before mechanical cervical dilatation for termination of pregnancy of up to 84 days gestation, by mouth, mifepristone 200 mg as a single dose under medical supervision 36–48 hours before procedure

- Termination of pregnancy of 13–24 weeks gestation (in combination with a prostaglandin), by mouth, mifepristone 600 mg (200 mg may be effective) as a single dose under medical supervision followed 36–48 hours later by gemeprost 1 mg by vagina every 3 hours up to max. 5 mg *or* misoprostol (see above [unlicensed]); if abortion does not occur, 24 hours after start of treatment repeat course of gemeprost 1 mg by vagina up to max. 5 mg; follow-up visit after appropriate interval to assess vaginal bleeding recommended

  Note Careful monitoring of blood pressure and pulse essential for 3 hours after administration of gemeprost pessary (risk of profound hypotension)

- Labour induction in fetal death *in utero* where prostaglandin or oxytocin inappropriate, by mouth, mifepristone 600 mg daily as a single dose for 2 days under medical supervision; if labour not started within 72 hours of first dose, another method should be used

Mifegyne® (Nordic) PoM

Tablets, yellow, mifepristone 200 mg, net price 3-tab pack = £52.66 (supplied to NHS hospitals and premises approved under Abortion Act 1967). Label: 10, patient information leaflet

7.1.3   Myometrial relaxants

Tocolytic drugs postpone *premature labour* and they are used with the aim of reducing harm to the child. However, there is no satisfactory evidence that the use of

these drugs reduces mortality. The greatest benefit is gained by using the delay to administer corticosteroid therapy or to implement other measures which improve perinatal health (including transfer to a unit with neonatal intensive care facility).

The oxytocin receptor antagonist, **atosiban**, is licensed for the inhibition of uncomplicated premature labour *between 24 and 33 weeks* of gestation. Atosiban may be preferable to a beta₂ agonist because it has fewer side-effects.

The dihydropyridine calcium-channel blocker **nifedipine** (section 2.6.2) also has fewer side-effects than a beta₂ agonist. Nifedipine [unlicensed indication] can be given initially in a dose of 20 mg followed by 10–20 mg 3–4 times daily adjusted according to uterine activity.

The beta₂ agonists **salbutamol** and **terbutaline** are licensed for inhibiting uncomplicated premature labour between 22 and 37 weeks of gestation to permit a delay in delivery of up to 48 hours. Use of high-dose short-acting beta₂ agonists in obstetric indications has been associated with serious, sometimes fatal cardiovascular events in the mother and fetus, particularly when used for a prolonged period of time. Oral therapy is no longer recommended and parenteral therapy should be restricted to a maximum duration of 48 hours, given under the supervision of a specialist, and with close monitoring (see under Beta₂ agonists).

Indometacin (section 10.1.1), a cyclo-oxygenase inhibitor, also inhibits labour [unlicensed indication] and it can be useful in situations where a beta₂ agonist is not appropriate; however, there are concerns about neonatal complications such as transient impairment of renal function and premature closure of ductus arteriosus.

Atosiban

ATOSIBAN

Indications   uncomplicated premature labour (see notes above)

Cautions   monitor blood loss after delivery; intra-uterine growth restriction; abnormal placental site

Contra-indications   eclampsia and severe pre-eclampsia, intra-uterine infection, intra-uterine fetal death, antepartum haemorrhage (requiring immediate delivery), placenta praevia, abruptio placenta, intra-uterine growth restriction with abnormal fetal heart rate, premature rupture of membranes after 30 weeks' gestation

Hepatic impairment   no information available

Renal impairment   no information available

Side-effects   nausea, vomiting, tachycardia, hypotension, headache, dizziness, hot flushes, hyperglycaemia, injection-site reaction; *less commonly* pruritus, rash, fever, insomnia

Dose

- By intravenous injection, initially 6.75 mg over 1 minute, then by intravenous infusion 18 mg/hour for 3 hours, then 6 mg/hour for up to 45 hours; max. duration of treatment 48 hours

Tractocile® (Ferring) PoM

Injection, atosiban (as acetate) 7.5 mg/mL, net price 0.9-mL (6.75-mg) vial = £18.41

Concentrate for intravenous infusion, atosiban (as acetate) 7.5 mg/mL, net price 5-mL vial = £52.82

Beta₂ agonists

Cautions   Beta agonists should be used with caution in patients with hypertension, mild to moderate pre-eclampsia, hyperthyroidism, and hypokalaemia (particular risk with potassium-depleting diuretics—see also Hypokalaemia, p. 189). Patients with suspected cardio-vascular disease should be assessed by a cardiologist before initiating therapy—see also Contra-indications, below). It is important to monitor blood pressure, pulse rate (should not exceed 120 beats per minute), ECG (discontinue treatment if signs of myocardial ischaemia develop), blood glucose and lactate concentrations, and the patient's fluid and electrolyte status (avoid over-hydration—discontinue drug immediately and initiate diuretic therapy if pulmonary oedema occurs). Beta₂ agonists should also be used with caution in dia-betes—monitor blood glucose (risk of hyperglycaemia and ketoacidosis, especially with intravenous beta₂ agonists).

Contra-indications   Beta₂ agonists are contra-indi-cated in patients with a history of cardiac disease and in patients with significant risk factors for myocardial ischaemia; they should also be avoided in pulmonary hypertension, antepartum haemorrhage, intra-uterine infection, intra-uterine fetal death, placenta praevia, abruptio placenta, threatened miscarriage, cord com-pression, and eclampsia or severe pre-eclampsia.

Side-effects   Side-effects of the beta₂ agonists include nausea, vomiting, pulmonary oedema (see Cau-tions above), palpitation, tachycardia, arrhythmias, myocardial ischaemia, hypotension, peripheral vasodi-lation, headache, tremor, hyperglycaemia, hypokal-aemia (see Cautions), muscle cramps and tension, and hypersensitivity reactions (including angioedema, urti-caria, rash, bronchospasm, hypotension, and collapse).

▌ SALBUTAMOL
    (Albuterol)

Indications   uncomplicated premature labour under specialist supervision (see notes above); asthma (section 3.1.1)

Cautions   see notes above; **interactions:** Appendix 1 (sympathomimetics, beta₂)

Contra-indications   see notes above

Side-effects   see notes above

Dose

- By intravenous infusion, initially 10 micrograms/minute, rate increased gradually according to response at 10-minute intervals until contractions diminish then increase rate slowly until contractions cease (max. rate 45 micrograms/minute); maintain rate for 1 hour after contractions have stopped, then gradually reduce by 50% every 6 hours; max. duration 48 hours

◢ **Preparations**
Section 3.1.1.1

▌ TERBUTALINE SULFATE

Indications   uncomplicated premature labour under specialist supervision (see notes above); asthma (section 3.1.1)

Cautions   see notes above; **interactions:** Appendix 1 (sympathomimetics, beta₂)

Contra-indications   see notes above

Side-effects   see notes above; also reported sleep disturbances and behavioural disturbances

Dose

- By intravenous infusion, 5 micrograms/minute for 20 minutes, increased every 20 minutes in steps of 2.5 micrograms/minute until contractions have ceased (more than 10 micrograms/minute should **seldom** be given—20 micrograms/minute should **not** be exceeded), continue for 1 hour then decrease every 20 minutes in steps of 2.5 micrograms/minute to lowest dose that maintains suppression; max. total duration 48 hours

◢ **Preparations**
Section 3.1.1.1

7.2 Treatment of vaginal and vulval conditions

7.2.1   Preparations for vaginal and vulval changes

7.2.2   Vaginal and vulval infections

Symptoms are often restricted to the vulva, but infec-tions almost invariably involve the vagina which should also be treated. Applications to the vulva alone are likely to give only symptomatic relief without cure.

Aqueous medicated douches may disturb normal vaginal acidity and bacterial flora.

Topical anaesthetic agents give only symptomatic relief and may cause sensitivity reactions. They are indicated only in cases of pruritus where specific local causes have been excluded.

Systemic drugs are required in the treatment of infections such as gonorrhoea and syphilis (section 5.1).

7.2.1 Preparations for vaginal and vulval changes

Topical HRT for vaginal atrophy

A cream containing an oestrogen may be applied on a short-term basis to improve the vaginal epithelium in *menopausal atrophic vaginitis*. It is **important** to bear in mind that topical oestrogens should be used in the **smallest effective** amount to minimise systemic effects. Modified-release vaginal tablets and an impregnated vaginal ring are now also available.

The risk of endometrial hyperplasia and carcinoma is increased when *systemic* oestrogens are administered alone for prolonged periods (section 6.4.1.1). The endo-metrial safety of long-term or repeated use of *topical* vaginal oestrogens is uncertain; treatment should be reviewed at least annually, with special consideration given to any symptoms of endometrial hyperplasia or carcinoma.

Topical oestrogens are also used in postmenopausal women before vaginal surgery for prolapse when there is epithelial atrophy.

For a general comment on hormone replacement ther-apy, including the role of topical oestrogens, see section 6.4.1.1.

7 Obstetrics, gynaecology, and urinary-tract disorders

▪ OESTROGENS, TOPICAL

Indications see notes above

Cautions see notes above; see also Oestrogens for HRT (section 6.4.1.1); interrupt treatment periodically to assess need for continued treatment

Contra-indications see notes above; see also Oestrogens for HRT (section 6.4.1.1)

Hepatic impairment see Combined Hormonal Contraceptives, section 7.3.1

Pregnancy see Combined Hormonal Contraceptives, section 7.3.1

Breast-feeding avoid; adverse effects on lactation; see also Combined Hormonal Contraceptives, section 7.3.1

Side-effects see notes above; see also Oestrogens for HRT (section 6.4.1.1); local irritation

Gynest® (Marlborough) (PoM)
Intravaginal cream, estriol 0.01%, net price 80 g with applicator = £4.67
Excipients include arachis (peanut) oil
Condoms may damage latex condoms and diaphragms
Dose insert 1 applicatorful daily, preferably in the evening until improvement occurs, reduced to 1 applicatorful twice a week; attempts to discontinue should be made at 3–6 month intervals with re-examination

Ortho-Gynest® (Janssen) (PoM)
Pessaries, estriol 500 micrograms, net price 15 pessaries = £4.73
Excipients include butylated hydroxytoluene
Condoms damages latex condoms and diaphragms
Dose insert 1 pessary daily, preferably in the evening, until improvement occurs; maintenance 1 pessary twice a week; attempts to reduce or discontinue should be made at 3–6 month intervals with re-examination

Ovestin® (Aspen) (PoM)
Intravaginal cream, estriol 0.1%, net price 15 g with applicator = £4.45
Excipients include cetyl alcohol, polysorbates, stearyl alcohol
Condoms effect on latex condoms and diaphragms not yet known
Dose insert 1 applicator-dose daily for 2–3 weeks, then reduce to twice a week (discontinue every 2–3 months for 4 weeks to assess need for further treatment); vaginal surgery, 1 applicator-dose daily for 2 weeks before surgery, resuming 2 weeks after surgery

Vagifem® (Novo Nordisk) (PoM)
Vaginal tablets, f/c, estradiol 10 micrograms in disposable applicators, net price 24-applicator pack = £16.72
Excipients none as listed in section 13.1.3
Condoms no evidence of damage to latex condoms and diaphragms
Dose insert 1 vaginal tablet daily for 2 weeks then reduce to 1 tablet twice weekly

◢ Vaginal ring

Estring® (Pharmacia) (PoM)
Vaginal ring, releasing estradiol approx. 7.5 micrograms/24 hours, net price 1-ring pack = £31.42
Label: 10, patient information leaflet
Dose for postmenopausal urogenital conditions (not suitable for vasomotor symptoms or osteoporosis prophylaxis), to be inserted into upper third of vagina and worn continuously; replace after 3 months; max. duration of continuous treatment 2 years

Non-hormonal preparations for vaginal atrophy

Replens MD® and *Sylk®* are acidic, non-hormonal vaginal moisturisers; *Replens MD®* provides a high moisture content for up to 3 days.

7.2.2 Vaginal and vulval infections

Effective specific treatments are available for the common vaginal infections.

Fungal infections

Candidal vulvitis can be treated locally with cream, but is almost invariably associated with vaginal infection which should also be treated. *Vaginal candidiasis* is treated primarily with antifungal pessaries or cream inserted high into the vagina (including during menstruation). Single-dose preparations offer an advantage when compliance is a problem. Local irritation may occur on application of vaginal antifungal products.

Imidazole drugs (clotrimazole, econazole, fenticonazole, and miconazole) are effective against candida in short courses of 1 to 14 days according to the preparation used; treatment can be repeated if initial course fails to control symptoms or if symptoms recur. Vaginal applications may be supplemented with antifungal cream for vulvitis and to treat other superficial sites of infection.

Oral treatment of vaginal infection with **fluconazole** or **itraconazole** (section 5.2.1) is also effective.

Vulvovaginal candidiasis in pregnancy Vulvovaginal candidiasis is common during pregnancy and can be treated with vaginal application of an imidazole (such as clotrimazole), and a topical imidazole cream for vulvitis. Pregnant women need a longer duration of treatment, usually about 7 days, to clear the infection. Oral antifungal treatment should be avoided during pregnancy.

Recurrent vulvovaginal candidiasis Recurrence of vulvovaginal candidiasis is particularly likely if there are predisposing factors, such as antibacterial therapy, pregnancy, diabetes mellitus, or possibly oral contraceptive use. Reservoirs of infection may also lead to recontamination and should be treated; these include other skin sites such as the digits, nail beds, and umbilicus as well as the gastro-intestinal tract and the bladder. The partner may also be the source of re-infection and, if symptomatic, should be treated with a topical imidazole cream at the same time.

Treatment against candida may need to be extended for 6 months in recurrent vulvovaginal candidiasis. Some recommended regimens [all unlicensed] include:

- initially, fluconazole (section 5.2.1) by mouth 150 mg every 72 hours for 3 doses, then 150 mg once every week for 6 months;

- initially, intravaginal application of a topical imidazole for 10–14 days, then clotrimazole vaginally 500-mg pessary once every week for 6 months;

- initially, intravaginal application of a topical imidazole for 10–14 days, then itraconazole (section 5.2.1) by mouth 50–100 mg daily for 6 months.

PREPARATIONS FOR VAGINAL AND VULVAL CANDIDIASIS

Indications   see notes above

Cautions   interactions: Appendix 1 (miconazole)

Pregnancy   see notes above

Side-effects   occasional local irritation

Dose

• See under preparations below

Clotrimazole (Non-proprietary)

Cream (topical), clotrimazole 1%, net price 20 g = £1.70; 50 g = £4.25

Condoms   check with manufacturer of cream for effect on latex condoms and diaphragms

Dose   apply to anogenital area 2–3 times daily

Pessary, clotrimazole 500 mg, net price 1 pessary with applicator = £3.45

Dose   insert 1 pessary at night as a single dose; can be repeated once if necessary

Canesten® (Bayer Consumer Care)

Cream (topical), clotrimazole 1%, net price 20 g = £2.14; 50 g = £3.50

Excipients   include benzyl alcohol, cetostearyl alcohol, polysorbates

Condoms   damages latex condoms and diaphragms

Dose   apply to anogenital area 2–3 times daily

Thrush Cream (topical), clotrimazole 2%, net price 20 g = £4.46

Excipients   include benzyl alcohol, cetostearyl alcohol, polysorbates

Condoms   damages latex condoms and diaphragms

Dose   apply to anogenital area 2–3 times daily

Intravaginal cream (*10% VC®*) [PoM], clotrimazole 10%, net price 5-g applicator pack = £4.50

Excipients   include benzyl alcohol, cetostearyl alcohol, polysorbates

Condoms   damages latex condoms and diaphragms

Dose   insert 5 g at night as a single dose; can be repeated once if necessary

Note   Brands for sale to the public include *Canesten® Internal Cream*

Cream Combi, clotrimazole 10% vaginal cream and 2% topical cream, net price 5-g vaginal cream (with applicator) and 10-g topical cream = £8.21

Excipients   include benzyl alcohol, cetostearyl alcohol, polysorbates

Condoms   damages latex condoms and diaphragms

Dose   see under individual components

Pessaries, clotrimazole 100 mg, net price 6 pessaries with applicator = £3.50; 200 mg, 3 pessaries with applicator = £3.10

Condoms   damages latex condoms and diaphragms

Dose   insert 200 mg for 3 nights or 100 mg for 6 nights; course can be repeated once if necessary

Pessary, clotrimazole 500 mg, net price 1 pessary with applicator = £2.00

Condoms   damages latex condoms and diaphragms

Dose   insert 1 pessary at night as a single dose; can be repeated once if necessary

Pessary Combi, clotrimazole 500-mg pessary and cream (topical) 2%, net price 1 pessary and 10-g cream = £8.21

Condoms   damages latex condoms and diaphragmsExcipients   include benzyl alcohol, cetostearyl alcohol, polysorbates

Dose   see under individual components

Soft Gel Pessary, clotrimazole 500 mg, net price 1 pessary with applicator = £6.41

Condoms   damages latex condoms and diaphragms

Dose   insert 1 pessary at night as a single dose; can be repeated once if necessary

Soft Gel Pessary Combi, clotrimazole 500-mg soft gel pessary and cream (topical) 2%, net price 1 pessary and 10-g cream = £5.73

Excipients   include benzyl alcohol, cetostearyl alcohol, polysorbates

Condoms   damages latex condoms and diaphragms

Dose   see under individual components

Gyno-Daktarin® (Janssen) [PoM]

Intravaginal cream, miconazole nitrate 2%, net price 78 g with applicators = £4.33

Excipients   include butylated hydroxyanisole

Condoms   damages latex condoms and diaphragms

Dose   insert 5-g applicatorful once daily for 10–14 days or twice daily for 7 days; course can be repeated once if necessary; topical, apply to anogenital area twice daily

Ovule (= vaginal capsule) (*Gyno-Daktarin 1®*), miconazole nitrate 1.2 g in a fatty basis, net price 1 ovule = £2.94

Excipients   include hydroxybenzoates (parabens)

Condoms   damages latex condoms and diaphragms

Dose   insert 1 ovule at night as a single dose; can be repeated once if necessary

Gyno-Pevaryl® (Janssen) [PoM]

Cream, econazole nitrate 1%, net price 15 g = £2.11; 30 g = £3.78

Excipients   none as listed in section 13.1.3

Condoms   damages latex condoms and diaphragms

Dose   insert 5-g applicatorful intravaginally and apply to vulva at night for at least 14 nights; course can be repeated once if necessary

Note   Applicator available separately from Marlborough

Pessaries, econazole nitrate 150 mg, net price 3 pessaries = £4.17

Excipients   none as listed in section 13.1.3

Condoms   damages latex condoms and diaphragms

Dose   ADULT and CHILD over 16 years, insert 1 pessary for 3 nights; course can be repeated once if necessary

Pessary (*Gyno-Pevaryl 1®*), econazole nitrate 150 mg, formulated for single-dose therapy, net price 1 pessary with applicator = £3.69

Excipients   none as listed in section 13.1.3

Condoms   damages latex condoms and diaphragms

Dose   ADULT and CHILD over 16 years, insert 1 pessary at night as a single dose; can be repeated once if necessary

Gynoxin® (Recordati) [PoM]

Intravaginal cream, fenticonazole nitrate 2%, net price 30 g with applicator = £3.74

Excipients   include cetyl alcohol, hydrogenated wool fat, propylene glycol

Condoms   damages latex condoms and diaphragms

Dose   insert 5-g applicatorful intravaginally twice daily for 3 days

Vaginal capsule, fenticonazole nitrate 200 mg, net price 3 vaginal capsules = £2.42

Excipients   include hydrobenzoates (parabens)

Condoms   damages latex condoms and diaphragms

Dose   insert 1 vaginal capsule at night for 3 nights

Vaginal capsule, fenticonazole nitrate 600 mg, net price 1 vaginal capsule = £2.62

Excipients   include hydrobenzoates (parabens)

Condoms   damages latex condoms and diaphragms

Dose   insert 1 vaginal capsule at night as a single dose

Nizoral® (Janssen) [PoM]

Cream (topical), ketoconazole 2%, net price 30 g = £4.24

Excipients   include polysorbates, propylene glycol, stearyl alcohol

Condoms   effect on latex condoms and diaphragms not yet known

Dose   ADULT over 18 years, apply to anogenital area once or twice daily

7

Obstetrics, gynaecology, and urinary-tract disorders

7 Obstetrics, gynaecology, and urinary-tract disorders

Other infections

Trichomonal infections commonly involve the lower urinary tract as well as the genital system and need systemic treatment with metronidazole or tinidazole (section 5.1.11).

Bacterial infections with Gram-negative organisms are particularly common in association with gynaecological operations and trauma. Metronidazole is effective against certain Gram-negative organisms, especially *Bacteroides* spp. and can be used prophylactically in gynaecological surgery.

Clindamycin cream and metronidazole gel are indicated for bacterial vaginosis.

Vaginal preparations intended to restore normal acidity may prevent recurrence of vaginal infections and permit the re-establishment of the normal vaginal flora.

The antiviral drugs aciclovir, famciclovir, and valaciclovir can be used in the treatment of genital infection due to *herpes simplex virus*, the HSV type 2 being a major cause of genital ulceration; they have a beneficial effect on virus shedding and healing, generally giving relief from pain and other symptoms. See section 5.3.2.1 for systemic preparations, and section 13.10.3 for topical preparations.

◼ PREPARATIONS FOR OTHER VAGINAL INFECTIONS

Balance Activ Rx® (BBI Healthcare)
Vaginal gel, lactic acid 4.9%, glycogen 0.1%, net price 7 x 5 mL-tube = £5.25
Excipients include propylene glycol
Dose prevention of bacterial vaginosis, insert contents of 1 tube once or twice weekly

Dalacin® (Pharmacia) [PoM]
Cream, clindamycin 2% (as phosphate), net price 40-g pack with 7 applicators = £10.86
Excipients include benzyl alcohol, cetostearyl alcohol, polysorbates, propylene glycol
Condoms damages latex condoms and diaphragms
Side-effects irritation, cervicitis, and vaginitis; poorly absorbed into the blood—low risk of systemic effects, see section 5.1.6
Dose bacterial vaginosis, insert 5-g applicatorful at night for 3–7 nights

Relactagel® (KoRa)
Vaginal gel, lactic acid 4.5%, glycogen 0.1%, net price 7 × 5 mL-tube = £5.25
Excipients include propylene glycol
Cautions not recommended if trying to conceive
Side-effects mild irritation
Dose prevention of bacterial vaginosis, ADULT over 18 years insert contents of 1 tube at night for 2–3 nights after menstruation

Zidoval® (Meda) [PoM]
Vaginal gel, metronidazole 0.75%, net price 40-g pack with 5 applicators = £4.31
Excipients include disodium edetate, hydroxybenzoates (parabens), propylene glycol
Cautions not recommended during menstruation; some absorption may occur, see section 5.1.11 for systemic effects
Side-effects local effects including irritation, candidiasis, abnormal discharge, pelvic discomfort
Dose bacterial vaginosis, insert 5-g applicatorful at night for 5 nights

7.3 Contraceptives

7.3.1	**Combined hormonal contraceptives**
7.3.2	**Progestogen-only contraceptives**
7.3.3	**Spermicidal contraceptives**
7.3.4	**Contraceptive devices**
7.3.5	**Emergency contraception**

The Fraser Guidelines[1] should be followed when prescribing contraception for women under 16 years. The UK Medical Eligibility Criteria for Contraceptive Use (available at www.fsrh.org) is published by the Faculty of Sexual and Reproductive Healthcare; it categorises the risks of using contraceptive methods with pre-existing medical conditions.

Hormonal contraception is the most effective method of fertility control, but can have major and minor side-effects, especially for certain groups of women.

Intra-uterine devices are a highly effective method of contraception but may produce undesirable local side-effects. They may be used in women of all ages irrespective of parity, but are less appropriate for those with an increased risk of pelvic inflammatory disease.

Barrier methods alone (condoms, diaphragms, and caps) are less effective but can be reliable for well-motivated couples if used in conjunction with a **spermicide**. Occasionally sensitivity reactions occur. A female condom (*Femidom®*) is also available; it is pre-lubricated but does not contain a spermicide.

7.3.1 Combined hormonal contraceptives

Oral contraceptives containing an oestrogen and a progestogen ('combined oral contraceptives') are effective preparations for general use. Advantages of combined oral contraceptives include:

* reliable and reversible;
* reduced dysmenorrhoea and menorrhagia;
* reduced incidence of premenstrual tension;
* less symptomatic fibroids and functional ovarian cysts;
* less benign breast disease;
* reduced risk of ovarian and endometrial cancer;
* reduced risk of pelvic inflammatory disease.

Combined oral contraceptives containing a fixed amount of an oestrogen and a progestogen in each active tablet are termed 'monophasic'; those with varying amounts of these two hormones are termed 'phasic'. A transdermal patch and a vaginal ring, both containing an oestrogen with a progestogen, are also available.

Choice The majority of combined oral contraceptives contain ethinylestradiol as the oestrogen component; mestranol and estradiol are also used. The ethinylestradiol content of combined oral contraceptives ranges from 20 to 40 micrograms. Generally a preparation with the lowest oestrogen and progestogen content

1. See Department of Health Guidance (July 2004): Best practice guidance for doctors and other health professionals on the provision of advice and treatment to young people under 16 on contraception, sexual and reproductive health. Available at tinyurl.com/bpg16

which gives good cycle control and minimal side-effects in the individual woman is chosen. It is recommended that combined hormonal contraceptives are not continued beyond 50 years of age since more suitable alternatives exist.

- *Low strength preparations* (containing ethinylestradiol 20 micrograms) are particularly appropriate for women with risk factors for circulatory disease, provided a combined oral contraceptive is otherwise suitable.

- *Standard strength preparations* (containing ethinylestradiol 30 or 35 micrograms or in 30–40 microgram *phased* preparations) are appropriate for standard use—but see Risk of Venous Thromboembolism below. Phased preparations are generally reserved for women who *either* do not have withdrawal bleeding *or* who have breakthrough bleeding with monophasic products.

The progestogens desogestrel, drospirenone, and gestodene (in combination with ethinylestradiol) may be considered for women who have side-effects (such as acne, headache, depression, breast symptoms, and breakthrough bleeding) with other progestogens. Drospirenone, a derivative of spironolactone, has anti-androgenic and anti-mineralocorticoid activity; it should be used with care if an increased plasma-potassium concentration might be hazardous.

The progestogen dienogest is combined with estradiol in the combined oral contraceptive *Qlaira*®. Nomegestrol is the progestogen contained in the combined oral contraceptive *Zoely*®, in combination with estradiol.

The progestogen norelgestromin is combined with ethinylestradiol in a transdermal patch (*Evra*®).

The vaginal contraceptive ring contains the progestogen etonogestrel combined with ethinylestradiol (*NuvaRing*®).

Risk of venous thromboembolism

There is an increased risk of venous thromboembolic disease in users of combined hormonal contraceptives particularly during the first year and possibly after restarting combined hormonal contraceptives following a break of four weeks or more. This risk is considerably smaller than that associated with pregnancy (about 60 cases of venous thromboembolic disease per 100 000 pregnancies). In all cases of venous thromboembolism increases with age and in the presence of other risk factors, such as obesity. The risk also varies depending on the type of progestogen, see the Combined Hormonal Contraception and Risk of Venous Thromboembolism table for details.

Provided that women are informed of the relative risks of venous thromboembolism and accept them, the choice of oral contraceptive is for the woman together with the prescriber jointly to make in light of her individual medical history and any contra-indications.

Combined hormonal contraceptives also slightly increase the risk of *arterial* thromboembolism; however, there is no evidence to suggest that this risk varies between different preparations.

Travel

Women taking oral contraceptives or using the patch or vaginal ring are at an increased risk of deep-vein thrombosis during travel involving long periods of immobility (over 3 hours). The risk may be reduced by appropriate exercise during the journey and possibly by wearing graduated compression hosiery.

Combined Hormonal Contraception and Risk of Venous Thromboembolism

Progestogen in Combined Hormonal Contraceptive	Estimated incidence per 10 000 women per year of use
Non-pregnant, not using combined hormonal contraception	2
Levonorgestrel[1]	
Norgestimate[1]	5–7
Norethisterone[1]	
Etonogestrel[1]	6–12
Norelgestromin[1]	
Gestodene[1]	
Desogestrel[1]	9–12
Drospirenone[1]	
Dienogest[2]	Not known—insufficient data
Nomegestrol acetate[2]	

1. Combined with ethinylestradiol
2. Combined with estradiol

Missed pill The critical time for loss of contraceptive protection is when a pill is omitted at the *beginning* or *end* of a cycle (which lengthens the pill-free interval).

If a woman forgets to take a pill, it should be taken as soon as she remembers, and the next one taken at the normal time (even if this means taking 2 pills together). A missed pill is one that is 24 or more hours late; for women taking *Qlaira*® or *Zoely*®, see below. If a woman misses only one pill, she should take an active pill as soon as she remembers and then resume normal pill-taking. No additional precautions are necessary.

If a woman misses 2 or more pills (especially from the first 7 in a packet), she may not be protected. She should take an active pill as soon as she remembers and then resume normal pill-taking. In addition, she must either abstain from sex or use an additional method of contraception such as a condom for the next 7 days. If these 7 days run beyond the end of the packet, the next packet should be started at once, omitting the pill-free interval (or, in the case of *everyday* (ED) pills, omitting the 7 inactive tablets).

A missed pill for a woman taking *Qlaira*® or *Zoely*® is one that is 12 hours or more late; for information on how to manage missed pills in women taking *Qlaira*® or *Zoely*®, refer to product literature.

Emergency contraception (section 7.3.5) is recommended if 2 or more combined oral contraceptive tablets are missed from the first 7 tablets in a packet and unprotected intercourse has occurred since finishing the last packet.

Delayed application or detached patch If a patch is partly detached for less than 24 hours, reapply to the same site or replace with a new patch immediately; no additional contraception is needed and the next patch should be applied on the usual 'change day'. If a patch remains detached for more than 24 hours or if the user is not aware when the patch became detached, then stop the current contraceptive cycle and start a new cycle by applying a new patch, giving a new 'Day 1'; an additional non-hormonal contraceptive must be used concurrently for the first 7 days of the new cycle. If application of a new patch at the start of a new cycle is delayed, contraceptive protection is lost. A new patch

7 Obstetrics, gynaecology, and urinary-tract disorders

should be applied as soon as remembered giving a new 'Day 1'; additional non-hormonal methods of contraception should be used for the first 7 days of the new cycle. If application of a patch in the middle of the cycle is delayed (i.e. the patch is not changed on day 8 or day 15):

- for up to 48 hours, apply a new patch immediately; next patch 'change day' remains the same and no additional contraception is required;

- for more than 48 hours, contraceptive protection may have been lost. Stop the current cycle and start a new 4-week cycle immediately by applying a new patch giving a new 'Day 1'; additional non-hormonal contraception should be used for the first 7 days of the new cycle.

If the patch is not removed at the end of the cycle (day 22), remove it as soon as possible and start the next cycle on the usual 'change day', the day after day 28; no additional contraception is required.

Expulsion, delayed insertion or removal, or broken vaginal ring If the vaginal ring is expelled for *less than 3 hours*, rinse the ring with cool water and reinsert immediately; no additional contraception is needed.

If the ring remains outside the vagina for *more than 3 hours* or if the user does not know when the ring was expelled, contraceptive protection may be reduced:

- If ring expelled during week 1 or 2 of cycle, rinse ring with cool water and reinsert; use additional precautions (barrier methods) for next 7 days;

- If ring expelled during week 3 of cycle, either insert a new ring to start a new cycle *or* allow a withdrawal bleed and insert a new ring no later than 7 days after ring was expelled; latter option only available if ring was used continuously for at least 7 days before expulsion.

If insertion of a new ring at the start of a new cycle is delayed, contraceptive protection is lost. A new ring should be inserted as soon as possible; additional precautions (barrier methods) should be used for the first 7 days of the new cycle. If intercourse occurred during the extended ring-free interval, pregnancy should be considered.

No additional contraception is required if removal of the ring is delayed by up to 1 week (4 weeks of continuous use). The 7-day ring-free interval should be observed and subsequently a new ring should be inserted. Contraceptive protection may be reduced with continuous use of the ring for more than 4 weeks—pregnancy should be ruled out before inserting a new ring.

If the ring breaks during use, remove it and insert a new ring immediately; additional precautions (barrier methods) should be used for the first 7 days of the new cycle.

Diarrhoea and vomiting Vomiting and persistent, severe diarrhoea can interfere with the absorption of combined oral contraceptives. If vomiting occurs within 2 hours of taking a combined oral contraceptive another pill should be taken as soon as possible. In cases of persistent vomiting or severe diarrhoea lasting more than 24 hours, additional precautions should be used during and for 7 days (9 days for *Qlaira*®) after recovery (see also under Missed pill, above). If the vomiting and diarrhoea occurs during the last 7 tablets, the next pill-free interval should be omitted (in the case of ED tablets the inactive ones should be omitted).

Interactions The effectiveness of *combined* oral contraceptives, *progestogen-only* oral contraceptives (section 7.3.2.1), contraceptive patches, and vaginal rings can be considerably reduced by interaction with drugs that induce hepatic enzyme activity (e.g. **carbamazepine, eslicarbazepine, nevirapine, oxcarbazepine, phenytoin, phenobarbital, primidone, ritonavir, St John's Wort, topiramate,** and, above all, **rifabutin** and **rifampicin**). A condom together with a long-acting method, such as an injectable contraceptive, may be more suitable for patients with HIV infection or at risk of HIV infection; advice on the possibility of interaction with antiretroviral drugs should be sought from HIV specialists.

Women taking combined hormonal contraceptives who require enzyme-inducing drugs should be advised to change to a contraceptive method that is unaffected by enzyme-inducers (e.g. some parenteral progestogen-only contraceptives (p. 555), intra-uterine devices) for the duration of treatment and for 4 weeks after stopping. If a change in contraceptive method is undesirable or inappropriate the following options should be discussed:

- For a *short course (2 months or less) of an enzyme-inducing drug*, continue with a combined oral contraceptive providing ethinylestradiol 30 micrograms or more daily and use a 'tricycling' regimen (i.e. taking 3 packets of monophasic tablets without a break followed by a shortened tablet-free interval of 4 days [unlicensed use]). Additional contraceptive precautions should also be used whilst taking the enzyme-inducing drug and for 4 weeks after stopping. Another option (except for rifampicin or rifabutin—see below) is to follow the advice for long-term courses, below.

  For women using combined hormonal contraceptive patches or vaginal rings, additional contraceptive precautions are also required whilst taking the enzyme-inducing drug and for 4 weeks after stopping. If concomitant administration runs beyond the 3 weeks of patch or vaginal ring use, a new treatment cycle should be started immediately, without a patch-free or ring-free break.

- For a *long-term course (over 2 months) of an enzyme-inducing drug* (except rifampicin or rifabutin—see below), adjust the dose of combined oral contraceptive to provide ethinylestradiol 50 micrograms or more daily [unlicensed use] and use a 'tricycling' regimen (as above); continue for the duration of treatment with the enzyme-inducing drug and for 4 weeks after stopping.

  If breakthrough bleeding occurs (and all other causes are ruled out) it is recommended that the dose of ethinylestradiol is increased by increments of 10 micrograms up to a maximum of 70 micrograms daily [unlicensed use], or to use additional precautions, or to change to a method unaffected by enzyme-inducing drugs.

  Contraceptive patches and vaginal rings are not recommended for women taking enzyme-inducing drugs over a long period.

- For a *long-term course (over 2 months) of rifampicin or rifabutin*, an alternative method of contraception (such as an IUD) is **always** recommended because they are such potent enzyme-inducing drugs; the alternative method of contraception should be continued for 4 weeks after stopping the enzyme-inducing drug.

For information on interactions of oral progestogen-only contraceptives, see also p. 551; for information on interactions of parenteral progestogen-only contraceptives, see also p. 555; for information on interactions of the intra-uterine progestogen-only device, see also p. 556; for information on interactions of hormonal emergency contraception, see also p. 559.

Antibacterials that do not induce liver enzymes Latest recommendations are that no additional contraceptive precautions are required when *combined* oral contraceptives are used with antibacterials that do not induce liver enzymes, unless diarrhoea or vomiting occur (see above). These recommendations should be discussed with the woman, who should also be advised that guidance in patient information leaflets may differ.

It is also currently recommended that no additional contraceptive precautions are required when contraceptive patches or vaginal rings are used with antibacterials that do not induce liver enzymes. There have been concerns that some antibacterials that do not induce liver enzymes (e.g. ampicillin, doxycycline) reduce the efficacy of *combined* oral contraceptives by impairing the bacterial flora responsible for recycling ethinylestradiol from the large bowel. However, there is a lack of evidence to support this interaction.

Surgery Oestrogen-containing contraceptives should preferably be discontinued (and adequate alternative contraceptive arrangements made) 4 weeks before major elective surgery and all surgery to the legs or surgery which involves prolonged immobilisation of a lower limb; they should normally be recommenced at the first menses occurring at least 2 weeks after full mobilisation. A progestogen-only contraceptive may be offered as an alternative and the oestrogen-containing contraceptive restarted after mobilisation, as above. When discontinuation of an oestrogen-containing contraceptive is not possible, e.g. after trauma or if a patient admitted for an elective procedure is still on an oestrogen-containing contraceptive, thromboprophylaxis (with unfractionated or low molecular weight heparin and graduated compression hosiery) is advised. These recommendations do not apply to minor surgery with short duration of anaesthesia, e.g. laparoscopic sterilisation or tooth extraction, or to women using oestrogen-free hormonal contraceptives.

Reason to stop immediately Combined hormonal contraceptives or hormone replacement therapy (HRT) should be stopped (pending investigation and treatment), if any of the following occur:

- sudden severe chest pain (even if not radiating to left arm);
- sudden breathlessness (or cough with blood-stained sputum);
- unexplained swelling or severe pain in calf of one leg;
- severe stomach pain;
- serious neurological effects including unusual severe, prolonged headache especially if first time or getting progressively worse *or* sudden partial or complete loss of vision *or* sudden disturbance of hearing or other perceptual disorders *or* dysphasia *or* bad fainting attack or collapse *or* first unexplained epileptic seizure *or* weakness, motor disturbances, very marked numbness suddenly affecting one side or one part of body;

- hepatitis, jaundice, liver enlargement;
- blood pressure above systolic 160 mmHg or diastolic 95 mmHg;
- prolonged immobility after surgery or leg injury;
- detection of a risk factor which contra-indicates treatment (see Cautions and Contra-indications under Combined Hormonal Contraceptives below or under Oestrogens for HRT (section 6.4.1.1)).

▌COMBINED HORMONAL CONTRACEPTIVES

Indications contraception; menstrual symptoms (section 6.4.1.2)

Cautions see notes above; risk factors for venous thromboembolism (see below and also notes above), arterial disease and migraine, see below; personal or family history of hypertriglyceridaemia (increased risk of pancreatitis); hyperprolactinaemia (seek specialist advice); history of severe depression especially if induced by hormonal contraceptive; undiagnosed breast mass; gene mutations associated with breast cancer (e.g. BRCA 1); sickle-cell disease; inflammatory bowel disease including Crohn's disease; reduced efficacy of contraceptive patch in women with body-weight ≥ 90 kg; active trophoblastic disease (until return to normal of urine- and plasma-gonadotrophin concentration)—seek specialist advice; **interactions:** see above and Appendix 1 (oestrogens, progestogens)

Risk factors for venous thromboembolism See also notes above. Use with **caution** if any of following factors present but **avoid** if two or more factors present:

- *family history of venous thromboembolism* in first-degree relative aged under 45 years (avoid contraceptive containing desogestrel or gestodene, *or* avoid if known prothrombotic coagulation abnormality e.g. factor V Leiden or antiphospholipid antibodies (including lupus anticoagulant));
- *obesity*—body mass index ≥ 30 kg/m² (avoid if body mass index ≥ 35 kg/m² unless no suitable alternative);
- *long-term immobilisation* e.g. in a wheelchair (avoid if confined to bed or leg in plaster cast);
- *history of superficial thrombophlebitis*;
- *age* over 35 years (avoid if over 50 years);
- *smoking*.

Risk factors for arterial disease Use with **caution** if any one of following factors present but **avoid** if two or more factors present:

- *family history of arterial disease* in first degree relative aged under 45 years (avoid if atherogenic lipid profile);
- *diabetes mellitus* (avoid if diabetes complications present);
- *hypertension*—blood pressure above *systolic 140 mmHg* or *diastolic 90 mmHg* (avoid if blood pressure above *systolic 160 mmHg* or *diastolic 95 mmHg*);
- *smoking* (avoid if smoking 40 or more cigarettes daily);
- *age* over 35 years (avoid if over 50 years);
- *obesity* (avoid if body mass index ≥ 35 kg/m² unless no suitable alternative);
- *migraine without aura* (avoid if *migraine with aura* (focal symptoms), *or* severe migraine frequently lasting over 72 hours despite treatment, *or* migraine treated with ergot derivatives).

Migraine Women should report any increase in headache frequency or onset of focal symptoms (discontinue immediately and refer urgently to neurology expert if focal neurological symptoms not typical of aura persist for more than 1 hour—see also Reason To Stop Immediately in notes above)

Contra-indications see notes above; personal history of venous or arterial thrombosis, severe or multiple risk factors for arterial disease or for venous thromboembolism (see above), heart disease associated with pulmonary hypertension or risk of embolus; sclerosing treatment for varicose veins; migraine with aura (see also above); transient cerebral ischaemic attacks without headaches; systemic lupus erythematosus with (or unknown) antiphospholipid antibodies; acute porphyria (section 9.8.2); gallstones; history of haemolytic uraemic syndrome or history during pregnancy of pruritus, cholestatic jaundice, chorea, pemphigoid gestationis; history of breast cancer but can be used after 5 years if no evidence of disease and non-hormonal methods unacceptable; undiagnosed vaginal bleeding

Hepatic impairment avoid in active liver disease including disorders of hepatic excretion (e.g. Dubin-Johnson or Rotor syndromes), infective hepatitis (until liver function returns to normal), and liver tumours

Pregnancy not known to be harmful; for *Zoely*®—toxicity in *animal* studies

Breast-feeding avoid until weaning or for 6 months after birth (adverse effects on lactation)

Side-effects see notes above; also nausea, vomiting, abdominal cramps, liver impairment, hepatic tumours; fluid retention, thrombosis (more common when factor V Leiden present or in blood groups A, B, and AB; see also notes above), hypertension, changes in lipid metabolism; headache, depression, chorea, nervousness, irritability; changes in libido, breast tenderness, enlargement, and secretion; reduced menstrual loss, 'spotting' in early cycles, absence of withdrawal bleeding, amenorrhoea after discontinuation, changes in vaginal discharge, cervical erosion; contact lenses may irritate, visual disturbances; leg cramps; skin reactions, chloasma, photosensitivity; rarely gallstones and systemic lupus erythematosus

Breast cancer There is a small increase in the risk of having breast cancer diagnosed in women taking the combined oral contraceptive pill; this relative risk may be due to an earlier diagnosis. In users of combined oral contraceptive pills the cancers are more likely to be localised to the breast. The most important factor for diagnosing breast cancer appears to be the age at which the contraceptive is stopped rather than the duration of use; any increase in the rate of diagnosis diminishes gradually during the 10 years after stopping and disappears by 10 years

Cervical cancer Use of combined oral contraceptives for 5 years or longer is associated with a small increased risk of cervical cancer; the risk diminishes after stopping and disappears by about 10 years. The risk of cervical cancer with transdermal patches and vaginal rings is not yet known

Note The possible small increase in the risk of breast cancer and cervical cancer should be weighed against the protective effect against cancers of the ovary and endometrium

Dose

- By mouth , each tablet should be taken at approximately same time each day; if delayed, contraceptive protection may be lost (see missed pill, p. 547)

21-day combined (monophasic) preparations, 1 tablet daily for 21 days; subsequent courses repeated after a 7-day interval (during which withdrawal bleeding occurs); if reasonably certain woman is not pregnant, first course can be started on any day of cycle—if starting on day 6 of cycle or later, additional precautions (barrier methods) necessary during first 7 days

Every day (ED) combined (monophasic) preparations, 1 *active* tablet daily for 21 days, followed by 1 *inactive* tablet daily for 7 days (see also Combined Oral Contraceptives table, below); subsequent courses repeated without interval (withdrawal bleeding occurs when *inactive* tablets being taken); if reasonably certain woman is not pregnant, first course can be started on any day of cycle—if starting on day 6 of cycle or later, additional precautions (barrier methods) necessary during first 7 days; for *Zoely*® see Combined Oral Contraceptives table, below

Phasic preparations, see Combined Oral Contraceptives table, below

Changing to combined preparation containing different progestogen If previous contraceptive used correctly, or pregnancy can reasonably be excluded, start the first *active* tablet of new brand immediately

Changing to Qlaira®: start the first *active* Qlaira® tablet on the day after taking the last active tablet of the previous brand

Changing to Zoely®: start the first *active Zoely*® tablet on the day after taking the last active tablet of the previous brand or, at the latest, the day after the tablet-free or inactive tablet interval of the previous brand

Changing from Qlaira® or *Zoely*®: start the new brand after taking the last active tablet; if the inactive tablets are taken before starting new brand, additional precautions (barrier methods) should be used during first 7 days of taking the new brand

Changing from progestogen-only tablet If previous contraceptive used correctly, or pregnancy can reasonably be excluded, start new brand immediately, additional precautions (barrier methods) necessary for first 7 days

Changing to Qlaira®: start any day, additional precautions (barrier methods) necessary for first 9 days

Secondary amenorrhoea (exclude pregnancy) Start any day, additional precautions (barrier methods) necessary during first 7 days (9 days for *Qlaira*®)

After childbirth (not breast-feeding) Start 3 weeks after birth (increased risk of thrombosis if started earlier); later than 3 weeks postpartum additional precautions (barrier methods) necessary for first 7 days (9 days for *Qlaira*®)

After abortion or miscarriage Start same day

- By transdermal application, apply first patch on day 1 of cycle, change patch on days 8 and 15; remove third patch on day 22 and apply new patch after 7-day patch-free interval to start subsequent contraceptive cycle

Note If first patch applied later than day 1, additional precautions (barrier methods) should be used for the next 7 days

Changing from combined oral contraception Apply patch on the first day of withdrawal bleeding; if no withdrawal bleeding within 5 days of taking last *active* tablet, rule out pregnancy before applying first patch. Unless patch is applied on first day of withdrawal bleeding, additional precautions (barrier methods) should be used concurrently for first 7 days

Changing from progestogen-only method From an implant, apply first patch on the day implant removed; from an injection, apply first patch when next injection due; from oral progestogen, first patch may be applied on any day after stopping pill. For all methods additional precautions (barrier methods) should be used concurrently for first 7 days

After childbirth (not breast-feeding) Start 4 weeks after birth; if started later than 4 weeks after birth additional precautions (barrier methods) should be used for first 7 days

After abortion or miscarriage Before 20 weeks' gestation start immediately; no additional contraception required if started immediately. After 20 weeks' gestation start on day 21 after abortion or on the first day of first spontaneous menstruation; additional precautions (barrier methods) should be used for first 7 days after applying the patch

- By vaginal ring, insert ring into vagina on day 1 of cycle and leave in for 3 weeks; remove ring on day 22; subsequent courses repeated after 7-day ring-free interval (during which withdrawal bleeding occurs)

Note If first ring inserted later than day 1, additional precautions (barrier methods) should be used for the next 7 days

Changing from combined hormonal contraception Insert ring at the latest on the day after the usual tablet-free, patch-free, or inactive-tablet interval. If previous contraceptive used correctly, or pregnancy can reasonably be excluded, can switch to ring on any day of cycle

Changing from progestogen-only method From an implant or intra-uterine progestogen-only device, insert ring on the day implant or intra-uterine progestogen-only device removed; from an injection, insert ring when next injection due; from oral preparation, first ring may be inserted on any day after stopping pill. For all methods additional precautions (barrier methods) should be used concurrently for first 7 days

After first trimester abortion Start immediately

After childbirth (not breast-feeding) or second trimester abortion Start 4 weeks after birth or abortion; if started later than 4 weeks after birth or abortion, additional precautions (barrier methods) should be used for first 7 days

▌Oral (low and standard strength)

For information on these preparations, see Combined Oral Contraceptives table, p. 552

▌Transdermal (standard strength)

◢**Ethinylestradiol with Norelgestromin**

See Risk of Venous Thromboembolism (in notes above) before prescribing

Evra® (Janssen) PoM

Patches, self-adhesive (releasing ethinylestradiol approx. 33.9 micrograms/24 hours and norelgestromin approx. 203 micrograms/24 hours); net price 9-patch pack = £19.51. Counselling, administration

Dose 1 patch to be applied once weekly for three weeks, followed by a 7-day patch-free interval; subsequent courses repeated after 7-day patch-free interval (during which withdrawal bleeding occurs); for starting routines see under Dose above

Note Adhesives or bandages should not be used to hold patch in place. If patch no longer sticky do not reapply but use a new patch.

The *Scottish Medicines Consortium* has advised (September 2003) that *Evra®* patches should be restricted for use in women who are likely to comply poorly with combined oral contraceptives

▌Vaginal (low strength)

◢**Ethinylestradiol with Etonogestrel**

See Risk of Venous Thromboembolism (in notes above) before prescribing

NuvaRing® (MSD) PoM

Vaginal ring, releasing ethinylestradiol approx. 15 micrograms/24 hours and etonogestrel approx. 120 micrograms/24 hours, net price 3-ring pack = £29.70. Counselling, administration

Dose 1 ring to be inserted into the vagina, removed on day 22; subsequent courses repeated after 7-day ring-free interval (during which withdrawal bleeding occurs); for starting routines see under Dose above

Counselling The presence of the ring should be checked regularly. In case of expulsion see Expulsion, Delayed Insertion or Removal, or Broken Vaginal Ring, p. 548

7.3.2 Progestogen-only contraceptives

7.3.2.1 Oral progestogen-only contraceptives
7.3.2.2 Parenteral progestogen-only contraceptives
7.3.2.3 Intra-uterine progestogen-only device

7.3.2.1 Oral progestogen-only contraceptives

Oral progestogen-only preparations alter cervical mucus to prevent sperm penetration and may inhibit ovulation in some women; oral desogestrel-only preparations consistently inhibit ovulation and this is their primary mechanism of action. There is insufficient clinical trial evidence to compare the efficacy of oral progestogen-only contraceptives with each other or with combined hormonal contraceptives. Progestogen-only contraceptives offer a suitable alternative to combined hormonal contraceptives when oestrogens are contra-indicated (including those with venous thrombosis or a past history or predisposition to venous thrombosis, heavy smokers, those with hypertension above systolic 160 mmHg or diastolic 95 mmHg, valvular heart disease, diabetes mellitus with complications, and migraine with aura). Menstrual irregularities (oligomenorrhoea, menorrhagia) are more common but tend to resolve on long-term treatment.

Interactions Effectiveness of oral progestogen-only preparations is not affected by antibacterials that do not induce liver enzymes. The efficacy of oral progestogen-only preparations is, however, reduced by enzyme-inducing drugs and an alternative contraceptive method, unaffected by the interacting drug, is recommended during treatment with an enzyme-inducing drug and for at least 4 weeks afterwards—see p. 548 and Appendix 1 (progestogens). For a short course of an enzyme-inducing drug, if a change in contraceptive method is undesirable or inappropriate, the progestogen-only oral method may be continued in combination with additional contraceptive precautions (e.g. barrier methods) for the duration of treatment with the enzyme-inducing drug and for 4 weeks after stopping.

Surgery All progestogen-only contraceptives (including those given by injection) are suitable for use as an alternative to combined hormonal contraceptives before major elective surgery, before all surgery to the legs, or before surgery which involves prolonged immobilisation of a lower limb.

Starting routine One tablet daily, on a continuous basis, starting on day 1 of cycle and taken at the same time each day (if delayed by longer than 3 hours (12 hours for desogestrel) contraceptive protection may be lost). Additional contraceptive precautions are not necessary when initiating treatment.

Changing from a combined oral contraceptive Start on the day following completion of the combined oral contraceptive course without a break (or in the case of ED tablets omitting the inactive ones).

Combined Oral Contraceptives

See Risk of Venous Thromboembolism (in notes above) before prescribing

Type of preparation	Oestrogen content	Progestogen content	Tablets per cycle	Brand	Net Price, 3-cycle pack (unless stated)	Manufacturer
[1]Monophasic low strength (21-day preparations)	Ethinylestradiol 20 micrograms	Desogestrel 150 micrograms	21	Gedarel® 20/150	£5.98	Consilient
				Mercilon®	£8.44	MSD
		Gestodene 75 micrograms	21	Femodette®	£8.85	Bayer
				Millinette® 20/75	£6.37	Consilient
				Sunya 20/75®	£6.62	Stragen
		Norethisterone acetate 1 mg	21	Loestrin 20®	£2.70	Galen
[1]Monophasic standard strength (21-day preparations)	Ethinylestradiol 30 micrograms	Desogestrel 150 micrograms	21	Gedarel® 30/150	£4.93	Consilient
				Marvelon®	£7.10	MSD
		Drospirenone 3 mg	21	[2]Yasmin®	£14.70	Bayer
		Gestodene 75 micrograms	21	Femodene®	£6.73	Bayer
				Katya 30/75®	£5.03	Stragen
				Millinette® 30/75	£4.85	Consilient
		Levonorgestrel 150 micrograms	21	Levest®	£1.80	Morningside
				Microgynon 30®	£2.82	Bayer
				Ovranette®	£2.20	Pfizer
				Rigevidon®	£1.89	Consilient
		Norethisterone acetate 1.5 mg	21	Loestrin 30®	£3.90	Galen
	Ethinylestradiol 35 micrograms	Norgestimate 250 micrograms	21	Cilest®	£7.16	Janssen
		Norethisterone 500 micrograms	21	Brevinor®	£1.99	Pharmacia
				Ovysmen®	£1.89	Janssen
		Norethisterone 1 mg	21	Norimin®	£2.28	Pharmacia
	Mestranol 50 micrograms	Norethisterone 1 mg	21	Norinyl-1®	£2.19	Pharmacia
[3]Monophasic standard strength (28-day 'Every day' preparations)	Ethinylestradiol 30 micrograms	Gestodene 75 micrograms	21 active / 7 inactive	Femodene® ED	£7.10	Bayer
	Ethinylestradiol 30 micrograms	Levonorgestrel 150 micrograms	21 active / 7 inactive	Microgynon 30 ED®	£2.99	Bayer
[4]Monophasic (28-day 'Every day' preparation)	Estradiol (as hemihydrate) 1.5 mg	Nomegestrol acetate 2.5 mg	24 active / 4 inactive	Zoely® ▼	£19.80	MSD

1. *Dose* 1 tablet daily for 21 days starting on day 1–5 of cycle (if reasonably certain woman is not pregnant, first course can be started on any day of cycle); subsequent courses repeated after 7-day tablet-free interval (during which withdrawal bleeding occurs); for starting and changing routines see under Dose above

2. *Caution* use with care if increased plasma-potassium concentration might be hazardous; *renal impairment* avoid if eGFR less than 30 mL/minute/1.73 m²

3. *Dose* 1 tablet daily for 28 days starting on day 1–5 of cycle with first active tablet (withdrawal bleeding occurs when inactive tablets being taken) (if reasonably certain woman is not pregnant, first course can be started on any day of cycle); subsequent courses repeated without interval; for starting and changing routines see under Dose above

4. *Dose* 1 tablet daily for 28 days starting on day 1 of cycle with first active tablet (withdrawal bleeding occurs when inactive tablets being taken); subsequent courses repeated without interval; for starting and changing routines see under Dose above

Combined Oral Contraceptives (*continued*)

See Risk of Venous Thromboembolism (in notes above) before prescribing

Type of preparation	Oestrogen content	Progestogen content	Tablets per cycle	Brand	Net Price, 3-cycle pack (unless stated)	Manufacturer
[1]Phasic standard strength (21-day preparations)	Ethinylestradiol 30 micrograms	Gestodene 50 micrograms	6	Triadene®	£10.40	Bayer
	Ethinylestradiol 40 micrograms	Gestodene 70 micrograms	5			
	Ethinylestradiol 30 micrograms	Gestodene 100 micrograms	10			
	Ethinylestradiol 30 micrograms	Levonorgestrel 50 micrograms	6	Logynon®	£3.82	Bayer
	Ethinylestradiol 40 micrograms	Levonorgestrel 75 micrograms	5	TriRegol®	£2.87	Consilient
	Ethinylestradiol 30 micrograms	Levonorgestrel 125 micrograms	10			
	Ethinylestradiol 35 micrograms	Norethisterone 500 micrograms	7	BiNovum®	£2.49	Janssen
	Ethinylestradiol 35 micrograms	Norethisterone 1 mg	14			
	Ethinylestradiol 35 micrograms	Norethisterone 500 micrograms	7	Synphase®	1-cycle pack = £1.20	Pharmacia
	Ethinylestradiol 35 micrograms	Norethisterone 1 mg	9			
	Ethinylestradiol 35 micrograms	Norethisterone 500 micrograms	5			
	Ethinylestradiol 35 micrograms	Norethisterone 500 micrograms	7	TriNovum®	£3.46	Janssen
	Ethinylestradiol 35 micrograms	Norethisterone 750 micrograms	7			
	Ethinylestradiol 35 micrograms	Norethisterone 1 mg	7			
[2]Phasic standard strength (28-day 'Every day' preparation)	Ethinylestradiol 30 micrograms	Levonorgestrel 50 micrograms	6 active	Logynon ED®	£4.00	Bayer
	Ethinylestradiol 40 micrograms	Levonorgestrel 75 micrograms	5 active			
	Ethinylestradiol 30 micrograms	Levonorgestrel 125 micrograms	10 active			
			7 inactive			
[3]Phasic (28-day 'Every day' preparation)	Estradiol valerate 3 mg		2 active	Qlaira®	£25.18	Bayer
	Estradiol valerate 2 mg	Dienogest 2 mg	5 active			
	Estradiol valerate 2 mg	Dienogest 3 mg	17 active			
	Estradiol valerate 1 mg		2 active			
			2 inactive			

1. *Dose* 1 tablet daily for 21 days starting on day 1–5 of cycle (if reasonably certain woman is not pregnant, first course can be started on any day of cycle); subsequent courses repeated after 7-day tablet-free interval (during which withdrawal bleeding occurs); for starting and changing routines see under Dose above
2. *Dose* 1 tablet daily for 28 days starting on day 1–5 of cycle with first active tablet (withdrawal bleeding occurs when inactive tablets being taken) (if reasonably certain woman is not pregnant, first course can be started on any day of cycle); subsequent courses repeated without interval; for starting and changing routines see under Dose above
3. *Dose* 1 tablet daily for 28 days starting on day 1 of cycle with first active tablet (withdrawal bleeding occurs when inactive tablets being taken); subsequent courses repeated without interval; for starting and changing routines see under Dose above

7

After childbirth Oral progestogen-only contraceptives can be started up to and including day 21 postpartum without the need for additional contraceptive precautions. If started more than 21 days postpartum, additional contraceptive precautions are required for 2 days.

Missed pill The following advice is recommended:

'If you forget a pill, take it as soon as you remember and carry on with the next pill at the right time. If the pill was more than 3 hours (12 hours for desogestrel) overdue you are not protected. Continue normal pill-taking but you must also use another method, such as the condom, for the next 2 days.'

The Faculty of Sexual and Reproductive Healthcare recommends emergency contraception (see p. 559) if one or more progestogen-only contraceptive tablets are missed or taken more than 3 hours (12 hours for desogestrel) late and unprotected intercourse has occurred before 2 further tablets have been correctly taken.

Diarrhoea and vomiting Vomiting and persistent, severe diarrhoea can interfere with the absorption of oral progestogen-only contraceptives. If vomiting occurs within 2 hours of taking an oral progestogen-only contraceptive, another pill should be taken as soon as possible. If a replacement pill is not taken within 3 hours (12 hours for desogestrel) of the normal time for taking the progestogen-only pill, or in cases of persistent vomiting or very severe diarrhoea, additional precautions should be used during illness and for 2 days after recovery (see also under Missed pill above).

ORAL PROGESTOGEN-ONLY CONTRACEPTIVES
(Progestogen-only pill, 'POP')

Indications contraception

Cautions arterial disease; sex-steroid dependent cancer; past ectopic pregnancy; malabsorption syndromes; active trophoblastic disease (until return to normal of urine- and plasma-gonadotrophin concentration)—seek specialist advice; systemic lupus erythematosus with positive (or unknown) antiphospholipid antibodies; functional ovarian cysts; history of jaundice in pregnancy; **interactions:** see notes above and Appendix 1 (progestogens)

Other conditions The product literature advises caution in patients with history of thromboembolism, hypertension, diabetes mellitus and migraine; evidence for caution in these conditions is unsatisfactory

Contra-indications undiagnosed vaginal bleeding; severe arterial disease; acute porphyria (section 9.8.2); history of breast cancer but can be used after 5 years if no evidence of disease and non-hormonal contraceptive methods unacceptable

Hepatic impairment caution in severe liver disease and recurrent cholestatic jaundice; avoid in liver tumour

Pregnancy not known to be harmful

Breast-feeding progestogen-only contraceptives do not affect lactation; see also After Childbirth above

Side-effects menstrual irregularities (see also notes above); nausea, vomiting, headache, dizziness, breast discomfort, depression, skin disorders, disturbance of appetite, changes in libido

Breast cancer There is a small increase in the risk of having breast cancer diagnosed in women using, or who have recently used, a progestogen-only contraceptive pill; this relative risk may be due to an earlier diagnosis. The most important risk factor appears to be the age at which the contraceptive is stopped rather than the duration of use; the risk disappears gradually during the 10 years after stopping and there is no excess risk by 10 years. A possible small increase in the risk of breast cancer should be weighed against the benefits

Dose

● 1 tablet daily at same time each day, starting on day 1 of cycle then continuously; if administration delayed for 3 hours (12 hours for desogestrel) or more it should be regarded as a 'missed pill', see notes above

Desogestrel (Non-proprietary) (PoM)

Tablets, desogestrel 75 micrograms, net price 3 × 28-tab pack = £3.56

Brands include *Aizea®, Cerelle®, Nacrez®*

Cerazette® (MSD) (PoM)

Tablets, f/c, desogestrel 75 micrograms, net price 3 × 28-tab pack = £9.55

The *Scottish Medicines Consortium* (p. 4) has advised (September 2003) that *Cerazette®* should be restricted for use in women who cannot tolerate oestrogen-containing contraceptives or in whom such preparations are contra-indicated

Micronor® (Janssen) (PoM)

Tablets, norethisterone 350 micrograms, net price 3 × 28-tab pack = £1.80

Norgeston® (Bayer) (PoM)

Tablets, s/c, levonorgestrel 30 micrograms, net price 35-tab pack = 92p

Noriday® (Pharmacia) (PoM)

Tablets, norethisterone 350 micrograms, net price 3 × 28-tab pack = £2.10

7.3.2.2 Parenteral progestogen-only contraceptives

Medroxyprogesterone acetate (*Depo-Provera®, SAYANA PRESS®*) is a long-acting progestogen given by injection; it is at least as effective as the combined oral preparations but because of its prolonged action it should never be given without *full counselling backed by the patient information leaflet*. It may be used as a short-term or long-term contraceptive for women who have been counselled about the likelihood of menstrual disturbance and the potential for a delay in return to full fertility. Delayed return of fertility and irregular cycles may occur after discontinuation of treatment but there is no evidence of permanent infertility. Troublesome bleeding has been reported in patients given medroxyprogesterone acetate in the immediate puerperium; delaying the first injection until 6 weeks after birth may minimise bleeding problems. If the woman is not breast-feeding, the first injection may be given within 5 days postpartum (she should be warned that the risk of troublesome bleeding may be increased). The manufacturers advise that in women who are breast-feeding, the first dose should be delayed until 6 weeks after birth; however, evidence suggests no harmful effect to infant if given earlier. The benefits of using medroxyprogesterone acetate in breast-feeding women outweigh any risks.

Reduction in bone mineral density and, rarely, osteoporosis and osteoporotic fractures have also been reported with medroxyprogesterone acetate. The reduction in bone mineral density occurs in the first 2–3 years of use and then stabilises. See also below.

> - In adolescents, medroxyprogesterone acetate (*Depo-Provera®, SAYANA PRESS®*) should be used only when other methods of contraception are inappropriate;
> - in all women, the benefits of using medroxyprogesterone acetate beyond 2 years should be evaluated against the risks;
> - in women with risk factors for osteoporosis, a method of contraception other than medroxyprogesterone acetate should be considered.

Norethisterone enantate (*Noristerat®*) is a long-acting progestogen given as an oily injection which provides contraception for 8 weeks; it is used as short-term interim contraception e.g. before vasectomy becomes effective.

An **etonogestrel-releasing implant** (*Nexplanon®*) is also available. It is a highly effective long-acting contraceptive, consisting of a single flexible rod that is inserted subdermally into the lower surface of the upper arm and provides contraception for up to 3 years. The manufacturer advises that in heavier women, blood-etonogestrel concentrations are lower and therefore the implant may not provide effective contraception during the third year; they advise that earlier replacement may be considered in such patients—however, evidence to support this recommendation is lacking. Local reactions such as bruising and itching can occur at the insertion site. The contraceptive effect of etonogestrel is rapidly reversed on removal of the implant. *The doctor or nurse administering (or removing) the system should be fully trained in the technique and should provide full counselling reinforced by the patient information leaflet.*

Implanon®, also an etonogestrel-releasing implant, has been discontinued (October 2010), but some women may have the implant in place until 2013.

Cautions, contra-indications, and side-effects

The cautions, contra-indications, and side-effects of oral progestogen-only contraceptives apply to parenteral progestogen-only contraceptives, except that parenteral preparations reliably inhibit ovulation and therefore protect against ectopic pregnancy and functional ovarian cysts.

Interactions   Effectiveness of parenteral progestogen-only contraceptives is not affected by antibacterials that do not induce liver enzymes. The effectiveness of norethisterone intramuscular injection and medroxyprogesterone acetate intramuscular and subcutaneous injections is not affected by enzyme-inducing drugs and they may be continued as normal during courses of these drugs. However, effectiveness of the etonogestrel-releasing implant may be reduced by enzyme-inducing drugs and an alternative contraceptive method, unaffected by the interacting drug, is recommended during treatment with the enzyme-inducing drug and for at least 4 weeks after stopping. For a short course of an enzyme-inducing drug, if a change in contraceptive method is undesirable or inappropriate, the implant may be continued in combination with additional contraceptive precautions (e.g. condom) for the duration of treatment with the enzyme-inducing drug and for 4 weeks after stopping it.

PARENTERAL PROGESTOGEN-ONLY CONTRACEPTIVES

Indications   contraception, see also notes above and under preparations (roles vary according to preparation)

Cautions   see notes above and under preparations; possible risk of breast cancer, see oral progestogen-only contraceptives (section 7.3.2.1); history during pregnancy of pruritus or of deterioration of otosclerosis, disturbances of lipid metabolism; **interactions:** see notes above and Appendix 1 (progestogens)

Counselling   Full counselling backed by *patient information leaflet* required before administration

Contra-indications   see notes above; history of breast cancer but can be used after 5 years if no evidence of disease and non-hormonal contraceptive methods unacceptable

Hepatic impairment   see Oral Progestogen-only Contraceptives, section 7.3.2.1

Pregnancy   not known to be harmful; for *Implanon®* or *Nexplanon®* if pregnancy occurs remove implant

Breast-feeding   progestogen-only contraceptives do not affect lactation; see also notes above and under preparations

Side-effects   see notes above; injection-site reactions; *with medroxyprogesterone acetate injection*, weight gain also reported

Cervical cancer   Use of injectable progestogen-only contraceptives may be associated with a small increased risk of cervical cancer, similar to that seen with combined oral contraceptives, see p. 550. The risk of cervical cancer with other progestogen-only contraceptives is not yet known.

Dose
- See under preparations

◢ Injectable preparations

Depo-Provera® (Pfizer) ▨PoM▨

Injection (aqueous suspension), medroxyprogesterone acetate 150 mg/mL, net price 1-mL prefilled syringe = £6.01, 1-mL vial = £6.01. Counselling, see patient information leaflet

Dose by deep intramuscular injection, 150 mg within first 5 days of cycle or within first 5 days after parturition (delay until 6 weeks after parturition if breast-feeding); for long-term contraception, repeated every 12 weeks (if interval greater than 12 weeks and 5 days, rule out pregnancy before next injection and advise patient to use additional contraceptive measures (e.g. barrier) for 14 days after the injection)

Noristerat® (Bayer) ▨PoM▨

Injection (oily), norethisterone enantate 200 mg/mL, net price 1-mL amp = £4.05. Counselling, see patient information leaflet

Dose by deep intramuscular injection given very slowly *into gluteal muscle*, short-term contraception, 200 mg within first 5 days of cycle or immediately after parturition (duration 8 weeks); may be repeated once after 8 weeks (withhold breast-feeding for neonates with severe or persistent jaundice requiring medical treatment)

SAYANA PRESS® (Pfizer) ▨PoM▨

Injection (suspension), medroxyprogesterone acetate 104 mg/0.65 mL, net price 0.65-mL prefilled injector device = £6.90. Counselling, see patient information leaflet

Dose by subcutaneous injection into anterior thigh or abdomen, no hormonal contraceptive use in previous month, 104 mg within first 5 days of cycle or within 5 days postpartum (delay until 6 weeks postpartum if breast-feeding); for long-term contraception, repeated every 13 weeks (if interval greater than 13 weeks and 7 days, rule out pregnancy before next injection); changing from other hormonal contraceptive, consult product literature

◢ **Implants**

Nexplanon® (MSD) [PoM]

Implant, containing etonogestrel 68 mg in radiopaque flexible rod, net price = £83.43. Counselling, see patient information leaflet

Dose by subdermal implantation, no hormonal contraceptive use in previous month, 1 implant inserted during first 5 days of cycle; postpartum, 1 implant inserted 21–28 days after delivery; in breast-feeding mothers, 1 implant inserted after 28 days postpartum; abortion or miscarriage in the second trimester, 1 implant inserted 21–28 days after abortion or miscarriage; abortion or miscarriage in first trimester, 1 implant inserted within 5 days; changing from other hormonal contraceptive, consult product literature; remove implant within 3 years of insertion

7.3.2.3 Intra-uterine progestogen-only device

The progestogen-only intra-uterine system, *Mirena*®, releases **levonorgestrel** directly into the uterine cavity. It is licensed for use as a contraceptive, for the treatment of primary menorrhagia and for the prevention of endometrial hyperplasia during oestrogen replacement therapy. This may therefore be a contraceptive method of choice for women who have excessively heavy menses.

The effects of the progestogen-only intra-uterine system are mainly local and hormonal including prevention of endometrial proliferation, thickening of cervical mucus, and suppression of ovulation in some women (in some cycles). In addition to the progestogenic activity, the intra-uterine system itself may contribute slightly to the contraceptive effect. Return of fertility after removal is rapid and appears to be complete. *The doctor or nurse administering (or removing) the system should be fully trained in the technique and should provide full counselling reinforced by the patient information leaflet.*

Advantages of the progestogen-only intra-uterine system over copper intra-uterine devices are that there may be an improvement in any dysmenorrhoea and a reduction in blood loss; there is also evidence that the frequency of pelvic inflammatory disease may be reduced (particularly in the youngest age groups who are most at risk).

In primary menorrhagia, menstrual bleeding is reduced significantly within 3–6 months of inserting the progestogen-only intra-uterine system, probably because it prevents endometrial proliferation. Another treatment should be considered if menorrhagia does not improve within this time (section 6.4.1.2).

Cautions and contra-indications Generally the cautions and contra-indications for the progestogen-only intra-uterine system are as for standard intra-uterine devices (section 7.3.4). Although the progestogen-only intra-uterine system produces little systemic progestogenic activity, it is usually avoided for 5 years after any evidence of breast cancer. However, the system can be considered for a woman in long-term remission from breast cancer who has menorrhagia and requires effective contraception. Since levonorgestrel is released close to the site of the main contraceptive action (on cervical mucus and endometrium) progestogenic side-effects and interactions are less likely; in particular, enzyme-inducing drugs are unlikely to significantly reduce the contraceptive effect of the progestogen-only intra-uterine system and additional contraceptive precautions are not required.

Side-effects Initially, changes in the pattern and duration of menstrual bleeding (spotting or prolonged bleeding) are common; endometrial disorders should be ruled out before insertion and the patient should be fully counselled (and provided with a patient information leaflet). Improvement in progestogenic side-effects, such as mastalgia and in the bleeding pattern usually occurs a few months after insertion and bleeding may often become very light or absent. Functional ovarian cysts (usually asymptomatic) can occur and usually resolve spontaneously (ultrasound monitoring recommended).

◢ **INTRA-UTERINE PROGESTOGEN-ONLY SYSTEM**

Indications see under preparation

Cautions see notes above; history of depression; advanced uterine atrophy; systemic lupus erythematosus with positive (or unknown) antiphospholipid antibodies; **interactions:** see notes above and Appendix 1 (progestogens)

Contra-indications see notes above; not suitable for emergency contraception

Hepatic impairment see Oral Progestogen-only Contraceptives, section 7.3.2.1

Pregnancy avoid; if pregnancy occurs remove system

Breast-feeding progestogen-only contraceptives do not affect lactation

Side-effects see notes above; also abdominal pain, expulsion, peripheral oedema, depression (sometimes severe), nervousness, salpingitis, pelvic inflammatory disease, pelvic pain, back pain; *rarely* uterine perforation, hirsutism, hair loss, pruritus, migraine, rash

Dose
- See under preparation

Mirena® (Bayer) [PoM]

Intra-uterine system, T-shaped plastic frame (impregnated with barium sulfate and with threads attached to base) with polydimethylsiloxane reservoir releasing levonorgestrel 20 micrograms/24 hours, net price = £88.00. Counselling, see patient information leaflet

Dose contraception and menorrhagia, insert into uterine cavity within 7 days of onset of menstruation, or any time if replacement, or any time if reasonably certain woman is not pregnant and there is no risk of conception (additional precautions (e.g. barrier methods) necessary for next 7 days), or immediately after first-trimester termination by curettage; postpartum insertions should be delayed until at least 4 weeks after delivery; effective for 5 years.

Prevention of endometrial hyperplasia during oestrogen replacement therapy, insert during last days of menstruation or withdrawal bleeding or any time if amenorrhoeic; effective for 4 years

Note When system is removed (and not immediately replaced) and pregnancy is not desired, remove during the first few days of menstruation, otherwise additional precautions (e.g. barrier methods) should be used for at least 7 days before removal

7.3.3 Spermicidal contraceptives

Spermicidal contraceptives are useful additional safeguards but do **not** give adequate protection if used alone unless fertility is already significantly diminished (section 6.4.1.1). They have two components: a spermicide and a vehicle which itself may have some inhibiting effect on sperm activity. They are suitable for use with barrier methods, such as diaphragms or caps; however, spermicidal contraceptives are not generally recommended for use with condoms, as there is no evidence of any additional protection compared with non-spermicidal lubricants.

Spermicidal contraceptives are not suitable for use in those with or at high risk of sexually transmitted infections (including HIV); high frequency use of the spermicide nonoxinol '9' has been associated with genital lesions, which may increase the risk of acquiring these infections.

> Products such as petroleum jelly (*Vaseline*®), baby oil and oil-based vaginal and rectal preparations are likely to damage condoms and contraceptive diaphragms made from latex rubber, and may render them less effective as a barrier method of contraception and as a protection from sexually transmitted infections (including HIV).

Gygel® (Marlborough)

Gel, nonoxinol '9' 2%, net price 30 g = £4.25
Excipients include hydroxybenzoates (parabens), propylene glycol, sorbic acid
Condoms no evidence of harm to latex condoms and diaphragms
Pregnancy toxicity in *animal* studies
Breast-feeding present in milk in *animal* studies

7.3.4 Contraceptive devices

Intra-uterine devices

The intra-uterine device (IUD) is a suitable contraceptive for women of all ages irrespective of parity; however, it is less appropriate for those with an increased risk of pelvic inflammatory disease (see below).

The most effective intra-uterine devices have at least 380 mm² of copper and have banded copper on the arms. Smaller devices have been introduced to minimise side-effects; these consist of a plastic carrier wound with copper wire or fitted with copper bands; some also have a central core of silver to prevent fragmentation of the copper.

Fertility declines with age and therefore a copper intra-uterine device which is fitted in a woman over the age of 40, may remain in the uterus until menopause.

A frameless, copper-bearing intra-uterine device (*Gyne-Fix*®) is also available. It consists of a knotted, polypropylene thread with 6 copper sleeves; the device is anchored in the uterus by inserting the knot into the uterine fundus.

The timing and technique of fitting an intra-uterine device are critical for its subsequent performance. *The healthcare professional inserting (or removing) the device should be fully trained in the technique and should provide full counselling backed, where available, by the patient information leaflet.* Devices should not be fitted during the heavy days of the period; they are best fitted after the end of menstruation and before the calculated time of implantation.

The main excess risk of infection occurs in the first 20 days after insertion and is believed to be related to

existing carriage of a sexually transmitted infection. Women are considered to be at a higher risk of sexually transmitted infections if:

- they are under 25 years old *or*
- they are over 25 years old *and*
  - have a new partner *or*
  - have had more than one partner in the past year *or*
  - their regular partner has other partners.

In these women, pre-insertion screening (for chlamydia and, depending on sexual history and local prevalence of disease, *Neisseria gonorrhoeae*) should be performed. If results are unavailable at the time of fitting an intra-uterine device for emergency contraception, appropriate prophylactic antibacterial cover should be given. The woman should be advised to attend *as an emergency* if she experiences sustained pain during the next 20 days.

An intra-uterine device should not be removed in mid-cycle unless an additional contraceptive was used for the previous 7 days. If removal is essential post-coital contraception should be considered.

If an intra-uterine device fails and the woman wishes to continue to full-term the device should be removed in the first trimester if possible.

INTRA-UTERINE CONTRACEPTIVE DEVICES

Indications see notes above

Cautions see notes above; also anaemia, menorrhagia (progestogen intra-uterine system might be preferable, section 7.3.2.3), endometriosis, severe primary dysmenorrhoea, history of pelvic inflammatory disease, diabetes, fertility problems, nulliparity and young age, severely scarred uterus (including after endometrial resection) or severe cervical stenosis; drug- or disease-induced immunosuppression (risk of infection—avoid if marked immunosuppression); epilepsy (risk of seizure at time of insertion); increased risk of expulsion if inserted before uterine involution; gynaecological examination before insertion, 6–8 weeks after then annually but counsel women to seek medical attention promptly in case of significant symptoms, especially pain; anticoagulant therapy (avoid if possible)

Contra-indications severe anaemia, recent sexually transmitted infection (if not fully investigated and treated), unexplained uterine bleeding, distorted or small uterine cavity, genital malignancy, active trophoblastic disease (until return to normal of urine- and plasma-gonadotrophin concentration), pelvic inflammatory disease, established or marked immunosuppression; *copper devices:* copper allergy, Wilson's disease, medical diathermy

Pregnancy remove device; if pregnancy occurs, increased likelihood that it may be ectopic

Breast-feeding not known to be harmful

Side-effects uterine or cervical perforation, displacement, expulsion; pelvic infection may be exacerbated, menorrhagia, dysmenorrhoea, allergy; *on insertion:* pain (alleviated by NSAID such as ibuprofen 30 minutes before insertion) and bleeding, occasionally epileptic seizure and vasovagal attack

Ancora® 375 Ag (RF Medical)

Intra-uterine device, copper wire with silver core, wound on vertical stem of U-shaped plastic carrier, surface area approx. 375 mm², impregnated with barium sulfate for radio-opacity, threads attached to base of vertical stem; preloaded in inserter, net price = £9.95

For uterine length over 6.5 cm; replacement every 5 years (see also notes above)

Ancora® 375 Cu (RF Medical)

Intra-uterine device, copper wire, wound on vertical stem of U-shaped plastic carrier, surface area approx. 375 mm², impregnated with barium sulfate for radio-opacity, threads attached to base of vertical stem; pre-loaded in inserter, net price = £7.95

For uterine length over 6.5 cm; replacement every 5 years (see also notes above)

Copper T 380A® (RF Medical)

Intra-uterine device, copper wire, wound on vertical stem of T-shaped plastic carrier with copper sleeve on each arm, total surface area approx. 380 mm², impregnated with barium sulfate for radio-opacity, threads attached to base of vertical stem; with loading capsule, net price = £8.95

For uterine length 6.5–9 cm; replacement every 10 years (see also notes above)

Cu-Safe® T300 (Williams) [NHS]

Intra-uterine device, copper wire, wound on vertical stem of T-shaped plastic carrier, surface area approx. 300 mm², impregnated with barium sulfate for radio-opacity, monofilament thread attached to base of vertical stem; preloaded in inserter, net price = £9.11

For uterine length over 5 cm; replacement every 5 years (see also notes above)

Flexi-T® 300 (Durbin)

Intra-uterine device, copper wire, wound on vertical stem of T-shaped plastic carrier, surface area approx. 300 mm², impregnated with barium sulfate for radio-opacity, monofilament thread attached to base of vertical stem; preloaded in inserter, net price = £9.47

For uterine length over 5 cm; replacement every 5 years (see also notes above)

Flexi-T® + 380 (Durbin)

Intra-uterine device, copper wire, wound on vertical stem of T-shaped plastic carrier with copper sleeve on each arm, total surface area approx. 380 mm², impregnated with barium sulfate for radio-opacity, monofilament thread attached to base of vertical stem; preloaded in inserter, net price = £10.06

For uterine length over 6 cm; replacement every 5 years (see also notes above)

GyneFix® (Williams)

Intra-uterine device, 6 copper sleeves with surface area of 330 mm² on polypropylene thread, net price = £27.11

Suitable for all uterine sizes; replacement every 5 years

Load® 375 (Durbin)

Intra-uterine device, copper wire, wound on vertical stem of U-shaped plastic carrier, surface area approx. 375 mm², impregnated with barium sulfate for radio-opacity, monofilament thread attached to base of vertical stem; preloaded in inserter, net price = £8.52

For uterine length over 7 cm; replacement every 5 years (see also notes above)

Mini TT 380® Slimline (Durbin)

Intra-uterine device, copper wire, wound on vertical stem of T-shaped plastic carrier with copper sleeves fitted flush on to distal portion of each horizontal arm, total surface area approx. 380 mm², impregnated with barium sulfate for radio-opacity, thread attached to base of vertical stem; easy-loading system, no capsule, net price = £12.46

For minimum uterine length 5 cm; replacement every 5 years (see also notes above)

Multiload® Cu375 (MSD)

Intra-uterine device, as Load® 375, with copper surface area approx. 375 mm² and vertical stem length 3.5 cm, net price = £9.24

For uterine length 6–9 cm; replacement every 5 years (see also notes above)

Multi-Safe® 375 (Williams)

Intra-uterine device, copper wire, wound on vertical stem of U-shaped plastic carrier, surface area approx. 375 mm², impregnated with barium sulfate for radio-opacity, monofilament thread attached to base of vertical stem; preloaded in inserter, net price = £8.96

For uterine length over 6–9 cm; replacement every 5 years (see also notes above)

Multi-Safe® 375 Short Stem (Williams) [NHS]

Intra-uterine device, copper wire, wound on vertical stem of U-shaped plastic carrier, surface area approx. 375 mm², impregnated with barium sulfate for radio-opacity, monofilament thread attached to base of vertical stem; preloaded in inserter, net price = £8.80

For uterine length 5–7 cm; replacement every 5 years (see also notes above)

Neo-Safe® T380 (Williams)

Intra-uterine device, copper wire, wound on vertical stem of T-shaped plastic carrier, surface area approx. 380 mm², impregnated with barium sulfate for radio-opacity, threads attached to base of vertical stem, net price = £13.31

For uterine length 6.5–9 cm; replacement every 5 years (see also notes above)

Novaplus T 380® Ag (RF Medical)

Intra-uterine device, copper wire with silver core, wound on vertical stem of T-shaped plastic carrier, surface area approx. 380 mm², impregnated with barium sulfate for radio-opacity, threads attached to base of vertical stem, net price = £12.50

'Mini' size for minimum uterine length 5 cm; 'Normal' size for uterine length 6.5–9 cm; replacement every 5 years (see also notes above)

Novaplus T 380® Cu (RF Medical)

Intra-uterine device, copper wire, wound on vertical stem of T-shaped plastic carrier, surface area approx. 380 mm², impregnated with barium sulfate for radio-opacity, threads attached to base of vertical stem, net price = £10.95

'Mini' size for minimum uterine length 5 cm; 'Normal' size for uterine length 6.5–9 cm; replacement every 5 years (see also notes above)

Nova-T® 380 (Bayer)

Intra-uterine device, copper wire with silver core, wound on vertical stem of T-shaped plastic carrier, surface area approx. 380 mm², impregnated with barium sulfate for radio-opacity, threads attached to base of vertical stem, net price = £15.20

For uterine length 6.5–9 cm; replacement every 5 years (see also notes above)

T-Safe® 380A QuickLoad (Williams)
Intra-uterine device, copper wire, wound on vertical stem of T-shaped plastic carrier with copper collar on the distal portion of each arm, total surface area approx. 380 mm^2, impregnated with barium sulfate for radio-opacity, threads attached to base of vertical stem, quick-loading system, net price = £10.29; also available with a capsule loading device (*T-Safe® 380A Capped* [NHS]), net price = £10.47
For uterine length 6.5–9 cm; replacement every 10 years (see also notes above)

TT 380® Slimline (Durbin)
Intra-uterine device, copper wire, wound on vertical stem of T-shaped plastic carrier, with copper sleeves fitted flush on to distal portion of each horizontal arm, total surface area approx. 380 mm^2, impregnated with barium sulfate for radio-opacity, thread attached to base of vertical stem; easy-loading system, no capsule, net price = £12.46
For uterine length 6.5–9 cm; replacement every 10 years (see also notes above)

UT 380 Short® (Durbin)
Intra-uterine device, copper wire, wound on vertical stem of T-shaped plastic carrier, surface area approx. 380 mm^2, impregnated with barium sulfate for radio-opacity, thread attached to base of vertical stem; net price = £11.22
For uterine length 5–7 cm; replacement every 5 years (see also notes above)

UT 380 Standard® (Durbin)
Intra-uterine device, copper wire, wound on vertical stem of T-shaped plastic carrier, surface area approx. 380 mm^2, impregnated with barium sulfate for radio-opacity, thread attached to base of vertical stem; net price = £11.22
For uterine length 6.5–9 cm; replacement every 5 years (see also notes above)

Other contraceptive devices

◢Silicone contraceptive caps

Silicone Contraceptive Pessary
Silicone, sizes 22, 26, and 30 mm, net price = £15.29
Brands include *FemCap®*

◢Rubber contraceptive diaphragms

Type A Diaphragm with Flat Metal Spring
Transparent rubber with flat metal spring, sizes 55–95 mm (rising in steps of 5 mm), net price = £6.22
Brands include *Reflexions®*

◢Silicone contraceptive diaphragms

Type B Diaphragm with Coiled Metal Spring
Silicone with coiled metal spring, sizes 60–90 mm (rising in steps of 5 mm), net price = £9.31
Brands include *Milex Omniflex®*

Type C Arcing Spring Diaphragm
Silicone with arcing spring, sizes 60–90 mm (rising in steps of 5 mm), net price = £8.35
Brands include *Milex Arcing Style®*, *Ortho All-flex®*

7.3.5 Emergency contraception

Hormonal methods

Hormonal emergency contraceptives include **levonorgestrel** and **ulipristal**; either drug should be taken as soon as possible after unprotected intercourse to increase efficacy.

Levonorgestrel is effective if taken within 72 hours (3 days) of unprotected intercourse and may also be used between 72 and 96 hours after unprotected intercourse [unlicensed use], but efficacy decreases with time. Ulipristal, a progesterone receptor modulator, is effective if taken within 120 hours (5 days) of unprotected intercourse.

Levonorgestrel is less effective than insertion of an intra-uterine device (see below). Ulipristal is as effective as levonorgestrel, but its efficacy compared to an intra-uterine device is not yet known.

If vomiting occurs within 2 hours of taking levonorgestrel or within 3 hours of taking ulipristal, a replacement dose should be given.

When prescribing or supplying hormonal emergency contraception, women should be advised:

- that their next period may be early or late;

- that a barrier method of contraception needs to be used until the next period;

- to seek medical attention promptly if any lower abdominal pain occurs because this could signify an ectopic pregnancy;

- to return in 3 to 4 weeks if the subsequent menstrual bleed is abnormally light, heavy or brief, or is absent, or if she is otherwise concerned (if there is any doubt as to whether menstruation has occurred, a pregnancy test should be performed at least 3 weeks after unprotected intercourse).

Interactions   The effectiveness of levonorgestrel, and possibly ulipristal, is reduced in women taking enzyme-inducing drugs (and possibly for 4 weeks after stopping); a copper intra-uterine device can be offered instead. If the copper intra-uterine device is undesirable or inappropriate, the dose of levonorgestrel should be increased to a total of 3 mg taken as a single dose [unlicensed dose—advise women accordingly]. There is no need to increase the dose for emergency contraception if the patient is taking antibacterials that are not enzyme inducers.

LEVONORGESTREL

Indications   emergency contraception

Cautions   see notes above; past ectopic pregnancy; severe malabsorption syndromes; active trophoblastic disease (until return to normal of urine- and plasma-gonadotrophin concentration)—seek specialist advice; **interactions:** see notes above and Appendix 1 (progestogens)

Contra-indications   acute porphyria (section 9.8.2)

Pregnancy   not known to be harmful

Breast-feeding   progestogen-only contraceptives do not affect lactation

Side-effects   menstrual irregularities (see also notes above), nausea, low abdominal pain, fatigue, headache, dizziness, breast tenderness, vomiting

7 Obstetrics, gynaecology, and urinary-tract disorders

Dose

- 1.5 mg as a single dose as soon as possible after coitus, preferably within 12 hours but no later than after 72 hours (but see also notes above)

¹Levonelle® One Step (Bayer)
Tablets, levonorgestrel 1.5 mg, net price 1-tab pack = £13.83

Levonelle® 1500 (Bayer) [PoM]
Tablets, levonorgestrel 1.5 mg, net price 1-tab pack = £5.20

ULIPRISTAL ACETATE

Indications emergency contraception; uterine fibroids, see section 6.4.1.2

Cautions see notes above; uncontrolled severe asthma; effectiveness of combined hormonal and progestogen-only contraceptives may be reduced—additional precautions (barrier methods) required for 14 days for combined and parenteral progestogen-only hormonal contraceptives (16 days for *Qlaira®*) and 9 days for oral progestogen-only contraceptives; **interactions:** see notes above and Appendix 1 (ulipristal)

Contra-indications repeated use within a menstrual cycle

Hepatic impairment manufacturer advises avoid in severe impairment—no information available

Pregnancy limited information available

Breast-feeding manufacturer advises avoid for 1 week after administration—present in milk

Side-effects gastro-intestinal disturbances (including nausea, vomiting, diarrhoea, and abdominal pain), dizziness, fatigue, headache, menstrual irregularities (see notes above), back pain, muscle spasms; *less commonly* tremor, hot flushes, uterine spasm, breast tenderness, dry mouth, blurred vision, pruritus, and rash

Dose

- 30 mg as a single dose as soon as possible after coitus, but no later than after 120 hours

ellaOne® (HRA Pharma) [PoM]
Tablets, ulipristal acetate 30 mg, net price 1-tab pack = £16.95

Intra-uterine device

Insertion of an intra-uterine device is more effective than oral levonorgestrel for emergency contraception. A copper intra-uterine contraceptive device (section 7.3.4) can be inserted up to 120 hours (5 days) after unprotected intercourse; sexually transmitted infections should be tested for and insertion of the device should usually be covered by antibacterial prophylaxis (e.g. azithromycin 1 g by mouth as a single dose). If intercourse has occurred more than 5 days previously, the device can still be inserted up to 5 days after the earliest likely calculated ovulation (i.e. within the minimum period before implantation), regardless of the number of episodes of unprotected intercourse earlier in the cycle.

1. Can be sold to women over 16 years; when supplying emergency contraception to the public, pharmacists should refer to guidance issued by the Royal Pharmaceutical Society

7.4 Drugs for genito-urinary disorders

7.4.1	Drugs for urinary retention
7.4.2	Drugs for urinary frequency, enuresis, and incontinence
7.4.3	Drugs used in urological pain
7.4.4	Bladder instillations and urological surgery
7.4.5	Drugs for erectile dysfunction

For drugs used in the treatment of urinary-tract infections see section 5.1.13.

7.4.1 Drugs for urinary retention

Acute retention is painful and is treated by catheterisation.

Chronic retention is painless and often long-standing. Catheterisation is unnecessary unless there is deterioration of renal function. After the cause has initially been established and treated, drugs may be required to increase detrusor muscle tone.

Benign prostatic hyperplasia is treated either surgically or medically with alpha-blockers (see below). Dutasteride and finasteride (section 6.4.2) are alternatives to alpha-blockers, particularly in men with a significantly enlarged prostate. Tadalafil (section 7.4.5), a phosphodiesterase type-5 inhibitor, may also be used in the management of benign prostatic hyperplasia.

Alpha-blockers

The alpha₁-selective alpha blockers, **alfuzosin, doxazosin, indoramin, prazosin, tamsulosin** and **terazosin** relax smooth muscle in benign prostatic hyperplasia producing an increase in urinary flow-rate and an improvement in obstructive symptoms.

Cautions Since alpha₁-selective alpha blockers reduce blood pressure, patients receiving antihypertensive treatment may require reduced dosage and specialist supervision. Caution is required in the elderly and in patients undergoing cataract surgery (risk of intra-operative floppy iris syndrome). For **interactions**, see Appendix 1 (alpha-blockers).

Contra-indications Alpha-blockers should be avoided in patients with a history of postural hypotension and micturition syncope.

Side-effects Side-effects of alpha₁-selective alpha blockers include drowsiness, hypotension (notably postural hypotension), syncope, asthenia, dizziness, depression, headache, dry mouth, gastro-intestinal disturbances, oedema, blurred vision, intra-operative floppy iris syndrome (most strongly associated with tamsulosin), rhinitis, erectile disorders (including priapism), tachycardia, and palpitations. Hypersensitivity reactions including rash, pruritus and angioedema have also been reported.

ALFUZOSIN HYDROCHLORIDE

Indications benign prostatic hyperplasia

Cautions see notes above; discontinue if angina worsens; acute heart failure; history of QT-interval prolongation; concomitant use with other drugs known to prolong QT interval

Driving May affect performance of skilled tasks e.g. driving

Contra-indications see notes above

Hepatic impairment initial dose 2.5 mg once daily, adjusted according to response to 2.5 mg twice daily in mild to moderate impairment—avoid if severe; avoid modified-release preparations

Renal impairment initial dose 2.5 mg twice daily and adjust according to response; manufacturers advise avoid use of modified-release preparations if eGFR less than 30 mL/minute/1.73 m^2 as limited experience

Side-effects see notes above; also *less commonly* flushes and chest pain; *also reported* liver damage and cholestasis

Dose

- 2.5 mg 3 times daily, max. 10 mg daily; ELDERLY initially 2.5 mg twice daily

First dose effect First dose may cause collapse due to hypotensive effect (therefore should be taken on retiring to bed). Patient should be warned to lie down if symptoms such as dizziness, fatigue or sweating develop, and to remain lying down until they abate completely

Alfuzosin hydrochloride (Non-proprietary) ▼ PoM
Tablets, f/c, alfuzosin hydrochloride 2.5 mg, net price 60-tab pack = £3.88. Counselling, initial dose, driving, see above

Xatral® (Sanofi-Aventis) PoM
Tablets, f/c, alfuzosin hydrochloride 2.5 mg, net price 60-tab pack = £20.37. Counselling, initial dose, driving, see above

◢ **Modified release**

Besavar® **XL** (Zentiva) PoM
Tablets, m/r, yellow/white, alfuzosin hydrochloride 10 mg, net price 30-tab pack = £12.51. Label: 21, 25, counselling, initial dose, driving, see above
Dose benign prostatic hyperplasia 10 mg once daily
Acute urinary retention associated with benign prostatic hyperplasia in men over 65 years, 10 mg once daily for 2–3 days during catheterisation and for one day after removal; max. 4 days

Vasran® **XL** (Ranbaxy) PoM
Tablets, m/r, alfuzosin hydrochloride 10 mg, net price 30-tab pack = £11.48. Label: 21, 25, counselling, initial dose, driving, see above
Dose benign prostatic hyperplasia 10 mg once daily

Xatral® **XL** (Sanofi-Aventis) PoM
Tablets, m/r, yellow/white, alfuzosin hydrochloride 10 mg, net price 10-tab pack = £4.17, 30-tab pack = £12.51. Label: 21, 25, counselling, initial dose, driving, see above
Dose benign prostatic hyperplasia 10 mg once daily
Acute urinary retention associated with benign prostatic hyperplasia in men over 65 years, 10 mg once daily for 2–3 days during catheterisation and for one day after removal; max. 4 days

◼ DOXAZOSIN

Indications benign prostatic hyperplasia; hypertension (section 2.5.4)

Cautions see notes above and section 2.5.4

Contra-indications see notes above

Hepatic impairment section 2.5.4

Side-effects see notes above and section 2.5.4

Dose

- Initially 1 mg daily; dose may be doubled at intervals of 1–2 weeks according to response, up to max. 8 mg daily; usual maintenance 2–4 mg daily

◢ **Preparations**
Section 2.5.4

◼ INDORAMIN

Indications benign prostatic hyperplasia; hypertension (section 2.5.4)

Cautions see notes above and section 2.5.4

Contra-indications see notes above and section 2.5.4

Hepatic impairment section 2.5.4

Renal impairment section 2.5.4

Side-effects see notes above and section 2.5.4

Dose

- 20 mg twice daily; increased if necessary by 20 mg every 2 weeks to max. 100 mg daily in divided doses; ELDERLY, 20 mg at night may be adequate

Doralese® (Chemidex) PoM
Tablets, yellow, f/c, indoramin 20 mg, net price 60-tab pack = £11.44. Label: 2

◼ PRAZOSIN

Indications benign prostatic hyperplasia; hypertension, congestive heart failure and Raynaud's syndrome (section 2.5.4)

Cautions see notes above and section 2.5.4

Contra-indications see notes above and section 2.5.4

Hepatic impairment section 2.5.4

Renal impairment section 2.5.4

Side-effects see notes above and section 2.5.4

Dose

- Initially 500 micrograms twice daily for 3–7 days, subsequently adjusted according to response; usual maintenance (and max.) 2 mg twice daily; ELDERLY initiate with lowest possible dose

First dose effect First dose may cause collapse due to hypotensive effect (therefore should be taken on retiring to bed). Patient should be warned to lie down if symptoms such as dizziness, fatigue or sweating develop, and to remain lying down until they abate completely

◢ **Preparations**
Section 2.5.4

◼ TAMSULOSIN HYDROCHLORIDE

Indications benign prostatic hyperplasia

Cautions see notes above

Driving May affect performance of skilled tasks e.g. driving

Contra-indications see notes above

Hepatic impairment avoid in severe impairment

Renal impairment use with caution if eGFR less than 10 mL/minute/1.73 m^2

Side-effects see notes above

Dose

- 400 micrograms daily

7 Obstetrics, gynaecology, and urinary-tract disorders

[1]**Tamsulosin hydrochloride** (Non-proprietary) PoM
Capsules, m/r, tamsulosin hydrochloride 400 micrograms, net price 30-cap pack = £4.64. Label: 25, counselling, driving
Brands include Bazetham® MR, Contiflo® XL, Diffundox® XL, Losinate® MR, Pinexel® PR, Prosurin® XL, Stronazon® MR, Tabphyn® MR

Flomaxtra® XL (Astellas) PoM
Tablets, m/r, tamsulosin hydrochloride 400 micrograms, net price 30-tab pack = £10.47. Label: 25, counselling, driving

◢**With dutasteride**
For prescribing information on dutasteride, see section 6.4.2

Combodart® (GSK) ▼ PoM
Capsules, m/r, brown/orange, tamsulosin hydrochloride 400 micrograms, dutasteride 500 micrograms, net price 30-cap pack = £19.80. Label: 25, counselling, driving
Dose benign prostatic hyperplasia, 1 capsule daily

◢**With solifenacin**
For prescribing information on solifenacin, see section 7.4.2

Vesomni® (Astellas) PoM
Tablets, m/r, f/c, red, tamsulosin hydrochloride 400 micrograms, solifenacin succinate 6 mg, net price 30-tab pack = £27.62. Label: 3, 25
Dose ADULT over 18 years, moderate to severe urinary frequency, urgency, and obstructive symptoms associated with benign prostatic hyperplasia when monotherapy ineffective, 1 tablet daily

TERAZOSIN

Indications   benign prostatic hyperplasia; hypertension (section 2.5.4)
Cautions   see notes above and section 2.5.4
Driving May affect performance of skilled tasks e.g. driving
Contra-indications   see notes above
Side-effects   see notes above and section 2.5.4
Dose
- Initially 1 mg at bedtime; if necessary dose may be doubled at intervals of 1–2 weeks according to response, up to max. 10 mg once daily; usual maintenance 5–10 mg daily
First dose effect First dose may cause collapse due to hypotensive effect (therefore should be taken on retiring to bed). Patient should be warned to lie down if symptoms such as dizziness, fatigue or sweating develop, and to remain lying down until they abate completely

Terazosin (Non-proprietary) PoM
Tablets, terazosin (as hydrochloride) 2 mg, net price 28-tab pack = £2.44; 5 mg, 28-tab pack = £2.76; 10 mg, 28-tab pack = £8.04. Counselling, initial dose, driving

Hytrin® (AMCo) PoM
Tablets, terazosin (as hydrochloride) 2 mg (yellow) net price, 28-tab pack = £2.20; 5 mg (tan), 28-tab pack = £4.13; 10 mg (blue), 28-tab pack = £8.24; starter pack (for benign prostatic hyperplasia) of 7 × 1-mg tab with 14 × 2-mg tab and 7 × 5-mg tab = £10.97. Counselling, initial dose, driving

1. Tamsulosin hydrochloride 400 microgram capsules can be sold to the public for the treatment of functional symptoms of benign prostatic hyperplasia in men aged 45–75 years to be taken for up to 6 weeks before clinical assessment by a doctor; a proprietary brand Flomax Relief® MR is on sale to the public

Parasympathomimetics

The parasympathomimetic **bethanechol** increases detrusor muscle contraction. However, it has only a limited role in the relief of urinary retention; its use has been superseded by catheterisation.

◢ BETHANECHOL CHLORIDE ◢

Indications   urinary retention, but see notes above
Cautions   autonomic neuropathy (use lower initial dose); **interactions:** Appendix 1 (parasympathomimetics)
Contra-indications   peptic ulcer; intestinal or urinary obstruction; conditions where increased motility of the urinary or gastro-intestinal tract could be harmful; cardiovascular disorders (including recent myocardial infarction, bradycardia, and heart block); hypotension; obstructive airways disease; epilepsy; parkinsonism; hyperthyroidism
Pregnancy   manufacturer advises avoid—no information available
Breast-feeding   manufacturer advises avoid; gastrointestinal disturbances in infant reported
Side-effects   nausea, vomiting, diarrhoea, abdominal pain, increased salivation, eructation; flushing, hypotension, bradycardia; bronchoconstriction, rhinorrhoea; headache; increased lacrimation; increased sweating
Dose
- 10–25 mg 3–4 times daily half an hour before food

Myotonine® (Glenwood) PoM ◢
Tablets, scored, bethanechol chloride 10 mg, net price 100-tab pack = £18.51; 25 mg, 100-tab pack = £27.26. Label: 22

7.4.2   Drugs for urinary frequency, enuresis, and incontinence

Urinary incontinence

Incontinence in adults which arises from detrusor instability is managed by combining drug therapy with conservative methods for managing urge incontinence such as pelvic floor exercises and bladder training; stress incontinence is generally managed by non-drug methods. **Duloxetine**, an inhibitor of serotonin and noradrenaline re-uptake can be added and is licensed for the treatment of moderate to severe stress incontinence in women; it may be more effective when used as an adjunct to pelvic floor exercises.

Antimuscarinic drugs reduce symptoms of urgency and urge incontinence and increase bladder capacity. **Oxybutynin** also has a direct relaxant effect on urinary smooth muscle. Side-effects limit the use of oxybutynin, but they may be reduced by starting at a lower dose. A modified-release preparation of oxybutynin is effective and has fewer side-effects; a transdermal patch is also available. The efficacy and side-effects of **tolterodine** are comparable to those of modified-release oxybutynin. **Flavoxate** has less marked side-effects but it is also less effective. **Darifenacin**, **fesoterodine**, **propiverine**, **solifenacin**, and **trospium** are newer antimuscarinic drugs licensed for urinary frequency, urgency, and incontinence. The need for continuing antimuscarinic drug therapy should be reviewed every 4–6 weeks until symptoms stabilise, and then every 6–12 months.

The *Scottish Medicines Consortium* (p. 4) has advised (June 2008) that fesoterodine (*Toviaz*®) is accepted for restricted use within NHS Scotland as a second-line treatment for overactive bladder syndrome.

Propantheline and tricyclic antidepressants were used for urge incontinence but they are little used now because of their side-effects. The use of imipramine is limited by its potential to cause cardiac side-effects.

Mirabegron, a selective beta$_3$ agonist, is licensed for the treatment of urinary frequency, urgency, and urge incontinence associated with overactive bladder syndrome.

> **NICE guidance**
> **Mirabegron for treating symptoms of overactive bladder (June 2013)**
> Mirabegron is recommended as an option only for patients in whom antimuscarinic drugs are ineffective, contra-indicated, or not tolerated; patients currently receiving mirabegron who do not meet these criteria should have the option to continue until they and their clinician consider it appropriate to stop.
> www.nice.org.uk/TA290

Purified bovine collagen implant (*Contigen*®, Bard) is indicated for *urinary incontinence* caused by intrinsic sphincter deficiency (poor or non-functioning bladder outlet mechanism). The implant should be inserted only by surgeons or physicians trained in the technique for injection of the implant.

Cautions Antimuscarinic drugs should be used with caution in the elderly (especially if frail), in those with autonomic neuropathy, and in those susceptible to angle-closure glaucoma. They should also be used with caution in hiatus hernia with reflux oesophagitis. Antimuscarinics can worsen hyperthyroidism, coronary artery disease, congestive heart failure, hypertension, prostatic hyperplasia, arrhythmias, and tachycardia. For **interactions**, see Appendix 1 (antimuscarinics).

Contra-indications Antimuscarinic drugs should be avoided in patients with myasthenia gravis, significant bladder outflow obstruction or urinary retention, severe ulcerative colitis, toxic megacolon, and in gastro-intestinal obstruction or intestinal atony.

Side-effects Side-effects of antimuscarinic drugs include dry mouth, gastro-intestinal disturbances including constipation, flatulence, taste disturbances, blurred vision, dry eyes, drowsiness, dizziness, fatigue, difficulty in micturition (less commonly urinary retention), palpitation, and skin reactions (including dry skin, rash, and photosensitivity); also headache, diarrhoea, angioedema, arrhythmias, and tachycardia. Central nervous system stimulation, such as restlessness, disorientation, hallucination, and convulsion may occur; children are at higher risk of these effects. Antimuscarinic drugs can reduce sweating, leading to heat sensations and fainting in hot environments or in patients with fever, and *very rarely* may precipitate angle-closure glaucoma.

DARIFENACIN

Indications urinary frequency, urgency, and incontinence

Cautions see notes above

Contra-indications see notes above

Hepatic impairment max. 7.5 mg daily in moderate impairment; avoid in severe impairment

Pregnancy manufacturer advises avoid—toxicity in *animal* studies

Breast-feeding present in milk in *animal* studies—manufacturer advises caution

Side-effects see notes above; also *less commonly* ulcerative stomatitis, oedema, hypertension, dyspnoea, cough, rhinitis, weakness, insomnia, impotence, and vaginitis

Dose

- ADULT over 18 years, 7.5 mg once daily, increased if necessary after 2 weeks to 15 mg once daily

Emselex® (Merus) [PoM]
Tablets, m/r, darifenacin (as hydrobromide) 7.5 mg (white), net price 28-tab pack = £25.48; 15 mg (peach), 28-tab pack = £25.48. Label: 3, 25

DULOXETINE

Indications moderate to severe stress urinary incontinence in women; major depressive disorder (section 4.3.4); diabetic neuropathy (section 4.3.4); generalised anxiety disorder (section 4.3.4)

Cautions elderly; cardiac disease; hypertension (avoid if uncontrolled); history of mania; history of seizures; raised intra-ocular pressure, susceptibility to angle-closure glaucoma; bleeding disorders or concomitant use of drugs that increase risk of bleeding; **interactions**: Appendix 1 (duloxetine)
Withdrawal Nausea, vomiting, headache, anxiety, dizziness, paraesthesia, sleep disturbances, and tremor are the most common features of abrupt withdrawal or marked reduction of the dose; dose should be reduced over at least 1–2 weeks

Hepatic impairment manufacturer advises avoid

Renal impairment avoid if eGFR less than 30 mL/minute/1.73 m^2

Pregnancy toxicity in *animal* studies—avoid in patients with stress urinary incontinence; risk of neonatal withdrawal symptoms if used near term

Breast-feeding present in milk—manufacturer advises avoid

Side-effects nausea, vomiting, dyspepsia, constipation, diarrhoea, abdominal pain, weight changes, decreased appetite, flatulence, dry mouth; palpitation, hot flush; insomnia, abnormal dreams, paraesthesia, drowsiness, anxiety, headache, dizziness, fatigue, weakness, tremor, nervousness, anorexia; sexual dysfunction; visual disturbances; sweating, pruritus; *less commonly* gastritis, halitosis, hepatitis, bruxism, dysphagia, tachycardia, hypertension, postural hypotension, syncope, raised cholesterol, vertigo, taste disturbance, cold extremities, impaired temperature regulation, impaired attention, movement disorders, muscle twitching, musculoskeletal pain, thirst, stomatitis, hypothyroidism, urinary disorders, and photosensitivity; *rarely* mania; *very rarely* angle-closure glaucoma; *also reported* supraventricular arrhythmia, chest pain, hallucinations, suicidal behaviour (see Suicidal Behaviour and Antidepressant Therapy, p. 253), seizures, hypersensitivity reactions including urticaria, angioedema, rash (including Stevens-Johnson syndrome) and anaphylaxis, hyponatraemia (see Hyponatraemia and Antidepressant Therapy, p. 253)

Dose

- ADULT over 18 years, 40 mg twice daily, assess for benefit and tolerability after 2–4 weeks

  Note Initial dose of 20 mg twice daily for 2 weeks can minimise side-effects

Yentreve® (Lilly) [PoM]

Capsules, duloxetine (as hydrochloride) 20 mg (blue), net price 28-cap pack = £18.48, 56-cap pack = £30.80; 40 mg (orange/blue), 56-cap pack = £36.96. Label: 2

Cymbalta® (Lilly) [PoM]

Section 4.3.4 (major depressive episode, generalised anxiety disorder, and diabetic neuropathy)

FESOTERODINE FUMARATE

Indications urinary frequency, urgency, and urge incontinence

Cautions see notes above; gastro-oesophageal reflux

Contra-indications see notes above

Hepatic impairment manufacturer advises increase dose cautiously; max. 4 mg daily in moderate impairment; avoid in severe impairment; consult product literature before concomitant use of cytochrome P450 enzyme inhibitors

Renal impairment increase dose cautiously if eGFR 30–80 mL/minute/1.73 m^2; max. 4 mg daily if eGFR less than 30 mL/minute/1.73 m^2; consult product literature before concomitant use of cytochrome P450 enzyme inhibitors

Pregnancy manufacturer advises avoid—toxicity in *animal* studies

Breast-feeding manufacturer advises avoid—no information available

Side-effects see notes above; also insomnia; *less commonly* nasal dryness, pharyngolaryngeal pain, cough, and vertigo

Dose

- ADULT over 18 years, 4 mg once daily, increased if necessary to max. 8 mg once daily

Note Max. 4 mg daily with concomitant atazanavir, clarithromycin, indinavir, itraconazole, ritonavir, saquinavir, or telithromycin; in patients with hepatic or renal impairment, consult product literature before concomitant use with amprenavir, aprepitant, atazanavir, clarithromycin, diltiazem, erythromycin, fluconazole, fosamprenavir, indinavir, itraconazole, ritonavir, saquinavir, telithromycin, verapamil, or grapefruit juice

Toviaz® (Pfizer) [PoM]

Tablets, m/r, f/c, fesoterodine fumarate 4 mg (light blue), net price 28-tab pack = £25.78; 8 mg (blue), 28-tab pack = £25.78. Label: 3, 25

FLAVOXATE HYDROCHLORIDE

Indications urinary frequency and incontinence, dysuria, urgency; bladder spasms due to catheterisation, cytoscopy, or surgery

Cautions see notes above

Contra-indications see notes above; gastro-intestinal haemorrhage

Pregnancy manufacturer advises avoid unless no safer alternative

Breast-feeding manufacturer advises caution—no information available

Side-effects see notes above; also vertigo, eosinophilia, leucopenia, urticaria, erythema, and pruritus

Dose

- ADULT and CHILD over 12 years, 200 mg 3 times daily

Urispas 200® (Recordati) [PoM]

Tablets, f/c, flavoxate hydrochloride 200 mg, net price 90-tab pack = £11.67. Label: 3

MIRABEGRON

Indications urinary frequency, urgency, and urge incontinence

Cautions history of QT-interval prolongation; concomitant use with drugs that prolong the QT interval; **interactions**: Appendix 1 (mirabegron)

Contra-indications severe hypertension

Hepatic impairment avoid in severe impairment—no information available; reduce dose to 25 mg once daily in moderate impairment; *with concomitant use of strong cytochrome P450 inhibitors such as itraconazole, ritonavir, or clarithromycin reduce dose to 25 mg once daily in mild impairment and avoid in moderate impairment*

Renal impairment avoid if eGFR less than 15 mL/minute/1.73 m^2—no information available; reduce dose to 25 mg once daily if eGFR 15–29 mL/minute/1.73 m^2; *with concomitant use of strong cytochrome P450 inhibitors such as itraconazole, ritonavir, or clarithromycin reduce dose to 25 mg once daily if eGFR 30–89 mL/minute/1.73 m^2 and avoid if eGFR less than 30 mL/minute/1.73 m^2*

Pregnancy avoid—toxicity in *animal* studies; contraception advised in women of child-bearing potential

Breast-feeding avoid—present in milk in *animal* studies

Side-effects tachycardia, urinary-tract infection; *less commonly* dyspepsia, gastritis, palpitation, atrial fibrillation, hypertension, vulvovaginal infection and pruritus, joint swelling, rash, pruritus

Dose

- ADULT over 18 years, 50 mg once daily

Betmiga® (Astellas) ▼ [PoM]

Tablets, m/r, mirabegron 25 mg (brown), net price 30-tab pack = £29.00; 50 mg (yellow), 30-tab pack = £29.00. Label: 25

OXYBUTYNIN HYDROCHLORIDE

Indications urinary frequency, urgency and incontinence, neurogenic bladder instability, and nocturnal enuresis associated with overactive bladder

Cautions see notes above; acute porphyria (section 9.8.2)

Contra-indications see notes above

Hepatic impairment manufacturer advises caution

Renal impairment manufacturer advises caution

Pregnancy manufacturers advise avoid unless essential—toxicity in *animal* studies

Breast-feeding manufacturers advise avoid—present in milk

Side-effects see notes above; also *less commonly* anorexia, facial flushing; *rarely* night terrors; applica-

7 **Obstetrics, gynaecology, and urinary-tract disorders**

tion site reactions with *patches*; also reported cognitive impairment

Dose

- ADULT and CHILD over 12 years, initially 5 mg 2–3 times daily, increased if necessary to max. 5 mg 4 times daily; ELDERLY initially 2.5–3 mg twice daily, increased to 5 mg twice daily according to response and tolerance; CHILD 5–12 years, neurogenic bladder instability, 2.5–3 mg twice daily, increased to 5 mg 2–3 times daily; CHILD under 5 years see *BNF for Children*; CHILD 5–18 years, nocturnal enuresis associated with overactive bladder, 2.5–3 mg twice daily increased to 5 mg 2–3 times daily (last dose before bedtime)

Oxybutynin Hydrochloride (Non-proprietary) PoM
Tablets, oxybutynin hydrochloride 2.5 mg, net price 56-tab pack = £2.03; 3 mg, 56-tab pack = £16.10; 5 mg, 56-tab pack = £2.89, 84-tab pack = £4.07. Label: 3

Cystrin® (Zentiva) PoM
Tablets, oxybutynin hydrochloride 5 mg (scored), net price 84-tab pack = £21.99. Label: 3

Ditropan® (Sanofi-Aventis) PoM
Tablets, both blue, scored, oxybutynin hydrochloride 2.5 mg, net price 84-tab pack = £1.60; 5 mg, 84-tab pack = £2.90. Label: 3

Elixir, oxybutynin hydrochloride 2.5 mg/5 mL, net price 150-mL pack = £6.88. Label: 3

◢**Modified release**

Lyrinel® XL (Janssen) PoM
Tablets, m/r, oxybutynin hydrochloride 5 mg (yellow), net price 30-tab pack = £13.77; 10 mg (pink), 30-tab pack = £27.54. Label: 3, 25
Dose ADULT over 18 years, initially 5 mg once daily, adjusted according to response in steps of 5 mg at weekly intervals; max. 20 mg once daily; CHILD 5–18 years see *BNF for Children*
Note Patients taking immediate-release oxybutynin may be transferred to the nearest equivalent daily dose of *Lyrinel® XL*

◢**Transdermal preparations**

Kentera® (Orion) PoM
Patches, self-adhesive, oxybutynin 36 mg (releasing oxybutynin approx. 3.9 mg/24 hours), net price 8-patch pack = £27.20. Label: 3, counselling, administration
Dose ADULT over 18 years, urinary frequency, urgency and incontinence, apply 1 patch twice weekly to clean, dry, unbroken skin on abdomen, hip or buttock, remove after every 3–4 days and site replacement patch on a different area (avoid using same area for 7 days)
Note The *Scottish Medicines Consortium* has advised (July 2005) that *Kentera®* should be restricted for use in patients who benefit from oral oxybutynin but cannot tolerate its side-effects

PROPANTHELINE BROMIDE

Indications adult enuresis
Cautions see notes above; ulcerative colitis
Contra-indications see notes above
Hepatic impairment manufacturer advises caution
Renal impairment manufacturer advises caution
Pregnancy manufacturer advises avoid—no information available
Breast-feeding may suppress lactation
Side-effects see notes above; also facial flushing

Dose

- Initially 15 mg 3 times daily at least one hour before food and 30 mg at bedtime, subsequently adjusted according to response (max. 120 mg daily)

◢**Preparations**
Section 1.2

PROPIVERINE HYDROCHLORIDE

Indications urinary frequency, urgency and incontinence associated with overactive bladder or neurogenic bladder instability
Cautions see notes above
Contra-indications see notes above
Hepatic impairment avoid in moderate to severe impairment
Renal impairment manfacturer advises caution in mild or moderate impairment; max. daily dose 30 mg if eGFR less than 30 mL/minute/1.73 m^2
Pregnancy manufacturer advises avoid (restriction of skeletal development in *animals*)
Breast-feeding manufacturer advises avoid—present in milk in *animal* studies
Side-effects see notes above

Dose

- Overactive bladder, ADULT over 18 years, 15 mg 1–2 times daily, increased if necessary to max. 15 mg 3 times daily
- Neurogenic bladder instability, ADULT over 18 years, 15 mg 3 times daily

Detrunorm® (AMCo) PoM
Tablets, pink, s/c, propiverine hydrochloride 15 mg, net price 56-tab pack = £18.00. Label: 3

◢**Modified release**

Detrunorm® XL (AMCo) PoM
Capsules, orange/white, m/r, propiverine hydrochloride 30 mg, net price 28-cap pack = £24.45. Label: 3, 25
Dose overactive bladder, ADULT over 18 years, urinary frequency, urgency, and incontinence, 30 mg once daily

SOLIFENACIN SUCCINATE

Indications urinary frequency, urgency and urge incontinence
Cautions see notes above; neurogenic bladder disorder; susceptibility to QT-interval prolongation
Contra-indications see notes above
Hepatic impairment max. 5 mg daily (in combination with tamsulosin, max. 1 *Vesomni®* tablet daily) in moderate impairment; avoid in moderate impairment in those already taking potent inhibitors of cytochrome P450 enzyme CYP3A4 (such as itraconazole or ritonavir); avoid in severe impairment
Renal impairment max. 5 mg daily (in combination with tamsulosin, max. 1 *Vesomni®* tablet daily) if eGFR less than 30 mL/minute/1.73 m^2; avoid if eGFR less than 30 mL/minute/1.73 m^2 in those already taking potent inhibitors of cytochrome P450 enzyme CYP3A4 (such as itraconazole or ritonavir)
Pregnancy manufacturer advises caution—no information available
Breast-feeding manufacturer advises avoid—present in milk in *animal* studies
Side-effects see notes above; also *less commonly* gastro-oesophageal reflux, oedema; *also reported* reduced appetite, hepatic impairment, torsade de pointes, dysphonia, hyperkalaemia, muscle weakness

7

Obstetrics, gynaecology, and urinary-tract disorders

Dose

- ADULT over 18 years, 5 mg daily, increased if necessary to 10 mg once daily

Note Max. 5 mg daily (in combination with tamsulosin, max. 1 *Vesomni*® tablet daily) with concomitant potent inhibitors of cytochrome P450 enzyme CYP3A4 (such as itraconazole or ritonavir)

Vesicare® (Astellas) [PoM]

Tablets, f/c, solifenacin succinate 5 mg (yellow), net price 30-tab pack = £27.62; 10 mg (pink), 30-tab pack = £35.91. Label: 3

◢ **With tamsulosin**

Section 7.4.1

▌ **TOLTERODINE TARTRATE**

Indications   see under Dose

Cautions   see notes above; history of QT-interval prolongation; concomitant use with other drugs known to prolong QT interval

Contra-indications   see notes above

Hepatic impairment   reduce dose to 1 mg twice daily; avoid modified-release preparations

Renal impairment   reduce dose to 1 mg twice daily and avoid modified-release preparations if eGFR less than 30 mL/minute/1.73 m^2

Pregnancy   manufacturer advises avoid—toxicity in *animal* studies

Breast-feeding   manufacturer advises avoid—no information available

Side-effects   see notes above; also chest pain, peripheral oedema; sinusitis, bronchitis; paraesthesia, fatigue, vertigo, weight gain; *less commonly* memory impairment; *also reported* flushing

Dose

- Urinary frequency, urgency, and incontinence, ADULT over 18 years, 2 mg twice daily; reduce to 1 mg twice daily if necessary to minimise side-effects; CHILD 2–18 years see *BNF for Children*
- Nocturnal enuresis associated with overactive bladder, CHILD 5–18 years see *BNF for Children*

Tolterodine Tartrate (Non-proprietary) [PoM]

Tablets, tolterodine tartrate 1 mg, net price 56-tab pack = £2.88; 2 mg, 56-tab pack = £2.92. Label: 3

Detrusitol® (Pfizer) [PoM]

Tablets, f/c, tolterodine tartrate 1 mg, net price 56-tab pack = £29.03; 2 mg, 56-tab pack = £30.56. Label: 3

◢ **Modified release**

Tolterodine Tartrate (Non-proprietary) [PoM]

Capsules, m/r, tolterodine tartrate 4 mg, net price 28-cap pack = £25.78. Label: 3, 25
Brands include *Santizor XL*®
Dose urinary frequency, urgency, and incontinence, ADULT over 18 years, 4 mg once daily

Detrusitol® XL (Pfizer) [PoM]

Capsules, blue, m/r, tolterodine tartrate 4 mg, net price 28-cap pack = £25.78. Label: 3, 25
Dose urinary frequency, urgency, and incontinence, ADULT over 18 years, 4 mg once daily

▌ **TROSPIUM CHLORIDE**

Indications   urinary frequency, urgency and incontinence

Cautions   see notes above

Contra-indications   see notes above

Hepatic impairment   manufacturer advises caution in mild to moderate impairment; avoid in severe impairment

Renal impairment   use with caution; reduce dose to 20 mg once daily or 20 mg on alternate days if eGFR 10–30 mL/minute/1.73 m^2; avoid *Regurin*® XL

Pregnancy   manufacturer advises caution

Breast-feeding   manufacturer advises caution

Side-effects   see notes above; *rarely* chest pain, dyspnoea, and asthenia; *very rarely* myalgia and arthralgia

Dose

- ADULT and CHILD over 12 years, 20 mg twice daily before food

Trospium Chloride (Non-proprietary) [PoM]

Tablets, f/c, trospium chloride 20 mg, net price 60-tab pack = £25.03. Label: 23
Brands include *Flotros*®

Regurin® (Speciality European) [PoM]

Tablets, brown-yellow, f/c, trospium chloride 20 mg, net price 60-tab pack = £26.00. Label: 23

◢ **Modified release**

Regurin® XL (Speciality European) [PoM]

Capsules, orange/white, m/r, trospium chloride 60 mg, net price 28-cap pack = £23.05. Label: 23, 25
Dose ADULT over 18 years, 60 mg once daily

Nocturnal enuresis in children

Nocturnal enuresis is common in young children, but persists in a small proportion by 10 years of age. For children under 5 years, reassurance and advice on the management of nocturnal enuresis can be useful for some families. Treatment may be considered in children over 5 years depending on their maturity and motivation, the frequency of nocturnal enuresis, and the needs of the child and their family.

Initially, advice should be given on fluid intake, diet, toileting behaviour, and reward systems; for children who do not respond to this advice, further treatment may be necessary. An **enuresis alarm** should be first-line treatment for motivated, well-supported children; alarms have a lower relapse rate than drug treatment when discontinued. Treatment should be reviewed after 4 weeks, and, if there are early signs of response, continued until a minimum of 2 weeks' uninterrupted dry nights have been achieved. If complete dryness is not achieved after 3 months, only continue if the condition is still improving and the child remains motivated to use the alarm. If initial alarm treatment is unsuccessful, consider combination treatment with desmopressin (see below), or **desmopressin** alone if the alarm is no longer appropriate or desirable.

Desmopressin (section 6.5.2), an analogue of vasopressin, is given by oral or by sublingual administration; it should not be given intranasally for nocturnal enuresis due to an increased incidence of side-effects. Desmopressin alone can be offered to children over 5 years of age if an alarm is inappropriate or undesirable, or when rapid or short-term results are the priority (for example to cover periods away from home); desmopressin alone can also be used if there has been a partial response to a combination of desmopressin and an alarm following initial treatment with an alarm. Treatment should be assessed after 4 weeks and continued for 3 months if there are signs of response. Desmopressin should be withdrawn at regular intervals (for 1 week every 3 months) for full reassessment. Particular care is needed to avoid fluid overload by restricting fluid intake from 1 hour before taking desmopressin until 8 hours after. When stopping treatment with desmopressin, gradual withdrawal should be considered.

Nocturnal enuresis associated with daytime symptoms (overactive bladder) can be managed with anti-muscarinic drugs (see Urinary incontinence, p. 562) in combination with desmopressin. Treatment should be prescribed only after specialist assessment and should be continued for 3 months; the course can be repeated if necessary.

The tricyclic antidepressant **imipramine** (section 4.3.1) may be considered for children who have not responded to all other treatments and have undergone specialist assessment, however, behavioural disturbances can occur and relapse is common after withdrawal. Treatment should not normally exceed 3 months unless a physical examination is made and the child is fully re-assessed; toxicity following overdosage with tricyclics is of particular concern.

7.4.3 Drugs used in urological pain

The acute pain of *ureteric colic* may be relieved with **pethidine** (section 4.7.2). **Diclofenac** by injection or as suppositories (section 10.1.1) is also effective and compares favourably with pethidine; other non-steroidal anti-inflammatory drugs are occasionally given by injection.

Lidocaine gel is a useful topical application in *urethral pain* or to relieve the discomfort of catheterisation (section 15.2).

Alkalinisation of urine

Alkalinisation of urine can be undertaken with **potassium citrate**. The alkalinising action may relieve the discomfort of *cystitis* caused by lower urinary tract infections. **Sodium bicarbonate** is used as a urinary alkalinising agent in some metabolic and renal disorders (section 9.2.1.3).

▌ POTASSIUM CITRATE

Indications   relief of discomfort in mild urinary-tract infections; alkalinisation of urine

Cautions   cardiac disease; elderly; **interactions:** Appendix 1 (potassium salts)

Renal impairment   close monitoring required—high risk of hyperkalaemia; avoid in severe impairment

Side-effects   hyperkalaemia on prolonged high dosage, mild diuresis

Dose
- See under preparation

Potassium Citrate Mixture BP
(Potassium Citrate Oral Solution)
Oral solution, potassium citrate 30%, citric acid monohydrate 5% in a suitable vehicle with a lemon flavour. Extemporaneous preparations should be recently prepared according to the following formula: potassium citrate 3 g, citric acid monohydrate 500 mg, syrup 2.5 mL, quillaia tincture 0.1 mL, lemon spirit 0.05 mL, double-strength chloroform

water 3 mL, water to 10 mL. Contains about 28 mmol K^+/10 mL. Label: 27
Dose 10 mL 3 times daily well diluted with water
Proprietary brands of potassium citrate are on sale to the public for the relief of discomfort in mild urinary-tract infections

▌ SODIUM BICARBONATE

Indications   relief of discomfort in mild urinary-tract infections; alkalinisation of urine

Cautions   cardiac disease; patients on sodium-restricted diet; elderly; avoid prolonged use; **interactions:** Appendix 1 (antacids)

Hepatic impairment   section 1.1.1

Renal impairment   avoid; specialised role in some forms of renal disease, see section 9.2.1.3

Pregnancy   use with caution

Side-effects   eructation, alkalosis on prolonged use

Dose
- 3 g in water every 2 hours until urinary pH exceeds 7; maintenance of alkaline urine 5–10 g daily

◢**Preparations**
Section 9.2.1.3

▌ SODIUM CITRATE

Indications   relief of discomfort in mild urinary-tract infections

Cautions   cardiac disease; hypertension; patients on a sodium-restricted diet; elderly; **interactions:** Appendix 1 (sodium citrate)

Renal impairment   section 1.1.1

Pregnancy   use with caution

Side-effects   mild diuresis

Note Proprietary brands of sodium citrate are on sale to the public for the relief of discomfort in mild urinary-tract infections

Other preparations for urinary disorders

A terpene mixture (*Rowatinex*®) is claimed to be of benefit in *urolithiasis* for the expulsion of calculi.

Rowatinex® (Rowa) PoM
Capsules, yellow, e/c, anethol 4 mg, borneol 10 mg, camphene 15 mg, cineole 3 mg, fenchone 4 mg, pinene 31 mg, net price 50 = £7.35. Label: 25
Dose 1–2 capsules 3–4 times daily before food; CHILD not recommended

7.4.4 Bladder instillations and urological surgery

Bladder infection   Various solutions are available as irrigations or washouts.

Aqueous **chlorhexidine** (section 13.11.2) can be used in the management of common infections of the bladder but it is ineffective against most *Pseudomonas* spp. Solutions containing chlorhexidine 1 in 5000 (0.02%) are used but they may irritate the mucosa and cause burning and haematuria (in which case they should be discontinued); sterile **sodium chloride solution 0.9%** (physiological saline) is usually adequate and is preferred as a mechanical irrigant.

Continuous bladder irrigation with **amphotericin** 50 micrograms/mL (section 5.2.3) may be of value in mycotic infections.

Dissolution of blood clots   Clot retention is usually treated by irrigation with sterile **sodium chloride solution 0.9%** but sterile **sodium citrate solution for bladder irrigation 3%** may also be helpful.

Bladder cancer   Bladder instillations of **doxorubicin** (section 8.1.2) and **mitomycin** (section 8.1.2) are used for recurrent superficial bladder tumours. Such instillations reduce systemic side-effects; adverse effects on the bladder (e.g. micturition disorders and reduction in bladder capacity) may occur.

Instillation of **epirubicin** (section 8.1.2) is used for treatment and prophylaxis of certain forms of superficial bladder cancer; instillation of **doxorubicin** (section 8.1.2) is also used for some papillary tumours.

Instillation of **BCG** (Bacillus Calmette-Guérin), a live attenuated strain derived from *Mycobacterium bovis* (section 8.2.4), is licensed for the treatment of primary or recurrent bladder carcinoma *in-situ* and for the prevention of recurrence following transurethral resection.

Interstitial cystitis   Dimethyl sulfoxide may be used for symptomatic relief in patients with interstitial cystitis (Hunner's ulcer). 50 mL of a 50% solution (*Rimso-50*®—available from 'special-order' manufacturers or specialist importing companies, p. 1124) is instilled into the bladder, retained for 15 minutes, and voided by the patient. Treatment is repeated at intervals of 2 weeks. Bladder spasm and hypersensitivity reactions may occur and long-term use requires ophthalmic, renal, and hepatic assessment at intervals of 6 months. **Interactions:** see Appendix 1 (dimethyl sulfoxide).

▌ SODIUM CITRATE

Indications   bladder washouts, see notes above

Sterile Sodium Citrate Solution for Bladder Irrigation
sodium citrate 3%, dilute hydrochloric acid 0.2%, in purified water, freshly boiled and cooled, and sterilised

Urological surgery

There is a high risk of fluid absorption from the irrigant used in endoscopic surgery within the urinary tract; if this occurs in excess, hypervolaemia, haemolysis, and renal failure may result. **Glycine irrigation solution 1.5%** is the irrigant of choice for transurethral resection of the prostate gland and bladder tumours; **sterile sodium chloride solution 0.9%** (physiological saline) is used for percutaneous renal surgery.

▌ GLYCINE

Indications   bladder irrigation during urological surgery; see notes above
Cautions   see notes above
Side-effects   see notes above

Glycine Irrigation Solution (Non-proprietary)
Irrigation solution, glycine 1.5% in water for injections

Maintenance of indwelling urinary catheters

The deposition which occurs in catheterised patients is usually chiefly composed of phosphate and to minimise this the catheter (if latex) should be changed at least as often as every 6 weeks. If the catheter is to be left for longer periods a silicone catheter should be used together with the appropriate use of catheter maintenance solutions. Repeated blockage usually indicates that the catheter needs to be changed.

▌ CATHETER PATENCY SOLUTIONS

Chlorhexidine 0.02%
Brands include *Uro-Tainer Chlorhexidine*®, net price 100-mL sachet = £2.70

Sodium chloride 0.9%
Brands include *OptiFlo S*®, net price 50- and 100-mL sachets = £3.30; *Uriflex S*®, 100-mL sachet = £3.45; *Uriflex SP*®, with integral drug additive port, 100-mL sachet = £3.45; *Uro-Tainer Sodium Chloride*®, 50- and 100-mL sachets = £3.45; *Uro-Tainer M*®, with integral drug additive port, 50- and 100-mL sachets = £2.90

Solution G
Citric acid 3.23%, magnesium oxide 0.38%, sodium bicarbonate 0.7%, disodium edetate 0.01%. Brands include *OptiFlo G*®, net price 50- and 100-mL sachets = £3.50; *Uriflex G*®, 100-mL sachet = £2.40; *Uro-Tainer*® Twin Suby G, 2 × 30-mL = £4.72

Solution R
Citric acid 6%, gluconolactone 0.6%, magnesium carbonate 2.8%, disodium edetate 0.01%. Brands include *OptiFlo R*®, net price 50- and 100-mL sachets = £3.50; *Uriflex R*®, 100-mL sachet = £2.40; *Uro-Tainer*® Twin Solutio R, 2 × 30-mL = £4.72

Diluents for bladder instillation

▌ SODIUM CHLORIDE

Indications   diluent for instillation of drugs to the bladder

Sodium Chloride 0.9% Solution for Intravesical Use (Non-proprietary)
Intravesical instillation, sodium chloride 0.9%, net price 50-mL bag = £9.66

7.4.5 Drugs for erectile dysfunction

Reasons for failure to produce a satisfactory erection include *psychogenic, vascular, neurogenic,* and *endocrine abnormalities*; impotence can also be drug-induced. Intracavernosal, urethral, or topical application of vasoactive drugs under careful medical supervision are used for the management of erectile dysfunction. Intracavernosal or intraurethral preparations can also be used in the diagnosis of erectile dysfunction.

Erectile disorders may also be treated with drugs given by mouth which increase the blood flow to the penis. Drugs should be used with caution if the penis is deformed (e.g. in angulation, cavernosal fibrosis, and Peyronie's disease).

7 Obstetrics, gynaecology, and urinary-tract disorders

Priapism If priapism occurs with alprostadil, treatment should not be delayed more than 6 hours and is as follows:

Initial therapy by penile aspiration—using aseptic technique a 19–21 gauge butterfly needle inserted into the corpus cavernosum and 20–50 mL of blood aspirated; if necessary the procedure may be repeated on the opposite side.

If initial aspiration is unsuccessful a second 19–21 gauge butterfly needle can be inserted into the opposite corpus cavernosum and sterile physiological saline introduced through the first needle and drained through the second.

If aspiration and lavage of corpora are unsuccessful, *cautious* intracavernosal injection of a sympathomimetic (section 2.7.2) with action on alpha-adrenergic receptors, continuously monitoring blood pressure and pulse (*extreme caution:* coronary heart disease, hypertension, cerebral ischaemia or if taking antidepressant) as follows:

- intracavernosal injections of phenylephrine 100–200 micrograms (0.5–1 mL of a 200 microgram/mL solution) every 5–10 minutes; max. total dose 1 mg [unlicensed indication] [*important:* if suitable strength of phenylephrine injection not available may be specially prepared by diluting 0.1 mL of the phenylephrine 1% (10 mg/mL) injection (section 2.7.2) to 5 mL with sodium chloride 0.9%]; *alternatively*

- intracavernosal injections of adrenaline 10–20 micrograms (0.5–1 mL of a 20 microgram/mL solution) every 5–10 minutes; max. total dose 100 micrograms [unlicensed indication] [*important:* if suitable strength of adrenaline not available may be specially prepared by diluting 0.1 mL of the adrenaline 1 in 1000 (1 mg/mL, section 3.4.3) injection to 5 mL with sodium chloride 0.9%]; *alternatively*

- intracavernosal injection of metaraminol (*caution: has been associated with fatal hypertensive crises*); metaraminol 1 mg (0.1 mL of 10 mg/mL metaraminol injection, section 2.7.2) is diluted to 50 mL with sodium chloride injection 0.9% and given carefully by slow injection into the corpora in 5-mL injections every 15 minutes [unlicensed indication].

If necessary the sympathomimetic injections can be followed by further aspiration of blood through the same butterfly needle.

If sympathomimetics unsuccessful, urgent surgical referral for management (possibly including shunt procedure).

Prescribing on the NHS Some drug treatments for erectile dysfunction may only be prescribed on the NHS under certain circumstances; for details see the criteria listed in part XVIIIB of the Drug Tariff (Part XIb of the Northern Ireland Drug Tariff, Part 12 of the Scottish Drug Tariff). The Drug Tariffs can be accessed online at: National Health Service Drug Tariff for England and Wales: www.ppa.org.uk/ppa/edt_intro.htm; Health and Personal Social Services for Northern Ireland Drug Tariff: www.dhsspsni.gov.uk/pas-tariff; Scottish Drug Tariff: www.isdscotland.org/Health-Topics/Prescribing-and-Medicines/Scottish-Drug-Tariff/

Alprostadil

Alprostadil (prostaglandin E$_1$) is given by intracavernosal injection, intraurethral application, or topical application for the management of erectile dysfunction (after exclusion of treatable medical causes). Intracavernosal or intraurethral preparations can also used in the diagnosis of erectile dysfunction.

◢ ALPROSTADIL

Indications erectile dysfunction (including aid to diagnosis)

Cautions priapism—patients should be instructed to report any erection lasting 4 hours or longer—for management, see section 7.4.5; anatomical deformations of penis (painful erection more likely)—follow up regularly to detect signs of penile fibrosis (consider discontinuation if angulation, cavernosal fibrosis or Peyronie's disease develop); **interactions:** Appendix 1 (prostaglandins)

Contra-indications predisposition to prolonged erection (as in thrombocythemia, polycythemia, sickle cell anaemia, multiple myeloma or leukaemia); not for use with other agents for erectile dysfunction, in patients with penile implants or when sexual activity medically inadvisable (e.g. orthostatic hypotension, myocardial infarction, and syncope); urethral and topical application also contra-indicated in urethral stricture, severe hypospadia, severe curvature, balanitis, urethritis

Side-effects hypotension, hypertension; dizziness, headache; penile pain, other localised pain (buttocks, leg, testicular, abdominal); influenza-like syndrome; urethral burning, urethral bleeding, urethral pain; injection site reactions including penile fibrosis, penile oedema, penile rash, haematoma, haemosiderin deposits; *less commonly* nausea, dry mouth, vasodilatation, syncope, supraventricular extrasystole, rapid pulse, asthenia, leg cramps, pelvic pain, scrotal or testicular oedema, scrotal erythema, scrotal pain, urethral stenosis, testicular thickening, micturition difficulties, haematuria, mydriasis, and sweating; local reactions including penile warmth, pruritus, irritation, penile numbness or sensitivity, balantitis, phimosis, priapism (see section 7.4.5 and under Cautions); abnormal ejaculation; *rarely* vertigo, urinary-tract infection, and hypersensitivity reactions (including rash, erythema, urticaria, and anaphylaxis)

Dose

- See under preparations below

◢ Intracavernosal injection

[1] Caverject® (Pharmacia) PoM NHS

Injection, powder for reconstitution, alprostadil, net price 5-microgram vial = £7.73; 10-microgram vial = £9.24; 20-microgram vial = £11.94; 40-microgram

---

1. NHS for treatment of erectile dysfunction except in men who meet the criteria listed in part XVIIIB of the Drug Tariff (Part XIb of the Northern Ireland Drug Tariff, Part 12 of the Scottish Drug Tariff). The prescription must be endorsed 'SLS'.
The Drug Tariffs can be accessed online at: National Health Service Drug Tariff for England and Wales: www.ppa.org.uk/ppa/edt_intro.htm; Health and Personal Social Services for Northern Ireland Drug Tariff: www.dhsspsni.gov.uk/pas-tariff; Scottish Drug Tariff: www.isdscotland.org/Health-Topics/Prescribing-and-Medicines/Scottish-Drug-Tariff/

7   Obstetrics, gynaecology, and urinary-tract disorders

vial = £21.58 (all with diluent-filled syringe, needles and swabs)

Caverject® Dual Chamber, double-chamber cartridges (containing alprostadil and diluent), net price 10-microgram cartridge (for doses 2.5–10 micrograms) = £7.35; 20-microgram cartridge (for doses 5–20 micrograms) = £9.50 (both with needles)

Dose by direct intracavernosal injection, ADULT over 18 years, erectile dysfunction, first dose 2.5 micrograms, second dose 5 micrograms (if some response to first dose) *or* 7.5 micrograms (if no response to first dose), increasing in steps of 5–10 micrograms to obtain dose suitable for producing erection lasting not more than 1 hour (neurological dysfunction, first dose 1.25 micrograms, second dose 2.5 micrograms, third dose 5 micrograms, increasing in steps of 5–10 micrograms to obtain suitable dose); if no response to dose then next higher dose can be given within 1 hour, if there is a response the next dose should not be given for at least 24 hours; usual dose 5–20 micrograms; max. 60 micrograms; max. frequency of injection not more than 3 times per week with at least 24 hour interval between injections

Note The first dose must be given by medically trained personnel; self-administration may only be undertaken after proper training

Aid to diagnosis, 10–20 micrograms as a single dose (where evidence of neurological dysfunction, initially 5 micrograms and max. 10 micrograms)—consult product literature for details

¹Viridal® Duo (UCB Pharma) PoM ⒩HS

Starter Pack (hosp. only), contents as for *Continuation Pack* below plus *Duoject* applicator, net price 10-microgram starter pack = £20.13, 20-microgram starter pack = £24.54, 40-microgram starter pack = £29.83; *Continuation Pack*, 2 double-chamber cartridges (containing alprostadil and diluent), 2 needles, swabs, 10-microgram continuation pack = £16.55, 20-microgram continuation pack = £21.39, 40-microgram continuation pack = £27.22; replacement *Duoject*® applicators available from UCB Pharma

Dose by direct intracavernosal injection, ADULT over 18 years, erectile dysfunction, initially 5 micrograms (2.5 micrograms in neurogenic erectile dysfunction) increasing in steps of 2.5–5 micrograms to obtain dose suitable for producing erection not lasting more than 1 hour; usual range 10–20 micrograms; max. 40 micrograms; max. frequency of injection not more than 2–3 times per week with at least 24 hour interval between injections; reduce dose if erection lasts longer than 2 hours

Note The first dose must be given by medically trained personnel; self-administration may only be undertaken after proper training

◢**Topical application**

Counselling Condoms should be used to avoid local reactions and exposure of alprostadil to women of childbearing age, pregnant, or lactating women

¹Vitaros® (Takeda) PoM ⒩HS

Cream, alprostadil, net price 300 microgram single-use container = £10.00

Condoms no evidence of damage to latex condoms

Dose ADULT over 18 years, erectile dysfunction, apply 300 micrograms to the tip of the penis, 5–30 minutes before sexual activity; max. 1 dose in 24 hours not more than 2-3 times per week

1. ⒩HS for treatment of erectile dysfunction except in men who meet the criteria listed in part XVIIIB of the Drug Tariff (Part XIb of the Northern Ireland Drug Tariff, Part 12 of the Scottish Drug Tariff). The prescription must be endorsed 'SLS'.
The Drug Tariffs can be accessed online at: National Health Service Drug Tariff for England and Wales: www.ppa.org.uk/ppa/edt_intro.htm; Health and Personal Social Services for Northern Ireland Drug Tariff: www.dhsspsni.gov.uk/pas-tariff; Scottish Drug Tariff: www.isdscotland.org/Health-Topics/Prescribing-and-Medicines/Scottish-Drug-Tariff/

◢**Urethral application**

Counselling If partner pregnant barrier contraception should be used

¹MUSE® (Meda) PoM ⒩HS

Urethral application, alprostadil, net price 250-microgram single-use applicator = £11.30, 500-microgram single-use applicator = £11.30, 1-mg single-use applicator = £11.56 (all strengths also available in packs of 6 applicators)

Condoms no evidence of harm to latex condoms and diaphragms

Dose by direct urethral application, ADULT over 18 years, erectile dysfunction, initially 250 micrograms adjusted according to response (usual range 0.125–1 mg); max. 2 doses in 24 hours and 7 doses in 7 days)

Note During initiation of treatment *MUSE*® should be used under medical supervision; self-administration may only be undertaken after proper training

Aid to diagnosis, 500 micrograms as a single dose

Phosphodiesterase type-5 inhibitors

Avanafil, **sildenafil**, **tadalafil**, and **vardenafil** are phosphodiesterase type-5 inhibitors licensed for the treatment of erectile dysfunction; they are not recommended for use with other treatments for erectile dysfunction. The patient should be assessed appropriately before prescribing avanafil, sildenafil, tadalafil or vardenafil. Since these drugs are given by mouth there is a potential for drug interactions.

Cautions Avanafil, sildenafil, tadalafil, and vardenafil should be used with caution in cardiovascular disease, left ventricular outflow obstruction, anatomical deformation of the penis (e.g. angulation, cavernosal fibrosis, Peyronie's disease), and in those with a predisposition to priapism (e.g. in sickle-cell disease, multiple myeloma, or leukaemia). Concomitant treatment with a phosphodiesterase type-5 inhibitor and an alpha-blocker (section 2.5.4 and section 7.4.1) can increase the risk of postural hypotension—initiate treatment with a phosphodiesterase type-5 inhibitor (at a low dose) only once the patient is stable on the alpha-blocker; see also **interactions**: Appendix 1 (avanafil, sildenafil, tadalafil, vardenafil).

Contra-indications Avanafil, sildenafil, tadalafil, and vardenafil are contra-indicated in patients receiving nitrates, in patients in whom vasodilation or sexual activity are inadvisable, or in patients with a previous history of non-arteritic anterior ischaemic optic neuropathy. In the absence of information, manufacturers contra-indicate these drugs in hypotension (avoid if systolic blood pressure below 90 mmHg), recent stroke, unstable angina, and myocardial infarction.

Side-effects The side-effects of avanafil, sildenafil, tadalafil, and vardenafil include dyspepsia, nausea, vomiting, headache (including migraine), flushing, dizziness, myalgia, back pain, visual disturbances (non-arteritic anterior ischaemic optic neuropathy has been reported—stop drug if sudden visual impairment occurs), and nasal congestion. *Less common* side-effects include painful red eyes, palpitation, tachycardia, hypotension, hypertension, epistaxis. Other side-effects reported rarely include syncope, hypersensitivity reactions (including rash, facial oedema, and Stevens-Johnson syndrome), and priapism. Serious cardiovascular events (including arrhythmia, unstable angina, and myocardial infarction), seizures, sudden hearing loss (discontinue drug and seek medical advice), and retinal vascular occlusion have also been reported.

■ AVANAFIL

Indications erectile dysfunction

Cautions see notes above; also bleeding disorders or active peptic ulceration; **interactions:** Appendix 1 (avanafil)

Contra-indications see notes above; also life-threatening arrhythmia in previous 6 months; blood pressure >170/100 mmHg; mild to severe heart failure; hereditary degenerative retinal disorders

Hepatic impairment use lowest effective initial dose in mild to moderate impairment, adjusted according to response; manufacturer advises avoid in severe impairment—no information available

Renal impairment avoid if eGFR less than 30 mL/minute/1.73 m^2

Side-effects see notes above; also *less commonly* malaise, drowsiness; *rarely* dry mouth, gastritis, abdominal pain, diarrhoea, hyperbilirubinaemia, peripheral oedema, hyperactivity, insomnia, weight gain, genital irritation, pollakiuria, increased serum creatinine, gout, muscle spasms, haematuria

Dose

● ADULT over 18 years, initially 100 mg (patients on alpha-blocker therapy 50 mg) approx. 30 minutes before sexual activity, subsequent doses adjusted according to response to 50–200 mg as a single dose as needed; max. 1 dose in 24 hours (max. single dose 200 mg)

Note Max. 100 mg once every 48 hours with concomitant moderate inhibitors of cytochrome P450 enzyme CYP3A4 e.g. aprepitant, diltiazem, erythromycin, fluconazole, fosamprenavir, or verapamil

Note Onset of effect may be delayed if taken with food

¹Spedra® (Menarini) ⒫ⓄⓂ ⒥ⒽⓈ
Tablets, all yellow, avanafil 50 mg, net price 4-tab pack = £10.94, 8-tab pack = £19.70; 100 mg, 4-tab pack = £14.08, 8-tab pack = £26.26; 200 mg, 4-tab pack = £21.90, 8-tab pack = £39.40

■ SILDENAFIL

Indications erectile dysfunction; pulmonary hypertension (section 2.5.1)

Cautions see notes above; also bleeding disorders or active peptic ulceration; **interactions:** Appendix 1 (sildenafil)

Contra-indications see notes above; also hereditary degenerative retinal disorders

Hepatic impairment initial dose 25 mg; manufacturer advises avoid in severe impairment

Renal impairment initial dose 25 mg if eGFR less than 30 mL/minute/1.73 m^2

Side-effects see notes above; also *less commonly* chest pain, drowsiness, hypoaesthesia, vertigo, tinnitus, dry mouth, fatigue; *rarely* cerebrovascular accident and atrial fibrillation

----

1. ⒥ⒽⓈ for treatment of erectile dysfunction except in men who meet the criteria listed in part XVIIIB of the Drug Tariff (Part XIb of the Northern Ireland Drug Tariff, Part 12 of the Scottish Drug Tariff). The prescription must be endorsed 'SLS'.
   The Drug Tariffs can be accessed online at: National Health Service Drug Tariff for England and Wales: www.ppa.org.uk/ppa/edt_intro.htm; Health and Personal Social Services for Northern Ireland Drug Tariff: www.dhsspsni.gov.uk/pas-tariff; Scottish Drug Tariff: www.isdscotland.org/Health-Topics/Prescribing-and-Medicines/Scottish-Drug-Tariff/

Dose

● ADULT over 18 years initially 50 mg approx. 1 hour before sexual activity, subsequent doses adjusted according to response to 25–100 mg as a single dose as needed; max. 1 dose in 24 hours (max. single dose 100 mg)

Note Onset of effect may be delayed if taken with food

Sildenafil (Non-proprietary) ⒫ⓄⓂ
Tablets, sildenafil (as citrate), 25 mg, net price 4-tab pack = £1.12, 8-tab pack = £2.09; 50 mg, 4-tab pack = £1.16, 8-tab pack = £2.23; 100 mg, 4-tab pack = £1.25, 8-tab pack = £2.32

Nipatra® (AMCo) ⒫ⓄⓂ
Chewable tablets, sildenafil (as citrate), 25 mg, net price 4-tab pack = £1.05, 8-tab pack = £2.10; 50 mg, 4-tab pack = £1.03, 8-tab pack = £2.06; 100 mg, 4-tab pack = £1.11, 8-tab pack = £2.22. Label: 24
Excipients include aspartame (section 9.4.1)

¹Viagra® (Pfizer) ⒫ⓄⓂ ⒥ⒽⓈ
Tablets, all blue, f/c, sildenafil (as citrate), 25 mg, net price 4-tab pack = £16.59, 8-tab pack = £33.19; 50 mg, 4-tab pack = £21.27, 8-tab pack = £42.54; 100 mg, 4-tab pack = £23.50, 8-tab pack = £46.99

Revatio® (Pfizer) ⒫ⓄⓂ
Section 2.5.1 (pulmonary hypertension)

■ TADALAFIL

Indications benign prostatic hyperplasia; erectile dysfunction; pulmonary hypertension (section 2.5.1)

Cautions see notes above; **interactions:** Appendix 1 (tadalafil)

Contra-indications see notes above; also mild to severe heart failure, uncontrolled arrhythmias, uncontrolled hypertension

Hepatic impairment max. dose 10 mg; manufacturer advises caution in severe impairment and for regular once-daily dosing—no information available

Renal impairment max. dose 10 mg if eGFR less than 30 mL/minute/1.73 m^2 (avoid regular once-daily dosing)

Side-effects see notes above; also increased sweating, abdominal pain, and transient amnesia reported

Dose

● Erectile dysfunction, ADULT over 18 years, initially 10 mg at least 30 minutes before sexual activity, subsequent doses adjusted according to response, up to 20 mg as a single dose; max. 1 dose in 24 hours (but daily dose of 10–20 mg not recommended); for patients who anticipate sexual activity at least twice weekly, 5 mg once daily can be taken, reduced to 2.5 mg once daily according to response

Note Effect of intermittent dosing may persist for longer than 24 hours

● Benign prostatic hyperplasia, ADULT over 18 years, 5 mg once daily

¹Cialis® (Lilly) ⒫ⓄⓂ ⒥ⒽⓈ
Tablets, f/c, tadalafil 2.5 mg (orange), net price 28-tab pack = £54.99; 5 mg (light yellow), 28-tab pack = £54.99; 10 mg (light yellow), 4-tab pack = £26.99; 20 mg (yellow), 4-tab pack = £26.99; 8-tab pack = £53.98

7 Obstetrics, gynaecology, and urinary-tract disorders

▌VARDENAFIL

Indications erectile dysfunction

Cautions see notes above; also elderly; bleeding disorders or active peptic ulceration; susceptibility to prolongation of QT interval (including concomitant use of drugs which prolong QT interval); **interactions**: Appendix 1 (vardenafil)

Contra-indications see notes above; also hereditary degenerative retinal disorders

Hepatic impairment initial dose 5 mg in mild to moderate impairment, increased subsequently according to response (max. 10 mg in moderate impairment); manufacturer advises avoid in severe impairment

Renal impairment initial dose 5 mg if eGFR less than 30 mL/minute/1.73 m^2

Side-effects see notes above; also *less commonly* drowsiness, dyspnoea, increased lacrimation, photosensitivity; *rarely* anxiety, transient amnesia, hypertonia, and raised intra-ocular pressure

Dose

● See under preparations

[1]**Levitra**® (Bayer) PoM NHS

Tablets, all orange, f/c, vardenafil (as hydrochloride trihydrate) 5 mg, net price 4-tab pack = £7.56, 8-tab pack = £15.12; 10 mg, 4-tab pack = £14.08, 8-tab pack = £28.16; 20 mg, 4-tab pack = £23.48, 8-tab pack = £46.96

Dose ADULT over 18 years, initially 10 mg (patients on alpha-blocker therapy 5 mg) approx. 25–60 minutes before sexual activity, subsequent doses adjusted according to response up to max. 20 mg as a single dose; max. 1 dose in 24 hours

Note Onset of effect may be delayed if taken with high-fat meal

Orodispersible tablets, vardenafil (as hydrochloride) 10 mg, net price 4–tab pack = £17.88

Excipients include aspartame

Dose ADULT over 18 years, 10 mg approx. 25–60 minutes before sexual activity; max. 10 mg in 24 hours (dose form not suitable for patients with moderate hepatic impairment, or for initiation of therapy in patients taking alpha-blockers, or if eGFR less than 30 mL/minute/1.73m^2)

The *Scottish Medicines Consortium* (p. 4) has advised (September 2011) that vardenafil orodispersible tablets (*Levitra*®) are accepted for restricted use within NHS Scotland for men for whom an orodispersible tablet is an appropriate formulation.

Important *Levitra*® *10 mg orodispersible* tablets and *Levitra*® *10 mg film coated tablets* are **not** bioequivalent

Papaverine and phentolamine

Although not licensed the smooth muscle relaxant **papaverine** has also been given by intracavernosal injection for erectile dysfunction. Patients with neurological or psychogenic impotence are more sensitive to the effect of papaverine than those with vascular abnormalities. **Phentolamine** is added if the response is inadequate [unlicensed indication].

1. NHS for treatment of erectile dysfunction except in men who meet the criteria listed in part XVIIIB of the Drug Tariff (Part XIb of the Northern Ireland Drug Tariff, Part 12 of the Scottish Drug Tariff). The prescription must be endorsed 'SLS'.

   The Drug Tariffs can be accessed online at: National Health Service Drug Tariff for England and Wales: www.ppa.org.uk/ppa/edt_intro.htm; Health and Personal Social Services for Northern Ireland Drug Tariff: www.dhsspsni.gov.uk/pas-tariff; Scottish Drug Tariff: www.isdscotland.org/Health-Topics/Prescribing-and-Medicines/Scottish-Drug-Tariff/

Persistence of the erection for longer than 4 hours is an emergency, see advice in section 7.4.5.

7.4.6 Drugs for premature ejaculation

Dapoxetine is a short-acting selective serotonin reuptake inhibitor licensed for use in the treatment of premature ejaculation in men who meet all the following criteria: poor control over ejaculation, a history of premature ejaculation over the past 6 months, marked distress or interpersonal difficulty as a consequence of premature ejaculation, and an intravaginal ejaculatory latency time of less than two minutes.

▌DAPOXETINE

Indications premature ejaculation (see notes above)

Cautions bleeding disorders; concomitant use of drugs that increase risk of bleeding; epilepsy (*avoid* if uncontrolled, discontinue if convulsions develop); susceptibility to angle-closure glaucoma; **interactions**: Appendix 1 (dapoxetine)

Postural hypotension and syncope Postural hypotension and syncope reported. Test for postural hypotension before starting treatment—avoid dapoxetine if postural hypotension occurs. Patients should be advised to maintain hydration and to sit or lie down until prodromal symptoms such as nausea, dizziness, and sweating abate

Contra-indications significant cardiac disease; history of syncope; history of mania, bipolar disorder, or severe depression; discontinue if psychiatric disorder develops

Hepatic impairment avoid in moderate to severe impairment

Renal impairment use with caution if eGFR 30–80 mL/minute/1.73 m^2; avoid if eGFR less than 30 mL/minute/1.73 m^2

Side-effects nausea, vomiting, diarrhoea, constipation, abdominal pain, abdominal distension, dyspepsia, dry mouth, flushing, sweating, hypertension, malaise, irritability, dizziness, headache, anxiety, agitation, abnormal dreams, sleep disturbances, drowsiness, tremor, paraesthesia, impaired attention, sexual dysfunction, visual disturbances, tinnitus; *less commonly* syncope, sinus arrest, bradycardia, tachycardia, hypotension (including postural hypotension), restlessness, taste disturbances, depression, mood disturbances (discontinue), confusion, abnormal thoughts, vertigo, bruxism, mydriasis, eye pain, pruritus; *rarely* defaecation urgency, sudden onset of sleep

Dose

● ADULT 18–64 years, initially 30 mg approx. 1–3 hours before sexual activity, subsequent doses adjusted according to response to max. 60 mg as a single dose; max. 1 dose in 24 hours; review treatment after 4 weeks (or 6 doses) and at least every 6 months thereafter

Note Max. single dose 30 mg with concomitant aprepitant, clarithromycin, diltiazem, erythromycin, fluconazole, fosamprenavir, and verapamil; use 60-mg dose with caution with concomitant potent inhibitors of cytochrome P450 enzyme CYP2D6

Priligy® (Menarini) PoM

Tablets, f/c, dapoxetine (as hydrochloride), 30 mg (light grey), net price 3-tab pack = £14.71, 6-tab pack = £26.48; 60 mg (grey), 3-tab pack = £19.12, 6-tab pack = £34.42. Label: 2, 25, counselling, postural hypotension

8 Malignant disease and immunosuppression

8.1 Cytotoxic drugs

8.1.1 Alkylating drugs

8.1.2 Anthracyclines and other cytotoxic antibiotics

8.1.3 Antimetabolites

8.1.4 Vinca alkaloids and etoposide

8.1.5 Other antineoplastic drugs

The chemotherapy of cancer is complex and should be confined to specialists in oncology. Cytotoxic drugs have both anti-cancer activity and the potential to damage normal tissue; most cytotoxic drugs are teratogenic. Chemotherapy may be given with a curative intent or it may aim to prolong life or to palliate symptoms. In an increasing number of cases chemotherapy may be combined with radiotherapy or surgery or both as either neoadjuvant treatment (initial chemotherapy aimed at shrinking the primary tumour, thereby rendering local therapy less destructive or more effective) or as adjuvant treatment (which follows definitive treatment of the primary disease, when the risk of subclinical metastatic disease is known to be high). All cytotoxic drugs cause side-effects and a balance has to be struck between likely benefit and acceptable toxicity.

Guidelines for handling cytotoxic drugs

- Trained personnel should reconstitute cytotoxics;
- Reconstitution should be carried out in designated pharmacy areas;
- Protective clothing (including gloves, gowns, and masks) should be worn;
- The eyes should be protected and means of first aid should be specified;
- Pregnant staff should avoid exposure to cytotoxic drugs (all females of child-bearing age should be informed of the reproductive hazard);
- Use local procedures for dealing with spillages and safe disposal of waste material, including syringes, containers, and absorbent material;
- Staff exposure to cytotoxic drugs should be monitored.

Combinations of cytotoxic drugs, as continuous or pulsed cycles of treatment, are frequently more toxic than single drugs but have the advantage in certain tumours of enhanced response, reduced development of drug resistance and increased survival. However for some tumours, single-agent chemotherapy remains the treatment of choice.

Cytotoxic drugs fall into a number of classes, each with characteristic antitumour activity, sites of action, and toxicity. A knowledge of sites of metabolism and excretion is important because impaired drug handling as a result of disease is not uncommon and may result in enhanced toxicity.

Intrathecal chemotherapy

A Health Service Circular (HSC 2008/001) provides guidance on the introduction of safe practice in NHS Trusts where intrathecal chemotherapy is administered; written local guidance covering all aspects of national guidance should be available. Support for training programmes is also available.

Copies, and further information may be obtained from:

Department of Health
PO Box 777
London SE1 6XH
Fax: 01623 724524

It is also available from the Department of Health website (www.dh.gov.uk)

Safe system requirements for cytotoxic medicines

- cytotoxic drugs for the treatment of cancer should be given as part of a wider pathway of care coordinated by a multidisciplinary team;

- cytotoxic drugs should be prescribed, dispensed, and administered only in the context of a written protocol or treatment plan;

- injectable cytotoxic drugs should only be dispensed if they are prepared for administration

- oral cytotoxic medicines should be dispensed with clear directions for use

Risks of incorrect dosing of oral anti-cancer medicines

The National Patient Safety Agency has advised (January 2008) that the prescribing and use of oral cytotoxic medicines should be carried out to the same standard as parenteral cytotoxic therapy. Standards to be followed to achieve this include:

- non-specialists who prescribe or administer on-going oral cytotoxic medication should have access to written protocols and treatment plans, including guidance on the monitoring and treatment of toxicity

- staff dispensing oral cytotoxic medicines should confirm that the prescribed dose is appropriate for the patient. Patients should have written information that includes details of the intended oral anti-cancer regimen, the treatment plan, and arrangements for monitoring, taken from the original protocol from the initiating hospital. Staff dispensing oral cytotoxic medicines should also have access to this information, and to advice from an experienced cancer pharmacist in the initiating hospital

Doses

Doses of cytotoxic drugs are determined using a variety of different methods including body-surface area or body-weight. Alternatively, doses may be fixed. Doses may be further adjusted following consideration of a patient's neutrophil count, renal and hepatic function, and history of previous adverse effects to the cytotoxic drug. Doses may also differ depending on whether a drug is used alone or in combination.

Because of the complexity of dosage regimens in the treatment of malignant disease, dose statements have been omitted from some of the drug entries in this chapter. However, even where dose statements have been provided, detailed specialist literature or individual hospital chemotherapy protocols should be consulted before prescribing, dispensing, or administering cytotoxic drugs.

Prescriptions should **not** be repeated except on the instructions of a specialist.

Side-effects of cytotoxic drugs

Side-effects common to most cytotoxic drugs are discussed below whilst side-effects characteristic of a particular drug or class of drugs (e.g. neurotoxicity with vinca alkaloids) are mentioned in the appropriate sections. Manufacturers' product literature, hospital-trust protocols, and cancer-network protocols should be consulted for full details of side-effects associated with individual drugs and specific chemotherapy regimes.

Many side-effects of cytotoxic drugs often do not occur at the time of administration, but days or weeks later. It is therefore important that patients and healthcare professionals can identify symptoms that cause concern and can contact an expert for advice. Toxicities should be accurately recorded using a recognised scoring system such as the Common Toxicity Criteria for Adverse Events (CTCAE) developed by the National Cancer Institute.

Extravasation of intravenous drugs A number of cytotoxic drugs will cause severe local tissue necrosis if leakage into the extravascular compartment occurs. To reduce the risk of extravasation injury it is recommended that cytotoxic drugs are administered by appropriately trained staff. For information on the prevention and management of extravasation injury, see section 10.3.

Oral mucositis A sore mouth is a common complication of cancer chemotherapy; it is most often associated with fluorouracil, methotrexate, and the anthracyclines. It is best to prevent the complication. Good oral hygiene (rinsing the mouth frequently and effective brushing of the teeth with a soft brush 2–3 times daily) is probably beneficial. For fluorouracil, sucking ice chips during short infusions of the drug is also helpful.

Once a sore mouth has developed, treatment is much less effective. Saline mouthwashes should be used but there is no good evidence to support the use of antiseptic or anti-inflammatory mouthwashes. In general, mucositis is self-limiting but with poor oral hygiene it can be a focus for blood-borne infection.

Tumour lysis syndrome Tumour lysis syndrome occurs secondary to spontaneous or treatment-related rapid destruction of malignant cells. Patients at risk of tumour lysis syndrome include those with non-Hodgkin's lymphoma (especially if high grade and bulky disease), Burkitt's lymphoma, acute lymphoblastic leukaemia and acute myeloid leukaemia (particularly if high white blood cell counts or bulky disease), and occasionally those with solid tumours. Pre-existing hyperuricaemia, dehydration, and renal impairment are also predisposing factors. Features include hyperkalaemia, hyperuricaemia (see below), and hyperphosphataemia with hypocalcaemia; renal damage and arrhythmias can follow. Early identification of patients at risk, and initiation of prophylaxis or therapy for tumour lysis syndrome, is essential.

Hyperuricaemia Hyperuricaemia, which may be present in high-grade lymphoma and leukaemia, can be markedly worsened by chemotherapy and is associated with acute renal failure. Allopurinol (section 10.1.4) should be started 24 hours before treating such tumours and patients should be adequately hydrated. The dose of mercaptopurine or azathioprine should be reduced if allopurinol needs to be given concomitantly (see Appendix 1).

Rasburicase (section 10.1.4), a recombinant urate oxidase, is licensed for hyperuricaemia in patients with haematological malignancy, for details, see p. 745. It rapidly reduces plasma-uric acid concentration and may be of particular value in preventing complications following treatment of leukaemias or bulky lymphomas.

Nausea and vomiting Nausea and vomiting cause considerable distress to many patients who receive chemotherapy and to a lesser extent abdominal radiotherapy, and may lead to refusal of further treatment; prophylaxis of nausea and vomiting is therefore extremely important. Symptoms may be acute (occurring within 24 hours of treatment), delayed (first occurring more than 24 hours after treatment), or anticipatory (occurring prior to subsequent doses). Delayed and anticipatory symptoms are more difficult to control than acute symptoms and require different management.

Patients vary in their susceptibility to drug-induced nausea and vomiting; those affected more often include women, patients under 50 years of age, anxious patients, and those who experience motion sickness. Susceptibility also increases with repeated exposure to the cytotoxic drug.

Drugs may be divided according to their emetogenic potential and some examples are given below, but the symptoms vary according to the dose, to other drugs administered and to individual susceptibility.

Mildly emetogenic treatment—fluorouracil, etoposide, methotrexate (less than 100 mg/m²), the vinca alkaloids, and abdominal radiotherapy.

Moderately emetogenic treatment—the taxanes, doxorubicin, intermediate and low doses of cyclophosphamide, mitoxantrone, and high doses of methotrexate (0.1–1.2 g/m²).

Highly emetogenic treatment—cisplatin, dacarbazine, and high doses of cyclophosphamide.

Prevention of acute symptoms For patients at *low risk of emesis*, pretreatment with dexamethasone (6–10 mg by mouth) or lorazepam (1–2 mg by mouth) may be used.

For patients at *high risk of emesis*, a 5HT₃-receptor antagonist (section 4.6), usually given by mouth in

combination with dexamethasone and the neurokinin receptor antagonist aprepitant is effective.

Prevention of delayed symptoms For delayed symptoms associated with moderately emetogenic chemotherapy, a combination of dexamethasone and 5HT₃-receptor antagonist is effective; for highly emetogenic chemotherapy, a combination of dexamethasone and aprepitant is effective. Metoclopramide is also licensed for delayed chemotherapy-induced nausea and vomiting.

Prevention of anticipatory symptoms Good symptom control is the best way to prevent anticipatory symptoms. Lorazepam can be helpful for its amnesic, sedative, and anxiolytic effects.

Bone-marrow suppression All cytotoxic drugs except vincristine and bleomycin cause bone-marrow suppression. This commonly occurs 7 to 10 days after administration, but is delayed for certain drugs, such as carmustine, lomustine, and melphalan. Peripheral blood counts must be checked before each treatment, and doses should be reduced or therapy delayed if bone-marrow has not recovered.

Cytotoxic drugs may be contra-indicated in patients with acute infection; any infection should be treated before, or when starting, cytotoxic drugs.

Fever in a neutropenic patient (neutrophil count less than 1.0×10^9/litre) requires immediate broad-spectrum antibacterial therapy. Appropriate bacteriological investigations should be conducted as soon as possible. Patients taking cytotoxic drugs who have signs or symptoms of infection should be advised to seek prompt medical attention. All patients should initially be investigated and treated under the supervision of the appropriate oncology or haematology specialist.

In selected patients, the duration and the severity of neutropenia can be reduced by the use of recombinant human granulocyte-colony stimulating factors, see section 9.1.6.

Symptomatic anaemia is usually treated with red blood cell transfusions. For guidance on the use of erythropoietins in patients with cancer, see MHRA/CHM advice (p. 667) and NICE guidance (p. 667).

For advice on the use of live vaccines in individuals with impaired immune response, see section 14.1.

Alopecia Reversible hair loss is a common complication, although it varies in degree between drugs and individual patients. No pharmacological methods of preventing this are available.

Pregnancy and reproductive function Most cytotoxic drugs are teratogenic and should not be administered during pregnancy, especially during the first trimester. Exclude pregnancy before treatment with cytotoxic drugs. Considerable caution is necessary if a pregnant woman presents with cancer requiring chemotherapy, and specialist advice should always be sought.

Contraceptive advice should be given to men and women before cytotoxic therapy begins (and should cover the duration of contraception required after therapy has ended).

Regimens that do not contain an alkylating drug or procarbazine may have less effect on fertility, but those with an alkylating drug or procarbazine carry the risk of causing permanent male sterility (there is no effect on potency). Pretreatment counselling and consideration of sperm storage may be appropriate. Women are less severely affected, though the span of reproductive life may be shortened by the onset of a premature menopause. No increase in fetal abnormalities or abortion rate has been recorded in patients who remain fertile after cytotoxic chemotherapy.

Thromboembolism Venous thromboembolism can be a complication of cancer itself, but chemotherapy increases the risk.

Treatment for cytotoxic-induced side-effects

Anthracycline side-effects

Anthracycline-induced cardiotoxicity The anthracycline cytotoxic drugs are associated with dose-related, cumulative, and potentially life-threatening cardiotoxic side-effects.

Dexrazoxane, an iron chelator, is licensed for the prevention of chronic cumulative cardiotoxicity caused by doxorubicin or epirubicin treatment in advanced or metastatic breast cancer patients who have received a prior cumulative dose of $300 \, mg/m^2$ of doxorubicin or a prior cumulative dose of $540 \, mg/m^2$ of epirubicin when further anthracycline treatment is required. Patients receiving dexrazoxane should still be monitored for cardiac toxicity. The myelosuppressive effects of dexrazoxane may be additive to those of chemotherapy. The use of dexrazoxane is restricted to adults with advanced or metastatic breast cancer. Dexrazoxane is contraindicated in children.

Anthracycline extravasation Dexrazoxane is licensed for the treatment of anthracycline extravasation. The first dose should be given as soon as possible and within six hours after the injury. For further information on the prevention and management of extravasation injury, see section 10.3.

> Local guidelines for the management of extravasation should be followed or specialist advice sought.

▌ DEXRAZOXANE

Indications see notes above and under preparations

Cautions see notes above; monitor full blood count and liver function; manufacturer of *Cardioxane®* advises caution in patients with myocardial infarction in previous 12 months, heart failure, uncontrolled angina, symptomatic valvular heart disease—no information available; **interactions:** Appendix 1 (dexrazoxane)

Hepatic impairment manufacturer of *Cardioxane®* advises that if anthracycline dose is reduced, reduce the *Cardioxane®* dose by a similar ratio; manufacturer of *Savene®* advises avoid—no information available

Renal impairment manufacturer of *Cardioxane®* advises reduce dose by 50% if creatinine clearance less than 40 mL/minute; manufacturer of *Savene®* advises avoid—risk of accumulation

Pregnancy avoid unless essential (toxicity in *animal* studies); ensure effective contraception during and for at least 3 months after treatment in men and women

Breast-feeding discontinue breast-feeding

Side-effects nausea, vomiting, diarrhoea, stomatitis, dry mouth, anorexia, oedema, dyspnoea, dizziness,

syncope, malaise, peripheral neuropathy, infection, pyrexia, blood disorders (including anaemia, leucopenia, and thrombocytopenia), alopecia, pruritus, erythema, injection-site reactions including phlebitis; *less commonly* thromboembolism (when given with cytotoxic drugs); *also with Cardioxane®*, dyspepsia, abdominal pain, constipation, reduced ejection fraction, tachycardia, cough, headache, nail disorder, lymphoedema, acute myeloid leukaemia; *also with Savene®*, tremor, drowsiness, weight loss, myalgia

Dose
- See under preparations

Cardioxane® (Clinigen) ▣PoM
Intravenous infusion, powder for reconstitution, dexrazoxane (as hydrochloride), net price 500-mg vial = £156.57
Dose prevention of anthracycline-induced cardiotoxicity, ADULT over 18 years, by intravenous infusion (30 minutes before anthracycline administration), 10 times the doxorubicin-equivalent dose or 10 times the epirubicin-equivalent dose

Savene® (Clinigen) ▣PoM
Intravenous infusion, powder for reconstitution, dexrazoxane (as hydrochloride), net price 10 x 500-mg vials (with diluent) = £6750.00
Electrolytes in *Savene®* diluent, K^+ 2.5 mmol/500 mL, Na^+ 70 mmol/500 mL
Dose anthracycline extravasation, ADULT over 18 years, by intravenous infusion, $1 \, g/m^2$ (max. 2 g) daily for 2 days, then $500 \, mg/m^2$ for 1 day
Note Local coolants such as ice packs should be removed at least 15 minutes before administration

---

Chemotherapy-induced mucositis and myelosuppression

Folinic acid (given as calcium folinate) is used to counteract the folate-antagonist action of methotrexate and thus speed recovery from methotrexate-induced mucositis or myelosuppression ('folinic acid rescue').

Folinic acid is also used in the management of methotrexate overdose, together with other measures to maintain fluid and electrolyte balance, and to manage possible renal failure.

Folinic acid does not counteract the antibacterial activity of folate antagonists such as trimethoprim.

When folinic acid and fluorouracil are used together in metastatic colorectal cancer the response-rate improves compared to that with fluorouracil alone.

The calcium salt of **levofolinic acid**, a single isomer of folinic acid, is also used for rescue therapy following methotrexate administration, for cases of methotrexate overdose, and for use with fluorouracil for colorectal cancer. The dose of calcium levofolinate is generally half that of calcium folinate.

The disodium salts of folinic acid and levofolinic acid are also used for rescue therapy following methotrexate therapy, and for use with fluorouracil for colorectal cancer.

Palifermin, a human keratinocyte growth factor, is licensed for the management of oral mucositis in patients with haematological malignancies receiving myeloablative radiochemotherapy with autologous haematopoietic stem-cell support.

FOLINIC ACID

Indications see notes above

Cautions avoid simultaneous administration of methotrexate; **not** indicated for pernicious anaemia or other megaloblastic anaemias caused by vitamin B_{12} deficiency; **interactions:** Appendix 1 (folates)

Contra-indications intrathecal injection

Pregnancy not known to be harmful; benefit outweighs risk

Breast-feeding presence in milk unknown but benefit outweighs risk

Side-effects *rarely* pyrexia after parenteral use; insomnia, agitation, and depression after high doses

Dose
- See under preparations

◢ **Calcium folinate**

(Calcium leucovorin)

Calcium Folinate (Non-proprietary) [PoM]
Tablets, scored, folinic acid (as calcium salt) 15 mg, net price 10-tab pack = £48.36, 30-tab pack = £85.74
Brands include *Refolinon*[®]
Note Not all strengths and pack sizes are available from all manufacturers

Injection, folinic acid (as calcium salt) 3 mg/mL, net price 1-mL amp = £4.00, 10-mL amp = £4.62; 7.5 mg/mL, net price 2-mL amp = £7.80; 10 mg/mL, net price 5-mL vial = £19.41, 10-mL vial = £34.94, 30-mL vial = £89.95, 35-mL vial = £90.98
Brands include *Refolinon*[®]
Note Not all strengths and pack sizes are available from all manufacturers

Injection, powder for reconstitution, folinic acid (as calcium salt), net price 15-mg vial = £4.46; 30-mg vial = £8.36

Dose
Note Doses expressed as folinic acid

Prevention of methotrexate-induced adverse effects, usually started 12–24 hours after start of methotrexate infusion, by intramuscular injection, *or* by intravenous injection, *or* by intravenous infusion, 15 mg, repeated every 6 hours for 24 hours (may be continued by mouth); consult local treatment protocol for further information

Suspected methotrexate overdosage, by intravenous injection *or* by intravenous infusion (at a max. rate of 160 mg/minute), initial dose equal to or exceeding dose of methotrexate; consult poisons information service (p. 33) for advice on continuing management

Adjunct to fluorouracil in colorectal cancer, consult product literature

◢ **Disodium folinate**

Sodiofolin[®] (Medac) [PoM]
Injection, folinic acid (as disodium salt) 50 mg/mL, net price 2-mL vial = £35.09, 8-mL vial = £126.25
Dose as an antidote to methotrexate, by intravenous injection or infusion, consult product literature

Adjunct to fluorouracil in colorectal cancer, consult product literature

LEVOFOLINIC ACID

Note Levofolinic acid is an isomer of folinic acid
Indications see notes above
Cautions see Folinic acid

Contra-indications see Folinic acid
Pregnancy see Folinic acid
Breast-feeding see Folinic acid
Side-effects see Folinic acid
Dose
- See under preparations

◢ **Calcium levofolinate**

Calcium Levofolinate (Non-proprietary) [PoM]
Injection, levofolinic acid (as calcium salt) 10 mg/mL, net price 17.5-mL vial = £84.63

Isovorin[®] (Pfizer) [PoM]
Injection, levofolinic acid (as calcium salt) 10 mg/mL, net price 2.5-mL vial = £11.62, 17.5-mL vial = £81.33
Dose
Note Doses expressed as levofolinic acid
Prevention of methotrexate-induced adverse effects, (usually started 12–24 hours after beginning of methotrexate infusion), by intramuscular injection, *or* by intravenous injection *or* by intravenous infusion, usually 7.5 mg every 6 hours for 10 doses
Suspected methotrexate overdosage, by intravenous injection *or* by intravenous infusion (at a max. rate of 160 mg/minute), initial dose at least 50% of the dose of methotrexate; consult poisons information service (p. 33) for advice on continuing management

Adjunct to fluorouracil in colorectal cancer, consult product literature

◢ **Disodium levofolinate**

Levofolinic Acid (Non-proprietary) [PoM]
Injection, levofolinic acid (as disodium salt) 50 mg/mL, net price 1-mL vial = £24.70, 4-mL vial = £80.40
Dose as an antidote to methotrexate, by intravenous injection or infusion, consult product literature
Adjunct to fluorouracil in colorectal cancer, consult product literature

PALIFERMIN

Indications see notes above
Pregnancy manufacturer advises avoid unless potential benefit outweighs risk—toxicity in *animal* studies
Breast-feeding manufacturer advises avoid—no information available
Side-effects oral paraesthesia, taste disturbance, thickening and discoloration of tongue; fever; oedema; arthralgia; rash, pruritus, erythema, skin hyperpigmentation
Dose
- By intravenous injection, 60 micrograms/kg once daily for 3 doses (third dose given 24–48 hours before myeloablative therapy) then 3 further doses at least 24 hours after myeloablative therapy, and more than 4 days after most recent palifermin injection, starting on same day as (but after) stem-cell infusion; CHILD not recommended

Kepivance[®] (Swedish Orphan) ▼ [PoM]
Injection, powder for reconstitution, palifermin, net price 6.25-mg vial = £544.24

Urothelial toxicity

Haemorrhagic cystitis is a common manifestation of urothelial toxicity which occurs with the oxazaphosphorines, cyclophosphamide and ifosfamide; it is caused by the metabolite acrolein. **Mesna** reacts specifically with this metabolite in the urinary tract, preventing toxicity. Mesna is used routinely (preferably by mouth) in patients receiving ifosfamide, and in patients receiving cyclophosphamide by the intravenous route at a high dose (e.g. more than 2 g) or in those who experienced urothelial toxicity when given cyclophosphamide previously.

MESNA

Indications   see notes above

Cautions   false positive urinary ketones; false positive or false negative urinary erythrocytes

Contra-indications   hypersensitivity to thiol-containing compounds

Pregnancy   not known to be harmful; see also Pregnancy and Reproductive Function, p. 575

Side-effects   nausea, vomiting, colic, diarrhoea, fatigue, headache, limb and joint pains, depression, irritability, rash, hypotension and tachycardia; *rarely* hypersensitivity reactions (more common in patients with auto-immune disorders)

Dose

● Calculated according to oxazaphosphorine (cyclophosphamide or ifosfamide) treatment—consult product literature

Mesna (Baxter) [PoM]
Tablets, f/c, mesna 400 mg, net price 10-tab pack = £42.90; 600 mg, 10-tab pack = £61.10
Injection, mesna 100 mg/mL, net price 4-mL amp = £3.95; 10-mL amp = £9.77
Note For oral administration contents of ampoule are taken in a flavoured drink such as orange juice or cola which may be stored in a refrigerator for up to 24 hours in a sealed container

8.1.1   Alkylating drugs

Extensive experience is available with these drugs, which are among the most widely used in cancer chemotherapy. They act by damaging DNA, thus interfering with cell replication. In addition to the side-effects common to many cytotoxic drugs (section 8.1), there are two problems associated with prolonged usage. Firstly, gametogenesis is often severely affected (section 8.1). Secondly, prolonged use of these drugs, particularly when combined with extensive irradiation, is associated with a marked increase in the incidence of acute non-lymphocytic leukaemia.

Cyclophosphamide is used mainly in combination with other agents for treating a wide range of malignancies, including some leukaemias, lymphomas, and solid tumours. It is given by mouth or intravenously; it is inactive until metabolised by the liver. A urinary metabolite of cyclophosphamide, acrolein, can cause haemorrhagic cystitis; this is a rare but serious complication; increased fluid intake for 24–48 hours after intravenous injection, can prevent this complication. When high-dose therapy (e.g. more than 2 g intravenously) is used or when the patient is considered to be at high risk of cystitis (e.g. because of pelvic irradiation), mesna (given initially intravenously then by mouth) can also help prevent cystitis—see under Urothelial Toxicity (section 8.1).

Ifosfamide is related to cyclophosphamide and is given intravenously; mesna (section 8.1) is routinely given with it to reduce urothelial toxicity.

Chlorambucil is used either alone or in combination therapy for some lymphomas and chronic leukaemias. It is given by mouth. Side-effects, apart from bone-marrow suppression, are uncommon. However, patients occasionally develop severe widespread rashes which can progress to Stevens-Johnson syndrome or to toxic epidermal necrolysis. If a rash occurs further chlorambucil is contra-indicated and cyclophosphamide is substituted.

Melphalan is licensed for the treatment of multiple myeloma, polycythaemia vera, childhood neuroblastoma, advanced ovarian adenocarcinoma, and advanced breast cancer. However, in practice, melphalan is rarely used for ovarian adenocarcinoma; it is no longer used for advanced breast cancer. Melphalan is also licensed for regional arterial perfusion in localised malignant melanoma of the extremities and localised soft-tissue sarcoma of the extremities. Interstitial pneumonitis and life-threatening pulmonary fibrosis are rarely associated with melphalan.

Busulfan is given by mouth to treat chronic myeloid leukaemia. Busulfan given by mouth or intravenously, followed by cyclophosphamide, is also licensed as conditioning treatment before haematopoietic stem-cell transplantation in adults and children. Frequent blood tests are necessary because excessive myelosuppression may result in irreversible bone-marrow aplasia. Rarely, progressive pulmonary fibrosis is associated with busulfan. Skin hyperpigmentation is a common side-effect of oral therapy.

Lomustine is a lipid-soluble nitrosourea and is given by mouth. It is used mainly to treat Hodgkin's disease resistant to conventional therapy, malignant melanoma and certain solid tumours. Bone-marrow toxicity is delayed, and the drug is therefore given at intervals of 4 to 6 weeks. Permanent bone-marrow damage can occur with prolonged use. Nausea and vomiting are common and moderately severe.

Bendamustine given intravenously is licensed for the treatment of chronic lymphocytic leukaemia, non-Hodgkin's lymphoma, and for the treatment of multiple myeloma.

The *Scottish Medicines Consortium* (p. 4) has advised (March 2011) that bendamustine (*Levact*®) is accepted for restricted use within NHS Scotland for the treatment of chronic lymphocytic leukaemia in patients for whom fludarabine combination chemotherapy is not appropriate.

> **NICE guidance**
> **Bendamustine for the first-line treatment of chronic lymphocytic leukaemia (February 2011)**
> Bendamustine is recommended as an option for the treatment of chronic lymphocytic leukaemia in patients for whom fludarabine combination chemotherapy is not appropriate.
> www.nice.org.uk/TA216

Carmustine given intravenously has similar activity to lomustine; it is given to patients with multiple myeloma, non-Hodgkin's lymphomas, and brain tumours. Cumulative renal damage and delayed pulmonary fibrosis may occur with intravenous use. Carmustine implants are licensed for intralesional use in adults for the treatment of recurrent glioblastoma multiforme as an adjunct to surgery. Carmustine implants are also licensed for high-grade malignant glioma as adjunctive treatment to surgery and radiotherapy.

> **NICE guidance (carmustine implants and temozolomide for the treatment of newly diagnosed high-grade glioma)**
> See p. 600

Estramustine is a combination of an oestrogen and chlormethine used predominantly in prostate cancer. It is given by mouth and has both an antimitotic effect and (by reducing testosterone concentration) a hormonal effect.

Treosulfan is given by mouth or by intravenous or intraperitoneal administration and is used to treat ovarian cancer. Skin pigmentation is a common side-effect and allergic alveolitis, pulmonary fibrosis and haemorrhagic cystitis occur rarely.

Thiotepa is licensed in combination with other chemotherapy as conditioning treatment in adults and children with haematological disease or solid tumours before haematopoietic stem cell transplantation.

Mitobronitol is occasionally used to treat chronic myeloid leukaemia; it is available on a named-patient basis from specialist importing companies, see p. 1124.

BENDAMUSTINE HYDROCHLORIDE

Indications　see notes above

Cautions　see section 8.1; cardiac disorders—monitor serum potassium and ECG; avoid in acute porphyria (but see section 9.8.2); **interactions**: see Appendix 1 (bendamustine)

Contra-indications　jaundice; severe bone marrow suppression, low leucocyte or platelet count; major surgery less than 30 days before start of treatment

Hepatic impairment　consider a 30% dose reduction in moderate impairment; avoid in severe impairment

Renal impairment　no information available on use in patients with creatinine clearance less than 10 mL/minute

Pregnancy　avoid (teratogenic and mutagenic in *animal* studies); effective contraception required during treatment in men or women, and for 6 months after treatment in men; see also Pregnancy and Reproductive function, p. 575

Breast-feeding　discontinue breast-feeding

Side-effects　see section 8.1; also anorexia, diarrhoea, constipation, haemorrhage, hypotension, hypertension, palpitation, angina, arrhythmias, respiratory dysfunction, insomnia, pain, chills, malaise, infection, pyrexia, amenorrhoea, dehydration, electrolyte disturbances (including hypokalaemia); *less commonly* pericardial effusion; *rarely* acute circulatory failure, drowsiness, voice changes, sweating; *very rarely* taste disturbance, tachycardia, myocardial infarction, cardiac failure, pulmonary fibrosis, paraesthesia, peripheral neuropathy, neurological disorders, ataxia, anticholinergic syndrome, encephalitis, phlebitis, multiple organ failure, haemolysis; *also reported* secondary tumours, Stevens-Johnson syndrome, toxic epidermal necrolysis

Dose
- See Doses, p. 574

Levact® (Napp) ▼ PoM
Injection, powder for reconstitution, bendamustine hydrochloride, net price 25-mg vial = £69.45; 100-mg vial = £275.81

BUSULFAN
(Busulphan)

Indications　see notes above

Cautions　see section 8.1 and notes above; monitor cardiac and liver function; ineffective once in blast crisis phase; high dose or history of seizures—anti-epileptic prophylaxis required; previous radiation therapy, three or more cycles of chemotherapy, or previous progenitor cell transplant—increased risk of hepatic veno-occlusive disease; discontinue if lung toxicity develops; risk of second malignancy; avoid in acute porphyria (but see section 9.8.2); **interactions**: Appendix 1 (busulfan)

Hepatic impairment　manufacturer advises caution and regular liver function tests—consult product literature

Pregnancy　avoid (teratogenic in *animals*); manufacturers advise effective contraception during and for 6 months after treatment in men or women; see also Pregnancy and Reproductive Function, p. 575

Breast-feeding　discontinue breast-feeding

Side-effects　see section 8.1 and notes above; also hepatotoxicity (including hepatic veno-occlusive disease, hyperbilirubinaemia, jaundice and fibrosis); cardiac tamponade in thalassaemia; pneumonia; skin hyperpigmentation; *rarely* seizures, aplastic anaemia, visual disturbances; *very rarely* myasthenia gravis, gynaecomastia

Dose

> Dose may need to be calculated based on body surface area or adjusted ideal body weight in obese patients—consult product literature

- Chronic myeloid leukaemia, induction of remission, by mouth, 60 micrograms/kg daily (max. 4 mg); maintenance, usually 0.5–2 mg daily
- Conditioning treatment before haematopoietic stem-cell transplantation, by mouth *or* by intravenous infusion, consult product literature

Myleran® (Alkopharma) PoM
Tablets, f/c, busulfan 2 mg, net price 25-tab pack = £65.22

Busilvex® (Fabre) PoM
Concentrate for intravenous infusion, busulfan 6 mg/mL, net price 10-mL vial = £201.25

CARMUSTINE

Indications　see notes above

Cautions　see section 8.1 and notes above; avoid in acute porphyria (but see section 9.8.2); **interactions**: Appendix 1 (carmustine)

Pregnancy　avoid (teratogenic and embryotoxic in *animals*); manufacturer advises effective contraception during treatment in men or women; see also Pregnancy and Reproductive Function, p. 575

Breast-feeding　discontinue breast-feeding

Side-effects　see section 8.1 and notes above; irritant to tissues

8　Malignant disease and immunosuppression

Malignant disease and immunosuppression *(side tab)*

8 *(side tab)*

Dose

● See Doses, p. 574

Gliadel® (Archimedes) PoM

Implant, carmustine 7.7 mg, net price = £650.38

CHLORAMBUCIL

Indications   see notes above

Cautions   see section 8.1 and notes above; history of epilepsy and children with nephrotic syndrome (increased risk of seizures); avoid in acute porphyria (but see section 9.8.2)

Hepatic impairment   manufacturer advises consider dose reduction in severe impairment—limited information available

Pregnancy   avoid; manufacturer advises effective contraception during treatment in men or women; see also Pregnancy and Reproductive Function, p. 575

Breast-feeding   discontinue breast-feeding

Side-effects   see section 8.1 and notes above

Dose

● See Doses, p. 574

Leukeran® (Alkopharma) PoM

Tablets, f/c, brown, chlorambucil 2 mg, net price 25-tab pack = £40.51

CYCLOPHOSPHAMIDE

Indications   see notes above; rheumatoid arthritis (section 10.1.3)

Cautions   see section 8.1 and notes above; previous or concurrent mediastinal irradiation—risk of cardiotoxicity; diabetes mellitus; avoid in acute porphyria (but see section 9.8.2); **interactions:** Appendix 1 (cyclophosphamide)

Contra-indications   haemorrhagic cystitis

Hepatic impairment   reduce dose—consult local treatment protocol for details

Renal impairment   reduce dose if serum creatinine concentration greater than 120 micromol/litre

Pregnancy   avoid (manufacturer advises effective contraception during and for at least 3 months after treatment in men or women); see also Pregnancy and Reproductive Function, p. 575

Breast-feeding   discontinue breast-feeding during and for 36 hours after stopping treatment

Side-effects   see section 8.1 and notes above; also anorexia; pancreatitis; cardiotoxicity at high doses; interstitial pulmonary fibrosis; inappropriate secretion of anti-diuretic hormone, disturbances of carbohydrate metabolism; urothelial toxicity; pigmentation of palms, nails, and soles; *rarely* hepatotoxicity and renal dysfunction

Dose

● See Doses, p. 574

Cyclophosphamide (Non-proprietary) PoM

Tablets, s/c, cyclophosphamide (anhydrous) 50 mg, net price 100 = £82.00. Label: 25, 27

Injection, powder for reconstitution, cyclophosphamide, net price 500-mg vial = £9.20; 1-g vial = £17.06

ESTRAMUSTINE PHOSPHATE

Indications   prostate cancer

Cautions   see section 8.1; cerebrovascular or cardiovascular disease; diabetes; hypertension; hypercalcaemia; congestive heart failure, epilepsy, migraine or other conditions which might be aggravated by fluid retention; avoid in acute porphyria (but see section 9.8.2); **interactions:** Appendix 1 (estramustine)

Contra-indications   peptic ulceration, severe cardiovascular disease, thromboembolic disorders

Hepatic impairment   manufacturer advises caution and regular liver function tests; avoid in severe impairment

Renal impairment   manufacturer advises caution

Pregnancy   men should use effective contraceptive methods during treatment

Side-effects   see section 8.1; also diarrhoea, congestive heart failure, ischaemic heart disease, myocardial infarction, oedema (rarely angioedema) impotence, gynaecomastia; altered liver function, altered endocrine function

Dose

● 0.14–1.4 g daily in divided doses (usual initial dose 560–840 mg daily)

Counselling   Each dose should be taken not less than 1 hour before or 2 hours after meals and should not be taken with products containing calcium, magnesium or aluminium, including dairy products and antacid medication

Estracyt® (Pharmacia) PoM

Capsules, estramustine phosphate 140 mg (as disodium salt), net price 100-cap pack = £171.28. Label: 5, 23, counselling, see above

---

IFOSFAMIDE

Indications   see notes above

Cautions   see section 8.1 and notes above; ensure satisfactory electrolyte balance and renal function before each course (risk of tubular dysfunction, Fanconi's syndrome or diabetes insipidus if renal toxicity not treated promptly); diabetes mellitus; avoid in acute porphyria (but see section 9.8.2); **interactions:** Appendix 1 (ifosfamide)

Contra-indications   urinary-tract obstruction; acute infection (including urinary-tract infection); urothelial damage

Hepatic impairment   avoid

Renal impairment   avoid if serum creatinine concentration greater than 120 micromol/litre

Pregnancy   avoid (teratogenic and carcinogenic in *animals*); manufacturer advises adequate contraception during and for at least 6 months after treatment in men or women; see also Pregnancy and Reproductive Function, p. 575

Breast-feeding   discontinue breast-feeding

Side-effects   see section 8.1 and notes above; also drowsiness, confusion, disorientation, restlessness, psychosis; urothelial toxicity, renal toxicity (see Cautions above); *less commonly* severe encephalopathy; *rarely* diarrhoea, constipation, convulsions, anorexia, *very rarely* jaundice, thrombophlebitis, syndrome of inappropriate antidiuretic hormone secretion; acute pancreatitis, arrhythmias, and heart failure also reported

Dose

● See Doses, p. 574

Ifosfamide (Non-proprietary) PoM

Injection, powder for reconstitution, ifosfamide, net price 1-g vial = £66.08; 2-g vial = £130.04 (hosp. only)

LOMUSTINE

Indications see notes above

Cautions see section 8.1 and notes above; avoid in acute porphyria (but see section 9.8.2); **interactions**: Appendix 1 (lomustine)

Contra-indications coeliac disease

Renal impairment avoid in severe impairment

Pregnancy avoid (manufacturer advises effective contraception during and for at least 6 months after treatment in men or women); see also Pregnancy and Reproductive Function, p. 575

Breast-feeding discontinue breast-feeding

Side-effects see section 8.1 and notes above

Dose

- Used alone, 120–130 mg/m^2 body-surface every 6–8 weeks

Lomustine (Medac) PoM

Capsules, blue/clear, lomustine 40 mg, net price 20-cap pack = £455.62

Note The brand name *CCNU*® has been used for lomustine capsules

MELPHALAN

Indications see notes above

Cautions see section 8.1 and notes above; avoid in acute porphyria (but see section 9.8.2); **interactions**: Appendix 1 (melphalan)

Renal impairment reduce dose initially (consult product literature)

Pregnancy avoid (manufacturer advises adequate contraception during treatment in men or women); see also Pregnancy and Reproductive Function, p. 575

Breast-feeding discontinue breast-feeding

Side-effects see section 8.1 and notes above

Dose

- By mouth, multiple myeloma, dose may vary according to regimen; typical dose 150 micrograms/kg daily for 4 days, repeated every 6 weeks

  Polycythaemia vera, initially, 6–10 mg daily reduced after 5–7 days to 2–4 mg daily until satisfactory response then further reduce to 2–6 mg **per week**
- By intravenous injection *or* infusion *or* regional arterial perfusion, consult product literature

Alkeran® (Genopharm) PoM

Tablets, melphalan 2 mg, net price 25-tab pack = £42.88

Injection, powder for reconstitution, melphalan 50 mg (as hydrochloride), net price 50-mg vial (with solvent-diluent) = £129.81

THIOTEPA

Indications see notes above

Cautions see section 8.1; avoid in acute porphyria (but see section 9.8.2); **interactions**: Appendix 1 (thiotepa)

Pregnancy avoid (teratogenic and embryotoxic in *animals*); see also Pregnancy and Reproductive Function, p. 575

Breast-feeding discontinue breast-feeding

Side-effects see section 8.1

Dose

- See Doses, p. 574

Tepadina® (Adienne) PoM

Injection, powder for reconstitution, thiotepa, net price 15-mg vial = £123.00; 100-mg vial = £736.00

Note The *Scottish Medicines Consortium* (p. 4) has advised (June 2012) that thiotepa (*Tepadina*®) is **not** recommended for use within NHS Scotland in combination with other chemotherapy as conditioning treatment in adults or children with haematological diseases, or solid tumours prior to haematopoietic stem cell transplantation.

TREOSULFAN

Indications see notes above

Cautions see section 8.1; avoid in acute porphyria (but see section 9.8.2)

Pregnancy avoid; see also Pregnancy and Reproductive Function, p. 575

Breast-feeding discontinue breast-feeding

Side-effects see section 8.1 and notes above

Dose

- Consult product literature

Treosulfan (Medac) PoM

Capsules, treosulfan 250 mg, net price 100-cap pack = £565.54. Label: 25

Injection, powder for reconstitution, treosulfan, net price 1 g = £39.44; 5 g = £152.41 (both in infusion bottle with transfer needle)

8.1.2 Anthracyclines and other cytotoxic antibiotics

Drugs in this group are widely used. Many cytotoxic antibiotics act as radiomimetics and simultaneous use of radiotherapy should be **avoided** because it may markedly increased toxicity.

Daunorubicin, **doxorubicin**, **epirubicin** and **idarubicin** are anthracycline antibiotics. Mitoxantrone is an anthracycline derivative.

Doxorubicin is available as both *conventional* and *liposomal* formulations. The different formulations vary in their licensed indications, pharmacokinetics, dosage and administration, and are not interchangeable. *Conventional* doxorubicin is used to treat the acute leukemias, Hodgkin's and non-Hodgkin's lymphomas, paediatric malignancies, and some solid tumours including breast cancer. It is given by injection into a fast-running infusion, commonly at 21-day intervals. Extravasation can cause severe tissue necrosis. Doxorubicin is largely excreted in the bile and an elevated bilirubin concentration is an indication for reducing the dose. Diarrhoea, dehydration, and red coloration of the urine can commonly occur, and renal damage has been reported. Supraventricular tachycardia related to drug administration is an uncommon complication. Higher cumulative doses are associated with cardiomyopathy and it is usual to limit total cumulative doses to 450 mg/m^2 because symptomatic and potentially fatal heart failure is common above this dose. Patients should be assessed before treatment by echocardiography; the elderly, and those with cardiac disease, hypertension, or who have received myocardial irradiation, should be treated cautiously. Cardiac monitoring may assist in determining safe dosage. Caution is necessary with concomitant use of cardiotoxic drugs, or drugs that reduce cardiac contractility. Some evidence suggests that weekly low-dose administration may be less cardiotoxic. Doxorubicin is also given by bladder instillation for the treatment of

8   Malignant disease and immunosuppression

transitional cell carcinoma, papillary bladder tumours and carcinoma *in-situ*.

Liposomal formulations of doxorubicin are also for intravenous use and differ in their licensed indications and doses. Liposomal formulations can not be used interchangeably. They may reduce the incidence of cardiotoxicity and lower the potential for local necrosis, but infusion reactions, sometimes severe, may occur. Hand-foot syndrome (painful, macular reddening skin eruptions) occurs commonly with liposomal doxorubicin and may be dose limiting. It can occur after 2–3 treatment cycles and may be prevented by cooling hands and feet and avoiding socks, gloves, or tight-fitting footwear for 4–7 days after treatment.

> ### NICE guidance (paclitaxel, pegylated liposomal doxorubicin and topotecan for second-line or subsequent treatment of advanced ovarian cancer)
> See p. 604

Epirubicin is structurally related to doxorubicin and clinical trials suggest that it is as effective in the treatment of breast cancer. A maximum cumulative dose of 0.9–$1 \, g/m^2$ is recommended to help avoid cardiotoxicity. Like doxorubicin it is given intravenously and by bladder instillation. Hyperpigmentation of skin, nails, and oral mucosa, and red coloration of the urine, may occur.

Idarubicin has general properties similar to those of doxorubicin; it is mostly used in the treatment of haematological malignancies. Diarrhoea, abdominal pain, haemorrhage, cardiac disorders, rash, and red pigmentation of the urine are commonly reported. Skin and nail hyperpigmentation have been reported less frequently. Idarubicin is given intravenously and it may also be given by mouth.

Daunorubicin also has general properties similar to those of doxorubicin. It should be given by intravenous infusion and is indicated for acute leukaemias. A liposomal formulation for intravenous use is licensed for advanced AIDS-related Kaposi's sarcoma.

> ### Use with trastuzumab
> Concomitant use of anthracyclines with trastuzumab (section 8.1.5) is associated with cardiotoxicity; for details, see p. 625.

Mitoxantrone is structurally related to doxorubicin; it is used for metastatic breast cancer. Mitoxantrone is also licensed for treatment of non-Hodgkin's lymphoma, adult acute non-lymphocytic leukaemia, and non-resectable primary hepatocellular carcinoma. It is given intravenously and is well tolerated, but myelosuppression and dose-related cardiotoxicity occur; cardiac examinations are recommended after a cumulative dose of $160 \, mg/m^2$.

Pixantrone is licensed as monotherapy for the treatment of refractory or multiply relapsed aggressive non-Hodgkin B-cell lymphomas, although the benefits of using it as a fifth-line or greater chemotherapy in refractory patients has not been established. Baseline investigations should include a full blood count, assessment of cardiac function measured by left ventricular ejection fraction, and measurement of serum concentrations of total bilirubin and total creatinine. Severe myelosuppression is a common side-effect, and cardiotoxicity

may occur during or following treatment; full blood count and cardiac function should be monitored throughout treatment. Patients with cardiac risk factors should have the risks and benefits of treatment carefully assessed. Photosensitivity is a theoretical risk and patients should be advised to follow sun protection strategies.

> ### NICE guidance
> ### Pixantrone monotherapy for treating multiply relapsed or refractory aggressive non-Hodgkin's B-cell lymphoma (February 2014)
> Pixantrone monotherapy is recommended as an option for treating adults with multiply relapsed or refractory aggressive non-Hodgkin's B-cell lymphoma in patients:
> - who have previously been treated with rituximab **and**
> - who are receiving third- or fourth-line treatment **and**
> - if the manufacturer provides pixantrone with the discount agreed in the patient access scheme
>
> www.nice.org.uk/TA306

Bleomycin is given intravenously or intramuscularly to treat metastatic germ cell cancer and, in some regimens, non-Hodgkin's lymphoma. It causes little bone-marrow suppression but dermatological toxicity is common and increased pigmentation particularly affecting the flexures and subcutaneous sclerotic plaques may occur. Mucositis is also relatively common and an association with Raynaud's phenomenon is reported. Hypersensitivity reactions manifest by chills and fevers commonly occur a few hours after drug administration and may be prevented by simultaneous administration of a corticosteroid, for example hydrocortisone intravenously. The principal problem associated with the use of bleomycin is progressive pulmonary fibrosis. This is dose-related, occurring more commonly at cumulative doses greater than 300 000 units (see Bleomycin, below) and in the elderly. Basal lung crepitations or suspicious chest X-ray changes are an indication to stop therapy with this drug. Patients who have received extensive treatment with bleomycin (e.g. cumulative dose more than 100 000 units—see Bleomycin below) may be at risk of developing respiratory failure if a general anaesthetic is given with high inspired oxygen concentrations. Anaesthetists should be warned of this.

Dactinomycin is principally used to treat paediatric cancers; it is given intravenously. Its side-effects are similar to those of doxorubicin, except that cardiac toxicity is not a problem.

Mitomycin is given intravenously to treat upper gastrointestinal and breast cancers and by bladder instillation for superficial bladder tumours. It causes delayed bone-marrow toxicity and therefore it is usually administered at 6-weekly intervals. Prolonged use may result in permanent bone-marrow damage. It may also cause lung fibrosis and renal damage.

▌ BLEOMYCIN

Indications squamous cell carcinoma; see also notes above

Cautions see section 8.1 and notes above; caution in handling—irritant to tissues; **interactions**: Appendix 1 (bleomycin)

Renal impairment reduce dose by half if serum-creatinine 177–354 micromol/litre; reduce dose further if serum-creatinine greater than 354 micromol/litre

Pregnancy   avoid (teratogenic and carcinogenic in *animal* studies); see also Pregnancy and Reproductive Function, p. 575

Breast-feeding   discontinue breast-feeding

Side-effects   see section 8.1 and notes above

Dose

• See Doses, p. 574

Bleomycin (Non-proprietary) PoM

Injection, powder for reconstitution, bleomycin (as sulfate), net price 15 000-unit vial = £15.56

Note To conform to the European Pharmacopoeia vials previously labelled as containing '15 units' of bleomycin are now labelled as containing 15 000 units. The amount of bleomycin in the vial has not changed.

Brands include *Bleo-Kyowa®*

DACTINOMYCIN

(Actinomycin D)

Indications   see notes above

Cautions   see section 8.1 and notes above; caution in handling—irritant to tissues; **interactions:** Appendix 1 (dactinomycin)

Pregnancy   avoid (teratogenic in *animal* studies); see also Pregnancy and Reproductive Function, p. 575

Breast-feeding   discontinue breast-feeding

Side-effects   see section 8.1 and notes above

Dose

• See Doses, p. 574

Dactinomycin (Non-proprietary) PoM

Injection, powder for reconstitution, dactinomycin Available from 'special-order' manufacturers or specialist importing companies, see p. 1124

DAUNORUBICIN

Indications   see notes above

Cautions   see section 8.1 and notes above; caution in handling—irritant to tissues; cardiac monitoring essential

Contra-indications   myocardial insufficiency, recent myocardial infarction, severe arrhythmia; previous treatment with maximum cumulative doses of daunorubicin or other anthracycline

Hepatic impairment   reduce dose according to serum bilirubin concentration—consult local protocol for details; avoid in severe impairment

Renal impairment   reduce dose by 25% if serum creatinine 105–265 micromol/litre and by 50% if serum creatinine greater than 265 micromol/litre; avoid in severe impairment

Pregnancy   avoid (teratogenic and carcinogenic in *animal* studies); see also Pregnancy and Reproductive Function, p. 575

Breast-feeding   discontinue breast-feeding

Side-effects   see section 8.1 and notes above

Dose

• See Doses, p. 574

Daunorubicin (Non-proprietary) PoM

Injection, powder for reconstitution, daunorubicin (as hydrochloride), net price 20-mg vial = £55.00

Note The brand name *Cerubidin®* was formerly used.

◄ Lipid formulation

DaunoXome® (Galen) PoM

Concentrate for intravenous infusion, daunorubicin encapsulated in liposomes. For dilution before use, net price 50-mg vial = £131.75

For advanced AIDS-related Kaposi's sarcoma

DOXORUBICIN HYDROCHLORIDE

Indications   see notes above and section 7.4.4

Cautions   see section 8.1, notes above and consult product literature; caution in handling—irritant to tissues; **interactions:** Appendix 1 (doxorubicin)

Contra-indications   see notes above; also consult product literature

Hepatic impairment   reduce dose according to bilirubin concentration—consult product literature; avoid in severe impairment

Renal impairment   consult product literature in severe impairment

Pregnancy   avoid (teratogenic and toxic in *animal* studies); manufacturers advise effective contraception during and for at least 6 months after treatment in men or women; see also Pregnancy and Reproductive Function, p. 575

Breast-feeding   discontinue breast-feeding

Side-effects   see section 8.1, notes above and product literature

Dose

• See Doses, p. 574

Doxorubicin (Non-proprietary) PoM

Injection, powder for reconstitution, doxorubicin hydrochloride, net price 10-mg vial = £18.72; 50-mg vial = £100.12

Injection, doxorubicin hydrochloride 2 mg/mL, net price 5-mL vial = £18.54, 25-mL vial = £92.70, 100-mL vial = £370.80

◄ Lipid formulation

Caelyx® (Janssen) PoM

Concentrate for intravenous infusion, pegylated doxorubicin hydrochloride 2 mg/mL encapsulated in liposomes. For dilution before use, net price 10-mL vial = £360.23, 25-mL vial = £712.49

For AIDS-related Kaposi's sarcoma in patients with low CD4 count and extensive mucocutaneous or visceral disease, for advanced ovarian cancer when platinum-based chemotherapy has failed, for progressive multiple myeloma (in combination with bortezomib) in patients who have received at least one prior therapy and who have undergone or are unsuitable for bone-marrow transplantation, and as monotherapy for metastatic breast cancer in patients with increased cardiac risk

Myocet® (TEVA UK) PoM

Injection, powder for reconstitution, doxorubicin hydrochloride (as doxorubicin–citrate complex) encapsulated in liposomes, net price 50-mg vial (with vials of liposomes and buffer) = £456.13

Electrolytes Contains approx. 4.7 mmol Na^+/vial

For use with cyclophosphamide for metastatic breast cancer

EPIRUBICIN HYDROCHLORIDE

Indications   see notes above and section 7.4.4

Cautions   see section 8.1 and notes above; caution in handling—irritant to tissues; **interactions:** Appendix 1 (epirubicin)

Contra-indications   severe myocardial insufficiency, recent myocardial infarction, severe arrhythmia, unstable angina, myocardiopathy; previous treatment with maximum cumulative doses of epirubicin or other anthracycline

Specific contra-indications for intravesical treatment urinary tract infections, bladder inflammation or contraction, haematuria, invasive tumours penetrating the bladder, catheterisation difficulties

Hepatic impairment reduce dose according to bilirubin concentration; avoid in severe impairment

Renal impairment dose reduction may be necessary in severe impairment

Pregnancy avoid (carcinogenic in *animal* studies); see also Pregnancy and Reproductive Function, p. 575

Breast-feeding discontinue breast-feeding

Side-effects see section 8.1 and notes above

Dose

● See Doses, p. 574

Epirubicin (Non-proprietary) ▢PoM▢
Injection, epirubicin hydrochloride 2 mg/mL, net price 5-mL vial = £17.38, 25-mL vial = £84.85, 50-mL vial = £95.54, 100-mL vial = £306.20

Injection, powder for reconstitution, epirubicin hydrochloride, net price 50-mg vial = £91.54

Pharmorubicin® Solution for Injection (Pharmacia) ▢PoM▢
Injection, epirubicin hydrochloride 2 mg/mL, net price 5-mL vial = £21.24, 25-mL vial = £106.19, 100-mL vial = £386.16

IDARUBICIN HYDROCHLORIDE

Indications acute leukaemias (see notes above); advanced breast cancer after failure of first-line chemotherapy (not including anthracyclines)

Cautions see section 8.1 and notes above; caution in handling—irritant to tissues; **interactions**: Appendix 1 (idarubicin)

Contra-indications severe myocardial insufficiency; recent myocardial infarction; severe arrhythmias; previous treatment with maximum cumulative dose of idarubicin or other anthracycline

Hepatic impairment reduce dose according to serum-bilirubin concentration; avoid in severe impairment

Renal impairment reduce dose; avoid in severe impairment

Pregnancy avoid (teratogenic and toxic in *animal* studies); see also Pregnancy and Reproductive Function, p. 575

Breast-feeding discontinue breast-feeding

Side-effects see section 8.1 and notes above

Dose

● By mouth, acute non-lymphocytic leukaemia, monotherapy, 30 mg/m² daily for 3 days *or* in combination therapy, 15–30 mg/m² daily for 3 days
Advanced breast cancer, monotherapy, 45 mg/m² as a single dose *or* 15 mg/m² daily for 3 consecutive days; repeat every 3–4 weeks

Note Max. cumulative dose by mouth (for all indications) 400 mg/m²

● By intravenous administration, consult product literature

Zavedos® (Pharmacia) ▢PoM▢
Capsules, idarubicin hydrochloride, 5 mg (red), net price 1-cap pack = £41.47; 10 mg (red/white), 1-cap pack = £69.12. Label: 25

Injection, powder for reconstitution, idarubicin hydrochloride, net price 5-mg vial = £87.36; 10-mg vial = £174.72

 MITOMYCIN

Indications see notes above and section 7.4.4

Cautions see section 8.1 and notes above; caution in handling—irritant to tissues

Pregnancy avoid (teratogenic in *animal* studies); see also Pregnancy and Reproductive Function, p. 575

Breast-feeding discontinue breast-feeding

Side-effects see section 8.1 and notes above

Dose

● See Doses, p. 574

Mitomycin C Kyowa® (ProStrakan) ▢PoM▢
Injection, powder for reconstitution, mitomycin, net price 2-mg vial = £5.88; 10-mg vial = £21.37; 20-mg vial = £39.94; 40-mg vial = £79.88 (hosp. only)

MITOXANTRONE
(Mitozantrone)

Indications see notes above

Cautions see section 8.1 and notes above; intrathecal administration not recommended; **interactions**: Appendix 1 (mitoxantrone)

Hepatic impairment use with caution—consult local treatment protocol

Pregnancy avoid; manufacturer advises effective contraception during and for at least 6 months after treatment in men or women; see also Pregnancy and Reproductive Function, p. 575

Breast-feeding discontinue breast-feeding

Side-effects see section 8.1 and notes above, anorexia, diarrhoea, abdominal pain, gastro-intestinal bleeding, constipation, dyspnoea, drowsiness, confusion, paraesthesia, anxiety, amenorrhoea, and transient blue-green discoloration of urine and blue discoloration of skin and nails also reported

Dose

● See Doses, p. 574

Mitoxantrone (Non-proprietary) ▢PoM▢
Concentrate for intravenous infusion, mitoxantrone (as hydrochloride) 2 mg/mL, net price 10-mL vial = £100.00

Onkotrone® (Baxter) ▢PoM▢
Concentrate for intravenous infusion, mitoxantrone (as hydrochloride) 2 mg/mL, net price 10-mL vial = £121.85, 12.5-mL vial = £152.33, 15-mL vial = £203.04

PIXANTRONE

Indications see notes above

Cautions see section 8.1 and notes above; history of, or active cardiovascular disease, previous therapy with anthracyclines or anthracenediones, previous or concurrent radiotherapy to the mediastinal area, or concurrent use of cardiotoxic drugs—increased risk of cardiotoxicity; **interactions**: Appendix 1 (pixantrone)

Contra-indications immunisation with live virus vaccines; active severe infection or risk factors for severe infection

Hepatic impairment no information available—manufacturer advises caution in mild to moderate impairment; avoid in severe impairment

Renal impairment no information available—manufacturer advises caution

Pregnancy manufacturer advises avoid—toxicity in *animal* studies; ensure effective contraception during and for at least 6 months after treatment in men or women; see also Pregnancy and Reproductive Function, p. 575

Breast-feeding manufacturer advises avoid—no information available

Side-effects see section 8.1 and notes above; loss of appetite, weight loss, taste disturbances, diarrhoea, constipation, abdominal pain, dyspepsia, dry mouth, abnormal liver function tests, cardiac toxicity and disorders, tachycardia, hypotension, pallor, vein discoloration, oedema, dyspnoea, cough, drowsiness, malaise, headache, paraesthesia, infection, pyrexia, biochemical and electrolyte disturbances, chromaturia, proteinuria, haematuria, bone pain, conjunctivitis, skin discoloration, pruritus, nail disorder; *less commonly* oesophagitis, rectal haemorrhage, arrhythmia, vein disorder, pleural effusion, pneumonitis, rhinorrhoea, anxiety, sleep disorder, dizziness, vertigo, spontaneous erection, tumour progression, oliguria, arthralgia, arthritis, musculoskeletal pain and weakness, dry eye, keratitis, night sweats, petechiae, skin ulcer, rash

Dose
- See Doses, p. 574

Pixuvri® (CTI) ▼ PoM
Injection, powder for reconstitution, pixantrone (as dimaleate), net price 29-mg vial = £553.50
Electrolytes Na⁺ 1.70 mmol/vial

8.1.3 Antimetabolites

Antimetabolites are incorporated into new nuclear material or combine irreversibly with cellular enzymes, preventing normal cellular division.

Methotrexate inhibits the enzyme dihydrofolate reductase, essential for the synthesis of purines and pyrimidines. It is given by mouth, intravenously, intramuscularly, or intrathecally.

Methotrexate is used as maintenance therapy for childhood acute lymphoblastic leukaemia. Other uses include choriocarcinoma, non-Hodgkin's lymphoma, and a number of solid tumours. Intrathecal methotrexate is used in the CNS prophylaxis of childhood acute lymphoblastic leukaemia, and as a therapy for established meningeal cancer or lymphoma.

Methotrexate causes myelosuppression, mucositis, and rarely pneumonitis. It is **contra-indicated** in significant renal impairment because it is excreted primarily by the kidney. It is also contra-indicated in patients with severe hepatic impairment. It should also be **avoided** in the presence of significant pleural effusion or ascites because it can accumulate in these fluids, and its subsequent return to the circulation may cause myelosuppression. Systemic toxicity may follow intrathecal administration and blood counts should be carefully monitored.

Folinic acid (section 8.1) following methotrexate administration helps to prevent methotrexate-induced mucositis or myelosuppression.

Capecitabine, which is metabolised to fluorouracil, is given by mouth. It is licensed as monotherapy or combination therapy for adjuvant treatment of advanced colon cancer following surgery, for mono-therapy or combination therapy of metastatic colorectal cancer, and for first-line treatment of advanced gastric cancer in combination with a platinum-based regimen. Capecitabine is also licensed for second-line treatment of locally advanced or metastatic breast cancer either in combination with docetaxel (where previous therapy included an anthracycline) or alone (after failure of a taxane and anthracycline regimen or where further anthracycline treatment is not indicated). For the role of capecitabine in the treatment of breast cancer, see section 8.3.4.1.

> **NICE guidance**
> **Capecitabine and oxaliplatin in the adjuvant treatment of stage III (Dukes' C) colon cancer (April 2006)**
> Capecitabine alone *or* oxaliplatin combined with fluorouracil and folinic acid are options for adjuvant treatment following surgery for stage III (Dukes' C) colon cancer.
> www.nice.org.uk/TA100

> **NICE guidance**
> **Capecitabine and tegafur with uracil for metastatic colorectal cancer (May 2003)**
> Capecitabine or tegafur with uracil [now discontinued] (in combination with folinic acid) is an option for the first-line treatment of metastatic colorectal cancer.
> www.nice.org.uk/TA61

> **NICE guidance**
> **Capecitabine for the treatment of advanced gastric cancer (July 2010)**
> Capecitabine in combination with a platinum-based regimen is recommended for the first-line treatment of inoperable advanced gastric cancer.
> www.nice.org.uk/TA191

Cytarabine acts by interfering with pyrimidine synthesis. It is given subcutaneously, intravenously, or intrathecally. Its predominant use is in the induction of remission of acute myeloblastic leukaemia. It is a potent myelosuppressant and requires careful haematological monitoring. A liposomal formulation of cytarabine for intrathecal use is licensed for lymphomatous meningitis.

Fludarabine is licensed for the initial treatment of advanced B-cell chronic lymphocytic leukaemia (CLL) or after first-line treatment in patients with sufficient bone-marrow reserves; it is usually given by mouth, but can be given by intravenous injection or infusion. Fludarabine is well tolerated but it does cause myelosuppression, which may be cumulative. Immunosuppression is also common (see panel on cladribine and fludarabine below), and co-trimoxazole is used to prevent pneumocystis infection. Immune-mediated haemolytic anaemia, thrombocytopenia, and neutropenia are less common side-effects.

The *Scottish Medicines Consortium* (p. 4) has advised (October 2006) that fludarabine is accepted for restricted use for the treatment of B-cell chronic lymphocytic leukaemia (CLL) in patients with sufficient bone marrow reserves. First-line treatment should only be initiated in patients with advanced disease, Rai stages III/IV (Binet stage C), or Rai stages I/II (Binet stage A/B) where the patient has disease-related symptoms or evidence of progressive disease.

NICE guidance
Fludarabine for the treatment of B-cell chronic lymphocytic leukaemia (September 2001)

Oral fludarabine is recommended for the second-line treatment of B-cell chronic lymphocytic leukaemia in patients who have either failed, or are intolerant of, first line chemotherapy, and who would otherwise have received combination chemotherapy of either:

- cyclophosphamide, doxorubicin, vincristine and prednisolone (CHOP)
- cyclophosphamide, doxorubicin and prednisolone (CAP) **or**
- cyclophosphamide, vincristine, and prednisolone (CVP)

Intravenous fludarabine should only be used when oral fludarabine is contra-indicated.
www.nice.org.uk/TA29

NICE guidance
Fludarabine monotherapy for the first-line treatment of chronic lymphocytic leukaemia (February 2007)

Fludarabine monotherapy is **not** recommended for the first-line treatment of chronic lymphocytic leukaemia.
www.nice.org.uk/TA119

Cladribine is given by intravenous infusion for the treatment of hairy cell leukaemia. It is also given for chronic lymphocytic leukaemia in patients who have failed to respond to standard regimens containing an alkylating agent. Cladribine produces severe myelosuppression, with neutropenia, anaemia, and thrombocytopenia; haemolytic anaemia has also been reported. High doses of cladribine have been associated with acute renal failure and severe neurotoxicity.

Cladribine and **fludarabine** have a potent and prolonged immunosuppressive effect. Patients treated with cladribine or fludarabine are more prone to serious bacterial, opportunistic fungal, and viral infections, and prophylactic therapy is recommended in those at risk. To prevent potentially fatal transfusion-related graft-versus-host reaction, only irradiated blood products should be administered. Prescribers should consult specialist literature when using highly immunosuppressive drugs.

Clofarabine is licensed for the treatment of acute lymphoblastic leukaemia in patients aged 1 to 21 years who have relapsed or are refractory after receiving at least two previous regimens. It is given by intravenous infusion.

Nelarabine is licensed for the treatment of T-cell acute lymphoblastic leukaemia and T-cell lymphoblastic lymphoma in patients who have relapsed or who are refractory after receiving at least two previous regimens. It is given by intravenous infusion. Neurotoxicity is common with nelarabine and close monitoring for neurological adverse events is strongly recommended—discontinue if neurotoxicity occurs.

The *Scottish Medicines Consortium* (p. 4) has advised (March 2008) that the use of nelarabine (*Atriance*®)

within NHS Scotland is restricted to bridging treatment before stem cell transplantation.

Gemcitabine is used intravenously; it is given alone for elderly patients or for palliative treatment, or with cisplatin as first-line treatment for locally advanced or metastatic non-small cell lung cancer. It is also used in the treatment of locally advanced or metastatic pancreatic cancer (see NICE guidance below). Combined with cisplatin, gemcitabine is also licensed for the treatment of advanced or metastatic bladder cancer. Combined with carboplatin, gemcitabine is licensed for the treatment of locally advanced or metastatic epithelial ovarian cancer which has relapsed after a recurrence-free interval of at least 6 months following previous platinum-based therapy. Combined with paclitaxel, gemcitabine is also licensed for the treatment of metastatic breast cancer which has relapsed after previous chemotherapy including an anthracycline (see NICE guidance below). Gemcitabine is generally well tolerated but it can cause mild gastro-intestinal side-effects, musculoskeletal pain, influenza-like symptoms and rashes; renal impairment and pulmonary toxicity have also been reported. Haemolytic uraemic syndrome has been reported rarely and gemcitabine should be discontinued if signs of microangiopathic haemolytic anaemia occur.

The *Scottish Medicines Consortium* has advised (November 2006) that gemcitabine is accepted for restricted use for the treatment of metastatic breast cancer, which has relapsed following previous chemotherapy including an anthracycline (unless contra-indicated).

NICE guidance
Gemcitabine for the treatment of metastatic breast cancer (January 2007)

Gemcitabine, in combination with paclitaxel, is an option for the treatment of metastatic breast cancer **only** when docetaxel monotherapy or docetaxel plus capecitabine are also considered appropriate.
www.nice.org.uk/TA116

NICE guidance
Gemcitabine for the treatment of pancreatic cancer (May 2001)

Gemcitabine is an option for first-line chemotherapy for patients with advanced or metastatic adenocarcinoma of the pancreas and a Karnofsky score of at least 50 [Karnofsky score is a measure of the ability to perform ordinary tasks].

Gemcitabine is not recommended for patients who can have potentially curative surgery. There is insufficient evidence about its use for second-line treatment of pancreatic adenocarcinoma.
www.nice.org.uk/TA25

Fluorouracil is used to treat a number of solid tumours, including gastro-intestinal tract cancers and breast cancer. It is commonly used with folinic acid in advanced colorectal cancer. It may also be used topically for certain malignant and pre-malignant skin lesions. Toxicity is unusual, but may include myelosuppression, mucositis, and rarely a cerebellar syndrome. On prolonged infusion, a desquamative hand–foot syndrome may occur.

NICE guidance
Aflibercept in combination with irinotecan and fluorouracil-based therapy for treating metastatic colorectal cancer that has progressed following prior oxaliplatin-based chemotherapy
See p. 594

Pemetrexed inhibits thymidylate transferase and other folate-dependent enzymes. It is licensed for use with cisplatin for the treatment of unresectable malignant pleural mesothelioma which has not previously been treated with chemotherapy (see NICE guidance, below). Pemetrexed is also licensed for use with cisplatin for the first-line treatment of locally advanced or metastatic non-small cell lung cancer other than predominantly squamous cell histology (see NICE guidance, below), and as monotherapy for its second-line treatment (but see NICE guidance, below). It is also licensed as monotherapy for maintenance treatment in locally advanced or metastatic non-small cell lung cancer other than predominantly squamous cell histology that has not progressed immediately following platinum-based chemotherapy (but see NICE guidance, below). Pemetrexed is given by intravenous infusion.

The *Scottish Medicines Consortium* (p. 4) has advised (July 2005) that pemetrexed (*Alimta*®) in combination with cisplatin is accepted for restricted use within NHS Scotland for previously untreated patients with stage III/IV unresectable malignant pleural mesothelioma.

The *Scottish Medicines Consortium* (p. 4) has advised (January 2010) that pemetrexed (*Alimta*®) is accepted for restricted use within NHS Scotland in combination with cisplatin for the first-line treatment of locally advanced or metastatic non-small cell lung cancer other than predominantly squamous cell histology; it is restricted to patients in whom the histology of the tumour has been confirmed as adenocarcinoma or large cell carcinoma.

The *Scottish Medicines Consortium* (p. 4) has advised (August 2008) that pemetrexed (*Alimta*®) is accepted for restricted use within NHS Scotland as monotherapy for the second-line treatment of locally advanced or metastatic non-small cell lung cancer without predominantly squamous cell histology; it is restricted for use in patients with good performance status who would otherwise be eligible for docetaxel treatment.

NICE guidance
Pemetrexed for the treatment of malignant pleural mesothelioma (January 2008)
Pemetrexed is an option for the treatment of malignant pleural mesothelioma only in patients who have a WHO performance status of 0 or 1 [WHO performance status is a measure of the ability to perform ordinary tasks], who are considered to have advanced disease and for whom surgical resection is considered inappropriate.
www.nice.org.uk/TA135

NICE guidance
Pemetrexed for the first-line treatment of non-small cell lung cancer (September 2009)
Pemetrexed, in combination with cisplatin, is an option for the first-line treatment of locally advanced or metastatic non-small cell lung cancer only if the histology of the tumour has been confirmed as adenocarcinoma or large-cell carcinoma.
www.nice.org.uk/TA181

NICE guidance
Pemetrexed for the treatment of non-small cell lung cancer (August 2007)
Pemetrexed is **not** recommended for the treatment of locally advanced or metastatic non-small cell lung cancer which has previously been treated with chemotherapy.
www.nice.org.uk/TA124

NICE guidance
Pemetrexed for the treatment of non-small cell lung cancer (June 2010)
Pemetrexed is an option for the maintenance treatment of locally advanced or metastatic non-small cell lung cancer other than predominantly squamous cell histology that has not progressed immediately following combination therapy of a platinum compound with either gemcitabine, paclitaxel, or docetaxel.
www.nice.org.uk/TA190

NICE guidance
Pemetrexed maintenance treatment following induction therapy with pemetrexed and cisplatin for non-squamous non-small-cell lung cancer (April 2014)
Pemetrexed is **not** recommended for the maintenance treatment of locally advanced or metastatic non-squamous non-small-cell lung cancer in patients whose disease has not progressed immediately following induction therapy with pemetrexed and cisplatin.
www.nice.org.uk/TA309

Raltitrexed, a thymidylate synthase inhibitor, is given intravenously for palliation of advanced colorectal cancer when fluorouracil and folinic acid cannot be used. It is probably of similar efficacy to fluorouracil. Raltitrexed is generally well tolerated, but can cause marked myelosuppression and gastro-intestinal side-effects.

NICE guidance (irinotecan, oxaliplatin and raltitrexed for advanced colorectal cancer)
See p. 604

Mercaptopurine is used as maintenance therapy for the acute leukaemias and in the management of ulcerative colitis and Crohn's disease (section 1.5.3). Azathioprine, which is metabolised to mercaptopurine, is generally used as an immunosuppressant (section 8.2.1 and section 10.1.3). The dose of both drugs should be reduced if the patient is receiving allopurinol since it interferes with their metabolism.

8 Malignant disease and immunosuppression

Tegafur is a prodrug of fluorouracil. Tegafur in combination with gimeracil and oteracil is given by mouth; gimeracil inhibits the degradation of fluorouracil and oteracil decreases the activity of fluorouracil in normal gastrointestinal mucosa. Tegafur in combination with gimeracil and oteracil is licensed for the treatment of advanced gastric cancer when used in combination with cisplatin.

Tioguanine is given by mouth for the treatment of acute leukaemias and chronic myeloid leukaemia. It can be given at various stages of treatment in short-term cycles. Tioguanine has a lower incidence of gastrointestinal side-effects than mercaptopurine. Long-term therapy is no longer recommended because of the high risk of liver toxicity; treatment with tioguanine should be discontinued if liver toxicity develops.

Azacitidine is a pyrimidine analogue that is given by subcutaneous injection. It is used in the treatment of intermediate-2 and high-risk myelodysplastic syndromes, chronic myelomonocytic leukaemia, and acute myeloid leukaemia, in adults who are not eligible for haemotopoietic stem cell transplantation.

> **NICE guidance**
> **Azacitidine for the treatment of myelodysplastic syndromes, chronic myelomonocytic leukaemia and acute myeloid leukaemia (March 2011)**
> Azacitidine is recommended in adults who are not eligible for haemotopoietic stem cell transplantation as an option for the treatment of intermediate-2 and high-risk myelodysplastic syndromes, chronic myelomonocytic leukaemia, or acute myeloid leukaemia.
> www.nice.org.uk/TA218

Decitabine is a pyrimidine analogue and is licensed for the treatment of newly diagnosed acute myeloid leukaemia in patients over 65 years who are not candidates for standard induction chemotherapy.

▌ AZACITIDINE

Indications see notes above

Cautions see section 8.1; history of severe congestive heart failure, unstable cardiac or pulmonary disease—consider cardiopulmonary assessment before and during treatment; monitor for bleeding; monitor liver function tests, serum creatinine, and serum bicarbonate before initiation of treatment and before each treatment cycle; monitor full blood count before initiation of treatment, before each treatment cycle, and as clinically indicated

Contra-indications advanced malignant hepatic tumour

Hepatic impairment caution in severe impairment

Renal impairment delay next treatment cycle if serum-creatinine or blood urea nitrogen greater than twice baseline value and above the upper level of normal until values return to normal or baseline, and then reduce dose by 50% on the next treatment cycle. Reduce dose by 50% on the next treatment cycle if serum-bicarbonate concentration less than 20 mmol/litre

Pregnancy avoid (toxicity in *animal* studies); manufacturer advises effective contraception during and for 3 months after treatment in men or women; see also Pregnancy and Reproductive Function, p. 575

Breast-feeding discontinue breast-feeding

Side-effects see section 8.1; also gastro-intestinal disturbances (including diarrhoea, constipation, abdominal pain, and dyspepsia), anorexia; hypertension, hypotension; dyspnoea, pneumonia; anxiety, insomnia, dizziness, headache, drowsiness; haematuria; hypokalaemia; arthralgia, myalgia; injection-site reactions, rash, haematoma; haemorrhage (including cerebral haemorrhage); *less commonly* hypersensitivity reactions (including anaphylactic reactions); hepatic coma, hepatic failure and renal failure also reported

Dose
● See Doses, p. 574

Vidaza® (Celgene) [PoM]
Injection, powder for reconstitution, azacitidine, net price 100-mg vial = £321.00

▌ CAPECITABINE

Indications see notes above

Cautions see section 8.1; history of significant cardiovascular disease, arrhythmias, angina pectoris; monitor plasma-calcium concentration; diabetes mellitus; electrolyte disturbances; nervous system disease; monitor for symptoms of severe skin reactions (including Stevens-Johnson syndrome and toxic epidermal necrolysis)—permanently discontinue treatment immediately if symptoms occur; monitor for symptoms of hand-foot syndrome—interrupt treatment if significant syndrome occurs and refer to product literature; diarrhoea or dehydration—consult product literature for guidance on dose modification and treatment interruption; monitor for eye disorders (including keratitis and corneal disorders); **interactions:** Appendix 1 (fluorouracil)

Contra-indications dihydropyrimidine dehydrogenase deficiency

Hepatic impairment manufacturer advises monitor liver function in mild to moderate impairment—consult product literature for guidance on treatment interruption; avoid in severe impairment

Renal impairment reduce starting dose of 1.25 g/m² to 75% if creatinine clearance 30–50 mL/minute; avoid if creatinine clearance less than 30 mL/minute

Pregnancy avoid (teratogenic in *animal* studies); see also Pregnancy and Reproductive Function, p. 575

Breast-feeding discontinue breast-feeding

Side-effects see section 8.1; also see product literature

Dose
● Stage III colon cancer, adjuvant following surgery, monotherapy, ADULT over 18 years 1.25 g/m² twice daily for 14 days, subsequent courses repeated after a 7-day interval; recommended duration of treatment 6 months
● Stage III colon cancer, adjuvant following surgery, in combination therapy, ADULT over 18 years 0.8–1 g/m² twice daily for 14 days, subsequent courses repeated after a 7-day interval; recommended duration of treatment 6 months
● Metastatic colorectal cancer, monotherapy, ADULT over 18 years 1.25 g/m² twice daily for 14 days, subsequent courses repeated after a 7-day interval
● Metastatic colorectal cancer, in combination therapy, ADULT over 18 years 0.8–1 g/m² twice daily for 14 days, subsequent courses repeated after a 7-day interval

- Advanced gastric cancer, in combination with a platinum-based regimen, ADULT over 18 years 0.8–1 g/m^2 twice daily for 14 days, subsequent courses repeated after a 7-day interval *or* 625 mg/m^2 twice daily given continuously
- Locally advanced or metastatic breast cancer, monotherapy or in combination with docetaxel, ADULT over 18 years 1.25 g/m^2 twice daily for 14 days, subsequent courses repeated after a 7-day interval

Note Adjust dose according to tolerability—consult product literature

Capecitabine (Non-proprietary) PoM
> Tablets, capecitabine 150 mg, net price 60-tab pack = £30.00; 500 mg, 120-tab pack = £225.72. Label: 21

Xeloda® (Roche) PoM
> Tablets, f/c, peach, capecitabine 150 mg, net price 60-tab pack = £40.02; 500 mg, 120-tab pack = £265.55. Label: 21

◼ CLADRIBINE

Indications   see notes above and under preparations

Cautions   see section 8.1 and notes above; use irradiated blood only; **interactions**: Appendix 1 (cladribine)

Hepatic impairment   regular monitoring recommended

Renal impairment   regular monitoring recommended

Pregnancy   avoid (teratogenic in *animal* studies); manufacturer advises that men should not father children during and for 6 months after treatment; see also Pregnancy and Reproductive Function, p. 575

Breast-feeding   discontinue breast-feeding

Side-effects   see section 8.1 and notes above; also constipation, diarrhoea, abdominal pain, flatulence; oedema, tachycardia; cough, dyspnoea; dizziness, insomnia, anxiety, headache; chills, asthenia, malaise; myalgia, arthralgia; sweating, rash, pruritus, and purpura

Dose
- See Doses, p. 574

Leustat® (Janssen) PoM
> Concentrate for intravenous infusion, cladribine 1 mg/mL, net price 10-mL vial = £159.70
> For hairy cell leukaemia and for B-cell chronic lymphocytic leukaemia in patients who have failed to respond to standard regimens containing an alkylating agent

Litak® (Lipomed) PoM
> Injection (for subcutaneous use only—no dilution required), cladribine 2 mg/mL, net price 5-mL vial = £165.00
> For hairy cell leukaemia

◼ CLOFARABINE

Indications   see notes above

Cautions   see section 8.1 and notes above; cardiac disease

Hepatic impairment   manufacturer advises caution in mild to moderate impairment; avoid in severe impairment

Renal impairment   manufacturer advises caution in mild to moderate impairment; avoid in severe impairment

Pregnancy   manufacturer advises avoid (teratogenic in *animal* studies); see also Pregnancy and Reproductive Function, p. 575

Breast-feeding   discontinue breast-feeding

Side-effects   see section 8.1; also diarrhoea, abdominal pain, jaundice; tachycardia, flushing, hypotension, pericardial effusion, oedema, haematoma; dyspnoea, cough; anxiety, agitation, dizziness, drowsiness, headache, paraesthesia, peripheral neuropathy, restlessness; haematuria; arthralgia, myalgia; rash, pruritus, hand-foot (desquamative) syndrome, sweating; pancreatitis also reported

Dose
- See Doses, p. 574

Evoltra® (Sanofi-Aventis) ▼ PoM
> Concentrate for intravenous infusion, clofarabine 1 mg/mL, net price 20-mL vial = £1326.18
> **Electrolytes** Na$^+$ 3.08 mmol/vial

◼ CYTARABINE

Indications   see notes above

Cautions   see section 8.1 and notes above; **interactions**: Appendix 1 (cytarabine)

Hepatic impairment   reduce dose—consult product literature

Pregnancy   avoid (teratogenic in *animal* studies); see also Pregnancy and Reproductive Function, p. 575

Breast-feeding   discontinue breast-feeding

Side-effects   see section 8.1 and notes above

Dose
- See Doses, p. 574

Cytarabine (Non-proprietary) PoM
> Injection (for intravenous, subcutaneous, or intrathecal use), cytarabine 20 mg/mL, net price 5-mL vial = £3.90

> Injection (for intravenous or subcutaneous use), cytarabine 20 mg/mL, net price 5-mL vial = £3.90, 25-mL vial = £19.50; 100 mg/mL, 1-mL vial = £6.00, 5-mL vial = £20.00, 10-mL vial = £39.00, 20-mL vial = £77.50

◢ Lipid formulation for intrathecal use

DepoCyte® (Napp) PoM
> Intrathecal injection, cytarabine encapsulated in liposomes, net price 50-mg vial = £1223.75
> For lymphomatous meningitis
> **Note** The *Scottish Medicines Consortium* (p. 4) has advised (July 2007) that liposomal cytarabine suspension (*DepoCyte*®) is not recommended for use within NHS Scotland for the intrathecal treatment of lymphomatous meningitis

◼ DECITABINE

Indications   see notes above

Cautions   see section 8.1; history of severe congestive heart failure or unstable cardiac disease; **interactions**: Appendix 1 (decitabine)

Hepatic impairment   manufacturer advises caution—no information available

Renal impairment   manufacturer advises caution if creatinine clearance less than 30 mL/minute—no information available

Pregnancy   avoid (teratogenic in *animal* studies); ensure effective contraception during treatment; men must avoid fathering a child during and for 3 months after treatment; see also Pregnancy and Reproductive Function, p. 575

Breast-feeding   discontinue breast-feeding

8   Malignant disease and immunosuppression

Side-effects see section 8.1; also diarrhoea, headache, epistaxis; *less commonly* acute febrile neutrophilic dermatosis

Dose

● See Doses, p. 574

Dacogen® (Janssen) ▼ PoM
Injection, powder for reconstitution, decitabine, net price 50-mg vial = £970.86
Electrolytes Na⁺ 0.29 mmol/vial, K⁺ 0.5 mmol/vial

FLUDARABINE PHOSPHATE

Indications see notes above

Cautions see section 8.1 and notes above; monitor for signs of haemolysis; monitor for neurological toxicity; worsening of existing and increased susceptibility to skin cancer; patients over 65 years—assess creatinine clearance before treatment initiation; **interactions:** Appendix 1 (fludarabine)

Contra-indications haemolytic anaemia

Renal impairment reduce dose by up to 50% if creatinine clearance 30–70 mL/minute; avoid if creatinine clearance less than 30 mL/minute

Pregnancy avoid (embryotoxic and teratogenic in *animal* studies); manufacturer advises effective contraception during and for at least 6 months after treatment in men or women; see also Pregnancy and Reproductive Function, p. 575

Breast-feeding discontinue breast-feeding

Side-effects see section 8.1 and notes above; also diarrhoea, anorexia, oedema, pneumonia, cough, peripheral neuropathy, chills, fever, malaise, weakness, myelodysplastic syndrome, acute myeloid leukaemia, visual disturbances, rash; *less commonly* pulmonary toxicity (including pneumonitis and fibrosis), confusion, haemorrhage, autoimmune disorder; *rarely* heart failure, arrhythmia, coma, seizures, agitation, skin cancer, optic neuropathy, blindness, Stevens-Johnson syndrome, toxic epidermal necrolysis; *also reported* haemorrhagic cystitis

Dose

● By mouth, ADULT 40 mg/m² for 5 days every 28 days usually for 6 cycles
● By intravenous injection *or* infusion, consult product literature

Fludarabine phosphate (Non-proprietary) PoM
Injection, powder for reconstitution, fludarabine phosphate, net price 50-mg vial = £155.00
Concentrate for intravenous injection or infusion, fludarabine phosphate 25 mg/mL, net price 2-mL vial = £155.00
Note Must be diluted before administration (consult product literature)

Fludara® (Sanofi-Aventis) PoM
Tablets, f/c, pink, fludarabine phosphate 10 mg, net price 15-tab pack = £302.48, 20-tab pack = £403.31
Injection, powder for reconstitution, fludarabine phosphate, net price 50-mg vial = £147.07

FLUOROURACIL

Indications see notes above; pre-malignant and malignant skin lesions (section 13.8.1)

Cautions see section 8.1 and notes above; caution in handling—irritant to tissues; **interactions:** Appendix 1 (fluorouracil)

Hepatic impairment manufacturer advises caution

Pregnancy avoid (teratogenic); see also Pregnancy and Reproductive Function, p. 575

Breast-feeding discontinue breast-feeding

Side-effects see section 8.1 and notes above; also local irritation with topical preparation

Dose

● By intravenous injection *or* infusion *or* by intra-arterial infusion, consult product literature

Fluorouracil (Non-proprietary) PoM
Injection, fluorouracil (as sodium salt) 25 mg/mL, net price 10-mL vial = £3.20, 20-mL vial = £6.40, 100-mL vial = £32.00; 50 mg/mL, 10-mL vial = £6.40, 20-mL vial = £12.80, 50-mL vial = £32.00, 100-mL vial = £64.00

GEMCITABINE

Indications see notes above

Cautions see section 8.1 and notes above; **interactions:** Appendix 1 (gemcitabine)

Hepatic impairment manufacturer advises caution

Renal impairment manufacturer advises caution

Pregnancy avoid (teratogenic in *animal* studies); manufacturer advises effective contraception during treatment; men must avoid fathering a child during and for 6 months after treatment; see also Pregnancy and Reproductive Function, p. 575

Breast-feeding discontinue breast-feeding

Side-effects see section 8.1 and notes above

Dose

● See Doses, p. 574

Gemcitabine (Non-proprietary) PoM
Injection, powder for reconstitution, gemcitabine (as hydrochloride), net price 200-mg vial = £29.80, 1-g vial = £154.62, 1.5-g vial = £213.93, 2-g vial = £324.00
Concentrate for intravenous infusion, gemcitabine (as hydrochloride) 38 mg/mL, net price 200-mg vial = £32.00, 1-g vial = £162.00, 2-g vial = £324.00

Gemzar® (Lilly) PoM
Injection, powder for reconstitution, gemcitabine (as hydrochloride), net price 200-mg vial = £32.55; 1-g vial = £162.76

MERCAPTOPURINE
(6-Mercaptopurine)

Indications acute leukaemias and chronic myeloid leukaemia; inflammatory bowel disease [unlicensed indication] (section 1.5.3)

Cautions see section 8.1 and notes above; thiopurine methyltransferase status (see section 8.2.1); monitor liver function; **interactions:** Appendix 1 (mercaptopurine)

Hepatic impairment may need dose reduction

Renal impairment reduce dose

Pregnancy avoid (teratogenic); see also Pregnancy and Reproductive Function, p. 575

Breast-feeding discontinue breast-feeding

Side-effects see section 8.1 and notes above; also hepatotoxicity, anorexia; *rarely* transient oligospermia, pancreatitis; *very rarely* intestinal ulceration, lymphoma

Dose

● See preparations below
Important *Puri-Nethol*® tablets and *Xaluprine*® oral suspension are **not** bioequivalent, haematological monitoring is advised when switching formulations

Puri-Nethol® (Alkopharma) (PoM)

Tablets, yellow, scored, mercaptopurine 50 mg, net price 25-tab pack = £50.47

Dose initially 2.5 mg/kg *or* 50–75 mg/m² daily, adjusted according to response

Xaluprine® (Nova) (PoM)

Oral suspension, mercaptopurine, 20 mg/1 mL, net price 100 mL (raspberry-flavoured)= £170.00

Excipients include aspartame (section 9.4.1)

Dose initially 25–75 mg/m² daily, adjusted according to response

METHOTREXATE

Indications see notes above and under Dose; Crohn's disease [unlicensed indication] (section 1.5.3); rheumatoid arthritis (section 10.1.3); psoriasis (section 13.5.3)

Cautions see section 8.1, notes above and section 10.1.3; **interactions:** Appendix 1 (methotrexate)

Hepatic impairment avoid in severe impairment

Renal impairment reduce dose; risk of nephrotoxicty at high doses; avoid in severe impairment

Pregnancy avoid (teratogenic; fertility may be reduced during therapy but this may be reversible); manufacturer advises effective contraception during and for at least 3 months after treatment in men or women; see also Pregnancy and Reproductive Function, p. 575

Breast-feeding discontinue breast-feeding—present in milk

Side-effects see section 8.1, notes above and section 10.1.3

Dose

- By mouth, leukaemia in children (maintenance), 15 mg/m² weekly in combination with other drugs

> **Important**
> Note that the above dose is a **weekly** dose.

- By intravenous injection *or* infusion, *or* by intra-arterial infusion, *or* by intramuscular injection, *or* intrathecal administration, consult product literature

Methotrexate (Non-proprietary) (PoM)

Injection, methotrexate (as sodium salt) 2.5 mg/mL, net price 2-mL vial = £4.80; 25 mg/mL, 2-mL vial = £2.62, 20-mL vial = £25.07

Injection, methotrexate 100 mg/mL (not for intrathecal use), net price 10-mL vial = £78.00, 50-mL vial = £380.00

◢**Oral preparations**

Section 10.1.3

NELARABINE

Indications see notes above

Cautions see section 8.1 and notes above; previous or concurrent intrathecal chemotherapy or craniospinal irradiation (increased risk of neurotoxicity)

Driving May affect performance of skilled tasks (e.g. driving)

Pregnancy avoid (toxicity in *animal* studies); manufacturer advises effective contraception during and for at least 3 months after treatment in men and women; see also Pregnancy and Reproductive Function, p. 575

Breast-feeding discontinue breast-feeding

Side-effects see section 8.1; also abdominal pain, constipation, taste disturbance, anorexia, diarrhoea; hypotension, oedema; pleural effusion, wheezing, dyspnoea, cough; confusion, seizures, amnesia, drowsiness, peripheral neurological disorders, hypoaesthesia, paraesthesia, ataxia, demyelination, tremor, dizziness, headache, asthenia, fatigue; pyrexia; electrolyte disturbances; blurred vision; muscle weakness, myalgia, arthralgia; benign and malignant tumours also reported

Dose

- See Doses, p. 574

Atriance® (GSK) ▼ (PoM)

Intravenous infusion, nelarabine 5 mg/mL, net price 50-mL vial = £222.00

Electrolytes Na⁺ 3.75 mmol/vial

PEMETREXED

Indications see notes above

Cautions see section 8.1 and notes above; history of cardiovascular disease; diabetes; prophylactic folic acid and vitamin B₁₂ supplementation required (consult product literature); concomitant nephrotoxic drugs including non-steroidal anti-inflammatory drugs (consult product literature); **interactions:** Appendix 1 (pemetrexed)

Renal impairment manufacturer advises avoid if creatinine clearance less than 45 mL/minute—no information available

Pregnancy avoid (toxicity in *animal* studies); manufacturer advises effective contraception during treatment; men must avoid fathering a child during and for 6 months after treatment; see also Pregnancy and Reproductive Function, p. 575

Breast-feeding discontinue breast-feeding

Side-effects see section 8.1; also gastro-intestinal disturbances; oedema; neuropathy; dehydration; conjunctivitis, increased lacrimation; skin disorders; *less commonly* colitis, arrhythmias, and interstitial pneumonitis; *rarely* hepatitis; peripheral ischaemia, acute renal failure, Stevens-Johnson syndrome and toxic epidermal necrolysis also reported

Dose

- See Doses, p. 574

Alimta® (Lilly) (PoM)

Injection, powder for reconstitution, pemetrexed (as disodium), net price 100-mg vial = £160.00; 500-mg vial = £800.00

Electrolytes Na⁺ <0.5 mmol/vial

RALTITREXED

Indications see notes above

Cautions see section 8.1 and notes above; **interactions:** Appendix 1 (raltitrexed)

Hepatic impairment caution in mild to moderate impairment; avoid if severe

Renal impairment reduce dose and increase dosing interval if creatinine clearance less than 65 mL/minute (consult product literature); avoid if creatinine clearance less than 25 mL/minute

Pregnancy pregnancy must be excluded before treatment; ensure effective contraception during and for at least 6 months after treatment in men or women; see also Pregnancy and Reproductive Function, p. 575

Breast-feeding discontinue breast-feeding

Side-effects see section 8.1 and notes above

Dose
• See Doses, p. 574

Tomudex® (Hospira) PoM
Injection, powder for reconstitution, raltitrexed, net price 2-mg vial = £175.00

▇ TEGAFUR WITH GIMERACIL AND OTERACIL

Indications see notes above

Cautions see section 8.1; **interactions**: Appendix 1 (fluorouracil)

Contra-indications dihydropyrimidine dehydrogenase deficiency

Renal impairment reduce dose if creatinine clearance 30–50 mL/minute—consult product literature; manufacturer advises avoid if creatinine clearance less than 30 mL/minute

Pregnancy avoid; manufacturer advises effective contraception during and for up to 6 months after treatment; see also Pregnancy and Reproductive Function, p. 575

Breast-feeding discontinue breast-feeding

Side-effects see section 8.1; also ocular toxicity and neuropathy

Dose
• See Doses, p. 574

Teysuno® (Nordic) ▼ PoM
Capsules, tegafur 15 mg, gimeracil 4.35 mg, oteracil (as potassium salt) 11.8 mg, net price 126-cap pack = £279.72; Label: 23

Capsules, tegafur 20 mg, gimeracil 5.8 mg, oteracil (as potassium salt) 15.8 mg, net price 84-cap pack = £248.40; Label: 23

Note The *Scottish Medicines Consortium* (p. 4) has advised (August 2012) that tegafur with gimeracil and oteracil (*Teysuno*®) is accepted for restricted use within NHS Scotland for the treatment of advanced gastric cancer, when given in combination with cisplatin, in patients who are unsuitable for an anthracycline, fluorouracil and platinum triplet first-line regimen.

▇ TIOGUANINE
(Thioguanine)

Indications see notes above

Cautions see section 8.1 and notes above; thiopurine methyltransferase status (see section 8.2.1); monitor liver function weekly—discontinue if liver toxicity develops; **interactions**: Appendix 1 (tioguanine)

Hepatic impairment reduce dose

Renal impairment reduce dose

Pregnancy avoid (teratogenicity reported when men receiving tioguanine have fathered children); ensure effective contraception during treatment in men or women; see also Pregnancy and Reproductive Function, p. 575

Breast-feeding discontinue breast-feeding

Side-effects see section 8.1; also stomatitis and hepatotoxicity; *rarely* intestinal necrosis and perforation

Dose
• 100–200 mg/m² daily

Lanvis® (Alkopharma) PoM
Tablets, yellow, scored, tioguanine 40 mg, net price 25-tab pack = £103.54

8.1.4 Vinca alkaloids and etoposide

The vinca alkaloids, **vinblastine**, **vincristine**, and **vindesine**, are used to treat a variety of cancers including leukaemias, lymphomas, and some solid tumours (e.g. breast and lung cancer). **Vinorelbine** is a semi-synthetic vinca alkaloid; it is given intravenously or orally for the treatment of advanced breast cancer and for advanced non-small cell lung cancer. For the role of vinorelbine in the treatment of breast cancer, see section 8.3.4.1. **Vinflunine** is licensed as monotherapy for the treatment of advanced or metastatic transitional cell carcinoma of the urothelial tract after failure of a platinum-containing regimen.

> **NICE guidance**
> **Vinflunine for the treatment of advanced or metastatic transitional cell carcinoma of the urothelial tract (January 2013)**
>
> Vinflunine is **not** recommended for the treatment of advanced or metastatic transitional cell carcinoma of the urothelial tract that has progressed after treatment with platinum-based chemotherapy.
> www.nice.org.uk/TA272

Neurotoxicity, usually as peripheral or autonomic neuropathy, occurs with all vinca alkaloids and is a limiting side-effect of vincristine; it occurs less often with vindesine, vinblastine, vinorelbine, and vinflunine. Patients with neurotoxicity commonly have peripheral paraesthesia, loss of deep tendon reflexes, abdominal pain, and constipation; ototoxicity has been reported. If symptoms of neurotoxicity are severe, doses should be reduced. Motor weakness can also occur, and increasing motor weakness calls for dose reduction or discontinuation of these drugs. Recovery from neurotoxic effects is usually slow but complete.

Myelosuppression is a dose-limiting side-effect of vinblastine, vindesine, vinorelbine, and vinflunine; vincristine causes negligible myelosuppression. The vinca alkaloids cause severe local irritation and care must be taken to avoid extravasation. Severe bronchospasm has been reported following administration of the vinca alkaloids (more commonly when used in combination with mitomycin-C).

> **Important**
> Vinblastine, vincristine, vindesine, vinflunine, and vinorelbine injections are for **intravenous administration only**. Inadvertent intrathecal administration can cause severe neurotoxicity, which is usually fatal.
>
> The National Patient Safety Agency has advised (August 2008) that adult and teenage patients treated in an adult or adolescent unit should receive their vinca alkaloid dose in a 50 mL minibag. Teenagers and children treated in a child unit may receive their vinca alkaloid dose in a syringe.

Etoposide may be given orally or by slow intravenous infusion, the oral dose being double the intravenous dose. A preparation containing etoposide phosphate can be given by intravenous injection or infusion. Etoposide is usually given daily for 3–5 days and courses should not be repeated more frequently than at intervals of 21 days. It has particularly useful activity in small cell carcinoma of the bronchus, the lymphomas, and testicular cancer.

ETOPOSIDE

Indications   see notes above

Cautions   see section 8.1 and notes above; **interactions**: Appendix 1 (etoposide)

Contra-indications   see section 8.1 and notes above

Hepatic impairment   avoid in severe impairment

Renal impairment   consider dose reduction—consult local treatment protocol for details

Pregnancy   avoid (teratogenic in *animal* studies); see also Pregnancy and Reproductive Function, p. 575

Breast-feeding   discontinue breast-feeding

Side-effects   see section 8.1; irritant to tissues

Dose

- By mouth, 120–240 mg/m^2 daily for 5 days
- By intravenous infusion, consult product literature

Etoposide (Non-proprietary) PoM
Concentrate for intravenous infusion, etoposide 20 mg/mL, net price 5-mL vial = £12.15, 10-mL vial = £29.00, 25-mL vial = £60.75
Brands include *Eposin*®

Etopophos® (Bristol-Myers Squibb) PoM
Injection, powder for reconstitution, etoposide (as phosphate), net price 100-mg vial = £26.17 (hosp. only)

Vepesid® (Bristol-Myers Squibb) PoM
Capsules, both pink, etoposide 50 mg, net price 20 = £99.82; 100 mg, 10-cap pack = £87.23 (hosp. only). Label: 23

VINBLASTINE SULFATE

Indications   see notes above

Cautions   see section 8.1 and notes above; caution in handling; **interactions**: Appendix 1 (vinblastine)

Contra-indications   see section 8.1 and notes above
Important Intrathecal injection **contra-indicated**

Hepatic impairment   dose reduction may be necessary

Pregnancy   avoid (limited experience suggests fetal harm; teratogenic in *animal* studies); see also Pregnancy and Reproductive Function, p. 575

Breast-feeding   discontinue breast-feeding

Side-effects   see section 8.1 and notes above; irritant to tissues

Dose

- See Doses, p. 574

Vinblastine (Non-proprietary) PoM
Injection, vinblastine sulfate 1 mg/mL, net price 10-mL vial = £13.09

Velbe® (Genus) PoM
Injection, powder for reconstitution, vinblastine sulfate, net price 10-mg amp = £14.15

VINCRISTINE SULFATE

Indications   see notes above

Cautions   see section 8.1 and notes above; neuromuscular disease; caution in handling; **interactions**: Appendix 1 (vincristine)

Contra-indications   see section 8.1 and notes above
Important Intrathecal injection **contra-indicated**

Hepatic impairment   dose reduction may be necessary

Pregnancy   avoid (teratogenicity and fetal loss in *animal* studies); see also Pregnancy and Reproductive Function, p. 575

Breast-feeding   discontinue breast-feeding

Side-effects   see section 8.1 and notes above; also *rarely* inappropriate secretion of antidiuretic hormone; diarrhoea, intestinal necrosis, paralytic ileus, seizures, urinary retention, muscle wasting, and eye disorders also reported; irritant to tissues

Dose

- See Doses, p. 574

Vincristine (Non-proprietary) PoM
Injection, vincristine sulfate 1 mg/mL, net price 1-mL vial = £10.92; 2-mL vial = £21.17; 5-mL vial = £44.16

Oncovin® (Genus) PoM
Injection, vincristine sulfate 1 mg/mL, net price 1-mL vial = £14.18; 2-mL vial = £28.05

VINDESINE SULFATE

Indications   see notes above

Cautions   see section 8.1 and notes above; neuromuscular disease; caution in handling; **interactions**: Appendix 1 (vindesine)

Contra-indications   see section 8.1 and notes above
Important Intrathecal injection **contra-indicated**

Hepatic impairment   dose reduction may be necessary

Pregnancy   avoid (teratogenic in *animal* studies); see also Pregnancy and Reproductive Function, p. 575

Breast-feeding   discontinue breast-feeding

Side-effects   see section 8.1 and notes above; irritant to tissues

Dose

- See Doses, p. 574

Eldisine® (Genus) PoM
Injection, powder for reconstitution, vindesine sulfate, net price 5-mg vial = £78.30 (hosp. only)

VINFLUNINE

Indications   see notes above

Cautions   see section 8.1 and notes above; cardiovascular disease; QT-interval prolongation (avoid hypokalaemia or concomitant use of drugs that prolong QT-interval); **interactions**: Appendix 1 (vinflunine)

Contra-indications   see notes above
Important Intrathecal injection **contra-indicated**

Hepatic impairment   reduce dose—consult product literature

Renal impairment   reduce dose if creatinine clearance less than 60 mL/minute—consult product literature

Pregnancy   avoid unless essential—teratogenicity and embryotoxicity in *animal* studies; manufacturer advises effective contraception during and for up to 3 months after treatment; see also Pregnancy and Reproductive Function, p. 575

Breast-feeding   discontinue breast-feeding

Side-effects   see section 8.1 and notes above; also anorexia, diarrhoea, dyspepsia; tachycardia, hypertension, hypotension, thrombosis; oedema; insomnia, fatigue; dehydration; cutaneous reactions, sweating; *less commonly* increased weight, myocardial infarction, renal failure; *also reported* QT-interval prolongation, inappropriate anti-diuretic hormone secretion, blurred vision

Dose

• See Doses, p. 574

Javlor® (Fabre) ▣PoM▣

Concentrate for intravenous infusion, vinflunine (as ditartrate) 25 mg/mL, net price 2-mL vial = £212.50, 10-mL vial = £1062.50

▮ VINORELBINE

Indications see notes above

Cautions see section 8.1 and notes above; ischaemic heart disease; caution in handling; **interactions**: Appendix 1 (vinorelbine)

Contra-indications see section 8.1 and notes above; *with capsules* previous significant surgical resection of stomach or small bowel, long-term oxygen therapy, concurrent radiotherapy if treating the liver

Important Intrathecal injection **contra-indicated**

Hepatic impairment reduce *oral* dose in moderate impairment, avoid *oral* use in severe impairment; reduce *intravenous* dose in severe impairment; consult product literature

Pregnancy avoid unless essential (teratogenicity, and fetal loss in *animal* studies); manufacturer advises effective contraception during and for 3 months after treatment; men must avoid fathering a child during and for at least 3 months after treatment; see also Pregnancy and Reproductive Function, p. 575

Breast-feeding discontinue breast-feeding

Side-effects see section 8.1 and notes above; also *rarely* pancreatitis; hyponatraemia and inappropriate secretion of antidiuretic hormone also reported; irritant to tissues

Dose

• By mouth, 60 mg/m^2 once weekly for 3 weeks, increased if tolerated to 80 mg/m^2 once weekly; max. 160 mg once weekly

• By intravenous injection *or* infusion, consult product literature

Vinorelbine (Non-proprietary) ▣PoM▣

Concentrate for intravenous infusion, vinorelbine (as tartrate) 10 mg/mL, net price 1-mL vial = £29.00, 5-mL vial = £139.00

Navelbine® (Fabre) ▣PoM▣

Concentrate for intravenous infusion, vinorelbine (as tartrate) 10 mg/mL, net price 1-mL vial = £29.75, 5-mL vial = £139.98

Capsules, vinorelbine (as tartrate) 20 mg (brown), net price 1-cap pack = £43.98; 30 mg (pink), 1-cap pack = £65.98; 80 mg (yellow), 1-cap pack = £175.92. Label: 21, 25

▮8.1.5 Other antineoplastic drugs

Aflibercept

Aflibercept is a recombinant fusion protein that acts as a soluble decoy receptor and binds to vascular endothelial growth factors A and B (VEGF-A, VEGF-B) and placental growth factor (PlGF). Aflibercept inhibits the activation of VEGF receptors and the proliferation of endothelial cells, thereby inhibiting the growth of new vessels

that supply tumours with oxygen and nutrients. It is licensed in combination with irinotecan, fluorouracil and folinic acid (FOLFIRI) chemotherapy, in adults with metastatic colorectal cancer that is resistant to, or has progressed after, an oxaliplatin-containing regimen. An intravitreal preparation is available for the treatment of neovascular age-related macular degeneration, see section 11.8.2

> **NICE guidance**
>
> **Aflibercept in combination with irinotecan and fluorouracil-based therapy for treating metastatic colorectal cancer that has progressed following prior oxaliplatin-based chemotherapy (March 2014)**
>
> Aflibercept in combination with irinotecan and fluorouracil-based therapy is **not** recommended within its marketing authorisation for treating metastatic colorectal cancer that is resistant to or has progressed after an oxaliplatin-containing regimen. www.nice.org.uk/TA307

▮ AFLIBERCEPT

Indications see notes above

Cautions see section 8.1; increased risk of hypertension; monitor blood pressure at initiation and at least fortnightly during treatment (do not initiate treatment if pre-existing hypertension is uncontrolled)—consult product literature if hypertension develops during treatment; history of cardiovascular disease (may be exacerbated by hypertension); increased risk of haemorrhage (including fatal events); monitor for signs of gastro-intestinal perforation (discontinue if perforation develops); risk of fistula formation (discontinue if fistula develops); risk of thrombocytopenia and neutropenia (including febrile neutropenia and neutropenic infection)—monitor full blood count, including differential count and platelets at baseline and before each treatment cycle; increased risk of thromboembolic events (consult product literature if event occurs); nephrotic syndrome and thrombotic microangiopathy reported—monitor for proteinuria before each treatment administration (consult product literature if symptoms develop); monitor for signs and symptoms of diarrhoea and dehydration, particularly in elderly—consult product literature if severe diarrhoea occurs; may impair wound healing—withhold treatment for at least 4 weeks before elective surgery and for at least 4 weeks after major surgery, or until wound fully healed; monitor for posterior reversible encephalopathy syndrome (presenting as seizures, altered mental status, nausea, vomiting, headache, or visual disturbance)

Contra-indications uncontrolled hypertension; moderate or severe congestive heart failure

Hepatic impairment caution in severe impairment—no information available

Renal impairment caution in severe impairment—no information available

Pregnancy manufacturer advises avoid—toxicity in *animal* studies; effective contraception required during and for at least 6 months after treatment in men and women; see also Pregnancy and Reproductive Function, p. 575

Breast-feeding avoid—no information available

Side-effects diarrhoea, stomatitis, abdominal pain, decreased appetite, weight loss, fistula, aphthous stomatitis, haemorrhoids, proctalgia, toothache, hypertension, haemorrhage (including nasal, rectal and gastro-intestinal), thromboembolic events (arterial and venous), dyspnoea, oropharyngeal pain, rhinorrhoea, nasopharyngitis, dysphonia, headache, malaise, infection, sepsis, urinary tract infection, leucopenia, neutropenia (including febrile neutropenia), thrombocytopenia, dehydration, proteinuria, hand-foot syndrome, skin hyperpigmentation; *less commonly* gastro-intestinal perforation, posterior reversible encephalopathy syndrome, nephrotic syndrome, thrombotic microangiopathy, impaired wound healing

Dose

- See Doses, p. 574

Zaltrap® (Sanofi-Aventis) ▼ PoM
Concentrate for intravenous infusion, aflibercept 25 mg/mL, net price 4-mL (100-mg) vial = £295.65, 8-mL (200-mg) vial = £591.30

Arsenic trioxide

Arsenic trioxide is licensed for acute promyelocytic leukaemia in patients who have relapsed or failed to respond to previous treatment with a retinoid and chemotherapy.

◼ ARSENIC TRIOXIDE

Indications see notes above

Cautions see section 8.1; correct electrolyte abnormalities before treatment; ECG required before and during treatment—consult product literature; avoid concomitant administration with drugs causing QT interval prolongation, hypokalaemia, and hypomagnesaemia; previous treatment with anthracyclines (increased risk of QT interval prolongation); **interactions**: Appendix 1 (arsenic trioxide)

Hepatic impairment manufacturer advises caution—limited information available

Renal impairment manufacturer advises caution—limited information available

Pregnancy avoid (teratogenic and embryotoxic in *animal* studies); manufacturer advises effective contraception during treatment in men and women; see also Pregnancy and Reproductive function, p. 575

Breast-feeding discontinue breast-feeding

Side-effects see section 8.1; diarrhoea, leucocyte activation syndrome (unexplained fever, dyspnoea, weight gain, pulmonary infiltrates, pleural or pericardial effusions, with or without leucocytosis—treat with high dose corticosteroids, consult product literature); hyperglycaemia, hypokalaemia, QT interval prolongation, atrial fibrillation, atrial flutter, haemorrhage, pleuritic pain, musculoskeletal pain, paraesthesia, fatigue; *less commonly* abdominal pain, tachycardia, vasculitis, hypotension, oedema, pneumonitis, seizures, renal failure, blurred vision, and rash

Dose

- See Doses, p. 574

Trisenox® (TEVA UK) PoM
Concentrate for intravenous infusion, arsenic trioxide 1 mg/mL, net price 10-mL amp = £292.00

Bevacizumab

Bevacizumab is a monoclonal antibody that inhibits vascular endothelial growth factor. It is licensed for the treatment of metastatic colorectal cancer in combination with fluoropyrimidine-based chemotherapy (but see NICE guidance below). It is also licensed for first-line treatment of metastatic breast cancer in combination with paclitaxel, or with capecitabine when treatment with other chemotherapy, including taxanes or anthracyclines is not appropriate; patients who have received adjuvant taxane or anthracyline-containing regimens in the previous 12 months should not be treated with bevacizumab in combination with capecitabine. Bevacizumab is also licensed for advanced or metastatic renal cell carcinoma in combination with interferon alfa-2a (but see NICE Guidance, p. 610). Bevacizumab, in combination with platinum-based chemotherapy, is licensed for first-line treatment of unresectable advanced, metastatic or recurrent non-small cell lung cancer other than predominantly squamous cell histology. It is also licensed, in combination with carboplatin and paclitaxel, for the first-line treatment of advanced (FIGO stages IIIB, IIIC and IV) epithelial ovarian, fallopian tube, or primary peritoneal cancer and, in combination with carboplatin and gemcitabine, for first recurrence of platinum-sensitive epithelial ovarian, fallopian tube, or primary peritoneal cancer in patients who have not been treated previously with bevacizumab or other drugs that target vascular endothelial growth factor. Bevacizumab is given by intravenous infusion.

> **MHRA/CHM advice**
> **Bevacizumab and sunitinib: risk of osteonecrosis of the jaw (January 2011)**
> Treatment with bevacizumab or sunitinib may be a risk factor for the development of osteonecrosis of the jaw.
> Patients treated with bevacizumab or sunitinib, who have previously received bisphosphonates, or are treated concurrently with bisphosphonates, may be particularly at risk.
> Dental examination and appropriate preventive dentistry should be considered before treatment with bevacizumab or sunitinib.
> If possible, invasive dental procedures should be avoided in patients treated with bevacizumab or sunitinib who have previously received, or who are currently receiving, intravenous bisphosphonates.

The *Scottish Medicines Consortium* (p. 4) has advised (April 2012) that bevacizumab (*Avastin®*) is **not** recommended for use within NHS Scotland for the first-line treatment of patients with metastatic breast cancer in whom treatment with other chemotherapy options including taxanes or anthracyclines is not considered appropriate, and (September 2012), in combination with carboplatin and paclitaxel, for the first-line treatment of advanced (FIGO stages IIIB, IIIC and IV) epithelial ovarian, fallopian tube, or primary peritoneal cancer.

8 Malignant disease and immunosuppression

NICE guidance
Bevacizumab and cetuximab for the treatment of metastatic colorectal cancer (January 2007)

Bevacizumab in combination with fluorouracil plus folinic acid, with or without irinotecan, is **not** recommended for the first-line treatment of metastatic colorectal cancer; see also NICE guidance Cetuximab, bevacizumab and panitimumab for the treatment of metastatic colorectal cancer after first-line chemotherapy, p. 599.
www.nice.org.uk/TA118

NICE guidance
Bevacizumab in combination with oxaliplatin and either fluorouracil plus folinic acid or capecitabine for the treatment of metastatic colorectal cancer (December 2010)

Bevacizumab in combination with oxaliplatin and either fluorouracil plus folinic acid or capecitabine is **not** recommended for the treatment of metastatic colorectal cancer.
www.nice.org.uk/TA212

NICE guidance
Bevacizumab in combination with a taxane for the first-line treatment of metastatic breast cancer (February 2011)

Bevacizumab in combination with a taxane is **not** recommended for the first-line treatment of metastatic breast cancer.
www.nice.org.uk/TA214

NICE guidance
Bevacizumab in combination with capecitabine for the first-line treatment of metastatic breast cancer (August 2012)

Bevacizumab in combinations with capecitabine is **not** recommended within its marketing authorisation for the first-line treatment of metastatic breast cancer, that is, when treatment with other chemotherapy options including taxanes or anthracyclines is not considered appropriate, or when taxanes or anthracyclines have been used as part of adjuvant treatment in the previous 12 months.
www.nice.org.uk/TA263

NICE guidance
Bevacizumab in combination with paclitaxel and carboplatin for the first-line treatment of advanced ovarian cancer (May 2013)

Bevacizumab in combination with paclitaxel and carboplatin is **not** recommended for the first-line treatment of advanced ovarian cancer (including fallopian tube and primary peritoneal cancer).
www.nice.org.uk/TA284

NICE guidance
Bevacizumab in combination with gemcitabine and carboplatin for the treatment of the first recurrence of platinum-sensitive advanced ovarian cancer (May 2013)

Bevacizumab in combination with gemcitabine and carboplatin is **not** recommended within its marketing authorisation, that is, for the treatment of the first recurrence of platinum-sensitive advanced ovarian cancer (including fallopian tube and primary peritoneal cancer) that has not been previously treated with bevacizumab or other vascular endothelial growth factor (VEGF) inhibitors or VEGF receptor-targeted agents.
www.nice.org.uk/TA285

BEVACIZUMAB

Indications see notes above

Cautions see section 8.1; intra-abdominal inflammation (risk of gastro-intestinal perforation and gall bladder perforation); increased risk of fistulas (discontinue permanently if tracheo-oesophageal or grade 4 fistula develops); withhold treatment for elective surgery and avoid for at least 28 days after major surgery or until wound fully healed; monitor for necrotising fasciitis (usually secondary to wound healing complications, gastro-intestinal perforation or fistula formation)—discontinue and initiate treatment promptly; history of hypertension (increased risk of proteinuria—discontinue if nephrotic syndrome); uncontrolled hypertension; monitor blood pressure; history of arterial thromboembolism; history of cardiovascular disease (increased risk of cardiovascular events especially in the elderly); monitor for congestive heart failure; increased risk of haemorrhage (especially tumour-associated haemorrhage); monitor for posterior reversible encephalopathy syndrome (presenting as seizures, headache, altered mental status, visual disturbance or cortical blindness, with or without hypertension); untreated CNS metastases; consider dental check-up before initiating treatment (risk of osteonecrosis of the jaw, see MHRA/CHM advice, above); **interactions:** Appendix 1 (bevacizumab)

Pregnancy avoid—toxicity in *animal* studies; effective contraception required during and for at least 6 months after treatment in women; see also Pregnancy and Reproductive Function, p. 575

Breast-feeding manufacturer advises avoid breast-feeding during and for at least 6 months after treatment

Side-effects see section 8.1; gastro-intestinal perforation, gall bladder perforation, intestinal obstruction, abdominal pain, diarrhoea, constipation, taste disturbances; mucocutaneous bleeding, haemorrhage, hypoxia, arterial thromboembolism, congestive heart failure, syncope, supraventricular tachycardia, hypertension (see also Cautions); dyspnoea, rhinitis; anorexia, drowsiness, headache, peripheral neuropathy, asthenia, lethargy, dysarthria, posterior reversible encephalopathy syndrome; pyrexia; infection, proteinuria; dehydration, neutropenia, thrombocytopenia, anaemia; eye disorders; fistulas, pulmonary hypertension, impaired wound healing, necrotising fasciitis (see Cautions) osteonecrosis of the jaw (see

MHRA/CHM advice, above), hand-foot syndrome, exfoliative dermatitis, dry skin, skin discoloration, and hypersensitivity reactions (including flushing, rash, hypotension, chest pain, and rigors) also reported

Dose
- See Doses, p. 574

Avastin® (Roche) ▼ PoM
Concentrate for intravenous infusion, bevacizumab 25 mg/mL, net price 4-ml (100-mg) vial = £242.66, 16-ml (400-mg) vial = £924.40

Bexarotene

Bexarotene is an agonist at the retinoid X receptor, which is involved in the regulation of cell differentiation and proliferation. It is associated with little myelosuppression or immunosuppression. Bexarotene can cause regression of cutaneous T-cell lymphoma. The main adverse effects are hyperlipidaemia, hypothyroidism, leucopenia, headache, rash, and pruritus.

The *Scottish Medicines Consortium* (p. 4) has advised (November 2002) that bexarotene is recommended for restricted use as a second-line treatment for patients with advanced cutaneous T-cell lymphoma.

■ BEXAROTENE

Indications   skin manifestations of cutaneous T-cell lymphoma refractory to previous systemic treatment

Cautions   see section 8.1 and notes above; hyperlipidaemia (avoid if uncontrolled); hypothyroidism (avoid if uncontrolled); hypersensitivity to retinoids; avoid in acute porphyria (section 9.8.2); **interactions:** Appendix 1 (bexarotene)

Contra-indications   see section 8.1 and notes above; history of pancreatitis, hypervitaminosis A

Hepatic impairment   avoid

Pregnancy   avoid; manufacturer advises effective contraception during and for at least 1 month after treatment in men or women; see also Pregnancy and Reproductive Function, p. 575

Breast-feeding   discontinue breast-feeding

Side-effects   see section 8.1 and notes above

Dose
- Initially 300 mg/m^2 daily as a single dose with a meal; adjust dose according to response

Targretin® (TEVA UK) PoM
Capsules, bexarotene 75 mg in a liquid suspension, net price 100-cap pack = £937.50

Bortezomib

Bortezomib, a proteasome inhibitor, is licensed as monotherapy, or in combination with pegylated liposomal doxorubicin or dexamethasone, for the treatment of multiple myeloma that has progressed despite the use of at least one therapy, and where the patient has already had, or is unable to have, haematopoietic stem cell transplantation. It is also licensed for use in combination with melphalan and prednisolone for the treatment of previously untreated multiple myeloma in patients who are not eligible for high-dose chemotherapy with haematopoietic stem cell transplantation. Bortezomib is also licensed in combination with dexamethasone, or with dexamethasone and thalidomide, for the induction treatment of previously untreated multiple myeloma in patients who are eligible for high-dose chemotherapy

with haematopoietic stem cell transplantation. Bortezomib is given by intravenous or subcutaneous injection.

> **Important**
> Bortezomib injection is for **intravenous or subcutaneous administration** only. Inadvertent intrathecal administration with fatal outcome has been reported.

The *Scottish Medicines Consortium*, p. 4 has advised (December 2013) that bortezomib (*Velcade®*) is accepted for restricted use within NHS Scotland in combination with dexamethasone and thalidomide for the induction treatment of adults with previously untreated multiple myeloma who are eligible for high-dose chemotherapy with haematopoietic stem cell transplantation.

> **NICE guidance**
> **Bortezomib monotherapy for relapsed multiple myeloma (October 2007)**
> Bortezomib monotherapy is an option for the treatment of progressive multiple myeloma in patients who are at first relapse having received one prior therapy and who have undergone, or are unsuitable for, bone-marrow transplantation, under the following circumstances:
> - the response to bortezomib is measured using serum M protein after a maximum of four cycles of treatment, and treatment is continued only in patients who have a reduction in serum M protein of 50% or more (where serum M protein is not measurable, an appropriate alternative biochemical measure of response should be used) and
> - the manufacturer rebates the full cost of bortezomib if there is an inadequate response (as defined above) after four cycles of treatment.
>
> www.nice.org.uk/TA129

> **NICE guidance**
> **Bortezomib and thalidomide for the first-line treatment of multiple myeloma (July 2011)**
> Bortezomib in combination with an alkylating drug and a corticosteroid is recommended as an option for the first-line treatment of multiple myeloma if:
> - high-dose chemotherapy with stem cell transplantation is considered inappropriate and
> - the person is unable to tolerate or has contra-indications to thalidomide.
>
> For thalidomide see under Lenalidomide and thalidomide, p. 645
>
> www.nice.org.uk/TA228

> **NICE guidance**
> **Bortezomib for induction therapy in multiple myeloma before high-dose chemotherapy and autologous stem cell transplantation (April 2014)**
> Bortezomib is recommended as an option within its marketing authorisation, in combination with dexamethasone, or with dexamethasone and thalidomide, for the induction treatment of adults with previously untreated multiple myeloma, who are eligible for high-dose chemotherapy with haematopoietic stem cell transplantation.
>
> www.nice.org.uk/TA311

Malignant disease and immunosuppression 8

■ BORTEZOMIB

Indications see notes above

Cautions see section 8.1; cardiovascular disease; pulmonary disease (chest x-ray recommended before treatment—discontinue if interstitial lung disease develops); consider antiviral prophylaxis for herpes zoster infection; risk factors for seizures; amyloidosis; history of syncope and concurrent use of medication which may cause hypotension; dehydration; risk of neuropathy—consult product literature; monitor blood-glucose concentration in patients on oral antidiabetics; monitor for symptoms of progressive multifocal leucoencephalopathy (presenting as new or worsening neurological signs or symptoms)—discontinue treatment if diagnosed; **interactions:** Appendix 1 (bortezomib)

Contra-indications acute diffuse infiltrative pulmonary disease; pericardial disease

Hepatic impairment reduce dose in moderate to severe impairment—consult product literature

Renal impairment no information available for creatinine clearance less than 20 mL/minute/1.73 m^2

Pregnancy manufacturer advises effective contraception during and for 3 months after treatment in men or women—toxicity in *animal* studies; see also Pregnancy and Reproductive Function, p. 575

Breast-feeding discontinue breast-feeding

Side-effects see section 8.1; also diarrhoea, constipation (cases of ileus reported), hypotension, dyspnoea, fatigue, pyrexia, peripheral neuropathy (including sensory), headache, paraesthesia, decreased appetite, herpes zoster (including reactivation), myalgia, rash; *less commonly* heart failure, pulmonary hypertension, acute diffuse infiltrative pulmonary disorders, seizures, posterior reversible encephalopathy syndrome (discontinue treatment); *rarely* autonomic neuropathy; *very rarely* progressive multifocal leucoencephalopathy; also consult product literature

Dose
● See Doses, p. 574

Velcade® (Janssen) PoM
Injection, powder for reconstitution, bortezomib (as mannitol boronic ester), net price 3.5-mg vial = £762.38

Brentuximab vedotin

Brentuximab vedotin is licensed for the treatment of relapsed or refractory CD-30 positive Hodgkin's disease following autologous stem cell transplant or following at least two prior therapies, when autologous stem cell transplant or muti-agent chemotherapy is not a treatment option. It is also licensed for relapsed or refractory systemic anaplastic large cell lymphoma.

■ BRENTUXIMAB VEDOTIN

Indications see notes above

Cautions see section 8.1; rapidly proliferating tumours and high tumour burden—risk of tumour lysis syndrome; elevated BMI—risk of hyperglycaemia; monitor for symptoms of progressive multifocal leucoencephalopathy (presenting as new or worsening neurological, cognitive or behavioural signs or symptoms); monitor for new or worsening abdominal pain—investigate and withhold treatment if acute

pancreatitis suspected and discontinue if confirmed (fatal cases reported); monitor for pulmonary toxicity—treat symptoms promptly; routinely monitor hepatic function; monitor for infusion-related (including anaphylactic) reactions; monitor for signs of peripheral neuropathy—consult product literature for treatment adjustment; **interactions:** Appendix 1 (brentuximab vedotin)

Pregnancy avoid unless potential benefit outweighs risk (toxicity in *animal* studies); effective contraception required during treatment and for 6 months after treatment in men and women

Breast-feeding avoid—no information available

Side-effects see section 8.1; diarrhoea, constipation, cough, dyspnoea, fatigue, infusion-related reactions (including anaphylaxis), pyrexia, dizziness, peripheral neuropathy, demyelinating polyneuropathy, hyperglycaemia, myalgia, arthralgia, back pain, pruritus, rash; *less commonly* acute pancreatitis, Stevens-Johnson syndrome; *also reported* progressive multifocal leucoencephalopathy

Dose
● See Doses, p. 574

Adcetris® (Takeda) ▼ PoM
Injection, powder for reconstitution, brentuximab vedotin, net price 50-mg vial = £2500.00
Electrolytes Na$^+$ 0.57 mmol/vial

Catumaxomab

Catumaxomab is licensed for the treatment of malignant ascites in patients with epithelial cell adhesion molecule (EpCAM) positive carcinomas, where standard therapy is not available or no longer feasible.

Catumaxomab is given by intraperitoneal infusion. Infusion related side-effects have been reported with catumaxomab; premedication with analgesics, antipyretics, or NSAIDs is recommended by the manufacturer.

■ CATUMAXOMAB

Indications see notes above

Cautions see section 8.1 and notes above; haemodynamic insufficiency, oedema, hypoproteinaemia; **interactions:** Appendix 1 (catumaxomab)

Pregnancy avoid—limited information available

Breast-feeding avoid—no information available

Side-effects see section 8.1 and notes above; also abdominal pain, diarrhoea, constipation, dyspepsia, flatulence, ileus, anorexia, dehydration, cholangitis, tachycardia, hypotension, hypertension, flushing, dyspnoea, pleural effusion, cough, hypoxia, insomnia, anxiety, headache, dizziness, infection, hyperglycaemia, electrolyte disturbances, proteinuria, haematuria, leucocyturia, myalgia, arthralgia, vertigo, rash, sweating, skin reactions, *less commonly* gastro-intestinal haemorrhage, intestinal obstruction, seizures, acute renal failure

Dose
● Consult product literature

Removab® (Fresenius Biotech) ▼ PoM
Concentrate for intraperitoneal infusion, catumaxomab 100 micrograms/mL, net price 10-microgram prefilled syringe = £510.00; 50-microgram prefilled syringe = £2550.00

Cetuximab

Cetuximab is licensed for the treatment of wild-type *RAS* metastatic colorectal cancer in patients with tumours expressing epidermal growth factor receptor, as combination therapy, or as monotherapy if oxaliplatin- and irinotecan-based therapy has failed or if irinotecan is not tolerated (but see NICE guidance below). Evidence of non-mutated (wild-type) *RAS* status (at exons 2, 3 and 4 of *KRAS* and *NRAS*) is required before cetuximab is initiated for the treatment of metastatic colorectal cancer, and should be determined by an experienced laboratory using a validated test method. The combination of cetuximab with oxaliplatin-containing chemotherapy is contra-indicated in patients with metastatic colorectal cancer who have mutant or unknown *RAS* status. Cetuximab is also licensed, in combination with radiotherapy, for the treatment of locally advanced squamous cell cancer of the head and neck and in combination with platinum-based chemotherapy for recurrent or metastatic squamous cell cancer of the head and neck (but see NICE guidance below).

Cetuximab is given by intravenous infusion. Patients must receive an antihistamine and a corticosteroid at least one hour before infusion. Resuscitation facilities should be available and treatment should be initiated by a specialist.

> **MHRA/CHM advice**
> **Epidermal growth factor receptor (EGFR) inhibitors: serious cases of keratitis and ulcerative keratitis (May 2012)**
> Keratitis and ulcerative keratitis have been reported following treatment with epidermal growth factor receptor (EGFR) inhibitors for cancer (cetuximab, erlotinib, gefitinib and panitumumab). In rare cases, this has resulted in corneal perforation and blindness. Patients undergoing treatment with EGFR inhibitors who present with acute or worsening signs and symptoms suggestive of keratitis should be referred promptly to an opthalmology specialist. Treatment should be interrupted or discontinued if ulcerative keratitis is diagnosed.

The *Scottish Medicines Consortium* (p. 4) has advised (January 2010) that cetuximab (*Erbitux*®) is accepted for restricted use within NHS Scotland, in combination with chemotherapy, for metastatic colorectal cancer in patients with tumours expressing epidermal growth factor; it is restricted to patients with non-resectable metastases confined to the liver, who have not previously received chemotherapy.

> **NICE guidance**
> **Cetuximab for the treatment of locally advanced squamous cell cancer of the head and neck (June 2008)**
> Cetuximab in combination with radiotherapy is an option for the treatment of locally advanced squamous cell cancer of the head and neck in patients who have a Karnofsky performance status of 90% or greater and when all forms of platinum-based chemoradiotherapy treatment are contra-indicated.
> www.nice.org.uk/TA145

> **NICE guidance**
> **Cetuximab for the treatment of recurrent or metastatic squamous cell cancer of the head and neck (June 2009)**
> Cetuximab in combination with platinum-based chemotherapy is **not** recommended for the treatment of recurrent or metastatic squamous cell cancer of the head and neck.
> www.nice.org.uk/TA172

> **NICE guidance**
> **Cetuximab for the first-line treatment of metastatic colorectal cancer (August 2009)**
> Cetuximab in combination with fluorouracil, folinic acid and oxaliplatin is an option for the first-line treatment of metastatic colorectal cancer under the following circumstances:
> - the primary tumour has been resected or is potentially operable;
> - the metastatic disease is confined to the liver and is unresectable; and
> - the patient is fit to undergo surgery to resect the primary colorectal tumour and to undergo liver surgery if the metastases become resectable after treatment with cetuximab.
>
> In patients unable to tolerate oxaliplatin, or in whom oxaliplatin is contra-indicated, cetuximab in combination with fluorouracil, folinic acid and irinotecan can be used as an alternative.
>
> In addition, the manufacturer is required to rebate 16% of the amount of cetuximab used per patient when used in combination with fluorouracil, folinic acid, and oxaliplatin.
>
> Patients who meet the above criteria should receive cetuximab for no more than 16 weeks. At 16 weeks, cetuximab should be stopped and the patient should be assessed for resection of liver metastases.
> www.nice.org.uk/TA176

> **NICE guidance**
> **Cetuximab, bevacizumab and panitumumab for the treatment of metastatic colorectal cancer after first-line chemotherapy (January 2012)**
> Cetuximab monotherapy or combination chemotherapy is **not** recommended for the treatment of patients with metastatic colorectal cancer that has progressed after first-line chemotherapy.
>
> Bevacizumab in combination with non-oxaliplatin (fluoropyrimidine-based) chemotherapy is **not** recommended for the treatment of patients with metastatic colorectal cancer that has progressed after first-line chemotherapy; see also NICE guidance Bevacizumab and cetuximab for the treatment of metastatic colorectal cancer (January 2007), p. 596
>
> Panitinumab monotherapy is **not** recommended for the treatment of patients with metastatic colorectal cancer that has progressed after first-line chemotherapy.
> www.nice.org.uk/TA242

8 Malignant disease and immunosuppression

Malignant disease and immunosuppression

8

CETUXIMAB

Indications   see notes above and product literature

Cautions   cardiovascular disease, cardiopulmonary disease, pulmonary disease—discontinue if interstitial lung disease; history of, or risk factors for keratitis, ulcerative keratitis (including contact lens use), or severe dry eye (see also MHRA/CHM advice above); **interactions**: Appendix 1 (cetuximab)

Contra-indications   *RAS* mutated colorectal tumours (or if *RAS* tumour status unknown)

Pregnancy   use only if potential benefit outweighs risk—no information available; see also Pregnancy and Reproductive Function, p. 575

Breast-feeding   avoid breast-feeding during and for 2 months after treatment—no information available

Side-effects   infusion-related reactions including dyspnoea, dizziness, chills, fever, and severe (sometimes fatal) hypersensitivity reactions (possibly delayed onset) such as rash, urticaria, bronchospasm, hypotension, hypertension, and shock; nausea, vomiting, diarrhoea, headache, aseptic meningitis, hypomagnesaemia, hypocalcaemia, conjunctivitis, blepharitis, keratitis, skin reactions including acne, pruritus, dry skin, desquamation, hypertrichosis, nail disorders; *very rarely* Stevens-Johnson syndrome, toxic epidermal necrolysis

Dose
- See Doses, p. 574

Erbitux® (Merck Serono) [PoM]
> Intravenous infusion, cetuximab 5 mg/mL, net price 20-mL vial = £178.10, 100-mL vial = £890.50

Crisantaspase

Crisantaspase is the enzyme asparaginase produced by *Erwinia chrysanthemi*. It is given *intramuscularly*, *intravenously*, or *subcutaneously* almost exclusively in acute lymphoblastic leukaemia. Facilities for the management of anaphylaxis should be available.

CRISANTASPASE

Indications   see notes above

Cautions   see notes above

Contra-indications   history of pancreatitis related to asparaginase therapy

Pregnancy   avoid; see also Pregnancy and Reproductive Function, p. 575

Breast-feeding   discontinue breast-feeding

Side-effects   see section 8.1; also liver dysfunction, pancreatitis, diarrhoea; coagulation disorders; lethargy, drowsiness, confusion, dizziness, neurotoxicity, convulsions, headache; *less commonly* changes in blood lipids, anaphylaxis, hyperglycaemia; *rarely* CNS depression; *very rarely* myalgia; abdominal pain and hypertension also reported

Dose
- See Doses, p. 574

Erwinase® (EUSA Pharma) [PoM]
> Injection, powder for reconstitution, crisantaspase, net price 10 000-unit vial = £613.00

Dacarbazine and temozolomide

Dacarbazine is used to treat metastatic melanoma and, in combination therapy, soft tissue sarcomas. It is also a component of a commonly used combination for Hodgkin's disease (ABVD—doxorubicin [previously *Adriamycin®*], bleomycin, vinblastine, and dacarbazine). It is given *intravenously*. The predominant side-effects are myelosuppression and severe nausea and vomiting.

Temozolomide is structurally related to dacarbazine. It is given by mouth and is licensed for the treatment of newly diagnosed glioblastoma multiforme in adults (in combination with radiotherapy) and subsequently as monotherapy. It is also licensed for second-line treatment of malignant glioma in adults and children over 3 years.

> **NICE guidance**
> **Temozolomide for the treatment of recurrent malignant glioma (brain cancer) (April 2001)**
>
> Temozolomide may be considered for the treatment of recurrent malignant glioma, which has not responded to first-line chemotherapy.
> www.nice.org.uk/TA23

> **NICE guidance**
> **Carmustine implants and temozolomide for the treatment of newly diagnosed high-grade glioma (June 2007)**
>
> Temozolomide is an option for the treatment of newly diagnosed glioblastoma multiforme in patients with a WHO performance status of 0 or 1.
> Carmustine implants are an option for the treatment of newly diagnosed high-grade (Grade 3 or 4) glioma **only** for patients in whom at least 90% of the tumour has been resected.
> Carmustine implants should only be used within specialist centres.
> www.nice.org.uk/TA121

DACARBAZINE

Indications   see notes above

Cautions   see section 8.1; caution in handling; **interactions**: Appendix 1 (dacarbazine)

Hepatic impairment   dose reduction may be required in combined renal and hepatic impairment; avoid in severe impairment

Renal impairment   dose reduction may be required in combined renal and hepatic impairment; avoid in severe impairment

Pregnancy   avoid (carcinogenic and teratogenic in *animal* studies); ensure effective contraception during and for at least 6 months after treatment in men or women; see also Pregnancy and Reproductive Function, p. 575

Breast-feeding   discontinue breast-feeding

Side-effects   see section 8.1 and notes above; *rarely* liver necrosis due to hepatic vein thrombosis; irritant to skin and tissues

Dose
- See Doses, p. 574

Dacarbazine (Non-proprietary) [PoM]
> Injection, powder for reconstitution, dacarbazine (as citrate), net price 100-mg vial = £5.05; 200-mg vial = £7.50; 500-mg vial = £16.50; 600-mg vial = £22.50; 1-g vial = £31.80

TEMOZOLOMIDE

Indications see notes above

Cautions see section 8.1; *Pneumocystis jirovecii* pneumonia—consult product literature for monitoring and prophylaxis requirements; monitor liver function before treatment initiation, after each treatment cycle and midway through 42-day treatment cycles—consider the balance of benefits and risks of treatment if results are abnormal at any point (fatal liver injury reported); monitor for myelodysplastic syndrome and secondary malignancies; **interactions**: Appendix 1 (temozolomide)

Hepatic impairment use with caution in severe impairment—no information available

Renal impairment manufacturer advises caution—no information available

Pregnancy avoid (teratogenic and embryotoxic in *animal* studies); manufacturer advises adequate contraception during treatment; men should avoid fathering a child during and for at least 6 months after treatment; see also Pregnancy and Reproductive Function, p. 575

Breast-feeding discontinue breast-feeding

Side-effects see section 8.1 and consult product literature

Dose

- Consult product literature; CHILD under 3 years not recommended

Temozolomide (Non-proprietary) ℗ℴ𝓂
Capsules, temozolomide 5 mg, net price 5-cap pack = £16.00; 20 mg, 5-cap pack = £60.30; 100 mg, 5-cap pack = £320.80; 140 mg, 5-cap pack = £451.40; 180 mg, 5-cap pack = £580.37; 250 mg, 5-cap pack = £806.08. Label: 23, 25
Brands include *Temomedac®*

Temodal® (MSD) ℗ℴ𝓂
Capsules, temozolomide 5 mg (green/white), net price 5-cap pack = £10.59; 20 mg (yellow/white), 5-cap pack = £42.35; 100 mg (pink/white), 5-cap pack = £211.77; 140 mg (blue/white), 5-cap pack = £296.48; 180 mg (orange/white), 5-cap pack = £381.19; 250 mg (white), 5-cap pack = £529.43. Label: 23, 25

Eribulin

Eribulin is licensed for the treatment of locally advanced or metastatic breast cancer when the disease has progressed after treatment with at least 1 chemotherapy regimen for advanced disease. Previous therapy should have included an anthracycline and a taxane in either the adjuvant or metastatic setting unless the patient is unsuitable for these treatments. It is given intravenously on day 1 and day 8 of a 21-day cycle. It can cause myelosuppression, peripheral neuropathy, and QT-interval prolongation.

> **NICE guidance**
> **Eribulin for the treatment of locally advanced or metastatic breast cancer (April 2012)**
>
> Eribulin is **not** recommended for the treatment of locally advanced or metastatic breast cancer that has progressed after at least two chemotherapy regimens for advanced disease.
> www.nice.org.uk/TA250

ERIBULIN

Indications see notes above

Cautions see section 8.1 and notes above; monitor for signs of peripheral neuropathy—severe peripheral neurotoxicity requires treatment delay or dose reduction (consult product literature); susceptibility to QT-interval prolongation (including congestive heart failure, bradyarrhythmias, electrolyte disturbances, concomitant use of drugs that prolong QT-interval)—ECG monitoring recommended; monitor electrolytes periodically; **interactions**: Appendix 1 (eribulin)

Contra-indications congenital long QT syndrome

Hepatic impairment reduce dose

Renal impairment consider dose reduction if creatinine clearance less than 40 mL/minute

Pregnancy avoid unless essential (teratogenic in *animal sudies*); ensure effective contraception during and for up to 3 months after treatment in men or women; see also Pregnancy and Reproductive Function, p. 575

Breast-feeding discontinue breast-feeding

Side-effects see section 8.1, notes above, and consult product literature

Dose

- See Doses, p. 574

Halaven® (Eisai) ▼ ℗ℴ𝓂
Injection, eribulin (as mesilate) 440 micrograms/mL, net price 2-mL vial = £361.00
Note Contains ethanol

Hydroxycarbamide

Hydroxycarbamide is an orally active drug used mainly in the treatment of chronic myeloid leukaemia. It is also licensed for the treatment of cancer of the cervix in conjunction with radiotherapy. It is occasionally used for polycythaemia (the usual treatment is venesection); patients receiving long-term therapy with hydroxycarbamide should be advised to protect skin from sun exposure and should be monitored for secondary malignancies. Myelosuppression, nausea, and skin reactions are the most common toxic effects.

HYDROXYCARBAMIDE
(Hydroxyurea)

Indications see notes above; sickle-cell disease (section 9.1.3)

Cautions see section 8.1 and notes above; **interactions**: Appendix 1 (hydroxycarbamide)

Hepatic impairment use with caution

Renal impairment use with caution

Pregnancy avoid (teratogenic in *animal* studies); manufacturer advises effective contraception before and during treatment; see also Pregnancy and Reproductive Function, p. 575

Breast-feeding discontinue breast-feeding

Side-effects see section 8.1 and notes above

Dose

- 20–30 mg/kg daily *or* 80 mg/kg every third day

Hydroxycarbamide (Non-proprietary) ℗ℴ𝓂
Capsules, hydroxycarbamide 500 mg, net price 100-cap pack = £11.08

Hydrea® (Squibb) ℗ℴ𝓂
Capsules, pink/green, hydroxycarbamide 500 mg, net price 100-cap pack = £10.47

Ipilimumab

Ipilimumab causes T-cell activation. It is licensed for the treatment of unresectable or metastatic advanced melanoma. Infusion-related side-effects have been reported with ipilimumab; premedication with paracetamol and an antihistamine is recommended. A corticosteroid can be used after starting ipilimumab, to treat immune-related reactions. The *Scottish Medicines Consortium* (p. 4) has advised (March 2013) that ipilimumab (*Yervoy*®) is accepted for restricted use within NHS Scotland for the treatment of advanced (unresectable or metastatic) melanoma in adults who have received prior therapy, only whilst ipilimumab is available at the price agreed in the patient access scheme.

> ### NICE guidance
> **Ipilimumab for previously untreated advanced (unresectable or metastatic) melanoma (July 2014)**
> Ipilimumab is recommended, within its marketing authorisation, as an option for treating adults with previously untreated advanced (unresectable or metastatic) melanoma, only if the manufacturer provides ipilimumab with the discount agreed in the patient access scheme.
> www.nice.org.uk/TA319

> ### NICE guidance
> **Ipilimumab for previously treated advanced (unresectable or metastatic) melanoma (December 2012)**
> Ipilimumab is recommended as an option for the treatment of advanced (unresectable or metastatic) melanoma in patients who have received prior therapy, only if the manufacturer provides ipilimumab with the discount agreed in the patient access scheme.
> www.nice.org.uk/TA268

◢ IPILIMUMAB

Indications see notes above

Cautions see notes above—for full details consult product literature; **interactions**: Appendix 1 (ipilimumab)

Hepatic impairment use with caution if plasma-bilirubin concentration greater than 3 times upper limit of normal range *or* if plasma-transaminase concentration 5 times or greater than the upper limit of normal range

Pregnancy avoid unless potential benefit outweighs risk (toxicity in *animal* studies); use effective contraception

Breast-feeding discontinue breast-feeding—no information available

Side-effects see notes above—for full details (including monitoring and management of side-effects) consult product literature

Dose
• Consult product literature

Yervoy® (Bristol-Myers Squibb) ▼ PoM
  Concentrate for intravenous infusion, ipilimumab 5 mg/mL, net price 10-mL vial = £3750.00, 40-mL vial = £15000.00
  Electrolytes Contains approx. 0.1 mmol Na⁺/mL

Mitotane

Mitotane is licensed for the symptomatic treatment of advanced or inoperable adrenocortical carcinoma. It selectively inhibits the activity of the adrenal cortex, necessitating corticosteroid replacement therapy (section 6.3.1); the dose of glucocorticoid should be increased in case of shock, trauma, or infection.

Gastro-intestinal side-effects such as anorexia, nausea, and vomiting, and endocrine side-effects, such as hypogonadism and thyroid disorders, are very common with mitotane; neurotoxicity occurs in many patients.

◢ MITOTANE

Indications see notes above

Cautions see section 8.1 and notes above; risk of accumulation in overweight patients; monitor plasma-mitotane concentration—consult product literature; avoid in acute porphyria (section 9.8.2); **interactions**: Appendix 1 (mitotane)
  Driving CNS effects may affect performance of skilled tasks (e.g. driving)
  Counselling Warn patient to contact doctor immediately if injury, infection, or illness occurs (because of risk of acute adrenal insufficiency)

Hepatic impairment manufacturer advises caution in mild to moderate impairment—monitoring of plasma-mitotane concentration recommended; avoid in severe impairment

Renal impairment manufacturer advises caution in mild to moderate impairment—monitoring of plasma-mitotane concentration recommended; avoid in severe impairment

Pregnancy manufacturer advises avoid—women of childbearing age should use effective contraception during and after treatment; see also Pregnancy and Reproductive Function, p. 575

Breast-feeding discontinue breast-feeding

Side-effects see section 8.1 and notes above; also gastro-intestinal disturbances (including nausea, vomiting, diarrhoea, epigastric discomfort), anorexia, liver disorders; hypercholesterolaemia, hypertriglyceridaemia; ataxia, confusion, asthenia, myasthenia, paraesthesia, drowsiness, neuropathy, cognitive impairment, movement disorder, dizziness, headache; gynaecomastia; prolonged bleeding time, leucopenia, thrombocytopenia, anaemia; rash; *rarely* hypersalivation, hypertension, postural hypotension, flushing, pyrexia, haematuria, proteinuria, haemorrhagic cystitis, hypouricaemia, visual disturbances, and ocular disorders

Dose
• ADULT over 18 years, initially 2–3 g daily, (up to 6 g daily in severe illness) in 2–3 divided doses, adjusted according to plasma-mitotane concentration; reduce dose or interrupt treatment if signs of toxicity; discontinue if inadequate response after 3 months
  Note Plasma-mitotane concentration for optimum response 14–20 mg/litre

Lysodren® (HRA Pharma) PoM
  Tablets, scored, mitotane 500 mg, net price 100-tab pack = £590.97. Label: 2, 10, 21, counselling, driving, adrenal suppression

Panitumumab

Panitumumab is a monoclonal antibody that binds to the epidermal growth factor receptor (EGFR). It is indicated as combination therapy for the treatment of non-mutated *RAS* metastatic colorectal cancer, or as monotherapy after failure of fluoropyrimidine-, oxaliplatin-, and irinotecan-containing chemotherapy regimens. Evidence of non-mutated *RAS* status (at exons 2, 3 and 4 of *KRAS* and *NRAS*) is required before panitumumab treatment is initiated, and should be determined by an experienced laboratory using a validated test method. The combination of panitumumab with oxaliplatin-containing chemotherapy is contra-indicated in patients with mutant *RAS* metastatic colorectal cancer or for whom *RAS* status is unknown. Panitumumab is given by intravenous infusion.

> **MHRA/CHM advice**
> **Severe skin reactions**
> Severe skin reactions have been reported very commonly in patients treated with panitumumab. Patients receiving panitumumab who have severe skin reactions or develop worsening skin reactions should be monitored for the development of inflammatory or infectious sequelae (including cellulitis, sepsis, and necrotising fasciitis). Appropriate treatment should be promptly initiated and panitumumab withheld or discontinued.

> **NICE guidance**
> **Cetuximab, bevacizumab and panitumumab for the treatment of metastatic colorectal cancer after first-line chemotherapy (January 2012)**
> See p. 599

▐ PANITUMUMAB

Indications see notes above

Cautions monitor for dermatological reactions including Stevens-Johnson syndrome and toxic epidermal necrolysis (see also Severe Skin Reactions above and consult product literature); pulmonary disease—discontinue if interstitial lung disease develops; monitor for hypomagnesaemia and hypocalcaemia; history of, or risk factors for keratitis, ulcerative keratitis (including contact lens use), or severe dry eye (see also MHRA/CHM advice Epidermal Growth Factor Receptor (EGFR) Inhibitors: Serious Cases of Keratitis and Ulcerative Keratitis, p. 599); **interactions:** Appendix 1 (panitumumab)

Contra-indications see notes above; interstitial pulmonary disease

Pregnancy avoid (toxicity in *animal* studies); manufacturer advises effective contraception during and for 6 months after treatment; see also Pregnancy and Reproductive Function, p. 575

Breast-feeding manufacturer advises avoid breast-feeding during and for 2 months after treatment

Side-effects see section 8.1; diarrhoea, abdominal pain, constipation, rectal haemorrhage, dehydration, cheilitis, dry mouth, anorexia, weight loss, dyspepsia, tachycardia, hypotension, hypertension, deep vein thrombosis, flushing, peripheral oedema, dyspnoea, cough, pulmonary embolism, epistaxis, malaise, insomnia, anxiety, pyrexia, dizziness, headache, biochemical and electrolyte disturbances, ocular disorders (including conjunctivitis, increased lacrimation, dry eyes, ocular hyperaemia and keratitis), eyelash growth, rash, cellulitis, erythema, pruritus, dry skin,

acne, hand-foot syndrome, mucosal inflammation, hypertrichosis, nail disorders; *less commonly* cyanosis, bronchospasm, nasal dryness, hirsutism, infusion-related reactions; *rarely* severe hypersensitivity reactions (possibly delayed onset), skin necrosis, Stevens-Johnson syndrome, toxic epidermal necrolysis; *also reported* interstitial lung disease

Dose
● See Doses, p. 574

Vectibix® (Amgen) ▼ PoM
Concentrate for intravenous infusion, panitumumab 20 mg/mL, net price 5-mL vial = £379.29, 20-mL vial = £1517.16
Electrolytes Na⁺ 0.75 mmol/vial

Pentostatin

Pentostatin is active in hairy cell leukaemia. It is given *intravenously* on alternate weeks and can induce prolonged complete remission. It can cause myelosuppression, immunosuppression, and a number of other side-effects that may be severe. Treatment should be withheld in patients who develop a severe rash, and withheld or discontinued in patients showing signs of neurotoxicity. Its use should be confined to specialist centres.

▐ PENTOSTATIN

Indications see notes above

Cautions see section 8.1 and notes above; **interactions:** Appendix 1 (pentostatin)

Hepatic impairment manufacturer advises caution—limited information available

Renal impairment avoid if creatinine clearance less than 60 mL/minute

Pregnancy avoid (teratogenic in *animal* studies); manufacturer advises that men should not father children during and for 6 months after treatment; see also Pregnancy and Reproductive Function, p. 575

Breast-feeding discontinue breast-feeding

Side-effects see section 8.1 and notes above

Dose
● See Doses, p. 574

Nipent® (Hospira) PoM
Injection, powder for reconstitution, pentostatin, net price 10-mg vial = £863.78

Pertuzumab

Pertuzumab is a recombinant humanised monoclonal antibody, and acts by inhibiting human epidermal growth factor receptor 2 protein (HER2) dimerisation. It is indicated for the treatment of HER2-positive metastatic or locally recurrent unresectable breast cancer in combination with trastuzumab and docetaxel, in patients who have not received previous anti-HER2 therapy or chemotherapy. Pertuzumab is given by intravenous infusion; resuscitation facilities should be available and treatment should be initiated by a specialist.

▐ PERTUZUMAB

Indications see notes above

Cautions see section 8.1 and notes above; history of congestive heart failure, impaired left ventricular function or conditions that could impair left ventricular function (including uncontrolled hypertension, recent myocardial infarction, serious cardiac arrhythmia, prior anthracycline exposure, or radio-therapy to the chest area); assess for signs and symptoms of congestive heart failure (including left ventricular ejection fraction) before and during treatment—consult product literature, and withhold treatment if necessary; monitor for febrile neutropenia; **interactions:** Appendix 1 (pertuzumab)

Hepatic impairment caution—no information available

Renal impairment caution in severe impairment—no information available

Pregnancy avoid (toxicity in *animal* studies); ensure effective contraception during and for six months after treatment in women of childbearing potential; see also Pregnancy and Reproductive Function

Breast-feeding avoid—no information available

Side-effects see section 8.1; also (when used in combination with trastuzumab and docetaxel) decreased appetite, diarrhoea, constipation, dyspepsia, left ventricular dysfunction, oedema, dyspnoea, cough, pleural effusion, nasopharyngitis, insomnia, peripheral neuropathy, headache, dizziness, taste disturbance, pain, malaise, pyrexia, chills, upper respiratory-tract infection, paronychia, neutropenia (including febrile neutropenia), leucopenia, anaemia, myalgia, arthralgia, increased lacrimation, rash, nail disorder, pruritus, dry skin; infusion-related reactions including severe hypersensitivity reactions; *less commonly* interstitial lung disease

Dose

* See Doses, p. 574

Perjeta (Roche) ▼ PoM
Concentrate for intravenous infusion, pertuzumab 30 mg/mL, net price 14-mL vial = £2395.00

Platinum compounds

Carboplatin is widely used in the treatment of advanced ovarian cancer and lung cancer (particularly the small cell type). It is given *intravenously*. The dose of carboplatin is determined according to renal function rather than body surface area. Carboplatin can be given on an outpatient basis and is better tolerated than cisplatin; nausea and vomiting are reduced in severity and nephrotoxicity, neurotoxicity, and ototoxicity are much less of a problem than with cisplatin. It is, however, more myelosuppressive than cisplatin.

Cisplatin is used alone or in combination for the treatment of testicular, lung, cervical, bladder, head and neck, and ovarian cancer (but carboplatin is preferred for ovarian cancer). It is given *intravenously*. Cisplatin requires intensive intravenous hydration and treatment may be complicated by severe nausea and vomiting. Cisplatin is toxic, causing nephrotoxicity (monitoring of renal function is essential), ototoxicity, peripheral neuropathy, hypomagnesaemia and myelosuppression. It is, however, increasingly given in a day-care setting.

Oxaliplatin is licensed in combination with fluorouracil and folinic acid, for the treatment of metastatic colorectal cancer and as adjuvant treatment of colon cancer after resection of the primary tumour; it is given by intravenous infusion. Neurotoxic side-effects (including sensory peripheral neuropathy) are dose limiting. Other side-effects include gastro-intestinal disturbances, ototoxicity, myelosuppression and transient vision loss (reversible on discontinuation). If unexplained respiratory symptoms occur, oxaliplatin should be discontinued until investigations exclude interstitial lung disease and pulmonary fibrosis. Posterior reversible encephalopathy syndrome has also been reported in patients receiving oxaliplatin combination chemotherapy.

NICE guidance
Irinotecan, oxaliplatin, and raltitrexed for advanced colorectal cancer (August 2005)
A combination of fluorouracil and folinic acid with either irinotecan or oxaliplatin are options for first-line treatment for advanced colorectal cancer.

Irinotecan alone or fluorouracil and folinic acid with oxaliplatin are options for patients who require further treatment subsequently.

Raltitrexed is **not** recommended for the treatment of advanced colorectal cancer. Its use should be confined to clinical studies.
www.nice.org.uk/TA93

NICE guidance (capecitabine and oxaliplatin in the adjuvant treatment of stage III (Dukes' C) colon cancer)
See p. 585

NICE guidance
Paclitaxel for ovarian cancer (January 2003)
Either paclitaxel in combination with a platinum compound (cisplatin or carboplatin) *or* a platinum compound alone are alternatives for the first-line treatment of ovarian cancer (usually following surgery).
www.nice.org.uk/TA55

NICE guidance
Paclitaxel, pegylated liposomal doxorubicin, and topotecan for second-line or subsequent treatment of advanced ovarian cancer (May 2005)
Paclitaxel, combined with a platinum compound (carboplatin or cisplatin), is an option for advanced cancer that relapses 6 months or more after completing initial platinum-based chemotherapy. Paclitaxel alone is an option for advanced ovarian cancer that does not respond to, or relapses within 6 months of completing initial platinum-based chemotherapy.

Pegylated liposomal doxorubicin is an option for advanced ovarian cancer that does not respond to, or relapses within 12 months of completing initial platinum-based chemotherapy.

Paclitaxel alone or pegylated liposomal doxorubicin are options for advanced ovarian cancer in patients who are allergic to platinum compounds. Topotecan alone is an option only for advanced ovarian cancer that does not respond to, or relapses within 6 months of completing initial platinum-based chemotherapy or in those allergic to platinum compounds *and* for whom paclitaxel alone or pegylated liposomal doxorubicin are inappropriate.
www.nice.org.uk/TA91

CARBOPLATIN

Indications see notes above

Cautions see section 8.1 and notes above; **interactions**: Appendix 1 (platinum compounds)

Renal impairment reduce dose and monitor haematological parameters and renal function; avoid if creatinine clearance less than 20 mL/minute

Pregnancy avoid (teratogenic and embryotoxic in *animal* studies); see also Pregnancy and Reproductive Function, p. 575

Breast-feeding discontinue breast-feeding

Side-effects see section 8.1 and notes above

Dose
- See Doses, p. 574

Carboplatin (Non-proprietary) [PoM]
Injection, carboplatin 10 mg/mL, net price 5-mL vial = £20.00, 15-mL vial = £50.00, 45-mL vial = £160.00, 60-mL vial = £260.00

CISPLATIN

Indications see notes above

Cautions see section 8.1 and notes above; **interactions**: Appendix 1 (platinum compounds)

Renal impairment avoid if possible; nephrotoxic

Pregnancy avoid (teratogenic and toxic in *animal* studies); see also Pregnancy and Reproductive Function, p. 575

Breast-feeding discontinue breast-feeding

Side-effects see section 8.1 and notes above

Dose
- See Doses, p. 574

Cisplatin (Non-proprietary) [PoM]
Injection, cisplatin 1 mg/mL, net price 10-mL vial = £5.90, 50-mL vial = £24.50, 100-mL vial = £50.22
Injection, powder for reconstitution, cisplatin, net price 50-mg vial = £17.00

OXALIPLATIN

Indications metastatic colorectal cancer in combination with fluorouracil and folinic acid; colon cancer—see notes above

Cautions see section 8.1 and notes above; **interactions**: Appendix 1 (platinum compounds)

Contra-indications see section 8.1; peripheral neuropathy with functional impairment

Renal impairment reduce dose in mild to moderate impairment (consult product literature); avoid if creatinine clearance less than 30 mL/minute

Pregnancy manufacturer advises avoid—toxicity in *animal* studies; effective contraception required during and for 4 months after treatment in women and 6 months after treatment in men; see also Pregnancy and Reproductive Function, p. 575

Breast-feeding discontinue breast-feeding

Side-effects see section 8.1 and notes above

Dose
- See Doses, p. 574

Oxaliplatin (Non-proprietary) [PoM]
Injection, powder for reconstitution, oxaliplatin, net price 50-mg vial = £150.00, 100-mg vial = £299.50
Concentrate for intravenous infusion, oxaliplatin 5 mg/mL, net price 10-mL vial = £155.00, 20-mL vial = £311.00, 40-mL vial = £622.38

Porfimer sodium and temoporfin

Porfimer sodium and **temoporfin** are used in the photodynamic treatment of various tumours. The drugs accumulate in malignant tissue and are activated by laser light to produce a cytotoxic effect.

Porfimer sodium is licensed for photodynamic therapy of non-small cell lung cancer and obstructing oesophageal cancer. Temoporfin is licensed for photodynamic therapy of advanced head and neck cancer.

PORFIMER SODIUM

Indications non-small cell lung cancer; oesophageal cancer; see notes above

Cautions see section 8.1; avoid exposure of skin and eyes to direct sunlight or bright indoor light for at least 30 days

Contra-indications see section 8.1; tracheo-oesophageal or broncho-oesophageal fistula; acute porphyria (section 9.8.2)

Hepatic impairment avoid in severe impairment

Pregnancy manufacturer advises avoid unless essential

Breast-feeding no information available—manufacturer advises avoid

Side-effects see section 8.1; photosensitivity (see Cautions above—sunscreens offer no protection), constipation

Dose
- See Doses, p. 574

Photofrin® (Pinnacle) [PoM]
Injection, powder for reconstitution, porfimer sodium, net price 15-mg vial = £154.00; 75-mg vial = £770.00

TEMOPORFIN

Indications advanced head and neck squamous cell carcinoma refractory to, or unsuitable for, other treatments

Cautions see section 8.1; avoid exposure of skin and eyes to direct sunlight or bright indoor light for at least 15 days after administration; avoid prolonged exposure of injection site arm to direct sunlight for 6 months after administration, if extravasation occurs protect area from light for at least 3 months; **interactions**: Appendix 1 (temoporfin)

Contra-indications see section 8.1; acute porphyria (section 9.8.2) or other diseases exacerbated by light; elective surgery or ophthalmic slit-lamp examination for 30 days after administration; concomitant photosensitising treatment

Pregnancy toxicity in *animal* studies—manufacturer advises avoid pregnancy for at least 3 months after treatment; see also Pregnancy and Reproductive Function, p. 575

Breast-feeding manufacturer advises avoid breast-feeding for at least 1 month after treatment—no information available

Side-effects see section 8.1; also constipation, dysphagia; haemorrhage, oedema, giddiness, trismus, facial pain; injection site pain, blistering, scarring, erythema, skin necrosis, hyperpigmentation, photosensitivity (see Cautions above; sunscreens ineffective)

Malignant disease and immunosuppression

8

Dose
• See Doses, p. 574

Foscan® (Biolitec) ▼ PoM
Injection, temoporfin 1 mg/mL, net price 3-mL vial = £1800.00, 6-mL vial = £3400.00

Procarbazine

Procarbazine is most often used in Hodgkin's disease. It is given *by mouth*. Toxic effects include nausea, myelosuppression, and a hypersensitivity rash preventing further use of this drug. It is a mild monoamine-oxidase inhibitor and dietary restriction is rarely considered necessary. Alcohol ingestion may cause a disulfiram-like reaction.

◢ PROCARBAZINE

Indications see notes above

Cautions see section 8.1 and notes above; cardiovascular or cerebrovascular disease; phaeochromocytoma; epilepsy; **interactions:** Appendix 1 (procarbazine)

Contra-indications pre-existing severe leucopenia or thrombocytopenia

Hepatic impairment caution in mild to moderate impairment; avoid in severe impairment

Renal impairment caution in mild to moderate impairment; avoid in severe impairment

Pregnancy avoid (teratogenic in *animal* studies and isolated reports in humans); see also Pregnancy and Reproductive Function, p. 575

Breast-feeding discontinue breast-feeding

Side-effects see section 8.1 and notes above; loss of appetite; *also reported* jaundice, hypersensitivity rash (discontinue treatment)

Dose
• See Doses, p. 574

Procarbazine (Non-proprietary) PoM
Capsules, procarbazine (as hydrochloride) 50 mg, net price 50-cap pack = £249.50. Label: 4

Protein kinase inhibitors

Afatinib is a protein kinase inhibitor licensed for the treatment of locally advanced or metastatic non-small cell lung cancer with activating epidermal growth factor receptor (EGFR) mutations, in patients who have not previously been treated with an EGFR tyrosine kinase inhibitor.

> **NICE guidance**
> **Afatinib for treating epidermal growth factor receptor mutation-positive locally advanced or metastatic non-small-cell lung cancer (April 2014)**
> Afatinib is recommended as an option, within its marketing authorisation, for treating locally advanced or metastatic non-small-cell lung cancer in adults:
> • whose tumour tests positive for the epidermal growth factor receptor tyrosine kinase (EGFR-TK) mutation, **and**
> • who have not previously had an EGFR-TK inhibitor, **and**
> • if the manufacturer provides afatinib with the discount agreed in the patient access scheme.
> www.nice.org.uk/TA310

Axitinib, a tyrosine kinase inhibitor, is licensed for the treatment of advanced renal cell carcinoma following failure of previous treatment with sunitinib or a cytokine (aldesleukin or interferon alfa).

Bosutinib is licensed for the treatment of chronic, accelerated and blast phase Philadelphia chromosome-positive chronic myeloid leukaemia, in those previously treated with one or more tyrosine kinase inhibitors, and for whom imatinib, nilotinib and dasatinib are not clinically appropriate.

> **NICE guidance**
> **Bosutinib for previously treated chronic myeloid leukaemia (November 2013)**
> Bosutinib is **not** recommended within its marketing authorisation for treating Philadelphia-chromosome-positive chronic myeloid leukaemia.
> www.nice.org.uk/TA299

Cabozantinib, an inhibitor of several protein kinases, is licensed for the treatment of progressive, unresectable locally advanced or metastatic medullary thyroid carcinoma.

Crizotinib, a tyrosine kinase inhibitor, is licensed for previously treated anaplastic lymphoma kinase (ALK)-positive advanced non-small cell lung cancer.

> **NICE guidance**
> **Crizotinib for previously treated non-small-cell lung cancer associated with an anaplastic lymphoma kinase fusion gene (September 2013)**
> Crizotinib is **not** recommended within its marketing authorisation, for treating adults with previously treated anaplastic-lymphoma-kinase-positive advanced non-small-cell lung cancer.
> www.nice.org.uk/TA296

Dabrafenib is a BRAF kinase inhibitor licensed as monotherapy for the treatment of unresectable or metastatic melanoma with a BRAF V600 mutation; it should not be used in patients with BRAF wild-type melanoma.

> **NICE guidance**
> **Dabrafenib for treating unresectable or metastatic BRAF V600 mutation-positive melanoma (October 2014)**
> Dabrafenib is recommended, within its marketing authorisation, as an option for treating unresectable or metastatic BRAF V600 mutation-positive melanoma only if the manufacturer provides dabrafenib with the discount agreed in the patient access scheme.
> www.nice.org.uk/TA321

Dasatinib, a tyrosine kinase inhibitor, is licensed for the treatment of chronic myeloid leukaemia in those who have resistance to or intolerance of previous therapy, including imatinib. It is also licensed for newly diagnosed Philadelphia chromosome-positive chronic myeloid leukaemia in the chronic phase and for acute lymphoblastic leukaemia (Philadelphia chromosome positive) in those who have resistance to or intolerance of previous therapy.

The *Scottish Medicines Consortium* (p. 4) has advised (April 2007) that the use of dasatinib (*Sprycel®*) in

NHS Scotland is restricted to patients in the chronic phase of chronic myeloid leukaemia.

> ### NICE guidance
> ### Dasatinib, nilotinib and standard-dose imatinib for the first-line treatment of chronic myeloid leukaemia (April 2012)
>
> Standard-dose imatinib is recommended as an option for the first-line treatment of adults with chronic phase Philadelphia-chromosome-positive chronic myeloid leukaemia (CML); see also NICE guidance Imatinib for chronic myeloid leukaemia (October 2003), p. 608.
>
> Nilotinib is recommended as an option for the first-line treatment of adults with chronic phase Philadelphia-chromosome-positive CML if the manufacturer makes nilotinib available with the discount agreed as part of the patient access scheme.
>
> Dasatinib is **not** recommended for the first-line treatment of chronic phase Philadelphia-chromosome-positive CML
>
> www.nice.org.uk/TA251

> ### NICE guidance
> ### Dasatinib, high-dose imatinib and nilotinib for the treatment of imatinib-resistant chronic myeloid leukaemia (CML), and dasatinib and nilotinib for people with CML for whom treatment with imatinib has failed because of intolerance (January 2012)
>
> Nilotinib is recommended for the treatment of chronic or accelerated phase Philadelphia-chromosome-positive chronic myeloid leukaemia (CML) in adults:
> - whose CML is resistant to treatment with standard-dose imatinib, **or**
> - who have imatinib intolerance, **and**
> - if the manufacturer makes nilotinib available with the discount agreed as part of the patient access scheme.
>
> Dasatinib is **not** recommended for the treatment of chronic, accelerated or blast-crisis phase CML in adults with imatinib intolerance or whose CML is resistant to treatment with standard-dose imatinib.
>
> High-dose imatinib is **not** recommended for the treatment of chronic, accelerated or blast-crisis phase Philadelphia-chromosome-positive CML that is resistant to standard-dose imatinib.
>
> www.nice.org.uk/TA241

Erlotinib, a tyrosine kinase inhibitor, is licensed in combination with gemcitabine for the treatment of metastatic pancreatic cancer. It is also licensed for the treatment of locally advanced or metastatic non-small cell lung cancer after failure of previous chemotherapy and as monotherapy for maintenance treatment of locally advanced or metastatic non-small cell lung cancer with stable disease after four cycles of platinum-based chemotherapy.

The *Scottish Medicines Consortium* (p. 4) has advised (May 2006) that erlotinib (*Tarceva*®) is accepted for restricted use within NHS Scotland for the treatment of locally advanced or metastatic non-small cell lung cancer, after failure of at least one chemotherapy regimen. Erlotinib is restricted to use in patients who would otherwise be eligible for treatment with docetaxel monotherapy. The *Scottish Medicines Consortium* (p. 4) has also advised (December 2011) that erlotinib (*Tarce-*

va®) is accepted for use within NHS Scotland for the first-line treatment of patients with locally advanced or metastatic non-small cell lung cancer (NSCLC) with epidermal growth factor receptor (EGFR) activating mutations.

> ### NICE guidance
> ### Erlotinib for non-small-cell lung cancer (November 2008)
>
> Erlotinib is recommended, as an alternative to docetaxel, as second-line treatment for locally advanced or metastatic non-small-cell lung cancer after failure of previous chemotherapy, on the basis that it is provided by the manufacturer at an overall treatment cost equal to that of docetaxel. Erlotinib is **not** recommended in patients for whom docetaxel is unsuitable or as third-line treatment after docetaxel.
>
> www.nice.org.uk/TA162

> ### NICE guidance
> ### Erlotinib monotherapy for maintenance treatment of non-small-cell lung cancer (June 2011)
>
> Erlotinib monotherapy is **not** recommended for maintenance treatment in people with locally advanced or metastatic non-small-cell lung cancer who have stable disease after platinum-based first-line chemotherapy.
>
> www.nice.org.uk/TA227

> ### NICE guidance
> ### Erlotinib for the first-line treatment of locally advanced or metastatic EGFR-TK mutation-positive non-small-cell lung cancer (June 2012)
>
> Erlotinib is recommended as an option for the first-line treatment of locally advanced or metastatic non-small-cell lung cancer if:
> - they test positive for the epidermal growth factor tyrosine kinase (EGFR-TK) mutation **and**
> - the manufacturer provides erlotinib at the discounted price agreed under the patient access scheme (as revised in 2012).
>
> www.nice.org.uk/TA258

Everolimus, a protein kinase inhibitor, is licensed for the treatment of advanced renal cell carcinoma when the disease has progressed despite treatment with vascular endothelial growth factor-targeted therapy (see NICE guidance below), and for the treatment of unresectable or metastatic, well- or moderately-differentiated neuroendocrine tumours of pancreatic origin. It is licensed for the treatment of subependymal giant cell astrocytoma associated with tuberous sclerosis complex in patients who require therapeutic intervention but are not amenable to surgery, and for renal angiomyolipoma associated with tuberous sclerosis complex in patients at risk of complications, but who do not require immediate surgery. Everolimus is also licensed for the treatment of hormone-receptor-positive, human epidermal growth factor-2 (HER-2) negative advanced breast cancer, in combination with exemestane, in postmenopausal women without symptomatic visceral disease after recurrence or progression following a non-steroidal aromatase inhibitor.

8 Malignant disease and immunosuppression

nosed acute lymphoblastic leukaemia in combination with other chemotherapy, and as monotherapy for relapsed or refractory acute lymphoblastic leukaemia. Imatinib is also licensed for the treatment of unresectable dermatofibrosarcoma protuberans and for patients with recurrent or metastatic dermatofibrosarcoma protuberans who cannot have surgery.

Imatinib is also licensed for the treatment of myelodysplastic/myeloproliferative diseases associated with platelet-derived growth factor receptor gene rearrangement and for the treatment of advanced hypereosinophilic syndrome and chronic eosinophilic leukaemia.

The *Scottish Medicines Consortium* (p. 4) has advised (March 2002) that imatinib (*Glivec*®) should be used for chronic myeloid leukaemia only under specialist supervision in accordance with British Society of Haematology guidelines (November 2001). The *Scottish Medicines Consortium* (p. 4) has also advised (February 2012) that imatinib (*Glivec*®) is accepted for restricted use within NHS Scotland for the treatment of adult patients who are at significant risk of relapse following resection of a KIT (CD117) positive gastrointestinal stromal tumour (GIST) and who are at high risk of recurrence following complete resection (according to the Armed Forces Institute of Pathology (AFIP) risk criteria).

> **NICE guidance**
> **Everolimus for the second-line treatment of advanced renal cell carcinoma (April 2011)**
> Everolimus is **not** recommended for the second-line treatment of advanced renal cell carcinoma.
> www.nice.org.uk/TA219

> **NICE guidance**
> **Everolimus in combination with exemestane for treating advanced HER2-negative hormone-receptor-positive breast cancer after endocrine therapy (August 2013)**
> Everolimus, in combination with exemestane, is **not** recommended within its marketing authorisation for treating postmenopausal women with advanced human epidermal growth factor receptor 2 (HER2) negative hormone-receptor-positive breast cancer that has recurred or progressed following treatment with a non-steroidal aromatase inhibitor.
> www.nice.org.uk/TA295

Gefitinib, a tyrosine kinase inhibitor, is licensed for the treatment of locally advanced or metastatic non-small cell lung cancer with activating mutations of epidermal growth factor receptor.

> **NICE guidance**
> **Gefitinib for the first-line treatment of locally advanced or metastatic non-small-cell lung cancer (July 2010)**
> Gefitinib is recommended as an option for the first-line treatment of locally advanced or metastatic non-small-cell lung cancer if the patient tests positive for the epidermal growth receptor tyrosine kinase (EGFR-TK) mutation and the manufacturer provides gefitinib at the fixed price agreed under the patient access scheme.
> www.nice.org.uk/TA192

Ibrutinib, a tyrosine kinase inhibitor, is licensed for the treatment of adults with relapsed or refractory mantle cell lymphoma. It is also licensed for the treatment of adults with chronic lymphocytic leukaemia, who have received at least one prior therapy, or as first-line treatment in patients with 17p deletion or TP53 mutation who are unsuitable for chemo-immunotherapy.

Idelalisib, a protein kinase inhibitor, is licensed in combination with rituximab for the treatment of chronic lymphocytic leukaemia in patients who have received at least one previous therapy, or as first-line treatment in the presence of 17p deletion or TP53 mutation in patients unsuitable for chemo-immunotherapy. It is also licensed as monotherapy for the treatment of follicular lymphoma refractory to two lines of treatment.

Imatinib, a tyrosine kinase inhibitor, is licensed for the treatment of newly diagnosed chronic myeloid leukaemia where bone marrow transplantation is not considered first-line treatment, and for chronic myeloid leukaemia in chronic phase after failure of interferon alfa, or in accelerated phase, or in blast crisis (see NICE guidance below). It is also licensed for the treatment of c-kit (CD117)-positive unresectable or metastatic malignant gastro-intestinal stromal tumours (GIST), and as adjuvant treatment following resection of c-kit (CD117)-positive GIST, in patients at significant risk of relapse. Imatinib is licensed for the treatment of newly diag-

> **NICE guidance**
> **Imatinib for chronic myeloid leukaemia (October 2003)**
> Imatinib is recommended as first-line treatment for Philadelphia-chromosome-positive chronic myeloid leukaemia in the chronic phase and as an option for patients presenting in the accelerated phase or with blast crisis, provided that imatinib has not been used previously.
> See also NICE guidance Dasatinib, nilotinib and standard-dose imatinib for the first-line treatment of chronic myeloid leukaemia (April 2012), p. 607 and NICE guidance Dasatinib, high-dose imatinib and nilotinib for the treatment of imatinib-resistant chronic myeloid leukaemia, and dasatinib and nilotinib for people with CML for whom treatment of imatinib has failed because of intolerance (January 2012), p. 607
> www.nice.org.uk/TA70

> **NICE guidance**
> **Imatinib for the adjuvant treatment of gastro-intestinal stromal tumours (November 2014)**
> Imatinib is recommended as an option for adjuvant treatment of adult patients who are at high risk of relapse after surgery for KIT (CD117)-positive gastro-intestinal stromal tumours, as defined by the Miettinen 2006 criteria (based on tumour size, location, and mitotic rate), for up to 3 years.
> Patients currently receiving treatment initiated within the NHS with imatinib that is not recommended for them by NICE in this guidance should be able to continue treatment until they and their NHS clinician consider it appropriate to stop.
> www.nice.org.uk/TA326

> **NICE guidance**
> **Imatinib for the treatment of unresectable and/or metastatic gastro-intestinal stromal tumours (October 2004)**
>
> Imatinib 400 mg daily is recommended as first-line management of KIT (CD117)-positive unresectable or metastatic, or both, gastro-intestinal stromal tumours. Continued therapy is recommended only if a response to initial treatment [as defined by Southwest Oncology Group criteria available at www.nice.org.uk/TA86] is achieved within 12 weeks. Patients who have responded should be assessed at 12-week intervals. Discontinue if tumour ceases to respond.
>
> www.nice.org.uk/TA86

> **NICE guidance**
> **Imatinib for the treatment of unresectable and/or metastatic gastro-intestinal stromal tumours (November 2010)**
>
> Imatinib 600 mg daily or 800 mg daily is **not** recommended for unresectable or metastatic, or both, gastro-intestinal stromal tumours whose disease has progressed after treatment with imatinib 400 mg daily.
>
> www.nice.org.uk/TA209

Lapatinib, a tyrosine kinase inhibitor, is licensed for the treatment of advanced or metastatic breast cancer in patients with tumours that overexpress human epidermal growth factor receptor-2 (HER2). It is indicated, in combination with capecitabine, for patients who have had previous treatment with an anthracycline, a taxane, and trastuzumab, in combination with trastuzumab, for patients with hormone-receptor-negative disease who have had previous treatment with trastuzumab in combination with chemotherapy, or for postmenopausal women with hormone-receptor-positive disease in combination with an aromatase inhibitor section 8.3.4.1.

> **NICE guidance**
> **Lapatinib or trastuzumab in combination with an aromatase inhibitor for the first-line treatment of metastatic hormone-receptor-positive breast cancer that overexpresses HER2 (June 2012)**
>
> Lapatinib or trastuzumab in combination with an aromatase inhibitor is **not** recommended for first-line treatment in postmenopausal women of metastatic hormone-receptor-positive breast cancer that overexpresses human epidermal growth factor receptor 2 (HER2).
>
> Postmenopausal women currently receiving lapatinib or trastuzumab in combination with an aromatase inhibitor for this indication should have the option to continue treatment until they and their clinician consider it appropriate to stop.
>
> www.nice.org.uk/TA257

Nilotinib, a tyrosine kinase inhibitor, is licensed for the treatment of newly diagnosed chronic myeloid leukaemia in the chronic phase, and also for patients with chronic or accelerated phase chronic myeloid leukaemia who have resistance to or intolerance of previous therapy, including imatinib.

The *Scottish Medicines Consortium* (p. 4) has advised (February 2008) that nilotinib (*Tasigna*®) is accepted for restricted use within NHS Scotland for the treatment of chronic-phase chronic myeloid leukaemia in adults resistant to or intolerant of at least one previous therapy, including imatinib, and (July 2011) for the treatment of adults with newly diagnosed chronic myeloid leukaemia in the chronic phase.

> **NICE guidance**
> **Dasatinib, nilotinib and standard-dose imatinib for the first-line treatment of chronic myeloid leukaemia (April 2012)**
> See p. 607

> **NICE guidance**
> **Dasatinib, high-dose imatinib and nilotinib for the treatment of imatinib-resistant chronic myeloid leukaemia (CML), and dasatinib and nilotinib for people with CML for whom treatment with imatinib has failed because of intolerance (January 2012)**
> See p. 607

Pazopanib, a tyrosine kinase inhibitor, is licensed for advanced renal cell carcinoma, as first-line treatment and for patients who have had previous treatment with cytokine therapy for advanced disease. It is also licensed for the treatment of selective subtypes of advanced soft tissue sarcoma (consult product literature for details).

The *Scottish Medicines Consortium* (p. 4) has advised (February 2011) that pazopanib (*Votrient*®) is accepted for restricted use within NHS Scotland for the first-line treatment of advanced renal cell carcinoma and (December 2012) is **not** recommended for use within NHS Scotland for the treatment of selective subtypes of advanced soft tissue sarcoma in patients who have received prior chemotherapy for metastatic disease, or who have progressed within 12 months after neoadjuvant therapy.

> **NICE guidance**
> **Pazopanib for the first-line treatment of advanced renal cell carcinoma (updated August 2013)**
>
> Pazopanib is recommended as a first-line treatment option for people with advanced renal cell carcinoma:
> - who have not received prior cytokine therapy and have an Eastern Cooperative Oncology Group performance status of 0 or 1 **and**
> - if the manufacturer provides pazopanib at the discounted price agreed under the patient access scheme.
>
> www.nice.org.uk/TA215

Ponatinib is licensed for the treatment of chronic, accelerated, or blast phase chronic myeloid leukaemia in patients who have the T315I mutation or who have resistance to or intolerance of dasatinib or nilotinib, and for whom subsequent treatment with imatinib is not clinically appropriate. It is also licensed for the treatment of Philadelphia chromosome-positive acute lymphoblastic leukaemia in patients who have the T315I mutation or who have resistance to or intolerance of dasatinib, and for whom subsequent treatment with imatinib is not clinically appropriate.

MHRA/CHM advice
Ponatinib: risk of vascular occlusive events (November 2014)

The benefits and risks of ponatinib have been reviewed by the European Medicines Agency's Committee on Medicinal Products for Human Use, which has recommended that strengthened warnings should be added to the product information aimed at minimising the risk of blood clots and blockages in the arteries. The review concluded that available evidence shows that the risk of blood vessel blockage with ponatinib is likely to be dose-dependent. However, the data is insufficient to recommend reducing the dose of ponatinib, and there is a risk that a lower dose might not be as effective as the current dose in all patients and in long-term treatment. Therefore, no change has been made to the recommended starting dose.

Prescribers may wish to consider reducing the dose in patients with chronic phase chronic myeloid leukaemia who are responding well to treatment, and who might be at high risk of blood vessel blockage. Stop ponatinib if a complete response has not occurred within 3 months of treatment, and monitor patients for high blood pressure or signs of heart problems.

Regorafenib, an inhibitor of several protein kinases, is licensed for the treatment of metastatic colorectal cancer in patients who have previously been treated with, or who are unsuitable for, standard treatment including fluoropyrimidine-based chemotherapy, a vascular endothelial growth factor inhibitor, and an epidermal growth factor receptor inhibitor.

Ruxolitinib is a selective inhibitor of the Janus-associated tyrosine kinases JAK1 and JAK2 and is licensed for the treatment of disease-related splenomegaly or symptoms in patients with primary myelofibrosis, post-polycythaemia vera myelofibrosis, or post-essential thrombocythaemia myelofibrosis.

NICE guidance
Ruxolitinib for disease-related splenomegaly or symptoms in adults with myelofibrosis (June 2013)

Ruxolitinib is **not** recommended for the treatment of disease-related splenomegaly or symptoms in adult patients with primary myelofibrosis (also known as chronic idiopathic myelofibrosis), post polycythaemia vera myelofibrosis or post essential thrombocythaemia myelofibrosis.
www.nice.org.uk/TA289

Sorafenib, an inhibitor of multiple kinases, is licensed for the treatment of progressive, locally advanced, or metastatic, differentiated thyroid carcinoma that is refractory to radioactive iodine. It is also licensed for the treatment of advanced renal cell carcinoma when treatment with interferon alfa or interleukin-2 has failed or is unsuitable, and for the treatment of hepatocellular carcinoma—see also NICE Guidance below.

NICE guidance
Sorafenib for the treatment of advanced hepatocellular carcinoma (May 2010)

Sorafenib is **not** recommended for the treatment of advanced hepatocellular carcinoma in patients for whom surgical or locoregional therapies have failed or are unsuitable.
www.nice.org.uk/TA189

Sunitinib, a tyrosine kinase inhibitor, is licensed for the treatment of advanced or metastatic renal cell carcinoma (but see NICE Guidance, below). It is also licensed for the treatment of unresectable or metastatic malignant gastro-intestinal stromal tumours, after failure of imatinib, and for the treatment of unresectable or metastatic pancreatic neuroendocrine tumours.

The *Scottish Medicines Consortium* (p. 4) has advised (October 2009 and April 2011) that sunitinib (*Sutent®*) is accepted for restricted use within NHS Scotland for the treatment of unresectable or metastatic malignant gastro-intestinal stromal tumours after failure of imatinib and for unresectable or metastatic pancreatic neuroendocrine tumours.

NICE guidance
Sunitinib for advanced or metastatic renal cell carcinoma (March 2009)

Sunitinib is recommended as first-line treatment for advanced or metastatic renal cell carcinoma in patients who are suitable for immunotherapy and have an Eastern Cooperative Oncology Group performance status of 0 or 1.
www.nice.org.uk/TA169

NICE guidance
Sunitinib for the treatment of gastro-intestinal stromal tumours (September 2009)

Sunitinib is recommended as an option for treatment in patients with unresectable or metastatic gastro-intestinal tumours if imatinib treatment has failed because of resistance or intolerance, and the cost of sunitinib for the first treatment cycle is met by the manufacturer.
www.nice.org.uk/TA179

NICE guidance
Bevacizumab (first-line), sorafenib (first- and second-line), sunitinib (second-line) and temsirolimus (first-line) for the treatment of advanced or metastatic renal cell carcinoma (August 2009)

Bevacizumab, sorafenib, and temsirolimus are **not** recommended as first-line treatments for people with advanced or metastatic renal cell carcinoma.

Sorafenib and sunitinib are not recommended as second-line treatments for people with advanced or metastatic renal cell carcinoma.
www.nice.org.uk/TA178

Temsirolimus is a protein kinase inhibitor licensed for the first-line treatment of advanced renal cell carcinoma (see NICE Guidance above), and for the treatment of relapsed or refractory mantle cell lymphoma. Hypersensitivity reactions, including some life-threatening and rare fatal reactions, are associated with temsirolimus therapy, usually during administration of the first dose. Symptoms include flushing, chest pain, dyspnoea, apnoea, hypotension, loss of consciousness, and anaphylaxis. Where possible, patients should receive an intravenous dose of antihistamine 30 minutes before starting the temsirolimus infusion. The infusion may have to be stopped temporarily for the treatment of infusion-related effects—consult product literature for appropriate management. If adverse reactions are not managed with dose delays, a dose reduction should be considered—consult product literature.

Vandetanib, a tyrosine kinase inhibitor, is licensed for the treatment of aggressive and symptomatic medullary thyroid cancer in patients with unresectable locally advanced or metastatic disease.

Vemurafenib, a BRAF kinase inhibitor, is licensed as a monotherapy for the treatment of BRAF V600 mutation-positive unresectable or metastatic melanoma.

The *Scottish Medicines Consortium* (p. 4) has advised (November 2013) that vemurafenib (*Zelboraf*®) is accepted for restricted use within NHS Scotland as monotherapy for the first-line treatment of BRAF V600 mutation-positive unresectable or metastatic melanoma.

> **NICE guidance**
> **Vemurafenib for treating locally advanced or metastatic BRAF V600 mutation-positive malignant melanoma (December 2012)**
> Vemurafenib is recommended as an option for the treatment of BRAF V600 mutation-positive unresectable or metastatic melanoma only if the manufacturer provides vemurafenib with the discount agreed in the patient access scheme.
> www.nice.org.uk/TA269

◢ AFATINIB

Indications   see notes above

Cautions   see section 8.1; diarrhoea—proactive management recommended (consult product literature); new or worsening pulmonary symptoms (including dyspnoea, cough, fever)—interrupt treatment until interstitial lung disease is excluded; history of keratitis, ulcerative keratitis, severe dry eyes or use of contact lenses; signs and symptoms of keratitis—promptly refer to ophthalmologist for assessment; cardiac risk factors and conditions which may affect left ventricular ejection fraction—consider cardiac monitoring, including assessment of left ventricular ejection fraction, at baseline and during treatment; protect skin from exposure to sun; signs and symptoms of skin reaction—treat promptly and interrupt afatinib treatment if severe or if Stevens-Johnson syndrome suspected (consult product literature); **interactions**: Appendix 1 (afatinib)

Driving   Ocular adverse reactions may affect performance of skilled tasks e.g. driving

Hepatic impairment   monitor hepatic function regularly and consult product literature for dose adjustment in worsening liver function; manufacturer advises avoid in severe hepatic impairment

Renal impairment   manufacturer advises avoid in severe renal impairment

Pregnancy   manufacturer advises avoid—ensure effective contraception during and for at least one

month after treatment in women of childbearing potential; see also Pregnancy and Reproductive Function, p. 575

Breast-feeding   manufacturer advises avoid—present in milk in *animal* studies

Side-effects   see section 8.1; also diarrhoea, dehydration, weight loss, decreased appetite, dyspepsia, dysgeusia, pyrexia, paronychia, cystitis, renal failure, hypokalaemia, muscle spasms, dry eyes, conjunctivitis, epistaxis, rhinorrhoea, rash (see Cautions), acne, pruritus, dry skin, hand-foot syndrome; *less commonly* interstitial lung disease, keratitis

Dose

- ADULT over 18 years, 40 mg once daily; if tolerated may be increased after 3 weeks to 50 mg once daily (but consult product literature); for dose adjustment due to side-effects, consult product literature

Giotrif® (Boehringer Ingelheim) ▼ PoM
Tablets, f/c, afatinib (as dimaleate) 20 mg (white-yellow), net price 28-tab pack = £2023.28; 30 mg (dark blue), 28-tab pack = £2023.28; 40 mg (light blue), 28-tab pack = £2023.28; 50 mg (dark blue), 28-tab pack = £2023.28. Label: 25, counselling, administration (see below), driving, see Cautions above
Counselling   Tablets should be taken whole on an empty stomach. Food should not be consumed for at least 3 hours before and at least 1 hour after each dose
Note   *Giotrif*® tablets may be dispersed in approximately 100 mL of noncarbonated water by stirring occasionally for up to 15 minutes (must not be crushed). The dispersion should be swallowed immediately, and the glass rinsed with the same volume of water which should also be swallowed. The dispersion can also be administered via a gastric tube

◢ AXITINIB

Indications   see notes above

Cautions   see section 8.1; hypertension (blood pressure should be well-controlled before starting and monitored during treatment); monitor for thyroid dysfunction; monitor haemoglobin or haematocrit before and during treatment; monitor for symptoms of gastro-intestinal perforation or fistula; monitor for proteinuria before and during treatment; monitor liver function before and during treatment; **interactions**: Appendix 1 (axitinib)

Contra-indications   untreated brain metastases; recent active gastro-intestinal bleeding

Hepatic impairment   reduce starting dose in moderate impairment; avoid in severe impairment—no information available

Pregnancy   manufacturer advises avoid unless potential benefit outweighs risk (toxicity in *animal* studies)—effective contraception required during and for up to 1 week after treatment; see also Pregnancy and Reproductive Function, p. 575

Side-effects   see section 8.1; also diarrhoea, constipation, abdominal pain, dyspepsia, flatulence, haemorrhoids, gastro-intestinal perforation, anal fistula, hypertension, haemorrhage (including gastro-intestinal, cerebral and haemoptysis), dysphonia, dyspnoea, cough, dysgeusia, headache, dizziness, fatigue, asthenia, decreased appetite, weight loss, hypothyroidism, hyperthyroidism, dehydration, proteinuria, hyperkalaemia, hypercalcaemia, renal failure, myalgia, arthralgia, tinnitus, hand-foot syndrome, rash, dry skin, pruritus, erythema; *less commonly* hypertensive crisis, posterior reversible encephalopathy syndrome, polycythaemia

Dose
- See Doses, p. 574

Inlyta® (Pfizer) ▼ PoM
Tablets, f/c, red, axitinib 1 mg, net price 56-tab pack = £703.40; 3 mg, 56-tab pack = £2110.20; 5 mg, 56-tab pack = £3517.00; 7 mg, 56-tab pack = £4923.80. Label: 25

BOSUTINIB

Indications   see notes above

Cautions   history or risk factors for QT prolongation (including recent cardiac event or concomitant use of drugs that prolong the QT interval)—monitor ECG and correct hypokalaemia and hypomagnesaemia before and during treatment; cardiac disease; significant gastrointestinal disorder; history of pancreatitis—withhold treatment if lipase elevated and abdominal symptoms occur; monitor liver function before treatment initiation, then monthly for the first 3 months and thereafter as clinically indicated—consult product literature for management of raised transaminases; monitor full blood count weekly for the first month and then monthly thereafter or as clinically indicated; monitor for signs and symptoms of fluid retention (including pericardial effusion, pleural effusion and pulmonary oedema); **interactions**: Appendix 1 (bosutinib)

Hepatic impairment   caution—no information available

Pregnancy   avoid—toxicity in *animal* studies; effective contraception required during treatment in women; see also Pregnancy and Reproductive Function, p. 575

Breast-feeding   manufacturer advises avoid—no information available

Side-effects   see section 8.1; also decreased appetite, dehydration, diarrhoea, abdominal pain, gastritis, hepatotoxicity, abnormal liver function, pericardial effusion, QT prolongation, oedema, cough, dyspnoea, pleural effusion, malaise, pyrexia, infection, biochemical and electrolyte disturbances, renal impairment and failure, arthralgia, myalgia, rash, urticaria, acne, pruritus; *less commonly* pancreatitis, gastric haemorrhage, pericarditis, pulmonary oedema, respiratory failure, pulmonary hypertension, tinnitus

Dose
- ADULT over 18 years, 500 mg once daily; for dose adjustment due to side-effects, or incomplete haematologic response by week 8, or incomplete cytogenetic response by week 12, consult product literature

Bosulif® (Pfizer) ▼ PoM
Tablets, f/c, bosutinib (as monohydrate) 100 mg (yellow), net price 28-tab pack = £859.17; 500 mg (red), 28-tab pack = £3436.67. Label: 21

CABOZANTINIB

Indications   see notes above

Cautions   see section 8.1; patients at increased risk of gastro-intestinal perforation, fistulas and intra-abdominal abscess—consult product literature for further details; patients at risk of thromboembolic events including myocardial infarction—discontinue if symptoms develop; patients at risk of haemorrhage (including tumour involvement of the trachea or bronchi)—discontinue if symptoms develop; withhold treatment for at least 28 days before elective surgery and restart only if adequate wound healing—discontinue in patients with wound healing complications requiring medical intervention; hypertension—discontinue treatment if uncontrolled despite medical intervention; concomitant use of drugs which increase the risk of osteonecrosis of the jaw e.g. bisphosphonates—discontinue treatment at least 28 days before elective invasive dental procedures—monitor for symptoms before and during treatment and discontinue if osteonecrosis develops; palmar-plantar erythrodysaesthesia syndrome—consider treatment interruption if severe and restart at a lower dose when resolved to grade 1; monitor urine protein regularly and discontinue if nephrotic syndrome develops; susceptibility to QT-interval prolongation (e.g. cardiac disease, electrolyte disturbances, bradycardia, concomitant use of drugs that prolong the QT interval)—monitor ECG and electrolytes periodically; **interactions**: Appendix 1 (cabozantinib)
Driving Fatigue and weakness may affect performance of skilled tasks e.g. driving

Contra-indications   Reversible Posterior Leukoencephalopathy Syndrome

Hepatic impairment   manufacturer advises avoid

Renal impairment   manufacturer advises caution in renal impairment; avoid in severe impairment

Pregnancy   manufacturer advises avoid unless potential benefit outweighs risk—toxicity in *animal* studies; patients and their sexual partners must use effective contraception (in addition to barrier method) during treatment and for at least 4 months after the last dose; see also Pregnancy and Reproductive Function, p. 575

Breast-feeding   manufacturer advises discontinue breast-feeding during treatment and for at least 4 months after the last dose

Side-effects   see section 8.1; also diarrhoea, nausea, stomatitis, constipation, vomiting, abdominal pain, dysphagia, dyspepsia, glossodynia, cholelithiasis, gastro-intestinal perforation, gastrointestinal haemorrhage, pancreatitis, haemorrhoids, anal fissure, cheilitis, decreased appetite, dehydration, atrial fibrillation, hypertension, lymphopenia, neutropenia, platelet disorders, hypotension, venous thrombosis, pallor, peripheral coldness, dysphonia, oropharyngeal pain, non-gastro-intestinal fistula, pulmonary embolism, respiratory tract haemorrhage, pneumonia, aspiration, dysgeusia, headache, dizziness, peripheral neuropathy, paraesthesia, tremor, anxiety, depression, abscess, folliculitis, fungal infection, hypothyroidism, proteinuria, dysuria, haematuria, hypocalcaemia, hypokalaemia, hypophosphataemia, hyperbilirubinaemia, hypoalbuminaemia, arthralgia, muscle spasms, musculoskeletal chest pain, osteonecrosis of the jaw, blurred vision, tinnitus, palmar-plantar erythrodysaesthesia syndrome, hair colour changes, rash, dry skin, alopecia, erythema, hyperkeratosis, acne, abnormal hair growth, skin exfoliation and hypopigmentation, impaired wound healing, chills, face oedema, mucosal inflammation; *less commonly* gastro-intestinal fistula, oesophagitis, angina, supraventricular tachycardia, arterial thrombosis, atelectasis, pharyngeal oedema, pneumonitis, delirium, ataxia, hepatic encephalopathy, loss of consciousness, speech disorder, transient ischaemic attack, posterior reversible encephalopathy syndrome, aspergilloma, amenorrhoea, vaginal haemorrhage, acute renal failure, rhabdomyolysis, cataract, conjunctivitis, hypoacusis, skin ulcer, telangiectasia, cyst, facial pain

Dose

- ADULT over 18 years, 140 mg once daily; for dose adjustment or treatment interruption due to side effects, consult product literature (closely monitor for first 8 weeks of therapy)

Cometriq® (Swedish Orphan) ▼ PoM
Capsules, cabozantinib 20 mg (grey), net price 28-cap pack = £4800.00; 80 mg (orange), 28-cap pack = £4800.00. Label: 25, counselling, driving, see Cautions above
Counselling Food should not be consumed for at least 2 hours before and at least 1 hour after each dose

CRIZOTINIB

Indications see notes above

Cautions see section 8.1; risk of gastrointestinal perforation (including history of diverticulitis, metastases of gastrointestinal tract, and concomitant use of drugs which may cause gastrointestinal perforation), inform all patients of early signs and symptoms and advise to seek immediate medical attention—discontinue treatment if gastrointestinal perforation occurs; monitor ECG and electrolytes (correct if abnormal) in all patients before starting treatment, then periodically and as clinically indicated thereafter—patients with susceptibility to QT-prolongation (including bradycardia, history of cardiac disease, concomitant use of drugs that prolong QT interval, and electrolyte disturbances) should also have periodic renal monitoring; monitor for signs and symptoms of treatment-emergent bradycardia (including syncope, dizziness and hypotension)—monitor blood pressure and heart rate regularly; monitor liver function once a week during the first 2 months of treatment, then at least monthly thereafter and as clinically indicted (sic); fatal interstitial lung disease and pneumonitis reported (monitor patients with pulmonary symptoms, withdraw treatment if suspected, and permanently discontinue treatment if diagnosed); vision disorders reported—consider full ophthalmological evaluation if vision disorder worsens or persists; **interactions**: Appendix 1 (crizotinib)
Driving Symptomatic bradycardia (including syncope, dizziness and hypotension), vision disorder and fatigue may affect performance of skilled tasks (e.g. driving or operating machinery)

Hepatic impairment manufacturer advises caution in mild to moderate impairment; avoid in severe impairment; also see Cautions

Renal impairment reduce dose to 250 mg once daily in severe impairment not requiring peritoneal dialysis or hemodialysis, may be increased to 200 mg twice daily after at least 4 weeks, based on individual assessment of safety and tolerability

Pregnancy avoid (toxicity in *animal* studies); ensure effective contraception during and for at least 90 days after treatment; see also Pregnancy and Reproductive Function, p. 575

Breast-feeding avoid—no information available

Side-effects see section 8.1; also diarrhoea, constipation, dyspepsia, bradycardia, syncope, QT-interval prolongation, oedema, interstitial lung disease (including pneumonitis), fatigue, neuropathy, dizziness, taste disturbance, decreased appetite, hypo-

phosphataemia, renal cyst, vision disorder; rash; *less commonly*; gastrointestinal perforation (fatalities reported), hepatotoxicity (including fatal hepatic failure)

Dose

- ADULT over 18 years, 250 mg twice daily; for dose adjustment due to side effects, consult product literature

Xalkori® (Pfizer) ▼ PoM
Capsules, crizotinib 200 mg (white/pink), net price 60-cap pack = £4689.00; 250 mg (pink), 60-cap pack = £4689.00. Label: 25

DABRAFENIB

Indications see notes above

Cautions pyrexia (interrupt treatment if ≥ 38.5°C and assess for signs and symptoms of infection—consult product literature); assess for cutaneous squamous cell carcinoma and new primary melanoma before treatment, monthly during treatment, and for 6 months after discontinuation or until initiation of alternative treatment; assess and monitor for non-cutaneous secondary or recurrent malignancy before, during, and for 6 months after discontinuation or until initiation of alternative treatment—consult product literature; monitor serum creatinine and other signs of renal failure—consult product literature and interrupt dose as appropriate; monitor for ophthalmologic reactions including uveitis and iritis; promptly investigate signs and symptoms of pancreatitis—consult product literature; monitor ECG and electrolytes (including magnesium) before and one month after treatment initiation and after each dose modification—consult product literature if abnormalities occur; **interactions**: Appendix 1 (dabrafenib)
Driving Ocular adverse reactions and fatigue may affect performance of skilled tasks e.g. driving

Contra-indications BRAF wild-type melanoma; uncorrectable electrolyte abnormalities (including magnesium); long QT syndrome, or concomitant use of drugs that prolong the QT interval

Hepatic impairment manufacturer advises caution in moderate to severe impairment; additional monitoring of ECG and electrolytes required—consult product literature

Renal impairment manufacturer advises caution in severe impairment—no information available

Pregnancy manufacturer advises avoid unless potential benefit outweighs risk (toxicity in *animal* studies)—effective non-hormonal contraception required during and for one month after treatment in women of childbearing potential; see also Pregnancy and Reproductive Function, p. 575

Breast-feeding manufacturer advises avoid

Side-effects see section 8.1; also decreased appetite, diarrhoea, constipation, decrease in left ventricular ejection fraction, cough, headache, malaise, pyrexia, chills, influenza-like symptoms, hyperglycaemia, basal cell carcinoma, cutaneous squamous cell carcinoma, hypophosphataemia, arthralgia, myalgia, papilloma, keratosis, hyperkeratosis, acrochordon, rash, hand-foot syndrome, dry skin, pruritus, skin lesions, erythema; *less commonly* pancreatitis, QT-interval prolongation, new primary melanoma, nephritis, renal failure, uveitis, panniculitis

Dose
* ADULT over 18 years, 150 mg every 12 hours; for dose adjustment due to side-effects, consult product literature

Tafinlar® (GSK) ▼ PoM
Capsules, dabrafenib (as mesilate) 50 mg (dark red), net price 28-cap pack = £933.33; 75 mg (dark pink), 28-cap pack = £1400.00. Label: 23, 25, counselling, driving, see Cautions above

DASATINIB

Indications see notes above

Cautions see section 8.1; susceptibility to QT-interval prolongation (correct hypokalaemia or hypomagnesaemia before starting treatment); risk of cardiac dysfunction (monitor closely); interactions: Appendix 1 (dasatinib)
Pulmonary arterial hypertension Patients should be evaluated for signs and symptoms of underlying cardiopulmonary disease before starting treatment; echocardiography should be performed at the start of treatment in patients with symptoms of cardiac disease and considered for patients with risk factors for cardiac or pulmonary disease.
Treatment should be interrupted or the dose reduced in patients who develop dyspnoea or fatigue, while they are evaluated for common aetiologies (e.g. pleural effusion, pulmonary oedema, anaemia or lung infiltration); pulmonary arterial hypertension should be considered in the absence of these conditions, and if there is no improvement following dose reduction or interruption.
If pulmonary arterial hypertension is confirmed, dasatinib should be permanently discontinued

Hepatic impairment manufacturer advises caution in hepatic impairment

Pregnancy manufacturer advises avoid unless potential benefit outweighs risk—toxicity in *animal* studies; effective contraception required during treatment; see also Pregnancy and Reproductive Function, p. 575

Breast-feeding discontinue breast-feeding

Side-effects see section 8.1; also diarrhoea, anorexia, weight changes, abdominal pain, taste disturbance, constipation, dyspepsia, colitis, gastritis; arrhythmias, congestive heart failure, hypertension, chest pain, flushing, haemorrhage (including gastro-intestinal and CNS haemorrhage), palpitation; dyspnoea, pulmonary hypertension, cough, oedema (more common in patients over 65 years old), pleural effusion; depression, dizziness, headache, insomnia, neuropathy; influenza-like symptoms; musculoskeletal pain; visual disturbances; tinnitus; acne, dry skin, sweating, pruritus, dermatitis, urticaria; *less commonly* pancreatitis, hepatitis, cholestasis, cholecystitis, oesophagitis, hypotension, transient ischaemic attack, thrombophlebitis, syncope, gynaecomastia, irregular menstruation, urinary frequency, proteinuria, hypocalcaemia, rhabdomyolysis, hypersensitivity reactions (including erythema nodosum), photosensitivity, and pigmentation and nail disorders; *rarely* cor pulmonale; thrombosis and interstitial lung disease also reported

Dose
* Chronic phase chronic myeloid leukaemia, ADULT over 18 years 100 mg once daily, increased if necessary to max. 140 mg once daily
* Accelerated and blast phase chronic myeloid leukaemia, acute lymphoblastic leukaemia, ADULT over 18 years 140 mg once daily, increased if necessary to max. 180 mg once daily

Sprycel® (Bristol-Myers Squibb) PoM
Tablets, f/c, dasatinib (as monohydrate) 20 mg, net price 60-tab pack = £1252.48; 50 mg, 60-tab pack = £2504.96; 80 mg, 30-tab pack = £2504.96; 100 mg, 30-tab pack = £2504.96; 140 mg, 30-tab pack = £2504.96. Label: 25

ERLOTINIB

Indications see notes above

Cautions see section 8.1; pre-existing liver disease or concomitant use with hepatotoxic drugs—monitor liver function; dose adjustment may be necessary if smoking started or stopped during treatment; see MHRA/CHM advice Epidermal Growth Factor Receptor (EGFR) Inhibitors: Serious Cases of Keratitis and Ulcerative Keratitis, p. 599; interactions: Appendix 1 (erlotinib)

Hepatic impairment manufacturer advises caution in mild to moderate impairment; avoid in severe impairment

Renal impairment manufacturer advises avoid in severe impairment

Pregnancy manufacturer advises avoid—toxicity in *animal* studies; effective contraception required during and for at least 2 weeks after treatment; see also Pregnancy and Reproductive Function, p. 575

Breast-feeding manufacturer advises avoid—no information available

Side-effects see section 8.1 and notes above; also diarrhoea, abdominal pain, dyspepsia, flatulence; anorexia, depression, neuropathy, headache; fatigue, rigor; conjunctivitis; pruritus, dry skin; *less commonly* gastro-intestinal perforation, interstitial lung disease—discontinue if unexplained symptoms such as dyspnoea, cough or fever occur; eyelash changes; *rarely* hepatic injury; *very rarely* corneal perforation or ulceration, Stevens-Johnson syndrome, and toxic epidermal necrolysis

Dose
* Non-small cell lung cancer, 150 mg once daily
* Pancreatic cancer, 100 mg once daily in combination with gemcitabine

Tarceva® (Roche) PoM
Tablets, f/c, white-yellow, erlotinib (as hydrochloride) 25 mg, net price 30-tab pack = £378.33; 100 mg, 30-tab pack = £1324.14; 150 mg, 30-tab pack = £1631.53. Label: 23

EVEROLIMUS

Indications see notes above

Cautions see section 8.1; monitor blood-glucose concentration, serum-triglycerides and serum-cholesterol before treatment and periodically thereafter; concomitant use of drugs that increase risk of bleeding; history of bleeding disorders; monitor renal function before treatment and periodically thereafter; reduce dose or discontinue if severe side-effects occur—consult product literature; interactions: Appendix 1 (everolimus)
Pneumonitis Non-infectious pneumonitis reported. Patients should be advised to seek urgent medical advice if new or worsening respiratory symptoms occur

Hepatic impairment consult product literature

Pregnancy manufacturer advises avoid (toxicity in *animal* studies); effective contraception must be used

(side margin) **Malignant disease and immunosuppression** **8**

during and for up to 8 weeks after treatment; see also Pregnancy and Reproductive Function, p. 575

Breast-feeding manufacturer advises avoid

Side-effects see section 8.1; also diarrhoea, dry mouth, abdominal pain, dysphagia, anorexia, taste disturbance, chest pain, hypertension, hyperlipidaemia, hypercholesterolaemia, peripheral oedema, pneumonitis (including interstitial lung disease), asthenia, fatigue, headache, insomnia, convulsions, irritability, increased susceptibility to infections (including pneumonia, aspergillosis, and candidiasis), hyperglycaemia, hypoglycaemia, dehydration, renal failure, electrolyte disturbance, arthralgia, eyelid oedema, epistaxis, skin and nail disorders (including hand-foot syndrome); *less commonly* congestive heart failure, flushing, agitation, aggression, rhabdomyolysis and impaired wound healing; hepatitis B reactivation and haemorrhage also reported

Dose

- See under preparations

Afinitor® (Novartis) PoM
Tablets, white-yellow, everolimus, 5 mg, net price 30-tab pack = £2250.00; 10 mg, 30-tab pack = £2970.00. Label: 25, counselling, pneumonitis
Dose renal cell carcinoma, neuroendocrine tumours of pancreatic origin, hormone-receptor-positive breast cancer, ADULT over 18 years, 10 mg once daily
The *Scottish Medicines Consortium* (p. 4) has advised (April 2012) that everolimus (*Afinitor®*) is accepted for restricted use within NHS Scotland for the treatment of unresectable or metastatic, well- or moderately-differentiated neuroendocrine tumours of pancreatic origin (pNET) in adults with progressive disease.

Votubia® (Novartis) ▼ PoM
Tablets, white-yellow, everolimus, 2.5 mg, net price 30-tab pack = £1200.00; 5 mg, 30-tab pack = £2250.00; 10 mg, 30-tab pack = £2970.00. Label: 25, counselling, pneumonitis
Dose subependymal giant cell astrocytoma or renal angiomyolipoma associated with tuberous sclerosis complex, consult product literature
Note Votubia® tablets may be dispersed in approximately 30 mL of water by gently stirring, immediately before drinking. After solution has been swallowed, any residue must be re-dispersed in the same volume of water and swallowed

GEFITINIB

Indications see notes above

Cautions monitor liver function—consider discontinuing if severe changes in liver function occur; monitor for worsening of dyspnoea, cough and fever—discontinue if interstitial lung disease confirmed; see MHRA/CHM advice Epidermal Growth Factor Receptor (EGFR) Inhibitors: Serious Cases of Keratitis and Ulcerative Keratitis, p. 599; **interactions**: Appendix 1 (gefitinib)

Hepatic impairment manufacturer advises caution in moderate to severe impairment due to cirrhosis

Renal impairment manufacturer advises caution if creatinine clearance less than 20 mL/minute

Pregnancy manufacturer advises avoid unless essential—toxicity in *animal* studies; see also Pregnancy and Reproductive Function, p. 575

Breast-feeding discontinue breast-feeding

Side-effects see section 8.1; also anorexia, diarrhoea, dry mouth; epistaxis, interstitial lung disease—discontinue if confirmed; asthenia; pyrexia; haematuria, proteinuria; dry eye, conjunctivitis, blepharitis; nail

disorder, skin reactions (including dry skin, rash, acne, and pruritus); *less commonly* pancreatitis, corneal erosion; *rarely* hepatitis, toxic epidermal necrolysis

Dose

- ADULT over 18 years, 250 mg once daily

Iressa® (AstraZeneca) PoM
Tablets, f/c, brown, gefitinib 250 mg, net price 30-tab pack = £2167.71

IBRUTINIB

Indications see notes above

Cautions see section 8.1; monitor full blood count once a month; increased lymphocytes—increased risk of leukostasis, consider withholding treatment temporarily and monitor closely; monitor for atrial fibrillation (increased risk in cardiac risk factors, acute infections and history of atrial fibrillation), monitor all patients periodically and complete ECG if arrhythmic symptoms or dyspnoea develop—consult product literature for treatment options; risk factors for shortening in QTc interval (including family or personal history of congenital short QT syndrome); risk of haemorrhagic events— withhold ibrutinib treatment for at least 3 to 7 days before and after surgery depending on risk of bleeding; avoid concomitant use of drugs that increase risk of bleeding but see also interactions Appendix 1 (ibrutinib)

Hepatic impairment reduce dose to 280 mg daily in mild impairment and reduce dose to 140 mg daily in moderate impairment—monitor for toxicity and adjust dose if necessary (consult product literature); avoid in severe impairment

Renal impairment maintain hydration and monitor serum creatinine periodically in mild to moderate impairment; use in severe impairment only if benefit outweighs risk and with close monitoring for toxicity

Pregnancy manufacturer advises avoid—toxicity in *animal* studies; highly effective contraception (must include a non-hormonal method) required during and for 3 months after stopping treatment; see also Pregnancy and Reproductive Function, p. 575

Breast-feeding manufacturer advises discontinue breastfeeding—no information available

Side-effects see section 8.1; also dry mouth, diarrhoea, constipation, peripheral oedema, atrial fibrillation, dizziness, headache, pyrexia, respiratory tract infection, sinusitis, sepsis, urinary tract infection, skin infection, dehydration, haemorrhage, bruising, petechiae, subdural haematoma, epistaxis, arthralgia, musculoskeletal pain, blurred vision, rash; *less commonly* leukostasis

Dose

- Relapsed or refractory mantle cell lymphoma ADULT 560 mg once daily; for dose adjustments due to side effects consult product literature
- Chronic lymphocytic leukaemia ADULT 420 mg once daily; for dose adjustments due to side effects consult product literature

Note 140 mg daily with concomitant potent CYP3A4 inhibitors (such as cobicistat, clarithromycin, darunavir boosted with ritonavir, indinavir, itraconazole, ritonavir, saquinavir, telithromycin, and voriconazole), alternatively temporarily stop ibrutinib if the potent CYP3A4 inhibitor is only required for 7 days or less; 140 mg daily with concomitant moderate CYP3A4 inhibitors (such as amiodarone, aprepitant, atazanavir, ciprofloxacin, crizotinib, diltiazem, dronedarone, erythromycin, fluconazole, fosamprenavir, imatinib, and verapamil); avoid concomitant use with these drugs unless unavoidable

Imbruvica® (Janssen) ▼ PoM
Capsules, ibrutinib 140 mg, net price 90-cap pack = £4599; 120-cap pack = £6132. Label: 25

IDELALISIB

Indications see notes above

Cautions see section 8.1; diarrhoea—symptomatic management recommended (consult product literature); pneumonitis—withhold treatment (consult product literature); active hepatitis; monitor liver function—consult product literature; **interactions:** Appendix 1 (idelalisib)

Hepatic impairment manufacturer advises caution in hepatic impairment

Pregnancy manufacturer advises avoid (toxicity in *animal* studies)—highly effective contraception (in addition to barrier method) required during and for one month after treatment; see also Pregnancy and Reproductive Function, p. 575

Breast-feeding manufacturer advises avoid—no information available

Side-effects see section 8.1; also diarrhoea, pneumonitis, infections, pyrexia, neutropenia, rash

Dose
- ADULT over 18 years, 150 mg twice daily; for dose adjustment due to side effects, consult product literature

Zydelig® (Gilead) ▼ PoM
Tablets, f/c, idelalisib 100 mg (orange), net price 60-tab pack = £3114.75; 150 mg (pink), 60-tab pack = £3114.75. Label: 25

IMATINIB

Indications see notes above

Cautions see section 8.1; cardiac disease; risk factors for heart failure; history of renal failure; monitor for fluid retention; monitor liver function (see also Hepatic Impairment, below); monitor growth in children (may cause growth retardation); **interactions:** Appendix 1 (imatinib)

Hepatic impairment max. 400 mg daily; reduce dose further if not tolerated

Renal impairment max. starting dose 400 mg daily if creatinine clearance less than 60 mL/minute; reduce dose further if not tolerated

Pregnancy manufacturer advises avoid unless potential benefit outweighs risk; effective contraception required during treatment; see also Pregnancy and Reproductive Function, p. 575

Breast-feeding discontinue breast-feeding

Side-effects see section 8.1; also abdominal pain, appetite changes, constipation, diarrhoea, flatulence, gastro-oesophageal reflux, taste disturbance, weight changes, dry mouth; oedema (including pulmonary oedema, pleural effusion, and ascites), flushing, haemorrhage; cough, dyspnoea; dizziness, headache, insomnia, hypoaesthesia, paraesthesia, fatigue; influenza-like symptoms; cramps, arthralgia; visual disturbances, increased lacrimation, conjunctivitis, dry eyes; epistaxis; dry skin, sweating, rash, pruritus, photosensitivity; *less commonly* gastric ulceration, pancreatitis, hepatic dysfunction (rarely hepatic failure, hepatic necrosis), dysphagia, heart failure, tachycardia, palpitation, syncope, haematoma, hypertension, hypotension, cold extremities, cough,

acute respiratory failure, depression, drowsiness, anxiety, peripheral neuropathy, tremor, migraine, impaired memory, vertigo, gynaecomastia, menorrhagia, irregular menstruation, sexual dysfunction, electrolyte disturbances, renal failure, urinary frequency, gout, tinnitus, hearing loss; skin hyperpigmentation; *rarely* intestinal obstruction, gastro-intestinal perforation, inflammatory bowel disease, arrhythmia, atrial fibrillation, myocardial infarction, angina, pulmonary fibrosis, pulmonary hypertension, increased intracranial pressure, convulsions, confusion, haemolytic anaemia, rhabdomyolysis, myopathy, aseptic necrosis of bone, cataract, glaucoma, angioedema, exfoliative dermatitis, and Stevens-Johnson syndrome; *also reported* drug rash with eosinophilia and systemic symptoms (DRESS), growth retardation in children

Dose
- Chronic phase chronic myeloid leukaemia, ADULT 400 mg once daily, increased if necessary to max. 800 mg daily (in 2 divided doses); CHILD consult product literature
- Accelerated phase and blast crisis chronic myeloid leukaemia, ADULT 600 mg once daily, increased if necessary to max. 800 mg daily (in 2 divided doses); CHILD consult product literature
- Acute lymphoblastic leukaemia, ADULT 600 mg once daily; CHILD consult product literature
- Gastro-intestinal stromal tumours, ADULT 400 mg once daily
- Dermatofibrosarcoma protuberans, ADULT 800 mg daily in 2 divided doses
- Myelodysplastic/myeloproliferative diseases, ADULT 400 mg once daily
- Advanced hypereosinophilic syndrome and chronic eosinophilic leukaemia, ADULT 100–400 mg once daily

Glivec® (Novartis) ▼ PoM
Tablets, f/c, imatinib (as mesilate) 100 mg (yellow-brown, scored), net price 60-tab pack = £862.19; 400 mg (yellow), 30-tab pack = £1724.39. Label: 21, 27

Counselling Tablets may be dispersed in water or apple juice

LAPATINIB

Indications see notes above

Cautions see section 8.1; diarrhoea—withold treatment if severe (consult product literature); low gastric pH (reduced absorption); susceptibility to QT-interval prolongation (including concomitant use of drugs that prolong QT-interval and electrolyte disturbances); monitor left ventricular function; monitor for pulmonary toxicity; monitor liver function before treatment and at monthly intervals; **interactions:** Appendix 1 (lapatinib)

Hepatic impairment caution in moderate to severe impairment—metabolism reduced

Renal impairment caution in severe impairment—no information available

Pregnancy avoid unless potential benefit outweighs risk—toxicity in *animal* studies; see also Pregnancy and Reproductive Function, p. 575

Breast-feeding discontinue breast-feeding

Side-effects see section 8.1; anorexia, diarrhoea (treat promptly), decreased left ventricular ejection fraction, cardiac failure (fatal cases reported), malaise, rash, nail disorders, hyperbilirubinaemia, hepatotoxicity (discontinue permanently if severe); *less commonly* interstitial lung disease; respiratory failure (including fatal cases) also reported

Dose

- In combination with capecitabine, ADULT over 18 years, 1.25 g once daily
- In combination with an aromatase inhibitor, ADULT over 18 years, 1.5 g once daily
- In combination with trastuzumab, ADULT over 18 years, 1 g once daily

Counselling Always take at the same time in relation to food: either one hour before or one hour after food. Patients should report unexpected changes in bowel habit

Tyverb® (GSK) ▼ PoM
Tablets, yellow, f/c, lapatinib 250 mg, net price 84-tab pack = £965.16, 105-tab pack = £1206.45. Counselling, administration

---

NILOTINIB

Indications   see notes above

Cautions   see section 8.1; history of pancreatitis; susceptibility to QT-interval prolongation (including electrolyte disturbances, concomitant use of drugs that prolong QT interval); **interactions:** Appendix 1 (nilotinib)

Hepatic impairment   manufacturer advises caution

Pregnancy   manufacturer advises avoid unless potential benefit outweighs risk—toxicity in *animal* studies; effective contraception required during treatment; see also Pregnancy and Reproductive Function, p. 575

Breast-feeding   manufacturer advises avoid—present in milk in *animal* studies

Side-effects   see section 8.1; also abdominal pain, constipation, diarrhoea, dyspepsia, flatulence, anorexia, weight changes; palpitation, QT-interval prolongation, hypertension, oedema, flushing; dyspnoea, cough, dysphonia; headache, fatigue, asthenia, dizziness, paraesthesia, insomnia, vertigo; hypomagnesaemia, hyperkalaemia, blood glucose changes; bone pain, arthralgia, muscle spasm; urticaria, erythema, hyperhidrosis, dry skin, rash, pruritus; *less commonly* hepatitis, pancreatitis, dry mouth, chest pain, cardiac failure, arrhythmias, pericardial effusion, coronary artery disease, cardiomegaly, cardiac murmur, bradycardia, hypertensive crisis, haemorrhage, melaena, haematoma, pleural effusion, interstitial lung disease, migraine, hypoaesthesia, hyperaesthesia, depression, anxiety, tremor, influenza-like symptoms, hyperthyroidism, breast pain, gynaecomastia, erectile dysfunction, dysuria, urinary frequency, hypokalaemia, hyponatraemia, hypocalcaemia, hypophosphataemia, dehydration, decreased visual acuity, conjunctivitis, dry eyes, epistaxis, and ecchymosis

Dose

- Newly diagnosed chronic myeloid leukaemia, chronic phase, ADULT over 18 years, 300 mg twice daily
- Chronic and accelerated phase chronic myeloid leukaemia (see notes above), ADULT over 18 years, 400 mg twice daily

Tasigna® (Novartis) PoM
Capsules, nilotinib (as hydrochloride monohydrate) 150 mg (red), net price 112-cap pack = £2432.85; 200 mg (yellow), 112-cap pack = £2432.85. Label: 23, 25, 27

PAZOPANIB

Indications   see notes above

Cautions   see section 8.1; monitor liver function before treatment and at weeks 3, 5, 7, and 9, then at months 3 and 4, and periodically thereafter as clinically indicated—consult product literature if elevated liver enzymes observed; control blood pressure before initiating and monitor blood pressure within 1 week of treatment initiation, then frequently throughout treatment (consider dose reduction or interruption if hypertension uncontrolled despite anti-hypertensive therapy; discontinue if blood pressure persistently elevated despite anti-hypertensive therapy and pazopanib dose reduction—consult product literature); susceptibility to QT-interval prolongation (including electrolyte disturbances, concomitant use of drugs that prolong QT-interval); patients at risk of thrombotic events including myocardial infarction, ischaemic stroke or transient ischaemic attack; cardiac disease (monitor for signs or symptoms of congestive heart failure—monitor left ventricular ejection fraction in patients at risk of heart failure before and during treatment); patients at increased risk of haemorrhage; patients at increased risk of gastro-intestinal perforation or fistulas; discontinue treatment 7 days before elective surgery and restart only if adequate wound healing; monitor thyroid function; monitor for proteinuria; increased risk of thrombotic microangiopathy—permanently discontinue if symptoms develop; monitor for signs and symptoms of posterior reversible encephalopathy syndrome (including headache, hypertension, seizure, lethargy, confusion, visual and neurological disturbances)—permanently discontinue treatment if symptoms occur **interactions:** Appendix 1 (pazopanib)

Contra-indications   cerebral or clinically significant gastro-intestinal haemorrhage or haemoptysis in the past 6 months

Hepatic impairment   use with caution in mild to moderate impairment—reduce dose to 200 mg once daily in moderate impairment; avoid in severe impairment

Renal impairment   use with caution if creatinine clearance less than 30 mL/minute—no information available

Pregnancy   avoid unless potential benefit outweighs risk—toxicity in *animal* studies; effective contraception advised during treatment; see also Pregnancy and Reproductive Function, p. 575

Breast-feeding   discontinue breast-feeding

Side-effects   see section 8.1; also abdominal pain, abdominal distension, dyspepsia, diarrhoea, weight loss, anorexia, dry mouth, taste disturbance, flatulence, hepatic dysfunction, hyperbilirubinaemia, hypertension, flushing, chest pain, oedema, venous thromboembolic events, dyspnoea, cough, pneumothorax, hiccups, epistaxis, voice changes, headache, dizziness, malaise, paraesthesia, insomnia, hypothyroidism, proteinuria (discontinue if grade 4), blood disorders (including thrombocytopenia), hyperalbuminaemia, increased amylase, dehydration, muscle spasm, myalgia, blurred vision, sweating, skin reactions, dry skin, hair and skin discoloration, nail disorders; *less commonly* hepatic failure, gastro-intestinal perforation, peritonitis, pancreatitis, fistula, cardiac dysfunction, transient ischaemic attack, stroke, myocardial infarction, myocardial ischaemia, bradycardia, haemorrhage, hypertensive crisis, QT-interval prolongation, pulmonary embolism, peripheral neuropathy, menstrual disturbances, hypomagnesaemia, arthralgia, oropharyngeal pain, photosensitivity reactions; *rarely* thrombotic microangiopathy

Dose

• ADULT over 18 years, 800 mg once daily; adjust dose in steps of 200 mg according to tolerability (max. 800 mg daily)

Votrient® (GSK)

Tablets, f/c, pazopanib (as hydrochloride) 200 mg (pink), net price 30-tab pack = £560.50; 400 mg (white), 30-tab pack = £1121.00. Label: 23, 25, counselling, see below

Counselling Do not take antacids for at least 1 hour before or 2 hours after *Votrient®*

▍ PONATINIB

Indications   see notes above

Cautions   history of pancreatitis, alcohol abuse or current severe hypertriglyceridaemia—increased risk of pancreatitis; monitor serum lipase every 2 weeks for the first 2 months and periodically thereafter for all patients—withhold treatment if lipase elevated and abdominal symptoms occur; monitor full blood count every 2 weeks for the first 3 months and then monthly thereafter or as clinically indicated; monitor liver function periodically; history of myocardial infarction or stroke—do not use unless potential benefit outweighs potential risk; assess cardiovascular status before treatment and regularly thereafter—manage risk factors before and during treatment; hypertension—medically control during treatment and interrupt treatment if uncontrolled; monitor for vascular occlusion or thromboembolism—interrupt treatment immediately if this occurs; discontinue treatment if a complete haematologic response has not occurred within 3 months; **interactions**: Appendix 1 (ponatinib)

Hepatic impairment   manufacturer advises caution in severe impairment

Renal impairment   no information available—manufacturer advises caution if creatinine clearance less than 50 mL/minute

Pregnancy   avoid—toxicity in *animal* studies; ensure effective contraception during treatment in men and women; effectiveness of hormonal contraception unknown—alternative or additional methods of contraception should be used; see also Pregnancy and Reproductive Function, p. 575

Breast-feeding   manufacturer advises discontinue breastfeeding—no information available

Side-effects   see section 8.1; also abdominal discomfort, gastro-oesophageal reflux disease, constipation, diarrhoea, pancreatitis, dyspepsia, dry mouth, dehydration, decreased appetite, weight loss, hypertension, cardiac disorders, cardiac events, cerebrovascular events, vascular occlusion, thromboembolic events, intermittent claudication, atrial fibrillation, pericardial effusion, oedema, flushing, dyspnoea, cough, pleural effusion, dysphonia, malaise, headache, insomnia, dizziness, peripheral neuropathy, altered sensations, pyrexia, infection, biochemistry and electrolyte disturbances, erectile dysfunction, arthralgia, musculoskeletal pain, muscle spasms, blurred vision, dry eyes, periorbital oedema, epistaxis, dry skin, rash, pruritus, exfoliative dermatitis, hyperhidrosis, bruising; *less commonly* gastric haemorrhage,

atrial flutter, cerebral infarction, cerebral artery stenosis, hepatotoxicity, jaundice, retinal vein thrombosis, retinal vein occlusion, visual impairment

Dose

• ADULT over 18 years, 45 mg once daily; for dose adjustment due to side-effects, consult product literature

Note See also MHRA/CHM advice above

Note Consider reducing the initial dose to 30 mg once daily with concomitant use of potent inhibitors of cytochrome P450 enzyme CYP3A4 (e.g. clarithromycin, indinavir, itraconazole, ritonavir, saquinavir, telithromycin or voriconazole)

Iclusig® (ARIAD) ▼

Tablets, ponatinib 15 mg, net price 60-tab pack = £5050.00; 45 mg, 30-tab pack = £5050.00. Label: 3, 25

▍ REGORAFENIB

Indications   see notes above

Cautions   predisposition to bleeding or concomitant treatment with drugs that may increase the risk of bleeding (increased risk of haemorrhagic events)—monitor blood count and coagulation parameters and consider permanent discontinuation in event of severe bleeding; history of ischaemic heart disease—monitor for signs and symptoms of myocardial ischaemia and interrupt treatment if signs of ischaemia or infarction develop; may impair wound healing—withhold treatment for major surgical procedures; hypertension—control blood pressure before treatment initiation and monitor as clinically indicated during treatment (review dose and consider treatment interruption if severe or persistent hypertension develops; discontinue treatment if hypertensive crisis occurs); Gilbert's syndrome—risk of hyperbilirubinaemia; monitor hepatic function before treatment, then at least every two weeks for the first 2 months, then at least monthly thereafter and as clinically indicated—consult product literature if changes in liver function observed; monitor for signs and symptoms of posterior reversible encephalopathy syndrome (including seizure, headache, altered mental status, visual disturbances or cortical blindness, with or without hypertension)—discontinue treatment if symptoms occur; monitor biochemical, electrolyte and metabolic parameters during treatment; ensure measures to prevent hand-foot skin reaction—consult product literature if signs or symptoms develop; **interactions**: Appendix 1 (regorafenib)

Hepatic impairment   manufacturer advises caution in moderate impairment; avoid in severe impairment

Renal impairment   caution in severe impairment—no information available

Pregnancy   manufacturer advises avoid unless potential benefit outweighs risk—toxicity in *animal* studies; women of childbearing potential and men must use effective contraception during treatment and up to 8 weeks after the last dose; see also Pregnancy and Reproductive Function, p. 575

Breast-feeding   avoid—present in milk in *animal* studies

Side-effects   see section 8.1; also decreased appetite, weight loss, diarrhoea, taste disorders, dry mouth, gastro-oesophageal reflux, gastro-enteritis, haemorrhage (including fatal), hypertension, headache, tremor, dysphonia, malaise, pain, pyrexia, infection, hypothyroidism, biochemical and electrolyte disturbances, abnormal international normalised ratio, musculoskeletal stiffness, hand-foot skin reaction, rash, dry skin, nail disorder, mucosal inflammation; *less commonly* gastro-intestinal perforation and fistula (discontinue treatment), myocardial infarction, myocardial ischaemia, hypertensive crisis, severe (including fatal) liver injury; *rarely* posterior reversible encephalopathy syndrome, keratoacanthoma, squamous cell carcinoma of the skin, Stevens-Johnson syndrome, toxic epidermal necrolysis

Dose
- ADULT over 18 years, 160 mg once daily for 21 consecutive days of repeated 28-day cycles; for dose adjustment due to side-effects, consult product literature

Stivarga® (Bayer) ▼ PoM
Tablets, f/c, pink, regorafenib 40 mg, net price 84-tab pack = £3744.00. Label: 21, counselling, administration
  Counselling Tablets should be taken at the same time each day, swallowed whole with water after a light meal that contains less than 30% fat
  Electrolytes Na⁺ 0.607 mmol/40 mg tablet

■ RUXOLITINIB

Indications see notes above

Cautions see section 8.1; monitor full blood count (including differential white cell count) before treatment, then every 2–4 weeks until dose stabilised, then as clinically indicated; assess risk of developing infection before treatment—do not initiate until active serious infections are resolved (see also under Tuberculosis below); monitor for infection during treatment; monitor for symptoms of progressive multifocal leucoencephalopathy (presenting as new or worsening neurological, cognitive or psychiatric signs or symptoms)—withhold treatment if suspected; **interactions**: Appendix 1 (ruxolitinib)
  Tuberculosis Patients should be evaluated for latent and active tuberculosis before starting treatment and monitored for signs and symptoms of tuberculosis during treatment

Hepatic impairment reduce dose (consult product literature)

Renal impairment reduce dose in severe impairment (consult product literature)

Pregnancy avoid—toxicity in *animal* studies

Breast-feeding avoid—present in milk in *animal* studies

Side-effects see section 8.1; also flatulence, hypercholesterolaemia, dizziness, headache, weight gain; *less commonly* tuberculosis; *also reported* progressive multifocal leucoencephalopathy

Dose
- See Doses, p. 574

Jakavi® (Novartis) ▼ PoM
Tablets, ruxolitinib (as phosphate) 5 mg, net price 56-tab pack = £1680.00; 15 mg, 56-tab pack = £3360.00; 20 mg, 56-tab pack = £3360.00

■ SORAFENIB

Indications see notes above

Cautions major surgical procedures; cardiac ischaemia; susceptibility to QT-interval prolongation—consider periodic monitoring of ECG and electrolytes; monitor blood pressure regularly and consider permanent discontinuation of sorafenib if resistant to antihypertensive therapy; potential risk of bleeding—

treat tracheal, bronchial, or oesophageal infiltration with localised therapy before initiating sorafenib in patients with differentiated thyroid carcinoma (DTC), and consider permanent withdrawal of sorafenib in any patient that requires medical intervention for bleeding; monitor plasma-calcium concentration (increased risk of hypocalcaemia if history of hypoparathyroidism) and thyroid stimulating hormone in patients with DTC; **interactions**: Appendix 1 (sorafenib)

Hepatic impairment manufacturer advises caution in severe impairment—no information available

Pregnancy manufacturer advises avoid unless essential—toxicity in *animal* studies; see also Pregnancy and Reproductive Function, p. 575

Breast-feeding discontinue breast-feeding

Side-effects see section 8.1; also diarrhoea, constipation, dyspepsia, gastro-oesophageal reflux disease, dysphagia, anorexia, myocardial ischaemia and infarction, congestive heart failure, hypertension, haemorrhage, flushing, malaise, dysgeusia, dysphonia, depression, peripheral neuropathy, fever, erectile dysfunction, thyroid dysfunction, proteinuria, renal failure, electrolyte disturbances (including hypophosphataemia), arthralgia, myalgia, muscle spasms, tinnitus, rhinorrhoea, rash, pruritus, erythema, dry skin, desquamation, acne, hand-foot skin reaction, keratoacanthoma, dermatitis, hyperkeratosis; *less commonly* dehydration, gastritis, pancreatitis, cholecystitis, cholangitis, gastro-intestinal perforations, hypertensive crisis, interstitial lung disease-like events, posterior reversible encephalopathy syndrome, gynaecomastia, altered prothrombin time or INR, eczema, erythema multiforme; *rarely* hepatitis, QT-interval prolongation, nephrotic syndrome, rhabdomyolysis, leucocytoclastic vasculitis, toxic epidermal necrolysis, Stevens-Johnson syndrome

Dose
- ADULT over 18 years, 400 mg twice daily; for dose adjustment due to side-effects, consult product literature

Nexavar® (Bayer) PoM
Tablets, f/c, red, sorafenib (as tosylate) 200 mg, net price 112-tab pack = £2980.47 Label: 23

■ SUNITINIB

Indications see notes above

Cautions see section 8.1; cardiovascular disease—discontinue if congestive heart failure develops; susceptibility to QT-interval prolongation; hypertension; increased risk of bleeding; monitor for thyroid dysfunction; consider dental check-up before initiating treatment (risk of osteonecrosis of the jaw, see MHRA/CHM advice, p. 595); **interactions**: Appendix 1 (sunitinib)

Pregnancy manufacturer advises avoid unless potential benefit outweighs risk—toxicity in *animal* studies; effective contraception required during treatment; see also Pregnancy and Reproductive Function, p. 575

Breast-feeding discontinue breast-feeding

Side-effects see section 8.1; also abdominal pain, diarrhoea, constipation, anorexia, taste disturbance, dehydration; hypertension, oedema; dyspnoea, cough; fatigue, dizziness, headache, insomnia, peripheral neuropathy, paraesthesia; hypothyroidism; arthralgia, myalgia; increased lacrimation; epistaxis; skin, hair, and urine discoloration, hand-foot syndrome, dry skin, and rash; gastro-intestinal perforation, fistula formation (interrupt treatment if occurs) pancreatitis, osteonecrosis of the jaw (see MHRA/CHM advice, p. 595), hepatic failure, proteinuria (*rarely* nephrotic syndrome) and seizures reported

Dose

- Gastro-intestinal stromal tumours and metastatic renal cell carcinoma, 50 mg once daily for 4 weeks, followed by a 2-week treatment-free period to complete 6-week cycle; adjust dose in steps of 12.5 mg according to tolerability; dose range 25–75 mg daily
- Pancreatic neuroendocrine tumours, 37.5 mg once daily, without a treatment-free period; adjust dose in steps of 12.5 mg according to tolerability; max. dose 50 mg daily

Sutent® (Pfizer) PoM

Capsules, sunitinib (as malate) 12.5 mg (orange), net price 28-cap pack = £784.70; 25 mg (caramel/orange), 28-cap pack = £1569.40; 50 mg (caramel), 28-cap pack = £3138.80. Label: 14

TEMSIROLIMUS

Indications see notes above

Cautions see notes above; monitor respiratory function; monitor blood lipids; **interactions:** Appendix 1 (temsirolimus)

Hepatic impairment use with caution; in renal cell carcinoma, reduce dose in severe impairment (consult product literature); in mantle cell lymphoma, avoid in moderate or severe impairment

Renal impairment manufacturer advises caution in severe impairment—no information available

Pregnancy manufacturer advises avoid (toxicity in *animal* studies); ensure effective contraception during treatment in men and women; see also Pregnancy and Reproductive Function, p. 575

Breast-feeding manufacturer advises discontinue breast-feeding

Side-effects see section 8.1; also abdominal pain, diarrhoea, anorexia, taste disturbance, gastro-intestinal haemorrhage, bowel perforation, dysphagia; hypertension, oedema, thrombosis, thrombophlebitis; cough, dyspnoea, chest pain, interstitial lung disease, hypersensitivity reactions (see notes above); insomnia, anxiety, depression, drowsiness, paraesthesia, dizziness, asthenia; increased susceptibility to infection (including urinary-tract infection and pneumonia), pyrexia; hyperglycaemia; renal failure; hypophosphataemia, hypokalaemia, hypercholesterolaemia, hyperlipidaemia; myalgia, arthralgia; eye disorders; rhinitis, epistaxis; skin disorders (including rash and acne), folliculitis, impaired wound healing; *less commonly* intracerebral bleeding

Dose

- See Doses, p. 574

Torisel® (Pfizer) PoM

Infusion, temsirolimus 30 mg concentrate (25 mg/mL), net price 1.2-mL amp (with diluent) = £620.00

Excipients include propylene glycol and ethanol

VANDETANIB

Indications see notes above

Cautions see section 8.1; susceptibility to QT-prolongation (including concomitant use of drugs that prolong QT interval and electrolyte disturbances)—monitor ECG, serum potassium, calcium, magnesium

and thyroid stimulating hormone before treatment, then 1, 3, 6 and 12 weeks after starting treatment and following dose adjustment or interruption, then every 3 months for at least 1 year; history of torsades de pointes; phototoxicity reactions reported (wear protective clothing and/or sunscreen); brain metastases (intracranial haemorrhage reported); hypertension; **interactions:** Appendix 1 (vandetanib)

Contra-indications congenital long QT syndrome; QT interval greater than 480 milliseconds

Hepatic impairment manufacturer advises avoid in severe impairment (serum bilirubin greater than 1.5 times the upper limit of normal)

Renal impairment reduce dose to 200 mg if creatinine clearance 30–49 mL/minute; avoid if creatinine clearance less than 30 mL/minute

Pregnancy manufacturer advises avoid unless potential benefit outweighs risk—effective contraception required during and for at least 4 months after treatment; see also Pregnancy and Reproductive Function, p. 575

Breast-feeding avoid—no information available

Side-effects see section 8.1; also abdominal pain, diarrhoea, constipation, dyspepsia, colitis, dry mouth, dysphagia, gastritis, gastrointestinal haemorrhage, cholelithiasis, QT-interval prolongation, hypertension, ischaemic cerebrovascular conditions, oedema, epistaxis, haemoptysis, pneumonitis, headache, paraesthesia, dysaesthesia, dizziness, tremor, lethargy, asthenia, pain, pyrexia, loss of consciousness, balance disorders, taste disturbance, insomnia, depression, anxiety, hypothyroidism, decreased appetite, hyperglycaemia, dehydration, electrolyte disturbances, proteinuria, nephrolithiasis, dysuria, haematuria, pollakiuria, micturition urgency, blurred vision, corneal changes (including corneal deposits and opacity), halo vision, photopsia, glaucoma, conjunctivitis, dry eye, keratopathy, photosensitivity reactions, hand-foot syndrome, alopecia; *less commonly* pancreatitis, peritonitis, ileus, intestinal perforation, faecal incontinence, heart failure, cardiac conduction, rate and rhythm disorders, ventricular arrhythmia, cardiac arrest, respiratory failure, aspiration pneumonia, interstitial lung disease (sometimes fatal), convulsions, clonus, brain oedema, posterior reversible encephalopathy syndrome, impaired healing, increased haemoglobin, chromaturia, anuria, cataract, accommodation disorders, bullous dermatitis, erythema multiforme and Stevens-Johnson syndrome

Dose

- ADULT, 300 mg once daily; for dose adjustment due to side-effects, consult product literature

Caprelsa® (AstraZeneca) ▼ PoM

Tablets, f/c, vandetanib 100 mg, net price 30-tab pack = £2500.00; 300 mg, 30-tab pack = £5000.00. Alert card

Note *Caprelsa®* tablets may be dispersed in half a glass of water by stirring until dispersed (approximately 10 minutes), immediately before drinking (do not crush). After solution has been swallowed, any residue must be re-dispersed in the same volume of water and swallowed. The solution can also be administered via nasogastric or gastrostomy tubes

VEMURAFENIB

Indications see notes above

Cautions see section 8.1; susceptibility to QT-prolongation (including concomitant use of drugs that prolong QT interval and electrolyte disturbances)—monitor ECG and electrolytes before treatment, after one month and following dose adjustment (treatment not recommended if QT interval greater than 500 milliseconds at baseline); monitor for cutaneous and non-cutaneous squamous cell carcinoma and new primary melanoma before, during and for up to 6 months after treatment—consult product literature; monitor liver function before treatment and periodically thereafter; monitor for uveitis, iritis and retinal vein occlusion; prior or concurrent cancer associated with RAS mutation—increased risk of tumour progression; **interactions**: Appendix 1 (vemurafenib)

Contra-indications wild-type BRAF malignant melanoma

Hepatic impairment manufacturer advises more frequent monitoring in moderate to severe impairment (including monthly ECG monitoring during first 3 months of treatment)

Renal impairment manufacturer advises caution in severe impairment

Pregnancy manufacturer advises avoid unless potential benefit outweighs risk—effective contraception required during and for at least 6 months after treatment; see also Pregnancy and Reproductive Function, p. 575

Breast-feeding avoid—no information available

Side-effects see section 8.1; also diarrhoea, constipation, decreased appetite, cough, peripheral oedema, QT-interval prolongation, fatigue, asthenia, pyrexia, headache, dizziness, taste disturbance, Bell's palsy, new primary melanoma, arthralgia, myalgia, pain in extremities, musculoskeletal pain, arthritis, uveitis, seborrhoeic keratosis, actinic keratosis, keratosis pilaris, skin papilloma, cutaneous squamous cell carcinoma, basal cell carcinoma, photosensitivity reactions, hyperkeratosis, erythema, alopecia, folliculitis, dry skin, hand-foot syndrome, erythema nodosum; *less commonly* vasculitis, peripheral neuropathy, non-cutaneous squamous cell carcinoma, retinal vein occlusion, toxic epidermal necrolysis, Stevens-Johnson syndrome; *rarely* progression of pre-existing NRAS mutated chronic myelomonocytic leukaemia; *also reported* hypersensitivity reactions

---

Drug rash with eosinophilia and systemic symptoms (DRESS syndrome)

DRESS syndrome has been reported in patients taking vemurafenib. DRESS syndrome starts with rash, fever, swollen glands, and increased white cell count, and it can affect the liver, kidneys and lungs; DRESS can also be fatal.

Patients should be advised to stop taking vemurafenib and consult their doctor immediately if skin rash develops. Treatment with vemurafenib should not be restarted.

Dose

- ADULT over 18 years, 960 mg twice daily; for dose adjustment due to side effects, consult product literature

Zelboraf® (Roche) ▼ PoM

Tablets, f/c, vemurafenib (as co-precipitate of vemurafenib and hypromellose acetate succinate) 240 mg, net price 56-tab pack = £1750.00. Label: 25, counselling

Counselling Food may affect absorption (take at the same time with respect to food)

Taxanes

Paclitaxel is a member of the taxane group of drugs. It is given by *intravenous infusion*, and is available as both conventional and albumin-bound formulations. The different formulations vary in their licensed indications, pharmacokinetics, dosage and administration, and are not interchangeable. *Conventional* paclitaxel given with carboplatin or cisplatin is used for the treatment of ovarian cancer (see NICE guidance p. 604); the combination is also considered appropriate for women whose ovarian cancer is initially considered inoperable; it is also licensed for the secondary treatment of metastatic breast cancer. There is limited evidence to support its use in non-small cell lung cancer. Routine premedication with a corticosteroid, an antihistamine and a histamine H_2-receptor antagonist is recommended to prevent severe hypersensitivity reactions; hypersensitivity reactions may occur rarely despite premedication, although more commonly only bradycardia or asymptomatic hypotension occur.

Other side-effects of *conventional* paclitaxel include myelosuppression, peripheral neuropathy, and cardiac conduction defects with arrhythmias (which are nearly always asymptomatic). It also causes alopecia and muscle pain; nausea and vomiting is mild to moderate.

Albumin-bound paclitaxel is licensed for monotherapy of metastatic breast cancer following failed first-line treatment for metastatic disease and when standard, anthracycline-containing therapy is not indicated. It is also licensed in combination with gemcitabine for the first-line treatment of metastatic adenocarcinoma of the pancreas. It causes myelosuppression (primarily neutropenia) and commonly febrile neutropenia. Other common side-effects include peripheral neuropathy, tachycardia, arrhythmia, myalgia, arthralgia and gastro-intestinal disorders; bradycardia, cardiac arrest, congestive heart failure, and left ventricular dysfunction are rare but cardiac monitoring should be undertaken, particularly if patients have underlying cardiac disease or previous exposure to anthracyclines. Patients aged over 75 years with metastatic adenocarcinoma of the pancreas should be treated with caution. Patients should also be monitored for signs and symptoms of pneumonitis and sepsis. Stevens-Johnson syndrome and toxic epidermal necrolysis have also been reported.

NICE guidance
Paclitaxel for the adjuvant treatment of early node-positive breast cancer (September 2006)

Paclitaxel, within its licensed indication, is **not** recommended for the adjuvant treatment of women with early node-positive breast cancer.
www.nice.org.uk/TA108

Docetaxel is licensed for use in locally advanced or metastatic breast cancer and non-small cell lung cancer resistant to other cytotoxic drugs or for initial chemotherapy in combination with other cytotoxic drugs. It is also licensed in combination with prednisone or prednisolone for hormone-resistant metastatic prostate cancer, for use with other cytotoxic drugs for gastric adenocarcinoma and head and neck cancer, and for adjuvant treatment of operable node-positive and operable node-negative breast cancer. Its side-effects are similar to those of paclitaxel but persistent fluid retention (commonly as leg oedema that worsens during

8 Malignant disease and immunosuppression

treatment) can be resistant to treatment; hypersensitivity reactions also occur. Severe skin reactions, gastrointestinal toxicity, peripheral neurotoxicity, heart failure, cystoid macular oedema, and fatal respiratory disorders have also been reported—consult product literature for monitoring and management. Pretreatment with dexamethasone by mouth is recommended for reducing fluid retention and hypersensitivity reactions (consult product literature).

For the role of taxanes in the treatment of breast cancer, see section 8.3.4.1.

The *Scottish Medicines Consortium* (p. 4) has advised that docetaxel (*Taxotere*®) in combination with cisplatin and fluorouracil is accepted for restricted use within NHS Scotland for the induction treatment of patients with unresectable (May 2007) and resectable (June 2008) locally advanced squamous cell carcinoma of the head and neck.

> **NICE guidance (paclitaxel, pegylated liposomal doxorubicin and topotecan for second-line or subsequent treatment of advanced ovarian cancer)**
>
> See p. 604

> **NICE guidance**
> **Docetaxel for the treatment of hormone-refractory metastatic prostate cancer (June 2006)**
>
> Docetaxel is an option for hormone-refractory metastatic prostate cancer and a Karnofsky score of at least 60% [Karnofsky score is a measure of the ability to perform ordinary tasks].
>
> www.nice.org.uk/TA101

> **NICE guidance**
> **Docetaxel for the adjuvant treatment of early node-positive breast cancer (September 2006)**
>
> Docetaxel, when given concurrently with doxorubicin and cyclophosphamide (TAC regimen), is recommended as an option for the adjuvant treatment of women with early node-positive breast cancer.
>
> www.nice.org.uk/TA109

Cabazitaxel, in combination with prednisone or prednisolone, is licensed for the treatment of hormone refractory metastatic prostate cancer in patients who have previously been treated with a docetaxel-containing regimen. Routine premedication with a corticosteroid, an antihistamine, and a histamine H₂-receptor antagonist is recommended to prevent severe hypersensitivity reactions. Hypersensitivity reactions are common.

Other side-effects of cabazitaxel include weight changes, diarrhoea, constipation, abdominal pain, dyspepsia, gastroesophageal reflux, haemorrhoids, rectal haemorrhage, taste disturbance, dry mouth, chest pain, atrial fibrillation, tachycardia, hypertension, hypotension, flushing, oedema, dyspnoea, cough, peripheral neuropathy, paraesthesia, hypoesthesia, anxiety, confusion, dizziness, headache, malaise, vertigo, chills, hyperglycaemia, urinary retention, urinary incontinence, renal disorders (fatal cases of renal failure reported), dehydration, electrolyte disturbances, sciatica, arthr-

algia, muscle spasm, myalgia, increased lacrimation, tinnitus, dry skin, erythema.

> **NICE guidance**
> **Cabazitaxel for hormone-refractory metastatic prostate cancer previously treated with a docetaxel-containing regimen (May 2012)**
>
> Cabazitaxel in combination with prednisone or prednisolone is **not** recommended for the treatment of hormone-refractory metastatic prostate cancer previously treated with a docetaxel-containing regimen.
>
> Patients currently receiving cabazitaxel in combination with prednisone or prednisolone for the treatment of hormone-refractory metastatic prostate cancer previously treated with a docetaxel-containing regimen should have the option to continue treatment until they and their clinicians consider it appropriate to stop.
>
> www.nice.org.uk/TA255

CABAZITAXEL

Indications   see notes above

Cautions   see section 8.1, notes above and consult product literature; monitor electrolytes—correct dehydration; avoid in acute porphyria (but see section 9.8.2); **interactions**: Appendix 1 (cabazitaxel)

Hepatic impairment   avoid

Renal impairment   use with caution if creatinine clearance less than 50 mL/minute

Pregnancy   ensure effective contraception during treatment (women) and for up to 6 months after treatment (men); see also Pregnancy and Reproductive Function, p. 575

Breast-feeding   discontinue breast-feeding

Side-effects   see section 8.1, notes above and consult product literature

Dose
● See Doses, p. 574

Jevtana® (Sanofi-Aventis) ▼ PoM
Concentrate for intravenous infusion, cabazitaxel 40 mg/mL, net price 1.5-mL vial (and solvent) = £3696.00
Note Incompatible with PVC. Solvent contains ethanol

DOCETAXEL

Indications   adjuvant treatment of operable node-positive and operable node-negative breast cancer, in combination with doxorubicin and cyclophosphamide; with doxorubicin for initial chemotherapy of locally advanced or metastatic breast cancer; monotherapy for locally advanced or metastatic breast cancer where cytotoxic chemotherapy with an anthracycline or an alkylating drug has failed; with capecitabine for locally advanced or metastatic breast cancer where cytotoxic chemotherapy with an anthracycline has failed; with trastuzumab for initial chemotherapy of metastatic breast cancer which overexpresses human epidermal growth factor-2; locally advanced or metastatic non-small cell lung cancer where previous chemotherapy has failed; with cisplatin for initial chemotherapy of unresectable, locally advanced or metastatic non-small cell lung cancer; with prednisone or prednisolone for hormone-refractory metastatic prostate cancer; with cisplatin and fluorouracil for initial treatment of metastatic gastric adenocarcinoma, including adenocarcinoma of the gastro-oesophageal junction; with cisplatin and fluorouracil for induction treatment of locally advanced squamous cell carcinoma of the head and neck

Cautions see section 8.1, notes above and consult product literature; avoid in acute porphyria (but see section 9.8.2); **interactions:** Appendix 1 (docetaxel)

Hepatic impairment monitor liver function—reduce dose according to liver enzymes (consult product literature); avoid in severe impairment

Pregnancy avoid (toxicity and reduced fertility in *animal* studies); manufacturer advises effective contraception for men and women during treatment, and for at least 6 months after stopping treatment in men; see also Pregnancy and Reproductive Function, p. 575

Breast-feeding discontinue breast-feeding

Side-effects see section 8.1, notes above and consult product literature

Dose
● See Doses, p. 574

Docetaxel (Non-proprietary) [PoM]
Infusion, docetaxel 10 mg/mL, net price 2-mL vial = £138.33, 8-mL vial = £454.53, 16-mL vial = £1069.50; 20 mg/mL, 1-mL vial = £160.00, 4-mL vial = £530.00, 7-mL vial = £900.00
Brands include *Taxceus*®

Taxotere® (Sanofi-Aventis) [PoM]
Infusion, docetaxel 20 mg/mL, net price 1-mL vial = £153.47, 4-mL vial = £504.27, 8-mL vial = £1008.54 (hosp. only)
Note Contains ethanol

▌ PACLITAXEL

Indications ovarian cancer (advanced or residual disease following laparotomy) in combination with cisplatin; metastatic ovarian cancer where platinum-containing therapy has failed; locally advanced or metastatic breast cancer (in combination with other cytotoxics or alone if other cytotoxics have failed or are inappropriate); adjuvant treatment of node-positive breast cancer following treatment with anthracycline and cyclophosphamide; non-small cell lung cancer (in combination with cisplatin) when surgery or radiotherapy not appropriate; advanced AIDS-related Kaposi's sarcoma where liposomal anthracycline therapy has failed; *albumin-bound* paclitaxel is licensed for monotherapy of metastatic breast cancer when first-line treatment has failed and standard, anthracycline-containing therapy is not indicated; first-line treatment of metastatic adenocarcinoma of the pancreas in combination with gemcitabine; also see Dose below

Cautions see section 8.1 and notes above, and consult product literature; avoid in acute porphyria (but see section 9.8.2); **interactions:** Appendix 1 (paclitaxel)

Contra-indications see section 8.1 and notes above

Hepatic impairment avoid in severe impairment

Pregnancy avoid (toxicity in *animal* studies); ensure effective contraception during and for at least 6 months after treatment in men or women; see also Pregnancy and Reproductive Function, p. 575

Breast-feeding discontinue breast-feeding

Side-effects see section 8.1, notes above, and consult product literature

Dose
● See Doses, p. 574
Note Different preparations of intravenous paclitaxel vary in their licensed indications, pharmacodynamics, pharmacokinetics, dosage, and administration; these preparations should **not** be considered interchangeable. To avoid confusion, prescribers should specify the brand to be dispensed.

Paclitaxel (Non-proprietary) [PoM]
Infusion, paclitaxel 6 mg/mL, net price 5-mL vial = £66.85, 16.7-mL vial = £200.35, 25-mL vial = £300.52, 50-mL vial = £601.03
Excipients include polyoxyl castor oil (risk of anaphylaxis, see Excipients, p. 2)

▲Albumin-bound formulation

Abraxane® (Celgene) [PoM]
Intravenous infusion, powder for reconstitution, paclitaxel as albumin bound nanoparticles, net price 100-mg vial = £246.00
Electrolytes Contains approx. 3.7 mmol Na+/vial
For monotherapy of metastatic breast cancer when first-line treatment for metastatic disease has failed and standard, anthracycline-containing therapy is not indicated; in combination with gemcitabine for the first-line treatment of metastatic adenocarcinoma of the pancreas

Topoisomerase I inhibitors

Irinotecan and topotecan inhibit topoisomerase I, an enzyme involved in DNA replication.

Irinotecan is licensed for metastatic colorectal cancer in combination with fluorouracil and folinic acid or as monotherapy when treatment containing fluorouracil has failed. It is also licensed in combination with cetuximab for the treatment of epidermal growth factor receptor-expressing metastatic colorectal cancer after failure of chemotherapy that has included irinotecan. Irinotecan is also licensed in combination with fluorouracil, folinic acid and bevacizumab for the first-line treatment of metastatic carcinoma of the colon or rectum. Irinotecan is also licensed in combination with capecitabine with or without bevacizumab for the first-line treatment of metastatic colorectal carcinoma. Irinotecan is given by intravenous infusion.

> **NICE guidance**
> Irinotecan, oxaliplatin and raltitrexed for advanced colorectal cancer (August 2005)
> See p. 604

> **NICE guidance**
> Aflibercept in combination with irinotecan and fluorouracil-based therapy for treating metastatic colorectal cancer that has progressed following prior oxaliplatin-based chemotherapy (March 2014)
> See p. 594

Topotecan is given by intravenous infusion or orally in relapsed small-cell lung cancer when retreatment with the first-line regimen is considered inappropriate. Topotecan injection is also licensed for metastatic ovarian cancer when first-line or subsequent treatment has failed. Topotecan injection is licensed in combination with cisplatin for treatment of recurrent carcinoma of the cervix, after radiotherapy, and for patients with stage IVB disease.

In addition to dose-limiting myelosuppression, side-effects of irinotecan and topotecan include gastro-intestinal effects (delayed diarrhoea requiring prompt treatment may follow irinotecan treatment), asthenia, alopecia, and anorexia.

The *Scottish Medicines Consortium* (p. 4) has advised (November 2007) that topotecan (*Hycamtin®*) is accepted for restricted use in combination with cisplatin for treatment of recurrent carcinoma of the cervix after radiotherapy and for stage IVB disease; it is restricted to patients who have not previously received cisplatin treatment.

The *Scottish Medicines Consortium* (p. 4) has advised (March 2009) that use of topotecan capsules within NHS Scotland is restricted to patients in whom standard intravenous chemotherapy is inappropriate and who would otherwise receive best supportive care.

> ### NICE guidance
> **Topotecan for the treatment of recurrent and stage IVB cervical cancer (October 2009)**
>
> Topotecan in combination with cisplatin is recommended as a treatment option for recurrent or stage IVB cervical cancer in patients who have not previously received cisplatin.
>
> www.nice.org.uk/TA183

> ### NICE guidance
> **Topotecan for the treatment of relapsed small-cell lung cancer (November 2009)**
>
> Oral topotecan is recommended as an option for treatment in patients with relapsed small-cell lung cancer only if re-treatment with the first-line regimen is not considered appropriate, and the combination of cyclophosphamide, doxorubicin and vincristine is contra-indicated. Intravenous topotecan is not recommended for people with relapsed small-cell lung cancer.
>
> www.nice.org.uk/TA184

> ### NICE guidance (paclitaxel, pegylated liposomal doxorubicin and topotecan for second-line or subsequent treatment of advanced ovarian cancer)
> See p. 604

▌ IRINOTECAN HYDROCHLORIDE

Indications see notes above

Cautions see section 8.1 and notes above; raised plasma-bilirubin concentration (see under Hepatic impairment); risk factors for cardiac disease; monitor respiratory function; **interactions**: Appendix 1 (irinotecan)

Contra-indications see section 8.1 and notes above; also chronic inflammatory bowel disease, bowel obstruction

Hepatic impairment monitor closely for neutropenia if plasma-bilirubin concentration 1.5–3 times upper limit of normal range (consult product literature); avoid if plasma-bilirubin concentration greater than 3 times upper limit of normal range

Renal impairment manufacturer advises avoid—no information available

Pregnancy avoid (teratogenic and toxic in *animal* studies); manufacturer advises effective contraception during and for up to 1 month after treatment in women and up to 3 months after treatment in men; see also Pregnancy and Reproductive Function, p. 575

Breast-feeding discontinue breast-feeding

Side-effects see section 8.1 and notes above; also acute cholinergic syndrome (with early diarrhoea) and delayed diarrhoea (consult product literature); *less commonly* interstitial pulmonary disease

Dose
● See Doses, p. 574

Irinotecan (Non-proprietary) ▢PoM▢
Infusion, irinotecan hydrochloride 20 mg/mL, net price 2-mL vial = £46.50, 5-mL vial = £114.00, 15-mL vial = £370.50, 25-mL vial = £601.25

Campto® (Pfizer) ▢PoM▢
Infusion, irinotecan hydrochloride 20 mg/mL, net price 2-mL vial = £53.00; 5-mL vial = £130.00; 15-mL vial = £390.00

▌ TOPOTECAN

Indications see notes above

Cautions see section 8.1 and notes above

Contra-indications see section 8.1 and notes above

Hepatic impairment avoid in severe impairment

Renal impairment reduce dose; avoid infusion if creatinine clearance less than 20 mL/minute; avoid oral route if creatinine clearance less than 60 mL/minute

Pregnancy avoid (teratogenicity and fetal loss in *animal* studies); see also Pregnancy and Reproductive Function, p. 575

Breast-feeding discontinue breast-feeding

Side-effects see section 8.1 and notes above

Dose
● See Doses, p. 574

Topotecan (Non-proprietary) ▢PoM▢
Concentrate for intravenous infusion, topotecan (as hydrochloride) 1 mg/mL, net price 1-mL vial = £87.88, 4-mL vial = £261.55

Intravenous infusion, powder for reconstitution, topotecan (as hydrochloride), net price 1-mg vial = £97.00, 4-mg vial = £290.00

Hycamtin® (GSK) ▢PoM▢
Capsules, topotecan (as hydrochloride) 250 micrograms (white), net price 10-cap pack = £75.00; 1 mg (pink), 10-cap pack = £360.00. Label: 25

Intravenous infusion, powder for reconstitution, topotecan (as hydrochloride), net price 1-mg vial = £97.65; 4-mg vial = £348.76

Trabectedin

Trabectedin is licensed for the treatment of advanced soft tissue sarcoma when treatment with anthracyclines and ifosfamide has failed or is contra-indicated and in combination with pegylated liposomal doxorubicin for the treatment of relapsed platinum-sensitive ovarian cancer.

Trabectedin is given by intravenous infusion. A corticosteroid, such as dexamethasone by intravenous infusion, must be given 30 minutes before therapy for its antiemetic and hepatoprotective effects (consult product literature).

◤ TRABECTEDIN

Indications   see notes above

Cautions   see section 8.1 and notes above; specific haematological, renal and hepatic parameters must be monitored and within certain ranges prior to starting treatment and repeated weekly during the first 2 cycles and at least once between treatments in subsequent cycles—consult product literature for full details; concomitant use with hepatotoxic drugs (avoid alcohol); monitor for signs and symptoms of rhabdomyolysis (including myelotoxicity, severe liver function disorder, renal failure, muscle weakness or pain)—monitor creatine phosphokinase closely and discontinue treatment (consult product literature)

Contra-indications   elevated creatine phosphokinase (consult product literature)

Hepatic impairment   manufacturer advises caution in impairment—monitor closely and consider dose reduction; avoid in patients with raised bilirubin

Renal impairment   avoid monotherapy if creatinine clearance less than 30 mL/minute; avoid combination regimens if creatinine clearance less than 60 mL/minute

Pregnancy   effective contraception recommended during and for at least 3 months after treatment in women and during and for at least 5 months after treatment in men; see also Pregnancy and Reproductive Function, p. 575

Breast-feeding   manufacturer advises avoid breast-feeding during and for 3 months after treatment

Side-effects   see section 8.1; also abdominal pain, constipation, diarrhoea, dehydration, anorexia, dyspepsia, hepatobiliary disorders, hypotension, oedema, flushing, dyspnoea, cough, headache, insomnia, peripheral neuropathy, taste disturbance; paraesthesia, dizziness, asthenia, fatigue, pyrexia, hypokalaemia, increased blood creatine kinase, myalgia, arthralgia, back pain; *less commonly* rhabdomyolysis (with raised creatine phosphokinase); *rarely* hepatic failure (fatal cases reported)

Dose
● See Doses, p. 574

Yondelis® (Pharma Mar) ▼ PoM
Injection, powder for reconstitution, trabectedin, net price 250-microgram vial = £363.00; 1-mg vial = £1366.00

Trastuzumab

Trastuzumab is licensed for the treatment of early breast cancer which overexpresses human epidermal growth factor receptor-2 (HER2).

Trastuzumab is also licensed, in combination with paclitaxel or docetaxel, for metastatic breast cancer in patients with HER2-positive tumours who have not received chemotherapy for metastatic breast cancer and in whom anthracycline treatment is inappropriate.

Trastuzumab is also licensed, in combination with an aromatase inhibitor, for metastatic breast cancer in postmenopausal patients with hormone-receptor positive HER2-positive tumours not previously treated with trastuzumab.

Trastuzumab is also licensed as monotherapy for metastatic breast cancer in patients with tumours that overexpress HER2 who have received at least 2 chemotherapy regimens including, where appropriate, an anthracycline and a taxane; women with oestrogen-receptor-positive breast cancer should also have received hormonal therapy.

Trastuzumab is also licensed (by intravenous infusion only), in combination with capecitabine or fluorouracil and cisplatin, for metastatic gastric cancer in patients with HER2-positive tumours who have not received treatment for metastatic gastric cancer.

Resuscitation facilities should be available during administration of trastuzumab and treatment should be initiated by a specialist. Trastuzumab is **not** interchangeable with trastuzumab emtansine. See section 8.3.4.1 for the role of trastuzumab in the treatment of breast cancer.

Use with anthracyclines   Concomitant use of trastuzumab with anthracyclines (section 8.1.2) is associated with cardiotoxicity. The use of anthracyclines even after stopping trastuzumab can increase the risk of cardiotoxicity and if possible should be avoided for up to 24 weeks. If an anthracycline needs to be used, cardiac function should be monitored closely.

8   Malignant disease and immunosuppression

NICE guidance
Trastuzumab for the adjuvant treatment of early-stage HER2-positive breast cancer (August 2006)

Trastuzumab, given at 3-week intervals for 1 year or until disease recurrence (whichever is the shorter period), is recommended as an option for women with early-stage HER2-positive breast cancer following surgery, chemotherapy (neoadjuvant or adjuvant) and radiotherapy (if applicable).
www.nice.org.uk/TA107

NICE guidance
Trastuzumab for the treatment of HER2-positive metastatic gastric cancer (November 2010)

Trastuzumab in combination with cisplatin and capecitabine or fluorouracil is recommended for human epidermal growth factor receptor-2-positive metastatic adenocarcinoma of the stomach or gastro-oesophageal junction in patients who:

● have not received treatment for metastatic disease
   and
● have tumours expressing high levels of HER2 as defined by a positive immunohistochemistry score of 3.

www.nice.org.uk/TA208

NICE guidance (lapatinib or trastuzumab in combination with an aromatase inhibitor for the first-line treatment of metastatic hormone-receptor-positive breast cancer that overexpresses HER2)
See p. 609

TRASTUZUMAB

Indications see notes above and product literature
Cautions see section 8.1 and notes above; symptomatic heart failure, history of hypertension, coronary artery disease, uncontrolled arrhythmias; **interactions**: Appendix 1 (trastuzumab)
Cardiotoxicity Monitor cardiac function before and during treatment—for details of monitoring and managing cardiotoxicity, consult product literature
Contra-indications see section 8.1 and notes above; severe dyspnoea at rest
Pregnancy manufacturer advises avoid—oligohydramnios reported; effective contraception must be used during treatment and for 6 months after stopping; see also Pregnancy and Reproductive Function, p. 575
Breast-feeding avoid breast-feeding during treatment and for 7 months afterwards
Side-effects see section 8.1; also infusion-related side-effects (possibly delayed onset, including chills, fever, hypersensitivity reactions such as anaphylaxis, urticaria, and angioedema), gastro-intestinal symptoms, hepatitis, cardiotoxicity (see also above), chest pain, hypertension, hypotension, pulmonary events (possibly delayed onset), headache, taste disturbance, anxiety, malaise, depression, insomnia, drowsiness, dizziness, paraesthesia, tremor, asthenia, peripheral neuropathy, hypertonia, paresis, mastitis, infection, ecchymosis, oedema, weight loss, arthralgia, myalgia, arthritis, bone pain, leg cramps, dry eye, increased lacrimation, rash, pruritus, sweating, dry skin, alopecia, acne, nail disorders

Dose
● See Doses, p. 574

Herceptin® (Roche) ▼ PoM
Intravenous infusion, powder for reconstitution, trastuzumab, net price 150-mg vial = £407.40
Injection (for subcutaneous use), trastuzumab 120 mg/mL, net price 5-mL vial = £1222.20
Note Subcutaneous preparation not licensed for use in metastatic gastric cancer
Note When prescribing, dispensing or administering, check that this is the correct preparation—trastuzumab and trastuzumab emtansine are **not** interchangeable
Note The *Scottish Medicines Consortium* p. 4 has advised (December 2013) that subcutaneous trastuzumab injection (*Herceptin®*) is accepted for restricted use within NHS Scotland for the treatment of adults with HER2 positive metastatic breast cancer and early breast cancer, when used within licensed indications excluding use in combination with an aromatase inhibitor for the treatment of postmenopausal patients with hormone-receptor positive metastatic breast cancer, not previously treated with trastuzumab

Trastuzumab emtansine

Trastuzumab emtansine is an antibody-drug conjugate that contains trastuzumab covalently linked to DM1, a cytotoxic microtubule inhibitor. Trastuzumab emtansine and trastuzumab are **not** interchangeable; trastuzumab emtansine is indicated as monotherapy for the treatment of HER2-positive, unresectable, locally advanced or metastatic breast cancer, in adult patients who have previously received trastuzumab and a taxane separately or in combination, or who have developed disease recurrence during or within 6 months of completing adjuvant therapy. Resuscitation facilities should be available during administration of trastuzumab emtansine and treatment should be initiated by a specialist. See section 8.3.4.1 for the role of trastuzumab emtansine in the treatment of breast cancer.

TRASTUZUMAB EMTANSINE

Indications see notes above
Cautions see section 8.1; patients over 75 years; dyspnoea at rest—increased risk of pulmonary events; monitor for dyspnoea, cough, fatigue and pulmonary infiltrates—discontinue if interstitial lung disease or pneumonitis confirmed (fatal cases reported); monitor hepatic function before each dose—see also Hepatic impairment; history of congestive heart failure, serious arrhythmias, recent history of myocardial infarction or unstable angina; risk of left ventricular dysfunction—consult product literature for specific risks with trastuzumab treatment; test cardiac function before treatment and regularly during treatment—delay or discontinue treatment in cases of left ventricular dysfunction; monitor closely for infusion-related and hypersensitivity reactions; monitor platelet count before each dose and as clinically indicated (consult product literature for treatment modification in thrombocytopenia); concomitant anticoagulant medication—increased risk of thrombocytopenia with haemorrhagic events; peripheral neuropathy (temporarily discontinue treatment—consult product literature); monitor for signs and symptoms of neurotoxicity; **interactions**: Appendix 1 (trastuzumab)
Hepatic impairment monitor hepatic function before each dose and consult product literature for initiating treatment, dose modification and discontinuation in cases of abnormal liver function tests

Renal impairment no information available—manufacturer advises caution in severe impairment

Pregnancy manufacturer advises avoid—oligohydramnios reported with trastuzumab; effective contraception must be used during and for 6 months after stopping treatment in women and men; see also Pregnancy and Reproductive Function, p. 575

Breast-feeding manufacturer advises avoid breast-feeding during and for 6 months after treatment

Side-effects see section 8.1; also diarrhoea, constipation, abdominal pain, dry mouth, dyspepsia, gingival bleeding, left ventricular dysfunction (see Cautions), hypertension, peripheral oedema, epistaxis, cough, dyspnoea, insomnia, peripheral neuropathy (see Cautions), headache, dizziness, dysgeusia, memory impairment, malaise, pyrexia, chills, urinary tract infection, thrombocytopenia (see Cautions), haemorrhage, hypokalaemia, infusion-related reactions, arthralgia, myalgia, dry eye, conjunctivitis, blurred vision, increased lacrimation, rash, pruritus, nail disorder, urticaria, hand-foot syndrome; *less commonly* interstitial lung disease including pneumonitis (see Cautions), hepatic toxicity and failure, nodular regenerative hyperplasia, portal hypertension

Dose
* See Doses, p. 574

Kadcyla® (Roche) ▼ PoM
Intravenous infusion, powder for reconstitution, trastuzumab emtansine, net price 100-mg vial = £1641.01; 160-mg vial = £2625.62
Note When prescribing, dispensing or administering, check that this is the correct preparation—trastuzumab emtansine and trastuzumab are **not** interchangeable

Tretinoin

Tretinoin is licensed for the induction of remission in acute promyelocytic leukaemia. It is used in previously untreated patients as well as in those who have relapsed after standard chemotherapy or who are refractory to it.

▌TRETINOIN

Note Tretinoin is the acid form of vitamin A

Indications see notes above; acne (section 13.6.1); photodamage (section 13.8.1)

Cautions exclude pregnancy before starting treatment; monitor haematological and coagulation profile, liver function, serum calcium and plasma lipids before and during treatment; increased risk of thromboembolism during first month of treatment; **interactions:** Appendix 1 (retinoids)

Hepatic impairment reduce dose to $25 \, \text{mg/m}^2$

Renal impairment reduce dose to $25 \, \text{mg/m}^2$

Pregnancy teratogenic; effective contraception must be used for at least 1 month before oral treatment, during treatment and for at least 1 month after stopping (oral progestogen-only contraceptives not considered effective); see also Pregnancy and Reproductive Function, p. 575

Breast-feeding avoid

Side-effects retinoic acid syndrome (fever, dyspnoea, acute respiratory distress, pulmonary infiltrates, pleural effusion, hyperleucocytosis, hypotension, oedema, weight gain, hepatic, renal and multi-organ failure) requires immediate treatment—consult product literature; gastro-intestinal disturbances, pancreatitis; arrhythmias, flushing, oedema; headache,

benign intracranial hypertension (mainly in children—consider dose reduction if intractable headache in children), shivering, dizziness, confusion, anxiety, depression, insomnia, paraesthesia, visual and hearing disturbances; raised liver enzymes, serum creatinine and lipids; bone and chest pain, alopecia, erythema, rash, pruritus, sweating, dry skin and mucous membranes, cheilitis; thromboembolism, hypercalcaemia, and genital ulceration reported

Dose
* ADULT and CHILD $45 \, \text{mg/m}^2$ daily in 2 divided doses, max. duration of treatment 90 days (consult product literature for details of concomitant chemotherapy)

Vesanoid® (Intrapharm) PoM
Capsules, yellow/brown, tretinoin 10 mg, net price 100-cap pack = £160.63. Label: 21, 25

Vismodegib

Vismodegib is a hedgehog pathway inhibitor used in the treatment of basal cell carcinoma. Vismodegib may cause severe birth defects and embryo-foetal death. For women of child-bearing potential, pregnancy must be excluded before initiation of treatment, and monthly during treatment. Women must use two contraceptive methods (including one highly effective method and one barrier method) during treatment and for 24 months after the final dose of vismodegib; men must use a condom during treatment and for 2 months after the final dose. Prescribers and pharmacists must comply with prescribing and dispensing restrictions as specified in the manufacturer's Pregnancy Prevention Programme, and ensure that the patient fully acknowledges the programme's pregnancy prevention measures—consult product literature for further information.

▌VISMODEGIB

Indications symptomatic metastatic basal cell carcinoma; locally advanced basal cell carcinoma not appropriate for surgery or radiotherapy

Cautions see notes above; **interactions:** Appendix 1 (vismodegib)

Hepatic impairment no information available—manufacturer advises caution in moderate to severe impairment

Renal impairment no information available—manufacturer advises caution in severe impairment

Pregnancy important: teratogenic risk; see also notes above

Breast-feeding avoid during treatment and for 24 months after final dose

Side-effects nausea, vomiting, diarrhoea, constipation, abdominal pain, decreased appetite, weight loss, dehydration, dyspepsia, taste disturbances, malaise, amenorrhoea, hyponatraemia, arthralgia, musculoskeletal pain, muscle spasms, alopecia, abnormal hair growth, pruritus, rash

Dose
* ADULT over 18 years, 150 mg once daily

Erivedge® (Roche) ▼ PoM
Capsules, pink/grey, vismodegib 150 mg, net price 28-cap pack = £6285.00. Label: 25, counselling, pregnancy and contraception
Note Patient, prescriber, and supplying pharmacy must comply with the manufacturer's pregnancy prevention programme

8 Malignant disease and immunosuppression

8.2 Drugs affecting the immune response

8.2.1 Antiproliferative immunosuppressants
8.2.2 Corticosteroids and other immunosuppressants
8.2.3 Anti-lymphocyte monoclonal antibodies
8.2.4 Other immunomodulating drugs

Immunosuppressant therapy

Immunosuppressants are used to suppress rejection in organ transplant recipients and to treat a variety of chronic inflammatory and autoimmune diseases. Solid organ transplant patients are maintained on drug regimens, which may include antiproliferative drugs (azathioprine or mycophenolate mofetil), calcineurin inhibitors (ciclosporin or tacrolimus), corticosteroids, or sirolimus. Choice is dependent on the type of organ, time after transplantation, and clinical condition of the patient. Specialist management is required and other immunomodulators may be used to initiate treatment or to treat rejection.

Impaired immune responsiveness Modification of tissue reactions caused by corticosteroids and other immunosuppressants may result in the rapid *spread of infection*. Corticosteroids may suppress clinical signs of infection and allow diseases such as septicaemia or tuberculosis to reach an advanced stage before being recognised—**important:** for advice on measles exposure, see section 14.5.1, and chickenpox (varicella) exposure, see section 14.5.2. For advice on the use of live vaccines in individuals with impaired immune response, see section 14.1. For general comments and warnings relating to corticosteroids and immunosuppressants, see section 6.3.2.

Pregnancy Transplant patients immunosuppressed with azathioprine should not discontinue it on becoming pregnant. However, there have been reports of premature birth and low birth-weight following exposure to azathioprine, particularly in combination with corticosteroids. Spontaneous abortion has been reported following maternal or paternal exposure. Azathioprine is teratogenic in *animal* studies.

There is less experience of ciclosporin in pregnancy but it does not appear to be any more harmful than azathioprine. The use of these drugs during pregnancy needs to be supervised in specialist units.

8.2.1 Antiproliferative immunosuppressants

Azathioprine is widely used for transplant recipients and it is also used to treat a number of auto-immune conditions, usually when corticosteroid therapy alone provides inadequate control. It is metabolised to mercaptopurine, and doses should be reduced when allopurinol is given concurrently. Blood tests and monitoring for signs of myelosuppression are essential in long-term treatment with azathioprine.

Thiopurine methyltransferase
The enzyme thiopurine methyltransferase (TPMT) metabolises thiopurine drugs (azathioprine, mercaptopurine, tioguanine); the risk of myelosuppression is increased in patients with reduced activity of the enzyme, particularly for the few individuals in whom TPMT activity is undetectable. Consider measuring TPMT activity before starting azathioprine, mercaptopurine, or tioguanine therapy. Patients with absent TPMT activity should not receive thiopurine drugs; those with reduced TPMT activity may be treated under specialist supervision.

Mycophenolate mofetil is metabolised to mycophenolic acid which has a more selective mode of action than azathioprine. It is licensed for the prophylaxis of acute rejection in renal, hepatic or cardiac transplantation when used in combination with ciclosporin and corticosteroids. There is evidence that compared with similar regimens incorporating azathioprine, mycophenolate mofetil reduces the risk of acute rejection episodes; the risk of opportunistic infections (particularly due to tissue-invasive cytomegalovirus) and the occurrence of blood disorders such as leucopenia may be higher.

Cases of pure red cell aplasia have been reported with azathioprine and with mycophenolate mofetil; dose reduction or discontinuation should be considered under specialist supervision.

Cyclophosphamide (section 8.1.1) is less commonly prescribed as an immunosuppressant.

▌ AZATHIOPRINE

Indications see notes above; inflammatory bowel disease (section 1.5.3); rheumatoid arthritis (section 10.1.3); severe refractory eczema [unlicensed indication] (section 13.5.3)

Cautions reduced thiopurine methyltransferase activity (see notes above); monitor for toxicity throughout treatment; monitor full blood count weekly (more frequently with higher doses or if severe hepatic or renal impairment) for first 4 weeks (manufacturer advises weekly monitoring for 8 weeks but evidence of practical value unsatisfactory), thereafter reduce frequency of monitoring to at least every 3 months; reduce dose in elderly; **interactions:** Appendix 1 (azathioprine)

Bone marrow suppression Patients should be warned to report immediately any signs or symptoms of bone marrow suppression e.g. inexplicable bruising or bleeding, infection

Contra-indications see notes above; hypersensitivity to mercaptopurine

Hepatic impairment reduce dose; monitor liver function; see also Cautions

Renal impairment reduce dose; see also Cautions

Pregnancy treatment should not generally be initiated during pregnancy; see also above

Breast-feeding present in milk in low concentration; no evidence of harm in small studies—use if potential benefit outweighs risk

Side-effects hypersensitivity reactions (including malaise, dizziness, vomiting, diarrhoea, fever, rigors, myalgia, arthralgia, rash, hypotension and interstitial nephritis—calling for immediate withdrawal); dose-related bone marrow suppression (see also Cautions); liver impairment, cholestatic jaundice, hair loss and increased susceptibility to infections and colitis in patients also receiving corticosteroids; nausea; *rarely* pancreatitis, pneumonitis, hepatic veno-occlusive disease, lymphoma, red cell aplasia—see notes above

Dose
* By mouth, *or* (if oral administration not possible—intravenous solution very irritant, see below) by intravenous injection over at least 1 minute (followed by 50 mL sodium chloride intravenous infusion), *or* by intravenous infusion

    Autoimmune conditions, 1–3 mg/kg daily, adjusted according to response (consider withdrawal if no improvement within 3 months)

    Suppression of transplant rejection, 1–2.5 mg/kg daily adjusted according to response

    Note Azathioprine doses in BNF may differ from those in product literature

    Note Intravenous injection is alkaline and very irritant, intravenous route should therefore be used **only** if oral route not feasible, see also Appendix 4

Azathioprine (Non-proprietary) PoM

Tablets, azathioprine 25 mg, net price 28-tab pack = £3.91; 50 mg, 56-tab pack = £3.54. Label: 21

Brands include *Azamune*®

Imuran® (Aspen) PoM

Tablets, both f/c, azathioprine 25 mg (orange), net price 100-tab pack = £10.99; 50 mg (yellow), 100-tab pack = £7.99. Label: 21

Injection, powder for reconstitution, azathioprine (as sodium salt), net price 50-mg vial = £15.38

▌ MYCOPHENOLATE MOFETIL

Indications prophylaxis of acute renal, cardiac, or hepatic transplant rejection (in combination with ciclosporin and corticosteroids) under specialist supervision

Cautions monitor full blood count every week for 4 weeks then twice a month for 2 months then every month in the first year (consider interrupting treatment if neutropenia develops); exclude pregnancy before starting treatment; elderly (increased risk of infection, gastro-intestinal haemorrhage and pulmonary oedema); children (higher incidence of side-effects may call for temporary reduction of dose or interruption); active serious gastro-intestinal disease (risk of haemorrhage, ulceration and perforation); delayed graft function; increased susceptibility to skin cancer (avoid exposure to strong sunlight); **interactions**: Appendix 1 (mycophenolate)

Bone marrow suppression Patients should be warned to report immediately any signs or symptoms of bone marrow suppression e.g. infection or inexplicable bruising or bleeding

Renal impairment no data available in cardiac or hepatic transplant patients with renal impairment

Pregnancy avoid—congenital malformations reported; effective contraception required before treatment, during treatment, and for 6 weeks after discontinuation of treatment; manufacturer of *Myfortic*® also advise that men should use condoms during treatment and for 13 weeks after last dose

Breast-feeding avoid—present in milk in *animal* studies

Side-effects taste disturbance, gingival hyperplasia, nausea, constipation, flatulence, anorexia, weight loss, vomiting, abdominal pain, gastro-intestinal inflammation, ulceration, and bleeding, hepatitis, jaundice, pancreatitis, stomatitis, oedema, tachycardia, hypertension, hypotension, vasodilatation, cough, dyspnoea, insomnia, agitation, confusion, depression, anxiety, convulsions, paraesthesia, myasthenic syndrome, tremor, dizziness, headache, influenza-like syndrome, infections, hyperglycaemia, renal impairment, malignancy (particularly of the skin), blood disorders (including leucopenia, anaemia, thrombocytopenia, pancytopenia, and red cell aplasia—see notes above), disturbances of electrolytes and blood lipids, arthralgia, alopecia, acne, skin hypertrophy, and rash; *also reported* intestinal villous atrophy, progressive multifocal leucoencephalopathy, interstitial lung disease, pulmonary fibrosis

Dose
* Renal transplantation, by mouth, 1 g twice daily starting within 72 hours of transplantation *or* by intravenous infusion, 1 g twice daily starting within 24 hours of transplantation for max. 14 days (then transfer to oral therapy); CHILD and ADOLESCENT 2–18 years, by mouth 600 mg/m² twice daily (max. 2 g daily)

    Note Tablets and capsules not appropriate for dose titration in children with body surface area less than 1.25 m²

* Cardiac transplantation, by mouth, ADULT over 18 years, 1.5 g twice daily starting within 5 days of transplantation

* Hepatic transplantation, by intravenous infusion, ADULT over 18 years, 1 g twice daily starting within 24 hours of transplantation for 4 days (up to max. 14 days), then by mouth, 1.5 g twice daily as soon as is tolerated

Mycophenolate Mofetil (Non-proprietary) PoM

Capsules, mycophenolate mofetil 250 mg, net price 100-cap pack = £82.26

Tablets, mycophenolate mofetil 500 mg, net price 50-tab pack = £17.80

Brands include Arzip®

CellCept® (Roche) PoM

Capsules, blue/brown, mycophenolate mofetil 250 mg, net price 100-cap pack = £82.26

Tablets, lavender, mycophenolate mofetil 500 mg, net price 50-tab pack = £82.26

Oral suspension, mycophenolate mofetil 1 g/5 mL when reconstituted with water, net price 175 mL = £115.16.

Excipients include aspartame (section 9.4.1)

Intravenous infusion, powder for reconstitution, mycophenolate mofetil (as hydrochloride), net price 500-mg vial = £9.12

▌Mycophenolic acid

Myfortic® (Novartis) PoM

Tablets, e/c, mycophenolic acid (as mycophenolate sodium) 180 mg (green), net price 120-tab pack = £96.72; 360 mg (orange), 120-tab pack = £193.43. Label: 25

Dose renal transplantation, 720 mg twice daily starting within 72 hours of transplantation

Equivalence to mycophenolate mofetil Mycophenolic acid 720 mg is approximately equivalent to mycophenolate mofetil 1 g but avoid unnecessary switching because of pharmacokinetic differences

8.2.2 Corticosteroids and other immunosuppressants

Prednisolone (section 6.3.2) is widely used in oncology. It has a marked antitumour effect in acute lymphoblastic leukaemia, Hodgkin's disease, and the non-Hodgkin lymphomas. It has a role in the palliation of symptomatic end-stage malignant disease when it may enhance appetite and produce a sense of well-being (see also Prescribing in Palliative Care, p. 21).

The corticosteroids are also powerful immunosuppressants. They are used to prevent organ transplant rejection, and in high dose to treat rejection episodes.

Ciclosporin a calcineurin inhibitor, is a potent immunosuppressant which is virtually non-myelotoxic but markedly nephrotoxic. It has an important role in organ and tissue transplantation, for prevention of graft rejection following bone marrow, kidney, liver, pancreas, heart, lung, and heart-lung transplantation, and for prophylaxis and treatment of graft-versus-host disease.

Tacrolimus is also a calcineurin inhibitor. Although not chemically related to ciclosporin it has a similar mode of action and side-effects, but the incidence of neurotoxicity appears to be greater; cardiomyopathy has also been reported. Disturbance of glucose metabolism also appears to be significant.

Sirolimus is a non-calcineurin inhibiting immunosuppressant licensed for renal transplantation.

Basiliximab is a monoclonal antibody that acts as an interleukin-2 receptor antagonist and prevents T-lymphocyte proliferation; it is used for prophylaxis of acute rejection in allogeneic renal transplantation. It is given with ciclosporin and corticosteroid immunosuppression regimens; its use should be confined to specialist centres.

Belatacept is a fusion protein and co-stimulation blocker that prevents T-cell activation; it is licensed for prophylaxis of graft rejection in adults undergoing renal transplantation who are seropositive for the Epstein-Barr virus. It is used with interleukin-2 receptor antagonist induction, in combination with corticosteroids and a mycophenolic acid.

Antithymocyte immunoglobulin (rabbit) is licensed for the prophylaxis of organ rejection in renal and heart allograft recipients and for the treatment of corticosteroid-resistant allograft rejection in renal transplantation. Tolerability is increased by pretreatment with an intravenous corticosteroid and antihistamine; an antipyretic drug such as paracetamol may also be beneficial.

NICE guidance
Immunosuppressive therapy for renal transplantation in adults (September 2004)
Immunosuppressive therapy for renal transplantation in children and adolescents (April 2006)

For induction therapy in the prophylaxis of organ rejection, either basiliximab or daclizumab [discontinued] are options for combining with a calcineurin inhibitor. For each individual, ciclosporin or tacrolimus is chosen as the calcineurin inhibitor on the basis of side-effects.

Mycophenolate mofetil [mycophenolic acid also available but not licensed for use in children, see p. 629] is recommended as part of an immunosuppressive regimen only if:

● the calcineurin inhibitor is not tolerated, particularly if nephrotoxicity endangers the transplanted kidney; or

● there is very high risk of nephrotoxicity from the calcineurin inhibitor, requiring a reduction in the dose of the calcineurin inhibitor or its avoidance.

Sirolimus is recommended as a component of immunosuppressive regimen only if intolerance necessitates the withdrawal of a calcineurin inhibitor.

These recommendations may not be consistent with the marketing authorisation of some of the products.
www.nice.org.uk/TA85

ANTITHYMOCYTE IMMUNOGLOBULIN (RABBIT)

Indications see notes above

Cautions see notes above; monitor blood count

Contra-indications infection

Pregnancy manufacturer advises use only if potential benefit outweighs risk—no information available

Breast-feeding manufacturer advises avoid—no information available

Side-effects nausea, vomiting, dysphagia, diarrhoea; hypotension; infusion-related reactions (including cytokine release syndrome and anaphylaxis, see notes above), serum sickness; fever, shivering, increased susceptibility to infection; increased susceptibility to malignancy; lymphopenia, neutropenia, thrombocytopenia; myalgia; pruritus, rash

Dose

● Heart transplantation, by intravenous infusion over at least 6 hours, 1–2.5 mg/kg daily for 3–5 days

● Renal transplantation, by intravenous infusion over at least 6 hours, 1–1.5 mg/kg daily for 3–9 days

● Corticosteroid-resistant renal graft rejection, by intravenous infusion over at least 6 hours, 1.5 mg/kg daily for 7–14 days

Note To avoid excessive dosage in obese patients, calculate dose on the basis of ideal body weight

Thymoglobuline® (Sanofi-Aventis) PoM
Intravenous infusion, powder for reconstitution, rabbit anti-human thymocyte immunoglobulin, net price 25-mg vial = £158.77

BASILIXIMAB

Indications see notes above

Cautions off-label use in cardiac transplantation—increased risk of serious cardiac side-effects including cardiac arrest, atrial flutter, and palpitations; **interactions**; Appendix 1 (basiliximab)

Pregnancy avoid—no information available; adequate contraception must be used during treatment and for 16 weeks after last dose

Breast-feeding avoid—no information available

Side-effects severe hypersensitivity reactions and cytokine release syndrome have been reported

Dose

• By intravenous injection *or* by intravenous infusion, 20 mg within 2 hours before transplant surgery and 20 mg 4 days after surgery; withhold second dose if severe hypersensitivity or graft loss occurs; CHILD and ADOLESCENT 1–17 years, body-weight under 35 kg, 10 mg within 2 hours before transplant surgery and 10 mg 4 days after surgery; body-weight over 35 kg, adult dose

Simulect® (Novartis) (PoM)
Injection, powder for reconstitution, basiliximab, net price 10-mg vial = £758.69, 20-mg vial = £842.38 (both with water for injections). For intravenous infusion

---

BELATACEPT

Indications see notes above

Cautions increased risk of infection; risk factors for post-transplant lymphoproliferative disorder; avoid excessive exposure to UV light including sunlight; tapering of corticosteroid, particularly in patients with high immunologic risk—increased risk of acute graft rejection
Tuberculosis Patients should be evaluated for latent and active tuberculosis before starting treatment, and monitored for signs and symptoms of tuberculosis during and after treatment

Pregnancy use only if essential; adequate contraception must be used during treatment and for up to 8 weeks after last dose

Breast-feeding avoid—no information available

Side-effects (reported when used in combination with basiliximab, mycophenolate mofetil and corticosteroids) diarrhoea, constipation, nausea, vomiting, hypertension, peripheral oedema, cough, headache, pyrexia, infection, malignancy, anaemia, leucopenia, dehydration, hypophosphataemia; *less commonly* infusion related reactions, progressive multifocal leucoencephalopathy

Dose

• Consult product literature

Nulojix® (Bristol-Myers Squibb) ▼(PoM)
Intravenous infusion, powder for reconstitution, belatacept, net price 250-mg vial = £354.52

CICLOSPORIN

(Cyclosporin)

Indications see notes above, and under Dose; severe acute ulcerative colitis [unlicensed indication] (section 1.5.3); rheumatoid arthritis (section 10.1.3); atopic dermatitis and psoriasis (section 13.5.3)

Cautions monitor kidney function—dose dependent increase in serum creatinine and urea during first few weeks may necessitate dose reduction in transplant patients (exclude rejection if kidney transplant) or discontinuation in non-transplant patients; monitor liver function (see Hepatic Impairment below); monitor blood pressure—discontinue if hypertension

develops that cannot be controlled by antihypertensives; hyperuricaemia; monitor serum potassium especially in renal dysfunction (risk of hyperkalaemia); monitor serum magnesium; measure blood lipids before treatment and after the first month of treatment; use with tacrolimus specifically contraindicated; for patients other than transplant recipients, preferably avoid other immunosuppressants (increased risk of infection and malignancies, including lymphoma and skin cancer); avoid excessive exposure to UV light, including sunlight; **interactions**: Appendix 1 (ciclosporin)
Additional cautions in nephrotic syndrome *Contraindicated* in uncontrolled hypertension, uncontrolled infections, and malignancy; in long-term management, perform renal biopsies at yearly intervals
Additional cautions Atopic Dermatitis and Psoriasis, section 13.5.3; Rheumatoid Arthritis, section 10.1.3

Hepatic impairment dosage adjustment based on bilirubin and liver enzymes may be needed

Renal impairment dose as in normal renal function but see Cautions above; in nephrotic syndrome reduce dose by 25–50% if serum creatinine more than 30% above baseline on more than one measurement; in patients with nephrotic syndrome and renal impairment initially 2.5 mg/kg daily

Pregnancy crosses placenta; see Immunosuppressant Therapy, p. 628

Breast-feeding present in milk—manufacturer advises avoid

Side-effects anorexia, nausea, vomiting, abdominal pain, diarrhoea, gingival hyperplasia, hepatic dysfunction, hypertension, tremor, headache, paraesthesia, fatigue, renal dysfunction (renal structural changes on long-term administration, see also under Cautions), hyperuricaemia, hyperkalaemia, hypomagnesaemia, hyperlipidaemia, hypercholesterolaemia, muscle cramps, myalgia, hypertrichosis; *less commonly* oedema, weight gain, signs of encephalopathy, anaemia, thrombocytopenia; *rarely* pancreatitis, motor polyneuropathy, menstrual disturbances, gynaecomastia, microangiopathic haemolytic anaemia, haemolytic uraemic syndrome, hyperglycaemia, muscle weakness, myopathy, visual disturbances secondary to benign intracranial hypertension (discontinue); *also reported with infusion* anaphylaxis

Dose

• Organ transplantation, used alone, ADULT and CHILD over 3 months 10–15 mg/kg by mouth 4–12 hours before transplantation followed by 10–15 mg/kg daily for 1–2 weeks postoperatively then reduced gradually to 2–6 mg/kg daily for maintenance (dose should be adjusted according to blood-ciclosporin concentration and renal function); dose lower if given concomitantly with other immunosuppressant therapy (e.g. corticosteroids); if necessary one-third corresponding oral dose can be given by intravenous infusion over 2–6 hours

• Bone-marrow transplantation, prevention and treatment of graft-versus-host disease, ADULT and CHILD over 3 months 3–5 mg/kg daily by intravenous infusion over 2–6 hours from day before transplantation to 2 weeks postoperatively (or 12.5–15 mg/kg daily by mouth) then 12.5 mg/kg daily by mouth for 3–6 months then tailed off (may take up to a year after transplantation)

• Nephrotic syndrome, by mouth, 5 mg/kg daily in 2 divided doses; CHILD 6 mg/kg daily in 2 divided doses; maintenance treatment reduce to lowest effective dose according to proteinuria and serum creatinine measurements; discontinue after 3 months if no improvement in glomerulonephritis or glomerulo-sclerosis (after 6 months in membranous glomerulonephritis)

Important

Patients should be stabilised on a particular brand of oral ciclosporin because switching between formulations without close monitoring may lead to clinically important changes in blood-ciclosporin concentration. Prescribing and dispensing of ciclosporin should be by brand name to avoid inadvertent switching. If it is necessary to switch a patient to a different brand of ciclosporin, the patient should be monitored closely for changes in blood-ciclosporin concentration, serum creatinine, blood pressure, and transplant function.

Capimune® (Mylan) ▣PoM▣

Capsules, ciclosporin 25 mg (grey), net price 30-cap pack = £13.05; 50 mg (white), 30-cap pack = £25.50; 100 mg (grey), 30-cap pack = £48.50. Counselling, administration

Excipients include propylene glycol (see Excipients, p. 2)

Note Contains ethanol

Counselling Total daily dose should be taken in 2 divided doses

Capsorin® (Morningside) ▣PoM▣

Capsules, ciclosporin 25 mg (grey), net price 30-cap pack = £13.05; 50 mg (white), 30-cap pack = £25.59; 100 mg (grey), 30-cap pack = £48.89. Counselling, administration

Note Contains ethanol

Counselling Total daily dose should be taken in 2 divided doses

Deximune® (Dexcel) ▣PoM▣

Capsules, grey, ciclosporin 25 mg, net price 30-cap pack = £13.06; 50 mg 30-cap pack = £25.60; 100 mg 30-cap pack = £48.90. Counselling, administration

Note Contains ethyl lactate which is metabolised to ethanol

Counselling Total daily dose should be taken in 2 divided doses

Neoral® (Novartis) ▣PoM▣

Capsules, ciclosporin 10 mg (yellow/white), net price 60-cap pack = £19.40; 25 mg (blue/grey), 30-cap pack = £19.52; 50 mg (yellow/white), 30-cap pack = £38.23; 100 mg (blue/grey), 30-cap pack = £72.57. Counselling, administration

Excipients include propylene glycol (see Excipients, p. 2)

Note Contains ethanol

Oral solution, yellow, sugar-free, ciclosporin 100 mg/mL, net price 50 mL = £108.73. Counselling, administration

Excipients include propylene glycol (see Excipients, p. 2)

Note Contains ethanol

Counselling Total daily dose should be taken in 2 divided doses

Mix solution with orange juice (or squash) or apple juice (to improve taste) or with water immediately before taking (and rinse with more to ensure total dose). Do not mix with grapefruit juice. Keep medicine measure away from other liquids (including water)

Sandimmun® (Novartis) ▣PoM▣

Concentrate for intravenous infusion (oily), ciclosporin 50 mg/mL. To be diluted before use, net price 1-mL amp = £1.94; 5-mL amp = £9.17

Excipients include polyoxyl castor oil (risk of anaphylaxis, see Excipients, p. 2)

Note Contains ethanol

Note Observe patients for signs of anaphylaxis for at least 30 minutes after starting infusion and at frequent intervals thereafter

Note Sandimmun® capsules and oral solution are available direct from Novartis for patients who cannot be transferred to a different oral preparation

◼ SIROLIMUS

Indications prophylaxis of organ rejection in kidney allograft recipients (initially in combination with ciclosporin and corticosteroid, then with corticosteroid only); see also under Dose

Cautions monitor kidney function when given with ciclosporin; monitor whole blood-sirolimus trough concentration (Afro-Caribbean patients may require higher doses); hyperlipidaemia (monitor lipids); monitor urine proteins; increased susceptibility to infection (especially urinary-tract infection); increased susceptibility to lymphoma and other malignancies, particularly of the skin (limit exposure to UV light); **interactions:** Appendix 1 (sirolimus)

Hepatic impairment monitor whole blood-sirolimus level closely and consult local treatment protocol; clearance reduced in mild to moderate impairment; in severe impairment decrease dose by 50% and monitor whole blood-sirolimus trough concentration every 5–7 days until 3 consecutive measurements have shown stable blood-sirolimus concentration

Pregnancy avoid unless essential—(toxicity in *animal* studies); effective contraception must be used during treatment and for 12 weeks after stopping

Breast-feeding discontinue breast-feeding

Side-effects abdominal pain, constipation, nausea, diarrhoea, ascites, stomatitis; oedema, tachycardia, hypertension, hypercholesterolaemia, hypertriglyceridaemia, venous thromboembolism; pleural effusion, pneumonitis; headache, pyrexia; proteinuria, haemolytic uraemic syndrome; anaemia, thrombocytopenia, thrombotic thrombocytopenic purpura, leucopenia, neutropenia, hypokalaemia, hypophosphataemia, hyperglycaemia, lymphocele; arthralgia, osteonecrosis; epistaxis; acne, rash, impaired healing; *less commonly* pancreatitis, pulmonary embolism, pulmonary haemorrhage, pericardial effusion, nephrotic syndrome, pancytopenia; *rarely* interstitial lung disease, alveolar proteinosis, hepatic necrosis, lymphoedema, and hypersensitivity reactions including anaphylactic reactions, angioedema, exfoliative dermatitis, and hypersensitivity vasculitis; focal segmental glomerulosclerosis and reversible impairment of male fertility also reported

Dose

• Initially 6 mg, after surgery (once wound has healed), then 2 mg once daily (dose adjusted according to whole blood-sirolimus trough concentration) in combination with ciclosporin and corticosteroid for 2–3 months (sirolimus given 4 hours after ciclosporin); ciclosporin should then be withdrawn over 4–8 weeks (if not possible, sirolimus should be discontinued and an alternate immunosuppressive regimen used)

Note Manufacturer advises pre-dose ('trough') whole blood-sirolimus concentration (using **chromatographic** assay) when used with ciclosporin should be 4–12 micrograms/litre (local treatment protocols may differ); after withdrawal of ciclosporin pre-dose whole blood-sirolimus concentration should be 12–20 micrograms/litre (local treatment protocols may differ); close monitoring of whole blood-sirolimus concentration required if concomitant treatment with potent inducers or inhibitors of metabolism and after discontinuing them, or if ciclosporin dose reduced significantly or stopped; see also Hepatic Impairment above

When changing between oral solution and tablets, measurement of whole blood 'trough' sirolimus concentration after 1–2 weeks is recommended

Therapeutic drug monitoring assays Sirolimus whole-blood concentration is measured using either high performance liquid chromatography (HPLC) or immunoassay. Switching between different immunoassays or between an immunoassay and HPLC can lead to clinically significant differences in results and therefore incorrect dose adjustments. Adjustment to the target therapeutic dose range should be made with knowledge of the assay used and corresponding reference range

Rapamune® (Pfizer) [PoM]
Tablets, coated, sirolimus 500 micrograms (tan), net price 30-tab pack = £69.00; 1 mg (white), 30-tab pack = £86.49; 2 mg (yellow), 30-tab pack = £172.98. Counselling, administration
Important The 500-microgram tablet is not bioequivalent to the 1-mg and 2-mg tablets. Multiples of 500 microgram tablets should **not** be used as a substitute for other tablet strengths

Oral solution, sirolimus 1 mg/mL, net price 60 mL = £162.41. Counselling, administration
Note Contains ethanol

Counselling Food may affect absorption (take at the same time with respect to food). Mix solution with at least 60 mL water or orange juice in a glass or plastic container immediately before taking; refill container with at least 120 mL of water or orange juice and drink immediately (to ensure total dose). Do not mix with any other liquids

▌ TACROLIMUS

Indications prophylaxis of organ rejection in liver, kidney, and heart allograft recipients and allograft rejection resistant to conventional immunosuppressive regimens, see also notes above; moderate to severe atopic eczema (section 13.5.3)

Cautions monitor blood pressure, ECG (**important:** see Cardiomyopathy below), fasting blood-glucose concentration, haematological and neurological (including visual) parameters, electrolytes, hepatic and renal function; monitor whole blood-tacrolimus trough concentration (especially during episodes of diarrhoea)—consult local treatment protocol for details; QT-interval prolongation; neurotoxicity; increased risk of infections, malignancies, and lymphoproliferative disorders; avoid excessive exposure to UV light including sunlight; **interactions:** Appendix 1 (tacrolimus)
Driving May affect performance of skilled tasks (e.g. driving)

Contra-indications hypersensitivity to macrolides; avoid concurrent administration with ciclosporin (care if patient has previously received ciclosporin)

Hepatic impairment dose reduction may be necessary in severe impairment

Pregnancy exclude before treatment; avoid unless potential benefit outweighs risk—risk of premature delivery, intra-uterine growth restriction, and hyperkalaemia

Breast-feeding avoid—present in breast milk

Side-effects nausea, vomiting, diarrhoea, constipation, dyspepsia, flatulence, bloating, weight changes, anorexia, gastro-intestinal inflammation, ulceration, and perforation, hepatic dysfunction, jaundice, cholestasis, ascites, bile-duct abnormalities, oedema, tachycardia, hypertension, haemorrhage, thromboembolic and ischaemic events, dyspnoea, pleural effusion, parenchymal lung disorders, sleep disturbances, tremor, headache, peripheral neuropathy, mood changes, depression, confusion, anxiety, psychosis, seizures, paraesthesia, dizziness, renal impairment, renal failure, renal tubular necrosis, urinary abnormalities, hyperglycaemia, electrolyte disturbances (including hyperkalaemia, hypokalaemia, and hyperuricaemia), blood disorders (including anaemia, leucopenia, pancytopenia, and thrombocytopenia), arthralgia, muscle cramp, visual disturbances, photophobia, tinnitus, impaired hearing, alopecia, sweating, acne; *less commonly* paralytic ileus, gastro-intestinal reflux disease, peritonitis, pancreatitis, heart failure, arrhythmia, cardiac arrest, cerebrovascular accident, cardiomyopathy (**important:** see Cardiomyopathy below), palpitation, respiratory failure, coma, speech disorder, amnesia, paralysis, influenza-like symptoms, encephalopathy, coagulation disorders, photosensitivity, cataract, hypoglycaemia, dysmenorrhoea, hypertonia, dermatitis; *rarely* pericardial effusion, respiratory distress syndrome, posterior reversible encephalopathy syndrome, dehydration, thrombotic thrombocytopenic purpura, blindness, toxic epidermal necrolysis, hirsutism; *very rarely* myasthenia, haemorrhagic cystitis, Stevens-Johnson syndrome; *also reported* pure red cell aplasia, agranulocytosis, haemolytic anaemia

Cardiomyopathy Cardiomyopathy has been reported in children. Patients should be monitored by echocardiography for hypertrophic changes—consider dose reduction or discontinuation if these occur

Dose
● See under preparations

MHRA/CHM advice
Oral tacrolimus products: prescribe and dispense by brand name only, to minimise the risk of inadvertent switching between products, which has been associated with reports of toxicity and graft rejection (June 2012)

Inadvertent switching between oral tacrolimus products has been associated with reports of toxicity and graft rejection. To ensure maintenance of therapeutic response when a patient is stabilised on a particular brand, oral tacrolimus products should be prescribed and dispensed by brand name only.

● *Adoport*®, *Prograf*®, *Capexion*®, *Tacni*®, and *Vivadex*® are immediate-release capsules that are taken twice daily, once in the morning and once in the evening;

● *Modigraf*® granules are used to prepare an immediate-release oral suspension which is taken twice daily, once in the morning and once in the evening;

● *Advagraf*® is a prolonged-release capsule that is taken once daily in the morning.

Switching between tacrolimus brands requires careful supervision and therapeutic monitoring by an appropriate specialist.

Adoport® (Sandoz) [PoM]
Capsules, tacrolimus (as monohydrate) 500 micrograms (white/ivory), net price 50-cap pack = £42.92; 1 mg (white/brown), 50-cap pack = £55.69,

100-cap pack = £111.36; 5 mg (white/orange), 50-cap pack = £205.74. Label: 23, counselling, driving

Note Tacrolimus is incompatible with PVC

Dose liver transplantation, starting 12 hours after transplantation, by mouth, 100–200 micrograms/kg daily in 2 divided doses; CHILD 300 micrograms/kg daily in 2 divided doses

Renal transplantation, starting within 24 hours of transplantation, by mouth, 200–300 micrograms/kg daily in 2 divided doses; CHILD 300 micrograms/kg daily in 2 divided doses

Heart transplantation with antibody induction (starting within 5 days of transplantation) or without antibody induction (starting within 12 hours of transplantation), by mouth, 75 micrograms/kg daily in 2 divided doses; CHILD, with antibody induction (starting within 5 days of transplantation), 100–300 micrograms/kg daily in 2 divided doses; without antibody induction (starting within 12 hours of transplantation), 300 micrograms/kg daily in 2 divided doses as soon as clinically possible (8–12 hours after discontinuing intravenous infusion)

Maintenance treatment, dose adjusted according to response and whole blood concentration

Rejection therapy, seek specialist advice

Capexion® (Generics) [PoM]

Capsules, tacrolimus 500 micrograms, (ivory), net price 50-cap pack = £52.50; 1 mg (white), 50-cap pack = £68.20, 100-cap pack = £136.20; 5 mg (red), 50-cap pack = £252.00. Label: 23, counselling, driving

Note Tacrolimus is incompatible with PVC

Dose liver transplantation, starting 12 hours after transplantation, by mouth, 100–200 micrograms/kg daily in 2 divided doses; CHILD 300 micrograms/kg daily in 2 divided doses

Renal transplantation, starting within 24 hours of transplantation, by mouth, 200–300 micrograms/kg daily in 2 divided doses; CHILD 300 micrograms/kg daily in 2 divided doses

Heart transplantation with antibody induction (starting within 5 days of transplantation) or without antibody induction (starting within 12 hours of transplantation), by mouth, 75 micrograms/kg daily in 2 divided doses; CHILD with antibody induction (starting within 5 days of transplantation), 100–300 micrograms/kg daily in 2 divided doses; without antibody induction (starting within 12 hours of transplantation), 300 micrograms/kg daily in 2 divided doses as soon as clinically possible (8–12 hours after discontinuing intravenous infusion)

Maintenance treatment, dose adjusted according to response and whole blood concentration

Rejection therapy, seek specialist advice

Modigraf® (Astellas) [PoM]

Granules, tacrolimus (as monohydrate), 200 micrograms, net price 50-sachet pack = £71.30; 1 mg, 50-sachet pack = £356.65. Label: 13, 23, counselling, driving

Note Tacrolimus is incompatible with PVC

Dose liver transplantation, starting 12 hours after transplantation, by mouth, 100–200 micrograms/kg daily in 2 divided doses; CHILD 300 micrograms/kg daily in 2 divided doses

Renal transplantation, starting within 24 hours of transplantation, by mouth, 200–300 micrograms/kg daily in 2 divided doses; CHILD 300 micrograms/kg daily in 2 divided doses

Heart transplantation with antibody induction (starting within 5 days of transplantation) or without antibody induction (starting within 12 hours of transplantation), by mouth, 75 micrograms/kg daily in 2 divided doses; CHILD, with antibody induction (starting within 5 days of transplantation), 100–300 micrograms/kg daily in 2 divided doses; without antibody induction (starting within 12 hours of transplantation), 300 micrograms/kg daily in 2 divided doses as soon as clinically possible (8–12 hours after discontinuing intravenous infusion)

Maintenance treatment, dose adjusted according to response and whole blood concentration

Rejection therapy, seek specialist advice

Note The *Scottish Medicines Consortium* (p. 4) has advised (November 2010) that tacrolimus granules for oral suspension (*Modigraf*®) are accepted for restricted use within NHS Scotland in patients for whom tacrolimus is an appropriate choice of immunosuppressive therapy and where small changes (less than 500 micrograms) in dosing increments are required (such as, in paediatric patients) or seriously ill patients who are unable to swallow tacrolimus capsules.

Prograf® (Astellas) [PoM]

Capsules, tacrolimus (as monohydrate) 500 micrograms (yellow), net price 50-cap pack = £61.88; 1 mg (white), 50-cap pack = £80.28, 100-cap pack = £160.54; 5 mg (greyish-red), 50-cap pack = £296.58. Label: 23, counselling, driving

Note Tacrolimus is incompatible with PVC

Concentrate for intravenous infusion, tacrolimus 5 mg/mL. To be diluted before use. Net price 1-mL amp = £58.45

Excipients include polyoxyl castor oil (risk of anaphylaxis, see Excipients, p. 2)

Note Tacrolimus is incompatible with PVC

Dose liver transplantation, starting 12 hours after transplantation, by mouth, 100–200 micrograms/kg daily in 2 divided doses *or* by intravenous infusion over 24 hours, 10–50 micrograms/kg daily for up to 7 days (then transfer to oral therapy); CHILD by mouth, 300 micrograms/kg daily in 2 divided doses *or* by intravenous infusion over 24 hours, 50 micrograms/kg daily for up to 7 days (then transfer to oral therapy)

Renal transplantation, starting within 24 hours of transplantation, by mouth, 200–300 micrograms/kg daily in 2 divided doses *or* by intravenous infusion over 24 hours, 50–100 micrograms/kg daily for up to 7 days (then transfer to oral therapy); CHILD by mouth, 300 micrograms/kg daily in 2 divided doses *or* by intravenous infusion over 24 hours, 75–100 micrograms/kg daily for up to 7 days (then transfer to oral therapy)

Heart transplantation with antibody induction (starting within 5 days of transplantation) or without antibody induction (starting within 12 hours of transplantation), by mouth, 75 micrograms/kg daily in 2 divided doses *or* by intravenous infusion over 24 hours, 10–20 micrograms/kg daily for up to 7 days (then transfer to oral therapy); CHILD, with antibody induction (starting within 5 days of transplantation), by mouth, 100–300 micrograms/kg daily in 2 divided doses; without antibody induction (starting within 12 hours of transplantation), initially by intravenous infusion over 24 hours, 30–50 micrograms/kg daily, then by mouth, 300 micrograms/kg daily in 2 divided doses as soon as clinically possible (8–12 hours after discontinuing intravenous infusion)

Maintenance treatment, dose adjusted according to response and whole blood concentration

Rejection therapy, seek specialist advice

Tacni® (TEVA UK) [PoM]

Capsules, tacrolimus 500 micrograms (ivory), net price 50-cap pack = £50.48; 1 mg (white), 50-cap pack = £65.49, 100-cap pack = £130.99; 5 mg (red), 50-cap pack = £242.01. Label: 23, counselling, driving

Note Tacrolimus is incompatible with PVC

Dose liver transplantation, starting 12 hours after transplantation, by mouth, 100–200 micrograms/kg daily in 2 divided doses; CHILD 300 micrograms/kg daily in 2 divided doses

Renal transplantation, starting within 24 hours of transplantation, by mouth, 200–300 micrograms/kg daily in 2 divided doses; CHILD 300 micrograms/kg daily in 2 divided doses

Heart transplantation with antibody induction (starting within 5 days of transplantation) or without antibody induction (starting within 12 hours of transplantation), by mouth, 75 micrograms/kg daily in 2 divided doses; CHILD

Maintenance treatment, dose adjusted according to response and whole blood concentration

Rejection therapy, seek specialist advice

with antibody induction (starting within 5 days of transplantation), 100–300 micrograms/kg daily in 2 divided doses; without antibody induction (starting within 12 hours of transplantation), 300 micrograms/kg daily in 2 divided doses as soon as clinically possible (8–12 hours after discontinuing intravenous infusion)

Maintenance treatment, dose adjusted according to response and whole blood concentration

Rejection therapy, seek specialist advice

Vivadex® (Dexcel) PoM

Capsules, tacrolimus 500 micrograms (ivory), net price 50-cap pack = £46.41; 1 mg (white), 50-cap pack = £60.21, 100-cap pack = £120.41; 5 mg (red), 50-cap pack = £222.44. Label: 23, counselling, driving

Note Tacrolimus is incompatible with PVC

Dose liver transplantation, starting 12 hours after transplantation, by mouth, 100–200 micrograms/kg daily in 2 divided doses; CHILD 300 micrograms/kg daily in 2 divided doses

Renal transplantation, starting within 24 hours of transplantation, by mouth, 200–300 micrograms/kg daily in 2 divided doses; CHILD 300 micrograms/kg daily in 2 divided doses

Heart transplantation with antibody induction (starting within 5 days of transplantation) or without antibody induction (starting within 12 hours of transplantation), by mouth, 75 micrograms/kg daily in 2 divided doses; CHILD, with antibody induction (starting within 5 days of transplantation), 100–300 micrograms/kg daily in 2 divided doses; without antibody induction (starting within 12 hours of transplantation), 300 micrograms/kg daily in 2 divided doses as soon as clinically possible (8–12 hours after discontinuing intravenous infusion)

Maintenance treatment, dose adjusted according to response and whole blood concentration

Rejection therapy, seek specialist advice

◢ Modified release

Advagraf® (Astellas) PoM

Capsules, m/r, tacrolimus (as monohydrate) 500 micrograms (yellow/orange), net price 50-cap pack = £35.79; 1 mg (white/orange), 50-cap pack = £71.59, 100-cap pack = £143.17; 3 mg (orange), 50-cap pack = £214.76; 5 mg (red/orange), 50-cap pack = £266.92. Label: 23, 25, counselling, driving

Note Tacrolimus is incompatible with PVC

Dose liver transplantation, starting 12–18 hours after transplantation, by mouth, 100–200 micrograms/kg once daily in the morning

Renal transplantation, starting within 24 hours of transplantation, by mouth, 200–300 micrograms/kg once daily in the morning

Rejection therapy, seek specialist advice

CHILD not recommended

8.2.3 Anti-lymphocyte monoclonal antibodies

The anti-lymphocyte monoclonal antibodies cause lysis of B lymphocytes. Infusion-related side-effects (including cytokine release syndrome) are reported commonly with anti-lymphocyte monoclonal antibodies and occur predominantly during the first infusion; they include fever and chills, nausea and vomiting, allergic reactions (such as rash, pruritus, angioedema, bronchospasm and dyspnoea), flushing, tumour pain and cardiac events. In rare cases infusion reactions may be fatal. Patients should receive premedication before administration of anti-lymphocyte monoclonal antibodies to reduce these effects—consult product literature for details of individual regimens. The infusion may have to be stopped

temporarily and the infusion-related effects treated—consult product literature for appropriate management. Evidence of pulmonary infiltration and features of tumour lysis syndrome should be sought if infusion-related effects occur. Patients should also be monitored for cytopenias—consult product literature for specific recommendations. All anti-lymphocyte monoclonal antibodies should be given under the supervision of an experienced specialist, in an environment where full resuscitation facilities are immediately available.

Fatalities following **severe** cytokine release syndrome (characterised by severe dyspnoea) and associated with features of tumour lysis syndrome have occurred after infusions of anti-lymphocyte monoclonal antibodies. Patients with a high tumour burden as well as those with pulmonary insufficiency or infiltration are at increased risk and should be monitored **very closely** (and a slower rate of infusion considered).

Hepatitis B infection and reactivation (including fatal cases) have been reported in patients taking **obinutuzumab**, **ofatumumab**, and **rituximab**. All patients should be screened before treatment. Patients with positive hepatitis B serology should be referred to a liver specialist for monitoring and initiation of antiviral therapy before treatment initiation; treatment should not be initiated in patients with evidence of current hepatitis B infection until the infection has been adequately treated. Patients should be closely monitored for clinical and laboratory signs of active hepatitis B infection during treatment and for up to a year following the last infusion (consult product literature).

Alemtuzumab is licensed for the treatment of adults with relapsing-remitting multiple sclerosis with active disease defined by clinical or imaging features. It is not recommended for inactive or stable disease. Pretreatment before administration is required (consult product literature) and all patients should receive oral prophylaxis for herpes infection starting on the first day of treatment and continuing for at least a month following each treatment course. Screening patients at high risk of hepatitis B or C is recommended before treatment—patients who are carriers should be treated with caution. HPV screening should be carried out annually in female patients. In patients with active infection, a delay in initiation of alemtuzumab treatment should be considered until the infection is fully controlled, and all patients should be evaluated for active or latent tuberculosis before starting alemtuzumab treatment. The risk of autoimmune mediated conditions may increase during treatment, including immune thrombocytopenic purpura, thyroid disorders, nephropathies, and cytopenias, and should be monitored for throughout the course of treatment (consult product literature). Patients with previous autoimmune conditions other than multiple sclerosis should be treated with caution. Alemtuzumab should be given under the care of a specialist with facilities for the management of hypersensitivity and anaphylactic reactions. Although no longer licensed for oncological and transplant indications, alemtuzumab is also available through a patient access programme for these indications.

8

Malignant disease and immunosuppression

Malignant disease and immunosuppression

8

NICE guidance
Alemtuzumab for treating relapsing-remitting multiple sclerosis (May 2014)

Alemtuzumab is recommended as an option, within its marketing authorisation, for treating adults with active relapsing-remitting multiple sclerosis
www.nice.org.uk/TA312

Rituximab is licensed, in combination with other chemotherapy, for the treatment of previously untreated stage III–IV follicular lymphoma, and for maintenance therapy in patients with follicular non-Hodgkin's lymphoma that has responded to induction therapy (see also NICE guidance below). It is also licensed, in combination with other chemotherapy, for the treatment of diffuse large B-cell non-Hodgkin's lymphoma (see also NICE guidance below). Rituximab is licensed by intravenous infusion for the treatment of chemotherapy-resistant or relapsed stage III–IV follicular non-Hodgkin's lymphoma, and for previously untreated or relapsed chronic lymphocytic leukaemia (see also NICE guidance below). The intravenous preparation of rituximab, in combination with glucocorticoids, is licensed for the induction of remission in patients with severe, active granulomatosis with polyangiitis (Wegener's) and microscopic polyangiitis (see SMC guidance and NICE guidance below). See section 10.1.3 for the role of rituximab in rheumatoid arthritis.

Rituximab should be used with caution in patients receiving cardiotoxic chemotherapy or with a history of cardiovascular disease because exacerbation of angina, arrhythmia, and heart failure have been reported. The use of rituximab for the treatment of granulomatosis with polyangiitis or microscopic polyangiitis is contra-indicated in patients with severe heart failure or severe, uncontrolled heart disease. Transient hypotension occurs frequently during infusion and anti-hypertensives may need to be withheld for 12 hours before infusion. Progressive multifocal leucoencephalopathy (which is usually fatal or causes severe disability) has been reported in association with rituximab; patients should be monitored for cognitive, neurological, or psychiatric signs and symptoms. If progressive multifocal leucoencephalopathy is suspected, suspend treatment until it has been excluded. Severe (including fatal) skin reactions, including toxic epidermal necrolysis and Stevens-Johnson syndrome have been reported—permanently discontinue treatment if severe skin reactions occur.

The *Scottish Medicines Consortium* (p. 4) has advised (August 2013) that intravenous rituximab (*MabThera*®) is accepted for restricted use within NHS Scotland, in combination with glucocorticoids for the induction of remission in adult patients with severe, active granulomatosis with polyangiitis (Wegener's) and microscopic polyangiitis. It is restricted to use in patients who have relapsed following treatment with cyclophosphamide or who are intolerant to or unable to receive cyclophosphamide.

The *Scottish Medicines Consortium* (p. 4) has advised (June 2014) that subcutaneous rituximab (*MabThera*®) is accepted for restricted use within NHS Scotland, in accordance with UK licensing, except in the maintenance setting, where use is restricted to patients who have responded to induction therapy with rituximab plus chemotherapy.

NICE guidance
Rituximab in combination with glucocorticoids for treating anti-neutrophil cytoplasmic antibody-associated vasculitis (March 2014)

[1]Rituximab, in combination with glucocorticoids, is recommended as an option for inducing remission in adults with anti-neutrophil cytoplasmic antibody [ANCA]-associated vasculitis (severely active granulomatosis with polyangiitis [Wegener's] and microscopic polyangiitis), only if:

- further cyclophosphamide treatment would exceed the maximum cumulative cyclophosphamide dose, **or**
- cyclophosphamide is contraindicated or not tolerated, **or**
- the patient has not completed their family, and treatment with cyclophosphamide may materially affect their fertility, **or**
- the disease has remained active or progressed despite a course of cyclophosphamide lasting 3–6 months, **or**
- the patient has had uroepithelial malignancy.

www.nice.org.uk/TA308

NICE guidance
Rituximab for the first-line treatment of stage III-IV follicular lymphoma (January 2012)

[1]Rituximab, in combination with:

- cyclophosphamide, vincristine and prednisolone (CVP);
- cyclophosphamide, doxorubicin, vincristine and prednisolone (CHOP);
- mitoxantrone, chlorambucil and prednisolone (MCP);
- cyclophosphamide, doxorubicin, etoposide, prednisolone and interferon-alfa (CHVPi); *or*
- chlorambucil

is recommended as an option for the treatment of symptomatic stage III and IV follicular lymphoma in previously untreated patients.
www.nice.org.uk/TA243

NICE guidance
Rituximab for the treatment of relapsed or refractory stage III or IV follicular non-Hodgkin's lymphoma (February 2008)

[1]Rituximab, in combination with chemotherapy, is an option for the induction of remission in patients with relapsed stage III or IV follicular non-Hodgkin's lymphoma.

Rituximab monotherapy as maintenance therapy is an option for the treatment of patients with relapsed stage III or IV follicular non-Hodgkin's lymphoma in remission induced with chemotherapy (with or without rituximab).

Rituximab monotherapy is an option for the treatment of patients with relapsed or refractory stage III or IV follicular non-Hodgkin's lymphoma, when all alternative treatment options have been exhausted (that is, if there is resistance to or intolerance of chemotherapy).
www.nice.org.uk/TA137

---

1. This NICE guidance was issued for rituximab by intravenous infusion.

NICE guidance
Rituximab for the treatment of relapsed or refractory chronic lymphocytic leukaemia (July 2010)

[1]Rituximab in combination with fludarabine and cyclophosphamide is recommended as a treatment option for people with relapsed or refractory chronic lymphocytic leukaemia except when the condition:

- is refractory to fludarabine (that is, it has not responded to fludarabine, or has relapsed within 6 months of treatment), or
- has previously been treated with rituximab, unless it was in the context of a clinical trial, at a dose lower than the dose currently licensed for chronic lymphocytic leukaemia or with chemotherapy other than fludarabine and cyclophosphamide.

Rituximab in combination with fludarabine and cyclophosphamide is recommended only in the context of research for patients with relapsed or refractory chronic lymphocytic leukaemia that has previously been treated with rituximab, unless rituximab has been given as specified above.

www.nice.org.uk/TA193

NICE guidance
Rituximab for the first-line maintenance treatment of follicular non-Hodgkin's lymphoma (June 2011)

[1]Rituximab maintenance therapy is recommended as an option for the treatment of people with follicular non-Hodgkins's lymphoma that has responded to first-line induction therapy with rituximab in combination with chemotherapy.

www.nice.org.uk/TA226

NICE guidance
Rituximab for the first-line treatment of chronic lymphocytic leukaemia (July 2009)

[1]Rituximab, in combination with fludarabine and cyclophosphamide, is recommended as an option for the first-line treatment of chronic lymphocytic leukaemia.

www.nice.org.uk/TA174

NICE guidance
Rituximab for aggressive non-Hodgkin's lymphoma (September 2003)

[1]Rituximab, in combination with cyclophosphamide, doxorubicin, vincristine, and prednisolone, is recommended for first-line treatment of CD20-positive diffuse large-B-cell lymphoma at clinical stage II, III or IV.

The use of rituximab for localised (stage I) disease should be limited to clinical trials.

www.nice.org.uk/TA65

Obinutuzumab is licensed for the treatment of previously untreated chronic lymphocytic leukaemia in patients for whom full-dose fludarabine-based therapy is unsuitable due to co-morbidities. Infusion-related side-effects have been reported with obinutuzumab.

Ofatumumab is licensed for treatment of chronic lymphocytic leukaemia (CLL) in patients refractory to

fludarabine and alemtuzumab. It is also licensed, in combination with chlorambucil or bendamustine for treatment of CLL in patients who have not received prior therapy and who are not eligible for fludarabine-based therapy. Infusion-related side-effects (including cytokine release syndrome—see above) have been reported with ofatumumab; premedication with paracetamol, an antihistamine, and a corticosteroid must be given—consult product literature.

NICE guidance
Ofatumumab for the treatment of chronic lymphocytic leukaemia refractory to fludarabine and alemtuzumab (October 2010)

Ofatumumab is **not** recommended for the treatment of chronic lymphocytic leukaemia that is refractory to fludarabine and alemtuzumab.

Patients currently receiving ofatumumab for this condition should have the option to continue treatment until they and their clinician consider it appropriate to stop.

www.nice.org.uk/TA202

▌ **ALEMTUZUMAB**

Indications see notes above

Cautions see notes above—for full details consult product literature; **interactions**: Appendix 1 (alemtuzumab)
Alert card Patients should be provided with a Patient Alert Card and Patient Guide

Contra-indications human immunodeficiency virus

Pregnancy manufacturer advises avoid unless potential benefit outweighs risk—toxicity in *animal* studies. Autoimmune thyroid disease during treatment may affect fetus (consult product literature); women of childbearing potential should use effective contraception during and for 4 months after treatment

Breast-feeding manufacturer advises avoid during and for 4 months after each treatment course unless potential benefit outweighs risk

Side-effects see notes above—for full details (including monitoring and management of side-effects) consult product literature

Dose
- Consult product literature
Important Patients should receive premedication before administration (consult product literature for details)

Lemtrada® (Genzyme) ▼ PoM
Concentrate for intravenous infusion, alemtuzumab 10 mg/mL, net price 1.2-mL vial = £7045.00

▌ **OBINUTUZUMAB**

Indications see notes above

Cautions see notes above—for full details consult product literature; **interactions**: Appendix 1 (obinutuzumab)

Contra-indications consult product literature

Pregnancy avoid unless potential benefit outweighs risk of B-lymphocyte depletion in fetus; use effective contraception during and for 18 months after treatment

Breast-feeding avoid breast-feeding during and for 18 months after treatment—present in milk in *animal* studies

---

1. This NICE guidance was issued for rituximab by intravenous infusion

Side-effects see notes above—for full details (including monitoring and management of side-effects) consult product literature

Dose

- See Doses, p. 574

  Important Patients should receive premedication before each dose (consult product literature for details)

Gazyvaro® (Roche) ▼ PoM

Concentrate for intravenous infusion, obinutuzumab 25 mg/mL, net price 40-mL vial = £3312.00

▌ OFATUMUMAB

Indications see notes above

Cautions history of cardiac disease—monitor closely and discontinue treatment if cardiac arrhythmias occur; monitor electrolytes (including potassium and magnesium) before and during administration and correct if abnormal; see also notes above— for full details consult product literature; **interactions**: Appendix 1 (ofatumumab)

Contra-indications consult product literature

Renal impairment no information available for creatinine clearance less than 30 mL/minute

Pregnancy avoid unless potential benefit outweighs risk; use effective contraception during and for 12 months after treatment

Breast-feeding discontinue breast-feeding during and for 12 months after treatment—no information available

Side-effects see notes above—for full details (including monitoring and management of side-effects) consult product literature

Dose

- See Doses, p. 574

  Important Premedication must be given 30 minutes to 2 hours before each dose—consult product literature for details; patients must be monitored closely during each infusion for the onset of infusion reactions

Arzerra® (GSK) ▼ PoM

Concentrate for intravenous infusion, ofatumumab 20 mg/mL, net price 5-mL vial = £182.00, 50-mL vial = £1820.00

Electrolytes Na⁺ 5.04 mmol/g

▌ RITUXIMAB

Indications see notes above; severe active rheumatoid arthritis (section 10.1.3)

Cautions see notes above—for full details consult product literature; **interactions**: Appendix 1 (rituximab)

Alert card Patients treated for granulomatosis with polyangiitis and microscopic polyangiitis should be provided with a patient alert card with each infusion

Contra-indications see notes above—for full details consult product literature

Pregnancy avoid unless potential benefit to mother outweighs risk of B-lymphocyte depletion in fetus—effective contraception required during and for 12 months after treatment

Breast-feeding avoid breast-feeding during and for 12 months after treatment

Side-effects see notes above—but for full details (including monitoring and management of side-effects) consult product literature

Dose

- See Doses, p. 574

  Important Patients should receive premedication before each dose (consult product literature for details)

MabThera® (Roche) PoM

Concentrate for intravenous infusion, rituximab 10 mg/mL, net price 10-mL vial = £174.63, 50-mL vial = £873.15

Solution for subcutaneous injection, rituximab 120 mg/mL, net price 11.7-mL vial = £1344.65

8.2.4 Other immunomodulating drugs

Interferon alfa

Interferon alfa has shown some antitumour effect in certain lymphomas and solid tumours. Interferon alfa preparations are also used in the treatment of chronic hepatitis B, and chronic hepatitis C ideally in combination with ribavirin (section 5.3.3). Side-effects are dose-related, but commonly include anorexia, nausea, diarrhoea, influenza-like symptoms, and lethargy. Ocular side-effects and depression (including suicidal behaviour) have also been reported. Myelosuppression may occur, particularly affecting granulocyte counts. Cardiovascular problems (hypotension, hypertension, palpitation, and arrhythmias), nephrotoxicity and hepatotoxicity have been reported. Hypertriglyceridaemia, sometimes severe, has been observed; monitoring of lipid concentration is recommended. Other side-effects include hypersensitivity reactions, thyroid abnormalities, hyperglycaemia, alopecia, psoriasiform rash, confusion, coma and seizures (usually with high doses in the elderly).

Polyethylene glycol-conjugated ('pegylated') derivatives of interferon alfa (**peginterferon alfa-2a** and **peginterferon alfa-2b**) are available; pegylation increases the persistence of the interferon in the blood. The peginterferons are licensed for the treatment of chronic hepatitis C, ideally in combination with ribavirin (see section 5.3.3.2). Peginterferon alfa-2a is also licensed for the treatment of chronic hepatitis B. For use of interferon alfa and peginterferon alfa in children see *BNF for Children*

> **NICE guidance (peginterferon alfa, interferon alfa, and ribavirin for chronic hepatitis C)**
> See p. 437

▌ INTERFERON ALFA

Indications see under preparations

Cautions consult product literature; **interactions**: Appendix 1 (interferons)

Contra-indications consult product literature; avoid injections containing benzyl alcohol in neonates (see under preparations below)

Hepatic impairment close monitoring in mild to moderate impairment; avoid if severe

Renal impairment close monitoring required; avoid in severe impairment

Pregnancy avoid unless potential benefit outweighs risk (toxicity in *animal* studies); effective contraception required during treatment—consult product literature

Breast-feeding unlikely to be harmful

Side-effects see notes above and consult product literature

Dose

- Consult product literature

IntronA® (MSD) (PoM)

Injection, interferon alfa-2b (rbe) 10 million units/mL, net price 1-mL vial = £41.55, 2.5-mL vial = £103.94. For subcutaneous injection or intravenous infusion

Injection pen, interferon alfa-2b (rbe), net price 15 million units/mL, 1.5-mL cartridge = £74.83; 25 million units/mL, 1.5-mL cartridge = £124.72; 50 million units/mL, 1.5-mL cartridge = £249.45. For subcutaneous injection

Note Each 1.5-mL multidose cartridge delivers 12 doses of 0.1 mL i.e. a total of 1.2 mL

For chronic myelogenous leukaemia (as monotherapy or in combination with cytarabine), hairy cell leukaemia, follicular lymphoma, lymph or liver metastases of carcinoid tumour, chronic hepatitis B, chronic hepatitis C, adjunct to surgery in malignant melanoma and maintenance of remission in multiple myeloma

Roferon-A® (Roche) (PoM)

Injection, interferon alfa-2a (rbe), net price 6 million units/mL, 0.5-mL (3 million-unit) prefilled syringe = £14.20; 9 million units/mL, 0.5-mL (4.5 million-unit) prefilled syringe = £21.29; 12 million units/mL, 0.5-mL (6 million-unit) prefilled syringe = £28.37; 18 million units/mL, 0.5-mL (9 million-unit) prefilled syringe = £42.57. For subcutaneous injection

Excipients include benzyl alcohol (avoid in neonates, see Excipients, p. 2)

For AIDS-related Kaposi's sarcoma, hairy cell leukaemia, chronic myelogenous leukaemia, advanced renal cell carcinoma, progressive cutaneous T-cell lymphoma, chronic hepatitis B and chronic hepatitis C, follicular non-Hodgkin's lymphoma, adjunct to surgery in malignant melanoma

---

PEGINTERFERON ALFA

Indications see under preparations

Cautions consult product literature; **interactions:** Appendix 1 (interferons)

Contra-indications consult product literature

Hepatic impairment avoid in severe impairment

Renal impairment close monitoring required—reduce dose in moderate to severe impairment; consult product literature

Pregnancy manufacturers recommend avoid unless potential benefit outweighs risk (toxicity in *animal* studies); effective contraception required during treatment—consult product literature

Breast-feeding manufacturers advise avoid—no information available

Side-effects see notes above and consult product literature

Dose

- Consult product literature

Pegasys® (Roche) (PoM)

Injection, peginterferon alfa-2a (rbe), net price 90-microgram prefilled syringe = £76.51, 135-microgram prefilled syringe = £107.76, 180-microgram prefilled syringe = £124.40; 135-microgram prefilled pen = £107.76, 180-microgram prefilled pen = £124.40. For subcutaneous injection

Excipients include benzyl alcohol (avoid in neonates, see Excipients, p)

Combined with ribavirin for chronic hepatitis C; as monotherapy for chronic hepatitis C if ribavirin not tolerated or contra-indicated (see section 5.3.3.2); as monotherapy for chronic hepatitis B

ViraferonPeg® (MSD) (PoM)

Injection, prefilled pen, powder for reconstitution, peginterferon alfa-2b (rbe), net price 50-microgram pen = £66.46, 80-microgram pen = £106.34, 100-microgram pen = £132.92, 120-microgram pen = £159.51, 150-microgram pen = £199.38 (all with needles and swabs). For subcutaneous injection

Combined with ribavirin for chronic hepatitis C; combined with ribavirin and boceprevir for chronic hepatitis C infection of genotype 1 in patients with compensated liver disease; as monotherapy for chronic hepatitis C if ribavirin not tolerated or contra-indicated (see section 5.3.3.2)

Interferon beta

Interferon beta is licensed for use in patients with *relapsing, remitting multiple sclerosis* (characterised by at least two attacks of neurological dysfunction over the previous 2 or 3 years, followed by complete or incomplete recovery) who are able to walk unaided. Not all patients respond and a deterioration in the bouts has been observed in some. It is also licensed for use in patients with a single demyelinating event with an active inflammatory process, if it is severe enough to require treatment with an intravenous corticosteroid, and they are at high risk of developing multiple sclerosis. Interferon beta-1b is also licensed for use in patients with *secondary progressive multiple sclerosis* but its role in this condition has not been confirmed.

Cautions Caution is advised in those with severe hepatic or renal impairment or a history of cardiac disorders, depressive disorders (avoid in severe depression or in those with suicidal ideation), seizures, or severe myelosupression. Patients should be monitored for clinical features of thrombotic microangiopathy (TMA), including thrombocytopenia, new onset hypertension, fever, central nervous system symptoms (e.g. confusion and paresis), and impaired renal function. Any signs of TMA should be investigated fully and, if diagnosed, interferon beta should be stopped immediately and treatment for TMA promptly initiated (consult product literature for details). Patients should also be monitored for signs and symptoms of nephrotic syndrome, including oedema, proteinuria, and impaired renal function—monitor renal function periodically. If nephrotic syndrome develops, treat promptly and consider stopping interferon beta treatment. Monitor for signs of hepatic injury—hepatic failure has been reported rarely.

Contra-indications Avoid treatment with interferon beta in patients with severe depressive illness or those with decompensated liver disease.

Side-effects Side-effects reported most frequently include irritation at injection site (including inflammation, hypersensitivity, necrosis) and influenza-like symptoms (fever, chills, myalgia, or malaise) but these decrease over time; nausea and vomiting occur occasionally. Other side-effects include hypersensitivity reactions (including anaphylaxis and urticaria), blood disorders, thrombotic microangiopathy, menstrual disorders, mood and personality changes, suicide attempts, confusion, convulsions, alopecia, hepatitis, nephrotic syndrome, and thyroid dysfunction (consult product literature for all side-effects).

8 Malignant disease and immunosuppression

NICE guidance
Interferon beta and glatiramer for multiple sclerosis (January 2002)

Interferon beta and glatiramer acetate are **not** recommended for the treatment of multiple sclerosis in the NHS in England and Wales.

Patients who are currently receiving interferon beta or glatiramer acetate for multiple sclerosis, whether as routine therapy or as part of a clinical trial, should have the option to continue treatment until they and their consultant consider it appropriate to stop, having regard to the established criteria for withdrawal from treatment.

www.nice.org.uk/TA32

A polyethylene glycol-conjugated ('pegylated') derivative of interferon beta (**peginterferon beta-1a**) is available; pegylation increases the persistence of interferon in the blood. Peginterferon beta-1a is licensed for the treatment of *relapsing, remitting multiple sclerosis.*

Provision of disease-modifying therapies for multiple sclerosis

The Department of Health, the National Assembly for Wales, the Scottish Executive, the Northern Ireland Department of Health, Social Services & Public Safety, and the manufacturers have reached agreement on a risk-sharing scheme for the NHS supply of interferon beta and glatiramer acetate for multiple sclerosis. Health Service Circular (HSC 2002/004) explains how patients can participate in the scheme. It is available on the Department of Health website (www.dh.gov.uk).

◢ INTERFERON BETA

Indications see notes above and under preparations

Cautions see notes above and consult product literature

Contra-indications see notes above and consult product literature

Hepatic impairment see notes above

Renal impairment see notes above

Pregnancy avoid unless potential benefit outweighs risk (toxicity in *animal* studies); effective contraception required during treatment—consult product literature

Breast-feeding avoid—no information available

Side-effects see notes above and consult product literature

Dose
● See under preparations

◢ Interferon beta-1a
Avonex® (Biogen) [PoM]

Injection, interferon beta-1a 60 micrograms (12 million units)/mL, net price 0.5-mL (30-microgram, 6 million-unit) prefilled syringe = £163.50; 0.5-mL (30-microgram, 6 million-unit) prefilled pen = £163.50

Note For intramuscular injection

Injection, powder for reconstitution, interferon beta-1a, net price 30-microgram (6 million-unit) vial with diluent = £163.50

Note For intramuscular injection

Dose for relapsing, remitting multiple sclerosis or for a single demyelinating event with an active inflammatory process (if it is severe enough to require intravenous corticosteroid and patient at high risk of developing multiple sclerosis), consult product literature

Rebif® (Merck Serono) [PoM]

Injection, interferon beta-1a, net price 22-microgram (6 million-unit) prefilled syringe = £48.16; 44-microgram (12 million-unit) prefilled syringe = £67.77; starter pack of 6 × 8.8-microgram (2.4 million-unit) prefilled syringes with 6 × 22-microgram (6 million-unit) prefilled syringes = £552.19

Note For subcutaneous injection

Excipients include benzyl alcohol (avoid in neonates, see Excipients, p. 2)

Injection, interferon beta-1a, 44 micrograms (12 million-units/mL), net price 1.5 mL (66-microgram, 18 million-unit) cartridge = £203.30; 88-micrograms (24 million-units/mL), 1.5 mL (132-microgram, 36 million-unit) cartridge = £171.97; starter pack of 2 × 1.5 mL (132-microgram, 36 million-unit) cartridge = £406.61

Note Cartridges for use with *RebiSmart®* auto-injector device. For subcutaneous injection

Excipients include benzyl alcohol (avoid in neonates, see Excipients, p. 2)

Injection (*RebiDose®*), interferon beta-1a, net price 22-microgram (6 million-unit) prefilled pen = £51.13; 44-microgram (12 million-unit) prefilled pen = £67.77; starter pack of 6 × 8.8-microgram (2.4 million-unit) prefilled pens with 6 × 22-microgram (6 million-unit) prefilled pens = £552.19

Note For subcutaneous injection

Excipients include benzyl alcohol (avoid in neonates, see Excipients, p. 2)

Dose for relapsing, remitting multiple sclerosis or for a single demyelinating event with an active inflammatory process (if alternative diagnoses have been excluded, and patient at high risk of developing multiple sclerosis), consult product literature

◢ Interferon beta-1b
Betaferon® (Bayer) [PoM]

Injection, powder for reconstitution, interferon beta-1b, net price 300-microgram (9.6 million-unit) vial with diluent = £39.78

Note For subcutaneous injection

Note An autoinjector device (*Betaject® Light*) is available from Bayer Schering

Dose for relapsing, remitting multiple sclerosis, for secondary progressive multiple sclerosis with active disease, or for a single demyelinating event with an active inflammatory process (if severe enough to require intravenous corticosteroid and patient at high risk of developing multiple sclerosis), consult product literature

Extavia® (Novartis) [PoM]

Injection, powder for reconstitution, interferon beta-1b. Net price 300-microgram (9.6 million-unit) vial with diluent = £39.78

Note For subcutaneous injection

Note An auto-injector device (*ExtaviPro® 30G*) is supplied as part of the *ExtaviPro® 30G* kit

Dose for relapsing, remitting multiple sclerosis, for secondary progressive multiple sclerosis with active disease, or for a single demyelinating event with an active inflammatory process (if severe enough to require intravenous corticosteroid and patient at high risk of developing multiple sclerosis), consult product literature

◢ PEGINTERFERON BETA-1a

Indications see notes above

Cautions see notes above and consult product literature

Contra-indications severe depression or suicidal ideation

Hepatic impairment see notes above

Renal impairment see notes above

Pregnancy do not initiate during pregnancy; avoid unless potential benefit outweighs risk; effective contraception required during treatment—consult product literature

Breast-feeding avoid—no information available

Side-effects consult product literature

Dose

- Consult product literature

Plegridy® (Biogen) ▼ PoM
Injection, prefilled pen, peginterferon beta-1a, net price 125-microgram pen = £327.00; treatment initiation pack, 63-microgram pen and 94-microgram pen = £654.00
Note For subcutaneous injection

Interferon gamma

Interferon gamma-1b is licensed to reduce the frequency of serious infection in chronic granulomatous disease and in severe malignant osteopetrosis.

■ INTERFERON GAMMA-1b
(Immune interferon)

Indications see notes above

Cautions seizure disorders (including seizures associated with fever); cardiac disease (including ischaemia, congestive heart failure, and arrhythmias); monitor before and during treatment: haematological tests (including full blood count, differential white cell count, and platelet count), blood chemistry tests (including renal and liver function tests) and urinalysis; avoid simultaneous administration of foreign proteins including immunological products (risk of exaggerated immune response); **interactions:** Appendix 1 (interferons)

Hepatic impairment manufacturer advises caution in severe impairment—risk of accumulation

Renal impairment manufacturer advises caution in severe impairment—risk of accumulation

Pregnancy manufacturers recommend avoid unless potential benefit outweighs risk (toxicity in *animal* studies); effective contraception required during treatment—consult product literature

Breast-feeding manufacturers advise avoid—no information available

Side-effects nausea, vomiting, diarrhoea, abdominal pain; headache, fatigue, fever, chills, depression; myalgia, arthralgia; rash, injection-site reactions; *rarely* confusion and systemic lupus erythematosus; also reported, neutropenia, thrombocytopenia, proteinuria and raised liver enzymes

Dose

- See under preparation

Immukin® (Boehringer Ingelheim) PoM
Injection, recombinant human interferon gamma-1b 200 micrograms/mL, net price 0.5-mL vial = £75.00
Dose By subcutaneous injection, 50 micrograms/m² 3 times a week; patients with body surface area of 0.5 m² or less, 1.5 micrograms/kg 3 times a week; not yet recommended for children under 6 months with chronic granulomatous disease

Aldesleukin

Aldesleukin (recombinant interleukin-2) is licensed for metastatic renal cell carcinoma **excluding** patients in whom all three of the following prognostic factors are present: performance status of Eastern Co-operative Oncology Group of 1 or greater, more than one organ with metastatic disease sites, and a period of less than 24 months between initial diagnosis of primary tumour and date of evaluation of treatment. It is usually given by subcutaneous injection. It is now rarely given by intravenous infusion because of an increased risk of capillary leak syndrome, which can cause pulmonary oedema and hypotension. Aldesleukin produces tumour shrinkage in a small proportion of patients, but it has not been shown to increase survival. Bone-marrow, hepatic, renal, thyroid, and CNS toxicity is common. It is for use in **specialist units only**.

■ ALDESLEUKIN

Indications see notes above

Cautions consult product literature; **interactions:** Appendix 1 (aldesleukin)

Contra-indications consult product literature

Pregnancy use only if potential benefit outweighs risk (toxicity in *animal* studies); ensure effective contraception during treatment in men and women; see also Pregnancy and Reproductive Function, p. 575

Breast-feeding discontinue breast-feeding

Side-effects see section 8.1, notes above, and consult product literature

Dose

- Consult product literature

Proleukin® (Novartis) PoM
Injection, powder for reconstitution, aldesleukin. Net price 18-million unit vial = £112.00. For subcutaneous injection *or* intravenous infusion (but see notes above)

BCG bladder instillation

BCG (Bacillus Calmette-Guérin) is a live attenuated strain derived from *Mycobacterium bovis*. It is licensed as a bladder instillation for the treatment of primary or recurrent bladder carcinoma and for the prevention of recurrence following transurethral resection.

■ BACILLUS CALMETTE-GUÉRIN

Indications see notes above; BCG immunisation (section 14.4)

Cautions screen for active tuberculosis (contra-indicated if tuberculosis confirmed); traumatic catheterisation or urethral or bladder injury (delay administration until mucosal damage healed)

Contra-indications impaired immune response, HIV infection, urinary-tract infection, severe haematuria, tuberculosis, fever of unknown origin

Pregnancy avoid

Breast-feeding avoid

Side-effects cystitis, dysuria, urinary frequency, haematuria, malaise, fever, influenza-like syndrome; also systemic BCG infection (with fatalities)—consult product literature; rarely hypersensitivity reactions (such as arthralgia and rash), orchitis, transient urethral obstruction, bladder contracture, renal abscess; ocular symptoms reported

Dose

- Consult product literature

8 Malignant disease and immunosuppression

ImmuCyst® (Alliance) [PoM]
Bladder instillation, freeze-dried powder containing attenuated *Mycobacterium bovis* prepared from the Connaught strain of bacillus of Calmette and Guérin, net price 81-mg vial = £79.23

OncoTICE® (MSD) [PoM]
Bladder instillation, freeze-dried powder containing attenuated *Mycobacterium bovis* prepared from the TICE strain of bacillus of Calmette and Guérin, net price 12.5-mg vial = £71.61

Canakinumab

Canakinumab is a recombinant human monoclonal antibody that selectively inhibits interleukin-1 beta receptor binding. It is licensed for the treatment of cryopyrin-associated periodic syndrome, including severe forms of familial cold auto-inflammatory syndrome (or familial cold urticaria), Muckle-Wells syndrome, and neonatal-onset multisystem inflammatory disease (also known as chronic infantile neurological cutaneous and articular syndrome). These are rare inherited auto-inflammatory disorders.

◼ CANAKINUMAB

Indications see notes above; acute gout (section 10.1.4)

Cautions history of recurrent infection or predisposition to infection; monitor full blood count including neutrophil count before starting treatment, 1–2 months after starting treatment, and periodically thereafter; patients should receive all recommended vaccinations (including pneumococcal and inactivated influenza vaccine) before starting treatment; avoid live vaccines unless potential benefit outweighs risk—consult product literature and section 14.1 (p. 842) for further information; **interactions:** Appendix 1 (canakinumab)
Tuberculosis Patients should be evaluated for latent and active tuberculosis before starting treatment and monitored for signs and symptoms of tuberculosis during and after treatment

Contra-indications active infection (see also Cautions); leucopenia; neutropenia; concomitant use with tumour necrosis factor inhibitors (possible increased risk of infections)

Hepatic impairment no information available

Renal impairment limited information available but manufacturer advises no dose adjustment required

Pregnancy manufacturer advises avoid unless potential benefit outweighs risk; effective contraception required during treatment and for up to 3 months after last dose

Breast-feeding consider if benefit outweighs risk—not known if present in human milk

Side-effects vertigo, malaise, increased susceptibility to infection (including serious infection), injection-site reactions, neutropenia, back pain; *less commonly* gastro-oesophageal reflux; *also reported* vomiting, malignancy

Dose
• See Doses, p. 574

Ilaris® (Novartis) ▼ [PoM]
Injection, powder for reconstitution, canakinumab, net price 150-mg vial = £9927.80

Dimethyl fumarate

Dimethyl fumarate has immunomodulatory and anti-inflammatory properties, and is licensed for the treatment of adults with relapsing-remitting multiple sclerosis. Treatment should be initiated by a physician experienced in the treatment of multiple sclerosis.

> **NICE guidance**
> **Dimethyl fumarate for treating relapsing-remitting multiple sclerosis (August 2014)**
> Dimethyl fumarate is recommended for the treatment of active relapsing-remitting multiple sclerosis, only if:
> • the patient does not have highly active or rapidly evolving severe relapsing-remitting multiple sclerosis **and**
> • the manufacturer provides dimethyl fumarate with the discount agreed in the patient access scheme
> Patients currently receiving dimethyl fumarate whose disease does not meet the above criteria should be able to continue treatment until they and their clinician consider it appropriate to stop.
> www.nice.org.uk/TA320

◼ DIMETHYL FUMARATE

Indications see notes above

Cautions reduced lymphocyte count; severe active gastro-intestinal disease; serious infection—do not start treatment until resolved and consider suspending treatment if infection develops during treatment; monitor full blood count before treatment (within 6 months before initiation), after 6 months of treatment, then every 6 to 12 months thereafter, and as clinically indicated; monitor renal and hepatic function before treatment, after 3 and 6 months of treatment, then every 6 to 12 months thereafter, and as clinically indicated

Hepatic impairment manufacturer advises caution in severe impairment

Renal impairment manufacturer advises caution in severe impairment

Pregnancy manufacturer advises avoid unless essential and potential benefit outweighs risk—toxicity in *animal* studies; contraception required in women of child-bearing potential (consider non-hormonal methods)

Breast-feeding manufacturer advises avoid

Side-effects nausea, vomiting, diarrhoea, abdominal pain, dyspepsia, gastritis, gastroenteritis, flushing (may be severe and indicate hypersensitivity), burning sensation, lymphopenia, leucopenia, proteinuria, pruritus, rash, erythema

Dose
• ADULT over 18 years, 120 mg twice daily; increased to 240 mg twice daily after 7 days; for dose adjustment due to side-effects, consult product literature

Tecfidera® (Biogen) [PoM]
Capsules, e/c, dimethyl fumarate 120 mg (green/white), net price 14-cap pack = £343.00; 240 mg (green), 56-cap pack = £1373.00. Label: 21, 25

Fingolimod

Fingolimod is an immunomodulating drug licensed for use in patients with highly active relapsing-remitting multiple sclerosis despite treatment with interferon beta or in those with rapidly evolving severe relapsing-remitting multiple sclerosis. Treatment with fingolimod should be initiated and supervised by a specialist.

MHRA/CHM advice
Fingolimod: not recommended for patients at known risk of cardiovascular events. Advice for extended monitoring for those with significant bradycardia or heart block after the first dose and following treatment interruption (January 2013)

Fingolimod is known to cause transient bradycardias and heart block after the first dose. Fingolimod is not recommended in the following patient groups who are at high risk of cardiovascular events unless the anticipated benefits outweigh the potential risks, and advice from a cardiologist is sought before initiation:

Patients with the following medical conditions:
- 2nd degree Mobitz Type II or higher degree atrioventricular block, sick sinus syndrome, or sino-atrial heart block
- significant QT prolongation (QT-interval greater than 470 milliseconds in women, or greater than 450 milliseconds in men)
- history of symptomatic bradycardia or recurrent syncope, known ischaemic heart disease, cerebrovascular disease, history of myocardial infarction, congestive heart failure, history of cardiac arrest, uncontrolled hypertension, or severe sleep apnoea.

Patients receiving the following antiarrhythmic or heart-rate lowering drugs:
- class Ia or class III antiarrhythmics
- beta blockers
- heart rate-lowering calcium channel blockers
- other substances which may decrease heart rate (e.g. digoxin, anticholinesteratic drugs or pilocarpine).

All patients receiving fingolimod should be monitored at treatment initiation, (first dose monitoring), and after treatment interruption (see note below); monitoring should include:

Pre-treatment
- a 12-lead ECG and blood pressure measurement before starting

During the first 6 hours of treatment
- continuous ECG monitoring for 6 hours
- blood pressure and heart rate measurement every hour

After 6 hours of treatment
- a further 12-lead ECG and blood pressure measurement

If heart rate at the end of the 6 hour period is at its lowest since fingolimod was first administered, monitoring should be extended by at least 2 hours and until heart rate increases.

Extended monitoring, (at least overnight), should be performed in patients with evidence of clinically important cardiac effects during first dose monitoring. Monitoring in patients requiring pharmacological intervention for bradyarrhythmia-related symptoms during first dose monitoring should be extended at least overnight, and first dose monitoring should be repeated after the second dose.

Note
First dose monitoring as above **should be repeated** in all patients whose treatment is interrupted for:
- 1 day or more during the first 2 weeks of treatment
- more than 7 days during weeks 3 and 4 of treatment
- more than 2 weeks after one month of treatment

If the treatment interruption is of shorter duration than the above, repeated monitoring is not required and treatment should be continued with the next dose as planned.

The *Scottish Medicines Consortium* (p. 4) has advised (August 2012) that fingolimod (*Gilenya*®) is accepted for restricted use within NHS Scotland as single disease modifying therapy in highly active relapsing-remitting multiple sclerosis despite treatment with interferon beta, with an unchanged or increased relapse rate or ongoing severe relapses, as compared to the previous year.

NICE guidance
Fingolimod for the treatment of highly active relapsing-remitting multiple sclerosis (April 2012)

Fingolimod is recommended as an option for the treatment of highly active relapsing-remitting multiple sclerosis in adults, only if:
- they have an unchanged or increased relapse rate or ongoing severe relapses compared with the previous year despite treatment with interferon beta, **and**
- the manufacturer provides fingolimod with the discount agreed as part of the patient access scheme.

Patients currently receiving fingolimod whose disease does not meet the above criteria should be able to continue treatment until they and their clinician consider it appropriate to stop.

www.nice.org.uk/TA254

▌ FINGOLIMOD

Indications   see notes above

Cautions   see MHRA/CHM advice above; susceptibility to QT-interval prolongation (including electrolyte disturbances, concomitant use of drugs that prolong QT interval); severe respiratory disease; pulmonary fibrosis; chronic obstructive pulmonary disease; risk of macular oedema—eye examination recommended 3–4 months after initiation of treatment (and before initiation of treatment in patients with diabetes or history of uveitis); monitor hepatic transaminases before treatment, then every 3 months for 1 year, then periodically thereafter; monitor full blood count before treatment, at 3 months, then at least yearly thereafter and if signs of infection—interrupt treatment if lymphocyte count reduced—consult product literature; monitor for signs and symptoms of haemophagocytic syndrome (including pyrexia, asthenia, hepato-splenomegaly and adenopathy—may be associated with hepatic failure and respiratory distress; also progressive cytopenia, elevated serum-ferritin concentrations, hypertriglyceridaemia, hypofibrinogenaemia, coagulopathy, hepatic cytolysis, hyponatraemia)—initiate treatment immediately; check varicella zoster virus status—consult product literature for further information; **interactions:** Appendix 1 (fingolimod)

Contra-indications   immunosuppression; active infection; active malignancies (except cutaneous basal cell carcinoma)

Hepatic impairment   use with caution in mild to moderate impairment; avoid in severe impairment

Pregnancy   avoid (toxicity in *animal* studies); exclude pregnancy before treatment and ensure effective contraception during and for at least 2 months after treatment

Breast-feeding   avoid

Side-effects   diarrhoea, weight loss, AV block, bradycardia, hypertension, cough, dyspnoea, depression, malaise, headache, migraine, dizziness, paraesthesia, influenza, herpes, bronchitis, sinusitis, gastro-enteritis, tinea, lymphopenia, leucopenia, back pain, blurred vision, eye pain, eczema, alopecia, pruritus; *less commonly* pneumonia, neutropenia, macular oedema; *also reported* haemophagocytic syndrome (see Cautions above), lymphoma

Dose

• ADULT over 18 years, 500 micrograms once daily

Gilenya® (Novartis) ▼ PoM
Capsules, fingolimod (as hydrochloride), 500 micrograms (yellow/white), net price 7-cap pack = £367.50, 28-cap pack = £1470.00

Glatiramer acetate

Glatiramer is an immunomodulating drug comprising synthetic polypeptides. It is licensed for treating initial symptoms in patients at high risk of developing multiple sclerosis, and also for reducing the frequency of relapses in ambulatory patients with relapsing-remitting multiple sclerosis who have had at least 2 clinical relapses in the past 2 years. Initiation of treatment with glatiramer should be supervised by a specialist.

> **NICE guidance (interferon beta and glatiramer for multiple sclerosis)**
> See p. 640

> **Provision of disease-modifying therapies for multiple sclerosis**
> See p. 640

■ GLATIRAMER ACETATE

Indications   see notes above
Cautions   cardiac disorders
Renal impairment   no information available—manufacturer advises caution
Pregnancy   manufacturer advises avoid—no information available
Breast-feeding   manufacturer advises caution—no information available
Side-effects   hypersensitivity reactions; flushing, chest pain, palpitation, tachycardia, and dyspnoea may occur within minutes of injection; nausea, constipation, dyspepsia; syncope, anxiety, asthenia, depression, headache, tremor, sweating; oedema, lymphadenopathy; hypertonia, back pain, arthralgia, influenza-like symptoms; injection-site reactions, rash; *rarely* seizures

Dose

• By subcutaneous injection, ADULT over 18 years, 20 mg daily

Copaxone® (Teva) PoM
Injection, glatiramer acetate 20 mg/mL, net price 1-mL prefilled syringe = £18.36

Histamine

Histamine is licensed for maintenance therapy, in combination with aldesleukin, in patients with acute myeloid leukaemia in first remission.

The *Scottish Medicines Consortium* (p. 4) has advised (December 2010) that histamine dihydrochloride (*Ceplene*®) is **not** recommended for use within NHS Scotland.

■ HISTAMINE DIHYDROCHLORIDE

Indications   see notes above
Cautions   consult product literature; **interactions**: Appendix 1 (histamine)
Contra-indications   consult product literature
Hepatic impairment   increased risk of tachycardia and hypotension in moderate to severe impairment
Renal impairment   increased risk of hypotension in severe impairment
Pregnancy   manufacturer advises avoid—no information available; ensure effective contraception during treatment in men and women
Breast-feeding   manufacturer advises avoid—no information available
Side-effects   consult product literature
Dose

• See Doses, p. 574

Ceplene® (Meda) ▼ PoM
Injection, histamine dihydrochloride 1 mg/mL, net price 0.5-mL vial = £84.38

Lenalidomide, pomalidomide, and thalidomide

Lenalidomide is an immunomodulating drug with anti-neoplastic, anti-angiogenic, and pro-erythropoietic properties. It is licensed for the treatment of transfusion-dependent anaemia due to low- or intermediate-1-risk myelodysplastic syndromes (MDS) associated with an isolated deletion 5q cytogenetic abnormality when other treatment options are insufficient or inadequate; it is also licensed in combination with dexamethasone, for the treatment of multiple myeloma in patients who have received at least one previous therapy.

The most serious side-effects of lenalidomide are venous thromboembolism, severe neutropenia, thrombocytopenia, and potentially fatal liver injuries. Lenalidomide is structurally related to thalidomide and there is a risk of peripheral neuropathy and teratogenesis.

> **NICE guidance**
> **Lenalidomide for treating myelodysplastic syndromes associated with an isolated deletion 5q cytogenetic abnormality (September 2014)**
> Lenalidomide is recommended as an option, within its marketing authorisation, for treating transfusion-dependent anaemia caused by low or intermediate-1-risk myelodysplastic syndromes associated with an isolated deletion 5q cytogenetic abnormality when other therapeutic options are insufficient or inadequate, with the following condition:
> • the drug cost of lenalidomide (excluding any related costs) for people who remain on treatment for more than 26 cycles (each of 28 days; normally a period of 2 years) will be met by the company.
> www.nice.org.uk/TA322

The *Scottish Medicines Consortium* (p. 4) has advised (April 2010) that lenalidomide, in combination with dexamethasone, is accepted for restricted use within NHS Scotland for patients with multiple myeloma who have received at least two prior therapies, and (March 2014) for those who have received prior treatment with bortezomib and for whom thalidomide has not been tolerated or is contra-indicated.

NICE guidance
Lenalidomide for the treatment of multiple myeloma (June 2009)

Lenalidomide in combination with dexamethasone is an option for the treatment of multiple myeloma in patients who have received two or more prior therapies. The drug cost of lenalidomide will be met by the manufacturer for patients who remain on treatment for more than 26 cycles.

www.nice.org.uk/TA171

Pomalidomide is structurally related to thalidomide and has immunomodulatory properties and direct anti-myeloma tumoricidal activity. It is licensed for use in combination with dexamethasone for the treatment of relapsed and refractory multiple myeloma in patients who have received at least two prior treatment regimens, including both lenalidomide and bortezomib, and who have had disease progression during the last treatment.

Thalidomide is used in combination with melphalan and prednisolone as first-line treatment for untreated multiple myeloma, in patients aged 65 years and over, or for those not eligible for high-dose chemotherapy (for example, patients with significant co-morbidity such as cardiac risk factors). It has immunomodulatory and anti-inflammatory activity. Thalidomide can cause drowsiness, neutropenia, thrombocytopenia, hepatic disorders, and thromboembolism. Patients should also be monitored for signs and symptoms of peripheral neuropathy.

NICE guidance
Bortezomib and thalidomide for the first-line treatment of multiple myeloma (July 2011)

Thalidomide in combination with an alkylating drug and a corticosteroid is recommended as an option for the first-line treatment of multiple myeloma in people for whom high-dose chemotherapy with stem cell transplantation is considered inappropriate.

For bortezomib, see p. 597
www.nice.org.uk/TA228

Pregnancy For women of child-bearing potential, pregnancy must be excluded before starting treatment with lenalidomide, pomalidomide, or thalidomide (perform pregnancy test on initiation or within 3 days prior to initiation). Women must practise effective contraception at least 1 month before, during, and for at least 1 month after treatment, including during dose interruptions (oral combined hormonal contraceptives and copper-releasing intrauterine devices not recommended) and men should use condoms during treatment, during dose interruption, and for at least 1 week after stopping if their partner is pregnant or is of child-bearing potential and not using effective contraception. Patients, prescribers and pharmacists must comply with pregnancy prevention measures as specified in the manufacturer's Pregnancy Prevention Programme.

◢ LENALIDOMIDE

Indications see notes above

Cautions see notes above; monitor full blood count (including differential white cell count, platelet count, haemoglobin, and haematocrit) and liver function before treatment, then every week for the first 8 weeks, then monthly thereafter (reduce dose or interrupt treatment if neutropenia, thrombocytopenia or impaired liver function develop—consult product literature); monitor for arterial or venous thromboembolism (if thromboembolic event occurs, discontinue lenalidomide and treat with standard anticoagulation therapy; lenalidomide may be restarted with continued anticoagulation therapy once thromboembolic event resolved—consult product literature); use caution with concomitant drugs that increase the risk of thromboembolism—see also Thromboembolism below; high tumour burden—risk of tumour lysis syndrome, see p. 574; monitor thyroid function; monitor for signs and symptoms of peripheral neuropathy; caution in patients with risk factors for myocardial infarction; discontinue permanently if angioedema, exfoliative or bullous rash, or if Stevens-Johnson syndrome or toxic epidermal necrolysis is suspected; **interactions:** Appendix 1 (lenalidomide)

Thromboembolism Risk factors for thromboembolism (such as smoking, hypertension, hyperlipidaemia) should be minimised and thromboprophylaxis should be considered in patients with multiple risk factors.

Patients and their carers should be made aware of the symptoms of thromboembolism and advised to report sudden breathlessness, chest pain, or swelling of a limb

Neutropenia and thrombocytopenia Patients and their carers should be made aware of the symptoms of neutropenia and advised to seek medical advice if symptoms suggestive of neutropenia (such as fever, sore throat) or of thrombocytopenia (such as bleeding) develop

Second primary malignancy Patients should be carefully evaluated before and during treatment with lenalidomide using routine cancer screening for occurrence of second primary malignancy and treatment should be instituted as indicated

Hepatic disorders Liver function should be monitored (see Cautions above), particularly when there is history of, or concurrent viral liver infection, or when lenalidomide is combined with drugs known to be associated with liver dysfunction (e.g. paracetamol)

Renal impairment reduce dose in renal impairment—consult product literature

Pregnancy important: **teratogenic risk**; see also notes above

Breast-feeding discontinue breast-feeding—no information available

Side-effects constipation, nausea, vomiting, diarrhoea, abdominal pain, dry mouth, dysphagia, dyspepsia, decreased appetite, stomatitis, cerebrovascular events, arrhythmias, bradycardia, tachycardia, myocardial infarction, chest pain, hypertension, hypotension, cardiac failure, oedema, pulmonary embolism, deep vein thrombosis, pneumonia, dyspnoea, respiratory tract infections, respiratory distress, tremor, malaise, mood changes, dizziness, syncope, falls, pyrexia, headache, ataxia, taste disturbance, peripheral neuropathy, sinusitis, sepsis, flu-like illness, hyperglycaemia, hypothyroidism, renal failure, urinary retention, urinary incontinence, haematuria, sexual dysfunction, haematoma, haemorrhagic disorders, iron-overload, neutropenia, thrombocytopenia, anaemia, leucopenia, dehydration, electrolyte disturbances, musculoskeletal disorders, visual disturbances, cataract, hearing disturbances, skin disorders, rash (if rash occurs, treatment should be discontinued and only restarted following appropriate clinical evaluation, see also Cautions above), hyperhidrosis, pruritus; *less commonly* hepatic failure, secondary malignancies; *rarely* Stevens-Johnson syndrome, toxic epidermal necrolysis, tumour lysis syndrome; *also reported* toxic hepatitis, cytolytic hepatitis, cholestatic hepatitis, pancreatitis, interstitial pneumonitis; also consult product literature

Dose

- Multiple myeloma, ADULT over 18 years, 25 mg once daily for 21 consecutive days of repeated 28-day cycles; for doses of dexamethasone, and dose adjustments due to side-effects, consult product literature
- Myelodysplastic syndromes, ADULT over 18 years, 10 mg once daily for 21 consecutive days of repeated 28-day cycles; for dose adjustments due to side-effects, consult product literature

Revlimid® (Celgene) ▼ PoM
Capsules, lenalidomide, 5 mg (white), net price 21-cap pack = £3570.00; 10 mg (blue/yellow), 21-cap pack = £3780.00; 15 mg (blue/white), 21-cap pack = £3969.00; 25 mg (white), 21-cap pack = £4368.00. Label: 25, counselling, pregnancy and contraception, symptoms of thromboembolism, neutropenia, and thrombocytopenia
Note Patient, prescriber, and supplying pharmacy must comply with a pregnancy prevention programme. Every prescription must be accompanied by a completed Prescription Authorisation Form

POMALIDOMIDE

Indications see notes above

Cautions monitor full blood count before treatment, then every week for the first 8 weeks, then monthly thereafter (reduce dose or interrupt treatment if neutropenia or thrombocytopenia develop—consult product literature); monitor for arterial or venous thromboembolism; use caution with concomitant drugs that increase the risk of bleeding or thromboembolism; peripheral neuropathy; significant cardiac dysfunction; high tumour burden—risk of tumour lysis syndrome, see p. 574; **interactions:** Appendix 1 (pomalidomide)

Thromboembolism Risk factors for thromboembolism (such as smoking, hypertension, hyperlipidaemia) should be minimised. Thromboprophylaxis should be considered, particularly in patients with additional risk factors. Patients and their carers should be made aware of the symptoms of thromboembolism and advised to report sudden breathlessness, chest pain, or swelling of a limb

Neutropenia and thrombocytopenia Patients and their carers should be made aware of the symptoms of neutropenia and advised to seek medical advice if symptoms suggestive of neutropenia (such as fever, sore throat) or of thrombocytopenia (such as bleeding) develop

Second primary malignancy Patients should be carefully evaluated before and during treatment with pomalidomide using routine cancer screening for occurrence of second primary malignancy and treatment should be instituted as indicated

Hepatic impairment manufacturer advises caution—no information available

Renal impairment manufacturer advises caution—no information available

Pregnancy important: teratogenic risk; see also notes above

Breast-feeding avoid—present in milk in *animal* studies

Side-effects decreased appetite, diarrhoea, nausea, vomiting, constipation, thromboembolic events, peripheral oedema, nasopharyngitis, dyspnoea, cough, impaired consciousness, malaise, confusion, peripheral neuropathy, dizziness, vertigo, tremor, pyrexia, pneumonia, respiratory tract infection, pelvic pain,

urinary retention, renal failure, leucopenia, neutropenia (including febrile neutropenia and neutropenic sepsis), thrombocytopenia, anaemia, hyperkalaemia, hyponatraemia, bone pain, muscle spasms, rash, pruritus

Dose

- ADULT over 18 years, 4 mg once daily for 21 consecutive days of repeated 28-day cycles; for doses of dexamethasone, and dose adjustments due to side-effects, consult product literature

Imnovid® (Celgene) ▼ PoM
Capsules, pomalidomide, 1 mg (blue/yellow), net price 21-cap pack = £8884.00; 2 mg (blue/orange), 21-cap pack = £8884.00; 3 mg (blue/green), 21-cap pack = £8884.00; 4 mg (blue), 21-cap pack = £8884.00. Label: 3, 25, counselling, pregnancy and contraception, symptoms of thromboembolism, neutropenia, and thrombocytopenia
Note Patient, prescriber, and supplying pharmacy must comply with a pregnancy prevention programme. Every prescription must be accompanied by a completed Prescription Authorisation Form
Excipients include propylene gylcol (see Excipients, p. 2)

THALIDOMIDE

Indications see notes above

Cautions see notes above; monitor white blood cell count (including differential count) and platelet count (reduce dose or interrupt treatment if neutropenia or thrombocytopenia develop - consult product literature); monitor liver function; high tumour burden—risk of tumour lysis syndrome, see p. 574; monitor for arterial or venous thromboembolism and use caution with concomitant drugs that increase the risk of peripheral neuropathy or thromboembolism—see also Thromboembolism, below

Thromboembolism Risk factors for thromboembolism (such as smoking, hypertension, hyperlipidaemia) should be minimised. Thromboprophylaxis is recommended for at least the first 5 months of treatment, especially in patients with additional thrombotic risk factors.

Patients and their carers should be made aware of the symptoms of thromboembolism and advised to report sudden breathlessness, chest pain, or swelling of a limb

Neutropenia and thrombocytopenia Patients and their carers should be made aware of the symptoms of neutropenia and advised to seek medical advice if symptoms suggestive of neutropenia (such as fever, sore throat) or of thrombocytopenia (such as bleeding) develop

Second primary malignancy Patients should be carefully evaluated before and during treatment with thalidomide using routine cancer screening for occurrence of second primary malignancy and treatment should be instituted as indicated

Hepatic disorder Liver function should be monitored, particularly when there is history of, or concurrent viral liver infection, or when thalidomide is combined with drugs known to be associated with liver dysfunction (e.g. paracetamol)

Peripheral neuropathy Monitor patients for signs and symptoms of peripheral neuropathy; patients and their carers should be advised to seek medical advice if symptoms such as paraesthesia, abnormal coordination, or weakness develop. Dose reduction, dose interruption, or treatment discontinuation may be necessary—consult product literature. Patients with pre-existing peripheral neuropathy should not be treated with thalidomide unless the potential clinical benefits outweigh the risk

Hepatic impairment caution in severe impairment—no information available

Renal impairment caution in severe impairment— no information available

Pregnancy important: teratogenic risk; see also notes above

Breast-feeding avoid—present in milk in *animal* studies

Side-effects vomiting, dry mouth, dyspepsia, constipation; bradycardia, cardiac failure, deep vein thrombosis; dyspnoea, interstitial lung disease, pulmonary embolism, peripheral oedema; asthenia, confusion, depression, dizziness, drowsiness, peripheral neuropathy, dysaesthesia, paraesthesia, syncope, tremor; pyrexia; pneumonia; anaemia, leucopenia, neutropenia, lymphopenia, thrombocytopenia; skin reactions including Stevens-Johnson syndrome (if rash occurs, treatment should be discontinued and only restarted following appropriate clinical evaluation); *also reported* atrial fibrillation, atrioventricular block, toxic epidermal necrolysis, intestinal obstruction, gastro-intestinal perforation and haemorrhage, worsening of Parkinson's disease symptoms, convulsions, hypothyroidism, sexual dysfunction, menstrual disorders, second primary malignancy, hepatic disorders, renal failure, hearing loss, myocardial infarction, cerebrovascular events

Dose
- ADULT over 18 years, 200 mg once daily at bedtime for 6-week cycle; max. 12 cycles

Thalidomide Celgene® (Celgene) PoM
Capsules, thalidomide 50 mg, net price 28-cap pack = £298.48. Label: 2, counselling, pregnancy and contraception, symptoms of peripheral neuropathy, thromboembolism, neutropenia,, and thrombocytopenia
Note Patient, prescriber, and supplying pharmacy must comply with a pregnancy prevention programme. Every prescription must be accompanied by a complete Prescription Authorisation Form.

Mifamurtide

Mifamurtide is licensed for high-grade, resectable, non-metastatic osteosarcoma after complete surgical resection, in patients 2 to 30 years of age at initial diagnosis. It is used in combination with chemotherapy.

> **NICE guidance**
> **Mifamurtide for the treatment of osteosarcoma (October 2011)**
>
> Mifamurtide in combination with postoperative multi-agent chemotherapy is recommended (within its licensed indication), as an option for the treatment of high-grade resectable non-metastatic osteosarcoma after macroscopically complete surgical resection in children, adolescents and young adults and when mifamurtide is made available at a reduced cost to the NHS under the patient access scheme.
> www.nice.org.uk/TA235

▌ MIFAMURTIDE

Indications see notes above
Cautions asthma and chronic obstructive pulmonary disease—consider prophylactic bronchodilator therapy; history of autoimmune, inflammatory, or collagen disease; monitor renal function, hepatic function and clotting parameters; monitor patients with history of venous thrombosis, vasculitis, or unstable

cardiovascular disorders for persistent or worsening symptoms during administration—consult product literature; **interactions:** Appendix 1 (mifamurtide)
Hepatic impairment use with caution—no information available
Renal impairment use with caution—no information available
Pregnancy avoid; effective contraception required
Breast-feeding avoid—no information available
Side-effects gastro-intestinal disturbances (including anorexia, nausea, vomiting, diarrhoea, constipation, abdominal pain, dyspepsia); tachycardia, hypertension, palpitations, hypotension, phlebitis, flushing; oedema, respiratory disorders (including dyspnoea, epistaxis, cough, tachypnoea, haemoptysis, pleural effusion); confusion, depression, insomnia, headache, dizziness, paraesthesia, hypoaesthesia, tremor, drowsiness, anxiety; hypokalaemia, anaemia, leucopenia, thrombocytopenia, granulocytopenia; haematuria, dysuria, pollakiuria; musculoskeletal pain; blurred vision; vertigo, tinnitus, hearing loss; sweating, alopecia, rash, dry skin

Dose
- See Doses, p. 574

Mepact® (Takeda) ▼ PoM
Intravenous infusion, powder for reconstitution, mifamurtide encapsulated in liposomes, net price 4-mg vial = £2375.00

Natalizumab

Natalizumab is a monoclonal antibody that inhibits the migration of leucocytes into the central nervous system, hence reducing inflammation and demyelination. It is licensed for use in patients with highly active *relapsing-remitting multiple sclerosis* despite treatment with interferon beta or glatiramer acetate, or those patients with rapidly evolving severe relapsing-remitting multiple sclerosis. Treatment with natalizumab should be initiated and supervised by a specialist.

Natalizumab is associated with an increased risk of opportunistic infection and progressive multifocal leucoencephalopathy (PML) caused by JC virus. The risk of developing PML increases with the presence of anti-JCV antibodies, previous use of immunosuppressant therapy, and treatment duration (especially beyond 2 years of treatment); the risk beyond 4 years of treatment is not known. Patients with all three risk factors should only be treated with natalizumab if the benefits of treatment outweigh the risks. Testing for serum anti-JCV antibodies before starting treatment or in those with unknown antibody status already receiving natalizumab is recommended and should be repeated every 6 months (consult product literature for full details). A magnetic resonance image (MRI) scan is recommended before starting treatment with natalizumab, and annually thereafter. Patients should be monitored for new or worsening neurological symptoms, and for cognitive and psychiatric signs of PML. Treatment should be suspended until PML has been excluded. If a patient develops an opportunistic infection or PML, natalizumab should be permanently discontinued. All patients should continue to be monitored for signs and symptoms that may be suggestive of PML for approximately 6 months following discontinuation of treatment.

Infusion-related side-effects include nausea, vomiting, flushing, headache, dizziness, fatigue, rigors, pyrexia, arthralgia, urticaria, and pruritus. Patients should be observed for hypersensitivity reactions, including anaphylaxis, during the infusion and for 1 hour after completion of the infusion. Natalizumab should be discontinued permanently if hypersensitivity reaction occurs.

The *Scottish Medicines Consortium* (p. 4) has advised (August 2007) that natalizumab is accepted for restricted use as single disease-modifying therapy in highly active relapsing-remitting multiple sclerosis only in patients with rapidly evolving severe relapsing-remitting multiple sclerosis defined by 2 or more disabling relapses in 1 year and with 1 or more gadolinium-enhancing lesions on brain magnetic resonance imaging (MRI) or a significant increase in T2 lesion load compared with a previous MRI.

> ### NICE guidance
> ### Natalizumab for the treatment of adults with highly active relapsing-remitting multiple sclerosis (August 2007)
> Natalizumab is an option for the treatment only of rapidly evolving severe relapsing-remitting multiple sclerosis (RES). RES is defined by 2 or more disabling relapses in 1 year, and 1 or more gadolinium-enhancing lesions on brain magnetic resonance imaging (MRI) or a significant increase in T2 lesion load compared with a previous MRI.
> www.nice.org.uk/TA127

NATALIZUMAB

Indications see notes above

Cautions see notes above and consult product literature; monitor liver function (see below); **interactions:** Appendix 1 (natalizumab)

> **Liver toxicity** Liver dysfunction reported; advise patients to seek immediate medical attention if symptoms such as jaundice or dark urine develop; discontinue treatment if significant liver injury occurs
>
> **Progressive multifocal leucoencephalopathy (PML)** Patients should be informed about the risks of PML before starting treatment with natalizumab and again after 2 years; they should be given an alert card which includes information about the symptoms of PML (see also notes above)
>
> **Hypersensitivity reactions** Patients should be told the importance of uninterrupted dosing, particularly in the early months of treatment (intermittent therapy may increase risk of sensitisation)

Contra-indications progressive multifocal leucoencephalopathy; active infection (see notes above); concurrent use of interferon beta or glatiramer acetate; immunosuppression; active malignancies (except cutaneous basal cell carcinoma)

Pregnancy avoid unless essential—toxicity in *animal* studies

Breast-feeding present in milk in *animal* studies—avoid

Side-effects see notes above; also urinary-tract infection, nasopharyngitis, autoantibodies, and arthralgia; *less commonly* hypersensitivity reactions (see above); liver toxicity also reported

Dose

- By intravenous infusion, ADULT over 18 years, 300 mg once every 4 weeks; discontinue if no response after 6 months

Tysabri® (Biogen) ▼ PoM
Concentrate for intravenous infusion, natalizumab 20 mg/mL, net price 15-mL vial = £1130.00. Counselling, liver toxicity, progressive multifocal leucoencephalopathy, and hypersensitivity, patient alert card
Electrolytes Na⁺ 2.3 mmol/vial

Siltuximab

Siltuximab is a monoclonal antibody that inhibits interleukin-6 receptor binding. It is licenced for the treatment of multicentric Castleman's disease (MCD) in patients who are human immunodeficiency virus (HIV) negative and human herpesvirus-8 (HHV-8) negative. Castleman's disease is a rare disorder of the lymphatic system that causes an abnormal cell growth in lymph nodes causing benign tumours.

Monitor neutrophil and platelet count, and haemoglobin levels prior to each dose of siltuximab treatment for the first 12 months and thereafter prior to every third dosing cycle. Consider delaying treatment if required neutrophil, platelet, and haemoglobin levels not achieved—consult product literature for details.

Infusion-related side-effects are reported commonly with siltuximab; resuscitation facilities should be available during treatment. Siltuximab therapy should be discontinued permanently in the event of a severe infusion-related reaction, anaphylaxis, a severe allergic reaction, or the occurence of cytokine-release syndrome. Mild to moderate infusion-related reactions may improve by temporarily reducing the rate or stopping the infusion. When restarting treatment, a reduced infusion rate and the administration of antihistamines, paracetamol, and corticosteroids should be considered. Consider discontinuation of siltuximab if more than 2 doses are delayed due to treatment-related toxicities during the first 48 weeks—for full details consult product literature.

SILTUXIMAB

Indications see notes above

Cautions see notes above and consult product literature; treat infection prior to treatment and monitor for infection during treatment; severe infection—withhold treatment until resolved; use with caution in patients at increased risk of gastrointestinal perforation; promptly investigate those presenting with symptoms suggestive of gastrointestinal perforation; hepatic impairment; live vaccines should not be given concurrently or within 4 weeks before starting siltuximab treatment; **interactions:** Appendix 1 (siltuximab)

Pregnancy manufacturer advises avoid unless potential benefit outweighs risk; women of childbearing potential should use effective contraception during and for 3 months after treatment

Breast-feeding manufacturer advises avoid—no information available

Side-effects see notes above; also abdominal pain, weight gain, hypertension, localised oedema, hypertriglyceridaemia, infections including upper respiratory tract infection and nasopharyngitis, renal impairment, hypoglobulinaemia, neutropenia, thrombocytopenia, maculopapular rash, pruritus, hypersensitivity reactions (including infusion-related reaction and anaphylaxis); *also reported* increased hae-moglobin levels, hepatitis B reactivation

Dose

• By intravenous infusion, ADULT over 18 years, 11 mg/kg every 3 weeks

Sylvant® (Janssen-Cilag) ▼ PoM

Intravenous infusion, powder for reconstitution, sil-tuximab, net price 100-mg vial =£415.00, 400-mg vial=£1661.00

Teriflunomide

Teriflunomide is a metabolite of leflunomide which has immunomodulating and anti-inflammatory properties. It is licensed for the treatment of adults with relapsing-remitting multiple sclerosis. Teriflunomide should be initiated and supervised by a physician experienced in the management of multiple sclerosis.

The *Scottish Medicines Consortium* (p. 4) has advised (February 2014) that the use of teriflunomide (*Auba-gio®*) in NHS Scotland is restricted to use in patients with relapsing-remitting multiple sclerosis who do not have highly active disease, and only as an alternative to treatment with interferon beta or glatiramer acetate.

NICE guidance
Teriflunomide for treating relapsing-remitting multiple sclerosis (January 2014)

Teriflunomide is recommended for the treatment of adults with active relapsing-remitting multiple sclerosis (normally defined as 2 clinically significant relapses in the previous 2 years), in adults who

• do not have highly active or rapidly evolving severe relapsing-remitting multiple sclerosis **and**

• the manufacturer provides teriflunomide with the dis-count agreed in the patient access scheme

www.nice.org.uk/TA303

■ **TERIFLUNOMIDE**

Note Teriflunomide is a metabolite of leflunomide

Indications see notes above

Cautions adult over 65 years; impaired bone-marrow function (avoid if severe) including anaemia, leuco-penia or thrombocytopenia; significant alcohol con-sumption; latent tuberculosis; hypoproteinaemia (avoid if severe); switching between other immuno-modulating drugs; persistent cough or dyspnoea—assess for interstitial lung disease and consider sus-pending treatment; severe infection—delay or sus-pend treatment until resolved; signs or symptoms of serious skin reactions (including ulcerative stomatitis, Stevens-Johnson syndrome, and toxic epidermal necrolysis)—discontinue treatment; monitor full blood count (including differential white cell count and platelet count) before treatment and as clinically indicated during treatment; monitor blood pressure before treatment and periodically thereafter; an accelerated elimination procedure is recommended following discontinuation due to serious adverse effects (consult product literature and see Accelerated Elimination Procedure below); **interactions:** Appen-dix 1 (teriflunomide)

Hepatic monitoring Monitor liver function before treatment and every 2 weeks for first 6 months then every 8 weeks thereafter or as clinically indicated (pre-existing liver disease may increase risk). Increase to weekly monitoring if alanine aminotransferase (ALT) is 2–3 times the upper limit of reference range; discontinue treatment if signs or

symptoms of hepatic injury, or if liver enzymes exceed 3 times the upper limit of reference range

Accelerated elimination procedure To aid drug elimination in case of serious adverse effect or before conception (see also Pregnancy below), stop treatment and give *either* colestyramine 8 g (reduce to 4 g if not tolerated) 3 times daily for 11 days *or* activated powdered charcoal 50 g every 12 hours for 11 days. After the accelerated elimination procedure a plasma concentration of less than 20 micrograms/litre (measured on 2 occasions at least 14 days apart) and a waiting period of one and a half months are necessary before conception. Use of non-oral contraception is recommended during the accelerated elimination procedure—consult product literature

Contra-indications significantly impaired bone-mar-row function (including anaemia, neutropenia, leuco-penia, or thrombocytopenia); severe immunodefi-ciency; severe hypoproteinaemia; serious infection

Hepatic impairment avoid in severe impairment; see also Hepatic Monitoring above

Pregnancy avoid—toxicity in *animal* studies; effective contraception essential for women of child-bearing potential during treatment and for up to 2 years after treatment (see also Accelerated Elimination Proce-dure above)

Breast-feeding present in milk in *animal* studies—manufacturer advises avoid

Side-effects diarrhoea, nausea, vomiting, gastroen-teritis, weight loss, hypertension, respiratory tract infection, laryngitis, anxiety, paraesthesia, peripheral neuropathy, sciatica, carpal tunnel syndrome, hyper-aesthesia, neuralgia, menorrhagia, urinary tract infection, cystitis, neutropenia, leucopenia, pollakiur-ia, elevated liver enzymes, musculoskeletal pain, myalgia, oral infection, alopecia, rash, acne, tinea pedis; *less commonly* anaemia, thrombocytopenia; *very rarely* interstitial lung disease, pancreatitis; **impor-tant:** accelerated elimination procedure recom-mended following discontinuation due to serious adverse effects (consult product literature and see Accelerated Elimination Procedure above)

Dose

• ADULT over 18 years, 14 mg once daily

Aubagio® (Genzyme) ▼ PoM

Tablets, f/c, pale blue, teriflunomide 14 mg, net price 28-tab pack = £1037.84.

8.3 Sex hormones and hormone antagonists in malignant disease

8.3.1 Oestrogens
8.3.2 Progestogens
8.3.3 Androgens
8.3.4 Hormone antagonists

Hormonal manipulation has an important role in the treatment of breast, prostate, and endometrial cancer, and a more marginal role in the treatment of hyperne-phroma. These treatments are not curative, but may provide excellent palliation of symptoms in selected patients, sometimes for a period of years. Tumour response, and treatment toxicity should be carefully monitored and treatment changed if progression occurs or side-effects exceed benefit.

Malignant disease and immunosuppression

8

8.3.1 Oestrogens

Diethylstilbestrol is sometimes used to treat prostate cancer, but it is not usually used first-line because of its side-effects. It is occasionally used in postmenopausal women with breast cancer. Toxicity is common and dose-related side-effects include nausea, fluid retention, and venous and arterial thrombosis. Impotence and gynaecomastia always occur in men, and withdrawal bleeding may be a problem in women. Hypercalcaemia and bone pain may also occur in breast cancer.

Ethinylestradiol is the most potent oestrogen available; unlike other oestrogens it is only slowly metabolised in the liver. Ethinylestradiol is licensed for the palliative treatment of prostate cancer.

DIETHYLSTILBESTROL
(Stilboestrol)

Indications   see notes above

Cautions   cardiovascular disease

Hepatic impairment   avoid; see also Combined Hormonal Contraceptives (section 7.3.1)

Pregnancy   in first trimester, high doses associated with vaginal carcinoma, urogenital abnormalities, and reduced fertility in female offspring; increased risk of hypospadias in male offspring

Side-effects   sodium retention with oedema, thromboembolism, jaundice, feminising effects in men; see also notes above

Dose
- Breast cancer, 10–20 mg daily
- Prostate cancer, 1–3 mg daily

Diethylstilbestrol (Non-proprietary) ᴾᵒᴹ
Tablets, diethylstilbestrol 1 mg, net price 28 = £107.79; 5 mg, 28 = £192.67

ETHINYLESTRADIOL
(Ethinyloestradiol)

Indications   see notes above; other indications (section 6.4.1.1)

Cautions   see section 6.4.1.1; **interactions:** Appendix 1 (oestrogens)

Contra-indications   see section 6.4.1.1

Hepatic impairment   avoid; see also Combined Hormonal Contraceptives (section 7.3.1)

Side-effects   see section 6.4.1.1

Dose
- Prostate cancer (palliative), 0.15–1.5 mg daily

◢**Preparations**
Section 6.4.1.1

8.3.2 Progestogens

Progestogens have a role in the treatment of endometrial cancer; their use in breast cancer and renal cell cancer has declined. Progestogens are now rarely used to treat prostate cancer. **Medroxyprogesterone** or **megestrol** are usually chosen and can be given orally; high-dose or parenteral treatment cannot be recommended. Side-effects are mild but may include nausea, fluid retention, and weight gain.

MEDROXYPROGESTERONE ACETATE

Indications   see notes above; contraception (section 7.3.2.2); other indications (section 6.4.1.2)

Cautions   see section 6.4.1.2; loss of vision during treatment (discontinue treatment if papilloedema or retinal vascular lesions); **interactions:** Appendix 1 (progestogens)

Contra-indications   see section 6.4.1.2 and notes above

Hepatic impairment   avoid; see also oral Progestogen-only Contraceptives (section 7.3.2.1)

Pregnancy   avoid—genital malformations and cardiac defects reported; see also Parenteral Progestogen-only Contraceptives (section 7.3.2.2)

Breast-feeding   present in milk—no adverse effects reported; see also Parenteral Progestogen-only Contraceptives (section 7.3.2.2)

Side-effects   see section 6.4.1.2 and notes above; glucocorticoid effects at high dose may lead to a cushingoid syndrome; also constipation, diarrhoea, dry mouth, vomiting, indigestion; adrenergic-like effects, congestive heart failure, hypertension, palpitation, tachycardia; confusion, euphoria, loss of concentration, nervousness, hyperpyrexia; hypercalcaemia; cervical erosions, galactorrhoea; raised white blood cell count, raised platelet count; vision disorders, retinal thrombosis

Dose
- See preparations below

Provera® (Pharmacia) ᴾᵒᴹ
Tablets, medroxyprogesterone acetate 100 mg (scored), net price 60-tab pack = £29.98, 100-tab pack = £49.94; 200 mg (scored), 30-tab pack = £29.65, 400 mg, 30-tab pack = £58.67
Dose endometrial and renal cell cancer, 200–600 mg daily; breast cancer, 0.4–1.5 g daily
Tablets, medroxyprogesterone acetate 2.5 mg, 5 mg and 10 mg, see section 6.4.1.2

MEGESTROL ACETATE

Indications   see notes above

Cautions   see under Medroxyprogesterone acetate (section 6.4.1.2) and notes above; **interactions:** Appendix 1 (progestogens)

Contra-indications   see under Medroxyprogesterone acetate (section 6.4.1.2) and notes above

Hepatic impairment   manufacturer advises caution in severe impairment

Pregnancy   avoid; reversible feminisation of male fetuses reported in *animal* studies; risk of hypospadias in male fetuses and masculinisation of female fetuses

Breast-feeding   discontinue breast-feeding

Side-effects   see under Medroxyprogesterone acetate (section 6.4.1.2) and notes above; vomiting, constipation, diarrhoea, carpal tunnel syndrome, adrenal insufficiency. Cushing's syndrome, urinary frequency, tumour flare (with or without hypercalcaemia), and asthenia

Dose
- Breast cancer, 160 mg once daily

Megace® (Swedish Orphan) ᴾᵒᴹ
Tablets, scored, megestrol acetate 160 mg (off-white), 30-tab pack = £19.52

▌ NORETHISTERONE

Indications see notes above; other indications (section 6.4.1.2)

Cautions see section 6.4.1.2 and notes above; **interactions:** Appendix 1 (progestogens)

Contra-indications see section 6.4.1.2 and notes above

Hepatic impairment avoid; see also oral Progestogen-only Contraceptives (section 7.3.2.1)

Pregnancy masculinisation of female fetuses and other defects reported; see also oral Progestogen-only Contraceptives (section 7.3.2.1)

Breast-feeding higher doses may suppress lactation and alter milk composition—use lowest effective dose; see also oral Progestogen-only Contraceptives (section 7.3.2.1)

Side-effects see section 6.4.1.2 and notes above

Dose
● Breast cancer, 40 mg daily, increased to 60 mg daily if required

◢ **Preparations**
Section 6.4.1.2

8.3.3 Androgens

Testosterone esters (section 6.4.2) have largely been superseded by other drugs for breast cancer.

8.3.4 Hormone antagonists

8.3.4.1 Breast cancer

8.3.4.2 Gonadorelin analogues and gonadotrophin-releasing hormone antagonists

8.3.4.3 Somatostatin analogues

8.3.4.1 Breast cancer

The management of patients with breast cancer involves surgery, radiotherapy, drug therapy, or a combination of these.

For operable breast cancer, treatment before surgery (neoadjuvant therapy) reduces the size of the tumour and facilitates breast-conserving surgery; hormone antagonist therapy (e.g. letrozole) is chosen for steroid hormone-receptor-positive breast cancer and chemotherapy for steroid hormone-receptor-negative tumours or for younger women.

Early breast cancer All women should be considered for adjuvant therapy following surgical removal of the tumour. Adjuvant therapy is used to eradicate the micrometastases that cause relapses. Choice of adjuvant treatment is determined by the risk of recurrence, steroid hormone-receptor status of the primary tumour, and menopausal status.

Adjuvant therapy comprises cytotoxic chemotherapy and hormone-antagonist therapy. Women with steroid hormone-receptor-positive breast cancer are considered for hormone-antagonist therapy (preceded by cytotoxic chemotherapy if necessary) whilst women with steroid hormone-receptor-negative breast cancer should be considered for cytotoxic chemotherapy.

Aromatase inhibitors act predominantly by blocking the conversion of androgens to oestrogens in the peripheral tissues. They do not inhibit ovarian oestrogen synthesis and should not be used in premenopausal women. **Anastrozole** and **letrozole** are non-steroidal aromatase inhibitors; **exemestane** is a steroidal aromatase inhibitor. Aromatase inhibitors are usually prescribed as initial adjuvant therapy in postmenopausal women with oestrogen-receptor-positive tumours; tamoxifen, an oestrogen-receptor antagonist, is used if an aromatase inhibitor is not appropriate. Adjuvant hormone antagonist therapy should generally be continued for 5 years following removal of the tumour. In postmenopausal women considered for extended adjuvant therapy, 5 years of tamoxifen is followed by letrozole for a further 2–3 years.

Trastuzumab (section 8.1.5) is licensed for use in early breast cancer which overexpresses human epidermal growth factor-2 (HER2) in women who have received surgery, chemotherapy and radiotherapy (as appropriate).

Premenopausal women with oestrogen-receptor-positive breast cancer who decline chemotherapy may benefit from treatment with goserelin (section 8.3.4.2) or ovarian ablation.

Advanced breast cancer Treatment of advanced breast cancer depends on the patient's drug history and an assessment of disease severity. Aromatase inhibitors, such as anastrozole or letrozole, are the preferred treatment in postmenopausal women with oestrogen-receptor-positive advanced breast cancer, a long disease-free interval following treatment for early breast cancer, and disease limited to bone or soft tissues; tamoxifen can be used if aromatase inhibitors are not suitable. Progestogens, such as medroxyprogesterone acetate (section 8.3.2), may be used after aromatase inhibitors and tamoxifen in postmenopausal women.

Tamoxifen should be considered for pre- and perimenopausal women with oestrogen-receptor-positive breast cancer not previously treated with tamoxifen. Ovarian suppression is used in pre- and perimenopausal women who have had disease progression despite treatment with tamoxifen. The gonadorelin analogue goserelin (section 8.3.4.2) is licensed for advanced breast cancer in pre- and perimenopausal women suitable for hormone manipulation.

Trastuzumab emtansine can be used alone for treating HER2-positive, unresectable, locally advanced breast cancer previously treated with trastuzumab and a taxane, or when there is disease recurrence during or following adjuvant therapy (section 8.1.5).

Cytotoxic chemotherapy is indicated for advanced steroid hormone-receptor-negative tumours and for aggressive disease, particularly when metastases involve visceral sites (e.g. the liver) or if the disease-free interval following treatment for early breast cancer is short.

Cytotoxic drugs used in breast cancer An anthracycline combined with fluorouracil (section 8.1.3) and cyclophosphamide (section 8.1.1), and sometimes also with methotrexate (section 8.1.3) is effective. Cyclophosphamide, methotrexate, and fluorouracil can be useful if an anthracycline is inappropriate (e.g. in cardiac disease).

Metastatic disease The choice of chemotherapy regimen will be influenced by whether the patient has previously received adjuvant treatment and the presence of any co-morbidity.

For women who have not previously received chemotherapy, an anthracycline (such as doxorubicin or epirubicin) alone or in combination with another cytotoxic drug is the standard initial therapy for metastatic breast disease.

Patients with anthracycline-refractory or resistant disease should be considered for treatment with a taxane (section 8.1.5) either alone or in combination with trastuzumab if they have tumours that overexpress HER2. Other cytotoxic drugs with activity against breast cancer include capecitabine (section 8.1.3), mitoxantrone, mitomycin (both section 8.1.2), and vinorelbine (section 8.1.4). Trastuzumab alone (section 8.1.5) is an option for chemotherapy-resistant cancers that overexpress HER2. Trastuzumab emtansine can be used as monotherapy in HER2-positive metastatic breast cancer previously treated with trastuzumab and a taxane, or when there is disease recurrence during or following adjuvant therapy (section 8.1.5). Trastuzumab and trastuzumab emtansine are **not** interchangeable.

The use of **bisphosphonates** (section 6.6.2) in patients with metastatic breast cancer may reduce pain and prevent skeletal complications of bone metastases.

ANASTROZOLE

Indications adjuvant treatment of oestrogen-receptor-positive early invasive breast cancer in postmenopausal women; adjuvant treatment of oestrogen-receptor-positive early breast cancer in postmenopausal women following 2–3 years of tamoxifen therapy; advanced breast cancer in postmenopausal women which is oestrogen-receptor-positive or responsive to tamoxifen

Cautions laboratory test for menopause if doubt; susceptibility to osteoporosis (assess bone mineral density before treatment and at regular intervals)

Contra-indications not for premenopausal women

Hepatic impairment avoid in moderate to severe impairment

Renal impairment avoid if creatinine clearance less than 20 mL/minute

Pregnancy avoid

Breast-feeding avoid

Side-effects hot flushes, vaginal dryness, vaginal bleeding, hair thinning, anorexia, nausea, vomiting, diarrhoea, headache, arthralgia, arthritis, bone fractures, bone pain, rash (including Stevens-Johnson syndrome), cutaneous vasculitis; asthenia and drowsiness—may initially affect ability to drive or operate machinery; slight increases in total cholesterol levels reported; very rarely allergic reactions including angioedema and anaphylaxis

Dose
● 1 mg daily

Anastrozole (Non-proprietary) (PoM)
Tablets, anastrozole 1 mg, net price 28-tab pack = £2.03
Brands include *Nastrosa*®

Arimidex® (AstraZeneca) (PoM)
Tablets, f/c, anastrozole 1 mg, net price 28-tab pack = £68.56
The *Scottish Medicines Consortium* (p. 4) has advised (August 2005 and October 2006) that anastrozole (*Arimidex*®) is accepted for restricted use within NHS Scotland, within the

licensed indications, for early breast cancer and early invasive breast cancer.

EXEMESTANE

Indications adjuvant treatment of oestrogen-receptor-positive early breast cancer in postmenopausal women following 2–3 years of tamoxifen therapy; advanced breast cancer in postmenopausal women in whom anti-oestrogen therapy has failed

Cautions interactions: Appendix 1 (exemestane)

Contra-indications not indicated for premenopausal women

Hepatic impairment manufacturer advises caution

Renal impairment manufacturer advises caution

Pregnancy avoid

Breast-feeding avoid

Side-effects nausea, vomiting, abdominal pain, dyspepsia, constipation, anorexia; dizziness, fatigue, headache, depression, insomnia; hot flushes, sweating; alopecia, rash; *less commonly* drowsiness, asthenia, and peripheral oedema; *rarely* thrombocytopenia, leucopenia

Dose
● 25 mg daily

Aromasin® (Pharmacia) (PoM)
Tablets, s/c, exemestane 25 mg, net price 30-tab pack = £88.80, 90-tab pack = £266.40. Label: 21
The *Scottish Medicines Consortium* (p. 4) has advised (October 2005) that exemestane (*Aromasin*®) is accepted for restricted use within NHS Scotland as an adjuvant treatment in postmenopausal women with oestrogen-receptor-positive invasive early breast cancer, following 2–3 years of initial adjuvant tamoxifen therapy.

FULVESTRANT

Indications treatment of oestrogen-receptor-positive metastatic or locally advanced breast cancer in postmenopausal women in whom disease progresses or relapses while on, or after, other anti-oestrogen therapy

Hepatic impairment manufacturer advises caution in mild to moderate impairment; avoid in severe impairment

Renal impairment manufacturer advises caution if creatinine clearance less than 30 mL/minute—no information available

Pregnancy manufacturer advises avoid—increased incidence of fetal abnormalities and death in *animal* studies

Breast-feeding manufacturer advises avoid—present in milk in *animal* studies

Side-effects nausea, vomiting, diarrhoea; venous thromboembolism; anorexia, headache, asthenia; urinary-tract infections; hot flushes; back pain; rash; injection-site reactions, hypersensitivity reactions; *less commonly* vaginal haemorrhage, vaginal candidiasis, and leucorrhoea

Dose
● By deep intramuscular injection into buttock, 500 mg every 2 weeks for the first 3 doses, then 500 mg every month
Note 500 mg dose should be administered as one 250-mg injection (slowly over 1–2 minutes) into each buttock

Faslodex® (AstraZeneca) (PoM)
Injection (oily), fulvestrant 50 mg/mL, net price 2 × 5-mL (250-mg) prefilled syringe = £522.41

LETROZOLE

Indications first-line treatment in postmenopausal women with hormone-dependent advanced breast cancer; adjuvant treatment of oestrogen-receptor-positive invasive early breast cancer in postmenopausal women; advanced breast cancer in postmenopausal women (naturally or artificially induced menopause) in whom other anti-oestrogen therapy has failed; extended adjuvant treatment of hormone-dependent invasive breast cancer in postmenopausal women who have received standard adjuvant tamoxifen therapy for 5 years; neo-adjuvant treatment in postmenopausal women with localised hormone-receptor-positive, human epidermal growth factor-2 negative breast cancer where chemotherapy is not suitable and surgery not yet indicated

Cautions susceptibility to osteoporosis (assess bone mineral density before treatment and at regular intervals)

Contra-indications not indicated for premenopausal women

Hepatic impairment manufacturer advises caution in severe impairment

Renal impairment manufacturer advises caution if creatinine clearance less than 10 mL/minute

Pregnancy avoid (isolated cases of birth defects reported); manufacturer advises effective contraception required until postmenopausal status fully established (return of ovarian function reported in postmenopausal women)

Breast-feeding manufacturer advises avoid

Side-effects nausea, vomiting, abdominal pain, hypertension, hot flushes, fatigue, dizziness, headache, dyspepsia, constipation, diarrhoea, depression, anorexia, appetite increase, weight changes, vaginal bleeding, hypercholesterolaemia, alopecia, increased sweating, rash, dry skin, peripheral oedema, arthralgia, musculoskeletal pain, osteoporosis, bone fracture; *less commonly* cerebrovascular events, cardiac events, palpitation, tachycardia, dyspnoea, cough, insomnia, anxiety, memory impairment, dysaesthesia, taste disturbance, pruritus, urticaria, thrombophlebitis, urinary frequency, urinary-tract infection, vaginal discharge, breast pain, pyrexia, mucosal dryness, stomatitis, cataract, eye irritation, blurred vision, tumour pain, arthritis, leucopenia, general oedema; *rarely* pulmonary embolism, arterial thrombosis; *also reported* hepatitis, toxic epidermal necrolysis

Dose
- 2.5 mg daily

Letrozole (Non-proprietary) [PoM]
Tablets, letrozole 2.5 mg, net price 14-tab pack = £1.88, 28-tab pack = £3.32

Femara® (Novartis) [PoM]
Tablets, f/c, letrozole 2.5 mg. Net price 30-tab pack = £90.92

TAMOXIFEN

Indications see under Dose and notes above; mastalgia [unlicensed indication] (section 6.7.2)

Cautions occasional cystic ovarian swellings in premenopausal women; increased risk of thromboembolic events, especially when used with cytotoxics (see also below); endometrial changes (**important:**

see below); porphyria, **interactions:** Appendix 1 (tamoxifen)
Endometrial changes Increased endometrial changes, including hyperplasia, polyps, cancer, and uterine sarcoma reported; prompt investigation required if abnormal vaginal bleeding including menstrual irregularities, vaginal discharge, and pelvic pain or pressure in those receiving (or who have received) tamoxifen. Patients should be informed of the risk of endometrial cancer and told to report relevant symptoms promptly

Contra-indications treatment of infertility contra-indicated if personal or family history of idiopathic venous thromboembolism or genetic predisposition to thromboembolism

Pregnancy avoid—possible effects on fetal development; effective contraception must be used during treatment and for 2 months after stopping

Breast-feeding suppresses lactation; avoid unless potential benefit outweighs risk

Side-effects hot flushes, vaginal bleeding and vaginal discharge (**important:** see also Endometrial Changes under Cautions), suppression of menstruation in some premenopausal women, pruritus vulvae, gastrointestinal disturbances, headache, light-headedness, tumour flare, decreased platelet counts; occasionally oedema, rarely hypercalcaemia if bony metastases, alopecia, rashes, uterine fibroids; also visual disturbances (including corneal changes, cataracts, retinopathy); leucopenia (sometimes with anaemia and thrombocytopenia), rarely neutropenia; hypertriglyceridaemia reported rarely (sometimes with pancreatitis); thromboembolic events reported (see below); liver enzyme changes (rarely fatty liver, cholestasis, hepatitis); rarely interstitial pneumonitis, hypersensitivity reactions including angioedema, Stevens-Johnson syndrome, bullous pemphigoid; see also notes above
Risk of thromboembolism Tamoxifen can increase the risk of thromboembolism particularly during and immediately after major surgery or periods of immobility (consider interrupting treatment to initiate anticoagulant measures). Patients should be made aware of the symptoms of thromboembolism and advised to report sudden breathlessness and any pain in the calf of one leg

Dose
- Breast cancer, 20 mg daily
- Anovulatory infertility, 20 mg daily on days 2, 3, 4 and 5 of cycle; if necessary the daily dose may be increased to 40 mg then 80 mg for subsequent courses; if cycles irregular, start initial course on any day, with subsequent course starting 45 days later *or* on day 2 of cycle if menstruation occurs

Tamoxifen (Non-proprietary) [PoM]
Tablets, tamoxifen (as citrate) 10 mg, net price 30-tab pack = £24.13; 20 mg, 30-tab pack = £2.27; 40 mg, 30-tab pack = £19.98
Oral solution, tamoxifen (as citrate) 10 mg/5 mL, net price 150 mL = £29.61
Brands include *Soltamox®*

TOREMIFENE

Indications hormone-dependent metastatic breast cancer in postmenopausal women

Cautions hypercalcaemia may occur (especially if bone metastases and usually at beginning of treatment); avoid in acute porphyria (but see section 9.8.2); history of severe thromboembolic disease; **interactions:** Appendix 1 (toremifene)
Endometrial changes Increased endometrial changes, including hyperplasia, polyps and cancer reported.

Abnormal vaginal bleeding including menstrual irregularities, vaginal discharge and symptoms such as pelvic pain or pressure should be promptly investigated

Contra-indications endometrial hyperplasia, QT prolongation (avoid concomitant administration of drugs that prolong QT interval), electrolyte disturbances (particularly uncorrected hypokalaemia), bradycardia, heart failure with reduced left-ventricular ejection fraction, history of arrhythmias

Hepatic impairment elimination decreased in hepatic impairment—avoid if severe

Pregnancy avoid

Breast-feeding avoid

Side-effects nausea, vomiting; oedema; depression, dizziness, fatigue; sweating, hot flushes, vaginal bleeding or discharge (**important**: see Cautions); rash; *less commonly* anorexia, constipation, increased weight, thromboembolic events, dyspnoea, insomnia, headache, endometrial hypertrophy; *very rarely* jaundice, transient corneal opacity, and alopecia

Dose
- 60 mg daily

Fareston® (Orion) [PoM]
Tablets, toremifene (as citrate) 60 mg. Net price 30-tab pack = £29.08

8.3.4.2 Gonadorelin analogues and gonadotrophin-releasing hormone antagonists

Metastatic cancer of the prostate usually responds to hormonal treatment aimed at androgen depletion. Standard treatments include bilateral subcapsular orchidectomy or use of a gonadorelin analogue (**buserelin, goserelin, histrelin, leuprorelin**, or **triptorelin**). The gonadotrophin-releasing hormone antagonist, **degarelix**, (p. 658) is also available. Response in most patients lasts for 12 to 18 months. No entirely satisfactory therapy exists for disease progression despite this treatment (hormone-refractory prostate cancer), but occasional patients respond to other hormone manipulation e.g. with an anti-androgen. Bone disease can often be palliated with irradiation or, if widespread, with strontium or prednisolone (section 6.3.2).

Gonadorelin analogues

Gonadorelin analogues are as effective as orchidectomy or **diethylstilbestrol** (section 8.3.1) but are expensive and require parenteral administration, at least initially. They cause initial stimulation then depression of luteinising hormone release by the pituitary. During the initial stage (1–2 weeks) increased production of testosterone may be associated with progression of prostate cancer. In susceptible patients this tumour 'flare' may cause spinal cord compression, ureteric obstruction or increased bone pain. When such problems are anticipated, alternative treatments (e.g. orchidectomy) or concomitant use of an anti-androgen such as cyproterone acetate or flutamide (see below) are recommended; anti-androgen treatment should be started before the gonadorelin analogue. Gonadorelin analogues are also used in women for breast cancer (section 8.3.4.1) and other indications (section 6.7.2).

The *Scottish Medicines Consortium* (p. 4) has advised (June 2009) that histrelin (*Vantas®*) is accepted for restricted use within NHS Scotland for the palliative treatment of advanced prostate cancer in patients with an anticipated life expectancy of at least one year in whom annual administration will offer advantages.

Cautions Men at risk of tumour 'flare' (see above) should be monitored closely during the first month of therapy. Caution is required in patients with metabolic bone disease because reduced bone mineral density can occur. The injection site should be rotated.

Side-effects The gonadorelin analogues cause side-effects similar to the menopause in women and orchidectomy in men and include hot flushes and sweating, sexual dysfunction, vaginal dryness or bleeding, and gynaecomastia or changes in breast size. Signs and symptoms of prostate or breast cancer may worsen initially (managed in prostate cancer with anti-androgens, see above). Other side-effects include hypersensitivity reactions (rashes, pruritus, asthma, and rarely anaphylaxis), injection site reactions (see Cautions), headache (rarely migraine), visual disturbances, dizziness, arthralgia and possibly myalgia, hair loss, peripheral oedema, gastro-intestinal disturbances, weight changes, sleep disorders, and mood changes.

■ BUSERELIN

Indications advanced prostate cancer; other indications (section 6.7.2)

Cautions diabetes, hypertension, depression; see also notes above

Side-effects see notes above; worsening hypertension, palpitation, glucose intolerance, altered blood lipids, thrombocytopenia, leucopenia, nervousness, fatigue, memory and concentration disturbances, anxiety, increased thirst, hearing disorders, musculoskeletal pain; nasal irritation, nose bleeds and altered sense of taste and smell (spray formulation only)

Dose
- By subcutaneous injection, 500 micrograms every 8 hours for 7 days, then intranasally, 1 spray into each nostril 6 times daily (see also notes above)
   Counselling Avoid use of nasal decongestants before and for at least 30 minutes after treatment.

Suprefact® (Sanofi-Aventis) [PoM]
Injection, buserelin (as acetate) 1 mg/mL. Net price 2 × 5.5-mL vial = £28.64

Nasal spray, buserelin (as acetate) 100 micrograms/metered spray. Net price treatment pack of 4 × 10-g bottle with spray pump = £101.87. Counselling, see above

■ GOSERELIN

Indications locally advanced prostate cancer as an alternative to surgical castration; adjuvant treatment to radiotherapy or radical prostatectomy in patients with high-risk localised or locally advanced prostate cancer; neoadjuvant treatment prior to radiotherapy in patients with high-risk localised or locally advanced prostate cancer; metastatic prostate cancer; advanced breast cancer; oestrogen-receptor-positive early breast cancer (section 8.3.4.1); endometriosis, endometrial thinning, uterine fibroids, assisted reproduction (section 6.7.2)

Cautions see notes above; diabetes; hypertension; depression; risk of ureteric obstruction and spinal cord compression in men

Contra-indications undiagnosed vaginal bleeding

Pregnancy see Goserelin, section 6.7.2

Breast-feeding see Goserelin, section 6.7.2

Side-effects see notes above; also transient changes in blood pressure, heart failure, myocardial infarction; paraesthesia; *rarely* hypercalcaemia (in patients with metastatic breast cancer)

Dose

- See under preparations below

Zoladex® (AstraZeneca) [PoM]

Implant, goserelin (as acetate) 3.6 mg in *SafeSystem®* syringe applicator, net price each = £65.00

Dose breast cancer and prostate cancer (see indications above) by subcutaneous injection into anterior abdominal wall, 3.6 mg every 28 days

Zoladex® LA (AstraZeneca) [PoM]

Implant, goserelin (as acetate) 10.8 mg in *SafeSystem®* syringe applicator, net price each = £235.00

Dose prostate cancer (see indications above), by subcutaneous injection into anterior abdominal wall, 10.8 mg every 12 weeks

■ HISTRELIN

Indications advanced prostate cancer

Cautions see notes above; monitor patients at high risk of metabolic disease (e.g. bone disease, worsening diabetes) or cardiovascular disease before and during treatment; risk of ureteric obstruction and spinal cord compression

Side-effects see notes above; also hepatic disorder, dyspnoea, depression, asthenia, elevated blood glucose-concentration, increased urinary frequency, hypertrichosis; *less commonly* hypercholesterolaemia, palpitation, ventricular extrasystole, haematoma, tremor, anaemia, renal failure, nephrolithiasis, hypercalcaemia

Dose

- By subcutaneous implantation into upper arm, 1 implant (50 mg) every 12 months; remove after 12 months of treatment

Counselling Avoid wetting arm containing implant for 24 hours and avoid lifting heavy objects or strenuous physical activity for 7 days after implantation

Vantas® (Orion) [PoM]

Implant, histrelin (as acetate) 50 mg, net price 1 pack (containing implantation device and implant) = £990.00

■ LEUPRORELIN ACETATE

Indications locally advanced prostate cancer as an alternative to surgical castration; adjuvant treatment to radiotherapy or radical prostatectomy in patients with high-risk localised or locally advanced prostate cancer; metastatic prostate cancer; endometriosis, endometrial thinning, uterine fibroids (section 6.7.2)

Cautions see notes above and section 6.7.2; risk of ureteric obstruction and spinal cord compression in men

Side-effects see notes above and section 6.7.2; also fatigue, muscle weakness, depression, paraesthesia, hypertension, palpitation, alteration of glucose tolerance and of blood lipids; hypotension, jaundice, thrombocytopenia and leucopenia reported

Dose

- See under preparations below

Prostap® SR DCS (Takeda) [PoM]

Injection, dual-chamber prefilled syringe containing powder for reconstitution, leuprorelin acetate and solvent, net price 3.75-mg prefilled syringe = £75.24

Dose prostate cancer (see indications), by subcutaneous or by intramuscular injection, 3.75 mg every month

Prostap® 3 DCS (Takeda) [PoM]

Injection, dual-chamber prefilled syringe containing powder for reconstitution, leuprorelin acetate and solvent, net price 11.25-mg prefilled syringe = £225.72

Dose prostate cancer (see indications), by subcutaneous injection, 11.25 mg every three months

■ TRIPTORELIN

Indications prostate cancer; endometriosis, precocious puberty, reduction in size of uterine fibroids; male hypersexuality with severe sexual deviation (section 6.7.2)

Cautions see notes above; risk of ureteric obstruction and spinal cord compression in men; risk factors for osteoporosis

Side-effects see notes above; also dry mouth, transient hypertension, paraesthesia, and increased dysuria

Dose

- See under preparations below

Decapeptyl® SR (Ipsen) [PoM]

Injection (powder for suspension), triptorelin (as acetate), net price 3-mg vial (with diluent) = £69.00

Dose locally advanced non-metastatic prostate cancer as an alternative to surgical castration, metastatic prostate cancer, as an adjuvant treatment to radiotherapy in high-risk localised or locally advanced prostate cancer, as neoadjuvant treatment prior to radiotherapy in patients with high-risk localised or locally advanced prostate cancer, as an adjuvant treatment to radical prostatectomy in patients with locally advanced prostate cancer at high risk of disease progression, by intramuscular injection, 3 mg every 4 weeks

Note Each vial includes an overage to allow accurate administration of a 3-mg dose

Injection (powder for suspension), triptorelin (as acetate), net price 11.25-mg vial (with diluent) = £207.00

Dose locally advanced non-metastatic prostate cancer as an alternative to surgical castration, metastatic prostate cancer, as an adjuvant treatment to radiotherapy in high-risk localised or locally advanced prostate cancer, as neoadjuvant treatment prior to radiotherapy in patients with high-risk localised or locally advanced prostate cancer, as an adjuvant treatment to radical prostatectomy in patients with locally advanced prostate cancer at high risk of disease progression, by intramuscular injection, 11.25 mg every 3 months (see also notes above)

Note Each vial includes an overage to allow accurate administration of an 11.25-mg dose

Injection (powder for suspension), triptorelin (as pamoate), net price 22.5-mg vial (with diluent) = £414.00

Dose locally advanced non-metastatic prostate cancer as an alternative to surgical castration, metastatic prostate cancer, as an adjuvant treatment to radiotherapy in high-risk localised or locally advanced prostate cancer, as neoadjuvant treatment prior to radiotherapy in patients with high-risk localised or locally advanced prostate cancer, as an adjuvant treatment to radical prostatectomy in patients with locally advanced prostate cancer at high risk of disease progression, by intramuscular injection, 22.5 mg every 6 months (see also notes above)

Note Each vial includes an overage to allow accurate administration of a 22.5-mg dose

Gonapeptyl Depot® (Ferring) [PoM]

Injection (powder for suspension), triptorelin (as acetate), net price 3.75-mg prefilled syringe (with prefilled syringe of vehicle) = £81.69

Dose advanced prostate cancer, by subcutaneous *or* deep intramuscular injection, 3.75 mg every 4 weeks (see also notes above)

Anti-androgens

Cyproterone acetate, **flutamide** and **bicalutamide** are anti-androgens that inhibit the tumour 'flare' which may occur after commencing gonadorelin analogue administration. Cyproterone acetate and flutamide are also licensed for use alone in patients with metastatic prostate cancer refractory to gonadorelin analogue therapy. Bicalutamide is used for prostate cancer either alone or as an adjunct to other therapy, according to the clinical circumstances.

Abiraterone (in combination with prednisone or prednisolone) and **enzalutamide** are licensed for metastatic castration-resistant prostate cancer in patients whose disease has progressed during or after treatment with a docetaxel-containing chemotherapy regimen. Abiraterone is also used to treat metastatic castration-resistant prostate cancer in patients who are asymptomatic or mildly symptomatic after failure of androgen deprivation therapy in whom chemotherapy is not yet clinically indicated. Medical castration with a luteinising hormone-releasing hormone analogue should be continued during treatment with abiraterone in patients not surgically castrated.

> **NICE guidance**
> **Enzalutamide for metastatic hormone-relapsed prostate cancer previously treated with a docetaxel-containing regimen** (July 2014)
>
> Enzalutamide is recommended, within its marketing authorisation, as an option for treating metastatic hormone-relapsed prostate cancer in adults only if:
> - their disease has progressed during or after docetaxel-containing chemotherapy, **and**
> - the manufacturer provides enzalutamide with the discount agreed in the patient access scheme.
>
> This guidance does not cover the use of enzalutamide for metastatic hormone-relapsed prostate cancer previously treated with abiraterone.
> www.nice.org.uk/TA316

The *Scottish Medicines Consortium* (p. 4) has advised (July 2012) that abiraterone (*Zytiga®*), in combination with prednisone or prednisolone, is accepted for restricted use within NHS Scotland for the treatment of metastatic castration-resistant prostate cancer in patients whose disease has progressed during or after treatment with docetaxel-containing chemotherapy regimen, and have received only one prior chemotherapy regimen.

> **NICE guidance**
> **Abiraterone for castration-resistant metastatic prostate cancer previously treated with a docetaxel-containing regimen** (June 2012)
>
> Abiraterone in combination with prednisone or prednisolone is recommended as an option for the treatment of castration-resistant metastatic prostate cancer only if:
> - their disease has progressed on or after one docetaxel-containing chemotherapy regimen, **and**
> - the manufacturer provides abiraterone with the discount agreed in the patient access scheme.
>
> Patients currently receiving abiraterone in combination with prednisone or prednisolone whose disease does not meet the first criteria should be able to continue therapy until they and their clinician consider it appropriate to stop.
> www.nice.org.uk/TA259

ABIRATERONE ACETATE

Indications   see notes above

Cautions   monitor blood pressure, serum potassium concentration, and fluid balance before treatment, and at least monthly during treatment—consult product literature for management of hypertension, hypokalaemia and oedema; history of cardiovascular disease—correct hypertension and hypokalaemia before treatment (if significant risk of congestive heart failure, such as history of cardiac failure, uncontrolled hypertension or cardiac events, consult product literature for management and increased monitoring); diabetes (increased risk of hyperglycaemia—monitor blood sugar frequently); concurrent chemotherapy—safety and efficacy not established; increased risk of myopathy and rhabdomyolysis with possible renal failure—caution with concomitant use of drugs known to be associated with myopathy or rhabdomyolysis; monitor liver function before treatment, then every 2 weeks for the first 3 months of treatment, then monthly thereafter—interrupt treatment if serum alanine aminotransferase or aspartate aminotransferase greater than 5 times the upper limit (consult product literature for details of restarting treatment at a lower dose) and discontinue permanently if 20 times the upper limit; **interactions**: Appendix 1 (abiraterone)

Hepatic impairment   use with caution in moderate impairment and only if benefit clearly outweighs risk; avoid in severe impairment; see also Cautions

Renal impairment   use with caution in severe impairment—no information available

Pregnancy   men should use condoms if their partner is pregnant, and use condoms in combination with another effective contraceptive method if their partner is of child-bearing potential—toxicity in *animal* studies

Side-effects   diarrhoea, dyspepsia, hepatotoxicity (see under Cautions, above), hypertension, hypertriglyceridaemia, heart failure, angina, arrhythmia, atrial fibrillation, tachycardia, peripheral oedema, urinary tract infection, sepsis, haematuria, hypokalaemia, fractures, rash; *less commonly* adrenal insufficiency, myopathy, rhabdomyolysis; *rarely* allergic alveolitis

Dose
- 1 g once daily

Note Consult product literature for dose of concurrent prednisone or prednisolone

Zytiga® (Janssen) ▼ PoM
Tablets, abiraterone actetate 250 mg, net price 120-tab pack = £2930.00. Label: 23

BICALUTAMIDE

Indications locally advanced prostate cancer at high risk of disease progression, either alone or as adjuvant treatment to prostatectomy or radiotherapy; locally advanced, non-metastatic prostate cancer when surgical castration or other medical intervention inappropriate; advanced prostate cancer in combination with gonadorelin analogue or surgical castration

Cautions consider periodic liver function tests; **interactions**: Appendix 1 (bicalutamide)

Hepatic impairment increased accumulation possible in moderate to severe impairment

Side-effects nausea, diarrhoea, cholestasis, jaundice; asthenia, weight gain; gynaecomastia, breast tenderness, hot flushes, impotence, decreased libido; anaemia; alopecia, dry skin, hirsutism, pruritus; *less commonly* vomiting, abdominal pain, dyspepsia, interstitial lung disease, pulmonary fibrosis, depression, haematuria, thrombocytopenia, hypersensitivity reactions including angioneurotic oedema and urticaria; *rarely* cardiovascular disorders (including angina, heart failure, and arrhythmias), and hepatic failure

Dose
* Locally advanced prostate cancer at high risk of disease progression, 150 mg once daily
* Locally advanced, non-metastatic prostate cancer when surgical castration or other medical intervention inappropriate, 150 mg once daily
* Advanced prostate cancer, in combination with gonadorelin analogue or surgical castration, 50 mg once daily (started at the same time as surgical castration or at least 3 days before gonadorelin therapy, see also notes above)

Bicalutamide (Non-proprietary) PoM
Tablets, bicalutamide 50 mg, net price 28-tab pack = £2.44; 150 mg, 28-tab pack = £6.17

Casodex® (AstraZeneca) PoM
Tablets, f/c, bicalutamide 50 mg, net price 28-tab pack = £119.79; 150 mg, 28-tab pack = £240.00

CYPROTERONE ACETATE

Indications prostate cancer, see under Dose and also notes above; other indications, see section 6.4.2

Cautions in prostate cancer, blood counts initially and throughout treatment; monitor hepatic function (liver function tests should be performed before treatment, see also under Side-effects below); monitor adrenocortical function regularly; risk of recurrence of thromboembolic disease; diabetes mellitus, sickle-cell anaemia, severe depression (in other indications some of these are contra-indicated, see section 6.4.2)
Driving Fatigue and lassitude may impair performance of skilled tasks (e.g. driving)

Contra-indications patients with meningioma or history of meningioma; for contra-indications relating to other indications see section 6.4.2

Hepatic impairment dose-related toxicity; see also under cautions (above) and side-effects (below)

Side-effects see section 6.4.2
Hepatotoxicity Direct hepatic toxicity including jaundice, hepatitis and hepatic failure have been reported (fatalities reported at dosages of 100 mg and above, usually in men treated for advanced prostate cancer). Liver function tests should be performed before and regularly during treatment and whenever symptoms suggestive of hepatotoxicity occur—if confirmed cyproterone should normally be withdrawn unless the hepatotoxicity can be explained by another cause such as metastatic disease (in which case cyproterone should be continued only if the perceived benefit exceeds the risk)

Dose
* Prevention of flare with initial gonadorelin analogue therapy, 200 mg daily in 2–3 divided doses for 5–7 days before initiation of gonadorelin analogue, followed by 200 mg daily in 2–3 divided doses for 3–4 weeks after initiation of gonadorelin analogue; max. 300 mg daily
* Long-term palliative therapy where gonadorelin analogues or orchidectomy contra-indicated, not tolerated, or where oral therapy preferred, 200–300 mg daily in 2–3 divided doses
* Hot flushes with gonadorelin analogue therapy or after orchidectomy, initially 50 mg daily, adjusted according to response to 50–150 mg daily in 1–3 divided doses

Cyproterone Acetate (Non-proprietary) PoM
Tablets, cyproterone acetate 50 mg, net price 56-tab pack = £29.00; 100 mg, 84-tab pack = £55.19. Label: 21, counselling, driving

Cyprostat® (Bayer) PoM
Tablets, scored, cyproterone acetate 50 mg, net price 168-tab pack = £87.00; 100 mg, 84-tab pack = £87.00. Label: 21, counselling, driving

ENZALUTAMIDE

Indications metastatic castration-resistant prostate cancer in patients whose disease has progressed during or after docetaxel therapy

Cautions history or risk of seizure (including brain injury, stroke, brain tumours, brain metastases, alcoholism, concurrent use of medication which may lower seizure threshold); recent cardiovascular disease; bradycardia; uncontrolled hypertension; concurrent chemotherapy—safety and efficacy not established; **interactions**: Appendix 1 (enzalutamide)

Hepatic impairment manufacturer advises caution in moderate impairment, avoid in severe impairment

Renal impairment caution in severe impairment—no information available

Pregnancy men should use condoms during treatment and for 3 months after stopping treatment if their partner is pregnant, and use condoms in combination with another effective contraceptive method if their partner is of child-bearing potential—toxicity in *animal* studies

Side-effects hot flush, hypertension, headache, visual hallucinations, anxiety, cognitive disorder, memory impairment, falls, neutropenia, fractures, dry skin, pruritus; *less commonly* seizure, leucopenia

Dose
* 160 mg once daily

Xtandi® (Astellas) ▼ PoM
Capsules, enzalutamide 40 mg, net price 112-cap pack = £2734.67. Label: 25

FLUTAMIDE

Indications advanced prostate cancer, see also notes above

Cautions cardiac disease (oedema reported); also liver function tests, monthly for first 4 months, periodically

Malignant disease and immunosuppression

8

thereafter and at the first sign or symptom of liver disorder (e.g. pruritus, dark urine, persistent anorexia, jaundice, abdominal pain, unexplained influenza-like symptoms); avoid excessive alcohol consumption; avoid in acute porphyria (section 9.8.2); **interactions:** Appendix 1 (flutamide)

Hepatic impairment use with caution (hepatotoxic)

Side-effects gynaecomastia (sometimes with galactorrhoea); nausea, vomiting, diarrhoea, increased appetite, insomnia, tiredness; other side-effects reported include decreased libido, reduced sperm count, gastric and chest pain, hypertension, headache, dizziness, oedema, blurred vision, thirst, rash, pruritus, haemolytic anaemia, systemic lupus erythematosus-like syndrome, and lymphoedema; hepatic injury (with transaminase abnormalities, cholestatic jaundice, hepatic necrosis, hepatic encephalopathy and occasional fatality) reported

Dose

• 250 mg 3 times daily (see also notes above)

Flutamide (Non-proprietary) ▢PoM

Tablets, flutamide 250 mg. Net price 84-tab pack = £52.72

Gonadotrophin-releasing hormone antagonists

Degarelix is a gonadotrophin-releasing hormone antagonist used to treat advanced hormone-dependent prostate cancer. It does not induce a testosterone surge or tumour 'flare', therefore anti-androgen therapy is not required.

▌ DEGARELIX

Indications see notes above

Cautions susceptibility to QT-interval prolongation (avoid concomitant use of drugs that prolong QT interval); monitor bone density; diabetes

Hepatic impairment manufacturer advises caution in severe impairment—no information available

Renal impairment manufacturer advises caution in severe impairment—no information available

Side-effects nausea; dizziness, headache, drowsiness, insomnia, asthenia; influenza-like symptoms; hot flushes, sweating (including night sweats), weight gain; injection-site reactions; *less commonly* diarrhoea, vomiting, abdominal discomfort, dry mouth, constipation, anorexia, atrio-ventricular block, QT-interval prolongation, fainting, hypertension, hypersensitivity reactions, depression, anxiety, oedema, gynaecomastia, micturition urgency, renal impairment, sexual dysfunction, pelvic pain, prostatitis, testicular pain, anaemia, musculoskeletal pain, tinnitus, urticaria, alopecia, and rash

Dose

• By subcutaneous injection into the abdominal region, ADULT over 18 years, initially 240 mg (administered as 2 injections of 120 mg), then 80 mg every 28 days

Firmagon® (Ferring) ▢PoM

Injection, powder for reconstitution, degarelix (as acetate), net price 80-mg vial (with diluent) = £129.37; 2 × 120-mg vials (with diluent) = £260.00

8.3.4.3 Somatostatin analogues

Lanreotide, **octreotide** and **pasireotide** are analogues of the hypothalamic release-inhibiting hormone somatostatin. Lanreotide and octreotide are indicated for the relief of symptoms associated with neuroendocrine (particularly carcinoid) tumours and acromegaly. Additionally, lanreotide is licensed for the treatment of thyroid tumours and octreotide is also licensed for the prevention of complications following pancreatic surgery. Octreotide long-acting depot injection is licensed for treatment of advanced neuroendocrine tumours of the midgut, or treatment where primary origin is not known but non-midgut sites of origin have been excluded. Octreotide may also be valuable in reducing vomiting in palliative care (see p. 23) and in stopping variceal bleeding [unlicensed indication]—see also vasopressin and terlipressin (section 6.5.2). Pasireotide is licensed for the treatment of Cushing's disease when surgery has failed or is inappropriate.

Cautions Growth hormone-secreting pituitary tumours can expand causing serious complications; during treatment with somatostatin analogues patients should be monitored for signs of tumour expansion (e.g. visual field defects). Ultrasound examination of the gallbladder is recommended before treatment and at intervals of 6–12 months during treatment (avoid abrupt withdrawal of short-acting octreotide—see Side-effects below). In insulinoma an increase in the depth and duration of hypoglycaemia may occur (observe patients when initiating treatment and changing doses); in diabetes mellitus, insulin or oral antidiabetic requirements may be reduced. Patients with carcinoid tumours must only receive lanreotide after excluding the presence of an obstructive intestinal tumour.

Side-effects Gastro-intestinal disturbances including anorexia, nausea, vomiting, abdominal pain and bloating, flatulence, diarrhoea, and steatorrhoea may occur (administering non-depot injections of octreotide between meals and at bedtime may reduce gastro-intestinal side-effects). Postprandial glucose tolerance may be impaired and rarely persistent hyperglycaemia occurs with chronic administration; hypoglycaemia has also been reported. Gallstones have been reported after long-term treatment (abrupt withdrawal of subcutaneous octreotide is associated with biliary colic and pancreatitis). Pain and irritation may occur at the injection site and sites should be rotated. Rarely, pancreatitis has been reported shortly after administration.

▌ LANREOTIDE

Indications see notes above

Cautions see notes above; cardiac disorders (including bradycardia); **interactions:** Appendix 1 (lanreotide)

Pregnancy manufacturer advises use only if potential benefit outweighs risk

Breast-feeding manufacturer advises caution—no information available

Side-effects see notes above; also reported constipation, dyspepsia, bradycardia, asthenia, dizziness, fatigue, raised bilirubin, biliary dilatation, alopecia; *less commonly* skin nodule, hot flushes, leg pain, malaise, headache, insomnia, tenesmus, decreased libido, drowsiness, pruritus, increased sweating; *rarely* hypothyroidism (monitor as necessary)

Dose

• See under preparations

Somatuline® LA (Ipsen) PoM

Injection (copolymer microparticles for aqueous suspension), lanreotide (as acetate) 30-mg vial (with vehicle) = £323.00

Dose by intramuscular injection, acromegaly and neuroendocrine (particularly carcinoid) tumours, initially 30 mg every 14 days, frequency increased to every 7–10 days according to response

Thyroid tumours, 30 mg every 14 days, frequency increased to every 10 days according to response

Somatuline Autogel® (Ipsen)

Injection, prefilled syringe, lanreotide (as acetate) 60 mg = £551.00; 90 mg = £736.00; 120 mg = £937.00

Dose by deep subcutaneous injection into the gluteal region, acromegaly (if somatostatin analogue not given previously), initially 60 mg every 28 days, adjusted according to response; for patients treated previously with somatostatin analogue, consult product literature for initial dose

Neuroendocrine (particularly carcinoid) tumours, initially 60–120 mg every 28 days, adjusted according to response

---

■ OCTREOTIDE

Indications see under Dose

Cautions see notes above; monitor thyroid function on long-term therapy; monitor liver function; **interactions**: Appendix 1 (octreotide)

Hepatic impairment adjustment of maintenance dose of non-depot preparations may be necessary in patients with liver cirrhosis

Pregnancy possible effect on fetal growth; manufacturer advises use only if potential benefit outweighs risk and effective contraception required during treatment

Breast-feeding manufacturer advises avoid—present in milk in *animal* studies

Side-effects see notes above; also arrhythmias, bradycardia, dyspnoea, headache, dizziness, dehydration, alopecia, rash; hepatitis also reported

Dose

• Symptoms associated with carcinoid tumours with features of carcinoid syndrome, VIPomas, glucagonomas, by subcutaneous injection, initially 50 micrograms once or twice daily, gradually increased according to response to 200 micrograms 3 times daily (higher doses required exceptionally); maintenance doses variable; in carcinoid tumours discontinue after 1 week if no effect; if rapid response required, initial dose by intravenous injection (with ECG monitoring and after dilution to a concentration of 10–50% with sodium chloride 0.9% injection)

• Acromegaly, short-term treatment before pituitary surgery *or* long-term treatment in those inadequately controlled by other treatment *or* until radiotherapy becomes fully effective by subcutaneous injection, 100–200 micrograms 3 times daily; discontinue if no improvement within 3 months

• Prevention of complications following pancreatic surgery, consult product literature

Octreotide (Non-proprietary) PoM

Injection, octreotide (as acetate) 50 micrograms/mL, net price 1-mL amp = £1.78; 100 micrograms/mL, 1-mL amp = £2.99; 200 micrograms/mL, 5-mL vial = £65.10; 500 micrograms/mL, 1-mL amp = £27.09

Sandostatin® (Novartis) PoM

Injection, octreotide (as acetate) 50 micrograms/mL, net price 1-mL amp = £2.97; 100 micrograms/mL, 1-mL amp = £5.59; 200 micrograms/mL 5-mL vial = £55.73; 500 micrograms/mL, 1-mL amp = £27.09

◀ Depot preparation

Sandostatin Lar® (Novartis) PoM

Injection (microsphere powder for aqueous suspension), octreotide (as acetate) 10-mg vial = £469.84; 20-mg vial = £776.05; 30-mg vial = £993.44 (all supplied with 2.5-mL diluent-filled syringe)

Dose acromegaly (test dose by subcutaneous injection 50–100 micrograms if subcutaneous octreotide not previously given), neuroendocrine (particularly carcinoid) tumour adequately controlled by subcutaneous octreotide, by deep intramuscular injection into gluteal muscle, initially 20 mg every 4 weeks for 3 months then adjusted according to response; max. 30 mg every 4 weeks

For acromegaly, start depot octreotide 1 day after the last dose of subcutaneous octreotide (for pituitary surgery give last dose of depot octreotide at least 3 weeks before surgery); for neuroendocrine tumours, continue subcutaneous octreotide for 2 weeks after first dose of depot octreotide

Advanced neuroendocrine tumours of the midgut, or tumours of unknown primary origin where non-midgut sites of origin have been excluded, 30 mg every 4 weeks

---

■ PASIREOTIDE

Indications see notes above

Cautions see notes above; diabetes mellitus (assess glycaemic status before treatment, weekly for the first 2–3 months of treatment, periodically thereafter, and 3 months after treatment is complete); monitor liver function before treatment and after 1, 2, 4, 8, and 12 weeks of treatment; cardiac disorders (including bradycardia); susceptibility to QT-interval prolongation (including concomitant use of drugs that prolong QT interval and electrolyte disturbances)—monitor ECG and electrolytes before treatment, after one week, and periodically thereafter; **interactions**: Appendix 1 (pasireotide)

Hepatic impairment reduce initial dose to 300 micrograms twice daily (increased if necessary after 2 months to max. 600 micrograms twice daily) in moderate impairment; avoid in severe impairment

Pregnancy avoid—toxicity in *animal* studies

Breast-feeding avoid—present in milk in *animal* studies

Side-effects see notes above; also bradycardia, QT-interval prolongation, hypotension, headache, fatigue, adrenal insufficiency, hyperglycaemia, decreased appetite, anaemia, alopecia, pruritus, myalgia, arthralgia

Dose

• By subcutaneous injection, ADULT over 18 years, initially 600 micrograms twice daily, increased if necessary after 2 months (according to response) to 900 micrograms twice daily; consider discontinuation if no response within 2 months; for dose adjustment due to side-effects, consult product literature

Signifor® (Novartis) ▼ PoM

Injection, pasireotide (as diaspartate) 300 micrograms/mL, net price 1-mL amp = £46.67; 600 micrograms/mL, 1-mL amp = £54.00; 900 micrograms/mL, 1-mL amp = £54.00

9 Nutrition and blood

9.1 Anaemias and some other blood disorders

9.1.1 Iron-deficiency anaemias
9.1.2 Drugs used in megaloblastic anaemias
9.1.3 Drugs used in hypoplastic, haemolytic, and renal anaemias
9.1.4 Drugs used in platelet disorders
9.1.5 G6PD deficiency
9.1.6 Drugs used in neutropenia
9.1.7 Drugs used to mobilise stem cells

Before initiating treatment for anaemia it is essential to determine which type is present. Iron salts may be harmful and result in iron overload if given alone to patients with anaemias other than those due to iron deficiency.

9.1.1 Iron-deficiency anaemias

9.1.1.1 Oral iron
9.1.1.2 Parenteral iron

Treatment with an iron preparation is justified only in the presence of a demonstrable iron-deficiency state. Before starting treatment, it is important to exclude any serious underlying cause of the anaemia (e.g. gastric erosion, gastro-intestinal cancer).

Prophylaxis with an iron preparation may be appropriate in malabsorption, menorrhagia, pregnancy, after subtotal or total gastrectomy, in haemodialysis patients, and in the management of low birth-weight infants such as preterm neonates.

9.1.1.1 Oral iron

Iron salts should be given by mouth unless there are good reasons for using another route.

Ferrous salts show only marginal differences between one another in efficiency of absorption of iron. Haemoglobin regeneration rate is little affected by the type of salt used provided sufficient iron is given, and in most patients the speed of response is not critical. Choice of preparation is thus usually decided by the incidence of side-effects and cost.

The oral dose of **elemental iron** for iron-deficiency anaemia should be 100 to 200 mg daily. It is customary to give this as **dried ferrous sulfate**, 200 mg ($\equiv$ 65 mg elemental iron) three times daily; for prophylaxis of iron-deficiency anaemia, a dose of ferrous sulfate 200 mg once or twice daily may be effective. For treatment of iron-deficiency anaemia in children and for prophylaxis of iron-deficiency anaemia in babies of low birth weight, see *BNF for Children*.

Iron content of different iron salts

Iron salt	Amount	Content of ferrous iron
Ferrous fumarate	200 mg	65 mg
Ferrous gluconate	300 mg	35 mg
Ferrous sulfate	300 mg	60 mg
Ferrous sulfate, dried	200 mg	65 mg

Therapeutic response The haemoglobin concentration should rise by about 100–200 mg/100 mL (1–2 g/litre) per day *or* 2 g/100 mL (20 g/litre) over 3–4 weeks. When the haemoglobin is in the reference range, treatment should be continued for a further 3 months to replenish the iron stores. Epithelial tissue changes such as atrophic glossitis and koilonychia are usually improved, but the response is often slow.

Side-effects Gastro-intestinal irritation can occur with iron salts. Nausea and epigastric pain are dose-related, but the relationship between dose and altered bowel habit (constipation or diarrhoea) is less clear. Oral iron, particularly modified-release preparations, can exacerbate diarrhoea in patients with inflammatory bowel disease; care is also needed in patients with intestinal strictures and diverticular disease.

Iron preparations taken orally can be constipating, particularly in older patients and occasionally lead to faecal impaction.

If side-effects occur, the dose may be reduced; alternatively, another iron salt may be used, but an improvement in tolerance may simply be a result of a lower content of elemental iron. The incidence of side-effects due to ferrous sulfate is no greater than with other iron salts when compared on the basis of equivalent amounts of elemental iron.

Iron preparations are a common cause of accidental overdose in children. For the treatment of **iron overdose**, see Emergency Treatment of Poisoning, p. 39.

Counselling Although iron preparations are best absorbed on an empty stomach they can be taken after food to reduce gastro-intestinal side-effects; they may discolour stools.

Compound preparations Preparations containing iron and **folic acid** are used during pregnancy in women who are at high risk of developing iron and folic acid deficiency; they should be distinguished from those used for the prevention of neural tube defects in women planning a pregnancy (see p. 665).

It is important to note that the small doses of folic acid contained in these preparations are inadequate for the treatment of megaloblastic anaemias.

Some oral preparations contain **ascorbic acid** to aid absorption of the iron but the therapeutic advantage of such preparations is minimal and cost may be increased.

There is no justification for the inclusion of other ingredients, such as the **B group of vitamins** (except folic acid for pregnant women, see notes above and on p. 665).

Modified-release preparations Modified-release preparations of iron are licensed for once-daily dosage, but have no therapeutic advantage and should not be used. These preparations are formulated to release iron gradually; the low incidence of side-effects may reflect the small amounts of iron available for absorption as the iron is carried past the first part of the duodenum into an area of the gut where absorption may be poor.

█ FERROUS SULFATE

Indications iron-deficiency anaemia

Cautions interactions: Appendix 1 (iron)

Side-effects see notes above

Dose

- See under preparations below and notes above

Ferrous Sulfate (Non-proprietary)

Tablets, coated, dried ferrous sulfate 200 mg (65 mg iron), net price 28-tab pack = £1.08

Dose prophylactic, 1 tablet daily; therapeutic, 1 tablet 2–3 times daily; CHILD, see *BNF for Children*

Ironorm® Drops (Wallace Mfg)

Oral drops, ferrous sulfate 125 mg (25 mg iron)/mL, net price 15-mL = £28.00

Dose prophylactic, 2.4–4.8 mL daily; therapeutic, 4 mL once or twice daily; CHILD see *BNF for Children*

◢ Modified-release preparations

Feospan® (Intrapharm) ᴺᴴˢ 🔲

Spansule® (= capsules m/r), clear/red, enclosing green and brown pellets, dried ferrous sulfate 150 mg (47 mg iron), net price 30-cap pack = £3.95. Label: 25

Dose 1–2 capsules daily; CHILD over 1 year, 1 capsule daily; can be opened and sprinkled on food

Ferrograd® (Teofarma) 🔲

Tablets, f/c, m/r, red, dried ferrous sulfate 325 mg (105 mg iron), net price 30-tab pack = £2.58. Label: 25

Dose ADULT and CHILD over 12 years, prophylactic and therapeutic, 1 tablet daily before food

◢ With folic acid

For prescribing information on folic acid, see section 9.1.2

Fefol® (Intrapharm) ᴺᴴˢ 🔲

Spansule® (= capsules m/r), clear/green, enclosing brown, yellow, and white pellets, dried ferrous sulfate 150 mg (47 mg iron), folic acid 500 micrograms, net price 30-cap pack = £4.25. Label: 25

Dose 1 capsule daily

Ferrograd Folic® (Teofarma) 🔲

Tablets, f/c, red/yellow, dried ferrous sulfate 325 mg (105 mg iron) for sustained release, folic acid 350 micrograms, net price 30-tab pack = £2.64. Label: 25

Dose ADULT and CHILD over 12 years, 1 tablet daily before food

9 Nutrition and blood

◢ **With ascorbic acid**

For prescribing information on ascorbic acid, see section 9.6.3

Ferrograd C® (Teofarma) ⬚S⬛

Tablets, f/c, red, dried ferrous sulfate 325 mg (105 mg iron) for sustained release, ascorbic acid 500 mg (as sodium salt), net price 30-tab pack = £3.20. Label: 25

Dose ADULT and CHILD over 12 years, 1 tablet daily before food

FERROUS FUMARATE

Indications   iron-deficiency anaemia
Cautions   interactions: Appendix 1 (iron)
Side-effects   see notes above
Dose

• See under preparations below and notes above

Fersaday® (AMCo)

Tablets, brown, f/c, ferrous fumarate 322 mg (100 mg iron), net price 28-tab pack = 95p

Dose prophylactic, 1 tablet daily; therapeutic, 1 tablet twice daily

Ferrous Fumarate (Non-proprietary)

Tablets, ferrous fumarate 210 mg (68 mg iron), net price 84 = £2.30

Dose ADULT and CHILD over 12 years, prophylactic, 1 tablet 1–2 times daily; therapeutic, 1 tablet 2–3 times daily

Syrup, ferrous fumarate approx. 140 mg (45 mg iron)/5 mL, net price 200 mL = £3.73

Dose prophylactic, 5 mL twice daily; therapeutic, 10 mL twice daily; CHILD see BNF for Children

Galfer® (Thornton & Ross)

Capsules, red/green, ferrous fumarate 305 mg (100 mg iron), net price 100 = £2.00

Dose ADULT and CHILD over 12 years, prophylactic, 1 capsule daily; therapeutic, 1 capsule twice daily

Syrup, brown, sugar-free ferrous fumarate 140 mg (45 mg iron)/5 mL, net price 300 mL = £5.33

Dose ADULT and CHILD over 12 years, prophylactic, 10 mL once daily; therapeutic, 10 mL 1–2 times daily; PRETERM NEONATE and NEONATE, see BNF for Children; CHILD 1 month–12 years, prophylactic and therapeutic, 0.5 mL/kg daily in 2–3 divided doses; max. 20 mL daily

◢ **With folic acid**

For prescribing information on folic acid, see section 9.1.2

Galfer FA® (Thornton & Ross)

Capsules, red/yellow, ferrous fumarate 305 mg (100 mg iron), folic acid 350 micrograms, net price 100 = £2.17

Dose 1 capsule daily before food

Pregaday® (RPH)

Tablets, brown, f/c, ferrous fumarate equivalent to 100 mg iron, folic acid 350 micrograms, net price 28-tab pack =£1.25

Dose 1 tablet daily

FERROUS GLUCONATE

Indications   iron-deficiency anaemia
Cautions   interactions: Appendix 1 (iron)
Side-effects   see notes above
Dose

• See under preparation below and notes above

Ferrous Gluconate (Non-proprietary)

Tablets, red, coated, ferrous gluconate 300 mg (35 mg iron), net price 28 = £1.95

Dose prophylactic, 2 tablets daily before food; therapeutic, 4–6 tablets daily in divided doses before food; CHILD 6–12 years, prophylactic and therapeutic, 1–3 tablets daily

POLYSACCHARIDE–IRON COMPLEX

Indications   iron-deficiency anaemia
Cautions   interactions: Appendix 1 (iron)
Side-effects   see notes above
Dose

• See under preparation below and notes above

Niferex® (Tillomed)

Elixir, brown, sugar-free, polysaccharide–iron complex equivalent to 100 mg of iron/5 mL, net price 240-mL pack = £6.06; ⬚S[1] 30-mL dropper bottle for paediatric use = £2.16. Counselling, use of dropper

Dose prophylactic, 2.5 mL daily; therapeutic, 5 mL 1–2 times daily (once daily if required during second and third trimester of pregnancy); PRETERM NEONATE, NEONATE, and INFANT (from dropper bottle) 1 drop (approx. 500 micrograms iron) per 450 g body-weight 3 times daily; CHILD 2–6 years 2.5 mL daily, 6–12 years 5 mL daily

SODIUM FEREDETATE

(Sodium ironedetate)

Indications   iron-deficiency anaemia
Cautions   interactions: Appendix 1 (iron)
Side-effects   see notes above
Dose

• See under preparation below and notes above

Sytron® (Forum)

Elixir, sugar-free, sodium feredetate 190 mg equivalent to 27.5 mg of iron/5 mL, net price 100 mL = £1.07

Dose therapeutic, 5 mL increasing gradually to 10 mL 3 times daily; CHILD under 1 year, see BNF for Children; CHILD 1–5 years, therapeutic, 2.5 mL 3 times daily, 6–12 years, therapeutic, 5 mL 3 times daily

9.1.1.2   Parenteral iron

Iron can be administered parenterally as **iron dextran**, **iron sucrose**, **ferric carboxymaltose**, **iron isomaltoside 1000**, or **ferumoxytol**. Parenteral iron is generally reserved for use when oral therapy is unsuccessful because the patient cannot tolerate oral iron, or does not take it reliably, or if there is continuing blood loss, or in malabsorption. Parenteral iron may also have a role in the management of chemotherapy-induced anaemia, when given with erythropoietins, in specific patient groups (see NICE guidance, p. 667).

The *Scottish Medicines Consortium* (p. 4) has advised (January 2013) that ferumoxytol (*Rienso*®) is accepted for restricted use within NHS Scotland for the treatment of iron deficiency anaemia in non-haemodialysis dependent adults with chronic kidney disease when oral iron preparations are ineffective or cannot be used.

Many patients with chronic renal failure who are receiving haemodialysis (and some who are receiving peritoneal dialysis) also require iron by the intravenous route

---

1. ⬚S except 30-mL paediatric dropper bottle for prophylaxis and treatment of iron deficiency in infants born prematurely; endorse prescription 'SLS'

on a regular basis (see also Erythropoietins, section 9.1.3).

With the exception of patients with severe renal failure receiving haemodialysis, parenteral iron does not produce a faster haemoglobin response than oral iron provided that the oral iron preparation is taken reliably and is absorbed adequately. If parenteral iron is necessary, the dose should be calculated according to the patient's body-weight and total iron deficit. Depending on the preparation used, parenteral iron is given as a total dose or in divided doses. Further treatment should be guided by monitoring haemoglobin and serum iron concentrations.

Anaphylactic reactions can occur with parenteral administration of iron complexes and facilities for cardiopulmonary resuscitation must be available—see MHRA/CHM advice, below.

> **MHRA/CHM advice**
> **Serious hypersensitivity reactions with intravenous iron (August 2013)**
> Serious hypersensitivity reactions, including life-threatening and fatal anaphylactic reactions, have been reported in patients receiving intravenous iron. These reactions can occur even when a previous administration has been tolerated (including a negative test dose). Test doses are no longer recommended and caution is needed with *every* dose of intravenous iron.
>
> Intravenous iron products should only be administered when appropriately trained staff and resuscitation facilities are immediately available; patients should be closely monitored for signs of hypersensitivity during and for at least 30 minutes after every administration. In the event of a hypersensitivity reaction, treatment should be stopped immediately and appropriate management initiated.
>
> The risk of hypersensitivity is increased in patients with known allergies, immune or inflammatory conditions, or those with a history of severe asthma, eczema, or other atopic allergy; in these patients, intravenous iron should only be used if the benefits outweigh the risks.
>
> Intravenous iron should be avoided in the first trimester of pregnancy and used in the second or third trimesters only if the benefit outweighs the potential risks for both mother and fetus.

FERRIC CARBOXYMALTOSE

A ferric carboxymaltose complex containing 5% (50 mg/mL) of iron

Indications iron-deficiency anaemia, see notes above

Cautions hypersensitivity can occur with parenteral iron and facilities for cardiopulmonary resuscitation must be available (see MHRA/CHM advice, p. 662); oral iron should not be given until 5 days after last injection; allergic disorders including asthma and eczema; infection (discontinue if ongoing bacteraemia)

Hepatic impairment use with caution; avoid in conditions where iron overload increases risk of impairment

Pregnancy avoid in first trimester; crosses the placenta in *animal* studies; may influence skeletal development

Side-effects gastro-intestinal disturbances; headache, dizziness; rash, injection-site reactions; *less commonly* hypertension, hypotension, flushing, chest pain, peripheral oedema, hypersensitivity reactions (including anaphylaxis), fatigue, paraesthesia, malaise, pyrexia, rigors, myalgia, arthralgia, back pain, pruritus, and urticaria; *rarely* dyspnoea

Dose

- By slow intravenous injection or by intravenous infusion, ADULT and CHILD over 14 years, calculated according to body-weight and iron deficit, consult product literature

Ferinject® (Vifor) ▼ PoM
Injection, iron (as ferric carboxymaltose) 50 mg/mL, net price 2-mL vial = £19.10, 10-mL vial = £95.50, 20-mL vial = £181.45
Electrolytes Na⁺ 0.24 mmol/mL

FERUMOXYTOL

A complex of iron oxide with polyglucose sorbitol-carboxymethylether containing 3% (30 mg/mL) of iron

Indications iron-deficiency anaemia in chronic renal failure, see notes above

Cautions hypersensitivity can occur with parenteral iron and facilities for cardiopulmonary resuscitation must be available (see MHRA/CHM advice, p. 662); oral iron should not be given until 5 days after last infusion; patients should recline or semi-recline during the infusion and for at least 30 minutes thereafter; allergic or immune conditions; infection (discontinue if ongoing bacteraemia)

Contra-indications history of drug allergy including hypersensitivity to other parenteral iron products

Hepatic impairment use with caution

Pregnancy avoid in first trimester; use only if benefits outweigh risks in second and third trimester—toxicity in *animal* studies

Breast-feeding avoid—present in milk in *animal* studies

Side-effects injection-site reactions; *less commonly* nausea, vomiting, constipation, diarrhoea, abdominal pain, appetite disorders, hypotension, hypertension, flushing, dyspnoea, dizziness, taste disturbances, headache, drowsiness, malaise, myalgia, arthralgia, back pain, pruritus, rash, hypersensitivity reactions (including anaphylaxis); *rarely* dry mouth, dyspepsia, epistaxis, blurred vision, paraesthesia, dehydration, hyperkalaemia, eosinophilia, gout; *also reported* arrhythmias, tachycardia, myocardial infarction, congestive heart failure, cough, bronchospasm, hypoxia, respiratory failure, syncope

Dose

- By intravenous infusion, ADULT over 18 years, calculated according to body-weight and iron deficit, consult product literature

Rienso® (Takeda) ▼ PoM
Injection, iron (as ferumoxytol) 30 mg/mL, net price 17-mL vial = £65.00

IRON DEXTRAN

A complex of ferric hydroxide with dextran containing 5% (50 mg/mL) of iron

Indications iron-deficiency anaemia, see notes above

9 Nutrition and blood

Cautions hypersensitivity can occur with parenteral iron and facilities for cardiopulmonary resuscitation must be available (see MHRA/CHM advice, p. 662); oral iron should not be given until 5 days after last injection

Contra-indications history of allergic disorders including asthma and eczema; infection; active rheumatoid arthritis

Hepatic impairment avoid in severe impairment

Renal impairment avoid in acute renal failure

Pregnancy avoid in first trimester

Side-effects *less commonly* nausea, vomiting, abdominal pain, flushing, dyspnoea, hypersensitivity reactions (including anaphylaxis), numbness, cramps, blurred vision, pruritus, and rash; *rarely* diarrhoea, chest pain, hypotension, angioedema, arrhythmias, tachycardia, dizziness, restlessness, fatigue, seizures, tremor, impaired consciousness, myalgia, arthralgia, sweating, and injection-site reactions; *very rarely* hypertension, palpitation, headache, paraesthesia, haemolysis, and transient deafness

Dose

- By deep intramuscular injection into the gluteal muscle *or* by slow intravenous injection *or* by intravenous infusion, calculated according to body-weight and iron deficit, consult product literature
  CHILD under 14 years, not recommended

CosmoFer® (Pharmacosmos) ▼ PoM
Injection, iron (as iron dextran) 50 mg/mL, net price 2-mL amp = £7.97, 10-mL amp = £39.85

IRON ISOMALTOSIDE 1000

A complex of ferric iron and isomaltosides containing 10% (100 mg/mL) of iron

Indications iron deficiency anaemia, see notes above

Cautions hypersensitivity can occur with parenteral iron and facilities for cardiopulmonary resuscitation must be available (see MHRA/CHM advice, p. 662); oral iron should not be given until 5 days after last injection; infection (discontinue if ongoing bacteraemia)

Contra-indications history of allergic disorders including asthma and eczema; active rheumatoid arthritis

Hepatic impairment avoid in decompensated liver disease and hepatitis

Pregnancy avoid in first trimester

Side-effects *less commonly* nausea, vomiting, constipation, abdominal pain, dyspnoea, dysphonia, flushing, numbness, fever, cramps, blurred vision, pruritus, rash, hypersensitivity reactions (including anaphylaxis), injection-site reactions; *rarely* diarrhoea, angioedema, tachycardia, arrhythmias, hypotension, chest pain, malaise, seizures, tremor, dizziness, restlessness, loss of consciousness, altered mental status, myalgia, arthralgia, sweating; *very rarely* hypertension, foetal bradycardia, palpitation, headache, paraesthesia, haemolysis, transient deafness

Dose

- By slow intravenous injection or by intravenous infusion, ADULT over 18 years, calculated according to body-weight and iron deficit, consult product literature

Monofer® (Pharmacosmos) ▼ PoM
Injection, iron (as iron isomaltoside 1000) 100 mg/mL, net price 1-mL vial = £16.95, 5-mL vial = £84.75, 10-mL vial = £169.50

IRON SUCROSE

A complex of ferric hydroxide with sucrose containing 2% (20 mg/mL) of iron

Indications iron-deficiency anaemia, see notes above

Cautions hypersensitivity reactions can occur with parenteral iron and facilities for cardiopulmonary resuscitation must be available (see MHRA/CHM advice, p. 662); oral iron should not be given until 5 days after last injection; infection (discontinue if ongoing bacteraemia)

Contra-indications history of allergic disorders including asthma, eczema, and anaphylaxis

Hepatic impairment use with caution; avoid in conditions where iron overload increases risk of impairment

Pregnancy avoid in first trimester

Side-effects taste disturbances; *less commonly* nausea, vomiting, abdominal pain, diarrhoea, hypotension, tachycardia, flushing, palpitation, chest pain, bronchospasm, dyspnoea, headache, dizziness, fever, myalgia, pruritus, rash, and injection-site reactions; *rarely* peripheral oedema, hypertension, hypersensitivity reactions (including anaphylaxis), fatigue, asthenia, and paraesthesia; bradycardia, confusion, arthralgia, and increased sweating also reported

Dose

- By slow intravenous injection *or* by intravenous infusion, calculated according to body-weight and iron deficit, consult product literature; CHILD not recommended but see *BNF for Children*

Venofer® (Vifor) ▼ PoM
Injection, iron (as iron sucrose) 20 mg/mL, net price 5-mL vial = £10.24

9.1.2 Drugs used in megaloblastic anaemias

Most megaloblastic anaemias result from a lack of either vitamin B_{12} or folate, and it is essential to establish in every case which deficiency is present and the underlying cause. In emergencies, when delay might be dangerous, it is sometimes necessary to administer both substances after the bone marrow test while plasma assay results are awaited. Normally, however, appropriate treatment should not be instituted until the results of tests are available.

One cause of megaloblastic anaemia in the UK is *pernicious anaemia* in which lack of gastric intrinsic factor resulting from an autoimmune gastritis causes malabsorption of vitamin B_{12}.

Vitamin B_{12} is also needed in the treatment of megaloblastosis caused by *prolonged nitrous oxide anaesthesia*, which inactivates the vitamin, and in the rare syndrome of *congenital transcobalamin II deficiency*.

Vitamin B_{12} should be given prophylactically after *total gastrectomy* or *total ileal resection* (or after *partial gastrectomy* if a vitamin B_{12} absorption test shows vitamin B_{12} malabsorption).

Nutrition and blood

9

Apart from dietary deficiency, all other causes of vitamin B_{12} deficiency are attributable to malabsorption. There is little place for the use of low-dose vitamin B_{12} orally and none for vitamin B_{12} intrinsic factor complexes given by mouth. Vitamin B_{12} in larger oral doses of 1–2 mg daily [unlicensed] may be effective.

Hydroxocobalamin has completely replaced cyanocobalamin as the form of vitamin B_{12} of choice for therapy; it is retained in the body longer than cyanocobalamin and thus for maintenance therapy can be given at intervals of up to 3 months. Treatment is generally initiated with frequent administration of intramuscular injections to replenish the depleted body stores. Thereafter, maintenance treatment, which is usually for life, can be instituted. There is no evidence that doses larger than those recommended provide any additional benefit in vitamin B_{12} neuropathy.

Folic acid has few indications for long-term therapy since most causes of folate deficiency are self-limiting or will yield to a short course of treatment. It should not be used in undiagnosed megaloblastic anaemia unless vitamin B_{12} is administered concurrently otherwise neuropathy may be precipitated (see above).

In *folate-deficient megaloblastic anaemia* (e.g. because of poor nutrition, pregnancy, or antiepileptic drugs), daily folic acid supplementation for 4 months brings about haematological remission and replenishes body stores.

For prophylaxis in *chronic haemolytic states, malabsorption,* or *in renal dialysis,* folic acid is given daily or sometimes weekly, depending on the diet and the rate of haemolysis.

For *prophylaxis in pregnancy,* see Prevention of Neural Tube Defects below.

Folic acid is also used for the prevention of methotrexate-induced side-effects in severe Crohn's disease (see section 1.5.3, p. 66), rheumatic disease (see section 10.1.3, p. 730), and severe psoriasis (see section 13.5.3, p. 816).

Folinic acid is also effective in the treatment of folate-deficient megaloblastic anaemia but it is generally used in association with cytotoxic drugs (see section 8.1); it is given as calcium folinate.

Prevention of neural tube defects   Folic acid supplements taken before and during pregnancy can reduce the occurrence of neural tube defects. The risk of a neural tube defect occurring in a child should be assessed and folic acid given as follows:

> Women at a low risk of conceiving a child with a neural tube defect should be advised to take folic acid as a medicinal or food supplement at a dose of 400 micrograms daily before conception and until week 12 of pregnancy. Women who have not been taking folic acid and who suspect they are pregnant should start at once and continue until week 12 of pregnancy.
>
> Couples are at a high risk of conceiving a child with a neural tube defect if either partner has a neural tube defect (or either partner has a family history of neural tube defects), if they have had a previous pregnancy affected by a neural tube defect, or if the woman has coeliac disease (or other malabsorption state), diabetes mellitus, sickle-cell anaemia, or is taking antiepileptic medicines (see also section 4.8.1).

> Women in the high-risk group who wish to become pregnant (or who are at risk of becoming pregnant) should be advised to take folic acid 5 mg daily and continue until week 12 of pregnancy (women with sickle-cell disease should continue taking their normal dose of folic acid 5 mg daily (or to increase the dose to 5 mg daily) and continue this throughout pregnancy).

> There is **no** justification for prescribing multiple-ingredient vitamin preparations containing vitamin B_{12} or folic acid.

▌HYDROXOCOBALAMIN

Indications   see under dose below; cyanide poisoning (see Emergency Treatment of Poisoning, p. 41)

Cautions   should not be given before diagnosis fully established but see also notes above; **interactions:** Appendix 1 (hydroxocobalamin)

Breast-feeding   present in milk but not known to be harmful

Side-effects   nausea, headache, dizziness; fever, hypersensitivity reactions (including rash and pruritus); injection-site reactions; hypokalaemia and thrombocytosis during initial treatment; chromaturia

Dose
- By intramuscular injection, pernicious anaemia and other macrocytic anaemias without neurological involvement, initially 1 mg 3 times a week for 2 weeks then 1 mg every 3 months

 Pernicious anaemia and other macrocytic anaemias with neurological involvement, initially 1 mg on alternate days until no further improvement, then 1 mg every 2 months

 Prophylaxis of macrocytic anaemias associated with vitamin B_{12} deficiency, 1 mg every 2–3 months

 Tobacco amblyopia and Leber's optic atrophy, initially 1 mg daily for 2 weeks, then 1 mg twice weekly until no further improvement, thereafter 1 mg every 1–3 months

 CHILD see *BNF for Children*

Hydroxocobalamin (Non-proprietary) ⒫ⓞⓜ
Injection, hydroxocobalamin 1 mg/mL. Net price 1-mL amp = £2.11
Note The BP directs that when vitamin B_{12} injection is prescribed or demanded hydroxocobalamin injection shall be dispensed or supplied
Brands include *Cobalin-H*® ⒣ⓢ, *Neo-Cytamen*® ⒣ⓢ

▌CYANOCOBALAMIN ◢

Indications   see notes above

Dose
- By mouth, vitamin B_{12} deficiency of dietary origin, 50–150 micrograms daily taken between meals; CHILD 50–105 micrograms daily in 1–3 divided doses
- By intramuscular injection, initially 1 mg repeated 10 times at intervals of 2–3 days, maintenance 1 mg every month, but see notes above

Cyanocobalamin (Non-proprietary) ◢
Tablets, cyanocobalamin 50 micrograms. Net price 50-tab pack = £6.24
Brands include *Cytacon*® ⒣ⓢ
Note Currently marketed brands may not be suitable for vegans

Liquid (JHS), cyanocobalamin 35 micrograms/5 mL. Net price 200 mL = £2.77
Brands include *Cytacon*® (JHS)

Injection (PoM), cyanocobalamin 1 mg/mL. Net price 1-mL amp = £2.90
Brands include *Cytamen*® (JHS)

Note The BP directs that when vitamin B_{12} injection is prescribed or demanded hydroxocobalamin injection shall be dispensed or supplied

▌ FOLIC ACID

Indications   see notes above and under dose
Cautions   should never be given alone for pernicious anaemia and other vitamin B_{12} deficiency states (may precipitate subacute combined degeneration of the spinal cord); **interactions:** Appendix 1 (folates)
Side-effects   *rarely* gastro-intestinal disturbances
Dose

- Folate-deficient megaloblastic anaemia, *by mouth*, ADULT and CHILD over 1 year, 5 mg daily for 4 months (until term in pregnant women); up to 15 mg daily may be required in malabsorption states; CHILD under 1 year, 500 micrograms/kg daily (max. 5 mg) for up to 4 months; up to 10 mg daily may be required in mal-absorption states
- Prevention of neural tube defects, *by mouth*, see notes above
- Prevention of methotrexate-induced side-effects in severe Crohn's disease [unlicensed], *by mouth*, see section 1.5.3
- Prevention of methotrexate-induced side-effects in rheumatic disease [unlicensed], *by mouth*, ADULT over 18 years 5 mg once weekly; CHILD 2–18 years see *BNF for Children*
- Prevention of methotrexate-induced side-effects in severe psoriasis [unlicensed], *by mouth*, see section 13.5.3
- Prophylaxis in chronic haemolytic states, *by mouth*, ADULT 5 mg every 1–7 days depending on underlying disease
- Prophylaxis of folate deficiency in dialysis, *by mouth*, ADULT 5 mg every 1–7 days; CHILD 1–12 years 250 micrograms/kg (max. 10 mg) once daily, CHILD 12–18 years 5–10 mg once daily

[1]**Folic Acid** (Non-proprietary) (PoM)
Tablets, folic acid 400 micrograms, net price 90-tab pack = £2.71; 5 mg, 28-tab pack = 99p
Syrup, folic acid 2.5 mg/5 mL, net price 150 mL = £9.16
Brands include *Lexpec*® (sugar-free)
Injection, folic acid 15 mg, net price 1-mL amp = £1.34
Available from 'special-order' manufacturers or specialist importing companies, see p. 1124

▌ 9.1.3 Drugs used in hypoplastic, haemolytic, and renal anaemias

Anabolic steroids (section 6.4.3), pyridoxine, anti-lymphocyte immunoglobulin, and various corticosteroids are used in hypoplastic and haemolytic anaemias.

Antilymphocyte immunoglobulin given intravenously through a central line over 12–18 hours each day for 5

1. Can be sold to the public provided daily doses do not exceed 500 micrograms

days produces a response in about 50% of cases of acquired *aplastic anaemia*; the response rate may be increased when ciclosporin is given as well. Severe reactions are common in the first 2 days and profound immunosuppression can occur; antilymphocyte immunoglobulin should be given under specialist supervision with appropriate resuscitation facilities. Alternatively, oxymetholone tablets (available from 'special-order' manufacturers or specialist importing companies, see p. 1124) can be used in aplastic anaemia at a dose of 1–5 mg/kg daily for 3 to 6 months.

It is unlikely that dietary deprivation of **pyridoxine** (section 9.6.2) produces clinically relevant haematological effects. However, certain forms of *sideroblastic anaemia* respond to pharmacological doses, possibly reflecting its role as a co-enzyme during haemoglobin synthesis. Pyridoxine is indicated in both *idiopathic acquired* and *hereditary sideroblastic anaemias*. Although complete cures have not been reported, some increase in haemoglobin can occur; the dose required is usually high, up to 400 mg daily. *Reversible sideroblastic anaemias* respond to treatment of the underlying cause but in pregnancy, haemolytic anaemias, and alcohol dependence, or during isoniazid treatment, pyridoxine is also indicated.

Corticosteroids (see section 6.3) have an important place in the management of a wide variety of haematological disorders. They include conditions with an immune basis such as *autoimmune haemolytic anaemia*, *immune thrombocytopenias* and *neutropenias*, and *major transfusion reactions*. They are also used in chemotherapy schedules for many types of *lymphoma*, *lymphoid leukaemias*, and *paraproteinaemias*, including *multiple myeloma*.

Erythropoietins

Epoetins (recombinant human erythropoietins) are used to treat symptomatic anaemia associated with erythropoietin deficiency in chronic renal failure, to increase the yield of autologous blood in normal individuals and to shorten the period of symptomatic anaemia in patients receiving cytotoxic chemotherapy. Epoetin beta is also used for the prevention of anaemia in preterm neonates of low birth-weight; only unpreserved formulations should be used in neonates because other preparations may contain benzyl alcohol (see Excipients, p. 2).

Darbepoetin is a hyperglycosylated derivative of epoetin; it has a longer half-life and can be administered less frequently than epoetin.

Methoxy polyethylene glycol-epoetin beta is a continuous erythropoietin receptor activator that is licensed for the treatment of symptomatic anaemia associated with chronic kidney disease. It has a longer duration of action than epoetin.

Other factors, such as iron or folate deficiency, that contribute to the anaemia of chronic renal failure should be corrected before treatment and monitored during therapy. Supplemental iron may improve the response in resistant patients. Aluminium toxicity, concurrent infection, or other inflammatory disease can impair the response to erythropoietin.

9 Nutrition and blood

MHRA/CHM advice (December 2007) Erythropoietins—haemoglobin concentration

Overcorrection of haemoglobin concentration in patients with chronic kidney disease may increase the risk of death and serious cardiovascular events, and in patients with cancer may increase the risk of thrombosis and related complications:

- patients should not be treated with erythropoietins for the licensed indications in chronic kidney disease or cancer in patients receiving chemotherapy *unless* symptoms of anaemia are present;
- the haemoglobin concentration should be maintained within the range 10–12 g/100 mL;
- haemoglobin concentrations higher than 12 g/100 mL should be avoided;
- the aim of treatment is to relieve symptoms of anaemia, and in patients with chronic kidney disease to avoid the need for blood transfusion; the haemoglobin concentration should not be increased beyond that which provides adequate control of symptoms of anaemia (in some patients, this may be achieved at concentrations lower than the recommended range).

See also MHRA/CHM advice below.

MHRA/CHM advice (December 2007 and July 2008) Erythropoietins—tumour progression and survival in patients with cancer

Clinical trial data show an unexplained excess mortality and increased risk of tumour progression in patients with anaemia associated with cancer who have been treated with erythropoietins. Many of these trials used erythropoietins *outside* of the licensed indications (i.e. overcorrected haemoglobin concentration or given to patients who have *not* received chemotherapy):

- erythropoietins licensed for the treatment of *symptomatic* anaemia associated with cancer, are licensed only for patients who are receiving chemotherapy;
- the decision to use erythropoietins should be based on an assessment of the benefits and risks for individual patients; blood transfusion may be the preferred treatment for anaemia associated with cancer chemotherapy, particularly in those with a good cancer prognosis.

See also MHRA/CHM advice above.

Pure red cell aplasia

There have been very rare reports of pure red cell aplasia in patients treated with erythropoietins. In patients who develop a lack of efficacy with erythropoietin therapy and with a diagnosis of pure red cell aplasia, treatment with erythropoietins must be discontinued and testing for erythropoietin antibodies considered. Patients who develop pure red cell aplasia should **not** be switched to another form of erythropoietin.

NICE guidance
Erythropoiesis-stimulating agents (epoetin and darbepoetin) for treating anaemia in people with cancer having chemotherapy (November 2014)

Erythropoiesis-stimulating agents (epoetin alfa, beta, theta and zeta, and darbepoetin alfa) are recommended, within their marketing authorisations, as options for treating anaemia in people with cancer who are having chemotherapy.

If different erythropoiesis-stimulating agents are equally suitable, the product with the lowest acquisition cost for the course of treatment should be used. www.nice.org.uk/TA323

◾ DARBEPOETIN ALFA

Indications   see under Dose below

Cautions   see Epoetin

Contra-indications   see Epoetin

Hepatic impairment   manufacturer advises caution

Pregnancy   no evidence of harm in *animal* studies—manufacturer advises caution

Breast-feeding   manufacturer advises avoid—no information available

Side-effects   see Epoetin; also, oedema, injection-site pain; isolated reports of pure red cell aplasia, particularly following subcutaneous administration in patients with chronic renal failure (discontinue therapy)—see also notes above

Dose

- Symptomatic anaemia associated with chronic renal failure in patients on dialysis (see also MHRA/CHM advice, above), ADULT and CHILD over 11 years, by subcutaneous *or* intravenous injection, initially 450 nanograms/kg once weekly, adjusted according to response by approx. 25% at intervals of at least 4 weeks; maintenance dose, given once weekly *or* once every 2 weeks

- Symptomatic anaemia associated with chronic renal failure in patients not on dialysis (see also MHRA/CHM advice, above), ADULT and CHILD over 11 years, by subcutaneous *or* intravenous injection, initially 450 nanograms/kg once weekly *or* by subcutaneous injection, initially 750 nanograms/kg once every 2 weeks; adjusted according to response by approx. 25% at intervals of at least 4 weeks; maintenance dose, given subcutaneously or intravenously once weekly *or* subcutaneously once every 2 weeks *or* subcutaneously once every month

Note Subcutaneous route preferred in patients not on haemodialysis. Reduce dose by approximately 25% if rise in haemoglobin concentration exceeds 2 g/100 mL over 4 weeks or if haemoglobin concentration exceeds 12 g/100 mL; if haemoglobin concentration continues to rise, despite dose reduction, suspend treatment until haemoglobin concentration decreases and then restart at a dose approximately 25% lower than the previous dose. When changing route give same dose then adjust according to weekly or fortnightly haemoglobin measurements. Adjust doses not more frequently than every 2 weeks during maintenance treatment

- Symptomatic anaemia in adults with non-myeloid malignancies receiving chemotherapy (see also MHRA/CHM advice, above), by subcutaneous injection, initially 6.75 micrograms/kg once every 3 weeks *or* 2.25 micrograms/kg once weekly (if response inadequate after 9 weeks further treatment may not be effective); if adequate response obtained, reduce dose by 25–50%

Note Reduce dose by approximately 25–50% if rise in haemoglobin concentration exceeds 2 g/100 mL over 4 weeks or if haemoglobin concentration exceeds 12 g/100 mL; if haemoglobin concentration continues to rise, despite dose reduction, suspend treatment until haemoglobin concentration decreases and restart at a dose approximately 25% lower than the previous dose. Discontinue approximately 4 weeks after ending chemotherapy

Aranesp® (Amgen) PoM

Injection, prefilled syringe, darbepoetin alfa, 25 micrograms/mL, net price 0.4 mL (10 micrograms) = £14.68; 40 micrograms/mL, 0.375 mL (15 micrograms) = £22.02, 0.5 mL (20 micrograms) = £29.36; 100 micrograms/mL, 0.3 mL (30 micrograms) = £44.04, 0.4 mL (40 micrograms) = £58.73, 0.5 mL (50 micrograms) = £73.41; 200 micrograms/mL, 0.3 mL (60 micrograms) = £88.09, 0.4 mL (80 micrograms) = £117.45, 0.5 mL (100 micrograms) = £146.81, 0.65 mL (130 micrograms) = £190.86; 500 micrograms/mL, 0.3 mL (150 micrograms) = £220.22, 0.6 mL (300 micrograms) = £440.43, 1 mL (500 micrograms) = £734.05

Injection (*Aranesp®SureClick*), prefilled disposable injection device, darbepoetin alfa, 40 micrograms/mL, net price 0.5 mL (20 micrograms) = £29.36; 100 micrograms/mL, 0.4 mL (40 micrograms) = £58.72; 200 micrograms/mL, 0.3 mL (60 micrograms) = £88.09, 0.4 mL (80 micrograms) = £117.45, 0.5 mL (100 micrograms) = £146.81; 500 micrograms/mL, 0.3 mL (150 micrograms) = £220.22, 0.6 mL (300 micrograms) = £440.43, 1 mL (500 micrograms) = £734.05

EPOETIN ALFA, BETA, THETA, and ZETA
(Recombinant human erythropoietins)

Note The prescriber must specify which epoetin is required, see also Biosimilar medicines, p. 1

Indications see under preparations, below

Cautions see notes above; also inadequately treated or poorly controlled blood pressure (monitor closely blood pressure, reticulocyte counts, haemoglobin, and electrolytes), interrupt treatment if blood pressure uncontrolled; sudden stabbing migraine-like pain is warning of a hypertensive crisis; sickle-cell disease (lower target haemoglobin concentration may be appropriate); ischaemic vascular disease; thrombocytosis (monitor platelet count for first 8 weeks); epilepsy; malignant disease; increase in unfractionated or low molecular weight heparin dose may be needed during dialysis; risk of thrombosis may be increased when used for anaemia in adults receiving cancer chemotherapy; risk of thrombosis may be increased when used for anaemia before orthopaedic surgery—avoid in cardiovascular disease including recent myocardial infarction or cerebrovascular accident

Contra-indications pure red cell aplasia following erythropoietin therapy (see also notes above); uncontrolled hypertension; patients unable to receive thromboprophylaxis; avoid injections containing benzyl alcohol in neonates (see under preparations, below)

Hepatic impairment manufacturers advise caution in chronic hepatic failure

Pregnancy no evidence of harm; benefits probably outweigh risk of anaemia and of transfusion in pregnancy

Breast-feeding unlikely to be present in milk; minimal effect on infant

Side-effects diarrhoea, nausea, vomiting; dose-dependent increase in blood pressure or aggravation of hypertension; in isolated patients with normal or low blood pressure, hypertensive crisis with encephalopathy-like symptoms and generalised tonic-clonic seizures requiring immediate medical attention; headache; dose-dependent increase in platelet count (but thrombocytosis rare) regressing during treatment; influenza-like symptoms (may be reduced if intravenous injection given over 5 minutes); cardiovascular events; shunt thrombosis especially if tendency to hypotension or arteriovenous shunt complications; *very rarely* sudden loss of efficacy because of pure red cell aplasia, particularly following subcutaneous administration in patients with chronic renal failure (discontinue erythropoietin therapy)—see also notes above, hyperkalaemia, hypersensitivity reactions (including anaphylaxis and angioedema), skin reactions, injection-site reactions, and peripheral oedema also reported

Dose
• See under preparations, below

◀ Epoetin alfa

Binocrit® (Sandoz) PoM

Injection, prefilled syringe, epoetin alfa, net price 1000 units = £4.33; 2000 units = £8.65; 3000 units = £12.98; 4000 units = £17.31; 5000 units = £21.64; 6000 units = £25.96; 8000 units = £40.73; 10 000 units = £43.27

Note Biosimilar medicine, p. 1

Dose symptomatic anaemia associated with chronic renal failure in patients on haemodialysis (see also MHRA/CHM advice, p. 667), by intravenous injection over 1–5 minutes, initially 50 units/kg 3 times weekly adjusted according to response in steps of 25 units/kg 3 times weekly at intervals of at least 4 weeks; maintenance dose, usually 25–100 units/kg 3 times weekly; CHILD by intravenous injection initially as for adults; maintenance dose, body-weight under 10 kg usually 75–150 units/kg 3 times weekly, body-weight 10–30 kg usually 60–150 units/kg 3 times weekly, body-weight over 30 kg usually 30–100 units/kg 3 times weekly

Symptomatic anaemia associated with chronic renal failure in adults on peritoneal dialysis (see also MHRA/CHM advice, p. 667), by intravenous injection over 1–5 minutes, initially 50 units/kg twice weekly; maintenance dose 25–50 units/kg twice weekly

Severe symptomatic anaemia of renal origin in adults with renal insufficiency not yet on dialysis (see also MHRA/CHM advice, p. 667), by intravenous injection over 1–5 minutes, initially 50 units/kg 3 times weekly increased according to response in steps of 25 units/kg 3 times weekly at intervals of at least 4 weeks; maintenance dose 17–33 units/kg 3 times weekly; max. 200 units/kg 3 times weekly

Note Reduce dose by approximately 25% if rise in haemoglobin concentration exceeds 2 g/100 mL over 4 weeks or if haemoglobin concentration exceeds 12 g/100 mL; if haemoglobin concentration continues to rise, despite dose reduction, suspend treatment until haemoglobin concentration decreases and then restart at a dose approximately 25% lower than the previous dose.

Symptomatic anaemia in adults receiving cancer chemotherapy (see also MHRA/CHM advice, p. 667), by subcutaneous injection (max. 1 mL per injection site), initially 150 units/kg 3 times weekly (or 450 units/kg once weekly), increased if appropriate rise in haemoglobin (or reticulocyte count) not achieved after 4 weeks to

300 units/kg 3 times weekly; discontinue if inadequate response after 4 weeks at higher dose

Note Reduce dose by approximately 25–50% if rise in haemoglobin concentration exceeds 2 g/100 mL over 4 weeks or if haemoglobin concentration exceeds 12 g/100 mL; if haemoglobin concentration continues to rise, despite dose reduction, suspend treatment until haemoglobin concentration decreases and then restart at a dose approximately 25% lower than the previous dose. Discontinue approximately 4 weeks after ending chemotherapy

To increase yield of autologous blood (to avoid homologous blood) in predonation programme in moderate anaemia *either* when large volume of blood required *or* when sufficient blood cannot be saved for elective major surgery, by intravenous injection over 1–5 minutes, 600 units/kg twice weekly for 3 weeks before surgery; consult product literature for details and advice on ensuring high iron stores

Moderate anaemia (haemoglobin concentration 10–13 g/100 mL) before elective orthopaedic surgery in adults with expected moderate blood loss to reduce exposure to allogeneic blood transfusion or if autologous transfusion unavailable, by subcutaneous injection (max. 1 mL per injection site), 600 units/kg every week for 3 weeks before surgery and on day of surgery *or* 300 units/kg daily for 15 days starting 10 days before surgery; consult product literature for details

Eprex® (Janssen) (PoM)

Injection, prefilled syringe, epoetin alfa, net price 1000 units = £5.53; 2000 units = £11.06; 3000 units = £16.59; 4000 units = £22.12; 5000 units = £27.65; 6000 units = £33.19; 8000 units = £44.25; 10 000 units = £55.31; 20 000 units = £110.62; 30 000 units = £199.11; 40 000 units = £265.48. An auto-injector device is available for use with pre-filled syringes

Dose symptomatic anaemia associated with chronic renal failure in patients on chronic haemodialysis (see also MHRA/CHM advice, p. 667), by intravenous injection over 1–5 minutes *or* by subcutaneous injection (max. 1 mL per injection site), initially 50 units/kg 3 times weekly adjusted according to response in steps of 25 units/kg 3 times weekly at intervals of at least 4 weeks; maintenance dose, usually a total of 75–300 units/kg weekly (as a single dose or in divided doses); CHILD by intravenous injection initially as for adults; maintenance dose, body-weight under 10 kg usually 75–150 units/kg 3 times weekly, body-weight 10–30 kg usually 60–150 units/kg 3 times weekly, body-weight over 30 kg usually 30–100 units/kg 3 times weekly

Symptomatic anaemia associated with chronic renal failure in adults on peritoneal dialysis (see also MHRA/CHM advice, p. 667), by intravenous injection over 1–5 minutes *or* by subcutaneous injection (max. 1 mL per injection site), initially 50 units/kg twice weekly; maintenance dose 25–50 units/kg twice weekly

Severe symptomatic anaemia of renal origin in adults with renal insufficiency not yet on dialysis (see also MHRA/CHM advice, p. 667), by intravenous injection over 1–5 minutes *or* by subcutaneous injection (max. 1 mL per injection site), initially 50 units/kg 3 times weekly increased according to response in steps of 25 units/kg 3 times weekly at intervals of at least 4 weeks; maintenance dose 17–33 units/kg 3 times weekly; max. 200 units/kg 3 times weekly

Note Intravenous route preferred; reduce dose by approximately 25% if rise in haemoglobin concentration exceeds 2 g/100 mL over 4 weeks or if haemoglobin concentration exceeds 12 g/100 mL; if haemoglobin concentration continues to rise, despite dose reduction, suspend treatment until haemoglobin concentration decreases and then restart at a dose approximately 25% lower than the previous dose.

Symptomatic anaemia in adults receiving cancer chemotherapy (see also MHRA/CHM advice, p. 667), by subcutaneous injection (max. 1 mL per injection site), initially 150 units/kg 3 times weekly (*or* 450 units/kg once weekly), increased if appropriate rise in haemoglobin (or reticulocyte count) not achieved after 4 weeks to

300 units/kg 3 times weekly; discontinue if inadequate response after 4 weeks at higher dose

Note Reduce dose by approximately 25–50% if rise in haemoglobin concentration exceeds 2 g/100 mL over 4 weeks or if haemoglobin concentration exceeds 12 g/100 mL; if haemoglobin concentration continues to rise, despite dose reduction, suspend treatment until haemoglobin concentration decreases and then restart at a dose approximately 25% lower than the previous dose. Discontinue approximately 4 weeks after ending chemotherapy

To increase yield of autologous blood (to avoid homologous blood) in predonation programme in moderate anaemia *either* when large volume of blood required *or* when sufficient blood cannot be saved for elective major surgery, by intravenous injection over 1–5 minutes, 600 units/kg twice weekly for 3 weeks before surgery; consult product literature for details and advice on ensuring high iron stores

Moderate anaemia (haemoglobin concentration 10–13 g/100 mL) before elective orthopaedic surgery in adults with expected moderate blood loss to reduce exposure to allogeneic blood transfusion or if autologous transfusion unavailable, by subcutaneous injection (max. 1 mL per injection site), 600 units/kg every week for 3 weeks before surgery and on day of surgery *or* 300 units/kg daily for 15 days starting 10 days before surgery; consult product literature for details

◀**Epoetin beta**

NeoRecormon® (Roche) (PoM)

Injection, prefilled syringe, epoetin beta, net price 500 units = £3.51; 2000 units = £14.03; 3000 units = £21.04; 4000 units = £28.06; 5000 units = £35.07; 6000 units = £42.08; 10 000 units = £70.14; 20 000 units = £140.29; 30 000 units = £210.43

Excipients include phenylalanine up to 300 micrograms/syringe (section 9.4.1)

Dose symptomatic anaemia associated with chronic renal failure (see also MHRA/CHM advice, p. 667), by subcutaneous injection, ADULT and CHILD, initially 20 units/kg 3 times weekly for 4 weeks, increased according to response at intervals of 4 weeks in steps of 20 units/kg 3 times weekly; total weekly dose may be divided into daily doses; maintenance dose, initially reduce dose by half then adjust according to response at intervals of 1–2 weeks; total weekly maintenance dose may be given as a single dose or in 3 or 7 divided doses; max. 720 units/kg weekly

By intravenous injection over 2 minutes, ADULT and CHILD, initially 40 units/kg 3 times weekly for 4 weeks, increased according to response to 80 units/kg 3 times weekly after 4 weeks, with further increases if needed at intervals of 4 weeks in steps of 20 units/kg 3 times weekly; maintenance dose, initially reduce dose by half then adjust according to response at intervals of 1–2 weeks; max. 720 units/kg weekly

Note Subcutaneous route preferred in patients not on haemodialysis. Reduce dose by approximately 25% if rise in haemoglobin concentration exceeds 2 g/100 mL over 4 weeks or if haemoglobin concentration approaches or exceeds 12 g/100 mL; if haemoglobin concentration continues to rise, despite dose reduction, suspend treatment until haemoglobin concentration decreases and then restart at a dose approximately 25% lower than the previous dose

Prevention of anaemia of prematurity in neonates with birth-weight of 0.75–1.5 kg and corrected gestational age of less than 34 weeks, by subcutaneous injection, 250 units/kg 3 times weekly preferably starting within 3 days of birth and continued for 6 weeks

Symptomatic anaemia in adults with non-myeloid malignancies receiving chemotherapy (see also MHRA/CHM advice, p. 667), by subcutaneous injection, initially 450 units/kg weekly (as a single dose or in 3–7 divided doses), increased if necessary after 4 weeks (if a rise in haemoglobin of at least 1 g/100 mL not achieved) to 900 units/kg weekly (as a single dose or in 3–7 divided doses); if adequate response obtained reduce dose by 25–50%; max. 60 000 units weekly

Note Discontinue treatment if haemoglobin concentration does not increase by at least 1 g/100 mL after 8 weeks of

9

Nutrition and blood

therapy (response unlikely). Reduce dose by approximately 25–50% if rise in haemoglobin concentration exceeds 2 g/100 mL over 4 weeks or if haemoglobin concentration exceeds 12 g/100 mL; if haemoglobin concentration continues to rise, despite dose reduction, suspend treatment until haemoglobin concentration decreases and then restart at a dose approximately 25% lower than the previous dose. Discontinue approximately 4 weeks after ending chemotherapy

To increase yield of autologous blood (to avoid homologous blood) in predonation programme in moderate anaemia when blood-conserving procedures are insufficient or unavailable, consult product literature

Multidose injection, powder for reconstitution, epoetin beta, net price 50 000-unit vial = £374.48 (with solvent)

Excipients include phenylalanine up to 5 mg/vial (section 9.4.1), benzyl alcohol (avoid in neonates, see Excipients p. 2)

Note Avoid contact of reconstituted injection with glass; use only plastic materials

Dose symptomatic anaemia associated with chronic renal failure (see also MHRA/CHM advice, p. 667), by subcutaneous injection, ADULT and CHILD over 3 years, initially 20 units/kg 3 times weekly for 4 weeks, increased according to response at intervals of 4 weeks in steps of 20 units/kg 3 times weekly; total weekly dose may be divided into daily doses; maintenance dose, initially reduce dose by half then adjust according to response at intervals of 1–2 weeks; total weekly maintenance dose may be given as a single dose or in 3 or 7 divided doses; max. 720 units/kg weekly

By intravenous injection over 2 minutes, ADULT and CHILD over 3 years, initially 40 units/kg 3 times weekly for 4 weeks, increased according to response to 80 units/kg 3 times weekly after 4 weeks, with further increases if needed at intervals of 4 weeks in steps of 20 units/kg 3 times weekly; maintenance dose, initially reduce dose by half then adjust according to response at intervals of 1–2 weeks; max. 720 units/kg weekly

Note Subcutaneous route preferred in patients not on haemodialysis. Reduce dose by approximately 25% if rise in haemoglobin concentration exceeds 2 g/100 mL over 4 weeks or if haemoglobin concentration approaches or exceeds 12 g/100 mL; if haemoglobin concentration continues to rise, despite dose reduction, suspend treatment until haemoglobin concentration decreases and then restart at a dose approximately 25% lower than the previous dose

Symptomatic anaemia in adults with non-myeloid malignancies receiving chemotherapy (see also MHRA/CHM advice, p. 667), by subcutaneous injection, initially 450 units/kg weekly (as a single dose or in 3–7 divided doses), increased if necessary after 4 weeks (if a rise in haemoglobin of at least 1 g/100 mL not achieved) to 900 units/kg weekly (as a single dose or in 3–7 divided doses); if adequate response obtained reduce dose by 25–50%; max. 60 000 units weekly

Note Discontinue treatment if haemoglobin concentration does not increase by at least 1 g/100 mL after 8 weeks of therapy (response unlikely). Reduce dose by approximately 25–50% if rise in haemoglobin concentration exceeds 2 g/100 mL over 4 weeks or if haemoglobin concentration exceeds 12 g/100 mL; if haemoglobin concentration continues to rise, despite dose reduction, suspend treatment until haemoglobin concentration decreases and then restart at a dose approximately 25% lower than the previous dose. Discontinue approximately 4 weeks after ending chemotherapy

To increase yield of autologous blood (to avoid homologous blood) in predonation programme in moderate anaemia when blood-conserving procedures are insufficient or unavailable, consult product literature

◢ Epoetin theta

Eporatio® (Ratiopharm UK) ▼ [PoM]
Injection, prefilled syringe, epoetin theta, net price 1000 units = £5.99; 2000 units = £11.98; 3000 units = £17.98; 4000 units = £23.97; 5000 units = £29.96; 10 000 units = £59.92; 20 000 units = £119.84; 30 000 units = £179.75

Note If epoetin theta is substituted for another epoetin the same route of administration should be used

Dose symptomatic anaemia associated with chronic renal failure (see also MHRA/CHM advice, p. 667), by subcutaneous injection, ADULT over 18 years, initially 20 units/kg 3 times weekly, increased after 4 weeks according to response to 40 units/kg 3 times weekly, with further increases if needed at 4-weekly intervals in steps of 25% of the previous dose; maintenance dose, adjusted if necessary in steps of 25%; weekly maintenance dose may be given as a single dose or in 3 divided doses; max. 700 units/kg weekly

By intravenous injection, ADULT over 18 years, initially 40 units/kg 3 times weekly, increased according to response to 80 units/kg 3 times weekly after 4 weeks, with further increases if needed at intervals of 4 weeks in steps of 25% of the previous dose; maintenance dose, adjusted if necessary in steps of 25%; weekly maintenance dose may be given in 2 divided doses in stable patients; max. 700 units/kg weekly

Note Subcutaneous route preferred in patients not on haemodialysis. Reduce dose by 25–50% if rise in haemoglobin concentration exceeds 2 g/100 mL over 4 weeks or if haemoglobin concentration approaches or exceeds 12 g/100 mL; if haemoglobin concentration continues to rise, despite dose reduction, suspend treatment until haemoglobin concentration decreases and then restart at a dose approximately 25% lower than the previous dose

Symptomatic anaemia in adults with non-myeloid malignancies receiving cancer chemotherapy (see also MHRA/CHM advice, p. 667), by subcutaneous injection, initially 20 000 units once weekly, increased if necessary after 4 weeks (if a rise in haemoglobin of at least 1 g/100 mL not achieved) to 40 000 units once weekly, with further increase if needed after 4 weeks to max. 60 000 units once weekly

Note Discontinue treatment if haemoglobin concentration does not increase by at least 1 g/100 mL after 12 weeks of therapy (response unlikely). Reduce dose by 25–50% if rise in haemoglobin concentration exceeds 2 g/100 mL over 4 weeks or if haemoglobin concentration exceeds 12 g/100 mL; if haemoglobin concentration continues to rise, despite dose reduction, suspend treatment until haemoglobin concentration decreases and then restart at a dose approximately 25% lower than the previous dose. Discontinue approximately 4 weeks after ending chemotherapy

◢ Epoetin zeta

Retacrit® (Hospira) [PoM]
Injection, prefilled syringe, epoetin zeta, net price 1000 units = £5.66; 2000 units = £11.31; 3000 units = £16.97; 4000 units = £22.63; 5000 units = £28.28; 6000 units = £33.94; 8000 units = £45.25; 10 000 units = £56.57; 20 000 units = £113.13; 30 000 units = £169.70; 40 000 units = £226.26

Excipients include phenylalanine up to 500 micrograms/syringe (section 9.4.1)

Note Biosimilar medicine, p. 1

Dose symptomatic anaemia associated with chronic renal failure in patients on haemodialysis (see also MHRA/CHM advice, p. 667), by intravenous injection over 1–5 minutes or by subcutaneous injection (max. 1 mL per injection site), initially 50 units/kg 3 times weekly adjusted according to response in steps of 25 units/kg 3 times weekly at intervals of at least 4 weeks; maintenance dose, usually 25–100 units/kg 3 times weekly; CHILD by intravenous injection initially as for adults; maintenance dose, body-weight under 10 kg usually 75–150 units/kg 3 times weekly, body-weight 10–30 kg usually 60–150 units/kg 3 times weekly, body-weight over 30 kg usually 30–100 units/kg 3 times weekly

Symptomatic anaemia associated with chronic renal failure in adults on peritoneal dialysis (see also MHRA/CHM advice, p. 667), by intravenous injection over 1–5 minutes or by subcutaneous injection (max. 1 mL per injection site), initially 50 units/kg twice weekly; maintenance dose 25–50 units/kg twice weekly

Severe symptomatic anaemia of renal origin in adults with renal insufficiency not yet on dialysis (see also MHRA/CHM advice, p. 667), by intravenous injection over 1–5 minutes *or* by subcutaneous injection (max. 1 mL per injection site), initially 50 units/kg 3 times weekly increased according to response in steps of 25 units/kg 3 times weekly at intervals of at least 4 weeks; maintenance dose 17–33 units/kg 3 times weekly; max. 200 units/kg 3 times weekly

Note Avoid increasing haemoglobin concentration at a rate exceeding 2 g/100 mL over 4 weeks

Symptomatic anaemia in adults receiving cancer chemotherapy (see also MHRA/CHM advice, p. 667), by subcutaneous injection (max. 1 mL per injection site), initially 150 units/kg 3 times weekly (*or* 450 units/kg once weekly), increased if appropriate rise in haemoglobin (or reticulocyte count) not achieved after 4 weeks to 300 units/kg 3 times weekly; discontinue if inadequate response after 4 weeks at higher dose

Note Reduce dose by approximately 25–50% if rise in haemoglobin concentration exceeds 2 g/100 mL over 4 weeks or if haemoglobin concentration exceeds 12 g/100 mL; if haemoglobin concentration continues to rise, despite dose reduction, suspend treatment until haemoglobin concentration decreases and then restart at a dose approximately 25% lower than the previous dose. Discontinue approximately 4 weeks after ending chemotherapy

To increase yield of autologous blood (to avoid homologous blood) in predonation programme in moderate anaemia *either* when large volume of blood required *or* when sufficient blood cannot be saved for elective major surgery, by intravenous injection over 1–5 minutes, 600 units/kg twice weekly for 3 weeks before surgery; consult product literature for details and advice on ensuring high iron stores

Moderate anaemia (haemoglobin concentration 10–13 g/100 mL) before elective orthopaedic surgery in adults with expected moderate blood loss to reduce exposure to allogeneic blood transfusion or if autologous transfusion unavailable, by subcutaneous injection (max. 1 mL per injection site), 600 units/kg every week for 3 weeks before surgery and on day of surgery *or* 300 units/kg daily for 15 days starting 10 days before surgery; consult product literature for details

▌ METHOXY POLYETHYLENE GLYCOL-EPOETIN BETA

Indications see under Dose below

Cautions see Epoetin

Contra-indications see Epoetin

Pregnancy no evidence of harm in *animal* studies—manufacturer advises caution

Breast-feeding manufacturer advises use only if potential benefit outweighs risk—present in milk in *animal* studies

Side-effects see Epoetin; also hot flushes reported

Dose

• Symptomatic anaemia associated with chronic kidney disease in patients on dialysis and *not* currently treated with erythropoietins (see also MHRA/CHM advice, p. 667), ADULT over 18 years, by subcutaneous *or* intravenous injection, initially 600 nanograms/kg once every 2 weeks; adjusted according to response at intervals of at least 4 weeks; maintenance dose of double the previous fortnightly dose may be given every 4 weeks

• Symptomatic anaemia associated with chronic kidney disease in patients *not* on dialysis and *not* currently treated with erythropoietins (see also MHRA/CHM advice, p. 667), ADULT over 18 years, by subcutaneous injection, initially 1.2 micrograms/kg once every 4 weeks, *alternatively* by subcutaneous *or* intravenous injection, initially 600 nanograms/kg once every 2 weeks; dose adjusted according to response at intervals of at least 4 weeks; patients treated once every 2

weeks may be given a maintenance dose of double the previous fortnightly dose every 4 weeks

• Symptomatic anaemia associated with chronic kidney disease in patients currently treated with erythropoietins (see also MHRA/CHM advice, p. 667), ADULT over 18 years, by subcutaneous *or* intravenous injection, consult product literature

Note Subcutaneous route preferred in patients not on haemodialysis. Reduce dose by approximately 25% if rise in haemoglobin concentration exceeds 2 g/100 mL over 4 weeks, or if haemoglobin concentration approaches or exceeds 12 g/100 mL; if haemoglobin concentration continues to rise, despite dose reduction, suspend treatment until haemoglobin concentration decreases and then restart at a dose approximately 25% lower than the previous dose

Mircera® (Roche) ▼ [PoM]

Injection, prefilled syringe, methoxy polyethylene glycol-epoetin beta, net price 30 micrograms/0.3 mL = £44.05; 50 micrograms/0.3 mL = £73.41; 75 micrograms/0.3 mL = £110.11; 100 micrograms/0.3 mL = £146.81; 120 micrograms/0.3 mL = £176.18; 150 micrograms/0.3 mL = £220.22; 200 micrograms/0.3 mL = £293.62; 250 micrograms/0.3 mL = £367.03; 360 micrograms/0.6 mL = £528.56

Sickle-cell disease

Sickle-cell disease is caused by a structural abnormality of haemoglobin resulting in deformed, less flexible red blood cells. Acute complications in the more severe forms include *sickle-cell crisis*, where infarction of the microvasculature and blood supply to organs results in severe pain. Sickle-cell crisis requires hospitalisation, intravenous fluids, analgesia (section 4.7), and treatment of any concurrent infection. Chronic complications include skin ulceration, renal failure, and increased susceptibility to infection. Pneumococcal vaccine (section 14.4), haemophilus influenzae type b vaccine (section 14.4), an annual influenza vaccine (section 14.4) and prophylactic penicillin (Table 2, section 5.1) reduce the risk of infection. Hepatitis B vaccine (section 14.4) should be considered if the patient is not immune.

In most forms of sickle-cell disease, varying degrees of haemolytic anaemia are present accompanied by increased erythropoiesis; this may increase folate requirements and folate supplementation may be necessary (section 9.1.2).

Hydroxycarbamide can reduce the frequency of crises and the need for blood transfusions in sickle-cell disease; it should be considered in consultation with a specialist centre. The beneficial effects of hydroxycarbamide may not become evident for several months. Myelosuppression and skin reactions are the most common side-effects.

▌ HYDROXYCARBAMIDE

(Hydroxyurea)

Indications sickle-cell disease (see notes above); chronic myeloid leukaemia, cancer of the cervix (section 8.1.5)

Cautions see section 8.1 and notes above; also monitor renal and hepatic function before and during treatment; monitor full blood count before treatment, then every 2 weeks for the first 2 months and then every 2 months thereafter (or every 2 weeks if on max. dose); leg ulcers (review treatment if cutaneous vasculitic ulcerations develop); **interactions:** Appendix 1 (hydroxycarbamide)

Hepatic impairment   manufacturer advises caution in mild to moderate impairment; avoid in severe impairment

Renal impairment   reduce initial dose by 50% if eGFR less than 60 mL/minute/1.73 m^2; avoid if eGFR less than 30 mL/minute/1.73 m^2

Pregnancy   section 8.1.5

Breast-feeding   section 8.1.5

Side-effects   see section 8.1 and notes above; also headache; *less commonly* dizziness and rash; *rarely* reduced sperm count and activity; fever, amenorrhoea, skin cancers (in elderly patients), bleeding and hypomagnesaemia also reported

Dose

- By mouth, initially 15 mg/kg daily, increased every 12 weeks in steps of 2.5–5 mg/kg daily according to response; usual dose 15–30 mg/kg daily (max. 35 mg/kg daily); CHILD under 18 years, see *BNF for Children*

Siklos® (Nordic) ▼ PoM

Tablets, scored, f/c, hydroxycarbamide 100 mg, net price 60-tab pack = £100.00; 1 g, 30-tab pack = £500.00

Iron overload

Severe tissue iron overload can occur in aplastic and other refractory anaemias, mainly as the result of repeated blood transfusions. It is a particular problem in refractory anaemias with hyperplastic bone marrow, especially *thalassaemia major*, where excessive iron absorption from the gut and inappropriate iron therapy can add to the tissue siderosis.

Iron overload associated with haemochromatosis can be treated with repeated venesection. Venesection may also be used for patients who have received multiple transfusions and whose bone marrow has recovered. Where venesection is contra-indicated, the long-term administration of the iron chelating compound **desferrioxamine mesilate** is useful. Subcutaneous infusions of desferrioxamine are given over 8–12 hours, 3–7 times a week. The dose should reflect the degree of iron overload. For children starting therapy (and who have low iron overload) the dose should not exceed 30 mg/kg. For established overload the dose is usually between 20 and 50 mg/kg daily. Desferrioxamine (up to 2 g per unit of blood) may also be given at the time of blood transfusion, provided that the desferrioxamine is **not** added to the blood and is **not** given through the same line as the blood (but the two may be given through the same cannula).

Iron excretion induced by desferrioxamine is enhanced by administration of ascorbic acid (vitamin C, section 9.6.3) 200 mg daily by mouth (100 mg in infants); it should be given separately from food since it also enhances iron absorption. Ascorbic acid should not be given to patients with cardiac dysfunction; in patients with normal cardiac function ascorbic acid should be introduced 1 month after starting desferrioxamine.

Desferrioxamine infusion can be used to treat *aluminium overload* in dialysis patients; theoretically 100 mg of desferrioxamine binds with 4.1 mg of aluminium.

Deferasirox, an oral iron chelator, is licensed for the treatment of chronic iron overload in adults and children over 6 years with thalassaemia major who receive frequent blood transfusions (more than 7 mL/kg/month of packed red blood cells). It is also licensed for transfusion-related chronic iron overload when desferrioxamine is contra-indicated or inadequate in children aged 2–5 years with thalassaemia major who receive frequent blood transfusions, adults and children over 2 years with thalassaemia major who receive infrequent blood transfusions (less than 7 mL/kg/month of packed red blood cells), and in adults and children over 2 years with other anaemias. Deferasirox is also licensed for the treatment of chronic iron overload when desferrioxamine is contra-indicated or inadequate in adults and children over 10 years with non-transfusion-dependent thalassaemia syndromes.

The *Scottish Medicines Consortium* (p. 4) has advised (January 2007) that deferasirox is accepted for restricted use within NHS Scotland for the treatment of chronic iron overload associated with the treatment of rare acquired or inherited anaemias requiring recurrent blood transfusions. It is not recommended for patients with myelodysplastic syndromes.

Deferiprone, an oral iron chelator, is licensed for the treatment of iron overload in patients with thalassaemia major in whom desferrioxamine is contra-indicated or is inadequate. Blood dyscrasias, particularly agranulocytosis, have been reported with deferiprone.

DEFERASIROX

Indications   see notes above

Cautions   eye and ear examinations required before treatment and annually during treatment; monitor body-weight, height, and sexual development in children annually; monitor serum-ferritin concentration monthly; elderly (increased risk of side-effects); risk of gastro-intestinal ulceration and haemorrhage; platelet count less than 50×10^9/litre; consider treatment interruption if unexplained cytopenia occurs; not recommended in conditions which may reduce life expectancy (e.g. high-risk myelodysplastic syndromes); history of liver cirrhosis; test liver function before treatment, then every 2 weeks during the first month, and then monthly; measure baseline serum creatinine and monitor renal function weekly during the first month of treatment and monthly thereafter; test for proteinuria monthly; **interactions:** Appendix 1 (deferasirox)

Hepatic impairment   use with caution in moderate impairment, reduce dose considerably then gradually increase to max. 50% of normal dose; avoid in severe impairment

Renal impairment   reduce dose by 10 mg/kg if eGFR 60–90 mL/minute/1.73 m^2 and if serum creatinine increased by more than 33% of baseline measurement on 2 consecutive occasions—interrupt treatment if deterioration in renal function persists after dose reduction; avoid if eGFR less than 60 mL/minute/1.73 m^2

Pregnancy   manufacturer advises avoid unless essential—toxicity in *animal* studies

Breast-feeding   manufacturer advises avoid—present in milk in *animal* studies

Side-effects   gastro-intestinal disturbances (including ulceration and fatal haemorrhage); headache; proteinuria; pruritus; rash; *less commonly* hepatitis, cholelithiasis, oedema, fatigue, anxiety, sleep disorder, dizziness, pyrexia, pharyngitis, glucosuria, renal tubulopathy, disturbances of hearing and vision (including lens opacity and maculopathy), and skin pigmentation; hepatic failure, acute renal failure, tubulointerstitial nephritis, blood disorders (including anaemia, agranulocytosis, neutropenia, pancytopenia, and thrombocytopenia), hypersensitivity reactions (including anaphylaxis and angioedema), alopecia also reported

Dose

- Transfusion-related chronic iron overload, ADULT and CHILD over 2 years initially 10–30 mg/kg once daily according to serum-ferritin concentration and amount of transfused blood (consult product literature); maintenance, adjust dose every 3–6 months in steps of 5–10 mg/kg according to serum-ferritin concentration; usual max. 30 mg/kg daily, but may be increased to max. 40 mg/kg daily and reduced in steps of 5–10 mg/kg once control achieved
- Chronic iron overload in non-transfusion-dependent thalassaemia syndromes, ADULT over 18 years initially 10 mg/kg once daily; maintenance, adjust dose every 3–6 months in steps of 5–10 mg/kg according to serum-ferritin concentration and liver-iron concentration (consult product literature); max. 20 mg/kg daily; CHILD under 18 years see *BNF for Children*

Exjade® (Novartis) ▼ PoM

Dispersible tablets, deferasirox 125 mg, net price 28-tab pack = £117.60; 250 mg, 28-tab pack = £235.20; 500 mg, 28-tab pack = £470.40. Label: 13, 22, counselling, administration

Counselling Tablets should be dispersed in water, orange juice, or apple juice; if necessary resuspend residue

▮ DEFERIPRONE

Indications   see notes above

Cautions   monitor neutrophil count weekly and discontinue treatment if neutropenia develops; monitor plasma-zinc concentration; **interactions:** Appendix 1 (deferiprone)

Blood disorders Patients or their carers should be told how to recognise signs of neutropenia and advised to seek immediate medical attention if symptoms such as fever or sore throat develop

Contra-indications   history of agranulocytosis or recurrent neutropenia

Hepatic impairment   manufacturer advises monitor liver function—interrupt treatment if persistent elevation in serum alanine aminotransferase

Renal impairment   manufacturer advises caution—no information available

Pregnancy   manufacturer advises avoid before intended conception and during pregnancy—teratogenic and embryotoxic in *animal* studies; contraception advised in women of child-bearing potential

Breast-feeding   manufacturer advises avoid—no information available

Side-effects   gastro-intestinal disturbances (reducing dose and increasing gradually may improve tolerance), increased appetite; headache; red-brown urine discoloration; neutropenia, agranulocytosis; zinc deficiency; arthropathy

Dose

- ADULT and CHILD over 6 years 25 mg/kg 3 times daily (max. 100 mg/kg daily)

Ferriprox® (Swedish Orphan) PoM

Tablets, f/c, scored, deferiprone 500 mg, net price 100-tab pack = £152.39; 1 g, 50-tab pack = £175.25. Label: 14, counselling, blood disorders

Oral solution, red, deferiprone 100 mg/mL, net price 500 mL = £152.39. Label: 14, counselling, blood disorders

▮ DESFERRIOXAMINE MESILATE
(Deferoxamine Mesilate)

Indications   see notes above; iron poisoning, see Emergency Treatment of Poisoning, p. 39

Cautions   eye and ear examinations before treatment and at 3-month intervals during treatment; monitor body-weight and height in children at 3-month intervals—risk of growth retardation with excessive doses; aluminium-related encephalopathy (may exacerbate neurological dysfunction); **interactions:** Appendix 1 (desferrioxamine)

Renal impairment   use with caution

Pregnancy   teratogenic in *animal* studies; manufacturer advises use only if potential benefit outweighs risk

Breast-feeding   manufacturer advises use only if potential benefit outweighs risk—no information available

Side-effects   nausea, vomiting, abdominal pain; headache; pyrexia; growth retardation and bone disorders (see Cautions); arthralgia, myalgia; hearing disturbances; injection-site reactions; *rarely* diarrhoea, hepatic impairment, hypotension (especially when given too rapidly by intravenous injection), anaphylaxis, Yersinia and mucormycosis infections, blood dyscrasias (including thrombocytopenia and leucopenia), leg cramps, bone pain, visual disturbances (including lens opacity and retinopathy), rash; *very rarely* acute respiratory distress, neurological disturbances (including dizziness, neuropathy, convulsions, and paraesthesia), renal impairment; muscle spasms also reported

Dose

- See notes above; iron poisoning, see Emergency Treatment of Poisoning, p. 39

Note For full details and warnings relating to administration, consult product literature

Desferrioxamine mesilate (Non-proprietary) PoM

Injection, powder for reconstitution, desferrioxamine mesilate, net price 500-mg vial = £4.26; 2-g vial = £17.65

Desferal® (Novartis) PoM

Injection, powder for reconstitution, desferrioxamine mesilate, net price 500-mg vial = £4.67; 2-g vial = £18.66

Paroxysmal nocturnal haemoglobinuria and atypical haemolytic uraemic syndrome

Eculizumab, a recombinant monoclonal antibody, inhibits terminal complement activation at the C5 protein and thereby reduces haemolysis and thrombotic microangiopathy. It is used to reduce haemolysis in paroxysmal nocturnal haemoglobinuria (PNH), a severe and disabling form of haemolytic anaemia. Eculizumab is also used to reduce thrombotic microangiopathy in atypical haemolytic uraemic syndrome (aHUS).

9

Nutrition and blood

ECULIZUMAB

Indications paroxysmal nocturnal haemoglobinuria, in those with a history of blood transfusions (under specialist supervision); atypical haemolytic uraemic syndrome (under specialist supervision)

Cautions active systemic infection; monitor for 1 hour after infusion; for *paroxysmal nocturnal haemoglobinuria*, monitor for intravascular haemolysis (including serum-lactate dehydrogenase concentration) during treatment and for at least 8 weeks after discontinuation; for *atypical haemolytic uraemic syndrome*, monitor for thrombotic microangiopathy (measure platelet count, serum-lactate dehydrogenase concentration, and serum creatinine) during treatment and for at least 12 weeks after discontinuation

Meningococcal infection Vaccinate against *Neisseria meningitidis* at least 2 weeks before treatment (tetravalent vaccine against serotypes A, C, W135 and Y recommended); revaccinate according to current medical guidelines. Patients receiving eculizumab less than 2 weeks after receiving meningococcal vaccine must be given prophylactic antibiotics until 2 weeks after vaccination. Advise patient to report promptly any signs of meningococcal infection. Other immunisations should also be up to date (section 14.1)

Contra-indications unresolved *Neisseria meningitidis* infection; patients unvaccinated against *Neisseria meningitidis* (see also Cautions above)

Pregnancy no information available—use only if potential benefit outweighs risk; human IgG antibodies known to cross placenta; manufacturer advises effective contraception during and for 5 months after treatment

Breast-feeding no information available—manufacturer advises avoid breast-feeding during and for 5 months after treatment

Side-effects gastro-intestinal disturbances; oedema; cough, nasopharyngitis; headache, dizziness, vertigo, fatigue, dysgeusia, paraesthesia; infection (including meningococcal infection); spontaneous erection, dysuria; arthralgia, myalgia; blood disorders (including thrombocytopenia, leucopenia); alopecia, pruritus, rash; influenza-like symptoms; infusion-related reactions; *less commonly* anorexia, gingival pain, jaundice, palpitation, haematoma, hypotension, chest pain, syncope, tremor, hot flushing, epistaxis, anxiety, depression, mood changes, sleep disturbances, Graves' disease, menstrual disorders, renal impairment, malignant melanoma, muscle spasms, myelodysplastic syndrome, visual disturbances, tinnitus, hyperhidrosis, petechiae, and skin depigmentation

Dose

* Paroxysmal nocturnal haemoglobinuria, by intravenous infusion, ADULT over 18 years, initially 600 mg once a week for 4 weeks, then 900 mg on week 5; maintenance, 900 mg once every 12–16 days; CHILD see *BNF for Children*

* Atypical haemolytic uraemic syndrome, by intravenous infusion, ADULT over 18 years, initially 900 mg once a week for 4 weeks, then 1200 mg on week 5; maintenance, 1200 mg once every 12–16 days; CHILD see *BNF for Children*

Note Consult product literature for details of supplemental doses with concomitant plasmapheresis, plasma exchange, or plasma infusion

Soliris® (Alexion) ▼PoM

Concentrate for intravenous infusion, eculizumab 10 mg/mL, net price 30-mL vial = £3150.00. Counselling, meningococcal infection, patient information card

Electrolytes Na⁺ 5 mmol/vial

9.1.4 Drugs used in platelet disorders

Idiopathic thrombocytopenic purpura

Acute idiopathic thrombocytopenic purpura is usually self-limiting in children. In adults, idiopathic thrombocytopenic purpura can be treated with a **corticosteroid**, e.g. prednisolone 1 mg/kg daily, gradually reducing the dose over several weeks. Splenectomy is considered if a satisfactory platelet count is not achieved or if there is a relapse on reducing the dose of corticosteroid or withdrawing it.

Immunoglobulin preparations (section 14.5.1), are also used in idiopathic thrombocytopenic purpura or where a temporary rapid rise in platelets is needed, as in pregnancy or pre-operatively; they are also used for children often in preference to a corticosteroid. **Anti-D (Rh₀) immunoglobulin** (section 14.5.3) is effective in raising the platelet count in about 80% of unsplenectomised rhesus-positive individuals; its effects may last longer than normal immunoglobulin for intravenous use, but further doses are usually required.

Other therapy that has been tried in refractory idiopathic thrombocytopenic purpura includes azathioprine (section 8.2.1), cyclophosphamide (section 8.1.1), vincristine (section 8.1.4), ciclosporin (section 8.2.2), and danazol (section 6.7.2). **Rituximab** (section 8.2.3) may also be effective and in some cases induces prolonged remission. For patients with chronic severe thrombocytopenia refractory to other therapy, tranexamic acid (section 2.11) may be given to reduce the severity of haemorrhage.

Eltrombopag and **romiplostim** are thrombopoietin receptor agonists licensed for the treatment of chronic idiopathic thrombocytopenic purpura in splenectomised patients refractory to other treatments, such as corticosteroids or immunoglobulins, or as a second-line treatment in non-splenectomised patients when surgery is contra-indicated (see also NICE guidance below). Eltrombopag is an oral preparation and romiplostim is an injection which is made biosynthetically by recombinant DNA technology; they should both be used under the supervision of a specialist.

The *Scottish Medicines Consortium* (p. 4) has advised (July 2010) that eltrombopag (*Revolade®*) is accepted for restricted use within NHS Scotland for the treatment of both splenectomised and non-splenectomised patients with severe symptomatic immune (idiopathic) thrombocytopenic purpura or a high risk of bleeding.

The *Scottish Medicines Consortium* (p. 4) has advised (September 2009) that romiplostim (*Nplate*®) is accepted for restricted use within NHS Scotland for patients with severe symptomatic idiopathic thrombocytopenic purpura or those at high risk of bleeding.

Eltrombopag is also used, under specialist supervision, to treat thrombocytopenia in patients with chronic hepatitis C infection, where the degree of thrombocytopenia is the main factor preventing the initiation or limiting the ability to maintain optimal interferon-based therapy. For the treatment of chronic hepatitis C, see section 5.3.3.2, p. 437.

ELTROMBOPAG

Indications   see notes above

Cautions   patients of East Asian origin (see under Dose for *idiopathic thrombocytopenic purpura*); risk factors for thromboembolism; monitor liver function before treatment, every two weeks when adjusting the dose, and monthly thereafter; regular ophthalmological examinations for cataract formation recommended; for *idiopathic thrombocytopenic purpura*, monitor full blood count including platelet count and peripheral blood smears every week during treatment until a stable platelet count is reached (50×10^9/litre or more for at least 4 weeks), then monthly thereafter; for *thrombocytopenia associated with chronic hepatitis C infection*, monitor platelet count every week before and during antiviral treatment until a stable platelet count is reached (50–75×10^9/litre), then monitor full blood count including platelet count and peripheral blood smears monthly thereafter; **interactions**: Appendix 1 (eltrombopag)

Hepatic impairment   for *idiopathic thrombocytopenic purpura*, avoid unless potential benefit outweighs risk—reduce initial dose to 25 mg once daily; for *thrombocytopenia associated with chronic hepatitis C infection*, in severe hepatic impairment use only if potential benefit outweighs risk and monitor closely—increased risk of hepatic decompensation and thromboembolic events

Renal impairment   use with caution

Pregnancy   avoid—toxicity in *animal* studies; ensure effective contraception during treatment

Breast-feeding   manufacturer advises avoid

Side-effects   gastro-intestinal disturbances (including nausea, diarrhoea, abdominal pain, and constipation), peripheral oedema, headache, insomnia, paraesthesia, fatigue, arthralgia, bone pain, myalgia, cataract, dry eye, pruritus, rash, alopecia; *less commonly* dry mouth, gingival bleeding, haemorrhoids, taste disturbances, cholestasis, hepatitis, anorexia, changes in appetite, weight gain, flushing, palpitation, QT-interval prolongation, hypertension, tachycardia, thromboembolic events (including deep vein thrombosis, pulmonary embolism, and acute myocardial infarction), cough, sleep disorders, mood changes, depression, anxiety, dizziness, migraine, hemiparesis, tremor, peripheral neuropathy, respiratory and urinary tract infections, renal failure, nocturia, rectosigmoid cancer, blood disorders (including anaemia, haemolysis, eosinophilia, myelocytosis), gout, eye disorders, vertigo, epistaxis, skin reactions including ecchymosis, sweating

Dose

- Idiopathic thrombocytopenic purpura, ADULT over 18 years, initially 50 mg once daily (patients of EAST ASIAN origin such as Chinese, Japanese, Taiwanese, or Korean, initially 25 mg once daily), adjusted to achieve a platelet count of 50×10^9/litre or more (consult product literature for dose adjustments); max. 75 mg once daily; discontinue if inadequate response after 4 weeks at maximum dose
- Thrombocytopenia associated with chronic hepatitis C infection (see also notes above), ADULT over 18 years, initially 25 mg once daily, adjusted to achieve a platelet count sufficient to initiate antiviral therapy then a platelet count of 50–75×10^9/litre during antiviral therapy (consult product literature for dose adjustments); max. 100 mg once daily; discontinue if inadequate response after 2 weeks at maximum dose

Counselling   Each dose should be taken at least 4 hours before or after any dairy products (or foods containing calcium), indigestion remedies, or medicines containing aluminium, calcium, iron, magnesium, zinc, or selenium to reduce possible interference with absorption

Revolade® (GSK) ▼ [PoM]
Tablets, f/c, eltrombopag (as olamine) 25 mg (white), net price 28-tab pack = £770.00; 50 mg (brown), 28-tab pack = £1540.00. Counselling, see above

ROMIPLOSTIM

Indications   see notes above

Cautions   monitor full blood count and peripheral blood smears for morphological abnormalities before and during treatment; monitor platelet count weekly until 50 × 10⁹/litre or more for at least 4 weeks without dose adjustment, then monthly thereafter

Driving Dizziness may affect performance of skilled tasks (e.g. driving)

Hepatic impairment　avoid in moderate or severe impairment unless potential benefit outweighs risk (e.g. of portal vein thrombosis)

Renal impairment　manufacturer advises caution—no information available

Pregnancy　manufacturer advises use only if essential—toxicity in *animal* studies

Breast-feeding　manufacturer advises avoid—no information available

Side-effects　gastro-intestinal disturbances; flushing, oedema; dizziness, migraine, insomnia, fatigue, asthenia, paraesthesia; influenza-like symptoms; arthralgia, myalgia, bone pain, muscle spasm; increased bone marrow reticulin; ecchymosis, rash; injection-site reactions

Dose

- By subcutaneous injection, ADULT over 18 years, initially 1 microgram/kg once weekly, adjusted in steps of 1 microgram/kg at weekly intervals until a stable platelet count of 50 × 10⁹/litre or more is reached (consult product literature for dose adjustments); max. 10 micrograms/kg once weekly; discontinue if inadequate response after 4 weeks at maximum dose

Nplate® (Amgen) ⒫ᴼᴹ
Injection, powder for reconstitution, romiplostim, net price 250-microgram vial (with solvent) = £482.00

Essential thrombocythaemia

Anagrelide inhibits platelet formation. It is licensed for essential thrombocythaemia in patients at risk of thrombo-haemorrhagic events who have not responded adequately to other drugs or who cannot tolerate other drugs. Anagrelide should be initiated under specialist supervision.

▋ ANAGRELIDE

Indications　see notes above

Cautions　cardiovascular disease—assess cardiac function before and during treatment; concomitant aspirin in patients at risk of haemorrhage; monitor full blood count (monitor platelet count every 2 days for 1 week, then weekly until maintenance dose established), liver function, serum creatinine and urea; **interactions:** Appendix 1 (anagrelide)

Driving Dizziness may affect performance of skilled tasks (e.g. driving)

Hepatic impairment　manufacturer advises caution in mild impairment; avoid in moderate to severe impairment

Renal impairment　manufacturer advises avoid if eGFR less than 50 mL/minute/1.73 m²

Pregnancy　manufacturer advises avoid (toxicity in *animal* studies)

Breast-feeding　manufacturer advises avoid—no information available

Side-effects　gastro-intestinal disturbances, palpitation, tachycardia, fluid retention, headache, dizziness, fatigue, anaemia, rash; *less commonly* pancreatitis, gastro-intestinal haemorrhage, congestive heart failure, hypertension, arrhythmias, syncope, chest pain, dyspnoea, sleep disturbances, paraesthesia, hypoaesthesia, depression, nervousness, confusion, amnesia, fever, weight changes, impotence, blood disorders, myalgia, arthralgia, epistaxis, dry mouth, alopecia, skin discoloration, pruritus; *rarely* gastritis, colitis, postural hypotension, angina, myocardial infarction, vasodilatation, pulmonary hypertension, pulmonary infiltrates, migraine, drowsiness, impaired coordination, dysarthria, asthenia, tinnitus, renal failure, nocturia, visual disturbances, gingival bleeding; *also reported* allergic alveolitis, interstitial lung disease, pneumonitis, hepatitis, tubulointerstitial nephritis

Dose

- Initially 500 micrograms twice daily adjusted according to response in steps of 500 micrograms daily at weekly intervals to max. 10 mg daily (max. single dose 2.5 mg); usual dose range 1–3 mg daily in divided doses; CHILD under 18 years see *BNF for Children*

Xagrid® (Shire) ▼ ⒫ᴼᴹ
Capsules, anagrelide (as hydrochloride), 500 micrograms, net price 100-cap pack = £404.57. Counselling, driving, see above

---

9.1.5　G6PD deficiency

Glucose 6-phosphate dehydrogenase (G6PD) deficiency is highly prevalent in individuals originating from most parts of Africa, from most parts of Asia, from Oceania, and from Southern Europe; it can also occur, rarely, in any other individuals. G6PD deficiency is more common in males than it is in females.

Individuals with G6PD deficiency are susceptible to developing acute haemolytic anaemia when they take a number of common drugs. They are also susceptible to developing acute haemolytic anaemia when they eat fava beans (broad beans, *Vicia faba*); this is termed *favism* and can be more severe in children or when the fresh fava beans are eaten raw.

When prescribing drugs for patients with G6PD deficiency, the following three points should be kept in mind:

- G6PD deficiency is genetically heterogeneous; susceptibility to the haemolytic risk from drugs varies; thus, a drug found to be safe in some G6PD-deficient individuals may not be equally safe in others;

- manufacturers do not routinely test drugs for their effects in G6PD-deficient individuals;

- the risk and severity of haemolysis is almost always dose-related.

The lists below should be read with these points in mind. Ideally, information about G6PD deficiency should be available before prescribing a drug listed below. However, in the absence of this information, the possibility of haemolysis should be considered, especially if the patient belongs to a group in which G6PD deficiency is common.

A very few G6PD-deficient individuals with chronic non-spherocytic haemolytic anaemia have haemolysis even in the absence of an exogenous trigger. These patients must be regarded as being at high risk of severe exacerbation of haemolysis following administration of any of the drugs listed below.

Drugs with definite risk of haemolysis in most G6PD-deficient individuals

Dapsone and other sulfones (higher doses for dermatitis herpetiformis more likely to cause problems)

Methylthioninium chloride

Niridazole [not on UK market]

Nitrofurantoin

Pamaquin [not on UK market]

Primaquine (30 mg weekly for 8 weeks has been found to be without undue harmful effects in African and Asian people, see section 5.4.1)

Quinolones (including ciprofloxacin, moxifloxacin, nalidixic acid, norfloxacin, and ofloxacin)

Rasburicase

Sulfonamides (including co-trimoxazole; some sulfonamides, e.g. sulfadiazine, have been tested and found not to be haemolytic in many G6PD-deficient individuals)

Drugs with possible risk of haemolysis in some G6PD-deficient individuals

Aspirin (acceptable up to a dose of at least 1 g daily in most G6PD-deficient individuals)

Chloroquine (acceptable in acute malaria and malaria chemoprophylaxis)

Menadione, water-soluble derivatives (e.g. menadiol sodium phosphate)

Quinidine (acceptable in acute malaria) [not on UK market]

Quinine (acceptable in acute malaria)

Sulfonylureas

Note Naphthalene in mothballs also causes haemolysis in individuals with G6PD deficiency

9.1.6 Drugs used in neutropenia

Recombinant human granulocyte-colony stimulating factor (rhG-CSF) stimulates the production of neutrophils and may reduce the duration of chemotherapy-induced neutropenia and thereby reduce the incidence of associated sepsis; there is as yet no evidence that it improves overall survival. **Filgrastim** (unglycosylated rhG-CSF) and **lenograstim** (glycosylated rhG-CSF) have similar effects; both have been used in a variety of clinical settings, but they do not have any clear-cut routine indications. In congenital neutropenia filgrastim usually increases the neutrophil count with an appropriate clinical response. Prolonged use may be associated with an increased risk of myeloid malignancy. **Pegfilgrastim** is a polyethylene glycol-conjugated ('pegylated') derivative of filgrastim; pegylation increases the duration of filgrastim activity.

Granulocyte-colony stimulating factors should only be prescribed by those experienced in their use.

Cautions Granulocyte-colony stimulating factors should be used with caution in patients with pre-malig-

nant or malignant myeloid conditions. Full blood counts including differential white cell and platelet counts should be monitored. Treatment should be withdrawn in patients who develop signs of pulmonary infiltration. There have been reports of pulmonary infiltrates leading to acute respiratory distress syndrome—patients with a recent history of pulmonary infiltrates or pneumonia may be at higher risk. Granulocyte-colony stimulating factors should be used with caution in patients with sickle-cell disease. Spleen size should be monitored during treatment because there is a risk of splenomegaly and rupture.

Pregnancy There have been reports of toxicity in *animal* studies and manufacturers advise not to use granulocyte-colony stimulating factors during pregnancy unless the potential benefit outweighs the risk.

Breast-feeding There is no evidence for the use of granulocyte-colony stimulating factors during breast-feeding and manufacturers advise avoiding their use.

Side-effects Side-effects of granulocyte-colony stimulating factors include gastro-intestinal disturbances, anorexia, headache, asthenia, fever, musculoskeletal pain, bone pain, rash, alopecia, injection-site reactions, thrombocytopenia, and leucocytosis. *Less commonly* chest pain can occur. Pulmonary side-effects, particularly interstitial pneumonia (see Cautions above), cutaneous vasculitis and acute febrile neutrophilic dermatosis have *rarely* been reported.

FILGRASTIM
(Recombinant human granulocyte-colony stimulating factor, G-CSF)

Indications (specialist use only) reduction in duration of neutropenia and incidence of febrile neutropenia in cytotoxic chemotherapy for malignancy (except chronic myeloid leukaemia and myelodysplastic syndromes); reduction in duration of neutropenia (and associated sequelae) in myeloablative therapy followed by bone-marrow transplantation; mobilisation of peripheral blood progenitor cells for harvesting and subsequent autologous or allogeneic infusion; severe congenital neutropenia, cyclic neutropenia, or idiopathic neutropenia and history of severe or recurrent infections (distinguish carefully from other haematological disorders, consult product literature); persistent neutropenia in advanced HIV infection

Cautions see notes above; also regular morphological and cytogenetic bone-marrow examinations recommended in severe congenital neutropenia (possible risk of myelodysplastic syndromes or leukaemia); secondary acute myeloid leukaemia; osteoporotic bone disease (monitor bone density if given for more than 6 months); **interactions:** Appendix 1 (filgrastim)

Contra-indications severe congenital neutropenia (Kostmann's syndrome) with abnormal cytogenetics

Pregnancy see notes above

Breast-feeding see notes above

Side-effects see notes above; also mucositis, splenic enlargement, hepatomegaly, transient hypotension, epistaxis, urinary abnormalities (including dysuria, proteinuria, and haematuria), osteoporosis, exacerbation of rheumatoid arthritis, anaemia, transient decrease in blood glucose, pseudogout, and raised uric acid; *less commonly* capillary leak syndrome (including fatal cases); *very rarely* splenic rupture

Nutrition and blood | **9**

Dose

- Cytotoxic-induced neutropenia, preferably by subcutaneous injection *or* by intravenous infusion (over 30 minutes), ADULT and CHILD, 500 000 units/kg daily started at least 24 hours after cytotoxic chemotherapy, continued until neutrophil count in normal range, usually for up to 14 days (up to 38 days in acute myeloid leukaemia)
- Myeloablative therapy followed by bone-marrow transplantation, by intravenous infusion over 30 minutes or over 24 hours *or* by subcutaneous infusion over 24 hours, 1 million units/kg daily, started at least 24 hours following cytotoxic chemotherapy (and within 24 hours of bone-marrow infusion), then adjusted according to neutrophil count (consult product literature)
- Mobilisation of peripheral blood progenitor cells for autologous infusion, used alone, by subcutaneous injection *or* by subcutaneous infusion over 24 hours, 1 million units/kg daily for 5–7 days; used following adjunctive myelosuppressive chemotherapy (to improve yield), by subcutaneous injection, 500 000 units/kg daily, started the day after completing chemotherapy and continued until neutrophil count in normal range; for timing of leucopheresis consult product literature
- Mobilisation of peripheral blood progenitor cells in normal donors for allogeneic infusion, by subcutaneous injection, ADULT under 60 years and CHILD over 16 years, 1 million units/kg daily for 4–5 days; for timing of leucopheresis consult product literature
- Severe chronic neutropenia, by subcutaneous injection, ADULT and CHILD, in severe congenital neutropenia, initially 1.2 million units/kg daily in single or divided doses (initially 500 000 units/kg daily in idiopathic or cyclic neutropenia), adjusted according to response (consult product literature)
- Persistent neutropenia in HIV infection, by subcutaneous injection, initially 100 000 units/kg daily, increased as necessary until neutrophil count in normal range (usual max. 400 000 units/kg daily), then adjusted to maintain neutrophil count in normal range (consult product literature)

Neupogen® (Amgen) PoM
Injection, filgrastim 30 million-units (300 micrograms)/mL, net price 1-mL vial = £52.70
Injection (Singleject®), filgrastim 60 million-units (600 micrograms)/mL, net price 0.5-mL prefilled syringe = £52.70; 96 million-units (960 micrograms)/mL, 0.5-mL prefilled syringe = £84.06

Nivestim® (Hospira) ▼ PoM
Injection, prefilled syringe, filgrastim, net price 12 million-units (120 micrograms)/0.2 mL = £36.00; 30 million-units (300 micrograms)/0.5 mL = £58.00; 48 million-units (480 micrograms)/0.5 mL = £93.00
Note Biosimilar medicine, p. 1

Ratiograstim® (Ratiopharm UK) ▼ PoM
Injection, prefilled syringe, filgrastim, net price 30 million-units (300 micrograms)/0.5 mL = £62.25; 48 million-units (480 micrograms)/0.8 mL = £99.29
Note Biosimilar medicine, p. 1

Zarzio® (Sandoz) PoM
Injection, prefilled syringe, filgrastim, net price 30 million-units (300 micrograms)/0.5 mL = £50.15; 48 million-units (480 micrograms)/0.5 mL = £79.90
Note Biosimilar medicine, p. 1

LENOGRASTIM
(Recombinant human granulocyte-colony stimulating factor, rHuG-CSF)

Indications (specialist use only) reduction in the duration of neutropenia and associated complications following peripheral stem cells or bone-marrow transplantation for non-myeloid malignancy, or following treatment with cytotoxic chemotherapy associated with a significant incidence of febrile neutropenia; mobilisation of peripheral blood progenitor cells for harvesting and subsequent infusion

Cautions see notes above

Pregnancy see notes above

Breast-feeding see notes above

Side-effects see notes above; also mucositis, splenic rupture, and toxic epidermal necrolysis

Dose

- Following bone-marrow transplantation, by intravenous infusion or subcutaneous injection, ADULT and CHILD over 2 years 19.2 million units/m² daily started the day after transplantation, continued until neutrophil count stable in acceptable range (max. 28 days)
- Following peripheral stem cells transplantation, by intravenous infusion or subcutaneous injection, ADULT 19.2 million units/m² daily started the day after transplantation, continued until neutrophil count stable in acceptable range (max. 28 days); CHILD see *BNF for Children*
- Cytotoxic-induced neutropenia, by subcutaneous injection, ADULT 19.2 million units/m² daily started the day after completion of chemotherapy, continued until neutrophil count stable in acceptable range (max. 28 days); CHILD see *BNF for Children*
- Mobilisation of peripheral blood progenitor cells, used alone, by subcutaneous injection, ADULT 1.28 million units/kg daily for 4–6 days (5–6 days in healthy donors); used following adjunctive myelosuppressive chemotherapy (to improve yield), by subcutaneous injection, 19.2 million units/m² daily, started 1–5 days after completion of chemotherapy and continued until neutrophil count in acceptable range; for timing of leucopheresis consult product literature; CHILD see *BNF for Children*

Granocyte® (Chugai) PoM
Injection, powder for reconstitution, lenograstim, net price 13.4 million-unit (105-microgram) vial = £40.11; 33.6 million-unit (263-microgram) vial = £62.54 (both with 1-mL prefilled syringe water for injections)
Excipients include phenylalanine (section 9.4.1)

PEGFILGRASTIM
(Pegylated recombinant methionyl human granulocyte-colony stimulating factor)

Indications (specialist use only) reduction in duration of neutropenia and incidence of febrile neutropenia in cytotoxic chemotherapy for malignancy (except chronic myeloid leukaemia and myelodysplastic syndromes)

Cautions see notes above; also acute leukaemia and myelosuppressive chemotherapy; **interactions:** Appendix 1 (filgrastim)

Pregnancy see notes above

Breast-feeding see notes above

Side-effects   see notes above; also *rarely* capillary leak syndrome (including fatal cases); *very rarely* splenic rupture

Dose

Note   Dose expressed as filgrastim

- By subcutaneous injection, ADULT over 18 years, 6 mg (0.6 mL) for each chemotherapy cycle, starting 24 hours after chemotherapy

Neulasta® (Amgen) [PoM]

Injection, pegfilgrastim (expressed as filgrastim) 10 mg/mL, net price 0.6-mL (6-mg) prefilled syringe = £686.38

9.1.7   Drugs used to mobilise stem cells

Plerixafor is a chemokine receptor antagonist licensed to mobilise haematopoietic stem cells to peripheral blood for collection and subsequent autologous transplantation in patients with lymphoma or multiple myeloma. Plerixafor should be given under specialist supervision following 4 days treatment with a granulocyte-colony stimulating factor (section 9.1.6)

PLERIXAFOR

Indications   see notes above

Cautions   monitor platelet and white blood cell count

Renal impairment   reduce dose to 160 micrograms/kg daily if creatinine clearance 20–50 mL/minute; no information available if creatinine clearance less than 20 mL/minute

Pregnancy   manufacturer advises avoid unless essential and use effective contraception during treatment—teratogenic in *animal* studies

Breast-feeding   manufacturer advises avoid—no information available

Side-effects   gastro-intestinal disturbances, dry mouth, oral hypoaesthesia; dizziness, headache, insomnia, fatigue; arthralgia, musculoskeletal pain; erythema, sweating; injection-site reactions; *less commonly* hypersensitivity reactions including dyspnoea and periorbital swelling

Dose

- By subcutaneous injection, ADULT over 18 years, 240 micrograms/kg daily 6–11 hours before initiation of apheresis; usual duration 2–4 days (max. 7 days)

Mozobil® (Genzyme) ▼ [PoM]

Injection, plerixafor 20 mg/mL, net price 1.2 mL-vial = £4882.77

Electrolytes   Na⁺<0.5 mmol/mL

9.2   Fluids and electrolytes

9.2.1   Oral preparations for fluid and electrolyte imbalance

9.2.2   Parenteral preparations for fluid and electrolyte imbalance

The following tables give a selection of useful electrolyte values:

Electrolyte concentrations—intravenous fluids

Intravenous infusion	Millimoles per litre				
	Na⁺	K⁺	HCO₃⁻	Cl⁻	Ca²⁺
Normal plasma values	142	4.5	26	103	2.5
Sodium Chloride 0.9%	150	—	—	150	—
Compound Sodium Lactate (Hartmann's)	131	5	29	111	2
Sodium Chloride 0.18% and Glucose 4%	30	—	—	30	—
Potassium Chloride 0.3% and Glucose 5%	—	40	—	40	—
Potassium Chloride 0.3% and Sodium Chloride 0.9%	150	40	—	190	—
To correct metabolic acidosis					
Sodium Bicarbonate 1.26%	150	—	150	—	—
Sodium Bicarbonate 8.4% for cardiac arrest	1000	—	1000	—	—
Sodium Lactate (m/6)	167	—	167	—	—

Electrolyte content—gastro-intestinal secretions

Type of fluid	Millimoles per litre				
	H⁺	Na⁺	K⁺	HCO₃⁻	Cl⁻
Gastric	40–60	20–80	5–20	—	100–150
Biliary	—	120–140	5–15	30–50	80–120
Pancreatic	—	120–140	5–15	70–110	40–80
Small bowel	—	120–140	5–15	20–40	90–130

Faeces, vomit, or aspiration should be saved and analysed where possible if abnormal losses are suspected; where this is impracticable the approximations above may be helpful in planning replacement therapy

9.2.1   Oral preparations for fluid and electrolyte imbalance

9.2.1.1   Oral potassium

9.2.1.2   Oral sodium and water

9.2.1.3   Oral bicarbonate

Sodium and potassium salts, which may be given by mouth to prevent deficiencies or to treat established deficiencies of mild or moderate degree, are discussed in this section. Oral preparations for removing excess potassium and preparations for oral rehydration therapy are also included here. Oral bicarbonate, for metabolic acidosis, is also described in this section.

For reference to calcium, magnesium, and phosphate, see section 9.5.

9   **Nutrition and blood**

9 Nutrition and blood

9.2.1.1 Oral potassium

Compensation for potassium loss is especially necessary:

- in those taking digoxin or anti-arrhythmic drugs, where potassium depletion may induce arrhythmias;

- in patients in whom secondary hyperaldosteronism occurs, e.g. renal artery stenosis, cirrhosis of the liver, the nephrotic syndrome, and severe heart failure;

- in patients with excessive losses of potassium in the faeces, e.g. chronic diarrhoea associated with intestinal malabsorption or laxative abuse.

Measures to compensate for potassium loss may also be required in the elderly since they frequently take inadequate amounts of potassium in the diet (but see below for **warning** on **renal insufficiency**). Measures may also be required during long-term administration of drugs known to induce potassium loss (e.g. corticosteroids). Potassium supplements are **seldom required** with the small doses of diuretics given to treat hypertension; **potassium-sparing diuretics** (rather than potassium supplements) are recommended for prevention of hypokalaemia due to diuretics such as furosemide or the thiazides when these are given to eliminate oedema.

Dosage If potassium salts are used for the *prevention of hypokalaemia*, then doses of potassium chloride 2 to 4 g (approx. 25 to 50 mmol) daily (in divided doses) by mouth are suitable in patients taking a normal diet. *Smaller doses* must be used if there is *renal insufficiency (common in the elderly)* to reduce the **risk** of **hyperkalaemia**. Potassium salts cause nausea and vomiting and poor compliance is a major limitation to their effectiveness; when appropriate, potassium-sparing diuretics are preferable (see also above). Regular monitoring of plasma-potassium concentration is essential in those taking potassium supplements. When there is *established potassium depletion* larger doses may be necessary, the quantity depending on the severity of any continuing potassium loss (monitoring of plasma-potassium concentration and specialist advice would be required). Potassium depletion is frequently associated with chloride depletion and with metabolic alkalosis, and these disorders require correction.

Administration Potassium salts are preferably given as a liquid (or effervescent) preparation, rather than modified-release tablets; they should be given as the chloride (the use of effervescent potassium tablets BPC 1968 should be restricted to *hyperchloraemic states*, section 9.2.1.3).

Salt substitutes A number of salt substitutes which contain significant amounts of potassium chloride are readily available as health food products (e.g. *LoSalt®* and *Ruthmol®*). These should not be used by patients with renal failure as potassium intoxication may result.

POTASSIUM CHLORIDE

Indications   potassium depletion (see notes above)

Cautions   see notes above; cardiac disease; elderly; *with modified-release preparations*, intestinal stricture, history of peptic ulcer, hiatus hernia; **interactions:** Appendix 1 (potassium salts)

Contra-indications   plasma-potassium concentration above 5 mmol/litre

Renal impairment   close monitoring required—risk of hyperkalaemia; avoid in severe impairment

Side-effects   nausea, vomiting, abdominal pain, diarrhoea, flatulence; *with modified-release preparations*, gastro-intestinal obstruction, ulceration and bleeding also reported

Dose

- See notes above

Note Do not confuse Effervescent Potassium Tablets BPC 1968 (section 9.2.1.3) with effervescent potassium chloride tablets. Effervescent Potassium Tablets BPC 1968 do not contain chloride ions and their use should be restricted to hyperchloraemic states (section 9.2.1.3).

Kay-Cee-L® (Geistlich)
Syrup, sugar-free, red, potassium chloride 7.5% (1 mmol/mL each of K+ and Cl−), net price 500 mL = £7.14. Label: 21

Sando-K® (HK Pharma)
Tablets, effervescent, potassium bicarbonate and chloride equivalent to potassium 470 mg (12 mmol of K+) and chloride 285 mg (8 mmol of Cl−). Net price 20 = £1.53. Label: 13, 21

◢**Modified-release preparations**
Avoid unless effervescent tablets or liquid preparations inappropriate

Slow-K® (Alliance) ◢
Tablets, m/r, orange, s/c, potassium chloride 600 mg (8 mmol each of K+ and Cl−), net price 100 = £5.95. Label: 25, 27, counselling, swallow whole with fluid during meals while sitting or standing
Note May be difficult to obtain

Management of hyperkalaemia

Acute severe hyperkalaemia (plasma-potassium concentration above 6.5 mmol/litre or in the presence of ECG changes) calls for urgent treatment with 10–20 mL of calcium gluconate 10% by slow intravenous injection, titrated and adjusted to ECG improvement, to temporarily protect against myocardial excitability. An intravenous injection of soluble insulin (5–10 units) with 50 mL glucose 50% given over 5–15 minutes, reduces serum-potassium concentration; this is repeated if necessary or a continuous infusion instituted. Salbutamol [unlicensed indication], by nebulisation or slow intravenous injection may also reduce plasma-potassium concentration; it should be used with caution in patients with cardiovascular disease. The correction of causal or compounding acidosis with sodium bicarbonate infusion (section 9.2.2) should be considered (**important:** preparations of sodium bicarbonate and calcium salts should not be administered in the same line—risk of precipitation). Drugs exacerbating hyperkalaemia should be reviewed and stopped as appropriate; occasionally haemodialysis is needed.

Ion-exchange resins may be used to remove excess potassium in *mild hyperkalaemia* or in *moderate hyperkalaemia* when there are no ECG changes.

POLYSTYRENE SULFONATE RESINS

Indications   hyperkalaemia associated with anuria or severe oliguria, and in dialysis patients

Cautions   children (impaction of resin with excessive dosage or inadequate dilution); monitor for electrolyte disturbances (stop if plasma-potassium concentration below 5 mmol/litre); *sodium-containing resin in con-*

gestive heart failure, hypertension, and oedema; **interactions:** Appendix 1 (polystyrene sulfonate resins)

Contra-indications obstructive bowel disease; neonates with reduced gut motility; *calcium-containing resin* in hyperparathyroidism, multiple myeloma, sarcoidosis, or metastatic carcinoma

Renal impairment use *sodium-containing resin* with caution

Pregnancy manufacturers advise use only if potential benefit outweighs risk—no information available

Breast-feeding manufacturers advise use only if potential benefit outweighs risk—no information available

Side-effects faecal impaction following rectal administration, gastro-intestinal concretions following oral administration, intestinal necrosis reported with concomitant use of sorbitol, gastric irritation, anorexia, nausea, vomiting, constipation (discontinue treatment—avoid magnesium-containing laxatives), diarrhoea, hypomagnesaemia; gastro-intestinal obstruction, ulceration, necrosis, and ischaemic colitis also reported; with *calcium-containing resin*, hypercalcaemia (including in dialysed patients and occasionally in those with renal impairment); with *sodium-containing resin*, sodium retention, hypocalcaemia

Dose

● See under preparations

Calcium Resonium® (Sanofi-Aventis)
Powder, buff, calcium polystyrene sulfonate. Net price 300 g = £68.47. Label: 13
Dose By mouth, 15 g 3–4 times daily in a small amount of water or syrup (not fruit juice which has a high potassium content); CHILD under 18 years see *BNF for Children*
By rectum, as an enema, 30 g in 150 mL of water or 10% glucose, retained for 9 hours followed by irrigation to remove resin from colon; NEONATE and CHILD under 18 years see *BNF for Children*

Resonium A® (Sanofi-Aventis)
Powder, buff, sodium polystyrene sulfonate. Net price 454 g = £67.50. Label: 13
Dose By mouth, 15 g 3–4 times daily in a small amount of water or syrup (not fruit juice which has a high potassium content); CHILD under 18 years see *BNF for Children*
By rectum, as an enema, 30 g in 150 mL of water or 10% glucose, retained for 9 hours followed by irrigation to remove resin from colon; NEONATE and CHILD under 18 years see *BNF for Children*

Sorbisterit® (Stanningley) [PoM]
Powder, buff, calcium polystyrene sulfonate 759–949 mg/g, net price 500 g = £49.95. Label: 13, 21
Excipients include sucrose 51–241 mg per 1 g of powder
Dose By mouth, 20 g 1–3 times daily in 150 mL of water or soft drink (not fruit juice which has a high potassium content); CHILD under 18 years see *BNF for Children*
By rectum, as an enema, 40 g in 150 mL of 5% glucose 1–3 times daily, retained for 6 hours followed by irrigation to remove resin from colon; NEONATE and CHILD under 18 years see *BNF for Children*

9.2.1.2 Oral sodium and water

Sodium chloride is indicated in states of sodium depletion and usually needs to be given intravenously (section 9.2.2). In chronic conditions associated with mild or moderate degrees of sodium depletion, e.g. in salt-losing bowel or renal disease, oral supplements of sodium

chloride or sodium bicarbonate (section 9.2.1.3), according to the acid-base status of the patient, may be sufficient.

SODIUM CHLORIDE

Indications sodium depletion—see also 9.2.2.1; nebuliser diluent (section 3.1.5); eye (section 11.8.1); oral hygiene (section 12.3.4); wound irrigation (section 13.11.1)

Slow Sodium® (HK Pharma)
Tablets, m/r, sodium chloride 600 mg (approx. 10 mmol each of Na^+ and Cl^-). Net price 100-tab pack = £6.05. Label: 25
Dose prophylaxis of sodium chloride deficiency 4–8 tablets daily with water (in severe depletion up to max. 20 tablets daily)
Chronic renal salt wasting, up to 20 tablets daily with appropriate fluid intake
CHILD see *BNF for Children*

Oral rehydration therapy (ORT)

As a worldwide problem *diarrhoea* is by far the most important indication for fluid and electrolyte replacement. Intestinal absorption of sodium and water is enhanced by glucose (and other carbohydrates). Replacement of fluid and electrolytes lost through diarrhoea can therefore be achieved by giving solutions containing sodium, potassium, and glucose or another carbohydrate such as rice starch.

Oral rehydration solutions should:

● enhance the absorption of water and electrolytes;

● replace the electrolyte deficit adequately and safely;

● contain an alkalinising agent to counter acidosis;

● be slightly hypo-osmolar (about 250 mmol/litre) to prevent the possible induction of osmotic diarrhoea;

● be simple to use in hospital and at home;

● be palatable and acceptable, especially to children;

● be readily available.

It is the policy of the World Health Organization (WHO) to promote a single oral rehydration solution but to use it flexibly (e.g. by giving extra water between drinks of oral rehydration solution to moderately dehydrated infants).

Oral rehydration solutions used in the UK are lower in sodium (50–60 mmol/litre) than the WHO formulation since, in general, patients suffer less severe sodium loss.

Rehydration should be rapid over 3 to 4 hours (except in hypernatraemic dehydration in which case rehydration should occur more slowly over 12 hours). The patient should be reassessed after initial rehydration and if still dehydrated rapid fluid replacement should continue.

Once rehydration is complete further dehydration is prevented by encouraging the patient to drink normal volumes of an appropriate fluid and by replacing continuing losses with an oral rehydration solution; in infants, breast-feeding or formula feeds should be offered between oral rehydration drinks.

For intravenous rehydration see section 9.2.2.

9

Nutrition and blood

ORAL REHYDRATION SALTS (ORS)

Indications fluid and electrolyte loss in diarrhoea, see notes above

Dose
- According to fluid loss, usually 200–400 mL solution after every loose motion; INFANT 1–1½ times usual feed volume; CHILD 200 mL after every loose motion

◢ **UK formulations**

Note After reconstitution any unused solution should be discarded no later than 1 hour after preparation unless stored in a refrigerator when it may be kept for up to 24 hours

Dioralyte® (Sanofi-Aventis)
Oral powder, sodium chloride 470 mg, potassium chloride 300 mg, disodium hydrogen citrate 530 mg, glucose 3.56 g/sachet, net price 6-sachet pack = £2.25, 20-sachet pack (black currant- or citrus-flavoured or natural) = £6.72
Note Reconstitute 1 sachet with 200 mL of water (freshly boiled and cooled for infants); 5 sachets reconstituted with 1 litre of water provide Na⁺ 60 mmol, K⁺ 20 mmol, Cl⁻ 60 mmol, citrate 10 mmol, and glucose 90 mmol

Dioralyte® Relief (Sanofi-Aventis)
Oral powder, sodium chloride 350 mg, potassium chloride 300 mg, sodium citrate 580 mg, cooked rice powder 6 g/sachet, net price 6-sachet pack (apricot-, black currant- or raspberry-flavoured) = £2.50, 20-sachet pack (apricot-flavoured) = £7.13
Note Reconstitute 1 sachet with 200 mL of water (freshly boiled and cooled for infants); 5 sachets when reconstituted with 1 litre of water provide Na⁺ 60 mmol, K⁺ 20 mmol, Cl⁻ 50 mmol and citrate 10 mmol; contains aspartame (section 9.4.1)

Electrolade® (Actavis)
Oral powder, sodium chloride 236 mg, potassium chloride 300 mg, sodium bicarbonate 500 mg, anhydrous glucose 4 g/sachet (banana-, black currant-, lemon and lime-, or orange-flavoured). Net price 6-sachet (plain or multiflavoured) pack = £1.33, 20-sachet (single- or multiflavoured) pack = £4.99
Note Reconstitute 1 sachet with 200 mL of water (freshly boiled and cooled for infants); 5 sachets when reconstituted with 1 litre of water provide Na⁺ 50 mmol, K⁺ 20 mmol, Cl⁻ 40 mmol, HCO₃⁻ 30 mmol, and glucose 111 mmol

◢ **WHO formulation**

Oral Rehydration Salts (Non-proprietary)
Oral powder, sodium chloride 2.6 g, potassium chloride 1.5 g, sodium citrate 2.9 g, anhydrous glucose 13.5 g. To be dissolved in sufficient water to produce 1 litre (providing Na⁺ 75 mmol, K⁺ 20 mmol, Cl⁻ 65 mmol, citrate 10 mmol, glucose 75 mmol/ litre)
Note Recommended by the WHO and the United Nations Children's Fund but not commonly used in the UK.

9.2.1.3 Oral bicarbonate

Sodium bicarbonate is given by mouth for *chronic acidotic states* such as uraemic acidosis or renal tubular acidosis. The dose for correction of metabolic acidosis is not predictable and the response must be assessed; sodium bicarbonate 4.8 g daily (57 mmol each of Na⁺ and HCO₃⁻) or more may be required. For severe *metabolic acidosis*, sodium bicarbonate can be given intravenously (section 9.2.2).

Sodium bicarbonate may also be used to increase the pH of the urine (see section 7.4.3); for use in dyspepsia see section 1.1.1.

Sodium supplements may increase blood pressure or cause fluid retention and pulmonary oedema in those at risk; hypokalaemia may be exacerbated.

Where *hyperchloraemic acidosis* is associated with potassium deficiency, as in some renal tubular and gastrointestinal disorders it may be appropriate to give oral **potassium bicarbonate**, although acute or severe deficiency should be managed by intravenous therapy.

◢ **SODIUM BICARBONATE**

Indications see notes above

Cautions see notes above; respiratory acidosis; **interactions:** Appendix 1 (antacids)

Dose
- See notes above

Sodium Bicarbonate (Non-proprietary)
Capsules, sodium bicarbonate 500 mg (approx. 6 mmol each of Na⁺ and HCO₃⁻), net price 56-cap pack = £2.93
Tablets, sodium bicarbonate 600 mg, net price 100 = £27.14
Important Oral solutions of sodium bicarbonate are required occasionally; these are available from 'special-order' manufacturers or specialist importing companies, see p. 1124; the strength of sodium bicarbonate should be stated on the prescription

◢ **POTASSIUM BICARBONATE**

Indications see notes above

Cautions elderly; cardiac disease; **interactions:** Appendix 1 (potassium salts)

Contra-indications hypochloraemia; plasma-potassium concentration above 5 mmol/litre

Renal impairment close monitoring required—high risk of hyperkalaemia; avoid in severe impairment

Side-effects nausea, vomiting, abdominal pain, diarrhoea, and flatulence

Dose
- See notes above

Potassium Tablets, Effervescent (Non-proprietary)
Effervescent tablets, potassium bicarbonate 500 mg, potassium acid tartrate 300 mg, each tablet providing 6.5 mmol of K⁺. To be dissolved in water before administration. Net price 56 = £91.31 Label: 13, 21
Note These tablets do not contain chloride; for effervescent tablets containing potassium and chloride, see under Potassium Chloride, section 9.2.1.1

9.2.2 Parenteral preparations for fluid and electrolyte imbalance

9.2.2.1 Electrolytes and water
9.2.2.2 Plasma and plasma substitutes

9.2.2.1 Electrolytes and water

Solutions of electrolytes are given intravenously, to meet normal fluid and electrolyte requirements or to replenish substantial deficits or continuing losses, when the patient is nauseated or vomiting and is unable to take adequate amounts by mouth. When intravenous administration is not possible, fluid (as sodium chloride

9 Nutrition and blood

0.9% or glucose 5%) can also be given by subcutaneous infusion (hypodermoclysis).

The nature and severity of the electrolyte imbalance must be assessed from the history and clinical and biochemical investigations. Sodium, potassium, chloride, magnesium, phosphate, and water depletion can occur singly and in combination with or without disturbances of acid-base balance; for reference to the use of magnesium and phosphates, see section 9.5.

Isotonic solutions may be infused safely into a peripheral vein. Solutions more concentrated than plasma, e.g. 20% glucose, are best given through an indwelling catheter positioned in a large vein.

Intravenous sodium

Sodium chloride in isotonic solution provides the most important extracellular ions in near physiological concentrations and is indicated in *sodium depletion*, which can arise from such conditions as gastro-enteritis, diabetic ketoacidosis, ileus, and ascites. In a severe deficit of 4 to 8 litres, 2 to 3 litres of isotonic sodium chloride may be given over 2 to 3 hours; thereafter the infusion can usually be at a slower rate. Excessive administration should be avoided; the jugular venous pressure should be assessed, the bases of the lungs should be examined for crepitations, and in elderly or seriously ill patients it is often helpful to monitor the right atrial (central) venous pressure.

Chronic hyponatraemia arising from inappropriate secretion of antidiuretic hormone should ideally be corrected by fluid restriction. However, if sodium chloride is required for acute or chronic hyponatraemia, regardless of the cause, the deficit should be corrected slowly to avoid the risk of osmotic demyelination syndrome and the rise in plasma-sodium concentration should not exceed 10 mmol/litre in 24 hours. In severe hyponatraemia, sodium chloride 1.8% may be used cautiously.

Compound sodium lactate (Hartmann's solution) can be used instead of isotonic sodium chloride solution during or after surgery, or in the initial management of the injured or wounded; it may reduce the risk of hyperchloraemic acidosis.

Sodium chloride and glucose solutions are indicated when there is combined *water and sodium depletion*. A 1:1 mixture of isotonic sodium chloride and 5% glucose allows some of the water (free of sodium) to enter body cells which suffer most from dehydration while the sodium salt with a volume of water determined by the normal plasma Na^+ remains extracellular. Maintenance fluid should accurately reflect daily requirements and close monitoring is required to avoid fluid and electrolyte imbalance. Illness or injury increase the secretion of anti-diuretic hormone and therefore the ability to excrete excess water may be impaired. Inappropriate use of hypotonic solutions such as sodium chloride 0.18% and glucose 4% may also cause dilutional hyponatraemia especially in children (see *BNF for Children*) and the elderly; if necessary, guidance should be sought from a clinician experienced in the management of fluid and electrolytes.

Combined sodium, potassium, chloride, and water depletion may occur, for example, with severe diarrhoea or persistent vomiting; replacement is carried out with sodium chloride intravenous infusion 0.9% and glucose intravenous infusion 5% with potassium as appropriate.

▌SODIUM CHLORIDE

Indications   electrolyte imbalance—see also section 9.2.1.2; nebuliser diluent (section 3.1.5); eye (section 11.8.1); oral hygiene (section 12.3.4); wound irrigation (section 13.11.1)

Cautions   restrict intake in impaired renal function, cardiac failure, hypertension, peripheral and pulmonary oedema, toxaemia of pregnancy

Side-effects   administration of large doses may give rise to sodium accumulation, oedema, and hyperchloraemic acidosis

Dose
● See notes above

Sodium Chloride Intravenous Infusion (Non-proprietary) PoM

Intravenous infusion, usual strength sodium chloride 0.9% (9 g, 150 mmol each of Na^+ and Cl^-/litre), this strength being supplied when normal saline for injection is requested. Net price 2-mL amp = 21p; 5-mL amp = 28p; 10-mL amp = 34p; 20-mL amp = £1.04; 50-mL amp = £4.27

In hospitals, 500- and 1000-mL packs, and sometimes other sizes, are available

Note The term 'normal saline' should **not** be used to describe sodium chloride intravenous infusion 0.9%; the term 'physiological saline' is acceptable but it is preferable to give the composition (i.e. sodium chloride intravenous infusion 0.9%).

◢With other ingredients

Sodium Chloride and Glucose Intravenous Infusion (Non-proprietary) PoM

Intravenous infusion, sodium chloride 0.18% (Na^+ and Cl^- each 30 mmol/litre), glucose 4%

In hospitals, usually 500-mL packs and sometimes other sizes are available

Intravenous infusion, sodium chloride 0.45% (Na^+ and Cl^- each 75 mmol/litre), glucose 2.5%

In hospitals, usually 500-mL packs and sometimes other sizes are available

Intravenous infusion, sodium chloride 0.45% (Na^+ and Cl^- each 75 mmol/litre), glucose 5%

In hospitals, usually 500-mL packs and sometimes other sizes are available

Intravenous infusion, sodium chloride 0.9% (Na^+ and Cl^- each 150 mmol/litre), glucose 5%

In hospitals, usually 500-mL packs and sometimes other sizes are available

Note See above for warning on hyponatraemia especially in children and elderly

Ringer's Solution for Injection PoM

Calcium chloride (dihydrate) 322 micrograms, potassium chloride 300 micrograms, sodium chloride 8.6 mg/mL, providing the following ions (in mmol/litre), Ca^{2+} 2.2, K^+ 4, Na^+ 147, Cl^- 156

In hospitals, 500- and 1000-mL packs, and sometimes other sizes, are available

Sodium Lactate Intravenous Infusion, Compound (Non-proprietary) PoM

(Hartmann's Solution for Injection; Ringer-Lactate Solution for Injection)

Intravenous infusion, sodium chloride 0.6%, sodium lactate 0.32%, potassium chloride 0.04%, calcium chloride 0.027% (containing Na^+ 131 mmol, K^+ 5 mmol, Ca^{2+} 2 mmol, HCO_3^- (as lactate) 29 mmol, Cl^- 111 mmol/litre)

In hospitals, 500- and 1000-mL packs, and sometimes other sizes, are available

9

Nutrition and blood

Intravenous glucose

Glucose solutions (5%) are used mainly to replace water deficit and should not be given alone except when there is no significant loss of electrolytes; prolonged administration of glucose solutions without electrolytes can lead to hyponatraemia and other electrolyte disturbances. Average water requirements in a healthy adult are 1.5 to 2.5 litres daily and this is needed to balance unavoidable losses of water through the skin and lungs and to provide sufficient for urinary excretion. Water depletion (dehydration) tends to occur when these losses are not matched by a comparable intake, as may occur in coma or dysphagia or in the elderly or apathetic who may not drink enough water on their own initiative.

Excessive loss of water without loss of electrolytes is uncommon, occurring in fevers, hyperthyroidism, and in uncommon water-losing renal states such as diabetes insipidus or hypercalcaemia. The volume of glucose solution needed to replace deficits varies with the severity of the disorder, but usually lies within the range of 2 to 6 litres.

Glucose solutions are also used to correct and prevent hypoglycaemia and to provide a source of energy in those too ill to be fed adequately by mouth; glucose solutions are a key component of parenteral nutrition (section 9.3).

Glucose solutions are given in regimens with calcium and insulin for the emergency management of *hyperkalaemia* (see p. 680). They are also given, after correction of hyperglycaemia, during treatment of diabetic ketoacidosis, when they must be accompanied by continuing insulin infusion.

GLUCOSE
(Dextrose Monohydrate)

Note Glucose BP is the monohydrate but Glucose Intravenous Infusion BP is a sterile solution of anhydrous glucose or glucose monohydrate, potency being expressed in terms of anhydrous glucose

Indications fluid replacement (see notes above), provision of energy (section 9.3); hypoglycaemia (section 6.1.4)

Side-effects glucose injections especially if hypertonic may have a low pH and may cause venous irritation and thrombophlebitis

Dose
- Water replacement, see notes above; energy source, 1–3 litres daily of 20–50% solution

Glucose Intravenous Infusion (Non-proprietary) PoM
Intravenous infusion, glucose or anhydrous glucose (potency expressed in terms of anhydrous glucose), usual strength 5% (50 mg/mL), 10% (100 mg/mL), and 20% (200 mg/mL); 20% solution, net price 20-mL amp = £2.04; 50% solution,[1] 20-mL amp = £1.00, 50-mL vial = £2.01
In hospitals, 500- and 1000-mL packs, and sometimes other sizes and strengths, are available; also available as *Minijet® Glucose*, 50% in 50-mL disposable syringe[1]

1. PoM restriction does not apply where administration is for saving life in emergency

Intravenous potassium

Potassium chloride and sodium chloride intravenous infusion is the initial treatment for the correction of *severe hypokalaemia* and when sufficient potassium cannot be taken by mouth. Ready-mixed infusion solutions should be used when possible; alternatively, potassium chloride concentrate, as ampoules containing 1.5 g (K+ 20 mmol) in 10 mL, is **thoroughly mixed** with 500 mL of sodium chloride 0.9% intravenous infusion and given slowly over 2 to 3 hours, with specialist advice and ECG monitoring in difficult cases. Higher concentrations of potassium chloride may be given in very severe depletion, but require specialist advice.

Repeated measurement of plasma-potassium concentration is necessary to determine whether further infusions are required and to avoid the development of hyperkalaemia, which is especially likely in renal impairment.

Initial potassium replacement therapy should **not** involve glucose infusions, because glucose may cause a further decrease in the plasma-potassium concentration.

POTASSIUM CHLORIDE

Indications electrolyte imbalance; see also oral potassium supplements, section 9.2.1.1

Cautions for intravenous infusion the concentration of solution should not usually exceed 3 g (40 mmol)/litre; specialist advice and ECG monitoring (see notes above); **interactions**: Appendix 1 (potassium salts)

Contra-indications plasma-potassium concentration above 5 mmol/litre

Renal impairment close monitoring required—high risk of hyperkalaemia; avoid in severe impairment

Side-effects rapid infusion toxic to heart

Dose
- By slow intravenous infusion, depending on the deficit or the daily maintenance requirements, see also notes above

Potassium Chloride and Glucose Intravenous Infusion (Non-proprietary) PoM
Intravenous infusion, usual strength potassium chloride 0.3% (3 g, 40 mmol each of K+ and Cl−/litre) or 0.15% (1.5 g, 20 mmol each of K+ and Cl−/litre) with 5% of anhydrous glucose
In hospitals, 500- and 1000-mL packs, and sometimes other sizes, are available

Potassium Chloride and Sodium Chloride Intravenous Infusion (Non-proprietary) PoM
Intravenous infusion, usual strength potassium chloride 0.15% (1.5 g/litre) with sodium chloride 0.9% (9 g/litre), containing K+ 20 mmol, Na+ 150 mmol, and Cl− 170 mmol/litre *or* potassium chloride 0.3% (3 g/litre) with sodium chloride 0.9% (9 g/litre), containing K+ 40 mmol, Na+ 150 mmol, and Cl− 190 mmol/litre
In hospitals, 500- and 1000-mL packs, and sometimes other sizes, are available

9 Nutrition and blood

Potassium Chloride, Sodium Chloride, and Glucose Intravenous Infusion (Non-proprietary) [PoM]

Intravenous infusion, sodium chloride 0.45% (4.5 g, Na⁺ 75 mmol/litre) with 5% of anhydrous glucose and usually sufficient potassium chloride to provide K⁺ 10–40 mmol/litre (to be specified by the prescriber)

In hospitals, 500- and 1000-mL packs, and sometimes other sizes, are available

Intravenous infusion, sodium chloride 0.18% (1.8 g, Na⁺ 30 mmol/litre) with 4% of anhydrous glucose and usually sufficient potassium chloride to provide K⁺ 10–40 mmol/litre (to be specified by the prescriber)

In hospitals, 500- and 1000-mL packs, and sometimes other sizes, are available

Potassium Chloride Concentrate, Sterile (Non-proprietary) [PoM]

Sterile concentrate, potassium chloride 15% (150 mg, approximately 2 mmol each of K⁺ and Cl⁻/mL). Net price 10-mL amp = 48p

Important Must be diluted with **not less** than 50 times its volume of sodium chloride intravenous infusion 0.9% or other suitable diluent and **mixed well**

Solutions containing 10 and 20% of potassium chloride are also available in both 5- and 10-mL ampoules

Bicarbonate and lactate

Sodium bicarbonate is used to control severe *metabolic acidosis* (pH < 7.1) particularly that caused by loss of bicarbonate (as in renal tubular acidosis or from excessive gastro-intestinal losses). Mild metabolic acidosis associated with volume depletion should first be managed by appropriate fluid replacement because acidosis usually resolves as tissue and renal perfusion are restored. In more severe metabolic acidosis or when the acidosis remains unresponsive to correction of anoxia or hypovolaemia, sodium bicarbonate (1.26%) can be infused over 3–4 hours with plasma-pH and electrolyte monitoring. In severe shock (section 2.7.1), for example in cardiac arrest, metabolic acidosis can develop without sodium or volume depletion; in these circumstances sodium bicarbonate is best given as a small volume of hypertonic solution, such as 50 mL of 8.4% solution intravenously; plasma-pH and electrolytes should be monitored.

Sodium lactate intravenous infusion is no longer used in metabolic acidosis because of the risk of producing lactic acidosis, particularly in seriously ill patients with poor tissue perfusion or impaired hepatic function.

For *chronic acidotic states*, sodium bicarbonate can be given by mouth (section 9.2.1.3).

▌ SODIUM BICARBONATE

Indications metabolic acidosis, see also notes above
Dose
- By slow intravenous injection, a strong solution (up to 8.4%), or by continuous intravenous infusion, a weaker solution (usually 1.26%), an amount appropriate to the body base deficit (see notes above)

Sodium Bicarbonate Intravenous Infusion [PoM]

Usual strength sodium bicarbonate 1.26% (12.6 g, 150 mmol each of Na⁺ and HCO₃⁻/litre); various other strengths available

In hospitals, 500- and 1000-mL packs, and sometimes other sizes, are available

Minijet® Sodium Bicarbonate (UCB Pharma) [PoM]

Intravenous injection, sodium bicarbonate in disposable syringe, net price 4.2%, 10 mL = £11.03; 8.4%, 10 mL = £11.10, 50 mL = £12.15

▌ SODIUM LACTATE ◢

Indications see notes above

Sodium Lactate (Non-proprietary) [PoM] ◢

Intravenous infusion, sodium lactate M/6, contains the following ions (in mmol/litre), Na⁺ 167, HCO₃⁻ (as lactate) 167

Water

Water for Injections [PoM]

Net price 1-mL amp = 18p; 2-mL amp = 14p; 5-mL amp = 24p; 10-mL amp = 25p, 10-mL vial = £1.40; 20-mL amp = 39p; 50-mL amp = £1.91; 100-mL vial = £3.00

Note Water for Injections can be sold or supplied by a pharmacist for a purpose other than parenteral administration, or when dry powder for parenteral administration has been prescribed without the Water for Injections that is needed as a diluent

9.2.2.2 Plasma and plasma substitutes

Plasma and plasma substitutes ('colloids') contain large molecules that do not readily leave the intravascular space where they exert osmotic pressure to maintain circulatory volume. Compared to fluids containing electrolytes such as sodium chloride and glucose ('crystalloids'), a smaller volume of colloid is required to produce the same expansion of blood volume, thereby shifting salt and water from the extravascular space. If resuscitation requires a volume of fluid that exceeds the maximum dose of the colloid then crystalloids may be given; packed red cells may also be required.

Albumin solutions, prepared from whole blood, contain soluble proteins and electrolytes but no clotting factors, blood group antibodies, or plasma cholinesterases; they may be given without regard to the recipient's blood group.

Albumin is usually used after the acute phase of illness, to correct a plasma-volume deficit; hypoalbuminaemia itself is not an appropriate indication. The use of albumin solutions in acute plasma or blood loss may be wasteful; plasma substitutes are more appropriate. Concentrated albumin solutions (20%) can be used under specialist supervision in patients with an intravascular fluid deficit and oedema because of interstitial fluid overload, to restore intravascular plasma volume with less exacerbation of the salt and water overload than isotonic solutions. Concentrated albumin solutions may also be used to obtain a diuresis in hypoalbuminaemic patients (e.g. in hepatic cirrhosis).

Recent evidence does not support the previous view that the use of albumin increases mortality.

> Plasma and plasma substitutes are often used in very ill patients whose condition is unstable. Therefore, close monitoring is required and fluid and electrolyte therapy should be adjusted according to the patient's condition at all times.

▌ ALBUMIN SOLUTION
(Human Albumin Solution)

A solution containing protein derived from plasma, serum, or normal placentas; at least 95% of the protein is albumin. The solution may be isotonic (containing 3.5–5% protein) or concentrated (containing 15–25% protein).

9

Nutrition and blood

Indications see under preparations, and also notes above

Cautions history of cardiac or circulatory disease (administer slowly to avoid rapid rise in blood pressure and cardiac failure, and monitor cardiovascular and respiratory function); increased capillary permeability; correct dehydration when administering concentrated solution

Contra-indications cardiac failure; severe anaemia

Side-effects hypersensitivity reactions (including anaphylaxis) with nausea, vomiting, increased salivation, fever, tachycardia, hypotension and chills reported

◢ **Isotonic solutions**

Indications: acute or sub-acute loss of plasma volume e.g. in burns, pancreatitis, trauma, and complications of surgery; plasma exchange

Available as: *Human Albumin Solution 4.5%* (50-, 100-, 250- and 400-mL bottles—Baxter); *Human Albumin Solution 5%* (250- and 500-mL bottles—Baxter); *Albunorm®* 5% (100-, 250-, and 500-mL bottles— Octapharm); *Zenalb®* 4.5% (50-, 100-, 250-, and 500-mL bottles—BPL)

◢ **Concentrated solutions (20%)**

Indications: severe hypoalbuminaemia associated with low plasma volume and generalised oedema where salt and water restriction with plasma volume expansion are required; adjunct in the treatment of hyperbilirubinaemia by exchange transfusion in the newborn; paracentesis of large volume ascites associated with portal hypertension

Available as: *Human Albumin Solution 20%* (50- and 100-mL vials—Baxter); *Albunorm®* 20% (50- and 100-mL bottles—Octapharm); *Flexbumin®* 20% (50- and 100-mL bags—Baxter); *Zenalb®* 20% (50- and 100-mL bottles—BPL)

Plasma substitutes

Dextran, **gelatin**, and the **hydroxyethyl starch, tetrastarch**, are macromolecular substances which are metabolised slowly. Dextran and gelatin may be used at the outset to expand and maintain blood volume in shock arising from conditions such as burns or septicaemia; they may also be used as an immediate short-term measure to treat haemorrhage until blood is available. Dextran and gelatin are rarely needed when shock is due to sodium and water depletion because, in these circumstances, the shock responds to water and electrolyte repletion; see also section 2.7.1 for the management of shock. Hydroxyethyl starches should be used at the lowest effective dose for the shortest duration, and they should only be used for the treatment of hypovolaemia due to acute blood loss when crystalloids alone are not sufficient.

Plasma substitutes should **not** be used to maintain plasma volume in conditions such as burns or peritonitis where there is loss of plasma protein, water, and electrolytes over periods of several days or weeks. In these situations, plasma or plasma protein fractions containing large amounts of albumin should be given.

Large volumes of *some* plasma substitutes can increase the risk of bleeding through depletion of coagulation factors.

Dextran 70 by intravenous infusion is used for volume expansion. Dextran may interfere with blood group cross-matching or biochemical measurements, and these should be carried out before infusion is begun.

> Plasma and plasma substitutes are often used in very ill patients whose condition is unstable. Therefore, close monitoring is required and fluid and electrolyte therapy should be adjusted according to the patient's condition at all times. Treatment with hydroxyethyl starches should be guided by continuous haemodynamic monitoring so that the infusion is stopped as soon as appropriate haemodynamic goals have been achieved.

Cautions Plasma substitutes should be used with caution in patients with cardiac disease, severe liver disease, or renal impairment; urine output should be monitored. Care should be taken to avoid haematocrit concentration from falling below 25–30% and the patient should be monitored for hypersensitivity reactions.

Side-effects Hypersensitivity reactions may occur including, rarely, severe anaphylactic reactions. Transient increase in bleeding time may occur.

▋ **DEXTRAN 70**

Dextrans of weight average molecular weight about '70 000'

Indications short-term blood volume expansion

Cautions see notes above; can interfere with some laboratory tests (see also above); where possible, monitor central venous pressure

Hepatic impairment use with caution in severe impairment

Pregnancy avoid—reports of anaphylaxis in mother causing fetal anoxia, neurological damage and death

Side-effects see notes above

Dose
● See under preparation below

◢ **Hypertonic solution**

RescueFlow® (Pharmacosmos) [PoM]
Intravenous infusion, dextran 70 intravenous infusion 6% in sodium chloride intravenous infusion 7.5%. Net price 250-mL bag = £28.50
Cautions see notes above; severe hyperglycaemia and hyperosmolality
Dose initial treatment of hypovolaemia with hypotension induced by traumatic injury, by intravenous infusion over 2–5 minutes, 250 mL, followed immediately by administration of isotonic fluids

▋ **GELATIN**

Note The gelatin is partially degraded

Indications low blood volume (but see notes above)

Cautions see notes above

Hepatic impairment use with caution in severe impairment

Pregnancy manufacturer of *Geloplasma®* advises avoid at the end of pregnancy

Side-effects see notes above

Dose
● By intravenous infusion, initially 500–1000 mL of a 3.5–4% solution (see notes above)

Gelaspan (B. Braun) PoM

Intravenous infusion, succinylated gelatin (modified fluid gelatin, average molecular weight 26 500) 40 g, Na$^+$ 151 mmol, K$^+$ 4 mmol, Mg^{2+} 1 mmol, Cl$^-$ 103 mmol, Ca^{2+} 1 mmol, acetate 24 mmol/litre, net price 500-mL bag = £6.80, 1-litre bag = £13.60

Gelofusine® (B. Braun) PoM

Intravenous infusion, succinylated gelatin (modified fluid gelatin, average molecular weight 30 000) 40 g (4%), Na$^+$ 154 mmol, Cl$^-$ 120 mmol/litre, net price 500-mL *Ecobag®* = £4.83, 1-litre *Ecobag®* = £9.04

Geloplasma® (Fresenius Kabi) PoM

Intravenous infusion, partially hydrolysed and succinylated gelatin (modified liquid gelatin) (as anhydrous gelatin) 30 g (3%), Na$^+$ 150 mmol, K$^+$ 5 mmol, Mg^{2+} 1.5 mmol, Cl$^-$ 100 mmol, lactate 30 mmol/litre, net price 500-mL bag = £5.05

Isoplex® (Beacon) PoM

Intravenous infusion, succinylated gelatin (modified fluid gelatin, average molecular weight 30 000) 40 g (4%), Na$^+$ 145 mmol, K$^+$ 4 mmol, Mg^{2+} 0.9 mmol, Cl$^-$ 105 mmol, lactate 25 mmol/litre, net price 500-mL bag = £7.53, 1-litre bag = £14.54

Volplex® (Beacon) PoM

Intravenous infusion, succinylated gelatin (modified fluid gelatin, average molecular weight 30 000) 40 g (4%), Na$^+$ 154 mmol, Cl$^-$ 125 mmol/litre, net price 500-mL bag = £4.70, 1-litre bag = £9.09

▌ HYDROXYETHYL STARCH

A starch composed of more than 90% of amylopectin that has been etherified with hydroxyethyl groups; the term tetrastarch reflects the degree of etherification

Indications   low blood volume (but see notes above)

Cautions   see notes above; surgery; trauma; monitor renal function; children

Contra-indications   sepsis; burns; intracranial or cerebral haemorrhage; critically ill patients; hyperhydration; dehydration; pulmonary oedema; severe coagulopathy

Hepatic impairment   avoid in severe impairment

Renal impairment   avoid

Side-effects   see notes above; also pruritus, raised serum amylase

Dose

- See under preparations below

◀ **Tetrastarch**

Volulyte® (Fresenius Kabi) PoM

Intravenous infusion, hydroxyethyl starch (weight average molecular weight 130 000) 6% in sodium chloride intravenous infusion 0.6%, containing Na$^+$ 137 mmol, K$^+$ 4 mmol, Mg^{2+} 1.5 mmol, Cl$^-$ 110 mmol, acetate 34 mmol/litre, net price 500-mL bag = £18.00

Dose by intravenous infusion, up to 50 mL/kg daily (see notes above)

Voluven® (Fresenius Kabi) PoM

Intravenous infusion, hydroxyethyl starch (weight average molecular weight 130 000) 6% in sodium chloride intravenous infusion 0.9%, net price 500-mL bag = £12.50

Dose by intravenous infusion, up to 50 mL/kg daily (see notes above)

9.3   Intravenous nutrition

When adequate feeding through the alimentary tract is not possible, nutrients may be given by intravenous infusion. This may be in addition to ordinary oral or tube feeding—**supplemental parenteral nutrition**, or may be the sole source of nutrition—**total parenteral nutrition** (TPN). Indications for this method include preparation of undernourished patients for surgery, chemotherapy, or radiation therapy; severe or prolonged disorders of the gastro-intestinal tract; major surgery, trauma, or burns; prolonged coma or refusal to eat; and some patients with renal or hepatic failure. The composition of proprietary preparations available is given under Proprietary Infusion Fluids for Parenteral Feeding, p. 689.

Parenteral nutrition requires the use of a solution containing amino acids, glucose, fat, electrolytes, trace elements, and vitamins. This is now commonly provided by the pharmacy in the form of a 3-litre bag. A single dose of vitamin B$_{12}$, as hydroxocobalamin, is given by intramuscular injection; regular vitamin B$_{12}$ injections are not usually required unless total parenteral nutrition continues for many months. Folic acid is given in a dose of 15 mg once or twice each week, usually in the nutrition solution. Other vitamins are usually given daily; they are generally introduced in the parenteral nutrition solution. Alternatively, if the patient is able to take small amounts by mouth, vitamins may be given orally.

The nutrition solution is infused through a central venous catheter inserted under full surgical precautions. Alternatively, infusion through a peripheral vein may be used for supplementary as well as total parenteral nutrition for periods of up to a month, depending on the availability of peripheral veins; factors prolonging cannula life and preventing thrombophlebitis include the use of soft polyurethane paediatric cannulas and use of feeds of low osmolality and neutral pH. Only nutritional fluids should be given by the dedicated intravenous line.

Before starting, the patient should be well oxygenated with a near normal circulating blood volume and attention should be given to renal function and acid-base status. Appropriate biochemical tests should have been carried out beforehand and serious deficits corrected. Nutritional and electrolyte status must be monitored throughout treatment.

Complications of long-term parenteral nutrition include gall bladder sludging, gall stones, cholestasis and abnormal liver function tests. For details of the prevention and management of parenteral nutrition complications, specialist literature should be consulted.

Protein is given as mixtures of essential and non-essential synthetic L-amino acids. Ideally, all essential amino acids should be included with a wide variety of non-essential ones to provide sufficient nitrogen together with electrolytes (see also section 9.2.2). Solutions vary in their composition of amino acids; they often contain an energy source (usually glucose) and electrolytes.

Energy is provided in a ratio of 0.6 to 1.1 megajoules (150–250 kcals) per gram of protein nitrogen. Energy requirements must be met if amino acids are to be utilised for tissue maintenance. A mixture of carbohydrate and fat energy sources (usually 30–50% as fat) gives better utilisation of amino acids than glucose alone.

Glucose is the preferred source of carbohydrate, but if more than 180 g is given per day frequent monitoring of blood glucose is required, and insulin may be necessary. Glucose in various strengths from 10 to 50% must be infused through a central venous catheter to avoid thrombosis.

In parenteral nutrition regimens, it is necessary to provide adequate **phosphate** in order to allow phosphorylation of glucose and to prevent hypophosphataemia; between 20 and 30 mmol of phosphate is required daily.

Fructose and sorbitol have been used in an attempt to avoid the problem of hyperosmolar hyperglycaemic non-ketotic acidosis but other metabolic problems may occur, as with xylitol and ethanol which are now rarely used.

Fat emulsions have the advantages of a high energy to fluid volume ratio, neutral pH, and iso-osmolarity with plasma, and provide essential fatty acids. Several days of adaptation may be required to attain maximal utilisation. Reactions include occasional febrile episodes (usually only with 20% emulsions) and rare anaphylactic responses. Interference with biochemical measurements such as those for blood gases and calcium may occur if samples are taken before fat has been cleared. Daily checks are necessary to ensure complete clearance from the plasma in conditions where fat metabolism may be disturbed. **Additives should not be mixed with fat emulsions unless compatibility is known.**

> **Administration**
>
> Because of the complex requirements relating to parenteral nutrition full details relating to administration have been omitted. In all cases *product literature and other specialist literature should be consulted.*

Supplementary preparations

> Compatibility with the infusion solution must be ascertained before adding supplementary preparations.

Addiphos® (Fresenius Kabi) PoM
Solution, sterile, phosphate 40 mmol, K^+ 30 mmol, Na^+ 30 mmol/20 mL. For addition to *Vamin®* solutions and glucose intravenous infusions. Net price 20-mL vial = £1.30

Additrace® (Fresenius Kabi) PoM
Solution, trace elements for addition to *Vamin®* solutions and glucose intravenous infusions, traces of Fe^{3+}, Zn^{2+}, Mn^{2+}, Cu^{2+}, Cr^{3+}, Se^{4+}, Mo^{6+}, F^-, I^-. For adults and children over 40 kg. Net price 10-mL amp = £1.96

Cernevit® (Baxter) PoM
Solution, *dl*-alpha tocopherol 11.2 units, ascorbic acid 125 mg, biotin 69 micrograms, colecalciferol 220 units, cyanocobalamin 6 micrograms, folic acid 414 micrograms, glycine 250 mg, nicotinamide 46 mg, pantothenic acid (as dexpanthenol) 17.25 mg, pyridoxine hydrochloride 5.5 mg, retinol (as palmitate) 3500 units, riboflavin (as dihydrated sodium phosphate) 4.14 mg, thiamine (as cocarboxylase tet-

rahydrate) 3.51 mg. Dissolve in 5 mL water for injections. Net price per vial = £4.64

Decan® (Baxter) PoM
Solution, trace elements for addition to infusion solutions, Fe^{2+}, Zn^{2+}, Cu^{2+}, Mn^{2+}, F^-, Co^{2+}, I^-, Se^{4+}, Mo^{6+}, Cr^{3+}. For adults over 40 kg. Net price 40-mL vial = £2.00

Dipeptiven® (Fresenius Kabi) PoM
Solution, $N(2)$-L-alanyl-L-glutamine 200 mg/mL (providing L-alanine 82 mg, L-glutamine 134.6 mg). For addition to infusion solutions containing amino acids. Net price 50 mL = £13.94, 100 mL = £25.93
Dose amino acid supplement for hypercatabolic or hypermetabolic states, 300–400 mg/kg daily; max. 400 mg/kg daily, dose not to exceed 20% of total amino acid intake

Glycophos® Sterile Concentrate (Fresenius Kabi) PoM
Solution, sterile, phosphate 20 mmol, Na^+ 40 mmol/20 mL. For addition to *Vamin®* and *Vaminolact®* solutions, and glucose intravenous infusions. Net price 20-mL vial = £3.91

Peditrace® (Fresenius Kabi) PoM
Solution, trace elements for addition to *Vaminolact®*, *Vamin® 14 Electrolyte-Free* solutions and glucose intravenous infusions, traces of Zn^{2+}, Cu^{2+}, Mn^{2+}, Se^{4+}, F^-, I^-. For use in neonates (when kidney function established, usually second day of life), infants, and children. Net price 10-mL vial = £3.55
Cautions reduced biliary excretion especially in cholestatic liver disease or in markedly reduced urinary excretion (careful biochemical monitoring required); total parenteral nutrition exceeding 1 month (measure serum manganese concentration and check liver function before commencing treatment and regularly during treatment)—discontinue if manganese concentration raised or if cholestasis develops

Solivito N® (Fresenius Kabi) PoM
Solution, powder for reconstitution, biotin 60 micrograms, cyanocobalamin 5 micrograms, folic acid 400 micrograms, glycine 300 mg, nicotinamide 40 mg, pyridoxine hydrochloride 4.9 mg, riboflavin sodium phosphate 4.9 mg, sodium ascorbate 113 mg, sodium pantothenate 16.5 mg, thiamine mononitrate 3.1 mg. Dissolve in water for injections or glucose intravenous infusion or *Intralipid®*; dissolve in *Vitlipid N®* or *Intralipid®* for adding to *Intralipid®* only. Net price per vial = £1.97

Tracutil® (B. Braun) PoM
Solution, trace elements for addition to infusion solutions, Fe^{2+}, Zn^{2+}, Mn^{2+}, Cu^{2+}, Cr^{3+}, Se^{4+}, Mo^{6+}, I^-, F^-. For adults. Net price 10-mL amp = 80p

Vitlipid N® (Fresenius Kabi) PoM
Emulsion, adult, vitamin A 330 units, ergocalciferol 20 units, *dl*-alpha tocopherol 1 unit, phytomenadione 15 micrograms/mL. For addition to *Intralipid®*. For adults and children over 11 years. Net price 10-mL amp = £1.97
Emulsion, infant, vitamin A 230 units, ergocalciferol 40 units, *dl*-alpha tocopherol 0.7 unit, phytomenadione 20 micrograms/mL. For addition to *Intralipid®*. Net price 10-mL amp = £1.97

Proprietary Infusion Fluids for Parenteral Feeding

Preparation	Nitrogen g/litre	[1,2]Energy kJ/litre	Electrolytes mmol/litre					Other components/litre
			K$^+$	Mg^{2+}	Na$^+$	Acet$^-$	Cl$^-$	
Aminoplasmal 5% E (B. Braun) Net price 500 mL = £9.02	8	—	25	2.6	43	59	29	dihydrogen phosphate 9 mmol, malic acid 1.01 g
Aminoplasmal 10% (B. Braun) Net price 500 mL = £17.06	16	—	—	—	—	—	57	—
Aminoven 25 (Fresenius Kabi) Net price 500 mL = £23.20	25.7	—	—	—	—	—	—	—
Clinimix N9G20E (Baxter) Net price (dual compartment bag of amino acids with electrolytes 1000 mL and glucose 20% with calcium 1000 mL) = £29.00	4.6	1680	30	2.5	35	50	40	Ca^{2+} 2.3 mmol, phosphate 15 mmol, anhydrous glucose 100 g
Clinimix N14G30E (Baxter) Net price (dual compartment bag of amino acids with electrolytes 1000 mL and glucose 30% with calcium 1000 mL) = £33.00	7	2520	30	2.5	35	70	40	Ca^{2+} 2.3 mmol, phosphate 15 mmol, anhydrous glucose 150 g
ClinOleic 20% (Baxter) Net price 100 mL = £6.28; 250 mL = £10.08; 500 mL = £13.88	—	8360	—	—	—	—	—	purified olive and soya oil 200 g, glycerol 22.5 g, egg phosphatides 12 g
Glamin (Fresenius Kabi) Net price 250 mL = £14.58; 500 mL = £27.20	22.4	—	—	—	—	62	—	—
Hyperamine 30 (B. Braun) Net price 500 mL = £23.67	30	—	—	—	5	—	—	—
Intralipid 10% (Fresenius Kabi) Net price 100 mL = £4.85; 500 mL = £10.60	—	4600	—	—	—	—	—	soya oil 100 g, glycerol 22 g, purified egg phospholipids 12 g, phosphate 15 mmol
Intralipid 20% (Fresenius Kabi) Net price 100 mL = £7.30; 250 mL = £11.95; 500 mL = £15.90	—	8400	—	—	—	—	—	soya oil 200 g, glycerol 22 g, purified egg phospholipids 12 g, phosphate 15 mmol
Intralipid 30% (Fresenius Kabi) Net price 333 mL = £17.80	—	12600	—	—	—	—	—	soya oil 300 g, glycerol 16.7 g, purified egg phospholipids 12 g, phosphate 15 mmol
Kabiven (Fresenius Kabi) Net price (triple compartment bag of amino acids and electrolytes 300 mL, 450 mL, 600 mL, or 750 mL; glucose 526 mL, 790 mL, 1053 mL, or 1316 mL; lipid emulsion 200 mL, 300 mL, 400 mL, or 500 mL) 1026 mL = £35.00, 1540 mL = £50.00, 2053 mL = £67.00, 2566 mL = £70.00	5.3	3275	23	4	31	38	45	Ca^{2+} 2 mmol, phosphate 9.7 mmol, anhydrous glucose 97 g, soya oil 39 g
Kabiven Peripheral (Fresenius Kabi) Net price (triple compartment bag of amino acids and electrolytes 300 mL, 400 mL, or 500 mL; glucose 885 mL, 1180 mL, or 1475 mL; lipid emulsion 255 mL, 340 mL, or 425 mL) 1440 mL = £35.00, 1920 mL = £50.00, 2400 mL = £64.00	3.75	2625	17	2.8	22	27	33	Ca^{2+} 1.4 mmol, phosphate 7.5 mmol, anhydrous glucose 67.5 g, soya oil 35.4 g
Lipidem (B. Braun) Net price 100 mL = £19.11; 250 mL = £31.85; 500 mL = £40.34	—	7900	—	—	—	—	—	omega-3-acid triglycerides 20 g, soya oil 80 g, medium-chain triglycerides 100 g
Lipofundin MCT/LCT 10% (B. Braun) Net price 100 mL = £7.70; 500 mL = £13.70	—	4430	—	—	—	—	—	soya oil 50 g, medium-chain triglycerides 50 g
Lipofundin MCT/LCT 20% (B. Braun) Net price 100 mL = £13.28; 250 mL = £11.30; 500 mL = £20.36	—	8000	—	—	—	—	—	soya oil 100 g, medium-chain triglycerides 100 g

1. *Note.* 1000 kcal = 4200 kJ; 1000 kJ = 238.8 kcal. All entries are PoM
2. Excludes protein- or amino acid-derived energy

Preparation	Nitrogen g/litre	[1,2]Energy kJ/litre	Electrolytes mmol/litre					Other components/litre
			K⁺	Mg²⁺	Na⁺	Acet⁻	Cl⁻	

Preparation	Nitrogen g/litre	Energy kJ/litre	K⁺	Mg²⁺	Na⁺	Acet⁻	Cl⁻	Other components/litre
Nutriflex basal (B. Braun) Net price (dual compartment bag of amino acids 400 mL or 800 mL; glucose 600 mL or 1200 mL) 1000 mL = £25.00, 2000 mL = £29.20	4.6	2095	30	5.7	49.9	35	50	Ca²⁺ 3.6 mmol, acid phosphate 12.8 mmol, anhydrous glucose 125 g
Nutriflex peri (B. Braun) Net price (dual compartment bag of amino acids 400 mL or 800 mL; glucose 600 mL or 1200 mL) 1000 mL = £26.00, 2000 mL = £30.47	5.7	1340	15	4	27	19.5	31.6	Ca²⁺ 2.5 mmol, acid phosphate 5.7 mmol, anhydrous glucose 80 g
Nutriflex plus (B. Braun) Net price (dual compartment bag of amino acids 400 mL or 800 mL; glucose 600 mL or 1200 mL) 1000 mL = £27.20, 2000 mL = £33.02	6.8	2510	25	5.7	37.2	22.9	35.5	Ca²⁺ 3.6 mmol, acid phosphate 20 mmol, anhydrous glucose 150 g
Nutriflex special (B. Braun) Net price (dual compartment bag of amino acids 500 mL or 750 mL; glucose 500 mL or 750 mL) 1000 mL = £28.60, 1500 mL = £27.60	10	4020	25.7	5	40.5	22	49.5	Ca²⁺ 4.1 mmol, acid phosphate 14.7 mmol, anhydrous glucose 240 g
NuTRIflex Lipid peri (B. Braun) Net price (triple compartment bag of amino acids 500 mL, 750 mL or 1000 mL; glucose 500 mL, 750 mL or 1000 mL; lipid emulsion 20% 250 mL, 375 mL or 500 mL) 1250 mL = £42.83, 1875 mL = £54.37, 2500 mL = £64.22	4.56	2664	24	2.4	40	32	38.4	Ca²⁺ 2.4 mmol, Zn²⁺ 24 micromol, phosphate 6 mmol, anhydrous glucose 64 g, soya oil 20 g, medium-chain triglycerides 20 g
NuTRIflex Lipid plus (B. Braun) Net price (triple compartment bag of amino acids 500 mL, 750 mL or 1000 mL; glucose 500 mL, 750 mL or 1000 mL; lipid emulsion 20% 250 mL, 375 mL or 500 mL) 1250 mL = £46.56, 1875 mL = £59.46, 2500 mL = £68.39	5.44	3600	28	3.2	40	36	36	Ca²⁺ 3.2 mmol, Zn²⁺ 24 micromol, phosphate 12 mmol, anhydrous glucose 120 g, soya oil 20 g, medium-chain triglycerides 20 g
NuTRIflex Lipid plus without Electrolytes (B. Braun) Net price (triple compartment bag of amino acids 500 mL, 750 mL or 1000 mL; glucose 500 mL, 750 mL or 1000 mL; lipid emulsion 20% 250 mL, 375 mL or 500 mL) 1250 mL = £46.56, 1875 mL = £59.45, 2500 mL = £68.39	5.44	3600	—	—	—	—	—	anhydrous glucose 120 g, soya oil 20 g, medium-chain triglycerides 20 g
NuTRIflex Lipid special (B. Braun) Net price (triple compartment bag of amino acids 500 mL, 750 mL or 1000 mL; glucose 500 mL, 750 mL or 1000 mL; lipid emulsion 20% 250 mL, 375 mL or 500 mL) 1250 mL = £56.96, 1875 mL = £74.62, 2500 mL = £83.00	8	4004	37.6	4.24	53.6	48	48	Ca²⁺ 4.24 mmol, Zn²⁺ 32 micromol, phosphate 16 mmol, anhydrous glucose 144 g, soya oil 20 g, medium-chain triglycerides 20 g

9 Nutrition and blood

1. *Note.* 1000 kcal = 4200 kJ; 1000 kJ = 238.8 kcal. All entries are (PoM)
2. Excludes protein- or amino acid-derived energy

Preparation	Nitrogen g/litre	[1,2]Energy kJ/litre	Electrolytes mmol/litre					Other components/litre
			K^+	Mg^{2+}	Na^+	$Acet^-$	Cl^-	
NuTRIflex Lipid special without Electrolytes (B. Braun) Net price (triple compartment bag of amino acids 500 mL, 750 mL or 1000 mL; glucose 500 mL, 750 mL or 1000 mL; lipid emulsion 20% 250 mL, 375 mL or 500 mL) 1250 mL = £56.96, 1875 mL = £74.62, 2500 mL = £79.80	8	4004	–	–	–	–	–	anhydrous glucose 144 g, soya oil 20 g, medium-chain triglycerides 20 g
NuTRIflex Omega plus (B. Braun) Net price (triple compartment bag of amino acids 500 mL, 750 mL or 1000 mL; glucose 500 mL, 750 mL or 1000 mL; lipid emulsion 250 mL, 375 mL or 500 mL) 1250 mL= £47.43, 1875 mL= £60.57, 2500 mL = £69.66	5.4	3600	28	3.2	40	36	36	Ca^{2+} 3.2 mmol, Zn^{2+} 24 micromol, phosphate 12 mmol, anhydrous glucose 120 g, refined soya oil 16 g, medium-chain triglycerides 20 g, omega-3-acid triglycerides 4 g
NuTRIflex Omega special (B. Braun) Net price (triple compartment bag of amino acids 250 mL, 500 mL, 750 mL or 1000 mL; glucose 250 mL, 500 mL, 750 mL or 1000 mL; lipid emulsion 125 mL, 250 mL, 375 mL or 500 mL) 625 mL = £43.62, 1250 mL= £59.02, 1875 mL= £76.01, 2500 mL = £89.71	8	4004	37.6	4.24	53.6	48	48	Ca^{2+} 4.24 mmol, Zn^{2+} 30 micromol, phosphate 16 mmol, anhydrous glucose 144 g, refined soya oil 16 g, medium-chain triglycerides 20 g, omega-3-acid triglycerides 4 g
OliClinomel N4-550E (Baxter) Net price (triple compartment bag of amino acids with electrolytes 1000 mL; glucose 20% 1000 mL; lipid emulsion 10% 500 mL) 2500 mL = £69.30	3.6	2184	16	2.2	21	30	33	Ca^{2+} 2 mmol, phosphate 8.5 mmol, refined olive and soya oil 20 g, anhydrous glucose 80 g
OliClinomel N4-720E (Baxter) Net price (triple compartment bag of amino acids with electrolytes 1000 mL; glucose 20% 1000 mL; lipid emulsion 20% 500 mL) 2500 mL = £69.30	3.64	3024	24	2	28	40	40	Ca^{2+} 1.8 mmol, phosphate 8 mmol, refined olive and soya oil 40 g, anhydrous glucose 80 g
OliClinomel N5-800E (Baxter) Net price (triple compartment bag of amino acids with electrolytes 800 mL or 1000 mL; glucose 25% 800 mL or 1000 mL; lipid emulsion 20% 400 mL or 500 mL) 2000 mL = £60.39, 2500 mL = £65.34	4.6	3360	24	2.2	32	49	44	Ca^{2+} 2 mmol, phosphate 10 mmol, refined olive and soya oil 40 g, anhydrous glucose 100 g
OliClinomel N6-900E (Baxter) Net price (triple compartment bag of amino acids with electrolytes 800 mL or 1000 mL; glucose 30% 800 mL or 1000 mL; lipid emulsion 20% 400 mL or 500 mL) 2000 mL = £70.40, 2500 mL = £75.90	5.6	3696	24	2.2	32	53	46	Ca^{2+} 2 mmol, phosphate 10 mmol, refined olive and soya oil 40 g, anhydrous glucose 120 g
OliClinomel N7-1000 (Baxter) Net price (triple compartment bag of amino acids 600 mL; glucose 40% 600 mL; lipid emulsion 20% 300 mL) 1500 mL = £43.70	6.6	4368	–	–	–	37	16	phosphate 3 mmol, refined olive and soya oil 40 g, anhydrous glucose 160 g
OliClinomel N7-1000E (Baxter) Net price (triple compartment bag of amino acids with electrolytes 800 mL; glucose 40% 800 mL; lipid emulsion 20% 400 mL) 2000 mL = £66.33	6.6	4368	24	2.2	32	57	48	Ca^{2+} 2 mmol, phosphate 10 mmol, refined olive and soya oil 40 g, anhydrous glucose 160 g

9 **Nutrition and blood**

1. *Note.* 1000 kcal = 4200 kJ; 1000 kJ = 238.8 kcal. All entries are PoM
2. Excludes protein- or amino acid-derived energy

Preparation	Nitrogen g/litre	[1,2]Energy kJ/litre	Electrolytes mmol/litre					Other components/litre
			K⁺	Mg²⁺	Na⁺	Acet⁻	Cl⁻	

Preparation	Nitrogen g/litre	Energy kJ/litre	K⁺	Mg²⁺	Na⁺	Acet⁻	Cl⁻	Other components/litre
OliClinomel N8-800 (Baxter) Net price (triple compartment bag of amino acids 800 mL; glucose 31.25% 800 mL; lipid emulsion 15% 400 mL) 2000 mL = £77.10	8.25	3360	—	—	—	42.5	20	phosphate 2.25 mmol, refined olive and soya oil 30 g, anhydrous glucose 125 g
Omegaven (Fresenius Kabi) Net price 100 mL = £22.50	—	4700	—	—	—	—	—	highly refined fish oil 100 g, glycerol 25 g, egg phosphatide 12 g
Plasma-Lyte 148 (water) (Baxter) Net price 1000 mL = £1.59	—		5	1.5	140	27	98	gluconate 23 mmol
Plasma-Lyte 148 (dextrose 5%) (Baxter) Net price 1000 mL = £1.59	—	840	5	1.5	140	27	98	gluconate 23 mmol, anhydrous glucose 50 g
Plasma-Lyte M (dextrose 5%) (Baxter) Net price 1000 mL = £1.33	—	840	16	1.5	40	12	40	Ca²⁺ 2.5 mmol, lactate 12 mmol, anhydrous glucose 50 g
[3]Primene 10% (Baxter) Net price 100 mL = £5.78, 250 mL = £7.92	15	—	—	—	—	—	19	—
SMOFlipid (Fresenius Kabi) Net price 500 mL = £20.50	—	8400	—	—	—	—	—	fish oil 30 g, olive oil 50 g, soya oil 60 g, medium-chain triglycerides 60 g
StructoKabiven Electrolyte Free (Fresenius Kabi) Net price (triple compartment bag of amino acids 500 mL, 750 mL or 1000 mL; glucose 42% 298 mL, 446 mL or 595 mL; lipid emulsion 188 mL, 281 mL or 375 mL) 986 mL = £66.50, 1477 mL = £69.00, 1970 mL = £74.00	8	3685	—	—	—	74.5	—	phosphate 2.8 mmol, anhydrous glucose 127 g, glycerol 4.23 g, egg phospholipids 4.56 g, purified structured triglyceride 38.5 g (contains coconut oil, palm kernel oil and soya oil triglycerides)
Structolipid 20% (Fresenius Kabi) Net price 500 mL = £16.09	—	8200	—	—	—	—	—	purified structured triglyceride 200 g (contains coconut oil, palm kernel oil, and soya oil triglycerides)
Synthamin 9 (Baxter) Net price 500 mL = £6.66; 1000 mL = £12.34	9.1		60	5	70	100	70	acid phosphate 30 mmol
Synthamin 9 EF (electrolyte-free) (Baxter) Net price 500 mL = £6.66; 1000 mL = £12.34	9.1		—	—	—	44	22	—
Synthamin 14 (Baxter) Net price 500 mL = £9.64; 1000 mL = £17.13; 3000 mL = £48.98	14		60	5	70	140	70	acid phosphate 30 mmol
Synthamin 14 EF (electrolyte–free) (Baxter) Net price 500 mL = £9.87; 1000 mL = £17.51	14		—	—	—	68	34	—
Synthamin 17 (Baxter) Net price 500 mL = £12.66; 1000 mL = £23.00	16.5		60	5	70	150	70	acid phosphate 30 mmol
Synthamin 17 EF (electrolyte–free) (Baxter) Net price 500 mL = £12.66; 1000 mL = £23.00	16.5		—	—	—	82	40	—
Vamin 9 Glucose (Fresenius Kabi) Net price 100 mL = £3.90; 500 mL = £7.95; 1000 mL = £13.80	9.4	1700	20	1.5	50	—	50	Ca²⁺ 2.5 mmol, anhydrous glucose 100 g
Vamin 14 (Fresenius Kabi) Net price 500 mL = £11.15; 1000 mL = £18.85	13.5	—	50	8	100	135	100	Ca²⁺ 5 mmol, SO₄²⁻ 8 mmol

1. *Note.* 1000 kcal = 4200 kJ; 1000 kJ = 238.8 kcal. All entries are (PoM)
2. Excludes protein- or amino acid-derived energy
3. For use in neonates and children only

Preparation	Nitrogen g/litre	[1,2]Energy kJ/litre	Electrolytes mmol/litre					Other components/litre
			K⁺	Mg²⁺	Na⁺	Acet⁻	Cl⁻	
Vamin 14 (Electrolyte-Free) (Fresenius Kabi) Net price 500 mL = £10.80; 1000 mL = £18.30	13.5	—	—	—	—	90	—	—
Vamin 18 (Electrolyte-Free) (Fresenius Kabi) Net price 500 mL = £13.70; 1000 mL = £26.70	18	—	—	—	—	110	—	—
[3]Vaminolact (Fresenius Kabi) Net price 100 mL = £4.35; 500 mL = £10.00	9.3	—	—	—	—	—	—	—

1. *Note.* 1000 kcal = 4200 kJ; 1000 kJ = 238.8 kcal. All entries are PoM
2. Excludes protein- or amino acid-derived energy
3. For use in neonates and children only

9.4 Oral nutrition

9.4.1 Foods for special diets
9.4.2 Enteral nutrition

9.4.1 Foods for special diets

These are preparations that have been modified to eliminate a particular constituent from a food or that are nutrient mixtures formulated as food substitutes for patients who either cannot tolerate or cannot metabolise certain common constituents of food. In certain clinical conditions, some food preparations are regarded as drugs and can be prescribed within the NHS if they have been approved by the Advisory Committee on Borderline Substances (ACBS)—see Appendix 2.

Phenylketonuria Phenylketonuria (hyperphenylalaninaemia), PKU, which results from the inability to metabolise phenylalanine, is managed by restricting dietary intake of phenylalanine to a small amount sufficient for tissue building and repair.

Sapropterin, a synthetic form of tetrahydrobiopterin, is licensed as an adjunct to dietary restriction of phenylalanine in the management of patients with phenylketonuria and tetrahydrobiopterin deficiency.

Aspartame (used as a sweetener in some foods and medicines) contributes to the phenylalanine intake and may affect control of phenylketonuria. Where the presence of aspartame is specified in the product literature this is indicated in the BNF against the preparation; the patient should be informed of this.

Coeliac disease Intolerance to gluten in coeliac disease is managed by completely eliminating gluten from the diet. A range of gluten-free products is available for prescription—see Appendix 2, p. 1042.

SAPROPTERIN DIHYDROCHLORIDE

Note Sapropterin is a synthetic form of tetrahydrobiopterin

Indications see under Dose below

Cautions monitor blood-phenylalanine concentration before and after first week of treatment—if unsatisfactory response increase dose at weekly intervals to max. dose and monitor blood-phenylalanine concentration weekly; discontinue treatment if unsatisfactory response after 1 month; monitor blood-phenylalanine and tyrosine concentrations 1–2 weeks after dose adjustment and during treatment; history of convulsions

Hepatic impairment manufacturer advises caution—no information available

Renal impairment manufacturer advises caution—no information available

Pregnancy manufacturer advises caution—consider only if strict dietary management inadequate

Breast-feeding manufacturer advises avoid—no information available

Side-effects diarrhoea, vomiting, abdominal pain, nasal congestion, cough, pharyngolaryngeal pain, headache; *also reported* hypersensitivity reactions

Dose
- Phenylketonuria (specialist use only), by mouth, ADULT and CHILD over 4 years, initially 10 mg/kg once daily, preferably in the morning, adjusted according to response; usual dose 5–20 mg/kg daily
- Tetrahydrobiopterin deficiency (specialist use only), by mouth, ADULT and CHILD initially 2–5 mg/kg once daily, preferably in the morning, adjusted according to response; max. 20 mg/kg daily; total daily dose may alternatively be given in 2–3 divided doses

Kuvan® (Merck Serono) PoM
Dispersible tablets, sapropterin dihydrochloride 100 mg, net price 30-tab pack = £597.22, 120-tab pack = £2388.88. Label: 13, 21
Counselling Tablets should be dissolved in water and taken within 20 minutes

9.4.2 Enteral nutrition

The body's reserves of protein rapidly become exhausted in severely ill patients, especially during chronic illness or in those with severe burns, extensive trauma, pancreatitis, or intestinal fistula. Much can be achieved by frequent meals and by persuading the patient to take supplementary snacks of ordinary food between the meals.

However, extra calories, protein, other nutrients, and vitamins are often best given by supplementing ordinary meals with enteral sip or tube feeds (preparations, see Appendix 2).

When patients cannot feed normally, for example, patients with severe facial injury, oesophageal obstruction, or coma, a nutritionally complete diet of enteral

9

Nutrition and blood

feeds must be given. The advice of a dietitian should be sought to determine the protein and total energy requirement of the patient and the form and relative contribution of carbohydrate and fat to the energy requirements.

Most enteral feeds contain protein derived from cows' milk or soya. Elemental feeds containing protein hydrolysates or free amino acids can be used for patients who have diminished ability to break down protein, for example in inflammatory bowel disease or pancreatic insufficiency.

Even when nutritionally complete feeds are given, water and electrolyte balance should be monitored. Haematological and biochemical parameters should also be monitored, particularly in clinically unstable patients. Extra minerals (e.g. magnesium and zinc) may be needed in patients where gastro-intestinal secretions are being lost. Additional vitamins may also be needed. Feeds containing vitamin K may affect the INR in patients receiving warfarin—see **interactions**: Appendix 1 (vitamins).

Children   Children have special requirements and in most situations liquid feeds prepared for adults are totally unsuitable—the advice of a paediatric dietitian should be sought; see also *BNF for Children*, section 9.4.2

◢**Preparations**

See Borderline Substances, Appendix 2.

9.5 Minerals

9.5.1 Calcium and magnesium
9.5.2 Phosphorus
9.5.3 Fluoride
9.5.4 Zinc
9.5.5 Selenium

See section 9.1.1 for iron salts.

9.5.1 Calcium and magnesium

9.5.1.1 Calcium supplements
9.5.1.2 Hypercalcaemia and hypercalciuria
9.5.1.3 Magnesium

9.5.1.1 Calcium supplements

Calcium supplements are usually only required where dietary calcium intake is deficient. This dietary requirement varies with age and is relatively greater in childhood, pregnancy, and lactation, due to an increased demand, and in old age, due to impaired absorption. In osteoporosis, a calcium intake which is double the recommended amount reduces the rate of bone loss. If the actual dietary intake is less than the recommended amount, a supplement of as much as 40 mmol is appropriate, see also Osteoporosis, p. 521 and Vitamin D, p. 703.

In severe acute hypocalcaemia or hypocalcaemic tetany, an initial slow intravenous injection of 10–20 mL of calcium gluconate injection 10% (providing approximately 2.25–4.5 mmol of calcium) should be given, with plasma-calcium and ECG monitoring (risk of arrhythmias if given too rapidly), and either repeated

as required or, if only temporary improvement, followed by a continuous intravenous infusion to prevent recurrence. For infusion, dilute 100 mL of calcium gluconate 10% in 1 litre of glucose 5% or sodium chloride 0.9% and give at an initial rate of 50 mL/hour adjusted according to response. Calcium chloride injection is also available, but is more irritant; care should be taken to prevent extravasation. Oral supplements of calcium and vitamin D may also be required in persistent hypocalcaemia (see also section 9.6.4). Concurrent hypomagnesaemia should be corrected with **magnesium sulphate** (section 9.5.1.3).

For the role of calcium gluconate in temporarily reducing the toxic effects of hyperkalaemia, see p. 680.

▌ CALCIUM SALTS

Indications   see notes above; calcium deficiency

Cautions   sarcoidosis; history of nephrolithiasis; avoid calcium chloride in respiratory acidosis or respiratory failure; **interactions**: Appendix 1 (antacids, calcium salts)

Contra-indications   conditions associated with hypercalcaemia and hypercalciuria (e.g. some forms of malignant disease)

Renal impairment   use with caution (but see also Calcium Gluconate injection, below)

Side-effects   *rarely* gastro-intestinal disturbances; *with injection*, bradycardia, arrhythmias, peripheral vasodilatation, fall in blood pressure, sweating, injection-site reactions, severe tissue damage with extravasation

Dose

● By mouth, daily in divided doses, see notes above
● By slow intravenous injection, acute hypocalcaemia, see notes above; CHILD see *BNF for Children*
● By continuous intravenous infusion, acute hypocalcaemia, see notes above

◢**Oral preparations**

Calcium Gluconate (Non-proprietary)
Effervescent tablets, calcium gluconate 1 g (calcium 89 mg or Ca^{2+} 2.23 mmol), net price 28-tab pack = £15.68. Label: 13
Note   Each tablet usually contains 4.46 mmol Na$^+$

Calcium Lactate (Non-proprietary)
Tablets, calcium lactate 300 mg (calcium 39 mg or Ca^{2+} 1 mmol), net price 84 = £4.57

Adcal® (ProStrakan)
Chewable tablets, fruit flavour, calcium carbonate 1.5 g (calcium 600 mg or Ca^{2+} 15 mmol), net price 100-tab pack = £8.70. Label: 24

Cacit® (Warner Chilcott)
Tablets, effervescent, pink, calcium carbonate 1.25 g, providing calcium citrate when dispersed in water (calcium 500 mg or Ca^{2+} 12.5 mmol), net price 76-tab pack = £11.81. Label: 13

Calcichew® (Takeda)
Tablets (chewable), orange flavour, calcium carbonate 1.25 g (calcium 500 mg or Ca^{2+} 12.5 mmol), net price 100-tab pack = £9.33. Label: 24
Forte tablets (chewable), orange flavour, scored, calcium carbonate 2.5 g (calcium 1 g or Ca^{2+} 25 mmol), net price 60-tab pack = £13.16. Label: 24
Excipients   include aspartame (section 9.4.1)

Nutrition and blood

9

Calcium-500 (Martindale)
Tablets, pink, f/c, calcium carbonate 1.25 g (calcium 500 mg or Ca^{2+} 12.5 mmol), net price 100-tab pack = £9.46. Label: 25

Calcium-Sandoz® (Alliance)
Syrup, orange flavour, calcium glubionate 1.09 g, calcium lactobionate 727 mg (calcium 108.3 mg or Ca^{2+} 2.7 mmol)/5 mL, net price 300 mL = £4.07

Sandocal® (Novartis Consumer Health)
Sandocal 1000 tablets, effervescent, orange flavour, calcium lactate gluconate 2.263 g, calcium carbonate 1.75 g, providing 1 g calcium (Ca^{2+} 25 mmol), net price 3 × 10-tab pack = £7.95. Label: 13
Excipients include aspartame (section 9.4.1)

◢**Parenteral preparations**

Calcium Gluconate (Non-proprietary) [PoM]
Injection, calcium gluconate 10% (Ca^{2+} approx. 225 micromol/mL), net price 10-mL amp = 65p
Note The MHRA has advised that repeated or prolonged administration of calcium gluconate injection packaged in 10 mL *glass* containers is contra-indicated in children under 18 years and in patients with renal impairment owing to the risk of aluminium accumulation; in these patients the use of calcium gluconate injection packaged in *plastic* containers is recommended

Calcium Chloride (Non-proprietary) [PoM]
Injection, calcium chloride dihydrate 10% (calcium 27.3 mg or Ca^{2+} 680 micromol/mL), net price 10-mL disposable syringe = £6.94
Brands include *Minijet® Calcium Chloride 10%*
Injection, calcium chloride dihydrate 13.4% (calcium 36 mg or Ca^{2+} 910 micromol/mL), net price 10-mL amp = £14.94

◢**With vitamin D**
Section 9.6.4

◢**With risedronate sodium and colecalciferol**
Section 6.6.2

9.5.1.2 Hypercalcaemia and hypercalciuria

Severe hypercalcaemia Severe hypercalcaemia calls for urgent treatment before detailed investigation of the cause. Dehydration should be corrected first with intravenous infusion of **sodium chloride 0.9%**. Drugs (such as thiazides and vitamin D compounds) which promote hypercalcaemia, should be discontinued and dietary calcium should be restricted.

If *severe hypercalcaemia persists* drugs which inhibit mobilisation of calcium from the skeleton may be required. The **bisphosphonates** are useful and pamidronate disodium (section 6.6.2) is probably the most effective.

Corticosteroids (section 6.3) are widely given, but may only be useful where hypercalcaemia is due to sarcoidosis or vitamin D intoxication; they often take several days to achieve the desired effect.

Calcitonin (section 6.6.1) can be used for the treatment of hypercalcaemia associated with malignancy; it is rarely effective where bisphosphonates have failed to reduce serum calcium adequately.

After treatment of severe hypercalcaemia the underlying cause must be established. *Further treatment* is governed by the same principles as for initial therapy.

Salt and water depletion and drugs promoting hypercalcaemia should be avoided; oral administration of a bisphosphonate may be useful.

Hyperparathyroidism Cinacalcet is licensed for the treatment of secondary hyperparathyroidism in dialysis patients with end-stage renal disease (but see NICE guidance below), for primary hyperparathyroidism in patients where parathyroidectomy is inappropriate, and for the treatment of hypercalcaemia in parathyroid carcinoma. Cinacalcet reduces parathyroid hormone which leads to a decrease in serum calcium concentrations.

Paricalcitol (section 9.6.4) is also licensed for the prevention and treatment of secondary hyperparathyroidism associated with chronic renal failure.

Parathyroidectomy may be indicated for hyperparathyroidism.

> **NICE guidance**
> **Cinacalcet for the treatment of secondary hyperparathyroidism in patients with end-stage renal disease on maintenance dialysis therapy (January 2007)**
> Cinacalcet is not recommended for the routine treatment of secondary hyperparathyroidism in patients with end-stage renal disease on maintenance dialysis therapy.
> Cinacalcet is recommended for the treatment of refractory secondary hyperparathyroidism in patients with end-stage renal disease (including those with calciphylaxis) **only** in those:
> - who have 'very uncontrolled' plasma concentration of intact parathyroid hormone (defined as greater than 85 picomol/litre) refractory to standard therapy, and a normal or high adjusted serum calcium concentration, **and**
> - in whom surgical parathyroidectomy is contraindicated, in that the risks of surgery outweigh the benefits.
>
> Response to treatment should be monitored regularly and treatment should be continued only if a reduction in the plasma concentration of intact parathyroid hormone of 30% or greater is seen within 4 months of treatment.
> www.nice.org.uk/TA117

Hypercalciuria Hypercalciuria should be investigated for an underlying cause, which should be treated. Where a cause is not identified (idiopathic hypercalciuria), the condition is managed by increasing fluid intake and giving bendroflumethiazide in a dose of 2.5 mg daily (a higher dose is not usually necessary). Reducing dietary calcium intake may be beneficial but severe restriction of calcium intake has not proved beneficial and may even be harmful.

◢ CINACALCET

Indications see under Dose and notes above

Cautions measure serum-calcium concentration before initiation of treatment and within 1 week after starting treatment or adjusting dose, then monthly for secondary hyperparathyroidism and every 2–3 months for primary hyperparathyroidism and parathyroid carcinoma; treatment should not be initiated in patients with hypocalcaemia; in secondary hyperparathyroidism measure parathyroid hormone concentration 1–4 weeks after starting treatment or adjusting dose, then every 1–3 months; dose adjustment may be necessary if smoking started or stopped during treatment; **interactions**: Appendix 1 (cinacalcet)

Hepatic impairment manufacturer advises caution in moderate to severe impairment—monitor closely especially when increasing dose

Pregnancy manufacturer advises use only if potential benefit outweighs risk—no information available

Breast-feeding manufacturer advises avoid—present in milk in *animal* studies

Side-effects nausea, vomiting, anorexia; dizziness, paraesthesia, asthenia; reduced testosterone concentrations; myalgia; rash; *less commonly* dyspepsia, diarrhoea, and seizures; hypotension, heart failure, and allergic reactions (including angioedema) also reported

Dose
- Secondary hyperparathyroidism in patients with end-stage renal disease on dialysis (but see notes above), ADULT over 18 years, initially 30 mg once daily, adjusted every 2–4 weeks to max. 180 mg daily
- Hypercalcaemia of primary hyperparathyroidism or parathyroid carcinoma, ADULT over 18 years, initially 30 mg twice daily, adjusted every 2–4 weeks according to response up to max. 90 mg 4 times daily

Mimpara® (Amgen) PoM

Tablets, green, f/c, cinacalcet (as hydrochloride) 30 mg, net price 28-tab pack = £125.75; 60 mg, 28-tab pack = £231.97; 90 mg, 28-tab pack = £347.96. Label: 21

9.5.1.3 Magnesium

Magnesium is an essential constituent of many enzyme systems, particularly those involved in energy generation; the largest stores are in the skeleton.

Magnesium salts are not well absorbed from the gastro-intestinal tract, which explains the use of magnesium sulfate (section 1.6.4) as an osmotic laxative.

Magnesium is excreted mainly by the kidneys and is therefore retained in renal failure, but significant *hypermagnesaemia* (causing muscle weakness and arrhythmias) is rare.

Hypomagnesaemia Since magnesium is secreted in large amounts in the gastro-intestinal fluid, excessive losses in diarrhoea, stoma or fistula are the most common causes of *hypomagnesaemia*; deficiency may also occur in alcoholism or as a result of treatment with certain drugs. Hypomagnesaemia often causes secondary hypocalcaemia, and also hypokalaemia and hyponatraemia.

Symptomatic *hypomagnesaemia* is associated with a deficit of 0.5–1 mmol/kg; up to 160 mmol Mg^{2+} over up to 5 days may be required to replace the deficit (allowing for urinary losses). Magnesium is given initially by intravenous infusion or by intramuscular injection of **magnesium sulfate**; the intramuscular injection is painful. Plasma magnesium concentration should be measured to determine the rate and duration of infusion and the dose should be reduced in renal impairment. To prevent *recurrence of the deficit*, magnesium may be given by mouth in a dose of 24 mmol Mg^{2+} daily in divided doses, but there is limited evidence of benefit; magnesium glycerophosphate tablets and liquid [unlicensed] are available from 'special-order' manufacturers

or specialist importing companies, see p. 1124. For maintenance (e.g. in intravenous nutrition), parenteral doses of magnesium are of the order of 10–20 mmol Mg^{2+} daily (often about 12 mmol Mg^{2+} daily).

Arrhythmias Magnesium sulfate injection has also been recommended for the emergency treatment of *serious arrhythmias*, especially in the presence of hypokalaemia (when hypomagnesaemia may also be present) and when salvos of rapid ventricular tachycardia show the characteristic twisting wave front known as *torsade de pointes* (see also section 2.3.1). The usual intravenous dose of magnesium sulfate injection is 8 mmol Mg^{2+} (2 g) over 10–15 minutes (repeated once if necessary).

Myocardial infarction Limited evidence that magnesium sulfate prevents arrhythmias and reperfusion injury in patients with suspected myocardial infarction has not been confirmed by large studies. Routine use of magnesium sulfate for this purpose is not recommended. For the management of myocardial infarction, see section 2.10.1.

Eclampsia and pre-eclampsia Magnesium sulfate injection is the drug of choice for the treatment of seizures and the prevention of recurrent seizures in women with *eclampsia*. Regimens may vary between hospitals. Calcium gluconate injection is used for the management of magnesium toxicity.

Magnesium sulfate injection is also of benefit in women with *pre-eclampsia* in whom there is concern about developing eclampsia. The patient should be monitored carefully (see under Magnesium Sulfate).

MAGNESIUM SULFATE

Note Magnesium Sulfate Injection BP is a sterile solution of Magnesium Sulfate Heptahydrate

Indications see notes above; constipation (section 1.6.4); severe acute asthma (section 3.1); paste for boils (section 13.10.5)

Cautions see notes above; in severe hypomagnesaemia administer initially via controlled infusion device (preferably syringe pump); monitor blood pressure, respiratory rate, urinary output and for signs of overdosage (loss of patellar reflexes, weakness, nausea, sensation of warmth, flushing, drowsiness, double vision, and slurred speech); **interactions**: Appendix 1 (magnesium, parenteral)

Hepatic impairment avoid in hepatic coma if risk of renal failure

Renal impairment avoid or reduce dose; increased risk of toxicity

Pregnancy not known to be harmful for short-term intravenous administration in eclampsia, but excessive doses in third trimester cause neonatal respiratory depression

Side-effects generally associated with hypermagnesaemia, nausea, vomiting, thirst, flushing of skin, hypotension, arrhythmias, coma, respiratory depression, drowsiness, confusion, loss of tendon reflexes, muscle weakness; colic and diarrhoea following oral administration

Dose
- Hypomagnesaemia, see notes above
- Arrhythmias, see notes above
- Prevention of seizures in pre-eclampsia [unlicensed indication], initially by intravenous injection over 5–15 minutes, 4 g (16 mmol Mg^{2+}) followed by intra-

venous infusion, 1 g/hour (4 mmol/hour Mg^{2+}) for 24 hours; if seizure occurs, additional dose by intravenous injection, 2 g (8 mmol Mg^{2+})

- Treatment of seizures and prevention of seizure recurrence in eclampsia, initially by intravenous injection over 5–15 minutes, 4 g (16 mmol Mg^{2+}), followed by intravenous infusion, 1 g/hour (4 mmol/hour Mg^{2+}) for 24 hours after seizure or delivery, whichever is later; if seizure recurs, increase the infusion rate to 1.5–2 g/hour (6–8 mmol/hour Mg^{2+}) or give an additional dose by intravenous injection, 2 g (8 mmol Mg^{2+})

Intravenous administration For intravenous injection, concentration of magnesium sulfate heptahydrate should not exceed 20% (200 mg/mL or 0.8 mmol/mL Mg^{2+}); dilute 1 part of magnesium sulfate injection 50% with at least 1.5 parts of water for injections

Note Magnesium sulfate heptahydrate 1 g equivalent to Mg^{2+} approx. 4 mmol

Magnesium Sulfate Injection, BP (Non-proprietary) [PoM]

Injection, magnesium sulfate heptahydrate 20% (Mg^{2+} approx. 0.8 mmol/mL), net price 20-mL (4-g) amp = £16.98; 50% (Mg^{2+} approx. 2 mmol/mL), 2-mL (1-g) amp = £1.18, 4-mL (2-g) prefilled syringe = £10.23, 5-mL (2.5-g) amp = £5.56, 10-mL (5-g) amp = £1.46; 10-mL (5-g) prefilled syringe = £4.95

Brands include *Minijet® Magnesium Sulfate Injection BP 50%*

Note The BP directs that the label states the strength as the % w/v of magnesium sulfate heptahydrate and as the approximate concentration of magnesium ions (Mg^{2+}) in mmol/mL

9.5.2 Phosphorus

9.5.2.1 Phosphate supplements
9.5.2.2 Phosphate-binding agents

9.5.2.1 Phosphate supplements

Oral phosphate supplements may be required in addition to vitamin D in a small minority of patients with hypophosphataemic vitamin D-resistant rickets. Diarrhoea is a common side-effect and should prompt a reduction in dosage.

Phosphate infusion is occasionally needed in alcohol dependence or in phosphate deficiency arising from use of parenteral nutrition deficient in phosphate supplements; phosphate depletion also occurs in severe diabetic ketoacidosis. For *established hypophosphataemia*, monobasic potassium phosphate may be infused at a rate of 9 mmol every 12 hours. In critically ill patients, the dose of phosphate can be increased up to 500 micromol/kg (approx. 30 mmol in adults, max. 50 mmol), infused over 6–12 hours, according to severity. Excessive doses of phosphates may cause hypocalcaemia and metastatic calcification; it is **essential** to monitor closely plasma concentrations of calcium, phosphate, potassium, and other electrolytes.

For phosphate requirements in *total parenteral nutrition* regimens, see section 9.3.

Phosphates (Fresenius Kabi) [PoM]

Intravenous infusion, phosphates (providing $PO_4{}^{3-}$ 100 mmol, K^+ 19 mmol, and Na^+ 162 mmol/litre), net price 500 mL (*Polyfusor®*) = £53.40.

For the treatment of moderate to severe hypophosphatemia

Phosphate-Sandoz® (HK Pharma)

Tablets, effervescent, anhydrous sodium acid phosphate 1.936 g, sodium bicarbonate 350 mg, potassium bicarbonate 315 mg, equivalent to phosphorus 500 mg (phosphate 16.1 mmol), sodium 468.8 mg (Na^+ 20.4 mmol), potassium 123 mg (K^+ 3.1 mmol). Net price 20 = £3.29. Label: 13

Dose vitamin D-resistant hypophosphataemic osteomalacia, 4–6 tablets daily; CHILD under 5 years 2–3 tablets daily

9.5.2.2 Phosphate-binding agents

Calcium-containing preparations are used as phosphate-binding agents in the management of hyperphosphataemia complicating renal failure. Aluminium-containing preparations are rarely used as phosphate-binding agents and can cause aluminium accumulation.

Sevelamer hydrochloride and **sevelamer carbonate** are both licensed for the treatment of hyperphosphataemia in patients on haemodialysis or peritoneal dialysis. Sevelamer carbonate is also licensed for the treatment of patients with chronic kidney disease not on dialysis who have a serum-phosphate concentration of 1.78 mmol/litre or more.

Lanthanum is licensed for the control of hyperphosphataemia in patients with chronic renal failure on haemodialysis or continuous ambulatory peritoneal dialysis (CAPD), and in patients with chronic kidney disease not on dialysis who have a serum-phosphate concentration of 1.78 mmol/litre or more that cannot be controlled by a low-phosphate diet.

The *Scottish Medicines Consortium* (p. 4) has advised (March 2007) that lanthanum (*Fosrenol®*) is accepted for restricted use within NHS Scotland for the control of hyperphosphataemia in patients with chronic renal failure on haemodialysis or continuous ambulatory peritoneal dialysis, as a second-line agent, where a non-aluminium, non-calcium phosphate binder is required.

Colestilan is licensed for the treatment of hyperphosphataemia in patients with chronic kidney disease receiving haemodialysis or peritoneal dialysis.

The *Scottish Medicines Consortium* (p. 4) has advised (July 2014) that colestilan (*BindRen®*) is **not** recommended for use within NHS Scotland.

ALUMINIUM HYDROXIDE

Indications hyperphosphataemia; dyspepsia (section 1.1)

Cautions see notes above; **interactions:** Appendix 1 (antacids)

Side-effects constipation; hyperaluminaemia

Alu-Cap® (Meda)

Capsules, green/red, dried aluminium hydroxide 475 mg (low Na^+), net price 120-cap pack = £13.71

Dose phosphate-binding agent in renal failure, 4–20 capsules daily in divided doses with meals

CALCIUM SALTS

Indications hyperphosphataemia

Cautions sarcoidosis; history of nephrolithiasis; **interactions:** Appendix 1 (antacids, calcium salts)

Contra-indications hypercalcaemia, hypercalciuria

Side-effects hypercalcaemia

9 Nutrition and blood

Adcal® section 9.5.1.1

Calcichew® section 9.5.1.1

Calcium-500 section 9.5.1.1

Phosex® (Pharmacosmos) PoM
Tablets, yellow, scored, calcium acetate 1 g (calcium 250 mg or Ca^{2+} 6.2 mmol), net price 180-tab pack = £19.79. Label: 25, counselling, with meals
Dose initially 1 tablet 3 times daily with meals, adjusted according to serum-phosphate concentration (usual dose 4–6 tablets daily (1 or 2 tablets with each meal)); max. 12 tablets daily

PhosLo® (Fresenius Medical Care) PoM
Capsules, calcium acetate (anhydrous) 667 mg (calcium 169 mg or Ca^{2+} 4.2 mmol), net price 200-cap pack = £14.40. Counselling, with meals
Excipients include propylene glycol (see Excipients, p. 2)
Dose initially 2 capsules with each meal, adjusted according to serum-phosphate concentration (usual dose 3 or 4 capsules with each meal)

Renacet® (KoRa) PoM
Tablets, f/c, calcium acetate 475 mg (calcium 120.25 mg or Ca^{2+} 3 mmol), net price 100-tab pack = £5.38, 200-tab pack = £9.71; 950 mg (calcium 240.5 mg or Ca^{2+} 6 mmol), scored, net price 100-tab pack = £10.25, 200-tab pack = £18.45. Label: 25, counselling, with meals, avoid other drugs at same time (see below)
Dose ADULT over 18 years, 475–950 mg with breakfast and with snacks, 0.95–2.85 g with main meals, 0.95–1.9 g with supper; adjusted according to serum-phosphate concentration; max. 6.65 g daily
Counselling Manufacturer advises that other drugs should be taken 1 to 2 hours before or after *Renacet®* to reduce possible interference with absorption of other drugs

◀With magnesium carbonate
Osvaren® (Fresenius Medical Care) PoM
Tablets, f/c, scored, calcium acetate 435 mg (calcium 110 mg or Ca^{2+} 2.7 mmol), heavy magnesium carbonate 235 mg (magnesium 60 mg), net price 180-tab pack = £24.00. Label: 25, counselling, with meals, avoid other drugs at same time (see below)
Contra-indications hypercalcaemia, hypermagnesaemia; third-degree AV block; myasthenia gravis
Dose ADULT over 18 years, initially 1 tablet 3 times daily with meals, adjusted according to serum-phosphate concentration (usual dose 3–10 tablets daily); max. 12 tablets daily
Counselling Manufacturer advises that other drugs should be taken at least 2 hours before or 3 hours after *Osvaren®* to reduce possible interference with absorption of other drugs

▌ **COLESTILAN**

Indications hyperphosphataemia in patients with chronic kidney disease on haemodialysis or peritoneal dialysis

Cautions constipation; predisposition to gastrointestinal haemorrhage; malabsorption syndromes; **interactions**: Appendix 1 (colestilan)

Contra-indications bowel obstruction; dysphagia; severe gastrointestinal disorders; biliary obstruction; seizure disorders; recent history of peritonitis in peritoneal dialysis patients; serum albumin less than 30 g/L

Hepatic impairment manufacturer advises avoid in severe impairment—no information available

Pregnancy no information available; not absorbed but supplements of fat-soluble vitamins and folic acid may be required

Breast-feeding no information available; not absorbed but supplements of fat-soluble vitamins and folic acid may be required

Side-effects constipation, diarrhoea, flatulence, nausea, vomiting, dyspepsia, gastritis, abdominal pain, decreased appetite; *less commonly* oesophagitis, gastrointestinal haemorrhage, taste disturbances; *rarely* intestinal obstruction

Dose
● ADULT over 18 years, initially 2–3 g 3 times daily with or immediately after meals, increased according to serum-phosphate concentration in steps of 3 g daily (in divided doses) every 2–3 weeks; max. 5 g 3 times daily

BindRen® (Mitsubishi) ▼ PoM
Tablets, f/c, colestilan 1 g, net price 198-tab pack = £143.00. Label: 21, 25, counselling, avoid other drugs at same time (see below)
Granules, f/c, colestilan 2 g/sachet, net price 90-sachet pack = £130.00; 3 g/sachet, net price 90-sachet pack = £195.00. Label: 21, counselling, avoid other drugs at same time (see below)
Counselling Manufacturer advises that other drugs should be taken at least 1 hour before or 3 hours after *BindRen®* to reduce possible interference with absorption of other drugs

▌ **LANTHANUM**

Indications see notes above

Cautions acute peptic ulcer; ulcerative colitis; Crohn's disease; bowel obstruction; **interactions**: Appendix 1 (lanthanum)

Hepatic impairment lanthanum excreted in bile—possible accumulation in obstructive jaundice

Pregnancy manufacturer advises avoid—toxicity in *animal* studies

Breast-feeding manufacturer advises caution—no information available

Side-effects gastro-intestinal disturbances, headache, hypocalcaemia; *less commonly* anorexia, increased appetite, taste disturbances, dry mouth, thirst, stomatitis, chest pain, peripheral oedema, dizziness, vertigo, asthenia, malaise, hyperglycaemia, hyperparathyroidism, hypercalcaemia, hypophosphataemia, eosinophilia, arthralgia, myalgia, osteoporosis, sweating, alopecia; accumulation of lanthanum in bone, and transient changes in QT interval also reported

Dose
● ADULT over 18 years, usual dose range 1.5–3 g daily in divided doses with or immediately after meals, adjusted according to serum-phosphate concentration every 2–3 weeks

Fosrenol® (Shire) PoM
Tablets (chewable), lanthanum (as carbonate hydrate) 500 mg, net price 90-tab pack = £124.06; 750 mg, 90-tab pack = £182.60; 1 g, 90-tab pack = £193.59. Label: 21, counselling, to be chewed
Powder, lanthanum (as carbonate hydrate) 750 mg, net price 90 sachets = £182.60; 1 g, 90 sachets = £193.59. Label: 21, counselling, administration
Counselling Each sachet to be mixed with soft food and consumed within 15 minutes

SEVELAMER HYDROCHLORIDE

Indications hyperphosphataemia in patients on haemodialysis or peritoneal dialysis

Cautions gastro-intestinal disorders; **interactions**: Appendix 1 (sevelamer)

Contra-indications bowel obstruction

Pregnancy manufacturer advises use only if potential benefit outweighs risk

Breast-feeding manufacturer advises use only if potential benefit outweighs risk

Side-effects nausea, vomiting, abdominal pain, constipation, diarrhoea, dyspepsia, flatulence; *very rarely* intestinal obstruction; *also reported* intestinal perforation, ileus, diverticulitis, pruritus, rash

Dose
- ADULT over 18 years, initially 2.4–4.8 g daily in 3 divided doses with meals, adjusted according to serum-phosphate concentration (usual dose range 2.4–12 g daily in 3 divided doses); CHILD see *BNF for Children*

Renagel® (Genzyme) [PoM]
Tablets, f/c, sevelamer hydrochloride 800 mg, net price 180-tab pack = £167.04. Label: 25, counselling, with meals
Excipients include propylene glycol (see Excipients, p. 2)

SEVELAMER CARBONATE

Indications hyperphosphataemia in patients on haemodialysis or peritoneal dialysis, and patients with chronic kidney disease not on dialysis who have a serum-phosphate concentration of 1.78 mmol/litre or more

Cautions gastro-intestinal disorders; **interactions**: Appendix 1 (sevelamer)

Contra-indications bowel obstruction

Pregnancy manufacturer advises use only if potential benefit outweighs risk

Breast-feeding unlikely to be present in milk (however, manufacturer advises avoid)

Side-effects nausea, vomiting, abdominal pain, constipation, diarrhoea, dyspepsia, flatulence; *also reported* intestinal obstruction and perforation, ileus, pruritus, rash

Dose
- ADULT over 18 years, initially 2.4–4.8 g daily in 3 divided doses with meals, adjusted according to serum-phosphate concentration every 2–4 weeks (usual dose approx. 6 g daily in 3 divided doses)

Renvela® (Genzyme) [PoM]
Tablets, f/c, sevelamer carbonate 800 mg, net price 180-tab pack = £167.04. Label: 25, counselling, with meals
Excipients include propylene glycol (see Excipients, p. 2)
Powder for oral suspension, pale yellow, sevelamer carbonate 2.4 g, net price 60-sachet pack (citrus-flavoured) = £167.04. Label: 13, counselling, with meals
Note Each sachet to be dispersed in 60 mL water

9.5.3 Fluoride

Availability of adequate fluoride confers significant resistance to dental caries. It is now considered that the topical action of fluoride on enamel and plaque is more important than the systemic effect.

When the fluoride content of drinking water is less than 700 micrograms per litre (0.7 parts per million), daily administration of fluoride tablets or drops provides suitable supplementation. Systemic fluoride supplements should not be prescribed without reference to the fluoride content of the local water supply. Infants need not receive fluoride supplements until the age of 6 months.

Dentifrices which incorporate sodium fluoride or monofluorophosphate are also a convenient source of fluoride.

Individuals who are either particularly caries prone or medically compromised may be given additional protection by use of fluoride rinses or by application of fluoride gels. Rinses may be used daily or weekly; daily use of a less concentrated rinse is more effective than weekly use of a more concentrated one. High-strength gels must be applied regularly under professional supervision; extreme caution is necessary to prevent children from swallowing any excess. Less concentrated gels are available for home use. Varnishes are also available and are particularly valuable for young or disabled children since they adhere to the teeth and set in the presence of moisture.

Fluoride mouthwash, oral drops, tablets and toothpaste are prescribable on form FP10D (GP14 in Scotland, WP10D in Wales); for details see preparations, p. 700).

There are also arrangements for health authorities to supply fluoride tablets in the course of pre-school dental schemes, and they may also be supplied in school dental schemes.

Fluoride gels are not prescribable on form FP10D (GP14 in Scotland, WP10D in Wales).

FLUORIDES

Note Sodium fluoride 2.2 mg provides approx. 1 mg fluoride ion

Indications prophylaxis of dental caries—see notes above

Contra-indications not for areas where drinking water is fluoridated

Side-effects occasional white flecks on teeth with recommended doses; *rarely* yellowish-brown discoloration if recommended doses are exceeded

Dose
Note Dose expressed as fluoride ion (F⁻)
- Water content less than F⁻ 300 micrograms/litre (0.3 parts per million), CHILD up to 6 months none; 6 months–3 years F⁻ 250 micrograms daily, 3–6 years F⁻ 500 micrograms daily, over 6 years F⁻ 1 mg daily
- Water content between F⁻ 300 and 700 micrograms/litre (0.3–0.7 parts per million), CHILD up to 3 years none, 3–6 years F⁻ 250 micrograms daily, over 6 years F⁻ 500 micrograms daily
- Water content above F⁻ 700 micrograms/litre (0.7 parts per million), supplements not advised

Note These doses reflect the recommendations of the British Dental Association, the British Society of Paediatric Dentistry and the British Association for the Study of Community Dentistry (*Br Dent J* 1997; **182**: 6–7)

9 **Nutrition and blood**

◢**Tablets**

Counselling Tablets should be sucked or dissolved in the mouth and taken preferably in the evening

En-De-Kay® (Manx)

Fluotabs 3–6 years, orange-flavoured, scored, sodium fluoride 1.1 mg (F⁻ 500 micrograms), net price 200-tab pack = £2.38

Dental prescribing on NHS May be prescribed as Sodium Fluoride Tablets

Fluotabs 6+ years, orange-flavoured, scored, sodium fluoride 2.2 mg (F⁻ 1 mg), net price 200-tab pack = £2.38

Dental prescribing on NHS May be prescribed as Sodium Fluoride Tablets

Fluor-a-day® (Dental Health)

Tablets, buff, sodium fluoride 1.1 mg (F⁻ 500 micrograms), net price 200-tab pack = £2.79; 2.2 mg (F⁻ 1 mg), 200-tab pack = £2.79

Dental prescribing on NHS May be prescribed as Sodium Fluoride Tablets

◢**Oral drops**

Note Fluoride supplements not considered necessary below 6 months of age (see notes above)

En-De-Kay® (Manx)

Fluodrops® (= paediatric drops), sugar-free, sodium fluoride 550 micrograms (F⁻ 250 micrograms)/ 0.15 mL. Net price 60 mL = £2.38

Dental prescribing on NHS May be prescribed as Sodium Fluoride Oral Drops

◢**Mouthwashes**

Rinse mouth for 1 minute and spit out

Counselling Avoid eating, drinking, or rinsing mouth for 15 minutes after use

En-De-Kay® (Manx)

Daily fluoride mouthrinse (= mouthwash), blue, sodium fluoride 0.05%. Net price 250 mL = £1.50

Dose CHILD 6 years and over, for *daily* use, rinse with 10 mL

Dental prescribing on NHS May be prescribed as Sodium Fluoride Mouthwash 0.05%

Fluorinse (= mouthwash), red, sodium fluoride 2%. Net price 100 mL = £4.97. Counselling, see above

Dose CHILD 8 years and over, for *daily* use, dilute 5 drops to 10 mL of water; for *weekly* use, dilute 20 drops to 10 mL

Dental prescribing on NHS May be prescribed as Sodium Fluoride Mouthwash 2%

FluoriGard® (Colgate-Palmolive)

Daily dental rinse (= mouthwash), blue, sodium fluoride 0.05%. Net price 400 mL = £2.99. Counselling, see above

Dose CHILD 6 years and over, for *daily* use, rinse with 10 mL

Dental prescribing on NHS May be prescribed as Sodium Fluoride Mouthwash 0.05%

◢**Toothpastes**

Duraphat® (Colgate-Palmolive) PoM

Duraphat® '2800 ppm' toothpaste, sodium fluoride 0.619%. Net price 75 mL = £3.26, dual pack (2 × 75 mL) = £5.54. Counselling, see below

Dose ADULT and CHILD over 10 years, apply 1 cm twice daily using a toothbrush

Counselling Brush teeth for 1 minute before spitting out. Avoid drinking or rinsing mouth for 30 minutes after use

Dental prescribing on NHS May be prescribed as Sodium Fluoride Toothpaste 0.619%

Duraphat® '5000 ppm' toothpaste, sodium fluoride 1.1%. Net price 51 g = £6.50. Counselling, see below

Dose ADULT and ADOLESCENT over 16 years, apply 2 cm 3 times daily after meals using a toothbrush

Counselling Brush teeth for 3 minutes before spitting out

Dental prescribing on NHS May be prescribed as Sodium Fluoride Toothpaste 1.1%

9.5.4 Zinc

Zinc supplements should not be given unless there is good evidence of deficiency (hypoproteinaemia spuriously lowers plasma-zinc concentration) or in zinc-losing conditions. Zinc deficiency can occur as a result of inadequate diet or malabsorption; excessive loss of zinc can occur in trauma, burns, and protein-losing conditions. A zinc supplement is given until clinical improvement occurs, but it may need to be continued in severe malabsorption, metabolic disease (section 9.8.1), or in zinc-losing states.

Parenteral nutrition regimens usually include trace amounts of zinc (section 9.3). If necessary, further zinc can be added to intravenous feeding regimens. A suggested dose for intravenous nutrition is elemental zinc 6.5 mg (Zn²⁺ 100 micromol) daily.

� **ZINC SULFATE**

Indications zinc deficiency or supplementation in zinc-losing conditions

Cautions interactions: Appendix 1 (zinc)

Renal impairment accumulation may occur in acute renal failure

Pregnancy crosses placenta; risk theoretically minimal, but no information available

Breast-feeding present in milk; risk theoretically minimal, but no information available

Side-effects abdominal pain, dyspepsia, nausea, vomiting, diarrhoea, gastric irritation; irritability, headache, lethargy

Dose

● See preparation below and notes above

Zinc Sulfate (Non-proprietary) PoM

Injection, zinc sulfate 14.6 mg/mL (zinc 50 micromol/mL), net price 10 mL vial = £2.50

Solvazinc® (Galen)

Effervescent tablets, zinc sulfate monohydrate 125 mg (45 mg zinc), net price 30 = £4.32. Label: 13, 21

Dose ADULT and CHILD over 30 kg, 1 tablet in water 1–3 times daily after food; CHILD under 10 kg, ½ tablet daily; 10–30 kg, ½ tablet 1–3 times daily

9.5.5 Selenium

Selenium deficiency can occur as a result of inadequate diet or prolonged parenteral nutrition. A selenium supplement should not be given unless there is good evidence of deficiency.

▰ **SELENIUM**

Indications selenium deficiency

Cautions interactions: Appendix 1 (selenium)

Dose

● By mouth *or* by intramuscular injection *or* by intravenous injection, 100–500 micrograms daily

Selenase® PoM

Oral solution, selenium (as sodium selenite pentahy-drate) 50 micrograms/mL, net price 2-mL amp = £1.03, 10-mL bottle = £4.05

Injection, selenium (as sodium selenite pentahy-drate) 50 micrograms/mL, net price 2-mL amp = £1.50, 10-mL vial = £4.25

Note May be difficult to obtain

9.6 Vitamins

9.6.1 Vitamin A
9.6.2 Vitamin B group
9.6.3 Vitamin C
9.6.4 Vitamin D
9.6.5 Vitamin E
9.6.6 Vitamin K
9.6.7 Multivitamin preparations

Vitamins are used for the prevention and treatment of specific deficiency states or where the diet is known to be inadequate; they may be prescribed in the NHS to prevent or treat deficiency but not as dietary supplements.

Their use as general 'pick-me-ups' is of unproven value and, in the case of preparations containing vitamin A or D, may actually be harmful if patients take more than the prescribed dose. The 'fad' for mega-vitamin therapy with water-soluble vitamins, such as ascorbic acid and pyridoxine, is unscientific and can be harmful.

Dietary reference values for vitamins are available in the Department of Health publication:

Dietary Reference Values for Food Energy and Nutrients for the United Kingdom: Report of the Panel on Dietary Reference Values of the Committee on Medical Aspects of Food Policy. *Report on Health and Social Subjects 41.* London: HMSO, 1991

Dental patients It is unjustifiable to treat stomatitis or glossitis with mixtures of vitamin preparations; this delays diagnosis and correct treatment.

Most patients who develop a nutritional deficiency despite an adequate intake of vitamins have malabsorption and if this is suspected the patient should be referred to a medical practitioner.

9.6.1 Vitamin A

Deficiency of vitamin A (retinol) is associated with ocular defects (particularly xerophthalmia) and an increased susceptibility to infections, but deficiency is rare in the UK (even in disorders of fat absorption).

Massive overdose can cause rough skin, dry hair, an enlarged liver, and a raised erythrocyte sedimentation rate and raised serum calcium and serum alkaline phosphatase concentrations.

Pregnancy In view of evidence suggesting that high levels of vitamin A may cause birth defects, women who are (or may become) pregnant are advised not to take vitamin A supplements (including tablets and fish-liver oil drops), except on the advice of a doctor or an antenatal clinic; nor should they eat liver or products such as liver paté or liver sausage.

◼ VITAMIN A
(Retinol)

Indications see notes above

Cautions see notes above; **interactions:** Appendix 1 (vitamins)

Pregnancy excessive doses may be teratogenic; see also notes above

Breast-feeding theoretical risk of toxicity in infants of mothers taking large doses

Side-effects see notes above

Dose

● See notes above and under preparations

◢Vitamins A and D

Halibut-liver Oil (Non-proprietary)

Capsules, vitamin A 4000 units [also contains vit-amin D], net price 100-cap pack = £1.05

Vitamins A and D (Non-proprietary)

Capsules, vitamin A 4000 units, vitamin D 400 units (10 micrograms), net price 84-cap pack = £8.42

Note May be difficult to obtain

◢Vitamins A, C and D

Healthy Start Children's Vitamin Drops (Non-proprietary)

Oral drops, vitamin A 5000 units, vitamin D 2000 units (50 micrograms), ascorbic acid 150 mg/mL

Available free of charge to children under 4 years in families on the Healthy Start Scheme, or alternatively may be available direct to the public—further information for healthcare professionals can be accessed at www.healthystart.nhs.uk. Beneficiaries can contact their midwife or health visitor for further information on where to obtain supplies.

Dose prevention of vitamin deficiency, CHILD 1 month–5 years, 5 drops daily (5 drops contain vitamin A approx. 700 units, vitamin D approx. 300 units (7.5 micrograms), ascorbic acid approx. 20 mg)

Note *Healthy Start Vitamins for women* (containing ascorbic acid, vitamin D, and folic acid) are also available free of charge to women on the Healthy Start Scheme during pregnancy and until their baby is one year old, or alternatively may be available direct to the public—further information for healthcare professionals can be accessed at www.healthystart.nhs.uk. Beneficiaries can contact their midwife or health visitor for further information on where to obtain supplies.

9.6.2 Vitamin B group

Deficiency of the B vitamins, other than vitamin B_{12} (section 9.1.2), is rare in the UK and is usually treated by preparations containing thiamine (B_1), riboflavin (B_2), and nicotinamide, which is used in preference to nicotinic acid, as it does not cause vasodilatation. Other members (or substances traditionally classified as members) of the vitamin B complex such as aminobenzoic acid, biotin, choline, inositol, and pantothenic acid or panthenol may be included in vitamin B preparations but there is no evidence of their value.

The severe deficiency states Wernicke's encephalopathy and Korsakoff's psychosis, especially as seen in chronic alcoholism (section 4.10.1), are best treated initially by the parenteral administration of B vitamins (*Pabrinex®*), followed by oral administration of **thiamine** in the longer term. Anaphylaxis has been reported

9

Nutrition and blood

with parenteral B vitamins (see MHRA/CHM advice, below).

As with other vitamins of the B group, **pyridoxine** (B_6) deficiency is rare, but it may occur during isoniazid therapy (section 5.1.9) or penicillamine treatment in Wilson's disease (section 9.8.1) and is characterised by peripheral neuritis. High doses of pyridoxine are given in some metabolic disorders, such as hyperoxaluria, and it is also used in sideroblastic anaemia (section 9.1.3). There is evidence to suggest that pyridoxine in a dose not exceeding 100 mg daily may provide some benefit in premenstrual syndrome. It has been tried for a wide variety of other disorders, but there is little sound evidence to support the claims of efficacy, and overdosage induces toxic effects.

Nicotinic acid inhibits the synthesis of cholesterol and triglyceride (see section 2.12). Folic acid and vitamin B_{12} are used in the treatment of megaloblastic anaemia (section 9.1.2). Folinic acid (available as calcium folinate) is used in association with cytotoxic therapy (section 8.1).

▌ RIBOFLAVIN
(Riboflavine, vitamin B_2)

Indications see notes above

◢**Preparations**
Injections of vitamins B and C, see under Thiamine

◢**Oral vitamin B complex preparations**
See p. 703

▌ THIAMINE
(Vitamin B_1)

Indications see notes above

Cautions anaphylaxis may occasionally follow injection (see MHRA/CHM advice below)

> **MHRA/CHM advice (September 2007)**
> Although potentially serious allergic adverse reactions may rarely occur during, or shortly after, parenteral administration, the CHM has recommended that:
> 1. This should not preclude the use of parenteral thiamine in patients where this route of administration is required, particularly in patients at risk of Wernicke-Korsakoff syndrome where treatment with thiamine is essential;
> 2. Intravenous administration should be by infusion over 30 minutes;
> 3. Facilities for treating anaphylaxis (including resuscitation facilities) should be available when parenteral thiamine is administered.

Breast-feeding severely thiamine-deficient mothers should avoid breast-feeding as toxic methyl-glyoxal present in milk

Dose
• Mild deficiency, by mouth, 25–100 mg daily; severe deficiency, 200–300 mg daily in divided doses

Thiamine (Non-proprietary)
Tablets, thiamine hydrochloride 50 mg, net price 100 = £4.80; 100 mg, 100 = £8.25
Brands include *Benerva*® ᴶᴴˢ

Pabrinex® (Archimedes) PoM
I/M High Potency injection, for intramuscular use only, ascorbic acid 500 mg, nicotinamide 160 mg, pyridoxine hydrochloride 50 mg, riboflavin 4 mg, thiamine hydrochloride 250 mg/7 mL. Net price 7 mL (in 2 amps) = £2.25
Excipients include benzyl alcohol (avoid in neonates, see Excipients, p. 2)

I/V High Potency injection, for intravenous use only, ascorbic acid 500 mg, anhydrous glucose 1 g, nicotinamide 160 mg, pyridoxine hydrochloride 50 mg, riboflavin 4 mg, thiamine hydrochloride 250 mg/ 10 mL. Net price 10 mL (in 2 × 5 mL amps) = £2.25
Parenteral vitamins B and C for rapid correction of severe depletion or malabsorption (e.g. in alcoholism, after acute infections, postoperatively, or in psychiatric states), maintenance of vitamins B and C in chronic intermittent haemodialysis
Dose see MHRA/CHM advice above

Treatment of Wernicke's encephalopathy, by intravenous infusion of *I/V High Potency*, 2–3 pairs 3 times daily for 2 days; if no response, discontinue; if symptoms respond after 2 days, give by intravenous infusion of *I/V High Potency* or by deep intramuscular injection into the gluteal muscle of *IM High Potency*, 1 pair once daily for 5 days or for as long as improvement continues

Prophylaxis of Wernicke's encephalopathy in alcohol dependence, by intravenous infusion of *I/V High Potency* or by deep intramuscular injection into the gluteal muscle of *I/M High Potency*, 1 pair once daily for at least 3–5 days

Psychosis following narcosis or electroconvulsive therapy, toxicity from acute infections, by intravenous infusion of *I/V High Potency* or by deep intramuscular injection into the gluteal muscle of *I/M High Potency*, 1 pair twice daily for up to 7 days

Haemodialysis, by intravenous infusion of *I/V High Potency* (in sodium chloride intravenous infusion 0.9%), 1 pair every 2 weeks
Note *Pabrinex*® doses in BNF may differ from those in product literature

◢**Oral vitamin B complex preparations**
See p. 703

▌ PYRIDOXINE HYDROCHLORIDE
(Vitamin B_6)

Indications see under Dose

Cautions interactions: Appendix 1 (vitamins)

Side-effects sensory neuropathy reported with high doses given for extended periods

Dose
• Deficiency states, 20–50 mg up to 3 times daily
• Isoniazid-induced neuropathy, prophylaxis 10 mg daily [or 20 mg daily if suitable product not available]; treatment, 50 mg three times daily; CHILD under 18 years see *BNF for Children*
• Idiopathic sideroblastic anaemia, 100–400 mg daily in divided doses
• Penicillamine-induced neuropathy, prophylaxis in Wilson's disease [unlicensed use] (see also notes above), 20 mg daily; CHILD under 18 years see *BNF for Children*
• Premenstrual syndrome [unlicensed use], 50–100 mg daily (see notes above)

> Prolonged use of pyridoxine in a dose of 10 mg daily is considered safe but the long-term use of pyridoxine in a dose of 200 mg or more daily has been associated with neuropathy. The safety of long-term pyridoxine supplementation with doses above 10 mg daily has not been established.

Pyridoxine (Non-proprietary)
Tablets, pyridoxine hydrochloride 10 mg, net price
500 = £8.48; 20 mg, 500 = £8.53; 50 mg, 28 = £3.68

◢ Injections of vitamins B and C
See under Thiamine

NICOTINAMIDE

Indications see notes above; acne vulgaris, see section 13.6.1

◢ Injections of vitamins B and C
See under Thiamine

Oral vitamin B complex preparations
Note Other multivitamin preparations are in section 9.6.7.

Vitamin B Tablets, Compound ◢
Tablets, nicotinamide 15 mg, riboflavin 1 mg, thiamine hydrochloride 1 mg, net price 28 = £24.22
Dose prophylactic, 1–2 tablets daily

Vitamin B Tablets, Compound, Strong ◢
Tablets, brown, f/c or s/c, nicotinamide 20 mg, pyridoxine hydrochloride 2 mg, riboflavin 2 mg, thiamine hydrochloride 5 mg. Net price 28-tab pack = £1.92
Dose treatment of vitamin-B deficiency, 1–2 tablets 3 times daily

Vigranon B® (Wallace Mfg) NHS ◢
Syrup, thiamine hydrochloride 5 mg, riboflavin 2 mg, nicotinamide 20 mg, pyridoxine hydrochloride 2 mg, panthenol 3 mg/5 mL. Net price 150 mL = £2.41

Other compounds

Potassium aminobenzoate has been used in the treatment of various disorders associated with excessive fibrosis such as scleroderma and Peyronie's disease. In Peyronie's disease there is some evidence to support efficacy in reducing progression when given early in the disease; however, there is no evidence for reversal of the condition. The therapeutic value of potassium aminobenzoate in scleroderma is doubtful.

Potaba® (Glenwood)
Capsules, potassium aminobenzoate 500 mg, net price 240 = £44.75. Label: 21
Envules® (= powder in sachets), potassium aminobenzoate 3 g, net price 40 sachets = £34.31. Label: 13, 21
Cautions interactions: Appendix 1 (potassium aminobenzoate)
Dose Peyronie's disease, scleroderma, 12 g daily in divided doses after food

9.6.3 Vitamin C
(Ascorbic acid)

Vitamin C therapy is essential in scurvy, but less florid manifestations of vitamin C deficiency are commonly found, especially in the elderly. It is rarely necessary to prescribe more than 100 mg daily except early in the treatment of scurvy.

Severe scurvy causes gingival swelling and bleeding margins as well as petechiae on the skin. This is, however, exceedingly rare and a patient with these signs is more likely to have leukaemia. Investigation should not be delayed by a trial period of vitamin treatment.

Claims that vitamin C ameliorates colds or promotes wound healing have not been proved.

ASCORBIC ACID

Indications prevention and treatment of scurvy
Cautions interactions: Appendix 1 (vitamins)
Dose
● Prophylactic, 25–75 mg daily; therapeutic, not less than 250 mg daily in divided doses

Ascorbic Acid (Non-proprietary)
Tablets, ascorbic acid 50 mg, net price 28 = £7.02; 100 mg, 28 = £7.95; 200 mg, 28 = £10.36; 500 mg (label: 24), 28 = £14.95
Brands include Redoxon® NHS
Injection, ascorbic acid 100 mg/mL. Net price 5-mL amp = £4.39
Available from UCB Pharma

9.6.4 Vitamin D

Note The term Vitamin D is used for a range of compounds which possess the property of preventing or curing rickets. They include ergocalciferol (calciferol, vitamin D₂), colecalciferol (vitamin D₃), dihydrotachysterol, alfacalcidol (1α-hydroxycholecalciferol), and calcitriol (1,25-dihydroxycholecalciferol).

Simple vitamin D deficiency can be prevented by taking an oral supplement of only 10 micrograms (400 units) of **ergocalciferol** (calciferol, vitamin D₂) or **colecalciferol** (vitamin D₃) daily. Vitamin D deficiency can occur in people whose exposure to sunlight is limited and in those whose diet is deficient in vitamin D. In these individuals, ergocalciferol or colecalciferol in a dose of 20 micrograms (800 units) daily by mouth may be given to treat vitamin D deficiency; higher doses may be necessary for *severe* deficiency. Patients who do not respond should be referred to a specialist.

Preparations containing **calcium with colecalciferol** are available for the management of combined calcium and vitamin D deficiency, or for those at high risk of deficiency (see also Osteoporosis, p. 521 and Calcium Supplements, p. 694).

Vitamin D deficiency caused by *intestinal malabsorption* or *chronic liver disease* usually requires vitamin D in pharmacological doses, such as ergocalciferol tablets up to 1 mg (40 000 units) daily; the hypocalcaemia of *hypoparathyroidism* often requires doses of up to 2.5 mg (100 000 units) daily in order to achieve normocalcaemia.

Vitamin D requires hydroxylation by the kidney to its active form, therefore the hydroxylated derivatives **alfacalcidol** or **calcitriol** should be prescribed if patients with *severe renal impairment* require vitamin D therapy. Calcitriol is also licensed for the management of postmenopausal osteoporosis.

Paricalcitol, a synthetic vitamin D analogue, is licensed for the prevention and treatment of secondary hyperparathyroidism associated with chronic renal failure (section 9.5.1.2).

Important. All patients receiving pharmacological doses of vitamin D should have their plasma-calcium concentration checked at intervals (initially once or twice weekly) and whenever nausea or vomiting occur.

9

Nutrition and blood

ERGOCALCIFEROL
(Calciferol, Vitamin D₂)

Indications see notes above

Cautions take care to ensure correct dose in infants; monitor plasma-calcium concentration in patients receiving high doses and in renal impairment (see notes above); **interactions**: Appendix 1 (vitamins)

Contra-indications hypercalcaemia; metastatic calcification

Pregnancy high doses teratogenic in *animals* but therapeutic doses unlikely to be harmful

Breast-feeding caution with high doses; may cause hypercalcaemia in infant—monitor serum-calcium concentration

Side-effects symptoms of overdosage include anorexia, lassitude, nausea and vomiting, diarrhoea, constipation, weight loss, polyuria, sweating, headache, thirst, vertigo, and raised concentrations of calcium and phosphate in plasma and urine

Dose
- See notes above

◢**With calcium**
For prescribing information on calcium, see section 9.5.1.1

Calcium and Ergocalciferol (Non-proprietary)
(Calcium and Vitamin D)
Tablets, calcium lactate 300 mg, calcium phosphate 150 mg (calcium 97 mg or Ca²⁺ 2.4 mmol), ergocalciferol 10 micrograms (400 units). Net price 28-tab pack = £11.26. Counselling, crush before administration or may be chewed

◢**Pharmacological strengths**
Note The BP directs that when calciferol is prescribed or demanded, colecalciferol or ergocalciferol should be dispensed or supplied

Ergocalciferol (Non-proprietary)
Tablets, ergocalciferol 250 micrograms (10 000 units), net price 100 = £21.99; 1.25 mg (50 000 units), 100 = £30.34
Note May be difficult to obtain
Important When the strength of the tablets ordered or prescribed is not clear, the intention of the prescriber with respect to the strength (expressed in micrograms or milligrams per tablet) should be ascertained.

Injection, for intramuscular use only, ergocalciferol, 7.5 mg (300 000 units)/mL in oil, net price 1-mL amp = £9.35, 2-mL amp = £10.84
Note Other formulations of ergocalciferol are available from 'special-order' manufacturers or specialist importing companies, see p. 1124

ALFACALCIDOL
(1α-Hydroxycholecalciferol)

Indications see notes above

Cautions see under Ergocalciferol; also nephrolithiasis

Contra-indications see under Ergocalciferol

Pregnancy see under Ergocalciferol

Breast-feeding see under Ergocalciferol

Side-effects see under Ergocalciferol; also *rarely* nephrocalcinosis, pruritus, rash, and urticaria

Dose
- By mouth *or* by intravenous injection over 30 seconds, ADULT and CHILD over 20 kg, initially 1 microgram daily (elderly 500 nanograms), adjusted to avoid hypercalcaemia; maintenance, usually 0.25–

1 microgram daily; NEONATE and PRETERM NEONATE initially 50–100 nanograms/kg daily, CHILD under 20 kg initially 50 nanograms/kg daily

Alfacalcidol (Non-proprietary) ℗ₒₘ
Capsules, alfacalcidol 250 nanograms, net price 30-cap pack = £2.67; 500 nanograms 30-cap pack = £5.80; 1 microgram 30-cap pack = £5.87

One-Alpha® (LEO) ℗ₒₘ
Capsules, alfacalcidol 250 nanograms (white), net price 30-cap pack = £3.37; 500 nanograms (red), 30-cap pack = £6.27; 1 microgram (brown), 30-cap pack = £8.75
Excipients include sesame oil

Oral drops, sugar-free, alfacalcidol 2 micrograms/mL (1 drop contains approx. 100 nanograms), net price 10 mL = £21.30
Excipients include alcohol
Note The concentration of alfacalcidol in *One-Alpha®* drops is **10 times greater** than that of the former preparation *One-Alpha®* solution.

Injection, alfacalcidol 2 micrograms/mL, net price 0.5-mL amp = £2.16, 1-mL amp = £4.11
Excipients include alcohol, propylene glycol (caution in neonates, see Excipients, p. 2)
Note Shake ampoule for at least 5 seconds before use

CALCITRIOL
(1,25-Dihydroxycholecalciferol)

Indications see notes above

Cautions see under Ergocalciferol; monitor plasma calcium, phosphate, and creatinine during dosage titration

Contra-indications see under Ergocalciferol

Pregnancy see under Ergocalciferol

Breast-feeding see under Ergocalciferol

Side-effects see under Ergocalciferol

Dose
- By mouth, renal osteodystrophy, initially 250 nanograms daily, or on alternate days (in patients with normal or only slightly reduced plasma-calcium concentration), increased if necessary in steps of 250 nanograms at intervals of 2–4 weeks; usual dose 0.5–1 microgram daily; CHILD not established
Established postmenopausal osteoporosis, 250 nanograms twice daily (monitor plasma-calcium concentration and creatinine, consult product literature)

Calcitriol (Non-proprietary) ℗ₒₘ
Capsules, calcitriol 250 nanograms, net price 30-cap pack = £5.41, 100-cap pack = £19.15; 500 nanograms, 30-cap pack = £9.68, 100-cap pack = £25.76

Rocaltrol® (Roche) ℗ₒₘ
Capsules, calcitriol 250 nanograms (red/white), net price 100 = £18.04; 500 nanograms (red), 100 = £32.25

COLECALCIFEROL
(Cholecalciferol, vitamin D₃)

Indications see notes above

Cautions see under Ergocalciferol

Contra-indications see under Ergocalciferol

Pregnancy see under Ergocalciferol

Breast-feeding see under Ergocalciferol

Side-effects see under Ergocalciferol

Dose

- See notes above

Desunin® (Meda) [PoM]
Tablets, colecalciferol 20 micrograms (800 units), net price 30-tab pack = £3.60

Fultium-D₃® (Internis) [PoM]
Capsules, colecalciferol 20 micrograms (800 units) (blue), net price 30-cap pack = £3.60, 90-cap pack = £10.80; 80 micrograms (3200 units) (green), 30-cap pack = £13.32, 90-cap pack = £39.96. Label: 25
Excipients include arachis (peanut) oil

InVita D3® (Consilient) [PoM]
Oral solution, colecalciferol 625 micrograms (25 000 units)/mL, net price 3 × 1-mL unit amp = £4.45. Label: 21
Note May be mixed with a small amount of cold or lukewarm food immediately before administration

Colecalciferol

Various formulations available from 'special-order' manufacturers or specialist importing companies, see p. 1124

◀With calcium

For prescribing information on calcium, see section 9.5.1.1

Accrete D3® (Internis)
Tablets, f/c, calcium carbonate 1.5 g (calcium 600 mg or Ca²⁺ 15 mmol), colecalciferol 10 micrograms (400 units), net price 60-tab pack = £2.95

Adcal-D₃® (ProStrakan)
Tablets (chewable) (lemon or tutti-frutti flavour), calcium carbonate 1.5 g (calcium 600 mg or Ca²⁺ 15 mmol), colecalciferol 10 micrograms (400 units), net price 56-tab pack = £3.65, 112-tab pack = £7.49. Label: 24
Dissolve (effervescent tablets), lemon flavour, calcium carbonate 1.5 g (calcium 600 mg or Ca²⁺ 15 mmol), colecalciferol 10 micrograms (400 units), net price 56-tab pack = £5.99. Label: 13
Caplets (= tablets), f/c, calcium carbonate 750 mg (calcium 300 mg or Ca²⁺ 7.5 mmol), colecalciferol 5 micrograms (200 units), net price 112-tab pack = £3.65

Cacit® D3 (Warner Chilcott)
Granules, effervescent, lemon flavour, calcium carbonate 1.25 g (calcium 500 mg or Ca²⁺ 12.5 mmol), colecalciferol 11 micrograms (440 units)/sachet, net price 30-sachet pack = £4.06. Label: 13

Calceos® (Galen)
Tablets (chewable), lemon flavour, calcium carbonate 1.25 g (calcium 500 mg or Ca²⁺ 12.5 mmol), colecalciferol 10 micrograms (400 units), net price 60-tab pack = £3.58. Label: 24

Calcichew-D₃® (Takeda)
Calcichew-D₃® Tablets (chewable), orange flavour, calcium carbonate 1.25 g (calcium 500 mg or Ca²⁺ 12.5 mmol), colecalciferol 5 micrograms (200 units), net price 100-tab pack = £7.68. Label: 24
Excipients include aspartame (section 9.4.1)
Calcichew-D₃® Forte Tablets (chewable), lemon flavour, calcium carbonate 1.25 g (calcium 500 mg or Ca²⁺ 12.5 mmol), colecalciferol 10 micrograms (400 units), net price 60-tab pack = £4.24, 100-tab pack = £7.08. Label: 24
Excipients include aspartame (section 9.4.1)

Calcichew-D₃® 500 mg/400 unit caplets, f/c, lemon flavour, calcium carbonate providing calcium 500 mg (Ca²⁺ 12.5 mmol), colecalciferol 10 micrograms (400 units), net price 100-tab pack = £7.43
Excipients include propylene glycol, see Excipients, p. 2

Calfovit D3® (Menarini)
Powder, lemon flavour, calcium phosphate 3.1 g (calcium 1.2 g or Ca²⁺ 30 mmol), colecalciferol 20 micrograms (800 units), net price 30-sachet pack = £4.32. Label: 13, 21

Kalcipos-D® (Meda) [PoM]
Tablets (chewable), calcium carbonate providing calcium 500 mg (Ca²⁺ 12.5 mmol), colecalciferol 20 micrograms (800 units), net price 30-tab pack = £4.21. Label: 24

Natecal D3® (Chiesi)
Tablets (chewable), (aniseed, peppermint, and molasses flavour), calcium carbonate 1.5 g (calcium 600 mg or Ca²⁺ 15 mmol), colecalciferol 10 micrograms (400 units), net price 60-tab pack = £3.63. Label: 24
Excipients include aspartame (section 9.4.1)

◀With alendronic acid
Section 6.6.2

◀With risedronate sodium and calcium
Section 6.6.2

DIHYDROTACHYSTEROL

Indications see notes above
Cautions see under Ergocalciferol
Contra-indications see under Ergocalciferol
Pregnancy see under Ergocalciferol
Breast-feeding see under Ergocalciferol
Side-effects see under Ergocalciferol

AT 10® (Intrapharm)
Oral solution, dihydrotachysterol 250 micrograms/mL. Net price 15-mL dropper bottle = £22.87
Excipients include arachis (peanut) oil
Dose acute, chronic, and latent forms of hypocalcaemic tetany due to hypoparathyroidism, consult product literature

PARICALCITOL

Indications see under preparations below
Cautions monitor plasma calcium and phosphate during dose titration and at least monthly when stabilised; monitor parathyroid hormone concentration; **interactions:** Appendix 1 (vitamins)
Contra-indications see under Ergocalciferol
Pregnancy toxicity in *animal* studies—manufacturer advises avoid unless potential benefit outweighs risk; see also under Ergocalciferol
Breast-feeding manufacturer advises caution—no information available; see also under Ergocalciferol
Side-effects see under Ergocalciferol; also dyspepsia, taste disturbance, breast tenderness, acne, pruritus, and rash
Dose
- Consult product literature

9

Nutrition and blood

Zemplar® (AbbVie) [PoM]

Capsules, paricalcitol 1 microgram (grey), net price 28-cap pack = £69.44; 2 micrograms (orange-brown), 28-cap pack = £138.88; 4 micrograms (gold), 28-cap pack = £277.76

For prevention and treatment of secondary hyperparathyroidism associated with chronic renal failure

Injection, paricalcitol 5 micrograms/mL, net price 1-mL amp = £12.40, 2-mL amp = £24.80. For injection via haemodialysis access

Excipients include propylene glycol, see Excipients, p. 2

For prevention and treatment of secondary hyperparathyroidism associated with chronic renal failure in patients on haemodialysis

9.6.5 Vitamin E
(Tocopherols)

The daily requirement of vitamin E has not been well defined but is probably about 3 to 15 mg daily. There is little evidence that oral supplements of vitamin E are essential in adults, even where there is fat malabsorption secondary to cholestasis. In young children with congenital cholestasis, abnormally low vitamin E concentrations may be found in association with neuromuscular abnormalities, which usually respond only to the parenteral administration of vitamin E.

Vitamin E has been tried for various other conditions but there is little scientific evidence of its value.

◼ ALPHA TOCOPHERYL ACETATE

Indications   see notes above

Cautions   predisposition to thrombosis; increased risk of necrotising enterocolitis in neonate weighing less than 1.5 kg; **interactions**: Appendix 1 (vitamins)

Pregnancy   no evidence of safety of high doses

Breast-feeding   excreted in milk; minimal risk, although caution with large doses

Side-effects   diarrhoea and abdominal pain with doses more than 1 g daily

Vitamin E Suspension (Non-proprietary)

Suspension, alpha tocopheryl acetate 500 mg/5 mL. Net price 100 mL = £42.12

Dose malabsorption in cystic fibrosis, 100–200 mg daily; CHILD 1 month–1 year 50 mg daily; 1–12 years, 100 mg daily

Malabsorption in abetalipoproteinaemia, ADULT and CHILD 50–100 mg/kg daily

Malabsorption in chronic cholestasis and severe liver disease, CHILD see BNF for Children

Note Tablets containing tocopheryl acetate are available from 'special-order' manufacturers or specialist importing companies, see p. 1124

◼ ALPHA TOCOPHEROL

Indications   vitamin E deficiency because of malabsorption in congenital or hereditary chronic cholestasis

Cautions   predisposition to thrombosis; **interactions**: Appendix 1 (Vitamin E)

Contra-indications   preterm neonates

Hepatic impairment   manufacturer advises caution and monitor closely—no information available

Renal impairment   manufacturer advises caution and monitor closely; risk of renal toxicity due to polyethylene glycol content

Pregnancy   manufacturer advises caution, no evidence of harm in *animal* studies

Breast-feeding   manufacturer advises use only if potential benefit outweighs risk—no information available

Side-effects   diarrhoea; *less commonly* asthenia, headache, disturbances in serum-potassium and serum-sodium concentrations, alopecia, pruritus, and rash

Vedrop® (Orphan Europe) ▼ [PoM]

Oral solution, yellow, D-alpha tocopherol (as tocofersolan) 50 mg/mL, net price 20 mL = £54.55, 60 mL = £163.65 (all with oral syringe)

Note Tocofersolan is a water-soluble form of D-alpha tocopherol

Dose CHILD under 18 years, 17 mg/kg daily, adjusted as necessary

9.6.6 Vitamin K

Vitamin K is necessary for the production of blood clotting factors and proteins necessary for the normal calcification of bone.

Because vitamin K is fat soluble, patients with fat malabsorption, especially in biliary obstruction or hepatic disease, may become deficient. **Menadiol sodium phosphate** is a water-soluble synthetic vitamin K derivative that can be given orally to prevent vitamin K deficiency in malabsorption syndromes.

Oral coumarin anticoagulants act by interfering with vitamin K metabolism in the hepatic cells and their effects can be antagonised by giving vitamin K; for advice on the use of vitamin K in haemorrhage, see section 2.8.2.

Vitamin K deficiency bleeding   Neonates are relatively deficient in vitamin K and those who do not receive supplements of vitamin K are at risk of serious bleeding including intracranial bleeding. The Chief Medical Officer and the Chief Nursing Officer have recommended that all newborn babies should receive vitamin K to prevent vitamin K deficiency bleeding (previously termed haemorrhagic disease of the newborn). An appropriate regimen should be selected after discussion with parents in the antenatal period.

Vitamin K (as **phytomenadione**) 1 mg may be given by a single intramuscular injection at birth; this prevents vitamin K deficiency bleeding in virtually all babies. For preterm neonates, see BNF for Children.

Alternatively, in healthy babies who are not at particular risk of bleeding disorders, vitamin K may be given by mouth, and arrangements must be in place to ensure the appropriate regimen is followed. Two doses of a colloidal (mixed micelle) preparation of phytomenadione 2 mg should be given by mouth in the first week, the first dose being given at birth and the second dose at 4–7 days. For exclusively breast-fed babies, a third dose of colloidal phytomenadione 2 mg is given by mouth at 1 month of age; the third dose is omitted in formula-fed babies because formula feeds contain adequate vitamin K. An alternative regimen is to give one dose of phytomenadione 1 mg by mouth at birth (using the contents of a phytomenadione capsule, see preparation below) to protect from the risk of vitamin K deficiency bleeding in the first week; for exclusively breast-fed babies, further doses of phytomenadione 1 mg are given by mouth (using the contents of a phytomenadione capsule) at weekly intervals for 12 weeks.

MENADIOL SODIUM PHOSPHATE

Indications see notes above

Cautions G6PD deficiency (section 9.1.5) and vitamin E deficiency (risk of haemolysis); **interactions:** Appendix 1 (vitamins)

Contra-indications neonates and infants

Pregnancy avoid in late pregnancy and labour unless benefit outweighs risk of neonatal haemolytic anaemia, hyperbilirubinaemia, and kernicterus in neonate

Dose

- 10–40 mg daily, adjusted as necessary; CHILD under 18 years see *BNF for Children*

Menadiol Phosphate (Non-proprietary)
Tablets, menadiol sodium phosphate equivalent to 10 mg of menadiol phosphate, net price 100-tab pack = £128.60

PHYTOMENADIONE
(Vitamin K₁)

Indications see notes above

Cautions intravenous injections should be given very slowly (see also below); **interactions:** Appendix 1 (vitamins)

Pregnancy use if potential benefit outweighs risk

Breast-feeding present in milk, but see notes above

Dose

- See notes above and section 2.8.2

Neokay® (Neoceuticals) [PoM]
Capsules, brown, phytomenadione 1 mg in an oily basis, net price 12-cap pack = £3.95; 100-cap pack = £34.00
Note The contents of one capsule should be administered by cutting the narrow tubular tip off and squeezing the liquid contents into the mouth; if the baby spits out the dose or is sick within three hours of administration a replacement dose should be given

◢Colloidal formulation

Konakion® MM (Roche) [PoM]
Injection, phytomenadione 10 mg/mL in a mixed micelles vehicle, net price 1-mL amp = 38p
Excipients include glycocholic acid 54.6 mg/amp, lecithin
Cautions reduce dose in elderly; liver impairment (glycocholic acid may displace bilirubin); reports of anaphylactoid reactions
Note *Konakion® MM* may be administered by slow intravenous injection or by intravenous infusion in glucose 5% (see Appendix 4); **not** for intramuscular injection

Konakion® MM Paediatric (Roche) ▼ [PoM]
Injection, phytomenadione 10 mg/mL in a mixed micelles vehicle, net price 0.2-mL amp = 94p
Excipients include glycocholic acid 10.9 mg/amp, lecithin
Cautions parenteral administration in neonate of less than 2.5 kg (increased risk of kernicterus)
Note *Konakion® MM Paediatric* may be administered by mouth or by intramuscular injection or by intravenous injection

9.6.7 Multivitamin preparations

Vitamins
Capsules, ascorbic acid 15 mg, nicotinamide 7.5 mg, riboflavin 500 micrograms, thiamine hydrochloride 1 mg, vitamin A 2500 units, vitamin D 300 units, net price 28-cap pack = £1.50

Abidec® (Chefaro UK)
Drops, vitamins A, B group, C, and D, net price 25 mL (with dropper) = £3.33
Excipients include arachis (peanut) oil
Note Contains 1333 units of vitamin A (as palmitate) per 0.6-mL dose

Dalivit® (LPC)
Oral drops, vitamins A, B group, C, and D, net price 25 mL = £3.28, 50 mL = £5.58
Note Contains 5000 units of vitamin A (as palmitate) per 0.6-mL dose

Vitamin and mineral supplements and adjuncts to synthetic diets

Forceval® (Alliance)
Capsules, brown/red, vitamins (ascorbic acid 60 mg, biotin 100 micrograms, cyanocobalamin 3 micrograms, folic acid 400 micrograms, nicotinamide 18 mg, pantothenic acid 4 mg, pyridoxine 2 mg, riboflavin 1.6 mg, thiamine 1.2 mg, vitamin A 2500 units, vitamin D₂ 400 units, vitamin E 10 mg, minerals and trace elements (calcium 100 mg, chromium 200 micrograms, copper 2 mg, iodine 140 micrograms, iron 12 mg, magnesium 30 mg, manganese 3 mg, molybdenum 250 micrograms, phosphorus 77 mg, potassium 4 mg, selenium 50 micrograms, zinc 15 mg), net price 15-cap pack = £3.40, 30-cap pack = £5.93, 90-cap pack = £14.32. Label: 25
Dose vitamin and mineral deficiency and as adjunct in synthetic diets, ADULT 1 capsule daily one hour after a meal

Ketovite® (Essential)
Tablets [PoM], yellow, ascorbic acid 16.6 mg, riboflavin 1 mg, thiamine hydrochloride 1 mg, pyridoxine hydrochloride 330 micrograms, nicotinamide 3.3 mg, calcium pantothenate 1.16 mg, alpha tocopheryl acetate 5 mg, inositol 50 mg, biotin 170 micrograms, folic acid 250 micrograms, acetomenaphthone 500 micrograms, net price 100-tab pack = £9.21
Dose prevention of vitamin deficiency in disorders of carbohydrate or amino-acid metabolism and adjunct in restricted, specialised, or synthetic diets, 1 tablet 3 times daily; use with *Ketovite® Liquid* for complete vitamin supplementation

Liquid, pink, sugar-free, vitamin A 2500 units, ergo-calciferol 400 units, choline chloride 150 mg, cyanocobalamin 12.5 micrograms/5 mL, net price 150-mL pack = £19.10
Dose prevention of vitamin deficiency in disorders of carbohydrate or amino-acid metabolism and adjunct in restricted, specialised, or synthetic diets, 5 mL daily; use with *Ketovite® Tablets* for complete vitamin supplementation

9.7 Bitters and tonics

Mixtures containing simple and aromatic bitters are traditional remedies for loss of appetite; there is no evidence to support their use.

9.8 Metabolic disorders

9.8.1 Drugs used in metabolic disorders
9.8.2 Acute porphyrias

This section covers drugs used in metabolic disorders and not readily classified elsewhere.

9 Nutrition and blood

9.8.1 Drugs used in metabolic disorders

Wilson's disease

Penicillamine (see also section 10.1.3) is used in Wilson's disease (hepatolenticular degeneration) to aid the elimination of copper ions. See below for other indications.

Trientine is used for the treatment of Wilson's disease only in patients intolerant of penicillamine; it is **not** an alternative to penicillamine for rheumatoid arthritis or cystinuria. Penicillamine-induced systemic lupus erythematosus may not resolve on transfer to trientine.

Zinc prevents the absorption of copper in Wilson's disease. Symptomatic patients should be treated initially with a chelating agent because zinc has a slow onset of action. When transferring from chelating treatment to zinc maintenance therapy, chelating treatment should be co-administered for 2–3 weeks until zinc produces its maximal effect.

◼ PENICILLAMINE

Indications see under Dose below

Cautions section 10.1.3; also neurological involvement in Wilson's disease

Contra-indications section 10.1.3

Renal impairment section 10.1.3

Pregnancy section 10.1.3

Breast-feeding section 10.1.3

Side-effects section 10.1.3; also neuropathy (especially if previous neurological involvement in Wilson's disease—prophylactic pyridoxine recommended, see section 9.6.2)

Dose
- Wilson's disease, 1.5–2 g daily in divided doses before food; max. 2 g daily for 1 year; maintenance 0.75–1 g daily; ELDERLY 20 mg/kg daily in divided doses, adjusted according to response; CHILD see *BNF for Children*
- Autoimmune hepatitis (used rarely; after disease controlled with corticosteroids), initially 500 mg daily in divided doses increased slowly over 3 months; usual maintenance dose 1.25 g daily; ELDERLY not recommended
- Cystinuria, therapeutic, 1–3 g daily in divided doses before food, adjusted to maintain urinary cystine below 200 mg/litre; prophylactic (maintain urinary cystine below 300 mg/litre) 0.5–1 g at bedtime; maintain adequate fluid intake (at least 3 litres daily); ELDERLY minimum dose to maintain urinary cystine below 200 mg/litre; CHILD see *BNF for Children*
- Severe active rheumatoid arthritis, section 10.1.3

◢**Preparations**
Section 10.1.3

◼ TRIENTINE DIHYDROCHLORIDE

Indications Wilson's disease in patients intolerant of penicillamine

Cautions see notes above; **interactions:** Appendix 1 (trientine)

Pregnancy manufacturer advises use only if potential benefit outweighs risk; monitor maternal and neonatal

serum-copper concentration; teratogenic in *animal* studies

Side-effects nausea, rash; *very rarely* anaemia; duodenitis and colitis also reported

Dose
- ADULT and CHILD over 12 years, 1.2–2.4 g daily in 2–4 divided doses before food; CHILD 2–12 years, initially 0.6–1.5 g daily in 2–4 divided doses before food, adjusted according to response

Trientine Dihydrochloride (Univar) ▱PoM▱
Capsules, trientine dihydrochloride 300 mg. Label: 6, 22

◼ ZINC ACETATE

Indications Wilson's disease (initiated under specialist supervision)

Cautions portal hypertension (risk of hepatic decompensation when switching from chelating agent); monitor full blood count and serum cholesterol; **interactions:** Appendix 1 (zinc)

Pregnancy reduce dose to 25 mg 3 times daily adjusted according to plasma-copper concentration and urinary copper excretion

Breast-feeding manufacturer advises avoid; present in milk—may cause zinc-induced copper deficiency in infant

Side-effects gastric irritation (usually transient; may be reduced if first dose taken mid-morning or with a little protein); *less commonly* sideroblastic anaemia and leucopenia

Dose
Note Dose expressed as elemental zinc
- Wilson's disease, 50 mg 3 times daily (max. 50 mg 5 times daily), adjusted according to response; CHILD 1–6 years, 25 mg twice daily; 6–16 years, body-weight under 57 kg, 25 mg 3 times daily, body-weight over 57 kg, 50 mg 3 times daily; ADOLESCENT 16–18 years, 50 mg 3 times daily

Wilzin® (Orphan Europe) ▱PoM▱
Capsules, zinc (as acetate) 25 mg (blue), net price 250-cap pack = £132.00; 50 mg (orange), 250-cap pack = £242.00. Label: 23

Carnitine deficiency

Levocarnitine is available for the management of primary carnitine deficiency due to inborn errors of metabolism or of secondary deficiency in haemodialysis patients.

◼ LEVOCARNITINE
(Carnitine)

Indications primary and secondary carnitine deficiency

Cautions diabetes mellitus; monitoring of free and acyl carnitine in blood and urine recommended

Renal impairment accumulation of metabolites may occur with chronic oral administration in severe impairment

Pregnancy appropriate to use; no evidence of teratogenicity in *animal* studies

Side-effects nausea, vomiting, abdominal pain, diarrhoea, body odour; side-effects may be dose-related—monitor tolerance during first week and after any dose increase

9 Nutrition and blood

Dose

- Primary deficiency, by mouth, up to 200 mg/kg daily in 2–4 divided doses; usual max. 3 g daily; by intravenous injection over 2–3 minutes, up to 100 mg/kg daily in 2–4 divided doses
- Secondary deficiency, by intravenous injection over 2–3 minutes, 20 mg/kg after each dialysis session (dosage adjusted according to plasma-carnitine concentration); maintenance (if benefit gained from first intravenous course), by mouth, 1 g daily

Levocarnitine (Non-proprietary) PoM

Paediatric oral solution, levocarnitine 300 mg/mL (30%), net price 20 mL = £55.55

Carnitor® (Sigma-Tau) PoM

Tablets, levocarnitine 330 mg, net price 90-tab pack = £103.95

Chewable tablets, levocarnitine 1 g, net price 10-tab pack = £35.00

Oral liquid, levocarnitine 100 mg/mL (10%), net price 10 × 10-mL (1-g) single-dose bottle = £35.00

Injection, levocarnitine 200 mg/mL, net price 5-mL amp = £11.90

Fabry's disease

Agalsidase alfa and **agalsidase beta**, enzymes produced by recombinant DNA technology, are licensed for long-term enzyme replacement therapy in Fabry's disease (a lysosomal storage disorder caused by deficiency of alpha-galactosidase A).

▍ AGALSIDASE ALFA and BETA

Indications Fabry's disease (specialist use only)

Cautions interactions: Appendix 1 (agalsidase alfa and beta)

Infusion-related reactions Infusion-related reactions very common; manage by slowing the infusion rate or interrupting the infusion, or minimise by pre-treatment with an antihistamine, antipyretic, or corticosteroid—consult product literature

Pregnancy use with caution

Breast-feeding use with caution—no information available

Side-effects gastro-intestinal disturbances, taste disturbances; tachycardia, bradycardia, palpitation, hypertension, hypotension, chest pain, oedema, flushing; dyspnoea, cough, rhinorrhoea; headache, fatigue, dizziness, asthenia, paraesthesia, syncope, neuropathic pain, tremor, sleep disturbances; influenza-like symptoms, nasopharyngitis; muscle spasms, myalgia, arthralgia; eye irritation; tinnitus; hypersensitivity reactions, angioedema, pruritus, urticaria, rash, acne; less commonly cold extremities, parosmia, ear pain and swelling, skin discoloration, and injection-site reactions

Fabrazyme® (Genzyme) PoM

Intravenous infusion, powder for reconstitution, agalsidase beta, net price 5-mg vial = £315.08; 35-mg vial = £2196.59

Dose By intravenous infusion, ADULT and CHILD over 8 years 1 mg/kg every 2 weeks

Replagal® (Shire HGT) PoM

Concentrate for intravenous infusion, agalsidase alfa 1 mg/mL, net price 3.5-mL vial = £1068.64

Dose By intravenous infusion, ADULT and CHILD over 7 years 200 micrograms/kg every 2 weeks

Gaucher's disease

Imiglucerase, an enzyme produced by recombinant DNA technology, is administered as enzyme replacement therapy for non-neurological manifestations of type I or type III Gaucher's disease, a familial disorder affecting principally the liver, spleen, bone marrow, and lymph nodes.

Velaglucerase alfa, an enzyme produced by recombinant DNA technology, is administered as enzyme replacement therapy for the treatment of type I Gaucher's disease.

Miglustat, an inhibitor of glucosylceramide synthase, is licensed for the treatment of mild to moderate type I Gaucher's disease in patients for whom enzyme replacement therapy is unsuitable; it is given by mouth; see p. 712.

▍ IMIGLUCERASE

Indications (specialist use only) non-neurological manifestations of type I or type III Gaucher's disease

Cautions monitor immunoglobulin G (IgG) antibody concentration; when stabilised, monitor all parameters and response to treatment at intervals of 6–12 months

Pregnancy manufacturer advises use with caution—limited information available

Breast-feeding no information available

Side-effects hypersensitivity reactions (including urticaria, angioedema, cyanosis, hypotension, flushing, tachycardia, paraesthesia, backache); less commonly nausea, vomiting, diarrhoea, abdominal cramps, headache, dizziness, fatigue, fever, arthralgia, and injection-site reactions

Dose

- By intravenous infusion, initially 60 units/kg once every 2 weeks (doses as low as 15 units/kg once every 2 weeks may improve haematological parameters and organomegaly); maintenance, adjust dose according to response; CHILD under 18 years see BNF for Children

Cerezyme® (Genzyme) PoM

Intravenous infusion, powder for reconstitution, imiglucerase, net price 200-unit vial = £535.65; 400-unit vial = £1071.29

Electrolytes Na⁺ 0.62 mmol/200-unit vial, 1.24 mmol/400-unit vial

▍ VELAGLUCERASE ALFA

Indications (specialist use only) type I Gaucher's disease

Cautions monitor immunoglobulin G (IgG) antibody concentration in severe infusion-related reactions or if there is a lack or loss of effect with velaglucerase alfa

Infusion-related reactions Infusion-related reactions very common; manage by slowing the infusion rate, or interrupting the infusion, or minimise by pre-treatment with an antihistamine, antipyretic, or corticosteroid—consult product literature

Pregnancy manufacturer advises use with caution—limited information available

Breast-feeding manufacturer advises use with caution—no information available

Side-effects nausea, abdominal pain, tachycardia, hypertension, hypotension, flushing, headache, dizziness, malaise, pyrexia, arthralgia, bone pain, back pain, hypersensitivity reactions, rash, urticaria

Dose

- By intravenous infusion, 60 units/kg once every 2 weeks; adjusted according to response to 15–60 units/kg once every 2 weeks; CHILD under 18 years see *BNF for Children*

VPRIV® (Shire HGT) ▼ PoM
Intravenous infusion, powder for reconstitution, velaglucerase alfa, net price 400-unit vial = £1410.20
Electrolytes Na⁺ 0.53 mmol/400-unit vial

Mucopolysaccharidosis

Laronidase, an enzyme produced by recombinant DNA technology, is licensed for long-term replacement therapy in the treatment of non-neurological manifestations of mucopolysaccharidosis I, a lysosomal storage disorder caused by deficiency of alpha-L-iduronidase.

Idursulfase, an enzyme produced by recombinant DNA technology, is licensed for long-term replacement therapy in mucopolysaccharidosis II (Hunter syndrome), a lysosomal storage disorder caused by deficiency of iduronate-2-sulfatase.

Galsulfase, a recombinant form of human N-acetylgalactosamine-4-sulfatase, is licensed for long-term replacement therapy in mucopolysaccharidosis VI (Maroteaux-Lamy syndrome).

Infusion-related reactions Infusion-related reactions often occur with administration of laronidase, idursulfase, and galsulfase; they can be managed by slowing the infusion rate or interrupting the infusion, and can be minimised by pre-treatment with an antihistamine and an antipyretic. Recurrent infusion-related reactions may require pre-treatment with a corticosteroid—consult product literature for details.

GALSULFASE

Indications (specialist use only) mucopolysaccharidosis VI

Cautions respiratory disease; acute febrile or respiratory illness (consider delaying treatment)
Infusion-related reactions See notes above

Pregnancy manufacturer advises avoid unless essential

Breast-feeding manufacturer advises avoid—no information available

Side-effects abdominal pain, umbilical hernia, gastroenteritis; chest pain, hypertension; dyspnoea, apnoea, nasal congestion; rigors, malaise, areflexia; pharyngitis; conjunctivitis, corneal opacity; ear pain; facial oedema

Dose

- By intravenous infusion, ADULT and CHILD over 5 years, 1 mg/kg once weekly

Naglazyme® (BioMarin) PoM
Concentrate for intravenous infusion, galsulfase 1 mg/mL, net price 5-mL vial = £982.00

IDURSULFASE

Indications (specialist use only) mucopolysaccharidosis II

Cautions severe respiratory disease; acute febrile respiratory illness (consider delaying treatment)
Infusion-related reactions See notes above

Contra-indications women of child-bearing potential

Pregnancy manufacturer advises avoid

Breast-feeding manufacturer advises avoid—present in milk in *animal* studies

Side-effects gastro-intestinal disturbances, swollen tongue; arrhythmia, tachycardia, chest pain, cyanosis, peripheral oedema, hypertension, hypotension, flushing; bronchospasm, hypoxia, cough, wheezing, tachypnoea, dyspnoea; headache, dizziness, tremor; pyrexia; arthralgia; facial oedema, urticaria, pruritus, rash, infusion-site swelling, erythema; pulmonary embolism and anaphylaxis also reported

Dose

- By intravenous infusion, ADULT and CHILD over 5 years, 500 micrograms/kg once weekly

Elaprase® (Shire HGT) ▼ PoM
Concentrate for intravenous infusion, idursulfase 2 mg/mL, net price 3-mL vial = £1985.00

LARONIDASE

Indications (specialist use only) non-neurological manifestations of mucopolysaccharidosis I

Cautions monitor immunoglobulin G (IgG) antibody concentration; **interactions:** Appendix 1 (laronidase)
Infusion-related reactions See notes above

Pregnancy manufacturer advises avoid unless essential—no information available

Breast-feeding manufacturer advises avoid—no information available

Side-effects nausea, vomiting, diarrhoea, abdominal pain; cold extremities, pallor, flushing, tachycardia, blood pressure changes; dyspnoea, cough, angioedema, anaphylaxis; headache, paraesthesia, dizziness, fatigue, restlessness; influenza-like symptoms; musculoskeletal pain, pain in extremities; rash, pruritus, urticaria, alopecia, infusion-site reactions; bronchospasm and respiratory arrest also reported

Dose

- By intravenous infusion, 100 units/kg once weekly; CHILD see *BNF for Children*

Aldurazyme® (Genzyme) PoM
Concentrate for intravenous infusion, laronidase 100 units/mL, net price 5-mL vial = £444.70
Electrolytes Na⁺ 1.29 mmol/5-mL vial

Nephropathic cystinosis

Mercaptamine is available for the treatment of nephropathic cystinosis.

MERCAPTAMINE
(Cysteamine)

Indications (specialist use only) nephropathic cystinosis

Cautions leucocyte-cystine concentration and haematological monitoring required—consult product literature; dose of phosphate supplement may need to be adjusted if transferring from phosphocysteamine to mercaptamine

Contra-indications hypersensitivity to penicillamine

Pregnancy avoid—teratogenic and toxic in *animal* studies

Breast-feeding avoid

Side-effects breath and body odour, nausea, vomiting, diarrhoea, anorexia, abdominal pain, gastroenteritis, dyspepsia, encephalopathy, headache, malaise, fever, rash; *less commonly* gastro-intestinal ulcer, seizures, hallucinations, drowsiness, nervousness, leucopenia, nephrotic syndrome

Dose

- Initial doses should be one-sixth to one-quarter of the expected maintenance dose, increased gradually over 4–6 weeks
- Maintenance, ADULT and CHILD over 50 kg bodyweight, 2 g daily in 4 divided doses
  CHILD up to 12 years, 1.3 g/m^2 (approx. 50 mg/kg) daily in 4 divided doses

Cystagon® (Orphan Europe) [PoM]
Capsules, mercaptamine (as bitartrate) 50 mg, net price 100-cap pack = £70.00; 150 mg, 100-cap pack = £190.00. Label: 21
Note CHILD under 6 years at risk of aspiration, capsules can be opened and contents sprinkled on food (at a temperature suitable for eating); avoid adding to acidic drinks (e.g. orange juice)

Pompe disease

Alglucosidase alfa, an enzyme produced by recombinant DNA technology, is licensed for long-term replacement therapy in Pompe disease, a lysosomal storage disorder caused by deficiency of acid alpha-glucosidase.

ALGLUCOSIDASE ALFA

Indications (specialist use only) Pompe disease

Cautions cardiac and respiratory dysfunction—monitor closely; monitor immunoglobulin G (IgG) antibody concentration

Infusion-related reactions Infusion-related reactions very common, calling for use of antihistamine, antipyretic, or corticosteroid; consult product literature for details

Pregnancy toxicity in *animal* studies, but treatment should not be withheld

Breast-feeding manufacturer advises avoid—no information available

Side-effects nausea, vomiting, diarrhoea; flushing, tachycardia, blood pressure changes, cold extremities, cyanosis, facial oedema, chest discomfort; cough, tachypnoea, bronchospasm; headache, agitation, tremor, irritability, restlessness, paraesthesia, dizziness, fatigue; pyrexia; antibody formation; myalgia, muscle spasm; sweating, rash, pruritus, urticaria, injection-site reactions; hypersensitivity reactions (including anaphylaxis); severe skin reactions (including ulcerative and necrotising skin lesions) also reported

Dose

- By intravenous infusion, ADULT and CHILD 20 mg/kg every 2 weeks

Myozyme® (Genzyme) [PoM]
Intravenous infusion, powder for reconstitution, alglucosidase alfa, net price 50-mg vial = £356.06

Tyrosinaemia type I

Nitisinone is licensed for the treatment of hereditary tyrosinaemia type I in combination with dietary restriction of tyrosine and phenylalanine.

NITISINONE
(NTBC)

Indications hereditary tyrosinaemia type I (specialist use only)

Cautions slit-lamp examination of eyes recommended before treatment; monitor liver function regularly; monitor platelet and white blood cell count every 6 months

Pregnancy manufacturer advises avoid unless potential benefit outweighs risk—toxicity in *animal* studies

Breast-feeding manufacturer advises avoid—adverse effects in *animal* studies

Side-effects thrombocytopenia, leucopenia, granulocytopenia; conjunctivitis, photophobia, corneal opacity, keratitis, eye pain; *less commonly* leucocytosis, blepharitis, pruritus, exfoliative dermatitis, and erythematous rash

Dose

- ADULT and CHILD initially 500 micrograms/kg twice daily, adjusted according to response; max. 2 mg/kg daily
  Note Capsules can be opened and the contents suspended in a small amount of water or formula diet and taken immediately

Orfadin® (Swedish Orphan) [PoM]
Capsules, nitisinone 2 mg, net price 60-cap pack = £564.00; 5 mg, 60-cap pack = £1127.00; 10 mg, 60-cap pack = £2062.00

Urea cycle disorders

Sodium phenylbutyrate is used in the management of urea cycle disorders. It is indicated as adjunctive therapy in all patients with neonatal-onset disease and in those with late-onset disease who have a history of hyperammonaemic encephalopathy.

Carglumic acid is licensed for the treatment of hyperammonaemia due to *N*-acetylglutamate synthase deficiency and organic acidaemia.

> **Emergency management**
> For further information on the emergency management of urea cycle disorders consult the British Inherited Metabolic Disease Group (BIMDG) website at www.bimdg.org.uk.

CARGLUMIC ACID

Indications hyperammonaemia due to *N*-acetylglutamate synthase deficiency and organic acidaemia under specialist supervision; see also notes above

Pregnancy manufacturer advises avoid unless essential—no information available

Breast-feeding manufacturer advises avoid—present in milk in *animal* studies

Side-effects sweating; *less commonly* diarrhoea, vomiting, bradycardia, pyrexia

Dose

- Hyperammonaemia due to *N*-acetylglutamate synthase deficiency, ADULT and CHILD initially 100–250 mg/kg daily in 2–4 divided doses immediately before food, adjusted according to plasma–ammonia concentration; maintenance 10–100 mg/kg daily in 2–4 divided doses
- Hyperammonaemia due to organic acidaemia, ADULT and CHILD initially 100–250 mg/kg daily in 2–4 divided doses immediately before food, adjusted according to plasma-ammonia concentration

9

Nutrition and blood

Carbaglu® (Orphan Europe) [PoM]
Dispersible tablets, carglumic acid 200 mg, net price 5-tab pack = £299.00, 60-tab pack = £3499.00.
Label: 13
Note Must be dispersed in at least 5–10 mL of water and taken orally immediately, or administered via a nasogastric tube

■ SODIUM PHENYLBUTYRATE

Indications adjunct in long-term treatment of urea cycle disorders (under specialist supervision); see also notes above

Cautions congestive heart failure; **interactions:** Appendix 1 (sodium phenylbutyrate)

Hepatic impairment manufacturer advises caution

Renal impairment manufacturer advises caution

Pregnancy avoid—toxicity in *animal* studies; manufacturer advises adequate contraception during administration

Breast-feeding manufacturer advises avoid—no information available

Side-effects gastro-intestinal disturbances, weight gain, taste disturbance, decreased appetite; syncope, oedema; headache, depression, irritability; renal tubular acidosis, menstrual disorders; blood disorders, metabolic acidosis, alkalosis; rash, body odour; *less commonly* rectal bleeding, peptic ulcer, pancreatitis, and arrhythmias

Dose
● ADULT 9.9–13 g/m² daily in divided doses with meals (max. 20 g daily); CHILD see *BNF for Children*

Ammonaps® (Swedish Orphan) [PoM]
Tablets, sodium phenylbutyrate 500 mg. Contains Na⁺ 2.7 mmol/tablet. Net price 250-tab pack = £493.00

Granules, sodium phenylbutyrate 940 mg/g. Contains Na⁺ 5.4 mmol/g of sodium phenylbutyrate. Net price 266-g pack = £860.00
Note Granules should be mixed with food before taking

Pheburane® (Lucane) [PoM]
Granules, sodium phenylbutyrate 483 mg/g. Contains Na⁺ 5.4 mmol/g of sodium phenylbutyrate, net price 174-g pack = £331.00
Note Granules should be mixed with food before taking orally and must not be administered by nasogastric or gastrostomy tubes

Homocystinuria

Betaine is licensed for the adjunctive treatment of homocystinuria involving deficiencies or defects in cystathionine beta-synthase, 5,10-methylene-tetrahydrofolate reductase, or cobalamin cofactor metabolism. Betaine should be used in conjunction with dietary restrictions and may be given with supplements of Vitamin B₁₂, pyridoxine, and folate under specialist advice.

The *Scottish Medicines Consortium* (p. 4) has advised (July 2010) that betaine anhydrous (*Cystadane®*) is accepted for restricted use within NHS Scotland for the adjunctive treatment of homocystinuria involving deficiencies or defects in cystathionine beta-synthase, 5,10-methylene-tetrahydrofolate reductase, or cobalamin cofactor metabolism in patients who are not responsive to pyridoxine treatment.

■ BETAINE

Indications (specialist use only) adjunctive treatment of homocystinuria

Cautions monitor plasma-methionine concentration before and during treatment—interrupt treatment if symptoms of cerebral oedema occur

Pregnancy manufacturer advises avoid unless essential—limited information available

Breast-feeding manufacturer advises caution—no information available

Side-effects *less commonly* gastro-intestinal disorders, anorexia, reversible cerebral oedema (see Cautions), agitation, depression, personality disorder, sleep disturbances, urinary incontinence, alopecia, and urticaria

Dose
● ADULT and CHILD over 10 years, 3 g twice daily, adjusted according to response; max. 20 g/day; CHILD under 10 years 50 mg/kg twice daily, dose and frequency adjusted according to response; max. 75 mg/kg twice daily

Cystadane® (Orphan Europe) [PoM]
Powder, betaine (anhydrous), net price 180 g = £347.00
Note Powder should be mixed with water, juice, milk, formula, or food until completely dissolved and taken immediately; measuring spoons are provided to measure 1 g, 150 mg, and 100 mg of powder

Other metabolic disorders

Miglustat is available for the treatment of progressive neurological manifestations of Niemann-Pick type C disease, a neurodegenerative disorder characterised by impaired intracellular lipid trafficking; it is also licensed for the treatment of mild to moderate type 1 Gaucher's disease for whom imiglucerase is unsuitable, see also p. 709.

■ MIGLUSTAT

Indications mild to moderate type I Gaucher's disease (specialist supervision only); Niemann-Pick type C disease (specialist supervision only)

Cautions monitor cognitive and neurological function; monitor growth and platelet count in Niemann-Pick type C disease

Hepatic impairment no information available—manufacturer advises caution

Renal impairment for Gaucher's disease initially 100 mg twice daily if eGFR 50–70 mL/minute/1.73 m²; initially 100 mg once daily if eGFR 30–50 mL/minute/1.73 m²; for Niemann-Pick type C disease, initially 200 mg twice daily if eGFR 50–70 mL/minute/1.73 m²; initially 100 mg twice daily if eGFR 30–50 mL/minute/1.73 m²; child under 12 years—consult product literature; avoid if eGFR less than 30 mL/minute/1.73 m²

Pregnancy manufacturer advises avoid (toxicity in *animal* studies)—effective contraception must be used during treatment; also men should avoid fathering a child during and for 3 months after treatment

Breast-feeding manufacturer advises avoid—no information available

Side-effects diarrhoea, flatulence, abdominal pain, dyspepsia, constipation, nausea, vomiting, anorexia,

weight changes, tremor, dizziness, headache, peripheral neuropathy, ataxia, amnesia, hypoaesthesia,
paraesthesia, insomnia, depression, chills, malaise,
decreased libido, thrombocytopenia, muscle spasm
and weakness

Dose
- Gaucher's disease, ADULT over 18 years, 100 mg 3
  times daily; reduced if not tolerated to 100 mg 1–2
  times daily
- Niemann-Pick type C disease, ADULT and CHILD over
  12 years, 200 mg 3 times daily; CHILD 4–12 years, body
  surface area less than 0.47 m^2, 100 mg once daily;
  body surface area 0.47–0.73 m^2, 100 mg twice daily;
  body surface area 0.73–0.88 m^2, 100 mg three times
  daily; body surface area 0.88–1.25 m^2, 200 mg twice
  daily; body surface area greater than 1.25 m^2, adult
  dose

Zavesca® (Actelion) PoM
Capsules, miglustat 100 mg, net price 84-cap pack =
£3934.17 (hospital only)

9.8.2 Acute porphyrias

The acute porphyrias (acute intermittent porphyria,
variegate porphyria, hereditary coproporphyria, and 5-
aminolaevulinic acid dehydratase deficiency porphyria)
are hereditary disorders of haem biosynthesis; they have
a prevalence of about 1 in 10 000 of the population.

Great care must be taken when prescribing for patients
with acute porphyria, since certain drugs can induce
acute porphyric crises. Since acute porphyrias are
hereditary, relatives of affected individuals should be
screened and advised about the potential danger of
certain drugs.

Treatment of serious or life-threatening conditions
should not be withheld from patients with acute porphyria. When there is no safe alternative, treatment
should be started and urinary porpholobilinogen excretion
should be measured regularly; if it increases or symptoms occur, the drug can be withdrawn and the acute
attack treated. If an acute attack of porphyria occurs
during pregnancy, contact an expert porphyria service
for further advice.

Haem arginate is administered by short intravenous
infusion as haem replacement in moderate, severe, or
unremitting acute porphyria crises.

In the United Kingdom the National Acute Porphyria
Service (NAPS) provides clinical support and treatment
with haem arginate from two centres (University Hospital of Wales in Cardiff, and King's College Hospital in
London). To access the service telephone (029) 2074
7747 and ask for the Acute Porphyria Service.

▌ HAEM ARGINATE
(Human hemin)

Indications   acute porphyrias (acute intermittent porphyria, porphyria variegata, hereditary coproporphyria)

Pregnancy   manufacturer advises avoid unless essential

Breast-feeding   manufacturer advises avoid unless
essential—no information available

Side-effects   pain and thrombophlebitis at injection
site; *rarely* hypersensitivity reactions and fever; *also
reported* headache

Dose
- By intravenous infusion, ADULT and CHILD 3 mg/kg
  once daily (max. 250 mg daily) for 4 days; if response
  inadequate, repeat 4-day course with close biochemical monitoring

Normosang® (Orphan Europe) ▼ PoM
Concentrate for intravenous infusion, haem arginate
25 mg/mL, net price 10-mL amp = £434.25

Drugs unsafe for use in acute porphyrias

The following list contains drugs on the UK market that
have been classified as 'unsafe' in porphyria because
they have been shown to be porphyrinogenic in animals
or *in vitro*, or have been associated with acute attacks in
patients. Absence of a drug from the following lists does
not necessarily imply that the drug is safe. For many
drugs no information about porphyria is available.

An up-to-date list of drugs considered **safe** in acute
porphyrias is available at www.wmic.wales.nhs.uk/
porphyria_info.php

Further information may be obtained from:
www.porphyria-europe.org

and also from:

Welsh Medicines Information Centre
University Hospital of Wales
Cardiff, CF14 4XW
Tel: (029) 2074 2979/3877
Note Quite modest changes in chemical structure can lead
to changes in porphyrinogenicity but where possible general
statements have been made about groups of drugs; these
should be checked first.

Unsafe Drug Groups (check first)

Alkylating drugs[1]	Calcium channel blockers[5]	Non-nucleoside reverse transcriptase inhibitors[1]	Taxanes[1]
Amfetamines	Contraceptives, hormonal[6]		Thiazolidinediones[1]
Anabolic steroids	Ergot derivatives[7]	Progestogens[6]	Triazole antifungals[8]
Antidepressants[2]	Hormone replacement therapy[6]	Protease inhibitors[1]	
Antihistamines[3]		Sulfonamides[9]	
Barbiturates[4]	Imidazole antifungals[8]	Sulfonylureas[10]	

Unsafe Drugs (check groups above first)

Aceclofenac	Disopyramide	Metolazone	Riluzole
Alcohol	Disulfiram	Metyrapone	Risperidone
Amiodarone	Erythromycin	Mifepristone	Selegiline
Aprepitant[1]	Etamsylate	Minoxidil[14]	Spironolactone
Artemether with lumefantrine	Ethosuximide	Mitotane	Sulfinpyrazone
Bexarotene	Etomidate	Nalidixic acid	Tamoxifen
Bosentan	Fenfluramine	Nitrazepam	Telithromycin
Bromocriptine	Flupentixol	Nitrofurantoin	Temoporfin
Buspirone	Flutamide	Orphenadrine	Tiagabine
Cabergoline	Fosaprepitant[1]	Oxcarbazepine	Tibolone
Carbamazepine	Fosphenytoin	Oxybutynin	Tinidazole
Chloral hydrate[11]	Griseofulvin	Pentazocine[15]	Topiramate
Chloramphenicol	Hydralazine	Pentoxifylline	Toremifene
Chloroform[12]	Indapamide	Phenoxybenzamine	Trimethoprim
Clindamycin	Isometheptene mucate	Phenytoin	Valproate
Cocaine	Isoniazid[13]	Pivmecillinam	Xipamide
Colistimethate sodium	Ketamine	Porfimer	Zidovudine[1]
Danazol	Mefenamic acid[14]	Raloxifene	Zuclopenthixol
Dapsone	Meprobamate	Rifabutin[13]	
Dexfenfluramine	Methyldopa	Rifampicin	

1. Contact Welsh Medicines Information Centre for further advice.
2. Includes tricyclic (and related) antidepressants and MAOIs; fluoxetine, duloxetine, venlafaxine, and trazodone thought to be safe.
3. Alimemazine, chlorphenamine, desloratadine, fexofenadine, ketotifen, loratadine, and promethazine thought to be safe.
4. Includes primidone and thiopental.
5. Amlodipine, felodipine, and nifedipine thought to be safe.
6. Progestogens are more porphyrinogenic than oestrogens; oestrogens may be safe at least in replacement doses. Progestogens should be avoided whenever possible by all women susceptible to acute porphyria; however, when non-hormonal contraception is inappropriate, progestogens may be used with extreme caution if the potential benefit outweighs risk. The risk of an acute attack is greatest in women who have had a previous attack or are aged under 30 years. Long-acting progestogen preparations should **never** be used in those at risk of acute porphyria.
7. Includes ergometrine (oxytocin probably safe) and pergolide.
8. Applies to oral and intravenous use; topical antifungals are thought to be safe due to low systemic exposure.
9. Includes co-trimoxazole and sulfasalazine.
10. Glipizide and glimepiride are thought to be safe.
11. Although evidence of hazard is uncertain, manufacturer advises avoid.
12. Small amounts in medicines probably safe.
13. Safety uncertain, contact Welsh Medicines Information Centre for further advice.
14. May be used with caution if safer alternative not available.
15. Buprenorphine, codeine, diamorphine, dihydrocodeine, fentanyl, methadone, morphine, oxycodone, pethidine, and tramadol are thought to be safe.

10 Musculoskeletal and joint diseases

This chapter also includes advice on the drug management of the following:

dental and orofacial pain, p. 717

extravasation, p. 750

gout, p. 742

myasthenia gravis, p. 745

osteoarthritis and soft-tissue disorders, below

rheumatic arthritis and other inflammatory disorders, below

For treatment of septic arthritis see Table 1, section 5.1.

10.1 Drugs used in rheumatic diseases and gout

Rheumatoid arthritis and other inflammatory disorders

A **non-steroidal anti-inflammatory drug** (NSAID) is indicated for pain and stiffness resulting from inflammatory rheumatic disease; analgesics such as **paracetamol** or **codeine** can also be used. For advice on the prophylaxis and treatment of NSAID-associated gastro-intestinal ulcers, see p. 51.

Drugs are also used to influence the rheumatic disease process itself (section 10.1.3). For *rheumatoid arthritis* these **disease-modifying antirheumatic drugs** (DMARDs) include methotrexate, cytokine modulators, azathioprine, ciclosporin, cyclophosphamide, leflunomide, penicillamine, gold, antimalarials (chloroquine and hydroxychloroquine), and sulfasalazine. **Corticosteroids** also have a significant role in the management of rheumatoid arthritis (section 10.1.2.1).

Drugs which may affect the disease process in *psoriatic arthritis* include sulfasalazine, gold, azathioprine, methotrexate, leflunomide, and cytokine modulators (section 10.1.3).

For long-term control of *gout*, xanthine-oxidase inhibitors or uricosuric drugs (section 10.1.4) can be used.

Osteoarthritis and soft-tissue disorders

For pain relief in osteoarthritis and soft-tissue disorders, **paracetamol** (section 4.7.1) should be used first and may need to be taken regularly. A **topical NSAID** (section 10.3.2) or topical **capsaicin** 0.025% (section 10.3.2) should also be considered, particularly in knee or hand osteoarthritis. An **oral NSAID** (section 10.1.1) can be substituted for, or used in addition to, paracetamol. If further pain relief is required in osteoarthritis, then the addition of an **opioid** analgesic (section 4.7.2) may be considered, but with a substantial risk of adverse effects; however, an opioid analgesic should be considered before a NSAID in patients taking low-dose aspirin. For advice on the prophylaxis and treatment of NSAID-associated gastro-intestinal ulcers, see p. 51.

Intra-articular **corticosteroid** injections (section 10.1.2.2) may produce temporary benefit in osteoarthritis, especially if associated with soft-tissue inflammation.

Non-drug measures, such as weight reduction and exercise, should also be encouraged.

Glucosamine (section 10.1.5) and **rubefacients** (section 10.3.2) are not recommended for the treatment of osteoarthritis.

Hyaluronic acid and its derivatives are available for osteoarthritis of the knee, but are not recommended. Sodium hyaluronate (*Durolane*®, *Euflexxa*®, *Fermathron*®, *Hyalgan*®, *Orthovisc*®, *Ostenil*®, *Ostenil Plus*®, *RenehaVis*®, *Suplasyn*®, *Synocrom*®, *Synopsis*®) or hylan G-F 20 (*Synvisc*®) is injected intra-articularly to supplement natural hyaluronic acid in the synovial fluid. These injections may reduce pain over 1–6 months, but are associated with a short-term increase in knee inflammation. Sodium hyaluronate (*SportVis*®) is also licensed for the relief of pain and optimisation of recovery following ankle sprain, and for the relief of chronic pain and disability associated with tennis elbow.

10.1.1 Non-steroidal anti-inflammatory drugs

In *single doses* non-steroidal anti-inflammatory drugs (NSAIDs) have analgesic activity comparable to that of paracetamol (section 4.7.1), but paracetamol is preferred, particularly in the elderly (see also Prescribing for the Elderly, p. 25).

In regular *full dosage* NSAIDs have both a lasting analgesic and an anti-inflammatory effect which makes them particularly useful for the treatment of continuous or regular pain associated with inflammation. Therefore, although paracetamol often gives adequate pain control in osteoarthritis, NSAIDs are more appropriate than paracetamol or the opioid analgesics in the *inflammatory arthritides* (e.g. rheumatoid arthritis) and in some cases of *advanced osteoarthritis*. NSAIDs can also be of benefit in the less well defined conditions of *back pain* and *soft-tissue disorders*.

Choice Differences in anti-inflammatory activity between NSAIDs are small, but there is considerable variation in individual response and tolerance to these drugs. About 60% of patients will respond to any NSAID; of the others, those who do not respond to one may well respond to another. Pain relief starts soon after taking the first dose and a full analgesic effect should normally be obtained within a week, whereas an anti-inflammatory effect may not be achieved (or may not be clinically assessable) for up to 3 weeks. If appropriate responses are not obtained within these times, another NSAID should be tried.

NSAIDs reduce the production of prostaglandins by inhibiting the enzyme cyclo-oxygenase. They vary in their selectivity for inhibiting different types of cyclo-oxygenase; selective inhibition of cyclo-oxygenase-2 is associated with less gastro-intestinal intolerance. Several other factors also influence susceptibility to gastro-intestinal effects, and a NSAID should be chosen on the basis of the incidence of gastro-intestinal and other side-effects.

Ibuprofen is a propionic acid derivative with anti-inflammatory, analgesic, and antipyretic properties. It has fewer side-effects than other non-selective NSAIDs but its anti-inflammatory properties are weaker. Doses of 1.6 to 2.4 g daily are needed for rheumatoid arthritis and it is unsuitable for conditions where inflammation is prominent, such as acute gout. **Dexibuprofen** is the active enantiomer of ibuprofen. It has similar properties to ibuprofen and is licensed for the relief of mild to moderate pain and inflammation.

Other propionic acid derivatives:

Naproxen is one of the first choices because it combines good efficacy with a low incidence of side-effects (but more than ibuprofen, see NSAIDs and Gastro-intestinal Events, below).

Fenoprofen is as effective as naproxen, and **flurbiprofen** may be slightly more effective. Both are associated with slightly more gastro-intestinal side-effects than ibuprofen.

Ketoprofen has anti-inflammatory properties similar to ibuprofen and has more side-effects (see also NSAIDs and Gastro-intestinal Events, below). **Dexketoprofen**, an isomer of ketoprofen, has been introduced for the short-term relief of mild to moderate pain.

Tiaprofenic acid is as effective as naproxen; it has more side-effects than ibuprofen (**important:** reports of severe cystitis, see CSM advice on p. 726).

Drugs with properties similar to those of propionic acid derivatives:

Diclofenac and **aceclofenac** are similar in efficacy to naproxen.

Etodolac is comparable in efficacy to naproxen; it is licensed for symptomatic relief of osteoarthritis and rheumatoid arthritis.

Indometacin has an action equal to or superior to that of naproxen, but with a high incidence of side-effects including headache, dizziness, and gastro-intestinal disturbances (see also NSAIDs and Gastro-intestinal Events, below).

Mefenamic acid has minor anti-inflammatory properties. It has occasionally been associated with diarrhoea and haemolytic anaemia which require discontinuation of treatment.

Meloxicam is licensed for the short-term relief of pain in osteoarthritis and for long-term treatment of rheumatoid arthritis and ankylosing spondylitis.

Nabumetone is comparable in effect to naproxen.

Phenylbutazone is licensed for ankylosing spondylitis, but is not recommended because it is associated with serious side-effects, in particular haematological reactions; it should be used only by a specialist in severe cases where other treatments have been found unsuitable.

Piroxicam is as effective as naproxen and has a long duration of action which permits once-daily administration. However, it has more gastro-intestinal side-effects than most other NSAIDs, and is associated with more frequent serious skin reactions (**important:** see CHMP advice, p. 725).

Sulindac is similar in tolerance to naproxen.

Tenoxicam is similar in activity and tolerance to naproxen. Its long duration of action allows once-daily administration.

Tolfenamic acid is licensed for the treatment of migraine (section 4.7.4.1).

Ketorolac and the selective inhibitor of cyclo-oxygenase-2, **parecoxib** are licensed for the short-term management of postoperative pain (section 15.1.4.2).

The selective inhibitors of cyclo-oxygenase-2, **etoricoxib** and **celecoxib**, are as effective as non-selective NSAIDs such as diclofenac and naproxen. Although selective inhibitors can cause serious gastro-intestinal events, available evidence appears to indicate that the risk of serious upper gastro-intestinal events is lower with selective inhibitors compared to non-selective NSAIDs; this advantage may be lost in patients who require concomitant low-dose aspirin.

Celecoxib and **etoricoxib** are licensed for the relief of pain in osteoarthritis, rheumatoid arthritis, and ankylosing spondylitis; etoricoxib is also licensed for the relief of pain from acute gout.

Dental and orofacial pain Most mild to moderate dental pain and inflammation is effectively relieved by NSAIDs. Those used for dental pain include **ibuprofen** and **diclofenac**.

For information on the risks of serious gastro-intestinal side-effects of NSAIDs, see p. 718.

For further information on the management of dental and orofacial pain, see p. 278.

Cautions and contra-indications NSAIDs should be used with caution in the elderly (risk of serious side-effects and fatalities, see also Prescribing for the Elderly p. 25), in allergic disorders (they are **contra-indicated** in patients with a history of hypersensitivity to aspirin or any other NSAID—which includes those in whom attacks of asthma, angioedema, urticaria or rhinitis have been precipitated by aspirin or any other NSAID), and in coagulation defects. Long-term use of some NSAIDs is associated with reduced female fertility, which is reversible on stopping treatment. Caution is also required in patients with connective-tissue disorders, see Side-effects below.

In patients with cardiac impairment, caution is required since NSAIDs may impair renal function (see also Side-effects, below). All NSAIDs are contra-indicated in severe heart failure. **Diclofenac** and the selective inhibitors of cyclo-oxygenase-2 (**celecoxib**, **etoricoxib**, and **parecoxib**) are contra-indicated in ischaemic heart disease, cerebrovascular disease, peripheral arterial disease, and mild to severe heart failure. They should be used with caution in patients with a history of cardiac failure, left ventricular dysfunction, hypertension, in patients with oedema for any other reason, and in patients with other risk factors for cardiovascular events. Other non-selective NSAIDs should be used with caution in uncontrolled hypertension, heart failure, ischaemic heart disease, peripheral arterial disease, cerebrovascular disease, and when used long term in patients with risk factors for cardiovascular events.

> **NSAIDs and cardiovascular events**
>
> All NSAID use (including cyclo-oxygenase-2 selective inhibitors) can, to varying degrees, be associated with a small increased risk of thrombotic events (e.g. myocardial infarction and stroke) independent of baseline cardiovascular risk factors or duration of NSAID use; however, the greatest risk may be in those receiving high doses long term.
>
> Cyclo-oxygenase-2 selective inhibitors, **diclofenac** (150 mg daily) and **ibuprofen** (2.4 g daily) are associated with an increased risk of thrombotic events. The increased risk for diclofenac is similar to that of licensed doses of **etoricoxib**. **Naproxen** (1 g daily) is associated with a lower thrombotic risk, and low doses of ibuprofen (1.2 g daily or less) have not been associated with an increased risk of myocardial infarction.
>
> The lowest effective dose of NSAID should be prescribed for the shortest period of time to control symptoms and the need for long-term treatment should be reviewed periodically.

All NSAIDs (including cyclo-oxygenase-2 selective inhibitors) are contra-indicated in patients with active gastro-intestinal ulceration or bleeding. Piroxicam, ketoprofen, and ketorolac are contra-indicated in patients with any history of gastro-intestinal bleeding, ulceration, or perforation. Other non-selective NSAIDs are contra-indicated in patients with a history of recurrent gastro-intestinal ulceration or haemorrhage (two or more distinct episodes), and in patients with a history of gastro-intestinal bleeding or perforation related to previous NSAID therapy (see also, p. 718). While it is preferable to avoid NSAIDs in patients with active or previous gastro-intestinal ulceration or bleeding, and to withdraw them if gastro-intestinal lesions develop, nevertheless patients with serious rheumatic diseases (e.g. rheumatoid arthritis) are usually dependent on NSAIDs for effective relief of pain and stiffness. Patients at risk of gastro-intestinal ulceration (including the elderly), who need NSAID treatment should receive gastroprotective treatment; for advice on the prophylaxis and treatment of NSAID-associated gastro-intestinal ulcers, see section 1.3. NSAIDs should also be used with caution in Crohn's disease or ulcerative colitis, as these conditions may be exacerbated.

For **interactions** of NSAIDs, see Appendix 1 (NSAIDs).

Hepatic impairment NSAIDs should be used with caution in patients with hepatic impairment; there is an increased risk of gastro-intestinal bleeding and fluid retention. NSAIDs should be avoided in severe liver disease; see also individual drugs.

Renal impairment NSAIDs should be avoided if possible or used with caution in patients with renal impairment; the **lowest effective dose** should be used for the **shortest possible duration**, and renal function should be **monitored**. Sodium and water retention may occur and renal function may deteriorate, possibly leading to renal failure; deterioration in renal function has also been reported after topical use; see also individual drugs.

Pregnancy Most manufacturers advise avoiding the use of NSAIDs during pregnancy or avoiding them unless the potential benefit outweighs the risk. NSAIDs should be avoided during the third trimester because use is associated with a risk of closure of fetal ductus arteriosus *in utero* and possibly persistent pulmonary hypertension of the newborn. In addition, the onset of labour may be delayed and its duration may be increased. See also individual monographs for celecoxib and etoricoxib.

Breast-feeding NSAIDs should be used with caution during breast-feeding; see also individual drugs.

Side-effects Gastro-intestinal disturbances including discomfort, nausea, diarrhoea, and occasionally bleeding and ulceration occur (see also NSAIDs and Gastro-intestinal Events, below and Cautions above). Systemic as well as local effects of NSAIDs contribute to gastro-intestinal damage; taking oral formulations with milk or food, or using enteric-coated formulations, or changing the route of administration may only partially reduce symptoms such as dyspepsia.

> ### NSAIDs and gastro-intestinal events
>
> All NSAIDs are associated with serious gastro-intestinal toxicity; the risk is higher in the elderly. Evidence on the relative safety of non-selective NSAIDs indicates differences in the risks of serious upper gastro-intestinal side-effects—piroxicam (see also CHMP advice, p. 725), ketoprofen, and ketorolac are associated with the highest risk; indometacin, diclofenac, and naproxen are associated with intermediate risk; and ibuprofen with the lowest risk (although high doses of ibuprofen have been associated with intermediate risk). **Selective inhibitors of cyclo-oxygenase-2** are associated with a *lower risk* of serious upper gastro-intestinal side-effects than non-selective NSAIDs.
>
> Recommendations are that NSAIDs associated with a low risk e.g. ibuprofen are *generally preferred*, to start at the *lowest recommended dose* and not to use more than one oral NSAID at a time. See also Cautions and Contra-indications, p. 717.
>
> The combination of a NSAID and low-dose aspirin can increase the risk of gastro-intestinal side-effects; this combination should be used only if absolutely necessary and the patient should be monitored closely.

Other side-effects include hypersensitivity reactions (particularly rashes, angioedema, and bronchospasm—see below), headache, dizziness, nervousness, depression, drowsiness, insomnia, vertigo, hearing disturbances such as tinnitus, photosensitivity, and haematuria. Blood disorders have also occurred. Fluid retention may occur (rarely precipitating congestive heart failure); blood pressure may be raised.

> ### Asthma
>
> Any degree of worsening of asthma may be related to the ingestion of NSAIDs, either prescribed or (in the case of ibuprofen and others) purchased over the counter.

Renal failure may be provoked by NSAIDs, especially in patients with pre-existing renal impairment (**important**, see Renal impairment, above). Rarely, papillary necrosis or interstitial fibrosis associated with NSAIDs can lead to renal failure.

Hepatic damage, alveolitis, pulmonary eosinophilia, pancreatitis, visual disturbances, Stevens-Johnson syndrome, and toxic epidermal necrolysis are other rare side-effects. Induction of or exacerbation of colitis

or Crohn's disease has been reported. Aseptic meningitis has been reported rarely with NSAIDs—patients with connective-tissue disorders such as systemic lupus erythematosus may be especially susceptible.

Overdosage: see Emergency Treatment of Poisoning, p. 35.

◤ ACECLOFENAC

Indications pain and inflammation in rheumatoid arthritis, osteoarthritis and ankylosing spondylitis

Cautions see notes above; avoid in acute porphyria (section 9.8.2)

Contra-indications see notes above

Hepatic impairment initially 100 mg daily; see also notes above

Renal impairment avoid in moderate to severe impairment; see also notes above

Pregnancy see notes above

Breast-feeding manufacturer advises avoid; see also notes above

Side-effects see notes above

Dose
• 100 mg twice daily; CHILD not recommended

Aceclofenac (Non-proprietary) [PoM]
Tablets, aceclofenac 100 mg, net price 60-tab pack = £9.63. Label: 21

Preservex® (Almirall) [PoM]
Tablets, f/c, aceclofenac 100 mg, net price 60-tab pack = £9.63. Label: 21

◤ ACEMETACIN

(Glycolic acid ester of indometacin)

Indications pain and inflammation in rheumatic disease and other musculoskeletal disorders; postoperative analgesia

Cautions see under Indometacin and notes above
Driving Dizziness may affect performance of skilled tasks (e.g. driving)

Contra-indications see notes above

Hepatic impairment see notes above

Renal impairment see notes above

Pregnancy see notes above

Breast-feeding manufacturer advises avoid; see also notes above

Side-effects see under Indometacin and notes above

Dose
• 120 mg daily in divided doses with food, increased if necessary to 180 mg daily; CHILD not recommended

Emflex® (Merck Serono) [PoM]
Capsules, yellow/orange, acemetacin 60 mg, net price 90-cap pack = £28.20. Label: 21, counselling, driving

◤ CELECOXIB

Indications pain and inflammation in osteoarthritis, rheumatoid arthritis, and ankylosing spondylitis

Cautions see notes above; monitor blood pressure before and during treatment

Contra-indications see notes above; sulfonamide sensitivity; inflammatory bowel disease

Hepatic impairment halve initial dose in moderate impairment; see also notes above

Musculoskeletal and joint diseases

10

Renal impairment avoid if eGFR less than 30 mL/minute/1.73 m^2; see also notes above

Pregnancy avoid (teratogenic in *animal* studies); see also notes above

Breast-feeding avoid—present in milk in *animal* studies; see also notes above

Side-effects see notes above; dyspnoea, influenza-like symptoms; *less commonly* stomatitis, palpitation, cerebral infarction, fatigue, paraesthesia, muscle cramps; *rarely* taste disturbance, alopecia; *very rarely* seizures; *also reported* chest pain

Dose

- Osteoarthritis, 200 mg daily in 1–2 divided doses, increased if necessary to max. 200 mg twice daily; CHILD not recommended
- Rheumatoid arthritis, 100 mg twice daily, increased if necessary to 200 mg twice daily; CHILD not recommended
- Ankylosing spondylitis, 200 mg daily in 1–2 divided doses, increased if necessary to max. 400 mg daily in 1–2 divided doses; CHILD not recommended

Note Discontinue if no improvement after 2 weeks on max. dose

Celebrex® (Pharmacia) PoM

Capsules, celecoxib 100 mg (white/blue), net price 60-cap pack = £21.55; 200 mg (white/gold), 30-cap pack = £21.55

DEXIBUPROFEN

Indications pain and inflammation associated with osteoarthritis and other musculoskeletal disorders; mild to moderate pain and inflammation including dysmenorrhoea and dental pain

Cautions see notes above

Contra-indications see notes above

Hepatic impairment see notes above

Renal impairment reduce initial dose; avoid if eGFR less than 30 mL/minute/1.73m^2; see also notes above

Pregnancy see notes above

Breast-feeding present in milk—but risk to infant minimal; see also notes above

Side-effects see notes above

Dose

- 600–900 mg daily in up to 3 divided doses; increased if necessary to max. 1.2 g daily (900 mg daily for dysmenorrhoea); max. single dose 400 mg (300 mg for dysmenorrhoea); CHILD not recommended

Seractil® (Genus) PoM

Tablets, f/c, dexibuprofen 300 mg, net price 60–tab pack = £9.47; 400 mg (scored) 60–tab pack = £9.97. Label: 21

DEXKETOPROFEN

Indications short-term treatment of mild to moderate pain including dysmenorrhoea

Cautions see notes above

Contra-indications see notes above

Hepatic impairment reduce initial dose to max. 50 mg daily in mild to moderate impairment; see also notes above

Renal impairment reduce initial dose to 50 mg daily; avoid in moderate to severe impairment; see also notes above

Pregnancy see notes above

Breast-feeding manufacturer advises avoid—no information available; see also notes above

Side-effects see notes above

Dose

- 12.5 mg every 4–6 hours *or* 25 mg every 8 hours; max. 75 mg daily; ELDERLY initially max. 50 mg daily; CHILD not recommended

Keral® (Menarini) PoM

Tablets, f/c, scored, dexketoprofen (as trometamol) 25 mg, net price 20-tab pack = £3.67, 50-tab pack = £9.18. Label: 22

DICLOFENAC POTASSIUM

Indications pain and inflammation in rheumatic disease and other musculoskeletal disorders; acute gout; postoperative pain; migraine; fever in ear, nose, or throat infection in children

Cautions see notes above

Contra-indications see notes above

Hepatic impairment see notes above

Renal impairment avoid in severe impairment; see also notes above

Pregnancy see notes above

Breast-feeding amount in milk too small to be harmful; see also notes above

Side-effects see notes above

Dose

- Rheumatic disease, musculoskeletal disorders, acute gout, 75–150 mg daily in 2–3 divided doses; CHILD over 14 years, 75–100 mg daily in 2–3 divided doses
- Postoperative pain, 75–150 mg daily in 2–3 divided doses; CHILD 9–14 years (body-weight 35 kg and over), up to 2 mg/kg (max. 100 mg) daily in 3 divided doses; CHILD over 14 years, 75–100 mg daily in 2–3 divided doses
- Migraine, 50 mg at onset, repeated after 2 hours if necessary then after 4–6 hours; max. 200 mg in 24 hours; CHILD not recommended
- Fever in ear, nose, or throat infection, CHILD over 9 years (body-weight 35 kg and over), up to 2 mg/kg (max. 100 mg) daily in 3 divided doses

Diclofenac Potassium (Non-proprietary) PoM

Tablets, diclofenac potassium 25 mg, net price 28-tab pack = £3.23; 50 mg, 28-tab pack = £6.18. Label: 21

[1]Voltarol® Rapid (Novartis) PoM

Tablets, s/c, diclofenac potassium 25 mg (red), net price 30-tab pack = £3.46; 50 mg (brown), 30-tab pack = £6.62. Label: 21

DICLOFENAC SODIUM

Indications pain and inflammation in rheumatic disease (including juvenile idiopathic arthritis) and other musculoskeletal disorders; acute gout; postoperative pain

Cautions see notes above

1. 12.5 mg tablets can be sold to the public for the treatment of headache, dental pain, period pain, rheumatic and muscular pain, backache and the symptoms of cold and flu (including fever), in patients aged over 14 years subject to max. single dose of 25 mg, max. daily dose of 75 mg for max. 3 days, and max. pack size of 18 × 12.5 mg

10

Musculoskeletal and joint diseases

Contra-indications see notes above; avoid suppositories in proctitis; avoid injections containing benzyl alcohol in neonates (see preparations below)
Intravenous use Additional contra-indications include concomitant NSAID or anticoagulant use (including low-dose heparins), history of haemorrhagic diathesis, history of confirmed or suspected cerebrovascular bleeding, operations with high risk of haemorrhage, history of asthma, moderate or severe renal impairment (see also Renal impairment below), hypovolaemia, dehydration;

Hepatic impairment see notes above

Renal impairment avoid in severe impairment; avoid intravenous use if serum creatinine greater than 160 micromol/litre; see also notes above

Pregnancy see notes above

Breast-feeding amount in milk too small to be harmful; see also notes above

Side-effects see notes above; suppositories may cause rectal irritation; injection site reactions

Dose
- By mouth, 75–150 mg daily in 2–3 divided doses
- By rectum in suppositories, 75–150 mg daily in divided doses
- Juvenile idiopathic arthritis, CHILD 6 months–18 years, by mouth, see *BNF for Children*
- Postoperative pain, CHILD 6 months–18 years, by rectum, see *BNF for Children*

Diclofenac Sodium (Non-proprietary) PoM
Tablets, e/c, diclofenac sodium 25 mg, net price 84-tab pack = £1.25; 50 mg, 84-tab pack = £1.61. Label: 5, 25
Brands include *Defenac®*, *Dicloflex®*, *Diclozip®*, *Fenactol®*, *Flamrase®*
Dental prescribing on NHS Diclofenac Sodium Tablets may be prescribed
Suppositories, diclofenac sodium 100 mg, net price 10 = £3.03
Brands include *Econac®*

Dyloject® (Therabel) PoM
Injection, diclofenac sodium 37.5 mg/mL, net price 2-mL vial = £4.80
Note May be difficult to obtain
Dose by deep intramuscular injection into the gluteal muscle, acute exacerbations of pain and postoperative pain, 75 mg once daily (twice daily in severe cases) for max. 2 days
Ureteric colic, 75 mg then a further 75 mg after 30 minutes if necessary
By intravenous injection (in supervised settings), acute postoperative pain, 75 mg repeated after 4–6 hours if necessary; max. 150 mg in 24 hours for 2 days
Prevention of postoperative pain, 25–50 mg after surgery; further doses given after 4–6 hours if necessary; max. 150 mg in 24 hours for 2 days
Note The *Scottish Medicines Consortium* (p. 4) has advised (February 2008) that *Dyloject®* is accepted for restricted use within NHS Scotland for the treatment or prevention of postoperative pain by intravenous injection in supervised healthcare settings

Voltarol® (Novartis) PoM
Tablets, e/c, diclofenac sodium 25 mg (yellow), net price 84-tab pack = £2.94; 50 mg (brown), 84-tab pack = £4.57. Label: 5, 25
Dispersible tablets, sugar-free, pink, diclofenac, equivalent to diclofenac sodium 50 mg, net price 21-tab pack = £6.19. Label: 13, 21
Note Voltarol Dispersible tablets are more suitable for **short-term** use in acute conditions for which treatment required for no more than 3 months (no information on use beyond 3 months)

Injection, diclofenac sodium 25 mg/mL, net price 3-mL amp = 83p
Excipients include benzyl alcohol (avoid in neonates unless there is no safer alternative, see Excipients, p. 2), propylene glycol
Dose by deep intramuscular injection into the gluteal muscle, acute exacerbations of pain and postoperative pain, 75 mg once daily (twice daily in severe cases) for max. 2 days; CHILD 2–18 years, see *BNF for Children*
Ureteric colic, 75 mg then a further 75 mg after 30 minutes if necessary
By intravenous infusion (in hospital setting), acute postoperative pain, 75 mg repeated if necessary after 4–6 hours; max. 150 mg in 24 hours for 2 days; CHILD 2–18 years, see *BNF for Children*
Prevention of postoperative pain, initially after surgery 25–50 mg over 15–60 minutes then 5 mg/hour; max. 150 mg in 24 hours for 2 days
Suppositories, diclofenac sodium 12.5 mg, net price 10 = 58p; 25 mg, 10 = £1.03; 50 mg, 10 = £1.70; 100 mg, 10 = £3.03

◢**Modified release**

Diclomax SR® (Galen) PoM
Capsules, m/r, yellow, diclofenac sodium 75 mg, net price 56-cap pack = £9.69. Label: 21, 25
Dose ADULT over 18 years, 1 capsule 1–2 times daily *or* 2 capsules once daily; CHILD 12–18 years see *BNF for Children*

Diclomax Retard® (Galen) PoM
Capsules, m/r, diclofenac sodium 100 mg, net price 28-cap pack = £6.97. Label: 21, 25
Dose ADULT over 18 years, 1 capsule once daily; CHILD 12–18 years see *BNF for Children*

Motifene® 75 mg (Daiichi Sankyo) PoM
Capsules, e/c, m/r, diclofenac sodium 75 mg (enclosing e/c pellets containing diclofenac sodium 25 mg and m/r pellets containing diclofenac sodium 50 mg), net price 56-cap pack = £8.00. Label: 25
Excipients include propylene glycol (see Excipients, p. 2)
Dose ADULT over 18 years, 1 capsule 1–2 times daily; CHILD 12–18 years see *BNF for Children*

Voltarol® 75 mg SR (Novartis) PoM
Tablets, m/r, f/c, pink, diclofenac sodium 75 mg, net price 28-tab pack = £6.46; 56-tab pack = £12.92. Label: 21, 25
Dose ADULT over 18 years, 1 tablet 1–2 times daily; CHILD 12–18 years see *BNF for Children*
Note Other brands of modified-release tablets containing diclofenac sodium 75 mg include *Defenac® SR*, *Dexomon® 75 SR*, *Dicloflex® 75 SR*, *Fenactol® 75 mg SR*, *Flamatak® 75 MR*, *Flamrase® SR*, *Flexotard® MR 75*, *Rheumatac® Retard 75*, *Rhumalgan® CR*, *Slofenac® SR*, *Volsaid® Retard 75*

Voltarol® Retard (Novartis) PoM
Tablets, m/r, f/c, red, diclofenac sodium 100 mg. Net price 28-tab pack = £9.47. Label: 21, 25
Dose ADULT over 18 years, 1 tablet once daily; CHILD 12–18 years see *BNF for Children*
Note Other brands of modified-release tablets containing diclofenac sodium 100 mg include *Defenac® Retard*, *Dexomon® Retard 100*, *Dicloflex® Retard*, *Fenactol® Retard 100 mg*, *Flamatak® 100 MR*, *Slofenac® SR*, *Volsaid® Retard 100*

◢**With misoprostol**

For prescribing information on misoprostol, see section 1.3.4

Arthrotec® (Pharmacia) PoM
Arthrotec® 50 tablets, diclofenac sodium (in e/c core) 50 mg, misoprostol 200 micrograms, net price 60-tab pack = £11.98; Label: 21, 25
Dose prophylaxis against NSAID-induced gastroduodenal ulceration in patients requiring diclofenac for rheumatoid

arthritis or osteoarthritis, 1 tablet 2–3 times daily with food; CHILD not recommended

Arthrotec® 75 tablets, diclofenac sodium (in e/c core) 75 mg, misoprostol 200 micrograms, net price 60-tab pack = £15.83. Label: 21, 25

Dose prophylaxis against NSAID-induced gastroduodenal ulceration in patients requiring diclofenac for rheumatoid arthritis or osteoarthritis, 1 tablet twice daily with food; CHILD not recommended

Note The BNF recommends a higher starting dose of misoprostol for prophylaxis against NSAID-induced gastroduodenal ulceration than that provided by *Arthrotec*® (see section 1.3.4)

Misofen® (Morningside) [PoM]

Tablets, diclofenac sodium (in e/c core) 50 mg, misoprostol 200 micrograms, net price 60-tab pack = £11.98. Label: 21, 25

Dose prophylaxis against NSAID-induced gastroduodenal ulceration in patients requiring diclofenac for rheumatoid arthritis or osteoarthritis, 1 tablet 2–3 times daily with food; CHILD not recommended

Tablets, diclofenac sodium (in e/c core) 75 mg, misoprostol 200 micrograms, net price 60-tab pack = £15.83. Label: 21, 25

Dose prophylaxis against NSAID-induced gastroduodenal ulceration in patients requiring diclofenac for rheumatoid arthritis or osteoarthritis, 1 tablet twice daily with food; CHILD not recommended

Note The BNF recommends a higher starting dose of misoprostol for prophylaxis against NSAID-induced gastroduodenal ulceration than that provided by *Misofen*® (see section 1.3.4)

◢ **Topical preparations**

Section 10.3.2

ETODOLAC

Indications pain and inflammation in rheumatoid arthritis and osteoarthritis

Cautions see notes above

Contra-indications see notes above

Hepatic impairment see notes above

Renal impairment avoid in severe impairment; see also notes above

Pregnancy see notes above

Breast-feeding manufacturer advises avoid; see also notes above

Side-effects see notes above; also stomatitis, vasculitis, palpitation, dyspnoea, confusion, fatigue, paraesthesia, tremor, urinary frequency, dysuria, pyrexia, and pruritus

Dose

• ADULT over 18 years, 300–600 mg daily in 1–2 divided doses

Etodolac (Non-proprietary) [PoM]

Capsules, etodolac 300 mg, net price 60-cap pack = £8.14

Brands include *Eccoxolac*®

◢ **Modified release**

Etopan XL® (Taro) [PoM]

Tablets, m/r, f/c, grey, etodolac 600 mg, net price 30-tab pack = £14.60. Label: 25

Dose 1 tablet daily; CHILD not recommended

Lodine SR® (Almirall) [PoM]

Tablets, m/r, f/c, light-grey, etodolac 600 mg, net price 30-tab pack = £15.50. Label: 25

Dose 1 tablet daily; CHILD not recommended

ETORICOXIB

Indications pain and inflammation in osteoarthritis, rheumatoid arthritis, and ankylosing spondylitis; acute gout

Cautions see notes above; also dehydration; monitor blood pressure before treatment, 2 weeks after initiation and periodically during treatment

Contra-indications see notes above; inflammatory bowel disease; uncontrolled hypertension (persistently above 140/90 mmHg)

Hepatic impairment max. 60 mg daily in mild impairment; max. 60 mg on alternate days or 30 mg once daily in moderate impairment; see also notes above

Renal impairment avoid if eGFR less than 30 mL/minute/1.73 m^2; see also notes above

Pregnancy manufacturer advises avoid (teratogenic in *animal* studies); see also notes above

Breast-feeding manufacturer advises avoid—present in milk in *animal* studies; see also notes above

Side-effects see notes above; also palpitation, fatigue, influenza-like symptoms, ecchymosis; *less commonly* dry mouth, taste disturbance, mouth ulcer, appetite and weight change, atrial fibrillation, transient ischaemic attack, chest pain, flushing, cough, dyspnoea, epistaxis, anxiety, mental acuity impaired, paraesthesia, electrolyte disturbance, myalgia and arthralgia; *very rarely* confusion and hallucinations

Dose

• Osteoarthritis, ADULT and CHILD over 16 years, 30 mg once daily, increased if necessary to 60 mg once daily

• Rheumatoid arthritis and ankylosing spondylitis, ADULT and CHILD over 16 years, 90 mg once daily

• Acute gout, ADULT and CHILD over 16 years, 120 mg once daily for max. 8 days

Arcoxia® (MSD) [PoM]

Tablets, f/c, etoricoxib 30 mg (blue-green), net price 28-tab pack = £13.99; 60 mg (dark green), 28-tab pack = £20.11; 90 mg (white), 28-tab pack = £22.96; 120 mg (pale green), 7-tab pack = £6.03, 28-tab pack = £24.11

FENOPROFEN

Indications pain and inflammation in rheumatic disease and other musculoskeletal disorders; mild to moderate pain

Cautions see notes above

Contra-indications see notes above

Hepatic impairment see notes above

Renal impairment see notes above

Pregnancy see notes above

Breast-feeding amount too small to be harmful; see also notes above

Side-effects see notes above; upper respiratory-tract infection, nasopharyngitis, and cystitis also reported

Dose

• 300–600 mg 3–4 times daily; max. 3 g daily; CHILD not recommended

Fenopron® 300 (Typharm) [PoM]

Tablets, orange, fenoprofen (as calcium salt) 300 mg, net price 100-tab pack = £9.45 Label: 21

Musculoskeletal and joint diseases *(left margin)*

10 *(left margin tab)*

■ FLURBIPROFEN

Indications pain and inflammation in rheumatic disease and other musculoskeletal disorders; mild to moderate pain including dysmenorrhoea; migraine; postoperative analgesia; sore throat (section 12.3.1)

Cautions see notes above

Contra-indications see notes above

Hepatic impairment see notes above

Renal impairment avoid in severe impairment; see also notes above

Pregnancy see notes above

Breast-feeding small amount present in milk—manufacturer advises avoid; see also notes above

Side-effects see notes above; also stomatitis; *less commonly* paraesthesia, confusion, hallucinations, and fatigue

Dose

● ADULT and CHILD over 12 years, 150–200 mg daily in 2–4 divided doses, increased in acute conditions to 300 mg daily

● Dysmenorrhoea, ADULT and CHILD over 12 years, initially 100 mg, then 50–100 mg every 4–6 hours; max. 300 mg daily

Flurbiprofen (Non-proprietary) [PoM]

Tablets, flurbiprofen 50 mg, net price 100 = £21.30; 100 mg, 100 = £38.10. Label: 21

Froben® (Abbott Healthcare) [PoM]

Tablets, yellow, s/c, flurbiprofen 50 mg, net price 100 = £10.27; 100 mg, 100 = £19.46. Label: 21

■ IBUPROFEN

Indications pain and inflammation in rheumatic disease (including juvenile idiopathic arthritis) and other musculoskeletal disorders; mild to moderate pain including dysmenorrhoea; postoperative analgesia; migraine; dental pain; fever with discomfort and pain in children; post-immunisation pyrexia (section 14.1)

Cautions see notes above

Contra-indications see notes above

Hepatic impairment see notes above

Renal impairment avoid in severe impairment; see also notes above

Pregnancy see notes above

Breast-feeding amount too small to be harmful but some manufacturers advise avoid (including topical use); see also notes above

Side-effects see notes above

Dose

● ADULT and CHILD over 12 years, initially 300–400 mg 3–4 times daily; increased if necessary to max. 2.4 g daily; maintenance dose of 0.6–1.2 g daily may be adequate

● Pain and fever in children, CHILD 1–3 months, see *BNF for Children*; CHILD 3–6 months (body-weight over 5 kg), 50 mg 3 times daily (max. 30 mg/kg daily in 3–4 divided doses); CHILD 6 months–1 year, 50 mg 3–4 times daily (max. 30 mg/kg daily in 3–4 divided doses); CHILD 1–4 years, 100 mg 3 times daily (max. 30 mg/kg daily in 3–4 divided doses); CHILD 4–7 years, 150 mg 3 times daily (max. 30 mg/kg daily in 3–4 divided doses); CHILD 7–10 years, 200 mg 3 times daily (up to 30 mg/kg daily (max. 2.4 g) in 3–4 divided doses); CHILD 10–12 years, 300 mg 3 times daily (up to 30 mg/kg daily (max. 2.4 g) in 3–4 divided doses)

● Rheumatic disease in children (including juvenile idiopathic arthritis), CHILD 3 months–18 years (body-weight over 5 kg), 30–40 mg/kg (max. 2.4 g) daily in 3–4 divided doses; in systemic juvenile idiopathic arthritis up to 60 mg/kg (max. 2.4 g) daily [unlicensed] in 4–6 divided doses

¹Ibuprofen (Non-proprietary) [PoM]

Tablets, coated, ibuprofen 200 mg, net price 84-tab pack = £3.54; 400 mg, 84-tab pack = £3.75; 600 mg, 84-tab pack = £3.50. Label: 21

Brands include *Arthrofen®, Ebufac®, Rimafen®*

Dental prescribing on NHS Ibuprofen Tablets may be prescribed

Oral suspension, ibuprofen 100 mg/5 mL, net price 100 mL = £1.37, 150 mL = £2.11, 500 mL = £8.88. Label: 21

Note Sugar-free versions are available and can be ordered by specifying 'sugar-free' on the prescription

Brands include *Calprofen®, Feverfen®, Nurofen® for Children, Orbifen® for Children*

Dental prescribing on NHS Ibuprofen Oral Suspension Sugar-free may be prescribed

Brufen® (Abbott Healthcare) [PoM]

Tablets, f/c, ibuprofen 200 mg, net price 100-tab pack = £3.92; 400 mg, 100-tab pack = £8.16; 600 mg, 100-tab pack = £12.24. Label: 21

Syrup, orange, ibuprofen 100 mg/5 mL, net price 500 mL (orange-flavoured) = £8.88. Label: 21

Granules, effervescent, ibuprofen 600 mg/sachet, net price 20-sachet pack = £6.80. Label: 13, 21

Electrolytes Na⁺ approx. 6.5 mmol/sachet

◢**Modified release**

Brufen Retard® (Abbott Healthcare) [PoM]

Tablets, m/r, ibuprofen 800 mg, net price 56-tab pack = £7.74. Label: 25, 27

Dose ADULT and CHILD over 12 years, 2 tablets daily as a single dose, preferably in the early evening, increased in severe cases to 3 tablets daily in 2 divided doses

◢**Topical preparations**

Section 10.3.2

■ INDOMETACIN
(Indomethacin)

Indications pain and moderate to severe inflammation in rheumatic disease and other acute musculoskeletal disorders; acute gout; dysmenorrhoea; premature labour (section 7.1.3)

Cautions see notes above; also epilepsy, parkinsonism, psychiatric disturbances; during prolonged therapy ophthalmic and blood examinations particularly advisable; avoid rectal administration in proctitis and haemorrhoids

Driving Dizziness may affect performance of skilled tasks (e.g. driving)

Contra-indications see notes above

Hepatic impairment see notes above

Renal impairment avoid in severe impairment; see also notes above

Pregnancy see notes above

Breast-feeding amount probably too small to be harmful—manufacturers advise avoid; see also notes above

Side-effects see notes above; *rarely* confusion, convulsions, psychiatric disturbances, syncope, blood

1. Can be sold to the public in certain circumstances

disorders (particularly thrombocytopenia), hyper-glycaemia, peripheral neuropathy, intestinal strictures; *also reported* hyperkalaemia; suppositories may cause rectal irritation and occasional bleeding

Dose

- By mouth, rheumatic disease, 50–200 mg daily in divided doses; CHILD see *BNF for Children*

  Acute gout, 150–200 mg daily in divided doses

  Dysmenorrhoea, up to 75 mg daily

- By rectum in suppositories, 100 mg at night and in the morning if required; CHILD not recommended

  Combined oral and rectal treatment, max. total daily dose 150–200 mg

Indometacin (Non-proprietary) PoM

Capsules, indometacin 25 mg, net price 28-cap pack = £1.32; 50 mg, 28-cap pack = £1.39. Label: 21, counselling, driving, see above

Suppositories, indometacin 100 mg, net price 10 = £17.61. Counselling, driving, see above

◢**Modified release**

Indometacin m/r preparations PoM

Capsules, m/r, indometacin 75 mg. Label: 21, 25, counselling, driving, see above

Brands include *Indolar SR®*, *Pardelprin®*

Dose 75 mg 1–2 times daily (once daily in dysmenorrhoea); CHILD not recommended

◼ KETOPROFEN

Indications pain and mild inflammation in rheumatic disease and other musculoskeletal disorders, and after orthopaedic surgery; acute gout; dysmenorrhoea

Cautions see notes above

Contra-indications see notes above

Hepatic impairment see notes above

Renal impairment avoid in severe impairment; see also notes above

Pregnancy see notes above

Breast-feeding amount probably too small to be harmful but manufacturers advise avoid; see also notes above

Side-effects see notes above; suppositories may cause rectal irritation

Dose

- By mouth, rheumatic disease, 100–200 mg daily in 2–4 divided doses; CHILD not recommended

  Pain and dysmenorrhoea, 50 mg up to 3 times daily; CHILD not recommended

- By rectum in suppositories, rheumatic disease, 100 mg at bedtime; CHILD not recommended

  Combined oral and rectal treatment, max. total daily dose 200 mg

Ketoprofen (Non-proprietary) PoM

Capsules, ketoprofen 50 mg, net price 28-cap pack = £9.32; 100 mg, 56-cap pack = £6.66. Label: 21

Orudis® (Sanofi-Aventis) PoM

Capsules, ketoprofen 50 mg (green/purple), net price 112-cap pack = £15.14; 100 mg (pink), 56-cap pack = £15.49. Label: 21

Suppositories, ketoprofen 100 mg. Net price 10 = £6.65

◢**Modified release**

Oruvail® (Sanofi-Aventis) PoM

Capsules, m/r, enclosing white pellets, ketoprofen 100 mg (pink/purple), net price 56-cap pack = £23.93; 150 mg (pink), 28-cap pack = £13.66; 200 mg (pink/white), 28-cap pack = £23.85. Label: 21, 25

Dose 100–200 mg once daily with food; CHILD not recommended

Note Other brands of modified-release capsules containing ketoprofen 100 mg and 200 mg include *Ketocid®* 200 mg, *Ketovail®*, *Tiloket®* CR

◢**With omeprazole**

For prescribing information on omeprazole, see section 1.3.5

Axorid® (Meda) PoM

Capsules, m/r, ketoprofen 100 mg, omeprazole 20 mg (yellow/white), net price 30-cap pack = £13.80; ketoprofen 200 mg, omeprazole 20 mg (white), 30-cap pack = £13.80. Label: 21, 25

Excipients include propylene glycol (see Excipients, p. 2)

Note Capsules enclose microgranules containing modified-release ketoprofen and gastro-resistant omeprazole

Dose (expressed as ketoprofen) patients requiring ketoprofen for osteoarthritis, rheumatoid arthritis, and ankylosing spondylitis, who are at risk of NSAID-associated duodenal or gastric ulcer or gastroduodenal erosions, ADULT and CHILD over 15 years, 100 mg (with omeprazole 20 mg) once daily increased to 200 mg (with omeprazole 20 mg) once daily depending on severity of symptoms

◢**Topical preparations**

Section 10.3.2

◼ MEFENAMIC ACID

Indications pain and inflammation in rheumatoid arthritis and osteoarthritis; postoperative pain; mild to moderate pain; dysmenorrhoea and menorrhagia

Cautions see notes above; epilepsy; acute porphyria (section 9.8.2)

Contra-indications see notes above; inflammatory bowel disease

Hepatic impairment see notes above

Renal impairment avoid in severe impairment; see also notes above

Pregnancy see notes above

Breast-feeding amount too small to be harmful but manufacturer advises avoid; see also notes above

Side-effects see notes above; also diarrhoea or rashes (withdraw treatment), stomatitis; *less commonly* paraesthesia and fatigue; *rarely* hypotension, palpitation, glucose intolerance, thrombocytopenia, haemolytic anaemia (positive Coombs' test), and aplastic anaemia

Dose

- ADULT over 18 years, 500 mg 3 times daily
- CHILD 12–18 years, acute pain including dysmenorrhoea, menorrhagia, 500 mg 3 times daily

Mefenamic Acid (Non-proprietary) PoM

Capsules, mefenamic acid 250 mg, net price 100-cap pack = £4.87. Label: 21

Tablets, mefenamic acid 500 mg, net price 28-tab pack = £2.62. Label: 21

Suspension, mefenamic acid 50 mg/5 mL, net price 125 mL = £79.98. Label: 21

Excipients include ethanol

10 Musculoskeletal and joint diseases

Ponstan® (Chemidex) [PoM]
Capsules, blue/ivory, mefenamic acid 250 mg, net price 100-cap pack = £8.17. Label: 21
Forte tablets, yellow, mefenamic acid 500 mg, net price 100-tab pack = £15.72. Label: 21

MELOXICAM

Indications pain and inflammation in rheumatic disease; exacerbation of osteoarthritis (short-term); ankylosing spondylitis

Cautions see notes above

Contra-indications see notes above

Hepatic impairment see notes above

Renal impairment avoid if eGFR less than 25 mL/minute/1.73m²; see also notes above

Pregnancy see notes above

Breast-feeding present in milk in *animal* studies—manufacturer advises avoid; see also notes above

Side-effects see notes above

Dose
- By mouth, osteoarthritis, ADULT and CHILD over 16 years, 7.5 mg once daily, increased if necessary to max. 15 mg once daily
  Rheumatoid arthritis, ankylosing spondylitis, ADULT and CHILD over 16 years, 15 mg once daily, may be reduced to 7.5 mg once daily; ELDERLY 7.5 mg daily
- CHILD over 12 years, see BNF for Children

Meloxicam (Non-proprietary) [PoM]
Tablets, meloxicam 7.5 mg, net price 30-tab pack = £1.18; 15 mg, 30-tab pack = £1.32. Label: 21

NABUMETONE

Indications pain and inflammation in osteoarthritis and rheumatoid arthritis

Cautions see notes above

Contra-indications see notes above

Hepatic impairment see notes above

Renal impairment avoid in severe impairment; see also notes above

Pregnancy see notes above

Breast-feeding manufacturer advises avoid; see also notes above

Side-effects see notes above

Dose
- 1 g at night; severe or persistent symptoms 0.5–1 g in morning and 1 g at night; ELDERLY 0.5–1 g daily; CHILD not recommended

Nabumetone (Non-proprietary) [PoM]
Tablets, nabumetone 500 mg, net price 56-tab pack = £8.56. Label: 21

Relifex® (Meda) [PoM]
Tablets, red, f /c, nabumetone 500 mg. Net price 56-tab pack = £6.18. Label: 21
Suspension, sugar-free, nabumetone 500 mg/5 mL. Net price 300-mL pack = £28.90. Label: 21

NAPROXEN

Indications pain and inflammation in rheumatic disease (including juvenile idiopathic arthritis) and other musculoskeletal disorders; dysmenorrhoea; acute gout

Cautions see notes above

Contra-indications see notes above

Hepatic impairment see notes above

Renal impairment avoid if eGFR less than 30 mL/minute/1.73 m²; see also notes above

Pregnancy see notes above

Breast-feeding amount too small to be harmful but manufacturer advises avoid; see also notes above

Side-effects see notes above

Dose
- Rheumatic disease, 0.5–1 g daily in 1–2 divided doses; CHILD 2–18 years, juvenile idiopathic arthritis, see BNF for Children
- Acute musculoskeletal disorders and dysmenorrhoea, 500 mg initially, then 250 mg every 6–8 hours as required; max. dose after first day 1.25 g daily; CHILD under 18 years, see BNF for Children
- Acute gout, 750 mg initially, then 250 mg every 8 hours until attack has passed; CHILD under 16 years not recommended

¹**Naproxen** (Non-proprietary) [PoM]
Tablets, naproxen 250 mg, net price 28-tab pack = £1.37; 500 mg, 28-tab pack = £1.99. Label: 21
Brands include *Arthroxen*®
Tablets, e/c, naproxen 250 mg, net price 56-tab pack = £4.35; 375 mg, 56-tab pack = £6.42; 500 mg, 56-tab pack = £11.73. Label: 5, 25

Naprosyn® (Roche) [PoM]
Tablets, yellow, scored, naproxen 250 mg, net price 56-tab pack = £4.29; 500 mg, 56-tab pack = £8.56. Label: 21
Tablets, e/c, (*Naprosyn EC*®), naproxen 250 mg, net price 56-tab pack = £4.29; 375 mg, 56-tab pack = £6.42; 500 mg, 56-tab pack = £8.56. Label: 5, 25

With esomeprazole

For prescribing information on esomeprazole, see section 1.3.5

Vimovo® (AstraZeneca) [PoM]
Tablets, f/c, m/r, naproxen 500 mg, esomeprazole (as magnesium trihydrate) 20 mg, net price 60-tab pack = £14.95. Label: 22, 25
Note Naproxen component is gastro-resistant
Dose patients requiring naproxen for osteoarthritis, rheumatoid arthritis, or ankylosing spondylitis, who are at risk of NSAID-associated duodenal or gastric ulcer and when treatment with lower doses of naproxen or other NSAIDs ineffective, ADULT over 18 years, 1 tablet twice daily

With misoprostol

For prescribing information on misoprostol, see section 1.3.4

Napratec® (Pharmacia) [PoM]
Combination pack, 56 yellow scored tablets, naproxen 500 mg; 56 white scored tablets, misoprostol 200 micrograms. Net price = £23.76. Label: 21
Dose patients requiring naproxen for rheumatoid arthritis, osteoarthritis, or ankylosing spondylitis, with prophylaxis against NSAID-induced gastroduodenal ulceration, 1 naproxen 500-mg tablet and 1 misoprostol 200-microgram tablet taken together twice daily with food; CHILD not recommended
Note The BNF recommends a higher starting dose of misoprostol for prophylaxis against NSAID-induced gastroduodenal ulceration than that provided by *Napratec*® (see section 1.3.4)

1. Can be sold to the public for the treatment of primary dysmenorrhoea in women aged 15–50 years subject to max. single dose of 500 mg, max. daily dose of 750 mg for max. 3 days, and a max. pack size of 9 × 250 mg tablets

� PIROXICAM

Indications   rheumatoid arthritis, osteoarthritis, and ankylosing spondylitis (see also CHMP advice below)

Cautions   see notes above and CHMP advice below

Contra-indications   inflammatory bowel disease; see also notes above

Hepatic impairment   see notes above

Renal impairment   see notes above

Pregnancy   see notes above

Breast-feeding   amount too small to be harmful; see also notes above

Side-effects   see notes above

Dose

- By mouth, max. 20 mg once daily (see also CHMP advice below); CHILD 6–18 years, juvenile idiopathic arthritis, see *BNF for Children*

> ### CHMP advice
> #### Piroxicam (June 2007)
> The CHMP has recommended restrictions on the use of piroxicam because of the increased risk of gastro-intestinal side effects and serious skin reactions. The CHMP has advised that:
>
> - piroxicam should be initiated only by physicians experienced in treating inflammatory or degenerative rheumatic diseases
> - piroxicam should not be used as first-line treatment
> - in adults, use of piroxicam should be limited to the symptomatic relief of osteoarthritis, rheumatoid arthritis, and ankylosing spondylitis
> - piroxicam dose should not exceed 20 mg daily
> - piroxicam should no longer be used for the treatment of acute painful and inflammatory conditions
> - treatment should be reviewed 2 weeks after initiating piroxicam, and periodically thereafter
> - concomitant administration of a gastro-protective agent (section 1.3) should be considered
>
> #### Note
> Topical preparations containing piroxicam are not affected by these restrictions

Piroxicam (Non-proprietary) ᴾᵒᴹ

Capsules, piroxicam 10 mg, net price 56-cap pack = £5.01; 20 mg, 28-cap pack = £4.84. Label: 21

Dispersible tablets, piroxicam 10 mg, net price 56-tab pack = £9.96; 20 mg, 28-tab pack = £32.41. Label: 13, 21

Brexidol® (Chiesi) ᴾᵒᴹ

Tablets, yellow, scored, piroxicam (as betadex) 20 mg, net price 30-tab pack = £13.82. Label: 21

Dose osteoarthritis, rheumatic disease and acute musculoskeletal disorders, 1 tablet daily (may be halved in elderly); CHILD not recommended

Feldene® (Pfizer) ᴾᵒᴹ

Capsules, piroxicam 10 mg (red/blue), net price 30-cap pack = £3.86; 20 mg (white), 30-cap pack = £7.71. Label: 21

Tablets, (*Feldene Melt®*), piroxicam 20 mg, net price 30-tab pack = £10.53. Label: 10, patient information leaflet, 21

Excipients include aspartame equivalent to phenylalanine 140 micrograms/tablet (section 9.4.1)

Note *Feldene Melt®* tablets can be taken by placing on tongue or by swallowing

◢ Topical preparations
Section 10.3.2

▰ SULINDAC

Indications   pain and inflammation in rheumatic disease and other musculoskeletal disorders; acute gout

Cautions   see notes above; also history of renal stones and ensure adequate hydration

Contra-indications   see notes above

Hepatic impairment   see notes above

Renal impairment   avoid in severe impairment; see also notes above

Pregnancy   see notes above

Breast-feeding   see notes above

Side-effects   see notes above; jaundice with fever, cholestasis, hepatitis, hepatic failure; also urine discoloration occasionally reported

Dose

- 200 mg twice daily (may be reduced according to response); max. 400 mg daily; acute gout should respond within 7 days; limit treatment of peri-articular disorders to 7–10 days; CHILD not recommended

Sulindac (Non-proprietary) ᴾᵒᴹ

Tablets, sulindac 100 mg, net price 56-tab pack = £29.78; 200 mg, 56-tab pack = £38.29. Label: 21

▰ TENOXICAM

Indications   pain and inflammation in rheumatic disease and other musculoskeletal disorders

Cautions   see notes above

Contra-indications   see notes above

Hepatic impairment   see notes above

Renal impairment   avoid in severe impairment; see also notes above

Pregnancy   see notes above

Breast-feeding   present in milk in *animal* studies; see also notes above

Side-effects   see notes above

Dose

- By mouth, rheumatic disease, ADULT over 18 years, 20 mg daily

  Acute musculoskeletal disorders, ADULT over 18 years, 20 mg daily for 7 days; max. duration of treatment 14 days (including treatment by intravenous or intramuscular injection)

- By intravenous *or* intramuscular injection, ADULT over 18 years, initial treatment for 1–2 days if oral administration not possible, 20 mg once daily

Tenoxicam (Non-proprietary) ᴾᵒᴹ

Tablets, f/c, tenoxicam 20 mg, net price 28-tab pack = £16.16. Label: 21

Injection, powder for reconstitution, tenoxicam, net price 20-mg vial = £3.98

Mobiflex® (Meda) ᴾᵒᴹ

Tablets, yellow, f/c, tenoxicam 20 mg, net price 30-tab pack = £13.42. Label: 21

▰ TIAPROFENIC ACID

Indications   pain and inflammation in rheumatic disease and other musculoskeletal disorders

Cautions   see notes above

Contra-indications   see notes above; also active bladder or prostate disease (or symptoms) and history of recurrent urinary-tract disorders—if urinary symptoms develop discontinue immediately and

10

Musculoskeletal and joint diseases

perform urine tests and culture; see also CSM advice below

Hepatic impairment reduce dose in mild or moderate impairment; see also notes above

Renal impairment reduce dose in mild or moderate impairment; avoid in severe impairment; see also notes above

Pregnancy see notes above

Breast-feeding amount too small to be harmful; see also notes above

Side-effects see notes above

Dose

• ADULT over 18 years, 300 mg twice daily

Surgam® (Sanofi-Aventis) PoM
Tablets, tiaprofenic acid 300 mg, net price 56-tab pack = £14.95. Label: 21

Aspirin

Aspirin (section 4.7.1) has been used in high doses to treat rheumatoid arthritis, but other NSAIDs are now preferred.

10.1.2 Corticosteroids

10.1.2.1 Systemic corticosteroids
10.1.2.2 Local corticosteroid injections

10.1.2.1 Systemic corticosteroids

The general actions, uses, and cautions of corticosteroids are described in section 6.3. Short-term treatment with corticosteroids can help to rapidly improve symptoms of rheumatoid arthritis. Long-term treatment in rheumatoid arthritis should be considered only after evaluating the risks and all other treatment options have been considered. Corticosteroids can induce osteoporosis, and prophylaxis should be considered on long-term treatment (section 6.6).

In severe, possibly life-threatening, situations a high initial dose of corticosteroid is given to induce remission and the dose is then reduced gradually and discontinued altogether. Relapse may occur as the dose of corticosteroid is reduced, particularly if the reduction is too rapid. The tendency is therefore to increase the maintenance dose and consequently the patient becomes dependent on corticosteroids. For this reason pulse doses of corticosteroids (e.g. methylprednisolone up to 1 g intravenously on 3 consecutive days) are used to suppress highly active inflammatory disease while longer-term treatment with a disease-modifying drug is commenced.

Prednisolone 7.5 mg daily may reduce the rate of joint destruction in moderate to severe *rheumatoid arthritis* of

less than 2 years' duration. The reduction in joint destruction must be distinguished from mere symptomatic improvement (which lasts only 6 to 12 months at this dose) and care should be taken to avoid increasing the dose above 7.5 mg daily. Evidence supports maintenance of this anti-erosive dose for 2–4 years only after which treatment should be tapered off to reduce long-term adverse effects.

A modified-release preparation of **prednisone** (section 6.3.2) is also available for the treatment of moderate to severe rheumatoid arthritis.

Polymyalgia rheumatica and *giant cell (temporal) arteritis* are always treated with corticosteroids. The usual initial dose of prednisolone in polymyalgia rheumatica is 10–15 mg daily and in giant cell arteritis 40–60 mg daily (the higher dose being used if visual symptoms occur). Treatment should be continued until remission of disease activity and doses are then reduced gradually to about 7.5–10 mg daily for maintenance. Relapse is common if therapy is stopped prematurely. Many patients require treatment for at least 2 years and in some patients it may be necessary to continue long-term low-dose corticosteroid treatment.

Polyarteritis nodosa and *polymyositis* are usually treated with corticosteroids. An initial dose of 60 mg of prednisolone daily is often used and reduced to a maintenance dose of 10–15 mg daily.

Systemic lupus erythematosus is treated with corticosteroids when necessary using a similar dosage regimen to that for polyarteritis nodosa and polymyositis (above). Patients with pleurisy, pericarditis, or other systemic manifestations will respond to corticosteroids. It may then be possible to reduce the dosage; alternate-day treatment is sometimes adequate, and the drug may be gradually withdrawn. In some mild cases corticosteroid treatment may be stopped after a few months. Many mild cases of systemic lupus erythematosus do not require corticosteroid treatment. Alternative treatment with anti-inflammatory analgesics, and possibly chloroquine or hydroxychloroquine, should be considered.

Ankylosing spondylitis should not be treated with long-term corticosteroids; rarely, pulse doses may be needed and may be useful in extremely active disease that does not respond to conventional treatment.

10.1.2.2 Local corticosteroid injections

Corticosteroids are injected locally for an anti-inflammatory effect. In inflammatory conditions of the joints, particularly in rheumatoid arthritis, they are given by *intra-articular injection* to relieve pain, increase mobility, and reduce deformity in one or a few joints; they can also provide symptomatic relief while waiting for DMARDs to take effect. Full aseptic precautions are essential; infected areas should be avoided. Occasionally an acute inflammatory reaction develops after an intra-articular or soft-tissue injection of a corticosteroid. This may be a reaction to the microcrystalline suspension of the corticosteroid used, but must be distinguished from sepsis introduced into the injection site.

Smaller amounts of corticosteroids may also be injected directly into soft tissues for the relief of inflammation in conditions such as *tennis* or *golfer's elbow* or *compression neuropathies*. In *tendinitis*, injections should be made into the tendon sheath and not directly into the tendon (due to the absence of a true tendon sheath and a high risk of rupture, the Achilles tendon should not be injected).

Musculoskeletal and joint diseases

10

Hydrocortisone acetate or one of the synthetic analogues is generally used for local injection. Intra-articular corticosteroid injections can cause flushing and may affect the hyaline cartilage. Each joint should not usually be treated more than 4 times in one year.

Corticosteroid injections are also injected into soft tissues for the treatment of skin lesions (see section 13.4).

LOCAL CORTICOSTEROID INJECTIONS

Indications   local inflammation of joints and soft tissues (for details, consult product literature)

Cautions   see notes above and consult product literature; see also section 6.3.2

Contra-indications   see notes above and consult product literature; avoid injections containing benzyl alcohol in neonates (see preparations below)

Side-effects   see notes above and consult product literature

Dose
- See under preparations

◢ Betamethasone

Betnesol® (RPH) [PoM]

Injection, betamethasone (as sodium phosphate) 4 mg/mL, net price 1-mL amp = £1.22.

◢ Dexamethasone

Dexamethasone (Non-proprietary) [PoM]

Injection, dexamethasone (as sodium phosphate) 3.8 mg/mL, net price 1-mL vial = £1.99

Note   Dexamethasone 3.8 mg/mL Injection has replaced Dexamethasone 4 mg/mL Injection

Dose   by intra-articular injection (for details consult product literature), 0.3–3 mg according to size; where appropriate may be repeated at intervals of 3–21 days according to response

Injection, dexamethasone (as sodium phosphate) 3.3 mg/mL, net price 1-mL amp = £1.20, 2-mL vial = £4.80

Dose   by intra-articular injection (for details consult product literature), 0.33–3.3 mg according to size (by soft-tissue infiltration 1.7–5 mg); where appropriate may be repeated at intervals of 3–21 days

◢ Hydrocortisone acetate

Hydrocortistab® (AMCo) [PoM]

Injection (aqueous suspension), hydrocortisone acetate 25 mg/mL, net price 1-mL amp = £6.87

Dose   by intra-articular injection (for details consult product literature), 5–50 mg according to size; where appropriate may be repeated at intervals of 21 days; not more than 3 joints should be treated on any one day; CHILD 5–30 mg (divided)

◢ Methylprednisolone acetate

Depo-Medrone® (Pharmacia) [PoM]

Injection (aqueous suspension), methylprednisolone acetate 40 mg/mL, net price 1-mL vial = £3.44; 2-mL vial = £6.18; 3-mL vial = £8.96

Dose   by intra-articular injection (for details consult product literature), 4–80 mg, according to size; where appropriate may be repeated at intervals of 7–35 days; also for intralesional injection

Depo-Medrone® **with Lidocaine** (Pharmacia) [PoM]

Injection (aqueous suspension), methylprednisolone acetate 40 mg, lidocaine hydrochloride 10 mg/mL, net price 1-mL vial = £3.94; 2-mL vial = £7.06

Dose   by intra-articular injection (for details consult product literature), 4–80 mg, according to size; where appropriate may be repeated at intervals of 7–35 days

◢ Prednisolone acetate

Deltastab® (AMCo) [PoM]

Injection (aqueous suspension), prednisolone acetate 25 mg/mL, net price 1-mL amp = £6.87

Dose   by intra-articular injection (for details consult product literature), 5–25 mg according to size; not more than 3 joints should be treated on any one day; where appropriate may be repeated when relapse occurs

For intramuscular injection, see section 6.3.2

◢ Triamcinolone acetonide

Adcortyl® **Intra-articular/Intradermal** (Squibb) [PoM]

Injection (aqueous suspension), triamcinolone acetonide 10 mg/mL, net price 1-mL amp = 89p; 5-mL vial = £3.63

Excipients   include benzyl alcohol (avoid in neonates, see Excipients, p. 2)

Dose   by intra-articular injection (for details consult product literature), 2.5–15 mg according to size (for larger doses use Kenalog®); where appropriate may be repeated when relapse occurs; CHILD under 18 years see BNF for Children

By intradermal injection, (for details consult product literature): 2–3 mg; max. 5 mg at any one site (total max. 30 mg); where appropriate may be repeated at intervals of 1–2 weeks; CHILD under 6 years not recommended

Kenalog® **Intra-articular/Intramuscular** (Squibb) [PoM]

Injection (aqueous suspension), triamcinolone acetonide 40 mg/mL, net price 1-mL vial = £1.49

Dose   by intra-articular injection (for details consult product literature), 5–40 mg according to size; total max. 80 mg (for doses below 5 mg use Adcortyl® Intra-articular/ Intradermal); where appropriate may be repeated when relapse occurs; CHILD under 18 years see BNF for Children

For intramuscular injection, see section 6.3.2

10.1.3   Drugs that suppress the rheumatic disease process

Certain drugs such as those affecting the immune response can suppress the disease process in *rheumatoid arthritis* and *psoriatic arthritis*; gold, penicillamine, hydroxychloroquine, chloroquine, and sulfasalazine can also suppress the disease process in *rheumatoid arthritis* while sulfasalazine and possibly gold can suppress the disease process in *psoriatic arthritis*. Unlike NSAIDs, which are used only for symptom control, disease-modifying anti-rheumatic drugs (DMARDs) can affect the progression of disease but may require 2–6 months of treatment for a full therapeutic response. Response to DMARDs may allow the NSAID dose to be reduced or withdrawn. All patients with suspected inflammatory joint disease should be referred to a specialist as soon as possible to confirm diagnosis and evaluate disease activity; early initiation of DMARDs is recommended to control the signs and symptoms, and to limit joint damage.

Choice   The choice of a disease-modifying anti-rheumatic drug should take into account co-morbidity and patient preference. Methotrexate, sulfasalazine, intramuscular gold, and penicillamine are similar in efficacy. However, **methotrexate** or **sulfasalazine** may be better tolerated.

A combination of **DMARDs** (including methotrexate and at least one other DMARD) and a short-term **corticosteroid** (section 10.1.2), should be given to patients with newly diagnosed active rheumatoid arthritis, ideally within 3 months of the onset of persistent symptoms. If the use of particular DMARDs is contra-

10 Musculoskeletal and joint diseases

Musculoskeletal and joint diseases *(side label)*

indicated and combination therapy is not possible, monotherapy with a suitable DMARD should be given and the dose rapidly increased until clinically effective. In patients with established and stable rheumatoid arthritis, cautiously reduce drug doses to the lowest that are clinically effective. Response to drug treatment often produces a reduction in requirements of both corticosteroids and other drugs.

Gold and penicillamine are effective in *palindromic rheumatism. Systemic* and *discoid lupus erythematosus* are sometimes treated with chloroquine or hydroxychloroquine.

If a disease-modifying anti-rheumatic drug does not lead to an objective benefit within 6 months, it should be replaced by a different one.

Juvenile idiopathic arthritis   Many children with *juvenile idiopathic arthritis* (juvenile chronic arthritis) do not require disease-modifying antirheumatic drugs. Methotrexate is effective (see *BNF for Children*); sulfasalazine is an alternative [unlicensed indication] but it should be avoided in *systemic-onset juvenile idiopathic arthritis* (see *BNF for Children*). Gold and penicillamine are no longer used. For the role of cytokine modulators in *juvenile idiopathic arthritis*, see *BNF for Children*.

Gold

Gold can be given as **sodium aurothiomalate** for active progressive rheumatoid arthritis; it must be given by deep intramuscular injection and the area gently massaged. A test dose of 10 mg must be given followed by doses of 50 mg at weekly intervals until there is definite evidence of remission. Benefit is not to be expected until about 300–500 mg has been given; it should be discontinued if there is no remission after 1 g has been given. In patients who do respond, the interval between injections is then gradually increased to 4 weeks and treatment is continued for up to 5 years after complete remission. If relapse occurs the dosage frequency may be immediately increased to 50 mg weekly and only once control has been obtained again should the dosage frequency be decreased; if no response is seen within 2 months, alternative treatment should be sought. It is important to avoid complete relapse since second courses of gold are not usually effective.

Sodium aurothiomalate should be discontinued in the presence of blood disorders, gastro-intestinal bleeding (associated with ulcerative enterocolitis), or unexplained proteinuria (associated with immune complex nephritis) which is repeatedly above 300 mg/litre. Urine tests and full blood counts (including total and differential white cell and platelet counts) must therefore be performed before starting treatment and before each intramuscular injection. Rashes with pruritus often occur after 2 to 6 months of treatment and may necessitate discontinuation.

▌ SODIUM AUROTHIOMALATE

Indications   active progressive rheumatoid arthritis

Cautions   see notes above; elderly, history of urticaria, eczema, colitis; monitor for pulmonary fibrosis with annual chest X-ray; **interactions**: Appendix 1 (sodium aurothiomalate)

> **Counselling**   Patients should be advised to seek prompt medical attention if diarrhoea, sore throat, fever, infection, non-specific illness, unexplained bleeding and bruising, purpura, mouth ulcers, metallic taste, rash, breathlessness, or cough develop

Contra-indications   history of blood disorders or bone marrow aplasia, exfoliative dermatitis, systemic lupus erythematosus, necrotising enterocolitis, pulmonary fibrosis

Hepatic impairment   caution in mild to moderate impairment, avoid in severe impairment

Renal impairment   caution in mild to moderate impairment; avoid in severe impairment

Pregnancy   manufacturer advises avoid but limited data suggests usually not necessary to withdraw if condition well controlled—consider reducing dose and frequency

Breast-feeding   manufacturer advises avoid—present in milk; theoretical possibility of rashes and idiosyncratic reactions

Side-effects   see notes above; also severe anaphylactic reactions; stomatitis, taste disturbances, colitis, hepatotoxicity with cholestatic jaundice, pulmonary fibrosis, peripheral neuropathy, mouth ulcers, proteinuria, blood disorders (sometimes sudden and fatal), nephrotic syndrome, gold deposits in eye, alopecia, and skin reactions (including, on prolonged parenteral treatment, irreversible pigmentation in sun-exposed areas)

Dose

- By deep intramuscular injection, administered on expert advice, see notes above

Myocrisin® (Sanofi-Aventis) [PoM]
Injection, sodium aurothiomalate 20 mg/mL, net price 0.5-mL (10-mg) amp = £4.56; 100 mg/mL, 0.5-mL (50-mg) amp = £13.48. Label: 11, counselling, blood disorder symptoms

Penicillamine

Penicillamine has a similar action to gold. More patients are able to continue treatment than with gold but side-effects are common.

Patients should be warned not to expect improvement for at least 6 to 12 weeks after treatment is initiated. Penicillamine should be discontinued if there is no improvement within 1 year.

Blood counts, including platelets, and urine examinations should be carried out before starting treatment and then every 1 or 2 weeks for the first 2 months then every 4 weeks to detect blood disorders and proteinuria (they should also be carried out in the week after any dose increase). A reduction in platelet count calls for discontinuation with subsequent re-introduction at a lower dosage and then, if possible, gradual increase. Proteinuria, associated with immune complex nephritis, occurs in up to 30% of patients, but may resolve despite continuation of treatment; treatment may be continued provided that renal function tests remain normal, oedema is absent, and the 24-hour urinary excretion of protein does not exceed 2 g.

Nausea may occur but is not usually a problem provided that penicillamine is taken before food or on retiring and that low initial doses are used and only gradually increased. Loss of taste can occur about 6 weeks after treatment is started but usually returns 6 weeks later irrespective of whether treatment is discontinued; mineral supplements are not recommended. Rashes are a common side-effect. Those that occur in the first few months of treatment disappear when the drug is stopped and treatment may then be re-introduced at a lower dose level and gradually increased.

Patients who are hypersensitive to penicillin may react rarely to penicillamine.

PENICILLAMINE

Indications   see notes above and under Dose

Cautions   see notes above; concomitant nephrotoxic drugs (increased risk of toxicity); gold treatment (avoid concomitant use if adverse reactions to gold); **interactions**: Appendix 1 (penicillamine)

Blood counts and urine tests See notes above. Longer intervals may be adequate in cystinuria and Wilson's disease. Consider withdrawal if platelet count falls below 120 000/mm³ or white blood cells below 2500/mm³ or if 3 successive falls within reference range (can restart at reduced dose when counts return to within reference range but permanent withdrawal necessary if recurrence of leucopenia or thrombocytopenia)

Counselling Warn patient to tell doctor promptly if sore throat, fever, infection, non-specific illness, unexplained bleeding and bruising, purpura, mouth ulcers, or rashes develop

Contra-indications   lupus erythematosus

Renal impairment   reduce dose and monitor renal function or avoid (consult product literature)

Pregnancy   fetal abnormalities reported rarely; avoid if possible

Breast-feeding   manufacturer advises avoid unless potential benefit outweighs risk—no information available

Side-effects   (see also notes above) initially nausea, anorexia, fever; proteinuria, thrombocytopenia; *rarely* mouth ulceration, stomatitis, male and female breast enlargement, haematuria (withdraw immediately if cause unknown), alopecia, pseudoxanthoma elasticum, elastosis perforans, skin laxity; *also reported* pancreatitis, vomiting, cholestatic jaundice, pulmonary haemorrhage, bronchiolitis, pneumonitis, blood disorders including neutropenia, agranulocytosis, aplastic anaemia, haemolytic anaemia and leucopenia, nephrotic syndrome, glomerulonephritis, Goodpasture's syndrome, septic arthritis in patients with rheumatoid arthritis, lupus erythematosus, myasthenia gravis, polymyositis, rheumatoid arthritis, urticaria, dermatomyositis, pemphigus, Stevens-Johnson syndrome, late rashes (consider dose reduction)

Dose

- Severe active rheumatoid arthritis, administered on expert advice, ADULT over 18 years, initially 125–250 mg daily for 1 month increased by similar amounts at intervals of not less than 4 weeks to usual maintenance of 500–750 mg daily in divided doses; max. 1.5 g daily; if remission sustained for 6 months, reduction of daily dose by 125–250 mg every 12 weeks may be attempted; ELDERLY initially up to 125 mg daily for 1 month increased by similar amounts at intervals of not less than 4 weeks; max. 1 g daily

- Wilson's disease, autoimmune hepatitis, and cystinuria, section 9.8.1

Penicillamine (Non-proprietary) ℞ℳ
Tablets, penicillamine 125 mg, net price 56-tab pack = £11.20; 250 mg, 56-tab pack = £21.46. Label: 6, 22, counselling, blood disorder symptoms (see above)

Distamine® (Alliance) ℞ℳ
Tablets, f/c, penicillamine 125 mg, net price 100-tab pack = £10.34; 250 mg, 250 mg, 100-tab pack= £17.78. Label: 6, 22, counselling, blood disorder symptoms (see above)

Antimalarials

The antimalarial **hydroxychloroquine** is used to treat rheumatoid arthritis of moderate inflammatory activity; **chloroquine** is also licensed for treating inflammatory disorders but is used much less frequently and is generally reserved for use if other drugs have failed. Chloroquine and hydroxychloroquine are effective for mild systemic lupus erythematosus, particularly involving the skin and joints. These drugs should not be used for psoriatic arthritis.

Chloroquine and hydroxychloroquine are better tolerated than gold or penicillamine. Retinopathy (see below) rarely occurs provided that the recommended doses are not exceeded; in the elderly it is difficult to distinguish drug-induced retinopathy from changes of ageing.

Mepacrine (section 5.4.4) is sometimes used in discoid lupus erythematosus [unlicensed].

Cautions   Manufacturers recommend regular ophthalmological examination but the evidence of practical value is unsatisfactory (see advice of the Royal College of Ophthalmologists, below). Chloroquine and hydroxychloroquine should be used with caution in neurological disorders (especially in those with a history of epilepsy), in severe gastro-intestinal disorders, in G6PD deficiency (section 9.1.5), in acute porphyria, and in the elderly (see also above). Chloroquine and hydroxychloroquine may exacerbate psoriasis and aggravate myasthenia gravis. Concurrent use of hepatotoxic drugs should be avoided; other **interactions**: Appendix 1 (chloroquine and hydroxychloroquine).

Screening for ocular toxicity A review group convened by the Royal College of Ophthalmologists has updated guidelines for screening to prevent ocular toxicity on long-term treatment with chloroquine and hydroxychloroquine (*Hydroxychloroquine and Ocular Toxicity: Recommendations on Screening 2009*). Chloroquine should be considered (for treating chronic inflammatory conditions) **only** if other drugs have failed. All patients taking chloroquine should receive ocular examination according to a protocol arranged locally between the prescriber and the ophthalmologist. The following recommendations relate to hydroxychloroquine, which is only rarely associated with toxicity.

Before treatment:

- Assess renal and liver function (adjust dose if impaired)

- Ask patient about visual impairment (not corrected by glasses). If impairment or eye disease present, assessment by an optometrist is advised and any abnormality should be referred to an ophthalmologist

- Record near visual acuity of each eye (with glasses where appropriate) using a standard reading chart

- Initiate hydroxychloroquine treatment if no abnormality detected (at a dose not exceeding hydroxychloroquine sulfate 6.5 mg/kg daily)

During treatment:

- Ask patient about visual symptoms and monitor visual acuity annually using the standard reading chart

- Refer to ophthalmologist if visual acuity changes or if vision blurred and warn patient to seek prescribing doctor's advice about stopping treatment

- A child treated for juvenile idiopathic arthritis should receive slit-lamp examination routinely to check for uveitis

- If long-term treatment is required (more than 5 years), individual arrangement should be agreed with the local ophthalmologist

Important

To avoid excessive dosage in obese patients, the doses of hydroxychloroquine and chloroquine should be calculated on the basis of ideal body-weight. Ocular toxicity is unlikely if the dose of chloroquine phosphate does not exceed 4 mg/kg daily (equivalent to chloroquine base approx. 2.5 mg/kg daily)

Hepatic impairment   Chloroquine and hydroxychloroquine should be used with caution in moderate to severe hepatic impairment.

Pregnancy   It is not necessary to withdraw an antimalarial drug during pregnancy if the rheumatic disease is well controlled; however, the manufacturer of hydroxychloroquine advises avoiding use.

Breast-feeding   Chloroquine and hydroxychloroquine are present in breast milk and breast-feeding should be avoided when they are used to treat rheumatic disease.

Side-effects   The side-effects of chloroquine and hydroxychloroquine include gastro-intestinal disturbances, headache and skin reactions (rashes, pruritus); those occurring less frequently include ECG changes, convulsions, visual changes, retinal damage (see above), keratopathy, ototoxicity, hair depigmentation, hair loss, and discoloration of skin, nails, and mucous membranes. Side-effects that occur rarely include blood disorders (including thrombocytopenia, agranulocytosis, and aplastic anaemia), mental changes (including emotional disturbances and psychosis), myopathy (including cardiomyopathy and neuromyopathy), angioedema, acute generalised exanthematous pustulosis, exfoliative dermatitis, Stevens-Johnson syndrome, photosensitivity, and hepatic damage; diffuse parenchymal lung disease, and drug rash with eosinophilia and systemic symptoms have also been reported. **Important**: very toxic in overdosage—immediate advice from poisons centres essential (see also p. 39).

CHLOROQUINE

Indications   active rheumatoid arthritis, systemic and discoid lupus erythematosus; malaria (section 5.4.1)

Cautions   see notes above

Hepatic impairment   see notes above

Renal impairment   manufacturer advises caution; reduce dose

Pregnancy   see notes above

Breast-feeding   see notes above

Side-effects   see notes above

Dose

- Administered on expert advice, by mouth, ADULT over 18 years, chloroquine (base) 150 mg daily; max.

2.5 mg/kg daily based on ideal body-weight, see also recommendations above

Note   Chloroquine base 150 mg ≡ chloroquine sulfate 200 mg ≡ chloroquine phosphate 250 mg (approx.).

◢**Preparations**

Section 5.4.1

HYDROXYCHLOROQUINE SULFATE

Indications   active rheumatoid arthritis (including juvenile idiopathic arthritis), systemic and discoid lupus erythematosus; dermatological conditions caused or aggravated by sunlight

Cautions   see notes above

Hepatic impairment   see notes above

Renal impairment   manufacturer advises caution and monitoring of plasma-hydroxychloroquine concentration in severe impairment

Pregnancy   see notes above

Breast-feeding   avoid—risk of toxicity in infant; see also notes above

Side-effects   see notes above; also reported bronchospasm

Dose

- Administered on expert advice, 200–400 mg daily (but not exceeding 6.5 mg/kg daily based on ideal body-weight, see also recommendations above); CHILD 1 month–18 years see BNF for Children

Hydroxychloroquine (Non-proprietary) PoM
Tablets, hydroxychloroquine sulfate 200 mg, net price 60-tab pack = £5.29. Label: 21, counselling, see below
Brands include Quinoric®
Counselling   Do not take antacids for at least 4 hours before or after hydroxychloroquine to reduce possible interference with hydroxychloroquine absorption

Plaquenil® (Sanofi-Aventis) PoM
Tablets, f/c, hydroxychloroquine sulfate 200 mg, net price 60-tab pack = £5.15. Label: 21, counselling, see below
Counselling   Do not take antacids for at least 4 hours before or after hydroxychloroquine to reduce possible interference with hydroxychloroquine absorption

Drugs affecting the immune response

Methotrexate is a disease-modifying antirheumatic drug suitable for moderate to severe rheumatoid arthritis. **Azathioprine**, **ciclosporin**, **cyclophosphamide**, **leflunomide**, and the **cytokine modulators** are considered more toxic and they are used in cases that have not responded to other disease-modifying drugs.

Methotrexate is usually given in an initial dose of 7.5 mg by mouth once a week, adjusted according to response to a maximum of 15 mg once a week (occasionally 20 mg once a week). Regular full blood counts (including differential white cell count and platelet count), renal and liver function tests are required. In patients who experience mucosal or gastro-intestinal side-effects with methotrexate, folic acid 5 mg every week [unlicensed indication], on a different day from the methotrexate, may help to reduce the frequency of such side-effects.

Azathioprine is usually given in a dose of up to 2.5 mg/kg daily in divided doses. Blood counts are needed to detect possible neutropenia or thrombocytopenia (usually resolved by reducing the dose). Nausea, vomiting, and diarrhoea may occur, usually starting early during the course of treatment, and may necessitate withdrawal of the drug; herpes zoster infection may also occur.

Leflunomide acts on the immune system as a disease-modifying antirheumatic drug. Its therapeutic effect starts after 4–6 weeks and improvement may continue for a further 4–6 months. Leflunomide, which is similar in efficacy to sulfasalazine and methotrexate, may be chosen when these drugs cannot be used. The active metabolite of leflunomide persists for a long period; active procedures to wash the drug out are required in case of serious adverse effects, or before starting treatment with another disease-modifying antirheumatic drug, or, in men or women, before conception. Side-effects of leflunomide include bone-marrow toxicity; its immunosuppressive effects increase the risk of infection and malignancy.

Ciclosporin is licensed for severe active rheumatoid arthritis when conventional second-line therapy is inappropriate or ineffective. There is some evidence that ciclosporin may retard the rate of erosive progression and improve symptom control in those who respond only partially to methotrexate.

Cyclophosphamide (section 8.1.1) may be used at a dose of 1 to 1.5 mg/kg daily by mouth for rheumatoid arthritis with severe systemic manifestations [unlicensed indication]; it is toxic and regular blood counts (including platelet counts) should be carried out. Cyclophosphamide can also be given intravenously in a dose of 0.5 to 1 g (with prophylactic mesna) for *severe systemic rheumatoid arthritis* and for other connective tissue diseases (especially with active vasculitis), repeated initially at fortnightly then at monthly intervals (according to clinical response and haematological monitoring).

Drugs that affect the immune response are also used in the management of severe cases of *systemic lupus erythematosus* and other connective tissue disorders. They are often given in conjunction with corticosteroids for patients with severe or progressive renal disease. They may be used in cases of *polymyositis* that are resistant to corticosteroids. They are used for their corticosteroid-sparing effect in patients whose corticosteroid requirements are excessive. **Azathioprine** is usually used.

In the specialist management of psoriatic arthritis affecting peripheral joints, leflunomide, methotrexate, or azathioprine [unlicensed indication] may be used.

▌ AZATHIOPRINE

Indications   see notes above; inflammatory bowel disease (section 1.5.3); autoimmune conditions and prophylaxis of transplantation rejection (section 8.2.1); severe refractory eczema [unlicensed indication] (section 13.5.3)

Cautions   section 8.2.1

Contra-indications   section 8.2.1

Hepatic impairment   section 8.2.1

Renal impairment   section 8.2.1

Pregnancy   section 8.2.1

Breast-feeding   section 8.2.1

Side-effects   section 8.2.1

Dose

● By mouth, initially, rarely more than 3 mg/kg daily, reduced according to response; maintenance 1–

3 mg/kg daily; consider withdrawal if no improvement within 3 months

▌**Preparations**

Section 8.2.1

▌ CICLOSPORIN
(Cyclosporin)

Indications   severe active rheumatoid arthritis when conventional second-line therapy inappropriate or ineffective; severe acute ulcerative colitis [unlicensed indication] (section 1.5.3); graft-versus-host disease (section 8.2.2); atopic dermatitis and psoriasis (section 13.5.3)

Cautions   section 8.2.2

Additional cautions in rheumatoid arthritis   *Contra-indicated* in abnormal renal function, uncontrolled hypertension (see also below), uncontrolled infections, and malignancy. Measure serum creatinine at least twice before treatment and monitor every 2 weeks for first 3 months, then every month for a further 3 months, then every 4–8 weeks depending on the stability of the disease, concomitant medication, and concomitant diseases, (or more frequently if dose increased or concomitant NSAIDs introduced or increased (see also *interactions:* Appendix 1 (ciclosporin)), reduce dose if serum creatinine increases more than 30% above baseline in more than 1 measurement; if above 50%, reduce dose by 50% (even if within normal range) and discontinue if reduction not successful within 1 month; monitor blood pressure (discontinue if hypertension develops that cannot be controlled by antihypertensive therapy); monitor hepatic function if concomitant NSAIDs given.

Hepatic impairment   section 8.2.2

Renal impairment   see Cautions above

Pregnancy   see section 8.2.2

Breast-feeding   section 8.2.2

Side-effects   section 8.2.2

Dose

● By mouth, administered in accordance with expert advice, initially 2.5 mg/kg daily in 2 divided doses, if necessary increased gradually after 6 weeks; max. 4 mg/kg daily (discontinue if response insufficient after 3 months); dose adjusted according to response for maintenance and treatment reviewed after 6 months (continue only if benefits outweigh risks); CHILD and under 18 years, not recommended

Important   For preparations and counselling and for advice on conversion between the preparations, see section 8.2.2

▌**Preparations**

Section 8.2.2

▌ LEFLUNOMIDE

Indications   (specialist use only) moderate to severe active rheumatoid arthritis; active psoriatic arthritis

Cautions   impaired bone-marrow function including anaemia, leucopenia or thrombocytopenia (avoid if significant and due to causes other than rheumatoid arthritis); recent treatment with other hepatotoxic or myelotoxic disease-modifying antirheumatic drugs; washout procedures recommended for serious adverse effects or before switching to other disease-modifying antirheumatic drugs (consult product literature and see Washout Procedure, below); history of tuberculosis; exclude pregnancy before treatment; effective contraception **essential** during treatment and for at least 2 years after treatment in women and at least 3 months after treatment in men (plasma concentration monitoring required); waiting time before conception may be reduced with washout procedure—consult product literature and see

Washout Procedure, below); monitor full blood count (including differential white cell count and platelet count) before treatment and every 2 weeks for 6 months then every 8 weeks; monitor liver function—see Hepatotoxicity, below; monitor blood pressure; **interactions**: Appendix 1 (leflunomide)

Hepatotoxicity Potentially life-threatening hepatotoxicity reported usually in the first 6 months; monitor liver function before treatment and every 2 weeks for first 6 months then every 8 weeks. Discontinue treatment (and institute washout procedure—consult product literature and see Washout Procedure below) or reduce dose according to liver-function abnormality; if liver-function abnormality persists after dose reduction, discontinue treatment and institute washout procedure

Washout procedure To aid drug elimination in case of serious adverse effect, or before starting another disease-modifying antirheumatic drug, or before conception (see also Pregnancy below), stop treatment and give *either* colestyramine 8 g 3 times daily for 11 days *or* activated charcoal 50 g 4 times daily for 11 days; the concentration of the active metabolite after washout should be less than 20 micrograms/litre (measured on 2 occasions 14 days apart) in men or women before conception—consult product literature. Procedure may be repeated as necessary

Contra-indications severe immunodeficiency; severe hypoproteinaemia; serious infection

Hepatic impairment avoid—active metabolite may accumulate; see also Cautions above

Renal impairment manufacturer advises avoid in moderate or severe impairment—no information available

Pregnancy avoid—active metabolite teratogenic in *animal* studies; effective contraception essential during treatment and for at least 2 years after treatment in women and at least 3 months after treatment in men (see also Cautions above)

Breast-feeding present in milk in *animal* studies—manufacturer advises avoid

Side-effects diarrhoea, nausea, vomiting, anorexia, oral mucosal disorders, abdominal pain; increased blood pressure; headache, dizziness, asthenia, paraesthesia; leucopenia; tenosynovitis; alopecia, rash, dry skin, pruritus; *less commonly* taste disturbance, anxiety, hyperlipidaemia, hypokalaemia, hypophosphataemia, anaemia, thrombocytopenia, and tendon rupture; *rarely* hepatitis, jaundice (see Hepatotoxicity, above), interstitial lung disease, severe infection, eosinophilia, and pancytopenia; *very rarely* pancreatitis, hepatic failure (see Hepatotoxicity, above), peripheral neuropathy, vasculitis, progressive multifocal leucoencephalopathy, Stevens-Johnson syndrome, and toxic epidermal necrolysis; hypouricaemia, reduced sperm count, and renal failure also reported; **important:** discontinue treatment and institute washout procedure (see Washout Procedure under Cautions) in case of serious side-effect

Dose
- Rheumatoid arthritis, ADULT over 18 years, initially 100 mg once daily for 3 days, then 10–20 mg once daily
- Psoriatic arthritis, ADULT over 18 years, initially 100 mg once daily for 3 days, then 20 mg once daily

Leflunomide (Non-proprietary) PoM
Tablets, leflunomide, 10 mg, net price 30-tab pack = £14.93; 20 mg, 30-tab pack = £15.42. Label: 4

Arava® (Sanofi-Aventis) PoM
Tablets, f/c, leflunomide 10 mg (white), net price 30-tab pack = £51.13; 20 mg (yellow), 30-tab pack = £61.36; 100 mg (white), 3-tab pack = £30.67. Label: 4

METHOTREXATE

Indications see under dose; Crohn's disease [unlicensed indication] (section 1.5.3); malignant disease (section 8.1.3); psoriasis (section 13.5.3)

Cautions section 8.1; see Monitoring, Blood Count, Liver Toxicity, and Pulmonary Toxicity below; extreme caution in blood disorders (avoid if severe); peptic ulceration, ulcerative colitis, diarrhoea and ulcerative stomatitis (withdraw if stomatitis develops—may be first sign of gastro-intestinal toxicity); risk of accumulation in pleural effusion or ascites—drain before treatment; acute porphyria (section 9.8.2); **interactions:** see below and Appendix 1 (methotrexate)

Monitoring

In view of reports of blood dyscrasias (including fatalities) and liver cirrhosis with low-dose methotrexate patients should:

- have full blood count and renal and liver function tests before starting treatment and repeated every 1–2 weeks until therapy stabilised; thereafter patients should be monitored every 2–3 months[1]
- be advised to report all symptoms and signs suggestive of infection, especially sore throat

Treatment with folinic acid (as calcium folinate, section 8.1) may be required in acute toxicity

Blood count Bone marrow suppression can occur abruptly; factors likely to increase toxicity include advanced age, renal impairment, and concomitant use with another anti-folate drug (e.g. trimethoprim). A clinically significant drop in white cell count or platelet count calls for immediate withdrawal of methotrexate and introduction of supportive therapy

Liver toxicity Liver cirrhosis reported. Treatment should not be started or should be discontinued if any abnormality of liver function tests or liver biopsy is present or develops during therapy. Abnormalities can return to normal within 2 weeks after which treatment may be recommenced if judged appropriate

Pulmonary toxicity Pulmonary toxicity may be a special problem in rheumatoid arthritis (patient to seek medical attention if dyspnoea, cough or fever); monitor for symptoms at each visit—discontinue if pneumonitis suspected.

Aspirin and other NSAIDs If aspirin or other NSAIDs are given concurrently the dose of methotrexate should be carefully monitored. Patients should be advised to avoid self-medication with over-the-counter aspirin or ibuprofen

Contra-indications see Cautions above; active infection and immunodeficiency syndromes

Hepatic impairment avoid—dose-related toxicity; see also Cautions above

Renal impairment reduce dose; risk of nephrotoxicity at high doses; avoid in severe impairment

Pregnancy avoid (teratogenic; fertility may be reduced during therapy but this may be reversible); effective contraception required during and for at least 3 months after treatment in men or women; see also section 8.1

Breast-feeding discontinue breast-feeding; present in milk

Side-effects section 8.1; also anorexia, abdominal discomfort, dyspepsia, gastro-intestinal ulceration and bleeding, diarrhoea, toxic megacolon, hepatotoxicity (see Cautions above); hypotension, pericarditis, pericardial tamponade; pulmonary oedema, pleuritic pain, pulmonary fibrosis, interstitial pneumonitis (see also Pulmonary Toxicity above); anaphylactic reactions, urticaria; dizziness, chills, fever, drowsiness, insomnia, malaise, headache, mood changes, neurotoxicity, confusion, paraesthesia; precipitation of diabetes; menstrual disturbances, vagin-

1. Local protocols for frequency of monitoring may vary

10 Musculoskeletal and joint diseases

itis, cystitis, reduced libido, impotence; blood disorders; haematuria, dysuria, renal failure; osteoporosis, arthralgia, myalgia, vasculitis; conjunctivitis, visual disturbance; rash, pruritus, Stevens-Johnson syndrome, toxic epidermal necrolysis, photosensitivity, changes in nail and skin pigmentation, telangiectasia, acne, furuncolosis, ecchymosis; injection-site reactions

Dose

- Moderate to severe active rheumatoid arthritis, by mouth, ADULT over 18 years, 7.5 mg once weekly, adjusted according to response; max. weekly dose 20 mg
- Severe active rheumatoid arthritis, by subcutaneous *or* by intramuscular *or* by intravenous injection, ADULT over 18 years, 7.5 mg once weekly, increased according to response by 2.5 mg weekly; max. weekly dose 25 mg
- CHILD under 18 years see *BNF for Children*

Important

Note that the above dose is a **weekly** dose. To avoid error with low-dose methotrexate, it is recommended that:

- the patient is carefully advised of the **dose** and **frequency** and the reason for taking methotrexate and any other prescribed medicine (e.g. folic acid);
- only one strength of methotrexate tablet (usually 2.5 mg) is prescribed and dispensed;
- the prescription and the dispensing label clearly show the dose and frequency of methotrexate administration;
- the patient is warned to report immediately the onset of any feature of blood disorders (e.g. sore throat, bruising, and mouth ulcers), liver toxicity (e.g. nausea, vomiting, abdominal discomfort, and dark urine), and respiratory effects (e.g. shortness of breath).

Methotrexate treatment booklets

Methotrexate treatment booklets should be issued where appropriate.

In **England**, **Wales**, and **Northern Ireland**, they are available for purchase from:

3M Security Print and Systems Limited
Gorse Street, Chadderton
Oldham
OL9 9QH
Tel: 0845 610 1112

GP practices can obtain supplies through their Local Area Team stores.

NHS Hospitals can order supplies from www. nhsforms.co.uk or by emailing nhsforms@mmm. com.

In **Scotland**, treatment booklets can be obtained by emailing stockorders.dppas@theapsgroup.com or by fax on 0131 629 9967.

These booklets include advice for adults taking oral methotrexate for inflammatory conditions, and a section for recording results of blood tests and dosage information.

Methotrexate (Non-proprietary) [PoM]

Tablets, yellow, methotrexate 2.5 mg, net price 24-tab pack = £2.22, 28-tab pack = £2.60. Counselling, dose, treatment booklet, NSAIDs
Brands include *Maxtrex*®

Tablets, yellow, methotrexate 10 mg, net price 100-tab pack = £34.48. Counselling, dose, treatment booklet, NSAIDs

---

◀**Parenteral preparations**

See also section 8.1.3

Metoject® (Medac) [PoM]
Injection, prefilled syringe, methotrexate (as disodium salt) 50 mg/mL, net price 0.15 mL (7.5 mg) = £14.85, 0.2 mL (10 mg) = £15.29, 0.25 mL (12.5 mg) = £16.50, 0.3 mL (15 mg) = £16.57, 0.35 mL (17.5 mg) = £17.50, 0.4 mL (20 mg) = £17.84, 0.45 mL (22.5 mg) = £18.45, 0.5 mL (25 mg) = £18.48, 0.55 mL (27.5 mg) = £18.89, 0.6 mL (30 mg) = £18.95

Cytokine modulators

Cytokine modulators should be used under specialist supervision.

Adalimumab, certolizumab pegol, etanercept, golimumab, and infliximab inhibit the activity of tumour necrosis factor alpha (TNF-α).

Adalimumab is licensed for moderate to severe active *rheumatoid arthritis* when response to other disease-modifying antirheumatic drugs (including methotrexate) has been inadequate (see also NICE guidance October 2007, p. 735 and August 2010, p. 735); it is also licensed for severe, active, and progressive disease in adults not previously treated with methotrexate. In the treatment of rheumatoid arthritis, adalimumab should be used in combination with methotrexate, but it can be given alone if methotrexate is inappropriate. Adalimumab is also licensed for the treatment of active and progressive *psoriatic arthritis* (see also NICE guidance, p. 736) and severe active *ankylosing spondylitis* (see also NICE guidance, p. 735) that have not responded adequately to other disease-modifying antirheumatic drugs. It is also licensed for the treatment of severe axial spondyloarthritis without radiographic evidence of ankylosing spondylitis but with objective signs of inflammation, in patients who have had an inadequate response to, or are intolerant of NSAIDs. For the role of adalimumab in inflammatory bowel disease, see section 1.5.3. For the role of adalimumab in plaque psoriasis, see section 13.5.3. For the role of adalimumab in juvenile idiopathic arthritis see *BNF for Children*.

Certolizumab pegol is licensed for use in patients with moderate to severe active *rheumatoid arthritis* when response to disease-modifying antirheumatic drugs (including methotrexate) has been inadequate (see also NICE guidance, below). Certolizumab pegol can be used in combination with methotrexate, or as a monotherapy if methotrexate is not tolerated or is contra-indicated. Certolizumab pegol is also licensed for the treatment of severe active *ankylosing spondylitis* in patients who have had an inadequate response to, or are intolerant of NSAIDs. It is also licensed for the treatment of severe active *axial spondyloarthritis*, without radiographic evidence of ankylosing spondylitis but with objective signs of inflammation, in patients who have had an inadequate response to, or are intolerant of NSAIDs.

10

Musculoskeletal and joint diseases

Musculoskeletal and joint diseases

10

Etanercept is licensed for the treatment of moderate to
severe active *rheumatoid arthritis* either alone or in
combination with methotrexate when the response to
other disease-modifying antirheumatic drugs is inadequate and in severe, active and progressive *rheumatoid
arthritis* in patients not previously treated with methotrexate (see also NICE guidance October 2007, p. 735
and August 2010, p. 735). It is also licensed for the
treatment of active and progressive *psoriatic arthritis*
inadequately responsive to other disease-modifying
antirheumatic drugs (see also NICE guidance, p. 736),
and for severe *ankylosing spondylitis* inadequately
responsive to conventional therapy (see also NICE
guidance, p. 735). For the role of etanercept in juvenile
idiopathic arthritis see *BNF for Children*. For the role of
etanercept in plaque psoriasis, see section 13.5.3.

Golimumab is licensed in combination with methotrexate for the treatment of moderate to severe active
rheumatoid arthritis when response to disease-modifying
antirheumatic drug (DMARD) therapy (including
methotrexate) has been inadequate (see also NICE
guidance below); it is also licensed in combination
with methotrexate for patients with severe, active, and
progressive rheumatoid arthritis not previously treated
with methotrexate. Golimumab is also licensed for the
treatment of active and progressive *psoriatic arthritis*, as
monotherapy or in combination with methotrexate,
when response to DMARD therapy has been inadequate
(see also NICE guidance below); it is also licensed for
the treatment of severe active *ankylosing spondylitis*
when there is an inadequate response to conventional
treatment (see also NICE guidance below).

The *Scottish Medicines Consortium* (p. 4) has advised
(June 2012) that golimumab (*Simponi*®) is accepted for
restricted use within NHS Scotland at a dose of 50 mg,
alone or in combination with methotrexate, for the
treatment of active and progressive psoriatic arthritis
in adults whose disease has not responded to adequate
trials of at least two standard DMARDs, administered
either individually or in combination.

Infliximab is licensed for the treatment of active *rheumatoid arthritis* in combination with methotrexate when
the response to other disease-modifying antirheumatic
drugs, including methotrexate, is inadequate (see also
NICE guidance October 2007, p. 735 and August 2010,

below); it is also licensed in combination with methotrexate for patients not previously treated with methotrexate or other DMARDs who have severe, active, and progressive rheumatoid arthritis. Infliximab is also licensed for the treatment of *ankylosing spondylitis*, in patients with severe axial symptoms who have not responded adequately to conventional therapy (but see also NICE guidance, below) and in combination with methotrexate (or alone if methotrexate is not tolerated or is contra-indicated) for the treatment of active and progressive *psoriatic arthritis* which has not responded adequately to disease-modifying antirheumatic drugs (see also NICE guidance, p. 736).

Rituximab is licensed in combination with methotrexate for the treatment of severe active *rheumatoid arthritis* in patients whose condition has not responded adequately to other disease-modifying antirheumatic drugs (including one or more tumour necrosis factor inhibitors) or who are intolerant of them (see also NICE guidance, below). For the role of rituximab in malignant disease, see section 8.2.3.

> ### NICE guidance
> **Adalimumab, etanercept, and infliximab for the treatment of rheumatoid arthritis (October 2007)**
>
> The tumour necrosis factor alpha (TNF-α) inhibitors adalimumab, etanercept, and infliximab are options for the treatment of adults with active rheumatoid arthritis who have failed to respond to at least 2 disease-modifying antirheumatic drugs (DMARDs), including methotrexate (unless contra-indicated). TNF-α inhibitors should be given in combination with methotrexate; however, when methotrexate cannot be used because of intolerance or contra-indications, adalimumab or etanercept can be given as monotherapy.
>
> Adalimumab, etanercept, and infliximab should be withdrawn if response is not adequate within 6 months. Response to treatment should be monitored at least every 6 months in patients who respond initially; treatment should be withdrawn if response is not maintained. An alternative TNF-α inhibitor may be considered for patients in whom treatment is withdrawn because of intolerance before the initial 6-month assessment of efficacy.
>
> Use of TNF-α inhibitors for the treatment of severe, active, and progressive rheumatoid arthritis in adults not previously treated with methotrexate or other DMARDs is not recommended.
> www.nice.org.uk/TA130

> ### NICE guidance
> **Adalimumab, etanercept, infliximab, rituximab, and abatacept for the treatment of rheumatoid arthritis after the failure of a TNF inhibitor (August 2010)**
>
> Rituximab, in combination with methotrexate, is an option for the treatment of severe active rheumatoid arthritis in adults who have had an inadequate response to, or are intolerant of, other disease-modifying antirheumatic drugs (DMARDs), including at least 1 tumour necrosis factor (TNF) inhibitor. Repeat courses of rituximab should be given no more frequently than every 6 months, and should only be continued if an adequate response is achieved and maintained.
>
> Adalimumab, etanercept, infliximab, or abatacept, in combination with methotrexate, are options for the treatment of severe active rheumatoid arthritis in adults who have had an inadequate response to, or have an intolerance of, other DMARDs including at least 1 TNF inhibitor, and who cannot use rituximab because of contra-indications or intolerance. In patients who cannot use methotrexate because of intolerance or contra-indications, adalimumab or etanercept can be given as monotherapy. Treatment should be continued only if there is adequate response. Patients should be monitored at least every 6 months.
> www.nice.org.uk/TA195

> ### NICE guidance
> **Adalimumab, etanercept, and infliximab for the treatment of ankylosing spondylitis (May 2008)**
>
> Adalimumab or etanercept are treatment options for adults with severe active ankylosing spondylitis whose disease satisfies specific criteria for diagnosis where there is confirmation of sustained active spinal disease, and where treatment with two or more NSAIDs taken sequentially at maximum tolerated or recommended doses for 4 weeks has failed to control symptoms.
>
> Response to adalimumab or etanercept treatment should be assessed at 12-week intervals and continued only if response is adequate. If response to treatment is not maintained, a repeat assessment should be made after a further 6 weeks and treatment discontinued if there is an inadequate response. Patients who are intolerant of adalimumab or etanercept during the initial 12 weeks may receive the alternative TNF-α inhibitor (adalimumab or etanercept). However an alternative TNF-α inhibitor is not recommended in patients who fail to respond initially or fail to maintain an adequate response.
>
> Infliximab is not recommended for the treatment of ankylosing spondylitis. Patients who are already receiving infliximab for the treatment of ankylosing spondylitis can continue treatment until they and their specialist consider it appropriate to stop.
>
> See full NICE guidance for specific criteria to diagnose severe active ankylosing spondylitis, confirm sustained active spinal disease, and assess response to treatment.
> www.nice.org.uk/TA143

10 Musculoskeletal and joint diseases

NICE guidance
Etanercept, infliximab, and adalimumab for the treatment of psoriatic arthritis (August 2010)

Etanercept, infliximab, or adalimumab are recommended for the treatment of active and progressive psoriatic arthritis in adults who have peripheral arthritis with at least 3 tender joints and at least 3 swollen joints, and who have not responded adequately to at least 2 standard disease-modifying antirheumatic drugs (used alone or in combination).

Etanercept, infliximab, and adalimumab should be discontinued if there is an inadequate response at 12 weeks.
www.nice.org.uk/TA199

Side-effects Adalimumab, certolizumab pegol, etanercept, golimumab, infliximab, and rituximab have been associated with infections, sometimes severe, including tuberculosis, septicaemia, and hepatitis B reactivation. Other side-effects include nausea, abdominal pain, worsening heart failure, hypersensitivity reactions, fever, headache, depression, antibody formation (including lupus erythematosus-like syndrome), pruritus, injection-site reactions, and blood disorders (including anaemia, leucopenia, thrombocytopenia, pancytopenia, and aplastic anaemia).

Abatacept prevents the full activation of T-lymphocytes. It is licensed for moderate to severe active *rheumatoid arthritis* in combination with methotrexate, in patients unresponsive to other disease-modifying antirheumatic drugs (including methotrexate or a tumour necrosis factor (TNF) inhibitor); see also NICE guidance (August 2010), p. 735 and (April 2013), below. For the role of abatacept in juvenile idiopathic arthritis see *BNF for Children*. Abatacept is not recommended for use in combination with TNF inhibitors.

The *Scottish Medicines Consortium* (p. 4) has advised (July 2013) that abatacept (*Orencia®*) is accepted for restricted use within NHS Scotland for adults with severe active rheumatoid arthritis, confirmed on at least two occasions, one month apart. This advice is contingent upon continuing availability of abatacept at the price agreed in the patient access scheme.

NICE guidance
Abatacept for the treatment of rheumatoid arthritis after the failure of conventional disease-modifying antirheumatic drugs (April 2013)

Abatacept, in combination with methotrexate, is an option for the treatment of highly active rheumatoid arthritis in adults who have had an inadequate response to at least two conventional disease-modifying antirheumatic drugs, including methotrexate, if:

- abatacept is used as described in the NICE guidance (October 2007) for other tumour necrosis factor (TNF) inhibitors (see Adalimumab, etanercept, and infliximab for the treatment of rheumatoid arthritis, *and*
- the manufacturer provides abatacept with the discount agreed in the patient access scheme

Patients already receiving abatacept for this indication, who do not fulfil the critera for treatment should continue treatment until they and their specialist consider it appropriate to stop.
www.nice.org.uk/TA280

Anakinra inhibits the activity of interleukin-1. Anakinra (in combination with methotrexate) is licensed for the treatment of *rheumatoid arthritis* which has not responded to methotrexate alone; it is not, however, recommended for routine management of *rheumatoid arthritis*, see NICE guidance below.

The *Scottish Medicines Consortium* (p. 4) has advised (July 2002) that anakinra is **not** recommended for the treatment of rheumatoid arthritis within NHS Scotland.

NICE guidance
Anakinra for the treatment of rheumatoid arthritis (February 2009)

Anakinra is **not** recommended for the treatment of rheumatoid arthritis except when used in a controlled long-term clinical study. Patients who are already receiving anakinra for rheumatoid arthritis should continue treatment until they and their specialist consider it appropriate to stop.

Belimumab inhibits the activity of B-lymphocyte stimulator. Belimumab is licensed as adjunctive therapy in patients with active, autoantibody-positive systemic lupus erythematosus with a high degree of disease activity despite standard therapy. Infusion-related side-effects are reported commonly with belimumab, including severe or life-threatening hypersensitivity and infusion reactions. These occur predominantly during the first 2 infusions. Delay in the onset of acute hypersensitivity reactions has been observed; patients should remain under clinical supervision for several hours following at least the first 2 infusions. Premedication with an antihistamine, with or without an antipyretic, may be considered.

Tocilizumab antagonises the actions of interleukin-6. Tocilizumab is licensed for use in patients with moderate to severe active *rheumatoid arthritis* when response to at least one disease-modifying antirheumatic drug or tumour necrosis factor inhibitor has been inadequate, or in those who are intolerant of these drugs. Tocilizumab can be used in combination with methotrexate, or as monotherapy if methotrexate is not tolerated or is contra-indicated (see also NICE guidance below). For the role of tocilizumab in juvenile idiopathic arthritis see *BNF for Children*.

The *Scottish Medicines Consortium* (p. 4) has advised (August 2012) that tocilizumab (*RoActemra*®) is accepted for restricted use within NHS Scotland as monotherapy in patients who are intolerant to methotrexate or where continued treatment with methotrexate is inappropriate, for the treatment of moderate to severe active rheumatoid arthritis in adults who have either responded inadequately to, or who were intolerant to, previous therapy with one or more disease-modifying anti-rheumatic drugs or tumour necrosis factor inhibitors, in accordance with the British Society for Rheumatology guidance on prescribing TNF-α blockers in adults with rheumatoid arthritis (2005).

NICE guidance
Tocilizumab for the treatment of rheumatoid arthritis (February 2012)

Tocilizumab, in combination with methotrexate, is recommended as an option for the treatment of rheumatoid arthritis in adults if:

- the disease has responded inadequately to disease-modifying anti-rheumatic drugs (DMARDs) and is used as described for tumour necrosis factor (TNF) inhibitor treatments (specifically the recommendations on disease activity and treatment) in the NICE guidance (October 2007) Adalimumab, etanercept and infliximab for the treatment of rheumatoid arthritis, p. 735 *or*

- the disease has responded inadequately to DMARDs and a TNF inhibitor and the patient cannot receive rituximab because of contra-indications or intolerance, **and** tocilizumab is used as described for TNF inhibitor treatments (specifically the recommendations on disease activity) in the NICE guidance (August 2010) Adalimumab, etanercept, infliximab, rituximab and abatacept for the treatment of rheumatoid arthritis after the failure of a TNF inhibitor, p. 735 *or*

- the disease has responded inadequately to one or more TNF inhibitor treatments and to rituximab

- **and** the manufacturer provides tocilizumab with the discount agreed as part of the patient access scheme.

Patients currently receiving tocilizumab for the treatment of rheumatoid arthritis who do not meet these criteria should have the option to continue treatment until they and their clinicians consider it appropriate to stop.

www.nice.org.uk/TA247

Ustekinumab inhibits the activity of interleukins 12 and 23. It is licensed for the treatment of active *psoriatic arthritis* (in combination with methotrexate or alone) in patients who have had an inadequate response to one or more disease-modifying antirheumatic drugs.

The *Scottish Medicines Consortium* (p. 4) has advised (February 2014) that ustekinumab (*Stelara*®) is accepted for restricted use within NHS Scotland either alone or in combination with methotrexate, for the treatment of active psoriatic arthritis in adults who have responded inadequately to previous therapy with a non-biological disease-modifying anti-rheumatic drug, and failed on, or are unsuitable for, treatment with a TNF inhibitor.

◢ ABATACEPT

Indications see under Cytokine Modulators, above

Cautions predisposition to infection (screen for latent tuberculosis and viral hepatitis); do not initiate until active infections are controlled; children should be

brought up to date with current immunisation schedule (section 14.1) before initiating therapy; progressive multifocal leucoencephalopathy—discontinue treatment if neurological symptoms present; elderly (increased risk of side-effects); **interactions:** Appendix 1 (abatacept)

Contra-indications severe infection (see also Cautions)

Pregnancy manufacturer advises avoid unless essential—effective contraception required during treatment and for 14 weeks after last dose

Breast-feeding present in milk in *animal* studies—manufacturer advises avoid breast-feeding during treatment and for 14 weeks after last dose

Side-effects abdominal pain, diarrhoea, dyspepsia, nausea, vomiting, stomatitis, flushing, hypertension, cough, dizziness, fatigue, headache, paraesthesia, infection, leucopenia, pain in extremities, conjunctivitis; *less commonly* gastritis, tachycardia, bradycardia, palpitation, hypotension, bronchospasm, dyspnoea, hyperhidrosis, weight gain, depression, anxiety, sleep disorder, menstrual disturbances, basal and squamous cell carcinoma, skin papilloma, thrombocytopenia, arthralgia, visual disturbance, dry eye, bruising, alopecia, dry skin, psoriasis; *also reported* lymphoma, lung cancer

Dose

- Rheumatoid arthritis (see notes above), by intravenous infusion, ADULT over 18 years, body-weight less than 60 kg, 500 mg, repeated 2 weeks and 4 weeks after initial infusion, then every 4 weeks; body-weight 60–100 kg, 750 mg repeated 2 weeks and 4 weeks after initial infusion, then every 4 weeks; body-weight over 100 kg, 1 g repeated 2 weeks and 4 weeks after initial infusion, then every 4 weeks; by subcutaneous injection (following intravenous infusion loading dose), ADULT over 18 years, 125 mg given within a day of the loading dose, then 125 mg weekly

  Note Patients who are unable to receive an infusion may initiate subcutaneous abatacept without receiving an intravenous loading dose

  Polyarticular juvenile idiopathic arthritis CHILD 6–17 years, see *BNF for Children*

  Note Review treatment if no response within 6 months

Orencia® (Bristol-Myers Squibb) ▼ PoM

Intravenous infusion, powder for reconstitution, abatacept, net price 250-mg vial = £302.40

Electrolytes Na⁺<0.5 mmol/vial

Injection, abatacept, net price 125-mg pre-filled syringe = £302.40

◢ ADALIMUMAB

Indications see under Cytokine Modulators above; inflammatory bowel disease (section 1.5.3); psoriasis (section 13.5.3)

Cautions predisposition to infection; monitor for infection before, during, and for 4 months after treatment (see also Tuberculosis below); do not initiate until active infections are controlled; discontinue if new serious infection develops; hepatitis B virus—monitor for active infection; children should be brought up to date with current immunisation schedule (section 14.1) before initiating therapy; mild heart failure (discontinue if symptoms develop or worsen—avoid in moderate or severe heart failure); demyelinating disorders (risk of exacerbation); history or development of malignancy; monitor for non-melanoma skin cancer before and during treatment, especially in patients with a history of PUVA treatment for psoriasis or extensive immunosuppressant therapy; **interactions**: Appendix 1 (adalimumab)

Tuberculosis Patients should be evaluated for tuberculosis before treatment. Active tuberculosis should be treated with standard treatment (section 5.1.9) for at least 2 months before starting adalimumab. Patients who have previously received adequate treatment for tuberculosis can start adalimumab but should be monitored every 3 months for possible recurrence. In patients without active tuberculosis but who were previously not treated adequately, chemoprophylaxis should ideally be completed before starting adalimumab. In patients at high risk of tuberculosis who cannot be assessed by tuberculin skin test, chemoprophylaxis can be given concurrently with adalimumab. Patients should be advised to seek medical attention if symptoms suggestive of tuberculosis (e.g. persistent cough, weight loss, and fever) develop

Blood disorders Patients should be advised to seek medical attention if symptoms suggestive of blood disorders (such as fever, sore throat, bruising, or bleeding) develop

Contra-indications severe infection (see also Cautions)

Pregnancy avoid; manufacturer advises effective contraception required during treatment and for at least 5 months after last dose

Breast-feeding avoid; manufacturer advises avoid for at least 5 months after last dose

Side-effects see under Cytokine Modulators (p. 736) and Cautions above; also vomiting, dyspepsia, gastro-intestinal haemorrhage, dizziness, hyperlipidaemia, hypertension, oedema, flushing, chest pain, tachycardia, cough, dyspnoea, mood changes, sleep disturbances, anxiety, paraesthesia, haematuria, renal impairment, benign tumours, skin cancer, electrolyte disturbances, hyperuricaemia, dehydration, musculoskeletal pain, eye disorders, rash, dermatitis, onycholysis, impaired healing; *less commonly* dysphagia, pancreatitis, cholelithiasis, hepatic steatosis, cholecystitis, arrhythmias, vascular occlusion, aortic aneurysm, interstitial lung disease, pneumonitis, tremor, neuropathy, erectile dysfunction, nocturia, malignancy (including solid tumours, lymphoma, and leukaemia), rhabdomyolysis, hearing loss, tinnitus; *rarely* autoimmune hepatitis, myocardial infarction, demyelinating disorders; *also reported* pulmonary embolism, pleural effusion, sarcoidosis, Stevens-Johnson syndrome, cutaneous vasculitis, new onset or worsening psoriasis

Dose
- By subcutaneous injection, rheumatoid arthritis, ADULT over 18 years, 40 mg on alternate weeks; if necessary increased to 40 mg weekly in patients receiving adalimumab alone; review treatment if no response within 12 weeks

  Psoriatic arthritis, ankylosing spondylitis, severe axial spondyloarthritis, ADULT over 18 years, 40 mg on alternate weeks; discontinue treatment if no response within 12 weeks

  Polyarticular juvenile idiopathic arthritis, CHILD 2–18 years, see *BNF for Children*

Humira® (AbbVie) [PoM]
Injection, adalimumab, net price 40-mg prefilled pen or prefilled syringe = £352.14; 40 mg/0.8-mL vial = £352.14. Label: 10, alert card, counselling, tuberculosis and blood disorders

ANAKINRA

Indications see under Cytokine Modulators above

Cautions predisposition to infection; history of asthma (risk of serious infection); **interactions**: Appendix 1 (anakinra)

Blood disorders Neutropenia reported commonly. Monitor neutrophil count before treatment, then every month for 6 months, then every 3 months—discontinue if neutropenia develops. Patients should be instructed to seek medical advice if symptoms suggestive of neutropenia (such as fever, sore throat, infection) develop

Contra-indications neutropenia

Renal impairment caution if eGFR 30–50 mL/minute/1.73 m^2; avoid if eGFR less than 30 mL/minute/1.73 m^2

Pregnancy manufacturer advises avoid; effective contraception must be used during treatment

Breast-feeding manufacturer advises avoid—no information available

Side-effects injection-site reactions; headache; infections, neutropenia (see also Cautions), and antibody formation; *also reported* malignancy

Dose
- By subcutaneous injection, ADULT over 18 years, 100 mg once daily

Kineret® (Swedish Orphan) [PoM]
Injection, anakinra, net price 100-mg prefilled syringe = £26.23. Counselling, blood disorder symptoms

BELIMUMAB

Indications see under Cytokine Modulators above

Cautions predisposition to infection; do not initiate until active infections controlled; history or development of malignancy; **interactions**: Appendix 1 (belimumab)

Renal impairment caution in severe impairment—no information available

Pregnancy avoid unless essential; manufacturer advises adequate contraception during treatment and for at least 4 months after last dose

Breast-feeding avoid—present in milk in *animal* studies

Side-effects see notes above; also diarrhoea, nausea, hypersensitivity reactions, vomiting, depression, insomnia, migraine, infections, pyrexia, leucopenia, pain in extremities

Dose
- By intravenous infusion, ADULT over 18 years, 10 mg/kg, repeated 2 weeks and 4 weeks after initial infusion, then every 4 weeks; review treatment if no response within 6 months

Benlysta® (GSK) ▼ [PoM]
Intravenous infusion, powder for reconstitution, belimumab, net price 120-mg vial = £121.50; 400-mg vial = £405.00

CERTOLIZUMAB PEGOL

Indications see under Cytokine Modulators above

Cautions predisposition to infection; monitor for infection before, during, and for 5 months after treatment (see also Tuberculosis below); do not initiate until active infections are controlled; discontinue if new serious infection develops until infection controlled; hepatitis B virus—monitor for active infection; mild heart failure (discontinue if symptoms develop or worsen—avoid in moderate to severe heart failure); demyelinating CNS disorders (risk of exacerbation); history or development of malignancy; **interactions**: Appendix 1 (certolizumab pegol)

Tuberculosis Patients should be evaluated for tuberculosis before treatment. Active tuberculosis should be treated with standard treatment (section 5.1.9) for at least 2 months before starting certolizumab pegol. Patients who have previously received adequate treatment for tuberculosis can start certolizumab pegol but should be monitored every 3 months for possible recurrence. In patients without active tuberculosis but who were previously not treated adequately, chemoprophylaxis should ideally be completed before starting certolizumab pegol. In patients at high risk of tuberculosis who cannot be assessed by tuberculin skin test, chemoprophylaxis can be given concurrently with certolizumab pegol. Patients should be advised to seek medical attention if symptoms suggestive of tuberculosis (e.g. persistent cough, weight loss, and fever) develop

Blood disorders Patients should be advised to seek medical attention if symptoms suggestive of blood disorders (such as fever, sore throat, bruising, or bleeding) develop

Contra-indications   severe active infection (see also Cautions)

Pregnancy   avoid; manufacturer advises adequate contraception during treatment and for at least 5 months after last dose

Breast-feeding   manufacturer advises use only if potential benefit outweighs risk—no information available

Side-effects   see under Cytokine Modulators (p. 736) and Cautions above; hypertension, sensory abnormalities, rash; *less commonly* ascites, cholestasis, gastrointestinal disorders (including perforation and ulcer), hepatic disorders, appetite disorders, cardiomyopathies (including heart failure), dyslipidaemia, syncope, oedema, dizziness, ischaemic coronary artery disorders, arrhythmias, asthma, pleural effusion, cough, peripheral neuropathy, tremor, anxiety, mood disorders, influenza-like illness, menstrual disorders, renal impairment, haematuria, malignancy (including solid tumours, lymphoma, and leukaemia), skin cancer, benign tumours, haemorrhage, electrolyte disorders, muscle disorders, visual disturbance, ocular inflammation, tinnitus, ecchymosis, impaired healing, alopecia, photosensitivity, acne, skin discoloration, nail disorders, new onset or worsening psoriasis, dermatitis; *rarely* cholelithiasis, splenomegaly, atrioventricular block, cerebrovascular accident, Raynaud's phenomenon, interstitial lung disease, impaired coordination, trigeminal neuralgia, seizures, thyroid disorders, sexual dysfunction, nephropathy; *also reported* multiple sclerosis

Dose

- By subcutaneous injection, rheumatoid arthritis, ADULT over 18 years, 400 mg, repeated 2 weeks and 4 weeks after initial injection, then 200 mg every 2 weeks; review treatment if no response within 12 weeks

  Severe ankylosing spondylitis, severe axial spondyloarthritis, ADULT over 18 years, 400 mg, repeated 2 weeks and 4 weeks after initial injection, then 200 mg every 2 weeks or 400 mg every 4 weeks; review treatment if no response within 12 weeks

Cimzia® (UCB Pharma) (PoM)

Injection, certolizumab pegol, net price 200-mg pre-filled syringe = £357.50. Label: 10, alert card, counselling, tuberculosis and blood disorders

---

ETANERCEPT

Indications   see under Cytokine Modulators above

Cautions   predisposition to infection (avoid if predisposition to septicaemia); significant exposure to herpes zoster virus—interrupt treatment and consider varicella-zoster immunoglobulin; hepatitis B virus—monitor for active infection; monitor for worsening hepatitis C infection; children should be brought up to date with current immunisation schedule (section 14.1) before initiating therapy; heart failure (risk of exacerbation); history or increased risk of demyelinating disorders; history or development of malignancy; monitor for skin cancer before and during treatment, particularly in those at risk (including patients with psoriasis or a history of PUVA treatment); history of blood disorders; diabetes mellitus; **interactions**: Appendix 1 (etanercept)

Tuberculosis Patients should be evaluated for tuberculosis before treatment. Active tuberculosis should be treated with standard treatment (section 5.1.9) for at least 2 months before starting etanercept. Patients who have previously received adequate treatment for tuberculosis can start etanercept but should be monitored every 3 months for possible recurrence. In patients without active tuberculosis but who were previously not treated adequately, chemoprophylaxis should ideally be completed before starting etanercept. In patients at high risk of tuberculosis who cannot be assessed by tuberculin skin test, chemoprophylaxis can be given concurrently with etanercept. Patients should be advised to seek medical attention if symptoms suggestive of tuberculosis (e.g. persistent cough, weight loss, and fever) develop

Blood disorders Patients should be advised to seek medical attention if symptoms suggestive of blood disorders (such as fever, sore throat, bruising, or bleeding) develop

Contra-indications   active infection; avoid injections containing benzyl alcohol in neonates (see preparations below)

Hepatic impairment   use with caution in moderate to severe alcoholic hepatitis

Pregnancy   avoid—limited information available; manufacturer advises effective contraception required during treatment and for 3 weeks after last dose

Breast-feeding   manufacturer advises avoid—present in milk in *animal* studies

Side-effects   see under Cytokine Modulators (p. 736); also *less commonly* interstitial lung disease, skin cancer, uveitis, rash, new onset or worsening psoriasis; *rarely* demyelinating disorders, seizures, lymphoma, Stevens-Johnson syndrome, vasculitis; *very rarely* toxic epidermal necrolysis; *also reported* appendicitis, gastritis, oesophagitis, inflammatory bowel disease, vomiting, diabetes mellitus, malignancy (including solid tumours and leukaemia), macrophage activation syndrome, and cutaneous ulcer

Dose

- By subcutaneous injection, rheumatoid arthritis, psoriatic arthritis, ankylosing spondylitis, ADULT over 18 years, 25 mg twice weekly or 50 mg once weekly

  Juvenile idiopathic arthritis, CHILD 2–17 years, see *BNF for Children*

Enbrel® (Pfizer) (PoM)

Injection, powder for reconstitution, etanercept, net price 25-mg vial (with solvent) = £89.38. Label: 10, alert card, counselling, tuberculosis and blood disorders

Paediatric injection, powder for reconstitution, etanercept, net price 10-mg vial (with solvent) = £35.75; 25-mg vial (with solvent) = £89.38. Label:

10, alert card, counselling, tuberculosis and blood disorders

Excipients include benzyl alcohol (avoid in neonates, see Excipients, p. 2)

Injection, etanercept, net price 25-mg prefilled syringe = £89.38; 50-mg prefilled pen or prefilled syringe = £178.75. Label: 10, alert card, counselling, tuberculosis and blood disorders

GOLIMUMAB

Indications see under Cytokine Modulators above; ulcerative colitis (section 1.5.3)

Cautions predisposition to infection; monitor for infection before, during, and for 5 months after treatment (see also Tuberculosis below); do not initiate until active infections are controlled; discontinue if new serious infection develops until infection controlled; hepatitis B virus—monitor for active infection; mild heart failure (discontinue if symptoms develop or worsen); demyelinating disorders (risk of exacerbation); history or development of malignancy; **interactions**: Appendix 1 (golimumab)

Tuberculosis Patients should be evaluated for tuberculosis before treatment. Active tuberculosis should be treated with standard treatment (section 5.1.9) for at least 2 months before starting golimumab. Patients who have previously received adequate treatment for tuberculosis can start golimumab but should be monitored every 3 months for possible recurrence. In patients without active tuberculosis but who were previously not treated adequately, chemoprophylaxis should ideally be completed before starting golimumab. In patients at high risk of tuberculosis who cannot be assessed by tuberculin skin test, chemoprophylaxis can be given concurrently with golimumab. Patients who have tested negative for latent tuberculosis, and those who are receiving or who have completed treatment for latent tuberculosis, should be monitored closely for symptoms of active infection. All patients should be advised to seek medical attention if symptoms suggestive of tuberculosis (e.g. persistent cough, weight loss, and fever) develop

Blood disorders Patients should be advised to seek medical attention if symptoms suggestive of blood disorders (such as fever, sore throat, bruising, or bleeding) develop

Contra-indications severe active infection (see also Cautions); moderate or severe heart failure

Hepatic impairment manufacturer advises caution—no information available

Pregnancy use only if essential; manufacturer advises adequate contraception during treatment and for at least 6 months after last dose

Breast-feeding manufacturer advises avoid during and for at least 6 months after treatment—present in milk in *animal* studies

Side-effects see under Cytokine Modulators (p. 736) and under Cautions above; also dyspepsia, hypertension, dizziness, asthenia; *less commonly* constipation, taste disturbance, gastritis, colitis, stomatitis, gastro-oesophageal reflux disease, cholelithiasis, hepatic disorders, hyperlipidaemia, arrhythmia, ischaemic coronary artery disease, Raynaud's syndrome, heart failure, thrombosis, flushing, bronchospasm, interstitial lung disease, demyelinating disorders, insomnia, paraesthesia, hyperglycaemia, thyroid disorders, menstrual disorders, malignancy (including lymphoma, melanoma), bone fractures, visual disturbance, eye irritation, new onset or worsening psoriasis, alopecia, dermatitis; *rarely* impaired wound healing

Dose
- By subcutaneous injection, ADULT over 18 years, 50 mg once a month on the same date each month, review treatment if no response after 3–4 doses; body-weight over 100 kg, if inadequate response to 3–4 doses of 50 mg once a month, dose can be increased to 100 mg once a month, review treatment if inadequate response to this higher dose after 3–4 doses

Note If dose administered more than 2 weeks late, subsequent doses should be administered on the new monthly due date

Simponi® (MSD) ▼PoM
Injection, golimumab, net price 50-mg prefilled pen or prefilled syringe = £762.97; 100-mg prefilled pen = £1525.94. Label: 10, alert card, counselling, tuberculosis and blood disorders

INFLIXIMAB

Indications see under Cytokine Modulators above; inflammatory bowel disease (section 1.5.3); psoriasis (section 13.5.3)

Cautions predisposition to infection; monitor for infection before, during, and for 6 months after treatment (see also Tuberculosis below); discontinue if new serious infection develops; hepatitis B virus—monitor for active infection; mild heart failure (discontinue if symptoms develop or worsen); demyelinating disorders (risk of exacerbation); history or development of malignancy; history of prolonged immunosuppressant or PUVA treatment in patients with psoriasis; **interactions**: Appendix 1 (infliximab)

Tuberculosis Patients should be evaluated for tuberculosis before treatment. Active tuberculosis should be treated with standard treatment (section 5.1.9) for at least 2 months before starting infliximab. Patients who have previously received adequate treatment for tuberculosis can start infliximab but should be monitored every 3 months for possible recurrence. In patients without active tuberculosis but who were previously not treated adequately, chemoprophylaxis should ideally be completed before starting infliximab. In patients at high risk of tuberculosis who cannot be assessed by tuberculin skin test, chemoprophylaxis can be given concurrently with infliximab. Patients should be advised to seek medical attention if symptoms suggestive of tuberculosis (e.g. persistent cough, weight loss, and fever) develop

Blood disorders Patients should be advised to seek medical attention if symptoms suggestive of blood disorders (such as fever, sore throat, bruising, or bleeding) develop

Hypersensitivity reactions Hypersensitivity reactions (including fever, chest pain, hypotension, hypertension, dyspnoea, transient visual loss, pruritus, urticaria, serum sickness-like reactions, angioedema, anaphylaxis) reported during or within 1–2 hours after infusion (risk greatest during first or second infusion or in patients who discontinue other immunosuppressants). All patients should be observed carefully for 1–2 hours after infusion and resuscitation equipment should be available for immediate use. Prophylactic antipyretics, antihistamines, or hydrocortisone may be administered. Monitor for symptoms of delayed hypersensitivity if readministered after a prolonged period. Patients should be advised to keep Alert card with them at all times and seek medical advice if symptoms of delayed hypersensitivity develop

Contra-indications severe infections (see also under Cautions); moderate or severe heart failure

Pregnancy use only if essential; manufacturer advises adequate contraception during and for at least 6 months after last dose

Breast-feeding amount probably too small to be harmful

Side-effects see under Cytokine Modulators (p. 736) and under Cautions above; also constipation, diarrhoea, dyspepsia, gastro-intestinal haemorrhage, gastro-oesophageal reflux, flushing, hypotension, hypertension, palpitation, tachycardia, sleep disturbances, dizziness, paraesthesia, hypoaesthesia, arthralgia, myalgia, epistaxis, alopecia, rash, ecchymosis, hyperhydrosis, new onset or worsening psoriasis, dry skin; *less commonly* hepatitis, cholecystitis, intestinal perforation, pancreatitis, heart failure, arrhythmia, bradycardia, syncope, peripheral ischaemia, pleurisy, pulmonary oedema, amnesia, agitation, confusion, nervousness, neuropathy, seizures, vaginitis, eye disorders, bullous eruption, cheilitis, seborrhoea, impaired healing, rosacea, hyperkeratosis, abnormal skin pigmentation; *rarely* pericardial effusion, vasospasm, interstitial lung disease, leukaemia, lymphoma, demyelinating disorders, Stevens-Johnson syndrome, toxic epidermal necrolysis; *also reported* hepatic failure

Dose

- By intravenous infusion, rheumatoid arthritis (in combination with methotrexate), ADULT over 18 years, 3 mg/kg, repeated 2 weeks and 6 weeks after initial infusion, then every 8 weeks; if response inadequate after 12 weeks, dose may be increased in steps of 1.5 mg/kg every 8 weeks, up to max. 7.5 mg/kg every 8 weeks; alternatively, 3 mg/kg may be given every 4 weeks; discontinue if no response by 12 weeks of initial infusion or after dose adjustment
  Ankylosing spondylitis, ADULT over 18 years, 5 mg/kg, repeated 2 weeks and 6 weeks after initial infusion, then every 6–8 weeks; discontinue if no response by 6 weeks of initial infusion
  Psoriatic arthritis (in combination with methotrexate), ADULT over 18 years, 5 mg/kg, repeated 2 weeks and 6 weeks after initial infusion, then every 8 weeks

Remicade® (MSD) ▭PoM▭
Intravenous infusion, powder for reconstitution, infliximab, net price 100-mg vial = £419.62. Label: 10, alert card, counselling, tuberculosis, blood disorders, and hypersensitivity reactions

▍RITUXIMAB

Indications   see under Cytokine Modulators above; malignant disease (section 8.2.3)

Cautions   section 8.2.3, p. 636; predisposition to infection
  Alert card Patients with rheumatoid arthritis should be provided with the patient alert card before administration

Contra-indications   section 8.2.3, p. 636; severe infection

Pregnancy   section 8.2.3, p. 638

Breast-feeding   section 8.2.3, p. 638

Side-effects   section 8.2.3, p. 636 and under Cytokine Modulators (p. 736); *also* dyspepsia; hypertension, hypotension; rhinitis, sore throat; asthenia, paraesthesia, migraine; arthralgia, muscle spasm; urticaria

Dose

- By intravenous infusion, ADULT, rheumatoid arthritis (in combination with methotrexate), 1 g, repeated 2 weeks after initial infusion
  Important Patients should receive premedication before each infusion (consult product literature for details) and be provided with a patient alert card

◢**Preparations**
Section 8.2.3

▍TOCILIZUMAB

Indications   see under Cytokine Modulators above

Cautions   predisposition to infection or history of recurrent or chronic infection; interrupt treatment if serious infection occurs; history of intestinal ulceration or diverticulitis; monitor hepatic transaminases every 4–8 weeks for first 6 months, then every 12 weeks; monitor neutrophil and platelet counts 4–8 weeks after starting treatment and then as indicated; low platelet or absolute neutrophil count (discontinue if absolute neutrophil count less than 0.5×10^9/litre or platelet count less than 50×10^3/microlitre); monitor lipid profile 4–8 weeks after starting treatment and then as indicated; monitor for demyelinating disorders; **interactions**: Appendix 1 (tocilizumab)
  Tuberculosis Patients should be evaluated for tuberculosis before treatment. Patients with latent tuberculosis should be treated with standard therapy (section 5.1.9) before starting tocilizumab

  Counselling Patients should be advised to seek immediate medical attention if symptoms of infection occur, or if symptoms of diverticular perforation such as abdominal pain, haemorrhage, or fever accompanying change in bowel habits occur

Contra-indications   severe active infection (see also Cautions); do not initiate if absolute neutrophil count less than 2×10^9/litre (see also Cautions)

Hepatic impairment   manufacturer advises caution (see also Dose below)

Renal impairment   manufacturer advises monitor renal function closely in moderate or severe impairment

Pregnancy   manufacturer advises avoid unless essential (toxicity in *animal* studies); effective contraception required during and for 3 months after treatment

Breast-feeding   manufacturer advises use only if potential benefit outweighs risk —no information available

Side-effects   abdominal pain, mouth ulceration, gastritis, raised hepatic transaminases; dizziness, peripheral oedema, hypertension, hypercholesterolaemia; headache; infection (including upper respiratory-tract infection); antibody formation, hypersensitivity, leucopenia, neutropenia; rash, pruritus; *less commonly* gastric ulcer, gastro-intestinal perforation, hypertriglyceridaemia, hypothyroidism, nephrolithiasis, infusion related reactions, anaphylaxis, and thrombocytopenia also reported

Dose

- Rheumatoid arthritis, by intravenous infusion, ADULT over 18 years, 8 mg/kg (max. 800 mg) once every 4 weeks; for details of dose adjustment in patients with liver enzyme abnormalities, or low absolute neutrophil or platelet count, consult product literature
- Juvenile idiopathic arthritis, CHILD 2–18 years, see *BNF for Children*

RoActemra® (Roche) ▭PoM▭
Concentrate for intravenous infusion, tocilizumab 20 mg/mL, net price 4 mL (80-mg) vial = £102.40, 10 mL (200-mg) vial = £256.00, 20 mL (400-mg) vial = £512.00. Alert card, counselling, see above

▍USTEKINUMAB

Indications   see under Cytokine Modulators above; plaque psoriasis (section 13.5.3)

Cautions   section 13.5.3, p. 819
  Important See section 13.5.3, p. 819 for information on tuberculosis

Contra-indications section 13.5.3, p. 819
Pregnancy section 13.5.3, p. 819
Breast-feeding section 13.5.3, p. 819
Side-effects section 13.5.3, p. 819
Dose
- By subcutaneous injection, ADULT over 18 years, body-weight under 100 kg, initially 45 mg, then 45 mg 4 weeks after initial dose, then 45 mg every 12 weeks; body-weight over 100 kg, initially 45–90 mg, then 45–90 mg 4 weeks after initial dose, then 45–90 mg every 12 weeks
  Note Review treatment if no response within 28 weeks

◢**Preparations**
Section 13.5.3

Sulfasalazine

Sulfasalazine has a beneficial effect in suppressing the inflammatory activity of rheumatoid arthritis. Sulfasalazine may also be used by specialists, in the management of psoriatic arthritis affecting peripheral joints [unlicensed indication]. Side-effects include rashes, gastrointestinal intolerance and, especially in patients with rheumatoid arthritis, occasional leucopenia, neutropenia, and thrombocytopenia. These haematological abnormalities occur usually in the first 3 to 6 months of treatment and are reversible on cessation of treatment. Close monitoring of full blood counts (including differential white cell count and platelet count) is necessary initially, and at monthly intervals during the first 3 months (liver function tests also being performed at monthly intervals for the first 3 months). Although the manufacturer recommends renal function tests, evidence of practical value is unsatisfactory.

◢ **SULFASALAZINE**
    (Sulphasalazine)

Indications active rheumatoid arthritis; inflammatory bowel disease, see section 1.5.1 and notes above
Cautions see section 1.5.1 and notes above
  Blood disorders Patients should be advised to report any unexplained bleeding, bruising, purpura, sore throat, fever or malaise. A blood count should be performed and the drug stopped immediately if there is suspicion of a blood dyscrasia.
Contra-indications see section 1.5.1 and notes above
Hepatic impairment section 1.5.1
Renal impairment section 1.5.1
Pregnancy section 1.5.1
Breast-feeding section 1.5.1
Side-effects see section 1.5.1 and notes above
Dose
- By mouth, administered on expert advice, as enteric-coated tablets, initially 500 mg daily, increased by 500 mg at intervals of 1 week to a max. of 2–3 g daily in divided doses

Sulfasalazine (Non-proprietary) ℗ⓄⓂ
Tablets, e/c, sulfasalazine 500 mg, net price 112-tab pack = £12.64 Label: 5, 14, 25, counselling, blood disorder symptoms (see recommendation above), contact lenses may be stained
Brands include *Sulazine EC*®

Salazopyrin EN-Tabs® (Pharmacia) ℗ⓄⓂ
Tablets, e/c, yellow, f/c, sulfasalazine 500 mg, net price 112-tab pack = £8.43. Label: 5, 14, 25, counselling, blood disorder symptoms (see recommendation above), contact lenses may be stained

10.1.4 Gout and cytotoxic-induced hyperuricaemia

It is important to distinguish drugs used for the treatment of acute attacks of gout from those used in the long-term control of the disease. The latter exacerbate and prolong the acute manifestations if started during an attack.

Acute attacks of gout

Acute attacks of gout are usually treated with high doses of **NSAIDs** such as diclofenac, etoricoxib, indometacin, ketoprofen, naproxen, or sulindac (section 10.1.1). **Colchicine** is an alternative in patients in whom NSAIDs are contra-indicated. Aspirin is *not* indicated in gout. Allopurinol, febuxostat, and uricosurics are not effective in treating an acute attack and may prolong it indefinitely if started during the acute episode.

The use of colchicine is limited by the development of toxicity at higher doses, but it is of value in patients with heart failure since, unlike NSAIDs, it does not induce fluid retention; moreover, it can be given to patients receiving anticoagulants.

Oral or parenteral **corticosteroids** are an effective alternative in those who cannot tolerate NSAIDs or who are resistant to other treatments. Intra-articular injection of a corticosteroid can be used in acute monoarticular gout [unlicensed indication]. A corticosteroid by intramuscular injection can be effective in podagra.

Canakinumab, a recombinant monoclonal antibody, can be used for the symptomatic treatment of frequent gouty arthritis attacks (at least 3 in the previous 12 months). It is licensed for use in patients whose condition has not responded adequately to treatment with NSAIDs or colchicine, or who are intolerant of them.

◢ **COLCHICINE**

Indications acute gout; short-term prophylaxis during initial therapy with allopurinol and uricosuric drugs; prophylaxis of familial Mediterranean fever (recurrent polyserositis)
Cautions see notes above; also elderly; gastro-intestinal disease; cardiac disease; **interactions**: Appendix 1 (colchicine)
Contra-indications blood disorders
Hepatic impairment use with caution
Renal impairment reduce dose or increase dosage interval if eGFR 10–50 mL/minute/1.73 m^2; avoid if eGFR less than 10 mL/minute/1.73 m^2
Pregnancy avoid—teratogenicity in *animal* studies
Breast-feeding present in milk but no adverse effects reported; manufacturers advise caution
Side-effects nausea, vomiting, and abdominal pain; excessive doses may cause profuse diarrhoea, gastrointestinal haemorrhage, rash, renal and hepatic damage; *rarely* peripheral neuritis, inhibition of spermatogenesis, myopathy, alopecia, and with prolonged treatment blood disorders

Dose
- Acute gout, 500 micrograms 2–4 times daily until symptoms relieved, max. 6 mg per course; course not to be repeated within 3 days
- Prevention of gout attacks during initial treatment with allopurinol or uricosuric drugs, 500 micrograms twice daily
- Prophylaxis of familial Mediterranean fever [unlicensed], 0.5–2 mg once daily

Note BNF doses may differ from those in the product literature

Colchicine (Non-proprietary) PoM
Tablets, colchicine 500 micrograms, net price 100 = £33.35

■ CANAKINUMAB

Indications   acute gout; malignant disease (section 8.2.4)
Cautions   section 8.2.4
Contra-indications   section 8.2.4
Hepatic impairment   section 8.2.4
Renal impairment   section 8.2.4
Pregnancy   section 8.2.4
Breast-feeding   section 8.2.4
Side-effects   section 8.2.4
Dose
- By subcutaneous injection, ADULT over 18 years, 150 mg as a single dose; may be repeated at least 12 weeks after initial response if symptoms recur

  Note Patients who do not respond to initial dose should not be retreated

◢**Preparations**
Section 8.2.4

Long-term control of gout

Frequent recurrence of acute attacks of gout, the presence of tophi, or signs of chronic gouty arthritis may call for the initiation of long-term ('interval') treatment. For long-term control of gout the formation of uric acid from purines may be reduced with the xanthine-oxidase inhibitors allopurinol or febuxostat; alternatively the uricosuric drug sulfinpyrazone may be used to increase the excretion of uric acid in the urine. Treatment should be continued indefinitely to prevent further attacks of gout by correcting the hyperuricaemia. These drugs should never be started during an acute attack; they are usually started 1–2 weeks after the attack has settled. The initiation of treatment may precipitate an acute attack, and therefore an anti-inflammatory analgesic or colchicine should be used as a prophylactic and continued for at least one month after the hyperuricaemia has been corrected. However, if an acute attack develops during treatment, then the treatment should continue at the same dosage and the acute attack treated in its own right.

Allopurinol is widely used and is especially useful in patients with renal impairment or urate stones when uricosuric drugs cannot be used; it is *not* indicated for the treatment of asymptomatic hyperuricaemia. It can cause rashes.

Febuxostat is licensed for the treatment of chronic hyperuricaemia where urate deposition has already occurred; it is *not* indicated for patients in whom the rate of urate formation is greatly increased, such as in malignant disease or in Lesch-Nyhan syndrome.

NICE guidance[1]
Febuxostat for the management of hyperuricaemia in patients with gout (December 2008)

Febuxostat is recommended as an option for the management of chronic hyperuricaemia in gout only for patients who are intolerant of allopurinol or for whom allopurinol is contra-indicated.

For the purposes of this guidance, intolerance of allopurinol is defined as adverse effects that are sufficiently severe to warrant discontinuation, or to prevent full dose escalation for optimal effectiveness.

www.nice.org.uk/TA164

Sulfinpyrazone can be used instead of allopurinol, or in conjunction with it in cases that are resistant to treatment.

Benzbromarone (available from 'special-order' manufacturers or specialist importing companies, see p. 1124) is a uricosuric drug that can be used in patients with mild renal impairment.

Crystallisation of urate in the urine can occur with the uricosuric drugs and it is important to ensure an adequate urine output especially in the first few weeks of treatment. As an additional precaution the urine may be rendered alkaline.

Aspirin and other salicylates antagonise the uricosuric drugs; they do not antagonise allopurinol but are nevertheless *not* indicated in gout.

■ ALLOPURINOL

Indications   prophylaxis of gout and of uric acid and calcium oxalate renal stones; prophylaxis of hyperuricaemia associated with cancer chemotherapy
Cautions   administer prophylactic NSAID (*not* aspirin or salicylates) or colchicine until at least 1 month after hyperuricaemia corrected (usually for first 3 months) to avoid precipitating an acute attack; ensure adequate fluid intake (2–3 litres/day); for hyperuricaemia associated with cancer therapy, allopurinol treatment should be started before cancer therapy; **interactions:** Appendix 1 (allopurinol)
Contra-indications   not a treatment for acute gout but continue if attack develops when already receiving allopurinol, and treat attack separately (see notes above)
Hepatic impairment   reduce dose
Renal impairment   max. 100 mg daily, increased only if response inadequate; in severe impairment, reduce daily dose below 100 mg, or increase dose interval; if facilities available, adjust dose to maintain plasma-oxipurinol concentration below 100 micromol/litre
Pregnancy   toxicity not reported; manufacturer advises use only if no safer alternative and disease carries risk for mother or child
Breast-feeding   present in milk—not known to be harmful
Side-effects   rashes (**withdraw** therapy; if rash mild re-introduce cautiously but **discontinue** promptly if recurrence—hypersensitivity reactions occur rarely and include exfoliation, fever, lymphadenopathy,

1. The *Scottish Medicines Consortium* issued similar advice in August 2010

10

Musculoskeletal and joint diseases

arthralgia, and eosinophilia resembling Stevens-Johnson syndrome or toxic epidermal necrolysis, vasculitis, hepatitis, renal impairment, and very rarely seizures); gastro-intestinal disorders; rarely malaise, headache, vertigo, drowsiness, visual and taste disturbances, hypertension, alopecia, hepatotoxicity, paraesthesia and neuropathy, gynaecomastia, blood disorders (including leucopenia, thrombocytopenia, haemolytic anaemia and aplastic anaemia)

Dose

- Initially 100 mg daily, preferably after food, then adjusted according to plasma or urinary uric acid concentration; usual maintenance dose in mild conditions 100–200 mg daily, in moderately severe conditions 300–600 mg daily, in severe conditions 700–900 mg daily; doses over 300 mg daily given in divided doses; CHILD under 15 years, (in neoplastic conditions, enzyme disorders) 10–20 mg/kg daily (max. 400 mg daily)

Allopurinol (Non-proprietary) PoM
Tablets, allopurinol 100 mg, net price 28-tab pack = £1.05; 300 mg, 28-tab pack = £1.16. Label: 8, 21, 27
Brands include Caplenal®, Cosuric®, Rimapurinol®

Zyloric® (Aspen) PoM
Tablets, allopurinol 100 mg, net price 100-tab pack = £10.19; 300 mg, 28-tab pack = £7.31. Label: 8, 21, 27

■ FEBUXOSTAT

Indications treatment of chronic hyperuricaemia in gout (but see also NICE guidance above)

Cautions administer prophylactic NSAID (*not* aspirin or salicylates) or colchicine for at least 6 months after starting febuxostat to avoid precipitating an acute attack; transplant recipients; monitor liver function tests before and periodically during treatment as indicated; thyroid disorders; ischaemic heart disease; congestive heart failure; **interactions**: Appendix 1 (febuxostat)

Contra-indications not a treatment for acute gout but continue if attack develops when already receiving febuxostat, and treat attack separately (see notes above)

Hepatic impairment max. 80 mg daily in mild impairment; no dose information available in moderate or severe impairment

Renal impairment use with caution if eGFR less than 30 mL/minute/1.73 m²—no information available

Pregnancy manufacturer advises avoid—limited information available

Breast-feeding manufacturer advises avoid—present in milk in *animal* studies

Side-effects gastro-intestinal disturbances, abnormal liver function tests, oedema, headache, rash; *less commonly* cholelithiasis, hyperlipidaemia, taste and smell disturbances, hypertension, chest pain, flushing, atrial fibrillation, ECG abnormalities, palpitation, dyspnoea, bronchitis, upper respiratory tract infection, cough, dizziness, paraesthesia, hypoaesthesia, hemiparesis, drowsiness, insomnia, appetite and weight change, diabetes mellitus, increased thyroid stimulating hormone, decreased libido, erectile dysfunction, haematuria, nephrolithiasis, increased urinary frequency, renal failure, proteinuria, myalgia, arthralgia, arthritis, muscle weakness, muscle spasm, bursitis, dermatitis; *rarely* pancreatitis, hepatitis, jaundice, thirst, asthenia, nervousness, tubulointerstitial nephritis, pancytopenia, thrombocytopenia, rhabdomyolysis, blurred vision, mouth ulceration, tinnitus

---

MHRA/CHM advice
Serious hypersensitivity reactions (June 2012)
There have been rare but serious reports of hypersensitivity reactions, including Stevens-Johnson syndrome and acute anaphylactic shock with febuxostat. Patients should be advised of the signs and symptoms of severe hypersensitivity; febuxostat must be stopped immediately if these occur (early withdrawal is associated with a better prognosis), and must not be restarted in patients who have ever developed a hypersensitivity reaction to febuxostat. Most cases occur during the first month of treatment; a prior history of hypersensitivity to allopurinol and/or renal disease may indicate potential hypersensitivity to febuxostat.

Dose

- ADULT over 18 years, 80 mg once daily, if after 2–4 weeks serum uric acid greater than 6 mg/100 mL, increase to 120 mg once daily

Adenuric® (Menarini) PoM
Tablets, both yellow, f/c, febuxostat 80 mg, net price 28-tab pack = £24.36; 120 mg 28-tab pack = £24.36

■ SULFINPYRAZONE
(Sulphinpyrazone)

Indications gout prophylaxis, hyperuricaemia

Cautions ensure adequate fluid intake (about 2–3 litres daily) and render urine alkaline during initial treatment; regular blood counts before treatment and at regular intervals during treatment; cardiac disease (may cause salt and water retention); **interactions**: Appendix 1 (sulfinpyrazone)

Contra-indications acute gout attack; history of blood disorders; acute porphyria (section 9.8.2); peptic ulceration; avoid in hypersensitivity to aspirin, salicylates, NSAIDs

Hepatic impairment avoid in severe impairment

Renal impairment reduce dose; avoid in severe impairment

Pregnancy manufacturer advises caution—no information available

Breast-feeding no information available

Side-effects gastro-intestinal disturbances, occasionally allergic skin reactions, salt and water retention; rarely blood disorders, gastro-intestinal ulceration and bleeding, acute renal failure, raised liver enzymes, jaundice and hepatitis

Dose

- Initially 100–200 mg daily with food (or milk) increasing over 2–3 weeks to 600 mg daily (rarely 800 mg daily), continued until serum uric acid concentration normal then reduced for maintenance (maintenance dose may be as low as 200 mg daily)

Sulfinpyrazone (Non-proprietary) PoM
Tablets, sulfinpyrazone 100 mg, net price 84-tab pack = £41.25; 200 mg, 84-tab pack = £79.00. Label: 12, 21

10 Musculoskeletal and joint diseases

Hyperuricaemia associated with cytotoxic drugs

Allopurinol is used to prevent hyperuricaemia associated with cytotoxic drugs—see section 8.1 (Hyperuricaemia) and Allopurinol above.

Rasburicase is licensed for the prophylaxis and treatment of acute hyperuricaemia, before and during initiation of chemotherapy, in patients with haematological malignancy and a high tumour burden at risk of rapid lysis.

▌ RASBURICASE

Indications prophylaxis and treatment of acute hyperuricaemia with initial chemotherapy for haematological malignancy

Cautions monitor closely for hypersensitivity; atopic allergies; may interfere with test for uric acid—consult product literature

Contra-indications G6PD deficiency (section 9.1.5)

Pregnancy manufacturer advises avoid—no information available

Breast-feeding manufacturer advises avoid—no information available

Side-effects fever; *less commonly* nausea, vomiting, diarrhoea, headache, hypersensitivity reactions (including rash, bronchospasm and anaphylaxis); haemolytic anaemia, methaemoglobinaemia

Dose
- By intravenous infusion, 200 micrograms/kg once daily for up to 7 days according to plasma-uric acid concentration

Fasturtec® (Sanofi-Aventis) [PoM]
Intravenous infusion, powder for reconstitution, rasburicase, net price 1.5-mg vial (with solvent) = £69.46; 7.5-mg vial (with solvent) = £289.44

10.1.5 Other drugs for rheumatic diseases

Glucosamine

Glucosamine is a natural substance found in mucopolysaccharides, mucoproteins, and chitin. It is licensed for symptomatic relief of mild to moderate osteoarthritis of the knee, but is not recommended. The mechanism of action is not understood and there is limited evidence to show it is effective.

The *Scottish Medicines Consortium* (p. 4) has advised (May 2008) that glucosamine (*Alateris®*) and (July 2011) glucosamine (*Glusartel®*) are **not** recommended for use within NHS Scotland for the symptomatic relief of mild to moderate osteoarthritis of the knee.

▌ GLUCOSAMINE

Indications symptomatic relief of mild to moderate osteoarthritis of the knee

Cautions impaired glucose tolerance (monitor blood-glucose concentration before treatment and periodically thereafter); predisposition to cardiovascular disease (monitor cholesterol); asthma; **interactions**: Appendix 1 (glucosamine)

Contra-indications shellfish allergy

Pregnancy manufacturers advise avoid—no information available

Breast-feeding manufacturers advise avoid—no information available

Side-effects nausea, abdominal pain, dyspepsia, flatulence, diarrhoea, constipation, drowsiness, headache, fatigue; *less commonly* flushing, rash, pruritus; *also reported* visual disturbances, hair loss

Dose
- See under preparations

Alateris® (Dee) [PoM]
Tablets, scored, glucosamine (as hydrochloride) 625 mg, net price 60-tab pack = £18.40
Dose ADULT over 18 years, 2 tablets once daily; review treatment if no benefit after 2–3 months

Dolenio® (Alissa) [PoM]
Tablets, f/c, scored, glucosamine sulfate (as sodium chloride) 1.5 g, net price 30-tab pack = £18.20
Electrolytes Na⁺ 6.52 mmol/tablet
Dose ADULT over 18 years, 1 tablet once daily; review treatment if no benefit after 2–3 months

Glusartel® (HFA Healthcare) [PoM]
Oral powder, sugar-free, glucosamine sulfate (as sodium chloride) 1.5 g/sachet, net price 30-sachet pack = £18.40. Label: 13
Electrolytes Na⁺ 6.6 mmol/sachet
Excipients include aspartame (section 9.4.1)
Dose ADULT over 18 years, 1 sachet (dissolved in at least 250 mL of water) once daily; review treatment if no benefit after 2–3 months

10.2 Drugs used in neuromuscular disorders

| 10.2.1 | Drugs that enhance neuromuscular transmission |
| 10.2.2 | Skeletal muscle relaxants |

10.2.1 Drugs that enhance neuromuscular transmission

Anticholinesterases are used as first-line treatment in *ocular myasthenia gravis* and as an adjunct to immunosuppressant therapy for *generalised myasthenia gravis*.

Corticosteroids are used when anticholinesterases do not control symptoms completely. A second-line immunosuppressant such as azathioprine is frequently used to reduce the dose of corticosteroid.

Plasmapheresis or infusion of intravenous immunoglobulin [unlicensed indication] may induce temporary remission in severe relapses, particularly where bulbar or respiratory function is compromised or before thymectomy.

Anticholinesterases

Anticholinesterase drugs enhance neuromuscular transmission in voluntary and involuntary muscle in myasthenia gravis. They prolong the action of acetylcholine by inhibiting the action of the enzyme acetylcholinesterase. Excessive dosage of these drugs can impair neuromuscular transmission and precipitate cholinergic crises by causing a depolarising block. This may be difficult to distinguish from a worsening myasthenic state.

10 Musculoskeletal and joint diseases

Muscarinic side-effects of anticholinesterases include increased sweating, increased salivary and gastric secretions, increased gastro-intestinal and uterine motility, and bradycardia. These parasympathomimetic effects are antagonised by atropine.

Neostigmine produces a therapeutic effect for up to 4 hours. Its pronounced muscarinic action is a disadvantage, and simultaneous administration of an antimuscarinic drug such as atropine or propantheline may be required to prevent colic, excessive salivation, or diarrhoea. In severe disease neostigmine can be given every 2 hours. The maximum that most patients can tolerate is 180 mg daily.

Pyridostigmine is less powerful and slower in action than neostigmine but it has a longer duration of action. It is preferable to neostigmine because of its smoother action and the need for less frequent dosage. It is particularly preferred in patients whose muscles are weak on waking. It has a comparatively mild gastro-intestinal effect but an antimuscarinic drug may still be required. It is inadvisable to exceed a total daily dose of 450 mg in order to avoid acetylcholine receptor down-regulation; patients requiring doses exceeding 450 mg daily will usually require input from a specialised neuro-muscular service. Immunosuppressant therapy is usually considered if the dose of pyridostigmine exceeds 360 mg daily.

Neostigmine is also used to reverse the actions of the non-depolarising neuromuscular blocking drugs (see section 15.1.6).

NEOSTIGMINE

Indications   myasthenia gravis; other indications (section 15.1.6)

Cautions   asthma (*extreme* caution), bradycardia, arrhythmias, recent myocardial infarction, epilepsy, hypotension, parkinsonism, vagotonia, peptic ulceration, hyperthyroidism; atropine or other antidote to muscarinic effects may be necessary (particularly when neostigmine is given by injection), but not given routinely because it may mask signs of overdosage; interactions: Appendix 1 (parasympathomimetics)

Contra-indications   intestinal or urinary obstruction

Renal impairment   may need dose reduction

Pregnancy   manufacturer advises use only if potential benefit outweighs risk

Breast-feeding   amount probably too small to be harmful

Side-effects   nausea, vomiting, increased salivation, diarrhoea, abdominal cramps (more marked with higher doses); signs of overdosage include broncho-constriction, increased bronchial secretions, lacrimation, excessive sweating, involuntary defaecation and micturition, miosis, nystagmus, bradycardia, heart block, arrhythmias, hypotension, agitation, excessive dreaming, and weakness eventually leading to fasci-culation and paralysis

Dose

- By mouth, neostigmine bromide 15–30 mg at suitable intervals throughout day, total daily dose 75–300 mg (but see also dose notes above); NEONATE 1–5 mg every 4 hours, half an hour before feeds; CHILD up to 6 years initially 7.5 mg, 6–12 years initially 15 mg, usual total daily dose 15–90 mg
- By subcutaneous *or* intramuscular injection, ADULT and CHILD over 12 years, neostigmine metilsulfate 1–

2.5 mg at suitable intervals throughout day (usual total daily dose 5–20 mg); NEONATE 150 micrograms/kg every 6–8 hours 30 minutes before feeds, increased to max. 300 micrograms/kg every 4 hours, if necessary [unlicensed]; CHILD 1 month–12 years 200–500 micrograms as required

Neostigmine (Non-proprietary) ▣PoM
Tablets, scored, neostigmine bromide 15 mg, net price 140 = £88.31

◢Injection
Section 15.1.6

▮ PYRIDOSTIGMINE BROMIDE

Indications   myasthenia gravis

Cautions   see under Neostigmine; weaker muscarinic action

Contra-indications   see under Neostigmine

Renal impairment   reduce dose; excreted by kidney

Pregnancy   see under Neostigmine

Breast-feeding   see under Neostigmine

Side-effects   see under Neostigmine

Dose

- By mouth, 30–120 mg at suitable intervals throughout day, total daily dose 0.3–1.2 g (but see also notes above); CHILD under 18 years, see *BNF for Children*

Mestinon® (Meda) ▣PoM
Tablets, scored, pyridostigmine bromide 60 mg, net price 200 = £45.57

Immunosuppressant therapy

Corticosteroids (section 6.3) are established as treatment for myasthenia gravis; although they are commonly given on alternate days there is little evidence of benefit over daily administration. Corticosteroid treatment is usually initiated under in-patient supervision and all patients should receive osteoporosis prophylaxis (section 6.6).

In *generalised myasthenia gravis* small initial doses of prednisolone (10 mg on alternate days) are increased in steps of 10 mg on alternate days to 1–1.5 mg/kg (max. 100 mg) on alternate days. When given daily, prednisolone is started at 5 mg daily and then increased in steps of 5 mg daily to 60 mg daily or occasionally up to 80 mg daily (0.75–1 mg/kg daily). About 10% of patients experience a transient but very serious worsening of symptoms in the first 2–3 weeks, especially if the corticosteroid is started at a high dose. However, ventilated patients may be started on 1.5 mg/kg (max. 100 mg) on alternate days. Smaller doses of corticosteroid are usually required in *ocular myasthenia*. Once clinical remission has occurred (usually after 2–6 months), the dose of prednisolone should be reduced slowly to the minimum effective dose (usually 10–40 mg on alternate days).

In generalised myasthenia gravis **azathioprine** (section 8.2.1) is usually started at the same time as the corticosteroid and it allows a lower maintenance dose of the corticosteroid to be used; azathioprine is initiated at a dose of 0.5–1 mg/kg daily, which is increased over 3–4 weeks to 2–2.5 mg/kg daily. **Ciclosporin** (section 8.2.2), **methotrexate** (section 8.1.3), or **mycophenolate mofetil** (section 8.2.1) can be used in patients unresponsive or intolerant to other treatments [unlicensed indications].

Acetylcholine-release enhancers

Amifampridine is licensed for the symptomatic treatment of Lambert-Eaton myasthenic syndrome (LEMS), a rare disorder of neuromuscular transmission.

The *Scottish Medicines Consortium* (p. 4) has advised (July 2012) that amifampridine phosphate (*Firdapse*®) is not recommended for use within NHS Scotland for the symptomatic treatment of Lambert-Eaton myasthenic syndrome (LEMS).

Fampridine is licensed for the improvement of walking in patients with multiple sclerosis who have a walking disability.

▌ AMIFAMPRIDINE

Indications (specialist use only) symptomatic treatment of Lambert-Eaton myasthenic syndrome

Cautions concomitant use of drugs that lower convulsive threshold; non-paraneoplastic form of Lambert-Eaton myasthenic syndrome; clinical and ECG monitoring required at treatment initiation and yearly thereafter

Contra-indications epilepsy; uncontrolled asthma; congenital QT syndromes; avoid concomitant use of drugs that prolong QT interval; avoid concomitant use of drugs with a narrow therapeutic index

Hepatic impairment use with caution; in mild impairment reduce initial dose to 10 mg daily in divided doses, increased in steps of 5 mg every 7 days; in moderate or severe impairment reduce initial dose to 5 mg daily in divided doses, increased in steps of 5 mg every 7 days

Renal impairment use with caution; in mild impairment reduce initial dose to 10 mg daily in divided doses, increased in steps of 5 mg every 7 days; in moderate or severe impairment reduce initial dose to 5 mg daily in divided doses, increased in steps of 5 mg every 7 days

Pregnancy manufacturer advises avoid—ensure effective contraception during treatment in men and women

Breast-feeding manufacturer advises avoid—no information available

Side-effects gastro-intestinal disorders; paraesthesia; palpitations, arrhythmias, Raynaud's syndrome, cough, bronchial hypersecretion, exacerbation or precipitation of asthma, sleep disturbances, convulsions, anxiety, drowsiness, dizziness, weakness, headache, chorea, myoclonia, and blurred vision also reported

Dose
● ADULT over 18 years, initially 15 mg daily in 3 divided doses, increased in steps of 5 mg every 4–5 days, to max. 60 mg daily in 3–4 divided doses; max. single dose 20 mg

Firdapse® (BioMarin) ▼ PoM
Tablets, scored, amifampridine (as phosphate) 10 mg, net price 100-tab pack = £1815.00. Label: 3, 21

▌ FAMPRIDINE

Indications (specialist use only) improvement of walking disability in multiple sclerosis

Cautions predisposition to seizures including concomitant use of drugs that lower seizure threshold;

symptomatic cardiac rhythm disorders, sinoatrial or atrioventricular conduction disorders; **interactions**: Appendix 1 (fampridine)

Contra-indications history of seizures (discontinue treatment if seizures occur)

Renal impairment avoid if eGFR less than 80 mL/minute/1.73 m^2

Pregnancy avoid—toxicity in *animal* studies

Breast-feeding avoid—no information available

Side-effects nausea, vomiting, constipation, dyspepsia, dyspnoea, pharyngolaryngeal pain, dizziness, headache, paraesthesia, tremor, malaise, insomnia, anxiety, urinary tract infection, back pain; *less commonly* seizures

Dose
● ADULT over 18 years, 10 mg every 12 hours; discontinue treatment if no improvement within 2 weeks

Fampyra® (Biogen) ▼ PoM
Tablets, f/c, m/r, fampridine 10 mg, net price 28-tab pack (2 × 14) = £181.00, 56-tab pack (4 × 14) = £362.00. Label: 23, 25
Note Dispense in original container (pack contains a desiccant) and discard any tablets remaining 7 days after opening

▌10.2.2 Skeletal muscle relaxants

The drugs described below are used for the relief of chronic muscle spasm or spasticity associated with multiple sclerosis or other neurological damage; they are not indicated for spasm associated with minor injuries. Baclofen, diazepam, and tizanidine act principally on the central nervous system. Dantrolene, has a peripheral site of action; cannabis extract has both a central and a peripheral action. Skeletal muscle relaxants differ in action from the muscle relaxants used in anaesthesia (section 15.1.5), which block transmission at the neuromuscular junction.

The underlying cause of spasticity should be treated and any aggravating factors (e.g. pressure sores, infection) remedied. Skeletal muscle relaxants are effective in most forms of spasticity except the rare alpha variety. The major disadvantage of treatment with these drugs is that reduction in muscle tone can cause a loss of splinting action of the spastic leg and trunk muscles and sometimes lead to an increase in disability.

Baclofen inhibits transmission at spinal level and also depresses the central nervous system. The dose should be increased slowly to avoid the major side-effects of sedation and muscular hypotonia (other adverse events are uncommon).

A **cannabis extract** containing dronabinol (delta-9-tetrahydrocannabinol) and cannabidiol is licensed as an adjunct treatment for moderate to severe spasticity associated with multiple sclerosis in patients who have not responded adequately to other skeletal muscle relaxants. The dose should be titrated over 2 weeks; response to treatment should be reviewed after 4 weeks and treatment stopped if an adequate response is not achieved.

Dantrolene acts directly on skeletal muscle and produces fewer central adverse effects making it a drug of choice. The dose should be increased slowly.

Diazepam can also be used. Sedation and occasionally extensor hypotonus are disadvantages. Other benzo-

10 Musculoskeletal and joint diseases

diazepines also have muscle-relaxant properties. Muscle-relaxant doses of benzodiazepines are similar to anxiolytic doses (section 4.1.2).

Tizanidine is an alpha$_2$-adrenoceptor agonist indicated for spasticity associated with multiple sclerosis or spinal cord injury.

BACLOFEN

Indications   chronic severe spasticity resulting from disorders such as multiple sclerosis or traumatic partial section of spinal cord

Cautions   psychiatric illness, Parkinson's disease, cerebrovascular disease, elderly; respiratory impairment; epilepsy; history of peptic ulcer (avoid oral route in active peptic ulceration); diabetes; hypertonic bladder sphincter; avoid abrupt withdrawal (risk of hyperactive state, may exacerbate spasticity, and precipitate autonomic dysfunction including hyperthermia, psychiatric reactions and convulsions, see also under Withdrawal below); **interactions**: Appendix 1 (muscle relaxants)

Withdrawal Serious side-effects can occur on abrupt withdrawal; to minimise risk, discontinue by gradual dose reduction over at least 1–2 weeks (longer if symptoms occur)

Driving Drowsiness may affect performance of skilled tasks (e.g. driving); effects of alcohol enhanced

Specific cautions for intrathecal treatment coagulation disorders; previous spinal fusion procedure; malnutrition (increased risk of post-surgical complications)

Contra-indications
Specific contra-indications for intrathecal treatment local or systemic infection

Hepatic impairment   manufacturer advises use by mouth with caution

Renal impairment   risk of toxicity—use smaller doses (e.g. 5 mg daily by mouth) and if necessary increase dosage interval; if eGFR less than 15 mL/minute/1.73m^2 manufacturer advises use by mouth only if potential benefit outweighs risk; excreted by kidney

Pregnancy   manufacturer advises use only if potential benefit outweighs risk (toxicity in *animal* studies)

Breast-feeding   present in milk—amount probably too small to be harmful

Side-effects   gastro-intestinal disturbances, dry mouth; hypotension, respiratory or cardiovascular depression; sedation, drowsiness, confusion, dizziness, ataxia, hallucinations, nightmares, headache, euphoria, insomnia, depression, anxiety, agitation, tremor; seizure; urinary disturbances; myalgia; visual disorders; rash, hyperhidrosis; *rarely* taste disturbances, abdominal pain, changes in hepatic function, paraesthesia, erectile dysfunction, dysarthria; *very rarely* hypothermia

Dose
- By mouth, ADULT over 18 years, initially 5 mg 3 times daily, gradually increased; usual maintenance dose up to 60 mg daily in divided doses (max. 100 mg daily); CHILD under 18 years, initially 300 micrograms/kg daily in 4 divided doses, increased gradually at weekly intervals until satisfactory response; usual maintenance dose 0.75–2 mg/kg daily in divided doses; CHILD up to 8 years, max. total daily dose 40 mg/day; CHILD 8–18 years, max. total daily dose 60 mg/day

  Note Review treatment if no benefit within 6 weeks of achieving maximum dose

- By intrathecal injection, specialist use only, severe chronic spasticity unresponsive to oral antispastic drugs (or where side-effects of oral therapy unac-

ceptable) *or* as alternative to ablative neurosurgical procedures, ADULT over 18 years, initial *test dose* 25–50 micrograms over at least 1 minute via catheter or lumbar puncture, increased in 25-microgram steps (not more often than every 24 hours) to max. 100 micrograms to determine appropriate dose, *then dose-titration phase*, most often using infusion pump (implanted into chest wall or abdominal wall tissues) to establish *maintenance dose* (ranging from 12 micrograms to 2 mg daily for spasticity of spinal origin *or* 22 micrograms to 1.4 mg daily for spasticity of cerebral origin) retaining some spasticity to avoid sensation of paralysis; CHILD 4–18 years (spasticity of cerebral or spinal origin only), initial *test dose* 25–50 micrograms then titrated as for ADULT, initial *maintenance dose* 25–200 micrograms daily, adjusted according to response

Important Consult product literature for details on test dose and titration—important to monitor patients closely in appropriately equipped and staffed environment during screening and immediately after pump implantation. Resuscitation equipment must be available for immediate use. Treatment with continuous pump-administered intrathecal baclofen should be initiated within 3 months of a satisfactory response to intrathecal baclofen testing.

Baclofen (Non-proprietary) PoM
Tablets, baclofen 10 mg, net price 84-tab pack = £1.86. Label: 2, 8, 21

Oral solution, baclofen 5 mg/5 mL, net price 300 mL = £4.83. Label: 2, 8, 21
Brands include *Lyflex*® (sugar-free)

Intrathecal injection, baclofen 50 micrograms/mL, net price 1-mL amp (for test dose) = £2.19; 500 micrograms/mL, 20-mL amp (for use with implantable pump) = £48.62; 2 mg/mL, 5-mL amp (for use with implantable pump) = £48.62

Lioresal® (Novartis) PoM
Tablets, scored, baclofen 10 mg, net price 100-tab pack = £12.38. Label: 2, 8, 21
Excipients include gluten

Liquid, sugar-free, raspberry-flavoured, baclofen 5 mg/5 mL, net price 300 mL = £8.59. Label: 2, 8, 21

Intrathecal injection, baclofen 50 micrograms/mL, net price 1-mL amp (for test dose) = £2.63; 500 micrograms/mL, 20-mL amp (for use with implantable pump) = £58.34; 2 mg/mL, 5-mL amp (for use with implantable pump) = £58.34

CANNABIS EXTRACT

Indications   adjunct in moderate to severe spasticity in multiple sclerosis (specialist use only)

Cautions   significant cardiovascular disease; history of epilepsy; monitor oral mucosa—interrupt treatment if lesions or persistent soreness; **interactions**: Appendix 1 (cannabis extract)

Driving May affect performance of skilled tasks (e.g. driving); effects of alcohol may be enhanced, see also Drugs and driving, p. 3

Contra-indications   personal or family history of psychosis; history of other severe psychiatric disorder

Hepatic impairment   manufacturer advises more frequent monitoring in significant impairment—possible risk of prolonged or enhanced effect

Renal impairment   manufacturer advises more frequent monitoring in significant impairment—possible risk of prolonged or enhanced effect

Pregnancy manufacturer advises use only if potential benefit outweighs risks, and recommends effective contraception during and for 3 months after treatment in men and women

Breast-feeding avoid—present in milk

Side-effects increased or decreased appetite, taste disturbance, constipation, diarrhoea, nausea, vomiting, dry mouth, mouth ulcers, oral pain, dizziness, vertigo, malaise, depression, disorientation, dissociation, mood disturbance, amnesia, impaired attention, drowsiness, dysarthria, blurred vision; *less commonly* abdominal pain, oromucosal and tooth discoloration, stomatitis, palpitation, tachycardia, hypertension, pharyngitis, syncope, hallucinations, paranoia, delusions, suicidal thoughts; *also reported* anxiety, seizures

Dose
- Consult product literature

Sativex® (Bayer) CD4-1
Oromucosal spray, *Cannabis sativa* extract (containing dronabinol (delta-9-tetrahydrocannabinol) 27 mg and cannabidiol 25 mg/mL), net price 3 × 10-mL units = £375.00. Counselling, driving see above
Excipients include propylene glycol

DANTROLENE SODIUM

Indications chronic severe spasticity of voluntary muscle; malignant hyperthermia (section 15.1.8)

Cautions impaired cardiac and pulmonary function; therapeutic effect may take a few weeks to develop—discontinue if no response within 6–8 weeks; **interactions:** Appendix 1 (muscle relaxants).
Hepatotoxicity Potentially life-threatening hepatotoxicity reported, usually if doses greater than 400 mg daily used, in females, patients over 30 years, if history of liver disorders, or concomitant use of hepatotoxic drugs; test liver function before and at intervals during therapy—discontinue if abnormal liver function tests or symptoms of liver disorder (counselling, see below); re-introduce only if complete reversal of hepatotoxicity
Counselling Patients should be told how to recognise signs of liver disorder and advised to seek prompt medical attention if symptoms such as anorexia, nausea, vomiting, fatigue, abdominal pain, dark urine, or pruritus develop
Driving Drowsiness may affect performance of skilled tasks (e.g. driving); effects of alcohol enhanced

Contra-indications acute muscle spasm; avoid when spasticity is useful, for example, locomotion

Hepatic impairment avoid—may cause severe liver damage; injection may be used in an emergency for malignant hyperthermia

Pregnancy avoid use in chronic spasticity—embryotoxic in *animal* studies

Breast-feeding present in milk—manufacturer advises avoid use in chronic spasticity

Side-effects diarrhoea (withdraw if severe, discontinue treatment if recurs on re-introduction), nausea, vomiting, anorexia, hepatotoxicity (see above), abdominal pain; pericarditis; pleural effusion, respiratory depression; headache, drowsiness, dizziness, asthenia, fatigue, seizures, fever, chills; speech and visual disturbances; rash; *less commonly* dysphagia, constipation, exacerbation of cardiac insufficiency, tachycardia, erratic blood pressure, dyspnoea, depression, confusion, nervousness, insomnia, increased urinary frequency, urinary incontinence or retention, haematuria, crystalluria, and increased sweating

Dose
- Initially 25 mg daily, may be increased at weekly intervals to max. 100 mg 4 times daily; usual dose 75 mg 3 times daily; CHILD 5–18 years see *BNF for Children*

Dantrium® (SpePharm) PoM
Capsules, orange/brown, dantrolene sodium 25 mg, net price 100 = £16.87; 100 mg, 100 = £43.07. Label: 2, counselling, driving, hepatotoxicity

DIAZEPAM

Indications muscle spasm of varied aetiology, including tetanus; other indications (section 4.1.2, section 4.8, section 15.1.4.1)

Cautions section 4.1.2; special precautions for intravenous injection (section 4.8.2)

Contra-indications section 4.1.2

Hepatic impairment section 4.1.2

Renal impairment section 4.1.2

Pregnancy section 4.1.2

Breast-feeding section 4.1.2

Side-effects section 4.1.2; also hypotonia

Dose
- Muscle spasm, by mouth, 2–15 mg daily in divided doses, increased if necessary in spastic conditions to 60 mg daily according to response

Cerebral spasticity in selected cases, CHILD 2–40 mg daily in divided doses

By intramuscular *or* by slow intravenous injection (into a large vein at a rate of not more than 5 mg/minute), in acute muscle spasm, 10 mg repeated if necessary after 4 hours
Note Only use intramuscular route when oral and intravenous routes not possible; emulsion formulation preferred for intravenous injection; special precautions for intravenous injection, see section 4.8.2
- Tetanus, ADULT and CHILD, by intravenous injection (emulsion preparation preferred), 100–300 micrograms/kg repeated every 1–4 hours; by intravenous infusion (*or* by nasoduodenal tube), 3–10 mg/kg over 24 hours, adjusted according to response

◢**Preparations**
Section 4.1.2

TIZANIDINE

Indications spasticity associated with multiple sclerosis or spinal cord injury or disease

Cautions elderly; monitor liver function monthly for first 4 months and in those who develop unexplained nausea, anorexia or fatigue; concomitant administration of drugs that prolong QT interval; avoid abrupt withdrawal (risk of rebound hypertension and tachycardia, see under Withdrawal, below); **interactions:** Appendix 1 (muscle relaxants)
Withdrawal Rebound hypertension and tachycardia can occur on abrupt withdrawal; to minimise risk, discontinue gradually and monitor blood pressure
Driving Drowsiness may affect performance of skilled tasks (e.g. driving); effects of alcohol enhanced

Hepatic impairment avoid in severe impairment; use in moderate impairment only if potential benefit outweighs risk

Renal impairment manufacturer advises caution

Pregnancy avoid (toxicity in *animal* studies)

10 Musculoskeletal and joint diseases

Breast-feeding avoid (present in milk in *animal* studies)

Side-effects dry mouth, nausea, gastro-intestinal disturbance, altered liver enzymes (discontinue if persistently raised—consult product literature), hypotension, drowsiness, fatigue, dizziness; *less commonly* bradycardia; *also reported* hepatitis, liver failure, insomnia, hallucinations, confusion, convulsions, syncope, asthenia, blurred vision

Dose

* ADULT over 18 years, initially 2 mg daily as a single dose increased according to response at intervals of at least 3–4 days in steps of 2 mg daily (and given in divided doses) usually up to 24 mg daily in 3–4 divided doses; max. 36 mg daily

Tizanidine (Non-proprietary) PoM
Tablets, tizanidine (as hydrochloride) 2 mg net price 120-tab pack = £23.34; 4 mg, 120-tab pack = £32.23. Label: 2, 8

Zanaflex® (TEVA UK) PoM
Tablets, scored, tizanidine (as hydrochloride) 2 mg, net price 120-tab pack = £30.41; 4 mg, 120-tab pack = £42.18. Label: 2, 8

Other muscle relaxants

The clinical efficacy of methocarbamol and meprobamate (section 4.1.2) as muscle relaxants is **not** well established, although they have been included in compound analgesic preparations.

METHOCARBAMOL

Indications short-term symptomatic relief of muscle spasm (but see notes above)

Cautions interactions: Appendix 1 (muscle relaxants)
Driving Drowsiness may affect performance of skilled tasks (e.g. driving); effects of alcohol enhanced

Contra-indications coma or pre-coma, brain damage, epilepsy, myasthenia gravis

Hepatic impairment manufacturer advises caution; half-life may be prolonged

Renal impairment manufacturer advises caution

Pregnancy manufacturer advises avoid unless potential benefit outweighs risk

Breast-feeding present in milk in *animal* studies—manufacturer advises caution

Side-effects nausea, vomiting, dyspepsia; hypersensitivity reactions (including urticaria, angioedema, anaphylaxis); fever, headache, drowsiness, dizziness, hypotension, bradycardia, confusion, amnesia, restlessness, anxiety, tremor, seizures; blurred vision, nasal congestion; rash, pruritus; leucopenia, cholestatic jaundice

Dose

* 1.5 g 4 times daily; may be reduced to 750 mg 3 times daily; ELDERLY up to 750 mg 4 times daily may be sufficient; CHILD not recommended

Robaxin® (Almirall) PoM
750 Tablets, f/c, scored, methocarbamol 750 mg, net price 100 = £12.65. Label: 2

Nocturnal leg cramps

Quinine salts (section 5.4.1), such as quinine sulfate 200–300 mg at bedtime, are effective in reducing the frequency of nocturnal leg cramps by about 25% in ambulatory patients; however, because of potential toxicity, quinine is not recommended for routine treatment and should not be used unless cramps cause regular disruption to sleep. Quinine should only be considered when cramps are very painful or frequent; when other treatable causes of cramp have been excluded; and when non-pharmacological treatments have not worked (e.g. passive stretching exercises). It may take up to 4 weeks for improvement to become apparent; if there is benefit, quinine treatment can be continued. Patients should be monitored closely during the early stages for adverse effects as well as for benefit. Treatment should be interrupted at intervals of approximately 3 months to assess the need for further quinine treatment. In patients taking quinine long term, a trial discontinuation may be considered. Quinine is toxic in overdosage and accidental fatalities have occurred (see also below).

QUININE

Indications see notes above; malaria (section 5.4.1)
Cautions see section 5.4.1 and notes above
Contra-indications section 5.4.1
Pregnancy section 5.4.1
Breast-feeding section 5.4.1
Side-effects section 5.4.1; **important:** very toxic in **overdosage**—immediate advice from poison centres essential (see also p. 39)

Dose

* See notes above

◢**Preparations**
Section 5.4.1

10.3 Drugs for the treatment of soft-tissue disorders and topical pain relief

10.3.1	Enzymes
10.3.2	Rubefacients, topical NSAIDs, capsaicin, and poultices

Extravasation

Local guidelines for the management of extravasation should be followed where they exist or specialist advice sought.

Extravasation injury follows leakage of drugs or intravenous fluids from the veins or inadvertent administration into the subcutaneous or subdermal tissue. It must be dealt with **promptly** to prevent tissue necrosis.

Acidic or alkaline preparations and those with an osmolarity greater than that of plasma can cause extravasation injury; excipients including alcohol and polyethylene glycol have also been implicated. Cytotoxic drugs commonly cause extravasation injury. In addition, certain patients such as the very young and the elderly are at increased risk. Those receiving anticoagulants are more likely to lose blood into surrounding tissues if extravasation occurs, while those receiving sedatives or analgesics may not notice the early signs or symptoms of extravasation.

Prevention of extravasation Precautions should be taken to avoid extravasation; ideally, drugs likely to cause extravasation injury should be given through a central line and patients receiving repeated doses of hazardous drugs peripherally should have the cannula resited at regular intervals. Attention should be paid to the manufacturers' recommendations for administration. Placing a glyceryl trinitrate patch (section 2.6.1) distal to the cannula may improve the patency of the vessel in patients with small veins or in those whose veins are prone to collapse.

Patients should be asked to report any pain or burning at the site of injection immediately.

Management of extravasation If extravasation is suspected the infusion should be stopped immediately but the cannula should not be removed until after an attempt has been made to aspirate the area (through the cannula) in order to remove as much of the drug as possible. Aspiration is sometimes possible if the extravasation presents with a raised bleb or blister at the injection site and is surrounded by hardened tissue, but it is often unsuccessful if the tissue is soft or soggy. **Corticosteroids** are usually given to treat inflammation, although there is little evidence to support their use in extravasation. Hydrocortisone or dexamethasone (section 6.3.2) can be given either locally by subcutaneous injection or intravenously at a site distant from the injury. **Antihistamines** (section 3.4.1) and **analgesics** (section 4.7) may be required for symptom relief.

The management of extravasation beyond these measures is not well standardised and calls for specialist advice. Treatment depends on the nature of the offending substance; one approach is to localise and neutralise the substance whereas another is to spread and dilute it. The first method may be appropriate following extravasation of vesicant drugs and involves administration of an antidote (if available) and the application of cold compresses 3–4 times a day (consult specialist literature for details of specific antidotes). Spreading and diluting the offending substance involves infiltrating the area with physiological saline, applying warm compresses, elevating the affected limb, and administering **hyaluronidase** (section 10.3.1). A saline flush-out technique (involving flushing the subcutaneous tissue with physiological saline) may be effective but requires specialist advice. Hyaluronidase should **not** be administered following extravasation of vesicant drugs (unless it is either specifically indicated or used in the saline flush-out technique). **Dexrazoxane** (section 8.1) is licensed for the treatment of anthracycline-induced extravasation.

10.3.1 Enzymes

Collagenase

Collagenases are proteolytic enzymes that are derived from the fermentation of *Clostridium histolyticum* and have the ability to break down collagen. A preparation containing a mixture of two collagenases is licensed for the treatment of Dupuytren's contracture; the preparation should be injected into a palpable cord with a contracture of a metacarpophalangeal joint or proximal interphalangeal joint.

The *Scottish Medicines Consortium* (p. 4) has advised (April 2012) that collagenase *Clostridium histolyticum* (*Xiapex*®) is accepted for restricted use within NHS Scotland as an alternative to limited fasciectomy, for the treatment of Dupuytren's contracture of moderate severity (as defined by the British Society for Surgery of the Hand) in patients with a palpable cord and up to two affected joints per hand, who are suitable for limited fasciectomy, but for whom percutaneous needle fasciectomy is not considered a suitable treatment option.

▌COLLAGENASE

Indications Dupuytren's contracture in patients with a palpable cord

Cautions coagulation disorders or use of anticoagulants

Contra-indications avoid injecting into other structures containing collagen (e.g. tendons, nerves, and blood vessels)—risk of tendon rupture or ligament damage

Pregnancy manufacturer advises avoid

Breast-feeding systemic absorption by mother negligible

Side-effects paraesthesia, hypoaesthesia, burning sensation, lymphadenopathy, arthralgia, myalgia, joint swelling, injection site reactions, ecchymosis, hyperhidrosis; *less commonly* complex regional pain syndrome, monoplegia, tremor, crepitus, muscle spasm and weakness, tendon rupture, ligament injury, wound dehiscence

Dose
- By intralesional injection into palpable cord, ADULT over 18 years, 580 micrograms; if necessary repeat at intervals of approx. 4 weeks; max. 3 injections per cord; max. 8 injections in total; only one cord may be treated at a time
  Note reconstitution and injected volumes vary with site of injection—consult product literature

Xiapex® (Auxilium) ▼ PoM
Injection, powder for reconstitution, collagenase *Clostridium histolyticum*, net price 900-microgram vial (with solvent) = £650.00

Hyaluronidase

Hyaluronidase is used to render the tissues more readily permeable to injected fluids, e.g. for introduction of fluids by subcutaneous infusion (termed hypodermoclysis).

▌HYALURONIDASE

Indications enhance permeation of subcutaneous or intramuscular injections, local anaesthetics and subcutaneous infusions; promote resorption of excess fluids and blood

Cautions infants or elderly (control speed and total volume and avoid overhydration especially in renal impairment)

Contra-indications do not apply direct to cornea; avoid sites where infection or malignancy; not for anaesthesia in unexplained premature labour; not to be used to reduce swelling of bites or stings; not for intravenous administration; not to be used to enhance the absorption and dispersion of dopamine and/or alpha-adrenoceptor agonists

Side-effects oedema; *rarely* local irritation, infection, bleeding, bruising; occasional severe allergy (including anaphylaxis)

Dose

- With subcutaneous or intramuscular injection, 1500 units dissolved directly in solution to be injected (ensure compatibility)
- With local anaesthetics, 1500 units mixed with local anaesthetic solution (ophthalmology, 15 units/mL)
- Hypodermoclysis, 1500 units dissolved in 1 mL water for injections or 0.9% sodium chloride injection, administered before start of 500–1000 mL infusion fluid
- Extravasation (see notes above) or haematoma, 1500 units dissolved in 1 mL water for injections or 0.9% sodium chloride injection, infiltrated into affected area (as soon as possible after extravasation)

Hyalase® (Wockhardt) PoM
Injection, powder for reconstitution, hyaluronidase (ovine). Net price 1500-unit amp = £7.60

10.3.2 Rubefacients, topical NSAIDs, capsaicin, and poultices

Rubefacients act by counter-irritation. Pain, whether superficial or deep-seated, is relieved by any method that itself produces irritation of the skin. Topical rubefacient preparations may contain nicotinate and salicylate compounds, essential oils, capsicum, and camphor. The evidence available does not support the use of topical rubefacients in acute or chronic musculoskeletal pain.

Topical NSAIDs

The use of a NSAID by mouth is effective for relieving musculoskeletal pain. **Topical NSAIDs** (e.g. felbinac, ibuprofen, ketoprofen, and piroxicam) may provide some relief of pain in musculoskeletal conditions; they can be considered as an adjunctive treatment in knee or hand osteoarthritis (see section 10.1).

Cautions Apply with gentle massage only. Avoid contact with eyes, mucous membranes, and inflamed or broken skin; discontinue if rash develops. Hands should be washed immediately after use. Not for use with occlusive dressings. Topical application of large amounts can result in systemic effects (see section 10.1.1), including hypersensitivity and asthma (renal disease has also been reported). Not generally suitable for children. Patient packs carry a **warning** to avoid during **pregnancy** or **breast-feeding**.

Hypersensitivity For NSAID hypersensitivity and asthma warning, see p. 717 and p. 718

Photosensitivity Patients should be advised against excessive exposure to sunlight of area treated in order to avoid possibility of photosensitivity. Patients using preparations containing ketoprofen should be advised not to expose area treated to sunbeds or sunlight (even on a bright but cloudy day) during, and for two weeks after stopping treatment; treated areas should be protected with clothing.

◢Non-proprietary preparations

Ibuprofen (Non-proprietary)
Gel, ibuprofen 5%, net price 30 g = £1.28, 50 g = £2.11, 100 g = £4.22. Counselling, photosensitivity, see above
Dose apply up to 3 times daily

Ketoprofen (Non-proprietary) PoM
Gel, ketoprofen 2.5%, net price 30 g = £4.47, 50 g = £1.88, 100 g = £3.76. Counselling, photosensitivity, see above
Dose apply 2–4 times daily for up to 7 days (usual max. 15 g daily)

Piroxicam (Non-proprietary) PoM
Gel, piroxicam 0.5%, net price 60 g = £7.20; 112 g = £13.44. Counselling, photosensitivity, see above
Dose apply 3–4 times daily

◢Proprietary preparations

Feldene® (Pfizer) PoM
Gel, piroxicam 0.5%, net price 60 g = £6.00; 112 g = £9.41 (also 7.5 g starter pack, hosp. only). Counselling, photosensitivity, see above
Excipients include benzyl alcohol, propylene glycol
Dose apply 3–4 times daily; therapy should be reviewed after 4 weeks

¹**Fenbid® Forte Gel** (AMCo) PoM
Gel, ibuprofen 10%, net price 100 g = £4.00. Counselling, photosensitivity, see above
Excipients include benzyl alcohol
Dose apply up to 4 times daily; therapy should be reviewed after 14 days

Ibugel® Forte (Dermal) PoM
Forte gel, ibuprofen 10%, net price 100 g = £5.79.
Counselling, photosensitivity, see above
Excipients none as listed in section 13.1.3
Dose apply up to 3 times daily

¹**Oruvail®** (Sanofi-Aventis) PoM
Gel, ketoprofen 2.5%, net price 100 g = £6.84. Counselling, photosensitivity, see above
Excipients include fragrance
Dose apply 2–4 times daily for up to 7 days (usual recommended dose 15 g daily)

Powergel® (Menarini) PoM
Gel, ketoprofen 2.5%, net price 50 g = £3.06; 100 g = £5.89. Counselling, photosensitivity, see above
Excipients include fragrance
Dose apply 2–3 times daily for up to max. 10 days

Traxam® (AMCo) PoM
Foam, felbinac 3.17%. Net price 100 g = £8.41.
Label: 15, counselling, photosensitivity, see above
Excipients include cetostearyl alcohol
Gel, felbinac 3%. Net price 100 g = £8.03. Counselling, photosensitivity, see above
Excipients none as listed in section 13.1.3
Dose apply 2–4 times daily; max. 25 g daily; therapy should be reviewed after 14 days
Note Felbinac is an active metabolite of the NSAID fenbufen

²**Voltarol Emulgel®** (Novartis) PoM
Gel, diclofenac diethylammonium salt 1.16% (equivalent to diclofenac sodium 1%), net price 20 g (hosp. only) = £1.55; 100 g = £5.63. Counselling, photosensitivity, see above
Excipients include propylene glycol, fragrance
Dose apply 3–4 times daily; therapy should be reviewed after 14 days (or after 28 days for osteoarthritis)

---

1. Smaller pack sizes available on sale to the public
2. Various pack sizes available on sale to the public

Voltarol Gel Patch® (Novartis) PoM

Gel patch, diclofenac epolamine (equivalent to 140 mg diclofenac sodium per patch), net price 10-patch pack = £14.09. Counselling, photosensitivity, see above

Excipients   include hydroxybenzoates (parabens), propylene glycol

Dose ADULT and CHILD over 15 years, ankle sprain, apply 1 patch daily for up to 3 days; epicondylitis, apply 1 patch twice daily for up to 14 days

Capsaicin

A preparation containing capsaicin 0.025% can be considered as an adjunct in hand or knee osteoarthritis (see section 10.1). It may need to be used for 1–2 weeks before pain is relieved.

A capsaicin 0.075% cream is licensed for the symptomatic relief of postherpetic neuralgia (section 4.7.3) after lesions have healed, and for the relief of painful diabetic neuropathy (section 6.1.5).

A self-adhesive patch containing capsaicin 8% is licensed for the treatment of peripheral neuropathic pain in non-diabetic patients.

The *Scottish Medicines Consortium* (p. 4) has advised (January 2011) that capsaicin 179 mg (8%) patch (*Qutenza*®) is accepted for restricted use within NHS Scotland for the treatment of postherpetic neuralgia in patients who have not achieved adequate pain relief from, or who have not tolerated conventional first and second-line treatments. Treatment should be under the supervision of a specialist in pain management.

Zacin® (TEVA UK) PoM

Cream, capsaicin 0.025%, net price 45 g = £17.71.

Excipients   include benzyl alcohol, cetyl alcohol

Cautions   avoid contact with eyes, inflamed or broken skin; wash hands immediately after use (or wash hands 30 minutes after application if hands treated); not to be used under tight bandages; avoid hot shower or bath just before or after application (burning sensation enhanced); avoid inhalation of vapours

Side-effects   transient burning sensation during initial treatment (particularly if too much used or if administered less than 4 times daily); *rarely* cough, sneezing, eye irritation; dyspnoea and exacerbation of asthma also reported

Dose symptomatic relief in osteoarthritis, apply sparingly 4 times daily (not more often than every 4 hours)

Axsain® (TEVA UK) PoM

Cream, capsaicin 0.075%, net price 45 g = £14.58.

Excipients   include benzyl alcohol, cetyl alcohol

Cautions   avoid contact with eyes, inflamed or broken skin; wash hands immediately after use (or wash hands 30 minutes after application if hands treated); not to be used under tight bandages; avoid hot shower or bath just before or after application (burning sensation enhanced); avoid inhalation of vapours

Side-effects   transient burning sensation during initial treatment (particularly if too much used or if administered less than 3–4 times daily); *rarely* cough, sneezing, eye irritation; dyspnoea and exacerbation of asthma also reported

Dose post-herpetic neuralgia (important: after lesions have healed), apply sparingly up to 3–4 times daily (not more often than every 4 hours)

Painful diabetic neuropathy, under specialist supervision, apply sparingly 3–4 times daily (not more often than every 4 hours) for 8 weeks then review

Qutenza® (Astellas) PoM

Patches, self-adhesive, capsaicin 179 mg (8%), net price 1 × 280 cm² patch (with cleansing gel) = £210.00.

Excipients   include butylated hydroxyanisole in cleansing gel (see section 13.1.3)

Cautions   avoid holding near eyes or mucous membranes; avoid contact with inflamed or broken skin, the face, scalp or in proximity to mucous membranes; monitor blood pressure during treatment procedure; uncontrolled hypertension; recent cardiovascular events

Side-effects   application site reactions including transient burning, erythema, pruritus; *less commonly* nausea; peripheral oedema, first degree AV block, tachycardia, palpitations, hypertension; cough, throat irritation; hypoaesthesia, burning sensation, dysgeusia; pain in extremities, muscle spasm; eye irritation; pruritus

Dose peripheral neuropathic pain in non-diabetic patients, applied under supervision of a physician, consult product literature

Note Nitrile gloves to be worn while handling patches and cleaning treatment areas (latex gloves do not provide adequate protection)

Poultices

Kaolin Poultice

Poultice, heavy kaolin 52.7%, thymol 0.05%, boric acid 4.5%, peppermint oil 0.05%, methyl salicylate 0.2%, glycerol 42.5%. Net price 200 g = £2.76

Dose warm and apply directly or between layers of muslin; avoid application of overheated poultice

Kaolin Poultice K/L Pack® (K/L)

Kaolin poultice Net price 4 × 100-g pouches = £6.40

11 Eye

11 Eye

11.1 Administration of drugs to the eye

Drugs are most commonly administered to the eye by topical application as eye drops or eye ointments. When a higher drug concentration is required within the eye, a local injection may be necessary, see Other Preparations, below.

Eye-drop dispenser devices are available to aid the instillation of eye drops from plastic bottles and some are prescribable on the NHS (consult Drug Tariff—see Appliances and Reagents, p. 1112 for links to online Drug Tariffs). Product-specific devices may be supplied by manufacturers—consult individual manufacturers for information. They are particularly useful for the elderly, visually impaired, arthritic, or otherwise physically limited patients.

Eye drops and eye ointments Eye drops are generally instilled into the pocket formed by gently pulling down the lower eyelid and keeping the eye closed for as long as possible after application; one drop is all that is needed. Instillation of more than one drop should be discouraged because it may increase systemic side-effects. A small amount of eye ointment is applied similarly; the ointment melts rapidly and blinking helps to spread it.

When two different eye-drop preparations are used at the same time of day, dilution and overflow may occur when one immediately follows the other. The patient should therefore leave an interval of at least 5 minutes between the two; the interval should be extended when eye drops with a prolonged contact time, such as gels and suspensions, are used. Eye ointment should be applied after drops.

Systemic effects may arise from absorption of drugs into the general circulation from conjunctival vessels or from the nasal mucosa after the excess preparation has drained down through the tear ducts. The extent of systemic absorption following ocular administration is highly variable; nasal drainage of drugs is associated with eye drops much more often than with eye ointments. Pressure on the lacrimal punctum for at least a minute after applying eye drops reduces nasolacrimal drainage and therefore decreases systemic absorption from the nasal mucosa.

After using eye drops or eye ointments, patients should be warned not to drive or perform other skilled tasks until vision is clear.

For warnings relating to eye drops and contact lenses, see section 11.9.

Eye lotions These are solutions for the irrigation of the conjunctival sac. They act mechanically to flush out irritants or foreign bodies as a first-aid treatment. Sterile sodium chloride 0.9% solution (section 11.8.1) is usually used. Clean water will suffice in an emergency.

Ophthalmic Specials The Royal College of Ophthalmologists and the UK Ophthalmic Pharmacy Group have produced the Ophthalmic Specials Guidance to help prescribers and pharmacists manage and restrict the use of unlicensed eye preparations. 'Specials' should only be prescribed in situations where a licensed product is not suitable for a patient's needs. The Ophthalmic Specials Guidance can be accessed on the Royal College of Ophthalmologists website (www. rcophth.ac.uk). The guidance will be reviewed every six months to ensure the most accurate and up-to-date information is available.

Other preparations Subconjunctival injection may be used to administer anti-infective drugs, mydriatics, or corticosteroids for conditions not responding to topical therapy; intracameral and intravitreal routes can also be used to administer certain drugs, for example antibacterials. These injections should only be used under specialist supervision.

Drugs such as antimicrobials and corticosteroids may be administered systemically to treat susceptible eye conditions.

Preservatives and sensitisers Information on preservatives and on substances identified as skin sensitisers (see section 13.1.3) is provided under Excipients statements in preparation entries. Very rarely, cases of corneal calcification have been reported with the use of phosphate-containing eye drops in patients with significantly damaged corneas—consult product literature for further information.

11.2 Control of microbial contamination

Preparations for the eye should be sterile when issued. Care should be taken to avoid contamination of the contents during use.

Eye drops in multiple-application containers for *domiciliary use* should not be used for more than 4 weeks after first opening (unless otherwise stated by the manufacturer).

Multiple application eye drops for use in *hospital wards* are normally discarded 1 week after first opening—local practice may vary. Individual containers should be provided for each patient. A separate container should be supplied for each eye only if there are special concerns about contamination. Containers used before an eye operation should be discarded at the time of the operation and fresh containers supplied postoperatively. A fresh supply should also be provided upon discharge from hospital; in specialist ophthalmology units, it may be acceptable to issue containers that have been dispensed to the patient on the day of discharge.

In *out-patient departments* single-application containers should be used; if multiple-application containers are used, they should be discarded after single patient use within one clinical session.

In *eye surgery* single-application containers should be used if possible; if a multiple-application container is used, it should be discarded after single use. Preparations used during intra-ocular procedures and others that may penetrate into the anterior chamber must be isotonic and without preservatives and buffered if necessary to a neutral pH. Specially formulated fluids should be used for intra-ocular surgery; intravenous infusion preparations are not usually suitable for this purpose (Hartmann's solution may be used in some ocular surgery). For all surgical procedures, a previously unopened container is used for each patient.

11.3 Anti-infective eye preparations

11.3.1   Antibacterials
11.3.2   Antifungals
11.3.3   Antivirals

Eye infections Most acute superficial eye infections can be treated topically. Blepharitis and conjunctivitis are often caused by staphylococci; keratitis and endophthalmitis may be bacterial, viral, or fungal.

Bacterial *blepharitis* is treated by application of an antibacterial eye ointment to the conjunctival sac or to the lid margins. Systemic treatment may occasionally be required and is usually undertaken after culturing organisms from the lid margin and determining their antimicrobial sensitivity; antibiotics such as the tetracyclines given for 3 months or longer may be appropriate.

Most cases of acute bacterial conjunctivitis are self-limiting; where treatment is appropriate, antibacterial eye drops or an eye ointment are used. A poor response might indicate viral or allergic conjunctivitis.

Corneal ulcer and *keratitis* require specialist treatment and may call for hospital admission for intensive therapy.

Endophthalmitis is a medical emergency which also calls for specialist management and requires intravitreal administration of antimicrobials; concomitant systemic treatment is required in some cases. Surgical intervention, such as vitrectomy, is sometimes indicated.

11.3.1 Antibacterials

Bacterial eye infections are generally treated topically with eye drops and eye ointments. Systemic administration is sometimes appropriate in blepharitis.

Chloramphenicol has a broad spectrum of activity and is the drug of choice for *superficial eye infections*. Chloramphenicol eye drops are well tolerated and the recommendation that chloramphenicol eye drops should be avoided because of an increased risk of aplastic anaemia is not well founded.

Other antibacterials with a broad spectrum of activity include the quinolones, **ciprofloxacin**, **levofloxacin**, **moxifloxacin**, and **ofloxacin**; the aminoglycosides, **gentamicin** and **tobramycin** are also active against a wide variety of bacteria. Gentamicin, tobramycin, quinolones (except moxifloxacin), and **polymyxin B** are effective for infections caused by *Pseudomonas aeruginosa*.

Ciprofloxacin eye drops are licensed for *corneal ulcers*; intensive application (especially in the first 2 days) is required throughout the day and night.

Azithromycin eye drops are licensed for trachomatous conjunctivitis caused by *Chlamydia trachomatis* and for purulent bacterial conjunctivitis. *Trachoma* which results from chronic infection with *Chlamydia trachomatis* can be treated with azithromycin by mouth [unlicensed indication].

Fusidic acid is useful for staphylococcal infections.

Propamidine isetionate is of little value in bacterial infections but is used by specialists to treat the rare, but

11   Eye

potentially sight-threatening, condition of *acanthamoeba keratitis* [unlicensed indication] (see also section 11.9).

Cefuroxime can be administered by intracameral injection for the prophylaxis of endophthalmitis following cataract surgery, see section 11.8.2.

With corticosteroids Many antibacterial preparations also incorporate a corticosteroid but such mixtures should **not** be used unless a patient is under close specialist supervision. In particular they should not be prescribed for undiagnosed 'red eye' which is sometimes caused by the herpes simplex virus and may be difficult to diagnose (section 11.4).

Administration Frequency of application depends on the severity of the infection and the potential for irreversible ocular damage; antibacterial eye preparations are usually administered as follows:

- *Eye drops*, apply 1 drop at least every 2 hours then reduce frequency as infection is controlled and continue for 48 hours after healing;
- *Eye ointment*, apply *either* at night (if eye drops used during the day) *or* 3–4 times daily (if eye ointment used alone).

◾ AZITHROMYCIN DIHYDRATE

Indications see notes above
Side-effects ocular discomfort (including pruritus, burning), blurred vision; *less commonly* eyelid eczema, eyelid erythema, eyelid oedema, conjunctival hyperaemia, keratitis
Dose
- Apply twice daily for 3 days; review if no improvement after 3 days

◢ **Single use**
Azyter® (Spectrum Thea) PoM
Eye drops, azithromycin dihydrate 1.5%, net price 6 × 0.25-g = £6.99

◾ CHLORAMPHENICOL

Indications see notes above
Pregnancy avoid unless essential—no information on *topical* use but risk of 'neonatal grey-baby syndrome' with *oral* use in third trimester
Breast-feeding avoid unless essential—*theoretical* risk of bone-marrow toxicity
Side-effects transient stinging; see also notes above
Dose
- See Administration in notes above

Chloramphenicol (Non-proprietary) PoM
Eye drops, chloramphenicol 0.5%. Net price 10 mL = £1.78
Eye ointment, chloramphenicol 1%. Net price 4 g = £1.76
Note Chloramphenicol 0.5% eye drops (in max. pack size 10 mL) and 1% eye ointment (in max. pack size 4 g) can be sold to the public for treatment of acute bacterial conjunctivitis in adults and children over 2 years; max. duration of treatment 5 days

Chloromycetin® (AMCo) PoM
Redidrops (= eye drops), chloramphenicol 0.5%. Net price 5 mL = £1.65; 10 mL = 90p
Excipients include phenylmercuric acetate
Ophthalmic ointment (= eye ointment), chloramphenicol 1%. Net price 4 g = £1.08

◢ **Single use**
Minims® Chloramphenicol (Bausch & Lomb) PoM
Eye drops, chloramphenicol 0.5%. Net price 20 × 0.5 mL = £10.53

◾ CIPROFLOXACIN

Indications superficial bacterial infections, see notes above; corneal ulcers
Pregnancy manufacturer advises use only if potential benefit outweighs risk
Breast-feeding manufacturer advises caution
Side-effects taste disturbance, ocular discomfort, ocular hyperaemia, corneal deposits (reversible after completion of treatment); *less commonly* nausea, headache, keratopathy, corneal infiltrates, corneal staining, photophobia, blurred vision, eyelid disorders (including oedema, exfoliation, erythema), eye irritation (including pain, swelling, pruritus, dryness), increased lacrimation, conjunctival hyperaemia; *rarely* diarrhoea, abdominal pain, dizziness, keratitis, corneal disorders including corneal epithelial defect, eye hypoaesthesia, asthenopia, diplopia, ear pain, paranasal sinus hypersecretion, rhinitis, dermatitis
Dose
- Superficial bacterial infection, ADULT and CHILD apply *eye drops* 4 times daily; in severe infection apply every 2 hours during waking hours for 2 days, then 4 times daily; max. duration of treatment 21 days
  ADULT and CHILD over 1 year, apply 1.25 cm *eye ointment* 3 times daily for 2 days, then twice daily for 5 days
- Corneal ulcer, ADULT and CHILD apply *eye drops* throughout day and night, day 1 apply every 15 minutes for 6 hours then every 30 minutes, day 2 apply every hour, days 3–14 apply every 4 hours; max. duration of treatment 21 days
  ADULT and CHILD over 1 year, apply *eye ointment* throughout day and night; apply 1.25 cm ointment every 1–2 hours for 2 days, then every 4 hours for next 12 days

Ciloxan® (Alcon) PoM
Ophthalmic solution (= eye drops), ciprofloxacin (as hydrochloride) 0.3%. Net price 5 mL = £4.70
Excipients include benzalkonium chloride
Eye ointment, ciprofloxacin (as hydrochloride) 0.3%. Net price 3.5 g = £5.22

◾ FUSIDIC ACID

Indications see notes above
Dose
- See under preparation below

Fucithalmic® (AMCo) PoM
Eye drops, fusidic acid 1% in gel basis (liquifies on contact with eye). Net price 5 g = £2.69
Excipients include benzalkonium chloride, disodium edetate
Dose apply twice daily

◾ GENTAMICIN

Indications see notes above
Dose
- See Administration in notes above

Genticin® (AMCo) PoM
Drops (for ear or eye), gentamicin (as sulfate) 0.3%. Net price 10 mL = £2.13
Excipients include benzalkonium chloride

11 Eye

LEVOFLOXACIN

Indications   see notes above

Pregnancy   manufacturer advises use only if potential benefit outweighs risk

Breast-feeding   manufacturer advises use only if potential benefit outweighs risk

Side-effects   ocular burning, visual disturbances; *less commonly* headache, ocular discomfort (including itching, pain, and dryness), conjunctival follicles, lid oedema, lid erythema, photophobia, rhinitis

Dose

- ADULT and CHILD over 1 year, apply every 2 hours (max. 8 times daily) for the first 2 days, then 4 times daily for 3 days

Oftaquix® (Kestrel Ophthalmics) PoM
Eye drops, levofloxacin 0.5%, net price 5 mL = £6.95
Excipients   include benzalkonium chloride
Unit dose eye drops, levofloxacin 0.5%, net price 30 × 0.5-mL single use units = £17.95

MOXIFLOXACIN

Indications   see notes above

Cautions   not recommended for neonates

Side-effects   taste disturbances, ocular discomfort (including pain, irritation and dryness), hyperaemia; *less commonly* vomiting, headache, paraesthesia, corneal disorders (including keratitis, erosion, and staining), conjunctival haemorrhage, eyelid erythema, visual disturbances, nasal discomfort, pharyngolaryngeal pain; *also reported* **nausea**, palpitation, dyspnoea, dizziness, raised intra-ocular pressure, photophobia, rash, pruritus

Dose

- ADULT and CHILD over 1 month, apply 3 times daily (continue treatment for 2–3 days after infection improves; review if no improvement within 5 days)

Moxivig® (Alcon) PoM
Eye drops, moxifloxacin (as hydrochloride) 0.5%, net price 5 mL = £9.80

OFLOXACIN

Indications   see notes above

Cautions   corneal ulcer or epithelial defect (risk of corneal perforation)

Pregnancy   manufacturer advises use only if benefit outweighs risk; systemic quinolones have caused arthropathy in *animal* studies

Breast-feeding   manufacturer advises avoid

Side-effects   ocular discomfort and irritation; *also reported* facial oedema, keratitis, visual disturbances, photophobia, increased lacrimation, ocular oedema, dry eyes, ocular hyperaemia

Dose

- ADULT and CHILD over 1 year, apply every 2–4 hours for the first 2 days, then reduce frequency to 4 times daily (max. 10 days treatment)

Exocin® (Allergan) PoM
Ophthalmic solution (= eye drops), ofloxacin 0.3%. Net price 5 mL = £2.17
Excipients   include benzalkonium chloride

PROPAMIDINE ISETIONATE

Indications   local treatment of infections (but see notes above)

Pregnancy   manufacturer advises avoid unless essential—no information available

Breast-feeding   manufacturer advises avoid unless essential—no information available

Side-effects   eye pain and irritation

Dose

- See preparations

Brolene® (Sanofi-Aventis)
Eye drops, propamidine isetionate 0.1%. Net price 10 mL = £2.80
Excipients   include benzalkonium chloride
Dose   apply up to 4 times daily
Eye ointment, dibrompropamidine isetionate 0.15%. Net price 5 g = £2.92
Dose   apply 1–2 times daily

Golden Eye® (Typharm)
Eye drops, propamidine isetionate 0.1%, net price 10 mL = £3.26
Excipients   include benzalkonium chloride
Dose   apply up to 4 times daily
Eye ointment, dibrompropamidine isetionate 0.15%, net price 5 g = £3.49
Dose   apply 1–2 times daily

TOBRAMYCIN

Indications   see notes above

Dose

- ADULT and CHILD over 1 year, apply twice daily for 6–8 days; in severe infection, apply 4 times daily on the first day, then twice daily for 5–7 days

Tobravisc® (Alcon) PoM
Eye drops, tobramycin 0.3%, net price 5 mL = £4.74
Excipients   include benzododecinium bromide

11.3.2 Antifungals

Fungal infections of the cornea are rare but can occur after agricultural injuries, especially in hot and humid climates. Orbital mycosis is rarer, and when it occurs it is usually because of direct spread of infection from the paranasal sinuses. Increasing age, debility, or immunosuppression can encourage fungal proliferation. The spread of infection through blood occasionally produces metastatic endophthalmitis.

Many different fungi are capable of producing ocular infection; they can be identified by appropriate laboratory procedures.

Antifungal preparations for the eye are not generally available. Treatment will normally be carried out at specialist centres, but requests for information about supplies of preparations not available commercially should be addressed to the Strategic Health Authority (or equivalent), or to the nearest hospital ophthalmology unit, or to Moorfields Eye Hospital, 162 City Road, London EC1V 2PD (tel. (020) 7253 3411) *or* www.moorfields.nhs.uk

11 Eye

11.3.3 Antivirals

Herpes simplex infections producing, for example, dendritic corneal ulcers can be treated with **aciclovir** or **ganciclovir**. Aciclovir eye ointment is used in combination with systemic treatment for ophthalmic zoster (section 5.3.2.1).

Slow-release ocular implants containing **ganciclovir** (available on a named-patient basis from specialist importing companies, see p. 1124) may be inserted surgically to treat immediate sight-threatening CMV retinitis. Local treatments do not protect against systemic infection or infection in the other eye. For systemic treatment of CMV retinitis, see section 5.3.2.2.

▌ ACICLOVIR

(Acyclovir)

Indications local treatment of herpes simplex infections

Side-effects local irritation and inflammation, superficial punctate keratopathy; *rarely* blepharitis; *very rarely* hypersensitivity reactions including angioedema

Dose
- Apply 1 cm ointment 5 times daily (continue for at least 3 days after complete healing)

Zovirax® (GSK) PoM
Eye ointment, aciclovir 3%, net price 4.5 g = £9.34

▌ GANCICLOVIR

Indications local treatment of herpes simplex infections

Side-effects burning sensation, tingling, superficial punctate keratitis

Dose
- Apply 5 times daily until healing complete, then apply 3 times daily for a further 7 days

Virgan® (Spectrum Thea) PoM
Ophthalmic gel, ganciclovir 0.15%, net price 5 g = £19.99
Excipients include benzalkonium chloride

11.4 Corticosteroids and other anti-inflammatory preparations

11.4.1 Corticosteroids

11.4.2 Other anti-inflammatory preparations

11.4.1 Corticosteroids

Corticosteroids administered locally to the eye or given by mouth are effective for treating anterior segment inflammation, including that which results from surgery.

Topical corticosteroids are applied frequently for the first 24–48 hours; once inflammation is controlled, the frequency of application is reduced. They should normally only be used under expert supervision; three main dangers are associated with their use:

- a 'red eye', when the diagnosis is unconfirmed, may be due to herpes simplex virus, and a corticosteroid may aggravate the condition, leading to corneal ulceration, with possible damage to vision and even loss of the eye. Bacterial, fungal, and amoebic infections pose a similar hazard;

- 'steroid glaucoma' can follow the use of corticosteroid eye preparations in susceptible individuals;

- a 'steroid cataract' can follow prolonged use.

Other side-effects of ocular corticosteroids include thinning of the cornea and sclera.

Combination products containing a corticosteroid with an anti-infective drug are sometimes used after ocular surgery to reduce inflammation and prevent infection; use of combination products is otherwise rarely justified.

Systemic corticosteroids (section 6.3.2) may be useful for ocular conditions. The risk of producing a 'steroid cataract' increases with the dose and duration of corticosteroid use.

▌ BETAMETHASONE

Indications local treatment of inflammation (short-term)

Cautions see notes above

Side-effects see notes above

Dose
- Apply eye drops every 1–2 hours until controlled then reduce frequency; apply eye ointment 2–4 times daily *or* at night when used with eye drops

Betnesol® (Focus) PoM
Drops (for ear, eye, or nose), betamethasone sodium phosphate 0.1%, net price 10 mL = £2.32
Excipients include benzalkonium chloride, disodium edetate
Eye ointment, betamethasone sodium phosphate 0.1%, net price 3 g = £1.41

Vistamethasone® (Martindale) PoM
Drops (for ear, eye, or nose), betamethasone sodium phosphate 0.1%, net price 5 mL = £1.02; 10 mL = £1.16
Excipients include benzalkonium chloride

◢With neomycin
Betnesol-N® (RPH) PoM ◢
Drops (for ear, eye, or nose), see section 12.1.1
Dose apply up to 6 times daily

▌ DEXAMETHASONE

Indications local treatment of inflammation (short-term)

Cautions see notes above

Side-effects see notes above

Dose
- Apply eye drops every 30–60 minutes until controlled then reduce frequency to 4–6 times daily

Maxidex® (Alcon) PoM
Eye drops, dexamethasone 0.1%, net price 5 mL = £1.42; 10 mL = £2.80
Excipients include benzalkonium chloride, disodium edetate, polysorbate 80

11 Eye

◢Single use

Dexafree® (Spectrum Thea) PoM

Eye drops, dexamethasone phosphate (as sodium phosphate) 0.1%, net price 30 × 0.4 mL = £9.70
Excipients include edetate

Dropodex® (Moorfields) PoM

Eye drops, dexamethasone (as sodium phosphate) 0.1%, net price 20 × 0.4 mL = £9.75
Excipients include disodium edetate

Minims® Dexamethasone (Bausch & Lomb) PoM

Eye drops, dexamethasone sodium phosphate 0.1%, net price 20 × 0.5 mL = £10.98
Excipients include disodium edetate

◢With antibacterials

Maxitrol® (Alcon) PoM ◢

Eye drops, dexamethasone 0.1%, neomycin sulfate 3500 units /g, polymyxin B sulfate 6000 units/mL, net price 5 mL = £1.68
Excipients include benzalkonium chloride, polysorbate 20

Eye ointment, dexamethasone 0.1%, neomycin sulfate 3500 units/g, polymyxin B sulfate 6000 units/g, net price 3.5 g = £1.44
Excipients include hydroxybenzoates (parabens), wool fat
Dose apply 3–4 times daily *or* at night when used with eye drops

Sofradex® (Sanofi-Aventis) PoM ◢

Drops (for ear or eye), see section 12.1.1

Tobradex® (Alcon) PoM ◢

Eye drops, dexamethasone 0.1%, tobramycin 0.3%, net price 5 mL = £5.37
Excipients include benzalkonium chloride, disodium edetate

◤ **FLUOROMETHOLONE**

Indications local treatment of inflammation (short-term)
Cautions see notes above
Side-effects see notes above
Dose

• ADULT and CHILD over 2 years, apply every hour for 24–48 hours, then reduce frequency to 2–4 times daily

FML® (Allergan) PoM

Ophthalmic suspension (= eye drops), fluorometholone 0.1%, polyvinyl alcohol (*Liquifilm®*) 1.4%, net price 5 mL = £1.71; 10 mL = £2.95
Excipients include benzalkonium chloride, disodium edetate, polysorbate 80

◤ **LOTEPREDNOL ETABONATE**

Indications treatment of post-operative inflammation following ocular surgery
Cautions see notes above
Side-effects see notes above
Dose

• Apply 4 times daily starting 24 hours after surgery; max. duration of treatment 14 days

Lotemax® (Bausch & Lomb) PoM

Opthalmic suspension (= eye drops), loteprednol etabonate 0.5%, net price 5 mL = £5.50
Excipients include benzalkonium chloride, disodium edetate

◤ **PREDNISOLONE**

Indications local treatment of inflammation (short-term)
Cautions see notes above
Side-effects see notes above
Dose

• Apply every 1–2 hours until controlled then reduce frequency

Predsol® (Focus) PoM

Drops (for ear or eye), prednisolone sodium phosphate 0.5%, net price 10 mL = £2.00
Excipients include benzalkonium chloride, disodium edetate

Pred Forte® (Allergan) PoM

Eye drops, prednisolone acetate 1%, net price 5 mL = £1.82; 10 mL = £3.66
Excipients include benzalkonium chloride, disodium edetate, polysorbate 80

◢Single use

Minims® Prednisolone Sodium Phosphate (Bausch & Lomb) PoM

Eye drops, prednisolone sodium phosphate 0.5%, net price 20 × 0.5 mL = £11.28
Excipients include disodium edetate

◤ **RIMEXOLONE**

Indications local treatment of inflammation (short-term)
Cautions see notes above
Side-effects see notes above
Dose

• Postoperative inflammation, apply 4 times daily for 2 weeks, beginning 24 hours after surgery
• Steroid-responsive inflammation, apply at least 4 times daily for up to 4 weeks
• Uveitis, apply every hour during daytime in week 1, then every 2 hours in week 2, then 4 times daily in week 3, then twice daily for first 4 days of week 4, then once daily for remaining 3 days of week 4

Vexol® (Alcon) PoM

Eye drops, rimexolone 1%, net price 5 mL = £5.66
Excipients include benzalkonium chloride, disodium edetate, polysorbate 80

Intravitreal corticosteroids

An intravitreal implant containing **dexamethasone** (*Ozurdex®*) is licensed for the treatment of adults with macular oedema following either branch retinal vein occlusion or central retinal vein occlusion; it is also licensed for the treatment of adult patients with inflammation of the posterior segment of the eye presenting as non-infectious uveitis. Dexamethasone is also indicated for the treatment of visual impairment due to diabetic macular oedema in adults who are pseudophakic, or who are insufficiently responsive to, or unsuitable for non-corticosteroid therapy. It should be administered by specialists experienced in the use of intravitreal injections.

The *Scottish Medicines Consortium*, (p. 4) has advised (May 2012) that dexamethasone intravitreal implant (*Ozurdex®*) is accepted for restricted use within NHS Scotland for the treatment of adults with macular oedema (i) following central retinal vein occlusion, and (ii) with branch retinal vein occlusion who are not

11 Eye

clinically suitable for laser treatment, including patients with dense macular haemorrhage, or patients who have received and failed on previous laser treatment.

NICE guidance
Dexamethasone intravitreal implant for the treatment of macular oedema secondary to retinal vein occlusion (July 2011)

Dexamethasone intravitreal implant is recommended as an option for the treatment of macular oedema following central retinal vein occlusion.

Dexamethasone intravitreal implant is also recommended as an option for the treatment of macular oedema following branch retinal vein occlusion when:

- treatment with laser photocoagulation has not been beneficial, or
- treatment with laser photocoagulation is not considered suitable because of the extent of macular haemorrhage.

www.nice.org.uk/TA229

An intravitreal implant containing **fluocinolone acetonide** (*Iluvien*®) is licensed for the treatment of visual impairment associated with chronic diabetic macular oedema which is insufficiently responsive to available therapies. It should be administered by specialists experienced in the use of intravitreal injections.

The *Scottish Medicines Consortium*, (p. 4) has advised (February 2014) that fluocinolone acetonide intravitreal implant (*Iluvien*®) is recommended for restricted use within NHS Scotland for the treatment of vision impairment associated with chronic diabetic macular oedema, considered insufficiently responsive to available therapies, only in patients in whom the affected eye is pseudophakic (has an artificial lens after cataract surgery), **and** retreatment would take place only if the patient had previously responded to treatment with fluocinolone acetonide and subsequently best corrected visual acuity had deteriorated to less than 20/32.

NICE guidance
Fluocinolone acetonide intravitreal implant for treating chronic diabetic macular oedema after an inadequate response to prior therapy (November 2013)

Fluocinolone acetonide intravitreal implant is recommended as an option for treating chronic diabetic macular oedema that is insufficiently responsive to available therapies only if:

- the implant is to be used in an eye with an intra-ocular (pseudophakic) lens and
- the manufacturer provides fluocinolone acetonide intravitreal implant with the discount agreed in the patient access scheme.

www.nice.org.uk/TA301

DEXAMETHASONE

Indications see notes above—specialist use only

Cautions monitor intra-ocular pressure and for signs of ocular infection; history of ocular viral infection including herpes simplex; posterior capsule tear or iris defect (risk of implant migration into the anterior chamber which may cause corneal oedema and, in persistent severe cases, the need for corneal transplantation—monitor for early diagnosis and man-

agement); retinal vein occlusion with significant retinal ischaemia; concomitant administration of anticoagulant or antiplatelet drugs—increased risk of haemorrhagic events

Contra-indications active or suspected ocular or peri-ocular infection (including active ocular herpes simplex); uncontrolled advanced glaucoma; rupture of the posterior lens capsule in patients with aphakia, iris or transscleral fixated intra-ocular lens or anterior chamber intra-ocular lens

Pregnancy manufacturer advises avoid unless potential benefit outweighs risk

Breast-feeding manufacturer advises avoid unless potential benefit outweighs risk—no information available

Side-effects headache, raised intra-ocular pressure, ocular hypertension, blepharitis, cataract, visual disturbance; *less commonly* migraine, necrotising retinitis, eyelid pruritus, glaucoma; *also reported* secondary ocular infection

Dose
- By intravitreal injection, 700 micrograms into the affected eye
  Note Concurrent administration to both eyes not recommended. For further information on pre-treatment, administration and repeat dosing, consult product literature

Ozurdex® (Allergan) ▼ PoM
Intravitreal implant, dexamethasone 700 micrograms in disposable applicator, net price = £870.00

FLUOCINOLONE ACETONIDE

Indications see notes above—specialist use only

Cautions raised baseline intra-ocular pressure (monitor intra-ocular pressure closely); monitor for raised intra-ocular pressure, retinal detachment, endophthalmitis, vitreous haemorrhage or detachment within 2–7 days following the procedure; monitor intra-ocular pressure at least every 3 months thereafter (for approximately 36 months); concomitant administration of anticoagulant or antiplatelet drugs (higher incidence of conjunctival haemorrhage)

Contra-indications pre-existing glaucoma; active or suspected ocular or peri-ocular infection

Pregnancy manufacturer advises avoid unless potential benefit outweighs risk—no information available

Breast-feeding manufacturer advises avoid unless essential

Side-effects cataract, raised intra-ocular pressure, vitreous floaters, glaucoma, ocular discomfort, vitreous haemorrhage, conjunctival haemorrhage, blurred vision, reduced visual acuity; *less commonly* headache, endophthalmitis, retinal vascular occlusion, optic nerve disorder, maculopathy, optic atrophy, conjunctival ulcer, iris neovascularisation or adhesions, retinal exudates, vitreous degeneration or detachment, posterior capsule opacification, ocular hyperaemia, sclera thinning, eye discharge or pruritus

Dose
- By intravitreal injection, 190 micrograms into the affected eye
  Note Concurrent administration to both eyes not recommended. For further information on administration and repeat dosing, consult product literature

Iluvien® (Alimera) ▼ PoM
Intravitreal implant, fluocinolone acetonide 190 micrograms in a disposable applicator, net price = £5500.00

11.4.2 Other anti-inflammatory preparations

Other preparations used for the topical treatment of inflammation and allergic conjunctivitis include antihistamines, lodoxamide, and sodium cromoglicate.

Eye drops containing antihistamines, such as **antazoline** (with xylometazoline as *Otrivine-Antistin*®), **azelastine**, **epinastine**, **ketotifen**, and **olopatadine**, can be used for allergic conjunctivitis.

Sodium cromoglicate (sodium cromoglycate) and **nedocromil sodium** eye drops can be useful for vernal keratoconjunctivitis and other allergic forms of conjunctivitis.

Lodoxamide eye drops are used for allergic conjunctival conditions including seasonal allergic conjunctivitis.

Diclofenac eye drops (section 11.8.2) and **emedastine** eye drops are also licensed for seasonal allergic conjunctivitis.

Non-steroidal anti-inflammatory eye drops (section 11.8.2) are used for the prophylaxis and treatment of inflammation of the eye following surgery or laser treatment.

ANTAZOLINE SULFATE

Indications   allergic conjunctivitis

Side-effects   transient stinging; *also reported* blurred vision, mydriasis, eye irritation

Otrivine-Antistin® (Spectrum Thea)
Eye drops, antazoline sulfate 0.5%, xylometazoline hydrochloride 0.05%. Net price 10 mL = £2.35
Excipients   include benzalkonium chloride, disodium edetate
Cautions   hypertension; hyperthyroidism; diabetes mellitus; angle-closure glaucoma; phaeochromocytoma; cardiovascular disease; urinary retention; **interactions**: Appendix 1 (antihistamines and sympathomimetics)
Dose   ADULT and CHILD over 12 years apply 2–3 times daily (max. 7 days)
Note   Xylometazoline is a sympathomimetic; absorption of antazoline and xylometazoline may result in systemic side-effects and the possibility of interaction with other drugs

AZELASTINE HYDROCHLORIDE

Indications   allergic conjunctivitis

Side-effects   mild transient irritation; bitter taste reported

Dose
• Seasonal allergic conjunctivitis, ADULT and CHILD over 4 years, apply twice daily, increased if necessary to 4 times daily
• Perennial conjunctivitis, ADULT and CHILD over 12 years, apply twice daily, increased if necessary to 4 times daily; max. duration of treatment 6 weeks

Optilast® (Meda) [PoM]
Eye drops, azelastine hydrochloride 0.05%. Net price 8 mL = £6.40
Excipients   include benzalkonium chloride, disodium edetate

EMEDASTINE

Indications   seasonal allergic conjunctivitis

Side-effects   transient burning or stinging; blurred vision, local oedema, keratitis, irritation, dry eye, lacrimation, corneal infiltrates (discontinue) and staining; photophobia; headache, and rhinitis occasionally reported

Dose
• ADULT and CHILD over 3 years, apply twice daily

Emadine® (Alcon) [PoM]
Eye drops, emedastine 0.05% (as difumarate), net price 5 mL = £7.31
Excipients   include benzalkonium chloride

EPINASTINE HYDROCHLORIDE

Indications   seasonal allergic conjunctivitis

Side-effects   burning; *less commonly* taste disturbance, headache, conjunctival hyperaemia, dry eye, eye pruritus, visual disturbance, increased lacrimation, eye pain, nasal irritation, rhinitis

Dose
• ADULT and CHILD over 12 years, apply twice daily; max. duration of treatment 8 weeks

Relestat® (Allergan) [PoM]
Eye drops, epinastine hydrochloride 500 micrograms/mL, net price 5 mL = £9.90
Excipients   include benzalkonium chloride, disodium edetate

KETOTIFEN

Indications   seasonal allergic conjunctivitis

Side-effects   transient burning or stinging, punctate corneal epithelial erosion; *less commonly* dry eye, subconjunctival haemorrhage, photophobia; headache, drowsiness, skin reactions, and dry mouth also reported

Dose
• ADULT and CHILD over 3 years, apply twice daily

Zaditen® (Spectrum Thea) [PoM]
Eye drops, ketotifen (as fumarate) 250 micrograms/mL, net price 5 mL = £7.80
Excipients   include benzalkonium chloride

LODOXAMIDE

Indications   allergic conjunctivitis

Side-effects   burning, stinging, itching, blurred vision, tear production disturbance, and ocular discomfort; *less commonly* flushing, nasal dryness, dizziness, drowsiness, headache, blepharitis and keratitis

Dose
• ADULT and CHILD over 4 years, apply 4 times daily; improvement of symptoms may sometimes require treatment for up to 4 weeks

Alomide® (Alcon) [PoM]
Ophthalmic solution (= eye drops), lodoxamide 0.1% (as trometamol). Net price 10 mL = £5.21
Excipients   include benzalkonium chloride, disodium edetate
Note   Lodoxamide 0.1% eye drops can be sold to the public for treatment of allergic conjunctivitis in adults and children over 4 years

NEDOCROMIL SODIUM

Indications   allergic conjunctivitis; seasonal keratoconjunctivitis

Side-effects   burning and stinging; distinctive taste reported

11 Eye

Dose
- Seasonal and perennial conjunctivitis, ADULT and CHILD over 6 years, apply twice daily increased if necessary to 4 times daily; max. 12 weeks treatment for seasonal allergic conjunctivitis
- Seasonal keratoconjunctivitis, ADULT and CHILD over 6 years, apply 4 times daily

Rapitil® (Sanofi-Aventis) PoM
Eye drops, nedocromil sodium 2%. Net price 5 mL = £2.86
Excipients include benzalkonium chloride, disodium edetate

◼ OLOPATADINE

Indications seasonal allergic conjunctivitis
Side-effects local irritation; less commonly keratitis, dry eye, local oedema, photophobia; headache, asthenia, dizziness; dry nose also reported
Dose
- ADULT and CHILD over 3 years, apply twice daily; max. duration of treatment 4 months

Opatanol® (Alcon) PoM
Eye drops, olopatadine (as hydrochloride) 1 mg/mL, net price 5 mL = £4.68
Excipients include benzalkonium chloride

◼ SODIUM CROMOGLICATE
(Sodium cromoglycate)

Indications allergic conjunctivitis; seasonal keratoconjunctivitis
Side-effects burning and stinging
Dose
- ADULT and CHILD apply eye drops 4 times daily

Sodium Cromoglicate (Non-proprietary) PoM
Eye drops, sodium cromoglicate 2%. Net price 13.5 mL = £1.98
Brands include Hay-Crom® Aqueous, Opticrom® Aqueous, Vividrin®
Note Sodium cromoglicate 2% eye drops can be sold to the public (in max. pack size of 10 mL) for treatment of acute seasonal and perennial allergic conjunctivitis

◀Single use
Catacrom® (Moorfields)
Eye drops, sodium cromoglicate 2%, net price 30 × 0.3 mL = £8.99

11.5 Mydriatics and cycloplegics

Antimuscarinics dilate the pupil and paralyse the ciliary muscle; they vary in potency and duration of action.

Short-acting, relatively weak mydriatics, such as **tropicamide** 0.5% (action lasts for 4–6 hours), facilitate the examination of the fundus of the eye. **Cyclopentolate** 1% (action up to 24 hours) or **atropine** (action up to 7 days) are preferable for producing cycloplegia for refraction in young children.

Mydriatics and cycloplegics are used in the treatment of anterior uveitis, usually as an adjunct to corticosteroids (section 11.4.1). Atropine is used in anterior uveitis mainly to prevent posterior synechiae and to relieve ciliary spasm; cyclopentolate or **homatropine** (action

up to 3 days) can also be used and may be preferred because they have a shorter duration of action.

Phenylephrine is used for mydriasis in diagnostic or therapeutic procedures; mydriasis occurs within 60–90 minutes and lasts up to 5–7 hours.

Cautions Darkly pigmented iris is more resistant to pupillary dilatation and caution should be exercised to avoid overdosage. Mydriasis can precipitate acute angle-closure glaucoma in a few patients, usually aged over 60 years and hypermetropic (long-sighted), who are predisposed to the condition because of a shallow anterior chamber. Phenylephrine may interact with systemically administered monoamine-oxidase inhibitors; other **interactions**: Appendix 1 (sympathomimetics).

Driving Patients should be warned not to drive until vision is clear after mydriasis.

Side-effects Ocular side-effects of mydriatics and cycloplegics include transient stinging and raised intra-ocular pressure; on prolonged administration, local irritation, hyperaemia, oedema and conjunctivitis can occur. Contact dermatitis can occur with the antimuscarinic mydriatic drugs, especially atropine.

Systemic side-effects of atropine and cyclopentolate can occur, particularly in children and the elderly; see section 1.2 for systemic side-effects of antimuscarinic drugs.

Antimuscarinics

◼ ATROPINE SULFATE

Indications see notes above
Cautions risk of systemic effects in infants under 3 months; see also notes above
Side-effects see notes above

Atropine (Non-proprietary) PoM
Eye drops, atropine sulfate 0.5%, net price 10 mL = £19.00; 1%, 10 mL = £13.25

◀Single use
Minims® Atropine Sulphate (Bausch & Lomb) PoM
Eye drops, atropine sulfate 1%. Net price 20 × 0.5 mL = £14.46

◼ CYCLOPENTOLATE HYDROCHLORIDE

Indications see notes above
Cautions see notes above
Side-effects see notes above

Mydrilate® (Intrapharm) PoM
Eye drops, cyclopentolate hydrochloride 0.5%, net price 5 mL = £6.73; 1%, 5 mL = £6.73
Excipients include benzalkonium chloride

◀Single use
Minims® Cyclopentolate Hydrochloride (Bausch & Lomb) PoM
Eye drops, cyclopentolate hydrochloride 0.5% and 1%. Net price 20 × 0.5 mL (both) = £9.95

◢ HOMATROPINE HYDROBROMIDE

Indications   see notes above
Cautions   see notes above
Side-effects   see notes above

Homatropine (Non-proprietary) PoM
Eye drops, homatropine hydrobromide, available from 'special-order' manufacturers, p. 1124

◢ TROPICAMIDE

Indications   see notes above
Cautions   see notes above
Side-effects   see notes above

Mydriacyl® (Alcon) PoM
Eye drops, tropicamide 0.5%, net price 5 mL = £1.29; 1%, 5 mL = £1.60
Excipients   include benzalkonium chloride, disodium edetate

◢ **Single use**

Minims® Tropicamide (Bausch & Lomb) PoM
Eye drops, tropicamide 0.5% and 1%. Net price 20 × 0.5 mL (both) = £10.00

◢ **With phenylephrine**
See under Phenylephrine Hydrochloride

Sympathomimetics

◢ PHENYLEPHRINE HYDROCHLORIDE

Indications   mydriasis; see also notes above
Cautions   corneal epithelial damage; ocular hyperaemia; susceptibility to angle-closure glaucoma; diabetes (avoid in long standing diabetes); cerebral arteriosclerosis; asthma; see also notes above
Contra-indications   10% strength in children and elderly; cardiovascular disease; hypertension; aneurysms; thyrotoxicosis
Pregnancy   use only if potential benefit outweighs risk
Breast-feeding   use only if potential benefit outweighs risk—no information available
Side-effects   see notes above; also blurred vision, photophobia; systemic effects include palpitations, tachycardia, extrasystoles, arrhythmias, hypertension; *also reported* coronary artery spasm, myocardial infarction (usually after use of 10% strength in patients with pre-existing cardiovascular disease)
Dose
- ADULT apply 1 drop before procedure; dose may be repeated after 60 minutes if necessary; CHILD apply 1 drop before procedure

◢ **Single use**

Minims® Phenylephrine Hydrochloride (Bausch & Lomb)
Eye drops, phenylephrine hydrochloride 2.5%, net price 20 × 0.5 mL = £10.93; 10%, 20 × 0.5 mL = £10.93
Excipients   include disodium edetate, sodium metabisulfite
Note   A drop of topical anaesthetic may be applied to the eye a few minutes before using phenylephrine to prevent stinging

◢ **With tropicamide**
For prescribing information on tropicamide, see notes above

Mydriasert® (Spectrum Thea) PoM
Ophthalmic insert, phenylephrine hydrochloride 5.4 mg, tropicamide 280 micrograms, net price 1 unit = £4.20
Dose   for pre-operative mydriasis, or for diagnostic procedures when monotherapy insufficient, ADULT over 18 years, apply 1 insert into the lower conjunctival sac up to max. 2 hours before procedure; remove insert within 30 minutes of satisfactory mydriasis, and within 2 hours of application
Note   Patients with severe dry eyes may require a drop of saline to improve insert tolerance

11.6   Treatment of glaucoma

Glaucoma describes a group of disorders characterised by a loss of visual field associated with cupping of the optic disc and optic nerve damage. While glaucoma is generally associated with raised intra-ocular pressure, it can occur when the intra-ocular pressure is within the normal range.

The most common form of glaucoma is primary open-angle glaucoma (chronic open-angle glaucoma), where drainage of the aqueous humour through the trabecular meshwork is restricted. The condition is often asymptomatic, but the patient may present with significant loss of visual-field. Patients with ocular hypertension are at high risk of developing primary open-angle glaucoma.

Drugs that reduce intra-ocular pressure by different mechanisms are available for managing ocular hypertension and glaucoma. A topical beta-blocker or a prostaglandin analogue is usually the drug of first choice for the treatment of ocular hypertension. A prostaglandin analogue should be used to manage patients with early or moderate primary open-angle glaucoma. After checking compliance and eye drop installation technique, it may be necessary to combine these drugs or add others, such as sympathomimetics, carbonic anhydrase inhibitors, or miotics to control intra-ocular pressure.

Acute angle-closure glaucoma   Acute angle-closure glaucoma occurs when the outflow of aqueous humour from the eye is obstructed by bowing of the iris against the trabecular meshwork; it is a medical emergency that requires urgent reduction of intra-ocular pressure to prevent loss of vision. Patients with acute angle-closure glaucoma should be referred immediately for specialist ophthalmology assessment and treatment.

Standard antiglaucoma therapy is used if supplementary treatment is required after iridotomy, iridectomy, laser treatment, or drainage surgery in either primary open-angle or acute angle-closure glaucoma.

Beta-blockers

Topical application of a beta-blocker to the eye reduces intra-ocular pressure effectively in *primary open-angle glaucoma*, probably by reducing the rate of production of aqueous humour. Administration by mouth also reduces intra-ocular pressure but this route is not used since side-effects may be troublesome.

Beta-blockers used as eye drops include **betaxolol**, **carteolol**, **levobunolol**, and **timolol**.

Cautions, contra-indications, and side-effects
Systemic absorption can follow topical application to the eyes; therefore, eye drops containing a beta-blocker are contra-indicated in patients with bradycardia, heart block, or uncontrolled heart failure. **Important:** for a

11
Eye

warning to avoid in asthma see below. Beta-blocker eye drops should be used with caution in patients with corneal diseases. Consider also other cautions, contra-indications, and side-effects of beta-blockers (p. 103). Local side-effects of eye drops include ocular stinging, burning, pain, itching, erythema, dry eyes and allergic reactions including anaphylaxis and blepharoconjuncti-vitis; occasionally corneal disorders have been reported. **Important** Beta-blockers, even those with apparent cardioselectivity, should not be used in patients with asthma or a history of obstructive airways disease, unless no alternative treatment is available. In such cases the risk of inducing bronchospasm should be appreciated and appropriate precautions taken.

Interactions Since systemic absorption may follow topical application the possibility of interactions, in particular, with drugs such as verapamil should be borne in mind. See also Appendix 1 (beta-blockers).

BETAXOLOL

Indications see notes above
Cautions see notes above
Contra-indications see notes above
Side-effects see notes above
Dose
- Apply twice daily

Betaxolol (Non-proprietary) [PoM]
 Eye drops, solution, betaxolol (as hydrochloride) 0.5%, net price 5 mL = £1.90
 Excipients may include benzalkonium chloride, disodium edetate

Betoptic® (Alcon) [PoM]
 Ophthalmic solution (= eye drops), betaxolol (as hydrochloride) 0.5%, net price 5 mL = £1.90
 Excipients include benzalkonium chloride, disodium edetate

 Ophthalmic suspension (= eye drops), betaxolol (as hydrochloride) 0.25%, net price 5 mL = £2.66
 Excipients include benzalkonium chloride, disodium edetate

 Unit dose eye drop suspension, betaxolol (as hydro-chloride) 0.25%, net price 50 × 0.25 mL = £13.77

CARTEOLOL HYDROCHLORIDE

Indications see notes above
Cautions see notes above
Contra-indications see notes above
Side-effects see notes above
Dose
- Apply twice daily

Teoptic® (Spectrum Thea) [PoM]
 Eye drops, carteolol hydrochloride 1%, net price 5 mL = £7.60; 2%, 5 mL = £8.40
 Excipients include benzalkonium chloride

LEVOBUNOLOL HYDROCHLORIDE

Indications see notes above
Cautions see notes above
Contra-indications see notes above
Side-effects see notes above; anterior uveitis occa-sionally reported
Dose
- Apply once or twice daily

Levobunolol (Non-proprietary) [PoM]
 Eye drops, levobunolol hydrochloride 0.5%. Net price 5 mL = £1.85
 Excipients may include benzalkonium chloride, disodium edetate, sodium metabisulfite

Betagan® (Allergan) [PoM]
 Eye drops, levobunolol hydrochloride 0.5%, poly-vinyl alcohol (*Liquifilm®*) 1.4%. Net price 5-mL = £1.85
 Excipients include benzalkonium chloride, disodium edetate, sodium metabisulfite

 Unit dose eye drops, levobunolol hydrochloride 0.5%, polyvinyl alcohol (*Liquifilm®*) 1.4%. Net price 30 × 0.4 mL = £9.98
 Excipients include disodium edetate

TIMOLOL

Indications see notes above
Cautions see notes above
Contra-indications see notes above
Side-effects see notes above
Dose
- Apply twice daily; long-acting preparations, apply once daily

Timolol (Non-proprietary) [PoM]
 Eye drops, timolol (as maleate) 0.25%, net price 5 mL = £1.30; 0.5%, 5 mL = £1.29

Timoptol® (MSD) [PoM]
 Eye drops, in *Ocumeter®* metered-dose unit, timolol (as maleate) 0.25%, net price 5 mL = £3.12; 0.5%, 5 mL = £3.12
 Excipients include benzalkonium chloride

 Unit dose eye drops, timolol (as maleate) 0.25%, net price 30 × 0.2 mL = £8.45; 0.5%, 30 × 0.2 mL = £9.65

◢**Once-daily preparations**

Timoptol®-LA (MSD) [PoM]
 Ophthalmic gel-forming solution (= eye drops), timolol (as maleate) 0.25%, net price 2.5 mL = £3.12; 0.5%, 2.5 mL = £3.12
 Excipients include benzododecinium bromide
 Dose apply once daily

Tiopex® (Spectrum Thea) [PoM]
 Unit dose eye gel (= eye drops), timolol (as maleate) 0.1%, net price 30 × 0.4 g = £7.49
 Dose apply once daily, in the morning
 Note The *Scottish Medicines Consortium* (p. 4) has advised (February 2014) that timolol gel eye drops (*Tiopex®*) are accepted for restricted use within NHS Scotland for the reduction of elevated intraocular pressure in patients with ocular hypertension or chronic open angle glaucoma who have proven sensitivity to preservatives.

◢**With bimatoprost**
 See under Bimatoprost

◢**With brimonidine**
 See under Brimonidine

◢**With brinzolomide**
 See under Brinzolomide

◢**With dorzolamide**
 See under Dorzolamide

◢**With latanoprost**
 See under Latanoprost

◢**With travoprost**
 See under Travoprost

Prostaglandin analogues and prostamides

The prostaglandin analogues **latanoprost**, **tafluprost**, and **travoprost**, and the synthetic prostamide, **bimatoprost**, increase uveoscleral outflow and subsequently reduce intra-ocular pressure. They are used to reduce intra-ocular pressure in ocular hypertension or open-angle glaucoma.

Cautions Use with caution in patients with aphakia, pseudophakia with torn posterior lens capsule or anterior chamber lenses, and in those with known risk factors for cystoid macular oedema, iritis, uveitis, or a history of significant ocular viral infections. Care is also needed in patients with COPD, asthma or compromised respiratory function. There is no experience of use in inflammatory ocular conditions, neovascular, angle-closure glaucoma, congenital glaucoma, or narrow-angle glaucoma. For use in contact lens wearers see Contact Lenses, p. 778.

> **Counselling** Before initiating treatment, patients should be warned of a possible change in eye colour as an increase in the brown pigment in the iris can occur, which may be permanent; particular care is required in those with mixed coloured irides and those receiving treatment to one eye only. Changes in eyelashes and vellus hair can also occur, and patients should also be advised to avoid repeated contact of the eye drop solution with skin as this can lead to hair growth or skin pigmentation.

Side-effects Side-effects of prostaglandin analogues and prostamides include changes in blood pressure, headache, ocular discomfort, conjunctival disorders, brown pigmentation particularly in those with mixed-colour irides, blepharitis, pigmentation of periocular skin, eyelash and vellus hair changes, reduced visual acuity, photophobia, punctuate keratitis, transient punctate epithelial erosion, corneal erosion; they may also cause, darkening, thickening and lengthening of eye lashes. Less frequent side-effects include dizziness, asthenopia, and skin rash. There have been rare reports of arthralgia, myalgia, iritis, uveitis, macular oedema, facial oedema, and darkening of palpebral skin. Very rarely chest pain, palpitation, exacerbation of angina, and periorbital changes resulting in deepening of the eyelid sulcus have occurred. Dyspnoea, asthma, exacerbation of asthma and COPD have also been reported.

◼ BIMATOPROST

Indications raised intra-ocular pressure in open-angle glaucoma; ocular hypertension

Cautions see notes above; also predisposition to hypotension or bradycardia

Hepatic impairment use with caution in moderate to severe impairment—no information available

Renal impairment use with caution—no information available

Pregnancy manufacturer advises use only if potential benefit outweighs risk

Breast-feeding manufacturer advises avoid—present in milk in *animal* studies

Side-effects see notes above; also nausea, bradycardia, malaise, retinal haemorrhage, blepharospasm, eyelid retraction, reactivation of previous corneal infiltrates or ocular infection

Dose

- ADULT over 18 years, apply once daily, preferably in the evening

Lumigan® (Allergan) (PoM)
Eye drops, bimatoprost 100 micrograms/mL, net price 3 mL = £11.71, triple pack (3 × 3 mL) = £35.13; 300 micrograms/mL, 3 mL = £10.30, triple pack (3 × 3 mL) = £30.90. Counselling, see Prostaglandin Analogues and Prostamides, above
Excipients include benzalkonium chloride

◼ Single use

Lumigan® (Allergan) (PoM)
Eye drops, bimatoprost 300 micrograms/mL, net price 30 × 0.4 mL = £13.75. Counselling, see Prostaglandin Analogues and Prostamides
Note The *Scottish Medicines Consortium* (p. 4) has advised (March 2013) that bimatoprost 300 micrograms/mL preservative-free eye drops (*Lumigan®* single-dose eye drops) are accepted for restricted use within NHS Scotland for the reduction of elevated intra-ocular pressure in chronic open-angle glaucoma and ocular hypertension (as monotherapy or as adjunctive therapy to beta-blockers) in adults who have proven sensitivity to benzalkonium chloride.

◼ With timolol

For prescribing information on timolol, see section 11.6, Beta-blockers

Ganfort® (Allergan) (PoM)
Eye drops, bimatoprost 300 micrograms/mL, timolol (as maleate) 5 mg/mL, net price 3-mL = £13.95, triple pack (3 × 3 mL) = £37.59. Counselling, see Prostaglandin Analogues and Prostamides, above
Excipients include benzalkonium chloride
Dose for raised intra-ocular pressure in patients with open-angle glaucoma or ocular hypertension when beta-blocker or prostaglandin analogue alone not adequate, ADULT over 18 years, apply once daily

◼ Single use

Ganfort® (Allergan) (PoM)
Eye drops, bimatoprost 300 micrograms/mL, timolol (as maleate) 5 mg/mL, net price 30 × 0.4 mL = £17.50. Counselling, see Prostaglandin Analogues and Prostamides, above
Dose for raised intra-ocular pressure in patients with open-angle glaucoma or ocular hypertension when beta-blocker or prostaglandin analogue alone not adequate, ADULT over 18 years, apply once daily
Note The *Scottish Medicines Consortium*, p. 4 has advised (October 2013) that *Ganfort®* unit dose eye drops are accepted for restricted use within NHS Scotland for the reduction of intra-ocular pressure in patients with open-angle glaucoma or ocular hypertension insufficiently responsive to topical beta-blockers or prostaglandin analogues who have proven sensitivity to preservatives

◼ LATANOPROST

Indications raised intra-ocular pressure in open-angle glaucoma; ocular hypertension

Cautions see notes above; peri-operative period of cataract surgery; do not use within 5 minutes of thiomersal-containing preparations

Contra-indications active herpes simplex keratitis; history of recurrent herpetic keratitis associated with prostaglandin analogues

Pregnancy manufacturer advises avoid

Breast-feeding may be present in milk—manufacturer advises avoid

Side-effects see notes above; *also reported* nasopharyngitis, pyrexia, (both in children), iris cyst

Dose

- Apply once daily, preferably in the evening

11 Eye

Latanoprost (Non-proprietary) PoM

Eye drops, latanoprost 50 micrograms/mL, net price 2.5 mL = £1.91. Counselling, see Prostaglandin Analogues and Prostamides, p. 765
Excipients may include benzalkonium chloride

Xalatan® (Pfizer) PoM

Eye drops, latanoprost 50 micrograms/mL, net price 2.5 mL = £12.48. Counselling, see Prostaglandin Analogues and Prostamides, p. 765
Excipients include benzalkonium chloride

◢**Single use**

Monopost® (Spectrum Thea) PoM

Eye drops, latanoprost 50 micrograms/mL, net price 30 × 0.2 mL = £8.49, 90 × 0.2 mL = £25.47. Counselling, see Prostaglandin Analogues and Prostamides, p. 765
Note The *Scottish Medicines Consortium*, p. 4 has advised (June 2013) that *Monopost®* is accepted for restricted use within NHS Scotland for the reduction of elevated intraocular pressure in patients with open-angle glaucoma and ocular hypertension who have proven sensitivity to benzalkonium chloride

◢**With timolol**

For prescribing information on timolol, see section 11.6, Beta-blockers

Latanoprost with Timolol (Non-proprietary) PoM

Eye drops, latanoprost 50 micrograms, timolol (as maleate) 5 mg/mL, net price 2.5 mL = £4.19. Counselling, see Prostaglandin Analogues and Prostamides, p. 765
Excipients may include benzalkonium chloride
Dose for raised intra-ocular pressure in patients with open-angle glaucoma and ocular hypertension when beta-blocker or prostaglandin analogue alone not adequate, ADULT over 18 years, apply once daily

Xalacom® (Pharmacia) PoM

Eye drops, latanoprost 50 micrograms, timolol (as maleate) 5 mg/mL, net price 2.5 mL = £14.32. Counselling, see Prostaglandin Analogues and Prostamides, p. 765
Excipients include benzalkonium chloride
Dose for raised intra-ocular pressure in patients with open-angle glaucoma and ocular hypertension when beta-blocker or prostaglandin analogue alone not adequate, ADULT over 18 years, apply once daily

◤ TAFLUPROST

Indications raised intra-ocular pressure in open-angle glaucoma; ocular hypertension

Cautions see notes above

Hepatic impairment use with caution—no information available

Renal impairment use with caution—no information available

Pregnancy manufacturer advises avoid unless potential benefit outweighs risk—toxicity in *animal* studies

Breast-feeding manufacturer advises avoid—present in milk in *animal* studies

Side-effects see notes above

Dose

● ADULT over 18 years, apply once daily, preferably in the evening

Saflutan® (MSD) PoM

Unit dose eye drops, tafluprost 15 micrograms/mL, net price 30 × 0.3 mL = £17.41. Counselling, see Prostaglandin Analogues and Prostamides, p. 765
Excipients include disodium edetate

◤ TRAVOPROST

Indications raised intra-ocular pressure in open-angle glaucoma; ocular hypertension

Cautions see notes above

Pregnancy manufacturer advises avoid unless potential benefit outweighs risk—toxicity in *animal* studies

Breast-feeding present in milk in *animal* studies; manufacturer advises avoid

Side-effects see notes above; also dry mouth, dysgeusia, peptic ulcer reactivation, gastro-intestinal disorders, constipation, bradycardia, oropharyngeal pain, cough, dysphonia, nasal congestion, throat irritation, malaise, herpes simplex, photopsia, mydriasis, cataract; *also reported* vertigo, tinnitus

Dose

● ADULT over 18 years, apply once daily, preferably in the evening

Travatan® (Alcon) PoM

Eye drops, travoprost 40 micrograms/mL, net price 2.5 mL = £10.95. Counselling, see Prostaglandin Analogues and Prostamides, p. 765
Excipients include propylene glycol

◢**With timolol**

For prescribing information on timolol, see section 11.6, Beta-blockers

DuoTrav® (Alcon) PoM

Eye drops, travoprost 40 micrograms, timolol (as maleate) 5 mg/mL, net price 2.5 mL = £13.95, triple pack (3 × 2.5 mL) = £39.68. Counselling, see Prostaglandin Analogues and Prostamides, p. 765
Excipients include propylene glycol
Dose for raised intra-ocular pressure in patients with open-angle glaucoma or ocular hypertension when beta-blocker or prostaglandin analogue alone not adequate, ADULT over 18 years, apply once daily

Sympathomimetics

Brimonidine, a selective alpha$_2$-adrenoceptor agonist, is thought to lower intra-ocular pressure by reducing aqueous humour formation and increasing uveoscleral outflow. It is licensed for the reduction of intra-ocular pressure in open-angle glaucoma or ocular hypertension in patients for whom beta-blockers are inappropriate; it may also be used as adjunctive therapy when intra-ocular pressure is inadequately controlled by other antiglaucoma therapy.

Apraclonidine (section 11.8.2) is another alpha$_2$-adrenoceptor agonist that lowers intra-ocular pressure by reducing aqueous humour formation. Eye drops containing apraclonidine 0.5% are used short-term to delay laser treatment or surgery in patients with glaucoma not adequately controlled by another drug; eye drops containing 1% are used for control of intra-ocular pressure after anterior segment laser surgery.

◤ BRIMONIDINE TARTRATE

Indications raised intra-ocular pressure, see notes above

Cautions severe cardiovascular disease; cerebral or coronary insufficiency, Raynaud's syndrome, thromboangiitis obliterans, postural hypotension, depression; children 2–12 years (increased risk of drowsiness); interactions: Appendix 1 (brimonidine)
Driving Drowsiness may affect performance of skilled tasks (e.g. driving)

11 Eye

Contra-indications neonate or child under 2 years

Hepatic impairment manufacturer advises use with caution

Renal impairment manufacturer advises use with caution

Pregnancy manufacturer advises use only if benefit outweighs risk

Breast-feeding manufacturer advises avoid

Side-effects dry mouth, gastro-intestinal disturbances, taste disturbances, upper respiratory symptoms, headache, drowsiness, dizziness, malaise, ocular disturbances (including hyperaemia, burning, stinging, pruritus, pain and dryness), visual disturbances, eyelid inflammation, photophobia, corneal erosion and staining, conjunctival disturbances (including blanching, follicles, and infection); *less commonly* palpitation, arrhythmia, bradycardia, tachycardia, depression, nasal dryness; *rarely* dyspnoea; *very rarely* hypertension, hypotension, syncope, insomnia, iritis, miosis

Dose

- Apply twice daily

Brimonidine Tartrate (Non-proprietary) [PoM]

Eye drops, brimonidine tartrate 0.2%, net price 5 mL = £2.28

Brands include *Brymont®*

Excipients may include benzalkonium chloride

Alphagan® (Allergan) [PoM]

Eye drops, brimonidine tartrate 0.2%, net price 5 mL = £6.85

Excipients include benzalkonium chloride

◢**With timolol**

For prescribing information on timolol, see section 11.6, Beta-blockers

Combigan® (Allergan) [PoM]

Eye drops, brimonidine tartrate 0.2%, timolol (as maleate) 0.5%, net price 5-mL = £10.00

Excipients include benzalkonium chloride

Dose for raised intra-ocular pressure in open-angle glaucoma and for ocular hypertension when beta-blocker alone not adequate, apply twice daily

Carbonic anhydrase inhibitors and systemic drugs

The **carbonic anhydrase inhibitors**, acetazolamide, brinzolamide, and dorzolamide, reduce intra-ocular pressure by reducing aqueous humour production. Systemic use also produces weak diuresis.

Acetazolamide is given by mouth or by intravenous injection (intramuscular injections are painful because of the alkaline pH of the solution). It is used as an adjunct to other treatment for reducing intra-ocular pressure. Acetazolamide is a sulfonamide derivative; blood disorders, rashes, and other sulfonamide-related side-effects occur occasionally—patients should be told to report any unusual skin rash. It is not generally recommended for long-term use; if electrolyte disturbances and metabolic acidosis occur, these can be corrected by administering potassium bicarbonate (as effervescent potassium tablets, section 9.2.1.3).

Dorzolamide and **brinzolamide** are topical carbonic anhydrase inhibitors. They are licensed for use in patients resistant to beta-blockers or those in whom beta-blockers are contra-indicated. They are used alone or as an adjunct to a topical beta-blocker. Brinzolamide

can also be used as an adjunct to a prostaglandin analogue. Systemic absorption can rarely cause sulfonamide-like side-effects and may require discontinuation if severe.

The **osmotic diuretics**, intravenous hypertonic **mannitol** (section 2.2.5) or **glycerol** by mouth are useful short-term ocular hypotensive drugs.

ACETAZOLAMIDE

Indications reduction of intra-ocular pressure in open-angle glaucoma, secondary glaucoma, and perioperatively in angle-closure glaucoma; diuresis (section 2.2.7); epilepsy

Cautions not generally recommended for prolonged use, but if given, monitor blood count and plasma-electrolyte concentrations; pulmonary obstruction and impaired alveolar ventilation (risk of acidosis); elderly; diabetes mellitus; renal calculi; avoid extravasation at injection site (risk of necrosis); **interactions**: Appendix 1 (diuretics)

Contra-indications hypokalaemia, hyponatraemia, hyperchloraemic acidosis; adrenocortical insufficiency; long-term administration in chronic angle-closure glaucoma; sulfonamide hypersensitivity

Hepatic impairment manufacturer advises avoid

Renal impairment avoid—risk of metabolic acidosis

Pregnancy manufacturer advises avoid, especially in first trimester (toxicity in *animal* studies)

Breast-feeding amount too small to be harmful

Side-effects see notes above; also nausea, vomiting, diarrhoea, taste disturbance, loss of appetite, paraesthesia, flushing, headache, dizziness, fatigue, irritability, excitement, ataxia, depression, thirst, polyuria, reduced libido; *less commonly* melaena, drowsiness, confusion, hearing disturbances, fever, glycosuria, metabolic acidosis and electrolyte disturbances on long-term therapy, haematuria, crystalluria, renal and ureteric colic, renal lesions or calculi, renal failure, blood disorders, bone marrow suppression, rash (including Stevens-Johnson syndrome and toxic epidermal necrosis); *rarely* fulminant hepatic necrosis, hepatitis, cholestatic jaundice, flaccid paralysis, convulsions, photosensitivity; *also reported* transient myopia

Dose

- Glaucoma, by mouth *or* by intravenous injection, 0.25–1 g daily in divided doses

- Epilepsy, by mouth *or* by intravenous injection, 0.25–1 g daily in divided doses; CHILD 8–30 mg/kg daily, max. 750 mg daily

Note Dose by intramuscular injection, as for intravenous injection but preferably avoided because of alkalinity

Diamox® (AMCo) [PoM]

Tablets, acetazolamide 250 mg. Net price 112-tab pack = £15.22. Label: 3

Injection, powder for reconstitution, acetazolamide (as sodium salt). Net price 500-mg vial = £14.76

◢**Modified release**

Diamox® SR (AMCo) [PoM]

Capsules, m/r, orange, enclosing orange f/c pellets, acetazolamide 250 mg. Net price 30-cap pack = £16.66 Label: 3, 25

Dose glaucoma, 1–2 capsules daily

■ BRINZOLAMIDE

Indications reduction of intra-ocular pressure in ocular hypertension and open-angle glaucoma *either* as adjunct to beta-blockers or prostaglandin analogues *or* used alone in patients unresponsive to beta-blockers or if beta-blockers contra-indicated

Cautions systemic absorption follows topical application; renal tubular immaturity or abnormality; **interactions:** Appendix 1 (brinzolamide)

Contra-indications hyperchloraemic acidosis; sulfonamide hypersensitivity

Hepatic impairment manufacturer advises avoid

Renal impairment see Cautions above; also avoid if eGFR less than 30 mL/minute/1.73 m²

Pregnancy avoid—toxicity in *animal* studies

Breast-feeding use only if benefit outweighs risk

Side-effects see notes above; also taste disturbances, dry mouth, headache, ocular disturbances (including corneal erosion, corneal oedema, photophobia, and reduced visual acuity); *less commonly* nausea, vomiting, diarrhoea, dyspepsia, oesophagitis, flatulence, oral hypoaesthesia and paraesthesia, chest pain, bradycardia, palpitation, dyspnoea, cough, upper respiratory tract congestion, pharyngitis, depression, sleep disturbances, nervousness, malaise, drowsiness, amnesia, dizziness, paraesthesia, sinusitis, decreased libido, erectile dysfunction, renal pain, epistaxis, nasal dryness, throat irritation, tinnitus, alopecia; *also reported* arrhythmia, tachycardia, hypertension, peripheral oedema, asthma, tremor, vertigo, rhinitis, dermatitis, erythema

Dose
- Apply twice daily increased to max. 3 times daily if necessary

Azopt® (Alcon) ⟨PoM⟩
Eye drops, brinzolamide 10 mg/mL, net price 5 mL = £6.92
Excipients include benzalkonium chloride, disodium edetate

◢**With timolol**
For prescribing information on timolol, see section 11.6, Beta blockers

Azarga® (Alcon) ⟨PoM⟩
Ophthalmic suspension (= eye drops), brinzolamide 10 mg, timolol (as maleate) 5 mg/mL, net price 5 mL = £11.05
Excipients include benzalkonium chloride, disodium edetate
Dose for raised intra-ocular pressure in open-angle glaucoma or ocular hypertension when beta-blocker alone not adequate, ADULT over 18 years apply twice daily

■ DORZOLAMIDE

Indications raised intra-ocular pressure in ocular hypertension, open-angle glaucoma, pseudo-exfoliative glaucoma *either* as adjunct to beta-blocker or used alone in patients unresponsive to beta-blockers or if beta-blockers contra-indicated

Cautions systemic absorption follows topical application; history of renal calculi; chronic corneal defects, low endothelial cell count, history of intra-ocular surgery; **interactions:** Appendix 1 (dorzolamide)

Contra-indications hyperchloraemic acidosis, sulfonamide hypersensitivity

Hepatic impairment manufacturer advises caution—no information available

Renal impairment avoid if eGFR less than 30 mL/minute/1.73 m²

Pregnancy manufacturer advises avoid—toxicity in *animal* studies

Breast-feeding manufacturer advises avoid—no information available

Side-effects see notes above; also nausea, bitter taste, headache, asthenia, ocular irritation, blurred vision, lacrimation, conjunctivitis, superficial punctuate keratitis, eyelid inflammation; *less commonly* iridocyclitis; *rarely* dry mouth, dizziness, paraesthesia, urolithiasis, eyelid crusting, transient myopia, corneal oedema, epistaxis, throat irritation, contact dermatitis, Stevens-Johnson syndrome, toxic epidermal necrolysis

Dose
- Used alone, apply 3 times daily
- With topical beta-blocker, apply twice daily

Dorzolamide (Non-proprietary) ⟨PoM⟩
Eye drops, dorzolamide (as hydrochloride) 2%, net price 5 mL = £2.44
Excipients may include benzalkonium chloride
Brands include *Dorzan*®

Trusopt® (MSD) ⟨PoM⟩
Ophthalmic solution (= eye drops), in *Ocumeter® Plus* metered-dose unit, dorzolamide (as hydrochloride) 2%, net price 5 mL = £6.33
Excipients include benzalkonium chloride
Unit dose eye drops, dorzolamide (as hydrochloride) 2%, net price 60 × 0.2 mL = £24.18

◢**With timolol**
For prescribing information on timolol, see section 11.6, Beta-blockers

Dorzolamide with Timolol (Non-proprietary) ⟨PoM⟩
Eye drops, dorzolamide (as hydrochloride) 2%, timolol (as maleate) 0.5%, net price 5 mL = £2.73
Excipients may include benzalkonium chloride

Cosopt® (MSD) ⟨PoM⟩
Ophthalmic solution (= eye drops), in *Ocumeter® Plus* metered-dose unit, dorzolamide (as hydrochloride) 2%, timolol (as maleate) 0.5%, net price 5 mL = £10.05
Excipients include benzalkonium chloride
Unit dose eye drops, dorzolamide (as hydrochloride) 2%, timolol (as maleate) 0.5%, net price 60 × 0.2 mL = £28.59

Miotics

Miotics act by opening the inefficient drainage channels in the trabecular meshwork.

Pilocarpine, a miotic, is not commonly used for the treatment of primary open-angle glaucoma because side-effects, such as pupil miosis, are poorly tolerated. It is used mainly in the treatment of primary angle-closure glaucoma and in some secondary glaucomas.

Cautions A darkly pigmented iris may require a higher concentration of the miotic or more frequent administration and care should be taken to avoid overdosage. Retinal detachment has occurred in susceptible individuals and those with retinal disease; therefore fundus examination is advised before starting treatment with a miotic. Care is also required in conjunctival or corneal damage. Intra-ocular pressure and visual fields should be monitored in those with chronic simple glaucoma and those receiving long-term treatment with a miotic. Miotics should be used with caution in patients with peptic ulceration, gastro-intestinal spasm, cardiac disease, hypertension, hypotension, marked vasomotor instability, asthma, epilepsy, Parkinson's disease, hyperthyroidism, and urinary-tract obstruction.

Counselling Blurred vision may affect performance of skilled tasks (e.g. driving) particularly at night or in reduced lighting

Contra-indications Miotics are contra-indicated in conditions where pupillary constriction is undesirable such as acute iritis, anterior uveitis and some forms of secondary glaucoma. They should be avoided in acute inflammatory disease of the anterior segment.

Pregnancy Miotics should be avoided during pregnancy unless the potential benefit outweighs risk—limited information available.

Breast-feeding Miotics should be avoided during breast-feeding unless the potential benefit outweighs risk—no information available.

Side-effects Ciliary spasm leads to headache and browache which may be more severe in the initial 2–4 weeks of treatment (a particular disadvantage in patients under 40 years of age). Ocular side-effects include burning, itching, smarting, blurred vision, conjunctival vascular congestion, myopia, lens changes with chronic use, vitreous haemorrhage, and pupillary block. Systemic side-effects (see under Parasympathomimetics, section 7.4.1) are rare following application to the eye.

▌ PILOCARPINE

Indications see notes above; dry mouth (section 12.3.5)

Cautions see notes above

Contra-indications see notes above

Side-effects see notes above

Dose

- Apply up to 4 times daily; long-acting preparations, see under preparations below

Pilocarpine Hydrochloride (Non-proprietary) PoM

Eye drops, pilocarpine hydrochloride 1%, net price 10 mL = £2.64; 2%, 10 mL = £3.65; 4%, 10 mL = £4.37

Excipients may include benzalkonium chloride

◢Single use

Minims® Pilocarpine Nitrate (Bausch & Lomb) PoM

Eye drops, pilocarpine nitrate 2%, net price 20 × 0.5 mL = £11.48

11.7 Local anaesthetics

Oxybuprocaine and **tetracaine** are widely used topical local anaesthetics. **Proxymetacaine** causes less initial stinging and is useful for children. Oxybuprocaine or a combined preparation of **lidocaine** and **fluorescein** is used for tonometry. Tetracaine produces a more profound anaesthesia and is suitable for use before minor surgical procedures, such as the removal of corneal sutures. It has a temporary disruptive effect on the corneal epithelium. Lidocaine (section 15.2), with or without adrenaline (epinephrine), is injected into the eyelids for minor surgery. Local anaesthetics should never be used for the management of ocular symptoms.

Local anaesthetic eye drops should be avoided in preterm neonates because of the immaturity of the metabolising enzyme system.

▌ LIDOCAINE HYDROCHLORIDE

(Lignocaine hydrochloride)

Indications local anaesthetic

Minims® Lidocaine and Fluorescein (Bausch & Lomb) PoM

Eye drops, lidocaine hydrochloride 4%, fluorescein sodium 0.25%. Net price 20 × 0.5 mL = £11.24

▌ OXYBUPROCAINE HYDROCHLORIDE

(Benoxinate hydrochloride)

Indications local anaesthetic

Minims® Oxybuprocaine Hydrochloride (Bausch & Lomb) PoM

Eye drops, oxybuprocaine hydrochloride 0.4%. Net price 20 × 0.5 mL = £9.72

▌ PROXYMETACAINE HYDROCHLORIDE

Indications local anaesthetic

Minims® Proxymetacaine (Bausch & Lomb) PoM

Eye drops, proxymetacaine hydrochloride 0.5%. Net price 20 × 0.5 mL = £11.05

▌ TETRACAINE HYDROCHLORIDE

(Amethocaine hydrochloride)

Indications local anaesthetic

Minims® Tetracaine Hydrochloride (Bausch & Lomb) PoM

Eye drops, tetracaine hydrochloride 0.5% and 1%. Net price 20 × 0.5 mL (both) = £9.73

11.8 Miscellaneous ophthalmic preparations

11.8.1 Tear deficiency, ocular lubricants, and astringents

11.8.2 Ocular diagnostic and peri-operative preparations and photodynamic treatment

Certain eye drops, e.g. amphotericin, ceftazidime, cefuroxime, colistimethate sodium, desferrioxamine, dexamethasone, gentamicin, and vancomycin can be prepared aseptically from material supplied for injection.

Botulinum toxin type A preparations are licensed for the treatment of blepharospasm (*Botox®*, *Dysport®*, and *Xeomin®*) and for the temporary improvement of moderate to severe wrinkles between the eyebrows in adults under 65 years (*Azzalure®*, *Bocouture®*, *Botox®*, and *Vistabel®*), see section 4.9.3; preparations are not interchangeable and should be used under specialist supervision.

11 Eye

11.8.1 Tear deficiency, ocular lubricants, and astringents

Chronic soreness of the eyes associated with reduced or abnormal tear secretion (e.g. in Sjögren's syndrome) often responds to tear replacement therapy or pilocarpine given by mouth (section 12.3.5). The severity of the condition and patient preference will often guide the choice of preparation.

Hypromellose is the traditional choice of treatment for tear deficiency. It may need to be instilled frequently (e.g. hourly) for adequate relief. Ocular surface mucin is often abnormal in tear deficiency and the combination of hypromellose with a mucolytic such as **acetylcysteine** can be helpful.

The ability of **carbomers** to cling to the eye surface may help reduce frequency of application to 4 times daily.

Polyvinyl alcohol increases the persistence of the tear film and is useful when the ocular surface mucin is reduced.

Sodium hyaluronate eye drops are also used in the management of tear deficiency.

Sodium chloride 0.9% drops are sometimes useful in tear deficiency, and can be used as 'comfort drops' by contact lens wearers, and to facilitate lens removal. They are also used to irrigate the eye. Special presentations of sodium chloride 0.9% and other irrigation solutions are used routinely for intra-ocular surgery. **Sodium chloride 5%** eye drops are used for the short-term treatment of corneal oedema.

Eye ointments containing a **paraffin** can be used to lubricate the eye surface, especially in cases of recurrent corneal epithelial erosion. They may cause temporary visual disturbance and are best suited for application before sleep. Ointments should not be used during contact lens wear.

ACETYLCYSTEINE

Indications tear deficiency, impaired or abnormal mucus production

Dose
- Apply 3–4 times daily

Ilube® (Moorfields) PoM
Eye drops, acetylcysteine 5%, hypromellose 0.35%. Net price 10 mL = £10.09
Excipients include benzalkonium chloride, disodium edetate

CARBOMERS

(Polyacrylic acid)

Note Synthetic high molecular weight polymers of acrylic acid cross-linked with either allyl ethers of sucrose or allyl ethers of pentaerithrityl

Indications dry eyes including keratoconjunctivitis sicca, unstable tear film

Dose
- Apply 3–4 times daily or as required

Carbomer Gel (Non-proprietary)
Gel (= eye drops), carbomer 980 (polyacrylic acid) 0.2%, net price 10 g = £2.80
Excipients include disodium edetate

Artelac® Nighttime Gel (Bausch & Lomb)
Gel (= eye drops), carbomer 2 mg, net price 10 g = £2.96

Clinitas Gel® (Altacor)
Gel (= eye drops), carbomer 980 (polyacrylic acid) 0.2%, net price 10 g = £1.49

GelTears® (Bausch & Lomb)
Gel (= eye drops), carbomer 980 (polyacrylic acid) 0.2%, net price 10 g = £2.80
Excipients include benzalkonium chloride

Liquivisc® (Spectrum Thea)
Gel (= eye drops), carbomer 974P (polyacrylic acid) 0.25%, net price 10 g = £4.50
Excipients include benzalkonium chloride

Lumecare® Carbomer Gel (Medicom)
Gel (= eye drops), carbomer 980 (polyacrylic acid) 0.2%, net price 10 g = £2.10
Excipients include cetrimide

Viscotears® (Alcon)
Liquid gel (= eye drops), carbomer 980 (polyacrylic acid) 0.2%, net price 10 g = £1.59
Excipients include cetrimide

◢ **Single use**
Viscotears® (Alcon)
Liquid gel (= eye drops), carbomer 980 (polyacrylic acid) 0.2%, net price 30 × 0.6-mL single-dose units = £5.42

CARMELLOSE SODIUM

Indications dry eye conditions
Dose
- Apply as required

Carmellose (Non-proprietary)
Eye drops, carmellose sodium 0.5%, net price 10 mL = £7.49

Carmize® (Aspire)
Eye drops, carmellose sodium 0.5%, net price 10 mL = £7.49

Optive® (Allergan)
Eye drops, carmellose sodium 0.5%, glycerol, net price 10 mL = £7.49

Optive® Plus (Allergan)
Eye drops, carmellose sodium 0.5%, glycerol 1%, castor oil 0.25%, net price 10 mL = £7.49

◢ **Single use**
Carmellose (Non-proprietary)
Eye drops, carmellose sodium 0.5%, net price 30 x 0.4 mL = £5.75; 1%, 30 x 0.4 mL = £3.00

Carmize® (Aspire)
Eye drops, carmellose sodium 0.5%, net price 30 × 0.4 mL = £5.75, 90 × 0.4 mL = £15.53; 1%, 30 × 0.4 mL = £3.00, 60 × 0.4 mL = £6.00

Celluvisc® (Allergan)
Eye drops, carmellose sodium 0.5%, net price 30 × 0.4 mL = £4.80, 90 × 0.4 mL = £15.53; 1%, 30 × 0.4 mL = £3.00, 60 × 0.4 mL = £10.99

Melophthal® (Martindale)
Eye drops, carmellose sodium 0.5%, net price 30 × 0.4 mL = £5.75; 1%, 30 × 0.4 mL = £3.00
Note Each unit is resealable and may be used for up to 12 hours

Eye

11

HYDROXYETHYLCELLULOSE

Indications   tear deficiency

Minims® Artificial Tears (Bausch & Lomb)
Eye drops, hydroxyethylcellulose 0.44%, sodium chloride 0.35%. Net price 20 × 0.5 mL = £8.97

HYPROMELLOSE

Indications   tear deficiency
Note The Royal Pharmaceutical Society has stated that where it is not possible to ascertain the strength of hypromellose prescribed, the prescriber should be contacted to clarify the strength intended.

Hypromellose (Non-proprietary)
Eye drops, hypromellose 0.3%, net price 10 mL = £1.15
Excipients may include benzalkonium chloride
Brands include Lumecare® Hypromellose, Mandanol®

Artelac® (Bausch & Lomb)
Eye drops, hypromellose 0.32%, net price 10 mL = £4.99
Excipients include cetrimide, disodium edetate

Isopto Alkaline® (Alcon)
Eye drops, hypromellose 1%, net price 10 mL = 94p
Excipients include benzalkonium chloride

Isopto Plain® (Alcon)
Eye drops, hypromellose 0.5%, net price 10 mL = 81p
Excipients include benzalkonium chloride

Tear-Lac® (Scope Ophthalmics)
Eye drops, hypromellose 0.3%, net price 10 mL = £5.75

Tears Naturale® (Alcon)
Eye drops, hypromellose 0.3%, dextran '70' 0.1%, net price 15 mL = £1.89
Excipients include benzalkonium chloride, disodium edetate

◢ **Single use**

Artelac® SDU (Bausch & Lomb)
Eye drops, hypromellose 0.32%, net price 30 × 0.5 mL = £16.95, 60 × 0.5 mL = £32.85

Hydromoor® (Moorfields)
Eye drops, hypromellose 0.3%, net price 30 × 0.4 mL = £5.75

Lumecare® Preservative Free Tear Drops (Medicom)
Eye drops, hypromellose 0.3%, net price 30 × 0.5 mL = £5.72

Tears Naturale® Single Dose (Alcon)
Eye drops, hypromellose 0.3%, dextran '70' 0.1%, net price 28 × 0.4 mL = £13.26

LIQUID PARAFFIN

Indications   dry eye conditions

Lacri-Lube® (Allergan)
Eye ointment, white soft paraffin 57.3%, liquid paraffin 42.5%, wool alcohols 0.2%. Net price 3.5 g = £2.94, 5 g = £3.88

VitA-POS® (Scope Ophthalmics)
Eye ointment, retinol palmitate 250 units/g, white soft paraffin, light liquid paraffin, liquid paraffin, wool fat, net price 5 g = £2.75

MACROGOLS
(Polyethylene glycols)

Indications   dry eye conditions
Dose
● Apply as required

Systane® (Alcon)
Eye drops, polyethylene glycol 400 0.4%, propylene glycol 0.3%, hydroxypropyl guar, net price 10 mL = £4.66

Systane® Ultra (Alcon)
Eye drops, polyethylene glycol 400 0.4%, propylene glycol 0.3%, hydroxypropyl guar, sorbitol, net price 10 mL = £6.69

◢ **Single use**

Systane® (Alcon)
Eye drops, polyethylene glycol 400 0.4%, propylene glycol 0.3%, hydroxypropyl guar, net price 28 × 0.8 mL = £4.66

Systane® Ultra (Alcon)
Eye drops, polyethylene glycol 400 0.4%, propylene glycol 0.3%, hydroxypropyl guar, sorbitol, net price 30 × 0.7 mL = £6.69

PARAFFIN, YELLOW, SOFT

Indications   see notes above

Simple Eye Ointment
Ointment, liquid paraffin 10%, wool fat 10%, in yellow soft paraffin. Net price 4 g = £3.47

POLYVINYL ALCOHOL

Indications   tear deficiency

Liquifilm Tears® (Allergan)
Ophthalmic solution (= eye drops), polyvinyl alcohol 1.4%, net price 15 mL = £1.93
Excipients include benzalkonium chloride, disodium edetate

Sno Tears® (Bausch & Lomb)
Eye drops, polyvinyl alcohol 1.4%. Net price 10 mL = £1.06
Excipients include benzalkonium chloride, disodium edetate

◢ **Single use**

Liquifilm Tears® (Allergan)
Ophthalmic solution (= eye drops), polyvinyl alcohol 1.4%, povidone 0.6%, net price 30 × 0.4 mL = £5.35

SODIUM CHLORIDE

Indications   see notes above

Sodium Chloride 0.9% Solutions
See section 13.11.1

Balanced Salt Solution PoM
Solution (sterile), sodium chloride 0.64%, sodium acetate 0.39%, sodium citrate 0.17%, calcium chloride 0.048%, magnesium chloride 0.03%, potassium chloride 0.075%
For intra-ocular or topical irrigation during surgical procedures

11   **Eye**

◢Single use

Minims® Saline (Bausch & Lomb)
Eye drops, sodium chloride 0.9%. Net price 20 × 0.5 mL = £7.14

NaCl® 5% (Essential)
Eye drops, Sodium chloride 5%, net price 20 × 0.45 mL = £73.58

◼ SODIUM HYALURONATE

Indications dry eye conditions
Dose
● Apply as required

Artelac Rebalance® (Bausch & Lomb)
Eye drops, sodium hyaluronate 0.15%, net price 10 mL = £4.00

Blink® Intensive Tears (AMO)
Eye drops, sodium hyaluronate 0.2%, polyethylene glycol 400 0.25%, net price 10 mL = £2.97

Hyabak® (Spectrum Thea)
Eye drops, sodium hyaluronate 0.15%, net price 10 mL = £7.99

Hylo-Care® (Scope Ophthalmics)
Eye drops, sodium hyaluronate 0.1%, dexpanthenol 2%, net price 10 mL = £10.30

Hylo-Forte® (Scope Opthalmics)
Eye drops, sodium hyaluronate 0.2%, net price 10 mL = £9.50

Hylo-Tear® (Scope Opthalmics)
Eye drops, sodium hyaluronate 0.1%, net price 10 mL = £8.50

Lumecare® Sodium Hyaluronate (Medicom)
Eye drops, sodium hyaluronate 0.15%, net price 10 mL = £3.97

Optive® Fusion (Allergan)
Eye drops, Sodium hyaluronate 0.1%, carmellose sodium 0.5%, glycerol 0.9%, net price 10 mL = £7.49

Oxyal® (Bausch & Lomb)
Eye drops, sodium hyaluronate 0.15%, net price 10 mL = £4.15

Vismed® Gel Multi (TRB Chemedica)
Eye drops, sodium hyaluronate 0.3%, net price 10 mL = £7.95

Vismed® Multi (TRB Chemedica)
Eye drops, sodium hyaluronate 0.18%, net price 10 mL = £6.81

◢Single use

Artelac® Splash (Bausch & Lomb)
Eye drops, sodium hyaluronate 0.2%, net price 30 × 0.5 mL = £7.00, 60 × 0.5 mL = £11.20

Blink® Intensive Tears (AMO)
Eye drops, sodium hyaluronate 0.2%, polyethylene glycol 400, net price 20 × 0.4 mL = £2.97

Clinitas® (Altacor)
Eye drops, sodium hyaluronate 0.4%, net price 30 × 0.4 mL = £5.70
Note Each unit is resealable and may be used for up to 12 hours

Lubristil® (Moorfields)
Eye drops, sodium hyaluronate 0.15%, net price 20 × 0.3 mL = £4.99

Lubristil® Gel (Moorfields)
Eye drops, sodium hyaluronate 0.15%, xanthan gum 1%, net price 20 × 0.4 mL = £6.49

Ocusan® (Agepha)
Eye drops, sodium hyaluronate 0.2%, net price 20 × 0.5 mL = £5.31

Vismed® (TRB Chemedica)
Eye drops, sodium hyaluronate 0.18%, net price 20 × 0.3 mL = £5.10

Vismed® Gel (TRB Chemedica)
Eye drops, sodium hyaluronate 0.3%, net price 20 × 0.45 mL = £5.98

◼ SOYBEAN OIL

Indications dry eye conditions
Dose
● Apply up to 4 times daily

Emustil® (Moorfields)
Eye drops, soybean oil 7%, natural phospholipids 3%, net price 20 × 0.3 mL = £6.22

11.8.2 Ocular diagnostic and peri-operative preparations and photodynamic treatment

Ocular diagnostic preparations

Fluorescein sodium is used in diagnostic procedures and for locating damaged areas of the cornea due to injury or disease.

◼ FLUORESCEIN SODIUM

Indications detection of lesions and foreign bodies

Minims® Fluorescein Sodium (Bausch & Lomb)
Eye drops, fluorescein sodium 1% or 2%. Net price 20 × 0.5 mL (both) = £8.52

◢With local anaesthetic
Section 11.7

Ocular peri-operative drugs

Drugs used to prepare the eye for surgery, drugs that are injected into the anterior chamber at the time of surgery, and those used after eye surgery, are included here.

Cefuroxime, administered by intra-ocular injection into the anterior chamber of the eye (intracameral use), is used for the prophylaxis of endophthalmitis after cataract surgery.

Non-steroidal anti-inflammatory eye drops such as **diclofenac**, **flurbiprofen**, **ketorolac**, and **nepafenac**, are used for the prophylaxis and treatment of inflammation, pain, and other symptoms associated with ocular surgery or laser treatment of the eye. **Bromfenac** is used for the treatment of postoperative inflammation following cataract surgery. Diclofenac and flurbiprofen are also used to prevent miosis during ocular surgery.

Apraclonidine, an alpha₂-adrenoceptor agonist, reduces intra-ocular pressure possibly by reducing the production of aqueous humour. It is used to control increases in intra-ocular pressure associated with ocular surgery and as short-term treatment to reduce intra-ocular pressure prior to surgery.

Acetylcholine, administered into the anterior chamber of the eye during surgery, rapidly produces miosis which lasts approximately 20 minutes. If prolonged miosis is required, it can be applied again.

Intra-ocular **sodium hyaluronate** and balanced salt solution (section 11.8.1) are used during surgical procedures on the eye.

Povidone-iodine is used for peri-ocular and conjunctival antisepsis before ocular surgery to support postoperative infection control.

ACETYLCHOLINE CHLORIDE

Indications   cataract surgery, penetrating keratoplasty, iridectomy, and other anterior segment surgery requiring rapid complete miosis

Cautions   gastro-intestinal spasm, peptic ulcer; heart failure; asthma; hyperthyroidism; urinary-tract obstruction; parkinsonism

Pregnancy   avoid unless potential benefit outweighs risk—no information available

Breast-feeding   avoid unless potential benefit outweighs risk—no information available

Side-effects   *rarely* bradycardia, hypotension, breathing difficulty, sweating, flushing

Miochol-E® (Bausch & Lomb) (PoM)
Intra-ocular irrigation, powder for reconstitution, acetylcholine chloride 10 mg/mL (1%) when reconstituted, net price 20-mg vial (with solvent) = £7.28

Miphtel® (Alan Pharmaceuticals) (PoM)
Intra-ocular irrigation, powder for reconstitution, acetylcholine chloride 10 mg/mL (1%) when reconstituted, net price 20-mg vial (with solvent) = £7.28

APRACLONIDINE

Note Apraclonidine is a derivative of clonidine

Indications   control of intra-ocular pressure

Cautions   history of angina, severe coronary insufficiency, recent myocardial infarction, heart failure, cerebrovascular disease, vasovagal attack, hypertension; Parkinson's syndrome; Raynaud's syndrome; thromboangiitis obliterans; depression; monitor intra-ocular pressure and visual fields; loss of effect may occur over time; suspend treatment if reduction in vision occurs in end-stage glaucoma; monitor for excessive reduction in intra-ocular pressure following peri-operative use; **interactions:** Appendix 1 (apraclonidine)
Driving Drowsiness may affect performance of skilled tasks (e.g. driving)

Contra-indications   history of severe or unstable and uncontrolled cardiovascular disease

Hepatic impairment   manufacturer advises caution

Renal impairment   use with caution in chronic renal failure

Pregnancy   manufacturer advises avoid—no information available

Breast-feeding   manufacturer advises avoid—no information available

Side-effects   taste disturbance, conjunctivitis, dry eye, ocular intolerance (withdraw if eye pruritus, ocular hyperaemia, increased lacrimation, or oedema of the eyelids and conjunctiva occur), rhinitis; *less commonly* chest pain, asthma, dyspnoea, throat irritation, nervousness, irritability, impaired co-ordination, myalgia, mydriasis, keratitis, keratopathy, photophobia, visual

impairment, corneal erosion and infiltrates, blepharospasm, blepharitis, eyelid ptosis or retraction, conjunctival vascular disorders, rhinorrhoea, parosmia; since absorption may follow topical application, systemic effects (see Clonidine, section 2.5.2) may occur

Dose
* See under preparations below

Iopidine® (Alcon) (PoM)
Ophthalmic solution (= eye drops), apraclonidine 1% (as hydrochloride), net price 12 × 2 single use 0.25-mL units = £77.85
Dose control or prevention of postoperative elevation of intra-ocular pressure after anterior segment laser surgery, apply 1 drop 1 hour before laser procedure then 1 drop immediately after completion of procedure; CHILD not recommended

Iopidine 0.5% ophthalmic solution (= eye drops), apraclonidine 0.5% (as hydrochloride), net price 5 mL = £10.88
Excipients include benzalkonium chloride
Dose short-term adjunctive treatment of chronic glaucoma in patients not adequately controlled by another drug (see note below), apply 1 drop 3 times daily usually for max. 1 month; CHILD not recommended
Note May not provide additional benefit if patient already using two drugs that suppress the production of aqueous humour

BROMFENAC

Indications   postoperative inflammation following cataract surgery

Yellox® (Bausch & Lomb) ▼ (PoM)
Eye drops, bromfenac (as sodium sesquihydrate) 0.09%, net price 5 mL = £8.50
Excipients include benzalkonium chloride, disodium edetate, sulfites

CEFUROXIME

Indications   prophylaxis of endophthalmitis after cataract surgery

Cautions   severe risk of infection; complicated cataracts or combined operations with cataract surgery; severe thyroid disease; reduced corneal endothelial cells (less than 2000)

Dose
* By intracameral injection, ADULT over 18 years, 1 mg into the anterior chamber of the eye at the end of cataract surgery
Note For information on administration, consult product literature

Aprokam® (Spectrum Thea) (PoM)
Injection for intracameral use, powder for reconstitution, cefuroxime (as sodium) 10 mg/mL when reconstituted with 5 mL sodium chloride 0.9%, net price 50-mg vial = £7.95

DICLOFENAC SODIUM

Indications   inhibition of intra-operative miosis during cataract surgery (but does not possess intrinsic mydriatic properties); postoperative inflammation in cataract surgery, strabismus surgery or argon laser trabeculoplasty; pain in corneal epithelial defects after photorefractive keratectomy, radial keratotomy or accidental trauma; seasonal allergic conjunctivitis (section 11.4.2)

11 Eye

Voltarol® Ophtha Multidose (Spectrum Thea) [PoM]
Eye drops, diclofenac sodium 0.1%, net price 5 mL = £6.68
Excipients include benzalkonium chloride, disodium edetate, propylene glycol

◀ Single use
Voltarol® Ophtha (Spectrum Thea) [PoM]
Eye drops, diclofenac sodium 0.1%, net price pack of 5 single-dose units = £4.00, 40 single-dose units = £32.00

FLURBIPROFEN SODIUM

Indications inhibition of intra-operative miosis (but does not possess intrinsic mydriatic properties); anterior segment inflammation following postoperative and post-laser trabeculoplasty when corticosteroids contra-indicated

Ocufen® (Allergan) [PoM]
Ophthalmic solution (= eye drops), flurbiprofen sodium 0.03%, polyvinyl alcohol (*Liquifilm®*) 1.4%, net price 40 × 0.4 mL = £37.15

KETOROLAC TROMETAMOL

Indications prophylaxis and reduction of inflammation and associated symptoms following ocular surgery

Acular® (Allergan) [PoM]
Eye drops, ketorolac trometamol 0.5%, net price 5 mL = £3.00
Excipients include benzalkonium chloride, disodium edetate

NEPAFENAC

Indications prophylaxis and treatment of postoperative pain and inflammation associated with cataract surgery; reduction in the risk of postoperative macular oedema associated with cataract surgery in diabetic patients

Cautions avoid sunlight; discontinue immediately if evidence of corneal epithelial breakdown

Side-effects punctuate keratitis; *less commonly* nausea, headache, corneal epithelium defect, iritis, keratitis, corneal deposits, choroidal effusion, ocular discomfort, blurred vision, dry eye, allergic conjunctivitis, eye pruritus, increased lacrimation, photophobia, conjunctival hyperaemia; *also reported* dizziness, impaired corneal healing, corneal opacity, reduced visual acuity, eye swelling, dermatochalasis

Nevanac® (Alcon) [PoM]
Ophthalmic suspension (= eye drops), nepafenac 1 mg/mL, net price 5 mL= £14.92
Excipients include benzalkonium chloride, disodium edetate

POVIDONE-IODINE

Indications cutaneous peri-ocular and conjunctival antisepsis before ocular surgery

Contra-indications concomitant use with ocular antimicrobial drugs, and ocular formulations containing mercury-based preservatives; preterm neonates

Side-effects *rarely* conjunctival hyperaemia, superficial punctuate keratitis; *also reported* residual yellow coloration of the conjunctiva, cytotoxicity on mucous

membranes and deep tissue, hypothyroidism in neonates

Dose
• Apply eye drops, leave for 2 minutes, then irrigate thoroughly with sodium chloride 0.9%

Minims® Povidone Iodine (Bausch & Lomb) [PoM]
Eye drops, povidone-iodine 5%, net price 20 × 0.4 mL = £16.00

Subfoveal choroidal neovascularisation

Aflibercept, **pegaptanib** and **ranibizumab** are vascular endothelial growth factor inhibitors licensed for the treatment of neovascular (wet) age-related macular degeneration. Aflibercept is also licensed for the treatment of macular oedema secondary to central retinal vein occlusion, and diabetic macular oedema; ranibizumab is also licensed for the treatment of visual impairment due to diabetic macular oedema, macular oedema secondary to branch or central retinal vein occlusion, and choroidal neovascularisation secondary to pathologic myopia. Ranibizumab can be administered concomitantly with laser photocoagulation for the treatment of diabetic macular oedema and for macular oedema secondary to branch retinal vein occlusion. They are given by intravitreal injection by specialists experienced in the management of this condition. There is a potential risk of arterial thromboembolic events and non-ocular haemorrhage following the intravitreal injection of vascular endothelial growth factor inhibitors. Endophthalmitis can occur after intravitreal injections—patients should be advised to report any signs of infection immediately.

The *Scottish Medicines Consortium* (p. 4) has advised (May 2007) that ranibizumab (*Lucentis®*) is accepted for use within NHS Scotland for the treatment of neovascular (wet) age-related macular degeneration. The *Scottish Medicines Consortium* (p. 4) has also advised (October 2011 and April 2013) that ranibizumab (*Lucentis®*) is accepted for use within NHS Scotland for the treatment of macular oedema secondary to branch or central retinal vein occlusion, and (November 2012) for restricted use for the treatment of visual impairment due to diabetic macular oedema in adults with best corrected visual acuity 75 Early Treatment Diabetic Retinopathy Study letters or less at baseline, and (October 2013) for the treatment of visual impairment due to choroidal neovascularisation secondary to pathologic myopia in adults; SMC advice is contingent upon the continuing availability of ranibizumab at the price agreed in the patient access scheme.

> **NICE guidance**
> **Aflibercept solution for injection for treating wet age-related macular degeneration (July 2013)**
>
> Aflibercept solution for injection is recommended as an option for treating wet age-related macular degeneration only if:
> • it is used in accordance with the recommendations for ranibizumab in NICE TA 155 **and**
> • the manufacturer provides aflibercept solution for injection with the discount agreed in the patient access scheme.
> www.nice.org.uk/TA294

11 Eye

NICE guidance
Aflibercept for treating visual impairment caused by macular oedema secondary to central retinal vein occlusion (February 2014)

Aflibercept solution for injection is recommended as an option for treating visual impairment caused by macular oedema secondary to central retinal vein occlusion only if the manufacturer provides aflibercept solution for injection with the discount agreed in the patient access scheme.
www.nice.org.uk/TA305

NICE guidance
Ranibizumab and pegaptanib for the treatment of age-related macular degeneration (updated May 2012)

Ranibizumab is recommended for the treatment of wet age-related macular degeneration if all of the following apply:

- the best corrected visual acuity is between 6/12 and 6/96;
- there is no permanent structural damage to the central fovea;
- the lesion size is less than or equal to 12 disc areas in greatest linear dimension;
- there is evidence of recent disease progression;
- the manufacturer provides ranibizumab with the discount agreed in the patient access scheme (as revised in 2012).

Ranibizumab should only be continued in patients who maintain adequate response to therapy.

Pegaptanib is not recommended for the treatment of wet age-related macular degeneration; patients currently receiving pegaptanib for any lesion type can continue therapy until they and their specialist consider it appropriate to stop.
www.nice.org.uk/TA155

NICE guidance
Ranibizumab for the treatment of diabetic macular oedema (February 2013)

Ranibizumab is recommended as an option for the treatment of visual impairment due to diabetic macular oedema only if:

- the eye has a central retinal thickness of 400 micrometres or more at the start of treatment **and**
- the manufacturer provides ranibizumab with the discount agreed in the patient access scheme (as revised in 2012).

Patients currently receiving ranibizumab for treating visual impairment due to diabetic macular oedema whose disease does not meet the criteria should be able to continue treatment until they and their clinician consider it appropriate to stop.
www.nice.org.uk/TA274

NICE guidance
Ranibizumab for the treatment of visual impairment caused by macular oedema secondary to retinal vein occlusion (May 2013)

Ranibizumab is recommended as an option for treating visual impairment caused by macular oedema:

- following central retinal vein occlusion **or**
- following branch retinal vein occlusion only if treatment with laser photocoagulation has not been beneficial, or when laser photocoagulation is not suitable because of the extent of macular haemorrhage **and**
- only if the manufacturer provides ranibizumab with the discount agreed in the patient access scheme revised in the context of NICE technology appraisal guidance 274.

www.nice.org.uk/TA283

NICE guidance
Ranibizumab for treating choroidal neovascularisation associated with pathological myopia (November 2013)

Ranibizumab is recommended as an option for treating visual impairment due to choroidal neovascularisation secondary to pathological myopia when the manufacturer provides ranibizumab with the discount agreed in the patient access scheme.
www.nice.org.uk/TA298

Verteporfin is licensed for use in the photodynamic treatment of age-related macular degeneration associated with predominantly classic subfoveal choroidal neovascularisation *or* with pathological myopia (see NICE guidance below). Following intravenous infusion, verteporfin is activated by local irradiation using non-thermal red light to produce cytotoxic derivatives. Only specialists experienced in the management of these conditions should use it.

NICE guidance
Verteporfin photodynamic therapy for wet age-related macular degeneration (September 2003)

Photodynamic therapy is recommended for wet age-related macular degeneration with a confirmed diagnosis of classic (no occult) subfoveal choroidal neovascularisation and best-corrected visual acuity of 6/60 or better.

Photodynamic therapy is **not** recommended for wet age-related macular degeneration with predominantly classic but partly occult subfoveal choroidal neovascularisation *except* in clinical studies.
www.nice.org.uk/TA68

11 Eye

▌ AFLIBERCEPT

Indications see notes above—specialist use only
Cautions see notes above; also monitor intra-ocular pressure following injection; patients at risk of retinal pigment epithelial tear; recent history of stroke, transient ischaemic attack, or myocardial infarction; poorly controlled glaucoma; active systemic infection, diabetic patients with uncontrolled hypertension; discontinue treatment in the event of a retinal break, rhegmatogenous retinal detachment, or development of stage 3 or 4 macular holes—consult product literature for full details

Contra-indications ocular or periocular infection; severe intra-ocular inflammation; clinical signs of irreversible ischaemic visual function loss

Pregnancy manufacturer advises avoid unless potential benefit outweighs risk and recommends women use effective contraception during and for at least 3 months after treatment

Breast-feeding manufacturer advises avoid—no information available

Side-effects see notes above; also conjunctival haemorrhage, reduced visual acuity, eye pain, vitreous haemorrhage, corneal erosion, retinal pigment epithelium tear, retinal pigment epithelium detachment, retinal degeneration, cataract formation, corneal abrasion or oedema, raised intra-ocular pressure, blurred vision, vitreous floaters, vitreous detachment, injection-site pain or haemorrhage, foreign body sensation in eye, increased lacrimation, eyelid oedema, punctate keratitis, conjunctival hyperaemia, ocular hyperaemia; *less commonly* blindness, retinal tear, retinal detachment, lenticular opacities, corneal epithelium defect, eyelid irritation, iritis, iridocyclitis, anterior chamber flare, uveitis; *rarely* vitritis, hypopyon

Dose

- Neovascular (wet) age-related macular degeneration, by intravitreal injection, ADULT over 18 years, 2 mg into the affected eye once a month for 3 months, then every 2 months thereafter; review treatment frequency after 12 months

- Macular oedema secondary to central retinal vein occlusion, by intravitreal injection, ADULT over 18 years, 2 mg into the affected eye once a month; monitor visual and anatomic outcomes monthly; continue treatment until visual and anatomic outcomes are stable for 3 monthly assessments (discontinue treatment if no improvement in visual and anatomic outcomes after initial 3 injections); if necessary subsequent doses may be given at least 1 month apart

- Diabetic macular oedema, by intravitreal injection, ADULT over 18 years, 2 mg into the affected eye once a month for 5 months, then every 2 months thereafter; review treatment frequency after 12 months (discontinue treatment if no improvement in visual and anatomic outcomes)

Note For further information on administration, consult product literature

Eylea® (Bayer) ▼ PoM
Solution for intravitreal injection, aflibercept 40 mg/mL, net price 0.1-mL vial = £816.00

PEGAPTANIB SODIUM

Indications see notes above—specialist use only

Cautions see notes above; also monitor intra-ocular pressure (transient increase may occur following injection, and small, sustained increases reported after repeated dosing); monitor for vitreous haemorrhage and for signs of ocular infection for 2 weeks following injection

Contra-indications ocular or periocular infection

Pregnancy manufacturer advises avoid unless potential benefit outweighs risk

Breast-feeding manufacturer advises avoid—no information available

Side-effects see notes above; also rhinorrhoea; headache; eye pain, anterior chamber inflammation, raised intra-ocular pressure, punctate keratitis, vitreous floaters, cataract, conjunctival and retinal haemorrhage, local oedema, conjunctivitis, corneal dystrophy, dry eye, eye discharge, eye irritation, macular degeneration, mydriasis, periorbital haematoma, photophobia, flashing lights, vitreous disorders; *less commonly* vomiting, dyspepsia, palpitation, chest pain, hypertension, aortic aneurysm, influenza-like symptoms, nightmares, depression, back pain, asthenopia, blepharitis, corneal deposits, vitreous haemorrhage, chalazion, retinal exudates, eyelid ptosis, decreased intra-ocular pressure, injection-site reactions, retinal detachment, occlusion of retinal blood vessels, ectropion, eye movement disorder, pupillary disorder, iritis, optic nerve cupping, nasopharyngitis, deafness, vertigo, eczema, changes in hair colour, rash, pruritus, night sweats

Dose

- By intravitreal injection, ADULT over 18 years, 300 micrograms once every 6 weeks into the affected eye

Note For further information on administration, consult product literature. Review treatment if no benefit after 2 consecutive injections

Macugen® (Pfizer) PoM
Solution for intravitreal injection, pegaptanib (as sodium salt), net price 300-microgram prefilled syringe = £514.00

RANIBIZUMAB

Indications see notes above—specialist use only

Cautions see notes above; also history of stroke or transient ischaemic attack; patients at risk of retinal pigment epithelial tear; monitor intra-ocular pressure, perfusion of the optic nerve head, and for signs of ocular infection following injection; retinal detachment or macular hole—discontinue treatment if rhegmatogenous retinal detachment or stage 3 or 4 macular hole develops; diabetic macular oedema due to type 1 diabetes (limited information available); previous intravitreal injections; active systemic infection; proliferative diabetic retinopathy; uncontrolled hypertension; diabetic patients with HbA_{1c} over 12%

Contra-indications ocular or periocular infection; severe intra-ocular inflammation; signs of irreversible ischaemic visual function loss in patients with retinal vein occlusion

Pregnancy manufacturer advises avoid unless potential benefit outweighs risk and recommends women use effective contraception during and for at least 3 months after treatment

Breast-feeding manufacturer advises avoid—no information available

Side-effects see notes above; also nausea, headache, nasopharyngitis, cough, anxiety, anaemia, urinary tract infection, arthralgia, raised intra-ocular pressure, visual disturbance, conjunctival, retinal, and vitreous disorders, ocular discomfort, eye haemorrhage, uveitis, iritis, blepharitis, iridocyclitis, cataract, posterior capsule opacification, punctuate keratitis, anterior chamber flare, conjunctivitis, photopsia, photophobia, eyelid oedema, allergic skin reactions; *less commonly* blindness, hypopyon, hyphaema, keratopathy, corneal disorders, iris adhesion

Dose

- Neovascular (wet) age-related macular degeneration, by intravitreal injection, ADULT over 18 years, 500 micrograms once a month into the affected eye; monitor visual acuity monthly; continue treatment until visual acuity is stable for 3 consecutive months; thereafter monitor visual acuity monthly; if necessary subsequent doses may be given at least 1 month apart
- Diabetic macular oedema, macular oedema secondary to retinal vein occlusion, by intravitreal injection, ADULT over 18 years, 500 micrograms once a month into the affected eye; monitor visual acuity monthly; continue treatment until visual acuity is stable for 3 consecutive months (discontinue treatment if no improvement in visual acuity after initial 3 injections); thereafter monitor visual acuity monthly; if necessary subsequent doses may be given at least 1 month apart
- Choroidal neovascularisation secondary to pathologic myopia, by intravitreal injection, ADULT over 18 years, initially 500 micrograms as a single injection into the affected eye; monitor for disease activity monthly for first 2 months, then at least every 3 months thereafter during the first year, then as required; if necessary subsequent doses may be given at least 1 month apart
- Concomitant treatment of diabetic macular oedema, or macular oedema secondary to branch retinal vein occlusion, with laser photocoagulation, by intravitreal injection, ADULT, 500 micrograms at least 30 minutes after laser photocoagulation

Note For further information on administration, consult product literature

Lucentis® (Novartis) ▼ PoM
Solution for intravitreal injection, ranibizumab 10 mg/mL, net price 0.23-mL vial = £742.17

■ **VERTEPORFIN**

Indications see notes above—specialist use only

Cautions photosensitivity—avoid exposure of unprotected skin and eyes to bright light during infusion and for 48 hours afterwards; concomitant use with other photosensitising drugs; biliary obstruction; avoid extravasation

Contra-indications acute porphyria

Hepatic impairment use with caution in moderate impairment; avoid in severe impairment

Pregnancy manufacturer advises use only if potential benefit outweighs risk (teratogenic in *animal* studies)

Breast-feeding no information available—manufacturer advises avoid breast-feeding for 48 hours after administration

Side-effects nausea, hypercholesterolaemia, malaise, back pain, photosensitivity, visual disturbances (including reduced visual acuity, flashing lights, visual-field defects), *less commonly* hypertension, hyperaesthesia, pyrexia, retinal detachment, subretinal, retinal or vitreous haemorrhage, *rarely* retinal or choroidal vessel non-perfusion; *also reported* chest pain, myocardial infarction, vasovagal reactions, macular oedema, retinal oedema

Dose

- By intravenous infusion over 10 minutes, 6 mg/m^2
  Note For information on administration and light activation, consult product literature

Visudyne® (Novartis) PoM
Injection, powder for reconstitution, verteporfin, net price 15-mg vial = £850.00
Excipients include butylated hydroxytoluene

Vitreomacular traction

Ocriplasmin is licensed for the treatment of vitreomacular traction, including when associated with a macular hole of diameter less than or equal to 400 microns. It is given by intravitreal injection by specialists experienced in the management of this condition.

The *Scottish Medicines Consortium* (p. 4) has advised (July 2014) that ocriplasmin (*Jetrea®*) is accepted for restricted use within NHS Scotland for the treatment of patients with vitreomacular traction plus macular hole, regardless of whether they have epiretinal membrane formation, and in patients with vitreomacular traction alone (no epiretinal membrane and no macular hole).

> **NICE guidance**
> **Ocriplasmin for treating vitreomacular traction (October 2013)**
>
> Ocriplasmin is recommended as an option for treating vitreomacular traction in adults, only if:
> - an epiretinal membrane is not present **and**
> - they have a stage II full-thickness macular hole with a diameter of 400 microns or less **and/or**
> - they have severe symptoms.
>
> www.nice.org.uk/TA297

■ **OCRIPLASMIN**

Indications see notes above—specialist use only

Cautions monitor intra-ocular pressure, visual acuity, and for signs of intra-ocular inflammation or infection following injection; non-proliferative diabetic retinopathy; history of uveitis (including severe active inflammation); significant eye trauma

Contra-indications active or suspected ocular or periocular infection; large diameter macular hole (> 400 microns); high myopia; aphakia; history of rhegmatogenous retinal detachment; lens zonule instability; recent ocular surgery or intra-ocular injection (including laser therapy); proliferative diabetic retinopathy; ischaemic retinopathies; retinal vein occlusions; exudative age-related macular degeneration; vitreous haemorrhage

Pregnancy manufacturer advises use only if potential benefit outweighs risk—no information available

Breast-feeding manufacturer advises use only if potential benefit outweighs risk—no information available

Side-effects conjunctival, retinal, and vitreous disorders, reduced visual acuity, raised intra-ocular pressure, macular hole, macular degeneration, macular oedema, metamorphopsia, eyelid oedema, anterior chamber cell or flare, iritis, photopsia, ocular hyperaemia, abnormal retinograph, ocular discomfort, photophobia, chromatopsia, retinal pigment epitheliopathy; *less commonly* transient blindness, lens subluxation, scotoma, visual field defect, diplopia, hyphaema, miosis, unequal pupils, corneal abrasion, anterior chamber inflammation, eye inflammation

Dose

- By intravitreal injection, ADULT over 18 years, 125 micrograms as a single dose into the affected eye
  Note Concurrent administration to both eyes not recommended. For further information on administration, consult product literature

Jetrea® (Alcon) ▼ PoM
Concentrate for solution for intravitreal injection, ocriplasmin 2.5 mg/mL, net price 0.2-mL vial = £2500.00

11 Eye

11.9 Contact lenses

For cosmetic reasons many people prefer to wear contact lenses rather than spectacles; contact lenses are also sometimes required for medical indications. Visual defects are corrected by either rigid ('hard' or gas permeable) lenses or soft (hydrogel or silicone hydrogel) lenses; soft lenses are the most popular type, because they are initially the most comfortable, but they may not give the best vision. Lenses should usually be worn for a specified number of hours each day and removed for sleeping. The risk of infectious and non-infectious keratitis is increased by extended continuous contact lens wear, which is not recommended, except when medically indicated.

Contact lenses require meticulous care. Poor compliance with directions for use, and with daily cleaning and disinfection, can result in complications including ulcerative keratitis or conjunctivitis. One-day disposable lenses, which are worn only once and therefore require no disinfection or cleaning, are becoming increasingly popular.

Acanthamoeba keratitis, a painful and sight-threatening condition, is associated with ineffective lens cleaning and disinfection, the use of contaminated lens cases, or tap water coming into contact with the lenses. The condition is especially associated with the use of soft lenses (including frequently replaced lenses) and should be treated by specialists.

Contact lenses and drug treatment Special care is required in prescribing eye preparations for contact lens users. Some drugs and preservatives in eye preparations can accumulate in hydrogel lenses and may induce toxic reactions. Therefore, unless medically indicated, the lenses should be removed before instillation of the eye preparation and not worn during the period of treatment. Alternatively, unpreserved drops can be used. Eye drops may, however, be instilled while patients are wearing rigid corneal contact lenses. Ointment preparations should never be used in conjunction with contact lens wear; oily eye drops should also be avoided.

Many drugs given systemically can also have adverse effects on contact lens wear. These include oral contraceptives (particularly those with a higher oestrogen content), drugs which reduce blink rate (e.g. anxiolytics, hypnotics, antihistamines, and muscle relaxants), drugs which reduce lacrimation (e.g. antihistamines, antimuscarinics, phenothiazines and related drugs, some beta-blockers, diuretics, and tricyclic antidepressants), and drugs which increase lacrimation (including ephedrine and hydralazine). Other drugs that may affect contact lens wear are isotretinoin (can cause conjunctival inflammation), aspirin (salicylic acid appears in tears and can be absorbed by contact lenses—leading to irritation), and rifampicin and sulfasalazine (can discolour lenses).

12 Ear, nose, and oropharynx

> This chapter also includes advice on the drug management of the following:
> allergic rhinitis, p. 783
> nasal polyps, p. 783
> oropharyngeal infections, p. 789
> periodontitis, p. 787

12.1   Drugs acting on the ear

12.1.1   Otitis externa

Otitis externa is an inflammatory reaction of the meatal skin. It is important to exclude an underlying chronic otitis media before treatment is commenced. Many cases recover after thorough cleansing of the external ear canal by suction or dry mopping. A frequent problem in resistant cases is the difficulty in applying lotions and ointments satisfactorily to the relatively inaccessible affected skin. The most effective method is to introduce a ribbon gauze dressing or sponge wick soaked with **corticosteroid** ear drops or with an astringent such as **aluminium acetate** solution. When this is not practical, the ear should be gently cleansed with a probe covered in cotton wool and the patient encouraged to lie with the affected ear uppermost for ten minutes after the canal has been filled with a liberal quantity of the appropriate solution.

If infection is present, a topical anti-infective which is not used systemically (such as **neomycin** or **clioquinol**) may be used, but for only about a week as excessive use may result in fungal infections; these may be difficult to treat and require expert advice. Sensitivity to the anti-infective or solvent may occur and resistance to antibacterials is a possibility with prolonged use. Aluminium acetate ear drops are also effective against bacterial infection and inflammation of the ear. **Chloramphenicol** may be used but the ear drops contain propylene glycol and cause hypersensitivity reactions in about 10% of patients. Solutions containing an anti-infective and a corticosteroid (such as *Locorten-Vioform*®) are used for treating cases where infection is present with inflammation and eczema.

In view of reports of ototoxicity, manufacturers contra-indicate treatment with topical **aminoglycosides** or **polymyxins** in patients with a perforated tympanic membrane (eardrum) or patent grommet. However, some specialists do use these drops cautiously in the presence of a perforation or patent grommet in patients with chronic suppurative otitis media (section 12.1.2) and when other measures have failed for otitis externa; treatment should be considered only **by specialists** in the following circumstance:

- drops should only be used in the presence of obvious infection;
- treatment should be for no longer than 2 weeks;
- patients should be counselled on the risk of ototoxicity and given justification for the use of these topical antibiotics;
- baseline audiometry should be performed, if possible, before treatment is commenced.

Clinical expertise and judgement should be used to assess the risk of treatment versus the benefit to the patient in such circumstances.

A solution of **acetic acid** 2% acts as an antifungal and antibacterial in the external ear canal. It may be used to treat mild otitis externa but in severe cases an anti-inflammatory preparation with or without an anti-infective drug is required. A proprietary preparation containing acetic acid 2% (*EarCalm*® spray) is on sale to the public.

For severe pain associated with otitis externa, a simple analgesic, such as **paracetamol** (section 4.7.1) or **ibuprofen** (section 10.1.1), can be used. A systemic antibacterial (Table 1, section 5.1) can be used if there is spreading cellulitis or if the patient is systemically unwell. When a resistant staphylococcal infection (a boil) is present in the external auditory meatus, **flucloxacillin** is the drug of choice; **ciprofloxacin** (or an aminoglycoside) may be needed in pseudomonal infections which may occur if the patient has diabetes or is immunocompromised.

The skin of the pinna adjacent to the ear canal is often affected by eczema. Topical corticosteroid creams and ointments (section 13.4) are then required, but prolonged use should be avoided.

Astringent preparations

◢ ALUMINIUM ACETATE

Indications   inflammation in otitis externa (see notes above)

Dose

- Insert into meatus or apply on a ribbon gauze dressing or sponge wick which should be kept saturated with the ear drops

Aluminium Acetate (Non-proprietary)

Ear drops 13%, aluminium sulfate 2.25 g, calcium carbonate 1 g, tartaric acid 450 mg, acetic acid (33%) 2.5 mL, purified water 7.5 mL

Available from manufacturers of 'special order' products

Ear drops 8%, dilute 8 parts aluminium acetate ear drops (13%) with 5 parts purified water. Must be freshly prepared

Anti-inflammatory preparations

Corticosteroids

Topical corticosteroids are used to treat inflammation and eczema in otitis externa.

Cautions   Prolonged use of topical corticosteroid ear preparations should be avoided.

Contra-indications   Corticosteroid ear preparations should be avoided in the presence of an untreated ear infection. If infection is present, the corticosteroid should be used in combination with a suitable anti-infective (see notes above).

Side-effects   Local sensitivity reactions may occur.

◢ BETAMETHASONE SODIUM PHOSPHATE

Indications   eczematous inflammation in otitis externa (see notes above)

Cautions   see notes above

Contra-indications   see notes above

Side-effects   see notes above

Betnesol® (RPH) [PoM]

Drops (for ear, eye, or nose), betamethasone sodium phosphate 0.1%. Net price 10 mL = £2.32

Excipients   include benzalkonium chloride, disodium edetate

Dose   ear, apply 2–3 drops every 2–3 hours; reduce frequency when relief obtained; eye, section 11.4.1; nose, section 12.2.1

Vistamethasone® (Martindale) [PoM]

Drops (for ear, eye, or nose), betamethasone sodium phosphate 0.1%. Net price 5 mL = £1.02; 10 mL = £1.16

Excipients   include benzalkonium chloride, disodium edetate

Dose   ear, apply 2–3 drops every 3–4 hours; reduce frequency when relief obtained; eye, section 11.4.1; nose, section 12.2.1

◢ With antibacterial

Betnesol-N® (RPH) [PoM]

Drops (for ear, eye, or nose), betamethasone sodium phosphate 0.1%, neomycin sulfate 0.5%. Net price 10 mL = £2.39

Excipients   include benzalkonium chloride, disodium edetate

Dose   ear, apply 2–3 drops 3–4 times daily; eye, section 11.4.1; nose, section 12.2.3

◢ DEXAMETHASONE

Indications   eczematous inflammation in otitis externa (see notes above)

Cautions   see notes above

Contra-indications   see notes above

Side-effects   see notes above

◢ With antibacterial

Otomize® (Forest) [PoM]

Ear spray, dexamethasone 0.1%, neomycin sulfate 3250 units/mL, glacial acetic acid 2%. Net price 5-mL pump-action aerosol unit = £3.27

Excipients   include hydroxybenzoates (parabens)

Dose   ADULT and CHILD over 2 years, apply 1 metered spray 3 times daily

Sofradex® (Sanofi-Aventis) [PoM] ◢

Drops (for ear or eye), dexamethasone (as sodium metasulphobenzoate) 0.05%, framycetin sulfate 0.5%, gramicidin 0.005%. Net price 10 mL = £6.25

Excipients   include polysorbate 80

Dose   ear, apply 2–3 drops 3–4 times daily; eye, section 11.4.1

◢ FLUMETASONE PIVALATE
(Flumethasone Pivalate)

Indications   eczematous inflammation in otitis externa (see notes above)

Cautions   see notes above

Contra-indications   see notes above

Side-effects   see notes above

◢ With antibacterial

Locorten-Vioform® (AMCo) [PoM]

Ear drops, flumetasone pivalate 0.02%, clioquinol 1%. Net price 7.5 mL = £1.76

Contra-indications   iodine sensitivity

Dose   ADULT and CHILD over 2 years apply 2–3 drops into the ear twice daily for 7–10 days

Note   Clioquinol stains skin and clothing

HYDROCORTISONE

Indications   eczematous inflammation in otitis externa (see notes above)

Cautions   see notes above

Contra-indications   see notes above

Side-effects   see notes above

◢ **With antibacterial**

Gentisone® HC (AMCo) [PoM]

> Ear drops, hydrocortisone acetate 1%, gentamicin 0.3% (as sulfate). Net price 10 mL = £4.76
> **Excipients** include benzalkonium chloride, disodium edetate
> **Dose** ear, apply 2–4 drops 3–4 times daily and at night

PREDNISOLONE SODIUM PHOSPHATE

Indications   eczematous inflammation in otitis externa (see notes above)

Cautions   see notes above

Contra-indications   see notes above

Side-effects   see notes above

Predsol® (RPH) [PoM]

> Drops (for ear or eye), prednisolone sodium phosphate 0.5%. Net price 10 mL = £2.00
> **Excipients** include benzalkonium chloride, disodium edetate
> **Dose** ear, apply 2–3 drops every 2–3 hours; reduce frequency when relief obtained; eye, section 11.4.1

Anti-infective preparations

CHLORAMPHENICOL ◢

Indications   bacterial infection in otitis externa (but see notes above)

Cautions   avoid prolonged use (see notes above)

Side-effects   high incidence of sensitivity reactions to vehicle

Chloramphenicol (Non-proprietary) [PoM] ◢

> Ear drops, chloramphenicol in propylene glycol, net price 5%, 10 mL = £40.92; 10%, 10 mL = £19.52
> **Dose** ear, apply 2–3 drops 2–3 times daily

CLIOQUINOL

Indications   mild bacterial or fungal infections in otitis externa (see notes above)

Cautions   avoid prolonged use (see notes above); manufacturer advises avoid in perforated tympanic membrane (but used by specialists for short periods)

Side-effects   local sensitivity; stains skin and clothing

◢ **With corticosteroid**

Locorten-Vioform®   see Flumetasone, p. 780

CLOTRIMAZOLE

Indications   fungal infection in otitis externa (see notes above)

Side-effects   occasional local irritation or sensitivity

Canesten® (Bayer Consumer Care)

> Solution, clotrimazole 1% in polyethylene glycol 400 (macrogol 400). Net price 20 mL = £2.30
> **Dose** ear, apply 2–3 times daily continuing for at least 14 days after disappearance of infection; skin, section 13.10.2

FRAMYCETIN SULFATE

Indications   bacterial infection in otitis externa (see notes above)

Cautions   avoid prolonged use (see notes above)

Contra-indications   perforated tympanic membrane (see p. 779)

Side-effects   local sensitivity

◢ **With corticosteroid**

Sofradex®   see Dexamethasone, p. 780

GENTAMICIN

Indications   bacterial infection in otitis externa (see notes above)

Cautions   avoid prolonged use (see notes above)

Contra-indications   perforated tympanic membrane (but see also p. 779 and section 12.1.2)

Side-effects   local sensitivity

Genticin® (AMCo) [PoM]

> Drops (for ear or eye), gentamicin 0.3% (as sulfate). Net price 10 mL = £2.13
> **Excipients** include benzalkonium chloride
> **Dose** ear, apply 2–3 drops 3–4 times daily and at night; eye, section 11.3.1

◢ **With corticosteroid**

Gentisone® HC   see Hydrocortisone, above

NEOMYCIN SULFATE

Indications   bacterial infection in otitis externa (see notes above)

Cautions   avoid prolonged use (see notes above)

Contra-indications   perforated tympanic membrane (see p. 779)

Side-effects   local sensitivity

◢ **With corticosteroid**

Betnesol-N®   see Betamethasone, p. 780

Otomize®   see Dexamethasone, p. 780

12.1.2 Otitis media

Acute otitis media   Acute otitis media is the commonest cause of severe aural pain in small children. Many infections, especially those accompanying coryza, are caused by viruses. Most uncomplicated cases resolve without antibacterial treatment and a **simple analgesic**, such as paracetamol, may be sufficient. In children without systemic features, a **systemic antibacterial** (Table 1, section 5.1) may be started after 72 hours if there is no improvement, or earlier if there is deterioration, if the patient is systemically unwell, if the patient is at high risk of serious complications (e.g. in immunosuppression, cystic fibrosis), if mastoiditis is present, or in children under 2 years of age with bilateral otitis media. Perforation of the tympanic membrane in patients with *acute otitis media* usually heals spontaneously without treatment; if there is no improvement, e.g. pain or discharge persists, a systemic antibacterial (Table 1, section 5.1) can be given. Topical treatment of acute otitis media is ineffective and there is no place for drops containing a local anaesthetic.

Otitis media with effusion Otitis media with effusion (glue ear) occurs in about 10% of children and in 90% of children with cleft palates. Systemic antibacterials are not usually required. If glue ear persists for more than a month or two, the child should be referred for assessment and follow up because of the risk of long-term hearing impairment which can delay language development. Untreated or resistant glue ear may be responsible for some types of *chronic otitis media*.

Chronic otitis media Opportunistic organisms are often present in the debris, keratin, and necrotic bone of the middle ear and mastoid in patients with chronic otitis media. The mainstay of treatment is thorough cleansing with aural microsuction which may completely resolve long-standing infection. Local cleansing of the meatal and middle ear may be followed by treatment with a sponge wick or ribbon gauze dressing soaked with corticosteroid ear drops or with an astringent such as aluminium acetate solution; this is particularly beneficial for discharging ears or infections of the mastoid cavity. An antibacterial ear ointment may also be used. Acute exacerbations of chronic infection may also require systemic treatment with amoxicillin (or erythromycin if penicillin-allergic); treatment is adjusted according to the results of sensitivity testing.

In view of reports of ototoxicity, manufacturers contraindicate topical treatment with ototoxic antibacterials in the presence of a tympanic perforation or patent grommet. Ciprofloxacin or ofloxacin eye drops used in the ear [unlicensed use] or ear drops [both unlicensed; available from 'special-order' manufacturers or specialist importing companies, see p. 1124] are an effective alternative to such ototoxic ear drops for chronic otitis media in patients with perforation of the tympanic membrane.

However, some specialists do use ear drops containing **aminoglycosides** or **polymyxins** [unlicensed indications] cautiously in patients with chronic suppurative otitis media and a perforation of the tympanic membrane, if the otitis media has failed to settle with systemic antibacterials; treatment should be considered only **by specialists** in the following circumstance:

- drops should only be used in the presence of obvious infection;
- treatment should be for no longer than 2 weeks;
- patients should be counselled on the risk of ototoxicity and given justification for the use of these topical antibiotics;
- baseline audiometry should be performed, if possible, before treatment is commenced.

Clinical expertise and judgement should be used to assess the risk of treatment versus the benefit to the patient in such circumstances. It is considered that the pus in the middle ear associated with otitis media also carries a risk of ototoxicity.

12.1.3 Removal of ear wax

Wax is a normal bodily secretion which provides a protective film on the meatal skin and need only be removed if it causes hearing loss or interferes with a proper view of the ear drum.

Wax can be softened using simple remedies such as **olive oil** ear drops or **almond oil** ear drops; **sodium bicarbonate** ear drops are also effective, but may cause dryness of the ear canal. If the wax is hard and impacted, the drops can be used twice daily for several days and this may reduce the need for mechanical removal of the wax. The patient should lie with the affected ear uppermost for 5 to 10 minutes after a generous amount of the softening remedy has been introduced into the ear. Some proprietary preparations containing organic solvents can irritate the meatal skin, and in most cases the simple remedies indicated above are just as effective and less likely to cause irritation. Docusate sodium or urea–hydrogen peroxide are ingredients in a number of proprietary preparations for softening ear wax.

If necessary, wax may be removed by irrigation with water (warmed to body temperature). Ear irrigation is generally best avoided in young children, in patients unable to co-operate with the procedure, in those with otitis media in the last six weeks, in otitis externa, in patients with cleft palate, a history of ear drum perforation, or previous ear surgery. A person who has hearing in one ear only should not have that ear irrigated because even a very slight risk of damage is unacceptable in this situation.

Almond Oil (Non-proprietary)

Ear drops, almond oil in a suitable container
Allow to warm to room temperature before use

Olive Oil (Non-proprietary)

Ear drops, olive oil in a suitable container
Allow to warm to room temperature before use

Sodium Bicarbonate (Non-proprietary)

Ear drops, sodium bicarbonate 5%, net price 10 mL = £1.25

Cerumol® (Thornton & Ross)

Ear drops, chlorobutanol 5%, arachis (peanut) oil 57.3%. Net price 11 mL = £2.05

Exterol® (Dermal)

Ear drops, urea–hydrogen peroxide complex 5% in glycerol. Net price 8 mL = £1.75

Molcer® (Wallace Mfg)

Ear drops, docusate sodium 5%. Net price 15 mL = £8.08
Excipients include propylene glycol

Otex® (DDD)

Ear drops, urea–hydrogen peroxide 5%. Net price 8 mL = £2.89

Waxsol® (Meda)

Ear drops, docusate sodium 0.5%. Net price 10 mL = £1.95

12.2 Drugs acting on the nose

12.2.1 Drugs used in nasal allergy
12.2.2 Topical nasal decongestants
12.2.3 Nasal preparations for infection

Rhinitis is often self-limiting but bacterial sinusitis may require treatment with antibacterials (Table 1, section 5.1). There are few indications for nasal sprays and drops except in allergic rhinitis and perennial rhinitis (section 12.2.1). Many nasal preparations contain sympathomimetic drugs which may damage the nasal cilia (section 12.2.2). **Sodium chloride 0.9%** solution may be used as a douche or 'sniff' following endonasal surgery.

Nasal polyps   Short-term use of corticosteroid nasal drops helps to shrink nasal polyps; to be effective, the drops must be administered with the patient in the 'head down' position. A short course of a systemic corticosteroid (section 6.3.2) may be required initially to shrink large polyps. A corticosteroid nasal spray can be used to maintain the reduction in swelling and also for the initial treatment of small polyps.

12.2.1 Drugs used in nasal allergy

Mild allergic rhinitis is controlled by **antihistamines** (see also section 3.4.1) or topical **nasal corticosteroids**; systemic nasal decongestants are of doubtful value (section 3.10). Topical nasal decongestants can be used for a short period to relieve congestion and allow penetration of a topical nasal corticosteroid.

More persistent symptoms and nasal congestion can be relieved by topical nasal **corticosteroids**; **sodium cromoglicate** is an alternative, but may be less effective. The topical antihistamine **azelastine** is useful for controlling breakthrough symptoms in allergic rhinitis. Topical antihistamines are considered less effective than topical corticosteroids but probably more effective than cromoglicate. In seasonal allergic rhinitis (e.g. hay fever), treatment should begin 2 to 3 weeks before the season commences and may have to be continued for several months; continuous treatment may be required for years in perennial rhinitis.

Montelukast (section 3.3.2) is less effective than topical nasal corticosteroids; montelukast can be used in patients with seasonal allergic rhinitis and concomitant asthma.

Sometimes allergic rhinitis is accompanied by vasomotor rhinitis. In this situation, the addition of topical nasal ipratropium bromide (section 12.2.2) can reduce watery rhinorrhoea.

Very disabling symptoms occasionally justify the use of **systemic corticosteroids** for short periods (section 6.3), for example, in students taking important examinations. They may also be used at the beginning of a course of treatment with a corticosteroid spray to relieve severe mucosal oedema and allow the spray to penetrate the nasal cavity.

Pregnancy   If a pregnant woman cannot tolerate the symptoms of allergic rhinitis, treatment with nasal beclometasone, budesonide, fluticasone, or sodium cromoglicate may be considered.

Antihistamines

▲ AZELASTINE HYDROCHLORIDE

Indications   allergic rhinitis
Side-effects   irritation of nasal mucosa; bitter taste (if applied incorrectly); *very rarely* hypersensitivity reactions including rash, pruritus, and urticaria

◢**With fluticasone propionate**
Dymista®
see Fluticasone propionate, p. 784

Corticosteroids

Nasal preparations containing corticosteroids (beclometasone, betamethasone, budesonide, fluticasone, mometasone, and triamcinolone) have a useful role in the prophylaxis and treatment of allergic rhinitis (see notes above).

Cautions   Corticosteroid nasal preparations should be avoided in the presence of untreated nasal infections, and also after nasal surgery (until healing has occurred); they should also be avoided in pulmonary tuberculosis. Patients transferred from systemic corticosteroids may experience exacerbation of some symptoms. Systemic absorption may follow nasal administration particularly if high doses are used or if treatment is prolonged; for cautions and side-effects of systemic corticosteroids, see section 6.3.2. The risk of systemic effects may be greater with nasal drops than with nasal sprays; drops are administered incorrectly more often than sprays. The height of children receiving prolonged treatment with nasal corticosteroids should be monitored; if growth is slowed, referral to a paediatrician should be considered.

Side-effects   Local side-effects include dryness, irritation of nose and throat, and epistaxis. Nasal ulceration has been reported, but occurs commonly with nasal preparations containing fluticasone furoate or mometasone furoate. Nasal septal perforation (usually following nasal surgery) occurs very rarely. Raised intra-ocular pressure or glaucoma may occur rarely. Headache, smell and taste disturbances may also occur. Hyperactivity, sleep disturbances, anxiety, depression, and aggression have been reported particularly in children. Hypersensitivity reactions, including bronchospasm, have been reported.

▌ BECLOMETASONE DIPROPIONATE
(Beclomethasone Dipropionate)

Indications   prophylaxis and treatment of allergic and vasomotor rhinitis
Cautions   see notes above
Side-effects   see notes above
Dose
● ADULT and CHILD over 6 years, 100 micrograms (2 sprays) into each nostril twice daily; max. total 400 micrograms (8 sprays) daily; when symptoms controlled, dose reduced to 50 micrograms (1 spray) into each nostril twice daily

Beclometasone (Non-proprietary) [PoM]
Nasal spray, beclometasone dipropionate 50 micrograms/metered spray. Net price 200-spray unit = £2.42
Brands include *Nasobec Aqueous*®
Note Preparations of beclometasone dipropionate can be sold to the public for nasal administration as a nasal spray if supplied for the prevention and treatment of allergic rhinitis in adults over 18 years subject to max. single dose of 100 micrograms per nostril, max. daily dose of 200 micrograms per nostril for max. 3 months, and a pack size of 20 mg

Beconase® (A&H) [PoM]
Nasal spray (aqueous suspension), beclometasone dipropionate 50 micrograms/metered spray. Net price 200-spray unit with applicator = £2.19
Excipients include benzalkonium chloride, polysorbate 80

BETAMETHASONE SODIUM PHOSPHATE

Indications non-infected inflammatory conditions of nose

Cautions see notes above

Side-effects see notes above

Betnesol® (RPH) [PoM]

Drops (for ear, eye, or nose), betamethasone sodium phosphate 0.1%, net price 10 mL = £2.32

Excipients include benzalkonium chloride, disodium edetate

Dose nose, 2–3 drops into each nostril 2–3 times daily; ear, section 12.1.1; eye, section 11.4.1

Vistamethasone® (Martindale) [PoM]

Drops (for ear, eye, or nose), betamethasone sodium phosphate 0.1%. Net price 5 mL = £1.02, 10 mL = £1.16

Excipients include benzalkonium chloride, disodium edetate

Dose nose, 2–3 drops into each nostril twice daily; ear, section 12.1.1; eye, section 11.4.1

BUDESONIDE

Indications prophylaxis and treatment of allergic and vasomotor rhinitis; nasal polyps

Cautions see notes above; **interactions:** Appendix 1 (corticosteroids)

Side-effects see notes above

Dose

- See preparations

Budesonide (Non-proprietary) [PoM]

Nasal spray, budesonide 100 micrograms/metered spray, net price 100-spray unit = £5.90

Dose rhinitis, ADULT and CHILD over 12 years, 200 micrograms (2 sprays) into each nostril once daily in the morning *or* 100 micrograms (1 spray) into each nostril twice daily; when control achieved reduce to 100 micrograms (1 spray) into each nostril once daily

Nasal polyps, ADULT and CHILD over 12 years, 100 micrograms (1 spray) into each nostril twice daily for up to 3 months

Note Preparations of budesonide can be sold to the public for nasal administration as a nasal spray if supplied for the prevention and treatment of seasonal allergic rhinitis in adults over 18 years subject to max. single dose of 200 micrograms per nostril, max. daily dose of 200 micrograms per nostril for max. period of 3 months, and a pack size of 10 mg

Rhinocort Aqua® (AstraZeneca) [PoM]

Nasal spray, budesonide 64 micrograms/metered spray. Net price 120-spray unit = £3.49

Excipients include disodium edetate, polysorbate 80, potassium sorbate

Dose rhinitis, ADULT and CHILD over 12 years, 128 micrograms (2 sprays) into each nostril once daily in the morning *or* 64 micrograms (1 spray) into each nostril twice daily; when control achieved reduce to 64 micrograms (1 spray) into each nostril once daily; max. duration of treatment 3 months

Nasal polyps, ADULT and CHILD over 12 years, 64 micrograms (1 spray) into each nostril twice daily for up to 3 months

FLUTICASONE PROPIONATE

Indications prophylaxis and treatment of allergic rhinitis and perennial rhinitis; nasal polyps

Cautions see notes above; **interactions:** Appendix 1 (corticosteroids)

Side-effects see notes above

Dose

- Rhinitis, 100 micrograms (2 sprays) into each nostril once daily, preferably in the morning, increased to max. twice daily if required; when control achieved reduce to 50 micrograms (1 spray) into each nostril once daily; CHILD 4–11 years, 50 micrograms (1 spray) into each nostril once daily, preferably in the morning, increased to max. twice daily if required

- Nasal polyps, see *Flixonase Nasule®* below

Flixonase® (A&H) [PoM]

Aqueous nasal spray, fluticasone propionate 50 micrograms/metered spray. Net price 150-spray unit with applicator = £11.01

Excipients include benzalkonium chloride, polysorbate 80

Note Preparations of fluticasone propionate can be sold to the public for nasal administration (other than by pressurised nasal spray) if supplied for the prevention and treatment of allergic rhinitis in adults over 18 years, subject to max. single dose of 100 micrograms per nostril, max. daily dose of 200 micrograms per nostril for max. 3 months, and a pack size of 3 mg

Flixonase Nasule® (A&H) [PoM]

Nasal drops, fluticasone propionate 400 micrograms/unit dose, net price 28 × 0.4-mL units = £12.99

Excipients include polysorbate 20

Dose nasal polyps, ADULT and ADOLESCENT over 16 years, 200 micrograms (approx. 6 drops) into each nostril once or twice daily; consider alternative treatment if no improvement after 4–6 weeks

Nasofan® (TEVA UK) [PoM]

Aqueous nasal spray fluticasone propionate 50 micrograms/metered spray. Net price 150-spray unit = £8.04

Excipients include benzalkonium chloride, polysorbate 80

◢With azelastine hydrochloride

Dymista® (Meda) [PoM]

Nasal spray, fluticasone propionate 50 micrograms, azelastine hydrochloride 137 micrograms/metered spray, net price 120-spray unit = £18.91

Excipients include benzalkonium chloride, polysorbate 80

Dose moderate to severe seasonal and perennial allergic rhinitis, if monotherapy with antihistamine or corticosteroid is inadequate, ADULT and CHILD over 12 years, 1 spray into each nostril twice daily

◢Fluticasone furoate

Avamys® (GSK) [PoM]

Nasal spray, fluticasone furoate 27.5 micrograms/metered spray, net price 120-spray unit = £6.44

Excipients include benzalkonium chloride, disodium edetate, polysorbate 80

Dose prophylaxis and treatment of allergic rhinitis, ADULT and CHILD over 12 years, 55 micrograms (2 sprays) into each nostril once daily; when control achieved reduce to minimum effective dose, 27.5 micrograms (1 spray) into each nostril once daily may be sufficient; CHILD 6–12 years, 27.5 micrograms (1 spray) into each nostril once daily, increased if necessary to 55 micrograms (2 sprays) into each nostril once daily; when control achieved reduce to 27.5 micrograms (1 spray) into each nostril once daily

MOMETASONE FUROATE

Indications prophylaxis and treatment of allergic rhinitis; nasal polyps

Cautions see notes above

Side-effects see notes above

Dose

- Rhinitis, ADULT and CHILD over 12 years, 100 micrograms (2 sprays) into each nostril once daily, increased if necessary to max. 200 micrograms (4 sprays) into each nostril once daily; when control achieved reduce to 50 micrograms (1 spray) into each nostril once daily; CHILD 6–12 years, 50 micrograms (1 spray) into each nostril once daily

- Nasal polyps, ADULT over 18 years, 100 micrograms (2 sprays) into each nostril once daily, increased if necessary after 5–6 weeks to 100 micrograms (2 sprays) into each nostril twice daily (consider alternative treatment if no improvement after further 5–6 weeks); reduce to the lowest effective dose when control achieved

Mometasone (Non-proprietary) [PoM]

Nasal spray, mometasone furoate 50 micrograms/metered spray, net price 140-spray unit = £5.79
Excipients include benzalkonium chloride, polysorbate 80

Nasonex® (MSD) [PoM]

Nasal spray, mometasone furoate 50 micrograms/metered spray, net price 140-spray unit = £7.68
Excipients include benzalkonium chloride, polysorbate 80

TRIAMCINOLONE ACETONIDE

Indications prophylaxis and treatment of allergic rhinitis

Cautions see notes above

Side-effects see notes above

Nasacort® (Sanofi-Aventis) [PoM]

Aqueous nasal spray, triamcinolone acetonide 55 micrograms/metered spray. Net price 120-spray unit = £7.39
Excipients include benzalkonium chloride, disodium edetate, polysorbate 80
Dose ADULT and CHILD over 12 years, 110 micrograms (2 sprays) into each nostril once daily; when control achieved, reduce to 55 micrograms (1 spray) into each nostril once daily; CHILD 6–12 years, 55 micrograms (1 spray) into each nostril once daily, increased if necessary to 110 micrograms (2 sprays) into each nostril once daily; when control achieved, reduce to 55 micrograms (1 spray) into each nostril once daily; max. duration of treatment 3 months; CHILD 2–6 years see BNF for Children
Note Preparations of triamcinolone acetonide can be sold to the public for nasal administration as a non-pressurised nasal spray if supplied for the symptomatic treatment of seasonal allergic rhinitis in adults over 18 years, subject to max. daily dose of 110 micrograms per nostril for max. 3 months, and a pack size of 3.575 mg

Cromoglicate

SODIUM CROMOGLICATE

(Sodium Cromoglycate)

Indications prophylaxis of allergic rhinitis

Side-effects local irritation; rarely transient bronchospasm

Rynacrom® (Sanofi-Aventis)

4% aqueous nasal spray, sodium cromoglicate 4% (5.2 mg/spray). Net price 22 mL (150-spray unit with pump) = £17.07
Excipients include benzalkonium chloride, disodium edetate
Dose ADULT and CHILD, 1 spray into each nostril 2–4 times daily

12.2.2 Topical nasal decongestants

The nasal mucosa is sensitive to changes in atmospheric temperature and humidity and these alone may cause slight nasal congestion. The nose and nasal sinuses produce a litre of mucus in 24 hours and much of this finds its way silently into the stomach via the nasopharynx. Slight changes in the nasal airway, accompanied by an awareness of mucus passing along the nasopharynx causes some patients to be inaccurately diagnosed as suffering from chronic sinusitis. These symptoms are particularly noticeable in the later stages of the common cold. **Sodium chloride** 0.9% given as nasal drops or spray may relieve nasal congestion by helping to liquefy mucous secretions.

Inhalation of **warm moist air** is useful in the treatment of symptoms of acute infective conditions. The addition of volatile substances such as menthol and eucalyptus may encourage the use of warm moist air (section 3.8).

Symptoms of nasal congestion associated with vasomotor rhinitis and the common cold can be relieved by the short-term use (usually not longer than 7 days) of decongestant nasal drops and sprays. These all contain sympathomimetic drugs which exert their effect by vasoconstriction of the mucosal blood vessels which in turn reduces oedema of the nasal mucosa. They are of limited value because they can give rise to a rebound congestion (rhinitis medicamentosa) on withdrawal, due to a secondary vasodilatation with a subsequent temporary increase in nasal congestion. This in turn tempts the further use of the decongestant, leading to a vicious cycle of events. **Ephedrine nasal drops** is the safest sympathomimetic preparation and can give relief for several hours. The more potent sympathomimetic drugs oxymetazoline and xylometazoline are more likely to cause a rebound effect. Sympathomimetics may cause a hypertensive crisis if used during treatment with a monoamine-oxidase inhibitor including moclobemide.

The CHM/MHRA has stated that non-prescription cough and cold medicines containing ephedrine, oxymetazoline, or xylometazoline can be continued for up to 5 days in children aged 6–12 years after basic principles of best care have been tried; these medicines should not be used in children under 6 years of age (section 3.9.1).

Non-allergic watery rhinorrhoea often responds well to treatment with the antimuscarinic **ipratropium bromide**.

Systemic nasal decongestants—see section 3.10.

Sinusitis and oral pain Sinusitis affecting the maxillary antrum can cause pain in the upper jaw. Where this is associated with blockage of the opening from the sinus into the nasal cavity, it may be helpful to relieve the congestion with inhalation of warm moist air (section 3.8) or with **ephedrine nasal drops** (see above). For antibacterial treatment of sinusitis, see Table 1, section 5.1.

Sympathomimetics

EPHEDRINE HYDROCHLORIDE

Indications nasal congestion

Cautions see section 3.1.1.2 and notes above; also avoid excessive or prolonged use; interactions: Appendix 1 (sympathomimetics)

12   Ear, nose, and oropharynx

Pregnancy   see section 3.1.1.2

Breast-feeding   see section 3.1.1.2

Side-effects   local irritation, nausea, headache; after excessive use tolerance with diminished effect, rebound congestion; cardiovascular effects also reported

Dose

- See below

[1]**Ephedrine** (Non-proprietary)

Nasal drops, ephedrine hydrochloride 0.5%, net price 10 mL = £1.49; 1%, 10 mL = £1.54

Note The BP directs that if no strength is specified 0.5% drops should be supplied

Dose ADULT and CHILD over 12 years, 1–2 drops into each nostril up to 4 times daily when required, max. duration 7 days

Dental prescribing on NHS Ephedrine nasal drops may be prescribed

XYLOMETAZOLINE HYDROCHLORIDE

Indications   nasal congestion

Cautions   see under Ephedrine Hydrochloride section 3.1.1.2 and notes above; also angle-closure glaucoma; avoid excessive or prolonged use

Pregnancy   manufacturer advises avoid

Breast-feeding   manufacturer advises caution—no information available

Side-effects   see under Ephedrine Hydrochloride and notes above; also reported transient visual disturbances; in small children, also restlessness, sleep disturbances, and hallucinations (discontinue treatment)

Dose

- See below

Xylometazoline (Non-proprietary)

Nasal drops, xylometazoline hydrochloride 0.1%, net price 10 mL = £2.10

Brands include Otradrops®, Otrivine® ᴊᴴꜱ

Dose 2–3 drops into each nostril 2–3 times daily when required; max. duration 7 days; not recommended for children under 12 years

Paediatric nasal drops, xylometazoline hydrochloride 0.05%, net price 10 mL = £1.91

Brands include Otradrops®, Otrivine® ᴊᴴꜱ

Dose CHILD 6–12 years 1–2 drops into each nostril 1–2 times daily when required; max. duration 5 days

Nasal spray, xylometazoline hydrochloride 0.1%, net price 10 mL = £2.10

Brands include Otrivine® ᴊᴴꜱ, Otrivine® Allergy Relief

Dose 1 spray into each nostril 1–3 times daily when required; max. duration 7 days; not recommended for children under 12 years

Antimuscarinic

IPRATROPIUM BROMIDE

Indications   rhinorrhoea associated with allergic and non-allergic rhinitis

Cautions   see section 3.1.2; avoid spraying near eyes

Side-effects   epistaxis, nasal dryness, and irritation; less frequently nausea, headache, and pharyngitis;

very rarely antimuscarinic effects such as gastro-intestinal motility disturbances, palpitations, and urinary retention

Dose

- ADULT and CHILD over 12 years, 42 micrograms (2 sprays) into each nostril 2–3 times daily

Rinatec® (Boehringer Ingelheim) ᴾᴼᴹ

Nasal spray 0.03%, ipratropium bromide 21 micrograms/metered spray. Net price 180-dose unit = £6.54

Excipients include benzalkonium chloride, disodium edetate

12.2.3   Nasal preparations for infection

There is no evidence that topical anti-infective nasal preparations have any therapeutic value in rhinitis or sinusitis; for elimination of nasal staphylococci, see below.

Systemic treatment of sinusitis—see Table 1 section 5.1.

Betnesol-N® (RPH) ᴾᴼᴹ ◢

Drops (for ear, eye, or nose), betamethasone sodium phosphate 0.1%, neomycin sulfate 0.5%. Net price 10 mL = £2.39

Excipients include benzalkonium chloride, disodium edetate

Dose nose, 2–3 drops into each nostril 2–3 times daily; eye, section 11.4.1; ear, section 12.1.1

Nasal staphylococci

Elimination of organisms such as staphylococci from the nasal vestibule can be achieved by the use of a cream containing **chlorhexidine and neomycin** (Naseptin®), but re-colonisation frequently occurs. Coagulase-positive staphylococci are present in the noses of 40% of the population.

A nasal ointment containing **mupirocin** is also available; it should probably be held in reserve for resistant cases. In hospital or in care establishments, mupirocin nasal ointment should be reserved for the eradication (in both patients and staff) of nasal carriage of meticillin-resistant *Staphylococcus aureus* (MRSA). The ointment should be applied 3 times daily for 5 days and a sample taken 2 days after treatment to confirm eradication. The course may be repeated if the sample is positive (and the throat is not colonised). To avoid the development of resistance, the treatment course should not exceed 7 days and the course should not be repeated on more than one occasion. If the MRSA strain is mupirocin-resistant or does not respond after 2 courses, consider alternative products such as chlorhexidine and neomycin cream.

Bactroban Nasal® (GSK) ᴾᴼᴹ

Nasal ointment, mupirocin 2% (as calcium salt) in white soft paraffin basis. Net price 3 g = £3.89

Dose for eradication of nasal carriage of staphylococci, including meticillin-resistant *Staphylococcus aureus* (MRSA), apply 2–3 times daily to the inner surface of each nostril

Naseptin® (Alliance) ᴾᴼᴹ

Cream, chlorhexidine hydrochloride 0.1%, neomycin sulfate 0.5%, net price 15 g = £1.90

Excipients include arachis (peanut) oil, cetostearyl alcohol

Dose for eradication of nasal carriage of staphylococci, apply to nostrils 4 times daily for 10 days; for preventing nasal carriage of staphylococci, apply to nostrils twice daily

12   Ear, nose, and oropharynx

---

1. Can be sold to the public provided no more than 180 mg of ephedrine base (or salts) are supplied at one time, and pseudoephedrine salts are not supplied at the same time; for conditions that apply to supplies made at the request of a patient, see *Medicines, Ethics and Practice*, London, Pharmaceutical Press (always consult latest edition)

12.3 Drugs acting on the oropharynx

12.3.1 Drugs for oral ulceration and inflammation

12.3.2 Oropharyngeal anti-infective drugs

12.3.3 Lozenges and sprays

12.3.4 Mouthwashes, gargles, and dentifrices

12.3.5 Treatment of dry mouth

12.3.1 Drugs for oral ulceration and inflammation

Ulceration of the oral mucosa may be caused by trauma (physical or chemical), recurrent aphthae, infections, carcinoma, dermatological disorders, nutritional deficiencies, gastro-intestinal disease, haematopoietic disorders, and drug therapy (see also Chemotherapy-induced mucositis and myelosuppression, section 8.1). It is important to establish the diagnosis in each case as the majority of these lesions require specific management in addition to local treatment. Local treatment aims to protect the ulcerated area, to relieve pain, to reduce inflammation, or to control secondary infection. Patients with an unexplained mouth ulcer of more than 3 weeks' duration require urgent referral to hospital to exclude oral cancer.

Simple mouthwashes   A saline mouthwash (section 12.3.4) may relieve the pain of traumatic ulceration. The mouthwash is made up with warm water and used at frequent intervals until the discomfort and swelling subsides.

Antiseptic mouthwashes   Secondary bacterial infection may be a feature of any mucosal ulceration; it can increase discomfort and delay healing. Use of chlorhexidine mouthwash (section 12.3.4) is often beneficial and may accelerate healing of recurrent aphthae.

Corticosteroids   Topical corticosteroid therapy may be used for some forms of oral ulceration. In the case of aphthous ulcers it is most effective if applied in the 'prodromal' phase.

Thrush or other types of candidiasis are recognised complications of corticosteroid treatment.

Hydrocortisone oromucosal tablets are allowed to dissolve next to an ulcer and are useful in recurrent aphthae and erosive lichenoid lesions.

Beclometasone dipropionate inhaler 50–100 micrograms sprayed twice daily on the oral mucosa is used to manage oral ulceration [unlicensed indication]. Alternatively, **betamethasone** soluble tablets dissolved in water can be used as a mouthwash to treat oral ulceration [unlicensed indication].

Systemic corticosteroid therapy (section 6.3.2) is reserved for severe conditions such as pemphigus vulgaris.

Local analgesics   Local analgesics have a limited role in the management of oral ulceration. When applied topically their action is of a relatively short duration so that analgesia cannot be maintained continuously throughout the day. The main indication for a topical local analgesic is to relieve the pain of otherwise intract-

able oral ulceration particularly when it is due to major aphthae. For this purpose lidocaine 5% ointment or lozenges containing a local anaesthetic are applied to the ulcer. Lidocaine 10% solution as spray (section 15.2) can be applied thinly to the ulcer [unlicensed indication] using a cotton bud. When local anaesthetics are used in the mouth care must be taken not to produce anaesthesia of the pharynx before meals as this might lead to choking.

Benzydamine and **Flurbiprofen** are non-steroidal anti-inflammatory drugs (NSAIDs). Benzydamine mouthwash or spray may be useful in reducing the discomfort associated with a variety of ulcerative conditions. It has also been found to be effective in reducing the discomfort of post-irradiation mucositis. Some patients find the full-strength mouthwash causes some stinging and, for them, it should be diluted with an equal volume of water. Flurbiprofen lozenges are licensed for the relief of sore throat.

Choline salicylate is a derivative of salicylic acid and has some analgesic action. The dental gel may provide relief for recurrent aphthae, but excessive application or confinement under a denture irritates the mucosa and can itself cause ulceration.

Other preparations   Doxycycline rinsed in the mouth may be of value for recurrent aphthous ulceration.

Periodontitis   Low-dose doxycycline (*Periostat*®) is licensed as an adjunct to scaling and root planing for the treatment of periodontitis; a low dose of doxycycline reduces collagenase activity without inhibiting bacteria associated with periodontitis. For anti-infectives used in the treatment of destructive (refractory) forms of periodontal disease, see section 12.3.2 and Table 1, section 5.1. For mouthwashes used for oral hygiene and plaque inhibition, see section 12.3.4.

BENZYDAMINE HYDROCHLORIDE

Indications   painful inflammatory conditions of oropharynx

Side-effects   occasional numbness or stinging; rarely hypersensitivity reactions

Dose

- As a mouthwash (benzydamine hydrochloride 0.15%), ADULT and CHILD over 13 years, rinse or gargle, using 15 mL (dilute with an equal volume of water if stinging occurs) every 1½–3 hours as required, usually for not more than 7 days

- As an oromucosal spray (benzydamine hydrochloride 0.15%), ADULT and CHILD over 12 years, 4–8 sprays onto affected area every 1½–3 hours; CHILD under 6 years 1 spray per 4 kg body-weight to max. 4 sprays every 1½–3 hours; 6–12 years 4 sprays every 1½–3 hours

Benzydamine hydrochloride (Non-proprietary)
Mouthwash, benzydamine hydrochloride 0.15%, net price 300 mL = £6.68
Brands include *Oroeze*®

Oromucosal spray, benzydamine hydrochloride 0.15%, net price 30 mL = £4.36
Brands include *Oroeze*®

Dental prescribing on NHS Benzydamine Oromucosal Spray 0.15% may be prescribed

Difflam® (Meda)

Mouthwash (oral rinse), green, benzydamine hydrochloride 0.15%, net price 200 mL (*Difflam® Sore Throat Rinse*) = £4.64; 300 mL = £6.50

Dental prescribing on NHS May be prescribed as Benzydamine Mouthwash 0.15%

Oromucosal spray, benzydamine hydrochloride 0.15%, net price 30-mL unit = £4.24

CORTICOSTEROIDS

Indications   oral and perioral lesions

Contra-indications   untreated oral infection

Side-effects   occasional exacerbation of local infection; thrush or other candidal infections

Betamethasone (Non-proprietary) PoM

Soluble tablets, betamethasone 500 micrograms (as sodium phosphate), net price 100-tab pack = £22.34. Label: 10, 13, counselling, administration

Dose oral ulceration, [unlicensed indication] ADULT and CHILD over 12 years, 500 micrograms dissolved in 20 mL water and rinsed around the mouth 4 times daily; not to be swallowed

Dental prescribing on NHS Betamethasone Soluble Tablets 500 micrograms may be prescribed

Hydrocortisone (Non-proprietary)

Mucoadhesive buccal tablets (= oromucosal tablets), hydrocortisone 2.5 mg (as sodium succinate). Net price 20 = £4.48

Dose ADULT and CHILD over 12 years, 1 lozenge 4 times daily, allowed to dissolve slowly in the mouth in contact with the ulcer; CHILD under 12 years, only on medical advice

Dental prescribing on NHS May be prescribed as Hydrocortisone Oromucosal Tablets

DOXYCYCLINE

Indications   see preparations; other indications (section 5.1.3)

Cautions   section 5.1.3; monitor for superficial fungal infection, particularly if predisposition to oral candidiasis

Contra-indications   section 5.1.3

Hepatic impairment   section 5.1.3

Renal impairment   section 5.1.3

Pregnancy   section 5.1.3

Breast-feeding   section 5.1.3

Side-effects   section 5.1.3; fungal superinfection

Dose

- See preparations

Note Doxycycline stains teeth; avoid in children under 12 years of age

Periostat® (Alliance) PoM

Tablets, f/c, doxycycline (as hyclate) 20 mg, net price 56-tab pack = £17.30. Label: 6, 11, 27, counselling, posture

Dose periodontitis (as an adjunct to gingival scaling and root planing), 20 mg twice daily for 3 months; CHILD under 12 years not recommended

Counselling Tablets should be swallowed whole with plenty of fluid (at least 100 mL), while sitting or standing

Dental prescribing on NHS May be prescribed as Doxycycline Tablets 20 mg

Note May be difficult to obtain

◢**Local application**

For recurrent aphthous ulceration, a 100 mg doxycycline dispersible tablet can be stirred into a small amount of water then rinsed around the mouth for 2–3 minutes 4 times daily usually for 3 days; it should preferably not be swallowed [unlicensed indication].

FLURBIPROFEN

Indications   relief of sore throat

Cautions   section 10.1.1

Contra-indications   section 10.1.1

Hepatic impairment   section 10.1.1

Renal impairment   section 10.1.1

Pregnancy   section 10.1.1

Breast-feeding   section 10.1.1

Side-effects   taste disturbance, mouth ulcers (move lozenge around mouth); see also section 10.1.1

Strefen® (Reckitt Benckiser)

Lozenges, flurbiprofen 8.75 mg, net price 16 = £2.58

Dose ADULT and CHILD over 12 years, allow 1 lozenge to dissolve slowly in the mouth every 3–6 hours, max. 5 lozenges in 24 hours, for max. 3 days

LOCAL ANAESTHETICS

Indications   relief of pain in oral lesions

Cautions   avoid prolonged use; hypersensitivity; avoid anaesthesia of the pharynx before meals—risk of choking

Hepatic impairment   see Lidocaine section 2.3.2

Renal impairment   see Lidocaine section 2.3.2

Pregnancy   see Lidocaine section 15.2

Breast-feeding   see Lidocaine section 2.3.2

Lidocaine (Non-proprietary)

Ointment, lidocaine 5% in a water-miscible basis, net price 15 g = £6.18

Dose rub sparingly and gently on affected areas

Dental prescribing on NHS Lidocaine 5% Ointment may be prescribed

Xylocaine® (AstraZeneca)

Spray (= pump spray), lidocaine 10% (100 mg/g) supplying 10 mg lidocaine/spray; 500 spray doses per container. Net price 50-mL bottle = £6.29

Dose apply thinly to the ulcer [unlicensed indication] using a cotton bud

Dental prescribing on NHS May be prescribed as Lidocaine Spray 10%

◢**Preparations on sale to the public**

Many mouth ulcer preparations, throat lozenges, and throat sprays on sale to the public contain a **local anaesthetic**. To identify the active ingredients in such preparations, consult the product literature of the manufacturer.

Note The correct proprietary name should be ascertained—many products have very similar names but different active ingredients

SALICYLATES

Indications   mild oral and perioral lesions

Cautions   not to be applied to dentures—leave at least 30 minutes before re-insertion of dentures; frequent application, especially in children, may give rise to salicylate poisoning

Contra-indications   children under 16 years

Reye's syndrome The CHM has advised that topical oral pain relief products containing salicylate salts should not be used in children under 16 years, as a cautionary measure due to the theoretical risk of Reye's syndrome

Side-effects   transient local burning sensation

◢Choline salicylate

Choline Salicylate Dental Gel, BP

Oral gel, choline salicylate 8.7% in a flavoured gel basis, net price 15 g = £2.26

Brands include *Bonjela®* (sugar-free)

Dose ADULT and CHILD over 16 years, apply ½-inch of gel with gentle massage not more often than every 3 hours

Dental prescribing on NHS Choline Salicylate Dental Gel may be prescribed

◢Salicylic acid

Pyralvex® (Meda)

Oral paint, brown, rhubarb extract (anthraquinone glycosides 0.5%), salicylic acid 1%. Net price 10 mL with brush = £3.25

Dose ADULT and CHILD over 16 years, apply 3–4 times daily; max. duration 7 days

Note May cause temporary discolouration of teeth and oral mucosa

12.3.2 Oropharyngeal anti-infective drugs

The most common cause of a sore throat is a viral infection which does not benefit from anti-infective treatment. Streptococcal sore throats require systemic **penicillin** therapy (Table 1, section 5.1). Acute ulcerative gingivitis (Vincent's infection) responds to systemic **metronidazole** (section 5.1.11).

Preparations administered in the dental surgery for the local treatment of periodontal disease include gels of metronidazole (*Elyzol®*, Colgate-Palmolive) and of minocycline (*Dentomycin®*, Blackwell).

Oropharyngeal fungal infections

Fungal infections of the mouth are usually caused by *Candida* spp. (candidiasis or candidosis). Different types of oropharyngeal candidiasis are managed as follows:

Thrush Acute pseudomembranous candidiasis (thrush), is usually an acute infection but it may persist for months in patients receiving inhaled corticosteroids, cytotoxics or broad-spectrum antibacterials. Thrush also occurs in patients with serious systemic disease associated with reduced immunity such as leukaemia, other malignancies, and HIV infection. Any predisposing condition should be managed appropriately. When thrush is associated with corticosteroid inhalers, rinsing the mouth with water (or cleaning a child's teeth) immediately after using the inhaler may avoid the problem. Treatment with **nystatin** or **miconazole** may be needed. **Fluconazole** (section 5.2.1) is effective for unresponsive infections or if a topical antifungal drug cannot be used or if the patient has dry mouth. Topical therapy may not be adequate in immunocompromised patients and an oral triazole antifungal is preferred (section 5.2.1).

Acute erythematous candidiasis Acute erythematous (atrophic) candidiasis is a relatively uncommon condition associated with corticosteroid and broad-spectrum antibacterial use and with HIV disease. It is usually treated with **fluconazole** (section 5.2.1).

Denture stomatitis Patients with denture stomatitis (chronic atrophic candidiasis), should cleanse their dentures thoroughly and leave them out as often as possible during the treatment period. To prevent recurrence of the problem, dentures should not normally be worn at night. New dentures may be required if these measures fail despite good compliance.

Miconazole oral gel can be applied to the fitting surface of the denture before insertion (for short periods only). Denture stomatitis is not always associated with candidiasis and other factors such as mechanical or chemical irritation, bacterial infection, or rarely allergy to the dental base material, may be the cause.

Chronic hyperplastic candidiasis Chronic hyperplastic candidiasis (candidal leucoplakia) carries an increased risk of malignancy; biopsy is essential—this type of candidiasis may be associated with varying degrees of dysplasia, with oral cancer present in a high proportion of cases. Chronic hyperplastic candidiasis is treated with a systemic antifungal such as **fluconazole** (section 5.2.1) to eliminate candidal overlay. Patients should avoid the use of tobacco.

Angular cheilitis Angular cheilitis (angular stomatitis) is characterised by soreness, erythema and fissuring at the angles of the mouth. It is commonly associated with denture stomatitis but may represent a nutritional deficiency or it may be related to orofacial granulomatosis or HIV infection. Both yeasts (*Candida* spp.) and bacteria (*Staphylococcus aureus* and beta-haemolytic streptococci) are commonly involved as interacting, infective factors. A reduction in facial height related to ageing and tooth loss with maceration in the deep occlusive folds that may subsequently arise, predisposes to such infection. While the underlying cause is being identified and treated, it is often helpful to apply **miconazole** cream (see p. 833) or **sodium fusidate** ointment (see p. 832); if the angular cheilitis is unresponsive to treatment, **miconazole** and **hydrocortisone** cream or ointment (see p. 802) can be used.

Immunocompromised patients For advice on prevention of fungal infections in immunocompromised patients see p. 412.

Drugs used in oropharyngeal candidiasis **Nystatin** is not absorbed from the gastro-intestinal tract and is applied locally (as a suspension) to the mouth for treating local fungal infections. **Miconazole** is applied locally (as an oral gel) in the mouth but it is absorbed to the extent that potential interactions need to be considered. Miconazole also has some activity against Gram-positive bacteria including streptococci and staphylococci. **Fluconazole** (section 5.2.1) is given by mouth for infections that do not respond to topical therapy or when topical therapy cannot be used. It is reliably absorbed and effective. **Itraconazole** (section 5.2.1) can be used for fluconazole-resistant infections.

If candidal infection fails to respond to 1 to 2 weeks of treatment with antifungal drugs the patient should be sent for investigation to eliminate the possibility of underlying disease. Persistent infection may also be caused by reinfection from the genito-urinary or gastro-intestinal tract. Infection can be eliminated from these sources by appropriate anticandidal therapy; the patient's partner may also require treatment to prevent reinfection.

For the role of antiseptic mouthwashes in the prevention of oral candidiasis in immunocompromised patients and treatment of denture stomatitis, see section 12.3.4.

12
Ear, nose, and oropharynx

� MICONAZOLE

Indications   see preparations

Cautions   avoid in acute porphyria (section 9.8.2); **interactions**: Appendix 1 (antifungals, imidazole)

Contra-indications   *with oral gel*, impaired swallowing reflex in infants, first 5–6 months of life of an infant born preterm

Hepatic impairment   avoid

Pregnancy   manufacturer advises avoid if possible— toxicity at high doses in *animal* studies

Breast-feeding   manufacturer advises caution—no information available

Side-effects   nausea, vomiting; rash; *with buccal tablets*, abdominal pain, taste disturbance, burning sensation at application site, pruritus, and oedema; *with oral gel, very rarely* diarrhoea (usually on long-term treatment), hepatitis, toxic epidermal necrolysis, and Stevens-Johnson syndrome

Dose

• See preparations

¹**Daktarin**® (Janssen) PoM

Oral gel, sugar-free, orange-flavoured, miconazole 24 mg/mL (20 mg/g). Net price 15-g tube = £2.97, 80-g tube = £4.38. Label: 9, counselling, hold in mouth, after food

Dose prevention and treatment of oral candidiasis, by mouth, ADULT and CHILD over 2 years, 2.5 mL 4 times daily after meals, retain near oral lesions before swallowing (dental prostheses should be removed at night and brushed with gel); CHILD under 2 years see *BNF for Children*

Prevention and treatment of intestinal candidiasis, by mouth, ADULT and CHILD over 4 months, 5 mg/kg 4 times daily; max. 250 mg (10 mL) 4 times daily

Note Treatment should be continued for at least 7 days after lesions have healed or symptoms have cleared

Dental prescribing on NHS May be prescribed as Miconazole Oromucosal Gel

◢**Buccal preparation**

Loramyc® (Therabel) PoM

Mucoadhesive buccal tablets, white-yellow, miconazole 50 mg, net price 14-tab pack = £52.12. Label: 10, counselling, administration

Dose oropharyngeal candidiasis in immunocompromised ADULT, 50 mg daily preferably taken in the morning for 7 days; if no improvement, continue treatment for a further 7 days

Counselling Place rounded side of tablet on upper gum above an incisor tooth and hold upper lip firmly over the gum for 30 seconds using a finger. If tablet detaches within 6 hours, replace with a new tablet. With each dose, use alternate sides of the gum

Note The Scottish Medicines Consortium (p. 4) has advised (January 2011) that miconazole mucoadhesive buccal tablets (*Loramyc*®) are not recommended for use within NHS Scotland.

▮ NYSTATIN

Indications   oral and perioral fungal infections

Side-effects   oral irritation and sensitisation, nausea reported

Dose

• Treatment, ADULT and CHILD, 100 000 units 4 times daily after food, usually for 7 days (continued for 48 hours after lesions have resolved)

Note Unlicensed for treating candidiasis in NEONATE

1. 15-g tube can be sold to the public

Nystatin (Non-proprietary) PoM

Oral suspension, nystatin 100 000 units/mL, net price 30 mL = £2.42. Label: 9, counselling, use of pipette, hold in mouth, after food

Dental prescribing on NHS Nystatin Oral Suspension may be prescribed

Nystan® (Squibb) PoM

Oral suspension, yellow, nystatin 100 000 units/mL, net price 30 mL with pipette = £1.80. Label: 9, counselling, use of pipette, hold in mouth, after food

Oropharyngeal viral infections

The management of primary herpetic gingivostomatitis is a soft diet, adequate fluid intake, and analgesics as required, including local use of **benzydamine** (section 12.3.1). The use of chlorhexidine mouthwash (section 12.3.4) will control plaque accumulation if toothbrushing is painful and will also help to control secondary infection in general.

In the case of severe herpetic stomatitis, a systemic antiviral such as aciclovir is required (section 5.3.2.1). Valaciclovir and famciclovir are suitable alternatives for oral lesions associated with herpes zoster. Aciclovir and valaciclovir are also used for the prevention of frequently recurring herpes simplex lesions of the mouth, particularly when implicated in the initiation of erythema multiforme. See section 13.10.3 for the treatment of labial herpes simplex infections.

12.3.3 Lozenges and sprays

There is no convincing evidence that antiseptic lozenges and sprays have a beneficial action and they sometimes irritate and cause sore tongue and sore lips. Some of these preparations also contain local anaesthetics which relieve pain but may cause sensitisation.

12.3.4 Mouthwashes, gargles, and dentifrices

Superficial infections of the mouth are often helped by warm mouthwashes which have a mechanical cleansing effect and cause some local hyperaemia. However, to be effective, they must be used frequently and vigorously. A warm saline mouthwash is ideal and can be prepared either by dissolving half a teaspoonful of salt in a glassful of warm water or by diluting **compound sodium chloride mouthwash** with an equal volume of warm water.

Mouthwashes containing an oxidising agent, such as **hydrogen peroxide**, may be useful in the treatment of acute ulcerative gingivitis (Vincent's infection) since the organisms involved are anaerobes. It also has a mechanical cleansing effect arising from frothing when in contact with oral debris.

Chlorhexidine is an effective antiseptic which has the advantage of inhibiting plaque formation on the teeth. It does not, however, completely control plaque deposition and is not a substitute for effective toothbrushing. Moreover, chlorhexidine preparations do not penetrate significantly into stagnation areas and are therefore of little value in the control of dental caries or of periodontal disease once pocketing has developed. Chlorhexidine mouthwash is used in the treatment of denture stomatitis. It is also used in the prevention of oral candidiasis in immunocompromised patients. Chlorhexidine mouthwash reduces the incidence of alveolar osteitis following tooth extraction. Chlorhexidine mouthwash should not be used for the prevention of endocarditis in patients undergoing dental procedures.

Chlorhexidine can be used as a mouthwash, spray or gel for secondary infection in mucosal ulceration and for controlling gingivitis, as an adjunct to other oral hygiene measures. These preparations may also be used instead of toothbrushing where there is a painful periodontal condition (e.g. primary herpetic stomatitis) or if the patient has a haemorrhagic disorder, or is disabled. Chlorhexidine preparations are of little value in the control of acute necrotising ulcerative gingivitis.

There is no convincing evidence that gargles are effective.

CHLORHEXIDINE GLUCONATE

Indications　see under preparations below

Side-effects　mucosal irritation (if desquamation occurs, discontinue treatment or dilute mouthwash with an equal volume of water); taste disturbance; reversible brown staining of teeth, and of silicate or composite restorations; tongue discoloration; parotid gland swelling and hypersensitivity (including anaphylaxis) reported

Note　Chlorhexidine gluconate may be incompatible with some ingredients in toothpaste; rinse the mouth thoroughly with water between using toothpaste and chlorhexidine-containing product

Chlorhexidine (Non-proprietary)
　Mouthwash, chlorhexidine gluconate 0.2%, net price 300 mL = £3.45
　Dose　oral hygiene and plaque inhibition, oral candidiasis, gingivitis, and management of aphthous ulcers, rinse mouth with 10 mL for about 1 minute twice daily
　Denture stomatitis, cleanse and soak dentures in mouthwash solution for 15 minutes twice daily

Corsodyl® (GSK Consumer Healthcare)
　Dental gel, chlorhexidine gluconate 1%. Net price 50 g = £1.21
　Dose　oral hygiene and plaque inhibition and gingivitis, brush on the teeth once or twice daily
　Oral candidiasis and management of aphthous ulcers, apply to affected areas once or twice daily
　Dental prescribing on NHS　May be prescribed as Chlorhexidine Gluconate Gel

　Mouthwash, chlorhexidine gluconate 0.2%, net price 300 mL (original or mint) = £2.28, 600 mL (mint) = £3.85, alcohol-free, 300 mL (mint) = £2.73
　Dose　oral hygiene and plaque inhibition, oral candidiasis, gingivitis, and management of aphthous ulcers, rinse mouth with 10 mL for about 1 minute twice daily
　Denture stomatitis, cleanse and soak dentures in mouthwash solution for 15 minutes twice daily
　Dental prescribing on NHS　May be prescribed as Chlorhexidine Mouthwash

　Oral spray, chlorhexidine gluconate 0.2% (mint-flavoured). Net price 60 mL = £4.10
　Dose　oral hygiene and plaque inhibition, oral candidiasis, gingivitis, and management of aphthous ulcers, apply as required to tooth, gingival, or ulcer surfaces using up to 12 actuations (approx. 0.14 mL/actuation) twice daily
　Dental prescribing on NHS　May be prescribed as Chlorhexidine Oral Spray

◢With chlorobutanol

Eludril® (Fabre)
　Mouthwash or *gargle*, chlorhexidine gluconate 0.1%, chlorobutanol 0.5% (mint-flavoured), net price 90 mL = £1.36, 250 mL = £2.83, 500 mL = £5.06
　Dose　oral hygiene and plaque inhibition, ADULT and CHILD over 6 years, use 10–15 mL (diluted with lukewarm water in measuring cup provided) 2–3 times daily
　Denture disinfection, soak previously cleansed dentures in mouthwash (diluted with 2 volumes of water) for 60 minutes

HEXETIDINE

Indications　oral hygiene

Side-effects　local irritation; *very rarely* taste disturbance and transient anaesthesia

Oraldene® (McNeil)
　Mouthwash or *gargle*, red or blue-green (mint-flavoured), hexetidine 0.1%. Net price 100 mL = £1.43; 200 mL = £2.21
　Dose　ADULT and CHILD over 6 years, use 15 mL undiluted 2–3 times daily

HYDROGEN PEROXIDE

Indications　oral hygiene, see notes above

Side-effects　hypertrophy of papillae of tongue on prolonged used

Hydrogen Peroxide Mouthwash, BP
　Mouthwash, consists of Hydrogen Peroxide Solution 6% (= approx. 20 volume) BP
　Dose　rinse the mouth for 2–3 minutes with 15 mL diluted in half a tumblerful of warm water 2–3 times daily
　Dental prescribing on NHS　Hydrogen Peroxide Mouthwash may be prescribed

Peroxyl® (Colgate-Palmolive)
　Mouthwash, hydrogen peroxide 1.5%, net price 300 mL = £2.94
　Dose　rinse the mouth with 10 mL for about 1 minute up to 4 times daily (after meals and at bedtime)

SODIUM CHLORIDE

Indications　oral hygiene, see notes above

Sodium Chloride Mouthwash, Compound, BP
　Mouthwash, sodium bicarbonate 1%, sodium chloride 1.5% in a suitable vehicle with a peppermint flavour.
　Dose　extemporaneous preparations should be prepared according to the following formula: sodium chloride 1.5 g, sodium bicarbonate 1 g, concentrated peppermint emulsion 2.5 mL, double-strength chloroform water 50 mL, water to 100 mL
　To be diluted with an equal volume of warm water
　Dental prescribing on NHS　Compound Sodium Chloride Mouthwash may be prescribed

12.3.5 Treatment of dry mouth

Dry mouth (xerostomia) may be caused by drugs with antimuscarinic (anticholinergic) side-effects (e.g. antispasmodics, tricyclic antidepressants, and some antipsychotics), by diuretics, by irradiation of the head and neck region or by damage to or disease of the salivary glands. Patients with a persistently dry mouth may develop a burning or scalded sensation and have poor oral hygiene; they may develop increased dental caries, periodontal disease, intolerance of dentures, and oral

12

Ear, nose, and oropharynx

infections (particularly candidiasis). Dry mouth may be relieved in many patients by simple measures such as frequent sips of cool drinks or sucking pieces of ice or sugar-free fruit pastilles. Sugar-free chewing gum stimulates salivation in patients with residual salivary function.

Artificial saliva can provide useful relief of dry mouth. A properly balanced artificial saliva should be of a neutral pH and contain electrolytes (including fluoride) to correspond approximately to the composition of saliva. The acidic pH of some artificial saliva products may be inappropriate. Of the proprietary preparations, *Aquoral*®, *Biotène Oralbalance*® gel, *AS Saliva Orthana*® Spray or *Xerotin*® can be used for any condition giving rise to a dry mouth. *BioXtra*®, *Glandosane*®, and *Saliveze*®, have ACBS approval for dry mouth associated only with radiotherapy or sicca syndrome. *Salivix*® pastilles, which act locally as salivary stimulants, are also available for any condition leading to a dry mouth and *SST* tablets may be prescribed for dry mouth in patients with salivary gland impairment (and patent salivary ducts).

Pilocarpine tablets are licensed for the treatment of xerostomia following irradiation for head and neck cancer and for dry mouth and dry eyes (xerophthalmia) in Sjögren's syndrome. They are effective only in patients who have some residual salivary gland function, and therefore should be withdrawn if there is no response.

Local treatment

Aquoral® (Sinclair IS)
Oral spray, oxidised glycerol triesters, silicon dioxide, flavouring agents, net price 40-mL bottle = £9.85

Excipients include aspartame (see section 9.4.1)

Dose symptomatic treatment of dry mouth, 1 spray onto the inside of each cheek 3–4 times daily

Dental Prescribing on NHS *Aquoral*® Oral Spray may be prescribed as Artificial Saliva Protective Spray

AS Saliva Orthana® (AS Pharma)
Oral spray, gastric mucin (porcine) 3.5%, xylitol 2%, sodium fluoride 4.2 mg/litre, with preservatives and flavouring agents, pH neutral. Net price 50-mL bottle = £4.92; 500-mL refill = £34.27

Dose Symptomatic treatment of dry mouth, spray 2–3 times onto oral and pharyngeal mucosa, when required

Dental prescribing on NHS *AS Saliva Orthana*® Oral Spray may be prescribed as Artificial Saliva Substitute Spray

Lozenges, mucin 65 mg, xylitol 59 mg, in a sorbitol basis, pH neutral. Net price 30-lozenge pack = £3.50

Dose Symptomatic treatment of dry mouth, allow 1 lozenge to dissolve slowly in the mouth when required

Note *AS Saliva Orthana*® lozenges do not contain fluoride

Biotène Oralbalance® (GSK)
Saliva replacement gel, lactoperoxidase, lactoferrin, lysozyme, glucose oxidase, xylitol in a gel basis, net price 50-g tube = £4.46

Dose symptomatic treatment of dry mouth, apply to gums and tongue as required

Note Avoid using with toothpastes containing detergents (including foaming agents)

Dental prescribing on NHS *Biotène Oralbalance*® Saliva Replacement Gel may be prescribed as Artificial Saliva Gel

BioXtra® (RIS Products)
Gel, lactoperoxidase, lactoferrin, lysozyme, whey colostrum, xylitol and other ingredients, net price 40-mL tube = £3.94, 50-mL spray = £3.94

Dose ACBS: patients suffering from dry mouth as a result of having (or having undergone) radiotherapy, or sicca syndrome, apply to oral mucosa as required

Dental prescribing on NHS *BioXtra*® Gel may be prescribed

Glandosane® (Fresenius Kabi)
Aerosol spray, carmellose sodium 500 mg, sorbitol 1.5 g, potassium chloride 60 mg, sodium chloride 42.2 mg, magnesium chloride 2.6 mg, calcium chloride 7.3 mg, and dipotassium hydrogen phosphate 17.1 mg/50 g, pH 5.75. Net price 50-mL unit (neutral, lemon or peppermint flavoured) = £5.38

Dose ACBS: patients suffering from dry mouth as a result of having (or having undergone) radiotherapy, or sicca syndrome, spray onto oral and pharyngeal mucosa as required

Dental prescribing on NHS *Glandosane*® Aerosol Spray may be prescribed

Saliveze® (Wyvern)
Oral spray, carmellose sodium (sodium carboxymethylcellulose), calcium chloride, magnesium chloride, potassium chloride, sodium chloride, and dibasic sodium phosphate, pH neutral. Net price 50-mL bottle (mint-flavoured) = £3.50

Dose ACBS: patients suffering from dry mouth as a result of having (or having undergone) radiotherapy, or sicca syndrome, 1 spray onto oral mucosa as required

Dental prescribing on NHS *Saliveze*® Oral Spray may be prescribed

Salivix® (Galen)
Pastilles, sugar-free, reddish-amber, acacia, malic acid and other ingredients. Net price 50-pastille pack = £3.55

Dose symptomatic treatment of dry mouth, suck 1 pastille when required

Dental prescribing on NHS *Salivix*® Pastilles may be prescribed as Artificial Saliva Pastilles

SST (Medac)
Tablets, sugar-free, citric acid, malic acid and other ingredients in a sorbitol base, net price 100-tab pack = £4.86

Dose symptomatic treatment of dry mouth in patients with impaired salivary gland function and patent salivary ducts, allow 1 tablet to dissolve slowly in the mouth when required

Dental prescribing on NHS May be prescribed as Saliva Stimulating Tablets

Xerotin® (SpePharm)
Oral spray, sugar-free, water, sorbitol, carmellose (carboxymethylcellulose), potassium chloride, sodium chloride, potassium phosphate, magnesium chloride, calcium chloride and other ingredients, pH neutral. Net price 100-mL unit = £6.86

Dose symptomatic treatment of dry mouth, spray as required

Dental prescribing on NHS *Xerotin*® Oral Spray may be prescribed as Artificial Saliva Oral Spray

Systemic treatment

PILOCARPINE HYDROCHLORIDE

Indications xerostomia following irradiation for head and neck cancer (see also notes above); dry mouth and dry eyes in Sjögren's syndrome

Cautions asthma and chronic obstructive pulmonary disease (avoid if uncontrolled, see Contra-indications), cardiovascular disease (avoid if uncontrolled); cholelithiasis or biliary-tract disease, peptic ulcer, risk of increased urethral smooth muscle tone and renal colic; maintain adequate fluid intake to avoid dehydration associated with excessive sweating; cognitive or psychiatric disturbances; susceptibility to angle-closure glaucoma; **interactions:** Appendix 1 (parasympathomimetics)

Counselling Blurred vision or dizziness may affect performance of skilled tasks (e.g. driving) particularly at night or in reduced lighting

Contra-indications uncontrolled asthma and chronic obstructive pulmonary disease (increased bronchial secretions and increased airways resistance); uncontrolled cardiorenal disease; acute iritis

Hepatic impairment reduce initial oral dose in moderate or severe cirrhosis

Renal impairment manufacturer advises caution with tablets

Pregnancy avoid—smooth muscle stimulant; toxicity in *animal* studies

Breast-feeding manufacturer advises avoid—present in milk in *animal* studies

Side-effects dyspepsia, diarrhoea, abdominal pain, nausea, vomiting, constipation; flushing, hypertension, palpitation, headache, dizziness, asthenia, influenza-like symptoms, sweating; increased urinary frequency; visual disturbances, lacrimation, ocular pain, conjunctivitis; rhinitis; rash, pruritus; *less commonly* flatulence, urinary urgency

Dose

- Xerostomia following irradiation for head and neck cancer, 5 mg 3 times daily with or immediately after meals (last dose always with evening meal); if tolerated but response insufficient after 4 weeks, may be increased to max. 30 mg daily in divided doses; max. therapeutic effect normally within 4–8 weeks; discontinue if no improvement after 2–3 months; CHILD not recommended

- Dry mouth and dry eyes in Sjögren's syndrome, 5 mg 4 times daily (with meals and at bedtime); if tolerated but response insufficient, may be increased to max. 30 mg daily in divided doses; discontinue if no improvement after 2–3 months; CHILD not recommended

Salagen® (Novartis) [PoM]
Tablets, f/c, pilocarpine hydrochloride 5 mg. Net price 84-tab pack = £41.14. Label: 21, 27, counselling, driving

12 Ear, nose, and oropharynx

13 Skin

This chapter also includes advice on the drug management of the following:

For information on wound management products and elasticated garments, see Appendix 5, p. 1081.

The British Association of Dermatologists list of preferred unlicensed dermatological preparations (specials) is available at www.bad.org.uk/specials.

13.1 Management of skin conditions

13.1.1 Vehicles

Both vehicle and active ingredients are important in the treatment of skin conditions; the vehicle alone may have more than a mere placebo effect. The vehicle affects the degree of hydration of the skin, has a mild anti-inflammatory effect, and aids the penetration of active drug.

Applications are usually viscous solutions, emulsions, or suspensions for application to the skin (including the scalp) or nails.

Collodions are painted on the skin and allowed to dry to leave a flexible film over the site of application.

Creams are emulsions of oil and water and are generally well absorbed into the skin. They may contain an antimicrobial preservative unless the active ingredient or basis is intrinsically bactericidal and fungicidal. Generally, creams are cosmetically more acceptable than ointments because they are less greasy and easier to apply.

Skin 13

Gels consist of active ingredients in suitable hydrophilic or hydrophobic bases; they generally have a high water content. Gels are particularly suitable for application to the face and scalp.

Lotions have a cooling effect and may be preferred to ointments or creams for application over a hairy area. Lotions in alcoholic basis can sting if used on broken skin. *Shake lotions* (such as calamine lotion) contain insoluble powders which leave a deposit on the skin surface.

Ointments are greasy preparations which are normally anhydrous and insoluble in water, and are more occlusive than creams. They are particularly suitable for chronic, dry lesions. The most commonly used ointment bases consist of soft paraffin or a combination of soft, liquid, and hard paraffin. Some ointment bases have both *hydrophilic and lipophilic* properties; they may have occlusive properties on the skin surface, encourage hydration, and also be miscible with water; they often have a mild anti-inflammatory effect. *Water-soluble ointments* contain macrogols which are freely soluble in water and are therefore readily washed off; they have a limited but useful role where ready removal is desirable.

Pastes are stiff preparations containing a high proportion of finely powdered solids such as zinc oxide and starch suspended in an ointment. They are used for circumscribed lesions such as those which occur in lichen simplex, chronic eczema, or psoriasis. They are less occlusive than ointments and can be used to protect inflamed, lichenified, or excoriated skin.

Dusting powders are used only rarely. They reduce friction between opposing skin surfaces. Dusting powders should not be applied to moist areas because they can cake and abrade the skin. Talc is a lubricant but it does not absorb moisture; it can cause respiratory irritation. Starch is less lubricant but absorbs water.

Dilution The BP directs that creams and ointments should not normally be diluted but that should dilution be necessary care should be taken, in particular, to prevent microbial contamination. The appropriate diluent should be used and heating should be avoided during mixing; excessive dilution may affect the stability of some creams. Diluted creams should normally be used within 2 weeks of preparation.

13.1.2   Suitable quantities for prescribing

Suitable quantities of dermatological preparations to be prescribed for specific areas of the body

Area of body	Creams and Ointments	Lotions
Face	15–30 g	100 mL
Both hands	25–50 g	200 mL
Scalp	50–100 g	200 mL
Both arms or both legs	100–200 g	200 mL
Trunk	400 g	500 mL
Groins and genitalia	15–25 g	100 mL

These amounts are usually suitable for an adult for twice daily application for 1 week. The recommendations do not apply to corticosteroid preparations—for suitable quantities of corticosteroid preparations, see section 13.4.

13.1.3   Excipients and sensitisation

Excipients in topical products rarely cause problems. If a patch test indicates allergy to an excipient, products containing the substance should be avoided (see also Anaphylaxis, p. 213). The following excipients in topical preparations are associated, rarely, with sensitisation; the presence of these excipients is indicated in the entries for topical products. See also Excipients, under General Guidance, p. 2.

Beeswax	Imidurea
Benzyl alcohol	Isopropyl palmitate
Butylated hydroxyanisole	*N*-(3-Chloroallyl)hexami-
Butylated hydroxytoluene	nium chloride (quater-
Cetostearyl alcohol	nium 15)
(including cetyl and	Polysorbates
stearyl alcohol)	Propylene glycol
Chlorocresol	Sodium metabisulfite
Edetic acid (EDTA)	Sorbic acid
Ethylenediamine	Wool fat and related sub-
Fragrances	stances including
Hydroxybenzoates (para-	lanolin[1]
bens)	

13.2   Emollient and barrier preparations

13.2.1   Emollients
13.2.2   Barrier preparations

Borderline substances The preparations marked 'ACBS' are regarded as drugs when prescribed in accordance with the advice of the Advisory Committee on Borderline Substances for the clinical conditions listed. Prescriptions issued in accordance with this advice and endorsed 'ACBS' will normally not be investigated. See Appendix 2 for listing by clinical condition.

13.2.1   Emollients

13.2.1.1   Emollient bath and shower preparations

Emollients soothe, smooth and hydrate the skin and are indicated for all dry or scaling disorders. Their effects are short-lived and they should be applied frequently even after improvement occurs. They are useful in dry and eczematous disorders, and to a lesser extent in psoriasis (section 13.5.2). The choice of an appropriate emollient will depend on the severity of the condition, patient preference, and the site of application. Emollient preparations contained in tubs should be removed with a clean spoon or spatula to reduce bacterial contamination of the emollient. Emollients should be applied in the direction of hair growth to reduce the risk of folliculitis. Ointments may exacerbate acne and folliculitis. Some ingredients rarely cause sensitisation (section 13.1.3) and this should be suspected if an eczematous reaction

1. Purified versions of wool fat have reduced the problem

occurs. The use of aqueous cream as a leave-on emollient may increase the risk of skin reactions, particularly in eczema.

> ### Fire hazard with paraffin-based emollients
>
> Emulsifying ointment *or* 50% Liquid Paraffin and 50% White Soft Paraffin Ointment in contact with dressings and clothing is easily ignited by a naked flame. The risk is greater when these preparations are applied to large areas of the body, and clothing or dressings become soaked with the ointment. Patients should be told to keep away from fire or flames, and not to smoke when using these preparations. The risk of fire should be considered when using large quantities of any paraffin-based emollient.

Preparations such as **aqueous cream** (section 13.2.1.1) and **emulsifying ointment** can be used as soap substitutes for hand washing and in the bath; the preparation is rubbed on the skin before rinsing off completely. The addition of a bath oil (section 13.2.1.1) may also be helpful.

Preparations containing an antibacterial (section 13.10) should be avoided unless infection is present or is a frequent complication.

Urea is a keratin softener and hydrating agent used in the treatment of dry, scaling conditions (including ichthyosis) and may be useful in elderly patients. It is occasionally used with other topical agents such as corticosteroids to enhance penetration of the skin.

◢ Non-proprietary emollient preparations

Emulsifying Ointment, BP
Ointment, emulsifying wax 30%, white soft paraffin 50%, liquid paraffin 20%, net price 500 g = £2.34
Excipients include cetostearyl alcohol

Hydrous Ointment, BP
Ointment, (oily cream), dried magnesium sulfate 0.5%, phenoxyethanol 1%, wool alcohols ointment 50%, in freshly boiled and cooled purified water, net price 500 g = £4.89

Liquid and White Soft Paraffin Ointment, NPF
Ointment, liquid paraffin 50%, white soft paraffin 50%, net price 500 g = £4.57

Paraffin, White Soft, BP
White petroleum jelly, net price 100 g = 50p

Paraffin, Yellow Soft, BP
Yellow petroleum jelly, net price 100 g = 54p

◢ Proprietary emollient preparations

Aquamax® (Dermato Logical)
Cream, light liquid paraffin 8%, white soft paraffin 20%, phenoxyethanol 1%, net price 100 g = £1.89, 500 g = £3.99
Excipients include cetostearyl alcohol, polysorbate 60
For dry skin conditions

Aquamol® (Thornton & Ross)
Cream, containing liquid paraffin, white soft paraffin, net price 50 g = £1.22, 500-g pump pack = £6.40
Excipients include cetostearyl alcohol, chlorocresol
For dry skin conditions

Aveeno® (J&J)
Cream, colloidal oatmeal in emollient basis, net price 100 mL = £3.97, 300-mL pump pack = £6.80
Excipients include benzyl alcohol, cetyl alcohol, isopropyl palmitate
ACBS: For endogenous and exogenous eczema, xeroderma, ichthyosis, and senile pruritus (pruritus of the elderly) associated with dry skin

Lotion, colloidal oatmeal in emollient basis, net price 500 mL = £6.66
Excipients include benzyl alcohol, cetyl alcohol, isopropyl palmitate, stearyl alcohol
ACBS: as for *Aveeno®* Cream

Cetraben® (Genus)
Emollient cream, white soft paraffin 13.2%, light liquid paraffin 10.5%, net price 50-g pump pack = £1.40, 150-g pump pack = £3.98, 500-g pump pack = £5.99, 1.05-kg pump pack = £11.62
Excipients include cetostearyl alcohol, hydroxybenzoates (parabens)
For inflamed, damaged, dry or chapped skin including eczema

Dermamist® (Alliance)
Spray application, white soft paraffin 10% in a basis containing liquid paraffin, fractionated coconut oil, net price 250-mL pressurised aerosol unit = £5.97
Excipients none as listed in section 13.1.3
For dry skin conditions including eczema, ichthyosis, pruritus of the elderly
Note Flammable

Diprobase® (MSD)
Cream, cetomacrogol 2.25%, cetostearyl alcohol 7.2%, liquid paraffin 6%, white soft paraffin 15%, water-miscible basis used for *Diprosone®* cream, net price 50 g = £1.28; 500-g pump pack = £6.32
Excipients include cetostearyl alcohol, chlorocresol
For dry skin conditions

Ointment, liquid paraffin 5%, white soft paraffin 95%, basis used for *Diprosone®* ointment, net price 50 g = £1.28, 500 g = £5.99
Excipients none as listed in section 13.1.3
For dry skin conditions

Doublebase® (Dermal)
Gel, isopropyl myristate 15%, liquid paraffin 15%, net price 100 g = £2.65, 500 g = £5.83
Excipients none as listed in section 13.1.3
For dry, chapped, or itchy skin conditions

Dayleve Gel, isopropyl myristate 15%, liquid paraffin 15%, net price 100 g = £2.65, 500-g pump pack = £6.29
Excipients none as listed in section 13.1.3
For dry, chapped, or itchy skin conditions

E45® (Reckitt Benckiser)
Cream, light liquid paraffin 12.6%, white soft paraffin 14.5%, hypoallergenic anhydrous wool fat (hypoallergenic lanolin) 1% in self-emulsifying monostearin, net price 50 g = £1.61, 125 g = £2.90, 350 g = £5.17, 500-g pump pack = £5.62
Excipients include cetyl alcohol, hydroxybenzoates (parabens)
For dry skin conditions

Lotion, light liquid paraffin 4%, cetomacrogol, white soft paraffin 10%, hypoallergenic anhydrous wool fat (hypoallergenic lanolin) 1% in glyceryl monostearate, net price 200 mL = £2.40, 500-mL pump pack = £4.50
Excipients include isopropyl palmitate, hydroxybenzoates (parabens), benzyl alcohol
ACBS: for symptomatic relief of dry skin conditions, such as those associated with atopic eczema and contact dermatitis

13 Skin

Emollin® (C D Medical)

Spray, liquid paraffin 50%, white soft paraffin 50% in aerosol basis, net price 150 mL = £3.97, 240 mL = £6.35

Excipients none as listed in section 13.1.3

For dry skin conditions

Epaderm® (Mölnlycke)

Cream, yellow soft paraffin 15%, liquid paraffin 10%, emulsifying wax 5%, net price 50-g pump pack = £1.70, 500-g pump pack = £6.95

Excipients include cetostearyl alcohol, chlorocresol

For use as an emollient or soap substitute

Ointment, emulsifying wax 30%, yellow soft paraffin 30%, liquid paraffin 40%, net price 125 g = £3.85, 500 g = £6.53, 1 kg = £12.02

Excipients include cetostearyl alcohol

For use as an emollient or soap substitute

Hydromol® (Alliance)

Cream, sodium pidolate 2.5%, liquid paraffin 13.8%, net price 50 g = £2.19, 100 g = £4.09, 500 g = £11.92

Excipients include cetostearyl alcohol, hydroxybenzoates (parabens)

For dry skin conditions

Ointment, yellow soft paraffin 30%, emulsifying wax 30%, liquid paraffin 40%, net price 125 g = £2.88, 500 g = £4.89, 1 kg = £9.09

Excipients include cetostearyl alcohol

For use as an emollient, bath additive, or soap substitute

Lipobase® (Astellas)

Cream, fatty cream basis used for *Locoid Lipocream®*, net price 50 g = £1.46

Excipients include cetostearyl alcohol, hydroxybenzoates (parabens)

For dry skin conditions, also for use during treatment with topical corticosteroid and as diluent for *Locoid Lipocream®*

Oilatum® (Stiefel)

Cream, light liquid paraffin 6%, white soft paraffin 15%, net price 50 g = £1.63, 150 g = £2.46, 500-mL pump pack = £4.99, 1.05-litre pump pack = £9.98

Excipients include benzyl alcohol, cetostearyl alcohol

For dry skin conditions

Oilatum® Junior Cream, light liquid paraffin 6%, white soft paraffin 15%, net price 150 g = £3.38, 350 mL = £4.65, 500 mL = £4.99, 1.05-litre pump pack = £9.98

Excipients include benzyl alcohol, cetostearyl alcohol

For dry skin conditions

QV® (Crawford)

Cream, glycerol 10%, light liquid paraffin 10%, white soft paraffin 5%, net price 100 g = £2.04, 500 g = £5.86, 1.05-kg pump pack = £11.94

Excipients include cetostearyl alcohol, hydroxybenzoates (parabens)

For dry skin conditions including eczema, psoriasis, ichthyosis, pruritus

Intensive ointment, light liquid paraffin 50.5%, white soft paraffin 20%, net price 450 g = £5.65

Excipients include cetostearyl alcohol

For dry skin conditions including eczema, psoriasis, ichthyosis, pruritus

Lotion, white soft paraffin 5%, net price 250 mL = £3.14, 500-mL pump pack = £5.24

Excipients include cetostearyl alcohol, hydroxybenzoates (parabens)

For dry skin conditions including eczema, psoriasis, ichthyosis, pruritus

Ultrabase® (Derma UK)

Cream, water-miscible, containing liquid paraffin and white soft paraffin, net price 50 g = £1.40, 500-g pump pack = £4.80

Excipients include fragrance, hydroxybenzoates (parabens), disodium edetate, stearyl alcohol

For dry skin conditions

Unguentum M® (Almirall)

Cream, containing saturated neutral oil, liquid paraffin, white soft paraffin, net price 50 g = £1.41, 100 g = £2.78, 200-mL pump pack = £5.50, 500 g = £8.48

Excipients include cetostearyl alcohol, polysorbate 40, propylene glycol, sorbic acid

For dry skin conditions and nappy rash

ZeroAQS® (Thornton & Ross)

Cream, macrogol cetostearyl ether 1.8%, liquid paraffin 6%, white soft paraffin 15%, net price 100 g = £1.65, 500 g = £3.29

Excipients include cetostearyl alcohol, chlorocresol

For use as an emollient or soap substitute

Zerobase® (Thornton & Ross)

Cream, liquid paraffin 11%, net price 50 g = £1.04, 500-g pump pack = £5.26

Excipients include cetostearyl alcohol, chlorocresol

For dry skin conditions

Zerocream® (Thornton & Ross)

Cream, liquid paraffin 12.6%, white soft paraffin 14.5%, net price 50 g = £1.17, 500-g pump pack = £4.08

Excipients include cetyl alcohol, hydroxybenzoates (parabens), lanolin anhydrous

For dry skin conditions

Zeroderm® (Thornton & Ross)

Ointment, liquid paraffin 40%, white soft paraffin 30%, net price 125 g = £2.41, 500 g = £4.10

Excipients include cetostearyl alcohol, polysorbate 60

For dry skin conditions

Zeroguent® (Thornton & Ross)

Cream, light liquid paraffin 8%, white soft paraffin 4%, refined soya bean oil 5%, net price 100 g = £2.33, 500 g = £6.99

Excipients include cetostearyl alcohol, polysorbate 40, propylene glycol, sorbic acid

For dry skin conditions

◢**Preparations containing urea**

Aquadrate® (Alliance)

Cream, urea 10%, net price 100 g = £4.37

Excipients none as listed in section 13.1.3

Dose for dry, scaling and itching skin, apply thinly twice daily

Balneum® (Almirall)

Cream, urea 5%, ceramide 0.1%, net price 50-g pump pack = £2.85, 500-g pump pack = £9.97

Excipients include cetostearyl alcohol, polysorbates, propylene glycol

Dose for dry skin conditions, apply twice daily

Balneum® Plus Cream, urea 5%, lauromacrogols 3%, net price 100 g = £3.29, 500-g pump pack = £14.99

Excipients include benzyl alcohol, polysorbates

Dose for dry, scaling and itching skin, apply twice daily

13

Skin

Calmurid® (Galderma)

Cream, urea 10%, lactic acid 5%, net price 100 g = £9.27, 500-g pump pack = £35.70

Excipients none as listed in section 13.1.3

Dose for dry, scaling and itching skin, apply a thick layer for 3–5 minutes, massage into area, and remove excess, usually twice daily. Use half-strength cream for 1 week if stinging occurs

Note Can be diluted with aqueous cream (life of diluted cream 14 days)

Dermatonics Once Heel Balm® (Dermatonics)

Cream, urea 25%, net price 75 mL = £3.60, 200 mL = £8.50

Excipients include beeswax, lanolin

Dose for dry skin on soles of feet, ADULT and CHILD over 12 years, apply once daily

E45® Itch Relief Cream (Reckitt Benckiser)

Cream, urea 5%, macrogol lauryl ether 3%, net price 50 g = £2.81, 100 g = £3.74, 500-g pump pack = £14.99

Excipients include benzyl alcohol, polysorbates

Dose for dry, scaling, and itching skin, apply twice daily

Eucerin® Intensive (Beiersdorf)

Cream, urea 10%, net price 100 mL = £7.59

Excipients include benzyl alcohol, isopropyl palmitate, wool fat

Dose for dry skin conditions including eczema, ichthyosis, xeroderma, hyperkeratosis, apply thinly and rub into area twice daily

Lotion, urea 10%, net price 250 mL = £7.93

Excipients include benzyl alcohol, isopropyl palmitate

Dose for dry skin conditions including eczema, ichthyosis, xeroderma, hyperkeratosis, apply sparingly and rub into area twice daily

Flexitol® (LaCorium)

Heel balm, urea 25%, net price 40 g = £2.75, 75 g = £3.80, 200 g = £9.40, 500 g = £14.75

Excipients include benzyl alcohol, cetostearyl alcohol, fragrance, lanolin

Dose for dry skin on soles of feet and heels, ADULT and CHILD over 12 years, apply 1–2 times daily

Hydromol® Intensive (Alliance)

Cream, urea 10%, net price 30 g = £1.64, 100 g = £4.37

Excipients none as listed in section 13.1.3

Dose for dry, scaling and itching skin, apply thinly twice daily

Nutraplus® (Galderma)

Cream, urea 10%, net price 100 g = £4.37

Excipients include hydroxybenzoates (parabens), propylene glycol

Dose for dry, scaling and itching skin, apply 2–3 times daily

◢**With antimicrobials**

Dermol® (Dermal)

Cream, benzalkonium chloride 0.1%, chlorhexidine hydrochloride 0.1%, isopropyl myristate 10%, liquid paraffin 10%, net price 100-g tube = £2.86, 500-g pump pack = £6.63

Excipients include cetostearyl alcohol

Dose for dry and pruritic skin conditions including eczema and dermatitis, apply to skin or use as soap substitute

Dermol® 500 Lotion, benzalkonium chloride 0.1%, chlorhexidine hydrochloride 0.1%, liquid paraffin 2.5%, isopropyl myristate 2.5%, net price 500-mL pump pack = £6.04

Excipients include cetostearyl alcohol

Dose for dry and pruritic skin conditions including eczema and dermatitis, apply to skin or use as soap substitute

Eczmol® (Genus)

Cream, chlorhexidine gluconate 1% in emollient basis, net price 250 mL = £3.70

Excipients include cetostearyl alcohol

Dose for dry and pruritic skin conditions including eczema and dermatitis, apply to skin or use as soap substitute

13.2.1.1 Emollient bath and shower preparations

Emollient bath additives should be added to bath water; hydration can be improved by soaking in the bath for 10–20 minutes. Some bath emollients can be applied to wet skin undiluted and rinsed off. In dry skin conditions soap should be avoided (see section 13.2.1 for soap substitutes). The quantities of bath additives recommended for adults are suitable for an adult-size bath. Proportionately less should be used for a child-size bath or a washbasin; recommended bath additive quantities for children reflect this.

These preparations make skin and surfaces slippery—particular care is needed when bathing

Aqueous Cream, BP

Cream, emulsifying ointment 30%, [1]phenoxyethanol 1% in freshly boiled and cooled purified water, net price 100 g = 97p, 500 g = £4.85

Excipients include cetostearyl alcohol

Aquamax® (Dermato Logical)

Cream wash, light liquid paraffin 8%, white soft paraffin 20%, phenoxyethanol 1%, net price 250 g = £2.99

Excipients include cetostearyl alcohol, polysorbate 60

Dose for dry skin conditions, apply to wet or dry skin and rinse

Aveeno® (J&J)

Aveeno® Bath oil, colloidal oatmeal, white oat fraction in emollient basis, net price 250 mL = £4.49

Excipients include beeswax, fragrance

Dose ACBS: for endogenous and exogenous eczema, xeroderma, ichthyosis, and senile pruritus (pruritus of the elderly) associated with dry skin, add 20–30 mL/bath or apply to wet skin and rinse

Balneum® (Almirall)

Balneum® bath oil, soya oil 84.75%, net price 200 mL = £2.48, 500 mL = £5.38, 1 litre = £10.39

Excipients include butylated hydroxytoluene, propylene glycol, fragrance

Dose for dry skin conditions including those associated with dermatitis and eczema; add 20–60 mL/bath (INFANT 5–15 mL); do not use undiluted

Balneum Plus® bath oil, soya oil 82.95%, mixed lauromacrogols 15%, net price 500 mL = £6.66

Excipients include butylated hydroxytoluene, propylene glycol, fragrance

Dose for dry skin conditions including those associated with dermatitis and eczema where pruritus also experienced; add 20 mL/bath (INFANT 5 mL) or apply to wet skin and rinse

---

1. The BP permits use of alternative antimicrobials provided their identity and concentration are stated on the label

Cetraben® (Genus)

Emollient bath additive, light liquid paraffin 82.8%, net price 500 mL = £5.75

Excipients none as listed in section 13.1.3

Dose for dry skin conditions, including eczema, add 1–2 capfuls/bath (CHILD ½–1 capful) or apply to wet skin and rinse

Dermalo® (Dermal)

Bath emollient, acetylated wool alcohols 5%, liquid paraffin 65%, net price 500 mL = £3.44

Excipients none as listed in section 13.1.3

Dose for dermatitis, dry skin conditions including ichthyosis and pruritus of the elderly; add 15–20 mL/bath (INFANT and CHILD 5–10 mL) or apply to wet skin and rinse

Doublebase® (Dermal)

Emollient bath additive, liquid paraffin 65%, net price 500 mL = £5.45

Excipients include cetostearyl alcohol

Dose for dry skin conditions including dermatitis, ichthyosis, and pruritus of the elderly; add 15–20 mL/bath, (INFANT and CHILD 5–10 mL)

Emollient shower gel, isopropyl myristate 15%, liquid paraffin 15%, net price 200 g = £5.21

Excipients none as listed in section 13.1.3

Dose for dry, chapped, or itchy skin conditions, apply to wet or dry skin and rinse, or apply to dry skin after showering

Note Also available as *Doublebase® Emollient Wash Gel*

E45® (Reckitt Benckiser)

Emollient bath oil, cetyl dimeticone 5%, liquid paraffin 91%, net price 250 mL = £3.19, 500 mL = £5.11

Excipients none as listed in section 13.1.3

Dose ACBS: for endogenous and exogenous eczema, xeroderma, ichthyosis, and senile pruritus (pruritus of the elderly) associated with dry skin; add 15 mL/bath (CHILD 5–10 mL) or apply to wet skin and rinse

Emollient wash cream, soap substitute, zinc oxide 5% in an emollient basis, net price 250-mL pump pack = £3.19

Excipients none as listed in section 13.1.3

Dose ACBS: for endogenous and exogenous eczema, xeroderma, ichthyosis and senile pruritus (pruritus of the elderly) associated with dry skin, use as soap substitute

Hydromol® (Alliance)

Bath and shower emollient, isopropyl myristate 13%, light liquid paraffin 37.8%, net price 350 mL = £3.88, 500 mL = £4.42, 1 litre = £8.80

Excipients none as listed in section 13.1.3

Dose for dry skin conditions including eczema, ichthyosis and pruritus of the elderly, add 1–3 capfuls/bath (INFANT ½–2 capfuls) or apply to wet skin and rinse

LPL 63.4® (Huxley)

Emollient bath additive, light liquid paraffin 63.4%, net price 500 mL = £3.10

Excipients include acetylated wool alcohols, isopropyl palmitate

Dose for dry skin conditions, add 1–3 capfuls/bath (CHILD 1 month–12 years, ½–2 capfuls) or apply to wet skin and rinse

Oilatum® (Stiefel)

Emollient bath additive (emulsion), light liquid paraffin 63.4%, net price 250 mL = £2.75, 500 mL = £4.57

Excipients include acetylated lanolin alcohols, palmitate, fragrance

Dose for dry skin conditions including dermatitis, pruritus of the elderly, and ichthyosis, add 1–3 capfuls/bath (INFANT 0.5–2 capfuls) or apply to wet skin and rinse

Junior bath additive, light liquid paraffin 63.4%, net price 150 mL = £2.82, 250 mL = £3.25, 300 mL = £5.10, 600 mL = £5.89

Excipients include acetylated lanolin alcohols, isopropyl palmitate

Dose for dry skin conditions including dermatitis, pruritus of the elderly, and ichthyosis, add 1–3 capfuls/bath (INFANT 0.5–2 capfuls) or apply to wet skin and rinse

Shower emollient (gel), light liquid paraffin 70%, net price (with fragrance or fragrance-free) 150 g = £5.15

Excipients none as listed in section 13.1.3

Dose for dry skin conditions including dermatitis, pruritus of the elderly, and ichthyosis, apply to wet skin and rinse

QV® (Crawford)

Bath oil, light liquid paraffin 85.13%, net price 200 mL = £2.20, 500 mL = £4.66

Excipients none as listed in section 13.1.3

Dose for dry skin conditions including eczema, psoriasis, ichthyosis, and pruritus, add 10 mL/bath (INFANT 5 mL) or apply to wet skin and rinse

Gentle wash, glycerol 15%, net price 250 mL = £3.14, 500-mL pump pack = £5.24

Excipients include hydroxybenzoates (parabens)

Dose for dry skin conditions including eczema, psoriasis, ichthyosis, and pruritus, use as soap substitute

Zerolatum® (Thornton & Ross)

Emollient medicinal bath oil, liquid paraffin 65%, acetylated wool alcohols 5%, net price 500 mL = £4.79

Excipients none as listed in section 13.1.3

Dose for dry skin conditions including dermatitis, pruritus of the elderly, and ichthyosis, add 15–20 mL/bath (CHILD 5–10 mL)

Zeroneum® (Thornton & Ross)

Bath oil, refined soya bean oil 83.35%, net price 500 mL = £4.48

Excipients include butylated hydroxytoluene, fragrance, propylene glycol

Dose for dry skin conditions including eczema, add 20 mL/bath (CHILD 5 mL)

◀**With antimicrobials**

Dermol® (Dermal)

Dermol 600® Bath Emollient, benzalkonium chloride 0.5%, liquid paraffin 25%, isopropyl myristate 25%, net price 600 mL = £7.55

Excipients include polysorbate 60

Dose for dry and pruritic skin conditions including eczema and dermatitis, add up to 30 mL/bath (INFANT up to 15 mL); do not use undiluted

Dermol® 200 Shower Emollient, benzalkonium chloride 0.1%, chlorhexidine hydrochloride 0.1%, liquid paraffin 2.5%, isopropyl myristate 2.5%, net price 200 mL = £3.55

Excipients include cetostearyl alcohol

Dose for dry and pruritic skin conditions including eczema and dermatitis, apply to skin or use as soap substitute

Dermol® Wash Emulsion, benzalkonium chloride 0.1%, chlorhexidine hydrochloride 0.1%, liquid paraffin 2.5%, isopropyl myristate 2.5%, net price 200-mL = £3.55

Excipients include cetostearyl alcohol

Dose for dry and pruritic skin conditions including eczema and dermatitis, apply to skin or use as soap substitute

Emulsiderm® (Dermal)

Liquid emulsion, benzalkonium chloride 0.5%, liquid paraffin 25%, isopropyl myristate 25%, net price 300 mL (with 15-mL measure) = £3.85, 1 litre (with 30-mL measure) = £12.00

Excipients include polysorbate 60

Dose for dry skin conditions including eczema and ichthyosis, add 7–30 mL/bath or rub into dry skin until absorbed

Oilatum® Plus (Stiefel)

Bath additive, benzalkonium chloride 6%, triclosan 2%, light liquid paraffin 52.5%, net price 500 mL = £6.98

Excipients include acetylated lanolin alcohols, isopropyl palmitate

Dose for topical treatment of eczema including eczema at risk from infection, add 1–2 capfuls/bath (INFANT over 6 months 1 mL); do not use undiluted

◢With tar

Section 13.5.2

13.2.2 Barrier preparations

Barrier preparations often contain water-repellent substances such as **dimeticone** or other silicones. They are used on the skin around stomas, bedsores, and pressure areas in the elderly where the skin is intact. Where the skin has broken down, barrier preparations have a limited role in protecting adjacent skin. Barrier preparations are not a substitute for adequate nursing care.

Nappy rash The first line of treatment is to ensure that nappies are changed frequently and that tightly fitting water-proof pants are avoided. The rash may clear when left exposed to the air and a barrier preparation, applied with each nappy change, can be helpful. A mild corticosteroid such as hydrocortisone 0.5% or 1% (section 13.4) can be used if inflammation is causing discomfort, but it should be avoided in neonates. The barrier preparation should be applied after the corticosteroid preparation to prevent further skin damage. Preparations containing hydrocortisone should be applied for no more than a week; the hydrocortisone should be discontinued as soon as the inflammation subsides. The occlusive effect of nappies and waterproof pants may increase absorption of corticosteroids (for cautions, see section 13.4). If the rash is associated with candidal infection, a topical antifungal such as clotrimazole cream (section 13.10.2) can be used. Topical antibacterial preparations (section 13.10.1) can be used if bacterial infection is present; treatment with an oral antibacterial may occasionally be required in severe or recurrent infection. Hydrocortisone may be used in combination with antimicrobial preparations if there is considerable inflammation, erosion, and infection.

◢Non-proprietary barrier preparations

Zinc and Castor Oil Ointment, BP

Ointment, zinc oxide 7.5%, castor oil 50%, arachis (peanut) oil 30.5%, white beeswax 10%, cetostearyl alcohol 2%, net price 500 g = £5.68

For nappy and urinary rash

◢Proprietary barrier preparations

Conotrane® (Astellas)

Cream, benzalkonium chloride 0.1%, dimeticone '350' 22%, net price 100 g = 88p, 500 g = £3.51

Excipients include cetostearyl alcohol, fragrance

For nappy and urinary rash and pressure sores

Drapolene® (Omega Pharma)

Cream, benzalkonium chloride 0.01%, cetrimide 0.2% in a basis containing white soft paraffin, cetyl alcohol and wool fat, net price 100 g = £1.76, 200 g = £2.86, 350 g = £4.28

Excipients include cetyl alcohol, chlorocresol, wool fat

For nappy and urinary rash; minor wounds

Medicaid® (LPC)

Cream, cetrimide 0.5% in a basis containing light liquid paraffin, white soft paraffin, cetostearyl alcohol, glyceryl monostearate, net price 50 g = £1.69

Excipients include cetostearyl alcohol, fragrance, hydroxybenzoates (parabens), wool fat

For nappy rash, minor burns, and abrasions

Metanium® (Thornton & Ross)

Ointment, titanium dioxide 20%, titanium peroxide 5%, titanium salicylate 3% in a basis containing dimeticone, light liquid paraffin, white soft paraffin, and benzoin tincture, net price 30 g = £2.24

Excipients none as listed in section 13.1.3

For nappy rash

Morhulin® (Actavis)

Ointment, cod-liver oil 11.4%, zinc oxide 38%, in a basis containing liquid paraffin and yellow soft paraffin, net price 50 g = £1.91

Excipients include wool fat derivative

For minor wounds, varicose ulcers, pressure sores, eczema, and nappy rash

Siopel® (Derma UK)

Barrier cream, dimeticone '1000' 10%, cetrimide 0.3%, arachis (peanut) oil, net price 50 g = £2.15

Excipients include butylated hydroxytoluene, cetostearyl alcohol, hydroxybenzoates (parabens)

For protection against water-soluble irritants

Sprilon® (Ayrton Saunders)

Spray application, dimeticone 1.04%, zinc oxide 12.5%, in a basis containing wool alcohols, cetostearyl alcohol, dextran, white soft paraffin, liquid paraffin, propellants, net price 115-g pressurised aerosol unit = £8.90

Excipients include cetostearyl alcohol, hydroxybenzoates (parabens), wool fat

For urinary rash, pressure sores, leg ulcers, moist eczema, fissures, fistulae and ileostomy care

Note Flammable

Sudocrem® (Forest)

Cream, benzyl alcohol 0.39%, benzyl benzoate 1.01%, benzyl cinnamate 0.15%, hydrous wool fat (hypoallergenic lanolin) 4%, zinc oxide 15.25%, net price 60 g = £1.45, 125 g = £2.15, 250 g = £3.67, 400 g = £5.25

Excipients include beeswax (synthetic), propylene glycol, butylated hydroxyanisole, fragrance

For nappy rash and pressure sores

13.3 Topical local anaesthetics and antipruritics

Pruritus may be caused by systemic disease (such as obstructive jaundice, endocrine disease, chronic renal disease, iron deficiency, and certain malignant diseases), skin disease (e.g. psoriasis, eczema, urticaria, and scabies), drug hypersensitivity, or as a side-effect of opioid analgesics. Where possible, the underlying causes should be treated. An **emollient** (section 13.2.1) may be of value where the pruritus is associated with dry skin. Pruritus that occurs in otherwise healthy elderly people can also be treated with an emollient. **Levomenthol cream** can be used to relieve pruritus; it exerts a cooling effect on the skin. For advice on the treatment of pruritus in palliative care, see p. 23.

13 Skin

Preparations containing **crotamiton** are sometimes used but are of uncertain value. Preparations containing **calamine** are often ineffective.

A topical preparation containing **doxepin** 5% is licensed for the relief of pruritus in eczema; it can cause drowsiness and there may be a risk of sensitisation.

Pruritus is common in biliary obstruction, especially in primary biliary cirrhosis and drug-induced cholestasis. Oral administration of **colestyramine** is the treatment of choice (section 1.9.2).

Topical antihistamines and local anaesthetics are only marginally effective and occasionally cause sensitisation. For *insect stings* and *insect bites*, a short course of a topical corticosteroid is appropriate. Short-term treatment with a **sedating antihistamine** (section 3.4.1) may help in insect stings and in intractable pruritus where sedation is desirable. Calamine preparations are of little value for the treatment of insect stings or bites.

For preparations used in *pruritus ani*, see section 1.7.1.

CALAMINE

Indications pruritus

Contra-indications avoid application prior to x-ray (zinc oxide may affect outcome of x-ray)

Calamine (Non-proprietary)
> Aqueous cream, calamine 4%, zinc oxide 3%, liquid paraffin 20%, self-emulsifying glyceryl monostearate 5%, cetomacrogol emulsifying wax 5%, phenoxyethanol 0.5%, freshly boiled and cooled purified water 62.5%, net price 100 mL = £1.28
>
> Lotion (= cutaneous suspension), calamine 15%, zinc oxide 5%, glycerol 5%, bentonite 3%, sodium citrate 0.5%, liquefied phenol 0.5%, in freshly boiled and cooled purified water, net price 200 mL = 88p
>
> Oily lotion (BP 1980), calamine 5%, arachis (peanut) oil 50%, oleic acid 0.5%, wool fat 1%, in calcium hydroxide solution, net price 200 mL = £1.57

CROTAMITON

Indications pruritus (including pruritus after scabies—section 13.10.4); see notes above

Cautions avoid use near eyes, in buccal mucosa, or on broken or very inflamed skin; use on doctor's advice for children under 3 years

Contra-indications acute exudative dermatoses

Pregnancy manufacturer advises avoid, especially during the first trimester—no information available

Breast-feeding no information available; avoid application to nipple area

Dose
- Pruritus, apply 2–3 times daily; CHILD under 3 years, apply once daily

Eurax® (Novartis Consumer Health)
> Cream, crotamiton 10%, net price 30 g = £2.38, 100 g = £4.15
> **Excipients** include beeswax, fragrance, hydroxybenzoates (parabens), stearyl alcohol
>
> Lotion, crotamiton 10%, net price 100 mL = £3.14
> **Excipients** include cetyl alcohol, fragrance, propylene glycol, sorbic acid, stearyl alcohol

DOXEPIN HYDROCHLORIDE

Indications pruritus in eczema; depressive illness (section 4.3.1)

Cautions susceptibility to angle-closure glaucoma; urinary retention; mania; cardiac arrhythmias; severe heart disease; avoid application to large areas; **interactions:** Appendix 1 (antidepressants, tricyclic)
> Driving Drowsiness may affect performance of skilled tasks (e.g. driving); effects of alcohol enhanced

Hepatic impairment manufacturer advises caution in severe liver disease

Pregnancy manufacturer advises use only if potential benefit outweighs risk

Breast-feeding manufacturer advises use only if potential benefit outweighs risk

Side-effects drowsiness; local burning, stinging, irritation, tingling and rash; systemic side-effects such as antimuscarinic effects, headache, fever, dizziness, gastro-intestinal disturbances also reported

Dose
- ADULT and CHILD over 12 years, apply thinly 3–4 times daily; usual max. 3 g per application; usual total max. 12 g daily; coverage should be less than 10% of body surface area

Xepin® (CHS) [PoM]
> Cream, doxepin hydrochloride 5%, net price 30 g = £11.70. Label: 2, 10, patient information leaflet
> **Excipients** include benzyl alcohol

LEVOMENTHOL

Indications pruritus

Levomenthol Cream, BP
(Menthol in Aqueous Cream)
> Cream, levomenthol 0.5%, net price 500 g = £16.07; 1% 100 g = £3.97, 500 g = £16.59; 2% 50 g = £1.53, 100 g = £3.67, 450 g = £17.99, 500 g = £16.97
> Dose apply 1–2 times daily

TOPICAL LOCAL ANAESTHETICS

Indications relief of local pain, see notes above. See section 15.2 for use in surface anaesthesia

Cautions occasionally cause hypersensitivity
> Note Topical local anaesthetic preparations may be absorbed, especially through mucosal surfaces, therefore excessive application should be avoided and they should preferably not be used for more than about 3 days; not generally suitable for young children

TOPICAL ANTIHISTAMINES

Indications see notes above

Cautions may cause hypersensitivity; avoid in eczema; photosensitivity (diphenhydramine); not recommended for longer than 3 days

13.4 Topical corticosteroids

Topical corticosteroids are used for the treatment of inflammatory conditions of the skin (other than those arising from an infection), in particular eczema (section 13.5.1), contact dermatitis, insect stings (p. 43), and eczema of scabies (section 13.10.4). Corticosteroids suppress the inflammatory reaction during use; they are not curative and on discontinuation a rebound

13 Skin

exacerbation of the condition may occur. They are generally used to relieve symptoms and suppress signs of the disorder when other measures such as emollients are ineffective.

Topical corticosteroids are not recommended in the routine treatment of urticaria; treatment should only be initiated and supervised by a specialist. Topical corticosteroids are **contra-indicated** in rosacea. They may worsen ulcerated or secondarily infected lesions. They should not be used indiscriminately in pruritus (where they will only benefit if inflammation is causing the itch) and are **not** recommended for acne vulgaris.

Systemic or very potent topical corticosteroids should be avoided or given only under specialist supervision in *psoriasis* because, although they may suppress the psoriasis in the short term, relapse or vigorous rebound occurs on withdrawal (sometimes precipitating severe pustular psoriasis). For the role of topical corticosteroids in the treatment of psoriasis, see section 13.5.2.

In general, the most potent topical corticosteroids should be reserved for recalcitrant dermatoses such as *chronic discoid lupus erythematosus, lichen simplex chronicus, hypertrophic lichen planus,* and *palmoplantar pustulosis.* Potent corticosteroids should generally be avoided on the face and skin flexures, but specialists occasionally prescribe them for use on these areas in certain circumstances.

When topical treatment has failed, intralesional corticosteroid injections (section 10.1.2.2) may be used. These are more effective than the very potent topical corticosteroid preparations and should be reserved for severe cases where there are localised lesions such as *keloid scars, hypertrophic lichen planus,* or *localised alopecia areata.*

Perioral lesions Hydrocortisone cream 1% can be used for up to 7 days to treat uninfected inflammatory lesions on the lips. **Hydrocortisone and miconazole** cream or ointment is useful where infection by susceptible organisms and inflammation co-exist, particularly for initial treatment (up to 7 days) e.g. in angular cheilitis (see also p. 789). Organisms susceptible to miconazole include *Candida* spp. and many Gram-positive bacteria including streptococci and staphylococci.

Children Children, especially infants, are particularly susceptible to side-effects. However, concern about the safety of topical corticosteroids in children should not result in the child being undertreated. The aim is to control the condition as well as possible; inadequate treatment will perpetuate the condition. A mild corticosteroid such as hydrocortisone 0.5% or 1% is useful for treating nappy rash (section 13.2.2) and hydrocortisone 1% for atopic eczema in childhood (section 13.5.1). A moderately potent or potent corticosteroid may be appropriate for severe atopic eczema on the limbs, for 1–2 weeks only, switching to a less potent preparation as the condition improves. In an acute flare-up of atopic eczema, it may be appropriate to use more potent formulations of topical corticosteroids for a short period to regain control of the condition. A very potent corticosteroid should be initiated under the supervision of a specialist. Continuous daily application of a mild corticosteroid such as hydrocortisone 1% is equivalent to a potent corticosteroid such as betamethasone 0.1% applied intermittently. Carers of young children should be advised that treatment should **not** necessarily be reserved to 'treat only the worst areas' and they may

need to be advised that patient information leaflets may contain inappropriate advice for the patient's condition.

Choice of formulation Water-miscible corticosteroid *creams* are suitable for moist or weeping lesions whereas *ointments* are generally chosen for dry, lichenified or scaly lesions or where a more occlusive effect is required. *Lotions* may be useful when minimal application to a large or hair-bearing area is required or for the treatment of exudative lesions. *Occlusive polythene or hydrocolloid dressings* increase absorption, but also increase the risk of side-effects; they are therefore used only under supervision on a short-term basis for areas of very thick skin (such as the palms and soles). The inclusion of urea or salicylic acid also increases the penetration of the corticosteroid.

In the BNF topical corticosteroids for the skin are categorised as 'mild', 'moderately potent', 'potent' or 'very potent' (see p. 803); the **least potent** preparation which is effective should be chosen but dilution should be avoided whenever possible.

Cautions Avoid prolonged use of a topical corticosteroid on the face (and keep away from eyes). In children avoid prolonged use and use potent or very potent corticosteroids under specialist supervision; extreme caution is required in dermatoses of infancy including nappy rash—treatment should be limited to 5–7 days.

Psoriasis The use of potent or very potent corticosteroids in psoriasis can result in rebound relapse, development of generalised pustular psoriasis, and local and systemic toxicity.

Contra-indications Topical corticosteroids are contra-indicated in untreated bacterial, fungal, or viral skin lesions, in acne, in rosacea, and in perioral dermatitis; potent corticosteroids are contra-indicated in widespread plaque psoriasis (see notes above).

Side-effects *Mild* and *moderately potent* topical corticosteroids are associated with few side-effects but care is required in the use of *potent* and *very potent* corticosteroids. Absorption through the skin can rarely cause adrenal suppression and even Cushing's syndrome (section 6.3.2), depending on the area of the body being treated and the duration of treatment. Absorption is greatest where the skin is thin or raw, and from intertriginous areas; it is increased by occlusion. Local side-effects include:

- spread and worsening of untreated infection;

- thinning of the skin which may be restored over a period after stopping treatment but the original structure may never return;

- irreversible striae atrophicae and telangiectasia;

- contact dermatitis;

- perioral dermatitis;

- acne, or worsening of acne or rosacea;

- mild depigmentation which may be reversible;

- hypertrichosis also reported.

> In order to minimise the side-effects of a topical corticosteroid, it is important to apply it **thinly** to affected areas **only**, no more frequently than **twice daily**, and to use the least potent formulation which is fully effective.

Application Topical corticosteroid preparations should be applied no more frequently than twice daily; once daily is often sufficient.

Topical corticosteroids should be spread thinly on the skin but in sufficient quantity to cover the affected areas. The length of cream or ointment expelled from a tube may be used to specify the quantity to be applied to a given area of skin. This length can be measured in terms of a *fingertip unit* (the distance from the tip of the adult index finger to the first crease). One fingertip unit (approximately 500 mg from a tube with a standard 5-mm diameter nozzle) is sufficient to cover an area that is twice that of the flat adult handprint (palm and fingers).

Suitable quantities of corticosteroid preparations to be prescribed for specific areas of the body

Area of body	Creams and Ointments
Face and neck	15 to 30 g
Both hands	15 to 30 g
Scalp	15 to 30 g
Both arms	30 to 60 g
Both legs	100 g
Trunk	100 g
Groins and genitalia	15 to 30 g

These amounts are usually suitable for an adult for a single daily application for 2 weeks

If a patient is using topical corticosteroids of different potencies, the patient should be told when to use each corticosteroid. The potency of each topical corticosteroid (see Topical Corticosteroid Preparation Potencies, below) should be included on the label with the directions for use. The label should be attached to the container (for example, the tube) rather than the outer packaging.

Mixing topical preparations on the skin should be avoided where possible; several minutes should elapse between application of different preparations.

Compound preparations The advantages of including other substances (such as antibacterials or antifungals) with corticosteroids in topical preparations are uncertain, but such combinations may have a place where inflammatory skin conditions are associated with bacterial or fungal infection, such as infected eczema. In these cases the antimicrobial drug should be chosen according to the sensitivity of the infecting organism and used regularly for a short period (typically twice daily for 1 week). Longer use increases the likelihood of resistance and of sensitisation.

The keratolytic effect of salicylic acid facilitates the absorption of topical corticosteroids; however, excessive and prolonged use of topical preparations containing salicylic acid may cause salicylism.

Topical corticosteroid preparation potencies

Potency of a topical corticosteroid preparation is a result of the formulation as well as the corticosteroid. Therefore, proprietary names are shown below.

Mild

Hydrocortisone 0.1–2.5%, *Dioderm, Mildison, Synalar 1 in 10 dilution*

- Mild with antimicrobials: *Canesten HC, Daktacort, Econacort, Fucidin H, Nystaform-HC, Terra-Cortril, Timodine*

Moderate

Betnovate-RD, Eumovate, Haelan, Modrasone, Synalar 1 in 4 Dilution, Ultralanum Plain

- Moderate with antimicrobials: *Trimovate*
- Moderate with urea: *Alphaderm, Calmurid HC*

Potent

Beclometasone dipropionate 0.025%, Betamethasone valerate 0.1%, *Betacap, Betesil, Bettamousse, Betnovate, Cutivate, Diprosone, Elocon,* Hydrocortisone butyrate, *Locoid, Locoid Crelo, Metosyn,* Mometasone furoate 0.1%, *Nerisone, Synalar*

- Potent with antimicrobials: *Aureocort,* Betamethasone and clioquinol, Betamethasone and neomycin, *Fucibet, Lotriderm, Synalar C, Synalar N*
- Potent with salicylic acid: *Diprosalic*

Very potent

Clarelux, Dermovate, Etrivex, Nerisone Forte

- Very potent with antimicrobials: Clobetasol with neomycin and nystatin

---

▌HYDROCORTISONE

Indications mild inflammatory skin disorders such as eczemas (but for over-the-counter preparations, see below); nappy rash (see also section 13.2.2)

Cautions see notes above

Contra-indications see notes above

Side-effects see notes above

Dose

- Apply thinly 1–2 times daily

Hydrocortisone (Non-proprietary) ▣POM▣
Cream, hydrocortisone 0.5%, net price, 15 g = £1.38, 30 g = £2.76; 1%, 15 g = £1.17, 30 g = £2.34, 50 g = £3.90; 2.5%, 15 g = £11.15. Label: 28, counselling, application, see above. Potency: mild
Dental prescribing on NHS Hydrocortisone Cream 1% 15 g may be prescribed

Ointment, hydrocortisone 0.5%, net price 15 g = £4.53, 30 g = £4.90; 1%, 15 g = £1.26, 30 g = £2.52, 50 g = £4.20; 2.5%, 15 g = £24.19. Label: 28, counselling, application, see above. Potency: mild
When hydrocortisone cream or ointment is prescribed and no strength is stated, the 1% strength should be supplied

◢**Over-the-counter hydrocortisone preparations**
Skin creams and ointments containing hydrocortisone (alone or with other ingredients) can be sold to the public for the treatment of allergic contact dermatitis, irritant dermatitis, insect bite reactions and mild to moderate eczema, to be applied sparingly over the affected area 1–2 times daily for max. 1 week. Over-the-counter hydrocortisone preparations should not be sold without medical advice for children under 10 years or for pregnant women; they should **not** be sold for application to the face, anogenital region, broken or infected skin (including cold sores, acne, and athlete's foot); over-the-counter hydrocortisone preparations containing clotrimazole or miconazole nitrate can be sold to the public for athlete's foot and candidal intertrigo

◾**Proprietary hydrocortisone preparations**

Dioderm® (Dermal) [PoM]

Cream, hydrocortisone 0.1%, net price 30 g = £2.39. Label: 28, counselling, application, see p. 803. Potency: mild

Excipients include cetostearyl alcohol, propylene glycol

Note Although this contains only 0.1% hydrocortisone, the formulation is designed to provide a clinical activity comparable to that of Hydrocortisone Cream 1% BP

Mildison® (Astellas) [PoM]

Lipocream, hydrocortisone 1%, net price 30 g = £1.71. Label: 28, counselling, application, see p. 803. Potency: mild

Excipients include benzyl alcohol, cetostearyl alcohol, hydroxybenzoates (parabens)

◾**Compound preparations**

Compound preparations with coal tar, see section 13.5.2

Alphaderm® (Alliance) [PoM]

Cream, hydrocortisone 1%, urea 10%, net price 30 g = £2.38; 100 g = £7.03. Label: 28, counselling, application, see p. 803. Potency: moderate

Excipients none as listed in section 13.1.3

Calmurid HC® (Galderma) [PoM]

Cream, hydrocortisone 1%, urea 10%, lactic acid 5%, net price 100 g = £10.51. Label: 28, counselling, application, see p. 803. Potency: moderate

Excipients none as listed in section 13.1.3

Note If stinging occurs, manufacturer advises dilute to half-strength with aqueous cream for 1 week then transfer to undiluted preparation (but see section 13.1.1 for advice to avoid dilution where possible)

◾**With antimicrobials**

See notes above for comment on compound preparations

Canesten HC® (Bayer Consumer Care) [PoM]

Cream, hydrocortisone 1%, clotrimazole 1%, net price 30 g = £2.42. Label: 28, counselling, application, see p. 803. Potency: mild

Excipients include benzyl alcohol, cetostearyl alcohol

Note A 15-g tube is on sale to the public for the treatment of athlete's foot and fungal infection of skin folds with associated inflammation

Daktacort® (Janssen) [PoM]

Cream, hydrocortisone 1%, miconazole nitrate 2%, net price 30 g = £2.49. Label: 28, counselling, application, see p. 803. Potency: mild

Excipients include butylated hydroxyanisole, disodium edetate

Cautions interactions: Appendix 1 (antifungals, imidazole)

Dental prescribing on NHS May be prescribed as Miconazole and Hydrocortisone Cream for max. 7 days

Note A 15-g tube is on sale to the public for the treatment of athlete's foot and candidal intertrigo

Ointment, hydrocortisone 1%, miconazole nitrate 2%, net price 30 g = £2.50. Label: 28, counselling, application, see p. 803. Potency: mild

Excipients none as listed in section 13.1.3

Cautions interactions: Appendix 1 (antifungals, imidazole)

Dental prescribing on NHS May be prescribed as Miconazole and Hydrocortisone Ointment for max. 7 days

Fucidin H® (LEO) [PoM]

Cream, hydrocortisone acetate 1%, fusidic acid 2%, net price 30 g = £5.02, 60 g = £10.04. Label: 28, counselling, application, see p. 803. Potency: mild

Excipients include butylated hydroxyanisole, cetyl alcohol, polysorbate 60, potassium sorbate

Nystaform-HC® (Typharm) [PoM]

Cream, hydrocortisone 0.5%, nystatin 100 000 units/g, chlorhexidine hydrochloride 1%, net price 30 g = £2.66. Label: 28, counselling, application, see p. 803. Potency: mild

Excipients include benzyl alcohol, cetostearyl alcohol, polysorbate '60'

Ointment, hydrocortisone 1%, nystatin 100 000 units/g, chlorhexidine acetate 1%, net price 30 g = £2.66. Label: 28, counselling, application, see p. 803. Potency: mild

Excipients none as listed in section 13.1.3

Terra-Cortril® (Alliance) [PoM]

Ointment, hydrocortisone 1%, oxytetracycline (as hydrochloride) 3%, net price 30 g = £5.01. Label: 28, counselling, application, see p. 803. Potency: mild

Excipients none as listed in section 13.1.3

Contra-indications children under 12 years

Pregnancy section 5.1.3

Breast-feeding section 5.1.3

Timodine® (Alliance) [PoM]

Cream, hydrocortisone 0.5%, nystatin 100 000 units/g, benzalkonium chloride solution 0.2%, dimeticone '350' 10%, net price 30 g = £2.86. Label: 28, counselling, application, see p. 803. Potency: mild

Excipients include butylated hydroxyanisole, cetostearyl alcohol, hydroxybenzoates (parabens), sodium metabisulfite, sorbic acid

---

HYDROCORTISONE BUTYRATE

Indications severe inflammatory skin disorders such as eczemas unresponsive to less potent corticosteroids; psoriasis, see notes above

Cautions see notes above

Contra-indications see notes above

Side-effects see notes above

Dose

• Apply thinly 1–2 times daily

Locoid® (Astellas) [PoM]

Cream, hydrocortisone butyrate 0.1%, net price 30 g = £1.60, 100 g = £4.93. Label: 28, counselling, application, see p. 803. Potency: potent

Excipients include cetostearyl alcohol, hydroxybenzoates (parabens)

Lipocream, hydrocortisone butyrate 0.1%, net price 30 g = £1.69, 100 g = £5.17. Label: 28, counselling, application, see p. 803. Potency: potent

Excipients include benzyl alcohol, cetostearyl alcohol, hydroxybenzoates (parabens)

Note For bland cream basis see *Lipobase®*, section 13.2.1

Ointment, hydrocortisone butyrate 0.1%, net price 30 g = £1.60, 100 g = £4.93. Label: 28, counselling, application, see p. 803. Potency: potent

Excipients none as listed in section 13.1.3

Scalp lotion, hydrocortisone butyrate 0.1%, in an aqueous isopropyl alcohol basis, net price 100 mL = £6.83. Label: 15, 28, counselling, application, see p. 803. Potency: potent

Excipients none as listed in section 13.1.3

Locoid Crelo® (Astellas) [PoM]

Lotion (topical emulsion), hydrocortisone butyrate 0.1% in a water-miscible basis, net price 100 g (with applicator nozzle) = £5.91. Label: 28, counselling, application, see p. 803. Potency: potent

Excipients include butylated hydroxytoluene, cetostearyl alcohol, hydroxybenzoates (parabens), propylene glycol

---

◼ ALCLOMETASONE DIPROPIONATE

Indications inflammatory skin disorders such as eczemas

Cautions see notes above

Contra-indications see notes above

Side-effects see notes above

Dose

• Apply thinly 1–2 times daily

Modrasone® (TEVA UK) [PoM]

Cream, alclometasone dipropionate 0.05%, net price 50 g = £2.68. Label: 28, counselling, application, see p. 803. Potency: moderate

Excipients include cetostearyl alcohol, chlorocresol, propylene glycol

---

◼ BECLOMETASONE DIPROPIONATE
(Beclomethasone dipropionate)

Indications severe inflammatory skin disorders such as eczemas unresponsive to less potent corticosteroids; psoriasis, see notes above

Cautions see notes above

Contra-indications see notes above

Side-effects see notes above

Dose

• Apply thinly 1–2 times daily

Beclometasone (Non-proprietary) [PoM]

Cream, beclometasone dipropionate 0.025%, net price 30 g = £68.00. Label: 28, counselling, application, see p. 803. Potency: potent

Ointment, beclometasone dipropionate 0.025%, net price 30 g = £68.00. Label: 28, counselling, application, see p. 803. Potency: potent

---

◼ BETAMETHASONE ESTERS

Indications severe inflammatory skin disorders such as eczemas unresponsive to less potent corticosteroids; psoriasis, see notes above

Cautions see notes above; use of more than 100 g per week of 0.1% preparation likely to cause adrenal suppression

Contra-indications see notes above

Side-effects see notes above

Dose

• Apply thinly 1–2 times daily

Betamethasone Valerate (Non-proprietary) [PoM]

Cream, betamethasone (as valerate) 0.1%, net price 30 g = £3.12, 100 g = £10.40. Label: 28, counselling, application, see p. 803. Potency: potent

Ointment, betamethasone (as valerate) 0.1%, net price 30 g = £2.43, 100 g = £8.10. Label: 28, counselling, application, see p. 803. Potency: potent

Betacap® (Dermal) [PoM]

Scalp application, betamethasone (as valerate) 0.1% in a water-miscible basis containing coconut oil derivative, net price 100 mL = £3.75. Label: 15, 28, counselling, application, see p. 803. Potency: potent

Excipients none as listed in section 13.1.3

Betesil® (Genus) [PoM]

Medicated plasters, betamethasone (as valerate) 2.25 mg, net price 4 = £9.92. Counselling, application. Potency: potent

Excipients include disodium edetate, hydroxybenzoates (parabens)

Dose ADULT over 18 years, apply plaster to clean, dry skin once daily; max. 6 plasters daily; max. duration of treatment 30 days

Counselling Leave at least 30 minutes between applications; plasters may be cut; avoid water contact with plaster—take bath or shower between applications; see also p. 803

Betnovate® (GSK) [PoM]

Cream, betamethasone (as valerate) 0.1% in a water-miscible basis, net price 30 g = £1.43, 100 g = £4.05. Label: 28, counselling, application, see p. 803. Potency: potent

Excipients include cetostearyl alcohol, chlorocresol

Ointment, betamethasone (as valerate) 0.1% in an anhydrous paraffin basis, net price 30 g = £1.43, 100 g = £4.05. Label: 28, counselling, application, see p. 803. Potency: potent

Excipients none as listed in section 13.1.3

Lotion, betamethasone (as valerate) 0.1%, net price 100 mL = £4.58. Label: 28, counselling, application, see p. 803. Potency: potent

Excipients include cetostearyl alcohol, hydroxybenzoates (parabens)

Scalp application, betamethasone (as valerate) 0.1% in a water-miscible basis, net price 100 mL = £4.99. Label: 15, 28, counselling, application, see p. 803. Potency: potent

Excipients none as listed in section 13.1.3

Betnovate-RD® (GSK) [PoM]

Cream, betamethasone (as valerate) 0.025% in a water-miscible basis (1 in 4 dilution of *Betnovate®* cream), net price 100 g = £3.15. Label: 28, counselling, application, see p. 803. Potency: moderate

Excipients include cetostearyl alcohol, chlorocresol

Ointment, betamethasone (as valerate) 0.025% in an anhydrous paraffin basis (1 in 4 dilution of *Betnovate®* ointment), net price 100 g = £3.15. Label: 28, counselling, application, see p. 803. Potency: moderate

Excipients none as listed in section 13.1.3

Bettamousse® (RPH) [PoM]

Foam (= scalp application), betamethasone valerate 0.12% (≡ betamethasone 0.1%), net price 100 g = £9.75. Label: 28, counselling, application, see p. 803. Potency: potent

Excipients include cetyl alcohol, polysorbate 60, propylene glycol, stearyl alcohol

Note Flammable

13 Skin

Diprosone® (MSD) PoM

Cream, betamethasone (as dipropionate) 0.05%, net price 30 g = £2.16, 100 g = £6.12. Label: 28, counselling, application, see p. 803. Potency: potent
Excipients include cetostearyl alcohol, chlorocresol

Ointment, betamethasone (as dipropionate) 0.05%, net price 30 g = £2.16, 100 g = £6.12. Label: 28, counselling, application, see p. 803. Potency: potent
Excipients none as listed in section 13.1.3

Lotion, betamethasone (as dipropionate) 0.05%, net price 30 mL = £2.73, 100 mL = £7.80. Label: 28, counselling, application, see p. 803. Potency: potent
Excipients none as listed in section 13.1.3

◢**With salicylic acid**

See notes above for comment on compound preparations
For prescribing information on salicylic acid, see, p. 814

Diprosalic® (MSD) PoM

Ointment, betamethasone (as dipropionate) 0.05%, salicylic acid 3%, net price 30 g = £3.18, 100 g = £9.14. Label: 28, counselling, application, see p. 803. Potency: potent
Excipients none as listed in section 13.1.3
Dose apply thinly 1–2 times daily; max. 60 g per week

Scalp application, betamethasone (as dipropionate) 0.05%, salicylic acid 2%, in an alcoholic basis, net price 100 mL = £10.10. Label: 28, counselling, application, see p. 803. Potency: potent
Excipients include disodium edetate
Dose apply a few drops 1–2 times daily

◢**With antimicrobials**

See notes above for comment on compound preparations

Betamethasone and clioquinol (Non-proprietary) PoM

Cream, betamethasone (as valerate) 0.1%, clioquinol 3%, net price 30 g = £18.88. Label: 28, counselling, application, see p. 803. Potency: potent
Excipients may include cetostearyl alcohol, chlorocresol
Note Stains clothing

Ointment, betamethasone (as valerate) 0.1%, clioquinol 3%, net price 30 g = £18.88. Label: 28, counselling, application, see p. 803. Potency: potent
Excipients may include cetostearyl alcohol, chlorocresol
Note Stains clothing

Betamethasone and neomycin (Non-proprietary) PoM

Cream, betamethasone (as valerate) 0.1%, neomycin sulfate 0.5%, net price 30 g = £18.88, 100 g = £38.00. Label: 28, counselling, application, see p. 803. Potency: potent
Excipients may include cetostearyl alcohol, chlorocresol

Ointment, betamethasone (as valerate) 0.1%, neomycin sulfate 0.5%, net price 30 g = £18.88, 100 g = £38.00. Label: 28, counselling, application, see p. 803. Potency: potent

Fucibet® (LEO) PoM

Cream, betamethasone (as valerate) 0.1%, fusidic acid 2%, net price 30 g = £5.32, 60 g = £10.63. Label: 28, counselling, application, see p. 803. Potency: potent
Excipients include cetostearyl alcohol, chlorocresol

Lipid cream, betamethasone (as valerate) 0.1%, fusidic acid 2%, net price 30 g = £5.62. Label: 28, counselling, application, see p. 803. Potency: potent
Excipients include cetostearyl alcohol, hydroxybenzoates (parabens)

Lotriderm® (TEVA UK) PoM

Cream, betamethasone dipropionate 0.064% (≡ betamethasone 0.05%), clotrimazole 1%, net price 30 g = £6.34. Label: 28, counselling, application, see p. 803. Potency: potent
Excipients include benzyl alcohol, cetostearyl alcohol, propylene glycol

---

▌CLOBETASOL PROPIONATE

Indications short-term treatment only of severe resistant inflammatory skin disorders such as recalcitrant eczemas unresponsive to less potent corticosteroids; psoriasis, see notes above

Cautions see notes above

Contra-indications see notes above

Side-effects see notes above

Dose
• Apply thinly 1–2 times daily for up to 4 weeks; max. 50 g of 0.05% preparation per week

Clarelux® (Fabre) PoM

Foam (= scalp application), clobetasol propionate 0.05%, net price 100 g = £11.06. Label: 15, 28, counselling, application, see p. 803. Potency: very potent
Excipients include cetyl alcohol, polysorbate 60, propylene glycol, stearyl alcohol
Caution flammable
Note Apply directly to scalp lesions (foam begins to subside immediately on contact with skin)

Dermovate® (GSK) PoM

Cream, clobetasol propionate 0.05%, net price 30 g = £2.69, 100 g = £7.90. Label: 28, counselling, application, see p. 803. Potency: very potent
Excipients include beeswax (or beeswax substitute), cetostearyl alcohol, chlorocresol, propylene glycol

Ointment, clobetasol propionate 0.05%, net price 30 g = £2.69, 100 g = £7.90. Label: 28, counselling, application, see p. 803. Potency: very potent
Excipients include propylene glycol

Scalp application, clobetasol propionate 0.05%, in a thickened alcoholic basis, net price 30 mL = £3.07, 100 mL = £10.42. Label: 15, 28, counselling, application, see p. 803. Potency: very potent
Excipients none as listed in section 13.1.3

Etrivex® (Galderma) PoM

Shampoo, clobetasol propionate 0.05%, net price 125 mL = £10.29. Label: 28, counselling, application, see p. 803. Potency: very potent
Excipients none as listed in section 13.1.3
Dose moderate scalp psoriasis, ADULT over 18 years, apply thinly once daily, rinse off after 15 minutes; reduce frequency of application after clinical improvement; max. duration of treatment 4 weeks

◢**With antimicrobials**

See notes above for comment on compound preparations

Clobetasol with neomycin and nystatin (Non-proprietary) PoM

Cream, clobetasol propionate 0.05%, neomycin sulfate 0.5%, nystatin 100 000 units/g, net price 30 g = £64.00. Label: 28, counselling, application, see p. 803. Potency: very potent

Ointment, clobetasol propionate 0.05%, neomycin sulfate 0.5%, nystatin 100 000 units/g, in a paraffin basis, net price 30 g = £64.00. Label: 28, counselling, application, see p. 803. Potency: very potent

CLOBETASONE BUTYRATE

Indications eczemas and dermatitis of all types; maintenance between courses of more potent corticosteroids

Cautions see notes above

Contra-indications see notes above

Side-effects see notes above

Dose

- Apply thinly 1–2 times daily

[1]**Eumovate**® (GSK) [PoM]

Cream, clobetasone butyrate 0.05%, net price 30 g = £1.86, 100 g = £5.44. Label: 28, counselling, application, see p. 803. Potency: moderate

Excipients include beeswax substitute, cetostearyl alcohol, chlorocresol

Ointment, clobetasone butyrate 0.05%, net price 30 g = £1.86, 100 g = £5.44. Label: 28, counselling, application, see p. 803. Potency: moderate

Excipients none as listed in section 13.1.3

◀**With antimicrobials**

See notes above for comment on compound preparations

Trimovate® (GSK) [PoM]

Cream, clobetasone butyrate 0.05%, oxytetracycline 3% (as calcium salt), nystatin 100 000 units/g, net price 30 g = £3.29. Label: 28, counselling, application, see p. 803. Potency: moderate

Excipients include cetostearyl alcohol, chlorocresol, sodium metabisulfite

Note Stains clothing

DIFLUCORTOLONE VALERATE

Indications severe inflammatory skin disorders such as eczemas unresponsive to less potent corticosteroids; high strength (0.3%), short-term treatment of severe exacerbations; psoriasis, see notes above

Cautions see notes above

Contra-indications see notes above

Side-effects see notes above

Dose

- Apply thinly 1–2 times daily for up to 4 weeks (0.1% preparations) or 2 weeks (0.3% preparations), reducing strength as condition responds; max. 60 g of 0.3% per week

Nerisone® (Meadow) [PoM]

Cream, diflucortolone valerate 0.1%, net price 30 g = £1.59. Label: 28, counselling, application, see p. 803. Potency: potent

Excipients include disodium edetate, hydroxybenzoates (parabens), stearyl alcohol

Oily cream, diflucortolone valerate 0.1%, net price 30 g = £2.56. Label: 28, counselling, application, see p. 803. Potency: potent

Excipients include beeswax

Ointment, diflucortolone valerate 0.1%, net price 30 g = £1.59. Label: 28, counselling, application, see p. 803. Potency: potent

Excipients none as listed in section 13.1.3

---

1. Cream can be sold to the public for short-term symptomatic treatment and control of patches of eczema and dermatitis (but not seborrhoeic dermatitis) in adults and children over 12 years provided pack does not contain more than 15 g

Nerisone Forte® (Meadow) [PoM]

Oily cream, diflucortolone valerate 0.3%, net price 15 g = £2.09. Label: 28, counselling, application, see p. 803. Potency: very potent

Excipients include beeswax

Ointment, diflucortolone valerate 0.3%, net price 15 g = £2.09. Label: 28, counselling, application, see p. 803. Potency: very potent

Excipients none as listed in section 13.1.3

FLUDROXYCORTIDE

(Flurandrenolone)

Indications inflammatory skin disorders such as eczemas

Cautions see notes above

Contra-indications see notes above

Side-effects see notes above

Dose

- Apply thinly 1–2 times daily

Haelan® (Typharm) [PoM]

Cream, fludroxycortide 0.0125%, net price 60 g = £3.26. Label: 28, counselling, application, see p. 803. Potency: moderate

Excipients include cetyl alcohol, propylene glycol

Ointment, fludroxycortide 0.0125%, net price 60 g = £3.26. Label: 28, counselling, application, see p. 803. Potency: moderate

Excipients include beeswax, cetyl alcohol, polysorbate

Tape, polythene adhesive film impregnated with fludroxycortide 4 micrograms /cm^2, net price 7.5 cm × 50 cm = £9.27, 7.5 cm × 200 cm = £24.95

Dose for chronic localised recalcitrant dermatoses (but not acute or weeping), cut tape to fit lesion, apply to clean, dry skin shorn of hair, usually for 12 hours daily

FLUOCINOLONE ACETONIDE

Indications inflammatory skin disorders such as eczemas; psoriasis, see notes above

Cautions see notes above

Contra-indications see notes above

Side-effects see notes above

Dose

- Apply thinly 1–2 times daily, reducing strength as condition responds

Synalar® (GP Pharma) [PoM]

Cream, fluocinolone acetonide 0.025%, net price 30 g = £4.14, 100 g = £11.75. Label: 28, counselling, application, see p. 803. Potency: potent

Excipients include benzyl alcohol, cetostearyl alcohol, polysorbates, propylene glycol

Gel, fluocinolone acetonide 0.025%, net price 30 g = £5.56, 60 g = £10.02. For use on scalp and other hairy areas. Label: 28, counselling, application, see p. 803. Potency: potent

Excipients include hydroxybenzoates (parabens), propylene glycol

Ointment, fluocinolone acetonide 0.025%, net price 30 g = £4.14, 100 g = £11.75. Label: 28, counselling, application, see p. 803. Potency: potent

Excipients include propylene glycol, wool fat

13 Skin

Synalar 1 in 4 Dilution® (GP Pharma) ℗ₒ𝙼

Cream, fluocinolone acetonide 0.00625%, net price 50 g = £4.84. Label: 28, counselling, application, see p. 803. Potency: moderate

Excipients include benzyl alcohol, cetostearyl alcohol, polysorbates, propylene glycol

Ointment, fluocinolone acetonide 0.00625%, net price 50 g = £4.84. Label: 28, counselling, application, see p. 803. Potency: moderate

Excipients include propylene glycol, wool fat

Synalar 1 in 10 Dilution® (GP Pharma) ℗ₒ𝙼

Cream, fluocinolone acetonide 0.0025%, net price 50 g = £4.58. Label: 28, counselling, application, see p. 803. Potency: mild

Excipients include benzyl alcohol, cetostearyl alcohol, polysorbates, propylene glycol

◢**With antimicrobials**
See notes above for comment on compound preparations

Synalar C® (GP Pharma) ℗ₒ𝙼

Cream, fluocinolone acetonide 0.025%, clioquinol 3%, net price 15 g = £2.66. Label: 28, counselling, application, see p. 803. Potency: potent

Excipients include cetostearyl alcohol, disodium edetate, hydroxybenzoates (parabens), polysorbates, propylene glycol

Ointment, fluocinolone acetonide 0.025%, clioquinol 3%, net price 15 g = £2.66. Label: 28, counselling, application, see p. 803. Potency: potent

Note stains clothing

Excipients include propylene glycol, wool fat

Synalar N® (GP Pharma) ℗ₒ𝙼

Cream, fluocinolone acetonide 0.025%, neomycin sulfate 0.5%, net price 30 g = £4.36. Label: 28, counselling, application, see p. 803. Potency: potent

Excipients include cetostearyl alcohol, hydroxybenzoates (parabens), polysorbates, propylene glycol

Ointment, fluocinolone acetonide 0.025%, neomycin sulfate 0.5%, in a greasy basis, net price 30 g = £4.36. Label: 28, counselling, application, see p. 803. Potency: potent

Excipients include propylene glycol, wool fat

◼ FLUOCINONIDE

Indications severe inflammatory skin disorders such as eczemas unresponsive to less potent corticosteroids; psoriasis, see notes above

Cautions see notes above

Contra-indications see notes above

Side-effects see notes above

Dose
- Apply thinly 1–2 times daily

Metosyn® (GP Pharma) ℗ₒ𝙼

FAPG cream, fluocinonide 0.05%, net price 25 g = £3.96, 100 g = £13.34. Label: 28, counselling, application, see p. 803. Potency: potent

Excipients include propylene glycol

Ointment, fluocinonide 0.05%, net price 25 g = £3.50, 100 g = £13.15. Label: 28, counselling, application, see p. 803. Potency: potent

Excipients include propylene glycol, wool fat

◼ FLUOCORTOLONE

Indications severe inflammatory skin disorders such as eczemas unresponsive to less potent corticosteroids; psoriasis, see notes above

Cautions see notes above

Contra-indications see notes above

Side-effects see notes above

Dose
- Apply thinly 1–2 times daily, reducing strength as condition responds

Ultralanum Plain® (Meadow) ℗ₒ𝙼

Cream, fluocortolone caproate 0.25%, fluocortolone pivalate 0.25%, net price 50 g = £2.95. Label: 28, counselling, application, see p. 803. Potency: moderate

Excipients include disodium edetate, fragrance, hydroxybenzoates (parabens), stearyl alcohol

Ointment, fluocortolone 0.25%, fluocortolone caproate 0.25%, net price 50 g = £2.95. Label: 28, counselling, application, see p. 803. Potency: moderate

Excipients include wool fat, fragrance

◼ FLUTICASONE PROPIONATE

Indications inflammatory skin disorders such as dermatitis and eczemas unresponsive to less potent corticosteroids

Cautions see notes above

Contra-indications see notes above

Side-effects see notes above

Dose
- Apply thinly 1–2 times daily

Cutivate® (GSK) ℗ₒ𝙼

Cream, fluticasone propionate 0.05%, net price 15 g = £2.27, 30 g = £4.24. Label: 28, counselling, application, see p. 803. Potency: potent

Excipients include cetostearyl alcohol, imidurea, propylene glycol

Ointment, fluticasone propionate 0.005%, net price 15 g = £2.27, 30 g = £4.24. Label: 28, counselling, application, see p. 803. Potency: potent

Excipients include propylene glycol

◼ MOMETASONE FUROATE

Indications severe inflammatory skin disorders such as eczemas unresponsive to less potent corticosteroids; psoriasis, see notes above

Cautions see notes above

Contra-indications see notes above

Side-effects see notes above

Dose
- Apply thinly once daily (to scalp in case of lotion)

Mometasone (Non-proprietary) ℗ₒ𝙼

Ointment, mometasone furoate 0.1%, net price 30 g = £3.53, 100 g = £11.77. Label: 28, counselling, application, see p. 803. Potency: potent

Elocon® (MSD) ℗ₒ𝙼

Cream, mometasone furoate 0.1%, net price 30 g = £4.36, 100 g = £12.58. Label: 28, counselling, application, see p. 803. Potency: potent

Excipients include beeswax

Ointment, mometasone furoate 0.1%, net price 30 g = £4.32, 100 g = £12.44. Label: 28, counselling, application, see p. 803. Potency: potent

Excipients include beeswax, propylene glycol

Scalp lotion, mometasone furoate 0.1% in an aqueous isopropyl alcohol basis, net price 30 mL = £4.36. Label: 28, counselling, application, see p. 803. Potency: potent

Excipients include propylene glycol

13 **Skin**

▌ TRIAMCINOLONE ACETONIDE

Indications   severe inflammatory skin disorders such
as eczemas unresponsive to less potent corticosteroids; psoriasis, see notes above

Cautions   see notes above

Contra-indications   see notes above

Side-effects   see notes above

Dose

• Apply thinly 1–2 times daily

▌**With antimicrobials**
See notes above for comment on compound preparations

Aureocort® (AMCo) [PoM]
Ointment, triamcinolone acetonide 0.1%, chlortetracycline hydrochloride 3%, in an anhydrous greasy
basis containing wool fat and white soft paraffin, net
price 15 g = £3.51. Label: 28, counselling, application, see p. 803. Potency: potent
Excipients   include wool fat
Note   Stains clothing

13.5 Preparations for eczema and psoriasis

13.5.1 Preparations for eczema
13.5.2 Preparations for psoriasis
13.5.3 Drugs affecting the immune response

13.5.1 Preparations for eczema

Eczema (dermatitis) has several causes, which may
influence treatment. The main types of eczema are
irritant, allergic contact, atopic, venous and discoid;
different types may co-exist. Lichenification, due to
scratching and rubbing, may complicate any chronic
eczema. *Atopic eczema* is the most common type and it
usually involves dry skin as well as infection and lichenification.

Management of eczema involves the removal or treatment of contributory factors including occupational and
domestic irritants. Known or suspected contact allergens should be avoided. Rarely, ingredients in topical
medicinal products may sensitise the skin; the BNF lists
active ingredients together with excipients that have
been associated with skin sensitisation.

Skin dryness and the consequent irritant eczema
requires **emollients** (section 13.2.1) applied regularly
(at least twice daily) and liberally to the affected area;
this can be supplemented with bath and shower emollients. The use of emollients should continue even if the
eczema improves or if other treatment is being used.

Topical corticosteroids (section 13.4) are also required
in the management of eczema; the potency of the
corticosteroid should be appropriate to the severity
and site of the condition. Mild corticosteroids are generally used on the face and on flexures; potent corticosteroids are generally required for use on adults with
discoid or lichenified eczema or with eczema on the
scalp, limbs, and trunk. Treatment should be reviewed
regularly, especially if a potent corticosteroid is
required. In patients with frequent flares (2–3 per
month), a topical corticosteroid can be applied on 2
consecutive days each week to prevent further flares.

Bandages (including those containing **zinc** and **ichthammol**) are sometimes applied over topical corticosteroids or emollients to treat eczema of the limbs. Dry-wrap dressings can be used to provide a physical barrier
to help prevent scratching and improve retention of
emollients.

For the role of topical **pimecrolimus** and **tacrolimus** in
atopic eczema see section 13.5.3.

Infection   Bacterial infection (commonly with *Staphylococcus aureus* and occasionally with *Streptococcus pyogenes*) can exacerbate eczema and requires treatment
with topical or systemic **antibacterial drugs** (section
13.10.1 and section 5.1). Antibacterial drugs should be
used in short courses (typically 1 week) to reduce the
risk of drug resistance or skin sensitisation. Associated
eczema is treated simultaneously with a topical corticosteroid which can be combined with a topical antimicrobial.

Eczema involving widespread or recurrent infection
requires the use of a systemic antibacterial that is active
against the infecting organism. Products that combine
an antiseptic with an emollient application (section
13.2.1) and with a bath emollient (section 13.2.1.1)
can also be used; antiseptic shampoos (section 13.9)
can be used on the scalp.

Intertriginous eczema commonly involves candida and
bacteria; it is best treated with a mild or moderately
potent topical corticosteroid and a suitable antimicrobial drug.

Widespread herpes simplex infection may complicate
atopic eczema and treatment with a systemic antiviral
drug (section 5.3.2.1) is indicated.

The management of *seborrhoeic dermatitis* is described
below.

Management of other features of eczema

Lichenification, which results from repeated scratching
is treated initially with a potent corticosteroid. Bandages
containing **ichthammol paste** (to reduce pruritus) and
other substances such as **zinc oxide** can be applied over
the corticosteroid or emollient. **Coal tar** (section 13.5.2)
and **ichthammol** can be useful in some cases of *chronic
eczema*.

A *non-sedating* **antihistamine** (section 3.4.1) may be of
some value in relieving severe itching or urticaria associated with eczema. A *sedating* antihistamine (section
3.4.1) can be used if itching causes sleep disturbance.

Exudative ('*weeping*') *eczema* requires a potent corticosteroid initially; infection may also be present and
require specific treatment (see above). **Potassium permanganate** solution (1 in 10 000) can be used in exudating eczema for its antiseptic and astringent effects;
treatment should be stopped when exudation stops.

Severe refractory eczema   *Severe refractory eczema*
is best managed under specialist supervision; it may
require phototherapy or drugs that act on the immune
system (section 13.5.3). **Alitretinoin** (p. 810) is licensed
for the treatment of severe chronic hand eczema refractory to potent topical corticosteroids; patients with
hyperkeratotic features are more likely to respond to
alitretinoin than those with pompholyx.

Seborrhoeic dermatitis   *Seborrhoeic dermatitis*
(*seborrhoeic eczema*) is associated with species of the
yeast *Malassezia* and affects the scalp, paranasal areas,
and eyebrows. Shampoos active against the yeast

13

Skin

(including those containing ketoconazole and coal tar, section 13.9) and combinations of mild corticosteroids with suitable antimicrobials (section 13.4) are used.

Topical preparations for eczema

 ICHTHAMMOL

Indications   chronic lichenified eczema
Side-effects   skin irritation
Dose
• Apply 1–3 times daily

Ichthammol Ointment, BP 1980
Ointment, ichthammol 10%, yellow soft paraffin 45%, wool fat 45%

Zinc and Ichthammol Cream, BP
Cream, ichthammol 5%, cetostearyl alcohol 3%, wool fat 10%, in zinc cream
Available from 'special-order' manufacturers or specialist importing companies, see p. 1124

Zinc Paste and Ichthammol Bandage, BP 1993
See Appendix 5 (section A5.8.9)

Oral retinoid for eczema

The retinoid, **alitretinoin**, is licensed for the treatment of severe chronic hand eczema refractory to potent topical corticosteroids; patients with hyperkeratotic features are more likely to respond to alitretinoin than those with pompholyx.

Alitretinoin should be prescribed **only** by, or under the supervision of, a consultant dermatologist.

Alitretinoin is **teratogenic** and must **not** be given to women of child-bearing potential unless they practise effective contraception and then only after detailed assessment and explanation by the physician. See also Pregnancy Prevention under Cautions, below.

> **NICE guidance**
> **Alitretinoin for the treatment of severe chronic hand eczema in adults (August 2009)**
> Alitretinoin is recommended for the treatment of severe chronic hand eczema that has not responded to potent topical corticosteroids. Treatment should be stopped as soon as an adequate response has been achieved (hands clear or almost clear), or if the eczema remains severe after 12 weeks, or if an adequate response has not been achieved by 24 weeks.
> www.nice.org.uk/TA177

 ALITRETINOIN

Indications   severe chronic hand eczema refractory to potent topical corticosteroids
Cautions   avoid blood donation during treatment and for at least 1 month after stopping treatment; monitor serum lipids (more frequently in those with diabetes, history of hyperlipidaemia, or risk factors for cardiovascular disease)—discontinue if uncontrolled hyperlipidaemia; history of depression; dry eye syndrome; **interactions:** Appendix 1 (retinoids)
Pregnancy prevention In women of child-bearing potential, exclude pregnancy 1 month before treatment, up to 3 days before treatment, every month during treatment (unless there are compelling reasons to indicate that there is

no risk of pregnancy), and 5 weeks after stopping treatment—perform pregnancy test in the first 3 days of the menstrual cycle. Women must practise effective contraception for at least 1 month before starting treatment, during treatment, and for at least 1 month after stopping treatment. Women should be advised to use at least 1 method of contraception but ideally they should use 2 methods of contraception. Oral progestogen-only contraceptives are not considered effective. Barrier methods should not be used alone but can be used in conjunction with other contraceptive methods. Each prescription for alitretinoin should be limited to a supply of up to 30 days' treatment and dispensed within 7 days of the date stated on the prescription. Women should be advised to discontinue treatment and to seek prompt medical attention if they become pregnant during treatment or within 1 month of stopping treatment

Contra-indications   uncontrolled hyperlipidaemia; uncontrolled hypothyroidism; hypervitaminosis A
Hepatic impairment   manufacturer advises avoid—no information available
Renal impairment   manufacturer advises avoid in severe impairment—no information available
Pregnancy   avoid—teratogenic; effective contraception must be used—see Pregnancy Prevention above
Breast-feeding   manufacturer advises avoid
Side-effects   raised serum concentration of triglycerides and of cholesterol (risk of pancreatitis if triglycerides above 9 mmol/litre), flushing; headache; changes in thyroid function tests; anaemia; myalgia; raised creatine kinase, arthralgia; conjunctivitis, dry eyes (may respond to lubricating eye ointment or tear replacement therapy)—sometimes decreased tolerance to contact lenses, eye irritation; dryness of skin and lips, cheilitis, erythema, alopecia; *less commonly* epistaxis, hyperostosis, ankylosing spondylitis, blurred vision, cataracts, pruritus, and asteotic eczema; *rarely* benign intracranial hypertension (discontinue if severe headache, nausea, vomiting, papilloedema, or visual disturbances occur) and vasculitis; also reported mood changes, depression, suicidal ideation, keratitis and impaired night vision
Dose
• ADULT over 18 years, 30 mg once daily, reduced to 10 mg once daily if not tolerated; patients with diabetes, history of hyperlipidaemia, or risk factors for cardiovascular disease, initially 10 mg once daily, increased if necessary up to max. 30 mg daily
  Note Duration of treatment 12–24 weeks; discontinue if no response after 12 weeks. Course may be repeated in those who relapse. See also Pregnancy Prevention, above

Toctino® (Basilea) PoM
Capsules, alitretinoin 10 mg (brown), net price 30-cap pack = £411.43; 30 mg (red-brown), 30-cap pack = £411.43. Label: 10, patient information leaflet, 11, 21

13.5.2 Preparations for psoriasis

Psoriasis is characterised by epidermal thickening and scaling. It commonly affects extensor surfaces and the scalp.

Occasionally, psoriasis is provoked or exacerbated by drugs such as lithium, chloroquine and hydroxychloroquine, beta-blockers, non-steroidal anti-inflammatory drugs, and ACE inhibitors. Psoriasis may not be seen until the drug has been taken for weeks or months.

Emollients (section 13.2.1), in addition to their effects on dryness, scaling and cracking, may have an anti-

13 Skin

proliferative effect in psoriasis, and may be the only treatment necessary for mild psoriasis. They are particularly useful in *inflammatory psoriasis* and in *plaque psoriasis of palms and soles*, in which irritant factors can perpetuate the condition. Emollients are useful adjuncts to other more specific treatment.

More specific topical treatment for *chronic stable plaque psoriasis* on extensor surfaces of trunk and limbs involves the use of **vitamin D analogues**, **coal tar**, **dithranol**, and the retinoid **tazarotene**. However, they can irritate the skin and they are not suitable for the more inflammatory forms of psoriasis; their use should be suspended during an inflammatory phase of psoriasis. The efficacy and the irritancy of each substance varies between patients. If a substance irritates significantly, it should be stopped or the concentration reduced; if it is tolerated, its effects should be assessed after 4 to 6 weeks and treatment continued if it is effective.

Scalp psoriasis is usually scaly, and the scale may be thick and adherent; this will require softening with an emollient cream, ointment, or oil. A tar-based shampoo is first-line treatment for scalp psoriasis; a keratolytic, such as salicylic acid, should also be used if there is significant scaling, to allow other treatments to work.

Some preparations prescribed for psoriasis affecting the scalp, combine salicylic acid with coal tar or sulfur. The product should be applied generously, and an adequate quantity should be prescribed. It should be left on for at least an hour, often more conveniently overnight, before washing off. The use of scalp preparations containing a potent corticosteroid or a vitamin D analogue, either alone or in combination, can also be helpful.

Facial, flexural and genital psoriasis can be managed with short-term use of a mild or moderate potency topical corticosteroid (a mild potency topical corticosteroid is preferred for the initial treatment of facial psoriasis). Calcitriol or tacalcitol can be used for longer-term treatment, or if the response to mild or moderate potency topical corticosteroids is inadequate; calcipotriol is more likely to cause irritation. Low strength tar preparations can also be used. Pimecrolimus or tacrolimus by topical application [unlicensed indication] can be used short-term, under specialist supervision, in patients whose condition has not responded adequately to other treatments, or who are intolerant of them.

Widespread *unstable psoriasis* of erythrodermic or generalised pustular type requires urgent specialist assessment. Initial topical treatment should be limited to using emollients frequently and generously; emollients should be prescribed in quantities of 1 kg or more. More localised acute or subacute *inflammatory psoriasis* with hot, spreading or itchy lesions, should be treated topically with emollients or with a corticosteroid of moderate potency.

Calcipotriol and **tacalcitol** are analogues of vitamin D that affect cell division and differentiation. **Calcitriol** is an active form of vitamin D. Vitamin D and its analogues are used first-line for the long-term treatment of plaque psoriasis; they do not smell or stain and they may be more acceptable than tar or dithranol products. Of the vitamin D analogues, tacalcitol and calcitriol are less likely to irritate.

Coal tar has anti-inflammatory properties that are useful in chronic plaque psoriasis; it also has antiscaling properties. Crude coal tar (coal tar, BP) is the most effective form, typically in a concentration of 1 to 10% in a soft paraffin base, but few outpatients tolerate the smell and mess. Cleaner extracts of coal tar included in proprietary preparations, are more practicable for home use but they are less effective and improvement takes longer. Contact of coal tar products with normal skin is not normally harmful and they can be used for widespread small lesions; however, irritation, contact allergy, and sterile folliculitis can occur. The milder tar extracts can be used on the face and flexures. Tar baths and tar shampoos are also helpful.

Dithranol is effective for chronic plaque psoriasis. Its major disadvantages are irritation (for which individual susceptibility varies) and staining of skin and of clothing. It should be applied to chronic extensor plaques only, carefully avoiding normal skin. Dithranol is not generally suitable for widespread small lesions nor should it be used in the flexures or on the face. Treatment should be started with a low concentration such as dithranol 0.1%, and the strength increased gradually every few days up to 3%, according to tolerance. Proprietary preparations are more suitable for home use; they are usually washed off after 5 to 60 minutes ('short contact'). Specialist nurses may apply intensive treatment with dithranol paste which is covered by stockinette dressings and usually retained overnight. Dithranol should be discontinued if even a low concentration causes acute inflammation; continued use can result in the psoriasis becoming unstable. When applying dithranol, hands should be protected by gloves or they should be washed thoroughly afterwards.

Tazarotene, a retinoid, has a similar efficacy to vitamin D and its analogues, but is associated with a greater incidence of irritation. Although irritation is common, it is minimised by applying tazarotene sparingly to the plaques and avoiding normal skin; application to the face and in flexures should also be avoided. Tazarotene does not stain and is odourless.

A topical **corticosteroid** (section 13.4) is not generally suitable for long-term use or as the sole treatment of extensive chronic plaque psoriasis; any early improvement is not usually maintained and there is a risk of the condition deteriorating or of precipitating an unstable form of psoriasis (e.g. erythrodermic psoriasis or generalised pustular psoriasis) on withdrawal. Topical use of potent corticosteroids on widespread psoriasis can also lead to systemic as well as local side-effects. However, topical corticosteroids used short-term may be appropriate to treat psoriasis in specific sites such as the face or flexures (with a mild or moderate corticosteroid), and psoriasis of the scalp, palms, and soles (with a potent corticosteroid). Very potent corticosteroids should only be used under specialist supervision.

Combining the use of a corticosteroid with another specific topical treatment may be beneficial in chronic plaque psoriasis; the drugs may be used separately at different times of the day or used together in a single formulation. *Eczema* co-existing with psoriasis may be treated with a corticosteroid, or coal tar, or both.

Phototherapy   Phototherapy is available in specialist centres under the supervision of a dermatologist. **Ultraviolet B** (UVB) radiation is usually effective for *chronic stable psoriasis* and for *guttate psoriasis*. It may be considered for patients with moderately severe psoriasis in whom topical treatment has failed, but it may irritate inflammatory psoriasis.

13 Skin

Photochemotherapy combining long-wave ultraviolet A radiation with a psoralen (PUVA) is available in specialist centres under the supervision of a dermatologist. The psoralen, which enhances the effect of irradiation, is administered either by mouth or topically. PUVA is effective in most forms of psoriasis, including *localised palmoplantar pustular psoriasis*. Early adverse effects include phototoxicity and pruritus. Higher cumulative doses exaggerate skin ageing, increase the risk of dysplastic and neoplastic skin lesions, especially squamous cancer, and pose a theoretical risk of cataracts.

Phototherapy combined with coal tar, dithranol, tazarotene, topical vitamin D or vitamin D analogues, or oral acitretin, allows reduction of the cumulative dose of phototherapy required to treat psoriasis.

Systemic treatment   Systemic treatment is required for severe, resistant, unstable or complicated forms of psoriasis, and it should be initiated only under specialist supervision. Systemic drugs for psoriasis include acitretin (see below) and drugs that affect the immune response (such as ciclosporin and methotrexate, section 13.5.3).

Systemic corticosteroids should be used only rarely in psoriasis because rebound deterioration may occur on reducing the dose.

Acitretin, a metabolite of etretinate, is a retinoid (vitamin A derivative); it is prescribed by specialists. The main indication for acitretin is *psoriasis*, but it is also used in disorders of keratinisation such as severe *Darier's disease* (keratosis follicularis), and some forms of *ichthyosis*. Although a minority of cases of psoriasis respond well to acitretin alone, it is only moderately effective in many cases and it is combined with other treatments. A therapeutic effect occurs after 2 to 4 weeks and the maximum benefit after 4 months. Consideration should be given to stopping acitretin if the response is inadequate after 4 months at the optimum dose. The manufacturers of acitretin do not recommend continuous treatment for longer than 6 months. However, some patients may benefit from longer treatment, provided that the lowest effective dose is used, patients are monitored carefully for adverse effects, and the need for treatment is reviewed regularly.

Apart from teratogenicity, which remains a risk for 3 years after stopping, acitretin is the least toxic systemic treatment for psoriasis; in women with a potential for child-bearing, the possibility of pregnancy must be excluded before treatment and effective contraception must be used during treatment and for at least 3 years afterwards (oral progestogen-only contraceptives not considered effective).

Topical preparations for psoriasis

Vitamin D and analogues

Calcitriol, calcitriol, and **tacalcitol** are used for the management of *plaque psoriasis*. They should be avoided by those with calcium metabolism disorders, and used with caution in *generalised pustular* or *erythrodermic exfoliative psoriasis* (enhanced risk of hypercalcaemia). Local skin reactions (itching, erythema, burning, paraesthesia, dermatitis) are common. Hands should be washed thoroughly after application to avoid inadvertent transfer to other body areas. Aggravation of psoriasis has also been reported.

CALCIPOTRIOL

Indications   see under Dose

Cautions   see notes above; avoid use on face; avoid excessive exposure to sunlight and sunlamps

Contra-indications   see notes above

Pregnancy   manufacturers advise avoid unless essential

Breast-feeding   no information available

Side-effects   see notes above; also photosensitivity, dry skin; *rarely* facial or perioral dermatitis

Dose

- Plaque psoriasis, apply ointment once or twice daily; max. 100 g weekly (less with *scalp solution*, see below); CHILD over 6 years, apply twice daily; 6–12 years max. 50 g weekly; over 12 years max. 75 g weekly
  Note Patient information leaflet for *Dovonex*® ointment advises liberal application (but note max. recommended weekly dose, above)

- Scalp psoriasis, apply scalp solution twice daily; max. 60 mL weekly (less with *ointment*, see below); CHILD under 18 years see *BNF for Children*
  Note When preparations used together max. total calcipotriol 5 mg in any one week (e.g. scalp solution 60 mL with ointment 30 g *or* scalp solution 30 mL with ointment 60 g)

Calcipotriol (Non-proprietary) ℞

Ointment, calcipotriol 50 micrograms/g, net price 120 g = £24.04

Note Not licensed for use in children under 18 years

Scalp solution, calcipotriol 50 micrograms/mL, net price 60 mL = £50.30, 120 mL = £100.59

Dovonex® (LEO) ℞

Ointment, calcipotriol 50 micrograms/g, net price 30 g = £6.65

Excipients include disodium edetate, propylene glycol

◢With betamethasone

For prescribing information and for comment on the limited role of corticosteroids in psoriasis, see section 13.4.

Dovobet® (LEO) ℞

Ointment, betamethasone (as dipropionate) 0.05%, calcipotriol (as monohydrate) 50 micrograms/g, net price 30 g = £19.02. Label: 28

Excipients include butylated hydroxytoluene

Dose stable plaque psoriasis, apply once daily to max. 30% of body surface (max. 15 g daily) for 4 weeks; if necessary, treatment may be continued beyond 4 weeks or repeated, on the advice of a specialist; CHILD under 18 years see *BNF for Children*

Gel, betamethasone (as dipropionate) 0.05%, calcipotriol (as monohydrate) 50 micrograms/g, net price 30 g = £16.54, 60 g = £33.08, 2 × 60 g = £61.43. Label: 28

Excipients include butylated hydroxytoluene

Dose scalp psoriasis, apply 1–4 g to scalp once daily, shampoo off after leaving on scalp overnight or during day; usual duration of therapy 4 weeks; if necessary, treatment may be continued beyond 4 weeks or repeated, on the advice of a specialist; CHILD under 18 years see *BNF for Children*

Mild to moderate plaque psoriasis, apply once daily to max. 30% of body surface (max. 15 g daily) for 8 weeks; if necessary, treatment may be continued beyond 8 weeks or repeated, on the advice of a specialist; CHILD under 18 years see *BNF for Children*

Note When different preparations containing calcipotriol used together, max. total calcipotriol 5 mg in any one week

13 Skin

CALCITRIOL
(1,25-Dihydroxycholecalciferol)

Indications   mild to moderate plaque psoriasis

Cautions   see notes above

Contra-indications   see notes above; do not apply under occlusion

Pregnancy   manufacturer advises use in restricted amounts only if clearly necessary and to monitor urine- and serum-calcium concentration

Breast-feeding   manufacturer advises avoid

Side-effects   see notes above

Dose

- ADULT and CHILD over 12 years, apply twice daily; not more than 35% of body surface to be treated daily, max. 30 g daily

Silkis® (Galderma) [PoM]

Ointment, calcitriol 3 micrograms/g, net price 100 g = £18.06

Excipients   none as listed in section 13.1.3

TACALCITOL

Indications   plaque psoriasis

Cautions   see notes above; avoid eyes; monitor serum calcium if risk of hypercalcaemia; if used in conjunction with UV treatment, UV radiation should be given in the morning and tacalcitol applied at bedtime

Contra-indications   see notes above

Pregnancy   manufacturer advises avoid unless no safer alternative—no information available

Breast-feeding   manufacturer advises avoid application to breast area; no information available on presence in milk

Side-effects   see notes above

Dose

- ADULT and CHILD over 12 years, apply once daily preferably at bedtime; max. 10 g *ointment* or 10 mL *lotion* daily

Note   When lotion and ointment used together, max. total tacalcitol 280 micrograms in any one week (e.g. lotion 30 mL with ointment 40 g)

Curatoderm® (Almirall) [PoM]

Lotion, tacalcitol (as monohydrate) 4 micrograms/g, net price 30 mL = £12.73

Excipients   include disodium edetate, propylene glycol

Ointment, tacalcitol (as monohydrate) 4 micrograms/g, net price 30 g = £13.40, 60 g = £23.14, 100 g = £30.86

Excipients   none as listed in section 13.1.3

Tazarotene

TAZAROTENE

Indications   mild to moderate plaque psoriasis affecting up to 10% of skin area

Cautions   wash hands immediately after use, avoid contact with eyes, face, intertriginous areas, hair-covered scalp, eczematous or inflamed skin; avoid excessive exposure to UV light (including sunlight, solariums, PUVA or UVB treatment); do not apply emollients or cosmetics within 1 hour of application

Pregnancy   avoid; effective contraception required (oral progestogen-only contraceptives not considered effective)

Breast-feeding   manufacturer advises avoid—present in milk in *animal* studies

Side-effects   local irritation (more common with higher concentration and may require discontinuation), pruritus, burning, erythema, desquamation, non-specific rash, contact dermatitis, and worsening of psoriasis; rarely stinging and inflamed, dry or painful skin

Dose

- Apply once daily in the evening usually for up to 12 weeks; CHILD under 18 years not recommended

Zorac® (Allergan) [PoM]

Gel, tazarotene 0.05%, net price 30 g = £14.09; 0.1%, 30 g = £14.80

Excipients   include benzyl alcohol, butylated hydroxyanisole, butylated hydroxytoluene, disodium edetate, polysorbate 40

Tars

TARS

Indications   psoriasis and occasionally chronic atopic eczema

Cautions   application to face and skin flexures; use suitable chemical protection gloves for extemporaneous preparation

Contra-indications   not for use in sore, acute, or pustular psoriasis or in presence of infection; avoid eyes, mucosa, genital or rectal areas; broken or inflamed skin

Side-effects   skin irritation and acne-like eruptions, photosensitivity; stains skin, hair, and fabric

Dose

- Apply 1–3 times daily starting with low-strength preparations

Note   For shampoo preparations see section 13.9; for use with dressings see Appendix 5 (section A5.8.9)

◢**Non-proprietary preparations**
May be difficult to obtain. Patients may find newer proprietary preparations more acceptable

Calamine and Coal Tar Ointment, BP

Ointment, calamine 12.5 g, strong coal tar solution 2.5 g, zinc oxide 12.5 g, hydrous wool fat 25 g, white soft paraffin 47.5 g

Excipients   include wool fat

Dose   apply 1–2 times daily

Coal Tar and Salicylic Acid Ointment, BP

Ointment, coal tar 2 g, salicylic acid 2 g, emulsifying wax 11.4 g, white soft paraffin 19 g, coconut oil 54 g, polysorbate '80' 4 g, liquid paraffin 7.6 g

Excipients   include cetostearyl alcohol

Dose   apply 1–2 times daily

Coal Tar Paste, BP

Paste, strong coal tar solution 7.5%, in compound zinc paste

Dose   apply 1–2 times daily

Zinc and Coal Tar Paste, BP

Paste, zinc oxide 6%, coal tar 6%, emulsifying wax 5%, starch 38%, yellow soft paraffin 45%

Excipients   include cetostearyl alcohol

Dose   apply 1–2 times daily

13 Skin

◢**Proprietary preparations**

Cocois® (RPH)

Scalp ointment, coal tar solution 12%, salicylic acid 2%, precipitated sulfur 4%, in a coconut oil emollient basis, net price 40 g (with applicator nozzle) = £6.22, 100 g = £11.69

Excipients include cetostearyl alcohol

Dose scaly scalp disorders including psoriasis, eczema, seborrhoeic dermatitis and dandruff, apply to scalp once weekly as necessary (if severe use daily for first 3–7 days), shampoo off after 1 hour; CHILD 6–12 years, medical supervision required (not recommended under 6 years)

Exorex® (Forest)

Lotion, coal tar solution 5% in an emollient basis, net price 100 mL = £8.11, 250 mL = £16.24

Excipients include hydroxybenzoates (parabens)

Dose psoriasis, apply to skin or scalp 2–3 times daily; CHILD under 12 years and ELDERLY, lotion can be diluted with a few drops of water before applying

Psoriderm® (Dermal)

Cream, coal tar 6%, lecithin 0.4%, net price 225 mL = £9.42

Excipients include isopropyl palmitate, propylene glycol

Dose psoriasis, apply to skin or scalp 1–2 times daily

Scalp lotion—section 13.9

Sebco® (Derma UK)

Scalp ointment, coal tar solution 12%, salicylic acid 2%, precipitated sulfur 4%, in a coconut oil emollient basis, net price 40 g = £4.54, 100 g = £8.52

Excipients include cetostearyl alcohol

Dose scaly scalp disorders including psoriasis, eczema, seborrhoeic dermatitis and dandruff, apply to scalp as necessary (if severe use daily for first 3–7 days), shampoo off after 1 hour; CHILD 6–12 years, medical supervision required (not recommended under 6 years)

◢**Bath preparations**

Coal Tar Solution, BP

Solution, coal tar 20%, polysorbate '80' 5%, in alcohol (96%), net price 500 mL = £11.20. Label: 15

Excipients include polysorbates

Dose use 100 mL in a bath

Note Strong Coal Tar Solution BP contains coal tar 40%

Polytar Emollient® (Stiefel)

Bath additive, coal tar solution 2.5%, arachis (peanut) oil extract of coal tar 7.5%, tar 7.5%, cade oil 7.5%, light liquid paraffin 35%, net price 500 mL = £5.78

Excipients include isopropyl palmitate

Dose psoriasis, eczema, atopic and pruritic dermatoses, use 2–4 capfuls (15–30 mL) in bath and soak for 20 minutes

Psoriderm® (Dermal)

Bath emulsion, coal tar 40%, net price 200 mL = £2.74

Excipients include polysorbate 20

Dose psoriasis, use 30 mL in a bath and soak for 5 minutes

Dithranol

▌ **DITHRANOL**
(Anthralin)

Indications subacute and chronic psoriasis, see notes above

Cautions avoid use near eyes and sensitive areas of skin; see also notes above

Contra-indications hypersensitivity; acute and pustular psoriasis

Side-effects local burning sensation and irritation; stains skin, hair, and fabrics

Dose
● See notes above and under preparations

Note Some of these dithranol preparations also contain coal tar or salicylic acid—for cautions, contra-indications, and side-effects see under Tars (above) or under Salicylic Acid

◢**Non-proprietary preparations**

[1]**Dithranol Ointment, BP** PoM

Ointment, dithranol, in yellow soft paraffin; usual strengths 0.1–2%. Part of basis may be replaced by hard paraffin if a stiffer preparation is required. Label: 28

Dithranol Paste, BP

Paste, dithranol in zinc and salicylic acid (Lassar's) paste. Usual strengths 0.1–1% of dithranol. Label: 28

◢**Proprietary preparations**

Dithrocream® (Dermal)

Cream, dithranol 0.1%, net price 50 g = £3.77; 0.25%, 50 g = £4.04; 0.5%, 50 g = £4.66; 1%, 50 g = £5.42; PoM 2%, 50 g = £6.79. Label: 28

Excipients include cetostearyl alcohol, chlorocresol

Dose for application to skin or scalp; 0.1–0.5% cream suitable for overnight treatment, 1–2% cream for max. 1 hour

Micanol® (GP Pharma)

Cream, dithranol 1% in a lipid-stabilised basis, net price 50 g = £16.18; PoM 3%, 50 g = £20.15. Label: 28

Excipients none as listed in section 13.1.3

Dose for application to skin or scalp, apply 1% cream for up to 30 minutes once daily, if necessary 3% cream can be used under medical supervision

Note At the end of contact time, use plenty of lukewarm (not hot) water to rinse off cream; soap may be used *after* the cream has been rinsed off; use shampoo before applying cream to scalp and if necessary after cream has been rinsed off

Psorin® (LPC)

Ointment, dithranol 0.11%, coal tar 1%, salicylic acid 1.6%, net price 50 g = £9.22, 100 g = £18.44. Label: 28

Excipients include beeswax, wool fat

Dose for application to skin up to twice daily

Scalp gel, dithranol 0.25%, salicylic acid 1.6% in gel basis containing methyl salicylate, net price 50 g = £7.03. Label: 28

Excipients none as listed in section 13.1.3

Dose for application to scalp, initially apply on alternate days for 10–20 minutes; may be increased to daily application for max. 1 hour and then wash off

Salicylic acid

▌ **SALICYLIC ACID**

For coal tar preparations containing salicylic acid, see under Tars, p. 813; for dithranol preparations containing salicylic acid see under Dithranol, above

Indications hyperkeratotic skin disorders; warts and calluses (section 13.7); scalp conditions (section 13.9); fungal nail infections (section 13.10.2)

Cautions see notes above; avoid broken or inflamed skin

Salicylate toxicity Salicylate toxicity may occur particularly if applied on large areas of skin or neonatal skin

---

1. PoM if dithranol content more than 1%, otherwise may be sold to the public

Side-effects sensitivity, excessive drying, irritation, systemic effects after widespread use (see under Cautions)

Dose

- See preparations

Zinc and Salicylic Acid Paste, BP

Paste, (Lassar's Paste), zinc oxide 24%, salicylic acid 2%, starch 24%, white soft paraffin 50%
Available from 'special-order' manufacturers or specialist importing companies, see p. 1124
Dose apply twice daily

Oral retinoids for psoriasis

▌ACITRETIN

Note Acitretin is a metabolite of etretinate

Indications severe extensive psoriasis resistant to other forms of therapy; palmoplantar pustular psoriasis; severe congenital ichthyosis; severe Darier's disease (keratosis follicularis)

Cautions avoid concomitant use of keratolytics; do not donate blood during and for 2 years after stopping therapy (teratogenic risk); check liver function at start, then every 2–4 weeks for first 2 months and then every 3 months; monitor serum-triglyceride and serum-cholesterol concentrations before treatment, 1 month after starting, then every 3 months; diabetes (can alter glucose tolerance—initial frequent blood glucose checks); investigate atypical musculoskeletal symptoms; in children use only in exceptional circumstances and monitor growth parameters and bone development (premature epiphyseal closure reported); avoid excessive exposure to sunlight and unsupervised use of sunlamps; **interactions:** Appendix 1 (retinoids)

Pregnancy prevention In women of child-bearing potential (including those with a history of infertility), exclude pregnancy up to 3 days before treatment, every month during treatment, and every 1–3 months for 3 years after stopping treatment. Treatment should be started on day 2 or 3 of menstrual cycle. Women must practise effective contraception for at least 1 month before starting treatment, during treatment, and for at least 3 years after stopping treatment. Women should be advised to use at least 1 method of contraception, but ideally they should use 2 methods of contraception. Oral progestogen-only contraceptives are not considered effective. Barrier methods should not be used alone but can be used in conjunction with other contraceptive methods. Each prescription for acitretin should be limited to a supply of up to 30 days' treatment and dispensed within 7 days of the date stated on the prescription. Women should be advised to seek medical attention immediately if they become pregnant during treatment or within 3 years of stopping treatment. They should also be advised to avoid alcohol during treatment and for 2 months after stopping treatment

Contra-indications hyperlipidaemia

Hepatic impairment avoid in severe impairment—risk of further impairment

Renal impairment avoid in severe impairment; increased risk of toxicity

Pregnancy avoid—teratogenic; effective contraception must be used—see Cautions above

Breast-feeding avoid

Side-effects abdominal pain, diarrhoea, nausea, vomiting, dryness and inflammation of mucous membranes, peripheral oedema, reversible increase in serum-cholesterol and serum-triglyceride concentrations (with high doses), headache, arthralgia, myalgia, dryness of conjunctiva (causing conjunctiv-

itis and decreased tolerance to contact lenses), alopecia (reversible on withdrawal), abnormal hair texture, skin exfoliation, pruritus, epidermal fragility, sticky skin, dermatitis, erythema, brittle nails, paronychia; *less commonly* hepatitis, dizziness, visual disturbances, photosensitivity; *rarely* peripheral neuropathy; *very rarely* benign intracranial hypertension (discontinue if severe headache, nausea, vomiting, or visual disturbances occur), bone pain, exostosis (skeletal hyperostosis and extra-osseous calcification reported following long-term treatment with etretinate, and premature epiphyseal closure in children, see Cautions above), night blindness, ulcerative keratitis; *also reported* taste disturbance, rectal haemorrhage, flushing, malaise, drowsiness, granulomatous lesions, impaired hearing, tinnitus, initial worsening of psoriasis, dry skin, sweating

Dose

- ADULT over 18 years (under expert supervision), initially 25–30 mg daily (Darier's disease 10 mg daily) for 2–4 weeks, then adjusted according to response, usual range 25–50 mg daily; up to 75 mg daily for short periods in psoriasis (see p. 812); CHILD under 18 years see *BNF for Children*

Neotigason® (Actavis) [PoM]

Capsules, acitretin 10 mg (brown/white), net price 60-cap pack = £17.30; 25 mg (brown/yellow), 60-cap pack = £43.00. Label: 10, patient information leaflet, 11, 21

▌13.5.3 Drugs affecting the immune response

Drugs affecting the immune response are used for eczema or psoriasis. Systemic drugs acting on the immune system are used under specialist supervision.

Pimecrolimus by topical application is licensed for *mild to moderate atopic eczema*. **Tacrolimus** is licensed for topical use in *moderate to severe atopic eczema*. Both are drugs whose long-term safety is still being evaluated and they should not usually be considered first-line treatments unless there is a specific reason to avoid or reduce the use of topical corticosteroids. Treatment of atopic eczema with topical pimecrolimus or topical tacrolimus should be initiated only by prescribers experienced in managing the condition. For the role of topical tacrolimus and pimecrolimus in the treatment of psoriasis, see section 13.5.2.

> **NICE guidance**
> **Tacrolimus and pimecrolimus for atopic eczema (August 2004)**
>
> Topical pimecrolimus and tacrolimus are options for atopic eczema not controlled by maximal topical corticosteroid treatment or if there is a risk of important corticosteroid side-effects (particularly skin atrophy).
>
> Topical pimecrolimus is recommended for moderate atopic eczema on the face and neck of children aged 2–16 years and topical tacrolimus is recommended for moderate to severe atopic eczema in adults and children over 2 years. Pimecrolimus and tacrolimus should be used within their licensed indications.
> www.nice.org.uk/TA82

The *Scottish Medicines Consortium* (p. 4) has advised (March 2010) that tacrolimus ointment (*Protopic®*) is accepted for restricted use within NHS Scotland for the prevention of flares in those with moderate to severe atopic eczema in accordance with the licensed indications; initiation of treatment is restricted to doctors (including general practitioners) with specialist interest and experience in treating atopic eczema with immunomodulatory therapy.

For the role of topical corticosteroids in eczema, see section 13.5.1, and for their role in psoriasis, see section 13.5.2. A short course of a systemic corticosteroid (section 6.3.2) can be given for eczema flares that have not improved despite appropriate topical treatment.

Ciclosporin by mouth can be used for *severe psoriasis* and for *severe eczema*. **Azathioprine** or **mycophenolate mofetil** (section 8.2.1) are used for severe refractory eczema [unlicensed indication].

Methotrexate can be used for *severe psoriasis*, the dose being adjusted according to severity of the condition and haematological and biochemical measurements. Folic acid (section 9.1.2) should be given to reduce the possibility of side-effects associated with methotrexate. Folic acid can be given at a dose of 5 mg once weekly [unlicensed indication], on a different day from the methotrexate; alternative regimens of folic acid may be used in some settings.

Etanercept, **adalimumab**, and **infliximab** inhibit the activity of tumour necrosis factor (TNFα). They are used for *severe plaque psoriasis* either refractory to at least 2 standard systemic treatments and photochemotherapy, or when standard treatments cannot be used because of intolerance or contra-indications; while either etanercept or adalimumab is considered to be the first choice in stable disease, infliximab or adalimumab may be useful when rapid disease control is required. **Ustekinumab** (a monoclonal antibody that inhibits interleukins 12 and 23) can be used for *severe plaque psoriasis* that has not responded to at least 2 standard systemic treatments and photochemotherapy, or when these treatments cannot be used because of intolerance or contra-indications (see also NICE guidance below). Adalimumab, etanercept, infliximab and ustekinumab are also licensed for psoriatic arthritis (section 10.1.3).

> **NICE guidance[1]**
> **Adalimumab for plaque psoriasis in adults (June 2008)**
> Adalimumab is recommended for the treatment of severe plaque psoriasis which has failed to respond to standard systemic treatments (including ciclosporin and methotrexate) and photochemotherapy, or when standard treatments cannot be used because of intolerance or contra-indications. Adalimumab should be withdrawn if the response is not adequate after 16 weeks.
> www.nice.org.uk/TA146

> **NICE guidance[2]**
> **Etanercept and efalizumab for plaque psoriasis in adults (July 2006)**
> Etanercept is recommended for severe plaque psoriasis which has failed to respond to standard systemic treatments (including ciclosporin and methotrexate) and to photochemotherapy, or when standard treatments cannot be used because of intolerance or contra-indications. Etanercept should be withdrawn if the response is not adequate after 12 weeks.
> Following suspension of the marketing authorisation for efalizumab, NICE has temporarily withdrawn its guidance on the use of efalizumab for plaque psoriasis.
> www.nice.org.uk/TA103

> **NICE guidance**
> **Infliximab for plaque psoriasis in adults (January 2008)**
> Infliximab is recommended for the treatment of very severe plaque psoriasis which has failed to respond to standard systemic treatments (including ciclosporin and methotrexate) or to photochemotherapy, or when standard treatments cannot be used because of intolerance or contra-indications. Infliximab should be withdrawn if the response is not adequate after 10 weeks.
> www.nice.org.uk/TA134

> **NICE guidance**
> **Ustekinumab for plaque psoriasis in adults (September 2009)**
> Ustekinumab is recommended for the treatment of severe plaque psoriasis which has failed to respond to standard systemic treatments (including ciclosporin and methotrexate) and to photochemotherapy, or when standard treatments cannot be used because of intolerance or contra-indications. Ustekinumab should be withdrawn if the response is not adequate after 16 weeks.
> For patients weighing over 100 kg, the manufacturer should provide the 90-mg dose of ustekinumab at the same price as the 45-mg dose
> www.nice.org.uk/TA180

AZATHIOPRINE

Indications   severe refractory eczema [unlicensed indication]; inflammatory bowel disease (section 1.5.3); autoimmune conditions and prophylaxis of transplant rejection (section 8.2.1); rheumatoid arthritis (section 10.1.3)

Cautions   section 8.2.1

Contra-indications   section 8.2.1; also very low or absent thiopurine methyltransferase (TPMT) activity

Hepatic impairment   section 8.2.1

Renal impairment   section 8.2.1

Pregnancy   section 8.2.1

Breast-feeding   section 8.2.1

Side-effects   section 8.2.1

1. The *Scottish Medicines Consortium* issued similar advice in May 2008.

2. The *Scottish Medicines Consortium* issued similar advice on the use of etanercept in adults (August 2009) and children over 6 years old (April 2012)

13 Skin

Dose

- Severe refractory eczema [unlicensed indication], by mouth, normal or high TPMT activity, 1–3 mg/kg daily; intermediate TPMT activity, 0.5–1.5 mg/kg daily

◢**Preparations**

Section 8.2.1

◼ **CICLOSPORIN**

(Cyclosporin)

Indications   see under Dose; severe acute ulcerative colitis (section 1.5.3); transplantation and graft-versus-host disease (section 8.2.2)

Cautions   section 8.2.2

Additional cautions in atopic dermatitis and psoriasis *Contra-indicated* in abnormal renal function, uncontrolled hypertension (see also below), infections not under control, and malignancy (see also below). Dermatological and physical examination, including blood pressure and renal function measurements required at least twice before starting. During treatment, monitor serum creatinine every 2 weeks for first 3 months then every month; reduce dose by 25–50% if serum creatinine increases more than 30% above baseline (even if within normal range) and discontinue if reduction not successful within 1 month. Discontinue if hypertension develops that cannot be controlled by dose reduction or antihypertensive therapy. Avoid excessive exposure to sunlight and avoid use of UVB or PUVA. *In atopic dermatitis*, also allow herpes simplex infections to clear before starting (if they occur during treatment withdraw if severe); *Staphylococcus aureus* skin infections not absolute contra-indication providing controlled (but avoid erythromycin unless no other alternative—see also **interactions**: Appendix 1 (ciclosporin)); investigate lymphadenopathy that persists despite improvement in atopic dermatitis. *In psoriasis*, also exclude malignancies (including those of skin and cervix) before starting (biopsy any lesions not typical of psoriasis) and treat patients with malignant or pre-malignant conditions of skin only after appropriate treatment (and if no other option); discontinue if lymphoproliferative disorder develops

Hepatic impairment   section 8.2.2

Renal impairment   see Cautions above

Pregnancy   see Immunosuppressant Therapy, p. 628

Breast-feeding   section 8.2.2

Side-effects   section 8.2.2

Dose

- Short-term treatment (usually for max. 8 weeks but can be longer under specialist supervision) of severe atopic dermatitis where conventional therapy ineffective or inappropriate, administered in accordance with expert advice, by mouth, ADULT and CHILD over 16 years, initially 2.5 mg/kg daily in 2 divided doses, if good initial response not achieved within 2 weeks, increase rapidly to max. 5 mg/kg daily; initial dose of 5 mg/kg daily in 2 divided doses if very severe; CHILD under 16 years see *BNF for Children*

- Severe psoriasis where conventional therapy ineffective or inappropriate, administered in accordance with expert advice, by mouth, ADULT and CHILD over 16 years, initially 2.5 mg/kg daily in 2 divided doses, increased gradually to max. 5 mg/kg daily if no improvement within 1 month; initial dose of 5 mg/kg daily justified if rapid control required; discontinue if inadequate response after 3 months at the optimum dose; max. duration of treatment usually 1 year unless other treatments cannot be used; CHILD under 16 years see *BNF for Children*

Important For preparations and counselling and for advice on conversion between the preparations, see section 8.2.2

◢**Preparations**

Section 8.2.2

◼ **METHOTREXATE**

Indications   severe psoriasis unresponsive to conventional therapy (specialist use only); Crohn's disease (section 1.5.3); malignant disease (section 8.1.3); rheumatoid arthritis (section 10.1.3)

Cautions   section 10.1.3; also photosensitivity—psoriasis lesions aggravated by UV radiation (skin ulceration reported)

Contra-indications   section 10.1.3

Hepatic impairment   avoid—dose-related toxicity

Renal impairment   section 10.1.3

Pregnancy   section 10.1.3

Breast-feeding   section 10.1.3

Side-effects   section 10.1.3

Dose

- By mouth *or* by intramuscular *or* intravenous *or* subcutaneous injection, 2.5–10 mg once weekly, increased according to response in steps of 2.5–5 mg at intervals of at least 1 week; usual dose 7.5–15 mg once weekly; max. weekly dose 30 mg; stop treatment if inadequate response after 3 months at the optimum dose; CHILD 2–18 years see *BNF for Children*

> **Important**
>
> Note that the above dose is a **weekly** dose. To avoid error with low dose methotrexate, it is recommended that:
>
> - the patient is carefully advised of the **dose** and **frequency** and the reason for taking methotrexate and any other prescribed medicine (e.g. folic acid);
> - only one **strength** of methotrexate tablet (usually 2.5 mg) is prescribed and dispensed;
> - the prescription and the dispensing label clearly show the dose and frequency of methotrexate administration;
> - the patient is warned to report immediately the onset of any feature of blood disorders (e.g. sore throat, bruising, and mouth ulcers), liver toxicity (e.g. nausea, vomiting, abdominal discomfort and dark urine), and respiratory effects (e.g. shortness of breath).

◢**Preparations**

Section 10.1.3

◼ **PIMECROLIMUS**

Indications   see Dose

Cautions   UV light (avoid excessive exposure to sunlight and sunlamps), avoid other topical treatments except emollients at treatment site; alcohol consumption (risk of facial flushing and skin irritation)

Contra-indications   contact with eyes and mucous membranes, application under occlusion, infection at treatment site; congenital epidermal barrier defects; generalised erythroderma; immunodeficiency; concomitant use with drugs that cause immunosuppression (may be prescribed in exceptional circumstances by specialists); application to malignant or potentially malignant skin lesions

Side-effects   burning sensation, pruritus, erythema, skin infections (including folliculitis and *less commonly* impetigo, herpes simplex and zoster, molluscum contagiosum); *rarely* papilloma, skin discoloration, local reactions including pain, paraesthesia, peeling, dryness, oedema, and worsening of eczema; skin malignancy reported

 13 Skin

Dose

- Short-term treatment of mild to moderate atopic eczema (including flares) when topical corticosteroids cannot be used (see also notes above), apply twice daily until symptoms resolve (stop treatment if eczema worsens or no response after 6 weeks); CHILD under 2 years not recommended
- Short-term treatment of facial, flexural, or genital psoriasis in patients unresponsive to, or intolerant of other topical therapy [unlicensed indication] (see also section 13.5.2), ADULT over 18 years, apply twice daily until symptoms resolve (max. duration of treatment 4 weeks)

Elidel® (Meda) PoM

Cream, pimecrolimus 1%, net price 30 g = £19.69, 60 g = £37.41, 100 g = £59.07. Label: 4, 11, 28
Excipients   include benzyl alcohol, cetyl alcohol, propylene glycol, stearyl alcohol

TACROLIMUS

Indications   see Dose; other indications section 8.2.2

Cautions   UV light (avoid excessive exposure to sunlight and sunlamps); alcohol consumption (risk of facial flushing and skin irritation)

Contra-indications   infection at treatment site; congenital epidermal barrier defects; generalised erythroderma; immunodeficiency; concomitant use with drugs that cause immunosuppression (may be prescribed in exceptional circumstances by specialists); application to malignant or potentially malignant skin lesions; avoid contact with eyes and mucous membranes; application under occlusion

Pregnancy   manufacturer advises avoid unless essential; toxicity in *animal* studies following systemic administration

Breast-feeding   manufacturer advises avoid—present in milk following systemic administration

Side-effects   application-site reactions including rash, irritation, pain and paraesthesia; herpes simplex infection, Kaposi's varicelliform eruption; application-site infections; *less commonly* acne; *also reported* rosacea, malignancies (including skin malignancy, cutaneous lymphoma and other types of lymphomas)

Dose

- Short-term treatment of moderate to severe atopic eczema (including flares) in patients unresponsive to, or intolerant of conventional therapy (see also notes above), ADULT and CHILD over 16 years, initially apply 0.1% ointment thinly twice daily until lesion clears (consider other treatment if eczema worsens or no improvement after 2 weeks); reduce to once daily or switch to 0.03% ointment if condition allows; CHILD 2–16 years, initially apply 0.03% ointment thinly twice daily for up to 3 weeks (consider other treatment if eczema worsens or if no improvement after 2 weeks) then reduce to once daily until lesion clears
- Prevention of flares in patients with moderate to severe atopic eczema and 4 or more flares a year who have responded to initial treatment with topical tacrolimus (see also notes above), ADULT and CHILD over 16 years, apply 0.1% ointment thinly twice weekly; use short-term treatment regimen during an acute flare; review need for preventative therapy after 1 year; CHILD 2–16 years, apply 0.03% ointment thinly twice weekly; use short-term treatment regimen during an acute flare; interrupt preventative therapy after 1 year to reassess condition

- Short-term treatment of facial, flexural, or genital psoriasis in patients unresponsive to, or intolerant of other topical therapy [unlicensed indication] (see also section 13.5.2), ADULT over 18 years, initially apply 0.1% ointment thinly twice daily until symptoms resolve; reduce to once daily or switch to 0.03% ointment if condition allows; max. duration of treatment 4 weeks

Protopic® (Astellas) PoM

Ointment, tacrolimus (as monohydrate) 0.03%, net price 30 g = £19.44, 60 g = £35.46; 0.1%, 30 g = £21.60, 60 g = £39.40. Label: 4, 11, 28
Excipients   include beeswax

Cytokine modulators

ADALIMUMAB

Indications   see notes above; Crohn's disease (section 1.5.3); ankylosing spondylitis, polyarticular juvenile idiopathic arthritis, psoriatic arthritis, rheumatoid arthritis (section 10.1.3)

Cautions   section 10.1.3, p. 737
Important   See section 10.1.3, p. 737 for information on tuberculosis and blood disorders

Contra-indications   section 10.1.3, p. 737

Pregnancy   section 10.1.3, p. 737

Breast-feeding   section 10.1.3, p. 737

Side-effects   section 10.1.3, p. 737

Dose

- By subcutaneous injection, plaque psoriasis, ADULT over 18 years, initially 80 mg, then 40 mg on alternate weeks starting 1 week after initial dose; discontinue treatment if no response within 16 weeks

Preparations
Section 10.1.3

ETANERCEPT

Indications   see notes above; ankylosing spondylitis, psoriatic arthritis, polyarticular course juvenile idiopathic arthritis, rheumatoid arthritis (section 10.1.3)

Cautions   section 10.1.3, p. 739
Important   See section 10.1.3, p. 739 for information on tuberculosis and blood disorders

Contra-indications   section 10.1.3, p. 739

Hepatic impairment   section 10.1.3, p. 739

Pregnancy   section 10.1.3, p. 739

Breast-feeding   section 10.1.3, p. 739

Side-effects   section 10.1.3, p. 739

Dose

- By subcutaneous injection, plaque psoriasis, 25 mg twice weekly or 50 mg once weekly for up to 24 weeks; discontinue if no response after 12 weeks; CHILD 6–18 years, 800 micrograms/kg (max. 50 mg) once weekly for up to 24 weeks; discontinue if no response after 12 weeks

Preparations
Section 10.1.3

13 Skin

▌ INFLIXIMAB

Indications see notes above; inflammatory bowel disease (section 1.5.3); ankylosing spondylitis, psoriatic arthritis, rheumatoid arthritis (section 10.1.3)

Cautions section 10.1.3, p. 740; monitor for non-melanoma skin cancer before and during treatment **Important** See section 10.1.3, p. 740 for information on tuberculosis, blood disorders, and hypersensitivity reactions

Contra-indications section 10.1.3, p. 740

Pregnancy section 10.1.3, p. 740

Breast-feeding section 10.1.3, p. 740

Side-effects section 10.1.3, p. 740

Dose

- By intravenous infusion, plaque psoriasis, ADULT over 18 years, 5 mg/kg, repeated 2 weeks and 6 weeks after initial infusion, then every 8 weeks; discontinue if no response within 14 weeks of initial infusion

◢**Preparations**

Section 10.1.3

▌ USTEKINUMAB

Indications see notes above; psoriatic arthritis (section 10.1.3)

Cautions predisposition to infection; history or development of malignancy; monitor for non-melanoma skin cancer, especially in patients with a history of PUVA treatment or prolonged immunosuppressant therapy, or those over 60 years of age; elderly; **interactions**: Appendix 1 (ustekinumab) **Tuberculosis** Patients should be evaluated for tuberculosis before treatment. Active tuberculosis should be treated with standard treatment (section 5.1.9) for at least 2 months before starting ustekinumab. Patients who have previously received adequate treatment for tuberculosis can start ustekinumab but should be monitored every 3 months for possible recurrence. In patients without active tuberculosis but who were previously not treated adequately, chemoprophylaxis should ideally be completed before starting ustekinumab. In patients at high risk of tuberculosis who cannot be assessed by tuberculin skin test, chemoprophylaxis can be given concurrently with ustekinumab. Patients should be advised to seek medical attention if symptoms suggestive of tuberculosis (e.g. persistent cough, weight loss, and fever) develop

Contra-indications active infection

Pregnancy avoid; manufacturer advises effective contraception during treatment and for 15 weeks after stopping treatment

Breast-feeding manufacturer advises avoid—present in milk in *animal* studies

Side-effects diarrhoea, nausea, headache, malaise, dizziness, infections (sometimes severe), arthralgia, myalgia, oropharyngeal pain, pruritus, injection-site reactions; *less commonly* depression, facial palsy, nasal congestion, hypersensitivity reactions (possibly delayed onset), pustular psoriasis

Dose

- By subcutaneous injection, plaque psoriasis, ADULT over 18 years, body-weight under 100 kg, initially 45 mg, then 45 mg 4 weeks after initial dose, then 45 mg every 12 weeks; body-weight over 100 kg, initially 45–90 mg, then 45–90 mg 4 weeks after initial dose, then 45–90 mg every 12 weeks **Note** Discontinue if no response within 16 weeks

Stelara® (Janssen) ⓅⓄⓂ

Injection, ustekinumab 90 mg/mL, net price 0.5-mL (45-mg) prefilled syringe = £2147.00. Label: 10, counselling, tuberculosis

13.6   Acne and rosacea

| 13.6.1 | Topical preparations for acne |
| 13.6.2 | Oral preparations for acne |

Acne Treatment of acne should be commenced early to prevent scarring. Patients should be counselled that an improvement may not be seen for at least a couple of months. The choice of treatment depends on whether the acne is predominantly inflammatory or comedonal and its severity.

Mild to moderate acne is generally treated with topical preparations (section 13.6.1). Systemic treatment (section 13.6.2) with oral antibacterials is generally used for *moderate to severe acne* or where topical preparations are not tolerated or are ineffective or where application to the site is difficult. Another oral preparation used for acne is the hormone treatment co-cyprindiol (cyproterone acetate with ethinylestradiol); it is for women only.

Severe acne, acne unresponsive to prolonged courses of oral antibacterials, scarring, or acne associated with psychological problems calls for early referral to a consultant dermatologist who may prescribe isotretinoin for administration by mouth.

Rosacea Brimonidine (section 13.6.3) is licensed for the treatment of facial erythema in rosacea. Rosacea is not comedonal (but may exist with acne which may be comedonal). The pustules and papules of rosacea respond to topical metronidazole (section 13.10.1.2) or to topical azelaic acid (section 13.6.1). Alternatively, oral administration of oxytetracycline or tetracycline 500 mg twice daily (section 5.1.3), or of erythromycin 500 mg twice daily (section 5.1.5), can be used; courses usually last 6–12 weeks and are repeated intermittently. Doxycycline (section 5.1.3) 100 mg once daily can be used [unlicensed indication] if oxytetracycline or tetracycline is inappropriate (e.g. in renal impairment). A modified-release preparation of doxycycline is licensed in low doses of 40 mg once daily for the treatment of facial rosacea (section 5.1.3). Isotretinoin is occasionally given in refractory cases [unlicensed indication]. Camouflagers (section 13.8.2) may be required for the redness.

13.6.1   Topical preparations for acne

In mild to moderate acne, comedones and inflamed lesions respond well to benzoyl peroxide (see below) or to a topical retinoid (see p. 821). Alternatively, topical application of an antibacterial such as erythromycin or clindamycin may be effective for inflammatory acne. If topical preparations prove inadequate, oral preparations may be needed (section 13.6.2).

Benzoyl peroxide and azelaic acid

Benzoyl peroxide is effective in mild to moderate acne. Both comedones and inflamed lesions respond well to benzoyl peroxide. The lower concentrations seem to be as effective as higher concentrations in reducing inflammation. It is usual to start with a lower strength and to increase the concentration of benzoyl peroxide gradually. Adverse effects include local skin irritation, particularly when therapy is initiated, but the scaling and redness often subside with treatment continued at a reduced frequency of application. If the acne does not respond after 2 months then use of a topical antibacterial should be considered.

Azelaic acid has antimicrobial and anticomedonal properties. It may be an alternative to benzoyl peroxide or to a topical retinoid for treating mild to moderate comedonal acne, particularly of the face. Some patients prefer azelaic acid because it is less likely to cause local irritation than benzoyl peroxide.

Quinoderm® (Alliance)

Cream, benzoyl peroxide 5%, potassium hydroxy-quinoline sulfate 0.5%, in an astringent vanishing-cream basis, net price 50 g = £2.43
Excipients include cetostearyl alcohol, edetic acid (EDTA)
Dose acne vulgaris, acneform eruptions, folliculitis, apply 2–3 times daily

Cream, benzoyl peroxide 10%, potassium hydroxy-quinoline sulfate 0.5%, in an astringent vanishing-cream basis, net price 25 g = £1.58, 50 g = £2.55
Excipients include cetostearyl alcohol, edetic acid (EDTA)
Dose acne vulgaris, acneform eruptions, folliculitis, apply 2–3 times daily

◢ BENZOYL PEROXIDE

Indications acne vulgaris

Cautions avoid contact with eyes, mouth, mucous membranes, and broken skin; may bleach fabrics and hair; avoid excessive exposure to sunlight

Side-effects skin irritation (reduce frequency or suspend use until irritation subsides and re-introduce at reduced frequency)

Dose
- Apply 1–2 times daily preferably after washing with soap and water, start treatment with lower-strength preparations
  Note May bleach clothing

Acnecide® (Galderma)

Gel, benzoyl peroxide 5% in an aqueous gel basis, net price 30 g = £5.44, 60 g = £10.88
Excipients include propylene glycol

Brevoxyl® (GSK)

Cream, benzoyl peroxide 4% in an aqueous basis, net price 50 g = £4.13
Excipients include cetyl alcohol, fragrance, stearyl alcohol

PanOxyl® (GSK)

Aquagel (= aqueous gel), benzoyl peroxide 2.5%, net price 40 g = £1.76; 5%, 40 g = £1.92; 10%, 40 g = £2.13
Excipients include propylene glycol

Cream, benzoyl peroxide 5% in a non-greasy basis, net price 40 g = £1.89
Excipients include isopropyl palmitate, propylene glycol

Gel, benzoyl peroxide 10% in an aqueous alcoholic basis, net price 40 g = £1.99
Excipients include fragrance

Wash, benzoyl peroxide 10% in a detergent basis, net price 150 mL = £4.00
Excipients include imidurea
Note May be difficult to obtain

◢With antimicrobials

See also Topical Antibacterials for Acne, below and Antibacterials, p. 821

Duac® Once Daily (GSK) (PoM)

Gel, benzoyl peroxide 3%, clindamycin 1% (as phosphate) in an aqueous basis, net price 30 g = £11.94
Excipients include disodium edetate
Dose ADULT and CHILD over 12 years, apply once daily in the evening

Gel, benzoyl peroxide 5%, clindamycin 1% (as phosphate) in an aqueous basis, net price 25 g = £10.95, 50 g = £21.89
Excipients include disodium edetate
Dose ADULT and CHILD over 12 years, apply once daily in the evening

◢ AZELAIC ACID

Indications see preparations

Cautions avoid contact with eyes, mouth, and mucous membranes

Side-effects local irritation (reduce frequency or discontinue temporarily); *less commonly* skin discoloration; *also reported* worsening of asthma

Finacea® (Bayer) (PoM)

Gel, azelaic acid 15%, net price 30 g = £7.48
Excipients include disodium edetate, polysorbate 80, propylene glycol
Dose facial acne vulgaris, ADULT and CHILD over 12 years, apply twice daily; discontinue if no improvement after 1 month

Papulopustular rosacea, ADULT over 18 years, apply twice daily; discontinue if no improvement after 2 months

Skinoren® (Bayer) (PoM)

Cream, azelaic acid 20%, net price 30 g = £3.74
Excipients include propylene glycol
Dose acne vulgaris, ADULT and CHILD over 12 years, apply twice daily (sensitive skin, once daily for first week)

Topical antibacterials for acne

For many patients with mild to moderate inflammatory acne, topical antibacterials may be no more effective than topical benzoyl peroxide or tretinoin. Topical antibacterials are probably best reserved for patients who wish to avoid oral antibacterials or who cannot tolerate them. Topical preparations of **erythromycin** and **clindamycin** are effective for inflammatory acne. Topical antibacterials can produce mild irritation of the skin, and on rare occasions cause sensitisation; gastro-intestinal disturbances have been reported with topical clindamycin.

Antibacterial resistance of *Propionibacterium acnes* is increasing; there is cross-resistance between erythromycin and clindamycin. To avoid development of resistance:

- when possible use non-antibiotic antimicrobials (such as benzoyl peroxide or azelaic acid);

- avoid concomitant treatment with different oral and topical antibacterials;

- if a particular antibacterial is effective, use it for repeat courses if needed (short intervening courses of benzoyl peroxide or azelaic acid may eliminate any resistant propionibacteria);

- do not continue treatment for longer than necessary (however, treatment with a topical preparation should be continued for at least 6 months).

ANTIBACTERIALS

Indications acne vulgaris

Cautions some manufacturers advise preparations containing alcohol are not suitable for use with benzoyl peroxide; discontinue clindamycin preparations immediately if diarrhoea or colitis occur

Dalacin T® (Pharmacia) PoM
Topical solution, clindamycin 1% (as phosphate), in an aqueous alcoholic basis, net price (both with applictor) 30 mL = £4.34, 50 mL = £7.23
Excipients include propylene glycol
Dose apply thinly twice daily

Lotion, clindamycin 1% (as phosphate) in an aqueous basis, net price 30 mL = £5.08, 60 mL = £10.16
Excipients include cetostearyl alcohol, hydroxybenzoates (parabens)
Dose apply thinly twice daily

Stiemycin® (Stiefel) PoM
Solution, erythromycin 2% in an alcoholic basis, net price 50 mL = £7.69
Excipients include propylene glycol
Dose ADULT and CHILD over 12 years, apply thinly twice daily

Zindaclin® (Crawford) PoM
Gel, clindamycin 1% (as phosphate), net price 30 g = £8.66
Excipients include propylene glycol
Dose ADULT and CHILD over 12 years, apply thinly once daily

Zineryt® (Astellas) PoM
Topical solution, powder for reconstitution, erythromycin 40 mg, zinc acetate 12 mg/mL when reconstituted with solvent containing ethanol, net price per pack of powder and solvent to provide 30 mL = £7.71, 90 mL = £16.68
Excipients none as listed in section 13.1.3
Dose apply twice daily

Topical retinoids and related preparations for acne

Topical **tretinoin**, its isomer **isotretinoin**, and **adapalene** (a retinoid-like drug), are useful for treating comedones and inflammatory lesions in mild to moderate acne. Patients should be warned that some redness and skin peeling can occur initially but settles with time. If undue irritation occurs, the frequency of application should be reduced or treatment suspended until the reaction subsides; if irritation persists, discontinue treatment. Several months of treatment may be needed to achieve an optimal response and the treatment should be continued until no new lesions develop.

Isotretinoin is given by mouth in severe acne; see section 13.6.2 for **warnings** relating to use by mouth.

Cautions Topical retinoids should be avoided in severe acne involving large areas. Contact with eyes, nostrils, mouth and mucous membranes, eczematous, broken or sunburned skin should be avoided. These drugs should be used with caution in sensitive areas such as the neck, and accumulation in angles of the nose should be avoided. Exposure to UV light (including sunlight, solariums) should be avoided; if sun exposure is unavoidable, an appropriate sunscreen or protective clothing should be used. Use of retinoids with abrasive cleaners, comedogenic or astringent cosmetics should

be avoided. Allow peeling (resulting from other irritant treatments) to subside before using a topical retinoid; alternating a preparation that causes peeling with a topical retinoid may give rise to contact dermatitis (reduce frequency of retinoid application).

Pregnancy Topical retinoids are contra-indicated in pregnancy; women of child-bearing age must use effective contraception (oral progestogen-only contraceptives not considered effective).

Side-effects Local reactions include burning, erythema, stinging, pruritus, dry or peeling skin (discontinue if severe). Increased sensitivity to UVB light or sunlight occurs. Temporary changes of skin pigmentation with tretinoin have been reported. Eye irritation and oedema, and blistering or crusting of skin have been reported rarely.

ADAPALENE

Indications mild to moderate acne

Cautions see notes above

Pregnancy see notes above

Breast-feeding amount of drug in milk probably too small to be harmful; ensure infant does not come in contact with treated areas

Side-effects see notes above

Dose
- ADULT and CHILD over 12 years, apply thinly once daily in the evening

Differin® (Galderma) PoM
Cream, adapalene 0.1%, net price 45 g = £16.43. Label: 11
Excipients include disodium edetate, hydroxybenzoates (parabens)

Gel, adapalene 0.1%, net price 45 g = £16.43. Label: 11
Excipients include disodium edetate, hydroxybenzoates (parabens), propylene glycol

◢With benzoyl peroxide
Epiduo® (Galderma) PoM
Gel, adapalene 0.1%, benzoyl peroxide 2.5%, net price 45 g = £17.91. Label: 11
Excipients include disodium edetate, polysorbate 80, propylene glycol
Dose ADULT and CHILD over 9 years, acne vulgaris, apply thinly once daily in the evening
Note May bleach clothing and hair
Note The *Scottish Medicines Consortium* (p. 4) has advised (March 2014) that *Epiduo*® should be restricted for use in mild to moderate facial acne when monotherapy with benzoyl peroxide or adapalene is inappropriate.

ISOTRETINOIN

Note Isotretinoin is an isomer of tretinoin
Important For prescribing information on isotretinoin **when given by mouth**, see p. 823

Indications see notes above; oral treatment (see section 13.6.2)

Cautions (*topical application* only) see notes above; also personal or familial history of non-melanoma skin cancer

Contra-indications (*topical application* only) rosacea, perioral dermatitis

Pregnancy (*topical application* only) see notes above

Breast-feeding avoid

Side-effects (*topical application* only) see notes above

13 Skin

Dose
• Apply thinly 1–2 times daily

Isotrex® (Stiefel) PoM
Gel, isotretinoin 0.05%, net price 30 g = £5.94.
Label: 11
Excipients include butylated hydroxytoluene

◢**With antibacterial**
Isotrexin® (Stiefel) PoM
Gel, isotretinoin 0.05%, erythromycin 2% in ethanolic basis, net price 30 g = £7.47. Label: 11
Excipients include butylated hydroxytoluene

◢ **TRETINOIN**

Note Tretinoin is the acid form of vitamin A

Indications see preparations; malignant disease (section 8.1.5)

Cautions see notes above

Contra-indications personal or familial history of non-melanoma skin cancer; rosacea; perioral dermatitis

Pregnancy see notes above

Breast-feeding amount of drug in milk after topical application probably too small to be harmful; ensure infant does not come in contact with treated areas

Side-effects see notes above

Dose
• See preparations

◢**With antibacterial**
See also Topical Antibacterials for Acne, p. 820 and Antibacterials, p. 821

Aknemycin® Plus (Almirall) PoM
Solution, tretinoin 0.025%, erythromycin 4% in an alcoholic basis, net price 25 mL = £7.05. Label: 11
Excipients none as listed in section 13.1.3
Dose acne, apply thinly 1–2 times daily

Treclin® (Meda) PoM
Gel, tretinoin 0.025%, clindamycin (as phosphate) 1%, net price 30 g = £11.94. Label: 11
Excipients include butylated hydroxytoluene, hydroxybenzoates (parabens), polysorbates
Dose ADULT and CHILD over 12 years, facial acne, apply thinly once daily at bedtime

Other topical preparations for acne

Preparations containing **abrasive agents** are not considered beneficial in acne.

A topical preparation of **nicotinamide** is available for inflammatory acne.

◢ **ABRASIVE AGENTS** ◢

Indications acne vulgaris (but see notes above)

Cautions avoid contact with eyes; discontinue use temporarily if skin becomes irritated

Contra-indications superficial venules, telangiectasia

Brasivol® (Stiefel) ◢
Paste No. 1, aluminium oxide 38.09% in fine particles, in a soap-detergent basis, net price 75 g = £2.76
Excipients include fragrance, N-(3-Chloroallyl) hexaminium chloride (quaternium 15)
Dose use instead of soap 1–3 times daily

◢ **NICOTINAMIDE**

Indications see under preparation

Cautions avoid contact with eyes and mucous membranes (including nose and mouth); reduce frequency of application if excessive dryness, irritation or peeling

Side-effects dry skin, pruritus, erythema, burning, irritation

Nicam® (Dermal)
Gel, nicotinamide 4%, net price 60 g = £7.10
Excipients none as listed in section 13.1.3
Dose inflammatory acne vulgaris, apply twice daily; reduce to once daily or on alternate days if irritation occurs

13.6.2 Oral preparations for acne

Oral antibacterials for acne

Systemic antibacterial treatment is useful for inflammatory acne if topical treatment is not adequately effective or if it is inappropriate. Anticomedonal treatment (e.g. with topical benzoyl peroxide) may also be required.

Either **oxytetracycline** or **tetracycline** (section 5.1.3) is usually given for acne in a dose of 500 mg twice daily. If there is no improvement after the first 3 months another oral antibacterial should be used. Maximum improvement usually occurs after 4 to 6 months but in more severe cases treatment may need to be continued for 2 years or longer.

Doxycycline and **lymecycline** (section 5.1.3) are alternatives to tetracycline. Doxycycline can be used in a dose of 100 mg daily. Lymecycline is given in a dose of 408 mg daily.

Although **minocycline** is as effective as other tetracyclines for acne, it is associated with a greater risk of lupus erythematosus-like syndrome. Minocycline sometimes causes irreversible pigmentation; it is given in a dose of 100 mg once daily or 50 mg twice daily.

Erythromycin (section 5.1.5) in a dose of 500 mg twice daily is an alternative for the management of acne but propionibacteria strains resistant to erythromycin are becoming widespread and this may explain poor response.

Trimethoprim (section 5.1.8) in a dose of 300 mg twice daily may be used for acne resistant to other antibacterials [unlicensed indication]. Prolonged treatment with trimethoprim may depress haematopoiesis; it should generally be initiated by specialists.

Concomitant use of different topical and systemic antibacterials is undesirable owing to the increased likelihood of the development of bacterial resistance.

Hormone treatment for acne

Co-cyprindiol (cyproterone acetate with ethinylestradiol) contains an anti-androgen. It is licensed for use in women with moderate to severe acne that has not responded to topical therapy or oral antibacterials, and for moderately severe hirsutism. Although it is an effective hormonal contraceptive, it should not be used solely for contraception.

13 Skin

Improvement of acne with co-cyprindiol probably occurs because of decreased sebum secretion which is under androgen control. Some women with moderately severe hirsutism may also benefit because hair growth is also androgen-dependent.

> There is an increased risk of venous thromboembolism in women taking co-cyprindiol, particularly during the first year of use. The incidence of venous thromboembolism is 1.5–2 times higher in women using co-cyprindiol than in women using combined oral contraceptives containing levonorgestrel, but the risk may be similar to that associated with use of combined oral contraceptives containing third-generation progestogens (desogestrel and gestodene) or drospirenone (see section 7.3.1). It is contra-indicated in those with a history of venous or arterial thromboembolism, or in those with severe or multiple risk factors for arterial disease or venous thromboembolism (see section 7.3.1). Women requiring co-cyprindiol may have an inherently increased risk of cardiovascular disease.

◤ CO-CYPRINDIOL

A mixture of cyproterone acetate and ethinylestradiol in the mass proportions 2000 parts to 35 parts, respectively

Indications moderate to severe acne in women refractory to topical therapy or oral antibacterials (but see notes above); moderately severe hirsutism

Cautions see under Combined Hormonal Contraceptives, section 7.3.1

Contra-indications see under Combined Hormonal Contraceptives, section 7.3.1 and notes above

Hepatic impairment see under Combined Hormonal Contraceptives, section 7.3.1

Pregnancy avoid—risk of feminisation of male fetus with cyproterone

Breast-feeding manufacturer advises avoid; possibility of anti-androgen effects in neonate with cyproterone

Side-effects see under Combined Hormonal Contraceptives, section 7.3.1

Dose

- 1 tablet daily for 21 days starting on day 1 of menstrual cycle; subsequent courses repeated after a 7-day interval (during which withdrawal bleeding occurs); time to symptom remission, at least 3 months; review need for treatment regularly

Co-cyprindiol (Non-proprietary) ▼ PoM
Tablets, co-cyprindiol 2000/35 (cyproterone acetate 2 mg, ethinylestradiol 35 micrograms), net price 63-tab pack = £5.42
Brands include Acnocin®, Cicafem®, Clairette®

Dianette® (Bayer) ▼ PoM
Tablets, beige, s/c, co-cyprindiol 2000/35 (cyproterone acetate 2 mg, ethinylestradiol 35 micrograms), net price 63-tab pack = £7.71

Oral retinoid for acne

The retinoid **isotretinoin** reduces sebum secretion. It is used for the systemic treatment of nodulo-cystic and conglobate acne, severe acne, scarring, acne which has not responded to an adequate course of a systemic

antibacterial, or acne which is associated with psychological problems. It is also useful in women who develop acne in the third or fourth decades of life, since late onset acne is frequently unresponsive to antibacterials.

Isotretinoin is a toxic drug that should be prescribed **only** by, or under the supervision of, a consultant dermatologist. It is given for at least 16 weeks; repeat courses are not normally required.

Side-effects of isotretinoin include severe dryness of the skin and mucous membranes, nose bleeds, and joint pains. The drug is **teratogenic** and must **not** be given to women of child-bearing age unless they practise effective contraception (oral progestogen-only contraceptives not considered effective) and then only after detailed assessment and explanation by the physician. Women must also be registered with a pregnancy prevention programme (see under Cautions below).

Although a causal link between isotretinoin use and psychiatric changes (including suicidal ideation) has not been established, the possibility should be considered before initiating treatment; if psychiatric changes occur during treatment, isotretinoin should be stopped, the prescriber informed, and specialist psychiatric advice should be sought.

◤ ISOTRETINOIN

Note Isotretinoin is an isomer of tretinoin

Indications see notes above

Cautions see notes above; also avoid blood donation during treatment and for at least 1 month after treatment; history of depression; monitor all patients for depression; measure hepatic function and serum lipids before treatment, 1 month after starting and then every 3 months (reduce dose or discontinue if transaminase or serum lipids persistently raised); discontinue if uncontrolled hypertriglyceridaemia or pancreatitis; diabetes; dry eye syndrome (associated with risk of keratitis); avoid keratolytics; **interactions:** Appendix 1 (retinoids)

Pregnancy prevention In women of child-bearing potential, exclude pregnancy up to 3 days before treatment (start treatment on day 2 or 3 of menstrual cycle), every month during treatment (unless there are compelling reasons to indicate that there is no risk of pregnancy), and 5 weeks after stopping treatment—perform pregnancy test in the first 3 days of the menstrual cycle. Women must practise effective contraception for at least 1 month before starting treatment, during treatment, and for at least 1 month after stopping treatment. Women should be advised to use at least 1 method of contraception, but ideally they should use 2 methods of contraception. Oral progestogen-only contraceptives are not considered effective. Barrier methods should not be used alone, but can be used in conjunction with other contraceptive methods. Each prescription for isotretinoin should be limited to a supply of up to 30 days' treatment and dispensed within 7 days of the date stated on the prescription; repeat prescriptions or faxed prescriptions are not acceptable. Women should be advised to discontinue treatment and to seek prompt medical attention if they become pregnant during treatment or within 1 month of stopping treatment.

Counselling Warn patient to avoid wax epilation (risk of epidermal stripping), dermabrasion, and laser skin treatments (risk of scarring) during treatment and for at least 6 months after stopping; patient should avoid exposure to UV light (including sunlight) and use sunscreen and emollient (including lip balm) preparations from the start of treatment.

Contra-indications hypervitaminosis A, hyperlipidaemia

Hepatic impairment avoid—further impairment of liver function may occur

Renal impairment in severe impairment, reduce initial dose (e.g. 10 mg daily) and increase gradually up to 1 mg/kg daily as tolerated

Pregnancy avoid—teratogenic; effective contraception must be used—see Pregnancy Prevention above

Breast-feeding avoid

Side-effects dryness of skin (with dermatitis, scaling, thinning, erythema, pruritus), epidermal fragility (trauma may cause blistering), dryness of lips (sometimes cheilitis), dryness of eyes (with blepharitis and conjunctivitis), dryness of pharyngeal mucosa (with hoarseness), dryness of nasal mucosa (with epistaxis), headache, myalgia and arthralgia, raised plasma-triglyceride concentration (risk of pancreatitis if triglycerides above 9 mmol/litre), raised serum-cholesterol concentration (with reduced high-density lipoprotein concentration), raised blood-glucose concentration, raised serum-transaminase concentration, haematuria and proteinuria, thrombocytopenia, thrombocytosis, neutropenia and anaemia; *rarely* mood changes (depression, aggressive behaviour, anxiety, and very rarely psychosis and suicidal ideation)—expert referral required, skin reactions (including reports of Stevens-Johnson syndrome and toxic epidermal necrolysis), alopecia; *very rarely* nausea, hepatitis, inflammatory bowel disease, gastrointestinal haemorrhage, haemorrhagic diarrhoea (discontinue treatment), benign intracranial hypertension (avoid concomitant tetracyclines), convulsions, malaise, drowsiness, dizziness, diabetes mellitus, lymphadenopathy, hyperuricaemia, glomerulonephritis, tendinitis, arthritis, raised serum-creatine kinase concentration, bone changes (including reduced bone density, early epiphyseal closure, and skeletal hyperostosis) and calcification of tendons and ligaments following long-term administration, visual disturbances (papilloedema, corneal opacities, cataracts, decreased night vision, photophobia, blurred vision, colour blindness)—expert referral required and consider withdrawal, decreased tolerance to contact lenses, keratitis, impaired hearing, Gram-positive infections of skin and mucous membranes, exacerbation of acne, acne fulminans, allergic vasculitis and granulomatous lesions, paronychia, hirsutism, nail dystrophy, skin hyperpigmentation, photosensitivity, increased sweating

Dose
- ADULT and CHILD over 12 years, 500 micrograms/kg daily (in 1–2 divided doses), increased if necessary to 1 mg/kg daily, for 16–24 weeks (repeat treatment course after a period of at least 8 weeks if relapse after first course); max. cumulative dose 150 mg/kg per course

Isotretinoin (Non-proprietary) ꜱPoM
Capsules, isotretinoin 5 mg, net price 56-cap pack = £14.78; 20 mg, 56-cap pack = £37.85. Label: 10, patient information leaflet, 11, 21

Roaccutane® (Roche) ꜱPoM
Capsules, isotretinoin 10 mg (brown-red), net price 30-cap pack = £14.54; 20 mg (brown-red/white), 30-cap pack = £20.02. Label: 10, patient information card, 11, 21

13.6.3 Topical preparations for rosacea

Brimonidine, a selective alpha$_2$-adrenoceptor agonist, reduces erythema in rosacea by cutaneous vasoconstriction. For advice on the management of rosacea, see Rosacea, p. 819.

▌ BRIMONIDINE TARTRATE

Indications facial erythema in rosacea

Cautions avoid contact with eyes, mouth, and mucous membranes; avoid use on irritated skin or open wounds; apply other topical preparations (including cosmetics) only after brimonidine gel has dried on skin; **interactions:** Appendix 1 (brimonidine)

Pregnancy manufacturer advises avoid—limited information available

Breast-feeding manufacturer advises avoid—no information available

Side-effects pruritus, burning sensation; *less commonly* dry mouth, headache, paraesthesia, skin irritation, dry skin

Dose
- ADULT over 18 years, apply thinly once daily until erythema subsides (max. 5 mg brimonidine tartrate daily divided over forehead, chin, nose, and cheeks)

Mirvaso® (Galderma) ꜱPoM
Gel, brimonidine tartrate 5 mg/g, net price 30 g = £33.69. Label: 28
Excipients include hydroxybenzoates (parabens), propylene glycol

13.7 Preparations for warts and calluses

Warts (verrucas) are caused by a human papillomavirus, which most frequently affects the hands, feet (plantar warts), and the anogenital region (see below); treatment usually relies on local tissue destruction. Warts may regress on their own and treatment is required only if the warts are painful, unsightly, persistent, or cause distress.

Preparations of **salicylic acid, formaldehyde, glutaraldehyde, or silver nitrate** are available for purchase by the public; they are suitable for the removal of warts on hands and feet. **Salicylic acid** is a useful keratolytic which may be considered first; it is also suitable for the removal of *corns and calluses*. Preparations of salicylic acid in a collodion basis are available but some patients may develop an allergy to colophony in the formulation. Cryotherapy causes pain, swelling, and blistering, and may be no more effective than topical salicylic acid in the treatment of warts.

▌ SALICYLIC ACID

Indications see under preparations; psoriasis (section 13.5.2); fungal nail infections (section 13.10.2)

Cautions significant peripheral neuropathy, patients with diabetes at risk of neuropathic ulcers; impaired peripheral circulation; protect surrounding skin and avoid broken skin; not suitable for application to face, anogenital region, or large areas

Side-effects skin irritation, skin ulceration (with high concentrations)

Dose
- See under preparations; advise patient to apply carefully to wart and to protect surrounding skin (e.g.

13 Skin

with soft paraffin or specially designed plaster); rub wart surface gently with file or pumice stone once weekly; treatment may need to be continued for up to 3 months

Cuplex® (Crawford)

Gel, salicylic acid 11%, lactic acid 4%, in a collodion basis, net price 5 g = £2.88. Label: 15

Dose for plantar and mosaic warts, corns, and calluses, apply twice daily

Note Contains colophony (see notes above)

Duofilm® (GSK)

Paint, salicylic acid 16.7%, lactic acid 16.7%, in flexible collodion, net price 15 mL (with applicator) = £2.25. Label: 15

Dose for plantar and mosaic warts, apply daily

Occlusal® (Alliance)

Cutaneous solution, salicylic acid 26% in polyacrylic solution, net price 10 mL (with applicator) = £3.56. Label: 15

Dose for common and plantar warts, apply daily

Salactol® (Dermal)

Paint, salicylic acid 16.7%, lactic acid 16.7%, in flexible collodion, net price 10 mL (with applicator) = £1.71. Label: 15

Dose for warts, particularly plantar warts, verrucas, corns, and calluses, apply daily

Note Contains colophony (see notes above)

Salatac® (Dermal)

Gel, salicylic acid 12%, lactic acid 4% in a collodion basis, net price 8 g (with applicator) = £2.98. Label: 15

Dose for warts, verrucas, corns, and calluses, apply daily

Verrugon® (Ransom)

Ointment, salicylic acid 50% in a paraffin basis, net price 6 g = £3.12

Dose for plantar warts, apply daily

▌ FORMALDEHYDE

Indications see under preparations

Cautions see under Salicylic Acid

Side-effects see under Salicylic Acid

Veracur® (Typharm)

Gel, formaldehyde 0.75% in a water-miscible gel basis, net price 15 g = £2.41

Dose for warts, particularly plantar warts, apply twice daily

▌ GLUTARALDEHYDE

Indications warts, particularly plantar warts

Cautions protect surrounding skin; not for application to face, mucosa, or anogenital areas

Side-effects rashes, skin irritation (discontinue if severe); stains skin brown

Dose

• Apply twice daily (see also under Salicylic acid)

Glutarol® (Dermal)

Solution (= application), glutaraldehyde 10%, net price 10 mL (with applicator) = £2.07

▌ SILVER NITRATE

Indications warts, verrucas, umbilical granulomas, over-granulating tissue, cauterisation

Cautions protect surrounding skin and avoid broken skin; not suitable for application to face, ano-genital region, or large areas

Side-effects chemical burns on surrounding skin; stains skin and fabric

Dose

• Common warts and verrucas, apply moistened caustic pencil tip for 1–2 minutes; repeat after 24 hours up to max. 3 applications for warts *or* max. 6 applications for verrucas

Note Instructions in proprietary packs generally incorporate advice to remove dead skin before use by gentle filing and to cover with adhesive dressing after application

• Umbilical granulomas, apply moistened caustic pencil tip (usually containing silver nitrate 40%) for 1–2 minutes while protecting surrounding skin with soft paraffin

AVOCA® (Bray)

Caustic pencil, tip containing silver nitrate 40%, potassium nitrate 60%, net price = 99p; silver nitrate 95%, potassium nitrate 5%, treatment pack (including emery file, 6 adhesive dressings and protector pads) = £2.40

Anogenital warts

The treatment of anogenital warts (condylomata acuminata) should be accompanied by screening for other sexually transmitted infections. **Podophyllotoxin** (the major active ingredient of podophyllum) may be used for *soft, non-keratinised* external anogenital warts. Patients with a limited number of external warts or *keratinised* lesions may be better treated with cryotherapy or other forms of physical ablation.

Imiquimod cream is licensed for the treatment of external anogenital warts; it may be used for both keratinised and non-keratinised lesions. It is also licensed for the treatment of superficial basal cell carcinoma and actinic keratosis (section 13.8.1).

Inosine pranobex (section 5.3.2.1) is licensed for adjunctive treatment of genital warts but it has been superseded by more effective drugs.

▌ IMIQUIMOD

Indications see preparations

Cautions avoid contact with eyes, lips, nostrils, or broken skin, and open wounds; not suitable for internal genital warts; uncircumcised males (risk of phimosis or stricture of foreskin); autoimmune disease; immunosuppressed patients

Pregnancy no evidence of teratogenicity or toxicity in *animal* studies; manufacturer advises caution

Breast-feeding no information available

Side-effects local reactions (including itching, burning sensation, erythema, erosion, oedema, excoriation, and scabbing); headache; influenza-like symptoms; myalgia; *less commonly* local ulceration and alopecia; *rarely* Stevens-Johnson syndrome and cutaneous lupus erythematosus-like effect; *very rarely* dysuria in women; permanent hypopigmentation or hyperpigmentation reported

Dose

• See preparations

Aldara® (Meda) [PoM]

Cream, imiquimod 5%, net price 12-sachet pack = £48.60. Label: 10, patient information leaflet

Excipients include benzyl alcohol, cetyl alcohol, hydroxybenzoates (parabens), polysorbate 60, stearyl alcohol

13

Skin

Condoms may damage latex condoms and diaphragms

Dose warts (external genital and perianal), apply thinly 3 times a week at night until lesions resolve (max. 16 weeks); CHILD under 18 years see *BNF for Children*

Superficial basal cell carcinoma, apply to lesion (and 1 cm beyond it) on 5 nights each week for 6 weeks; assess response 12 weeks after completing treatment

Actinic keratosis, apply to lesion 3 times a week at night for 4 weeks; assess response after a 4 week treatment-free interval; repeat 4-week course if lesions persist; max. 2 courses

Important Should be rubbed in and allowed to stay on the treated area for 6–10 hours for warts or for 8 hours for basal cell carcinoma and actinic keratosis, then washed off with mild soap and water (uncircumcised males treating warts under foreskin should wash the area daily). The cream should be washed off before sexual contact

Zyclara® (Meda) PoM

Cream, imiquimod 3.75%, net price 28-sachet pack = £113.00. Label: 10, patient information leaflet

Excipients include benzyl alcohol, cetyl alcohol, hydroxybenzoates (parabens), polysorbate 60, stearyl alcohol

Dose Actinic keratosis, apply to lesion on face or balding scalp at bedtime for 2 weeks (max. 2 sachets daily); repeat course after a 2-week treatment-free interval; assess response 8 weeks after second course

Important Should be rubbed in and allowed to stay on the treated area for 8 hours, then washed off with mild soap and water

PODOPHYLLOTOXIN

Indications see under preparations

Cautions avoid normal skin and open wounds; keep away from face; very irritant to eyes

Pregnancy avoid

Breast-feeding avoid

Side-effects local irritation

Condyline® (Takeda) PoM

Solution, podophyllotoxin 0.5% in alcoholic basis, net price 3.5 mL (with applicators) = £14.49. Label: 15

Dose condylomata acuminata affecting the penis or the female external genitalia, apply twice daily for 3 consecutive days; treatment may be repeated at weekly intervals if necessary for a total of five 3-day treatment courses; direct medical supervision for lesions in the female and for lesions greater than 4 cm² in the male; max. 50 single applications ('loops') per session (consult product literature); CHILD 2–18 years see *BNF for Children*

Warticon® (GSK) PoM

Cream, podophyllotoxin 0.15%, net price 5 g (with mirror) = £17.83

Excipients include butylated hydroxyanisole, cetyl alcohol, hydroxybenzoates (parabens), sorbic acid, stearyl alcohol

Dose condylomata acuminata affecting the penis or the female external genitalia, apply twice daily for 3 consecutive days; treatment may be repeated at weekly intervals if necessary for a total of four 3-day treatment courses; direct medical supervision for lesions greater than 4 cm²; CHILD 2–18 years see *BNF for Children*

Solution, blue, podophyllotoxin 0.5% in alcoholic basis, net price 3 mL (with applicators) = £14.86. Label: 15

Dose condylomata acuminata affecting the penis or the female external genitalia, apply twice daily for 3 consecutive days; treatment may be repeated at weekly intervals if necessary for a total of four 3-day treatment courses; direct medical supervision for lesions greater than 4 cm²; max. 50 single applications ('loops') per session (consult product literature); CHILD 2–18 years see *BNF for Children*

13.8 Sunscreens and camouflagers

13.8.1   Sunscreen preparations

13.8.2   Camouflagers

13.8.1   Sunscreen preparations

Solar ultraviolet irradiation can be harmful to the skin. It is responsible for disorders such as *polymorphic light eruption, solar urticaria,* and it provokes the various *cutaneous porphyrias.* It also provokes (or at least aggravates) skin lesions of *lupus erythematosus* and may aggravate *rosacea* and some other *dermatoses.* Certain drugs, such as demeclocycline, phenothiazines, or amiodarone, can cause photosensitivity. All these conditions (as well as *sunburn*) may occur after relatively short periods of exposure to the sun. Solar ultraviolet irradiation may provoke attacks of recurrent herpes labialis (but it is not known whether the effect of sunlight exposure is local or systemic).

The effects of exposure over longer periods include *ageing changes* and more importantly the initiation of *skin cancer.*

Solar ultraviolet radiation is approximately 200–400 nm in wavelength. The medium wavelengths (290–320 nm, known as UVB) cause *sunburn.* The long wavelengths (320–400 nm, known as UVA) are responsible for many *photosensitivity reactions* and *photodermatoses.* Both UVA and UVB contribute to long-term *photodamage* and to the changes responsible for *skin cancer* and ageing.

Sunscreen preparations contain substances that protect the skin against UVA and UVB radiation, but they are no substitute for covering the skin and avoiding sunlight. The sun protection factor (SPF, usually indicated in the preparation title) provides guidance on the degree of protection offered against UVB; it indicates the multiples of protection provided against burning, compared with unprotected skin; for example, an SPF of 8 should enable a person to remain 8 times longer in the sun without burning. However, in practice, users do not apply sufficient sunscreen product and the protection is lower than that found in experimental studies.

Some manufacturers use a star rating system to indicate the protection against UVA relative to protection against UVB for sunscreen products. However, the usefulness of the star rating system remains controversial. The EU Commission (September 2006) has recommended that the UVA protection factor for a sunscreen should be at least one-third of the sun protection factor (SPF); products that achieve this requirement will be labelled with a UVA logo alongside the SPF classification. Preparations that also contain reflective substances, such as titanium dioxide, provide the most effective protection against UVA.

Sunscreen preparations may rarely cause allergic reactions.

> For optimum photoprotection, sunscreen preparations should be applied **thickly** and **frequently** (approximately 2 hourly). In photodermatoses, they should be used from spring to autumn. As maximum protection from sunlight is desirable, preparations with the highest SPF should be prescribed.

13 Skin

Ingredient nomenclature in sunscreen preparations	
rINN	INCI
amiloxate	isoamyl *p*-methoxycinnamate
avobenzone	butyl methoxydibenzoylmethane
bemotrizinol	bis-ethylhexyloxyphenol methoxyphenyl triazine
bisoctrizole	methylene bis-benzotriazolyl tetramethylbutylphenol
ecamsule	terephthalylidene dicamphor sulfonic acid
ensulizole	phenylbenzimidazole sulfonic acid
enzacamene	4-methylbenzylidene camphor
octinoxate	octyl (*or* ethylhexyl) methoxycinnamate
octocrilene	octocrylene
oxybenzone	benzophenone-3

The European Commission Cosmetic Products Regulation (EC) 1223/2009 requires the use of INCI (International Nomenclature of Cosmetic Ingredients) for cosmetics and sunscreens. This table includes the rINN and the INCI synonym for the active ingredients of sunscreen preparations in the BNF.

Borderline substances   The preparations marked 'ACBS' are regarded as drugs when prescribed for skin protection against ultraviolet radiation in abnormal cutaneous photosensitivity resulting from genetic disorders or photodermatoses, including vitiligo and those resulting from radiotherapy; chronic or recurrent herpes simplex labialis. Preparations with SPF less than 30 should not normally be prescribed. See also Appendix 2.

Anthelios® (L'Oréal Active)
XL SPF 50+ Melt-in cream (UVA and UVB protection; UVB-SPF 50+), avobenzone 3.5%, bemotrizinol 3%, drometrizole trisiloxane 0.5%, ecamsule 1%, octocrilene 2.5%, titanium dioxide 4.2%, net price 50 mL = £3.63. ACBS
Excipients   include disodium edetate, stearyl alcohol
Note   For INCI synonyms, see table above

Sunsense® Ultra (Crawford)
Lotion (UVA and UVB protection; UVB-SPF 50+), octinoxate 6%, enzacamene 4%, avobenzone 2%, oxybenzone 2%, ensulizole 2%, titanium dioxide 3%, net price 50-mL bottle with roll-on applicator = £5.01, 125 mL = £8.14, 500-mL pump pack = £18.17. ACBS
Excipients   include butylated hydroxytoluene, cetyl alcohol, fragrance, hydroxybenzoates (parabens), propylene glycol
Note   For INCI synonyms, see table above

Uvistat® (LPC)
Cream (UVA and UVB protection; UVB-SPF 30), avobenzone 5%, bisoctrizole 1.5%, octinoxate 7.5%, octocrilene 4%, titanium dioxide 5.2%, net price 125 mL = £7.45. ACBS
Excipients   include disodium edetate, hydroxybenzoates (parabens), propylene glycol
Note   For INCI synonyms, see table above
Cream (UVA and UVB protection; UVB-SPF 50), amiloxate 2%, avobenzone 5%, bisoctrizole 6%, octinoxate 10%, octocrilene 4%, titanium dioxide 4.8%, net price 125 mL = £8.45. ACBS
Excipients   include disodium edetate, polysorbate 60, propylene glycol
Note   For INCI synonyms, see table above

Lipscreen (UVA and UVB protection; UVB-SPF 50), avobenzone 5%, bemotrizinol 3%, octinoxate 10%, octocrilene 4%, titanium dioxide 3%, net price 5 g = £2.99. ACBS
Excipients   include butylated hydroxytoluene, hydroxybenzoates (parabens)
Note   For INCI synonyms, see table above

Photodamage

Patients should be advised to use a high-SPF sunscreen and to minimise exposure of the skin to direct sunlight or sun lamps.

Topical treatments can be used for *actinic keratosis*. An **emollient** may be sufficient for mild lesions. **Diclofenac** gel is suitable for the treatment of superficial lesions in mild disease. **Fluorouracil** cream is effective against most types of non-hypertrophic actinic keratosis; a solution containing fluorouracil and salicylic acid is available for the treatment of low or moderately thick hyperkeratotic actinic keratosis. **Imiquimod** (section 13.7) is used for lesions on the face and scalp when cryotherapy or other topical treatments cannot be used. Fluorouracil and imiquimod produce a more marked inflammatory reaction than diclofenac but lesions resolve faster. A short course of **ingenol mebutate** is licensed for the treatment of non-hypertrophic actinic keratosis; response to treatment can usually be assessed 8 weeks after the course. **Photodynamic therapy** in combination with methyl-5-aminolevulinate cream (*Metvix®*, available from Galderma) or 5-aminolaevulinic acid gel (*Ameluz®▼*, available from Spirit Healthcare) is used in specialist centres for treating superficial and confluent, non-hypertrophic actinic keratosis when other treatments are inadequate or unsuitable; it is particularly suitable for multiple lesions, for periorbital lesions, or for lesions located at sites of poor healing.

Imiquimod or topical fluorouracil is used for treating superficial *basal cell carcinomas*. Photodynamic therapy in combination with methyl-5-aminolevulinate cream is used in specialist centres for treating superficial, nodular basal cell carcinomas when other treatments are unsuitable.

▌ DICLOFENAC SODIUM

Indications   actinic keratosis
Cautions   as for topical NSAIDs, see section 10.3.2
Contra-indications   as for topical NSAIDs, see section 10.3.2
Side-effects   as for topical NSAIDs, see section 10.3.2; also paraesthesia; application of large amounts may result in systemic effects, see section 10.1
Dose
• Apply thinly twice daily for 60–90 days; max. 8 g daily

Solaraze® (Almirall) ▒PoM▒
Gel, diclofenac sodium 3% in a sodium hyaluronate basis, net price 50 g = £38.30, 100 g = £76.60
Excipients   include benzyl alcohol

▌ FLUOROURACIL

Indications   superficial malignant and pre-malignant skin lesions; other malignant disease (section 8.1.3)
Cautions   avoid contact with eyes and mucous membranes; do not apply to bleeding lesions; caution in handling—irritant to tissues
Pregnancy   manufacturers advise avoid (teratogenic)

13   **Skin**

Breast-feeding   manufacturers advise avoid

Side-effects   local irritation (use a topical cortico-steroid for severe discomfort associated with inflammatory reactions), photosensitivity, erythema multiforme

Dose

- See under preparations

Efudix® (Meda) [PoM]

Cream, fluorouracil 5%, net price 40 g = £32.90

Excipients   include hydroxybenzoates (parabens), polysorbate 60, propylene glycol, stearyl alcohol

Dose superficial malignant and pre-malignant skin lesions, apply thinly to the affected area once or twice daily; max. area of skin treated at one time, 500 cm² (e.g. 23 cm × 23 cm); usual duration of initial therapy, 3–4 weeks

Note Alternative regimens may be in use in some settings

◢**With salicylic acid**

For prescribing information on salicylic acid, see section 13.5.2

Actikerall® (Almirall) [PoM]

Solution, fluorouracil 0.5%, salicylic acid 10%, net price 25 mL = £38.30. Label: 15

Excipients   none as listed in section 13.1.3

Dose low or moderately thick hyperkeratotic actinic keratosis, apply to affected area once daily for up to 12 weeks; if severe side-effects occur, reduce frequency to 3 times a week until side-effects improve; if treating area with thin epidermis, reduce frequency of application and monitor response more often; max. area of skin treated at one time, 25 cm² (e.g. 5 cm x 5 cm)

INGENOL MEBUTATE

Indications   see under Dose

Cautions   avoid contact with eyes, lips, broken skin, or inside of nostrils and ears; avoid occlusive dressings on treated area

Pregnancy   not absorbed from skin, but manufacturer advises avoid

Breast-feeding   not absorbed from skin; ensure infant does not come in contact with treated area for 6 hours after application

Side-effects   local reactions (including erythema, blistering, crusting, erosion, exfoliation, pain, pruritus, oedema, infection), headache; *less commonly* local ulceration, paraesthesia

Dose

- Actinic keratosis on face and scalp, apply 150 micrograms/g gel once daily for 3 days
- Actinic keratosis on trunk and extremities, apply 500 micrograms/g gel once daily for 2 days

Note One tube covers skin area of 25 cm². Allow gel to dry on treatment area for 15 minutes. Avoid washing or touching the treated area for 6 hours after application; after this time, area may be washed with mild soap and water. Avoid use immediately after shower or less than 2 hours before bedtime.

Picato® (LEO) ▼ [PoM]

Gel, ingenol mebutate 150 micrograms/g, net price 3 × 0.47-g single-use tubes = £65.00; 500 micrograms/g, 2 × 0.47-g single-use tubes = £65.00

Excipients   include benzyl alcohol

Note Flammable

13.8.2 Camouflagers

Disfigurement of the skin can be very distressing to patients and may have a marked psychological effect. In

skilled hands, or with experience, camouflage cosmetics can be very effective in concealing scars and birthmarks. The depigmented patches in vitiligo are also very disfiguring and camouflage creams are of great cosmetic value.

Borderline substances   The preparations marked 'ACBS' are regarded as drugs when prescribed for postoperative scars and other deformities and as an adjunctive therapy in the relief of emotional disturbances due to disfiguring skin disease, such as vitiligo. See also Appendix 2.

Covermark® (Derma UK)

Classic foundation (masking cream), net price 15 mL (10 shades) = £11.86. ACBS

Excipients   include beeswax, hydroxybenzoates (parabens), fragrance

Finishing powder, net price 25 g = £11.86. ACBS

Excipients   include beeswax, hydroxybenzoates (parabens), fragrance

Dermablend® (L'Oréal Active)

Ultra corrective foundation, (7 shades), net price 12 g = £5.60. ACBS

Excipients   include beeswax, isopropyl palmitate

Dermacolor® (Fox)

Camouflage creme, (100 shades), net price 25 mL = £10.52. ACBS

Excipients   include beeswax, butylated hydroxytoluene, fragrance, propylene glycol, stearyl alcohol, wool fat

Fixing powder, (7 shades), net price 60 g = £9.05. ACBS

Excipients   include fragrance

Keromask® (Lornamead)

Masking cream, (24 shades), net price 15 mL = £5.68. ACBS

Excipients   include butylated hydroxyanisole, hydroxybenzoates (parabens), wool fat, propylene glycol

Finishing powder, (4 shades), net price 20 g = £5.68. ACBS

Excipients   include butylated hydroxytoluene, hydroxybenzoates (parabens)

Veil® (Thomas Blake)

Cover cream, (40 shades), net price 19 g = £22.42, 44 g = £33.35, 70 g = £42.10. ACBS

Excipients   include hydroxybenzoates (parabens), wool fat derivative

Finishing powder, translucent, net price 35 g = £24.58. ACBS

Excipients   include butylated hydroxyanisole, hydroxybenzoates (parabens)

13.9 Shampoos and other preparations for scalp and hair conditions

Dandruff is considered to be a mild form of seborrhoeic dermatitis (see also section 13.5.1). Shampoos containing antimicrobial agents such as **pyrithione zinc** (which are widely available) and **selenium sulfide** may have beneficial effects. Shampoos containing **tar** extracts may be useful and they are also used in *psoriasis*. **Ketoconazole** shampoo should be considered for more persistent or severe dandruff or for seborrhoeic dermatitis of the scalp.

Corticosteroid gels and lotions (section 13.4) can also be used.

13 Skin

Shampoos containing **coal tar** and **salicylic acid** may also be useful. A cream or an ointment containing coal tar and salicylic acid is very helpful in *psoriasis* that affects the scalp (section 13.5.2). Patients who do not respond to these treatments may need to be referred to exclude the possibility of other skin conditions.

Cradle cap in infants may be treated with **coconut oil** or **olive oil** applications followed by shampooing.

See below for male-pattern baldness and also section 13.5 (psoriasis and eczema), section 13.10.4 (lice), and section 13.10.2 (ringworm).

◢ Shampoos

[1]Ketoconazole (Non-proprietary) PoM

Cream—section 13.10.2

Shampoo, ketoconazole 2%, net price 120 mL = £3.50

Excipients include imidurea

Brands include *Dandrazol® 2% Shampoo, Nizoral®*

Dose ADULT and CHILD over 12 years, treatment of seborrhoeic dermatitis and dandruff apply twice weekly for 2–4 weeks (prophylaxis apply once every 1–2 weeks); treatment of pityriasis versicolor apply once daily for max. 5 days (prophylaxis apply once daily for up to 3 days before sun exposure); leave preparation on for 3–5 minutes before rinsing

Alphosyl 2 in 1® (GSK Consumer Healthcare)

Shampoo, alcoholic coal tar extract 5%, net price 125 mL = £1.89, 250 mL = £4.52

Excipients include hydroxybenzoates (parabens), fragrance

Dose dandruff, use once or twice weekly as necessary; psoriasis, seborrhoeic dermatitis, scaling and itching, use every 2–3 days

Capasal® (Dermal)

Shampoo, coal tar 1%, coconut oil 1%, salicylic acid 0.5%, net price 250 mL = £4.69

Excipients none as listed in section 13.1.3

Dose scaly scalp disorders including psoriasis, seborrhoeic dermatitis, dandruff, and cradle cap, apply daily as necessary

Ceanel Concentrate® (Alliance)

Shampoo, cetrimide 10%, undecenoic acid 1%, net price 150 mL = £3.40, 500 mL = £9.80

Excipients none as listed in section 13.1.3

Dose scalp psoriasis, seborrhoeic dermatitis, dandruff, apply 3 times in first week then twice weekly

Dermax® (Dermal)

Shampoo, benzalkonium chloride 0.5%, net price 250 mL = £5.69

Excipients none as listed in section 13.1.3

Dose seborrhoeic scalp conditions associated with dandruff and scaling, apply as necessary

Psoriderm® (Dermal)

Scalp lotion (= shampoo), coal tar 2.5%, lecithin 0.3%, net price 250 mL = £4.74

Excipients include disodium edetate

Dose scalp psoriasis, use as necessary

1. Can be sold to the public for the prevention and treatment of dandruff and seborrhoeic dermatitis of the scalp as a shampoo formulation containing ketoconazole max. 2%, in a pack containing max. 120 mL and labelled to show a max. frequency of application of once every 3 days

Selsun® (Chattem UK)

Shampoo, selenium sulfide 2.5%, net price 50 mL = £1.44, 100 mL = £1.96, 150 mL = £2.75

Excipients include fragrance

Cautions avoid using 48 hours before or after applying hair colouring, straightening or waving preparations

Dose seborrhoeic dermatitis and dandruff, apply twice weekly for 2 weeks then once weekly for 2 weeks and then as necessary; CHILD under 5 years not recommended; pityriasis versicolor, section 13.10.2 [unlicensed indication]

T/Gel® (J&J)

Shampoo, coal tar extract 2%, net price 125 mL = £3.61, 250 mL = £5.12

Excipients include fragrance, hydroxybenzoates (parabens), imidurea

Dose scalp psoriasis, seborrhoeic dermatitis, dandruff, apply 2–3 times weekly

◢ Other scalp preparations

Cocois®

Section 13.5.2

Etrivex®

Section 13.4

Polytar® (GSK)

Liquid, tar blend 1%, net price 250 mL = £2.23

Excipients include arachis (peanut) oil, fragrance, imidurea, polysorbate 80

Dose scalp disorders including psoriasis, seborrhoea, eczema, pruritus, and dandruff, apply 1–2 times weekly

Polytar Plus® (GSK)

Liquid, tar blend 1%, net price 500 mL = £3.91

Excipients include arachis (peanut) oil, fragrance, imidurea, polysorbate 80

Dose scalp disorders including psoriasis, seborrhoea, pruritus, and dandruff, apply 1–2 times weekly

Sebco®

Section 13.5.2

Hirsutism

Hirsutism may result from hormonal disorders or as a side-effect of drugs such as minoxidil, corticosteroids, anabolic steroids, androgens, danazol, and progestogens.

Weight loss can reduce hirsutism in obese women.

Women should be advised about local methods of hair removal, and in the mildest cases this may be all that is required.

Eflornithine, an antiprotozoal drug, inhibits the enzyme ornithine decarboxylase in hair follicles. Topical eflornithine can be used as an adjunct to laser therapy for facial hirsutism in women. Eflornithine should be discontinued in the absence of improvement after treatment for 4 months.

Co-cyprindiol (section 13.6.2) may be effective for moderately severe hirsutism. **Metformin** (section 6.1.2.2) is an alternative in women with polycystic ovary syndrome [unlicensed indication]. Systemic treatment is required for 6–12 months before benefit is seen.

▮ EFLORNITHINE

Indications see notes above

Pregnancy toxicity in *animal* studies—manufacturer advises avoid

Breast-feeding manufacturer advises avoid—no information available

13 Skin

Side-effects acne, application site reactions including burning and stinging sensation, rash; *less commonly* abnormal hair texture and growth

Dose

- ADULT over 18 years, apply thinly twice daily

  Note Preparation must be rubbed in thoroughly; cosmetics may be applied over treated area 5 minutes after eflornithine; do not wash treated area for 4 hours after application

Vaniqa® (Almirall) [PoM]

Cream, eflornithine (as hydrochloride monohydrate) 11.5%, net price 60 g = £56.87

Excipients include cetostearyl alcohol, hydroxybenzoates, stearyl alcohol

Note The *Scottish Medicines Consortium* has advised (September 2005) that eflornithine for facial hirsutism be restricted for use in women in whom alternative drug treatment cannot be used

---

Androgenetic alopecia

Finasteride is licensed for the treatment of androgenetic alopecia in men. Continuous use for 3–6 months is required before benefit is seen, and effects are reversed 6–12 months after treatment is discontinued.

Topical application of **minoxidil** may stimulate limited hair growth in a small proportion of adults but only for as long as it is used.

▌ FINASTERIDE

Indications androgenetic alopecia in men; benign prostatic hyperplasia (section 6.4.2)

Cautions section 6.4.2

Side-effects section 6.4.2

Dose

- By mouth 1 mg daily

Propecia® (MSD) [PoM] [NHS]

Tablets, f/c, beige, finasteride 1 mg, net price 28-tab pack = £26.99, 84-tab pack = £81.55

▌ MINOXIDIL

Indications androgenetic alopecia (men and women)

Cautions section 2.5.1 (but only about 1–2% absorbed); avoid contact with eyes, mouth and mucous membranes, broken, infected, shaved, or inflamed skin; avoid inhalation of spray mist; avoid occlusive dressings and topical drugs which enhance absorption

Contra-indications section 2.5.1

Pregnancy section 2.5.1

Breast-feeding section 2.5.1

Side-effects section 2.5.1; also headache, local irritation; *less commonly* hypotension, changes in hair colour or texture (discontinue if increased hair loss persists for more than 2 weeks)

Dose

- See under preparations below

Regaine® (McNeil) [NHS]

Regaine® for Women Regular Strength cutaneous solution, minoxidil 2% in an aqueous alcoholic basis, net price 60-mL bottle with applicators = £14.16

Excipients include propylene glycol

Cautions flammable; wash hands after application

Dose apply 1 mL twice daily to affected areas of scalp; discontinue if no improvement after 1 year

Regaine® for Men Extra Strength cutaneous solution, minoxidil 5% in an aqueous alcoholic basis, net price 60-mL bottle with applicators = £19.84, 3 × 60-mL bottles = £39.71

Excipients include propylene glycol

Cautions flammable; wash hands after application

Dose apply 1 mL twice daily to affected areas of scalp; discontinue if no improvement after 1 year

Regaine® for Men Extra Strength cutaneous foam, minoxidil 5%, net price 60 g = £21.84, 3 × 60 g = £43.69

Excipients include butylated hydroxytoluene. cetyl alcohol, stearyl alcohol, polysorbate 60

Cautions flammable; wash hands after application

Dose apply half a capful twice daily to affected areas of scalp; discontinue if no improvement after 16 weeks

Note Ensure hair and scalp dry before application

13.10 Anti-infective skin preparations

- **13.10.1** Antibacterial preparations
- **13.10.2** Antifungal preparations
- **13.10.3** Antiviral preparations
- **13.10.4** Parasiticidal preparations
- **13.10.5** Preparations for minor cuts and abrasions

13.10.1 Antibacterial preparations

- **13.10.1.1** Antibacterial preparations only used topically
- **13.10.1.2** Antibacterial preparations also used systemically

Cellulitis, a rapidly spreading deeply seated inflammation of the skin and subcutaneous tissue, requires systemic antibacterial treatment (see Table 1, section 5.1). Lower leg infections or infections spreading around wounds are almost always cellulitis. *Erysipelas*, a superficial infection with clearly defined edges (and often affecting the face), is also treated with a systemic antibacterial (see Table 1, section 5.1).

In the community, acute *impetigo* on small areas of the skin may be treated by short-term topical application of **fusidic acid**; **mupirocin** should be used only to treat meticillin-resistant *Staphylococcus aureus*. If the impetigo is extensive or longstanding, an oral antibacterial such as **flucloxacillin** (or **clarithromycin** in penicillin-allergy) (Table 1, section 5.1) should be used. Mild antiseptics (section 13.11) can be used to soften crusts.

Although many antibacterial drugs are available in topical preparations, some are potentially hazardous and frequently their use is not necessary if adequate hygienic measures can be taken. Moreover, not all skin conditions that are oozing, crusted, or characterised by pustules are actually infected. Topical antibacterials should be **avoided** on *leg ulcers* unless used in short courses for defined infections; treatment of bacterial colonisation is generally inappropriate.

To minimise the development of resistant organisms it is advisable to limit the choice of antibacterials applied topically to those not used systemically. Unfortunately some of these, for example neomycin, may cause sensitisation, and there is cross-sensitivity with other aminoglycoside antibiotics, such as gentamicin. If *large areas of skin* are being treated, ototoxicity may also be a hazard with aminoglycoside antibiotics (and also with polymyxins), particularly in children, in the elderly, and in those with renal impairment. *Resistant organisms* are more common in hospitals, and whenever possible swabs should be taken for bacteriological examination before beginning treatment.

Mupirocin is not related to any other antibacterial in use; it is effective for skin infections, particularly those due to Gram-positive organisms but it is not indicated for pseudomonal infection. Although *Staphylococcus aureus* strains with low-level resistance to mupirocin are emerging, it is generally useful in infections resistant to other antibacterials. To avoid the development of resistance, mupirocin or fusidic acid should not be used for longer than 10 days and local microbiology advice should be sought before using it in hospital. In the presence of mupirocin-resistant MRSA infection, a topical antiseptic such as povidone–iodine, chlorhexidine, or alcohol can be used; their use should be discussed with the local microbiologist.

Retapamulin can be used for impetigo and other superficial bacterial skin infections caused by *Staphylococcus aureus* and *Streptococcus pyogenes* that are resistant to first-line topical antibacterials. However, it is not effective against MRSA. The *Scottish Medicines Consortium* (p. 4) has advised (March 2008) that retapamulin (*Altargo*®) is **not** recommended for use within NHS Scotland for the treatment of superficial skin infections.

Silver sulfadiazine is used in the treatment of infected burns.

13.10.1.1 Antibacterial preparations only used topically

MUPIROCIN

Indications   bacterial skin infections (see also notes above)

Renal impairment   manufacturer advises caution when mupirocin ointment used in moderate or severe impairment because it contains macrogols (polyethylene glycol)

Pregnancy   manufacturer advises avoid unless potential benefit outweighs risk—no information available

Breast-feeding   no information available

Side-effects   local reactions including urticaria, pruritus, burning sensation, rash

Dose

- ADULT and CHILD over 1 year, apply up to 3 times daily for up to 10 days; CHILD under 1 year see *BNF for Children*

Mupirocin (Non-proprietary) PoM
Ointment, mupirocin 2%, net price 15 g = £5.35

Bactroban® (GSK) PoM
Cream, mupirocin (as mupirocin calcium) 2%, net price 15 g = £5.26
Excipients   include benzyl alcohol, cetyl alcohol, stearyl alcohol
Ointment, mupirocin 2%, net price 15 g = £4.38
Excipients   none as listed in section 13.1.3
Nasal ointment—section 12.2.3

NEOMYCIN SULFATE

Indications   bacterial skin infections

Cautions   large areas, see below
Large areas   If large areas of skin are being treated ototoxicity may be a hazard, particularly in children, in the elderly, and in those with renal impairment

Contra-indications   neonates

Renal impairment   see Cautions above

Side-effects   sensitisation (see also notes above)

Neomycin Cream BPC PoM
Cream, neomycin sulfate 0.5%, cetomacrogol emulsifying ointment 30%, chlorocresol 0.1%, disodium edetate 0.01%, in freshly boiled and cooled purified water, net price 15 g = £2.17
Excipients   include cetostearyl alcohol, edetic acid (EDTA)
Dose   apply up to 3 times daily (short-term use)

POLYMYXINS

Indications   bacterial skin infections

Cautions   large areas, see below
Large areas   If large areas of skin are being treated nephrotoxicity and neurotoxicity may be a hazard, particularly in children, in the elderly, and in those with renal impairment

Renal impairment   see Cautions above

Side-effects   sensitisation (see also notes above)

Polyfax® (TEVA UK) PoM
Ointment, polymyxin B sulfate 10 000 units, bacitracin zinc 500 units/g, net price 4 g = £3.26, 20 g = £4.62
Excipients   none as listed in section 13.1.3
Dose   apply twice daily or more frequently if required

RETAPAMULIN

Indications   superficial bacterial skin infections (see also notes above)

Contra-indications   contact with eyes and mucous membranes

Side-effects   local reactions including irritation, erythema, pain, contact dermatitis, and pruritus

Dose

- ADULT over 18 years, apply thinly twice daily for 5 days; max. area of skin treated 100 cm^2 or lesion length 10 cm; CHILD 9 months–18 years, apply thinly twice daily for 5 days; max. area of skin treated 2% of body surface area
Note   Review treatment if no response within 2–3 days

Altargo® (GSK) PoM
Ointment, retapamulin 1%, net price 5 g = £7.89.
Label: 28
Excipients   include butylated hydroxytoluene

SILVER SULFADIAZINE

Indications   prophylaxis and treatment of infection in burn wounds; as an adjunct to short-term treatment of infection in leg ulcers and pressure sores; as an adjunct to prophylaxis of infection in skin graft donor sites and extensive abrasions; for conservative management of finger-tip injuries

Cautions   G6PD deficiency; may inactivate enzymatic debriding agents—concomitant use may be inappropriate; for large amounts see also **interactions**: Appendix 1 (sulfonamides)
Large areas   Plasma-sulfadiazine concentrations may approach therapeutic levels with *side-effects* and *interactions*

13 Skin

as for sulfonamides (see section 5.1.8) if large areas of skin are treated. Owing to the association of sulfonamides with severe blood and skin disorders, treatment should be stopped immediately if blood disorders or rashes develop—but leucopenia developing 2–3 days after starting treatment of burns patients is reported usually to be self-limiting and silver sulfadiazine need not usually be discontinued provided blood counts are monitored carefully to ensure return to normality within a few days. Argyria may also occur if large areas of skin are treated (or if application is prolonged).

Contra-indications sensitivity to sulfonamides; not recommended for neonates

Hepatic impairment manufacturer advises caution if significant impairment; see also Large Areas, above

Renal impairment manufacturer advises caution if significant impairment; see also Large Areas, above

Pregnancy risk of neonatal haemolysis and methaemoglobinaemia in third trimester

Breast-feeding small risk of kernicterus in jaundiced infants and of haemolysis in G6PD-deficient infants

Side-effects allergic reactions including burning, itching and rashes; argyria reported following prolonged use; leucopenia reported (monitor blood levels)

Flamazine® (S&N Hlth.) PoM
Cream, silver sulfadiazine 1%, net price 20 g = £2.91, 50 g = £3.85, 250 g = £10.32, 500 g = £18.27
Excipients include cetyl alcohol, polysorbates, propylene glycol
Dose burns, apply daily or more frequently if very exudative; leg ulcers or pressure sores, apply daily or on alternate days (not recommended if ulcer very exudative); finger-tip injuries, apply every 2–3 days; consult product literature for details
Note Apply with sterile applicator

13.10.1.2 Antibacterial preparations also used systemically

Sodium fusidate is a narrow-spectrum antibacterial used for staphylococcal infections. For the role of sodium fusidate in the treatment of impetigo see p. 830.

Metronidazole is used topically for rosacea and to reduce the odour associated with anaerobic infections; oral metronidazole (section 5.1.11) is used to treat wounds infected with anaerobic bacteria.

Angular cheilitis An ointment containing sodium fusidate is used in the fissures of angular cheilitis when associated with staphylococcal infection. For further information on angular cheilitis, see section 12.3.2.

FUSIDIC ACID

Indications staphylococcal skin infections; penicillin-resistant staphylococcal infections (section 5.1.7); staphylococcal eye infections (section 11.3.1)

Cautions see notes above; avoid contact with eyes

Side-effects rarely hypersensitivity reactions

Dose
• Apply 3–4 times daily

Fucidin® (LEO) PoM
Cream, fusidic acid 2%, net price 15 g = £1.92, 30 g = £3.59
Excipients include butylated hydroxyanisole, cetyl alcohol
Ointment, sodium fusidate 2%, net price 15 g = £2.23, 30 g = £3.79
Excipients include cetyl alcohol, wool fat
Dental prescribing on NHS May be prescribed as Sodium Fusidate ointment

METRONIDAZOLE

Indications see preparations; rosacea (see also section 13.6); *Helicobacter pylori* eradication (section 1.3); anaerobic infections (section 5.1.11 and section 7.2.2); protozoal infections (section 5.4.2)

Cautions avoid exposure to strong sunlight or UV light

Side-effects skin irritation

Dose
• See preparations

Acea® (Ferndale) PoM
Gel, metronidazole 0.75%, net price 40 g = £9.95
Excipients include disodium edetate, hydroxybenzoates (parabens)
Dose acute inflammatory exacerbation of rosacea, apply thinly twice daily for 8 weeks

Anabact® (CHS) PoM
Gel, metronidazole 0.75%, net price 15 g = £4.47, 30 g = £7.89
Excipients include hydroxybenzoates (parabens), propylene glycol
Dose malodorous fungating tumours and malodorous gravitational and decubitus ulcers, apply to clean wound 1–2 times daily and cover with non-adherent dressing

Metrogel® (Galderma) PoM
Gel, metronidazole 0.75%, net price 40 g = £22.63
Excipients include hydroxybenzoates (parabens), propylene glycol
Dose acute inflammatory exacerbation of rosacea, apply thinly twice daily for 8–9 weeks
Malodorous fungating tumours, apply to clean wound 1–2 times daily and cover with non-adherent dressing

Metrosa® (Linderma) PoM
Gel, metronidazole 0.75%, net price 40 g = £19.90
Excipients include propylene glycol
Dose acute exacerbation of rosacea, apply thinly twice daily for up to 8 weeks

Rosiced® (Fabre) PoM
Cream, metronidazole 0.75%, net price 30 g = £7.50
Excipients include propylene glycol
Dose inflammatory papules and pustules of rosacea, apply twice daily for 6 weeks (longer if necessary)

Rozex® (Galderma) PoM
Cream, metronidazole 0.75%, net price 30 g = £6.60, 40 g = £9.88
Excipients include benzyl alcohol, isopropyl palmitate
Gel, metronidazole 0.75%, net price 30 g = £6.60, 40 g = £9.88
Excipients include disodium edetate, hydroxybenzoates (parabens), propylene glycol
Dose inflammatory papules, pustules and erythema of rosacea, apply twice daily for 3–4 months

Zyomet® (AMCo) PoM
Gel, metronidazole 0.75%, net price 30 g = £12.00
Excipients include benzyl alcohol, disodium edetate, propylene glycol
Dose acute inflammatory exacerbation of rosacea, apply thinly twice daily for 8–9 weeks

13.10.2 Antifungal preparations

Most localised fungal infections are treated with topical preparations. To prevent relapse, local antifungal treatment should be continued for 1–2 weeks after the disappearance of all signs of infection. Systemic therapy (section 5.2) is necessary for scalp infection or if the skin infection is widespread, disseminated, or intractable; although topical therapy may be used to treat some

13 Skin

nail infections, systemic therapy (section 5.2) is more effective. Skin scrapings should be examined if systemic therapy is being considered or where there is doubt about the diagnosis.

Dermatophytoses Ringworm infection can affect the scalp (tinea capitis), body (tinea corporis), groin (tinea cruris), hand (tinea manuum), foot (tinea pedis, athlete's foot), or nail (tinea unguium). Scalp infection requires systemic treatment (section 5.2); additional application of a topical antifungal, during the early stages of treatment, may reduce the risk of transmission. A topical antifungal can also be used to treat asymptomatic carriers of scalp ringworm. Most other local ringworm infections can be treated adequately with topical antifungal preparations (including shampoos, section 13.9). The imidazole antifungals **clotrimazole, econazole, ketoconazole**, and **miconazole** are all effective. **Terbinafine** cream is also effective but it is more expensive. Other topical antifungals include **griseofulvin** and the **undecenoates**. **Compound benzoic acid ointment** (Whitfield's ointment) has been used for ringworm infections but it is cosmetically less acceptable than proprietary preparations. Topical preparations for athlete's foot containing **tolnaftate** are on sale to the public.

Antifungal dusting powders are of little therapeutic value in the treatment of fungal skin infections and may cause skin irritation; they may have some role in preventing re-infection.

Antifungal treatment may not be necessary in asymptomatic patients with tinea infection of the nails. If treatment is necessary, a systemic antifungal (section 5.2) is more effective than topical therapy. However, topical application of **amorolfine** or **tioconazole** may be useful for treating early onychomycosis when involvement is limited to mild distal disease, or for superficial white onychomycosis, or where there are contra-indications to systemic therapy.

Pityriasis versicolor Pityriasis (tinea) versicolor can be treated with **ketoconazole** shampoo (section 13.9). Alternatively, **selenium sulfide** shampoo [unlicensed indication] (section 13.9) can be used as a lotion (diluting with a small amount of water can reduce irritation) and left on the affected area for 10 minutes before rinsing off; it should be applied once daily for 7 days, and the course repeated if necessary.

Topical imidazole antifungals such as **clotrimazole, econazole, ketoconazole**, and **miconazole**, or topical **terbinafine** are alternatives, but large quantities may be required.

If topical therapy fails, or if the infection is widespread, pityriasis versicolor is treated systemically with a triazole antifungal (section 5.2). Relapse is common, especially in the immunocompromised.

Candidiasis Candidal skin infections can be treated with a topical imidazole antifungal, such as **clotrimazole, econazole, ketoconazole**, or **miconazole**; topical **terbinafine** is an alternative. Topical application of **nystatin** is also effective for candidiasis but it is ineffective against dermatophytosis. Refractory candidiasis requires systemic treatment (section 5.2) generally with a triazole such as fluconazole; systemic treatment with terbinafine is **not appropriate** for refractory candidiasis.

Angular cheilitis Miconazole cream is used in the fissures of angular cheilitis when associated with *Candi-*

da. For further information on angular cheilitis, see p. 789.

Compound topical preparations Combination of an imidazole and a mild corticosteroid (such as hydrocortisone 1%) (section 13.4) may be of value in the treatment of eczematous intertrigo and, in the first few days only, of a severely inflamed patch of ringworm. Combination of a mild corticosteroid with either an imidazole or nystatin may be of use in the treatment of intertrigo associated with candida.

Cautions Contact with eyes and mucous membranes should be avoided.

Side-effects Occasional local irritation and hypersensitivity reactions include mild burning sensation, erythema, and itching. Treatment should be discontinued if these are severe.

▌ AMOROLFINE

Indications fungal nail infections

Cautions see notes above; also avoid contact with ears; use with caution in child likely to suck affected digits

Side-effects see notes above

Dose

- Apply to infected nails 1–2 times weekly after filing and cleansing; allow to dry (approx. 3 minutes); treat finger nails for 6 months, toe nails for 9–12 months (review at intervals of 3 months); avoid nail varnish or artificial nails during treatment

Amorolfine (Non-proprietary) [PoM]
Nail lacquer, amorolfine (as hydrochloride) 5%, net price 5-mL pack = £6.50, 2 × 2.5-mL pack = £19.53. Label: 10, patient information leaflet
Brands include *Omicur*®
Note Amorolfine nail lacquer can be sold to the public if supplied for the treatment of mild cases of distal and lateral subungual onychomycoses caused by dermatophytes, yeasts and moulds; subject to treatment of max. 2 nails, max. strength of nail lacquer amorolfine 5% and a pack size of 3 mL

Loceryl® (Galderma) [PoM]
Nail lacquer, amorolfine (as hydrochloride) 5%, net price 5-mL pack (with nail files, spatulas, and cleansing swabs) = £9.08. Label: 10, patient information leaflet
Excipients none as listed in section 13.1.3

▌ BENZOIC ACID

Indications ringworm (tinea), but see notes above

Benzoic Acid Ointment, Compound, BP
(Whitfield's ointment)
Ointment, benzoic acid 6%, salicylic acid 3%, in emulsifying ointment
Excipients include cetostearyl alcohol
Dose apply twice daily

▌ CLOTRIMAZOLE

Indications fungal skin infections; vaginal candidiasis (section 7.2.2); otitis externa (section 12.1.1)

Cautions see notes above

Pregnancy minimal absorption from skin; not known to be harmful

Side-effects see notes above

13 Skin

Dose
- Apply 2–3 times daily

Clotrimazole (Non-proprietary)
Cream, clotrimazole 1%, net price 20 g = £1.70

Canesten® (Bayer Consumer Care)
Cream, clotrimazole 1%, net price 20 g = £2.14, 50 g = £3.50
Excipients include benzyl alcohol, cetostearyl alcohol, polysorbate 60
Solution, clotrimazole 1% in macrogol 400 (poly-ethylene glycol 400), net price 20 mL = £2.30. For hairy areas
Excipients none as listed in section 13.1.3
Spray, clotrimazole 1%, in 30% isopropyl alcohol, net price 40-mL atomiser = £4.72. Label: 15. For large or hairy areas
Excipients include propylene glycol

ECONAZOLE NITRATE

Indications fungal skin infections; vaginal candidiasis (section 7.2.2)

Cautions see notes above

Pregnancy minimal absorption from skin; not known to be harmful

Side-effects see notes above

Dose
- Skin infections apply twice daily; nail infections, apply once daily under occlusive dressing

Pevaryl® (Janssen)
Cream, econazole nitrate 1%, net price 30 g = £3.71
Excipients include butylated hydroxyanisole, fragrance

GRISEOFULVIN

Indications tinea pedis; resistant fungal infections (section 5.2.5)

Cautions see notes above

Pregnancy manufacturer advises avoid unless poten-tial benefit outweighs risk

Breast-feeding manufacturer advises avoid unless potential benefit outweighs risk

Side-effects see notes above

Dose
- Apply 400 micrograms (1 spray) to an area approx. 13 cm^2 once daily, increased to 1.2 mg (3 sprays, allowing each spray to dry between applications) once daily if necessary; max. treatment duration 4 weeks

Grisol AF® (Transdermal)
Spray, griseofulvin 400 micrograms/metered spray, net price 20-mL (400-dose) spray = £3.35. Label: 15
Excipients include benzyl alcohol

KETOCONAZOLE

Indications fungal skin infections; vulval candidiasis (section 7.2.2)

Cautions see notes above

Side-effects see notes above

Dose
- ADULT over 18 years, tinea pedis, apply twice daily; other fungal infections, apply 1–2 times daily

Nizoral® (Janssen) [PoM]
[1]Cream, ketoconazole 2%, net price 30 g = £4.24
Excipients include cetyl alcohol, polysorbates, propylene glycol, stearyl alcohol
Note A 15-g tube is available for sale to the public for the treatment of tinea pedis, tinea cruris, and candidal intertrigo
Shampoo—section 13.9

MICONAZOLE NITRATE

Indications fungal skin infections; oral and intestinal fungal infections (section 12.3.2); vaginal candidiasis (section 7.2.2)

Cautions see notes above; **interactions**: Appendix 1 (antifungals, imidazole)

Pregnancy absorbed from skin in small amounts; manufacturer advises caution

Side-effects see notes above

Dose
- Apply twice daily continuing for 10 days after lesions have healed; nail infections, apply 1–2 times daily

Miconazole (Non-proprietary)
Cream, miconazole nitrate 2%, net price 20 g = £2.05, 45 g = £1.97
Dental prescribing on NHS Miconazole cream may be prescribed

Daktarin® (Janssen)
Cream, miconazole nitrate 2%, net price 30 g = £1.82
Excipients include butylated hydroxyanisole
Note A 15-g tube [DHS] is on sale to the public
Powder [DHS], miconazole nitrate 2%, net price 20 g = £2.37
Excipients none as listed in section 13.1.3
Aktiv Spray powder, miconazole nitrate 0.16%, in an aerosol basis, net price 100 g = £3.11. Label: 15
Excipients none as listed in section 13.1.3

NYSTATIN

Indications skin infections due to *Candida* spp.; oral fungal infections (section 12.3.2)

Cautions see notes above

Side-effects see notes above

Nystaform® (Typharm) [PoM]
Cream, nystatin 100 000 units/g, chlorhexidine hydrochloride 1%, net price 30 g = £2.62
Excipients include benzyl alcohol, cetostearyl alcohol, polysorbate 60
Dose apply 2–3 times daily continuing for 7 days after lesions have healed.

SALICYLIC ACID

Indications fungal nail infections, particularly tinea; hyperkeratotic skin disorders (section 13.5.2); warts and calluses (section 13.7)

Cautions avoid broken or inflamed skin

Salicylate toxicity Salicylate toxicity can occur particularly if applied on large areas of skin

Pregnancy avoid

Side-effects see notes above

Dose
- ADULT and CHILD over 5 years, apply twice daily and after washing

---

1. [DHS] except for seborrhoeic dermatitis and pityriasis versicolor and endorsed 'SLS'

Phytex® (Wynlit) ◢

Paint, salicylic acid 1.46% (total combined), tannic acid 4.89% and boric acid 3.12% (as borotannic complex), in a vehicle containing alcohol and ethyl acetate, net price 25 mL (with brush) = £2.97

Excipients none as listed in section 13.1.3

Note Flammable

TERBINAFINE

Indications fungal skin infections

Cautions avoid contact with eyes

Pregnancy manufacturer advises use only if potential benefit outweighs risk—*animal* studies suggest no adverse effects

Breast-feeding manufacturer advises avoid—present in milk, but less than 5% of the dose is absorbed after topical application of terbinafine; avoid application to mother's chest

Side-effects see notes above

Dose

• Apply thinly 1–2 times daily for up to 1 week in tinea pedis, 1–2 weeks in tinea corporis and tinea cruris, 2 weeks in cutaneous candidiasis and pityriasis versicolor; review after 2 weeks; CHILD see *BNF for Children*

¹Terbinafine (Non-proprietary) ℗ℴ𝕄

Cream, terbinafine hydrochloride 1%, net price 15 g = £1.75, 30 g = £3.50

Lamisil® (Novartis Consumer Health) ℗ℴ𝕄

Cream, terbinafine hydrochloride 1%, net price 15 g = £4.86, 30 g = £8.76

Excipients include benzyl alcohol, cetyl alcohol, polysorbate 60, stearyl alcohol

Tablets—section 5.2.5

TIOCONAZOLE

Indications fungal nail infections

Cautions see notes above

Pregnancy manufacturer advises avoid

Side-effects see notes above; also local oedema, dry skin, nail discoloration, periungual inflammation, nail pain, rash, exfoliation

Dose

• Apply to nails and surrounding skin twice daily usually for up to 6 months (may be extended to 12 months)

Trosyl® (Pfizer) ℗ℴ𝕄

Cutaneous solution, tioconazole 28%, net price 12 mL (with applicator brush) = £27.38

Excipients none as listed in section 13.1.3

UNDECENOATES

Indications see under preparations below

Cautions see notes above; avoid broken skin

Side-effects see notes above

Dose

• See under preparations below

1. Preparations of terbinafine hydrochloride (max. 1%) can be sold to the public for external use for the treatment of tinea pedis as a cutaneous solution in a pack containing max. 15 g, *or* for the treatment of tinea pedis and cruris as a cream in a pack containing max. 15 g, *or* for the treatment of tinea pedis, cruris, and corporis as a spray in a pack containing max. 30 mL spray or as a gel in a pack containing max. 30 g gel

Mycota® (Thornton & Ross)

Cream, zinc undecenoate 20%, undecenoic acid 5%, net price 25 g = £2.01

Excipients include cetostearyl alcohol, fragrance

Dose treatment of athlete's foot, apply twice daily continuing for 7 days after lesions have healed

Prevention of athlete's foot, apply once daily

Powder, zinc undecenoate 20%, undecenoic acid 2%, net price 70 g = £2.71

Excipients include fragrance

Dose treatment of athlete's foot, apply twice daily continuing for 7 days after lesions have healed

Prevention of athlete's foot, apply once daily

Spray application, undecenoic acid 3.9%, dichlorophen 0.4% (pressurised aerosol pack), net price 100 mL = £2.50

Excipients include fragrance

Dose treatment of athlete's foot, apply twice daily continuing for 7 days after lesions have healed

Prevention of athlete's foot, apply once daily

Note flammable

13.10.3 Antiviral preparations

Aciclovir cream is licensed for the treatment of initial and recurrent labial and genital *herpes simplex infections*; treatment should begin as early as possible. Systemic treatment is necessary for buccal or vaginal infections and for *herpes zoster (shingles)* (for details of systemic use see section 5.3.2.1).

Herpes labialis Aciclovir cream can be used for the treatment of initial and recurrent labial herpes simplex infections (cold sores). It is best applied at the earliest possible stage, usually when prodromal changes of sensation are felt in the lip and before vesicles appear.

Systemic treatment is necessary if cold sores recur frequently or for infections in the mouth (see p. 431).

ACICLOVIR

(Acyclovir)

Indications see notes above; herpes simplex and varicella–zoster infections (section 5.3.2.1); eye infections (section 11.3.3)

Cautions avoid contact with eyes and mucous membranes

Pregnancy not known to be harmful—manufacturers advise use only when potential benefit outweighs risk; limited absorption from topical aciclovir preparations

Side-effects transient stinging or burning; occasionally erythema, itching or drying of the skin

Dose

• Apply to lesions every 4 hours (5 times daily) for 5–10 days, starting at first sign of attack

Aciclovir (Non-proprietary) ℗ℴ𝕄

Cream, aciclovir 5%, net price 2 g = £1.13, 10 g = £5.65

Dental prescribing on NHS Aciclovir Cream may be prescribed

Note A 2-g tube and a pump pack are on sale to the public for the treatment of cold sores

Zovirax® (GSK) ℗ℴ𝕄

Cream, aciclovir 5%, net price 2 g = £4.63, 10 g = £13.96

Excipients include cetostearyl alcohol, propylene glycol

Eye ointment—section 11.3.3

Tablets—section 5.3.2.1

13

Skin

13.10.4 Parasiticidal preparations

Suitable quantities of parasiticidal preparations

Area of body	Skin creams	Lotions	Cream rinses
Scalp (head lice)	—	50–100 mL	50–100 mL
Body (scabies)	30–60 g	100 mL	—
Body (crab lice)	30–60 g	100 mL	—

These amounts are usually suitable for an adult for single application.

Scabies

Permethrin is used for the treatment of *scabies* (*Sarcoptes scabiei*); **malathion** can be used if permethrin is inappropriate.

Benzyl benzoate is an irritant and should be avoided in children; it is less effective than malathion and permethrin.

Ivermectin (available on a named patient basis from 'special-order' manufacturers or specialist importing companies, see p. 1124) in a dose of 200 micrograms/kg by mouth has been used, in combination with topical drugs, for the treatment of hyperkeratotic (crusted or 'Norwegian') scabies that does not respond to topical treatment alone; further doses of 200 micrograms/kg may be required.

Application   Although acaricides have traditionally been applied after a hot bath, this is **not** necessary and there is even evidence that a hot bath may increase absorption into the blood, removing them from their site of action on the skin.

All members of the affected household should be treated simultaneously. Treatment should be applied to the whole body including the scalp, neck, face, and ears. Particular attention should be paid to the webs of the fingers and toes and lotion brushed under the ends of nails. It is now recommended that malathion and permethrin should be applied twice, one week apart; in the case of benzyl benzoate up to 3 applications on consecutive days may be needed. It is important to warn users to reapply treatment to the hands if they are washed. Patients with hyperkeratotic scabies may require 2 or 3 applications of acaricide on consecutive days to ensure that enough penetrates the skin crusts to kill all the mites.

Itching   The *itch* and *eczema* of scabies persists for some weeks after the infestation has been eliminated and treatment for pruritus and eczema (section 13.5.1) may be required. Application of **crotamiton** can be used to control itching after treatment with more effective acaricides. A topical corticosteroid may help to reduce itch and inflammation after scabies has been treated successfully; however, persistent symptoms suggest that scabies eradication was not successful. Oral administration of a **sedating antihistamine** (section 3.4.1) at night may also be useful.

Head lice

Dimeticone is effective against head lice (*Pediculus humanus capitis*) and acts on the surface of the organism. **Malathion**, an organophosphorus insecticide, is an alternative, but resistance has been reported. Benzyl benzoate is licensed for the treatment of head lice but it is less effective than other drugs.

Head lice infestation (pediculosis) should be treated using lotion or liquid formulations only if live lice are present. Shampoos are diluted too much in use to be effective. A contact time of 8–12 hours or overnight treatment is recommended for lotions and liquids; a 2-hour treatment is not sufficient to kill eggs.

In general, a course of treatment for head lice should be 2 applications of product 7 days apart to kill lice emerging from any eggs that survive the first application. All affected household members should be treated simultaneously.

Wet combing methods   Head lice can be mechanically removed by combing wet hair meticulously with a plastic detection comb (probably for at least 30 minutes each time) over the whole scalp at 4-day intervals for a minimum of 2 weeks, and continued until no lice are found on 3 consecutive sessions; hair conditioner or vegetable oil can be used to facilitate the process.

Several devices for the removal of head lice such as combs and topical solutions, are available and some are prescribable on the NHS (consult Drug Tariff—see Appliances and Reagents, p. 1112 for links to online Drug Tariffs).

Crab lice

Permethrin and **malathion** are used to eliminate *crab lice* (*Pthirus pubis*). An aqueous preparation should be applied, allowed to dry naturally and washed off after 12 hours; a second treatment is needed after 7 days to kill lice emerging from surviving eggs. All surfaces of the body should be treated, including the scalp, neck, and face (paying particular attention to the eyebrows and other facial hair). A different insecticide should be used if a course of treatment fails.

Benzyl benzoate

Benzyl benzoate is effective for *scabies* but is not a first-choice for *scabies* (see notes above).

▶ BENZYL BENZOATE

Indications   scabies (but see notes above)

Cautions   children (not recommended, see also under Dose, below), avoid contact with eyes and mucous membranes; do not use on broken or secondarily infected skin

Breast-feeding   suspend feeding until product has been washed off

Side-effects   skin irritation, burning sensation especially on genitalia and excoriations, occasionally rashes

Dose

• Apply over the whole body; repeat without bathing on the following day and wash off 24 hours later; a third application may be required in some cases

   Note Not recommended for children—dilution to reduce irritant effect also reduces efficacy. Some manufacturers recommend application to the body but to exclude the head and neck. However, application should be extended to the scalp, neck, face, and ears

13 Skin

Benzyl Benzoate Application, BP (Non-proprietary) ◢
    Application, benzyl benzoate 25% in an emulsion basis, net price 500 mL = £2.50

Dimeticone

Dimeticone coats head lice and interferes with water balance in lice by preventing the excretion of water; it is less active against eggs and treatment should be repeated after 7 days.

▮ DIMETICONE

Indications   head lice

Cautions   avoid contact with eyes; children under 6 months, medical supervision required

Side-effects   skin irritation

Dose
- Rub into dry hair and scalp, allow to dry naturally, shampoo after minimum 8 hours (or overnight); repeat application after 7 days

Hedrin® (Thornton & Ross)
    Lotion, dimeticone 4%, net price 50 mL = £2.98, 120 mL spray pack = £7.13, 150 mL = £6.92
    Note Patients should be told to keep hair away from fire and flames during treatment

Malathion

Malathion is recommended for *scabies, head lice* and *crab lice* (for details see notes above).

The risk of systemic effects associated with 1–2 applications of malathion is considered to be very low; however, applications of malathion liquid repeated at intervals of less than 1 week *or* application for more than 3 consecutive weeks should be **avoided** since the likelihood of eradication of lice is not increased.

▮ MALATHION

Indications   see notes above and under preparations

Cautions   avoid contact with eyes; do not use on broken or secondarily infected skin; children under 6 months, medical supervision required

Side-effects   skin irritation and hypersensitivity reactions; chemical burns also reported

Dose
- Head lice, rub 0.5% preparation into dry hair and scalp, allow to dry naturally, remove by washing after 12 hours (see also notes above); repeat application after 7 days
- Crab lice, apply 0.5% aqueous preparation over whole body, allow to dry naturally, wash off after 12 hours or overnight; repeat application after 7 days
- Scabies, apply 0.5% preparation over whole body, and wash off after 24 hours; if hands are washed with soap within 24 hours, they should be retreated; see also notes above; repeat application after 7 days
    Note For scabies, manufacturer recommends application to the body but not necessarily to the head and neck. However, application should be extended to the scalp, neck, face, and ears

Derbac-M® (SSL)
    Liquid, malathion 0.5% in an aqueous basis, net price 50 mL = £3.05, 200 mL = £7.33
    Excipients include cetostearyl alcohol, fragrance, hydroxybenzoates (parabens)
    For crab lice, head lice, and scabies

Permethrin

Permethrin is effective for *scabies* and *crab lice* (for details see notes above). Permethrin is active against *head lice* but the formulation and licensed methods of application of the current products make them unsuitable for the treatment of head lice.

▮ PERMETHRIN

Indications   see notes above and under Dose

Cautions   avoid contact with eyes; do not use on broken or secondarily infected skin; children under 6 months, medical supervision required for cream rinse (head lice); children aged 2 months–2 years, medical supervision required for dermal cream (scabies)

Side-effects   pruritus, erythema, and stinging; rarely rashes and oedema

Dose
- Scabies, apply 5% preparation over whole body and wash off after 8–12 hours; CHILD (see also Cautions, above) apply over whole body including face, neck, scalp and ears; if hands washed with soap within 8 hours of application, they should be treated again with cream (see notes above); repeat application after 7 days
    Note Manufacturer recommends application to the body but to exclude head and neck. However, application should be extended to the scalp, neck, face, and ears
    Larger patients may require up to two 30-g packs for adequate treatment
- Crab lice, ADULT over 18 years, apply 5% cream over whole body, allow to dry naturally and wash off after 12 hours or after leaving on overnight; repeat application after 7 days

Permethrin (Non-proprietary)
    Cream, permethrin 5%, net price 30 g = £7.34

Lyclear® Creme Rinse (Omega Pharma) ◢
    Cream rinse, permethrin 1% in basis containing isopropyl alcohol 20%, net price 59 mL = £3.55, 2 × 59-mL pack = £6.46
    Excipients include cetyl alcohol
    Dose head lice, not recommended, therefore no dose stated (insufficient contact time)

Lyclear® Dermal Cream (Omega Pharma)
    Dermal cream, permethrin 5%, net price 30 g = £5.71. Label: 10, patient information leaflet
    Excipients include butylated hydroxytoluene, wool fat derivative

�__13.10.5__ Preparations for minor cuts and abrasions

Some of the preparations listed are used in minor burns, and abrasions. They are applied as necessary but should not be used on large wounds or for prolonged periods because of the possibility of hypersensitivity. The effervescent effect of hydrogen peroxide (section 13.11.6) is used to clean minor cuts and abrasions. Preparations containing camphor and sulfonamides should be **avoided**. Preparations such as magnesium sulfate paste are also listed but are now rarely used to treat carbuncles and boils as these are best treated with antibiotics (section 5.1.1.2).

Cetrimide Cream, BP
    Cream, cetrimide 0.5% in a suitable water-miscible basis such as cetostearyl alcohol 5%, liquid paraffin 50% in freshly boiled and cooled purified water, net price 50 g = £1.11

13 Skin

Proflavine Cream, BPC
Cream, proflavine hemisulfate 0.1%, yellow beeswax 2.5%, chlorocresol 0.1%, liquid paraffin 67.3%, freshly boiled and cooled purified water 25%, wool fat 5%, net price 100 mL = £2.40
Excipients   include beeswax, wool fat
Note   Stains clothing

◢Preparations for boils
Magnesium Sulfate Paste, BP
Paste, dried magnesium sulfate 45 g, glycerol 55 g, phenol 500 mg, net price 25 g = 97p, 50 g = £2.01
Note   Should be stirred before use
Dose   apply under dressing

Collodion

Flexible collodion may be used to seal minor cuts and wounds that have partially healed.

Collodion, Flexible, BP
Collodion, castor oil 2.5%, colophony 2.5% in a collodion basis, prepared by dissolving pyroxylin (10%) in a mixture of 3 volumes of ether and 1 volume of alcohol (90%), net price 10 mL = 30p. Label: 15
Contra-indications   allergy to colophony in elastic adhesive plasters and tape

Skin tissue adhesive

Tissue adhesives are used for closure of minor skin wounds and for additional suture support. They should be applied by an appropriately trained healthcare professional. Skin tissue adhesives may cause skin sensitisation.

Dermabond ProPen® (Ethicon)
Topical Skin Adhesive, sterile, octyl 2-cyanoacrylate, net price 0.5 mL = £18.92

Epiglu® (Schuco)
Tissue adhesive, sterile, ethyl-2-cyanoacrylate 954.5 mg/g, polymethylmethacrylate, net price 4 × 3-g vials = £149.50 (with dispensing pipettes and pallete)

Histoacryl® (B. Braun)
Tissue adhesive, sterile, enbucrilate, net price 5 × 200-mg unit (blue) = £32.00, 10 × 200-mg unit (blue) = £67.20, 5 × 500-mg unit (clear or blue) = £34.65, 10 × 500-mg unit (blue) = £69.30

LiquiBand® (MedLogic)
Tissue adhesive, sterile, enbucrilate, net price 0.5-g amp = £5.50

13.11   Skin cleansers, antiseptics, and desloughing agents

Soap or detergent is used with water to cleanse intact skin; emollient preparations such as aqueous cream (section 13.2.1.1) or emulsifying ointment (section 13.2.1) can be used in place of soap or detergent for cleansing dry skin.

An antiseptic is used for skin that is infected or that is susceptible to recurrent infection. Detergent preparations containing **chlorhexidine** or **povidone–iodine**, which should be thoroughly rinsed off, are used. Emollients may also contain antiseptics (section 13.2.1).

Antiseptics such as **chlorhexidine** or **povidone–iodine** are used on intact skin before surgical procedures; their antiseptic effect is enhanced by an alcoholic solvent. Antiseptic solutions containing **cetrimide** can be used if a detergent effect is also required.

Hydrogen peroxide, an oxidising agent, can be used in solutions of up to 6% for skin disinfection, such as cleansing and deodorising wounds and ulcers; hydrogen peroxide is also available as a cream for superficial bacterial skin infections.

For irrigating ulcers or wounds, lukewarm sterile sodium chloride 0.9% solution is used, but tap water is often appropriate.

Potassium permanganate solution 1 in 10 000, a mild antiseptic with astringent properties, can be used for exudative eczematous areas; treatment should be stopped when the skin becomes dry. It can stain skin and nails especially with prolonged use.

13.11.1   Alcohols and saline

ALCOHOL

Indications   skin preparation before injection
Cautions   flammable; avoid broken skin; patients have suffered severe burns when diathermy has been preceded by application of alcoholic skin disinfectants

Industrial Methylated Spirit, BP
Solution, 19 volumes of ethanol and 1 volume approved wood naphtha, net price '66 OP' (containing 95% by volume alcohol) 100 mL = 50p; '74 OP' (containing 99% by volume alcohol) 100 mL = 39p. Label: 15

Surgical Spirit, BP
Spirit, methyl salicylate 0.5 mL, diethyl phthalate 2%, castor oil 2.5%, in industrial methylated spirit, net price 100 mL = 20p. Label: 15

SODIUM CHLORIDE

Indications   see notes above; nebuliser diluent (section 3.1.5); sodium depletion (section 9.2.1.2); electrolyte imbalance (section 9.2.2.1); eye (section 11.8.1); oral hygiene (section 12.3.4)

Sodium Chloride (Non-proprietary)
Solution (sterile), sodium chloride 0.9%, net price 25 × 20-mL unit = £4.95, 200-mL can = £2.65, 1 litre = 80p

Flowfusor® (Fresenius Kabi)
Solution (sterile), sodium chloride 0.9%, net price 120-mL Bellows Pack = £1.53

Irriclens® (ConvaTec)
Solution in aerosol can (sterile), sodium chloride 0.9%, net price 240-mL can = £3.49

13   Skin

Irripod® (C D Medical)
Solution (sterile), sodium chloride 0.9%, net price 25 × 20-mL sachet = £5.84

Miniversol® (Aguettant)
Solution (sterile), sodium chloride 0.9%, net price 30 × 45-mL unit = £13.20; 30 × 100-mL unit = £19.50

Normasol® (Mölnlycke)
Solution (sterile), sodium chloride 0.9%, net price 25 × 25-mL sachet = £6.42; 10 × 100-mL sachet = £7.80

Stericlens® (C D Medical)
Solution in aerosol can (sterile), sodium chloride 0.9%, net price 100-mL can = £2.06, 240-mL can = £3.13

Steripod® Sodium Chloride (Medlock)
Solution (sterile), sodium chloride 0.9%, net price 25 × 20-mL sachet = £7.90

13.11.2 Chlorhexidine salts

CHLORHEXIDINE

Indications see under preparations; bladder irrigation and catheter patency solutions (see section 7.4.4)

Cautions avoid contact with eyes, brain, meninges and middle ear; not for use in body cavities; alcoholic solutions not suitable before diathermy or for use on neonatal skin; in preterm neonates, use sparingly, do not allow solution to pool, and monitor for skin reactions—risk of severe chemical burns

Side-effects occasional sensitivity; *also reported* chemical burns in preterm neonates

Chlorhexidine 0.05% (Baxter)
2000 Solution (sterile), pink, chlorhexidine acetate 0.05%, net price 1000 mL = 77p
For cleansing and disinfecting wounds and burns

Cepton® (LPC)
Skin wash (= solution), red, chlorhexidine gluconate 1%, net price 150 mL = £3.64
For use as skin wash in acne
Lotion, blue, chlorhexidine gluconate 0.1%, net price 150 mL = £2.48
For skin disinfection in acne

ChloraPrep® (CareFusion)
Cutaneous solution, sterile, chlorhexidine gluconate 2% in isopropyl alcohol 70%, net price (all with single applicator) 0.67 mL (with *SEPP®* applicator) = 30p, 1.5 mL (with *FREPP®* applicator) = 55p, 1.5 mL = 55p, 3 mL = 85p, 10.5 mL = £2.92, 26 mL = £6.50; (all with single applicator, with tint) 3 mL = 89p, 10.5 mL = £3.07, 26 mL = £6.83
For skin disinfection before invasive procedures; CHILD under 2 months, not recommended
Note Flammable

CX Antiseptic Dusting Powder® (Ecolab)
Dusting powder, sterile, chlorhexidine acetate 1%, net price 15 g = £3.93
For skin disinfection

Hibiscrub® (Mölnlycke)
Cleansing solution, red, chlorhexidine gluconate 4%, perfumed, in a surfactant solution, net price 250 mL = £4.25, 500 mL = £5.25, 5 litres = £24.00
Excipients include fragrance
Use instead of soap for pre-operative hand and skin preparation and for general hand and skin disinfection

Hibi® Liquid Hand Rub+ (Mölnlycke)
Solution, chlorhexidine gluconate 0.5%, in isopropyl alcohol 70%, net price 500 mL = £5.25
To be used undiluted for hand and skin disinfection

Hibitane Obstetric® (Derma UK)
Cream, chlorhexidine gluconate solution 5% (≡ 1% chlorhexidine gluconate), in a pourable water-miscible basis, net price 250 mL = £9.00
For use in obstetrics and gynaecology as an antiseptic and lubricant (for application to skin around vulva and perineum and to hands of midwife or doctor)

Hydrex® (Ecolab)
Solution, chlorhexidine gluconate solution 2.5% (≡ chlorhexidine gluconate 0.5%), in denatured ethanol 70%, net price 600 mL (clear) = £3.49; 600 mL (pink) = £3.49, 200-mL spray = £1.77, 500-mL spray = £3.01
For pre-operative skin disinfection
Note Flammable
Surgical scrub, chlorhexidine gluconate 4% in a surfactant solution, net price 250 mL = £3.39, 500 mL = £3.59
Excipients include fragrance
For pre-operative hand and skin preparation and for general hand disinfection

Unisept® (Medlock)
Solution (sterile), pink, chlorhexidine gluconate 0.05%, net price 25 × 25-mL sachet = £5.54; 10 × 100-mL sachet = £6.83
For cleansing and disinfecting wounds and burns and swabbing in obstetrics

◢**With cetrimide**

Tisept® (Medlock)
Solution (sterile), yellow, chlorhexidine gluconate 0.015%, cetrimide 0.15%, net price 25 × 25-mL sachet = £5.33; 10 × 100-mL sachet = £6.85
To be used undiluted for general skin disinfection and wound cleansing

Travasept 100® (Baxter)
Solution (sterile), yellow, chlorhexidine acetate 0.015%, cetrimide 0.15%, net price 500 mL = 72p, 1 litre = 77p
To be used undiluted in skin disinfection such as wound cleansing and obstetrics

13.11.3 Cationic surfactants and soaps

CETRIMIDE

Indications skin disinfection

Cautions avoid contact with eyes; avoid use in body cavities

Side-effects skin irritation and occasionally sensitisation

◢**Preparations**
Ingredient of *Tisept®* and *Travasept® 100*, see above

13.11.4 Iodine

POVIDONE–IODINE

Indications skin disinfection

Cautions broken skin (see below)

Large open wounds The application of povidone–iodine to large wounds or severe burns may produce systemic adverse effects such as metabolic acidosis, hypernatraemia and impairment of renal function.

Contra-indications corrected gestational age under 32 weeks; avoid regular use in patients with thyroid disorders or those receiving lithium therapy

Renal impairment avoid regular application to inflamed or broken mucosa

Pregnancy sufficient iodine may be absorbed to affect the fetal thyroid in the second and third trimester

Breast-feeding avoid

Side-effects rarely sensitivity; may interfere with thyroid function tests

Betadine® (Ayrton Saunders)

Dry powder spray, povidone–iodine 2.5% in a pressurised aerosol unit, net price 150-g unit = £2.63

For skin disinfection, particularly minor wounds and infections; CHILD under 2 years not recommended

Note Not for use in serous cavities

Savlon® Dry (Novartis Consumer Health)

Powder spray, povidone–iodine 1.14% in a pressurised aerosol unit, net price 50-mL unit = £2.51

For minor wounds

Videne® (Ecolab)

Alcoholic tincture, povidone–iodine 10%, net price 500 mL = £5.43

To be applied undiluted in pre-operative skin disinfection

Antiseptic solution, povidone–iodine 10% in aqueous solution, net price 500 mL = £5.43

To be applied undiluted in pre-operative skin disinfection and general antisepsis

Surgical scrub, povidone–iodine 7.5% in aqueous solution, net price 500 mL = £5.43

To be used as a pre-operative scrub for hand and skin disinfection

13.11.5 Phenolics

Triclosan has been used for disinfection of the hands and wounds, and for disinfection of the skin before surgery.

13.11.6 Oxidisers and dyes

HYDROGEN PEROXIDE

Indications see under preparations below

Cautions large or deep wounds; avoid on healthy skin and eyes; bleaches fabric; incompatible with products containing iodine or potassium permanganate

Hydrogen Peroxide Solution, BP

Solution 6% (20 vols), net price 200 mL = 54p

Solution 3% (10 vols), net price 200 mL = 53p

For skin disinfection, particularly cleansing and deodorising wounds and ulcers

Note The BP directs that when hydrogen peroxide is prescribed, hydrogen peroxide solution 6% (20 vols) should be dispensed.

Important Strong solutions of hydrogen peroxide which contain 27% (90 vols) and 30% (100 vols) are only for the preparation of weaker solutions

Crystacide® (Derma UK)

Cream, hydrogen peroxide 1%, net price 25 g = £8.07, 40 g = £11.62

Excipients include edetic acid (EDTA), propylene glycol

Dose superficial bacterial skin infection, apply 2–3 times daily for up to 3 weeks

POTASSIUM PERMANGANATE

Indications cleansing and deodorising suppurating eczematous reactions and wounds

Cautions irritant to mucous membranes

Dose

● Wet dressings or baths, approx. 0.01% solution

Note Stains skin and clothing

Potassium Permanganate Solution

Solution, potassium permanganate 0.1% (1 in 1000) in water

Dose to be diluted 1 in 10 to provide a 0.01% (1 in 10 000) solution

Permitabs® (Alliance)

Solution tablets, for preparation of topical solution, potassium permanganate 400 mg, net price 30-tab pack = £15.95

Note 1 tablet dissolved in 4 litres of water provides a 0.01% (1 in 10 000) solution

13.11.7 Desloughing agents

Alginate, hydrogel and hydrocolloid dressings (Appendix 5) are effective at wound debridement. Sterile larvae (maggots) (available from BioMonde) are also used for managing sloughing wounds and are prescribable on the NHS.

Desloughing solutions and creams are of little clinical value. Substances applied to an open area are easily absorbed and perilesional skin is easily sensitised; gravitational dermatitis may be complicated by superimposed contact sensitivity to substances such as neomycin or lanolin.

For further information on wound management products see Appendix 5, p. 1081.

13.12 Antiperspirants

Aluminium chloride is a potent antiperspirant used in the treatment of hyperhidrosis. Aluminium salts are also incorporated in preparations used for minor fungal skin infections associated with hyperhidrosis.

In more severe cases specialists use **glycopyrronium bromide** as a 0.05% solution in the iontophoretic treatment of hyperhidrosis of plantar and palmar areas. *Botox®* contains **botulinum toxin type A complex** and is licensed for use intradermally for severe hyperhidrosis of the axillae unresponsive to topical antiperspirant or other antihidrotic treatment (section 4.9.3).

ALUMINIUM SALTS

Indications see under Dose below

Cautions avoid contact with eyes or mucous membranes; avoid use on broken or irritated skin; do not shave axillae or use depilatories within 12 hours of application; avoid contact with clothing

Side-effects skin irritation

Dose

- Hyperhidrosis affecting axillae, hands or feet, apply liquid formulation at night to dry skin, wash off the following morning, initially daily then reduce frequency as condition improves—do not bathe immediately before use
- Hyperhidrosis, bromidrosis, intertrigo, and prevention of tinea pedis and related conditions, apply powder to dry skin

Anhydrol® Forte (Dermal)

Solution (= application), aluminium chloride hexahydrate 20% in an alcoholic basis, net price 60-mL bottle with roll-on applicator = £2.51. Label: 15
Excipients none as listed in section 13.1.3

Driclor® (Stiefel)

Application, aluminium chloride hexahydrate 20% in an alcoholic basis, net price 75-mL bottle with roll-on applicator = £3.01. Label: 15
Excipients none as listed in section 13.1.3
Note A 30-mL pack is on sale to the public

ZeaSORB® (Stiefel)

Dusting powder, aldioxa 0.22%, chloroxylenol 0.5%, net price 50 g = £2.61
Excipients include fragrance

▊ GLYCOPYRRONIUM BROMIDE

Indications iontophoretic treatment of hyperhidrosis; drying secretions (see Prescribing in Palliative Care, p. 21); maintenance treatment of chronic obstructive pulmonary disease (section 3.1.2); other indications, see section 15.1.3

Cautions see notes (Antimuscarinics) in section 1.2 (but poorly absorbed and systemic effects unlikely)

Contra-indications see notes (Antimuscarinics) in section 1.2 (but poorly absorbed and systemic effects unlikely); also infections affecting the treatment site

Side-effects see notes (Antimuscarinics) in section 1.2 (but poorly absorbed and systemic effects unlikely); also tingling at administration site

Dose

- Consult product literature; only 1 site to be treated at a time, max. 2 sites treated in any 24 hours, treatment not to be repeated within 7 days

Robinul® (AMCo) [PoM]

Powder, glycopyrronium bromide, net price 3 g = £266.00

▊13.13 Topical circulatory preparations

These preparations are used to improve circulation in conditions such as bruising, superficial thrombophlebitis, chilblains and varicose veins but are of little value. Chilblains are best managed by avoidance of exposure to cold; neither systemic nor topical vasodilator therapy is established as being effective. Sclerotherapy of varicose veins is described in section 2.13.

Rubefacients are described in section 10.3.2.

Hirudoid® (Genus) ▱

Cream, heparinoid 0.3% in a vanishing-cream basis, net price 50 g = £3.99
Excipients include cetostearyl alcohol, hydroxybenzoates (parabens)

Gel, heparinoid 0.3%, net price 50 g = £3.99
Excipients include propylene glycol, fragrance
Dose apply up to 4 times daily in superficial soft-tissue injuries and superficial thrombophlebitis

14 Immunological products and vaccines

14.1 Active immunity

Active immunity can be acquired by natural disease or by vaccination. **Vaccines** stimulate production of antibodies and other components of the immune mechanism; they consist of either:

1. a *live attenuated* form of a virus (e.g. measles, mumps and rubella vaccine) or bacteria (e.g. BCG vaccine), or

2. *inactivated* preparations of the virus (e.g. influenza vaccine) or bacteria, or

3. *detoxified exotoxins* produced by a micro-organism (e.g. tetanus vaccine), or

4. *extracts of* a micro-organism, which may be derived from the organism (e.g. pneumococcal vaccine) or produced by recombinant DNA technology (e.g. hepatitis B vaccine).

Live attenuated vaccines usually produce a durable immunity, but not always as long-lasting as that resulting from natural infection.

Inactivated vaccines may require a primary series of injections of vaccine to produce an adequate antibody response, and in most cases booster (reinforcing) injections are required; the duration of immunity varies from months to many years. Some inactivated vaccines are adsorbed onto an adjuvant (such as aluminium hydroxide) to enhance the antibody response.

Advice in this chapter reflects that in the handbook *Immunisation against Infectious Disease* (2006), which in turn reflects the guidance of the Joint Committee on Vaccination and Immunisation (JCVI).
Chapters from the handbook are available at www.immunisation.dh.gov.uk
The advice in this chapter also incorporates changes announced by the Chief Medical Officer and Health Department Updates.

Cautions Most individuals can safely receive the majority of vaccines. Vaccination may be postponed if the individual is suffering from an acute illness; however, it is not necessary to postpone immunisation in patients with minor illnesses without fever or systemic upset. See also Predisposition to Neurological Problems, below. For individuals with bleeding disorders, see Route of Administration, below. If alcohol or disinfectant is used for cleansing the skin it should be allowed to evaporate before vaccination to prevent possible inactivation of live vaccines.

When 2 or more live vaccines are required (and are not available as a combined preparation), they can be administered at any time before or after each other at different sites, preferably in a different limb; if more than one injection is to be given in the same limb, they should be administered at least 2.5 cm apart (but see also BCG Vaccines, p. 846). Yellow fever and MMR vaccines should **not** be administered on the same day; there should be a 4-week minimum interval between the vaccines. When protection is rapidly required, the vaccines can be given at any interval and an additional dose of MMR may be considered. Varicella–zoster and MMR vaccines can be given on the same day or separated by a 4-week minimum interval. When protection is rapidly required, the vaccines can be given at any interval and an additional dose of the vaccine given second may be considered. For **interactions** see Appendix 1 (vaccines).

See also Cautions under individual vaccines.

Contra-indications Vaccines are contra-indicated in those who have a confirmed anaphylactic reaction to a preceding dose of a vaccine containing the same antigens or vaccine component (such as antibacterials in viral vaccines). The presence of the following excipients in vaccines and immunological products has been noted under the relevant entries:

Gelatin	Penicillins
Gentamicin	Polymyxin B
Kanamycin	Streptomycin
Neomycin	Thiomersal

Hypersensitivity to egg Individuals with evidence of previous anaphylactic reaction to egg should not be given tick-borne encephalitis vaccine, and yellow fever vaccine should only be considered under the guidance of a specialist. Individuals with a history of egg allergy can be immunised with either an egg free influenza vaccine, if available, or an influenza vaccine with an ovalbumin content less than 120 nanograms/mL (facilities should be available to treat anaphylaxis). Vaccines with an ovalbumin content more than 120 nanograms/mL or where content is not stated should not be used in individuals with egg allergy. If an influenza vaccine containing ovalbumin is being considered in those with a history of anaphylaxis to egg or egg allergy with uncontrolled asthma, these individuals should be referred to a specialist in hospital. See also Cautions under MMR vaccine.

See also Vaccines and HIV infection, below.

Live vaccines may be contra-indicated temporarily in individuals who are:

- immunosuppressed (see Impaired Immune Response, below);

- pregnant (see Pregnancy and Breast-feeding, below).

See also Contra-indications under individual vaccines.

Impaired immune response Immune response to vaccines may be reduced in immunosuppressed patients and there is also a risk of generalised infection with live vaccines. Severely immunosuppressed patients should not be given live vaccines (including those with severe primary immunodeficiency). Specialist advice should be sought for those being treated with high doses of corticosteroids (dose equivalents of prednisolone: **adults**, at least 40 mg daily for more than 1 week; **children**, 2 mg/kg daily for at least 1 week or 1 mg/kg daily for 1 month), or other immunosuppressive drugs[1], and those being treated for malignant conditions with chemotherapy or generalised radiotherapy[1,2]. However, with the exception of severe combined immunodeficiency, the benefit from rotavirus vaccination is likely to outweigh the risk in other types of immunosuppression; if there is any doubt, advice should be sought from a specialist. For special reference to *HIV infection*, see below.

The Royal College of Paediatrics and Child Health has produced a statement, *Immunisation of the Immunocompromised Child (2002)* (available at www.rcpch.ac.uk).

Pregnancy Live vaccines should not be administered routinely to *pregnant women* because of the theoretical risk of fetal infection but where there is a significant risk of exposure to disease (e.g. to yellow fever), the need for vaccination usually outweighs any possible risk to the fetus. Termination of pregnancy following inadvertent immunisation is not recommended. There is no evidence of risk from vaccinating pregnant women with inactivated viral or bacterial vaccines or toxoids. For use of specific vaccines during pregnancy, see under individual vaccines.

Breast-feeding Although there is a theoretical risk of live vaccine being present in breast milk, vaccination is not contra-indicated for women who are breast-feeding when there is significant risk of exposure to disease. There is no evidence of risk from vaccinating women who are breast-feeding, with inactivated viral or bacterial vaccines or toxoids. For use of specific vaccines during breast-feeding, see under individual vaccines.

Side-effects Injection of a vaccine may be followed by local reactions such as pain, inflammation, redness, and lymphangitis. An induration or sterile abscess may develop at the injection site. Gastro-intestinal disturbances, fever, headache, irritability, loss of appetite, fatigue, myalgia, and malaise are among the most commonly reported side-effects. Other side-effects include influenza-like symptoms, dizziness, paraes-

---

1. Live vaccines should be postponed until at least 3 months after stopping high-dose systemic corticosteroids and at least 6 months after stopping other immunosuppressive drugs or generalised radiotherapy (at least 12 months after discontinuing immunosuppressants following bone-marrow transplantation).
2. Use of normal immunoglobulin should be considered after exposure to measles (see p. 867) and varicella–zoster immunoglobulin considered after exposure to chickenpox or herpes zoster (see p. 870).

thesia, asthenia, drowsiness, arthralgia, rash, and lymphadenopathy. Hypersensitivity reactions, such as bronchospasm, angioedema, urticaria, and anaphylaxis, are very rare but can be fatal (see section 3.4.3 for management of allergic emergencies).

Oral vaccines such as cholera, live poliomyelitis, rotavirus, and live typhoid can also cause gastro-intestinal disturbances such as nausea, vomiting, abdominal pain and cramps, and diarrhoea.

See also Predisposition to Neurological Problems, below.

Some vaccines (e.g. poliomyelitis) produce very few reactions, while others (e.g. measles, mumps and rubella) may cause a very mild form of the disease. Occasionally more serious adverse reactions can occur—these should always be reported to the CHM (see Adverse Reactions to Drugs, p. 12).

See also Preterm Birth, p. 844.

Post-immunisation pyrexia in infants

The parent should be advised that if pyrexia develops after childhood immunisation, and the infant seems distressed, a dose of paracetamol can be given and, if necessary, a second dose can be given 4–6 hours later. Ibuprofen can be used if paracetamol is unsuitable, but if a second dose of ibuprofen is required, it is given 6 hours after the first dose. The parent should be warned to seek medical advice if the pyrexia persists.

For post-immunisation pyrexia in an infant aged 2–3 months, the dose of paracetamol is 60 mg; the dose of ibuprofen is 50 mg (on a doctor's advice). An oral syringe can be obtained from any pharmacy to give the small volume required.

Predisposition to neurological problems

When there is a personal or family history of *febrile* convulsions, there is an increased risk of these occurring during fever from any cause including immunisation, but this is not a contra-indication to immunisation. In children who have had a seizure associated with fever without neurological deterioration, immunisation is *recommended*; advice on the *management of fever* (see Post-immunisation pyrexia in infants, above) should be given before immunisation. When a child has had a convulsion not associated with fever, and the neurological condition is not deteriorating, immunisation is *recommended*.

Children with stable neurological disorders (e.g. spina bifida, congenital brain abnormality, and perinatal hypoxic-ischaemic encephalopathy) should be immunised according to the recommended schedule.

When there is a *still evolving neurological problem*, including poorly controlled epilepsy, immunisation should be *deferred* and the child referred to a specialist. Immunisation is recommended if a cause for the neurological disorder is identified. If a cause is not identified, immunisation should be deferred until the condition is stable.

Further information on adverse effects associated with specific vaccines can be found under individual vaccines.

Immunisation schedule

Vaccines for the childhood immunisation schedule should be obtained from **local health organisations** or from ImmForm (www.immform.dh.gov.uk)—not to be prescribed on FP10 (HS21 in Northern Ireland; GP10 in Scotland; WP10 in Wales).

Preterm birth

Babies born preterm should receive all routine immunisations based on their actual date of birth. The risk of apnoea following vaccination is increased in preterm babies, particularly in those born at or before 28 weeks gestational age. If babies at risk of apnoea are in hospital at the time of their first immunisation, they should be monitored for 48 hours after immunisation. If a baby develops apnoea, bradycardia, or desaturation after the first immunisation, the second immunisation should also be given in hospital with similar monitoring. Seroconversion may be unreliable in babies born earlier than 28 weeks' gestation or in babies treated with corticosteroids for chronic lung disease; consideration should be given to testing for antibodies against *Haemophilus influenzae* type b, meningococcal C, and hepatitis B after primary immunisation.

When to immunise (for preterm infants—see note above)	Vaccine given and dose schedule (for details of dose, see under individual vaccines)
Neonates at risk only	• **BCG Vaccine** See section 14.4, BCG Vaccines • **Hepatitis B Vaccine** See section 14.4, Hepatitis B Vaccine
2 months	• **Diphtheria, Tetanus, Pertussis (Acellular, Component), Poliomyelitis (Inactivated), and Haemophilus Type b Conjugate Vaccine (Adsorbed)** First dose • **Pneumococcal Polysaccharide Conjugate Vaccine (Adsorbed)** First dose • **Rotavirus vaccine** First dose
3 months	• **Diphtheria, Tetanus, Pertussis (Acellular, Component), Poliomyelitis (Inactivated), and Haemophilus Type b Conjugate Vaccine (Adsorbed)** Second dose • **Meningococcal Group C Conjugate Vaccine** First dose • **Rotavirus vaccine** Second dose
4 months	• **Diphtheria, Tetanus, Pertussis (Acellular, Component), Poliomyelitis (Inactivated), and Haemophilus Type b Conjugate Vaccine (Adsorbed)** Third dose • **Pneumococcal Polysaccharide Conjugate Vaccine (Adsorbed)** Second dose
12–13 months	• **Measles, Mumps and Rubella Vaccine, Live (MMR)** First dose • **Pneumococcal Polysaccharide Conjugate Vaccine (Adsorbed)** Single booster dose • **Haemophilus Type b Conjugate Vaccine and Meningococcal Group C Conjugate Vaccine** Single booster dose
Between 3 years and 4 months, and 5 years	• **Adsorbed Diphtheria [low dose], Tetanus, Pertussis (Acellular, Component) and Poliomyelitis (Inactivated) Vaccine** *or* **Adsorbed Diphtheria, Tetanus, Pertussis (Acellular, Component) and Poliomyelitis (Inactivated) Vaccine** Single booster dose **Note:** Preferably allow interval of at least 3 years after completing primary course • **Measles, Mumps and Rubella Vaccine, Live (MMR)** Second dose
11–14 years (females only)[1]	• **Human Papillomavirus Vaccine** 2 doses; second dose 12 months after first dose[2,3]
13–15 years	• **Meningococcal Group C Conjugate Vaccine** Single booster dose
13–18 years	• **Adsorbed Diphtheria [low dose], Tetanus, and Poliomyelitis (Inactivated) Vaccine** Single booster dose **Note:** Can be given at the same time as the booster dose of meningococcal group C conjugate vaccine at 13–15 years of age
During adult life, women of child-bearing age susceptible to rubella	• **Measles, Mumps and Rubella Vaccine, Live (MMR)** Women of child-bearing age who have not received 2 doses of a rubella-containing vaccine or who do not have a positive antibody test for rubella should be offered rubella immunisation (using the MMR vaccine)—exclude pregnancy before immunisation, but see also section 14.4, Measles, Mumps and Rubella Vaccine

Immunological products and vaccines

14

---

1. First dose of HPV vaccine will be offered to females aged 12–13 years of age in England, Wales, and Northern Ireland, and 11–14 years of age in Scotland.
2. If a 3-dose course of HPV vaccine has been started under the 2013/2014 programme, where possible, the course should be completed.
3. The two human papillomavirus vaccines are not interchangeable and, ideally, one vaccine product should be used for the entire course. However, for those females who started the schedule with *Cervarix*® under the national immunisation programme, but did not complete the vaccination course, the course can be completed with *Gardasil*®.

Immunisation schedule (*continued*)

When to immunise (for preterm infants—see note above)	Vaccine given and dose schedule (for details of dose, see under individual vaccines)
During adult life, those entering or being at university who are at risk of meningococcal group C disease	• **Meningococcal Group C Conjugate Vaccine** Single dose **Note:** Should be offered to those of any age entering or being at university who have never been vaccinated against meningocccal group C disease, or those born after September 1995 who are entering university and only received meningococcal group C vaccine under the age of 10 years
During adult life, if not previously immunised	• **Adsorbed Diphtheria [low dose], Tetanus, and Poliomyelitis (Inactivated) Vaccine** 3 doses at intervals of 1 month Booster dose at least 1 year after primary course and again 5–10 years later
70 years	• **Shingles (Herpes Zoster) Vaccine, Live** Single dose

Vaccines and HIV infection HIV-positive individuals with or without symptoms can receive the following live vaccines:

MMR (but avoid if immunity significantly impaired), varicella-zoster vaccine against chickenpox (but avoid if immunity significantly impaired—consult product literature)[1], rotavirus;

and the following inactivated vaccines:

anthrax, cholera (oral), diphtheria, haemophilus influenzae type b, hepatitis A, hepatitis B, human papillomavirus, influenza (injection), meningococcal, pertussis, pneumococcal, poliomyelitis, rabies, tetanus, tick-borne encephalitis, typhoid (injection).

HIV-positive individuals should **not** receive:

BCG, influenza nasal spray (unless stable HIV infection and receiving antiretroviral therapy), typhoid (oral), yellow fever[2]

Note The above advice differs from that for other immunocompromised patients; *Immunisation Guidelines for HIV-infected Adults* issued by British HIV Association (BHIVA) are available at www.bhiva.org and, *Immunisation of HIV-infected Children* issued by Children's HIV Association (CHIVA) are available at www.chiva.org.uk

Vaccines and asplenia The following vaccines are recommended for asplenic patients or those with splenic dysfunction:

haemophilus influenzae type b; influenza; meningococcal A, C, W135, and Y conjugate; pneumococcal.

For antibiotic prophylaxis in asplenia see p. 363.

Route of administration Vaccines should not be given intravenously. Most vaccines are given by the intramuscular route, although some are given by either the intradermal, deep subcutaneous, or oral route. The intramuscular route should not be used in patients with **bleeding disorders** such as haemophilia or thrombocytopenia, vaccines usually given by the intramuscular route should be given by deep subcutaneous injection instead.

Note The Department of Health has advised *against the use of jet guns* for vaccination owing to the risk of transmitting blood-borne infections, such as HIV.

1. Use of normal immunoglobulin should be considered after exposure to measles (see p. 867) and varicella–zoster immunoglobulin considered after exposure to chickenpox or herpes zoster (see p. 870).
2. If yellow fever risk is unavoidable, specialist advice should be sought.

High-risk groups

For information on high-risk groups, see section 14.4 under individual vaccines

BCG Vaccines

Hepatitis A Vaccine

Hepatitis B Vaccine

Influenza Vaccine

Pneumococcal Vaccines

Tetanus Vaccines

14.2 Passive immunity

Immunity with immediate protection against certain infective organisms can be obtained by injecting preparations made from the plasma of immune individuals with adequate levels of antibody to the disease for which protection is sought (see under Immunoglobulins, section 14.5). The duration of this passive immunity varies according to the dose and the type of immunoglobulin. Passive immunity may last only a few weeks; when necessary, passive immunisation can be repeated.

Antibodies of human origin are usually termed *immunoglobulins*. The term *antiserum* is applied to material prepared in animals. Because of serum sickness and other allergic-type reactions that may follow injections of antisera, this therapy has been replaced wherever possible by the use of immunoglobulins. Reactions are theoretically possible after injection of human immunoglobulins but reports of such reactions are very rare.

14.3 Storage and use

Care must be taken to store all vaccines and other immunological products under the conditions recommended in the product literature, otherwise the preparation may become ineffective. **Refrigerated storage** is usually necessary; many vaccines and immunoglobulins need to be stored at 2–8°C and not allowed to freeze. Vaccines and immunoglobulins should be protected from light. Reconstituted vaccines and opened multidose vials must be used within the period recommended in the product literature. Unused vaccines should be disposed of by incineration at a registered disposal contractor.

Particular attention must be paid to instructions on the use of diluents. Vaccines which are liquid suspensions or are reconstituted before use should be adequately mixed to ensure uniformity of the material to be injected.

14.4 Vaccines and antisera

Availability   Anthrax and yellow fever vaccines, botulism antitoxin, diphtheria antitoxin, and snake and spider venom antitoxins are available from local designated holding centres.

For antivenom, see Emergency Treatment of Poisoning, p. 43.

Enquiries for vaccines not available commercially can also be made to:

Vaccines and Countermeasures Response Department
Public Health England
Wellington House
133–155 Waterloo Road
London, SE1 8UG
vaccinesupply@phe.gov.uk

In Scotland information about availability of vaccines can be obtained from a Specialist in Pharmaceutical Public Health.

In Wales enquiries for vaccines not available commercially should be directed to:

Welsh Medicines Information Centre
University Hospital of Wales
Cardiff, CF14 4XW
Tel: (029) 2074 2979

In Northern Ireland:

Pharmacy and Medicines Management Centre
Beech House
Antrim Hospital Site
Northern Health and Social Care Trust
Bush Road
Antrim, BT41 2RL
rphps.admin@northerntrust.hscni.net

For further details of availability, see under individual vaccines.

Anthrax vaccine

Anthrax vaccine is made from antigens from *B. anthracis*. Anthrax immunisation is indicated for individuals who handle infected animals, for those exposed to imported infected animal products, and for laboratory staff who work with *Bacillus anthracis*. A 4-dose regimen is used for primary immunisation; booster doses should be given annually to workers at continued risk of exposure to anthrax.

In the event of possible contact with *B. anthracis*, post-exposure immunisation may be indicated, in addition to antimicrobial prophylaxis (section 5.1.12). Advice on the use of anthrax vaccine for post-exposure prophylaxis must be obtained from Public Health England Colindale (tel. 020 8200 4400).

◤ ANTHRAX VACCINE

Indications   pre-exposure immunisation against anthrax; post-exposure immunisation (see notes above)

Cautions   see section 14.1

Contra-indications   see section 14.1

Pregnancy   see p. 843

Breast-feeding   see p. 843

Side-effects   see section 14.1

Dose

- By intramuscular injection in deltoid region, initial course 3 doses of 0.5 mL at intervals of 3 weeks followed by a fourth dose after an interval of 6 months; booster, 0.5 mL every 12 months

Anthrax Vaccine [PoM]
Injection, suspension of anthrax antigens (not less than 0.125 mL/0.5 mL dose), sterile filtrate, adsorbed on to aluminium potassium sulfate
Excipients   include thiomersal
Available from Public Health England's Centre for Emergency Preparedness and Response (Porton Down)

BCG vaccines

BCG (Bacillus Calmette-Guérin) is a live attenuated strain derived from *Mycobacterium bovis* which stimulates the development of immunity to *M. tuberculosis*. BCG vaccine should be given intradermally by operators skilled in the technique (see below).

The expected reaction to successful BCG vaccination is induration at the site of injection followed by a local lesion which starts as a papule 2 or more weeks after vaccination; the lesion may ulcerate then subside over several weeks or months, leaving a small, flat scar. A dry dressing may be used if the ulcer discharges, but air should **not** be excluded.

Apart from children under 6 years, any person being considered for BCG immunisation must first be given a skin test for hypersensitivity to tuberculoprotein (see under Diagnostic Agents, below). A skin test is not necessary for a child under 6 years provided that the child has not stayed for longer than 3 months in a country with an incidence of tuberculosis greater than 40 per 100 000, the child has not had contact with a person with tuberculosis, and there is no family history of tuberculosis within the last 5 years.

BCG is recommended for the following groups if BCG immunisation has not previously been carried out:

- neonates with a family history of tuberculosis in the last 5 years;

- all neonates and infants (0–12 months) born in areas where the incidence[1] of tuberculosis is greater than 40 per 100 000;

- neonates, infants, and children under 16 years with a parent or grandparent born in a country with an incidence[1] of tuberculosis greater than 40 per 100 000;

- new immigrants aged under 16 years who were born in, or lived for more than 3 months in a country with an incidence[1] of tuberculosis greater than 40 per 100 000;

- new immigrants aged 16–35 years from Sub-Saharan Africa or a country with an incidence[1] of tuberculosis greater than 500 per 100 000

- contacts aged under 36 years of those with active respiratory tuberculosis (for healthcare or laboratory workers who have had contact with clinical materials or patients with tuberculosis, age limit does not apply);

1. List of countries or primary care trusts where the incidence of tuberculosis is greater than 40 cases per 100 000 is available at www.hpa.org.uk

- healthcare workers and laboratory staff (irrespective of age) who are likely to have contact with patients, clinical materials, or derived isolates; other individuals under 35 years[1] at occupational risk including veterinary and other staff who handle animal species susceptible to tuberculosis, and staff working directly with prisoners, in care homes for the elderly, or in hostels or facilities for the homeless or refugees;

- individuals under 16 years intending to live with local people for more than 3 months in a country with an incidence[2] of tuberculosis greater than 40 per 100 000 (section 14.6).

BCG vaccine can be given simultaneously with another live vaccine (see also section 14.1), but if they are not given at the same time an interval of 4 weeks should normally be allowed. When BCG is given to infants, there is no need to delay routine primary immunisations. No further vaccination should be given in the arm used for BCG vaccination for at least 3 months because of the risk of regional lymphadenitis.

Bladder instillations of BCG are licensed for the management of bladder carcinoma (section 8.2.4).

For advice on chemoprophylaxis against tuberculosis, see section 5.1.9; for the treatment of infection following vaccination, seek expert advice.

BACILLUS CALMETTE-GUÉRIN VACCINE
BCG Vaccine

Indications immunisation against tuberculosis

Cautions see section 14.1

Contra-indications see section 14.1; *also* neonate in household contact with known or suspected case of active tuberculosis; generalised septic skin conditions (for patients with eczema, lesion-free site should be used)

Pregnancy see p. 843

Breast-feeding see p. 843

Side-effects see section 14.1 and notes above; *also* at the injection site, subcutaneous abscess, prolonged ulceration; *rarely* disseminated complications such as osteitis or osteomyelitis

Dose

- By intradermal injection ADULT and CHILD over 1 year, 0.1 mL; NEONATE and CHILD under 1 year, 0.05 mL
  Intradermal injection technique Skin is stretched between thumb and forefinger and needle (size 25G or 26G) inserted (bevel upwards) for about 3 mm into superficial layers of dermis (almost parallel with surface). Needle should be short with short bevel (can usually be seen through epidermis during insertion). Tense raised blanched bleb showing tips of hair follicles is sign of correct injection; 7 mm bleb ≡ 0.1 mL injection, 3 mm bleb ≡ 0.05 mL injection; if considerable resistance not felt, needle too deep and should be removed and reinserted before giving more vaccine.
  To be injected at insertion of deltoid muscle onto humerus (keloid formation more likely with sites higher on arm); tip of shoulder should be **avoided**.

1. There is inadequate evidence of protection by BCG vaccine in adults aged over 35 years; however, vaccination is recommended for healthcare workers irrespective of age because of the increased risk to them or their patients
2. List of countries or primary care trusts where the incidence of tuberculosis is greater than 40 cases per 100 000 is available at www.hpa.org.uk

◄**Intradermal**

Bacillus Calmette-Guérin Vaccine [PoM]
BCG Vaccine, Dried/Tub/BCG
Injection (powder for suspension), freeze-dried preparation of live bacteria of a strain derived from the bacillus of Calmette and Guérin.
Available from health organisations or direct from ImmForm (SSI brand, multidose vial with diluent)

Diagnostic agents

The *Mantoux test* is recommended for tuberculin skin testing, but no licensed preparation is currently available. Guidance for healthcare professionals is available at www.dh.gov.uk/immunisation.

In the Mantoux test, the diagnostic dose is administered by intradermal injection of Tuberculin Purified Protein Derivative (PPD).

The *Heaf test* (involving the use of multiple-puncture apparatus) is no longer available.

Note Response to tuberculin may be suppressed by live viral vaccines, viral infection, sarcoidosis, corticosteroid therapy, or immunosuppression due to disease or treatment. Tuberculin testing should not be carried out within 4 weeks of receiving a live viral vaccine.

Two interferon gamma release assay (IGRA) tests are also available as an aid in the diagnosis of tuberculosis infection: *QuanitFERON®* TB Gold and *T-SPOT®.TB*. Both tests measure T-cell mediated immune response to synthetic antigens. For further information on the use of interferon gamma release assay tests for tuberculosis, see www.hpa.org.uk.

Tuberculin Purified Protein Derivative [PoM] (Tuberculin PPD)

Injection, heat-treated products of growth and lysis of appropriate *Mycobacterium* spp. 20 units/mL (2 units/0.1-mL dose) (for routine use), 1.5-mL vial; 100 units/mL (10 units/0.1-mL dose), 1.5-mL vial
Dose by intradermal injection, for Mantoux test, 2 units (0.1 mL of 20 units/mL strength) for routine Mantoux test; if first test is negative and a further test is considered appropriate 10 units (0.1 mL of 100 units/mL strength)
Available from ImmForm (SSI brand)
Note The strength of tuberculin PPD in this product may be different to the strengths of products used previously for the Mantoux test; care is required to select the correct strength

Botulism antitoxin

A polyvalent botulism antitoxin is available for the post-exposure prophylaxis of botulism and for the treatment of persons thought to be suffering from botulism. It specifically neutralises the toxins produced by *Clostridium botulinum* types A, B, and E. It is not effective against infant botulism as the toxin (type A) is seldom, if ever, found in the blood in this type of infection.

Hypersensitivity reactions are a problem. It is essential to read the contra-indications, warnings, and details of sensitivity tests on the package insert. Prior to treatment checks should be made regarding previous administration of any antitoxin and history of any allergic condition, e.g. asthma, hay fever, etc. All patients should be tested for sensitivity (diluting the antitoxin if history of allergy).

14 **Immunological products and vaccines**

Botulism Antitoxin PoM

A preparation containing the specific antitoxic globulins that have the power of neutralising the toxins formed by types A, B, and E of *Clostridium botulinum*.

Note The BP title Botulinum Antitoxin is not used because the preparation currently in use may have a different specification.

Dose prophylaxis, consult product literature

Available from local designated centres, for details see TOXBASE (requires registration) www.toxbase.org. For supplies outside working hours apply to other designated centres or to the Public Health England Colindale duty doctor (Tel (020) 8200 6868). For major incidents, obtain supplies from the local blood bank

Cholera vaccine

Cholera vaccine (oral) contains inactivated Inaba (including El-Tor biotype) and Ogawa strains of *Vibrio cholerae*, serotype O1 together with recombinant B-subunit of the cholera toxin produced in Inaba strains of *V.cholerae*, serotype O1.

Oral cholera vaccine is licensed for travellers to endemic or epidemic areas on the basis of current recommendations (see also section 14.6). Immunisation should be completed at least 1 week before potential exposure. However, there is no requirement for cholera vaccination for international travel.

Immunisation with cholera vaccine does not provide complete protection and all travellers to a country where cholera exists should be warned that scrupulous attention to food, water, and personal hygiene is **essential**.

Injectable cholera vaccine provides unreliable protection and is no longer available in the UK.

▌CHOLERA VACCINE

Indications see notes above

Cautions see section 14.1 and notes above

Contra-indications see section 14.1; also acute gastro-intestinal illness

Pregnancy see p. 843

Breast-feeding see p. 843

Side-effects see section 14.1; also *rarely* respiratory symptoms such as rhinitis and cough; *very rarely* sore throat, insomnia

Dose

- ADULT and CHILD over 6 years, 2 doses separated by an interval of 1–6 weeks; CHILD 2–6 years, 3 doses each separated by an interval of 1–6 weeks
  Note If more than 6 weeks have elapsed between doses, the primary course should be restarted

- A single booster dose can be given within 2 years after primary course for adults and children over 6 years, and within 6 months after primary course for children 2–6 years. If more than 2 years have elapsed since the last vaccination (more than 6 months for children 2–6 years), the primary course should be repeated
  Counselling Dissolve effervescent sodium bicarbonate granules in a glassful of water *or* chlorinated water (approximately 150 mL). For adults and children over 6 years, add vaccine suspension to make one dose. For child 2–6 years, discard half (approximately 75 mL) of the solution, then add vaccine suspension to make one dose. Drink within 2 hours. Food, drink, and other oral medicines should be avoided for 1 hour before and after vaccination

Dukoral® (Crucell) PoM

Oral suspension, for dilution with solution of effervescent sodium bicarbonate granules, heat- and formaldehyde-inactivated Inaba (including El-Tor biotype) and Ogawa strains of *Vibrio cholerae* bacteria and recombinant cholera toxin B-subunit produced in *V. cholerae*, net price 2-dose pack = £23.42. Counselling, administration

Diphtheria vaccines

Diphtheria vaccines are prepared from the toxin of *Corynebacterium diphtheriae* and adsorption on aluminium hydroxide or aluminium phosphate improves antigenicity. The vaccine stimulates the production of the protective antibody. The quantity of diphtheria toxoid in a preparation determines whether the vaccine is defined as 'high dose' or 'low dose'. Vaccines containing the higher dose of diphtheria toxoid are used for primary immunisation of children under 10 years of age. Vaccines containing the lower dose of diphtheria toxoid are used for primary immunisation in adults and children over 10 years. Single-antigen diphtheria vaccine is not available and adsorbed diphtheria vaccine is given as a combination product containing other vaccines.

For primary immunisation *of children aged between 2 months and 10 years* vaccination is recommended usually in the form of 3 doses (separated by 1-month intervals) of **diphtheria, tetanus, pertussis (acellular, component), poliomyelitis (inactivated) and haemophilus type b conjugate vaccine (adsorbed)** (see Immunisation schedule, section 14.1). In unimmunised individuals aged *over 10 years* the primary course comprises of 3 doses of **adsorbed diphtheria** [low dose], **tetanus and poliomyelitis (inactivated) vaccine**.

A booster dose should be given 3 years after the primary course (this interval can be reduced to a minimum of 1 year if the primary course was delayed). Children *under 10 years* should receive *either* **adsorbed diphtheria, tetanus, pertussis (acellular, component) and poliomyelitis (inactivated) vaccine** *or* **adsorbed diphtheria** [low dose], **tetanus, pertussis (acellular, component) and poliomyelitis (inactivated) vaccine**. Individuals aged *over 10 years* should receive **adsorbed diphtheria** [low dose], **tetanus, and poliomyelitis (inactivated) vaccine**.

A second booster dose, of adsorbed diphtheria [low dose], tetanus and poliomyelitis (inactivated) vaccine, should be given 10 years after the previous booster dose (this interval can be reduced to a minimum of 5 years if previous doses were delayed).

Travel Those intending to travel to areas with a risk of diphtheria infection should be fully immunised according to the UK schedule (see also section 14.6). If more than 10 years have lapsed since completion of the UK schedule, a dose of **adsorbed diphtheria** [low dose], **tetanus and poliomyelitis (inactivated) vaccine** should be administered.

Contacts Staff in contact with diphtheria patients or with potentially pathogenic clinical specimens or working directly with *C. diphtheriae* or *C. ulcerans* should receive a booster dose if fully immunised (with 5 doses of diphtheria-containing vaccine given at appropriate intervals); further doses should be given at 10-year intervals if risk persists. Individuals at risk who are not fully immunised should complete the primary course; a booster dose should be given after 5 years and then at 10-year intervals. **Adsorbed diphtheria** [low dose], **tetanus and poliomyelitis (inactivated) vaccine** is used for this purpose; immunity should be checked by antibody testing at least 3 months after completion of immunisation.

Advice on the management of cases, carriers, contacts and outbreaks must be sought from health protection units. The immunisation history of infected individuals and their contacts should be determined; those who have been incompletely immunised should complete their immunisation and fully immunised individuals should receive a reinforcing dose. For advice on antibacterial treatment to prevent a secondary case of diphtheria in a non-immune individual, see Table 2, section 5.1.

◼ DIPHTHERIA-CONTAINING VACCINES

Indications see notes above

Cautions see section 14.1 and see also individual components of vaccines

Contra-indications see section 14.1 and see also individual components of vaccines

Pregnancy see p. 843

Breast-feeding see p. 843

Side-effects see section 14.1; also restlessness, sleep disturbances, and unusual crying in infants

Dose

• See under preparations

◢ Diphtheria-containing vaccines for children under 10 years

Important For persons aged 10 years or over see Diphtheria-containing Vaccines for Children over 10 years and Adults, below, and see Diphtheria-containing Vaccines for Immunisation of Pregnant Women Against Pertussis, below

Diphtheria, Tetanus, Pertussis (Acellular, Component), Poliomyelitis (Inactivated) and Haemophilus Type b Conjugate Vaccine (Adsorbed) (PoM)

Injection, suspension of diphtheria toxoid, tetanus toxoid, acellular pertussis, inactivated poliomyelitis and *Haemophilus influenzae* type b (conjugated to tetanus protein), net price 0.5-mL prefilled syringe = £32.00

Excipients may include neomycin, polymyxin B and streptomycin

Brands include *Infanrix®-IPV+Hib* and *Pediacel®*; available as part of childhood immunisation schedule from health organisations or ImmForm

Dose by intramuscular injection, CHILD 2 months–10 years, primary immunisation, 3 doses each of 0.5 mL separated by intervals of 1 month; see also notes on booster doses, above

Adsorbed Diphtheria, Tetanus, Pertussis (Acellular, Component) and Poliomyelitis (Inactivated) Vaccine (PoM)

Injection, suspension of diphtheria toxoid, tetanus toxoid, acellular pertussis and inactivated poliomyelitis vaccine components adsorbed on a mineral carrier, net price 0.5-mL prefilled syringe = £17.56

Excipients may include neomycin and polymyxin B

Brands include *Infanrix-IPV®*; available as part of childhood immunisation schedule from health organisations or ImmForm

Dose by intramuscular injection, CHILD 3–10 years, first booster dose 3 years after primary immunisation, 0.5 mL; *see also* notes on booster doses, above

Adsorbed Diphtheria [low dose], Tetanus, Pertussis (Acellular, Component) and Poliomyelitis (Inactivated) Vaccine (PoM)

Injection, suspension of diphtheria toxoid [low dose], tetanus toxoid, acellular pertussis and inactivated poliomyelitis vaccine components adsorbed on a mineral carrier, net price 0.5-mL prefilled syringe = £20.00

Excipients may include neomycin, polymyxin B and streptomycin

Brands include *Repevax®*; available as part of childhood immunisation schedule from health organisations or ImmForm

Dose by intramuscular injection, CHILD 3–10 years, first booster dose 3 years after primary immunisation, 0.5 mL; *see also* notes on booster doses, above

◢ Diphtheria-containing vaccines for children over 10 years and adults

A **low dose** of diphtheria toxoid is sufficient to recall immunity in individuals previously immunised against diphtheria but whose immunity may have diminished with time; it is insufficient to cause serious reactions in an individual who is already immune. Preparations containing low dose diphtheria should be used for adults and children *over 10 years*, for both primary immunisation and booster doses. For immunisation of pregnant women against pertussis see Diphtheria-containing Vaccines for Immunisation of Pregnant Women Against Pertussis, below.

Adsorbed Diphtheria [low dose], Tetanus and Poliomyelitis (Inactivated) Vaccine (PoM)

Injection, suspension of diphtheria toxoid [low dose], tetanus toxoid and inactivated poliomyelitis vaccine components adsorbed on a mineral carrier, net price 0.5-mL prefilled syringe = £6.50

Excipients may include neomycin, polymyxin B and streptomycin

Brands include *Revaxis®*; available as part of immunisation schedule from health organisations or ImmForm

Dose by intramuscular injection, ADULT and CHILD over 10 years, primary immunisation, 3 doses each of 0.5 mL separated by intervals of 1 month; second booster dose, 0.5 mL given 10 years after first booster dose (may also be used as first booster dose in those over 10 years who have received only 3 previous doses of a diphtheria-containing vaccine); see also notes on booster doses and contacts, above

◢ Diphtheria-containing vaccines for immunisation of pregnant women against pertussis

For immunisation of children over 10 years and adults against diphtheria see Diphtheria-containing Vaccines for Children over 10 years and Adults, above

Adsorbed Diphtheria [low dose], Tetanus, Pertussis (Acellular, Component) and Poliomyelitis (Inactivated) Vaccine (PoM)

Injection, suspension of diphtheria toxoid [low dose], tetanus toxoid, acellular pertussis and inactivated poliomyelitis vaccine components adsorbed on a mineral carrier, net price 0.5-mL prefilled syringe = £16.32

Excipients may include neomycin, polymyxin B

Brands include *Boostrix-IPV®*; available from Immform

Contra-indications section 14.1; see also individual components of vaccine; also pregnant women with a history of encephalopathy of unknown origin within 7 days of previous immunisation with a pertussis-containing vaccine, pregnant women with a history of transient thrombocytopenia or neurological complications following previous immunisation against diphtheria or tetanus

Dose Vaccination of pregnant women against pertussis (see p. 859), by intramuscular injection, 0.5 mL as a single dose

◢**Diphtheria antitoxin**

Diphtheria antitoxin is used for passive immunisation in suspected cases of diphtheria only (without waiting for bacteriological confirmation); tests for hypersensitivity should be first carried out. It is derived from horse serum, and reactions are common after administration; resuscitation facilities should be available immediately.

It is no longer used for prophylaxis because of the risk of hypersensitivity; unimmunised contacts should be promptly investigated and given antibacterial prophylaxis (section 5.1, table 2) and vaccine (see Contacts above).

Diphtheria Antitoxin PoM
Dip/Ser
Dose prophylaxis, not recommended therefore no dose stated (see notes above)
Treatment, consult product literature
Available from Centre for Infections (Tel (020) 8200 6868) or in Northern Ireland from Public Health Laboratory, Belfast City Hospital (Tel (028) 9032 9241)

Haemophilus type b conjugate vaccine

Haemophilus influenzae type b (Hib) vaccine is made from capsular polysaccharide; it is conjugated with a protein such as tetanus toxoid to increase immunogenicity, especially in young children. Haemophilus influenzae type b vaccine immunisation is given in combination with diphtheria, tetanus, pertussis (acellular, component) and poliomyelitis (inactivated) vaccine, as a component of the primary course of childhood immunisation (see Immunisation schedule, section 14.1) (see under Diphtheria-containing Vaccines). For infants under 1 year, the course consists of 3 doses of a vaccine containing *Haemophilus influenzae* type b component with an interval of 1 month between doses. A booster dose of haemophilus influenzae type b vaccine (combined with meningococcal group C conjugate vaccine) should be given at 12–13 months of age.

Children 1–10 years who have not been immunised against *Haemophilus influenzae* type b need to receive only 1 dose of Haemophilus influenzae type b vaccine (combined with meningococcal group C conjugate vaccine). However, if a primary course of immunisation has not been completed, these children should be given 3 doses of diphtheria, tetanus, pertussis (acellular, component), poliomyelitis (inactivated) and haemophilus type b conjugate vaccine (adsorbed). The risk of infection falls sharply in older children and the vaccine is not normally required for children over 10 years.

Haemophilus influenzae type b vaccine may be given to those over 10 years who are considered to be at increased risk of invasive *H. influenzae* type b disease (such as those with sickle-cell disease or complement deficiency, or those receiving treatment for malignancy).

Invasive *Haemophilus influenzae* type b disease
After recovery from infection, unimmunised and partially immunised index cases under 10 years of age should complete their age-specific course of immunisation. Previously vaccinated cases under 10 years of age should be given an additional dose of haemophilus influenzae type b vaccine (combined with meningococcal group C conjugate vaccine) if Hib antibody concentrations are low or if it is not possible to measure antibody concentrations. Index cases of any age with asplenia or splenic dysfunction should complete their immunisation according to the recommendations below; fully vaccinated cases with asplenia or splenic dysfunction should be given an additional dose of haemophilus influenzae type b vaccine (combined with meningococcal group C conjugate vaccine) if they received their previous dose over 1 year ago.

For use of rifampicin in the prevention of secondary cases of *Haemophilus influenzae* type b disease, see Table 2, section 5.1.

Asplenia, splenic dysfunction or complement deficiency Individuals diagnosed with asplenia, splenic dysfunction, or complement deficiency at:

● *under 2 years of age* should be vaccinated according to the Immunisation Schedule (section 14.1). The booster dose of haemophilus influenzae type b vaccine (combined with meningococcal group C conjugate vaccine), given at 12–13 months of age, should be followed at least 1 month later by one dose of meningococcal A, C, W135, and Y conjugate vaccine. An additional dose of haemophilus influenzae type b vaccine (combined with meningococcal group C conjugate vaccine) should be given after the second birthday;

● *over 2 years of age* should receive one dose of haemophilus influenzae type b vaccine (combined with meningococcal group C conjugate vaccine), followed 1 month later by one dose of meningococcal A, C, W135, and Y conjugate vaccine.

▇ **HAEMOPHILUS TYPE B CONJUGATE VACCINE**

Indications see notes above
Cautions see section 14.1
Contra-indications see section 14.1
Pregnancy see p. 843
Breast-feeding see p. 843
Side-effects see section 14.1; also atopic dermatitis, hypotonia
Dose
● Primary immunisation, see under Diphtheria
● Booster dose, see notes above and under preparation below

Menitorix® (GSK) PoM
Injection, powder for reconstitution, capsular polysaccharide of *Haemophilus influenzae* type b and capsular polysaccharide of *Neisseria meningitidis* group C (both conjugated to tetanus protein), net price single-dose vial (with syringe containing 0.5 mL diluent) = £37.76
Dose by intramuscular injection, CHILD 1–10 years, 0.5 mL
ADULT and CHILD over 1 year, with asplenia or splenic dysfunction (see notes above), 0.5 mL
Available as part of the childhood immunisation schedule from ImmForm

◢**Combined vaccines**
See also under Diphtheria-containing Vaccines

Hepatitis A vaccine

Hepatitis A vaccine is prepared from formaldehyde-inactivated hepatitis A virus grown in human diploid cells.

14 Immunological products and vaccines

Immunisation is recommended for:

- laboratory staff who work directly with the virus;
- staff and residents of homes for those with severe learning difficulties;
- workers at risk of exposure to untreated sewage;
- individuals who work with primates;
- patients with haemophilia or other conditions treated with plasma-derived clotting factors;
- patients with severe liver disease;
- travellers to high-risk areas (see p. 872);
- individuals who are at risk due to their sexual behaviour;
- parenteral drug abusers.

Immunisation should be considered for:

- patients with chronic liver disease including chronic hepatitis B or chronic hepatitis C;
- prevention of secondary cases in close contacts of confirmed cases of hepatitis A, within 14 days of exposure to the primary case (within 8 weeks of exposure to the primary case where there is more than 1 contact in the household).

A booster dose is usually given 6–12 months after the initial dose. A second booster dose can be given 20 years after the previous booster dose to those who continue to be at risk. Specialist advice should be sought on re-immunisation of immunocompromised individuals.

For rapid protection against hepatitis A after exposure or during an outbreak, in adults a single dose of a monovalent vaccine is recommended; for children under 16 years, a single dose of the combined vaccine *Ambirix*® can also be used.

Intramuscular **normal immunoglobulin** (section 14.5.1) is recommended for use in addition to Hepatitis A vaccine for close contacts (of confirmed cases of hepatitis A) who have chronic liver disease or HIV infection, or who are immunosuppressed or over 50 years of age.

Post-exposure prophylaxis is not required for healthy children under 1 year of age, so long as all those involved in nappy changing are vaccinated against hepatitis A. However, children 2–12 months of age can be given a dose of hepatitis A vaccine if it is not possible to vaccinate their carers, or if the child becomes a source of infection to others [unlicensed use]; in these cases, if the child goes on to require long-term protection against hepatitis A after the first birthday, the full course of 2 doses should be given.

▌ HEPATITIS A VACCINE

Indications   immunisation against hepatitis A infection
Cautions   see section 14.1
Contra-indications   see section 14.1
Pregnancy   see p. 843
Breast-feeding   see p. 843
Side-effects   see section 14.1; for combination vaccines, see also Typhoid vaccine, p. 864
Dose

- See under preparations

◢ Single component

Avaxim® (Sanofi Pasteur) ⒫ⓄⓂ
Injection, suspension of formaldehyde-inactivated hepatitis A virus (GBM grown in human diploid cells) 320 antigen units/mL adsorbed onto aluminium hydroxide, net price 0.5-mL prefilled syringe = £18.10
Excipients   include neomycin
Dose   by intramuscular injection (see note below), ADULT and CHILD over 16 years, 0.5 mL as a single dose; booster dose 0.5 mL 6–12 months after initial dose
Note   Booster dose may be delayed by up to 3 years if not given after recommended interval following primary dose with *Avaxim*®. The deltoid region is the preferred site of injection. The subcutaneous route may be used for patients with bleeding disorders; not to be injected into the buttock (vaccine efficacy reduced)

Epaxal® (Crucell) ⒫ⓄⓂ
Injection, suspension of formaldehyde-inactivated hepatitis A virus (RG-SB grown in human diploid cells) at least 48 units/mL, net price 0.5-mL prefilled syringe = £23.81
Dose   by intramuscular injection (see note below), ADULT and CHILD over 1 year, 0.5 mL as a single dose; booster dose 0.5 mL 6–12 months after initial dose (1–6 months if splenectomised)
Note   Booster dose may be delayed by up to 4 years in adults if not given after recommended interval following primary dose. The deltoid region is the preferred site of injection. The subcutaneous route may be used for patients with bleeding disorders
Important   *Epaxal*® contains influenza virus haemagglutinin grown in the allantoic cavity of chick embryos, therefore contra-indicated in those hypersensitive to eggs or chicken protein.

Havrix Monodose® (GSK) ⒫ⓄⓂ
Injection, suspension of formaldehyde-inactivated hepatitis A virus (HM 175 grown in human diploid cells) 1440 ELISA units/mL adsorbed onto aluminium hydroxide, net price 1-mL prefilled syringe = £22.14, 0.5-mL (720 ELISA units) prefilled syringe (*Havrix Junior Monodose*®) = £16.77
Excipients   include neomycin
Dose   by intramuscular injection (see note below), ADULT and CHILD over 16 years, 1 mL as a single dose; booster dose, 1 mL 6–12 months after initial dose; CHILD 1–15 years 0.5 mL; booster dose, 0.5 mL 6–12 months after initial dose
Note   Booster dose may be delayed by up to 3 years if not given after recommended interval following primary dose with *Havrix Monodose*®. The deltoid region is the preferred site of injection. The subcutaneous route may be used for patients with bleeding disorders

Vaqta® **Paediatric** (Sanofi Pasteur) ⒫ⓄⓂ
Injection, suspension of formaldehyde-inactivated hepatitis A virus (grown in human diploid cells) 50 antigen units/mL adsorbed onto aluminium hydroxyphosphate sulfate, net price 0.5-mL prefilled syringe = £14.74
Excipients   include neomycin
Dose   by intramuscular injection (see note below) CHILD 1–17 years, 0.5 mL as a single dose; booster dose 0.5 mL 6–18 months after initial dose; under 1 year, not recommended
Note   The deltoid region is the preferred site of injection. The subcutaneous route may be used for patients with bleeding disorders (but immune response may be reduced)

14   Immunological products and vaccines

Vaqta® Adult (Sanofi Pasteur) [PoM]

Injection, suspension of formaldehyde-inactivated hepatitis A virus (grown in human diploid cells) 50 antigen units/mL adsorbed onto aluminium hydroxyphosphate sulfate, net price 1-mL prefilled syringe = £18.10

Excipients include neomycin

Dose by intramuscular injection (see note below), ADULT over 18 years, 1 mL as a single dose; booster dose 1 mL 6–18 months after initial dose

Note The deltoid region is the preferred site of injection. The subcutaneous route may be used for patients with bleeding disorders (but immune response may be delayed)

◀**With hepatitis B vaccine**

Ambirix® (GSK) [PoM]

Injection, suspension of inactivated hepatitis A virus (grown in human diploid cells) 720 ELISA units/mL adsorbed onto aluminium hydroxide, and recombinant (DNA) hepatitis B surface antigen (grown in yeast cells) 20 micrograms/mL adsorbed onto aluminium phosphate, net price 1-mL prefilled syringe = £31.18

Excipients include neomycin

Dose CHILD 1–15 years, by intramuscular injection (see note below); primary course, 2 doses of 1 mL, the second 6–12 months after initial dose

Note Primary course should be completed with *Ambirix®* (single component vaccines given at appropriate intervals may be used for booster dose); the deltoid region is the preferred site of injection in older children; anterolateral thigh is the preferred site in infants; not to be injected into the buttock (vaccine efficacy reduced); subcutaneous route used for patients with bleeding disorders (but immune response may be reduced)

Important *Ambirix®* is **not** recommended for post-exposure prophylaxis following percutaneous (needle-stick), ocular, or mucous membrane exposure to hepatitis B virus

Twinrix® (GSK) [PoM]

Injection, inactivated hepatitis A virus (grown in human diploid cells) 720 ELISA units/mL adsorbed onto aluminium hydroxide and recombinant (DNA) hepatitis B surface antigen (grown in yeast cells) 20 micrograms/mL adsorbed onto aluminium phosphate, net price 1-mL prefilled syringe (*Twinrix® Adult*) = £33.31, 1-mL vial (*Twinrix® Adult*) = £26.44, 0.5-mL prefilled syringe (*Twinrix® Paediatric*) = £20.79

Excipients include neomycin

Dose by intramuscular injection (see note below); ADULT and CHILD over 16 years, primary course of 3 doses of 1 mL (*Twinrix® Adult*), the second 1 month and the third 6 months after the first dose; CHILD 1–15 years, 3 doses of 0.5 mL (*Twinrix® Paediatric*)

Accelerated schedule (e.g. for travellers departing within 1 month), ADULT over 16 years, second dose 7 days and third dose 21 days after the first dose, and fourth dose 12 months after the first dose

Note Primary course should be completed with *Twinrix®* (single component vaccines given at appropriate intervals may be used for booster dose); the deltoid region is the preferred site of injection in adults and older children; anterolateral thigh is preferred site in infants; not to be injected into the buttock (vaccine efficacy reduced); subcutaneous route used for patients with bleeding disorders (but immune response may be reduced).

Important *Twinrix®* **not** recommended for post-exposure prophylaxis following percutaneous (needle-stick), ocular or mucous membrane exposure to hepatitis B virus.

◀**With typhoid vaccine**

Hepatyrix® (GSK) [PoM]

Injection, suspension of inactivated hepatitis A virus (grown in human diploid cells) 1440 ELISA units/mL adsorbed onto aluminium hydroxide, combined with typhoid vaccine containing 25 micrograms/mL virulence polysaccharide antigen of *Salmonella typhi*, net price 1-mL prefilled syringe = £32.08

Excipients include neomycin

Note May be difficult to obtain

Dose by intramuscular injection (see note below), ADULT and CHILD over 15 years, 1 mL as a single dose; booster doses, see under single component hepatitis A vaccine (above) and under polysaccharide typhoid vaccine, p. 864

Note The deltoid region is the preferred site of injection. The subcutaneous route may be used for patients with bleeding disorders; not to be injected into the buttock (vaccine efficacy reduced)

ViATIM® (Sanofi Pasteur) [PoM]

Injection, suspension of inactivated hepatitis A virus (grown in human diploid cells) 160 antigen units/mL adsorbed onto aluminium hydroxide, combined with typhoid vaccine containing 25 micrograms/mL virulence polysaccharide antigen of *Salmonella typhi*, net price 1-mL prefilled syringe = £29.80

Excipients include neomycin

Dose by intramuscular injection (see note below), ADULT and CHILD over 16 years, 1 mL as a single dose; booster doses, see under single component hepatitis A vaccine (above) and under polysaccharide typhoid vaccine, p. 864

Note The deltoid region is the preferred site of injection. The subcutaneous route may be used for patients with bleeding disorders; not to be injected into the buttock (vaccine efficacy reduced)

Hepatitis B vaccine

Hepatitis B vaccine contains inactivated hepatitis B virus surface antigen (HBsAg) adsorbed onto aluminium hydroxide adjuvant. It is made biosynthetically using recombinant DNA technology. The vaccine is used in individuals at high risk of contracting hepatitis B.

In the UK, groups at high-risk of hepatitis B include:

- parenteral drug misusers, their sexual partners, and household contacts; other drug misusers who are likely to 'progress' to injecting;

- individuals who change sexual partners frequently;

- close family contacts of a case or individual with chronic hepatitis B infection;

- babies whose mothers have had acute hepatitis B during pregnancy *or* are positive for hepatitis B surface antigen (regardless of e-antigen markers); hepatitis B vaccination is started immediately on delivery and *hepatitis B immunoglobulin* (see p. 869) given at the same time (but preferably at a different site). Babies whose mothers are positive for hepatitis B surface antigen and for e-antigen antibody should receive the vaccine only (but babies weighing 1.5 kg or less should also receive the immunoglobulin regardless of the mother's e-antigen antibody status);

- individuals with haemophilia, those receiving regular blood transfusions or blood products, and carers responsible for the administration of such products;

- patients with chronic renal failure including those on haemodialysis. Haemodialysis patients should be monitored for antibodies annually and re-immunised if necessary. Home carers (of dialysis patients) should be vaccinated;

- individuals with chronic liver disease;

- healthcare personnel (including trainees) who have direct contact with blood or blood-stained body fluids or with patients' tissues;

- laboratory staff who handle material that may contain the virus;

- other occupational risk groups such as morticians and embalmers;

- staff and patients of day-care or residential accommodation for those with severe learning difficulties;

- staff and inmates of custodial institutions;

- those travelling to areas of high or intermediate prevalence who are at increased risk or who plan to remain there for lengthy periods (see p. 872);

- families adopting children from countries with a high or intermediate prevalence of hepatitis B;

- foster carers and their families.

Different immunisation schedules for hepatitis B vaccine are recommended for specific circumstances (see under individual preparations). Generally, three or four doses are required for primary immunisation; an 'accelerated schedule' is recommended for pre-exposure prophylaxis in high-risk groups where rapid protection is required, and for post-exposure prophylaxis (see below).

Immunisation may take up to 6 months to confer adequate protection; the duration of immunity is not known precisely, but a single booster 5 years after the primary course may be sufficient to maintain immunity for those who continue to be at risk.

Immunisation does not eliminate the need for commonsense precautions for avoiding the risk of infection from known carriers by the routes of infection which have been clearly established, consult *Guidance for Clinical Health Care Workers: Protection against Infection with Blood-borne Viruses* (available at www.dh.gov.uk). Accidental inoculation of hepatitis B virus-infected blood into a wound, incision, needle-prick, or abrasion may lead to infection, whereas it is unlikely that indirect exposure to a carrier will do so.

Following significant exposure to hepatitis B, an accelerated schedule, with the second dose given 1 month, and the third dose 2 months after the first dose, is recommended. For those at continued risk, a fourth dose should be given 12 months after the first dose. More detailed guidance is given in the handbook *Immunisation against Infectious Disease* see p. 842.

Specific **hepatitis B immunoglobulin** ('HBIG') is available for use with the vaccine in those accidentally inoculated and in neonates at special risk of infection (section 14.5.2).

A combined hepatitis A and hepatitis B vaccine is also available.

■ HEPATITIS B VACCINE

Indications immunisation against hepatitis B infection
Cautions see section 14.1

Contra-indications see section 14.1
Pregnancy see p. 843
Breast-feeding see p. 843
Side-effects see section 14.1
Dose
- See under preparations

◢Single component

Engerix B® (GSK) ꟼoM

Injection, suspension of hepatitis B surface antigen (prepared from yeast cells by recombinant DNA technique) 20 micrograms/mL adsorbed onto aluminium hydroxide, net price 0.5-mL (paediatric) pre-filled syringe = £9.67, 1-mL vial = £12.34, 1-mL pre-filled syringe = £12.99

Dose by intramuscular injection (see note below), ADULT and CHILD over 16 years, 3 doses of 20 micrograms, the second 1 month and the third 6 months after the first dose; NEONATE (except if born to hepatitis B surface antigen positive mother, see below) and CHILD 1 month–16 years, 3 doses of 10 micrograms

Accelerated schedule (all ages), second dose 1 month after first dose, third dose 2 months after first dose and fourth dose 12 months after first dose; *exceptionally* (e.g. for travellers departing within 1 month), ADULT over 18 years, second dose 7 days after first dose, third dose 21 days after first dose, and fourth dose 12 months after first dose

Alternative schedule for CHILD 11–15 years, 2 doses of 20 micrograms, the second dose 6 months after the first dose (this schedule not suitable if high risk of infection between doses or if compliance with second dose uncertain)

NEONATE born to hepatitis B surface antigen-positive mother (see also notes above), 4 doses of 10 micrograms, first dose at birth with hepatitis B immunoglobulin injection (separate site) the second 1 month, the third 2 months and the fourth 12 months after the first dose

Renal insufficiency (including haemodialysis patients), by intramuscular injection (see note below), ADULT and CHILD over 16 years, 4 doses of 40 micrograms, the second 1 month, the third 2 months and the fourth 6 months after the first dose; immunisation schedule and booster doses may need to be adjusted in those with low antibody concentration; NEONATE (except if born to hepatitis B surface antigen positive mother, see above) and CHILD 1 month–16 years 3 doses of 10 micrograms, second dose 1 month and third dose 6 months after first dose *or* accelerated schedule, 4 doses of 10 micrograms, second dose 1 month, third dose 2 months and fourth dose 12 months after first dose; immunisation schedule and booster doses may need to be adjusted in those with low antibody concentration

Note Deltoid muscle is preferred site of injection in adults and older children; anterolateral thigh is preferred site in neonates, infants and young children; not to be injected into the buttock (vaccine efficacy reduced)

Fendrix® (GSK) ꟼoM

Injection, suspension of hepatitis B surface antigen (prepared from yeast cells by recombinant DNA technique) 40 micrograms/mL adsorbed onto aluminium phosphate, net price 0.5-mL prefilled syringe = £38.10

Excipients include traces of thiomersal

Dose ADULT and CHILD over 15 years with renal insufficiency (including pre-haemodialysis and haemodialysis patients), by intramuscular injection (see note below) 4 doses of 20 micrograms, the second 1 month, the third 2 months and the fourth 6 months after the first dose; immunisation schedule and booster doses may need to be adjusted in those with low antibody concentration

Note Deltoid muscle is preferred site of injection; not to be injected into the buttock (vaccine efficacy reduced)

HBvaxPRO® (Sanofi Pasteur) [PoM]

Injection, suspension of hepatitis B surface antigen (prepared from yeast cells by recombinant DNA technique) 10 micrograms/mL adsorbed onto aluminium hydroxyphosphate sulfate, net price 0.5-mL (5-microgram) prefilled syringe = £8.95, 1-mL (10-microgram) prefilled syringe = £12.20; 40 micrograms/mL, 1-mL (40-microgram) vial = £27.60

Dose by intramuscular injection (see note below), ADULT and CHILD over 16 years, 3 doses of 10 micrograms, the second 1 month and the third 6 months after the first dose; CHILD under 16 years, 3 doses of 5 micrograms

Accelerated schedule (all ages), second dose 1 month after first dose, third dose 2 months after first dose with fourth dose at 12 months

Booster doses may be required in immunocompromised patients with low antibody concentration

NEONATE born to hepatitis B surface antigen-positive mother (see also notes above), 4 doses of 5 micrograms, first dose at birth with hepatitis B immunoglobulin injection (separate site), the second 1 month, the third 2 months and the fourth 12 months after the first dose

Chronic haemodialysis patients, by intramuscular injection (see note below) 3 doses of 40 micrograms, the second 1 month and the third 6 months after the first dose; booster doses may be required in those with low antibody concentration

Note Deltoid muscle is preferred site of injection in adults and older children; anterolateral thigh is preferred site in neonates and infants; not to be injected into the buttock (vaccine efficacy reduced)

◢**With hepatitis A vaccine**

See Hepatitis A Vaccine

Human papillomavirus vaccines

Human papillomavirus vaccine is available as a bivalent vaccine (*Cervarix*®) or a quadrivalent vaccine (*Gardasil*®). *Cervarix*® is licensed for use in females for the prevention of cervical cancer and other pre-cancerous lesions caused by human papillomavirus types 16 and 18. *Gardasil*® is licensed for use in females for the prevention of cervical and anal cancers, genital warts, and pre-cancerous genital (cervical, vulvar, and vaginal) and anal lesions caused by human papillomavirus types 6, 11, 16, and 18. The vaccines may also provide limited protection against disease caused by other types of human papillomavirus. The two vaccines are not interchangeable and one vaccine product should be used for an entire course.

Human papillomavirus vaccine will be most effective if given before sexual activity starts. From September 2014, a 2-dose schedule is recommended, as long as the first dose is received before the age of 15 years. The first dose is given to females aged 11 to 14 years, and the second dose is given 6–24 months after the first dose (for the purposes of planning the national immunisation programme, it is appropriate to give the second dose 12 months after the first—see Immunisation schedule, section 14.1). If the course is interrupted, it should be resumed (using the same vaccine) but not repeated, even if more than 24 months have elapsed since the first dose or if the girl is then aged 15 years or more. Females receiving their first dose aged 15 years or older require a 3-dose schedule (see *Cervarix*® and *Gardasil*®), with the second and third doses given 1 and 4–6 months after the first dose; all 3 doses should be given within a 12-month period. If the course is interrupted, it should be resumed (using the same vaccine) but not repeated, allowing the appropriate interval between the remaining doses. If a 3-dose course of vaccination has been started before September 2014, then where possible this should be completed; if the course is interrupted, it should be resumed (using the same vaccine) but not repeated, allowing the appropriate interval between the remaining doses. Under the national programme in England, females remain eligible to receive the vaccine up to the age of 18 years if they did not receive the vaccine when scheduled. Where appropriate, immunisation with human papillomavirus vaccine should be offered to females coming into the UK as they may not have been offered protection in their country of origin. The duration of protection has not been established, but current studies suggest that protection is maintained for at least 6 years after completion of the primary course.

As the vaccines do not protect against all strains of human papillomavirus, routine cervical screening should continue.

◼ HUMAN PAPILLOMAVIRUS VACCINES

Indications see notes above and under preparations

Cautions see section 14.1

Contra-indications see section 14.1

Pregnancy not known to be harmful, but vaccination should be postponed until completion of pregnancy

Breast-feeding see p. 843

Side-effects see section 14.1

Dose
- See notes above and under preparations

Note To avoid confusion, prescribers should specify the brand to be dispensed

Cervarix® (GSK) [PoM]

Injection, suspension of virus-like particles of human papillomavirus type 16 (40 micrograms/mL), type 18 (40 micrograms/mL) capsid protein (prepared by recombinant DNA technique using a Baculovirus expression system) in monophosphoryl lipid A adjuvant adsorbed onto aluminium hydroxide, net price 0.5-mL prefilled syringe = £80.50

Dose prevention of premalignant genital lesions and cervical cancer, by intramuscular injection into deltoid region, ADULT and CHILD over 15 years, 3 doses of 0.5 mL, the second 1–2.5 months, and the third 5–12 months after the first dose; CHILD 9–14 years, 2 doses of 0.5 mL, the second 5–7 months after the first dose (if second dose administered earlier than 5 months after the first, a third dose should be administered)

Gardasil® (Sanofi Pasteur) [PoM]

Injection, suspension of virus-like particles of human papillomavirus type 6 (40 micrograms/mL), type 11 (80 micrograms/mL), type 16 (80 micrograms/mL), type 18 (40 micrograms/mL) capsid protein (prepared from yeast cells by recombinant DNA technique) adsorbed onto aluminium hydroxyphosphate sulfate, net price 0.5-mL prefilled syringe = £86.50

Dose prevention of premalignant genital (cervical, vulvar, and vaginal) and anal lesions, cervical and anal cancers, and genital warts, by intramuscular injection preferably into deltoid region or higher anterolateral thigh, ADULT and CHILD over 9 years, 3 doses of 0.5 mL, the second at least 1 month after the first dose, and the third at least 3 months after the second dose, schedule should be completed within 12 months after the first dose; alternative schedule for CHILD 9–13 years, 2 doses of 0.5 mL, the second 6 months after the first dose (if administered earlier than 6 months, a third dose should be administered)

Influenza vaccines

While most viruses are antigenically stable, the influenza viruses A and B (especially A) are constantly altering their antigenic structure as indicated by changes in the haemagglutinins (H) and neuraminidases (N) on the surface of the viruses. It is essential that influenza vaccines in use contain the H and N components of the prevalent strain or strains as recommended each year by the World Health Organization.

Immunisation is recommended *for persons at high risk*, and to reduce transmission of infection. Annual immunisation is strongly recommended for individuals aged over 6 months with the following conditions:

- chronic respiratory disease (includes asthma treated with continuous or repeated use of inhaled or systemic corticosteroids or asthma with previous exacerbations requiring hospital admission);
- chronic heart disease;
- chronic liver disease;
- chronic renal disease;
- chronic neurological disease;
- diabetes mellitus;
- immunosuppression because of disease (including asplenia or splenic dysfunction) or treatment (including prolonged systemic corticosteroid treatment [for over 1 month at dose equivalents of prednisolone: *adult and child over 20 kg*, 20 mg or more daily; *child under 20 kg*, 1 mg/kg or more daily] and chemotherapy);
- HIV infection (regardless of immune status).

Seasonal influenza vaccine is also recommended for all pregnant women, for all persons aged over 65 years, for residents of nursing or residential homes for the elderly and other long-stay facilities, and for carers of persons whose welfare may be at risk if the carer falls ill. Influenza immunisation should also be considered for household contacts of immunocompromised individuals.

As part of winter planning, NHS employers should offer vaccination to healthcare workers who are directly involved in patient care. Employers of social care workers should consider similar action.

Unless contra-indicated, the live influenza vaccine, *Fluenz Tetra*®, is preferred in children aged 2–18 years because it provides a higher level of protection than inactivated influenza vaccine. From 1 September 2014, seasonal influenza vaccine will be offered to all children aged 2–4 years (i.e. those born between 2 September 2009 and 1 September 2012).

Information on pandemic influenza, avian influenza and swine influenza may be found at www.dh.gov.uk/pandemicflu and at www.phe.org.uk.

◢ INFLUENZA VACCINES

Indications   annual immunisation against seasonal influenza

Cautions   see section 14.1; increased risk of fever in child under 5 years with *Inflexal*® *V*, and in child 5–9 years with *Enzira*® or preparations marketed by Pfizer or CSL Biotherapies

Contra-indications   see section 14.1 and also *Fluenz Tetra*® below; avoid *Enzira*® or preparations marketed by Pfizer, or CSL Biotherapies in child under 5 years—increased risk of febrile convulsions

Pregnancy   see section 14.1; inactivated vaccines not known to be harmful; avoid *Fluenz Tetra*®

Breast-feeding   see section 14.1; inactivated vaccines not known to be harmful; avoid *Fluenz Tetra*®

Side-effects   see section 14.1; also reported vasculitis, febrile convulsions and transient thrombocytopenia; *with intranasal spray*, rhinorrhoea and *less commonly* epistaxis

Dose

- By intramuscular injection, ADULT and CHILD over 9 years, 0.5 mL as a single dose; CHILD 6 months–9 years, 0.5 mL; for children 6 months to 9 years who have not received seasonal influenza vaccine previously, repeat after at least 4 weeks
- By intradermal injection, see under *Intanza*® below
- Intranasally, see under *Fluenz Tetra*® below

◢ Trivalent seasonal influenza vaccines for intramuscular use

Inactivated Influenza Vaccine (Split Virion) [PoM]
Flu
Injection, suspension of formaldehyde-inactivated influenza virus (split virion grown in fertilised hens' egg's), net price 0.25-mL prefilled syringe = £6.29; 0.5-mL prefilled syringe = £6.59
Excipients   may include neomycin and polymyxin
Available from Sanofi Pasteur
Cautions   increased risk of fever in child 5–9 years with preparations marketed by Pfizer or CSL Biotherapies—use alternative influenza vaccine if available
Contra-indications   avoid preparations marketed by Pfizer or CSL Biotherapies in child under 5 years—increased risk of febrile convulsions

Inactivated Influenza Vaccine (Surface Antigen) [PoM]
Flu or Flu(adj)
Injection, suspension of propiolactone-inactivated influenza virus (surface antigen, grown in fertilised hens' eggs), net price 0.5-mL prefilled syringe = £4.15
Excipients   may include neomycin and polymyxin B, and traces of thiomersal
Available from Novartis Vaccines
Note   Not licensed for children under 4 years

Agrippal® (Novartis Vaccines) [PoM]
Injection, suspension of formaldehyde-inactivated influenza virus (surface antigen, grown in fertilised hens' eggs), net price 0.5-mL prefilled syringe = £5.85
Excipients   include kanamycin and neomycin

Enzira® (Pfizer) [PoM]
Injection, suspension of inactivated influenza virus (split virion, grown in fertilised hens' eggs), net price 0.5-mL prefilled syringe = £5.25
Excipients   include neomycin and polymyxin B
Cautions   child 5–9 years (increased risk of fever)—use alternative influenza vaccine if available
Contra-indications   child under 5 years—increased risk of febrile convulsions

Fluarix® (GSK) [PoM]
Injection, suspension of formaldehyde-inactivated influenza virus (split virion, grown in fertilised hens' eggs), net price 0.5-mL prefilled syringe = £5.39
Excipients   include gentamicin
Note   Ovalbumin content less than 100 nanograms/mL

Fluvirin® (Novartis Vaccines) [PoM]
Injection, suspension of formaldehyde-inactivated influenza virus (surface antigen, grown in fertilised hens' eggs), net price 0.5-mL prefilled syringe = £5.55
Excipients   include neomycin, polymyxin B, and traces of thiomersal
Note   Not licensed for use in children under 4 years

Imuvac® (Abbott Healthcare) [PoM]

Injection, suspension of formaldehyde-inactivated influenza virus (surface antigen, grown in fertilised hens' eggs), net price 0.5-mL prefilled syringe = £6.59

Excipients include gentamicin

Influvac Desu® (Abbott Healthcare) [PoM]

Injection, suspension of formaldehyde-inactivated influenza virus (surface antigen, grown in fertilised hens' eggs), net price 0.5-mL prefilled syringe = £5.22

Excipients include gentamicin

Optaflu® (Novartis Vaccines) [PoM]

Injection, suspension of inactivated influenza virus (surface antigen, grown in canine kidney cells), net price 0.5-mL prefilled syringe = £6.59

Note Not licensed for use in children and adolescents under 18 years

◢**Tetravalent seasonal influenza vaccine for intramuscular use**

Fluarix Tetra® (GSK) ▼ [PoM]

Injection, suspension of formaldehyde-inactivated influenza virus (split virion, grown in fertilised hens' eggs) net price 0.5-mL prefilled syringe = £9.94

Excipients include gentamicin

Note Ovalbumin content less than 100 nanograms/mL

Note Not licensed for use in children under 3 years of age

◢**Trivalent seasonal influenza vaccine for intradermal use**

Intanza® (Sanofi Pasteur) [PoM]

Injection, suspension of formaldehyde-inactivated influenza virus (split virion, grown in fertilised hens' eggs), net price, prefilled syringe, 9 micrograms (0.1 mL) = £9.05; prefilled syringe, 15 micrograms (0.1 mL) = £9.05

Excipients include neomycin

Dose by intradermal injection into deltoid region, ADULT 18–60 years, 9 micrograms as a single dose; ADULT over 60 years, 15 micrograms as a single dose

◢**Tetravalent seasonal influenza vaccine for intranasal use**

Fluenz Tetra® (AstraZeneca) ▼ [PoM]

Nasal spray, suspension of live, attenuated influenza virus (produced in vero cells and grown in fertilised hens' eggs), net price 0.2 mL nasal applicator = £14.00

Excipients include gelatin and gentamicin

Contra-indications see section 14.1; also severe asthma, active wheezing; avoid close contact with severely immunocompromised patients for 1–2 weeks after vaccination; concomitant use with antiviral therapy for influenza (avoid antiviral for at least 2 weeks after *Fluenz Tetra®*; avoid *Fluenz Tetra®* for at least 48 hours after stopping the antiviral); concomitant use with salicylates in children

Dose CHILD 2–18 years, 0.1 mL into each nostril as a single dose; for children 2–9 years in the clinical risk groups, who have not received seasonal influenza vaccine previously, repeat after at least 4 weeks

Japanese encephalitis vaccine

Japanese encephalitis vaccine is indicated for travellers to areas in Asia and the Far East where infection is endemic and for laboratory staff at risk of exposure to the virus. The primary immunisation course of 2 doses should be completed at least one week before potential exposure to Japanese encephalitis virus.

Up-to-date information on the risk of Japanese encephalitis in specific countries can be obtained from the National Travel Health Network and Centre (www.nathnac.org)

◢ **JAPANESE ENCEPHALITIS VACCINE**

Indications immunisation against Japanese encephalitis

Cautions see section 14.1

Contra-indications see section 14.1

Pregnancy although manufacturer advises avoid because of limited information, miscarriage has been associated with Japanese encephalitis virus infection acquired during the first 2 trimesters of pregnancy

Breast-feeding see

Side-effects see section 14.1; also *less commonly* migraine, vertigo; *rarely* dyspnoea, palpitation, tachycardia, thrombocytopenia, neuritis

Dose

• See under preparation

Ixiaro® (Novartis Vaccines) ▼ [PoM]

Injection, suspension, inactivated Japanese encephalitis virus (produced in Vero cells), adsorbed onto aluminium hydroxide, net price 0.5-mL (6 micrograms) prefilled syringe = £59.50

Dose by intramuscular injection in deltoid region, ADULT over 18 years, 2 doses of 0.5 mL separated by interval of 28 days; booster dose 1–2 years after completing primary course, but for those at continued risk the booster dose should be given 1 year after completing the primary course; CHILD 2 months–3 years, 2 doses of 0.25 mL separated by interval of 28 days; CHILD 3–18 years, 2 doses of 0.5 mL separated by interval of 28 days

Note Anterolateral thigh is preferred site in infants. The subcutaneous route may be used for patients with bleeding disorders see section 14.1

Measles vaccine

Measles vaccine has been replaced by a combined live measles, mumps and rubella vaccine (MMR vaccine).

MMR vaccine may be used in the control of outbreaks of measles (see under MMR Vaccine).

◢**Single antigen vaccine**

No longer available in the UK

◢**Combined vaccines**

See MMR vaccine

Measles, Mumps and Rubella (MMR) vaccine

A combined live **measles, mumps, and rubella vaccine** (MMR vaccine) aims to eliminate measles, mumps, and rubella (and congenital rubella syndrome). Every child should receive two doses of MMR vaccine by entry to primary school, unless there is a valid contra-indication (see section 14.1). MMR vaccine should be given irrespective of previous measles, mumps, or rubella infection or vaccination.

The first dose of MMR vaccine is given to children aged 12–13 months. A second dose is given before starting school at 3 years and 4 months–5 years of age (see Immunisation Schedule, section 14.1).

Children presenting for pre-school booster who have not received the first dose of MMR vaccine should be given a dose of MMR vaccine followed 3 months later by a second dose.

At school-leaving age or at entry into further education, MMR immunisation should be offered to individuals of both sexes who have not received 2 doses during childhood. In those who have received only a single dose of MMR in childhood, a second dose is recommended to achieve full protection. If 2 doses of MMR vaccine are required, the second dose should be given one month after the initial dose. The decision on whether to vaccinate adults should take into consideration their vaccination history, the likelihood of the individual remaining susceptible, and the future risk of exposure and disease.

MMR vaccine should be used to protect against rubella in *seronegative women of child-bearing age* (see Immunisation Schedule, section 14.1); unimmunised healthcare workers who might put pregnant women and other vulnerable groups at risk of rubella or measles should be vaccinated. MMR vaccine may also be offered to previously *unimmunised and seronegative post-partum women* (see MMR Vaccine, section 14.5.3)—vaccination a few days after delivery is important because about 60% of congenital abnormalities from rubella infection occur in babies of women who have borne more than one child. Immigrants arriving after the age of school immunisation are particularly likely to require immunisation.

Contacts   MMR vaccine may also be used in the control of outbreaks of measles and should be offered to susceptible children aged over 6 months who are contacts of a case, within 3 days of exposure to infection. Children immunised before 12 months of age should still receive two doses of MMR vaccine at the recommended ages. If one dose of MMR vaccine has already been given to a child, then the second dose may be brought forward to at least one month after the first, to ensure complete protection. If the child is under 18 months of age and the second dose is given within 3 months of the first, then the routine dose before starting school at 3 years and 4 months–5 years should still be given. Children aged under 9 months for whom avoidance of measles infection is particularly important (such as those with history of recent severe illness) can be given normal immunoglobulin (section 14.5.1) after exposure to measles; routine MMR immunisation should then be given after at least 3 months at the appropriate age.

MMR vaccine is **not suitable** for prophylaxis following exposure to mumps or rubella since the antibody response to the mumps and rubella components is too slow for effective prophylaxis.

Children and adults with impaired immune response should not receive live vaccines (for advice on HIV see section 14.1). If they have been exposed to measles infection they should be given normal immunoglobulin (section 14.5.1).

Travel   Unimmunised travellers, including children over 6 months, to areas where measles is endemic or epidemic should receive MMR vaccine. Children immunised before 12 months of age should still receive two doses of MMR vaccine at the recommended ages. If one dose of MMR vaccine has already been given to a child, then the second dose should be brought forward to at least one month after the first, to ensure complete protection. If the child is under 18 months of age and the second dose is given within 3 months of the first,

then the routine dose before starting school at 3 years and 4 months–5 years should still be given.

Side-effects   See section 14.1; also malaise, fever, or a rash can occur after the first dose of MMR vaccine, most commonly about a week after vaccination and lasting about 2 to 3 days. Leaflets are available for parents on advice for reducing fever (including the use of paracetamol). Febrile seizures occur rarely 6 to 11 days after MMR vaccination; the incidence of febrile seizures is lower than that following measles infection. Parotid swelling occurs occasionally, usually in the third week, and rarely, arthropathy 2 to 3 weeks after immunisation. Adverse reactions are considerably less frequent after the second dose of MMR vaccine than after the first dose.

Idiopathic thrombocytopenic purpura has occurred rarely following MMR vaccination, usually within 6 weeks of the first dose. The risk of idiopathic thrombocytopenic purpura after MMR vaccine is much less than the risk after infection with wild measles or rubella virus. Children who develop idiopathic thrombocytopenic purpura within 6 weeks of the first dose of MMR should undergo serological testing before the second dose is due; if the results suggest incomplete immunity against measles, mumps or rubella then a second dose of MMR is recommended. The Specialist and Reference Microbiology Division, Health Protection Agency offers free serological testing for children who develop idiopathic thrombocytopenic purpura *within 6 weeks* of the first dose of MMR.

Post-vaccination aseptic meningitis was reported (rarely and with complete recovery) following vaccination with MMR vaccine containing Urabe mumps vaccine, which has now been discontinued; no cases have been confirmed in association with the currently used Jeryl Lynn mumps vaccine. Children with post-vaccination symptoms are not infectious.

> Reviews undertaken on behalf of the CSM, the Medical Research Council, and the Cochrane Collaboration, have not found any evidence of a link between MMR vaccination and bowel disease or autism. The Chief Medical Officers have advised that the MMR vaccine is the safest and best way to protect children against measles, mumps, and rubella. Information (including fact sheets and a list of references) may be obtained from:
> www.dh.gov.uk/immunisation

MEASLES, MUMPS AND RUBELLA VACCINE, LIVE

Indications   immunisation against measles, mumps, and rubella

Cautions   see section 14.1; also, after immunoglobulin administration or blood transfusion, leave an interval of at least 3 months before MMR immunisation as antibody response to measles component may be reduced—see also p. 870
Hypersensitivity to egg   MMR vaccine can be given safely even when the child has had an anaphylactic reaction to food containing egg. Dislike of eggs, refusal to eat egg, or confirmed anaphylactic reactions to egg-containing food is not a contra-indication to MMR vaccination. Children with a confirmed anaphylactic reaction to the MMR vaccine should be assessed by a specialist.

Contra-indications   see section 14.1

Pregnancy   avoid pregnancy for at least 1 month after vaccination; see also, p. 843

Breast-feeding   see p. 843

Side-effects   see section 14.1 and notes above; also *less commonly* sleep disturbances, unusual crying in infants; also reported peripheral and optic neuritis

Dose

• By intramuscular or deep subcutaneous injection, ADULT and CHILD over 9 months (but see also notes above), primary immunisation, 2 doses each of 0.5 mL, see Immunisation Schedule, section 14.1, p. 844; see also notes above for use in outbreaks, for contacts of cases, and for travel

◀**Combined vaccines**

MMRvaxPro® (Sanofi Pasteur) PoM

Injection, powder for reconstitution, live attenuated, measles virus (Enders' Edmonston strain) and mumps virus (Jeryl Lynn strain) prepared in chick embryo cells, and rubella virus (Wistar RA 27/3 strain); single-dose vial (with syringe containing solvent)

Excipients   include gelatin and neomycin

Only available as part of childhood immunisation schedule from health organisations or ImmForm

Priorix® (GSK) PoM

Injection, powder for reconstitution, live attenuated, measles virus (Schwarz strain) and mumps virus (RIT 4385 strain) prepared in chick embryo cells, and rubella virus (Wistar RA 27/3 strain); net price single-dose vial (with syringe containing solvent) = £7.64

Excipients   include neomycin

Also available as part of childhood immunisation schedule from health organisations or ImmForm

Meningococcal vaccines

Almost all childhood meningococcal disease in the UK is caused by *Neisseria meningitidis* serogroups B and C. **Meningococcal group C conjugate vaccine** protects only against infection by serogroup C. The risk of meningococcal disease declines with age—immunisation is not generally recommended after the age of 25 years.

Tetravalent meningococcal vaccines that cover serogroups A, C, W135, and Y are available. Although the duration of protection has not been established, the **meningococcal groups A, C, W135, and Y conjugate vaccine** is likely to provide longer-lasting protection than the unconjugated meningococcal polysaccharide vaccine. The antibody response to serogroup C in unconjugated meningococcal polysaccharide vaccines in young children may be suboptimal [not currently available in the UK].

A **meningococcal group B vaccine**, *Bexsero*®, is licensed in the UK against infection caused by *Neisseria meningitidis* serogroup B. *Bexsero*® contains 3 recombinant *Neisseria meningitidis* serogroup B proteins and the outer membrane vesicles from the NZ 98/254 strain, in order to achieve broad protection against *Neisseria meningitidis* serogroup B; the proteins are adsorbed onto an aluminium compound to stimulate an enhanced immune response.

Childhood immunisation   Meningococcal group C conjugate vaccine provides long-term protection against infection by serogroup C of *Neisseria meningitidis*. Immunisation consists of 1 dose given at 3 months

of age; 2 booster doses are recommended, the first is given at 12–13 months of age (combined with haemophilus influenzae type b vaccine), and the second at 13–15 years of age (see Immunisation Schedule, section 14.1, p. 844).

Unimmunised children aged 4–12 months should be given 1 dose of meningococcal group C conjugate vaccine and then they should be vaccinated according to the Immunisation Schedule (section 14.1, p. 844). Unimmunised children aged 1–10 years should be given 1 dose of meningococcal group C conjugate vaccine, followed by a booster dose at 13–15 years of age. Unimmunised individuals aged 10–25 years should be given 1 dose of meningococcal group C conjugate vaccine, but a booster dose is not required.

From August 2014 there will be a catch-up programme for individuals aged under 25 years who are attending university for the first time and who did not receive a dose of meningococcal group C conjugate vaccine at 13–15 years of age.

Patients under 25 years of age with confirmed serogroup C disease, who have previously been immunised with meningococcal group C vaccine, should be offered meningococcal group C conjugate vaccine before discharge from hospital.

Asplenia, splenic dysfunction, or complement deficiency   See p. 850.

Travel   Individuals travelling to countries of risk (see below) should be immunised with **meningococcal groups A, C, W135, and Y conjugate vaccine**, even if they have previously received meningococcal group C conjugate vaccine. If an individual has recently received meningococcal group C conjugate vaccine, an interval of at least 4 weeks should be allowed before administration of the tetravalent (meningococcal groups A, C, W135, and Y) vaccine.

Vaccination is particularly important for those living or working with local people or visiting an area of risk during outbreaks.

Immunisation recommendations and requirements for visa entry for individual countries should be checked before travelling, particularly to countries in Sub-Saharan Africa, Asia, and the Indian sub-continent where epidemics of meningococcal outbreaks and infection are reported. Country-by-country information is available from the National Travel Health Network and Centre (www.nathnac.org).

Proof of vaccination with the tetravalent (meningococcal groups A, C, W135, and Y) vaccine is required for those travelling to Saudi Arabia during the Hajj and Umrah pilgrimages (where outbreaks of the W135 strain have occurred).

Contacts   For advice on the immunisation of *laboratory workers and close contacts* of cases of meningococcal disease in the UK and on the role of the vaccine in the control of *local outbreaks*, consult Guidance for Public Health Management of Meningococcal Disease in the UK at www.hpa.org.uk. See Table 2, section 5.1 for antibacterial prophylaxis for prevention of secondary cases of meningococcal meningitis.

The need for immunisation of laboratory staff who work directly with *Neisseria meningitidis* should be considered.

MENINGOCOCCAL VACCINES

Indications immunisation against *Neisseria meningitidis*

Cautions see section 14.1

Contra-indications see section 14.1

Pregnancy see p. 843

Breast-feeding see p. 843

Side-effects see section 14.1; also *rarely* symptoms of meningitis reported (but no evidence that the vaccine causes meningococcal C meningitis); also reported in children with meningococcal group B vaccine (*Bexsero*®) unusual crying and *rarely* Kawasaki disease

Dose

● See under preparations

◢Meningococcal group C conjugate vaccine

Menjugate Kit® (Novartis Vaccines) PoM

Injection, powder for reconstitution, capsular polysaccharide antigen of *Neisseria meningitidis* group C (conjugated to *Corynebacterium diphtheriae* protein), adsorbed onto aluminium hydroxide, single-dose vial with diluent

Dose by intramuscular injection, ADULT and CHILD 3 months–25 years 0.5 mL, see notes above and Immunisation Schedule, section 14.1

Available as part of childhood immunisation schedule from ImmForm

NeisVac-C® (Baxter) PoM

Injection, suspension of polysaccharide antigen of *Neisseria meningitidis* group C (conjugated to tetanus toxoid protein), adsorbed onto aluminium hydroxide, 0.5-mL prefilled syringe

Dose by intramuscular injection, ADULT and CHILD 3 months–25 years 0.5 mL, see notes above and Immunisation Schedule, section 14.1

Available as part of childhood immunisation schedule from ImmForm

◢Meningococcal group C conjugate vaccine with Haemophilus Influenzae type B vaccine

See Haemophilus Influenzae type B vaccine

◢Meningococcal groups A, C, W135, and Y conjugate vaccine

Menveo® (Novartis Vaccines) PoM

Injection, powder for reconstitution, capsular oligosaccharide antigens of *Neisseria meningitidis* groups A, C, W135, and Y (conjugated to *Corynebacterium diphtheriae* protein), net price single-dose vial (with vial or prefilled syringe containing diluent) = £30.00

Dose by intramuscular injection preferably into deltoid region, ADULT and CHILD over 1 year 0.5 mL as a single dose; CHILD 3 months–1 year 2 doses of 0.5 mL separated by an interval of 1 month

Note Advice in BNF may differ from that in product literature

Nimenrix® (GSK) ▼ PoM

Injection, powder for reconstitution, capsular polysaccharide antigens of *Neisseria meningitidis* groups A, C, W135, and Y (conjugated to tetanus toxoid protein), net price single-dose vial (with syringe containing diluent) = £30.00

Dose by intramuscular injection preferably into deltoid region (or anterolateral thigh in child 1–2 years), ADULT and CHILD over 1 year 0.5 mL as a single dose; a second dose may be considered after 1 year in those who continue to be at risk of *Neisseria meningitidis* serogroup A infection

◢Meningococcal group B vaccine

Bexsero® (Novartis) ▼ PoM

Injection, suspension of antigen of *Neisseria meningitidis* group B (produced in *E. Coli* cells by recombinant DNA technology), adsorbed onto aluminium hydroxide, net price 0.5 mL prefilled syringe = £75.00

Excipients may include traces of kanamycin

Dose by deep intramuscular injection preferably into deltoid region (or anterolateral thigh in infants), ADULT and CHILD over 11 years (unimmunised), 2 doses of 0.5 mL separated by an interval of at least 1 month; CHILD 2–6 months, primary immunisation 3 doses of 0.5 mL separated by an interval of at least 1 month, booster dose of 0.5 mL given between 1–2 years of age; CHILD 6 months–1 year (unimmunised), primary immunisation 2 doses of 0.5 mL separated by an interval of at least 2 months, booster dose of 0.5 mL given between 1–2 years of age and at least 2 months after completion of primary immunisation; CHILD 1–2 years (unimmunised), primary immunisation 2 doses of 0.5 mL separated by an interval of at least 2 months, booster dose of 0.5 mL given 12–24 months after completion of primary immunisation; CHILD 2–11 years (unimmunised), 2 doses of 0.5 mL separated by an interval of at least 2 months

Mumps vaccine

◢Single antigen vaccine

No longer available in the UK

◢Combined vaccines

See MMR Vaccine

Pertussis vaccine

Pertussis vaccine is given as a combination preparation containing other vaccines (see Diphtheria containing Vaccines). Acellular vaccines are derived from highly purified components of *Bordetella pertussis*. Primary immunisation against pertussis (whooping cough) requires 3 doses of an acellular pertussis-containing vaccine (see Immunisation schedule, section 14.1), given at intervals of 1 month from the age of 2 months.

All children up to the age of 10 years should receive primary immunisation with diphtheria, tetanus, pertussis (acellular, component), poliomyelitis (inactivated) and haemophilus type b conjugate vaccine (adsorbed).

A booster dose of an acellular pertussis-containing vaccine should ideally be given 3 years after the primary course, although, the interval can be reduced to 1 year if the primary course was delayed.

Children aged 1–10 years who have not received a *pertussis-containing* vaccine as part of their primary immunisation should be offered 1 dose of a suitable pertussis-containing vaccine; after an interval of at least 1 year, a booster dose of a suitable pertussis-containing vaccine should be given. Immunisation against pertussis is not routinely recommended in individuals over 10 years of age.

Vaccination of pregnant women against pertussis In reponse to the pertussis outbreak, the UK health departments introduced a temporary programme (October 2012) to vaccinate pregnant women against pertussis, and this programme will continue until further notice. The aim of the programme is to boost the levels of pertussis-specific antibodies that are transferred through the placenta, from the mother to the fetus, so that the newborn is protected before routine immunisation begins at 2 months of age.

Pregnant women should be offered a single dose of acellular pertussis-containing vaccine (as adsorbed diphtheria [low dose], tetanus, pertussis (acellular, component) and poliomyelitis (inactivated) vaccine; *Boostrix-IPV®*) between 28 to 38 weeks of pregnancy; the optimal time for vaccination is between 28–32 weeks of pregnancy. Pregnant women should be offered a single dose of acellular pertussis-containing vaccine up to the onset of labour if they missed the opportunity for vaccination at 28–38 weeks of pregnancy. A single dose of acellular pertussis-containing vaccine may also be offered to new mothers, who have never previously been vaccinated against pertussis, until the child receives the first vaccination.

While this programme is in place, women who become pregnant again should be offered vaccination during each pregnancy to maximise transplacental transfer of antibody.

Contacts   Vaccination against pertussis should be considered for close contacts of cases with pertussis who have been offered antibacterial prophylaxis (Table 2, section 5.1). Unimmunised or partially immunised contacts under 10 years of age should complete their vaccination against pertussis. A booster dose of an acellular pertussis-containing vaccine is recommended for contacts aged over 10 years who have not received a pertussis-containing vaccine in the last 5 years and who have not received adsorbed diphtheria [low dose], tetanus, and poliomyelitis (inactivated) vaccine in the last month.

Cautions   Section 14.1.

Contra-indications   Section 14.1.

Pregnancy   See p. 843 and also Vaccination of Pregnant Women Against Pertussis above.

Breast-feeding   See p. 843.

Side-effects   See also section 14.1. The incidence of local and systemic effects is generally lower with vaccines containing acellular pertussis components than with the whole-cell pertussis vaccine used previously. However, compared with primary vaccination, booster doses with vaccines containing acellular pertussis are reported to increase the risk of injection-site reactions (some of which affect the entire limb); local reactions do not contra-indicate further doses (see below).

The vaccine should not be withheld from children with a history to a preceding dose of:

- fever, irrespective of severity;
- persistent crying or screaming for more than 3 hours;
- severe local reaction, irrespective of extent.

◢ **Combined vaccines**

Combined vaccines, see under Diphtheria-containing vaccines

Pneumococcal vaccines

Pneumococcal vaccines protect against infection with *Streptococcus pneumoniae* (pneumococcus); the vaccines contain polysaccharide from capsular types of pneumococci. **Pneumococcal polysaccharide vaccine** contains purified polysaccharide from 23 capsular types of pneumococci, whereas **pneumococcal polysaccharide conjugate vaccine (adsorbed)** contains polysaccharide from

either 10 capsular types (*Synflorix®*) or 13 capsular types (*Prevenar 13®*) and the polysaccharide is conjugated to protein.

The 13-valent conjugate vaccine (*Prevenar 13®*) is used in the childhood immunisation schedule. The recommended schedule consists of 3 doses, the first at 2 months of age, the second at 4 months, and the third at 12–13 months (see Immunisation Schedule, section 14.1).

Pneumococcal vaccination is recommended for individuals at increased risk of pneumococcal infection as follows:

- age over 65 years;
- asplenia or splenic dysfunction (including homozygous sickle cell disease and coeliac disease which could lead to splenic dysfunction);
- chronic respiratory disease (includes asthma treated with continuous or frequent use of a systemic corticosteroid);
- chronic heart disease;
- chronic renal disease;
- chronic liver disease;
- diabetes mellitus requiring insulin or oral hypoglycaemic drugs;
- immune deficiency because of disease (e.g. HIV infection) or treatment (including prolonged systemic corticosteroid treatment for over 1 month at dose equivalents of prednisolone: *adult and child over 20 kg*, 20 mg or more daily; *child under 20 kg*, 1 mg/kg or more daily);
- presence of cochlear implant;
- conditions where leakage of cerebrospinal fluid may occur;
- child under 5 years with a history of invasive pneumococcal disease;
- at risk of occupational exposure to metal fume (e.g. welders).

Where possible, the vaccine should be given at least 2 weeks before splenectomy, cochlear implant surgery, chemotherapy, or radiotherapy; patients should be given advice about increased risk of pneumococcal infection. If it is not practical to vaccinate at least 2 weeks before splenectomy, chemotherapy, or radiotherapy, the vaccine should be given at least 2 weeks after the splenectomy or, where possible, at least 3 months after completion of chemotherapy or radiotherapy. Prophylactic antibacterial therapy against pneumococcal infection (Table 2, section 5.1) should not be stopped after immunisation. A patient card and information leaflet for patients with asplenia are available from the Department of Health or in Scotland from the Scottish Executive, Public Health Division 1 (Tel (0131) 244 2501).

Choice of vaccine   Children under 2 years at increased risk of pneumococcal infection (see list above) should receive the 13-valent pneumococcal polysaccharide conjugate vaccine (adsorbed) at the recommended ages, followed by a single dose of the 23-valent pneumococcal polysaccharide vaccine after their second birthday (see below). Children at increased risk of pneumococcal infection presenting late for vaccination should receive 2 doses (separated by at least 1 month) of the 13-valent pneumococcal polysaccharide conjugate vaccine (adsorbed) before the age of 12 months, and a third dose at 12–13 months. Children over 12 months and under 5 years (who have not been vaccinated or not completed the primary course) should receive a single dose of the 13-valent pneumococcal polysaccharide conjugate vaccine (adsorbed) (2 doses separated by an interval of 2 months in the immunocompromised or those with asplenia or splenic dysfunction). All children under 5 years at increased risk of pneumococcal infection should receive a single dose of the 23-valent pneumococcal polysaccharide vaccine after their second birthday and at least 2 months after the final dose of the 13-valent pneumococcal polysaccharide conjugate vaccine (adsorbed).

Children over 5 years and adults who are at increased risk of pneumococcal disease should receive a single dose of the 23-valent unconjugated pneumococcal polysaccharide vaccine.

Revaccination In individuals with higher concentrations of antibodies to pneumococcal polysaccharides, revaccination with the 23-valent pneumococcal polysaccharide vaccine more commonly produces adverse reactions. Revaccination is therefore not recommended, except every 5 years in individuals in whom the antibody concentration is likely to decline rapidly (e.g. asplenia, splenic dysfunction and nephrotic syndrome). If there is doubt, the need for revaccination should be discussed with a haematologist, immunologist, or microbiologist.

▌ PNEUMOCOCCAL VACCINE

Indications immunisation against pneumococcal infection
Cautions see section 14.1
Contra-indications see section 14.1
Pregnancy see p. 843
Breast-feeding see p. 843
Side-effects see section 14.1; *also* Revaccination, above
Dose
● See under preparations

◢Pneumococcal polysaccharide vaccine

Pneumovax® II (Sanofi Pasteur) ⒫ℴ🄼
Injection, polysaccharide from each of 23 capsular types of pneumococcus, net price 0.5-mL vial = £8.32
Contra-indications concomitant use with the high potency varicella-zoster vaccine (*Zostavax®*)
Dose by intramuscular or subcutaneous injection, ADULT and CHILD over 2 years, 0.5 mL; revaccination, see notes above

◢Pneumococcal polysaccharide conjugate vaccine (adsorbed)

Prevenar 13® (Pfizer) ⒫ℴ🄼
Injection, polysaccharide from each of 13 capsular types of pneumococcus (conjugated to carrier protein) adsorbed onto aluminium phosphate, net price 0.5-mL prefilled syringe = £49.10
Dose by intramuscular injection, CHILD 2 months–5 years, 0.5 mL (see notes above and Immunisation Schedule, section 14.1)
Note Deltoid muscle is preferred site of injection in young children; anterolateral thigh is preferred site in infants.
The dose in the BNF may differ from that in product literature.
Available as part of childhood immunisation schedule from ImmForm

Synflorix® (GSK) ⒫ℴ🄼
Injection, polysaccharide from each of 10 capsular types of pneumococcus (conjugated to carrier proteins) adsorbed onto aluminium phosphate, net price 0.5-mL prefilled syringe = £27.60
Dose by intramuscular injection, CHILD 6 weeks–5 years, consult product literature
Note Deltoid muscle is preferred site of injection in young children; anterolateral thigh is preferred site in infants

Poliomyelitis vaccines

Two types of poliomyelitis vaccine (containing strains of poliovirus types 1, 2, and 3) are available, inactivated poliomyelitis vaccine (for injection) and live (oral) poliomyelitis vaccine. **Inactivated poliomyelitis vaccine**, only available in combined preparation (see under Diphtheria Vaccines), is recommended for routine immunisation.

A course of primary immunisation consists of 3 doses of a combined preparation containing inactivated poliomyelitis vaccine, starting at 2 months of age with intervals of 1 month between doses (see Immunisation schedule, section 14.1). A course of 3 doses should also be given to all unimmunised adults; no adult should remain unimmunised against poliomyelitis.

Two booster doses of a preparation containing inactivated poliomyelitis vaccine are recommended, the first before school entry and the second before leaving school (see Immunisation schedule, section 14.1). Further booster doses are only necessary for adults at special risk, such as travellers to endemic areas, or laboratory staff likely to be exposed to the viruses, or healthcare workers in possible contact with cases; booster doses should be given to such individuals every 10 years.

Live (oral) poliomyelitis vaccine is no longer available for routine use; its use may be considered during large outbreaks, but advice should be sought from Public Health England. The live (oral) vaccine poses a very rare risk of vaccine-associated paralytic polio because the attenuated strain of the virus can revert to a virulent form. For this reason the live (oral) vaccine must **not** be used for immunosuppressed individuals or their household contacts. The use of inactivated poliomyelitis vaccine removes the risk of vaccine-associated paralytic polio altogether.

Travel Unimmunised travellers to areas with a high incidence of poliomyelitis should receive a full 3-dose course of a preparation containing inactivated poliomyelitis vaccine. Those who have not been vaccinated in the last 10 years should receive a booster dose of **adsorbed diphtheria [low dose], tetanus and poliomyelitis (inactivated) vaccine**. Information about countries with a high incidence of poliomyelitis can be obtained from www.travax.nhs.uk or from the National Travel Health Network and Centre (www.nathnac.org).

▌ POLIOMYELITIS VACCINES

Indications immunisation against poliomyelitis
Cautions see section 14.1
Contra-indications see notes above and section 14.1
Pregnancy see p. 843
Breast-feeding see p. 843
Side-effects see notes above and section 14.1
Dose
● See under preparations

◢**Combined vaccines**
See under Diphtheria-containing Vaccines

◢**Inactivated (Salk) vaccine**
See under Diphtheria-containing vaccines

Rabies vaccine

Rabies vaccine contains inactivated rabies virus cultivated in either human diploid cells or purified chick embryo cells; vaccines are used for pre- and post-exposure prophylaxis.

Pre-exposure prophylaxis Immunisation should be offered to those at high risk of exposure to rabies—laboratory staff who handle the rabies virus, those working in quarantine stations, animal handlers, veterinary surgeons and field workers who are likely to be bitten by infected wild animals, certain port officials, and bat handlers. Transmission of rabies by humans has not been recorded but it is advised that those caring for patients with the disease should be vaccinated.

Immunisation against rabies is also recommended where there is limited access to prompt medical care for those living in areas where rabies is enzootic, for those travelling to such areas for longer than 1 month, and for those on shorter visits who may be exposed to unusual risk.

Immunisation against rabies is indicated during pregnancy if there is substantial risk of exposure to rabies and rapid access to post-exposure prophylaxis is likely to be limited.

Up-to-date country-by-country information on the incidence of rabies can be obtained from the National Travel Health Network and Centre (www.nathnac.org) and, in Scotland, from Health Protection Scotland (www.hps.scot.nhs.uk).

Immunisation against rabies requires 3 doses of rabies vaccine, with further booster doses for those who remain at frequent risk. To ensure continued protection in persons at high risk (e.g. laboratory workers), the concentration of antirabies antibodies in plasma is used to determine the intervals between doses.

Post-exposure management Following potential exposure to rabies, the wound or site of exposure (e.g. mucous membrane) should be cleansed under running water and washed for several minutes with soapy water as soon as possible after exposure. Disinfectant and a simple dressing can be applied, but suturing should be delayed because it may increase the risk of introducing rabies virus into the nerves.

Post-exposure prophylaxis against rabies depends on the level of risk in the country, the nature of exposure, and the individual's immunity. In each case, expert risk assessment and advice on appropriate management should be obtained from the local Public Health England Centre or Public Health England's Virus Reference Department, Colindale (tel. (020) 8200 4400) or the PHE Colindale Duty Doctor (tel. (020) 8200 6868), in Wales from the Public Health Wales local Health Protection Team or Public Health Wales Virus Reference Laboratory (tel. (029) 2074 7747), in Scotland from the local on-call infectious diseases consultant, and in Northern Ireland from the Public Health Agency Duty Room (tel (028) 9055 3997/ (028) 9063 2662) or the Regional Virology Service (tel. (028) 9024 0503).

There are no specific contra-indications to the use of rabies vaccine for post-exposure prophylaxis and its use should be considered whenever a patient has been attacked by an animal in a country where rabies is enzootic, even if there is no direct evidence of rabies in the attacking animal. Because of the potential consequences of untreated rabies exposure and because rabies vaccination has not been associated with fetal abnormalities, pregnancy is not considered a contra-indication to post-exposure prophylaxis.

For post-exposure prophylaxis of *fully immunised* individuals (who have previously received pre-exposure or post-exposure prophylaxis with cell-derived rabies vaccine), 2 doses of cell-derived vaccine are likely to be sufficient; the first dose is given on day 0 and the second dose is given between day 3–7. Rabies immunoglobulin is not necessary in such cases.

Post-exposure treatment for *unimmunised individuals* (or those whose prophylaxis is possibly incomplete) comprises 5 doses of rabies vaccine given over 1 month (on days 0, 3, 7, 14, and the fifth dose is given bween day 28–30); also, depending on the level of risk (determined by factors such as the nature of the bite and the country where it was sustained), rabies immunoglobulin (section 14.5.2) is given to unimmunised individuals on day 0 or within 7 days of starting the course of rabies vaccine. The immunisation course can be discontinued if it is proved that the individual was not at risk.

◤ RABIES VACCINE

Indications immunisation against rabies
Cautions see section 14.1
Contra-indications see section 14.1; but see also Post-exposure Management in notes above
Pregnancy see p. 843
Breast-feeding see p. 843
Side-effects see section 14.1; also reported paresis
Dose
- Pre-exposure prophylaxis, by intramuscular injection in deltoid region or anterolateral thigh in infants, 1 mL on days 0, 7, and 28 (3rd dose can be given from day 21 if insufficient time before travel); for those at continous risk, measure plasma-concentration of antirabies antibodies every 6 months and give a booster dose if the titre is less than 0.5 units/mL; for those at frequent risk, give a single reinforcing dose 1 year after the primary course is completed, and then give booster doses every 3–5 years or determine the frequency of booster doses according to plasma concentration of antirabies antibodies; for those at infrequent risk, consider giving a booster dose 10 years after the primary course is completed
- Post-exposure prophylaxis, by intramuscular injection in deltoid region or anterolateral thigh in infants, 1 mL (see notes above)

Rabies Vaccine (Sanofi Pasteur) PoM
Rab
Injection, powder for reconstitution, freeze-dried inactivated Wistar rabies virus strain PM/ WI 38 1503-3M cultivated in human diploid cells, net price single-dose vial with syringe containing diluent = £33.90
Excipients include neomycin

Rabipur® (Novartis Vaccines) [PoM]
Injection, powder for reconstitution, freeze-dried inactivated Flury LEP rabies virus strain cultivated in chick embryo cells, net price single-dose vial = £28.80
Excipients include neomycin

Rotavirus vaccine

Rotavirus vaccine is a live, oral vaccine that protects young children against gastro-enteritis caused by rota-virus infection. The recommended schedule consists of 2 doses, the first at 2 months of age, and the second at 3 months of age (see Immunisation schedule, section 14.1). The first dose of rotavirus vaccine must be given between 6–15 weeks of age and the second dose should be given after an interval of at least 4 weeks; the vaccine should not be started in children 15 weeks of age or older. Ideally, the full course should be completed before 16 weeks of age to provide protection before the main burden of disease, and to avoid a temporal association between vaccination and intussus-ception; the course must be completed before 24 weeks of age.

The rotavirus vaccine virus is excreted in the stool and may be transmitted to close contacts; however, vaccin-ation of those with *immunosuppressed* close contacts may protect the contacts from wild-type rotavirus dis-ease and outweigh any risk from transmission of vaccine virus. Carers of a recently vaccinated baby should be advised of the need to wash their hands after changing the baby's nappies.

■ ROTAVIRUS VACCINE

Indications immunisation against gastro-enteritis caused by rotavirus
Cautions see section 14.1; *also* diarrhoea or vomiting (postpone vaccination); immunosuppressed close contacts (see notes above)
Contra-indications see section 14.1, however, with the exception of severe combined immunodeficiency, benefit from vaccination is likely to outweigh the risk in other types of immunosuppression–if there is any doubt, seek specialist advice; *also* predisposition to, or history of, intussusception
Side-effects see section 14.1
Dose
- By mouth, CHILD over 6 weeks, 2 doses of 1.5 mL, separated by an interval of at least 4 weeks; first dose must be given between 6–15 weeks of age; course should be completed before 24 weeks of age (prefer-ably before 16 weeks)

Rotarix® (GSK) [PoM]
Oral suspension, live attenuated rotavirus (RIX4414 strain), net price 1.5 mL prefilled oral syringe = £34.76

Rubella vaccine

A combined measles, mumps and rubella vaccine (MMR vaccine) aims to eliminate rubella (German measles) and congenital rubella syndrome. MMR vaccine is used for childhood vaccination as well as for vaccinating adults (including women of child-bearing age) who do not have immunity against rubella (see MMR vaccine, p. 856)

◢ Single antigen vaccine

No longer available in the UK; the combined live measles, mumps and rubella vaccine is a suitable alter-native

◢ Combined vaccines

see MMR vaccine

Smallpox vaccine

Limited supplies of **smallpox vaccine** are held at the Specialist and Reference Microbiology Division, Public Health England Colindale (Tel. (020) 8200 4400) for the exclusive use of workers in laboratories where pox viruses (such as vaccinia) are handled.

If a wider use of the vaccine is being considered, *Guide-lines for smallpox response and management in the post-eradication era* should be consulted at www.hpa.org.uk.

Tetanus vaccines

Tetanus vaccine contains a cell-free purified toxin of *Clostridium tetani* adsorbed on aluminium hydroxide or aluminium phosphate to improve antigenicity.

Primary immunisation for children under 10 years con-sists of 3 doses of a combined preparation containing adsorbed tetanus vaccine (see Diphtheria-containing Vaccines), with an interval of 1 month between doses. Following routine childhood vaccination, 2 booster doses of a preparation containing adsorbed tetanus vaccine are recommended, the first before school entry and the second before leaving school (see Immunisation schedule, section 14.1).

The recommended schedule of tetanus vaccination not only gives protection against tetanus in childhood but also gives the basic immunity for subsequent booster doses. In most circumstances, a total of 5 doses of tetanus vaccine is considered sufficient for long term protection.

For primary immunisation of adults and children over 10 years previously unimmunised against tetanus, 3 doses of **adsorbed diphtheria [low dose], tetanus and poliomyelitis (inactivated) vaccine** are given with an interval of 1 month between doses (see Diph-theria-containing Vaccines).

Cautions See also section 14.1. When an individual presents for a booster dose but has been vaccinated following a tetanus-prone wound, the vaccine prepara-tion administered at the time of injury should be deter-mined. If this is not possible, the booster should still be given to ensure adequate protection against all antigens in the booster vaccine.

Very rarely, tetanus has developed after abdominal surgery; patients awaiting elective surgery should be asked about tetanus immunisation and immunised if necessary.

Parenteral drug abuse is also associated with tetanus; those abusing drugs by injection should be vaccinated if unimmunised—booster doses should be given if there is any doubt about their immunisation status.

All laboratory staff should be offered a primary course if unimmunised.

Travel recommendations see section 14.6.

Contra-indications See section 14.1.

Pregnancy See p. 843.

Breast-feeding   See p. 843.

Side effects   See section 14.1.

Wounds   Wounds are considered to be tetanus-prone if they are sustained more than 6 hours before surgical treatment *or* at any interval after injury and are puncture-type (particularly if contaminated with soil or manure) *or* show much devitalised tissue *or* are septic *or* are compound fractures *or* contain foreign bodies. All wounds should receive thorough cleansing.

- For *clean wounds*: fully immunised individuals (those who have received a total of 5 doses of a tetanus-containing vaccine at appropriate intervals) and those whose primary immunisation is complete (with boosters up to date), do not require tetanus vaccine; individuals whose primary immunisation is incomplete or whose boosters are not up to date require a reinforcing dose of a tetanus-containing vaccine (followed by further doses as required to complete the schedule); non-immunised individuals (or those whose immunisation status is not known or who have been fully immunised but are now immunocompromised) should be given a dose of the appropriate tetanus-containing vaccine immediately (followed by completion of the full course of the vaccine if records confirm the need).

- For *tetanus-prone wounds*: management is as for clean wounds with the addition of a dose of tetanus immunoglobulin (section 14.5.2) given at a different site; in fully immunised individuals and those whose primary immunisation is complete (with boosters up to date) the immunoglobulin is needed only if the risk of infection is especially high (e.g. contamination with manure). Antibacterial prophylaxis (with benzylpenicillin, co-amoxiclav, or metronidazole) may also be required for tetanus-prone wounds.

◢**Combined vaccines**

See Diphtheria-containing Vaccines

Tick-borne encephalitis vaccine

Tick-borne encephalitis vaccine contains inactivated tick-borne encephalitis virus cultivated in chick embryo cells. It is recommended for immunisation of those working in, or visiting, high-risk areas (see International Travel, section 14.6). Those working, walking or camping in warm forested areas of Central and Eastern Europe, Scandinavia, Northern and Eastern China, and some parts of Japan, particularly from April to November when ticks are most prevalent, are at greatest risk of tick-borne encephalitis. For full protection, 3 doses of the vaccine are required; booster doses are required every 3–5 years for those still at risk. Ideally, immunisation should be completed at least one month before travel.

▌ TICK-BORNE ENCEPHALITIS VACCINE, INACTIVATED

Indications   immunisation against tick-borne encephalitis

Cautions   see section 14.1

Contra-indications   see section 14.1

Pregnancy   see p. 843

Breast-feeding   see p. 843

Side-effects   see section 14.1

Dose

- Initial immunisation, by intramuscular injection in deltoid region or anterolateral thigh in infants, ADULT and CHILD over 16 years, 3 doses each of 0.5 mL, second dose after 1–3 months and third dose after further 5–12 months; CHILD 1–16 years 3 doses of 0.25 mL, second dose after 1–3 months and third dose after further 5–12 months; ELDERLY over 60 years and immunocompromised (including those receiving immunosuppressants), antibody concentration may be measured 4 weeks after second dose and dose repeated if protective levels not achieved
  Note   To achieve more rapid protection, second dose may be given 14 days after first dose

- Booster doses, give first dose within 3 years after initial course completed, then every 3–5 years

TicoVac® (MASTA) [PoM]
Injection, suspension, formaldehyde-inactivated Neudörfl tick-borne encephalitis virus strain (cultivated in chick embryo cells) adsorbed onto hydrated aluminium hydroxide, net price 0.25-mL prefilled syringe (*TicoVac Junior®*) = £28.00, 0.5-mL prefilled syringe = £32.00
Excipients   include gentamicin and neomycin

Typhoid vaccines

Typhoid vaccine is available as Vi capsular polysaccharide (from *Salmonella typhi*) vaccine for injection and as live attenuated *Salmonella typhi* for oral use.

Typhoid immunisation is advised for :

- travellers to areas where typhoid is endemic, especially if staying with or visiting local people;

- travellers to endemic areas where frequent or prolonged exposure to poor sanitation and poor food hygiene is likely;

- laboratory personnel who, in the course of their work, may be exposed to *Salmonella typhi*.

Typhoid vaccination is not a substitute for scrupulous personal hygiene (see p. 872).

Capsular **polysaccharide typhoid vaccine** is usually given by *intramuscular injection*. Children under 2 years may respond suboptimally to the vaccine, but children aged between 1–2 years should be immunised if the risk of typhoid fever is considered high (immunisation is not recommended for infants under 12 months). Revaccination is needed every 3 years on continued exposure.

Oral typhoid vaccine is a **live attenuated** vaccine contained in an enteric-coated capsule. One capsule taken on alternate days for a total of 3 doses, provides protection 7–10 days after the last dose. Protection may persist for up to 3 years in those constantly (or repeatedly) exposed to *Salmonella typhi*, but those who only occasionally travel to endemic areas require further courses at intervals of 1 year.

Interactions   Oral typhoid vaccine is inactivated by concomitant administration of antibacterials or antimalarials:

- Antibacterials should be avoided for 3 days before and after oral typhoid vaccination;

- *Mefloquine* should be avoided for at least 12 hours before or after oral typhoid;

- For other antimalarials vaccination with oral typhoid vaccine should be completed at least 3 days before the first dose of the antimalarial (except proguanil hydrochloride with atovaquone, which may be given concomitantly).

14   **Immunological products and vaccines**

▄ TYPHOID VACCINE

Indications immunisation against typhoid fever

Cautions section 14.1; **interactions:** see above and Appendix 1 (vaccines)

Contra-indications section 14.1; also for *oral* vaccine, acute gastro-intestinal illness

Pregnancy see p. 843

Breast-feeding see p. 843

Side-effects section 14.1

Dose
● See under preparations

▄Typhoid polysaccharide vaccine for injection

Typherix® (GSK) ꟼoᴍ

Injection, Vi capsular polysaccharide typhoid vaccine, 50 micrograms/mL virulence polysaccharide antigen of *Salmonella typhi*, net price 0.5-mL prefilled syringe = £9.93

Dose by intramuscular injection, 0.5 mL at least 2 weeks before potential exposure to typhoid infection; CHILD under 2 years (see notes above)

Note May be difficult to obtain

Typhim Vi® (Sanofi Pasteur) ꟼoᴍ

Injection, Vi capsular polysaccharide typhoid vaccine, 50 micrograms/mL virulence polysaccharide antigen of formaldehyde-inactivated *Salmonella typhi*, net price 0.5-mL prefilled syringe = £9.30

Dose by intramuscular injection, 0.5 mL, at least 2 weeks before potential exposure to typhoid infection CHILD under 2 years (see notes above)

▄Polysaccharide vaccine with hepatitis A vaccine

See Hepatitis A Vaccine

▄Typhoid vaccine, live (oral)

Vivotif® (Crucell) ꟼoᴍ

Capsules, e/c, live attenuated *Salmonella typhi* (Ty21a), net price 3-cap pack = £14.77. Label: 25, counselling, administration

Dose ADULT and CHILD over 6 years, 1 capsule on days 1, 3, and 5

Counselling Take one hour before a meal. Swallow as soon as possible after placing in mouth with a cold or lukewarm drink; it is important to store capsules in a refrigerator

Varicella–zoster vaccines

The live varicella–zoster vaccines, *Varilrix®* and *Varivax®*, are licensed for immunisation against *varicella* (chickenpox) in seronegative individuals. They are not recommended for routine use in children, but can be given to seronegative healthy children over 1 year who come into close contact with individuals at high risk of severe varicella infections. The Department of Health recommends these vaccines for seronegative healthcare workers who come into direct contact with patients. Those with a history of chickenpox or shingles can be considered immune, but healthcare workers with a negative or uncertain history should be tested.

Rarely, the varicella–zoster vaccine virus has been transmitted from the vaccinated individual to close contacts. Therefore, contact with the following should be avoided if a vaccine-related cutaneous rash develops within 4–6 weeks of the first or second dose:

● varicella-susceptible pregnant women;

● individuals at high risk of severe varicella, including those with immunodeficiency or those receiving immunosuppressive therapy.

Healthcare workers who develop a generalised papular or vesicular rash on vaccination should avoid contact with patients until the lesions have crusted. Those who develop a localised rash after vaccination should cover the lesions and be allowed to continue working unless in contact with patients at high risk of severe varicella.

The high potency, live varicella–zoster vaccine, *Zostavax®*, is recommended for the prevention of *herpes zoster* (shingles) in adults who are, or were, 70 years of age on 1 September 2014. The 2014-15 catch-up programme with *Zostavax®* will be offered to all who are, or were, 78 or 79 years of age on 1 September 2014. A single dose of *Zostavax®* is likely to give protection for at least 7 years, but the need for, or timing of, a booster dose has not been established. Although *Zostavax®* is not recommended for the treatment of shingles or post-herpetic neuralgia, it can be given to those with a previous history of shingles; ideally the vaccine should be delayed until systemic antiviral therapy has been completed.

Varicella–zoster immunoglobulin is used to protect susceptible individuals at increased risk of varicella infection, see p. 870.

▄ VARICELLA-ZOSTER VACCINE

Indications see notes above and preparations below

Cautions see section 14.1; *also* post-vaccination close-contact with susceptible individuals (see notes above)

Contra-indications see section 14.1

Pregnancy avoid pregnancy for 3 months after vaccination; see also p. 843

Breast-feeding see p. 843

Side-effects see section 14.1; also conjunctivitis and varicella-like rash; *rarely* thrombocytopenia

Dose
● See under preparations

Varilrix® (GSK) ꟼoᴍ

Injection, powder for reconstitution, live attenuated varicella–zoster virus (Oka strain) in human diploid cells, net price 0.5-mL vial (with diluent) = £27.31

Excipients include neomycin

Dose prevention of varicella infection (chickenpox), by subcutaneous injection preferably into deltoid region, ADULT and CHILD over 1 year (see notes above), 2 doses of 0.5 mL separated by an interval of at least 6 weeks (minimum 4 weeks)

Varivax® (Sanofi Pasteur) ꟼoᴍ

Injection powder for reconstitution, live attenuated varicella–zoster virus (Oka/Merck strain) propagated in human diploid cells, net price 0.5-mL vial (with diluent) = £30.28

Excipients include gelatin and neomycin

Dose prevention of varicella infection (chickenpox), by intramuscular or subcutaneous injection into deltoid region (or higher anterolateral thigh in children), ADULT and CHILD over 13 years (see notes above), 2 doses of 0.5 mL separated by 4–8 weeks; CHILD 1–13 years (see notes above) 2 doses of 0.5 mL separated by an interval of at least 4 weeks (two doses separated by 12 weeks in children with asymptomatic HIV infection)

Zostavax® (Sanofi Pasteur) PoM
Injection, powder for reconstitution, live attenuated varicella–zoster virus (Oka/Merck strain) propagated in human diploid cells, net price single-dose vial (with syringe containing diluent) = £99.96
Excipients include gelatin and neomycin
Dose prevention of herpes zoster (shingles), by subcutaneous injection preferably into deltoid region, ADULT 70–80 years, 0.65 mL as a single dose
Note Advice in BNF may differ from that in product literature

Yellow fever vaccine

Live yellow fever vaccine is indicated for those travelling or living in areas where infection is endemic (see p. 871) and for laboratory staff who handle the virus or who handle clinical material from suspected cases. Infants under 6 months of age should not be vaccinated because there is a small risk of encephalitis; infants aged 6–9 months should be vaccinated only if the risk of yellow fever is high and unavoidable (seek expert advice). The immunity which probably lasts for life is officially accepted for 10 years starting from 10 days after primary immunisation and for a further 10 years immediately after revaccination.

Very rare, vaccine-associated adverse effects have been reported, such as viscerotropic disease (yellow fever vaccine-associated viscerotropic disease, YEL-AVD), a syndrome which may include metabolic acidosis, muscle and liver cytolysis, and multi-organ failure. Neurological disorders (yellow fever vaccine-associated neurotropic disease, YEL-AND) such as encephalitis have also been reported. These *very rare* adverse effects usually have occurred after the first dose of yellow fever vaccine in those with no previous immunity.

Pregnancy Live yellow fever vaccine should not be given during pregnancy because there is a theoretical risk of fetal infection. Pregnant women should be advised not to travel to areas at high risk of yellow fever. If exposure cannot be avoided during pregnancy, then the vaccine should be given if the risk from disease in the mother outweighs the risk to the fetus from vaccination.

Breast-feeding Avoid; seek specialist advice if exposure to virus cannot be avoided.

■ YELLOW FEVER VACCINE, LIVE

Indications immunisation against yellow fever
Cautions see section 14.1; *also* individuals over 60 years—greater risk of vaccine-associated adverse effects, see notes above
Contra-indications see section 14.1 and notes above; *also* children under 6 months; history of thymus dysfunction
Pregnancy see notes above
Breast-feeding see notes above
Side-effects see section 14.1; also reported neurotropic disease and viscerotropic disease (see notes above)
Dose
• By deep subcutaneous injection, ADULT and CHILD over 9 months, 0.5 mL (see also notes above)

Yellow Fever Vaccine, Live PoM
Yel(live)
Injection, powder for reconstitution, live, attenuated 17D-204 strain of yellow fever virus, cultivated in chick embryos; single dose vial with syringe containing 0.5 mL diluent
Available (only to designated Yellow Fever Vaccination centres) as *Stamaril®*

14.5 Immunoglobulins

14.5.1　Normal immunoglobulin
14.5.2　Disease-specific immunoglobulins
14.5.3　Anti-D (Rh₀) immunoglobulin

Two types of human immunoglobulin preparation are available, **normal immunoglobulin** and **disease-specific immunoglobulins**.

Human immunoglobulin is a sterile preparation of concentrated antibodies (immune globulins) recovered from pooled human plasma or serum obtained from outside the UK, tested and found non-reactive for hepatitis B surface antigen and for antibodies against hepatitis C virus and human immunodeficiency virus (types 1 and 2). A global shortage of human immunoglobulin and the rapidly increasing range of clinical indications for treatment with immunoglobulins has resulted in the need for a Demand Management programme in the UK (for further information consult www.ivig.nhs.uk and *Clinical Guidelines for Immunoglobulin Use*, www.gov.uk/dh).

Immunoglobulins of animal origin (antisera were frequently associated with hypersensitivity reactions and are no longer used.

Further information on the use of immunoglobulins is included in the Health Protection Agency's *Immunoglobulin Handbook* www.hpa.org.uk, and in the Department of Health's publication, *Immunisation against Infectious Disease*, www.gov.uk/dh.

Availability Normal immunoglobulin for intramuscular administration is available from some regional Public Health laboratories for protection of contacts and the control of outbreaks of hepatitis A, measles, and rubella only. For other indications, subcutaneous or intravenous normal immunoglobulin should be purchased from the manufacturer.

Disease-specific immunoglobulins (section 14.5.2) are available from some regional Public Health laboratories, with the exception of **tetanus immunoglobulin** which is available from BPL, hospital pharmacies, or blood transfusion departments. **Rabies immunoglobulin** is available from the Specialist and Reference Microbiology Division, Public Health England, Colindale. **Hepatitis B immunoglobulin** required by transplant centres should be obtained commercially.

In Scotland all immunoglobulins are available from the *Scottish National Blood Transfusion Service* (SNBTS).

In Wales all immunoglobulins are available from the *Welsh Blood Service* (WBS).

In Northern Ireland all immunoglobulins are available from the *Northern Ireland Blood Transfusion Service* (NIBTS).

14.5.1 Normal immunoglobulin

Human **normal immunoglobulin** ('HNIG') is prepared from pools of at least 1000 donations of human plasma; it contains immunoglobulin G (IgG) and antibodies to hepatitis A, measles, mumps, rubella, varicella, and other viruses that are currently prevalent in the general population.

Normal immunoglobulin may **interfere with the immune response to live virus vaccines** which should therefore only be given **at least 3 weeks before or 3 months after** an injection of normal immunoglobulin (this does not apply to yellow fever vaccine since normal immunoglobulin does not contain antibody to this virus).

Uses Normal immunoglobulin (containing 10%–18% protein) is administered by *intramuscular injection* for the protection of susceptible contacts against **hepatitis A** virus (infectious hepatitis), **measles** and, to a lesser extent, **rubella**. Injection of immunoglobulin produces immediate protection lasting several weeks.

Normal immunoglobulin (containing 3%–12% protein) for *intravenous administration* is used as *replacement therapy* for patients with congenital agammaglobulinaemia and hypogammaglobulinaemia, and for the short-term treatment of idiopathic thrombocytopenic purpura and Kawasaki disease; it is also used for the prophylaxis of infection following bone-marrow transplantation and in children with symptomatic HIV infection who have recurrent bacterial infections. Normal immunoglobulin for replacement therapy may also be given intramuscularly or subcutaneously, but intravenous formulations are normally preferred. Intravenous immunoglobulin is also used in the treatment of Guillain-Barré syndrome as an alternative to plasma exchange.

For guidance on the use of intravenous normal immunoglobulins and alternative therapies for certain conditions, consult *Clinical Guidelines for Immunoglobulin Use* (www.gov.uk/dh).

Hepatitis A Hepatitis A vaccine is preferred for individuals at risk of infection (see p. 850) including those visiting areas where the disease is highly endemic (all countries excluding Northern and Western Europe, North America, Japan, Australia, and New Zealand). In unimmunised individuals, transmission of hepatitis A is reduced by good hygiene. Intramuscular normal immunoglobulin is no longer recommended for routine prophylaxis in travellers, but it may be indicated for immunocompromised patients if their antibody response to the vaccine is unlikely to be adequate.

Intramuscular normal immunoglobulin is recommended for prevention of infection in close contacts (of confirmed cases of hepatitis A) who have chronic liver disease or HIV infection, or who are immunosuppressed or over 50 years of age; normal immunoglobulin should be given as soon as possible, preferably within 14 days of exposure to the primary case. However, normal immunoglobulin can still be given to contacts at risk of severe disease up to 28 days after exposure to the primary case. Hepatitis A vaccine can be given at the same time, but it should be given at a separate injection site.

Measles Intravenous or subcutaneous normal immunoglobulin may be given to prevent or attenuate an attack of measles in individuals who do not have adequate immunity. Children and adults with compromised immunity who have come into contact with measles should receive intravenous or subcutaneous normal immunoglobulin as soon as possible after exposure. It is most effective if given within 72 hours but can be effective if given within 6 days.

Subcutaneous or intramuscular normal immunoglobulin should also be considered for the following individuals if they have been in contact with a confirmed case of measles or with a person associated with a local outbreak:

- non-immune pregnant women;
- infants under 9 months.

Further advice should be sought from the Centre for Infections, Public Health England (tel. (020) 8200 6868).

Individuals with normal immunity who are not in the above categories and who have not been fully immunised against measles, can be given MMR vaccine (section 14.4) for prophylaxis following exposure to measles.

Rubella Intramuscular immunoglobulin after exposure to rubella does **not** prevent infection in non-immune contacts and is **not** recommended for protection of pregnant women exposed to rubella. It may, however, reduce the likelihood of a clinical attack which may possibly reduce the risk to the fetus. Risk of intrauterine transmission is greatest in the first 11 weeks of pregnancy, between 16 and 20 weeks there is minimal risk of deafness only, after 20 weeks there is no increased risk. Intramuscular normal immunoglobulin should be used only if termination of pregnancy would be unacceptable to the pregnant woman—it should be given as soon as possible after exposure. Serological follow-up of recipients is essential to determine if the woman has become infected despite receiving immunoglobulin.

For routine prophylaxis against Rubella, see MMR vaccine (p. 856).

NORMAL IMMUNOGLOBULIN

Indications see notes above

Cautions hypo- or agammaglobulinaemia with or without IgA deficiency; interference with live virus vaccines—see above

Intravenous use thrombophilic disorders, or risk factors for arterial or venous thromboembolic events; obesity; ensure adequate hydration, renal insufficiency

Contra-indications patients with selective IgA deficiency who have known antibody against IgA

Renal impairment monitor for acute renal failure; consider discontinuation if renal function deteriorates. Intravenous preparations with added sucrose have been associated with cases of renal dysfunction and acute renal failure

Side-effects nausea, diarrhoea, chills, fever, headache, dizziness, arthralgia, myalgia, muscle spasms, low back pain; *rarely* hypotension, anaphylaxis, cutaneous skin reactions, aseptic meningitis, acute renal failure; also reported with *intravenous use*, injection site reactions, abdominal pain and distension, blood pressure fluctuations, haemolytic anaemia, thromboembolic events including myocardial infarction, stroke, pulmonary embolism, and deep vein thrombosis

Note Adverse reactions are more likely to occur in patients receiving normal immunoglobulin for the first time, or following a prolonged period between treatments, or when a different brand of normal immunoglobulin is administered.

14 Immunological products and vaccines

Dose

● See under preparations

Note Antibody titres can vary widely between normal immunoglobulin preparations from different manufacturers—formulations are **not interchangeable**; patients should be maintained on the same formulation throughout long-term treatment to avoid adverse effects

◢**For intramuscular use**

Normal Immunoglobulin (PoM)

Normal immunoglobulin injection. 250-mg vial; 750-mg vial

Dose by deep intramuscular injection, to control outbreaks of hepatitis A (see notes above), 500 mg; CHILD under 10 years 250 mg

Rubella in pregnancy, prevention of clinical attack, 750 mg

Available from the Centre for Infections and other regional Health Protection Agency offices (for contacts and control of outbreaks only, see above)

◢**For subcutaneous use**

Gammanorm® (Octapharma) (PoM)

Normal immunoglobulin (protein 16.5%) injection, net price 1.65 g (10 mL) = £96.77, 3.3 g (20 mL) = £193.55

Electrolytes Na$^+$ 1.09 mmol/10-mL vial

Dose by subcutaneous infusion, antibody deficiency syndromes, consult product literature

Note May be administered by intramuscular injection (if subcutaneous route not possible) but **not** for patients with thrombocytopenia or other bleeding disorders

Hizentra® (CSL Behring) ▼ (PoM)

Normal immunoglobulin (protein 20%) injection, net price 1 g (5 mL) = £45.90, 2 g (10 mL) = £91.80, 4 g (20 mL) = £183.60

Note Contains L-proline; contra-indicated in patients with hyperprolinaemia

Dose by subcutaneous infusion, antibody deficiency syndromes, consult product literature

Subcuvia® (Baxter) (PoM)

Normal immunoglobulin (protein 16%) injection, net price 800 mg (5 mL) = £32.56, 1.6 g (10 mL) = £65.12

Dose by subcutaneous infusion, ADULT and CHILD over 12 years antibody deficiency syndromes, consult product literature

Note May be administered by intramuscular injection (if subcutaneous route not possible) but **not** for patients with thrombocytopenia or other bleeding disorders

Subgam® (BPL) (PoM)

Normal immunoglobulin (protein 14%-18%) injection, net price 250-mg vial = £11.20, 750-mg vial = £34.20, 1.5-g vial = £68.40

Dose by subcutaneous infusion, antibody deficiency syndromes, consult product literature

By intramuscular injection, Hepatitis A prophylaxis in outbreaks (see notes above), ADULT and CHILD over 10 years, 750 mg, CHILD under 10 years, 500 mg

Rubella, in pregnancy, prevention of clinical attack (see also notes above), 750 mg

Note *Subgam®* is not licensed for prophylactic use, but due to difficulty in obtaining suitable immunoglobulin products, the Health Protection Agency recommends intramuscular use for prophylaxis against Hepatitis A or rubella

◢**For intravenous use**

Note Dose recommendation for Kawasaki disease, see *BNF for Children*; other indications—consult product literature for dosage regimens

Aragam® (Oxbridge) (PoM)

Intravenous infusion, human normal immunoglobulin, protein 5%, net price 2.5 g (50 mL) = £145.00, 5 g (100 mL) = £290.00, 10 g (200 mL) = £580.00, 20 g (400 mL) = £1160.00

Excipients include glucose 50 mg/mL

Flebogamma® DIF (Grifols) (PoM)

Intravenous infusion, human normal immunoglobulin, protein 5%, net price 0.5 g (10 mL) = £30.00, 2.5 g (50 mL) = £127.50, 5 g (100 mL) = £255.00, 10 g (200 mL) = £510.00, 20 g (400 mL) = £1020.00; protein 10%, 5 g (50 mL) = £300.00, 10 g (100 mL) = £600.00, 20 g (200 mL) = £1200.00

Note Both strengths contain sorbitol 50 mg/mL; contra-indicated in patients with hereditary fructose intolerance

Gammagard S/D® (Baxter) (PoM)

Intravenous infusion, (providing protein 5% or 10%), net price 5 g (with diluent) = £200.50, 10 g (with diluent) = £401.00

Gammaplex® (BPL) (PoM)

Intravenous infusion, human normal immunoglobulin (protein 5%), net price 2.5 g (50 mL) = £104.50, 5 g (100 mL) = £209.00, 10 g (200 mL) = £418.00

Note Contains sorbitol 50 mg/mL; contra-indicated in patients with hereditary fructose intolerance

Gamunex® (Grifols) (PoM)

Intravenous infusion, human normal immunoglobulin (protein 10%), net price 5 g (50 mL) = £212.50, 10 g (100 mL) = £425.00, 20 g (200 mL) = £850.00

Note Use Glucose 5% intravenous infusion if dilution prior to infusion is required

Intratect® (Biotest UK) (PoM)

Intravenous infusion, human normal immunoglobulin, protein 5%, net price 1 g (20 mL) = £45.00, 2.5 g (50 mL) = £112.50, 5 g (100 mL) = £225.00, 10 g (200 mL) = £450.00; protein 10%, 1 g (10 mL) = £45.00, 5 g (50 mL) = £225.00, 10 g (100 mL) = £450.00, 20 g (200 mL) = £900.00

Kiovig® (Baxter) (PoM)

Intravenous infusion, human normal immunoglobulin (protein 10%), net price 1 g (10 mL) = £49.00, 2.5 g (25 mL) = £122.50, 5 g (50 mL) = £245.00, 10 g (100 mL) = £490.00, 20 g (200 mL) = £980.00, 30 g (300 mL) = £1470.00

Note Use Glucose 5% intravenous infusion, if dilution prior to administration is required

Octagam® (Octapharma) (PoM)

Intravenous infusion, human normal immunoglobulin, protein 5%, net price 2.5 g (50 mL) = £102.00, 5 g (100 mL) = £204.00, 10 g (200 mL) = £408.00; protein 10%, 2 g (20 mL) = £117.30, 5 g (50 mL) = £293.25, 10 g (100 mL) = £586.50, 20 g (200 mL) = £1173.00

Note Contains maltose (may cause falsely elevated results with blood glucose testing systems)

Privigen® (CSL Behring) (PoM)

Intravenous infusion, human normal immunoglobulin (protein 10%), net price 2.5 g (25 mL) = £114.75, 5 g (50 mL) = £229.50, 10 g (100 mL) = £459.00, 20 g (200 mL) = £918.00

Note Contains L-proline; contra-indicated in patients with hyperprolinaemia

Vigam® (BPL) (PoM)

Intravenous infusion, human normal immunoglobulin (protein 5%), net price 2.5 g (50 mL) = £95.00, 5 g (100 mL) = £209.00, 10 g (200 mL) = £418.00

Note Contains sucrose (see Renal impairment, above)

14 Immunological products and vaccines

14.5.2 Disease-specific immunoglobulins

Specific immunoglobulins are prepared by pooling the plasma of selected human donors with high levels of the specific antibody required. For further information, see Immunoglobulin Handbook (www.hpa.org.uk).

There are no specific immunoglobulins for hepatitis A, measles, or rubella—normal immunoglobulin, section 14.5.1 is used in certain circumstances. There is no specific immunoglobulin for mumps; neither normal immunoglobulin nor MMR vaccine is effective as post-exposure prophylaxis.

Hepatitis B

Disease-specific **hepatitis B immunoglobulin** ('HBIG') is available for use in association with hepatitis B vaccine for the prevention of infection in laboratory and other personnel who have been accidentally inoculated with hepatitis B virus, and in infants born to mothers who have become infected with this virus in pregnancy or who are high-risk carriers (see Hepatitis B Vaccine, p. 852). Hepatitis B immunoglobulin will not inhibit the antibody response when given at the same time as hepatitis B vaccine but should be given at different sites.

An intravenous and subcutaneous preparation of hepatitis B-specific immunoglobulin is licensed for the prevention of hepatitis B recurrence in HBV-DNA negative patients who have undergone liver transplantation for liver failure caused by the virus.

▌ HEPATITIS B IMMUNOGLOBULIN

Indications prophylaxis against hepatitis B infection

Cautions IgA deficiency; interference with live virus vaccines see under Normal Immunoglobulin, p. 867.

Side-effects injection site reactions; less frequently, buccal ulceration, glossitis, abdominal pain, chest pain, dyspnoea, anaphylaxis, tremor, dizziness, headache, arthralgia; for side-effects associated with intravenous immunoglobulin, see section 14.5.1

Dose
- See under preparations and see also notes above

◢For intramuscular use

Hepatitis B Immunoglobulin PoM

Injection, hepatitis B-specific immunoglobulin, 100 units/mL. Vials containing 200 units or 500 units, available from selected Health Protection Agency and NHS laboratories (except for Transplant Centres, see p. 866), also available from BPL

Dose by intramuscular injection (as soon as possible after exposure; ideally within 12–48 hours, but no later than 7 days after exposure), ADULT and CHILD over 10 years 500 units; CHILD under 5 years 200 units, 5–9 years 300 units; NEONATE 200 units

Prevention of transmitted infection at birth, NEONATE 200 units as soon as possible after birth; for full details consult *Immunisation against Infectious Disease* (www.dh. gov.uk)

◢For intravenous use

Hepatect®CP (Biotest UK) PoM

Intravenous infusion, hepatitis B-specific immunoglobulin 50 units/mL, net price 500 units (10 mL) = £300.00, 2000 units (40 mL) = £1100.00, 5000 units (100 mL) = £3000.00

Dose by intravenous infusion, after exposure to hepatitis B virus-contaminated material—consult product literature

Prevention of transmitted infection at birth—consult product literature

Prevention of hepatitis B in haemodialysed patients, prophylaxis against re-infection of transplanted liver—consult product literature

◢For subcutaneous use

Zutectra® (Biotest UK) PoM

Injection, hepatitis B-specific immunoglobulin, 500 units/mL, net price 5 × 1-mL prefilled syringes = £1500.00

Dose prevention of hepatitis B re-infection more than 6 months after liver transplantation in stable HBV-DNA negative patients starting 2–3 weeks after last dose of intravenous hepatitis B immunoglobulin, by subcutaneous injection, ADULT body-weight under 75 kg 500 units once weekly, increased if necessary up to 1000 units once weekly; body-weight over 75 kg 1000 units once weekly

Rabies

Following exposure of an unimmunised individual to an animal in or from a country where the risk of rabies is high the site of the bite should be washed with soapy water and specific rabies immunoglobulin of human origin administered. All of the dose should be injected around the site of the wound; if this is difficult or the wound has completely healed it can be given in the anterolateral thigh (remote from the site used for vaccination).

Rabies vaccine should also be given intramuscularly at a different site (for details see Rabies vaccine p. 862). If there is delay in giving the rabies immunoglobulin, it should be given within 7 days of starting the course of rabies vaccine.

▌ RABIES IMMUNOGLOBULIN

Indications post-exposure prophylaxis against rabies infection

Cautions IgA deficiency; interference with live virus vaccines—see p. 867 under Normal Immunoglobulin

Side-effects injection site swelling and pain; *very rarely* anaphylaxis; buccal ulceration, glossitis, chest tightness, dyspnoea, tremor, dizziness, arthralgia, and facial oedema also reported

Dose
- See under preparation

Rabies Immunoglobulin PoM
(Antirabies Immunoglobulin Injection)
See notes above

Dose 20 units/kg by infiltration in and around the cleansed wound; if wound not visible or healed or if infiltration of whole volume not possible, give remainder by intramuscular injection into anterolateral thigh (remote from vaccination site)

Note The potency of individual batches of rabies immunoglobulin from the manufacturer may vary; potency may also be described differently by different manufacturers. It is therefore critical to know the potency of the batch to be used and the weight of the patient in order to calculate the specific volume required to provide the necessary dose

Available from Specialist and Reference Microbiology Division, Public Health England (see section 14.5 under availability) (also from BPL)

Tetanus

For the management of tetanus-prone wounds, **tetanus immunoglobulin** should be used in addition to wound cleansing and, where appropriate, antibacterial prophylaxis and a tetanus-containing vaccine (see Diphtheria-containing Vaccines, section 14.4). Tetanus immunoglobulin, together with metronidazole (section 5.1.11) and wound cleansing, should also be used for the treatment of established cases of tetanus.

▌ TETANUS IMMUNOGLOBULIN

Indications   post-exposure prophylaxis and treatment of tetanus infection

Cautions   IgA deficiency; interference with live virus vaccines—see p. 867

Side-effects   injection site swelling and pain; *rarely* anaphylaxis

Dose

- Post-exposure prophylaxis, by intramuscular injection 250 units, increased to 500 units if more than 24 hours have elapsed or there is risk of heavy contamination or following burns
- Treatment of tetanus infection, by intramuscular injection 150 units/kg (multiple sites)

Tetanus Immunoglobulin PoM
(Antitetanus Immunoglobulin Injection)
Available from BPL
Note   May be difficult to obtain

Varicella–zoster

Varicella–zoster immunoglobulin (VZIG) is recommended for individuals who are at increased risk of severe varicella *and* who have no antibodies to varicella–zoster virus *and* who have significant exposure to chickenpox or herpes zoster. Those at increased risk include:

- neonates whose mothers develop chickenpox in the period 7 days before to 7 days after delivery;
- susceptible neonates exposed in the first 7 days of life;
- susceptible neonates or infants exposed whilst requiring intensive or prolonged special care nursing;
- susceptible women exposed at any stage of pregnancy (but when supplies of VZIG are short, may only be issued to those exposed in the first 20 weeks' gestation or to those near term) providing VZIG is given within 10 days of contact;
- immunocompromised individuals including those who have received corticosteroids in the previous 3 months at the following dose equivalents of prednisolone; *children* 2 mg/kg daily for at least 1 week or 1 mg/kg daily for 1 month; *adults* about 40 mg daily for more than 1 week.

Important: for full details consult *Immunisation against Infectious Disease*. **Varicella–zoster vaccine** is available—see section 14.4. For treatment of varicella–zoster infections, see section 5.3.2.1

▌ VARICELLA–ZOSTER IMMUNOGLOBULIN

Indications   prophylaxis against varicella infection

Cautions   IgA deficiency; interference with live virus vaccines—see p. 867

Side-effects   injection site swelling and pain; *rarely* anaphylaxis

Dose

- By intramuscular injection, prophylaxis (as soon as possible—not later than 10 days after exposure), ADULT and CHILD 15 years and over, 1 g; NEONATE, INFANT and CHILD up to and including 5 years 250 mg, 6–10 years 500 mg, 11–14 years 750 mg; give second dose if further exposure occurs more than 3 weeks after first dose

Note   No evidence that effective in treatment of severe disease. Normal immunoglobulin for intravenous use (section 14.5.1) may be used in those unable to receive intramuscular injections

Varicella–Zoster Immunoglobulin PoM
(Antivaricella–zoster Immunoglobulin)
Available from selected Health Protection Agency and NHS laboratories; (see section 14.5 under Availability); also from BPL

14.5.3   Anti-D (Rh₀) immunoglobulin

Anti-D (Rh₀) immunoglobulin is prepared from plasma taken from rhesus-negative donors who have been immunised against the anti-D-antigen. Anti-D (Rh₀) immunoglobulin is used to prevent a rhesus-negative mother from forming antibodies to fetal rhesus-positive cells which may pass into the maternal circulation. The objective is to protect any subsequent child from the hazard of haemolytic disease of the newborn.

Anti-D immunoglobulin should be administered to the mother following any sensitising episode (e.g. abortion, miscarriage and birth); it should be injected within 72 hours of the episode but even if a longer period has elapsed it may still give protection and should be administered. Anti-D (Rh₀) immunoglobulin is also given when significant feto-maternal haemorrhage occurs in rhesus-negative women during delivery. The dose of anti-D immunoglobulin is determined according to the level of exposure to rhesus-positive blood.

For routine antenatal prophylaxis NICE recommends that two doses of either 500 units *or* 1000–1650 units of anti-D immunoglobulin should be given, the first at 28 weeks' gestation and the second at 34 weeks; alternatively a single dose of 1500 units given between 28 and 30 weeks gestation can be used (see also NICE guidance below).

Use of routine *antenatal* anti-D prophylaxis should be given irrespective of previous anti-D prophylaxis for a sensitising event early in the same pregnancy. Similarly, *postpartum* anti-D prophylaxis should be given irrespective of previous routine antenatal anti-D prophylaxis or antenatal anti-D prophylaxis for a sensitising event in the same pregnancy.

MMR vaccine

MMR vaccine may be given in the postpartum
period with anti-D (Rh$_0$) immunoglobulin injection
provided that separate syringes are used and the
products are administered into different limbs. If
blood is transfused, the antibody response to the
vaccine may be inhibited—measure rubella antibodies after 6–8 weeks and revaccinate if necessary.

Anti-D (Rh$_0$) immunoglobulin is also given to women of
child-bearing potential after the inadvertent transfusion
of rhesus-incompatible blood components and is used
for the treatment of idiopathic thrombocytopenia
purpura.

ANTI-D (Rh$_0$) IMMUNOGLOBULIN

Indications see notes above

Cautions immunoglobulin A deficiency; possible
interference with live virus vaccines, see under p. 867,
but see notes above about administration with MMR
vaccine

Contra-indications treatment of idiopathic thrombocytopenia purpura in rhesus negative or splenectomised patients

Side-effects nausea, vomiting, diarrhoea, abdominal
pain; hypotension, hypertension, headache, fever,
malaise, asthenia, drowsiness, dizziness, back pain,
arthralgia, myalgia; pruritus, rash, sweating, injection
site pain; *rarely* tachycardia, anaphylaxis, dyspnoea,
hypotension, and urticaria; (for side-effects associated
with *intravenous* immunoglobulins, see section 14.5.1

Dose
● See preparations below

Anti-D (Rh$_0$) Immunoglobulin [PoM]
Injection, anti-D (Rh$_0$) immunoglobulin, net price
250-unit vial = £23.75, 500-unit vial = £33.75, 1500-
unit vial = £58.00, 2500-unit vial = £94.40
Dose by deep intramuscular injection, to rhesus-negative
woman for prevention of Rh$_0$(D) sensitisation:

Following birth of rhesus-positive infant, 500 units
immediately or within 72 hours; for transplacental bleed of
over 4 mL fetal red cells, extra 100–125 units per mL fetal
red cells

Following any potentially sensitising episode (e.g. stillbirth,
abortion, amniocentesis) up to 20 weeks' gestation
250 units per episode (after 20 weeks, 500 units)
immediately or within 72 hours

Antenatal prophylaxis, 500 units given at weeks 28 and 34
of pregnancy; if infant rhesus-positive, a further dose is still
needed immediately or within 72 hours of delivery

Following Rh$_0$(D) incompatible blood transfusion, 100–
125 units per mL transfused rhesus-positive red cells
Note Subcutaneous route used for patients with bleeding
disorders

Available from Blood Centres and from BPL (*D-Gam*®)

Rhophylac® (CSL Behring) [PoM]
Injection, anti-D (Rh$_0$) immunoglobulin 750 units/
mL (150 micrograms/mL), net price 2-mL (1500-
unit) prefilled syringe = £39.52.
Dose by intramuscular *or* intravenous injection, to rhesus-
negative woman for prevention of Rh$_0$(D) sensitisation:

Following birth of rhesus-positive infant, 1000–1500 units
immediately or within 72 hours; for large transplacental
bleed, extra 100 units per mL fetal red cells (preferably by
intravenous injection)

Following any potentially sensitising episode (e.g. abortion,
amniocentesis, chorionic villous sampling) up to 12 weeks'
gestation 1000 units per episode (after 12 weeks, higher
doses may be required) immediately or within 72 hours

Antenatal prophylaxis, 1500 units given between weeks
28–30 of pregnancy; if infant rhesus-positive, a further
dose is still needed immediately or within 72 hours of
delivery

Following Rh$_0$(D) incompatible blood transfusion, by
intravenous injection, 50 units per mL transfused rhesus-
positive blood (or 100 units per mL of erythrocyte
concentrate)

Note Intravenous route recommended for patients with
bleeding disorders.

14.6 International travel

Note For advice on **malaria chemoprophylaxis**, see section
5.4.1.

No special immunisation is required for travellers to the
United States, Europe, Australia, or New Zealand,
although all travellers should have immunity to tetanus
and poliomyelitis (and childhood immunisations should
be up to date); see also Tick-borne Encephalitis, p. 864,
Certain special precautions are required in non-Eur-
opean areas surrounding the Mediterranean, in Africa,
the Middle East, Asia, and South America.

Travellers to areas that have a high incidence of **poliomyelitis** or **tuberculosis** should be immunised with the
appropriate vaccine; in the case of poliomyelitis previously immunised adults may be given a booster dose of
a preparation containing inactivated poliomyelitis
vaccine (see p. 861). BCG immunisation (see p. 846) is
recommended for travellers aged under 16 years[1] pro-
posing to stay for longer than 3 months (or in close
contact with the local population) in countries with an
incidence of tuberculosis greater than 40 per 100 000[2]; it
should preferably be given 3 months or more before
departure.

Yellow fever immunisation (see p. 866) is recommended for travel to the endemic zones of Africa and
South America. Many countries require an International
Certificate of Vaccination from individuals arriving
from, or who have been travelling through, endemic
areas; other countries require a certificate from all
entering travellers (consult the Department of Health
handbook, *Health Information for Overseas Travel*, www.
dh.gov.uk).

Immunisation against **meningococcal meningitis** is
recommended for a number of areas of the world (for
details, see p. 858).

---

1. There is inadequate evidence of protection by BCG
vaccine in adults aged over 35 years; however, vaccination is recommended for healthcare workers irrespective of age because of the increased risk to them or their
patients
2. List of countries where the incidence of tuberculosis is
greater than 40 cases per 100 000 is available at www.
hpa.org.uk

14 Immunological products and vaccines

Protection against **hepatitis A** is recommended for travellers to high-risk areas outside Northern and Western Europe, North America, Japan, Australia and New Zealand. Hepatitis A vaccine (see p. 850) is preferred and it is likely to be effective even if given shortly before departure; normal immunoglobulin is no longer given routinely but may be indicated in the immunocompromised (see p. 867). Special care must also be taken with food hygiene (see below).

Hepatitis B vaccine (see p. 852) is recommended for those travelling to areas of high or intermediate prevalence who intend to seek employment as healthcare workers or who plan to remain there for lengthy periods and who may therefore be at increased risk of acquiring infection as the result of medical or dental procedures carried out in those countries. Short-term tourists or business travellers are not generally at increased risk of infection but may put themselves at risk by their sexual behaviour when abroad.

Prophylactic immunisation against **rabies** (see p. 862) is recommended for travellers to enzootic areas on long journeys or to areas out of reach of immediate medical attention.

Travellers who have not had a **tetanus** booster in the last 10 years and are visiting areas where medical attention may not be accessible should receive a booster dose of adsorbed diphtheria [low dose], tetanus and poliomyelitis (inactivated) vaccine (see p. 848), even if they have received 5 doses of a tetanus-containing vaccine previously.

Typhoid vaccine (see p. 864) is indicated for travellers to countries where typhoid is endemic, but the vaccine is no substitute for personal precautions (see below).

There is no requirement for cholera vaccination as a condition for entry into any country, but **oral cholera vaccine** (see p. 848) should be considered for backpackers and those travelling to situations where the risk is greatest (e.g. refugee camps). Regardless of vaccination, travellers to areas where cholera is endemic should take special care with food hygiene (see below).

Advice on **diphtheria** (see p. 848), on **Japanese encephalitis** (see p. 856), and on **tick-borne encephalitis** (see p. 864) is included in *Health Information for Overseas Travel*, see below.

Food hygiene In areas where sanitation is poor, good food hygiene is important to help prevent hepatitis A, typhoid, cholera, and other diarrhoeal diseases (including travellers' diarrhoea). Food should be freshly prepared and hot, and uncooked vegetables (including green salads) should be avoided; only fruits which can be peeled should be eaten. Only suitable bottled water, or tap water that has been boiled or treated with sterilising tablets, should be used for drinking.

Information on health advice for travellers

Health professionals and travellers can find the latest information on immunisation requirements and precautions for avoiding disease while travelling from: www.nathnac.org

The handbook, *Health Information for Overseas Travel* (2010), which draws together essential information *for healthcare professionals* regarding health advice for travellers, can also be obtained from this website.

Immunisation requirements change from time to time, and information on the current requirements for any particular country may be obtained from the embassy or legation of the appropriate country or from:

National Travel Health Network and Centre
UCLH NHS Foundation Trust
3rd Floor Central
250 Euston Road
London, NW1 2PG
Tel: 0845 602 6712
(8.30–11.45 a.m, 1–3.15 p.m. weekdays for healthcare professionals **only**)
www.nathnac.org

Travel Medicine Team
Health Protection Scotland
Meridian Court
5 Cadogan Street
Glasgow, G2 6QE
Tel: (0141) 300 1130
(2-4 p.m. Monday and Wednesday, 9.30-11.30 a.m. Friday; for registered TRAVAX users **only**)
www.travax.nhs.uk (free for NHS Scotland users, registration required; subscription fee may be payable for users outside NHS Scotland)

Welsh Assembly Government
Tel: (029) 2082 5397
(9 a.m.–5.30 p.m. weekdays)

Department of Health, Social Services and Public Safety
Castle Buildings
Stormont
Belfast, BT4 3SQ
Tel: (028) 9052 2118
(9 a.m.–5 p.m. weekdays)
www.dhsspsni.gov.uk

15 Anaesthesia

15.1 General anaesthesia

- **15.1.1** Intravenous anaesthetics
- **15.1.2** Inhalational anaesthetics
- **15.1.3** Antimuscarinic drugs
- **15.1.4** Sedative and analgesic peri-operative drugs
- **15.1.5** Neuromuscular blocking drugs
- **15.1.6** Drugs for reversal of neuromuscular blockade
- **15.1.7** Antagonists for central and respiratory depression
- **15.1.8** Drugs for malignant hyperthermia

Important

The drugs in section 15.1 should only be administered by, or under the direct supervision of, personnel experienced in their use, with adequate training in anaesthesia and airway management, and when resuscitation equipment is available.

Several different types of drug are given together during general anaesthesia. Anaesthesia is induced with either a volatile drug given by inhalation (section 15.1.2) or with an intravenously administered drug (section 15.1.1); anaesthesia is maintained with an intravenous or inhalational anaesthetic. Analgesics (section 15.1.4), usually short-acting opioids, are also used. The use of neuromuscular blocking drugs (section 15.1.5) necessitates intermittent positive-pressure ventilation. Following surgery, anticholinesterases (section 15.1.6) can be given to reverse the effects of neuromuscular blocking drugs; specific antagonists (section 15.1.7) can be used to reverse central and respiratory depression caused by some drugs used in surgery. A local topical anaesthetic (section 15.2) can be used to reduce pain at the injection site.

Individual requirements vary considerably and the recommended doses are only a guide. Smaller doses are indicated in ill, shocked, or debilitated patients and in significant hepatic impairment, while robust individuals may require larger doses. The required dose of induction agent may be less if the patient has been premedicated with a sedative agent or if an opioid analgesic has been used.

Surgery and long-term medication The risk of losing disease control on stopping long-term medication before surgery is often greater than the risk posed by continuing it during surgery. It is vital that the anaesthetist knows about all drugs that a patient is (or has been) taking.

Patients with adrenal atrophy resulting from long-term corticosteroid use (section 6.3.2) may suffer a precipitous fall in blood pressure unless corticosteroid cover is provided during anaesthesia and in the immediate post-operative period. Anaesthetists must therefore know whether a patient is, or has been, receiving corticosteroids (including high-dose inhaled corticosteroids).

15 Anaesthesia

Other drugs that should normally not be stopped before surgery include antiepileptics, antiparkinsonian drugs, antipsychotics, anxiolytics, bronchodilators, cardiovascular drugs (but see potassium-sparing diuretics, angiotensin-converting enzyme inhibitors, and angiotensin-II receptor antagonists below), glaucoma drugs, immunosuppressants, drugs of dependence, and thyroid or antithyroid drugs. Expert advice is required for patients receiving antivirals for HIV infection. For general advice on surgery in diabetic patients see section 6.1.1, p. 467.

Patients taking antiplatelet medication or an oral anticoagulant present an increased risk for surgery. In these circumstances, the anaesthetist and surgeon should assess the relative risks and decide jointly whether the antiplatelet or the anticoagulant drug should be stopped or replaced with unfractionated or low molecular weight heparin therapy.

Drugs that should be stopped before surgery include combined oral contraceptives (see Surgery, section 7.3.1 for details); for advice on hormone replacement therapy, see section 6.4.1.1. If antidepressants need to be stopped, they should be withdrawn gradually to avoid withdrawal symptoms. MAOIs can have important interactions with some drugs used during surgery, such as pethidine (for interactions of MAOIs, see Appendix 1, MAOIs). Tricyclic antidepressants need not be stopped, but there may be an increased risk of arrhythmias and hypotension (and dangerous interactions with vasopressor drugs); therefore, the anaesthetist should be informed if they are not stopped. Lithium should be stopped 24 hours before major surgery but the normal dose can be continued for minor surgery (with careful monitoring of fluids and electrolytes). Potassium-sparing diuretics may need to be withheld on the morning of surgery because hyperkalaemia may develop if renal perfusion is impaired or if there is tissue damage. Angiotensin-converting enzyme (ACE) inhibitors and angiotensin-II receptor antagonists can be associated with severe hypotension after induction of anaesthesia; these drugs may need to be discontinued 24 hours before surgery. Herbal medicines may be associated with adverse effects when given with anaesthetic drugs and consideration should be given to stopping them before surgery.

Anaesthesia and driving   Patients given sedatives and analgesics during minor outpatient procedures should be very carefully warned about the risk of driving afterwards. For intravenous benzodiazepines and for a short general anaesthetic the risk extends to **at least 24 hours** after administration. Responsible persons should be available to take patients home. The dangers of taking **alcohol** should also be emphasised. See also Drugs and Driving, p. 3.

Prophylaxis of acid aspiration   Regurgitation and aspiration of gastric contents (Mendelson's syndrome) can be an important complication of general anaesthesia, particularly in obstetrics and during emergency surgery, and requires prophylaxis against acid aspiration. Prophylaxis is also needed in those with gastro-oesophageal reflux disease and in circumstances where gastric emptying may be delayed.

A H_2-receptor antagonist (section 1.3.1) can be used before surgery to increase the pH and reduce the volume of gastric fluid. It does not affect the pH of fluid already in the stomach and this limits its value in emergency procedures; an oral H_2-receptor antagonist can be given 1–2 hours before the procedure. Antacids

are frequently used to neutralise the acidity of the fluid already in the stomach; 'clear' (non-particulate) antacids such as sodium citrate are preferred. Sodium citrate 300 mmol/litre (88.2 mg/mL) oral solution is licensed for use before general anaesthesia for caesarean section (available from Viridian).

Anaesthesia, sedation, and resuscitation in dental practice

> For details see *A Conscious Decision: A review of the use of general anaesthesia and conscious sedation in primary dental care*; report by a group chaired by the Chief Medical Officer and Chief Dental Officer, July 2000 and associated documents. Further details can also be found in *Conscious Sedation in the Provision of Dental Care*; report of an Expert Group on Sedation for Dentistry (commissioned by the Department of Health), 2003.
>
> Guidance is also included in *Conscious Sedation in Dentistry: Dental Clinical Guidance*, Scottish Dental Clinical Effectiveness Programme, June 2012 (www.sdcep.org.uk).

15.1.1   Intravenous anaesthetics

> **Important**
> The drugs in this section should only be administered by, or under the direct supervision of, personnel experienced in their use, with adequate training in anaesthesia and airway management, and when resuscitation equipment is available.

Intravenous anaesthetics may be used either to induce anaesthesia or for maintenance of anaesthesia throughout surgery. Intravenous anaesthetics nearly all produce their effect in one arm-brain circulation time and can cause apnoea and hypotension, and so adequate resuscitative facilities **must** be available. They are **contra-indicated** if the anaesthetist is not confident of being able to maintain the airway (e.g. in the presence of a tumour in the pharynx or larynx). Extreme care is required in surgery of the mouth, pharynx, or larynx and in patients with acute circulatory failure (shock) or fixed cardiac output.

To facilitate tracheal intubation, induction is usually followed by a neuromuscular blocking drug (section 15.1.5) or a short-acting opioid (section 15.1.4.3).

The doses of all intravenous anaesthetic drugs should be titrated to effect (except when using 'rapid sequence induction'). The doses and rates of administration should be reduced in the elderly, and particularly in those with hypovolaemia or cardiovascular disease; lower doses may also be required in premedicated patients.

Total intravenous anaesthesia   This is a technique in which major surgery is carried out with all drugs given intravenously. Respiration can be spontaneous, or controlled with oxygen-enriched air. Neuromuscular blocking drugs can be used to provide relaxation and prevent reflex muscle movements. The main problem to be overcome is the assessment of depth of anaesthesia. Target Controlled Infusion (TCI) systems can be used to titrate intravenous anaesthetic infusions to predicted plasma-drug concentrations in ventilated adult patients.

Anaesthesia and driving   See section 15.1.

Drugs used for intravenous anaesthesia

Propofol, the most widely used intravenous anaesthetic, can be used for induction or maintenance of anaesthesia in adults and children, but it is not commonly used in neonates.

Propofol is associated with rapid recovery and less hangover effect than other intravenous anaesthetics. It causes pain on intravenous injection, which can be reduced by intravenous lidocaine. Significant extraneous muscle movements can occur. Rarely, convulsions, anaphylaxis, and delayed recovery from anaesthesia can occur after propofol administration; the onset of convulsions can be delayed. Propofol is associated with bradycardia, occasionally profound; intravenous administration of an antimuscarinic drug is used to treat this.

Propofol can be used for sedation during diagnostic procedures. In adults, it can be used for sedation in intensive care, but it is contra-indicated in children under 16 years receiving intensive care because of the risk of propofol infusion syndrome (potentially fatal effects, including metabolic acidosis, arrhythmias, cardiac failure, rhabdomyolysis, hyperlipidaemia, hyperkalaemia, hepatomegaly, and renal failure).

Thiopental sodium is a barbiturate that is used for induction of anaesthesia, but has no analgesic properties. Induction is generally smooth and rapid, but dose-related cardiovascular and respiratory depression can occur. Awakening from a moderate dose of thiopental is rapid because the drug redistributes into other tissues, particularly fat. However, metabolism is slow and sedative effects can persist for 24 hours. Repeated doses have a cumulative effect and recovery is much slower.

Etomidate is an intravenous agent associated with rapid recovery without a hangover effect. Etomidate causes less hypotension than thiopental and propofol during induction. It produces a high incidence of extraneous muscle movements, which can be minimised by an opioid analgesic or a short-acting benzodiazepine given just before induction. Pain on injection can be reduced by injecting into a larger vein or by giving an opioid analgesic just before induction. Etomidate suppresses adrenocortical function, particularly during continuous administration, and it should not be used for maintenance of anaesthesia. It should be used with caution in patients with underlying adrenal insufficiency, for example, those with sepsis.

Ketamine is used rarely. Ketamine causes less hypotension than thiopental and propofol during induction. It is used mainly for paediatric anaesthesia, particularly when repeated administration is required (such as for serial burns dressings); recovery is relatively slow and there is a high incidence of extraneous muscle movements. The main disadvantage of ketamine is the high incidence of hallucinations, nightmares, and other transient psychotic effects; these can be reduced by a benzodiazepine such as diazepam or midazolam.

◢ ETOMIDATE

Indications   induction of anaesthesia

Cautions   see under Intravenous Anaesthetics and notes above; avoid in acute porphyria (section 9.8.2); **interactions**: Appendix 1 (anaesthetics, general)

Contra-indications   see under Intravenous Anaesthetics and notes above

Hepatic impairment   reduce dose in liver cirrhosis

Pregnancy   may depress neonatal respiration if used during delivery

Breast-feeding   breast-feeding can be resumed as soon as mother has recovered sufficiently from anaesthesia

Side-effects   see notes above; also nausea, vomiting, hypotension, apnoea, hyperventilation, stridor, rash; *less commonly* hypersalivation, arrhythmias, hypertension, hiccups, cough, phlebitis; AV block, cardiac arrest, respiratory depression, seizures, shivering, and Stevens-Johnson syndrome also reported

Dose
- ADULT, by slow intravenous injection over 30–60 seconds, 150–300 micrograms/kg (max. total dose 60 mg); ELDERLY 150–200 micrograms/kg (max. total dose 60 mg); CHILD see *BNF for Children*
  Note Administer over 60 seconds in patients in whom hypotension might be hazardous

Etomidate-Lipuro® (B. Braun) ▣PoM▣
Injection (emulsion), etomidate 2 mg/mL, net price 10-mL amp = £1.56

Hypnomidate® (Janssen) ▣PoM▣
Injection, etomidate 2 mg/mL, net price 10-mL amp = £1.38
Excipients include propylene glycol (see Excipients, p. 2)

◢ KETAMINE

Indications   induction and maintenance of anaesthesia (but rarely used)

Cautions   see under Intravenous Anaesthetics and notes above; dehydration; hypertension; respiratory tract infection; increased cerebrospinal fluid pressure; predisposition to seizures, hallucinations, or nightmares; psychotic disorders; head injury or intracranial mass lesions; thyroid dysfunction; raised intra-ocular pressure; **interactions**: Appendix 1 (anaesthetics, general)

Contra-indications   see under Intravenous Anaesthetics; hypertension, pre-eclampsia or eclampsia, severe cardiac disease; stroke; raised intracranial pressure; head trauma; acute porphyria (section 9.8.2)

Hepatic impairment   consider dose reduction

Pregnancy   may depress neonatal respiration if used during delivery

Breast-feeding   avoid for at least 12 hours after last dose

Side-effects   see notes above; also nausea, vomiting, tachycardia, hypertension, diplopia, nystagmus, rash; *less commonly* arrhythmias, hypotension, bradycardia, respiratory depression, laryngospasm; *rarely* hypersalivation, apnoea, insomnia, cystitis (including haemorrhagic); raised intra-ocular pressure also reported

Dose
- By intramuscular injection, short procedures, ADULT, initially 6.5–13 mg/kg, adjusted according to response (10 mg/kg usually produces 12–25 minutes of surgical anaesthesia); CHILD under 18 years see *BNF for Children*

  Diagnostic manoeuvres and procedures not involving intense pain, initially 4 mg/kg
- By intravenous injection over at least 60 seconds, short procedures, ADULT, initially 1–4.5 mg/kg, adjusted according to response (2 mg/kg usually

15

Anaesthesia

produces 5–10 minutes of surgical anaesthesia); CHILD under 18 years see *BNF for Children*

- By intravenous infusion of a solution containing 1 mg/mL, longer procedures, ADULT, induction, total dose of 0.5–2 mg/kg; maintenance, 10–45 micrograms/kg/minute, rate adjusted according to response; CHILD under 18 years see *BNF for Children*

Ketalar® (Pfizer) CD4-1

Injection, ketamine (as hydrochloride) 10 mg/mL, net price 20-mL vial = £5.06; 50 mg/mL, 10-mL vial = £8.77; 100 mg/mL, 10-mL vial = £16.10

Administration For *intravenous injection*, dilute 100 mg/mL strength to a concentration of not more than 50 mg/mL with Glucose 5% *or* Sodium Chloride 0.9% *or* Water for Injections

Note May be difficult to obtain

PROPOFOL

Indications see under Dose

Cautions see under Intravenous Anaesthetics and notes above; cardiac impairment; respiratory impairment; elderly; hypovolaemia; epilepsy; hypotension; raised intracranial pressure; monitor blood-lipid concentration if risk of fat overload or if sedation longer than 3 days; **interactions**: Appendix 1 (anaesthetics, general)

Contra-indications see under Intravenous Anaesthetics and notes above

Hepatic impairment use with caution

Renal impairment use with caution

Pregnancy may depress neonatal respiration if used during delivery; max. dose for maintenance of anaesthesia 6 mg/kg/hour

Breast-feeding breast-feeding can be resumed as soon as mother has recovered sufficiently from anaesthesia

Side-effects see notes above; also hypotension, tachycardia, transient apnoea, headache; *less commonly* thrombosis, phlebitis; *rarely* arrhythmia, euphoria; *very rarely* pancreatitis, pulmonary oedema, sexual disinhibition, and discoloration of urine; propofol infusion syndrome (potentially fatal effects, including metabolic acidosis, arrhythmias, cardiac failure, rhabdomyolysis, hyperlipidaemia, hyperkalaemia, hepatomegaly, and renal failure) reported with prolonged infusion of doses exceeding 4 mg/kg/hour

Dose

- Induction of anaesthesia using 0.5% *or* 1% injection, by slow intravenous injection *or* infusion, ADULT under 55 years, 1.5–2.5 mg/kg at a rate of 20–40 mg every 10 seconds until response; ADULT over 55 years or debilitated, 1–1.5 mg/kg at a rate of 20 mg every 10 seconds until response; CHILD 1 month–18 years see *BNF for Children*
- Induction of anaesthesia using 2% injection, by intravenous infusion, ADULT under 55 years, 1.5–2.5 mg/kg at a rate of 20–40 mg every 10 seconds; ADULT over 55 years or debilitated, 1–1.5 mg/kg at a rate of 20 mg every 10 seconds until response; CHILD 3–18 years see *BNF for Children*
- Maintenance of anaesthesia using 1% injection, by intravenous infusion, 4–12 mg/kg/hour (3–6 mg/kg/hour in ELDERLY or debilitated) *or* by slow intravenous injection, 25–50 mg repeated according to response; CHILD 1 month–18 years see *BNF for Children*
- Maintenance of anaesthesia using 2% injection, by intravenous infusion, 4–12 mg/kg/hour (3–6 mg/kg/

hour in ELDERLY or debilitated); CHILD 3–18 years see *BNF for Children*

- Sedation of ventilated patients in intensive care using 1% *or* 2% injection, by intravenous infusion, ADULT and CHILD over 16 years, 0.3–4 mg/kg/hour
- Induction of sedation for surgical and diagnostic procedures using 0.5% *or* 1% injection, ADULT, initially by slow intravenous injection over 1–5 minutes, 0.5–1 mg/kg, dose and rate of administration adjusted according to desired level of sedation and response; CHILD 1 month–18 years see *BNF for Children*
- Maintenance of sedation for surgical and diagnostic procedures using 0.5% injection, by intravenous infusion, ADULT, 1.5–4.5 mg/kg/hour, dose and rate of administration adjusted according to desired level of sedation and response (additionally, if rapid increase in sedation required, by slow intravenous injection, 10–20 mg); patients over 55 years or debilitated may require lower dose and rate of administration; CHILD 17–18 years see *BNF for Children*
- Maintenance of sedation for surgical and diagnostic procedures using 1% injection, by intravenous infusion, ADULT, 1.5–4.5 mg/kg/hour, dose and rate of administration adjusted according to desired level of sedation and response (additionally, if rapid increase in sedation required, by slow intravenous injection, 10–20 mg); patients over 55 years or debilitated may require lower dose and rate of administration; CHILD 1 month–18 years see *BNF for Children*
- Maintenance of sedation for surgical and diagnostic procedures using 2% injection, by intravenous infusion, ADULT, 1.5–4.5 mg/kg/hour, dose and rate of administration adjusted according to desired level of sedation and response (additionally, if rapid increase in sedation required, by slow intravenous injection using 0.5% *or* 1% injection, 10–20 mg); patients over 55 years or debilitated may require lower dose and rate of administration; CHILD 3–18 years see *BNF for Children*

Propofol (Non-proprietary) PoM

0.5% injection (emulsion), propofol 5 mg/mL, net price 20-mL amp = £3.46

Brands include *Propofol-Lipuro®*

1% injection (emulsion), propofol 10 mg/mL, net price 20-mL amp = £4.18, 50-mL bottle = £10.10, 100-mL bottle = £19.40

Brands include *Propofol-Lipuro®*, *Propoven®*

2% injection (emulsion), propofol 20 mg/mL, net price 50-mL vial = £21.30

Brands include *Propofol-Lipuro®*, *Propoven®*

Diprivan® (AstraZeneca) PoM

1% injection (emulsion), propofol 10 mg/mL, net price 20-mL amp = £3.07, 50-mL prefilled syringe (for use with *Diprifusor® TCI* system) = £10.68

2% injection (emulsion), propofol 20 mg/mL, net price 50-mL prefilled syringe (for use with *Diprifusor® TCI* system) = £15.16

THIOPENTAL SODIUM
(Thiopentone sodium)

Indications induction of general anaesthesia; anaesthesia of short duration; reduction of raised intracranial pressure if ventilation controlled; status epilepticus (see also section 4.8.2)

Cautions see under Intravenous Anaesthetics and notes above; cardiovascular disease; reconstituted solution is highly alkaline—extravasation causes tissue necrosis and severe pain; avoid intra-arterial injection; **interactions:** Appendix 1 (anaesthetics, general)

Contra-indications see notes above; acute porphyria (section 9.8.2); myotonic dystrophy

Hepatic impairment use with caution—reduce dose

Renal impairment caution in severe impairment

Pregnancy may depress neonatal respiration when used during delivery

Breast-feeding breast-feeding can be resumed as soon as mother has recovered sufficiently from anaesthesia

Side-effects hypotension, arrhythmias, myocardial depression, laryngeal spasm, cough, headache, sneezing, hypersensitivity reactions, rash

Dose

- Induction of general anaesthesia, by slow intravenous injection usually as a 2.5% (25 mg/mL) solution, ADULT, fit and premedicated, initially 100–150 mg (reduced in elderly or debilitated) over 10–15 seconds (longer in elderly or debilitated), followed by further quantity if necessary according to response after 30–60 seconds; *or* up to 4 mg/kg (max. 500 mg); CHILD under 18 years see *BNF for Children*

- Raised intracranial pressure, by slow intravenous injection, 1.5–3 mg/kg, repeated as required

- Status epilepticus (only if other measures fail, see section 4.8.2), by slow intravenous injection as a 2.5% (25 mg/mL) solution, ADULT, 75–125 mg as a single dose; CHILD under 18 years see *BNF for Children*

Thiopental (Archimedes) [PoM]
Injection, powder for reconstitution, thiopental sodium, net price 500-mg vial = £5.75

15.1.2 Inhalational anaesthetics

Important
The drugs in this section should only be administered by, or under the direct supervision of, personnel experienced in their use, with adequate training in anaesthesia and airway management, and when resuscitation equipment is available.

Inhalational anaesthetics include gases and volatile liquids. *Gaseous anaesthetics* require suitable equipment for storage and administration. *Volatile liquid anaesthetics* are administered using calibrated vaporisers, using air, oxygen, or nitrous oxide-oxygen mixtures as the carrier gas. To prevent hypoxia, the inspired gas mixture should contain a minimum of 25% oxygen at all times. Higher concentrations of oxygen (greater than 30%) are usually required during inhalational anaesthesia when nitrous oxide is being administered, see Nitrous Oxide, p. 878.

Anaesthesia and driving See section 15.1.

Volatile liquid anaesthetics

Volatile liquid anaesthetics can be used for induction and maintenance of anaesthesia, and following induction with an intravenous anaesthetic (section 15.1.1).

Volatile liquid anaesthetics can trigger malignant hyperthermia (section 15.1.8) and are contra-indicated in those susceptible to malignant hyperthermia. They can increase cerebrospinal pressure and should be

used with caution in those with raised intracranial pressure. They can also cause hepatotoxicity in those sensitised to halogenated anaesthetics. In children with neuromuscular disease, inhalational anaesthetics are very rarely associated with hyperkalaemia, resulting in cardiac arrhythmias and death. Cardiorespiratory depression, hypotension, and arrhythmias are common side-effects of volatile liquid anaesthetics; convulsions have also been reported. They may also cause mood changes that can last for several days.

Isoflurane is a volatile liquid anaesthetic. Heart rhythm is generally stable during isoflurane anaesthesia, but heart-rate can rise, particularly in younger patients. Systemic arterial pressure and cardiac output can fall, owing to a decrease in systemic vascular resistance. Muscle relaxation occurs and the effects of muscle relaxant drugs are potentiated. Isoflurane can irritate mucous membranes, causing cough, breath-holding, and laryngospasm. Isoflurane is the preferred inhalational anaesthetic for use in obstetrics.

Desflurane is a rapid acting volatile liquid anaesthetic; it is reported to have about one-fifth the potency of isoflurane. Emergence and recovery from anaesthesia are particularly rapid because of its low solubility. Desflurane is not recommended for induction of anaesthesia as it is irritant to the upper respiratory tract; cough, breath-holding, apnoea, laryngospasm, and increased secretions can occur.

Sevoflurane is a rapid acting volatile liquid anaesthetic and is more potent than desflurane. Emergence and recovery are particularly rapid, but slower than desflurane. Sevoflurane is non-irritant and is therefore often used for inhalational induction of anaesthesia; it has little effect on heart rhythm compared with other volatile liquid anaesthetics. Sevoflurane can interact with carbon dioxide absorbents to form compound A, a potentially nephrotoxic vinyl ether. However, in spite of extensive use, no cases of sevoflurane-induced permanent renal injury have been reported and the carbon dioxide absorbents used in the UK produce very low concentrations of compound A, even in low-flow anaesthetic systems.

DESFLURANE

Indications see notes above

Cautions see notes above; **interactions:** Appendix 1 (anaesthetics, general)

Contra-indications see notes above

Pregnancy may depress neonatal respiration if used during delivery

Breast-feeding breast-feeding can be resumed as soon as mother has recovered sufficiently from anaesthesia

Side-effects see notes above

Dose

- Induction of anaesthesia (but not recommended—see notes above), by inhalation through specifically calibrated vaporiser, ADULT 4–11%

- Maintenance of anaesthesia, by inhalation through specifically calibrated vaporiser, ADULT 2–6% in nitrous oxide–oxygen; 2.5–8.5% in oxygen or oxygen-enriched air; CHILD 1 month–18 years see *BNF for Children*

ISOFLURANE

Indications   see notes above

Cautions   see notes above; **interactions**: Appendix 1 (anaesthetics, general)

Contra-indications   see notes above

Pregnancy   may depress neonatal respiration if used during delivery

Breast-feeding   breast-feeding can be resumed as soon as mother has recovered sufficiently from anaesthesia

Side-effects   see notes above

Dose

- Induction of anaesthesia, by inhalation using specifically calibrated vaporiser, in oxygen or nitrous oxide–oxygen, increased gradually according to response from 0.5% to 3%
- Maintenance of anaesthesia, by inhalation using specifically calibrated vaporiser, 1–2.5% in nitrous oxide–oxygen; an additional 0.5–1% may be required when given with oxygen alone; caesarean section, 0.5–0.75% in nitrous oxide–oxygen

SEVOFLURANE

Indications   see notes above

Cautions   see notes above; susceptibility to QT-interval prolongation; **interactions**: Appendix 1 (anaesthetics, general)

Contra-indications   see notes above

Renal impairment   use with caution

Pregnancy   may depress neonatal respiration if used during delivery

Breast-feeding   breast-feeding can be resumed as soon as mother has recovered sufficiently from anaesthesia

Side-effects   see notes above; also urinary retention, leucopenia, agitation in children; cardiac arrest, torsade de pointes, and dystonia also reported

Dose

- Induction of anaesthesia, by inhalation using a specifically calibrated vaporiser, in oxygen or nitrous oxide–oxygen, adjusted according to response, ADULT and CHILD over 1 month initially 0.5–1% then increased gradually up to 8%
- Maintenance of anaesthesia, by inhalation using a specifically calibrated vaporiser, in oxygen or nitrous oxide–oxygen, adjusted according to response, ADULT and CHILD over 1 month 0.5–3%

Nitrous oxide

Nitrous oxide is used for maintenance of anaesthesia and, in sub-anaesthetic concentrations, for analgesia. For *anaesthesia*, nitrous oxide is commonly used in a concentration of 50 to 66% in oxygen as part of a balanced technique in association with other inhalational or intravenous agents. Nitrous oxide is unsatisfactory as a sole anaesthetic owing to lack of potency, but is useful as part of a combination of drugs since it allows a significant reduction in dosage.

For *analgesia* (without loss of consciousness), a mixture of nitrous oxide and oxygen containing 50% of each gas (*Entonox*®, *Equanox*®) is used. Self-administration using a demand valve is popular in obstetric practice, for changing painful dressings, as an aid to postoperative physiotherapy, and in emergency ambulances.

Nitrous oxide may have a deleterious effect if used in patients with an air-containing closed space since nitrous oxide diffuses into such a space with a resulting increase in pressure. This effect may be dangerous in conditions such as pneumothorax, which may enlarge to compromise respiration, or in the presence of intracranial air after head injury, entrapped air following recent underwater dive, or recent intra-ocular gas injection.

Hypoxia can occur immediately following the administration of nitrous oxide; additional oxygen should always be given for several minutes after stopping the flow of nitrous oxide.

Exposure of patients to nitrous oxide for prolonged periods, either by continuous or by intermittent administration, may result in megaloblastic anaemia owing to interference with the action of vitamin B_{12}; neurological toxic effects can occur without preceding overt haematological changes. For the same reason, exposure of theatre staff to nitrous oxide should be minimised. Depression of white cell formation may also occur.

Assessment of plasma-vitamin B_{12} concentration should be considered in those at risk of deficiency, including the elderly, those who have a poor, vegetarian, or vegan diet, and those with a history of anaemia. Nitrous oxide should **not** be given continuously for longer than 24 hours or more frequently than every 4 days without close supervision and haematological monitoring.

NITROUS OXIDE

Indications   see notes above

Cautions   see notes above; **interactions**: Appendix 1 (anaesthetics, general)

Pregnancy   may depress neonatal respiration if used during delivery

Breast-feeding   breast-feeding can be resumed as soon as mother has recovered sufficiently from anaesthesia

Side-effects   see notes above

Dose

- Maintenance of anaesthesia in conjunction with other anaesthetic agents, by inhalation using suitable anaesthetic apparatus, 50–66% in oxygen
- Analgesia, by inhalation using suitable apparatus, up to 50% in oxygen, according to the patient's needs

15.1.3   Antimuscarinic drugs

> **Important**
> The drugs in this section should only be administered by, or under the direct supervision of, personnel experienced in their use.

Antimuscarinic drugs are used (less commonly nowadays) as premedicants to dry bronchial and salivary secretions which are increased by intubation, upper airway surgery, or some inhalational anaesthetics. They are also used before or with neostigmine (section 15.1.6) to prevent bradycardia, excessive salivation, and other muscarinic actions of neostigmine. They also prevent bradycardia and hypotension associated with drugs such as propofol and suxamethonium.

Atropine sulfate is now rarely used for premedication but still has an emergency role in the treatment of vagotonic side-effects. For its role in acute arrhythmias after myocardial infarction, see section 2.3.1.

Hyoscine hydrobromide reduces secretions and also provides a degree of amnesia, sedation, and anti-emesis. Unlike atropine it may produce bradycardia rather than tachycardia. In some patients, especially the elderly, hyoscine may cause the central anticholinergic syndrome (excitement, ataxia, hallucinations, behavioural abnormalities, and drowsiness).

Glycopyrronium bromide reduces salivary secretions. When given intravenously it produces less tachycardia than atropine. It is widely used with neostigmine for reversal of non-depolarising neuromuscular blocking drugs (section 15.1.5).

Phenothiazines do not effectively reduce secretions when used alone.

ATROPINE SULFATE

Indications premedication; intra-operative brady-cardia; with anticholinesterases for reversal of non-depolarising neuromuscular block; antidote to organophosphorous poisoning (see Emergency Treatment of Poisoning p. 42); symptomatic relief of gastro-intestinal disorders characterised by smooth muscle spasm (section 1.2); bradycardia (section 2.3.1); cardiopulmonary resuscitation (section 2.7.3); cycloplegia, anterior uveitis (section 11.5)

Cautions see notes in section 1.2
Duration of action Since atropine has a shorter duration of action than neostigmine, late unopposed bradycardia may result; close monitoring of the patient is necessary

Contra-indications see notes in section 1.2

Pregnancy not known to be harmful; manufacturer advises caution

Breast-feeding small amount present in milk—manufacturer advises caution

Side-effects see notes in section 1.2

Dose
- Premedication, by intravenous injection, 300–600 micrograms immediately before induction of anaesthesia; CHILD under 12 years see *BNF for Children*
By subcutaneous or intramuscular injection, 300–600 micrograms 30–60 minutes before induction of anaesthesia; CHILD under 12 years see *BNF for Children*
- Intra-operative bradycardia, by intravenous injection, 300–600 micrograms (larger doses in emergencies); CHILD under 12 years see *BNF for Children*
- Control of muscarinic side-effects of neostigmine in reversal of competitive neuromuscular block, by intravenous injection, 0.6–1.2 mg; CHILD under 12 years see *BNF for Children*
- Arrhythmias after myocardial infarction, see section 2.3.1

[1]Atropine (Non-proprietary) PoM
Injection, atropine sulfate 600 micrograms/mL, net price 1-mL amp = £1.16
Note Other strengths also available
Injection, prefilled disposable syringe, atropine sulfate 100 micrograms/mL, net price 5 mL = £4.58, 10 mL = £5.39, 30 mL = £8.95
Injection, prefilled disposable syringe, atropine sulfate 200 micrograms/mL, net price 5 mL = £6.78; 300 micrograms/mL, 10 mL = £6.47; 600 micrograms/mL, 1 mL = £6.78

1. PoM restriction does not apply where administration is for saving life in emergency

[1]Minijet® Atropine (UCB Pharma) PoM
Injection, atropine sulfate 100 micrograms/mL, net price 5 mL = £6.34, 10 mL = £7.11, 30 mL = £11.19

GLYCOPYRRONIUM BROMIDE
(Glycopyrrolate)

Indications drying secretions (see Prescribing in Palliative Care, p. 21); premedication; intra-operative bradycardia; with neostigmine for reversal of non-depolarising neuromuscular block; maintenance treatment of chronic obstructive pulmonary disease (section 3.1.2); hyperhidrosis (section 13.12)

Cautions see notes in section 1.2 (Antimuscarinics)

Contra-indications see notes in section 1.2 (Antimuscarinics)

Side-effects see notes in section 1.2 (Antimuscarinics)

Dose
- Premedication, by intramuscular or intravenous injection, 200–400 micrograms or 4–5 micrograms/kg (max. 400 micrograms); CHILD 1 month–12 years, 4–8 micrograms/kg (max. 200 micrograms)
- Intra-operative bradycardia, by intravenous injection, 200–400 micrograms or 4–5 micrograms/kg (max. 400 micrograms), repeated if necessary; CHILD 1 month–18 years, 4–8 micrograms/kg (max. 200 micrograms), repeated if necessary
- Control of muscarinic side-effects of neostigmine in reversal of non-depolarising neuromuscular block, by intravenous injection, 200 micrograms per 1 mg of neostigmine, or 10–15 micrograms/kg; CHILD 1 month–12 years, 10 micrograms/kg (max. 500 micrograms)

Glycopyrronium bromide (Non-proprietary) PoM
Injection, glycopyrronium bromide 200 micrograms/mL, net price 1-mL amp = 54p, 3-mL amp = £1.50

◢**With neostigmine metilsulfate**
Section 15.1.6

HYOSCINE HYDROBROMIDE
(Scopolamine hydrobromide)

Indications premedication, motion sickness, hypersalivation associated with clozapine therapy (section 4.6); excessive respiratory secretions (see Prescribing in Palliative Care, p. 21)

Cautions see notes in section 1.2 and notes above; also epilepsy

Contra-indications see notes in section 1.2

Hepatic impairment use with caution

Renal impairment use with caution

Pregnancy use only if potential benefit outweighs risk; injection may depress neonatal respiration

Breast-feeding amount too small to be harmful

Side-effects see notes in section 1.2

Dose
- Premedication, by subcutaneous or intramuscular injection, 200–600 micrograms 30–60 minutes before induction of anaesthesia; CHILD 15 micrograms/kg

Hyoscine (Non-proprietary) PoM
Injection, hyoscine hydrobromide 400 micrograms/mL, net price 1-mL amp = £3.05; 600 micrograms/mL, 1-mL amp = £2.53

◢**With papaveretum**
Section 4.7.2

15 Anaesthesia

15.1.4 Sedative and analgesic peri-operative drugs

15.1.4.1 Benzodiazepines
15.1.4.2 Non-opioid analgesics
15.1.4.3 Opioid analgesics
15.1.4.4 Other drugs for sedation

Important
The drugs in this section should only be administered by, or under the direct supervision of, personnel experienced in their use, with adequate training in anaesthesia and airway management.

Premedication   Fear and anxiety before a procedure (including the night before) can be minimised by using a sedative drug, usually a **benzodiazepine**. Premedication may also augment the action of anaesthetics and provide some degree of pre-operative amnesia. The choice of drug depends on the individual, the nature of the procedure, the anaesthetic to be used, and other prevailing circumstances such as outpatients, obstetrics, and availability of recovery facilities. Sedative premedication with benzodiazepines should be avoided in patients with a compromised airway, CNS depression, or a history of sleep apnoea.

Premedicants can be given the night before major surgery; a further, smaller dose may be required before surgery. Alternatively, the first dose may be given on the day of the procedure.

Premedication in children   Oral administration is preferred; the rectal route should only be used in exceptional circumstances. For further details, consult *BNF for Children*.

Conscious sedation for clinical procedures
Sedation of patients during diagnostic and therapeutic procedures is used to reduce fear and anxiety, to control pain, and to minimise excessive movement. The choice of sedative drug will depend upon the intended procedure; some procedures are safer and more successful under anaesthesia. The patient should be *monitored carefully*; monitoring should begin as soon as the sedative is given or when the patient becomes drowsy, and should be continued until the patient wakes up.

For details on sedation for clinical procedures in children, see *BNF for Children*.

Dental procedures   Sedation for dental procedures should be limited to conscious sedation. Diazepam and temazepam are effective anxiolytics for dental treatment in adults. For further information on hypnotics used for dental procedures, see section 4.1.1.

For details on sedation for dental procedures in children, see *BNF for Children*.

Anaesthesia and driving   See section 15.1.

15.1.4.1 Benzodiazepines

Benzodiazepines possess useful properties for premedication including relief of anxiety, sedation, and amnesia; short-acting benzodiazepines taken by mouth are the most common premedicants. Benzodiazepines are also used in intensive care units for sedation, particularly in those receiving assisted ventilation.

Benzodiazepines may occasionally cause marked respiratory depression and facilities for its treatment are essential; flumazenil (section 15.1.7) is used to antagonise the effects of benzodiazepines.

Diazepam is used to produce mild sedation with amnesia. It is a long-acting drug with active metabolites and a second period of drowsiness can occur several hours after its administration. Peri-operative use of diazepam in children is not recommended; its effect and timing of response are unreliable and paradoxical effects may occur.

Diazepam is relatively insoluble in water and preparations formulated in organic solvents are painful on intravenous injection and give rise to a high incidence of venous thrombosis (which may not be noticed for several days after the injection). Intramuscular injection of diazepam is painful and absorption is erratic. An emulsion formulated for intravenous injection is less irritant and reduces the risk of venous thrombosis; it is not suitable for intramuscular injection.

Temazepam is given by mouth for premedication and has a shorter duration of action and a more rapid onset than oral diazepam; anxiolytic and sedative effects last about 90 minutes although there may be residual drowsiness.

Lorazepam produces more prolonged sedation than temazepam and it has marked amnesic effects.

Midazolam is a water-soluble benzodiazepine that is often used in preference to intravenous diazepam; recovery is faster than from diazepam, but may be significantly longer in the elderly, in patients with a low cardiac output, or after repeated dosing. Midazolam is associated with profound sedation when high doses are given intravenously or when it is used with certain other drugs.

Drugs and driving   See Drugs and Driving in general guidance, p. 3

Overdosage with midazolam
There have been reports of overdosage when high strength midazolam has been used for conscious sedation. The use of high-strength midazolam (5 mg/mL in 2 mL and 10 mL ampoules, or 2 mg/mL in 5 mL ampoules) should be restricted to general anaesthesia, intensive care, palliative care, or other situations where the risk has been assessed. It is advised that flumazenil (section 15.1.7) is available when midazolam is used, to reverse the effects if necessary.

DIAZEPAM

Indications   premedication; conscious sedation for procedures, and in conjunction with local anaesthesia; short-term use in anxiety or insomnia, adjunct in acute alcohol withdrawal (section 4.1.2); status epilepticus (section 4.8.2); muscle spasms (section 10.2.2)

Cautions   see notes above, section 4.1.2, and section 4.8.2; **interactions**: Appendix 1 (anxiolytics and hypnotics)

Contra-indications   see section 4.1.2

Hepatic impairment   see Benzodiazepines, section 4.1.2

Renal impairment   see Benzodiazepines, section 4.1.2

15 Anaesthesia

Pregnancy see Benzodiazepines, section 4.1.2

Breast-feeding see Benzodiazepines, section 4.1.2

Side-effects see notes above and section 4.1.2

Dose

- By mouth, ADULT over 18 years, 5–10 mg 1–2 hours before procedure (up to max. 20 mg for dental procedures carried out in hospital); ELDERLY (or debilitated), half adult dose

- By intravenous injection into a large vein (emulsion preparation preferred), sedative cover for minor surgical and medical procedures, ADULT over 18 years, 10–20 mg over 2–4 minutes, immediately before procedure; premedication 100–200 micrograms/kg

◢ **Preparations**

Section 4.1.2

▊ LORAZEPAM

Indications conscious sedation for procedures; premedication; short-term use in anxiety or insomnia (section 4.1.2); status epilepticus (section 4.8.2)

Cautions see notes above and section 4.1.2; **interactions:** Appendix 1 (anxiolytics and hypnotics)

Contra-indications see Diazepam, section 4.1.2

Hepatic impairment see Benzodiazepines, section 4.1.2

Renal impairment see Benzodiazepines, section 4.1.2

Pregnancy see Benzodiazepines, section 4.1.2

Breast-feeding see Benzodiazepines, section 4.1.2

Side-effects see notes above and Diazepam, section 4.1.2

Dose

- By mouth, 2–3 mg the night before operation; 2–4 mg 1–2 hours before operation

- By slow intravenous injection, preferably diluted with an equal volume of sodium chloride intravenous infusion 0.9% or water for injections, 50 micrograms/kg 30–45 minutes before operation

- By intramuscular injection, diluted as above, 50 micrograms/kg 60–90 minutes before operation

◢ **Preparations**

Section 4.1.2

▊ MIDAZOLAM

Indications conscious sedation for procedures; sedation in intensive care; sedation in anaesthesia; premedication; induction of anaesthesia; status epilepticus (section 4.8.2)

Cautions see notes above; cardiac disease; respiratory disease; myasthenia gravis; neonates; children (particularly if cardiovascular impairment); risk of airways obstruction and hypoventilation in children under 6 months (monitor respiratory rate and oxygen saturation); history of drug or alcohol abuse; reduce dose in elderly and debilitated; risk of severe hypotension in hypovolaemia, vasoconstriction, hypothermia; avoid prolonged use (and abrupt withdrawal thereafter); concentration of midazolam in children under 15 kg not to exceed 1 mg/mL; **interactions:** Appendix 1 (anxiolytics and hypnotics)

Contra-indications marked neuromuscular respiratory weakness including unstable myasthenia gravis; severe respiratory depression; acute pulmonary insufficiency; sleep apnoea syndrome

Hepatic impairment use with caution; can precipitate coma

Renal impairment use with caution in chronic renal failure—increased cerebral sensitivity

Pregnancy avoid regular use (risk of neonatal withdrawal symptoms); use only if clear indication such as seizure control (high doses during late pregnancy or labour may cause neonatal hypothermia, hypotonia, and respiratory depression)

Breast-feeding small amount present in milk—avoid breast-feeding for 24 hours after administration (although amount probably too small to be harmful after single doses)

Side-effects see notes above; gastro-intestinal disturbances, dry mouth, hiccups, increased appetite, jaundice; hypotension, cardiac arrest, heart rate changes, anaphylaxis, thrombosis; laryngospasm, bronchospasm, respiratory depression and respiratory arrest (particularly with high doses or on rapid injection); drowsiness, confusion, ataxia, amnesia, headache, euphoria, hallucinations, convulsions (more common in neonates), dizziness, vertigo, involuntary movements, paradoxical excitement and aggression (especially in children and elderly), dysarthria; urinary retention, incontinence, changes in libido; blood disorders; muscle weakness; visual disturbances; salivation changes; skin reactions; injection-site reactions

Dose

- Conscious sedation for procedures, by slow intravenous injection (approx. 2 mg/minute) 5–10 minutes before procedure, initially 2–2.5 mg (ELDERLY 0.5–1 mg), increased if necessary in steps of 1 mg (ELDERLY 0.5–1 mg); usual total dose 3.5–5 mg (max. 7.5 mg), ELDERLY max. 3.5 mg; CHILD 1 month–18 years see *BNF for Children*

  By rectum, CHILD 6 months–18 years see *BNF for Children*

  By mouth, CHILD 1 month–18 years see *BNF for Children*

  By buccal administration, CHILD 6 months–18 years see *BNF for Children*

- Sedative in combined anaesthesia, by intravenous injection, 30–100 micrograms/kg repeated as required or by continuous intravenous infusion, 30–100 micrograms/kg/hour (ELDERLY lower doses needed); CHILD not recommended

- Premedication, by deep intramuscular injection, ADULT over 18 years, 70–100 micrograms/kg (ELDERLY or debilitated 25–50 micrograms/kg) 20–60 minutes before induction

  By intravenous injection, ADULT over 18 years, 1–2 mg 5–30 minutes before procedure, repeated as required (ELDERLY or debilitated 0.5 mg, repeat dose slowly as required)

  By rectum, CHILD 6 months–12 years see *BNF for Children*

  By mouth, CHILD 1 month–18 years see *BNF for Children*

- Induction (but rarely used), by slow intravenous injection, 150–200 micrograms/kg (ELDERLY or debilitated 50–150 micrograms/kg) given in divided doses (max. 5 mg) at intervals of 2 minutes; max. total dose 600 micrograms/kg; CHILD 7–18 years initially 150 micrograms/kg (max. 7.5 mg) given in steps of 50 micrograms/kg (max. 2.5 mg) over 2–5 minutes; wait for 2–5 minutes then give additional doses of 50 micrograms/kg (max. 2.5 mg) every 2 minutes if necessary; max. total dose 500 micrograms/kg (not exceeding 25 mg)

- Sedation of patients receiving intensive care, by slow intravenous injection, initially 30–300 micrograms/kg given in steps of 1–2.5 mg every 2 minutes, then by slow intravenous injection *or* by continuous intravenous infusion, 30–200 micrograms/kg/hour; reduce dose (or reduce or omit initial dose) in hypovolaemia, vasoconstriction, or hypothermia; lower doses may be adequate if opioid analgesic also used; CHILD under 12 years see *BNF for Children*

Midazolam (Non-proprietary) CD3
Injection, midazolam (as hydrochloride) 1 mg/mL, net price 2-mL amp = 45p, 5-mL amp = 60p, 50-mL vial = £9.56; 2 mg/mL, 5-mL amp = 65p; 5 mg/mL, 2-mL amp = 63p, 10-mL amp = £2.50

Hypnovel® (Roche) CD3
Injection, midazolam (as hydrochloride) 5 mg/mL, 2-mL amp = 71p

▎ TEMAZEPAM

Indications premedication before surgery or investigatory procedures; conscious sedation for dental procedures [unlicensed]; hypnotic (section 4.1.1)

Cautions see notes above and Diazepam, section 4.1.2; **interactions:** Appendix 1 (anxiolytics and hypnotics)

Contra-indications see Diazepam, section 4.1.2

Hepatic impairment see Benzodiazepines, section 4.1.1

Renal impairment see Benzodiazepines, section 4.1.1

Pregnancy see Benzodiazepines, section 4.1.1

Breast-feeding see Benzodiazepines, section 4.1.1

Side-effects see notes above and Diazepam, section 4.1.2

Dose
- By mouth, premedication, ADULT, 10–20 mg (up to 30 mg in exceptional circumstances) 1–2 hours before procedure; ELDERLY 10 mg (up to 20 mg in exceptional circumstances); CHILD 12–18 years see *BNF for Children*
- By mouth, conscious sedation for dental procedures, ADULT over 18 years, 15–30 mg 30–60 minutes before procedure

Note Temazepam doses in BNF may differ from those in product literature

▎**Preparations**
Section 4.1.1

15.1.4.2 Non-opioid analgesics

Since non-steroidal anti-inflammatory drugs (NSAIDs) do not depress respiration, do not impair gastro-intestinal motility, and do not cause dependence, they may be useful alternatives or adjuncts to opioids for the relief of postoperative pain. NSAIDs may be inadequate for the relief of severe pain.

Acemetacin, **diclofenac**, **flurbiprofen**, **ibuprofen**, **ketoprofen** (section 10.1.1), **paracetamol** (section 4.7.1), **parecoxib**, and **ketorolac** are licensed for postoperative use. Diclofenac and paracetamol can be given by injection as well as by mouth. Diclofenac can be given by intravenous infusion for the treatment or prevention of postoperative pain. Intramuscular injections of diclofenac and ketoprofen are rarely used; they are given deep into the gluteal muscle to minimise pain and tissue damage. Ketorolac is less irritant on intramuscu-

lar injection but pain has been reported; it can also be given by intravenous injection.

Parecoxib (a selective inhibitor of cyclo-oxygenase-2) can be given by intramuscular or intravenous injection (but see also NSAIDs and Cardiovascular Events, section 10.1.1). The *Scottish Medicines Consortium* (p. 4) has advised (January 2003) that parecoxib is **not** recommended for use within NHS Scotland.

Suppositories of diclofenac and ketoprofen may be effective alternatives to the parenteral use of these drugs.

▎ KETOROLAC TROMETAMOL

Indications short-term management of moderate to severe acute postoperative pain only

Cautions section 10.1.1; **interactions:** Appendix 1 (NSAIDs)

Contra-indications section 10.1.1; also complete or partial syndrome of nasal polyps; haemorrhagic diatheses (including coagulation disorders) and following operations with high risk of haemorrhage or incomplete haemostasis; confirmed or suspected cerebrovascular bleeding; hypovolaemia or dehydration

Hepatic impairment section 10.1.1

Renal impairment max. 60 mg daily by intramuscular or intravenous injection; avoid if serum creatinine greater than 160 micromol/litre; see also section 10.1.1

Pregnancy section 10.1.1

Breast-feeding amount too small to be harmful

Side-effects section 10.1.1; also gastro-intestinal disturbances, taste disturbances, dry mouth; flushing, bradycardia, palpitation, chest pain, hypertension, pallor; dyspnoea, asthma; malaise, euphoria, psychosis, paraesthesia, convulsions, abnormal dreams, hyperkinesia, confusion, hallucinations; urinary frequency, thirst, sweating; hyponatraemia, hyperkalaemia, myalgia; visual disturbances (including optic neuritis); purpura, pain at injection site

Dose
- ADULT and CHILD over 16 years, by intramuscular injection *or* by intravenous injection over at least 15 seconds, initially 10 mg, then 10–30 mg every 4–6 hours as required (up to every 2 hours during initial postoperative period); max. 90 mg daily (ELDERLY and patients weighing less than 50 kg max. 60 mg daily); max. duration of treatment 2 days; CHILD 6 months–16 years see *BNF for Children*

Ketorolac (Non-proprietary) PoM
Injection, ketorolac trometamol 30 mg/mL, net price 1-mL amp = £1.09

Toradol® (Roche) PoM
Injection, ketorolac trometamol 30 mg/mL, net price 1-mL amp = £1.07

▎ PARECOXIB

Indications short-term management of acute postoperative pain

Cautions section 10.1.1; dehydration; following coronary artery bypass graft surgery; **interactions:** Appendix 1 (NSAIDs)

Contra-indications section 10.1.1; also history of allergic drug reactions including sulfonamide hypersensitivity; inflammatory bowel disease

Hepatic impairment halve dose in moderate impairment (max. 40 mg daily); see also section 10.1.1

Renal impairment section 10.1.1

Pregnancy section 10.1.1

Breast-feeding avoid—present in milk

Side-effects section 10.1.1; also flatulence, hypotension, hypoaesthesia, alveolar osteitis, postoperative anaemia, hypokalaemia, sweating; *less commonly* bradycardia, cardiovascular events, pulmonary embolism, anorexia, malaise, hyperglycaemia, arthralgia, ecchymosis; also reported tachycardia, circulatory collapse

Dose

- By deep intramuscular injection *or* by intravenous injection, initially 40 mg, then 20–40 mg every 6–12 hours when required for up to 3 days; max. 80 mg daily; ELDERLY weighing less than 50 kg, initially 20 mg, then max. 40 mg daily; CHILD under 18 years, not recommended

Dynastat® (Pharmacia) [PoM]
Injection, powder for reconstitution, parecoxib (as sodium salt), net price 40-mg vial = £4.96, 40-mg vial (with solvent) = £5.67

15.1.4.3 Opioid analgesics

Opioid analgesics are now rarely used as premedicants; they are more likely to be administered at induction. Pre-operative use of opioid analgesics is generally limited to those patients who require control of existing pain. The main side-effects of opioid analgesics are respiratory depression, cardiovascular depression, nausea, and vomiting; for general notes on opioid analgesics and their use in postoperative pain, see section 4.7.2.

For the management of opioid-induced respiratory depression, see section 15.1.7.

Intra-operative analgesia Opioid analgesics given in small doses before or with induction reduce the dose requirement of some drugs used during anaesthesia.

Alfentanil, fentanyl, and **remifentanil** are particularly useful because they act within 1–2 minutes and have short durations of action. The initial doses of alfentanil or fentanyl are followed either by successive intravenous injections or by an intravenous infusion; prolonged infusions increase the duration of effect. Repeated intra-operative doses of alfentanil or fentanyl should be given with care since the resulting respiratory depression can persist postoperatively and occasionally it may become apparent for the first time postoperatively when monitoring of the patient might be less intensive. Alfentanil, fentanyl, and remifentanil can cause muscle rigidity, particularly of the chest wall or jaw; this can be managed by the use of neuromuscular blocking drugs.

In contrast to other opioids which are metabolised in the liver, remifentanil undergoes rapid metabolism by non-specific blood and tissue esterases; its short duration of action allows prolonged administration at high dosage, without accumulation, and with little risk of residual postoperative respiratory depression. Remifentanil should not be given by intravenous injection intra-operatively, but it is well suited to continuous infusion; a supplementary analgesic is given before stopping the infusion of remifentanil.

▌ ALFENTANIL

Indications analgesia especially during short operative procedure and outpatient surgery; enhancement of anaesthesia; analgesia and suppression of respiratory activity in patients receiving intensive care, with assisted ventilation, for up to 4 days

Cautions section 4.7.2 and notes above

Contra-indications section 4.7.2

Hepatic impairment section 4.7.2

Renal impairment section 4.7.2

Pregnancy section 4.7.2

Breast-feeding present in milk—withhold breast-feeding for 24 hours

Side-effects section 4.7.2 and notes above; also hypertension, myoclonic movements; *less commonly* arrhythmias, hiccup, laryngospasm; *rarely* epistaxis; also reported cardiac arrest, cough, convulsions, and pyrexia

Dose

> To avoid excessive dosage in obese patients, dose may need to be calculated on the basis of ideal body-weight

- Spontaneous respiration: analgesia and enhancement of anaesthesia for short procedures, by intravenous injection, ADULT, initially up to 500 micrograms over 30 seconds; supplemental doses 250 micrograms
- Assisted ventilation: analgesia and enhancement of anaesthesia for short procedures, by intravenous injection, ADULT, initially 30–50 micrograms/kg; supplemental doses 15 micrograms/kg; CHILD under 18 years see *BNF for Children*
- Assisted ventilation: analgesia and enhancement of anaesthesia during maintenance of anaesthesia for longer procedures, by intravenous infusion, ADULT, initially 50–100 micrograms/kg over 10 minutes *or as* a bolus, followed by maintenance of 30–60 micrograms/kg/hour; CHILD under 18 years see *BNF for Children*
- Assisted ventilation: analgesia and suppression of respiratory activity during intensive care, by intravenous infusion, ADULT over 18 years, initially 2 mg/hour subsequently adjusted according to response (usual range 0.5–10 mg/hour); more rapid initial control may be obtained with an intravenous dose of 5 mg given in divided portions over 10 minutes (reduce rate of administration if hypotension or bradycardia occur); additional doses of 0.5–1 mg may be given by intravenous injection during short painful procedures

Alfentanil (Non-proprietary) [CD2]
Injection, alfentanil (as hydrochloride) 500 micrograms/mL, net price 2-mL amp = 70p, 10-mL amp = £3.20
Injection, alfentanil (as hydrochloride) 5 mg/mL, net price 1-mL amp = £2.50
Note To be diluted before use

Rapifen® (Janssen) [CD2]
Injection, alfentanil (as hydrochloride) 500 micrograms/mL, net price 2-mL amp = 63p; 10-mL amp = £2.90
Intensive care injection, alfentanil (as hydrochloride) 5 mg/mL, net price 1-mL amp = £2.32
Note To be diluted before use

FENTANYL

Indications analgesia during operation, enhancement of anaesthesia; analgesia and respiratory depression in assisted respiration in intensive care; analgesia in other situations (section 4.7.2)

Cautions see Fentanyl, section 4.7.2 and notes above

Contra-indications see notes in section 4.7.2

Hepatic impairment see notes in section 4.7.2

Renal impairment see notes in section 4.7.2

Pregnancy see notes in section 4.7.2

Breast-feeding see Fentanyl, section 4.7.2

Side-effects see Fentanyl, section 4.7.2 and notes above; also myoclonic movements; *less commonly* laryngospasm; *rarely* asystole and insomnia

Dose

> To avoid excessive dosage in obese patients, dose may need to be calculated on the basis of ideal body-weight

- Spontaneous respiration: analgesia and enhancement of anaesthesia during operation, by slow intravenous injection, ADULT, initially 50–100 micrograms (max. 200 micrograms on specialist advice), then 25–50 micrograms as required, by intravenous infusion, ADULT, 3–4.8 micrograms/kg/hour adjusted according to response; CHILD 1 month–18 years see *BNF for Children*
- Assisted ventilation: analgesia and enhancement of anaesthesia during operation, analgesia and respiratory depression in intensive care, by slow intravenous injection, ADULT, initially 300–3500 micrograms, then 100–200 micrograms as required, by intravenous infusion, ADULT, initially 10 micrograms/kg over 10 minutes, then 6 micrograms/kg/hour adjusted according to response; may require up to 180 micrograms/kg/hour during cardiac surgery; CHILD under 18 years see *BNF for Children*

Fentanyl (Non-proprietary) CD2
Injection, fentanyl (as citrate) 50 micrograms/mL, net price 2-mL amp = 45p, 10-mL amp = 75p

Sublimaze® (Janssen) CD2
Injection, fentanyl (as citrate) 50 micrograms/mL, net price 10-mL amp = £1.31

REMIFENTANIL

Indications analgesia and enhancement of anaesthesia during induction and maintenance of anaesthesia (consult product literature for use in patients undergoing cardiac surgery); analgesia and sedation in ventilated, intensive care patients

Cautions section 4.7.2 (but no dose adjustment necessary in renal impairment) and notes above

Contra-indications section 4.7.2 and notes above; analgesia in conscious patients

Hepatic impairment section 4.7.2

Pregnancy no information available: see also section 4.7.2

Breast-feeding avoid breast-feeding for 24 hours after administration—present in milk in *animal* studies

Side-effects section 4.7.2 and notes above; also hypertension; *less commonly* hypoxia; *rarely* asystole, AV block and convulsions also reported

Dose

> To avoid excessive dosage in obese patients, dose should be calculated on the basis of ideal body-weight

- Analgesia and enhancement of anaesthesia at induction, by intravenous infusion, ADULT, 30–60 micrograms/kg/hour, *with or without* an initial dose by intravenous injection of 0.25–1 micrograms/kg over at least 30 seconds; CHILD 12–18 years see *BNF for Children*

  Note If patient to be intubated more than 8 minutes after start of intravenous infusion, initial intravenous injection dose is not necessary

- Assisted ventilation: analgesia and enhancement of anaesthesia during maintenance of anaesthesia, by intravenous infusion, ADULT, 3–120 micrograms/kg/hour, *with or without* an initial dose by intravenous injection of 0.25–1 micrograms/kg over at least 30 seconds, according to anaesthetic technique and adjusted according to response; in light anaesthesia supplemental doses by intravenous injection every 2–5 minutes; CHILD under 18 years see *BNF for Children*
- Spontaneous respiration: analgesia and enhancement of anaesthesia during maintenance of anaesthesia, by intravenous infusion, ADULT, initially 2.4 micrograms/kg/hour adjusted according to response, usual range 1.5–6 micrograms/kg/hour; CHILD 12–18 years see *BNF for Children*
- Assisted ventilation: analgesia and sedation in intensive-care patients, for max. 3 days, by intravenous infusion, ADULT over 18 years, initially 6–9 micrograms/kg/hour adjusted according to response in steps of 1.5 micrograms/kg/hour (allow at least 5 minutes between dose adjustments); usual range 0.36–44.4 micrograms/kg/hour; if an infusion rate of 12 micrograms/kg/hour does not produce adequate sedation add another sedative (consult product literature for details)
- Assisted ventilation: additional analgesia during stimulating or painful procedures in intensive-care patients, by intravenous infusion, ADULT over 18 years, maintain infusion rate of at least 6 micrograms/kg/hour for at least 5 minutes before procedure and adjust every 2–5 minutes according to requirements, usual range 15–45 micrograms/kg/hour
- Cardiac surgery, consult product literature

Note Remifentanil doses in BNF may differ from those in product literature

Remifentanil (Non-proprietary) CD2
Injection, powder for reconstitution, remifentanil (as hydrochloride), net price 1-mg vial = £4.61; 2-mg vial = £9.21; 5-mg vial = £25.40

Ultiva® (GSK) CD2
Injection, powder for reconstitution, remifentanil (as hydrochloride), net price 1-mg vial = £5.12; 2-mg vial = £10.23; 5-mg vial = £25.58

15.1.4.4   Other drugs for sedation

Dexmedetomidine and clonidine (section 2.5.2) are alpha$_2$-adrenergic agonists with sedative properties. Dexmedetomidine is licensed for the sedation of patients receiving intensive care who need to remain responsive to verbal stimulation. Clonidine [unlicensed indication] can be used by mouth or by intravenous injection as a sedative agent when adequate sedation cannot be achieved with standard treatment.

15 Anaesthesia

◢ DEXMEDETOMIDINE

Indications maintenance of sedation during intensive care

Cautions monitor cardiac function; monitor respiratory function in non-intubated patients; severe neurological disorders; bradycardia; ischaemic heart disease or severe cerebrovascular disease (especially at higher doses); spinal cord injury; abrupt withdrawal after prolonged use; malignant hyperthermia

Contra-indications second- or third-degree AV block (unless pacemaker fitted); uncontrolled hypotension; acute cerebrovascular disorders

Hepatic impairment manufacturer advises caution—dose reduction may be required

Pregnancy manufacturer advises avoid unless potential benefit outweighs risk—toxicity in *animal* studies

Breast-feeding manufacturer advises avoid unless potential benefit outweighs risk—present in milk in *animal* studies

Side-effects nausea, vomiting, dry mouth, bradycardia, myocardial ischaemia, myocardial infarction, tachycardia, blood pressure changes, agitation, changes in blood sugar, hyperthermia; *less commonly* abdominal distension, AV block, decreased cardiac output, dyspnoea, hallucination, metabolic acidosis, hypoalbuminaemia, thirst

Dose

- By intravenous infusion, ADULT over 18 years, 0.7 micrograms/kg/hour adjusted according to response (usual range 0.2–1.4 micrograms/kg/hour)

Dexdor® (Orion) ⓅⓄⓂ

Injection, dexmedetomidine (as hydrochloride) 100 micrograms/mL, net price 2-mL amp = £15.66; 4-mL vial = £31.32; 10-mL vial = £78.30
Note To be diluted before use

15.1.5 Neuromuscular blocking drugs

> **Important**
> The drugs in this section should only be administered by, or under direct supervision of, personnel experienced in their use, with adequate training in anaesthesia and airway management.

Neuromuscular blocking drugs used in anaesthesia are also known as **muscle relaxants**. By specific blockade of the neuromuscular junction they enable light anaesthesia to be used with adequate relaxation of the muscles of the abdomen and diaphragm. They also relax the vocal cords and allow the passage of a tracheal tube. Their action differs from the muscle relaxants used in musculoskeletal disorders (section 10.2.2) that act on the spinal cord or brain.

Patients who have received a neuromuscular blocking drug should **always** have their respiration assisted or controlled until the drug has been inactivated or antagonised (section 15.1.6). They should also receive sufficient concomitant inhalational or intravenous anaesthetic or sedative drugs to prevent awareness.

Non-depolarising neuromuscular blocking drugs

Non-depolarising neuromuscular blocking drugs (also known as competitive muscle relaxants) compete with acetylcholine for receptor sites at the neuromuscular junction and their action can be reversed with anticholinesterases such as neostigmine (section 15.1.6). Non-depolarising neuromuscular blocking drugs can be divided into the **aminosteroid** group, comprising pancuronium, rocuronium, and vecuronium, and the **benzylisoquinolinium** group, comprising atracurium, cisatracurium, and mivacurium.

Non-depolarising neuromuscular blocking drugs have a slower onset of action than suxamethonium. These drugs can be classified by their duration of action as short-acting (15–30 minutes), intermediate-acting (30–40 minutes), and long-acting (60–120 minutes), although duration of action is dose-dependent. Drugs with a shorter or intermediate duration of action, such as atracurium and vecuronium, are more widely used than those with a longer duration of action, such as pancuronium.

Non-depolarising neuromuscular blocking drugs have no sedative or analgesic effects and are not considered to trigger malignant hyperthermia.

For patients receiving intensive care and who require tracheal intubation and mechanical ventilation, a non-depolarising neuromuscular blocking drug is chosen according to its onset of effect, duration of action, and side-effects. Rocuronium, with a rapid onset of effect, may facilitate intubation. Atracurium or cisatracurium may be suitable for long-term neuromuscular blockade since their duration of action is not dependent on elimination by the liver or the kidneys.

Cautions Allergic cross-reactivity between neuromuscular blocking drugs has been reported; caution is advised in cases of hypersensitivity to these drugs. Their activity is prolonged in patients with myasthenia gravis and in hypothermia, and lower doses are required. Non-depolarising neuromuscular blocking drugs should be used with great care in those with other neuromuscular disorders and those with fluid and electrolyte disturbances, as response is unpredictable. Resistance can develop in patients with burns, who may require increased doses; low plasma cholinesterase activity in these patients requires dose titration for mivacurium. The rate of administration of neuromuscular blocking drugs should be reduced in patients with cardiovascular disease. **Interactions:** Appendix 1 (muscle relaxants).

Pregnancy Non-depolarising neuromuscular blocking drugs are highly ionised at physiological pH and are therefore unlikely to cross the placenta in significant amounts.

Breast-feeding Because they are ionised at physiological pH, non-depolarising neuromuscular blocking drugs are unlikely to be present in milk in significant amounts. Breast-feeding may be resumed once the mother has recovered from neuromuscular block.

Side-effects Benzylisoquinolinium non-depolarising neuromuscular blocking drugs (except cisatracurium) are associated with histamine release, which can cause skin flushing, hypotension, tachycardia, bronchospasm, and very rarely anaphylactoid reactions. Most aminosteroid neuromuscular blocking drugs produce minimal histamine release. Drugs with vagolytic activity can counteract any bradycardia that occurs during surgery. Acute myopathy has also been reported after prolonged use in intensive care.

Atracurium, a mixture of 10 isomers, is a benzylisoquinolinium neuromuscular blocking drug with an inter-

15 Anaesthesia

mediate duration of action. It undergoes non-enzymatic metabolism which is independent of liver and kidney function, thus allowing its use in patients with hepatic or renal impairment. Cardiovascular effects are associated with significant histamine release; histamine release can be minimised by administering slowly or in divided doses over at least 1 minute.

Cisatracurium is a single isomer of atracurium. It is more potent and has a slightly longer duration of action than atracurium and provides greater cardiovascular stability because cisatracurium lacks histamine-releasing effects.

Mivacurium, a benzylisoquinolinium neuromuscular blocking drug, has a short duration of action. It is metabolised by plasma cholinesterase and muscle paralysis is prolonged in individuals deficient in this enzyme. It is not associated with vagolytic activity or ganglionic blockade although histamine release can occur, particularly with rapid injection.

Pancuronium, an aminosteroid neuromuscular blocking drug, has a long duration of action and is often used in patients receiving long-term mechanical ventilation in intensive care units. It lacks a histamine-releasing effect, but vagolytic and sympathomimetic effects can cause tachycardia and hypertension.

Rocuronium exerts an effect within 2 minutes and has the most rapid onset of any of the non-depolarising neuromuscular blocking drugs. It is an aminosteroid neuromuscular blocking drug with an intermediate duration of action. It is reported to have minimal cardiovascular effects; high doses produce mild vagolytic activity.

Vecuronium, an aminosteroid neuromuscular blocking drug, has an intermediate duration of action. It does not generally produce histamine release and lacks cardiovascular effects.

ATRACURIUM BESILATE
(Atracurium besylate)

Indications neuromuscular blockade (short to inter-mediate duration) for surgery or during intensive care

Cautions see notes above

Pregnancy see notes above

Breast-feeding see notes above

Side-effects see notes above; seizures also reported

Dose

> To avoid excessive dosage in obese patients, dose should be calculated on the basis of ideal body-weight

- Intubation and surgery, ADULT, by intravenous injection, initially 300–600 micrograms/kg, then 100–200 micrograms/kg as required or initially by intravenous injection, 300–600 micrograms/kg followed by intravenous infusion, 300–600 micrograms/kg/hour; CHILD under 18 years see *BNF for Children*
- Intensive care, ADULT, by intravenous injection, initially 300–600 micrograms/kg (optional) then by intravenous infusion 270–1770 micrograms/kg/hour (usual dose 650–780 micrograms/kg/hour); CHILD under 18 years see *BNF for Children*

Atracurium (Non-proprietary) PoM
Injection, atracurium besilate 10 mg/mL, net price 2.5-mL amp = £1.70; 5-mL amp = £3.00; 25-mL vial = £14.45

Tracrium® (GSK) PoM
Injection, atracurium besilate 10 mg/mL, net price 2.5-mL amp = £1.66; 5-mL amp = £3.00; 25-mL vial = £12.91

CISATRACURIUM

Indications neuromuscular blockade (intermediate duration) for surgery or during intensive care

Cautions see notes above

Pregnancy see notes above

Breast-feeding see notes above

Side-effects see notes above; also bradycardia

Dose

> To avoid excessive dosage in obese patients, dose should be calculated on the basis of ideal body-weight

- Intubation and surgery, ADULT, by intravenous injection, initially 150 micrograms/kg; maintenance, by intravenous injection, 30 micrograms/kg approx. every 20 minutes or by intravenous infusion, initially 180 micrograms/kg/hour, *then after stabilisation*, 60–120 micrograms/kg/hour; CHILD 1 month–18 years see *BNF for Children*
- Intensive care, ADULT, by intravenous injection, initially 150 micrograms/kg (optional), then by intravenous infusion 180 micrograms/kg/hour adjusted according to response (usual range 30–600 micrograms/kg/hour)

Cisatracurium (Non-proprietary) PoM
Injection, cisatracurium (as besilate) 2 mg/mL, net price 10-mL vial = £7.55; 5 mg/mL, 30-mL vial = £31.09

Nimbex® (GSK) PoM
Injection, cisatracurium (as besilate) 2 mg/mL, net price 10-mL amp = £7.55
Forte injection, cisatracurium (as besilate) 5 mg/mL, net price 30-mL vial = £31.09

MIVACURIUM

Indications neuromuscular blockade (short duration) for surgery

Cautions see notes above; low plasma cholinesterase activity; elderly

Hepatic impairment reduce dose in severe impairment

Renal impairment clinical effect prolonged in renal failure—reduce dose according to response

Pregnancy see notes above

Breast-feeding see notes above

Side-effects see notes above

Dose

> To avoid excessive dosage in obese patients, dose should be calculated on the basis of ideal body-weight

- Intubation and surgery, ADULT, by intravenous injection, 70–250 micrograms/kg; maintenance, by intravenous injection, 100 micrograms/kg every 15 minutes or by intravenous infusion, 8–10 micrograms/kg/minute, adjusted if necessary every 3 minutes by 1 microgram/kg/minute to usual dose of 6–7 micrograms/kg/minute; CHILD 2 months–18 years see *BNF for Children*

Note Doses up to 150 micrograms/kg may be given over 5–15 seconds, higher doses should be given over 30 seconds. In patients with asthma, cardiovascular disease or those who are sensitive to falls in arterial blood pressure give over 60 seconds

Mivacron® (GSK) PoM

Injection, mivacurium (as chloride) 2 mg/mL, net price 5-mL amp = £2.79; 10-mL amp = £4.51

PANCURONIUM BROMIDE

Indications neuromuscular blockade (long duration) for surgery or during intensive care

Cautions see notes above

Hepatic impairment possibly slower onset, higher dose requirement, and prolonged recovery time

Renal impairment use with caution; prolonged duration of block

Pregnancy see notes above

Breast-feeding see notes above

Side-effects see notes above

Dose

> To avoid excessive dosage in obese patients, dose should be calculated on the basis of ideal body-weight

- Intubation and surgery, ADULT, by intravenous injection, initially 100 micrograms/kg then 20 micrograms/kg as required; CHILD under 18 years see *BNF for Children*
- Intensive care, ADULT, by intravenous injection, initially 100 micrograms/kg (optional) then 60 micrograms/kg every 60–90 minutes

Pancuronium (Non-proprietary) PoM

Injection, pancuronium bromide 2 mg/mL, net price 2-mL amp = £4.00

ROCURONIUM BROMIDE

Indications neuromuscular blockade (intermediate duration) for surgery or during intensive care

Cautions see notes above

Hepatic impairment reduce dose

Renal impairment reduce maintenance dose; prolonged paralysis

Pregnancy see notes above

Breast-feeding see notes above

Side-effects see notes above

Dose

> To avoid excessive dosage in obese patients, dose should be calculated on the basis of ideal body-weight

- Intubation and surgery, ADULT, by intravenous injection, initially 600 micrograms/kg; maintenance, by intravenous injection, 150 micrograms/kg (ELDERLY 75–100 micrograms/kg) *or* by intravenous infusion, 300–600 micrograms/kg/hour (ELDERLY up to 400 micrograms/kg/hour) adjusted according to response; CHILD under 18 years see *BNF for Children*
- Intensive care, ADULT, by intravenous injection, initially 600 micrograms/kg (optional); maintenance by intravenous infusion, 300–600 micrograms/kg/hour for first hour, then adjusted according to response; CHILD 1 month–18 years see *BNF for Children*

Rocuronium (Non-proprietary) PoM

Injection, rocuronium bromide 10 mg/mL, net price 5-mL vial = £3.00, 10-mL vial = £6.00

Esmeron® (MSD) PoM

Injection, rocuronium bromide 10 mg/mL, net price 5-mL vial = £2.89, 10-mL vial = £5.79

VECURONIUM BROMIDE

Indications neuromuscular blockade (intermediate duration) for surgery

Cautions see notes above

Hepatic impairment use with caution in significant impairment

Renal impairment use with caution in renal failure

Pregnancy see notes above

Breast-feeding see notes above

Side-effects see notes above

Dose

> To avoid excessive dosage in obese patients, dose should be calculated on the basis of ideal body-weight

- Intubation and surgery, ADULT, by intravenous injection, 80–100 micrograms/kg; maintenance, by intravenous injection, 20–30 micrograms/kg, adjusted according to response (max. 100 micrograms/kg in caesarian section) *or* by intravenous infusion, 0.8–1.4 micrograms/kg/minute, adjusted according to response; CHILD under 18 years see *BNF for Children*

Norcuron® (MSD) PoM

Injection, powder for reconstitution, vecuronium bromide, net price 10-mg vial = £3.37 (with water for injections)

Depolarising neuromuscular blocking drugs

Suxamethonium has the most rapid onset of action of any of the neuromuscular blocking drugs and is ideal if fast onset and brief duration of action are required, e.g. with tracheal intubation.

Suxamethonium acts by mimicking acetylcholine at the neuromuscular junction but hydrolysis is much slower than for acetylcholine; depolarisation is therefore prolonged, resulting in neuromuscular blockade. Unlike the non-depolarising neuromuscular blocking drugs, its action cannot be reversed and recovery is spontaneous; anticholinesterases such as neostigmine potentiate the neuromuscular block.

Suxamethonium should be given after anaesthetic induction because paralysis is usually preceded by painful muscle fasciculations. While tachycardia occurs with single use, bradycardia may occur with repeated doses in adults and with the first dose in children. Premedication with atropine reduces bradycardia as well as the excessive salivation associated with suxamethonium use.

Prolonged paralysis may occur in **dual block**, which occurs with high or repeated doses of suxamethonium and is caused by the development of a non-depolarising block following the initial depolarising block. Individuals with myasthenia gravis are resistant to suxamethonium but can develop dual block resulting in delayed recovery. Prolonged paralysis may also occur in those with

15

Anaesthesia

low or atypical plasma cholinesterase. Assisted ventilation should be continued until muscle function is restored.

 SUXAMETHONIUM CHLORIDE
(Succinylcholine chloride)

Indications neuromuscular blockade (short duration) for surgery

Cautions see notes above; hypersensitivity to other neuromuscular blocking drugs; patients with cardiac, respiratory, or neuromuscular disease; raised intra-ocular pressure (avoid in penetrating eye injury); severe sepsis (risk of hyperkalaemia); **interactions:** Appendix 1 (muscle relaxants)

Contra-indications family history of malignant hyperthermia, hyperkalaemia; major trauma, severe burns, neurological disease involving acute wasting of major muscle, prolonged immobilisation—risk of hyperkalaemia, personal or family history of congenital myotonic disease, Duchenne muscular dystrophy, low plasma-cholinesterase activity (including severe liver disease, see Hepatic Impairment)

Hepatic impairment prolonged apnoea may occur in severe liver disease because of reduced hepatic synthesis of pseudocholinesterase

Pregnancy mildly prolonged maternal neuromuscular blockade may occur

Breast-feeding unlikely to be present in breast milk in significant amounts (ionised at physiological pH); breast-feeding may be resumed once the mother recovered from neuromuscular block

Side-effects see notes above; also increased gastric pressure; hyperkalaemia; postoperative muscle pain, myoglobinuria, myoglobinaemia; increased intra-ocular pressure; flushing, rash; *rarely* arrhythmias, cardiac arrest; bronchospasm, apnoea, prolonged respiratory depression; limited jaw mobility; *very rarely* anaphylactic reactions, malignant hyperthermia; *also reported* hypertension, hypotension, rhabdomyolysis

Dose

● Intubation and surgery, ADULT, by intravenous injection, 1–1.5 mg/kg; CHILD under 18 years, see *BNF for Children*

Note Doses of suxamethonium in BNF may differ from those in product literature

Suxamethonium Chloride (Non-proprietary) [PoM]
Injection, suxamethonium chloride 50 mg/mL, net price 2-mL amp = 58p, 2-mL prefilled syringe = £8.45

Anectine® (GSK) [PoM]
Injection, suxamethonium chloride 50 mg/mL, net price 2-mL amp = 71p

Anticholinesterases

Anticholinesterases reverse the effects of the non-depolarising (competitive) neuromuscular blocking drugs such as pancuronium but they prolong the action of the depolarising neuromuscular blocking drug suxamethonium.

Neostigmine is used specifically for reversal of non-depolarising (competitive) blockade. It acts within one minute of intravenous injection and its effects last for 20 to 30 minutes; a second dose may then be necessary. Glycopyrronium or alternatively atropine (section 15.1.3), given before or with neostigmine, prevent bradycardia, excessive salivation, and other muscarinic effects of neostigmine.

 NEOSTIGMINE METILSULFATE
(Neostigmine methylsulfate)

Indications see under Dose

Cautions section 10.2.1 and notes above; glycopyrronium or atropine should also be given

Contra-indications section 10.2.1 and notes above

Renal impairment section 10.2.1

Pregnancy section 10.2.1

Breast-feeding section 10.2.1

Side-effects section 10.2.1 and notes above

Dose

● Reversal of non-depolarising neuromuscular blockade, by intravenous injection over 1 minute, ADULT over 18 years, 2.5 mg repeated if necessary (max. 5 mg) after or with glycopyrronium or atropine; CHILD under 18 years see *BNF for Children*

● Myasthenia gravis, see section 10.2.1

Neostigmine (Non-proprietary) [PoM]
Injection, neostigmine metilsulfate 2.5 mg/mL, net price 1-mL amp = 50p

◢**With glycopyrronium bromide**

Glycopyrronium–Neostigmine (Non-proprietary) [PoM]
Injection, neostigmine metilsulfate 2.5 mg, glycopyrronium bromide 500 micrograms/mL, net price 1-mL amp = £1.15

Dose reversal of non-depolarising neuromuscular blockade, by intravenous injection over 10–30 seconds, 1–2 mL *or* 0.02 mL/kg, dose may be repeated if required (total max. 2 mL); CHILD 0.02 mL/kg (or 0.2 mL/kg of a 1 in 10 dilution using water for injections or sodium chloride injection 0.9%), dose may be repeated if required (total max. 2 mL)

Other drugs for reversal of neuromuscular blockade

Sugammadex is a modified gamma cyclodextrin that can be used for rapid reversal of neuromuscular blockade induced by rocuronium or vecuronium (section 15.1.5). In practice, sugammadex is used mainly for rapid reversal of neuromuscular blockade in an emergency.

The *Scottish Medicines Consortium*, p. 4 has advised (February 2013) that sugammadex (*Bridion®*) is accepted for restricted use within NHS Scotland for the routine reversal of neuromuscular blockade in high-risk patients only, or where prompt reversal of neuromuscular block is required.

15.1.6   Drugs for reversal of neuromuscular blockade

> **Important**
> The drugs in this section should only be administered by, or under the direct supervision of, personnel experienced in their use.

15 Anaesthesia

SUGAMMADEX

Indications reversal of neuromuscular blockade induced by rocuronium or vecuronium

Cautions recurrence of neuromuscular blockade—monitor respiratory function until fully recovered; recovery may be delayed in cardiovascular disease and elderly; pre-existing coagulation disorders or use of anticoagulants (unrelated to surgery); wait 24 hours before re-administering rocuronium or vecuronium; **interactions:** Appendix 1 (sugammadex)

Renal impairment avoid if eGFR less than 30 mL/minute/1.73 m^2

Pregnancy use with caution—no information available

Side-effects bronchospasm, bradycardia, cardiac arrest, hypersensitivity reactions

Dose
- Routine reversal of neuromuscular blockade induced by rocuronium or vecuronium, by intravenous injection, ADULT over 18 years, 2–4 mg/kg (consult product literature); a further dose of 4 mg/kg may be required if recurrence of neuromuscular blockade occurs
- Routine reversal of neuromuscular blockade induced by rocuronium, by intravenous injection, CHILD 2–18 years, 2 mg/kg (consult product literature)
- Immediate reversal of neuromuscular blockade induced by rocuronium, by intravenous injection, ADULT over 18 years, 16 mg/kg (consult product literature)

Bridion® (MSD) (PoM)
Injection, sugammadex (as sodium salt) 100 mg/mL, net price 2-mL amp = £59.64, 5-mL amp = £149.10
Electrolytes Na$^+$ 0.42 mmol/mL

15.1.7 Antagonists for central and respiratory depression

> **Important**
> The drugs in this section should only be administered by, or under the direct supervision of, personnel experienced in their use.

Respiratory depression is a major concern with opioid analgesics and it may be treated by artificial ventilation or be reversed by **naloxone**. Naloxone will immediately reverse opioid-induced respiratory depression but the dose may have to be repeated because of the short duration of action of naloxone; however, naloxone will also antagonise the analgesic effect.

Flumazenil is a benzodiazepine antagonist for the reversal of the central sedative effects of benzodiazepines after anaesthetic and similar procedures. Flumazenil has a shorter half-life and duration of action than diazepam or midazolam so patients may become resedated.

Doxapram (section 3.5.1) is a central and respiratory stimulant but is of limited value in anaesthesia.

FLUMAZENIL

Indications reversal of sedative effects of benzodiazepines in anaesthetic, intensive care, and clinical procedures; overdosage with benzodiazepines (see Emergency Treatment of Poisoning)

Cautions short-acting (repeat doses may be necessary—benzodiazepine effects may persist for at least 24 hours); benzodiazepine dependence (may precipitate withdrawal symptoms); prolonged benzodiazepine therapy for epilepsy (risk of convulsions); history of panic disorders (risk of recurrence); ensure neuromuscular blockade cleared before giving; avoid rapid injection in high-risk or anxious patients and following major surgery; head injury (rapid reversal of benzodiazepine sedation may cause convulsions); elderly; children

Contra-indications life-threatening condition (e.g. raised intracranial pressure, status epilepticus) controlled by benzodiazepines

Hepatic impairment carefully titrate dose

Pregnancy not known to be harmful

Breast-feeding avoid breast-feeding for 24 hours

Side-effects nausea and vomiting; *less commonly* palpitation, anxiety, fear; *also reported* transient hypertension, tachycardia, flushing, agitation, convulsions (particularly in those with epilepsy), dizziness, sensory disturbance, chills, sweating

Dose
- Anaesthesia and clinical procedures, by intravenous injection, 200 micrograms over 15 seconds, then 100 micrograms at 60-second intervals if required; usual dose range, 300–600 micrograms; max. total dose 1 mg; CHILD 1 month–18 years see *BNF for Children*
- Intensive care, by intravenous injection, 300 micrograms over 15 seconds, then 100 micrograms at 60-second intervals if required; max. total dose 2 mg; then if drowsiness recurs *either*, by intravenous injection, 300 micrograms, *or* by intravenous infusion, 100–400 micrograms/hour, adjusted according to response; CHILD 1 month–18 years see *BNF for Children*

Flumazenil (Non-proprietary) (PoM)
Injection, flumazenil 100 micrograms/mL, net price 5-mL amp = £13.50

NALOXONE HYDROCHLORIDE

Indications see under Dose

Cautions cardiovascular disease or those receiving cardiotoxic drugs (serious adverse cardiovascular effects reported); physical dependence on opioids (precipitates withdrawal); pain (see also under Titration of Dose, below); has short duration of action (repeated doses or infusion may be necessary to reverse effects of opioids with longer duration of action)

Titration of dose In postoperative use, the dose should be titrated for each patient in order to obtain sufficient respiratory response; however, naloxone antagonises analgesia

Pregnancy use only if potential benefit outweighs risk

Breast-feeding not orally bioavailable

Side-effects nausea, vomiting, hypotension, hypertension, tachycardia, headache, dizziness; *less commonly* diarrhoea, dry mouth, bradycardia, arrhythmia, hyperventilation, tremor, sweating; *rarely* seizures; *very rarely* ventricular fibrillation, cardiac arrest, pulmonary oedema, erythema multiforme, and hypersensitivity reactions including anaphylaxis; *also reported* agitation

15 Anaesthesia

Dose

- Reversal of postoperative respiratory depression, ADULT and CHILD over 12 years, by intravenous injection, 100–200 micrograms (1.5–3 micrograms/kg); if response inadequate, give subsequent dose of 100 micrograms every 2 minutes; alternatively, subsequent doses can be given by intramuscular injection every 1–2 hours; CHILD 1 month–12 years see *BNF for Children*

- Reversal of respiratory and CNS depression resulting from opioid administration to mother during labour, NEONATE, by intramuscular injection, 200 micrograms (60 micrograms/kg) as a single dose at birth; alternatively by subcutaneous *or* intravenous injection, 10 micrograms/kg, repeated every 2–3 minutes

- Opioid overdose, see Emergency Treatment of Poisoning, p. 38

Note Naloxone doses in BNF may differ from those in product literature

◢**Preparations**

See Emergency Treatment of Poisoning, p. 38

15.1.8 Drugs for malignant hyperthermia

> **Important**
> The drugs in this section should only be administered by, or under the direct supervision of, personnel experienced in their use.

Malignant hyperthermia is a rare but potentially lethal complication of anaesthesia. It is characterised by a rapid rise in temperature, increased muscle rigidity, tachycardia, and acidosis. The most common triggers of malignant hyperthermia are the volatile anaesthetics. Suxamethonium has also been implicated, but malignant hyperthermia is more likely if it is given following a volatile anaesthetic. Volatile anaesthetics and suxamethonium should be avoided during anaesthesia in patients at high risk of malignant hyperthermia.

Dantrolene is used in the treatment of malignant hyperthermia. It acts on skeletal muscle cells by interfering with calcium efflux, thereby stopping the contractile process.

▉ DANTROLENE SODIUM

Indications malignant hyperthermia; chronic severe spasticity of voluntary muscle (section 10.2.2)

Cautions avoid extravasation (risk of tissue necrosis); **interactions:** Appendix 1 (muscle relaxants)

Pregnancy use only if potential benefit outweighs risk

Breast-feeding present in milk—use only if potential benefit outweighs risk

Side-effects hepatotoxicity, pulmonary oedema, dizziness, weakness, and injection-site reactions including erythema, rash, swelling, and thrombophlebitis

Dose

- By rapid intravenous injection, ADULT, initially 2–3 mg/kg, then 1 mg/kg repeated as required to a cumulative max. of 10 mg/kg; CHILD 1 month–18 years see *BNF for Children*

Dantrium Intravenous® (SpePharm) [PoM]
Injection, powder for reconstitution, dantrolene sodium, net price 20-mg vial = £51.00 (hosp. only)

15.2 Local anaesthesia

> **Important**
> The drugs in section 15.2 should only be administered by, or under the direct supervision of, personnel experienced in their use, with adequate training in anaesthesia and airway management, and should not be administered parenterally unless adequate resuscitation equipment is available.

The use of local anaesthetics by injection or by application to mucous membranes to produce local analgesia is discussed in this section.

See also section 1.7 (anus), section 11.7 (eye), section 12.3 (oropharynx), and section 13.3 (skin).

Use of local anaesthetics Local anaesthetic drugs act by causing a reversible block to conduction along nerve fibres. They vary widely in their potency, toxicity, duration of action, stability, solubility in water, and ability to penetrate mucous membranes. These factors determine their application, e.g. topical (surface), infiltration, peripheral nerve block, intravenous regional anaesthesia (Bier's block), plexus, epidural (extradural), or spinal (intrathecal or subarachnoid) block. Local anaesthetics may also be used for postoperative pain relief, thereby reducing the need for analgesics such as opioids.

Administration The dose of local anaesthetic depends on the injection site and the procedure used. In determining the safe dosage, it is important to take account of the rate of absorption and excretion, and of the potency. The patient's age, weight, physique, and clinical condition, and the vascularity of the administration site and the duration of administration, must also be considered.

Uptake of local anaesthetics into the systemic circulation determines their duration of action and produces toxicity.

Great care must be taken to avoid accidental intravascular injection; local anaesthetic injections should be given slowly in order to detect inadvertent intravascular administration. When prolonged analgesia is required, a long-acting local anaesthetic is preferred to minimise the likelihood of cumulative systemic toxicity. Local anaesthesia around the oral cavity may impair swallowing and therefore increases the risk of aspiration.

Following most regional anaesthetic procedures, maximum arterial plasma concentration of anaesthetic develops within about 10 to 25 minutes, so **careful surveillance** for toxic effects (see Toxicity and Side-effects, p. 891) is necessary during the first 30 minutes after injection.

Epidural anaesthesia is commonly used during surgery, often combined with general anaesthesia, because of its protective effect against the stress response of surgery. It is often used when good postoperative pain relief is essential (e.g. major thoracic or intra-abdominal surgery).

Use of vasoconstrictors Local anaesthetics cause dilatation of blood vessels. The addition of a vasoconstrictor such as **adrenaline (epinephrine)** to the local anaesthetic preparation diminishes local blood flow, slowing the rate of absorption and thereby prolonging the anaesthetic effect. Great care should be taken to avoid inadvertent intravenous administration of a preparation containing adrenaline, and it is **not** advisable to give adrenaline with a local anaesthetic injection in digits or appendages because of the risk of ischaemic necrosis.

Adrenaline must be used in a low concentration when administered with a local anaesthetic (but see also Dental Anaesthesia, below). The total dose of adrenaline should **not** exceed 500 micrograms and it is essential not to exceed a concentration of 1 in 200 000 (5 micrograms/mL) if more than 50 mL of the mixture is to be injected. Care must also be taken to calculate a safe maximum dose of local anaesthetic when using combination products. For prescribing information on adrenaline, see section 2.7.3. For drug interactions of adrenaline, see Appendix 1 (sympathomimetics).

In patients with severe hypertension or unstable cardiac rhythm, the use of adrenaline with a local anaesthetic may be hazardous. For these patients an anaesthetic without adrenaline should be used.

Dental anaesthesia Lidocaine is widely used in dental procedures; it is most often used in combination with **adrenaline** (epinephrine). Lidocaine 2% combined with adrenaline 1 in 80 000 (12.5 micrograms/mL) is a safe and effective preparation; there is no justification for using higher concentrations of adrenaline. See also Use of Vasoconstrictors, p. 890.

The local anaesthetics **articaine** and **mepivacaine** are also used in dentistry; they are available in cartridges suitable for dental use. Mepivacaine is available with or without adrenaline and articaine is available with adrenaline.

In patients with severe hypertension or unstable cardiac rhythm, mepivacaine without adrenaline may be used. Alternatively, **prilocaine** with or without felypressin can be used but there is no evidence that it is any safer. Felypressin can cause coronary vasoconstriction when used at high doses; limit dose in patients with coronary artery disease.

Cautions of local anaesthetics Local anaesthetics should be administered with caution in children, elderly or debilitated patients (consider dose reduction), or in patients with impaired cardiac conduction, cardiovascular disease, hypovolaemia, shock, impaired respiratory function, epilepsy, or myasthenia gravis. See also Administration and Use of Vasoconstrictors, above.

Contra-indications of local anaesthetics Local anaesthetics should not be injected into inflamed or infected tissues nor should they be applied to damaged skin. In such circumstances, increased absorption into the blood increases the possibility of systemic side-effects, and the local anaesthetic effect may also be reduced by altered local pH. See also Use of Vasoconstrictors, p. 890.

Local anaesthetic preparations containing preservatives should not be used for caudal, epidural, or spinal block, or for intravenous regional anaesthesia (Bier's block).

Local anaesthetics can cause ototoxicity and should not be applied to the middle ear. They are also contra-indicated in patients with complete heart block.

Toxicity and side-effects A single application of a topical lidocaine preparation does not generally cause systemic side-effects. Toxic effects after administration of local anaesthetics are a result of excessively high plasma concentrations; severe toxicity usually results from inadvertent intravascular injection or too rapid injection.

The systemic toxicity of local anaesthetics mainly involves the central nervous and cardiovascular systems. CNS effects include a feeling of inebriation and lightheadedness followed by drowsiness, numbness of the tongue and perioral region, restlessness, paraesthesia (including sensations of hot and cold), dizziness, blurred vision, tinnitus, headache, nausea and vomiting, muscle twitching, tremors, and convulsions. Transient excitation may also occur, followed by depression with drowsiness, respiratory failure, unconsciousness, and coma. Effects on the cardiovascular system include myocardial depression and peripheral vasodilatation resulting in hypotension and bradycardia; arrhythmias and cardiac arrest can occur.

Hypersensitivity reactions occur mainly with the ester-type local anaesthetics, such as tetracaine and chloroprocaine; reactions are less frequent with the amide types, such as articaine, bupivacaine, levobupivacaine, lidocaine, mepivacaine, prilocaine, and ropivacaine. Cross-sensitivity reactions may be avoided by using the alternative chemical type.

Management of severe local anaesthetic-induced cardiovascular toxicity

After injection of a bolus of local anaesthetic, toxicity may develop at any time in the following hour. In the event of signs of toxicity during injection, the administration of the local anaesthetic must be stopped immediately.

Cardiovascular status must be assessed and cardiopulmonary resuscitation procedures must be followed, see section 2.7.3 (Cardiopulmonary Resuscitation).

In the event of local anaesthetic-induced cardiac arrest, standard cardiopulmonary resuscitation should be initiated immediately. Lidocaine must not be used as anti-arrhythmic therapy.

If the patient does not respond rapidly to standard procedures, 20% lipid emulsion such as *Intralipid*® [unlicensed indication] should be given intravenously at an initial bolus dose of 1.5 mL/kg over 1 minute, followed by an infusion of 15 mL/kg/hour. After 5 minutes, if cardiovascular stability has not been restored *or* circulation deteriorates, give a maximum of two further bolus doses of 1.5 mL/kg over 1 minute, 5 minutes apart, and increase the infusion rate to 30 mL/kg/hour. Continue infusion until cardiovascular stability and adequate circulation are restored *or* maximum cumulative dose of 12 mL/kg is given.

Standard cardiopulmonary resuscitation must be maintained throughout lipid emulsion treatment.

Propofol is not a suitable alternative to lipid emulsion.

Further advice on ongoing treatment should be obtained from the **National Poisons Information Service**, p. 33.

Detailed treatment algorithms and accompanying notes are available at www.toxbase.org *or* www.aagbi.org (search site for: local anaesthetic toxicity).

Articaine

Articaine is an amide-type local anaesthetic used for dental anaesthesia (see Dental Anaesthesia, above). It is available in a preparation that also contains adrenaline (see Use of Vasoconstrictors, p. 890).

▌ ARTICAINE HYDROCHLORIDE WITH ADRENALINE

(Carticaine hydrochloride with adrenaline)

Indications infiltration anaesthesia in dentistry

Cautions see Cautions of Local Anaesthetics, p. 891 and Adrenaline, section 2.7.3

Contra-indications see Contra-indications of Local Anaesthetics, p. 891 and Adrenaline, section 2.7.3

Hepatic impairment use with caution; increased risk of side-effects in severe impairment

Renal impairment see Adrenaline, section 2.7.3

Pregnancy use only if potential benefit outweighs risk—no information available

Breast-feeding avoid breast-feeding for 48 hours after administration

Side-effects see Toxicity and Side-effects, p. 891 and Adrenaline, section 2.7.3; also methaemoglobinaemia (see Prilocaine (p. 896) for treatment)

Dose

> To avoid excessive dosage in obese patients, dose may need to be calculated on the basis of ideal body-weight

- ADULT and CHILD over 4 years, consult expert dental sources; **important**: see also Administration, p. 890

Septanest® (Septodont) [PoM]
Injection, articaine hydrochloride 40 mg/mL, adrenaline 1 in 200 000 (5 micrograms/mL), net price 2.2-mL cartridge = 41p
Excipients include sulfites

Injection, articaine hydrochloride 40 mg/mL, adrenaline 1 in 100 000 (10 micrograms/mL), net price 2.2-mL cartridge = 41p
Excipients include sulfites

Bupivacaine

Bupivacaine has a longer duration of action than other local anaesthetics. It has a slow onset of action, taking up to 30 minutes for full effect. It is often used in lumbar epidural blockade and is particularly suitable for continuous epidural analgesia in labour, or for postoperative pain relief. It is the principal drug used for spinal anaesthesia. Hyperbaric solutions containing glucose may be used for spinal block.

▌ BUPIVACAINE HYDROCHLORIDE

Indications see under Dose

Cautions see Cautions of Local Anaesthetics, p. 891; myocardial depression may be more severe and more resistant to treatment; cardiovascular disease; hypertension; hypotension; cerebral atheroma; **interactions**: Appendix 1 (bupivacaine)

Contra-indications see Contra-indications of Local Anaesthetics, p. 891

Hepatic impairment use with caution in severe impairment

Renal impairment use with caution in severe impairment

Pregnancy large doses during delivery can cause neonatal respiratory depression, hypotonia, and

bradycardia after epidural block; use lower doses for intrathecal use during late pregnancy

Breast-feeding amount too small to be harmful

Side-effects see Toxicity and Side-effects, p. 891

Dose

> To avoid excessive dosage in obese patients, dose may need to be calculated on the basis of ideal body-weight

Note Doses should be adjusted according to patient's physical status and nature of procedure—**important**: see also under Administration, p. 890

- Surgical anaesthesia

  Lumbar epidural block, ADULT and CHILD over 12 years, 75–150 mg using a 5 mg/mL (0.5%) solution

  Thoracic epidural block, ADULT and CHILD over 12 years, 12.5–50 mg using a 2.5 mg/mL (0.25%) or 5 mg/mL (0.5%) solution

  Caudal epidural block, ADULT and CHILD over 12 years, 50–150 mg using a 2.5 mg/mL (0.25%) or 5 mg/mL (0.5%) solution

  Major nerve block, ADULT and CHILD over 12 years, 50–175 mg using a 5 mg/mL (0.5%) solution

  Field block, ADULT and CHILD over 12 years, up to max. 150 mg using a 2.5 mg/mL (0.25%) or 5 mg/mL (0.5%) solution

  Intrathecal injection, see *Marcain Heavy*®

- Acute pain

  Lumbar epidural block, ADULT and CHILD over 12 years, by intermittent injection, 15–37.5 mg using a 2.5 mg/mL (0.25%) solution, repeated when required (at intervals of at least 30 minutes) *or* by continuous epidural infusion, 12.5–18.8 mg/hour using a 1.25 mg/mL (0.125%) or 2.5 mg/mL (0.25%) solution; labour pain, by continuous epidural infusion, 6.25–12.5 mg/hour using a 1.25 mg/mL (0.125%) solution; max. 400 mg in 24 hours

  Thoracic epidural block, ADULT and CHILD over 12 years, by continuous epidural infusion, 6.3–18.8 mg/hour using a 1.25 mg/mL (0.125%) or 2.5 mg/mL (0.25%) solution; max. 400 mg in 24 hours

  Intra-articular block, ADULT and CHILD over 12 years, up to max. 100 mg using a 2.5 mg/mL (0.25%) solution; when co-administered with bupivacaine by another route, total max. 150 mg

  Field block, ADULT and CHILD over 12 years, up to max. 150 mg using a 2.5 mg/mL (0.25%) solution

  With fentanyl, see *Bufyl*®

> **Important**
> The licensed doses stated above may not be appropriate in some settings and expert advice should be sought

Bupivacaine (Non-proprietary) [PoM]
Injection, anhydrous bupivacaine hydrochloride 2.5 mg/mL (0.25%), net price 10 mL = 88p; 5 mg/mL (0.5%), 10 mL = 92p

Infusion (epidural), anhydrous bupivacaine hydrochloride 1 mg/mL (0.1%), net price 100 mL = £8.41; 250 mL = £10.59; 1.25 mg/mL (0.125%), 250 mL = £10.80

Marcain® (AstraZeneca) [PoM]
Injection, anhydrous bupivacaine hydrochloride 2.5 mg/mL (*Marcain*® *0.25%*), net price 10-mL *Polyamp*® = £1.06; 5 mg/mL (*Marcain*® *0.5%*), 10-mL *Polyamp*® = £1.21

Marcain Heavy® (AstraZeneca) [PoM]

Injection, anhydrous bupivacaine hydrochloride 5 mg/mL (0.5%), glucose 80 mg/mL, net price 4-mL amp = £1.45

Dose ADULT and CHILD over 12 years, intrathecal anaesthesia for surgery, 10–20 mg bupivacaine hydrochloride; dose may need to be reduced in elderly and in late pregnancy

◢**With adrenaline**

For prescribing information on adrenaline, see section 2.7.3; see also Use of Vasoconstrictors, p. 890.

Bupivacaine and Adrenaline (Non-proprietary) [PoM]

Injection, anhydrous bupivacaine hydrochloride 2.5 mg/mL (0.25%), adrenaline 1 in 200 000 (5 micrograms/mL), net price 10-mL amp = £1.40

Injection, anhydrous bupivacaine hydrochloride 5 mg/mL (0.5%), adrenaline 1 in 200 000 (5 micrograms/mL), net price 10-mL amp = £2.10

◢**With fentanyl**

For prescribing information on fentanyl, see section 15.1.4.3

Bufyl® (AMCo) [CD2]

Infusion (epidural), bupivacaine hydrochloride 1 mg/mL (0.1%), fentanyl (as citrate) 2 micrograms/ mL, net price 250 mL = £8.50, 500 mL= £9.20

Infusion (epidural), bupivacaine hydrochloride 1.25 mg/mL (0.125%), fentanyl (as citrate) 2 micrograms/mL, net price 250 mL= £9.05, 500 mL = £9.20

Electrolytes Na$^+$ < 0.5 mmol/mL

Dose ADULT, continuous lumbar epidural infusion during labour (once epidural block established), 10–18.75 mg/ hour bupivacaine, 16–30 micrograms/hour fentanyl; continuous thoracic, upper abdominal, or lower abdominal epidural infusion for postoperative pain (once epidural block established), 4–18.75 mg/hour bupivacaine, 8– 30 micrograms/hour fentanyl; max. 400 mg bupivacaine or 720 micrograms fentanyl in 24 hours; not recommended for use in children

Chloroprocaine

Chloroprocaine, a para-aminobenzoic acid ester, is used for spinal anaesthesia in adults where the planned procedure should not exceed 40 minutes.

◢ CHLOROPROCAINE HYDROCHLORIDE

Indications intrathecal anaesthesia for surgical procedures lasting up to 40 minutes

Cautions see Cautions of Local Anaesthetics, p. 891; also acute porphyria (section 9.8.2); **interactions:** Appendix 1 (chloroprocaine)

Contra-indications see Contra-indications of Local Anaesthetics, p. 891; also severe anaemia

Hepatic impairment use with caution in severe impairment

Renal impairment use with caution in severe impairment

Pregnancy avoid—no information available

Breast-feeding avoid—no information available

Side-effects see Toxicity and Side-effects, p. 891; also *less commonly* hypertension

Dose

> To avoid excessive dosage in obese patients, dose may need to be calculated on the basis of ideal body-weight

> **Note** Doses should be adjusted according to patient's physical status and nature of the procedure—**important:** see also under Administration, p. 890

● ADULT over 18 years, by slow intrathecal injection, 40–50 mg depending on desired length of block

> **Important**
> The licensed doses stated above may not be appropriate in some settings and expert advice should be sought

Ampres® (AMCo) ▼ [PoM]

Injection, chloroprocaine hydrochloride 10 mg/mL, net price 5-mL amp = £8.75

Levobupivacaine

Levobupivacaine, an isomer of bupivacaine, has anaesthetic and analgesic properties similar to bupivacaine, but is thought to have fewer adverse effects.

◢ LEVOBUPIVACAINE

Note Levobupivacaine is an isomer of bupivacaine

Indications see under Dose

Cautions see Cautions of Local Anaesthetics, p. 891; cardiovascular disease; **interactions:** Appendix 1 (levobupivacaine)

Contra-indications see Contra-indications of Local Anaesthetics, p. 891

Hepatic impairment use with caution

Pregnancy large doses during delivery can cause neonatal respiratory depression, hypotonia, and bradycardia after epidural block; avoid if possible in the first trimester—toxicity in *animal* studies; may cause fetal distress syndrome; do not use for paracervical block in obstetrics; do not use 7.5 mg/mL strength in obstetrics

Breast-feeding amount too small to be harmful

Side-effects see Toxicity and Side-effects, p. 891; also sweating, pyrexia, anaemia

Dose

> To avoid excessive dosage in obese patients, dose may need to be calculated on the basis of ideal body-weight

Note Doses should be adjusted according to patient's physical status and nature of procedure—**important:** see also under Administration, p. 890

● Surgical anaesthesia

Lumbar epidural, ADULT, 50–150 mg using a 5 mg/mL (0.5%) or 7.5 mg/mL (0.75%) solution, given over 5 minutes; caesarean section, 75–150 mg using a 5 mg/ mL (0.5%) solution, given over 15–20 minutes

Intrathecal injection, ADULT, 15 mg using a 5 mg/mL (0.5%) solution

Peripheral nerve block, ADULT, 2.5–150 mg using a 2.5 mg/mL (0.25%) or 5 mg/mL (0.5%) solution

Peribulbar block, ADULT, 37.5–112.5 mg using a 7.5 mg/mL (0.75%) solution

Local infiltration, ADULT, 2.5–150 mg using a 2.5 mg/ mL (0.25%) solution

- Acute pain

  Lumbar epidural, ADULT, labour pain, by intermittent injection, 15–25 mg using a 2.5 mg/mL (0.25%) solution, repeated as required at intervals of at least 15 minutes *or* by continuous epidural infusion, 5–12.5 mg/hour using a 1.25 mg/mL (0.125%) solution; postoperative pain, by continuous epidural infusion, 12.5–18.75 mg/hour using a 1.25 mg/mL (0.125%) or 2.5 mg/mL (0.25%) solution; max. 400 mg in 24 hours

> **Important**
>
> The licensed doses stated above may not be appropriate in some settings and expert advice should be sought

Chirocaine® (AbbVie) PoM

Injection, levobupivacaine (as hydrochloride) 2.5 mg/mL, net price 10-mL amp = £1.41; 5 mg/mL, 10-mL amp = £1.62; 7.5 mg/mL, 10-mL amp = £2.42

Note For 1.25 mg/mL concentration dilute standard solutions with sodium chloride 0.9%

Epidural infusion, levobupivacaine (as hydrochloride) 1.25 mg/mL, net price 100 mL = £7.26, 200 mL = £12.20

Lidocaine

Lidocaine is effectively absorbed from mucous membranes and is a useful surface anaesthetic in concentrations up to 10%. Except for surface anaesthesia and dental anaesthesia, solutions should **not** usually exceed 1% in strength. The duration of the block (with adrenaline) is about 90 minutes.

▐ LIDOCAINE HYDROCHLORIDE
(Lignocaine hydrochloride)

Indications see under Dose; ventricular arrhythmias (section 2.3.2); eye (section 11.7); oral lesions (section 12.3.1)

Cautions See Cautions of Local Anaesthetics, p. 891 and section 2.3.2; hypertension; topical preparations can damage plastic cuffs of endotracheal tubes

Contra-indications see notes above, Contra-indications of Local Anaesthetics, p. 891, and section 2.3.2

Hepatic impairment section 2.3.2

Renal impairment section 2.3.2

Pregnancy large doses can cause fetal bradycardia; large doses during delivery can cause neonatal respiratory depression, hypotonia, or bradycardia after paracervical or epidural block

Breast-feeding section 2.3.2

Side-effects see Toxicity and Side-effects, p. 891 and section 2.3.2; also methaemoglobinaemia (see under Prilocaine (p. 896) for treatment), nystagmus, rash; hypoglycaemia also reported following intrathecal or extradural administration

Dose

> To avoid excessive dosage in obese patients, dose may need to be calculated on the basis of ideal body-weight

- Infiltration anaesthesia, ADULT, according to patient's weight and nature of procedure, max. 200 mg (or 500 mg if given in solutions containing adrenaline)—see also Administration, p. 890 and **important** warning below; CHILD under 18 years see *BNF for Children*

- Intravenous regional anaesthesia and nerve blocks, seek expert advice
- Surface anaesthesia, see preparations below

> **Important**
>
> The licensed doses stated above may not be appropriate in some settings and expert advice should be sought

▐ Lidocaine hydrochloride injections

Lidocaine (Non-proprietary) PoM

Injection, lidocaine hydrochloride 5 mg/mL (0.5%), net price 10-mL amp = 50p; 10 mg/mL (1%), 2-mL amp = 27p, 5-mL amp = 27p, 10-mL amp = 40p, 10-mL prefilled syringe = £8.48; 20-mL amp = 79p; 20 mg/mL (2%), 2-mL amp = 31p, 5-mL amp = 31p

▐ With adrenaline

For prescribing information on adrenaline see section 2.7.3; see also Use of Vasoconstrictors, p. 890.

Xylocaine® (AstraZeneca) PoM

Injection, anhydrous lidocaine hydrochloride 10 mg/mL (1%), adrenaline 1 in 200 000 (5 micrograms/mL), net price 20-mL vial = £1.93

Excipients include sulfites

Injection, anhydrous lidocaine hydrochloride 20 mg/mL (2%), adrenaline 1 in 200 000 (5 micrograms/mL), net price 20-mL vial = £1.77

Excipients include sulfites

▐ Lidocaine injections for dental use

A variety of lidocaine injections with adrenaline is available in dental cartridges; brands include *Lignospan Special®*, *Rexocaine®*, and *Xylocaine®*.

For prescribing information on adrenaline see section 2.7.3; see also Use of Vasoconstrictors, p. 890.

Note Consult expert dental sources for specific advice in relation to dose of lidocaine for dental anaesthesia

▐ Lidocaine for surface anaesthesia

Lidocaine (Non-proprietary)

Ointment, lidocaine 5%, net price 15 g = £6.18

Dose dental practice, rub gently into dry gum

Sore nipples from breast-feeding, apply using gauze and wash off immediately before next feed

Pain relief (in anal fissures, haemorrhoids, pruritus ani, pruritus vulvae, herpes zoster, or herpes labialis), lubricant in cystoscopy or proctoscopy, apply 1–2 mL when necessary; avoid long-term use

Dental prescribing on NHS Lidocaine Ointment, 5% may be prescribed

Instillagel® (CliniMed)

Gel, lidocaine hydrochloride 2%, chlorhexidine gluconate solution 0.25%, in a sterile lubricant basis in disposable syringe, net price 6-mL syringe = 23p, 11-mL syringe = 14p

Excipients include hydroxybenzoates (parabens)

Dose urethral sounding and catheterisation, 6–11 mL into urethra

Cystoscopy, 11 mL (a further instillation of 6–11 mL may be required)

Laryngojet® (UCB Pharma) PoM

Solution, lidocaine hydrochloride 40 mg/mL (4%), net price per unit (4-mL vial and disposable sterile cannula with cover and vial injector) = £5.10

Note May be difficult to obtain

Dose anaesthesia of mucous membranes of oropharynx, trachea, or respiratory tract, 40–200 mg (1–5 mL) as a single dose sprayed, instilled (if a cavity), or applied with a swab (reduce dose according to size, age and condition of patient), usual dose 160 mg (4 mL); CHILD up to 3 mg/kg

LMX 4® (Ferndale)

Cream, lidocaine 4%, net price 5-g tube = £2.98, 30-g tube = £14.90; 12 × 5-g tube with 24 waterproof dressings = £38.16

Excipients include benzyl alcohol and propylene glycol

Dose ADULT and CHILD over 1 month, anaesthesia before venous cannulation or venepuncture, apply thick layer (1–2.5 g; CHILD under 1 year max. 1 g) to small area (2.5 cm × 2.5 cm) of non–irritated skin at least 30 minutes before procedure; may be applied under an occlusive dressing; max. application time 5 hours (CHILD 1–3 months, 60 minutes; CHILD 3 months–1 year, 4 hours); remove cream with gauze and perform procedure after approximately 5 minutes

Versatis® (Grünenthal) PoM

Plasters, lidocaine 5% (700 mg/medicated plaster), net price 30 = £72.40

Excipients include hydroxybenzoates (parabens), propylene glycol

Dose postherpetic neuralgia, ADULT over 18 years, apply to intact, dry, non-hairy, non-irritated skin once daily for up to 12 hours, followed by a 12-hour plaster-free period; discontinue if no response after 4 weeks

Note Up to 3 plasters may be used to cover large areas; plasters may be cut

Note The *Scottish Medicines Consortium* (p. 4) has advised (July 2008) that *Versatis*® is accepted for restricted use within NHS Scotland for the treatment of postherpetic neuralgia in patients who are intolerant of first-line systemic therapies or when they have been ineffective

Xylocaine® (AstraZeneca)

Spray, lidocaine 10% (100 mg/g) supplying 10 mg lidocaine/dose; 500 spray doses per container, net price 50-mL bottle = £6.29

Dose dental practice, 1–5 doses

Maxillary sinus puncture, 3 doses

During delivery in obstetrics, up to 20 doses

Bronchoscopy, laryngoscopy, oesophagoscopy, endotracheal intubation, up to 20 doses; CHILD up to 3 mg/kg

◢**With prilocaine**

For prescribing information on prilocaine, see p. 896

Lidocaine with prilocaine (Non-proprietary)

Cream, lidocaine 2.5%, prilocaine 2.5%, net price 5-g tube = £2.84; 30-g tube (surgical pack) = £14.75; 5-g tube with 2 occlusive dressings = £3.29; 5 5-g tube with 12 occlusive dressings (premedication pack) = £12.99

Brands include *Denela*®

Contra-indications use in child less than 37 weeks corrected gestational age

Dose ADULT and CHILD over 1 year, anaesthesia before minor skin procedures including venepuncture, apply thick layer under occlusive dressing 1–5 hours before procedure (2–5 hours before procedures on large areas e.g. split skin grafting); max. 2 doses in 24 hours for CHILD 1–12 years; CHILD under 3 months, apply max. 1 g under occlusive dressing for max. 1 hour before procedure, max. 1 dose in 24 hours; CHILD 3–12 months, apply max. 2 g under occlusive dressing for max. 4 hours before procedure, max. 2 doses in 24 hours

Note Shorter application time of 15–30 minutes is recommended for children with atopic dermatitis (30 minutes before removal of mollusca)

Anaesthesia on genital skin before injection of local anaesthetics, apply under occlusive dressing for 15 minutes (in adult men) and 60 minutes (in adult women)

Anaesthesia before surgical treatment of lesions on genital mucosa in adults, apply up to 10 g 5–10 minutes before procedure

Anaesthesia before cervical curettage in adults, administer 10 g in lateral vaginal fornices for 10 minutes

Anaesthesia before mechanical cleansing or debridement of leg ulcer in adults, apply up to 10 g under occlusive dressing for 30–60 minutes

EMLA® (AstraZeneca)

Cream, lidocaine 2.5%, prilocaine 2.5%, net price 5-g tube = £2.25; 30-g tube (surgical pack) = £12.30; 5 × 5-g tube with 12 occlusive dressings (premedication pack) = £11.70

Contra-indications use in child less than 37 weeks corrected gestational age

Dose ADULT and CHILD over 1 year, anaesthesia before minor skin procedures including venepuncture, apply thick layer under occlusive dressing 1–5 hours before procedure (2–5 hours before procedures on large areas e.g. split skin grafting); max. 2 doses in 24 hours for CHILD 1–12 years; CHILD under 3 months, apply max. 1 g under occlusive dressing for max. 1 hour before procedure, max. 1 dose in 24 hours; CHILD 3–12 months, apply max. 2 g under occlusive dressing for max. 4 hours before procedure, max. 2 doses in 24 hours

Note Shorter application time of 15–30 minutes is recommended for children with atopic dermatitis (30 minutes before removal of mollusca)

Anaesthesia on genital skin before injection of local anaesthetics, apply under occlusive dressing for 15 minutes (in adult men) and 60 minutes (in adult women)

Anaesthesia before surgical treatment of lesions on genital mucosa in adults, apply up to 10 g 5–10 minutes before procedure

Anaesthesia before cervical curettage in adults, administer 10 g in lateral vaginal fornices for 10 minutes

Anaesthesia before mechanical cleansing or debridement of leg ulcer in adults, apply up to 10 g under occlusive dressing for 30–60 minutes

◢**With tetracaine**

For prescribing information on tetracaine, see p. 897

Pliaglis® (Galderma) PoM

Cream, lidocaine 7% (70 mg/g), tetracaine 7% (70 mg/g), net price 15-g tube = £22.95

Excipients include hydroxybenzoates (parabens)

Dose ADULT anaesthesia before dermatological procedures and venepuncture, apply 1 mm layer using a spatula 30 minutes before procedure, then peel off immediately before procedure; max. application area 400 cm²

Note Application time of 60 minutes indicated for certain procedures, such as laser–assisted tattoo removal and laser leg vein ablation

◢**Lidocaine for ear, nose, and oropharyngeal use**

For prescribing information on phenylephrine, see section 2.7.2

Lidocaine with phenylephrine (Non-proprietary)

Topical solution, lidocaine hydrochloride 5%, phenylephrine hydrochloride 0.5%, net price 2.5 mL (with nasal applicator) = £11.48

Dose anaesthesia before nasal surgery, endoscopy, laryngoscopy, or removal of foreign bodies from the nose, ADULT and CHILD over 12 years, up to max. 8 sprays

Mepivacaine

Mepivacaine is an amide-type local anaesthetic used for dental anaesthesia (see Dental Anaesthesia, p. 891).

◤ **MEPIVACAINE HYDROCHLORIDE**

Indications infiltration anaesthesia and nerve block in dentistry

Cautions see Cautions of Local Anaesthetics, p. 891

Contra-indications see Contra-indications of Local Anaesthetics, p. 891

15 Anaesthesia

Hepatic impairment use with caution; increased risk of side-effects in severe impairment

Renal impairment use with caution; increased risk of side-effects

Pregnancy use with caution in early pregnancy

Breast-feeding use with caution

Side-effects see Toxicity and Side-effects, p. 891

Dose

> To avoid excessive dosage in obese patients, dose may need to be calculated on the basis of ideal body-weight

- ADULT and CHILD over 3 years, consult expert dental sources; **important**: see also Administration, p. 890

Scandonest® 3% Plain (Septodont) PoM
Injection, mepivacaine hydrochloride 30 mg/mL, net price 2.2-mL cartridge = 36p

◢**With adrenaline**

For prescribing information on adrenaline, see section 2.7.3; see also Use of Vasoconstrictors, p. 890.

Scandonest® 2% Special (Septodont) PoM
Injection, mepivacaine hydrochloride 20 mg/mL, adrenaline 1 in 100 000 (10 micrograms/mL), net price 2.2-mL cartridge = 36p
Excipients include sulfites

Prilocaine

Prilocaine is a local anaesthetic of low toxicity which is similar to lidocaine. If used in high doses, methaemoglobinaemia may occur, which can be treated with an intravenous injection of **methylthioninium chloride** (see Emergency Treatment of Poisoning, p. 34). Infants under 6 months are particularly susceptible to methaemoglobinaemia. A hyperbaric solution of prilocaine (containing glucose) may be used for spinal anaesthesia.

▮ PRILOCAINE HYDROCHLORIDE

Indications see under preparations

Cautions see Cautions of Local Anaesthetics, p. 891; severe or untreated hypertension; concomitant use of drugs that cause methaemoglobinaemia; acute porphyria (section 9.8.2); **interactions**: Appendix 1 (prilocaine)

Contra-indications see Contra-indications of Local Anaesthetics, p. 891; anaemia or congenital or acquired methaemoglobinaemia

Hepatic impairment use with caution; lower doses may be required for intrathecal anaesthesia

Renal impairment use with caution; lower doses may be required for intrathecal anaesthesia

Pregnancy large doses during delivery can cause neonatal respiratory depression, hypotonia, and bradycardia after epidural block; avoid paracervical or pudendal block in obstetrics (neonatal methaemoglobinaemia reported); use lower doses for intrathecal use during late pregnancy

Breast-feeding present in milk but not known to be harmful

Side-effects see notes above and Toxicity and Side-effects, p. 891; also hypertension

Dose

> To avoid excessive dosage in obese patients, dose may need to be calculated on the basis of ideal body-weight

- See under preparations—**important**: see also Administration, p. 890

Citanest 1%® (AstraZeneca) PoM
Injection, prilocaine hydrochloride 10 mg/mL, net price 50-mL multidose vial = £5.06
Dose infiltration anaesthesia and nerve block, adjusted according to site of administration and response, 100–200 mg/minute, or in incremental doses, to max. total dose 400 mg (dose may need to be adjusted in ELDERLY or debilitated patients); CHILD over 6 months up to 5 mg/kg

Prilotekal® (AMCo) PoM
Injection, prilocaine hydrochloride 20 mg/mL (2%), glucose 60 mg/mL, net price 5-mL amp = £7.88
Dose spinal anaesthesia, by intrathecal injection, ADULT over 18 years, usually 40–60 mg, max. 80 mg (dose may need to be reduced in ELDERLY or debilitated patients, or in late pregnancy)
Note The *Scottish Medicines Consortium* (p. 4) has advised (December 2010) that prilocaine 2% hyperbaric solution for injection (*Prilotekal®*) is accepted for restricted use within NHS Scotland for use in spinal anaesthesia in ambulatory surgery settings.

◢**With lidocaine**
See Lidocaine, p. 895

◢**For dental use**
Note Consult expert dental sources for specific advice in relation to dose of prilocaine for dental anaesthesia.

Citanest 3% with Octapressin® (Dentsply) PoM
Injection, prilocaine hydrochloride 30 mg/mL, felypressin 0.03 unit/mL, net price 2.2-mL cartridge and self-aspirating cartridge (both) = 47p

Ropivacaine

Ropivacaine is an amide-type local anaesthetic agent similar to bupivacaine. It is less cardiotoxic than bupivacaine, but also less potent.

▮ ROPIVACAINE HYDROCHLORIDE

Indications see under Dose

Cautions see Cautions of Local Anaesthetics, p. 891; also acute porphyria (section 9.8.2); **interactions**: Appendix 1 (ropivacaine)

Contra-indications see Contra-indications of Local Anaesthetics, p. 891

Hepatic impairment use with caution in severe impairment

Renal impairment caution in severe impairment; increased risk of systemic toxicity in chronic renal failure

Pregnancy not known to be harmful; do not use for paracervical block in obstetrics

Breast-feeding not known to be harmful

Side-effects see Toxicity and Side-effects, p. 891; also hypertension, pyrexia; *less commonly* syncope and hypothermia

Dose

> To avoid excessive dosage in obese patients, dose may need to be calculated on the basis of ideal body-weight

Note Doses should be adjusted according to patient's physical status and nature of procedure—**important** see also under Administration, p. 890

- Surgical anaesthesia

  Lumbar epidural block, ADULT and CHILD over 12 years, 113–200 mg using a 7.5 mg/mL (0.75%) *or* 10 mg/mL (1%) solution; caesarean section, 113–150 mg in incremental doses using a 7.5 mg/mL (0.75%) solution

  Thoracic epidural block (to establish block for post-operative pain), ADULT and CHILD over 12 years, 38–113 mg using a 7.5 mg/mL (0.75%) solution

  Major nerve block (brachial plexus block), ADULT and CHILD over 12 years, 225–300 mg using a 7.5 mg/mL (0.75%) solution

  Field block, ADULT and CHILD over 12 years, 7.5–225 mg using a 7.5 mg/mL (0.75%) solution

- Acute pain, using a 2 mg/mL (0.2%) solution

  Lumbar epidural block, ADULT and CHILD over 12 years, 20–40 mg followed by 20–30 mg at intervals of at least 30 minutes; *or* as a continuous epidural infusion (labour pain) 12–20 mg/hour (up to 28 mg/hour for postoperative pain)

  Thoracic epidural block (for postoperative pain), ADULT and CHILD over 12 years, 12–28 mg/hour as a continuous epidural infusion

  Field block, ADULT and CHILD over 12 years, 2–200 mg

  Peripheral nerve block, ADULT and CHILD over 12 years, 10–20 mg/hour as a continuous infusion *or* by intermittent injection

Ropivacaine (Non-proprietary) ▢PoM

Injection, ropivacaine hydrochloride 2 mg/mL, net price 10 mL = £1.65; 7.5 mg/mL, 10 mL = £2.50; 10 mg/mL, 10 mL = £3.00

Infusion, ropivacaine hydrochloride 2 mg/mL, net price 200 mL = £13.70

Naropin® (AstraZeneca) ▢PoM

Injection, ropivacaine hydrochloride 2 mg/mL, net price 10-mL *Polyamp*® = £1.37; 7.5 mg/mL, 10-mL *Polyamp*® = £2.65; 10 mg/mL, 10-mL *Polyamp*® = £3.20

Electrolytes Na⁺ <0.5 mmol/mL

Infusion, ropivacaine hydrochloride 2 mg/mL, net price 200-mL *Polybag*® = £17.34

Electrolytes Na⁺ <0.5 mmol/mL

Tetracaine

Tetracaine, a para-aminobenzoic acid ester, is an effective local anaesthetic for topical application; a 4% gel is indicated for anaesthesia before venepuncture or venous cannulation. It is rapidly absorbed from mucous membranes and should **never** be applied to inflamed, traumatised, or highly vascular surfaces. It should never be used to provide anaesthesia for bronchoscopy or cystoscopy because lidocaine is a safer alternative.

 TETRACAINE
(Amethocaine)

Indications see under preparation; eye (section 11.7)

Cautions see Cautions of Local Anaesthetics, p. 891

Contra-indications see Contra-indications of Local Anaesthetics, p. 891

Breast-feeding not known to be harmful

Side-effects see Toxicity and Side-effects, p. 891
Important Rapid and extensive absorption may result in systemic side-effects (see also notes above)

Ametop® (S&N Hlth.)

Gel, tetracaine 4%, net price 1.5-g tube = £1.08

Excipients include hydroxybenzoates (parabens)

Dose ADULT and CHILD over 1 month, apply contents of tube to site of venepuncture or venous cannulation and cover with occlusive dressing; remove gel and dressing after 30 minutes for venepuncture and after 45 minutes for venous cannulation; NEONATE see *BNF for Children*

Note ADULT and CHILD over 5 years, contents of max. 5 tubes applied at separate sites at a single time; CHILD 1 month–5 years, contents of max. 1 tube applied at separate sites at a single time

◢**With lidocaine**

See Lidocaine, p. 895

A1 Interactions

Two or more drugs given at the same time may exert their effects independently or may interact. The interaction may be potentiation or antagonism of one drug by another, or occasionally some other effect. Adverse drug interactions should be reported to the Medicines and Healthcare products Regulatory Agency (MHRA), through the Yellow Card Scheme (see Adverse Reactions to Drugs, p. 12), as for other adverse drug reactions.

Drug interactions may be **pharmacodynamic** or **pharmacokinetic**.

Pharmacodynamic interactions

These are interactions between drugs which have similar or antagonistic pharmacological effects or side-effects. They may be due to competition at receptor sites, or occur between drugs acting on the same physiological system. They are usually predictable from a knowledge of the pharmacology of the interacting drugs; in general, those demonstrated with one drug are likely to occur with related drugs. They occur to a greater or lesser extent in most patients who receive the interacting drugs.

Pharmacokinetic interactions

These occur when one drug alters the absorption, distribution, metabolism, or excretion of another, thus increasing or reducing the amount of drug available to produce its pharmacological effects. They are not easily predicted and many of them affect only a small proportion of patients taking the combination of drugs. Pharmacokinetic interactions occurring with one drug cannot be assumed to occur with related drugs unless their pharmacokinetic properties are known to be similar.

Pharmacokinetic interactions are of several types:

Affecting absorption The rate of absorption or the total amount absorbed can both be altered by drug interactions. Delayed absorption is rarely of clinical importance unless high peak plasma concentrations are required (e.g. when giving an analgesic). Reduction in the total amount absorbed, however, may result in ineffective therapy.

Due to changes in protein binding To a variable extent most drugs are loosely bound to plasma proteins. Protein-binding sites are non-specific and one drug can displace another thereby increasing its proportion free to diffuse from plasma to its site of action. This only produces a detectable increase in effect if it is an extensively bound drug (more than 90%) that is not widely distributed throughout the body. Even so displacement rarely produces more than transient potentiation because this increased concentration of free drug results in an increased rate of elimination.

Displacement from protein binding plays a part in the potentiation of warfarin by sulfonamides and tolbutamide but the importance of these interactions is due mainly to the fact that warfarin metabolism is also inhibited.

Affecting metabolism Many drugs are metabolised in the liver. Induction of the hepatic microsomal enzyme system by one drug can gradually increase the rate of metabolism of another, resulting in lower plasma concentrations and a reduced effect. On withdrawal of the inducer plasma concentrations increase and toxicity may occur. Barbiturates, griseofulvin, many antiepileptics, and rifampicin are the most important enzyme inducers. Drugs affected include warfarin and the oral contraceptives.

Conversely when one drug inhibits the metabolism of another higher plasma concentrations are produced, rapidly resulting in an increased effect with risk of toxicity. Some drugs which potentiate warfarin and phenytoin do so by this mechanism.

Isoenzymes of the hepatic cytochrome P450 system interact with a wide range of drugs. Drugs may be substrates, inducers or inhibitors of the different isoenzymes. A great deal of *in-vitro* information is available on the effect of drugs on the isoenzymes; however, since drugs are eliminated by a number of different metabolic routes as well as renal excretion, the clinical effects of interactions cannot be predicted accurately from laboratory data on the cytochrome P450 isoenzymes. Except where a combination of drugs is specifically contra-indicated, the BNF presents only interactions that have been reported in clinical practice. In all cases the possibility of an interaction must be considered if toxic effects occur or if the activity of a drug diminishes.

Affecting renal excretion Drugs are eliminated through the kidney both by glomerular filtration and by active tubular secretion. Competition occurs between those which share active transport mechanisms in the proximal tubule. For example, salicylates and some other NSAIDs delay the excretion of methotrexate; serious methotrexate toxicity is possible.

Relative importance of interactions

Many drug interactions are harmless and many of those which are potentially harmful only occur in a small proportion of patients; moreover, the severity of an interaction varies from one patient to another. Drugs with a small therapeutic ratio (e.g. phenytoin) and those which require careful control of dosage (e.g. anticoagulants, antihypertensives, and antidiabetics) are most often involved.

Patients at increased risk from drug interactions include the elderly and those with impaired renal or liver function.

Serious interactions The symbol • has been placed against interactions that are **potentially serious** and where concomitant administration of the drugs involved should be **avoided** (or only undertaken with caution and appropriate monitoring).

Interactions that have no symbol do not usually have serious consequences.

List of drug interactions

The following is an alphabetical list of drugs and their interactions; to avoid excessive cross-referencing each drug or group is listed twice: in the alphabetical list and also against the drug or group with which it interacts. For explanation of symbol • see above

Abacavir

Analgesics: abacavir possibly reduces plasma concentration of methadone

Antibacterials: plasma concentration of abacavir possibly reduced by rifampicin

Antiepileptics: plasma concentration of abacavir possibly reduced by phenobarbital and phenytoin

• Antivirals: abacavir possibly reduces effects of •ribavirin; plasma concentration of abacavir reduced by •tipranavir

• Orlistat: absorption of abacavir possibly reduced by •orlistat

Abatacept

• Cytotoxics: increased risk of side-effects when abatacept given with adalimumab; avoid concomitant use of abatacept with •certolizumab pegol, •golimumab or •infliximab

• Etanercept: avoid concomitant use of abatacept with •etanercept

• Vaccines: avoid concomitant use of abatacept with live •vaccines (see p. 842)

Abiraterone

Analgesics: abiraterone increases plasma concentration of dextromethorphan

• Antibacterials: plasma concentration of abiraterone possibly reduced by •rifabutin—manufacturer of abiraterone advises avoid concomitant use; plasma concentration of abiraterone reduced by •rifampicin—manufacturer of abiraterone advises avoid concomitant use

• Antidepressants: plasma concentration of abiraterone possibly reduced by •St John's wort—manufacturer of abiraterone advises avoid concomitant use

• Antiepileptics: plasma concentration of abiraterone possibly reduced by •carbamazepine, •phenobarbital and •phenytoin—manufacturer of abiraterone advises avoid concomitant use

Acarbose see Antidiabetics

ACE Inhibitors

Alcohol: enhanced hypotensive effect when ACE inhibitors given with alcohol

Aldesleukin: enhanced hypotensive effect when ACE inhibitors given with aldesleukin

• Aliskiren: avoid concomitant use of ACE inhibitors with •aliskiren (see also under Renin inhibitors, p. 129)

Allopurinol: manufacturers state possible increased risk of leucopenia and hypersensitivity reactions when ACE inhibitors given with allopurinol especially in renal impairment

Alpha-blockers: enhanced hypotensive effect when ACE inhibitors given with alpha-blockers

Anaesthetics, General: enhanced hypotensive effect when ACE inhibitors given with general anaesthetics

Analgesics: increased risk of renal impairment when ACE inhibitors given with NSAIDs, also hypotensive effect antagonised

• Angiotensin-II Receptor Antagonists: increased risk of hyperkalaemia, hypotension, and impaired renal function when ACE inhibitors given with •angiotensin-II receptor antagonists (see also under Concomitant Use of Drugs Affecting the Renin-Angiotensin System, p. 119)

ACE Inhibitors (continued)

Antacids: absorption of ACE inhibitors possibly reduced by antacids; absorption of captopril, enalapril and fosinopril reduced by antacids

Antibacterials: plasma concentration of active metabolite of imidapril reduced by rifampicin (reduced antihypertensive effect); quinapril tablets reduce absorption of tetracyclines (quinapril tablets contain magnesium carbonate); possible increased risk of hyperkalaemia when ACE inhibitors given with trimethoprim

Anticoagulants: increased risk of hyperkalaemia when ACE inhibitors given with heparins

Antidepressants: hypotensive effect of ACE inhibitors possibly enhanced by MAOIs

Antidiabetics: ACE inhibitors possibly enhance hypoglycaemic effect of insulin, metformin and sulfonylureas

Antipsychotics: enhanced hypotensive effect when ACE inhibitors given with antipsychotics

Anxiolytics and Hypnotics: enhanced hypotensive effect when ACE inhibitors given with anxiolytics and hypnotics

Avanafil: hypotensive effect of enalapril possibly enhanced by avanafil

Azathioprine: increased risk of anaemia or leucopenia when captopril given with azathioprine especially in renal impairment; increased risk of anaemia when enalapril given with azathioprine especially in renal impairment

Beta-blockers: enhanced hypotensive effect when ACE inhibitors given with beta-blockers

Calcium-channel Blockers: enhanced hypotensive effect when ACE inhibitors given with calcium-channel blockers

Cardiac Glycosides: captopril possibly increases plasma concentration of digoxin

• Ciclosporin: increased risk of hyperkalaemia when ACE inhibitors given with •ciclosporin

Clonidine: enhanced hypotensive effect when ACE inhibitors given with clonidine; antihypertensive effect of captopril possibly delayed by previous treatment with clonidine

Corticosteroids: hypotensive effect of ACE inhibitors antagonised by corticosteroids

• Cytotoxics: increased risk of angioedema when ACE inhibitors given with •everolimus

Diazoxide: enhanced hypotensive effect when ACE inhibitors given with diazoxide

• Diuretics: enhanced hypotensive effect when ACE inhibitors given with •diuretics; increased risk of severe hyperkalaemia when ACE inhibitors given with •potassium-sparing diuretics and aldosterone antagonists

Dopaminergics: enhanced hypotensive effect when ACE inhibitors given with levodopa

• Gold: flushing and hypotension reported when ACE inhibitors given with •sodium aurothiomalate

• Lithium: ACE inhibitors reduce excretion of •lithium (increased plasma concentration)

Methyldopa: enhanced hypotensive effect when ACE inhibitors given with methyldopa

Moxisylyte: enhanced hypotensive effect when ACE inhibitors given with moxisylyte

Moxonidine: enhanced hypotensive effect when ACE inhibitors given with moxonidine

Muscle Relaxants: enhanced hypotensive effect when ACE inhibitors given with baclofen or tizanidine

Nitrates: enhanced hypotensive effect when ACE inhibitors given with nitrates

Oestrogens: hypotensive effect of ACE inhibitors antagonised by oestrogens

• Potassium Salts: increased risk of severe hyperkalaemia when ACE inhibitors given with •potassium salts

ACE Inhibitors *(continued)*

Prostaglandins: enhanced hypotensive effect when ACE inhibitors given with alprostadil

Vasodilator Antihypertensives: enhanced hypotensive effect when ACE inhibitors given with hydralazine, minoxidil or sodium nitroprusside

Acebutolol *see* Beta-blockers

Aceclofenac *see* NSAIDs

Acemetacin *see* NSAIDs

Acenocoumarol *see* Coumarins

Acetazolamide *see* Diuretics

Aciclovir

Note Interactions do not apply to topical aciclovir preparations

Note Valaciclovir interactions as for aciclovir

Ciclosporin: increased risk of nephrotoxicity when aciclovir given with ciclosporin

Mycophenolate: plasma concentration of aciclovir increased by mycophenolate, also plasma concentration of inactive metabolite of mycophenolate increased

Tacrolimus: possible increased risk of nephrotoxicity when aciclovir given with tacrolimus

Theophylline: aciclovir possibly increases plasma concentration of theophylline

Acitretin *see* Retinoids

Aclidinium *see* Antimuscarinics

Acrivastine *see* Antihistamines

Adalimumab

Abatacept: increased risk of side-effects when adalimumab given with abatacept

- Anakinra: avoid concomitant use of adalimumab with ●anakinra
- Antipsychotics: avoid concomitant use of cytotoxics with ●clozapine (increased risk of agranulocytosis)
- Vaccines: avoid concomitant use of monoclonal antibodies with live ●vaccines (see p. 842)

Adefovir

Antivirals: avoidance of adefovir advised by manufacturer of tenofovir

Interferons: manufacturer of adefovir advises caution with peginterferon alfa

Adenosine

Note Possibility of interaction with drugs tending to impair myocardial conduction

Anaesthetics, Local: increased myocardial depression when anti-arrhythmics given with bupivacaine, levobupivacaine, prilocaine or ropivacaine

- Anti-arrhythmics: increased myocardial depression when anti-arrhythmics given with other ●anti-arrhythmics
- Antipsychotics: increased risk of ventricular arrhythmias when anti-arrhythmics that prolong the QT interval given with ●antipsychotics that prolong the QT interval
- Beta-blockers: increased myocardial depression when anti-arrhythmics given with ●beta-blockers

Caffeine citrate: anti-arrhythmic effect of adenosine antagonised by caffeine citrate—manufacturer of adenosine advises avoid caffeine citrate for at least 12 hours before adenosine

- Dipyridamole: effect of adenosine enhanced and extended by ●dipyridamole (important risk of toxicity)—reduce dose of adenosine, see Dose under Adenosine, p. 96

Nicotine: effects of adenosine possibly enhanced by nicotine

Theophylline: anti-arrhythmic effect of adenosine antagonised by theophylline—manufacturer of adenosine advises avoid theophylline for 24 hours before adenosine

Adrenaline (epinephrine) *see* Sympathomimetics

Adrenergic Neurone Blockers

Alcohol: enhanced hypotensive effect when adrenergic neurone blockers given with alcohol

Adrenergic Neurone Blockers *(continued)*

Alpha-blockers: enhanced hypotensive effect when adrenergic neurone blockers given with alpha-blockers

- Anaesthetics, General: enhanced hypotensive effect when adrenergic neurone blockers given with ●general anaesthetics

Analgesics: hypotensive effect of adrenergic neurone blockers antagonised by NSAIDs

Angiotensin-II Receptor Antagonists: enhanced hypotensive effect when adrenergic neurone blockers given with angiotensin-II receptor antagonists

Antidepressants: enhanced hypotensive effect when adrenergic neurone blockers given with MAOIs; hypotensive effect of adrenergic neurone blockers antagonised by tricyclics

Antipsychotics: hypotensive effect of adrenergic neurone blockers antagonised by haloperidol; hypotensive effect of adrenergic neurone blockers antagonised by higher doses of chlorpromazine; enhanced hypotensive effect when adrenergic neurone blockers given with phenothiazines

Anxiolytics and Hypnotics: enhanced hypotensive effect when adrenergic neurone blockers given with anxiolytics and hypnotics

Beta-blockers: enhanced hypotensive effect when adrenergic neurone blockers given with beta-blockers

Calcium-channel Blockers: enhanced hypotensive effect when adrenergic neurone blockers given with calcium-channel blockers

Clonidine: enhanced hypotensive effect when adrenergic neurone blockers given with clonidine

Corticosteroids: hypotensive effect of adrenergic neurone blockers antagonised by corticosteroids

Diazoxide: enhanced hypotensive effect when adrenergic neurone blockers given with diazoxide

Diuretics: enhanced hypotensive effect when adrenergic neurone blockers given with diuretics

Dopaminergics: enhanced hypotensive effect when adrenergic neurone blockers given with levodopa

Methyldopa: enhanced hypotensive effect when adrenergic neurone blockers given with methyldopa

Moxisylyte: enhanced hypotensive effect when adrenergic neurone blockers given with moxisylyte

Moxonidine: enhanced hypotensive effect when adrenergic neurone blockers given with moxonidine

Muscle Relaxants: enhanced hypotensive effect when adrenergic neurone blockers given with baclofen or tizanidine

Nitrates: enhanced hypotensive effect when adrenergic neurone blockers given with nitrates

Oestrogens: hypotensive effect of adrenergic neurone blockers antagonised by oestrogens

Pizotifen: hypotensive effect of adrenergic neurone blockers antagonised by pizotifen

Prostaglandins: enhanced hypotensive effect when adrenergic neurone blockers given with alprostadil

- Sympathomimetics: increased risk of hypertension when guanethidine given with ●adrenaline (epinephrine); hypotensive effect of guanethidine antagonised by ●dexamfetamine and ●lisdexamfetamine; hypotensive effect of adrenergic neurone blockers antagonised by ●ephedrine, ●isometheptene, ●metaraminol, ●methylphenidate, ●noradrenaline (norepinephrine), ●oxymetazoline, ●phenylephrine, ●pseudoephedrine and ●xylometazoline

Vasodilator Antihypertensives: enhanced hypotensive effect when adrenergic neurone blockers given with hydralazine, minoxidil or sodium nitroprusside

Adsorbents *see* Kaolin

Afatinib

Anti-arrhythmics: plasma concentration of afatinib possibly increased by amiodarone—manufacturer of afatinib advises separating administration of amiodarone by 6 to 12 hours

Afatinib (continued)

Antibacterials: plasma concentration of afatinib possibly increased by **erythromycin**—manufacturer of afatinib advises separating administration of erythromycin by 6 to 12 hours; plasma concentration of afatinib reduced by **rifampicin**

Antifungals: plasma concentration of afatinib possibly increased by **itraconazole**—manufacturer of afatinib advises separating administration of itraconazole by 6 to 12 hours

● Antipsychotics: avoid concomitant use of cytotoxics with ●**clozapine** (increased risk of agranulocytosis)

Antivirals: plasma concentration of afatinib increased by **ritonavir**—manufacturer of afatinib advises separating administration of ritonavir by 6 to 12 hours; plasma concentration of afatinib possibly increased by **saquinavir**—manufacturer of afatinib advises separating administration of saquinavir by 6 to 12 hours

Calcium-channel Blockers: plasma concentration of afatinib possibly increased by **verapamil**—manufacturer of afatinib advises separating administration of verapamil by 6 to 12 hours

Ciclosporin: plasma concentration of afatinib possibly increased by **ciclosporin**—manufacturer of afatinib advises separating administration of ciclosporin by 6 to 12 hours

Tacrolimus: plasma concentration of afatinib possibly increased by **tacrolimus**—manufacturer of afatinib advises separating administration of tacrolimus by 6 to 12 hours

Agalsidase Alfa and Beta

Anti-arrhythmics: effects of agalsidase alfa and beta possibly inhibited by **amiodarone** (manufacturers of agalsidase alfa and beta advise avoid concomitant use)

Antibacterials: effects of agalsidase alfa and beta possibly inhibited by **gentamicin** (manufacturers of agalsidase alfa and beta advise avoid concomitant use)

Antimalarials: effects of agalsidase alfa and beta possibly inhibited by **chloroquine and hydroxychloroquine** (manufacturers of agalsidase alfa and beta advise avoid concomitant use)

Agomelatine

● Antibacterials: manufacturer of agomelatine advises avoid concomitant use with ●**ciprofloxacin**

● Antidepressants: metabolism of agomelatine inhibited by ●**fluvoxamine** (increased plasma concentration)

● Antimalarials: avoidance of antidepressants advised by manufacturer of ●**artemether with lumefantrine** and ●**piperaquine with artenimol**

Atomoxetine: possible increased risk of convulsions when antidepressants given with **atomoxetine**

Alcohol

ACE Inhibitors: enhanced hypotensive effect when alcohol given with **ACE inhibitors**

Adrenergic Neurone Blockers: enhanced hypotensive effect when alcohol given with **adrenergic neurone blockers**

Alpha-blockers: increased sedative effect when alcohol given with **indoramin**; enhanced hypotensive effect when alcohol given with **alpha-blockers**

Analgesics: enhanced hypotensive and sedative effects when alcohol given with **opioid analgesics**

Angiotensin-II Receptor Antagonists: enhanced hypotensive effect when alcohol given with **angiotensin-II receptor antagonists**

● Antibacterials: disulfiram-like reaction when alcohol given with **metronidazole**; possibility of disulfiram-like reaction when alcohol given with **tinidazole**; increased risk of convulsions when alcohol given with ●**cycloserine**

● Anticoagulants: major changes in consumption of alcohol may affect anticoagulant control with ●**coumarins** or ●**phenindione**

Alcohol (continued)

● Antidepressants: some beverages containing alcohol and some dealcoholised beverages contain tyramine which interacts with ●**MAOIs** (hypertensive crisis)—if no tyramine, enhanced hypotensive effect; sedative effects possibly increased when alcohol given with **SSRIs**; increased sedative effect when alcohol given with ●**mirtazapine**, ●**tricyclic-related antidepressants** or ●**tricyclics**

Antidiabetics: alcohol enhances hypoglycaemic effect of **antidiabetics**; increased risk of lactic acidosis when alcohol given with **metformin**

Antiepileptics: alcohol possibly increases CNS side-effects of **carbamazepine**; increased sedative effect when alcohol given with **phenobarbital**; chronic heavy consumption of alcohol possibly reduces plasma concentration of **phenytoin**; increased risk of blurred vision when alcohol given with **retigabine**

Antifungals: effects of alcohol possibly enhanced by **griseofulvin**

Antihistamines: increased sedative effect when alcohol given with **antihistamines** (possibly less effect with non-sedating antihistamines)

Antimuscarinics: increased sedative effect when alcohol given with **hyoscine**

Antipsychotics: increased sedative effect when alcohol given with **antipsychotics**

Anxiolytics and Hypnotics: increased sedative effect when alcohol given with **anxiolytics and hypnotics**

Avanafil: possible enhanced hypotensive effect when alcohol given with **avanafil**

Beta-blockers: enhanced hypotensive effect when alcohol given with **beta-blockers**

Calcium-channel Blockers: enhanced hypotensive effect when alcohol given with **calcium-channel blockers**; plasma concentration of alcohol possibly increased by **verapamil**

Clonidine: enhanced hypotensive effect when alcohol given with **clonidine**

● Cytotoxics: disulfiram-like reaction when alcohol given with **procarbazine**; avoidance of alcohol advised by manufacturer of ●**trabectedin**

● Dapoxetine: increased sedative effect when alcohol given with ●**dapoxetine**

Diazoxide: enhanced hypotensive effect when alcohol given with **diazoxide**

Disulfiram: disulfiram reaction when alcohol given with **disulfiram** (see p. 339)

Diuretics: enhanced hypotensive effect when alcohol given with **diuretics**

Dopaminergics: alcohol reduces tolerance to **bromocriptine**

Levamisole: possibility of disulfiram-like reaction when alcohol given with **levamisole**

Lipid-regulating Drugs: avoidance of alcohol advised by manufacturer of **lomitapide**

Lofexidine: increased sedative effect when alcohol given with **lofexidine**

Methyldopa: enhanced hypotensive effect when alcohol given with **methyldopa**

Metoclopramide: absorption of alcohol possibly increased by **metoclopramide**

Moxonidine: enhanced hypotensive effect when alcohol given with **moxonidine**

Muscle Relaxants: increased sedative effect when alcohol given with **baclofen**, **methocarbamol** or **tizanidine**

Nicorandil: alcohol possibly enhances hypotensive effect of **nicorandil**

Nitrates: enhanced hypotensive effect when alcohol given with **nitrates**

● Paraldehyde: increased sedative effect when alcohol given with ●**paraldehyde**

● Retinoids: presence of alcohol causes etretinate to be formed from ●**acitretin** (increased risk of teratogenicity in women of child-bearing potential)

Appendix 1: Interactions

Alcohol (continued)

Sympathomimetics: alcohol possibly enhances effects of methylphenidate

Vasodilator Antihypertensives: enhanced hypotensive effect when alcohol given with hydralazine, minoxidil or sodium nitroprusside

Aldesleukin

ACE Inhibitors: enhanced hypotensive effect when aldesleukin given with ACE inhibitors

Alpha-blockers: enhanced hypotensive effect when aldesleukin given with alpha-blockers

Angiotensin-II Receptor Antagonists: enhanced hypotensive effect when aldesleukin given with angiotensin-II receptor antagonists

Antivirals: aldesleukin possibly increases plasma concentration of indinavir

Beta-blockers: enhanced hypotensive effect when aldesleukin given with beta-blockers

Calcium-channel Blockers: enhanced hypotensive effect when aldesleukin given with calcium-channel blockers

Clonidine: enhanced hypotensive effect when aldesleukin given with clonidine

• Corticosteroids: manufacturer of aldesleukin advises avoid concomitant use with •corticosteroids

• Cytotoxics: manufacturer of aldesleukin advises avoid concomitant use with •cisplatin, •dacarbazine and •vinblastine

Diazoxide: enhanced hypotensive effect when aldesleukin given with diazoxide

Diuretics: enhanced hypotensive effect when aldesleukin given with diuretics

Methyldopa: enhanced hypotensive effect when aldesleukin given with methyldopa

Moxonidine: enhanced hypotensive effect when aldesleukin given with moxonidine

Nitrates: enhanced hypotensive effect when aldesleukin given with nitrates

Vasodilator Antihypertensives: enhanced hypotensive effect when aldesleukin given with hydralazine, minoxidil or sodium nitroprusside

Alemtuzumab

• Antipsychotics: avoid concomitant use of cytotoxics with •clozapine (increased risk of agranulocytosis)

• Vaccines: avoid concomitant use of monoclonal antibodies with live •vaccines (see p. 842)

Alendronic Acid see Bisphosphonates

Alfentanil see Opioid Analgesics

Alfuzosin see Alpha-blockers

Alimemazine see Antihistamines

Aliskiren

• ACE Inhibitors: avoid concomitant use of aliskiren with •ACE inhibitors (see also under Renin inhibitors, p. 129)

Analgesics: hypotensive effect of aliskiren possibly antagonised by NSAIDs

• Angiotensin-II Receptor Antagonists: avoid concomitant use of aliskiren with •angiotensin-II receptor antagonists (see also under Renin inhibitors, p. 129); plasma concentration of aliskiren possibly reduced by irbesartan

Antibacterials: plasma concentration of aliskiren reduced by rifampicin

Anticoagulants: increased risk of hyperkalaemia when aliskiren given with heparins

• Antifungals: plasma concentration of aliskiren increased by •itraconazole—avoid concomitant use

Calcium-channel Blockers: plasma concentration of aliskiren increased by verapamil

• Ciclosporin: plasma concentration of aliskiren increased by •ciclosporin—avoid concomitant use

Diuretics: aliskiren reduces plasma concentration of furosemide; increased risk of hyperkalaemia when aliskiren given with potassium-sparing diuretics and aldosterone antagonists

Aliskiren (continued)

• Grapefruit Juice: plasma concentration of aliskiren reduced by •grapefruit juice—avoid concomitant use

Potassium Salts: increased risk of hyperkalaemia when aliskiren given with potassium salts

Alitretinoin see Retinoids

Alkylating Drugs see Bendamustine, Busulfan, Carmustine, Cyclophosphamide, Estramustine, Ifosfamide, Lomustine, Melphalan, and Thiotepa

Allopurinol

ACE Inhibitors: manufacturers state possible increased risk of leucopenia and hypersensitivity reactions when allopurinol given with ACE inhibitors especially in renal impairment

Antibacterials: increased risk of rash when allopurinol given with amoxicillin or ampicillin

Anticoagulants: allopurinol possibly enhances anticoagulant effect of coumarins

• Antivirals: allopurinol increases plasma concentration of •didanosine (risk of toxicity)—avoid concomitant use

• Azathioprine: allopurinol enhances effects and increases toxicity of •azathioprine (reduce dose of azathioprine to one quarter of usual dose)

Ciclosporin: allopurinol possibly increases plasma concentration of ciclosporin (risk of nephrotoxicity)

• Cytotoxics: allopurinol enhances effects and increases toxicity of •mercaptopurine (reduce dose of mercaptopurine to one quarter of usual dose); avoidance of allopurinol advised by manufacturer of •capecitabine

Diuretics: increased risk of hypersensitivity when allopurinol given with thiazides and related diuretics especially in renal impairment

Theophylline: allopurinol possibly increases plasma concentration of theophylline

Almotriptan see 5HT$_1$-receptor Agonists (under HT)

Alogliptin see Antidiabetics

Alpha$_2$-adrenoceptor Stimulants see Apraclonidine, Brimonidine, Clonidine, and Methyldopa

Alpha-blockers

ACE Inhibitors: enhanced hypotensive effect when alpha-blockers given with ACE inhibitors

Adrenergic Neurone Blockers: enhanced hypotensive effect when alpha-blockers given with adrenergic neurone blockers

Alcohol: enhanced hypotensive effect when alpha-blockers given with alcohol; increased sedative effect when indoramin given with alcohol

Aldesleukin: enhanced hypotensive effect when alpha-blockers given with aldesleukin

• Anaesthetics, General: enhanced hypotensive effect when alpha-blockers given with •general anaesthetics

Analgesics: hypotensive effect of alpha-blockers antagonised by NSAIDs

Angiotensin-II Receptor Antagonists: enhanced hypotensive effect when alpha-blockers given with angiotensin-II receptor antagonists

• Antidepressants: manufacturer of indoramin advises avoid concomitant use with •MAOIs; enhanced hypotensive effect when alpha-blockers given with MAOIs

Antipsychotics: enhanced hypotensive effect when alpha-blockers given with antipsychotics

• Antivirals: plasma concentration of doxazosin and tamsulosin possibly increased by boceprevir—manufacturer of boceprevir advises avoid concomitant use; plasma concentration of alfuzosin possibly increased by •ritonavir—avoid concomitant use; avoidance of alfuzosin advised by manufacturer of •telaprevir

Anxiolytics and Hypnotics: enhanced hypotensive and sedative effects when alpha-blockers given with anxiolytics and hypnotics

Alpha-blockers *(continued)*

- Avanafil: enhanced hypotensive effect when alpha-blockers given with ●avanafil—see also p. 570
- Beta-blockers: enhanced hypotensive effect when alpha-blockers given with ●beta-blockers, also increased risk of first-dose hypotension with post-synaptic alpha-blockers such as prazosin
- Calcium-channel Blockers: enhanced hypotensive effect when alpha-blockers given with ●calcium-channel blockers, also increased risk of first-dose hypotension with post-synaptic alpha-blockers such as prazosin; plasma concentration of tamsulosin increased by verapamil

Cardiac Glycosides: prazosin increases plasma concentration of digoxin

Clonidine: enhanced hypotensive effect when alpha-blockers given with clonidine
- Cobicistat: plasma concentration of alfuzosin possibly increased by ●cobicistat—manufacturer of cobicistat advises avoid concomitant use

Corticosteroids: hypotensive effect of alpha-blockers antagonised by corticosteroids

Cytotoxics: avoidance of alfuzosin advised by manufacturer of idelalisib

Diazoxide: enhanced hypotensive effect when alpha-blockers given with diazoxide
- Diuretics: enhanced hypotensive effect when alpha-blockers given with ●diuretics, also increased risk of first-dose hypotension with post-synaptic alpha-blockers such as prazosin

Dopaminergics: enhanced hypotensive effect when alpha-blockers given with levodopa

Methyldopa: enhanced hypotensive effect when alpha-blockers given with methyldopa
- Moxisylyte: possible severe postural hypotension when alpha-blockers given with ●moxisylyte

Moxonidine: enhanced hypotensive effect when alpha-blockers given with moxonidine

Muscle Relaxants: enhanced hypotensive effect when alpha-blockers given with baclofen or tizanidine

Nitrates: enhanced hypotensive effect when alpha-blockers given with nitrates

Oestrogens: hypotensive effect of alpha-blockers antagonised by oestrogens

Prostaglandins: enhanced hypotensive effect when alpha-blockers given with alprostadil
- Sildenafil: enhanced hypotensive effect when alpha-blockers given with ●sildenafil (avoid alpha-blockers for 4 hours after sildenafil)—see also p. 570
- Sympathomimetics: avoid concomitant use of tolazoline with ●adrenaline (epinephrine) or ●dopamine
- Tadalafil: enhanced hypotensive effect when alpha-blockers given with ●tadalafil—see also p. 570; enhanced hypotensive effect when doxazosin given with ●tadalafil—manufacturer of tadalafil advises avoid concomitant use
- Ulcer-healing Drugs: effects of tolazoline antagonised by ●cimetidine and ●ranitidine
- Vardenafil: enhanced hypotensive effect when alpha-blockers given with ●vardenafil—separate doses by 6 hours (except with tamsulosin)—see also p. 570

Vasodilator Antihypertensives: enhanced hypotensive effect when alpha-blockers given with hydralazine, minoxidil or sodium nitroprusside

Alpha-blockers (post-synaptic) *see* Alpha-blockers

Alprazolam *see* Anxiolytics and Hypnotics

Alprostadil *see* Prostaglandins

Aluminium Hydroxide *see* Antacids

Amantadine

Antimalarials: plasma concentration of amantadine possibly increased by quinine

Antipsychotics: increased risk of extrapyramidal side-effects when amantadine given with antipsychotics

Bupropion: increased risk of side-effects when amantadine given with bupropion

Amantadine *(continued)*

- Memantine: increased risk of CNS toxicity when amantadine given with ●memantine (manufacturer of memantine advises avoid concomitant use); effects of dopaminergics possibly enhanced by memantine

Methyldopa: increased risk of extrapyramidal side-effects when amantadine given with methyldopa; antiparkinsonian effect of dopaminergics antagonised by methyldopa

Tetrabenazine: increased risk of extrapyramidal side-effects when amantadine given with tetrabenazine

Ambrisentan

Antibacterials: plasma concentration of ambrisentan possibly increased by rifampicin
- Ciclosporin: plasma concentration of ambrisentan increased by ●ciclosporin (see Dose under Ambrisentan, p. 111)

Amikacin *see* Aminoglycosides

Amiloride *see* Diuretics

Aminoglycosides

Agalsidase Alfa and Beta: gentamicin possibly inhibits effects of agalsidase alfa and beta (manufacturers of agalsidase alfa and beta advise avoid concomitant use)

Analgesics: plasma concentration of amikacin and gentamicin in neonates possibly increased by indometacin
- Antibacterials: neomycin reduces absorption of phenoxymethylpenicillin; increased risk of nephrotoxicity when aminoglycosides given with colistimethate sodium or polymyxins; increased risk of nephrotoxicity and ototoxicity when aminoglycosides given with capreomycin or ●vancomycin; possible increased risk of nephrotoxicity when aminoglycosides given with cephalosporins
- Anticoagulants: experience in anticoagulant clinics suggests that INR possibly altered when neomycin (given for local action on gut) is given with ●coumarins or ●phenindione

Antidiabetics: neomycin possibly enhances hypoglycaemic effect of acarbose, also severity of gastro-intestinal effects increased

Antifungals: increased risk of nephrotoxicity when aminoglycosides given with amphotericin

Bisphosphonates: increased risk of hypocalcaemia when aminoglycosides given with bisphosphonates

Cardiac Glycosides: gentamicin possibly increases plasma concentration of digoxin; neomycin reduces absorption of digoxin
- Ciclosporin: increased risk of nephrotoxicity when aminoglycosides given with ●ciclosporin
- Cytotoxics: neomycin possibly reduces absorption of methotrexate; neomycin reduces bioavailability of sorafenib; increased risk of nephrotoxicity and possibly of ototoxicity when aminoglycosides given with ●platinum compounds
- Diuretics: increased risk of ototoxicity when aminoglycosides given with ●loop diuretics

Mannitol: manufacturer of tobramycin advises avoid concomitant use with mannitol
- Muscle Relaxants: aminoglycosides enhance effects of ●non-depolarising muscle relaxants and ●suxamethonium
- Parasympathomimetics: aminoglycosides antagonise effects of ●neostigmine and ●pyridostigmine
- Tacrolimus: increased risk of nephrotoxicity when aminoglycosides given with ●tacrolimus

Vaccines: antibacterials inactivate oral typhoid vaccine—see p. 864

Vitamins: neomycin possibly reduces absorption of vitamin A

Aminophylline *see* Theophylline

Aminosalicylates *see* individual drugs

Amiodarone

Note Amiodarone has a long half-life; there is a potential for drug interactions to occur for several weeks (or even months) after treatment with it has been stopped

Agalsidase Alfa and Beta: amiodarone possibly inhibits effects of agalsidase alfa and beta (manufacturers of agalsidase alfa and beta advise avoid concomitant use)

Anaesthetics, Local: increased myocardial depression when anti-arrhythmics given with bupivacaine, levobupivacaine, prilocaine or ropivacaine

- Anti-arrhythmics: increased myocardial depression when anti-arrhythmics given with other ●anti-arrhythmics; increased risk of ventricular arrhythmias when amiodarone given with ●disopyramide or ●dronedarone—avoid concomitant use; amiodarone increases plasma concentration of ●flecainide (halve dose of flecainide)

- Antibacterials: increased risk of ventricular arrhythmias when amiodarone given with *parenteral* ●erythromycin—avoid concomitant use; increased risk of ventricular arrhythmias when amiodarone given with ●levofloxacin or ●moxifloxacin—avoid concomitant use; possible increased risk of ventricular arrhythmias when amiodarone given with sulfamethoxazole and trimethoprim (as co-trimoxazole)—manufacturer of amiodarone advises avoid concomitant use of co-trimoxazole; increased risk of ventricular arrhythmias when amiodarone given with ●delamanid; possible increased risk of ventricular arrhythmias when amiodarone given with ●telithromycin

- Anticoagulants: amiodarone inhibits metabolism of ●coumarins and ●phenindione (enhanced anticoagulant effect); amiodarone increases plasma concentration of ●dabigatran (see Dose under Dabigatran, p. 156)

- Antidepressants: avoidance of amiodarone advised by manufacturer of ●citalopram and ●escitalopram (risk of ventricular arrhythmias); increased risk of ventricular arrhythmias when amiodarone given with ●tricyclics—avoid concomitant use

- Antiepileptics: amiodarone inhibits metabolism of ●phenytoin (increased plasma concentration)

- Antihistamines: increased risk of ventricular arrhythmias when amiodarone given with ●mizolastine—avoid concomitant use

- Antimalarials: avoidance of amiodarone advised by manufacturer of ●piperaquine with artenimol (possible risk of ventricular arrhythmias); avoidance of amiodarone advised by manufacturer of ●artemether with lumefantrine (risk of ventricular arrhythmias); increased risk of ventricular arrhythmias when amiodarone given with ●chloroquine and hydroxychloroquine, ●mefloquine or ●quinine—avoid concomitant use

- Antimuscarinics: increased risk of ventricular arrhythmias when amiodarone given with ●tolterodine

- Antipsychotics: increased risk of ventricular arrhythmias when anti-arrhythmics that prolong the QT interval given with ●antipsychotics that prolong the QT interval; increased risk of ventricular arrhythmias when amiodarone given with ●benperidol—manufacturer of benperidol advises avoid concomitant use; increased risk of ventricular arrhythmias when amiodarone given with ●amisulpride, ●droperidol, ●haloperidol, ●phenothiazines, ●pimozide or ●zuclopenthixol—avoid concomitant use; increased risk of ventricular arrhythmias when amiodarone given with ●sulpiride

- Antivirals: plasma concentration of amiodarone possibly increased by ●atazanavir, plasma concentration of amiodarone possibly increased by ●fosamprenavir (increased risk of ventricular arrhythmias)—avoid concomitant use; plasma concentration of amiodarone possibly increased by ●indinavir—avoid

Amiodarone

- Antivirals *(continued)*
  concomitant use; plasma concentration of amiodarone increased by ●ritonavir (increased risk of ventricular arrhythmias)—avoid concomitant use; increased risk of ventricular arrhythmias when amiodarone given with ●saquinavir—avoid concomitant use; avoidance of amiodarone advised by manufacturer of ●telaprevir (risk of ventricular arrhythmias)

- Atomoxetine: increased risk of ventricular arrhythmias when amiodarone given with ●atomoxetine

- Beta-blockers: increased risk of bradycardia, AV block and myocardial depression when amiodarone given with ●beta-blockers; increased myocardial depression when anti-arrhythmics given with ●beta-blockers; increased risk of ventricular arrhythmias when amiodarone given with ●sotalol—avoid concomitant use

- Calcium-channel Blockers: increased risk of bradycardia, AV block and myocardial depression when amiodarone given with ●diltiazem or ●verapamil

- Cardiac Glycosides: amiodarone increases plasma concentration of ●digoxin (halve dose of digoxin)

Ciclosporin: amiodarone possibly increases plasma concentration of ciclosporin

- Cobicistat: plasma concentration of amiodarone possibly increased by ●cobicistat—manufacturer of cobicistat advises avoid concomitant use

- Colchicine: amiodarone possibly increases risk of ●colchicine toxicity

- Cytotoxics: amiodarone possibly increases the plasma concentration of afatinib—manufacturer of afatinib advises separating administration of amiodarone by 6 to 12 hours; possible increased risk of ventricular arrhythmias when amiodarone given with ●bosutinib; amiodarone possibly increases the plasma concentration of ●ibrutinib—reduce dose of ibrutinib (see Dose under Ibrutinib, p. 615); avoidance of amiodarone advised by manufacturer of idelalisib; possible increased risk of ventricular arrhythmias when amiodarone given with ●vandetanib—avoid concomitant use; increased risk of ventricular arrhythmias when amiodarone given with ●arsenic trioxide

Diuretics: increased cardiac toxicity with amiodarone if hypokalaemia occurs with acetazolamide, loop diuretics or thiazides and related diuretics; amiodarone increases plasma concentration of eplerenone (reduce dose of eplerenone)

Fidaxomicin: avoidance of amiodarone advised by manufacturer of fidaxomicin

- Fingolimod: possible increased risk of bradycardia when amiodarone given with ●fingolimod

Grapefruit Juice: plasma concentration of amiodarone increased by grapefruit juice

- Ivabradine: increased risk of ventricular arrhythmias when amiodarone given with ●ivabradine

- Lipid-regulating Drugs: increased risk of myopathy when amiodarone given with ●simvastatin (see Dose under Simvastatin, p. 177)

- Lithium: manufacturer of amiodarone advises avoid concomitant use with ●lithium (risk of ventricular arrhythmias)

Orlistat: plasma concentration of amiodarone possibly reduced by orlistat

- Pentamidine Isetionate: increased risk of ventricular arrhythmias when amiodarone given with ●pentamidine isetionate—avoid concomitant use

Thyroid Hormones: for concomitant use of amiodarone and thyroid hormones see p. 98

Ulcer-healing Drugs: plasma concentration of amiodarone increased by cimetidine

Amisulpride *see* Antipsychotics

Amitriptyline *see* Antidepressants, Tricyclic

Amlodipine *see* Calcium-channel Blockers

Amoxicillin see Penicillins

Amphotericin

Note Close monitoring required with concomitant administration of nephrotoxic drugs or cytotoxics

Antibacterials: increased risk of nephrotoxicity when amphotericin given with aminoglycosides or polymyxins; possible increased risk of nephrotoxicity when amphotericin given with vancomycin

Antifungals: amphotericin reduces renal excretion and increases cellular uptake of flucytosine (toxicity possibly increased); effects of amphotericin possibly antagonised by imidazoles and triazoles; plasma concentration of amphotericin possibly increased by micafungin

• Cardiac Glycosides: hypokalaemia caused by amphotericin increases cardiac toxicity with ●cardiac glycosides

• Ciclosporin: increased risk of nephrotoxicity when amphotericin given with ●ciclosporin

• Corticosteroids: increased risk of hypokalaemia when amphotericin given with ●corticosteroids—avoid concomitant use unless corticosteroids needed to control reactions

• Cytotoxics: increased risk of ventricular arrhythmias when amphotericin given with ●arsenic trioxide

Diuretics: increased risk of hypokalaemia when amphotericin given with loop diuretics or thiazides and related diuretics

Pentamidine Isetionate: possible increased risk of nephrotoxicity when amphotericin given with pentamidine isetionate

• Sodium Stibogluconate: possible increased risk of arrhythmias when amphotericin given after ●sodium stibogluconate—manufacturer of sodium stibogluconate advises giving 14 days apart

• Tacrolimus: increased risk of nephrotoxicity when amphotericin given with ●tacrolimus

Ampicillin see Penicillins

Anabolic Steroids

• Anticoagulants: anabolic steroids enhance anticoagulant effect of ●coumarins and ●phenindione

Antidiabetics: anabolic steroids possibly enhance hypoglycaemic effect of antidiabetics

Anaesthetics, General

Note See also Surgery and Long-term Medication, p. 873

ACE Inhibitors: enhanced hypotensive effect when general anaesthetics given with ACE inhibitors

• Adrenergic Neurone Blockers: enhanced hypotensive effect when general anaesthetics given with ●adrenergic neurone blockers

• Alpha-blockers: enhanced hypotensive effect when general anaesthetics given with ●alpha-blockers

Analgesics: metabolism of etomidate inhibited by fentanyl (consider reducing dose of etomidate); effects of thiopental possibly enhanced by aspirin; effects of intravenous general anaesthetics and volatile liquid general anaesthetics possibly enhanced by opioid analgesics

Angiotensin-II Receptor Antagonists: enhanced hypotensive effect when general anaesthetics given with angiotensin-II receptor antagonists

Antibacterials: increased risk of hepatotoxicity when isoflurane given with isoniazid; effects of thiopental enhanced by sulfonamides; hypersensitivity-like reactions can occur when general anaesthetics given with intravenous vancomycin

Antidepressants: increased risk of arrhythmias and hypotension when general anaesthetics given with tricyclics

• Antipsychotics: enhanced hypotensive effect when general anaesthetics given with ●antipsychotics; effects of thiopental enhanced by droperidol

Anxiolytics and Hypnotics: increased sedative effect when general anaesthetics given with anxiolytics and hypnotics

Anaesthetics, General (continued)

Beta-blockers: enhanced hypotensive effect when general anaesthetics given with beta-blockers

• Calcium-channel Blockers: enhanced hypotensive effect when general anaesthetics or isoflurane given with calcium-channel blockers; general anaesthetics enhance hypotensive effect of ●verapamil (also AV delay)

Clonidine: enhanced hypotensive effect when general anaesthetics given with clonidine

• Cytotoxics: nitrous oxide increases antifolate effect of ●methotrexate—avoid concomitant use

Diazoxide: enhanced hypotensive effect when general anaesthetics given with diazoxide

Diuretics: enhanced hypotensive effect when general anaesthetics given with diuretics

• Dopaminergics: increased risk of arrhythmias when volatile liquid general anaesthetics given with ●levodopa

• Doxapram: increased risk of arrhythmias when volatile liquid general anaesthetics given with ●doxapram (avoid doxapram for at least 10 minutes after volatile liquid general anaesthetics)

• Memantine: increased risk of CNS toxicity when ketamine given with ●memantine (manufacturer of memantine advises avoid concomitant use)

Methyldopa: enhanced hypotensive effect when general anaesthetics given with methyldopa

Metoclopramide: effects of thiopental enhanced by metoclopramide

Moxonidine: enhanced hypotensive effect when general anaesthetics given with moxonidine

• Muscle Relaxants: increased risk of myocardial depression and bradycardia when propofol given with ●suxamethonium; volatile liquid general anaesthetics enhance effects of non-depolarising muscle relaxants and suxamethonium; ketamine enhances effects of atracurium

Nitrates: enhanced hypotensive effect when general anaesthetics given with nitrates

Oxytocin: oxytocic effect possibly reduced, also ●enhanced hypotensive effect and risk of arrhythmias when volatile liquid general anaesthetics given with oxytocin

• Sympathomimetics: manufacturer of isoflurane advises avoid concomitant use with ●sympathomimetics (risk of ventricular arrhythmias); increased risk of arrhythmias when volatile liquid general anaesthetics given with ●adrenaline (epinephrine) or ●noradrenaline (norepinephrine); increased risk of hypertension when volatile liquid general anaesthetics given with ●methylphenidate

Theophylline: increased risk of convulsions when ketamine given with theophylline

Vasodilator Antihypertensives: enhanced hypotensive effect when general anaesthetics given with hydralazine, minoxidil or sodium nitroprusside

Anaesthetics, General (intravenous) see Anaesthetics, General

Anaesthetics, General (volatile liquids) see Anaesthetics, General

Anaesthetics, Local see Bupivacaine, Chloroprocaine, Levobupivacaine, Lidocaine, Prilocaine, and Ropivacaine

Anagrelide

• Cilostazol: manufacturer of anagrelide advises avoid concomitant use with ●cilostazol

• Phosphodiesterase Type-3 Inhibitors: manufacturer of anagrelide advises avoid concomitant use with ●enoximone and ●milrinone

Anakinra

• Cytotoxics: avoid concomitant use of anakinra with ●adalimumab, ●certolizumab pegol, ●golimumab or ●infliximab

• Etanercept: avoid concomitant use of anakinra with ●etanercept

Anakinra *(continued)*
- Vaccines: avoid concomitant use of anakinra with live ●vaccines (see p. 842)

Analgesics *see* Aspirin, Nefopam, NSAIDs, Opioid Analgesics, and Paracetamol

Angiotensin-II Receptor Antagonists
- ACE Inhibitors: increased risk of hyperkalaemia, hypotension, and impaired renal function when angiotensin-II receptor antagonists given with ●ACE inhibitors (see also under Concomitant Use of Drugs Affecting the Renin-Angiotensin System, p. 119)

Adrenergic Neurone Blockers: enhanced hypotensive effect when angiotensin-II receptor antagonists given with adrenergic neurone blockers

Alcohol: enhanced hypotensive effect when angiotensin-II receptor antagonists given with alcohol

Aldesleukin: enhanced hypotensive effect when angiotensin-II receptor antagonists given with aldesleukin

- Aliskiren: avoid concomitant use of angiotensin-II receptor antagonists with ●aliskiren (see also under Renin inhibitors, p. 129); irbesartan possibly reduces plasma concentration of aliskiren

Alpha-blockers: enhanced hypotensive effect when angiotensin-II receptor antagonists given with alpha-blockers

Anaesthetics, General: enhanced hypotensive effect when angiotensin-II receptor antagonists given with general anaesthetics

Analgesics: increased risk of renal impairment when angiotensin-II receptor antagonists given with NSAIDs, also hypotensive effect antagonised

Antibacterials: plasma concentration of losartan and its active metabolite reduced by rifampicin; possible increased risk of hyperkalaemia when angiotensin-II receptor antagonists given with trimethoprim

Anticoagulants: increased risk of hyperkalaemia when angiotensin-II receptor antagonists given with heparins

Antidepressants: hypotensive effect of angiotensin-II receptor antagonists possibly enhanced by MAOIs

Antipsychotics: enhanced hypotensive effect when angiotensin-II receptor antagonists given with antipsychotics

Anxiolytics and Hypnotics: enhanced hypotensive effect when angiotensin-II receptor antagonists given with anxiolytics and hypnotics

Beta-blockers: enhanced hypotensive effect when angiotensin-II receptor antagonists given with beta-blockers

Calcium-channel Blockers: enhanced hypotensive effect when angiotensin-II receptor antagonists given with calcium-channel blockers

- Ciclosporin: increased risk of hyperkalaemia when angiotensin-II receptor antagonists given with ●ciclosporin

Clonidine: enhanced hypotensive effect when angiotensin-II receptor antagonists given with clonidine

Corticosteroids: hypotensive effect of angiotensin-II receptor antagonists antagonised by corticosteroids

Diazoxide: enhanced hypotensive effect when angiotensin-II receptor antagonists given with diazoxide

- Diuretics: enhanced hypotensive effect when angiotensin-II receptor antagonists given with ●diuretics; increased risk of hyperkalaemia when angiotensin-II receptor antagonists given with ●potassium-sparing diuretics and aldosterone antagonists

Dopaminergics: enhanced hypotensive effect when angiotensin-II receptor antagonists given with levodopa

- Lithium: angiotensin-II receptor antagonists reduce excretion of ●lithium (increased plasma concentration)

Methyldopa: enhanced hypotensive effect when angiotensin-II receptor antagonists given with methyldopa

Angiotensin-II Receptor Antagonists *(continued)*
Moxisylyte: enhanced hypotensive effect when angiotensin-II receptor antagonists given with moxisylyte

Moxonidine: enhanced hypotensive effect when angiotensin-II receptor antagonists given with moxonidine

Muscle Relaxants: enhanced hypotensive effect when angiotensin-II receptor antagonists given with baclofen or tizanidine

Nitrates: enhanced hypotensive effect when angiotensin-II receptor antagonists given with nitrates

Oestrogens: hypotensive effect of angiotensin-II receptor antagonists antagonised by oestrogens

- Potassium Salts: increased risk of hyperkalaemia when angiotensin-II receptor antagonists given with ●potassium salts

Prostaglandins: enhanced hypotensive effect when angiotensin-II receptor antagonists given with alprostadil

Tacrolimus: increased risk of hyperkalaemia when angiotensin-II receptor antagonists given with tacrolimus

Vasodilator Antihypertensives: enhanced hypotensive effect when angiotensin-II receptor antagonists given with hydralazine, minoxidil or sodium nitroprusside

Antacids
Note Antacids should preferably not be taken at the same time as other drugs since they may impair absorption

ACE Inhibitors: antacids possibly reduce absorption of ACE inhibitors; antacids reduce absorption of captopril, enalapril and fosinopril

Analgesics: antacids possibly reduce absorption of acemetacin; alkaline urine due to some antacids increases excretion of aspirin

Antibacterials: antacids reduce absorption of azithromycin, cefaclor, ciprofloxacin, isoniazid, levofloxacin, moxifloxacin, norfloxacin, ofloxacin, rifampicin and tetracyclines; avoid concomitant use of antacids with methenamine; oral magnesium salts (as magnesium trisilicate) reduce absorption of nitrofurantoin

Antiepileptics: antacids reduce absorption of gabapentin and phenytoin

Antifungals: antacids reduce absorption of itraconazole

Antihistamines: antacids reduce absorption of fexofenadine

Antimalarials: antacids reduce absorption of chloroquine and hydroxychloroquine; oral magnesium salts (as magnesium trisilicate) reduce absorption of proguanil

Antipsychotics: antacids reduce absorption of phenothiazines and sulpiride

Antivirals: antacids reduce absorption of atazanavir (give at least 2 hours before or 1 hour after antacids); aluminium hydroxide reduces absorption of dolutegravir—manufacturer of dolutegravir advises give at least 2 hours before or 6 hours after aluminium hydroxide; oral magnesium salts reduce absorption of dolutegravir—manufacturer of dolutegravir advises give at least 2 hours before or 6 hours after oral magnesium salts; antacids reduce absorption of elvitegravir (give at least 4 hours apart); antacids possibly reduce absorption of raltegravir (give at least 2 hours apart); manufacturer of rilpivirine advises give antacids 2 hours before or 4 hours after rilpivirine; antacids reduce absorption of tipranavir (give at least 2 hours apart)

Bile Acids: antacids possibly reduce absorption of bile acids

Bisphosphonates: antacids reduce absorption of bisphosphonates

Cardiac Glycosides: antacids possibly reduce absorption of digoxin

Antacids (continued)
  Corticosteroids: antacids reduce absorption of deflaza-
    cort
- Cytotoxics: aluminium hydroxide and oral magnesium
    salts possibly reduce absorption of estramustine—
    manufacturer of estramustine advises avoid conco-
    mitant administration; separating administration
    with antacids by about 12 hours advised by manu-
    facturer of bosutinib; antacids possibly reduce
    plasma concentration of ●erlotinib—give antacids at
    least 4 hours before or 2 hours after erlotinib
  Deferasirox: antacids containing aluminium possibly
    reduce absorption of deferasirox (manufacturer of
    deferasirox advises avoid concomitant use)
  Deferiprone: antacids containing aluminium possibly
    reduce absorption of deferiprone (manufacturer of
    deferiprone advises avoid concomitant use)
  Dipyridamole: antacids possibly reduce absorption of
    dipyridamole
  Eltrombopag: antacids reduce absorption of eltrombo-
    pag (give at least 4 hours apart)
  Folates: antacids possibly reduce absorption of folic
    acid (manufacturer of folic acid advises give at least
    2 hours apart)
  Iron: oral magnesium salts (as magnesium trisilicate)
    reduce absorption of *oral* iron
  Lipid-regulating Drugs: antacids reduce absorption of
    rosuvastatin
  Lithium: sodium bicarbonate increases excretion of
    lithium (reduced plasma concentration)
  Mycophenolate: antacids reduce absorption of myco-
    phenolate
  Penicillamine: antacids reduce absorption of penicill-
    amine
  Polystyrene Sulfonate Resins: risk of intestinal
    obstruction when aluminium hydroxide given with
    polystyrene sulfonate resins; risk of metabolic alka-
    losis when oral magnesium salts given with poly-
    styrene sulfonate resins
  Riociguat: antacids reduce absorption of riociguat
    (give at least 2 hours before or 1 hour after rioci-
    guat)
  Sympathomimetics: aluminium hydroxide possibly
    increases absorption of pseudoephedrine
  Thyroid Hormones: antacids possibly reduce absorp-
    tion of levothyroxine
  Ulcer-healing Drugs: antacids possibly reduce absorp-
    tion of lansoprazole
Antazoline *see* Antihistamines
Anthrax vaccine *see* Vaccines
Anti-arrhythmics *see* Adenosine, Amiodarone, Diso-
  pyramide, Dronedarone, Flecainide, Lidocaine, and
  Propafenone
Antibacterials *see* individual drugs
Antibiotics (cytotoxic) *see* Bleomycin, Doxorubicin,
  Epirubicin, Idarubicin, Mitomycin, Mitoxantrone,
  and Pixantrone
Anticoagulants *see* Apixaban, Argatroban, Bivalirudin,
  Coumarins, Dabigatran, Danaparoid, Fondaparinux,
  Heparins, Phenindione, and Rivaroxaban
Antidepressants *see* Agomelatine; Antidepressants,
  SSRI; Antidepressants, Tricyclic; Antidepressants,
  Tricyclic (related); MAOIs; Mirtazapine; Moclobe-
  mide; Reboxetine; St John's Wort; Venlafaxine
**Antidepressants, Noradrenaline Re-uptake Inhi-
bitors** *see* Reboxetine
Antidepressants, SSRI
  Note *see also* Dapoxetine
  Alcohol: sedative effects possibly increased when
    SSRIs given with alcohol
  Anaesthetics, Local: fluvoxamine inhibits metabolism
    of ropivacaine—avoid prolonged administration of
    ropivacaine
- Analgesics: increased risk of bleeding when SSRIs
    given with ●NSAIDs or ●aspirin; possible increased
    serotonergic effects when SSRIs given with fentanyl;

Antidepressants, SSRI
- Analgesics (continued)
    fluoxetine, fluvoxamine, paroxetine and sertraline
    possibly increase plasma concentration of metha-
    done; increased risk of CNS toxicity when SSRIs
    given with ●tramadol
- Anti-arrhythmics: manufacturer of citalopram and esci-
    talopram advises avoid concomitant use with
    ●amiodarone (risk of ventricular arrhythmias); man-
    ufacturer of citalopram and escitalopram advises
    avoid concomitant use with ●disopyramide (risk of
    ventricular arrhythmias); manufacturer of citalopram
    and escitalopram advises avoid concomitant use
    with ●dronedarone (risk of ventricular arrhythmias);
    fluoxetine increases plasma concentration of fle-
    cainide; fluoxetine and paroxetine possibly inhibit
    metabolism of propafenone
- Antibacterials: manufacturer of citalopram and escita-
    lopram advises avoid concomitant use with *intra-
    venous* ●erythromycin (risk of ventricular arrhyth-
    mias); manufacturer of citalopram and escitalopram
    advises avoid concomitant use with ●moxifloxacin
    (risk of ventricular arrhythmias); possible increased
    risk of ventricular arrhythmias when citalopram
    given with ●telithromycin
- Anticoagulants: SSRIs possibly enhance anticoagulant
    effect of ●coumarins; possible increased risk of
    bleeding when SSRIs given with ●dabigatran
- Antidepressants: avoidance of fluvoxamine advised
    by manufacturer of ●reboxetine; possible increased
    serotonergic effects when SSRIs given with duloxe-
    tine; fluvoxamine inhibits metabolism of ●duloxe-
    tine—avoid concomitant use; fluoxetine should not
    be started until 2 weeks after stopping ●MAOIs,
    also MAOIs should not be started until at least 5
    weeks after stopping fluoxetine; citalopram, escita-
    lopram, fluvoxamine, paroxetine or sertraline should
    not be started until 2 weeks after stopping ●MAOIs,
    also MAOIs should not be started until at least 1
    week after stopping citalopram, escitalopram, flu-
    voxamine, paroxetine or sertraline; CNS effects of
    SSRIs increased by ●MAOIs (risk of serious toxi-
    city); increased risk of CNS toxicity when escitalo-
    pram given with ●moclobemide, preferably avoid
    concomitant use; after stopping citalopram, fluvox-
    amine, paroxetine or sertraline do not start ●moclo-
    bemide for at least 1 week; after stopping fluoxetine
    do not start ●moclobemide for 5 weeks; increased
    serotonergic effects when SSRIs given with ●St
    John's wort—avoid concomitant use; fluvoxamine
    inhibits metabolism of ●agomelatine (increased
    plasma concentration); possible increased seroto-
    nergic effects when fluoxetine or fluvoxamine given
    with mirtazapine; manufacturer of citalopram and
    escitalopram advises avoid concomitant use with
    ●tricyclics (risk of ventricular arrhythmias); SSRIs
    increase plasma concentration of some ●tricyclics
- Antiepileptics: SSRIs antagonise anticonvulsant effect
    of ●antiepileptics (convulsive threshold lowered);
    fluoxetine and fluvoxamine increase plasma con-
    centration of ●carbamazepine; plasma concentra-
    tion of paroxetine reduced by phenobarbital and
    phenytoin; fluoxetine and fluvoxamine increase
    plasma concentration of ●phenytoin; plasma con-
    centration of sertraline possibly reduced by pheny-
    toin, also plasma concentration of phenytoin possi-
    bly increased
  Antifungals: plasma concentration of paroxetine possi-
    bly increased by terbinafine
- Antihistamines: manufacturer of citalopram and esci-
    talopram advises avoid concomitant use with
    ●mizolastine (risk of ventricular arrhythmias); anti-
    depressant effect of SSRIs possibly antagonised by
    cyproheptadine
- Antimalarials: manufacturer of citalopram and escita-
    lopram advises avoid concomitant use with

Appendix 1: Interactions

Antidepressants, SSRI

- Antimalarials (continued)
  - •antimalarials (risk of ventricular arrhythmias); avoidance of antidepressants advised by manufacturer of •artemether with lumefantrine and •piperaquine with artenimol

  Antimuscarinics: paroxetine increases plasma concentration of darifenacin and procyclidine

- Antipsychotics: avoidance of fluoxetine, fluvoxamine and sertraline advised by manufacturer of •droperidol (risk of ventricular arrhythmias); manufacturer of citalopram and escitalopram advises avoid concomitant use with •haloperidol (risk of ventricular arrhythmias); fluoxetine increases plasma concentration of •clozapine, •haloperidol and risperidone; fluvoxamine possibly increases plasma concentration of asenapine and haloperidol; paroxetine inhibits metabolism of perphenazine (reduce dose of perphenazine); fluoxetine and paroxetine possibly increase plasma concentration of •aripiprazole (reduce dose of aripiprazole—consult aripiprazole product literature); plasma concentration of paroxetine possibly increased by asenapine; fluvoxamine, paroxetine and sertraline increase plasma concentration of •clozapine; citalopram possibly increases plasma concentration of clozapine (increased risk of toxicity); fluvoxamine increases plasma concentration of olanzapine; manufacturer of citalopram and escitalopram advises avoid concomitant use with •phenothiazines (risk of ventricular arrhythmias); SSRIs possibly increase plasma concentration of •pimozide (increased risk of ventricular arrhythmias—avoid concomitant use); manufacturer of citalopram and escitalopram advises avoid concomitant use with •pimozide (risk of ventricular arrhythmias); paroxetine possibly increases plasma concentration of risperidone (increased risk of toxicity)

- Antivirals: plasma concentration of paroxetine and sertraline possibly reduced by darunavir; plasma concentration of SSRIs possibly increased by •ritonavir; plasma concentration of paroxetine possibly reduced by ritonavir

- Anxiolytics and Hypnotics: fluoxetine increases plasma concentration of alprazolam; fluvoxamine increases plasma concentration of some benzodiazepines; fluvoxamine increases plasma concentration of •melatonin—avoid concomitant use; sedative effects possibly increased when sertraline given with zolpidem

  Atomoxetine: possible increased risk of convulsions when antidepressants given with atomoxetine; fluoxetine and paroxetine possibly inhibit metabolism of atomoxetine

- Beta-blockers: paroxetine possibly increases the plasma concentration of •metoprolol—increased risk of AV block (manufacturer of paroxetine advises avoid concomitant use in cardiac insufficiency); citalopram and escitalopram increase plasma concentration of metoprolol; fluvoxamine increases plasma concentration of propranolol; increased risk of ventricular arrhythmias when citalopram given with •sotalol—avoid concomitant use; manufacturer of escitalopram advises avoid concomitant use with •sotalol (risk of ventricular arrhythmias)

  Bupropion: plasma concentration of citalopram possibly increased by bupropion

  Calcium-channel Blockers: fluoxetine possibly inhibits metabolism of nifedipine (increased plasma concentration)

- Clopidogrel: fluoxetine and fluvoxamine possibly reduce antiplatelet effect of •clopidogrel

- Dapoxetine: possible increased risk of serotonergic effects when SSRIs given with •dapoxetine (manufacturer of dapoxetine advises SSRIs should not be

Antidepressants, SSRI

- Dapoxetine (continued)
  started until 1 week after stopping dapoxetine, avoid dapoxetine for 2 weeks after stopping SSRIs)

- Dopaminergics: fluvoxamine should not be started until 2 weeks after stopping •rasagiline; fluoxetine should not be started until 2 weeks after stopping •rasagiline, also rasagiline should not be started until at least 5 weeks after stopping fluoxetine; increased risk of CNS toxicity when SSRIs given with •rasagiline; increased risk of hypertension and CNS excitation when fluvoxamine or sertraline given with •selegiline (selegiline should not be started until 1 week after stopping fluvoxamine or sertraline, avoid fluvoxamine or sertraline for 2 weeks after stopping selegiline); increased risk of hypertension and CNS excitation when fluoxetine given with •selegiline (selegiline should not be started until 5 weeks after stopping fluoxetine, avoid fluoxetine for 2 weeks after stopping selegiline); avoidance of citalopram and escitalopram advised by manufacturer of selegiline; increased risk of hypertension and CNS excitation when paroxetine given with •selegiline (selegiline should not be started until 2 weeks after stopping paroxetine, avoid paroxetine for 2 weeks after stopping selegiline)

  Grapefruit Juice: plasma concentration of sertraline possibly increased by grapefruit juice

- Hormone Antagonists: fluoxetine and paroxetine possibly inhibit metabolism of •tamoxifen to active metabolite (avoid concomitant use)

- 5HT$_1$-receptor Agonists: increased risk of CNS toxicity when citalopram given with •5HT$_1$ agonists (manufacturer of citalopram advises avoid concomitant use); fluvoxamine inhibits the metabolism of frovatriptan; possible increased serotonergic effects when SSRIs given with naratriptan; increased risk of CNS toxicity when citalopram, escitalopram, fluoxetine, fluvoxamine or paroxetine given with •sumatriptan; CNS toxicity reported when sertraline given with sumatriptan; fluvoxamine possibly inhibits metabolism of zolmitriptan (reduce dose of zolmitriptan)

  5HT$_3$-receptor Antagonists: possible increased serotonergic effects when SSRIs given with 5HT$_3$ antagonists

- Lithium: Increased risk of CNS effects when SSRIs given with •lithium (lithium toxicity reported)

- Methylthioninium: risk of CNS toxicity when SSRIs given with •methylthioninium—avoid concomitant use (if avoidance not possible, use lowest possible dose of methylthioninium and observe patient for up to 4 hours after administration)

  Metoclopramide: CNS toxicity reported when SSRIs given with metoclopramide

- Muscle Relaxants: fluvoxamine increases plasma concentration of •tizanidine (increased risk of toxicity)—avoid concomitant use

  Parasympathomimetics: paroxetine increases plasma concentration of galantamine

- Pentamidine Isetionate: manufacturer of citalopram and escitalopram advises avoid concomitant use with •pentamidine isetionate (risk of ventricular arrhythmias)

- Pirfenidone: fluvoxamine increases plasma concentration of •pirfenidone—manufacturer of pirfenidone advises avoid concomitant use

- Pomalidomide: fluvoxamine increases plasma concentration of •pomalidomide

  Ranolazine: paroxetine increases plasma concentration of ranolazine

  Roflumilast: fluvoxamine inhibits the metabolism of roflumilast

  Sympathomimetics: metabolism of SSRIs possibly inhibited by methylphenidate

Antidepressants, SSRI (continued)

- Theophylline: fluvoxamine increases plasma concentration of ●theophylline (concomitant use should usually be avoided, but where not possible halve theophylline dose and monitor plasma-theophylline concentration)

  Ticagrelor: possible increased risk of bleeding when citalopram, paroxetine or sertraline given with ticagrelor

  Ulcer-healing Drugs: plasma concentration of citalopram, escitalopram and sertraline increased by cimetidine; fluvoxamine possibly increases plasma concentration of lansoprazole; plasma concentration of escitalopram increased by omeprazole

Antidepressants, SSRI (related) see Duloxetine and Venlafaxine

Antidepressants, Tricyclic

  Adrenergic Neurone Blockers: tricyclics antagonise hypotensive effect of adrenergic neurone blockers

- Alcohol: increased sedative effect when tricyclics given with ●alcohol

  Alpha$_2$-adrenoceptor Stimulants: avoidance of tricyclics advised by manufacturer of apraclonidine and brimonidine

  Anaesthetics, General: increased risk of arrhythmias and hypotension when tricyclics given with general anaesthetics

- Analgesics: increased risk of CNS toxicity when tricyclics given with ●tramadol; side-effects possibly increased when tricyclics given with nefopam; sedative effects possibly increased when tricyclics given with opioid analgesics

- Anti-arrhythmics: increased risk of ventricular arrhythmias when tricyclics given with ●amiodarone—avoid concomitant use; increased risk of ventricular arrhythmias when tricyclics given with ●disopyramide or ●flecainide; avoidance of tricyclics advised by manufacturer of ●dronedarone (risk of ventricular arrhythmias); increased risk of arrhythmias when tricyclics given with ●propafenone

- Antibacterials: increased risk of ventricular arrhythmias when tricyclics given with ●moxifloxacin—avoid concomitant use; possible increased risk of ventricular arrhythmias when tricyclics that prolong the QT interval given with ●delamanid; possible increased risk of ventricular arrhythmias when tricyclics given with ●telithromycin

- Anticoagulants: tricyclics may enhance or reduce anticoagulant effect of ●coumarins

- Antidepressants: avoidance of tricyclics advised by manufacturer of ●citalopram and ●escitalopram (risk of ventricular arrhythmias); possible increased serotonergic effects when amitriptyline or clomipramine given with duloxetine; increased risk of hypertension and CNS excitation when tricyclics given with ●MAOIs, tricyclics should not be started until 2 weeks after stopping MAOIs (3 weeks if starting clomipramine or imipramine), also MAOIs should not be started for at least 1–2 weeks after stopping tricyclics (3 weeks in the case of clomipramine or imipramine); after stopping tricyclics do not start ●moclobemide for at least 1 week; plasma concentration of some tricyclics increased by ●SSRIs; plasma concentration of amitriptyline reduced by St John's wort

- Antiepileptics: tricyclics antagonise anticonvulsant effect of ●antiepileptics (convulsive threshold lowered); metabolism of tricyclics accelerated by ●carbamazepine (reduced plasma concentration and reduced effect); metabolism of tricyclics possibly accelerated by ●phenobarbital (reduced plasma concentration); plasma concentration of tricyclics possibly reduced by ●phenytoin

  Antifungals: plasma concentration of amitriptyline and nortriptyline possibly increased by fluconazole;

Antidepressants, Tricyclic

  Antifungals (continued)
  plasma concentration of tricyclics possibly increased by terbinafine

  Antihistamines: increased antimuscarinic and sedative effects when tricyclics given with antihistamines

- Antimalarials: avoidance of antidepressants advised by manufacturer of ●artemether with lumefantrine and ●piperaquine with artenimol

  Antimuscarinics: increased risk of antimuscarinic side-effects when tricyclics given with antimuscarinics

- Antipsychotics: avoidance of tricyclics advised by manufacturer of ●droperidol, ●fluphenazine, ●haloperidol, ●sulpiride and ●zuclopenthixol (risk of ventricular arrhythmias); possible increased antimuscarinic side-effects when tricyclics given with clozapine; increased risk of antimuscarinic side-effects when tricyclics given with phenothiazines; possible increased risk of ventricular arrhythmias when tricyclics given with ●risperidone

- Antivirals: plasma concentration of tricyclics possibly increased by ●ritonavir; increased risk of ventricular arrhythmias when tricyclics given with ●saquinavir—avoid concomitant use

  Anxiolytics and Hypnotics: increased sedative effect when tricyclics given with anxiolytics and hypnotics

- Atomoxetine: increased risk of ventricular arrhythmias when tricyclics given with ●atomoxetine; possible increased risk of convulsions when antidepressants given with atomoxetine

- Beta-blockers: plasma concentration of imipramine increased by labetalol and propranolol; increased risk of ventricular arrhythmias when tricyclics given with ●sotalol

  Bupropion: plasma concentration of tricyclics possibly increased by bupropion (possible increased risk of convulsions)

  Calcium-channel Blockers: plasma concentration of imipramine increased by diltiazem and verapamil; plasma concentration of tricyclics possibly increased by diltiazem and verapamil

  Cannabis Extract: possible increased risk of hypertension and tachycardia when tricyclics given with cannabis extract

- Clonidine: tricyclics antagonise hypotensive effect of ●clonidine, also increased risk of hypertension on clonidine withdrawal

- Cytotoxics: increased risk of ventricular arrhythmias when amitriptyline or clomipramine given with ●arsenic trioxide

- Dapoxetine: possible increased risk of serotonergic effects when tricyclics given with ●dapoxetine (manufacturer of dapoxetine advises tricyclics should not be started until 1 week after stopping dapoxetine, avoid dapoxetine for 2 weeks after stopping tricyclics)

  Disulfiram: metabolism of tricyclics inhibited by disulfiram (increased plasma concentration); concomitant amitriptyline reported to increase disulfiram reaction with alcohol

  Diuretics: increased risk of postural hypotension when tricyclics given with diuretics

- Dopaminergics: caution with tricyclics advised by manufacturer of entacapone; increased risk of CNS toxicity when tricyclics given with ●rasagiline; CNS toxicity reported when tricyclics given with ●selegiline

  Histamine: tricyclics theoretically antagonise effects of histamine—manufacturer of histamine advises avoid concomitant use

  Lithium: risk of toxicity when tricyclics given with lithium

- Methylthioninium: risk of CNS toxicity when clomipramine given with ●methylthioninium—avoid concomitant use (if avoidance not possible, use lowest

Antidepressants, Tricyclic

- Methylthioninium *(continued)*
possible dose of methylthioninium and observe patient for up to 4 hours after administration)
Moxonidine: tricyclics possibly antagonise hypotensive effect of moxonidine (manufacturer of moxonidine advises avoid concomitant use)
Muscle Relaxants: tricyclics enhance muscle relaxant effect of baclofen
Nicorandil: tricyclics possibly enhance hypotensive effect of nicorandil
Nitrates: tricyclics reduce effects of sublingual tablets of nitrates (failure to dissolve under tongue owing to dry mouth)
Oestrogens: antidepressant effect of tricyclics antagonised by oestrogens (but side-effects of tricyclics possibly increased due to increased plasma concentration)
- Pentamidine Isetionate: increased risk of ventricular arrhythmias when tricyclics given with ●pentamidine isetionate
Sodium Oxybate: increased risk of side-effects when tricyclics given with sodium oxybate
- Sympathomimetics: increased risk of hypertension and arrhythmias when tricyclics given with ●adrenaline (epinephrine) (but local anaesthetics with adrenaline appear to be safe); metabolism of tricyclics possibly inhibited by methylphenidate; increased risk of hypertension and arrhythmias when tricyclics given with ●noradrenaline (norepinephrine) or phenylephrine
Thyroid Hormones: effects of tricyclics possibly enhanced by thyroid hormones; effects of amitriptyline and imipramine enhanced by thyroid hormones
Ulcer-healing Drugs: plasma concentration of tricyclics possibly increased by cimetidine; metabolism of amitriptyline, doxepin, imipramine and nortriptyline inhibited by cimetidine (increased plasma concentration)

Antidepressants, Tricyclic (related)

- Alcohol: increased sedative effect when tricyclic-related antidepressants given with ●alcohol
Alpha$_2$-adrenoceptor Stimulants: avoidance of tricyclic-related antidepressants advised by manufacturer of apraclonidine and brimonidine
Antibacterials: plasma concentration of trazodone possibly increased by clarithromycin
Anticoagulants: trazodone may enhance or reduce anticoagulant effect of warfarin
- Antidepressants: tricyclic-related antidepressants should not be started until 2 weeks after stopping ●MAOIs, also MAOIs should not be started until at least 1–2 weeks after stopping tricyclic-related antidepressants; after stopping tricyclic-related antidepressants do not start ●moclobemide for at least 1 week
- Antiepileptics: tricyclic-related antidepressants possibly antagonise anticonvulsant effect of ●antiepileptics (convulsive threshold lowered); plasma concentration of mianserin and trazodone reduced by ●carbamazepine; metabolism of mianserin accelerated by ●phenobarbital (reduced plasma concentration); plasma concentration of mianserin reduced by ●phenytoin
Antihistamines: possible increased antimuscarinic and sedative effects when tricyclic-related antidepressants given with antihistamines
- Antimalarials: avoidance of antidepressants advised by manufacturer of ●artemether with lumefantrine and ●piperaquine with artenimol
Antimuscarinics: possible increased antimuscarinic side-effects when tricyclic-related antidepressants given with antimuscarinics
- Antivirals: plasma concentration of trazodone increased by ●ritonavir (increased risk of toxicity); increased risk of ventricular arrhythmias when

Antidepressants, Tricyclic (related)

- Antivirals *(continued)*
trazodone given with ●saquinavir—avoid concomitant use; plasma concentration of trazodone possibly increased by telaprevir
Anxiolytics and Hypnotics: increased sedative effect when tricyclic-related antidepressants given with anxiolytics and hypnotics
Atomoxetine: possible increased risk of convulsions when antidepressants given with atomoxetine
Diazoxide: enhanced hypotensive effect when tricyclic-related antidepressants given with diazoxide
Nitrates: tricyclic-related antidepressants possibly reduce effects of sublingual tablets of nitrates (failure to dissolve under tongue owing to dry mouth)
Vasodilator Antihypertensives: enhanced hypotensive effect when tricyclic-related antidepressants given with hydralazine or sodium nitroprusside

Antidiabetics

Note Other drugs administered orally may need to be taken at least 1 hour before or 4 hours after lixisenatide injection, or taken with a meal when lixisenatide is not administered, to minimise possible interference with absorption

Note Other drugs administered orally may need to be taken at least 1 hour before or 4 hours after exenatide injection, or taken with a meal when exenatide is not administered, to minimise possible interference with absorption

ACE Inhibitors: hypoglycaemic effect of insulin, metformin and sulfonylureas possibly enhanced by ACE inhibitors
Alcohol: hypoglycaemic effect of antidiabetics enhanced by alcohol; increased risk of lactic acidosis when metformin given with alcohol
Anabolic Steroids: hypoglycaemic effect of antidiabetics possibly enhanced by anabolic steroids
- Analgesics: effects of sulfonylureas possibly enhanced by ●NSAIDs; lixisenatide possibly reduces the absorption of paracetamol when given 1 to 4 hours before paracetamol
Anti-arrhythmics: hypoglycaemic effect of gliclazide, insulin and metformin possibly enhanced by disopyramide
- Antibacterials: hypoglycaemic effect of acarbose possibly enhanced by neomycin, also severity of gastro-intestinal effects increased; effects of repaglinide enhanced by clarithromycin; effects of glibenclamide possibly enhanced by norfloxacin; plasma concentration of canagliflozin and nateglinide reduced by ●rifampicin; effects of linagliptin possibly reduced by rifampicin; hypoglycaemic effect of repaglinide possibly antagonised by rifampicin; effects of sulfonylureas enhanced by ●chloramphenicol; metabolism of tolbutamide accelerated by ●rifamycins (reduced effect); metabolism of sulfonylureas possibly accelerated by ●rifamycins (reduced effect); effects of sulfonylureas rarely enhanced by sulfonamides and trimethoprim; hypoglycaemic effect of sulfonylureas possibly enhanced by tetracyclines; hypoglycaemic effect of repaglinide possibly enhanced by trimethoprim—manufacturer advises avoid concomitant use
- Anticoagulants: exenatide possibly enhances anticoagulant effect of warfarin; hypoglycaemic effect of sulfonylureas possibly enhanced by ●coumarins, also possible changes to anticoagulant effect
Antidepressants: hypoglycaemic effect of antidiabetics possibly enhanced by MAOIs; hypoglycaemic effect of insulin, metformin and sulfonylureas enhanced by MAOIs
Antidiabetics: manufacturer of dapagliflozin advises avoid concomitant use with pioglitazone
Antiepileptics: tolbutamide transiently increases plasma concentration of phenytoin (possibility of toxicity); plasma concentration of glibenclamide possibly reduced by topiramate; plasma concentration of metformin possibly increased by topiramate

Antidiabetics *(continued)*

- Antifungals: plasma concentration of sulfonylureas increased by ●fluconazole and ●miconazole; hypoglycaemic effect of gliclazide and glipizide enhanced by ●miconazole—avoid concomitant use; hypoglycaemic effect of nateglinide possibly enhanced by fluconazole; hypoglycaemic effect of repaglinide possibly enhanced by itraconazole; hypoglycaemic effect of glipizide possibly enhanced by posaconazole; plasma concentration of sulfonylureas possibly increased by voriconazole

Antihistamines: thrombocyte count depressed when metformin given with ketotifen (manufacturer of ketotifen advises avoid concomitant use)

Antipsychotics: hypoglycaemic effect of sulfonylureas possibly antagonised by phenothiazines

Antivirals: plasma concentration of tolbutamide possibly increased by ritonavir; plasma concentration of metformin increased by telaprevir (consider reducing dose of metformin)

Aprepitant: plasma concentration of tolbutamide reduced by aprepitant

Beta-blockers: warning signs of hypoglycaemia (such as tremor) with antidiabetics may be masked when given with beta-blockers; hypoglycaemic effect of insulin enhanced by beta-blockers

- Bosentan: increased risk of hepatotoxicity when glibenclamide given with ●bosentan—avoid concomitant use

Calcium-channel Blockers: glucose tolerance occasionally impaired when insulin given with nifedipine

Cardiac Glycosides: canagliflozin and sitagliptin increase plasma concentration of digoxin; acarbose possibly reduces plasma concentration of digoxin

Ciclosporin: hypoglycaemic effect of repaglinide possibly enhanced by ciclosporin

Corticosteroids: hypoglycaemic effect of antidiabetics antagonised by corticosteroids

- Cytotoxics: avoidance of repaglinide advised by manufacturer of ●lapatinib; plasma concentration of metformin possibly increased by vandetanib (consider reducing dose of metformin)

Deferasirox: plasma concentration of repaglinide increased by deferasirox

Diazoxide: hypoglycaemic effect of antidiabetics antagonised by diazoxide

Diuretics: canagliflozin possibly enhances diuretic effect of diuretics; manufacturer of canagliflozin advises avoid concomitant use with loop diuretics; hypoglycaemic effect of antidiabetics antagonised by loop diuretics and thiazides and related diuretics; dapagliflozin possibly enhances diuretic effect of loop diuretics and thiazides and related diuretics

Hormone Antagonists: requirements for antidiabetics possibly reduced by lanreotide, octreotide and pasireotide

Leflunomide: hypoglycaemic effect of tolbutamide possibly enhanced by leflunomide

- Lipid-regulating Drugs: absorption of glibenclamide and glipizide reduced by colesevelam; absorption of glimepiride reduced by colesevelam—manufacturer of glimepiride advises give at least 4 hours before colesevelam; hypoglycaemic effect of acarbose possibly enhanced by colestyramine; hypoglycaemic effect of nateglinide possibly enhanced by gemfibrozil; increased risk of severe hypoglycaemia when repaglinide given with ●gemfibrozil—avoid concomitant use; plasma concentration of glibenclamide possibly increased by fluvastatin; manufacturer of canagliflozin advises give at least 1 hour before or 4–6 hours after bile acid sequestrants; may be improved glucose tolerance and an additive effect when insulin or sulfonylureas given with fibrates

Oestrogens: hypoglycaemic effect of antidiabetics antagonised by oestrogens

Antidiabetics *(continued)*

Orlistat: avoidance of acarbose advised by manufacturer of orlistat

Pancreatin: hypoglycaemic effect of acarbose antagonised by pancreatin

Progestogens: hypoglycaemic effect of antidiabetics antagonised by progestogens

- Sulfinpyrazone: effects of sulfonylureas enhanced by ●sulfinpyrazone

Teriflunomide: plasma concentration of repaglinide increased by teriflunomide

Testosterone: hypoglycaemic effect of antidiabetics possibly enhanced by testosterone

Ulcer-healing Drugs: excretion of metformin reduced by cimetidine (increased plasma concentration); hypoglycaemic effect of sulfonylureas enhanced by cimetidine

Antiepileptics *see* Carbamazepine, Eslicarbazepine, Ethosuximide, Gabapentin, Lacosamide, Lamotrigine, Levetiracetam, Oxcarbazepine, Perampanel, Phenobarbital, Phenytoin, Pregabalin, Retigabine, Rufinamide, Stiripentol, Tiagabine, Topiramate, Valproate, Vigabatrin, and Zonisamide

Antifungals *see* Amphotericin; Antifungals, Imidazole; Antifungals, Triazole; Caspofungin; Flucytosine; Griseofulvin; Micafungin; Terbinafine

Antifungals, Imidazole

- Anticoagulants: miconazole enhances anticoagulant effect of ●coumarins (miconazole oral gel and possibly vaginal and topical formulations absorbed)

- Antidepressants: avoidance of imidazoles advised by manufacturer of ●reboxetine

- Antidiabetics: miconazole enhances hypoglycaemic effect of ●gliclazide and glipizide—avoid concomitant use; miconazole increases plasma concentration of ●sulfonylureas

- Antiepileptics: miconazole possibly increases plasma concentration of carbamazepine; miconazole enhances anticonvulsant effect of ●phenytoin (plasma concentration of phenytoin increased)

Antifungals: imidazoles possibly antagonise effects of amphotericin

- Antihistamines: imidazoles possibly inhibit metabolism of ●mizolastine (avoid concomitant use)

- Antimalarials: avoidance of imidazoles advised by manufacturer of ●piperaquine with artenimol (possible risk of ventricular arrhythmias); avoidance of imidazoles advised by manufacturer of ●artemether with lumefantrine

- Antipsychotics: increased risk of ventricular arrhythmias when imidazoles given with ●pimozide—avoid concomitant use; imidazoles possibly increase plasma concentration of ●quetiapine—manufacturer of quetiapine advises avoid concomitant use

Antivirals: imidazoles possibly increase plasma concentration of saquinavir

- Ciclosporin: miconazole possibly inhibits metabolism of ●ciclosporin (increased plasma concentration)

- Ergot Alkaloids: increased risk of ergotism when imidazoles given with ●ergotamine—avoid concomitant use

- Lipid-regulating Drugs: possible increased risk of myopathy when imidazoles given with atorvastatin; possible increased risk of myopathy when miconazole given with ●simvastatin

Oestrogens: anecdotal reports of contraceptive failure when imidazoles given with oestrogens

- Sirolimus: miconazole increases plasma concentration of ●sirolimus

- Tacrolimus: miconazole *oral gel* possibly increases plasma concentration of ●tacrolimus

Vitamins: miconazole possibly reduces effects of vitamin D

Antifungals, Polyene *see* Amphotericin

Antifungals, Triazole

Note In general, fluconazole interactions relate to multiple-dose treatment

- Aliskiren: itraconazole increases plasma concentration of ●aliskiren—avoid concomitant use
- Analgesics: fluconazole increases plasma concentration of celecoxib (halve dose of celecoxib); voriconazole increases plasma concentration of diclofenac, ibuprofen and ●oxycodone; fluconazole increases plasma concentration of flurbiprofen, ibuprofen and methadone; fluconazole increases plasma concentration of parecoxib (reduce dose of parecoxib); voriconazole increases plasma concentration of ●alfentanil and ●methadone (consider reducing dose of alfentanil and methadone); fluconazole inhibits metabolism of alfentanil (risk of prolonged or delayed respiratory depression); itraconazole possibly inhibits metabolism of alfentanil; triazoles possibly increase plasma concentration of ●fentanyl; itraconazole possibly increases plasma concentration of ●methadone (increased risk of ventricular arrhythmias); itraconazole increases plasma concentration of oxycodone
- Antacids: absorption of itraconazole reduced by antacids
- Anti-arrhythmics: manufacturer of itraconazole advises avoid concomitant use with ●disopyramide; avoidance of itraconazole, posaconazole and voriconazole advised by manufacturer of ●dronedarone
- Antibacterials: plasma concentration of itraconazole increased by clarithromycin; manufacturer of fluconazole advises avoid concomitant use with erythromycin; triazoles possibly increase plasma concentration of ●rifabutin (increased risk of uveitis—reduce rifabutin dose); posaconazole increases plasma concentration of ●rifabutin (also plasma concentration of posaconazole reduced); voriconazole increases plasma concentration of ●rifabutin, also rifabutin reduces plasma concentration of voriconazole (increase dose of voriconazole and also monitor for rifabutin toxicity); fluconazole increases plasma concentration of ●rifabutin (increased risk of uveitis—reduce rifabutin dose); plasma concentration of itraconazole reduced by ●rifabutin and ●rifampicin—manufacturer of itraconazole advises avoid concomitant use; plasma concentration of posaconazole reduced by ●rifampicin; plasma concentration of voriconazole reduced by ●rifampicin—avoid concomitant use; metabolism of fluconazole accelerated by ●rifampicin (reduced plasma concentration); fluconazole possibly increases plasma concentration of bedaquiline—avoid concomitant use if fluconazole given for more than 14 days
- Anticoagulants: avoidance of itraconazole, posaconazole and voriconazole advised by manufacturer of apixaban; fluconazole, itraconazole and voriconazole enhance anticoagulant effect of ●coumarins; avoidance of itraconazole advised by manufacturer of dabigatran and rivaroxaban; avoidance of posaconazole and voriconazole advised by manufacturer of rivaroxaban
- Antidepressants: avoidance of triazoles advised by manufacturer of ●reboxetine; fluconazole possibly increases plasma concentration of amitriptyline and nortriptyline; plasma concentration of voriconazole reduced by ●St John's wort—avoid concomitant use
- Antidiabetics: posaconazole possibly enhances hypoglycaemic effect of glipizide; fluconazole possibly enhances hypoglycaemic effect of nateglinide; itraconazole possibly enhances hypoglycaemic effect of repaglinide; voriconazole possibly increases plasma concentration of sulfonylureas; fluconazole increases plasma concentration of ●sulfonylureas
- Antiepileptics: plasma concentration of itraconazole and posaconazole possibly reduced by

Antifungals, Triazole

- Antiepileptics (continued)
  ●carbamazepine; fluconazole possibly increases plasma concentration of carbamazepine; plasma concentration of voriconazole possibly reduced by ●carbamazepine and ●phenobarbital—avoid concomitant use; plasma concentration of itraconazole and posaconazole possibly reduced by ●phenobarbital; plasma concentration of itraconazole reduced by ●phenytoin—avoid concomitant use; fluconazole increases plasma concentration of ●phenytoin (consider reducing dose of phenytoin); voriconazole increases plasma concentration of ●phenytoin, also phenytoin reduces plasma concentration of voriconazole (increase dose of voriconazole and also monitor for phenytoin toxicity); plasma concentration of posaconazole reduced by ●phenytoin
- Antifungals: triazoles possibly antagonise effects of amphotericin; monitoring for increased voriconazole side effects advised by manufacturer of fluconazole if voriconazole given after fluconazole; plasma concentration of itraconazole increased by micafungin (consider reducing dose of itraconazole); plasma concentration of fluconazole increased by terbinafine
- Antihistamines: itraconazole inhibits metabolism of ●mizolastine—avoid concomitant use
- Antimalarials: avoidance of triazoles advised by manufacturer of ●piperaquine with artenimol (possible risk of ventricular arrhythmias); avoidance of triazoles advised by manufacturer of ●artemether with lumefantrine
- Antimuscarinics: avoidance of itraconazole advised by manufacturer of darifenacin and tolterodine; manufacturer of fesoterodine advises dose reduction when itraconazole given with fesoterodine—consult fesoterodine product literature; itraconazole possibly increases plasma concentration of ●solifenacin—see Dose under Solifenacin, p. 565
- Antipsychotics: itraconazole possibly increases plasma concentration of haloperidol; itraconazole possibly increases plasma concentration of ●aripiprazole (reduce dose of aripiprazole—consult aripiprazole product literature); itraconazole, posaconazole and voriconazole possibly increase plasma concentration of ●lurasidone—avoid concomitant use; fluconazole possibly increases the plasma concentration of ●lurasidone (see Dose under Lurasidone, p. 243); increased risk of ventricular arrhythmias when triazoles given with ●pimozide—avoid concomitant use; triazoles possibly increase plasma concentration of ●quetiapine—manufacturer of quetiapine advises avoid concomitant use; itraconazole possibly increases side-effects of risperidone
- Antivirals: plasma concentration of voriconazole increased or decreased by ●atazanavir and plasma concentration of atazanavir also reduced; posaconazole increases plasma concentration of ●atazanavir; itraconazole, posaconazole and voriconazole possibly increase the plasma concentration of ●daclatasvir—reduce dose of daclatasvir (see Dose under Daclatasvir, p. 438); plasma concentration of itraconazole and posaconazole reduced by ●efavirenz; plasma concentration of voriconazole reduced by ●efavirenz, also plasma concentration of efavirenz increased (increase voriconazole dose and reduce efavirenz dose); plasma concentration of both drugs may increase when itraconazole given with fosamprenavir; plasma concentration of posaconazole possibly reduced by fosamprenavir; itraconazole increases plasma concentration of ●indinavir (consider reducing dose of indinavir); fluconazole increases plasma concentration of ●nevirapine, ritonavir and tipranavir; plasma concentration of itraconazole possibly reduced by nevirapine—consider increasing dose of itraconazole; plasma concentra-

Antifungals, Triazole

- Antivirals *(continued)*

tion of voriconazole reduced by ●ritonavir—avoid concomitant use; combination of itraconazole with ●ritonavir may increase plasma concentration of either drug (or both); triazoles possibly increase plasma concentration of saquinavir; fluconazole, itraconazole, posaconazole and voriconazole possibly increase plasma concentration of ●simeprevir—manufacturer of simeprevir advises avoid concomitant use; plasma concentration of voriconazole possibly affected by ●telaprevir (possible increased risk of ventricular arrhythmias); plasma concentration of posaconazole possibly increased by ●telaprevir (increased risk of ventricular arrhythmias); plasma concentration of itraconazole possibly increased by telaprevir; fluconazole increases plasma concentration of ●zidovudine (increased risk of toxicity)

- Anxiolytics and Hypnotics: itraconazole increases plasma concentration of alprazolam; fluconazole and voriconazole increase plasma concentration of ●diazepam (risk of prolonged sedation); fluconazole, itraconazole, posaconazole and voriconazole increase plasma concentration of ●midazolam (risk of prolonged sedation); itraconazole increases plasma concentration of buspirone (reduce dose of buspirone)

- Avanafil: itraconazole and voriconazole possibly increase plasma concentration of ●avanafil—manufacturer of avanafil advises avoid concomitant use; fluconazole possibly increases plasma concentration of ●avanafil—see Dose under Avanafil, p. 571

- Bosentan: fluconazole possibly increases plasma concentration of ●bosentan—avoid concomitant use; itraconazole possibly increases plasma concentration of bosentan

- Calcium-channel Blockers: negative inotropic effect possibly increased when itraconazole given with calcium-channel blockers; itraconazole inhibits metabolism of ●felodipine (increased plasma concentration); avoidance of itraconazole advised by manufacturer of lercanidipine; itraconazole possibly inhibits metabolism of dihydropyridines (increased plasma concentration)

- Cardiac Glycosides: itraconazole increases plasma concentration of ●digoxin

- Ciclosporin: fluconazole, itraconazole, posaconazole and voriconazole inhibit metabolism of ●ciclosporin (increased plasma concentration)

- Cilostazol: itraconazole possibly increases plasma concentration of ●cilostazol (see Dose under Cilostazol, p. 141)

- Clopidogrel: fluconazole, itraconazole and voriconazole possibly reduce antiplatelet effect of ●clopidogrel

  Cobicistat: plasma concentration of itraconazole possibly increased by cobicistat—manufacturer of cobicistat advises reduce dose of itraconazole

- Colchicine: itraconazole possibly increases risk of ●colchicine toxicity—suspend or reduce dose of colchicine (avoid concomitant use in hepatic or renal impairment)

- Corticosteroids: itraconazole possibly inhibits metabolism of corticosteroids and methylprednisolone; itraconazole increases the plasma concentration of *inhaled* and *oral* (and possibly also *intranasal* and *rectal*) ●budesonide; itraconazole increases plasma concentration of *inhaled* fluticasone

- Cytotoxics: itraconazole inhibits metabolism of busulfan (increased risk of toxicity); fluconazole and itraconazole possibly increase side-effects of cyclophosphamide; itraconazole possibly increases the plasma concentration of afatinib—manufacturer of afatinib advises separating administration of itraconazole by 6 to 12 hours; itraconazole possibly increases plasma concentration of axitinib (reduce

Antifungals, Triazole

- Cytotoxics *(continued)*

dose of axitinib—consult axitinib product literature); fluconazole, itraconazole, posaconazole and voriconazole possibly increase the plasma concentration of ●bosutinib—manufacturer of bosutinib advises avoid or consider reducing dose of bosutinib; itraconazole possibly increases plasma concentration of cabozantinib; itraconazole and voriconazole possibly increase plasma concentration of ●crizotinib—manufacturer of crizotinib advises avoid concomitant use; itraconazole, posaconazole and voriconazole possibly increase plasma concentration of ●everolimus—manufacturer of everolimus advises avoid concomitant use; itraconazole increases plasma concentration of gefitinib; fluconazole, itraconazole and voriconazole possibly increase the plasma concentration of ●ibrutinib (see Dose under Ibrutinib, p. 615); avoidance of itraconazole, posaconazole and voriconazole advised by manufacturer of ●lapatinib; avoidance of itraconazole and voriconazole advised by manufacturer of ●nilotinib; itraconazole and voriconazole possibly increase plasma concentration of ●pazopanib (reduce dose of pazopanib); itraconazole and voriconazole possibly increase plasma concentration of ●ponatinib—consider reducing initial dose of ponatinib (see Dose under Ponatinib, p. 618); manufacturer of ruxolitinib advises dose reduction when fluconazole, itraconazole, posaconazole and voriconazole given with ●ruxolitinib—consult ruxolitinib product literature; avoidance of itraconazole advised by manufacturer of ●temsirolimus (plasma concentration of temsirolimus possibly increased); itraconazole and voriconazole possibly increase the plasma concentration of ●cabazitaxel—manufacturer of cabazitaxel advises avoid or consider reducing dose of cabazitaxel; itraconazole and voriconazole possibly increase plasma concentration of ●docetaxel—manufacturer of docetaxel advises avoid concomitant use or consider reducing docetaxel dose; increased risk of toxicity when itraconazole given with ●irinotecan—avoid concomitant use; posaconazole possibly inhibits metabolism of ●vinblastine and ●vincristine (increased risk of neurotoxicity); itraconazole possibly increases risk of ●vinblastine, ●vindesine, ●vinflunine and ●vinorelbine toxicity; itraconazole increases risk of ●vincristine toxicity

- Dapoxetine: manufacturer of dapoxetine advises dose reduction when fluconazole given with dapoxetine (see Dose under Dapoxetine, p. 572); avoidance of itraconazole advised by manufacturer of ●dapoxetine (increased risk of toxicity)

- Diuretics: fluconazole increases plasma concentration of eplerenone (reduce dose of eplerenone); itraconazole increases plasma concentration of ●eplerenone—avoid concomitant use; plasma concentration of fluconazole increased by hydrochlorothiazide

- Domperidone: possible increased risk of ventricular arrhythmias when itraconazole or voriconazole given with ●domperidone—avoid concomitant use

- Ergot Alkaloids: increased risk of ergotism when voriconazole given with ●ergometrine—avoid concomitant use; manufacturer of itraconazole advises avoid concomitant use with ●ergometrine (increased risk of ergotism); increased risk of ergotism when triazoles given with ●ergotamine—avoid concomitant use

- 5HT$_1$-receptor Agonists: itraconazole increases plasma concentration of ●eletriptan (risk of toxicity)—avoid concomitant use

- Ivabradine: fluconazole increases plasma concentration of ivabradine—reduce initial dose of ivabra-

Antifungals, Triazole

- Ivabradine (continued)
  dine; itraconazole possibly increases plasma concentration of ●ivabradine—avoid concomitant use
- Ivacaftor: itraconazole, posaconazole and voriconazole possibly increase plasma concentration of ●ivacaftor (see Dose under Ivacaftor, p. 220); fluconazole increases plasma concentration of ●ivacaftor (see Dose under Ivacaftor, p. 220)
- Lenalidomide: itraconazole possibly increases plasma concentration of ●lenalidomide (increased risk of toxicity)
  Leukotriene Receptor Antagonists: fluconazole increases plasma concentration of zafirlukast
- Lipid-regulating Drugs: increased risk of myopathy when itraconazole, posaconazole or voriconazole given with ●atorvastatin; possible increased risk of myopathy when fluconazole given with ●atorvastatin or ●simvastatin; fluconazole increases plasma concentration of fluvastatin—possible increased risk of myopathy; itraconazole increases plasma concentration of ●rosuvastatin—adjust dose of rosuvastatin (consult product literature); increased risk of myopathy when itraconazole or posaconazole given with ●simvastatin (avoid concomitant use); increased risk of myopathy when voriconazole given with ●simvastatin; avoidance of triazoles advised by manufacturer of ●lomitapide (plasma concentration of lomitapide possibly increased)
  Mirabegron: when given with itraconazole avoid or reduce dose of mirabegron in hepatic or renal impairment—see Mirabegron, p. 564
  Oestrogens: plasma concentration of voriconazole increased by oestrogens
  Progestogens: plasma concentration of voriconazole possibly increased by progestogens
- Ranolazine: itraconazole, posaconazole and voriconazole possibly increase plasma concentration of ●ranolazine—manufacturer of ranolazine advises avoid concomitant use
- Retinoids: fluconazole and voriconazole possibly increase risk of ●tretinoin toxicity
  Riociguat: avoidance of itraconazole and voriconazole advised by manufacturer of riociguat
  Sildenafil: itraconazole increases plasma concentration of sildenafil—reduce initial dose of sildenafil
- Sirolimus: fluconazole and posaconazole possibly increase plasma concentration of sirolimus; itraconazole and voriconazole increase plasma concentration of ●sirolimus—avoid concomitant use
- Tacrolimus: fluconazole, itraconazole, posaconazole and voriconazole increase plasma concentration of ●tacrolimus (consider reducing dose of tacrolimus)
  Tadalafil: itraconazole possibly increases plasma concentration of tadalafil
- Theophylline: fluconazole possibly increases plasma concentration of ●theophylline
- Ulcer-healing Drugs: plasma concentration of posaconazole reduced by ●cimetidine and ●esomeprazole—manufacturer of posaconazole suspension advises avoid concomitant use; plasma concentration of posaconazole possibly reduced by ●famotidine, ●lansoprazole, ●nizatidine, ●omeprazole, ●pantoprazole, ●rabeprazole and ●ranitidine—manufacturer of posaconazole suspension advises avoid concomitant use; voriconazole possibly increases plasma concentration of esomeprazole; voriconazole increases plasma concentration of omeprazole (consider reducing dose of omeprazole); absorption of itraconazole reduced by histamine H$_2$-antagonists and proton pump inhibitors
  Ulipristal: avoidance of itraconazole advised by manufacturer of ulipristal

Antifungals, Triazole (continued)

- Vardenafil: itraconazole possibly increases plasma concentration of ●vardenafil—avoid concomitant use

Antihistamines

Note Sedative interactions apply to a lesser extent to the non-sedating antihistamines. Interactions do not generally apply to antihistamines used for topical action (including inhalation)

Alcohol: increased sedative effect when antihistamines given with alcohol (possibly less effect with non-sedating antihistamines)

- Analgesics: sedative effects possibly increased when sedating antihistamines given with ●opioid analgesics
  Antacids: absorption of fexofenadine reduced by antacids
- Anti-arrhythmics: increased risk of ventricular arrhythmias when mizolastine given with ●amiodarone, ●disopyramide or ●flecainide—avoid concomitant use; manufacturer of mizolastine advises avoid concomitant use with propafenone (possible risk of ventricular arrhythmias)
- Antibacterials: plasma concentration of rupatadine increased by erythromycin; manufacturer of loratadine advises plasma concentration possibly increased by erythromycin; metabolism of mizolastine inhibited by ●erythromycin—avoid concomitant use; increased risk of ventricular arrhythmias when mizolastine given with ●moxifloxacin—avoid concomitant use; effects of fexofenadine possibly reduced by rifampicin; metabolism of mizolastine possibly inhibited by ●macrolides (avoid concomitant use)
- Antidepressants: avoidance of mizolastine advised by manufacturer of ●citalopram and ●escitalopram (risk of ventricular arrhythmias); manufacturer of promethazine advises avoid for 2 weeks after stopping MAOIs; manufacturer of hydroxyzine advises avoid concomitant use with MAOIs; increased antimuscarinic and sedative effects when antihistamines given with MAOIs or tricyclics; cyproheptadine possibly antagonises antidepressant effect of SSRIs; possible increased antimuscarinic and sedative effects when antihistamines given with tricyclic-related antidepressants
  Antidiabetics: thrombocyte count depressed when ketotifen given with metformin (manufacturer of ketotifen advises avoid concomitant use)
- Antifungals: metabolism of mizolastine inhibited by ●itraconazole—avoid concomitant use; metabolism of mizolastine possibly inhibited by ●imidazoles (avoid concomitant use)
- Antimalarials: avoidance of mizolastine advised by manufacturer of ●piperaquine with artenimol (possible risk of ventricular arrhythmias)
  Antimuscarinics: increased risk of antimuscarinic side-effects when antihistamines given with antimuscarinics
- Antivirals: plasma concentration of chlorphenamine possibly increased by lopinavir; plasma concentration of non-sedating antihistamines possibly increased by ritonavir; increased risk of ventricular arrhythmias when mizolastine given with ●saquinavir—avoid concomitant use
  Anxiolytics and Hypnotics: increased sedative effect when antihistamines given with anxiolytics and hypnotics
- Beta-blockers: increased risk of ventricular arrhythmias when mizolastine given with ●sotalol—avoid concomitant use
  Betahistine: antihistamines theoretically antagonise effect of betahistine
- Cytotoxics: possible increased risk of ventricular arrhythmias when mizolastine given with ●vandetanib—avoid concomitant use

Antihistamines *(continued)*

- Grapefruit Juice: plasma concentration of bilastine reduced by grapefruit juice; plasma concentration of rupatadine increased by ●grapefruit juice—avoid concomitant use

  Histamine: antihistamines theoretically antagonise effects of histamine—manufacturer of histamine advises avoid concomitant use

  Ulcer-healing Drugs: manufacturer of loratadine advises plasma concentration possibly increased by cimetidine; plasma concentration of hydroxyzine increased by cimetidine

  Ulipristal: manufacturer of ulipristal advises give fexofenadine at least 1.5 hours before or after ulipristal

Antihistamines, Non-sedating *see* Antihistamines

Antihistamines, Sedating *see* Antihistamines

Antimalarials *see* Artemether with Lumefantrine, Chloroquine and Hydroxychloroquine, Mefloquine, Piperaquine with Artenimol, Primaquine, Proguanil, Pyrimethamine, and Quinine

Antimetabolites *see* Cladribine, Cytarabine, Decitabine, Fludarabine, Fluorouracil, Gemcitabine, Mercaptopurine, Methotrexate, Pemetrexed, Raltitrexed, and Tioguanine

Antimuscarinics

Note Many drugs have antimuscarinic effects; concomitant use of two or more such drugs can increase side-effects such as dry mouth, urine retention, and constipation; concomitant use can also lead to confusion in the elderly. Interactions do not generally apply to antimuscarinics used by inhalation

Alcohol: increased sedative effect when hyoscine given with alcohol

Analgesics: possible increased risk of antimuscarinic side-effects when antimuscarinics given with codeine; increased risk of antimuscarinic side-effects when antimuscarinics given with nefopam

- Anti-arrhythmics: increased risk of ventricular arrhythmias when tolterodine given with ●amiodarone, ●disopyramide or ●flecainide; increased risk of antimuscarinic side-effects when antimuscarinics given with disopyramide

  Antibacterials: manufacturer of fesoterodine advises dose reduction when fesoterodine given with clarithromycin and telithromycin—consult fesoterodine product literature; manufacturer of tolterodine advises avoid concomitant use with clarithromycin and erythromycin; plasma concentration of darifenacin possibly increased by erythromycin; plasma concentration of active metabolite of fesoterodine reduced by rifampicin

  Antidepressants: plasma concentration of darifenacin and procyclidine increased by paroxetine; increased risk of antimuscarinic side-effects when antimuscarinics given with MAOIs or tricyclics; possible increased antimuscarinic side-effects when antimuscarinics given with tricyclic-related antidepressants

- Antifungals: manufacturer of fesoterodine advises dose reduction when fesoterodine given with itraconazole—consult fesoterodine product literature; manufacturer of darifenacin and tolterodine advises avoid concomitant use with itraconazole; plasma concentration of solifenacin possibly increased by ●itraconazole—see Dose under Solifenacin, p. 565

  Antihistamines: increased risk of antimuscarinic side-effects when antimuscarinics given with antihistamines

  Antipsychotics: antimuscarinics possibly reduce effects of haloperidol; increased risk of antimuscarinic side-effects when antimuscarinics given with clozapine; antimuscarinics reduce plasma concentration of phenothiazines, but risk of antimuscarinic side-effects increased

- Antivirals: manufacturer of fesoterodine advises dose reduction when fesoterodine given with atazanavir, indinavir, ritonavir and saquinavir—consult fesoter-

Antimuscarinics

- Antivirals *(continued)*

  odine product literature; manufacturer of darifenacin advises avoid concomitant use with atazanavir, fosamprenavir, indinavir, lopinavir, ritonavir, saquinavir and tipranavir; manufacturer of tolterodine advises avoid concomitant use with fosamprenavir, indinavir, lopinavir, ritonavir and saquinavir; plasma concentration of solifenacin possibly increased by ●ritonavir—see Dose under Solifenacin, p. 565

- Beta-blockers: increased risk of ventricular arrhythmias when tolterodine given with ●sotalol

  Calcium-channel Blockers: plasma concentration of solifenacin increased by verapamil; manufacturer of darifenacin advises avoid concomitant use with verapamil

  Cardiac Glycosides: darifenacin possibly increases plasma concentration of digoxin

  Ciclosporin: manufacturer of darifenacin advises avoid concomitant use with ciclosporin

  Domperidone: antimuscarinics antagonise effects of domperidone on gastro-intestinal activity

  Dopaminergics: antimuscarinics possibly reduce absorption of levodopa

  Hormone Antagonists: possible increased risk of bradycardia when ipratropium or oxybutynin given with pasireotide

  Memantine: effects of antimuscarinics possibly enhanced by memantine

  Metoclopramide: antimuscarinics antagonise effects of metoclopramide on gastro-intestinal activity

  Nitrates: antimuscarinics possibly reduce effects of sublingual tablets of nitrates (failure to dissolve under tongue owing to dry mouth)

  Parasympathomimetics: antimuscarinics antagonise effects of parasympathomimetics

Antipsychotics

Note Increased risk of toxicity with myelosuppressive drugs

Note Avoid concomitant use of clozapine with drugs that have a substantial potential for causing agranulocytosis

ACE Inhibitors: enhanced hypotensive effect when antipsychotics given with ACE inhibitors

Adrenergic Neurone Blockers: enhanced hypotensive effect when phenothiazines given with adrenergic neurone blockers; higher doses of chlorpromazine antagonise hypotensive effect of adrenergic neurone blockers; haloperidol antagonises hypotensive effect of adrenergic neurone blockers

Adsorbents: absorption of phenothiazines possibly reduced by kaolin

Alcohol: increased sedative effect when antipsychotics given with alcohol

Alpha-blockers: enhanced hypotensive effect when antipsychotics given with alpha-blockers

- Anaesthetics, General: droperidol enhances effects of thiopental; enhanced hypotensive effect when antipsychotics given with ●general anaesthetics

- Analgesics: possible severe drowsiness when haloperidol given with acemetacin or indometacin; increased risk of ventricular arrhythmias when antipsychotics that prolong the QT interval given with ●methadone; increased risk of ventricular arrhythmias when amisulpride given with ●methadone—avoid concomitant use; increased risk of convulsions when antipsychotics given with tramadol; enhanced hypotensive and sedative effects when antipsychotics given with opioid analgesics

  Angiotensin-II Receptor Antagonists: enhanced hypotensive effect when antipsychotics given with angiotensin-II receptor antagonists

  Antacids: absorption of phenothiazines and sulpiride reduced by antacids

- Anti-arrhythmics: increased risk of ventricular arrhythmias when antipsychotics that prolong the QT interval given with ●anti-arrhythmics that prolong the QT interval; increased risk of ventricular arrhyth-

Antipsychotics

- **Anti-arrhythmics** *(continued)*
mias when amisulpride, droperidol, haloperidol, phenothiazines, pimozide or zuclopenthixol given with ●amiodarone—avoid concomitant use; increased risk of ventricular arrhythmias when benperidol given with ●amiodarone—manufacturer of benperidol advises avoid concomitant use; increased risk of ventricular arrhythmias when sulpiride given with ●amiodarone or ●disopyramide; increased risk of ventricular arrhythmias when amisulpride, droperidol, pimozide or zuclopenthixol given with ●disopyramide—avoid concomitant use; possible increased risk of ventricular arrhythmias when haloperidol given with ●disopyramide—avoid concomitant use; increased risk of ventricular arrhythmias when phenothiazines given with ●disopyramide—avoidance of phenothiazines advised by manufacturer of ●dronedarone (risk of ventricular arrhythmias); increased risk of arrhythmias when clozapine given with ●flecainide

- **Antibacterials:** plasma concentration of lurasidone possibly increased by ●clarithromycin and ●telithromycin—avoid concomitant use; increased risk of ventricular arrhythmias when pimozide given with ●clarithromycin, ●moxifloxacin or ●telithromycin—avoid concomitant use; plasma concentration of quetiapine possibly increased by ●clarithromycin—manufacturer of quetiapine advises avoid concomitant use; plasma concentration of lurasidone possibly increased by ●erythromycin (see Dose under Lurasidone, p. 243); increased risk of ventricular arrhythmias when amisulpride given with ●erythromycin—avoid concomitant use; plasma concentration of clozapine possibly increased by ●erythromycin (possible increased risk of convulsions); possible increased risk of ventricular arrhythmias when pimozide given with ●erythromycin—avoid concomitant use; plasma concentration of quetiapine increased by ●erythromycin—manufacturer of quetiapine advises avoid concomitant use; increased risk of ventricular arrhythmias when sulpiride given with *parenteral* ●erythromycin; increased risk of ventricular arrhythmias when zuclopenthixol given with *parenteral* ●erythromycin—avoid concomitant use; plasma concentration of clozapine increased by ciprofloxacin; plasma concentration of olanzapine possibly increased by ciprofloxacin; increased risk of ventricular arrhythmias when droperidol, haloperidol, phenothiazines or zuclopenthixol given with ●moxifloxacin—avoid concomitant use; increased risk of ventricular arrhythmias when benperidol given with ●moxifloxacin—manufacturer of benperidol advises avoid concomitant use; plasma concentration of aripiprazole possibly reduced by ●rifabutin and ●rifampicin (avoid concomitant use or consider increasing the dose of aripiprazole—consult aripiprazole product literature); plasma concentration of lurasidone reduced by ●rifampicin—avoid concomitant use; plasma concentration of clozapine possibly reduced by rifampicin; metabolism of haloperidol accelerated by ●rifampicin (reduced plasma concentration); avoid concomitant use of clozapine with ●chloramphenicol or ●sulfonamides (increased risk of agranulocytosis); increased risk of ventricular arrhythmias when droperidol, haloperidol or pimozide given with ●delamanid; increased risk of ventricular arrhythmias when phenothiazines that prolong the QT interval given with ●delamanid; manufacturer of droperidol advises avoid concomitant use with ●macrolides (risk of ventricular arrhythmias); possible increased risk of ventricular arrhythmias when chlorpromazine given with ●telithromycin; plasma concentration of quetiapine possibly increased by telithromycin

Antipsychotics *(continued)*

- **Antidepressants:** plasma concentration of clozapine possibly increased by citalopram (increased risk of toxicity); avoidance of haloperidol, phenothiazines and pimozide advised by manufacturer of ●citalopram (risk of ventricular arrhythmias); avoidance of haloperidol, phenothiazines and pimozide advised by manufacturer of ●escitalopram (risk of ventricular arrhythmias); plasma concentration of aripiprazole possibly increased by ●fluoxetine and ●paroxetine (reduce dose of aripiprazole—consult aripiprazole product literature); plasma concentration of clozapine, haloperidol and risperidone increased by ●fluoxetine; manufacturer of droperidol advises avoid concomitant use with ●fluoxetine, ●fluvoxamine, ●sertraline and ●tricyclics (risk of ventricular arrhythmias); plasma concentration of asenapine and haloperidol possibly increased by fluvoxamine; plasma concentration of clozapine and olanzapine increased by ●fluvoxamine; asenapine possibly increases plasma concentration of paroxetine; plasma concentration of clozapine increased by ●paroxetine and ●sertraline; plasma concentration of risperidone possibly increased by paroxetine (increased risk of toxicity); metabolism of perphenazine inhibited by paroxetine (reduce dose of perphenazine); plasma concentration of haloperidol increased by venlafaxine; clozapine possibly increases CNS effects of ●MAOIs; plasma concentration of pimozide possibly increased by ●SSRIs (increased risk of ventricular arrhythmias—avoid concomitant use); plasma concentration of lurasidone possibly reduced by ●St John's wort—avoid concomitant use; plasma concentration of aripiprazole possibly reduced by ●St John's wort (avoid concomitant use or consider increasing the dose of aripiprazole—consult aripiprazole product literature); increased risk of antimuscarinic side-effects when phenothiazines given with tricyclics; manufacturer of fluphenazine, haloperidol, sulpiride and zuclopenthixol advises avoid concomitant use with ●tricyclics (risk of ventricular arrhythmias); possible increased risk of ventricular arrhythmias when risperidone given with ●tricyclics; possible increased antimuscarinic side-effects when clozapine given with tricyclics

Antidiabetics: phenothiazines possibly antagonise hypoglycaemic effect of sulfonylureas

- **Antiepileptics:** antipsychotics antagonise anticonvulsant effect of ●antiepileptics (convulsive threshold lowered); plasma concentration of lurasidone possibly reduced by ●carbamazepine, ●phenobarbital and ●phenytoin—avoid concomitant use; metabolism of haloperidol, olanzapine, quetiapine and risperidone accelerated by carbamazepine (reduced plasma concentration); metabolism of clozapine accelerated by ●carbamazepine (reduced plasma concentration), also avoid concomitant use of drugs with substantial potential for causing agranulocytosis; plasma concentration of aripiprazole reduced by ●carbamazepine (avoid concomitant use or consider increasing the dose of aripiprazole —consult aripiprazole product literature); plasma concentration of paliperidone reduced by carbamazepine; plasma concentration of aripiprazole possibly reduced by ●phenobarbital and ●phenytoin (avoid concomitant use or consider increasing the dose of aripiprazole—consult aripiprazole product literature); metabolism of haloperidol accelerated by phenobarbital (reduced plasma concentration); plasma concentration of both drugs reduced when chlorpromazine given with phenobarbital; plasma concentration of clozapine possibly reduced by phenobarbital; plasma concentration of haloperidol reduced by phenytoin; chlorpromazine possibly increases or decreases

Antipsychotics

- **Antiepileptics** *(continued)*
  plasma concentration of phenytoin; metabolism of clozapine and quetiapine accelerated by phenytoin (reduced plasma concentration); increased risk of side-effects including neutropenia when olanzapine given with ●valproate; plasma concentration of clozapine possibly increased or decreased by valproate

- **Antifungals**: plasma concentration of lurasidone possibly increased by ●fluconazole (see Dose under Lurasidone, p. 243); plasma concentration of lurasidone possibly increased by ●itraconazole, ●posaconazole and ●voriconazole—avoid concomitant use; plasma concentration of aripiprazole possibly increased by ●itraconazole (reduce dose of aripiprazole—consult aripiprazole product literature); side-effects of risperidone possibly increased by itraconazole; plasma concentration of haloperidol possibly increased by itraconazole; plasma concentration of quetiapine possibly increased by ●imidazoles and ●triazoles—manufacturer of quetiapine advises avoid concomitant use; increased risk of ventricular arrhythmias when pimozide given with ●imidazoles or ●triazoles—avoid concomitant use

- **Antimalarials**: avoidance of droperidol, haloperidol, phenothiazines and pimozide advised by manufacturer of ●piperaquine with artenimol (possible risk of ventricular arrhythmias); avoidance of antipsychotics advised by manufacturer of ●artemether with lumefantrine; increased risk of ventricular arrhythmias when droperidol given with ●chloroquine and hydroxychloroquine or ●quinine—avoid concomitant use; manufacturer of risperidone advises possible risk of ventricular arrhythmias when risperidone given with ●mefloquine; increased risk of ventricular arrhythmias when pimozide given with ●mefloquine or ●quinine—avoid concomitant use; manufacturer of amisulpride advises avoid concomitant use with mefloquine; possible increased risk of ventricular arrhythmias when haloperidol given with ●mefloquine or ●quinine—avoid concomitant use; possible increased risk of ventricular arrhythmias when risperidone given with ●quinine

  Antimuscarinics: increased risk of antimuscarinic side-effects when clozapine given with antimuscarinics; plasma concentration of phenothiazines reduced by antimuscarinics, but risk of antimuscarinic side-effects increased; effects of haloperidol possibly reduced by antimuscarinics

- **Antipsychotics**: increased risk of ventricular arrhythmias when amisulpride, pimozide or sulpiride given with ●droperidol—avoid concomitant use; increased risk of ventricular arrhythmias when phenothiazines that prolong the QT interval given with ●droperidol—avoid concomitant use; avoid concomitant use of clozapine with depot formulation of ●flupentixol, ●fluphenazine, ●haloperidol, ●pipotiazine, ●risperidone or ●zuclopenthixol as cannot be withdrawn quickly if neutropenia occurs; increased risk of ventricular arrhythmias when sulpiride given with ●haloperidol; chlorpromazine possibly increases plasma concentration of haloperidol; increased risk of ventricular arrhythmias when droperidol given with ●haloperidol—avoid concomitant use; increased risk of ventricular arrhythmias when pimozide given with ●phenothiazines—avoid concomitant use; lurasidone possibly increases plasma concentration of pimozide (increased risk of toxicity); possible increased risk of ventricular arrhythmias when antipsychotics that prolong the QT interval given with ●risperidone; increased risk of ventricular arrhythmias when pimozide given with ●sulpiride

- **Antivirals**: plasma concentration of pimozide possibly increased by ●atazanavir—avoid concomitant use;

Antipsychotics

- **Antivirals** *(continued)*
  plasma concentration of aripiprazole possibly increased by ●atazanavir, ●darunavir, ●fosamprenavir, ●indinavir, ●lopinavir, ●ritonavir, ●saquinavir and ●tipranavir (reduce dose of aripiprazole—consult aripiprazole product literature); plasma concentration of quetiapine possibly increased by ●atazanavir, ●boceprevir, ●darunavir, ●fosamprenavir, ●indinavir, ●lopinavir, ●ritonavir, ●saquinavir, ●telaprevir and ●tipranavir—manufacturer of quetiapine advises avoid concomitant use; avoidance of pimozide advised by manufacturer of ●boceprevir and ●telaprevir; plasma concentration of lurasidone possibly increased by ●boceprevir, ●indinavir, ●ritonavir, ●saquinavir and ●telaprevir—avoid concomitant use; plasma concentration of aripiprazole possibly reduced by ●efavirenz and ●nevirapine (avoid concomitant use or consider increasing the dose of aripiprazole—consult aripiprazole product literature); plasma concentration of pimozide possibly increased by ●efavirenz, ●indinavir and ●saquinavir (increased risk of ventricular arrhythmias—avoid concomitant use); plasma concentration of pimozide increased by ●fosamprenavir and ●ritonavir (increased risk of ventricular arrhythmias—avoid concomitant use); plasma concentration of olanzapine reduced by ritonavir—consider increasing dose of olanzapine; avoidance of clozapine advised by manufacturer of ●ritonavir (increased risk of toxicity); plasma concentration of antipsychotics possibly increased by ●ritonavir; increased risk of ventricular arrhythmias when clozapine, haloperidol or phenothiazines given with ●saquinavir—avoid concomitant use

- **Anxiolytics and Hypnotics**: increased sedative effect when antipsychotics given with anxiolytics and hypnotics; plasma concentration of haloperidol possibly increased by alprazolam; lurasidone increases plasma concentration of midazolam; serious adverse events reported with concomitant use of clozapine and ●benzodiazepines (causality not established); increased risk of hypotension, bradycardia and respiratory depression when *intramuscular* olanzapine given with *parenteral* ●benzodiazepines; plasma concentration of haloperidol increased by buspirone

- **Aprepitant**: avoidance of pimozide advised by manufacturer of ●aprepitant

- **Atomoxetine**: increased risk of ventricular arrhythmias when antipsychotics that prolong the QT interval given with ●atomoxetine

- **Beta-blockers**: enhanced hypotensive effect when phenothiazines given with beta-blockers; plasma concentration of both drugs may increase when chlorpromazine given with ●propranolol; increased risk of ventricular arrhythmias when amisulpride, phenothiazines, pimozide or sulpiride given with ●sotalol; possible increased risk of ventricular arrhythmias when risperidone given with ●sotalol; increased risk of ventricular arrhythmias when droperidol or zuclopenthixol given with ●sotalol—avoid concomitant use; possible increased risk of ventricular arrhythmias when haloperidol given with ●sotalol—avoid concomitant use

- **Calcium-channel Blockers**: enhanced hypotensive effect when antipsychotics given with calcium-channel blockers; plasma concentration of lurasidone increased by ●diltiazem (see Dose under Lurasidone, p. 243); plasma concentration of lurasidone possibly increased by ●verapamil (see Dose under Lurasidone, p. 243)

  Clonidine: enhanced hypotensive effect when phenothiazines given with clonidine

- **Cobicistat**: plasma concentration of lurasidone possibly increased by ●cobicistat—avoid concomitant

Antipsychotics

- Cobicistat *(continued)*
  use; plasma concentration of pimozide possibly
  increased by ●cobicistat—manufacturer of cobicistat advises avoid concomitant use
- Cytotoxics: avoid concomitant use of clozapine with
  ●cytotoxics (increased risk of agranulocytosis); possible increased risk of ventricular arrhythmias when
  haloperidol given with ●bosutinib; caution with
  pimozide advised by manufacturer of ●crizotinib;
  avoidance of pimozide and quetiapine advised by
  manufacturer of idelalisib; avoidance of pimozide
  advised by manufacturer of ●lapatinib; possible
  increased risk of ventricular arrhythmias when amisulpride, chlorpromazine, haloperidol, pimozide, sulpiride or zuclopenthixol given with ●vandetanib—
  avoid concomitant use; increased risk of ventricular
  arrhythmias when antipsychotics that prolong the
  QT interval given with ●arsenic trioxide; increased
  risk of ventricular arrhythmias when haloperidol
  given with ●arsenic trioxide
  Deferasirox: avoidance of clozapine advised by manufacturer of deferasirox
  Desferrioxamine: manufacturer of levomepromazine
  advises avoid concomitant use with desferrioxamine; avoidance of prochlorperazine advised by
  manufacturer of desferrioxamine
  Diazoxide: enhanced hypotensive effect when phenothiazines given with diazoxide
- Diuretics: risk of ventricular arrhythmias with amisulpride increased by hypokalaemia caused by ●diur-
  etics; risk of ventricular arrhythmias with pimozide
  increased by hypokalaemia caused by ●diuretics
  (avoid concomitant use); enhanced hypotensive
  effect when phenothiazines given with diuretics
  Dopaminergics: increased risk of extrapyramidal side-
  effects when antipsychotics given with amantadine;
  antipsychotics antagonise effects of apomorphine,
  levodopa and pergolide; antipsychotics antagonise
  hypoprolactinaemic and antiparkinsonian effects of
  bromocriptine and cabergoline; manufacturer of
  amisulpride advises avoid concomitant use of levodopa (antagonism of effect); avoidance of antipsychotics advised by manufacturer of pramipexole,
  ropinirole and rotigotine (antagonism of effect)
  Ergot Alkaloids: lurasidone possibly increases plasma
  concentration of ergot alkaloids (increased risk of
  toxicity)
- Grapefruit Juice: manufacturer of lurasidone advises
  avoid concomitant use with grapefruit juice; plasma
  concentration of quetiapine possibly increased by
  ●grapefruit juice—manufacturer of quetiapine
  advises avoid concomitant use
  Histamine: antipsychotics theoretically antagonise
  effects of histamine—manufacturer of histamine
  advises avoid concomitant use
- Hormone Antagonists: manufacturer of droperidol
  advises avoid concomitant use with ●tamoxifen
  (risk of ventricular arrhythmias)
- Ivabradine: increased risk of ventricular arrhythmias
  when pimozide given with ●ivabradine
- Lithium: increased risk of extrapyramidal side-effects
  and possibly neurotoxicity when clozapine, flupentixol, haloperidol, phenothiazines, risperidone or
  zuclopenthixol given with ●lithium; possible risk of
  toxicity when olanzapine given with lithium; extrapyramidal side-effects of quetiapine possibly
  increased by lithium; increased risk of extrapyramidal side-effects when sulpiride given with lithium
  Memantine: effects of antipsychotics possibly reduced
  by memantine
  Methyldopa: enhanced hypotensive effect when antipsychotics given with methyldopa (also increased
  risk of extrapyramidal effects)

Antipsychotics *(continued)*

  Metoclopramide: increased risk of extrapyramidal
  side-effects when antipsychotics given with metoclopramide
  Moxonidine: enhanced hypotensive effect when
  phenothiazines given with moxonidine
  Muscle Relaxants: promazine possibly enhances
  effects of suxamethonium
  Nitrates: enhanced hypotensive effect when phenothiazines given with nitrates
- Penicillamine: avoid concomitant use of clozapine
  with ●penicillamine (increased risk of agranulocytosis)
- Pentamidine Isetionate: increased risk of ventricular
  arrhythmias when amisulpride or droperidol given
  with ●pentamidine isetionate—avoid concomitant
  use; increased risk of ventricular arrhythmias when
  phenothiazines given with ●pentamidine isetionate
  Sodium Benzoate: haloperidol possibly reduces effects
  of sodium benzoate
  Sodium Oxybate: antipsychotics possibly enhance
  effects of sodium oxybate
  Sodium Phenylbutyrate: haloperidol possibly reduces
  effects of sodium phenylbutyrate
  Sympathomimetics: antipsychotics antagonise hypertensive effect of sympathomimetics; antipsychotic
  effects of chlorpromazine possibly antagonised by
  dexamfetamine; chlorpromazine possibly reduces
  effects of lisdexamfetamine; side-effects of risperidone possibly increased by methylphenidate
- Tacrolimus: manufacturer of droperidol advises avoid
  concomitant use with ●tacrolimus (risk of ventricular arrhythmias)
  Tetrabenazine: increased risk of extrapyramidal side-
  effects when antipsychotics given with tetrabenazine
  Ulcer-healing Drugs: effects of antipsychotics, chlorpromazine and clozapine possibly enhanced by
  cimetidine; plasma concentration of clozapine possibly reduced by omeprazole; absorption of sulpiride reduced by sucralfate
  Vasodilator Antihypertensives: enhanced hypotensive
  effect when phenothiazines given with hydralazine,
  minoxidil or sodium nitroprusside

Antivirals *see individual drugs*

Anxiolytics and Hypnotics

  ACE Inhibitors: enhanced hypotensive effect when
  anxiolytics and hypnotics given with ACE inhibitors
  Adrenergic Neurone Blockers: enhanced hypotensive
  effect when anxiolytics and hypnotics given with
  adrenergic neurone blockers
  Alcohol: increased sedative effect when anxiolytics
  and hypnotics given with alcohol
  Alpha-blockers: enhanced hypotensive and sedative
  effects when anxiolytics and hypnotics given with
  alpha-blockers
  Anaesthetics, General: increased sedative effect when
  anxiolytics and hypnotics given with general anaesthetics
  Analgesics: metabolism of midazolam possibly inhibited by fentanyl; increased sedative effect when
  anxiolytics and hypnotics given with opioid analgesics
  Angiotensin-II Receptor Antagonists: enhanced hypotensive effect when anxiolytics and hypnotics given
  with angiotensin-II receptor antagonists
- Antibacterials: metabolism of midazolam inhibited by
  ●clarithromycin, ●erythromycin and ●telithromycin
  (increased plasma concentration with increased
  sedation); plasma concentration of buspirone
  increased by erythromycin (reduce dose of buspirone); metabolism of zopiclone inhibited by erythromycin; manufacturer of zolpidem advises avoid concomitant use with ciprofloxacin; metabolism of
  benzodiazepines possibly accelerated by rifampicin
  (reduced plasma concentration); metabolism of

Anxiolytics and Hypnotics

- Antibacterials *(continued)*

    diazepam and zaleplon accelerated by rifampicin (reduced plasma concentration); metabolism of buspirone possibly accelerated by rifampicin; metabolism of zolpidem accelerated by rifampicin (reduced plasma concentration and reduced effect); plasma concentration of zopiclone significantly reduced by rifampicin; metabolism of diazepam inhibited by isoniazid

    Anticoagulants: chloral may transiently enhance anticoagulant effect of coumarins

- Antidepressants: plasma concentration of alprazolam increased by fluoxetine; plasma concentration of melatonin increased by ●fluvoxamine—avoid concomitant use; plasma concentration of some benzodiazepines increased by fluvoxamine; sedative effects possibly increased when zolpidem given with sertraline; manufacturer of buspirone advises avoid concomitant use with MAOIs; avoidance of buspirone for 14 days after stopping ●tranylcypromine advised by manufacturer of tranylcypromine; plasma concentration of *oral* midazolam possibly reduced by St John's wort; increased sedative effect when anxiolytics and hypnotics given with mirtazapine, tricyclic-related antidepressants or tricyclics

    Antiepileptics: plasma concentration of clonazepam often reduced by carbamazepine, phenobarbital and phenytoin; plasma concentration of midazolam reduced by carbamazepine and perampanel; increased sedative effect when anxiolytics and hypnotics given with phenobarbital; benzodiazepines possibly increase or decrease plasma concentration of phenytoin; diazepam increases or decreases plasma concentration of phenytoin; plasma concentration of clobazam increased by stiripentol; plasma concentration of diazepam and lorazepam possibly increased by valproate; increased risk of side-effects when clonazepam given with valproate; clobazam possibly increases plasma concentration of valproate

- Antifungals: plasma concentration of diazepam and midazolam increased by ●fluconazole (risk of prolonged sedation); plasma concentration of alprazolam increased by itraconazole; plasma concentration of midazolam increased by ●itraconazole, ●posaconazole and ●voriconazole (risk of prolonged sedation); plasma concentration of buspirone increased by itraconazole (reduce dose of buspirone); plasma concentration of diazepam increased by ●voriconazole (risk of prolonged sedation)

    Antihistamines: increased sedative effect when anxiolytics and hypnotics given with antihistamines

- Antipsychotics: increased sedative effect when anxiolytics and hypnotics given with antipsychotics; alprazolam possibly increases plasma concentration of haloperidol; buspirone increases plasma concentration of haloperidol; serious adverse events reported with concomitant use of benzodiazepines and ●clozapine (causality not established); plasma concentration of midazolam increased by lurasidone; increased risk of hypotension, bradycardia and respiratory depression when *parenteral* benzodiazepines given with *intramuscular* ●olanzapine

- Antivirals: plasma concentration of midazolam possibly increased by ●atazanavir—avoid concomitant use of *oral* midazolam; plasma concentration of *oral* midazolam increased by ●boceprevir—manufacturer of boceprevir advises avoid concomitant use; increased risk of prolonged sedation when midazolam given with ●efavirenz—avoid concomitant use; plasma concentration of midazolam possibly increased by ●fosamprenavir, ●indinavir, ●ritonavir and ●telaprevir (risk of prolonged sedation—avoid concomitant use of *oral* midazolam); increased risk

Anxiolytics and Hypnotics

- Antivirals *(continued)*

    of prolonged sedation when alprazolam given with ●indinavir—avoid concomitant use; plasma concentration of alprazolam, diazepam, flurazepam and zolpidem possibly increased by ●ritonavir (risk of extreme sedation and respiratory depression—avoid concomitant use); plasma concentration of buspirone increased by ritonavir (increased risk of toxicity); plasma concentration of anxiolytics and hypnotics possibly increased by ●ritonavir; plasma concentration of midazolam increased by ●saquinavir (risk of prolonged sedation—avoid concomitant use of *oral* midazolam); plasma concentration of *oral* midazolam increased by simeprevir

    Aprepitant: plasma concentration of midazolam increased by aprepitant (risk of prolonged sedation)

    Beta-blockers: enhanced hypotensive effect when anxiolytics and hypnotics given with beta-blockers

    Calcium-channel Blockers: enhanced hypotensive effect when anxiolytics and hypnotics given with calcium-channel blockers; midazolam increases absorption of lercanidipine; plasma concentration of buspirone increased by diltiazem and verapamil (reduce dose of buspirone); metabolism of midazolam inhibited by diltiazem and verapamil (increased plasma concentration with increased sedation)

    Cardiac Glycosides: alprazolam increases plasma concentration of digoxin (increased risk of toxicity)

    Clonidine: enhanced hypotensive effect when anxiolytics and hypnotics given with clonidine

- Cobicistat: avoidance of *oral* midazolam advised by manufacturer of ●cobicistat

- Cytotoxics: plasma concentration of midazolam increased by ●crizotinib and nilotinib; avoidance of *oral* midazolam advised by manufacturer of idelalisib

    Deferasirox: plasma concentration of midazolam possibly reduced by deferasirox

    Diazoxide: enhanced hypotensive effect when anxiolytics and hypnotics given with diazoxide

    Disulfiram: metabolism of benzodiazepines inhibited by disulfiram (increased sedative effects); increased risk of temazepam toxicity when given with disulfiram

    Diuretics: enhanced hypotensive effect when anxiolytics and hypnotics given with diuretics; administration of chloral with *parenteral* furosemide may displace thyroid hormone from binding sites

    Dopaminergics: benzodiazepines possibly antagonise effects of levodopa

    Grapefruit Juice: plasma concentration of *oral* midazolam possibly increased by grapefruit juice; plasma concentration of buspirone increased by grapefruit juice

    Ivacaftor: plasma concentration of midazolam increased by ivacaftor

    Lipid-regulating Drugs: plasma concentration of midazolam possibly increased by atorvastatin

    Lithium: increased risk of neurotoxicity when clonazepam given with lithium

    Lofexidine: increased sedative effect when anxiolytics and hypnotics given with lofexidine

    Methyldopa: enhanced hypotensive effect when anxiolytics and hypnotics given with methyldopa

- Methylthioninium: possible risk of CNS toxicity when buspirone given with ●methylthioninium—avoid concomitant use (if avoidance not possible, use lowest possible dose of methylthioninium and observe patient for up to 4 hours after administration)

    Moxonidine: enhanced hypotensive effect when anxiolytics and hypnotics given with moxonidine; sedative effects possibly increased when benzodiazepines given with moxonidine

Anxiolytics and Hypnotics *(continued)*

Muscle Relaxants: increased sedative effect when anxiolytics and hypnotics given with baclofen or tizanidine

Nitrates: enhanced hypotensive effect when anxiolytics and hypnotics given with nitrates

Oestrogens: plasma concentration of melatonin increased by oestrogens; plasma concentration of chlordiazepoxide, diazepam and nitrazepam possibly increased by oestrogens; plasma concentration of lorazepam, oxazepam and temazepam possibly reduced by oestrogens

Progestogens: plasma concentration of chlordiazepoxide, diazepam and nitrazepam possibly increased by progestogens; plasma concentration of lorazepam, oxazepam and temazepam possibly reduced by progestogens

- Sodium Oxybate: benzodiazepines enhance effects of ●sodium oxybate (avoid concomitant use)

Theophylline: effects of benzodiazepines possibly reduced by theophylline

Ulcer-healing Drugs: plasma concentration of melatonin increased by cimetidine; metabolism of benzodiazepines, clomethiazole and zaleplon inhibited by cimetidine (increased plasma concentration); metabolism of diazepam possibly inhibited by esomeprazole and omeprazole (increased plasma concentration)

Vasodilator Antihypertensives: enhanced hypotensive effect when anxiolytics and hypnotics given with hydralazine, minoxidil or sodium nitroprusside

Apixaban

- Analgesics: increased risk of haemorrhage when anticoagulants given with *intravenous* ●diclofenac (avoid concomitant use, including low-dose heparins); increased risk of haemorrhage when anticoagulants given with ●ketorolac (avoid concomitant use, including low-dose heparins)

- Antibacterials: manufacturer of apixaban advises avoid concomitant use with clarithromycin and telithromycin; plasma concentration of apixaban possibly reduced by ●rifampicin—manufacturer of apixaban advises avoid concomitant use when given for treatment of deep-vein thrombosis or pulmonary embolism

- Anticoagulants: increased risk of haemorrhage when apixaban given with other ●anticoagulants (avoid concomitant use except when switching with other anticoagulants or using heparin to maintain catheter patency); increased risk of haemorrhage when other anticoagulants given with ●dabigatran and ●rivaroxaban (avoid concomitant use except when switching with other anticoagulants or using heparin to maintain catheter patency)

- Antidepressants: plasma concentration of apixaban possibly reduced by ●St John's wort—manufacturer of apixaban advises avoid concomitant use when given for treatment of deep-vein thrombosis or pulmonary embolism

- Antiepileptics: plasma concentration of apixaban possibly reduced by ●carbamazepine—manufacturer of apixaban advises avoid concomitant use when given for treatment of deep-vein thrombosis or pulmonary embolism; plasma concentration of apixaban possibly reduced by ●phenobarbital and ●phenytoin

Antifungals: manufacturer of apixaban advises avoid concomitant use with itraconazole, posaconazole and voriconazole

Antivirals: manufacturer of apixaban advises avoid concomitant use with atazanavir, boceprevir, darunavir, fosamprenavir, indinavir, lopinavir, ritonavir, saquinavir, telaprevir and tipranavir

Cobicistat: manufacturer of apixaban advises avoid concomitant use with cobicistat

Apixaban *(continued)*

Sulfinpyrazone: increased risk of bleeding when apixaban given with sulfinpyrazone

Apomorphine

Antipsychotics: effects of apomorphine antagonised by antipsychotics

Dopaminergics: effects of apomorphine possibly enhanced by entacapone

- 5HT₃-receptor Antagonists: possible increased hypotensive effect when apomorphine given with ●ondansetron—avoid concomitant use

Memantine: effects of dopaminergics possibly enhanced by memantine

Methyldopa: antiparkinsonian effect of dopaminergics antagonised by methyldopa

Apraclonidine

Antidepressants: manufacturer of apraclonidine advises avoid concomitant use with MAOIs, tricyclic-related antidepressants and tricyclics

Sympathomimetics: manufacturer of apraclonidine advises avoid concomitant use with sympathomimetics

Aprepitant

Note Fosaprepitant is a prodrug of aprepitant

Antibacterials: plasma concentration of aprepitant possibly increased by clarithromycin and telithromycin; plasma concentration of aprepitant reduced by rifampicin

Anticoagulants: aprepitant possibly reduces anticoagulant effect of warfarin

- Antidepressants: manufacturer of aprepitant advises avoid concomitant use with ●St John's wort

Antidiabetics: aprepitant reduces plasma concentration of tolbutamide

Antiepileptics: plasma concentration of aprepitant possibly reduced by carbamazepine, phenobarbital and phenytoin

- Antipsychotics: manufacturer of aprepitant advises avoid concomitant use with ●pimozide

Antivirals: plasma concentration of aprepitant possibly increased by ritonavir

Anxiolytics and Hypnotics: aprepitant increases plasma concentration of midazolam (risk of prolonged sedation)

- Avanafil: aprepitant possibly increases plasma concentration of ●avanafil—see Dose under Avanafil, p. 571

Calcium-channel Blockers: plasma concentration of both drugs may increase when aprepitant given with diltiazem

Corticosteroids: aprepitant inhibits metabolism of dexamethasone and methylprednisolone (reduce dose of dexamethasone and methylprednisolone)

- Cytotoxics: aprepitant possibly increases the plasma concentration of ●bosutinib—manufacturer of bosutinib advises avoid or consider reducing dose of bosutinib; aprepitant possibly increases the plasma concentration of ●ibrutinib—reduce dose of ibrutinib (see Dose under Ibrutinib, p. 615)

Dapoxetine: manufacturer of dapoxetine advises dose reduction when aprepitant given with dapoxetine (see Dose under Dapoxetine, p. 572)

Lipid-regulating Drugs: manufacturer of lomitapide advises dose reduction when fosaprepitant given with lomitapide (see Dose under Lomitapide, p. 180)

- Oestrogens: aprepitant possibly causes contraceptive failure of hormonal contraceptives containing ●oestrogens (alternative contraception recommended)

- Progestogens: aprepitant possibly causes contraceptive failure of hormonal contraceptives containing ●progestogens (alternative contraception recommended)

Argatroban

- Analgesics: increased risk of haemorrhage when anti-coagulants given with *intravenous* ●diclofenac (avoid concomitant use, including low-dose heparins); increased risk of haemorrhage when anticoagulants given with ●ketorolac (avoid concomitant use, including low-dose heparins)
- Anticoagulants: increased risk of haemorrhage when other anticoagulants given with ●apixaban, ●dabiga-tran and ●rivaroxaban (avoid concomitant use except when switching with other anticoagulants or using heparin to maintain catheter patency)

Aripiprazole *see* Antipsychotics

Arsenic Trioxide

- Anti-arrhythmics: increased risk of ventricular arrhyth-mias when arsenic trioxide given with ●amiodarone or ●disopyramide
- Antibacterials: increased risk of ventricular arrhyth-mias when arsenic trioxide given with ●delamanid, ●erythromycin, ●levofloxacin or ●moxifloxacin
- Antidepressants: increased risk of ventricular arrhyth-mias when arsenic trioxide given with ●amitripty-line or ●clomipramine
- Antifungals: increased risk of ventricular arrhythmias when arsenic trioxide given with ●amphotericin
- Antimalarials: avoidance of arsenic trioxide advised by manufacturer of ●piperaquine with artenimol (possible risk of ventricular arrhythmias)
- Antipsychotics: increased risk of ventricular arrhyth-mias when arsenic trioxide given with ●antipsy-chotics that prolong the QT interval; increased risk of ventricular arrhythmias when arsenic trioxide given with ●haloperidol; avoid concomitant use of cytotoxics with ●clozapine (increased risk of agranulocytosis)
- Beta-blockers: increased risk of ventricular arrhyth-mias when arsenic trioxide given with ●sotalol
- Cytotoxics: possible increased risk of ventricular arrhy-thmias when arsenic trioxide given with ●vandeta-nib—avoid concomitant use
- Diuretics: risk of ventricular arrhythmias with arsenic trioxide increased by hypokalaemia caused by ●acetazolamide, ●loop diuretics or ●thiazides and related diuretics
- Lithium: increased risk of ventricular arrhythmias when arsenic trioxide given with ●lithium

Artemether with Lumefantrine

- Anti-arrhythmics: manufacturer of artemether with lumefantrine advises avoid concomitant use with ●amiodarone, ●disopyramide and ●flecainide (risk of ventricular arrhythmias)
- Antibacterials: manufacturer of artemether with lume-fantrine advises avoid concomitant use with ●macrolides and ●quinolones
- Antidepressants: avoidance of antimalarials advised by manufacturer of ●citalopram and ●escitalopram (risk of ventricular arrhythmias); manufacturer of artemether with lumefantrine advises avoid conco-mitant use with ●antidepressants
- Antifungals: manufacturer of artemether with lumefan-trine advises avoid concomitant use with ●imida-zoles and ●triazoles
- Antimalarials: manufacturer of artemether with lume-fantrine advises avoid concomitant use with ●anti-malarials; increased risk of ventricular arrhythmias when artemether with lumefantrine given with ●quinine
- Antipsychotics: manufacturer of artemether with lumefantrine advises avoid concomitant use with ●antipsychotics
- Antivirals: manufacturer of artemether with lumefan-trine advises caution with atazanavir, fosamprena-vir, indinavir, lopinavir, ritonavir, saquinavir and tipranavir; avoidance of artemether with lumefan-trine advised by manufacturer of ●boceprevir; plasma concentration of lumefantrine increased by

Artemether with Lumefantrine

- Antivirals *(continued)*
  darunavir; plasma concentration of artemether with lumefantrine reduced by ●efavirenz and etravirine
- Beta-blockers: manufacturer of artemether with lume-fantrine advises avoid concomitant use with ●metoprolol and ●sotalol
- Cytotoxics: possible increased risk of ventricular arrhy-thmias when artemether with lumefantrine given with ●vandetanib—avoid concomitant use
  Grapefruit Juice: plasma concentration of artemether with lumefantrine possibly increased by grapefruit juice
  Histamine: avoidance of antimalarials advised by manufacturer of histamine
- Ulcer-healing Drugs: manufacturer of artemether with lumefantrine advises avoid concomitant use with ●cimetidine
  Vaccines: antimalarials inactivate oral typhoid vaccine—see p. 864

Ascorbic acid *see* Vitamins

Asenapine *see* Antipsychotics

Aspirin

  Adsorbents: absorption of aspirin possibly reduced by kaolin
  Anaesthetics, General: aspirin possibly enhances effects of thiopental
- Analgesics: avoid concomitant use of aspirin with ●NSAIDs (increased side-effects); antiplatelet effect of aspirin possibly reduced by ibuprofen
  Antacids: excretion of aspirin increased by alkaline urine due to some antacids
- Anticoagulants: increased risk of bleeding when aspirin given with ●coumarins or ●phenindione (due to antiplatelet effect); aspirin enhances anti-coagulant effect of ●heparins
- Antidepressants: increased risk of bleeding when aspirin given with ●SSRIs or ●venlafaxine
  Antiepileptics: aspirin enhances effects of phenytoin and valproate
  Clopidogrel: increased risk of bleeding when aspirin given with clopidogrel
  Corticosteroids: increased risk of gastro-intestinal bleeding and ulceration when aspirin given with corticosteroids, also corticosteroids reduce plasma concentration of salicylate
- Cytotoxics: aspirin reduces excretion of ●methotrexate (increased risk of toxicity)—but for concomitant use in rheumatic disease see p. 732; aspirin possibly reduces renal excretion of pemetrexed—consult product literature
- Diuretics: increased risk of toxicity when high-dose aspirin given with ●acetazolamide; aspirin antago-nises diuretic effect of spironolactone; possible increased risk of toxicity when high-dose aspirin given with loop diuretics (also possible reduced effect of loop diuretics)
  Iloprost: increased risk of bleeding when aspirin given with iloprost
  Leukotriene Receptor Antagonists: aspirin increases plasma concentration of zafirlukast
  Metoclopramide: rate of absorption of aspirin increased by metoclopramide (enhanced effect)
  Sulfinpyrazone: aspirin antagonises effects of sulfin-pyrazone

Atazanavir

  Antacids: absorption of atazanavir reduced by antacids (give at least 2 hours before or 1 hour after antacids)
- Anti-arrhythmics: atazanavir possibly increases plasma concentration of ●amiodarone and ●lidocaine
- Antibacterials: plasma concentration of both drugs increased when atazanavir given with clarithro-mycin; atazanavir increases plasma concentration of ●rifabutin (reduce dose of rifabutin); plasma con-centration of atazanavir reduced by ●rifampicin—

Atazanavir

- Antibacterials *(continued)*
  avoid concomitant use; avoidance of concomitant atazanavir in severe renal and hepatic impairment advised by manufacturer of ●telithromycin

  Anticoagulants: atazanavir may enhance or reduce anticoagulant effect of warfarin; avoidance of atazanavir advised by manufacturer of apixaban and rivaroxaban

- Antidepressants: plasma concentration of atazanavir reduced by ●St John's wort—avoid concomitant use

- Antifungals: plasma concentration of atazanavir increased by ●posaconazole; atazanavir increases or decreases the plasma concentration of ●voriconazole and plasma concentration of atazanavir also reduced

- Antimalarials: caution with atazanavir advised by manufacturer of artemether with lumefantrine; atazanavir possibly increases plasma concentration of ●quinine (increased risk of toxicity)

  Antimuscarinics: avoidance of atazanavir advised by manufacturer of darifenacin; manufacturer of fesoterodine advises dose reduction when atazanavir given with fesoterodine—consult fesoterodine product literature

- Antipsychotics: atazanavir possibly increases plasma concentration of ●aripiprazole (reduce dose of aripiprazole—consult aripiprazole product literature); atazanavir possibly increases plasma concentration of ●pimozide—avoid concomitant use; atazanavir possibly increases plasma concentration of ●quetiapine—manufacturer of quetiapine advises avoid concomitant use

- Antivirals: plasma concentration of atazanavir reduced by ●boceprevir; atazanavir increases the plasma concentration of ●daclatasvir—reduce dose of daclatasvir (see Dose under Daclatasvir, p. 438); absorption of atazanavir reduced by didanosine *tablets* (give at least 2 hours before or 1 hour after didanosine *tablets*); manufacturer of atazanavir advises avoid concomitant use with ●efavirenz (plasma concentration of atazanavir reduced); atazanavir boosted with ritonavir increases plasma concentration of ●elvitegravir (reduce dose of elvitegravir); avoid concomitant use of atazanavir with ●indinavir; atazanavir increases plasma concentration of ●maraviroc (consider reducing dose of maraviroc); plasma concentration of atazanavir possibly reduced by ●nevirapine—avoid concomitant use; increased risk of ventricular arrhythmias when atazanavir given with ●saquinavir—avoid concomitant use; atazanavir possibly reduces plasma concentration of telaprevir, also plasma concentration of atazanavir possibly increased; plasma concentration of atazanavir reduced by tenofovir, also plasma concentration of tenofovir possibly increased; atazanavir increases plasma concentration of tipranavir (also plasma concentration of atazanavir reduced)

- Anxiolytics and Hypnotics: atazanavir possibly increases plasma concentration of ●midazolam—avoid concomitant use of *oral* midazolam

- Avanafil: atazanavir possibly increases plasma concentration of ●avanafil—manufacturer of avanafil advises avoid concomitant use

- Calcium-channel Blockers: atazanavir increases plasma concentration of ●diltiazem (reduce dose of diltiazem); atazanavir possibly increases plasma concentration of verapamil

- Ciclosporin: atazanavir possibly increases plasma concentration of ●ciclosporin

- Colchicine: atazanavir possibly increases risk of ●colchicine toxicity—suspend or reduce dose of colchicine (avoid concomitant use in hepatic or renal impairment)

Atazanavir *(continued)*

- Cytotoxics: atazanavir possibly increases plasma concentration of axitinib (reduce dose of axitinib—consult axitinib product literature); atazanavir possibly increases the plasma concentration of ●bosutinib—manufacturer of bosutinib advises avoid or consider reducing dose of bosutinib; atazanavir possibly increases plasma concentration of ●crizotinib and ●everolimus—manufacturer of crizotinib and everolimus advises avoid concomitant use; atazanavir possibly increases the plasma concentration of ●ibrutinib—reduce dose of ibrutinib (see Dose under Ibrutinib, p. 615); atazanavir possibly increases plasma concentration of ●pazopanib (reduce dose of pazopanib); avoidance of atazanavir advised by manufacturer of ●cabazitaxel; atazanavir possibly inhibits metabolism of ●irinotecan (increased risk of toxicity)

- Dapoxetine: avoidance of atazanavir advised by manufacturer of ●dapoxetine (increased risk of toxicity)

- Ergot Alkaloids: atazanavir possibly increases plasma concentration of ●ergot alkaloids—avoid concomitant use

- Lipid-regulating Drugs: possible increased risk of myopathy when atazanavir given with ●atorvastatin or pravastatin; atazanavir increases plasma concentration of ●rosuvastatin—adjust dose of rosuvastatin (consult product literature); increased risk of myopathy when atazanavir given with ●simvastatin (avoid concomitant use)

  Oestrogens: atazanavir increases plasma concentration of ethinylestradiol

- Orlistat: absorption of atazanavir possibly reduced by ●orlistat

  Progestogens: atazanavir increases plasma concentration of norethisterone

- Ranolazine: atazanavir possibly increases plasma concentration of ●ranolazine—manufacturer of ranolazine advises avoid concomitant use

- Sildenafil: atazanavir possibly increases side-effects of ●sildenafil

- Sirolimus: atazanavir possibly increases plasma concentration of ●sirolimus

- Tacrolimus: atazanavir possibly increases plasma concentration of ●tacrolimus

- Ticagrelor: atazanavir possibly increases plasma concentration of ●ticagrelor—manufacturer of ticagrelor advises avoid concomitant use

- Ulcer-healing Drugs: manufacturer of atazanavir advises adjust doses of both drugs when atazanavir given with cimetidine and nizatidine—consult atazanavir product literature; plasma concentration of atazanavir reduced by ●famotidine and ●ranitidine (adjust doses of both drugs—consult atazanavir product literature); plasma concentration of atazanavir reduced by ●proton pump inhibitors—avoid or adjust dose of both drugs (consult product literature)

Atenolol *see* Beta-blockers

Atomoxetine

- Analgesics: increased risk of ventricular arrhythmias when atomoxetine given with ●methadone; possible increased risk of convulsions when atomoxetine given with tramadol

- Anti-arrhythmics: increased risk of ventricular arrhythmias when atomoxetine given with ●amiodarone or ●disopyramide

- Antibacterials: increased risk of ventricular arrhythmias when atomoxetine given with *parenteral* ●erythromycin; increased risk of ventricular arrhythmias when atomoxetine given with ●moxifloxacin

- Antidepressants: metabolism of atomoxetine possibly inhibited by fluoxetine and paroxetine; possible increased risk of convulsions when atomoxetine given with antidepressants; atomoxetine should not be started until 2 weeks after stopping ●MAOIs,

Atomoxetine

- Antidepressants *(continued)*
  also MAOIs should not be started until at least 2 weeks after stopping atomoxetine; increased risk of ventricular arrhythmias when atomoxetine given with ●tricyclics
- Antimalarials: increased risk of ventricular arrhythmias when atomoxetine given with ●mefloquine
- Antipsychotics: increased risk of ventricular arrhythmias when atomoxetine given with ●antipsychotics that prolong the QT interval
- Beta-blockers: increased risk of ventricular arrhythmias when atomoxetine given with ●sotalol
  Bupropion: possible increased risk of convulsions when atomoxetine given with bupropion
- Diuretics: risk of ventricular arrhythmias with atomoxetine increased by hypokalaemia caused by ●diuretics
  Sympathomimetics, Beta$_2$: Increased risk of cardiovascular side-effects when atomoxetine given with *parenteral* salbutamol

Atorvastatin *see* Statins

Atovaquone

- Antibacterials: manufacturer of atovaquone advises avoid concomitant use with rifabutin (plasma concentration of both drugs reduced); plasma concentration of atovaquone reduced by ●rifampicin (and concentration of rifampicin increased)—avoid concomitant use; plasma concentration of atovaquone reduced by tetracycline
- Antivirals: plasma concentration of atovaquone reduced by ●efavirenz—avoid concomitant use; atovaquone possibly reduces plasma concentration of indinavir; plasma concentration of atovaquone possibly reduced by ritonavir—manufacturer of atovaquone advises avoid concomitant use; atovaquone increases plasma concentration of zidovudine (increased risk of toxicity)
  Cytotoxics: atovaquone possibly increases plasma concentration of etoposide
  Histamine: avoidance of atovaquone advised by manufacturer of histamine
  Metoclopramide: plasma concentration of atovaquone reduced by metoclopramide—avoid concomitant use

Atracurium *see* Muscle Relaxants

Atropine *see* Antimuscarinics

Avanafil

ACE Inhibitors: avanafil possibly enhances hypotensive effect of enalapril
  Alcohol: possible enhanced hypotensive effect when avanafil given with alcohol
- Alpha-blockers: enhanced hypotensive effect when avanafil given with ●alpha-blockers—see also p. 570
- Antibacterials: plasma concentration of avanafil possibly increased by ●clarithromycin and ●telithromycin—manufacturer of avanafil advises avoid concomitant use; plasma concentration of avanafil increased by ●erythromycin—see Dose under Avanafil, p. 571; plasma concentration of avanafil possibly reduced by rifampicin—manufacturer of avanafil advises avoid concomitant use
  Antiepileptics: plasma concentration of avanafil possibly reduced by carbamazepine and phenobarbital—manufacturer of avanafil advises avoid concomitant use
- Antifungals: plasma concentration of avanafil possibly increased by ●fluconazole—see Dose under Avanafil, p. 571; plasma concentration of avanafil possibly increased by ●itraconazole and ●voriconazole—manufacturer of avanafil advises avoid concomitant use
- Antivirals: plasma concentration of avanafil possibly increased by ●atazanavir, ●indinavir and ●saquinavir—manufacturer of avanafil advises avoid conco-

Avanafil

- Antivirals *(continued)*
  mitant use; plasma concentration of avanafil possibly reduced by efavirenz—manufacturer of avanafil advises avoid concomitant use; plasma concentration of avanafil possibly increased by ●fosamprenavir—see Dose under Avanafil, p. 571; plasma concentration of avanafil significantly increased by ●ritonavir—avoid concomitant use
- Aprepitant: plasma concentration of avanafil possibly increased by ●aprepitant—see Dose under Avanafil, p. 571
  Bosentan: plasma concentration of avanafil possibly reduced by bosentan—manufacturer of avanafil advises avoid concomitant use
- Calcium-channel Blockers: plasma concentration of avanafil possibly increased by ●diltiazem and ●verapamil—see Dose under Avanafil, p. 571
  Grapefruit Juice: plasma concentration of avanafil possibly increased by grapefruit juice— manufacturer of avanafil advises avoid grapefruit juice for 24 hours before avanafil
- Nicorandil: avanafil significantly enhances hypotensive effect of ●nicorandil (avoid concomitant use)
- Nitrates: avanafil significantly enhances hypotensive effect of ●nitrates (avoid concomitant use)
- Riociguat: possible enhanced hypotensive effect when avanafil given with ●riociguat—avoid concomitant use

Axitinib

Antibacterials: plasma concentration of axitinib possibly increased by clarithromycin, erythromycin and telithromycin (reduce dose of axitinib—consult axitinib product literature); plasma concentration of axitinib possibly decreased by rifabutin (increase dose of axitinib—consult axitinib product literature); plasma concentration of axitinib decreased by rifampicin (increase dose of axitinib—consult axitinib product literature)
  Antidepressants: plasma concentration of axitinib possibly reduced by St John's wort—consider increasing dose of axitinib
  Antiepileptics: plasma concentration of axitinib possibly decreased by carbamazepine, phenobarbital and phenytoin (increase dose of axitinib—consult axitinib product literature)
  Antifungals: plasma concentration of axitinib possibly increased by itraconazole (reduce dose of axitinib—consult axitinib product literature)
- Antipsychotics: avoid concomitant use of cytotoxics with ●clozapine (increased risk of agranulocytosis)
  Antivirals: plasma concentration of axitinib possibly increased by atazanavir, indinavir, ritonavir and saquinavir (reduce dose of axitinib—consult axitinib product literature)
  Corticosteroids: plasma concentration of axitinib possibly decreased by dexamethasone (increase dose of axitinib—consult axitinib product literature)
  Grapefruit Juice: plasma concentration of axitinib possibly increased by grapefruit juice

Azathioprine

ACE Inhibitors: increased risk of anaemia or leucopenia when azathioprine given with captopril especially in renal impairment; increased risk of anaemia when azathioprine given with enalapril especially in renal impairment
- Allopurinol: enhanced effects and increased toxicity of azathioprine when given with ●allopurinol (reduce dose of azathioprine to one quarter of usual dose)
- Antibacterials: increased risk of haematological toxicity when azathioprine given with ●sulfamethoxazole (as co-trimoxazole); increased risk of haematological toxicity when azathioprine given with ●trimethoprim (also with co-trimoxazole)
- Anticoagulants: azathioprine possibly reduces anticoagulant effect of ●coumarins

Azathioprine (continued)
- Antivirals: myelosuppressive effects of azathioprine possibly enhanced by ●ribavirin
- Febuxostat: avoidance of azathioprine advised by manufacturer of ●febuxostat

Azilsartan see Angiotensin-II Receptor Antagonists

Azithromycin see Macrolides

Aztreonam
- Anticoagulants: aztreonam possibly enhances anticoagulant effect of ●coumarins
  Vaccines: antibacterials inactivate oral typhoid vaccine—see p. 864

Baclofen see Muscle Relaxants

Bambuterol see Sympathomimetics, Beta₂

Basiliximab
- Antipsychotics: avoid concomitant use of cytotoxics with ●clozapine (increased risk of agranulocytosis)
- Vaccines: avoid concomitant use of monoclonal antibodies with live ●vaccines (see p. 842)

BCG vaccine see Vaccines

Beclometasone see Corticosteroids

Bedaquiline
- Antibacterials: plasma concentration of bedaquiline possibly increased by ciprofloxacin, clarithromycin and erythromycin—avoid concomitant use if ciprofloxacin, clarithromycin and erythromycin given for more than 14 days; manufacturer of bedaquiline advises avoid concomitant use with moxifloxacin; plasma concentration of bedaquiline possibly reduced by rifabutin—manufacturer of bedaquiline advises avoid concomitant use; plasma concentration of bedaquiline reduced by ●rifampicin—manufacturer of bedaquiline advises avoid concomitant use; possible increased risk of ventricular arrhythmias when bedaquiline given with ●clofazimine
  Antidepressants: plasma concentration of bedaquiline possibly reduced by St John's wort—manufacturer of bedaquiline advises avoid concomitant use
- Antiepileptics: plasma concentration of bedaquiline possibly reduced by ●carbamazepine and ●phenytoin—manufacturer of bedaquiline advises avoid concomitant use
  Antifungals: plasma concentration of bedaquiline possibly increased by fluconazole—avoid concomitant use if fluconazole given for more than 14 days
  Antivirals: plasma concentration of bedaquiline possibly reduced by efavirenz and etravirine—manufacturer of bedaquiline advises avoid concomitant use; plasma concentration of bedaquiline possibly increased by ritonavir—avoid concomitant use if ritonavir given for more than 14 days
  Vaccines: antibacterials inactivate oral typhoid vaccine—see p. 864

Belimumab
- Antipsychotics: avoid concomitant use of cytotoxics with ●clozapine (increased risk of agranulocytosis)
- Vaccines: avoid concomitant use of monoclonal antibodies with live ●vaccines (see p. 842)

Bendamustine
- Antipsychotics: avoid concomitant use of cytotoxics with ●clozapine (increased risk of agranulocytosis)

Bendroflumethiazide see Diuretics

Benperidol see Antipsychotics

Benzodiazepines see Anxiolytics and Hypnotics

Benzthiazide see Diuretics

Benzylpenicillin see Penicillins

Beta-blockers
Note Since systemic absorption may follow topical application of beta-blockers to the eye the possibility of interactions, in particular, with drugs such as verapamil should be borne in mind
ACE Inhibitors: enhanced hypotensive effect when beta-blockers given with ACE inhibitors
Adrenergic Neurone Blockers: enhanced hypotensive effect when beta-blockers given with adrenergic neurone blockers

Beta-blockers (continued)
Alcohol: enhanced hypotensive effect when beta-blockers given with alcohol
Aldesleukin: enhanced hypotensive effect when beta-blockers given with aldesleukin
- Alpha-blockers: enhanced hypotensive effect when beta-blockers given with ●alpha-blockers, also increased risk of first-dose hypotension with post-synaptic alpha-blockers such as prazosin
  Anaesthetics, General: enhanced hypotensive effect when beta-blockers given with general anaesthetics
- Anaesthetics, Local: propranolol increases risk of ●bupivacaine toxicity
  Analgesics: hypotensive effect of beta-blockers antagonised by NSAIDs; plasma concentration of esmolol possibly increased by morphine
  Angiotensin-II Receptor Antagonists: enhanced hypotensive effect when beta-blockers given with angiotensin-II receptor antagonists
- Anti-arrhythmics: increased myocardial depression when beta-blockers given with ●anti-arrhythmics; increased risk of ventricular arrhythmias when sotalol given with ●amiodarone, ●disopyramide or ●dronedarone—avoid concomitant use; increased risk of bradycardia, AV block and myocardial depression when beta-blockers given with ●amiodarone; plasma concentration of metoprolol and propranolol possibly increased by dronedarone; increased risk of myocardial depression and bradycardia when beta-blockers given with ●flecainide; nadolol possibly increases risk of lidocaine toxicity; propranolol increases risk of ●lidocaine toxicity; plasma concentration of metoprolol and propranolol increased by propafenone
- Antibacterials: increased risk of ventricular arrhythmias when sotalol given with ●moxifloxacin—avoid concomitant use; metabolism of bisoprolol and propranolol accelerated by rifampicin (plasma concentration significantly reduced); plasma concentration of carvedilol, celiprolol and metoprolol reduced by rifampicin; plasma concentration of oral timolol possibly reduced by rifampicin; increased risk of ventricular arrhythmias when sotalol given with ●delamanid
- Antidepressants: plasma concentration of metoprolol increased by citalopram and escitalopram; increased risk of ventricular arrhythmias when sotalol given with ●citalopram—avoid concomitant use; avoidance of sotalol advised by manufacturer of ●escitalopram (risk of ventricular arrhythmias); plasma concentration of propranolol increased by fluvoxamine; plasma concentration of metoprolol possibly increased by ●paroxetine—increased risk of AV block (manufacturer of paroxetine advises avoid concomitant use in cardiac insufficiency); labetalol and propranolol increase plasma concentration of imipramine; enhanced hypotensive effect when beta-blockers given with MAOIs; increased risk of ventricular arrhythmias when sotalol given with ●tricyclics
  Antidiabetics: beta-blockers may mask warning signs of hypoglycaemia (such as tremor) with antidiabetics; beta-blockers enhance hypoglycaemic effect of insulin
  Antiepileptics: plasma concentration of propranolol possibly reduced by phenobarbital
- Antihistamines: increased risk of ventricular arrhythmias when sotalol given with ●mizolastine—avoid concomitant use
- Antimalarials: avoidance of sotalol advised by manufacturer of ●piperaquine with artenimol (possible risk of ventricular arrhythmias); avoidance of metoprolol and sotalol advised by manufacturer of ●artemether with lumefantrine; increased risk of bradycardia when beta-blockers given with mefloquine

Beta-blockers *(continued)*

- Antimuscarinics: increased risk of ventricular arrhythmias when sotalol given with ●tolterodine
- Antipsychotics: increased risk of ventricular arrhythmias when sotalol given with ●droperidol or ●zuclopenthixol—avoid concomitant use; possible increased risk of ventricular arrhythmias when sotalol given with ●haloperidol—avoid concomitant use; plasma concentration of both drugs may increase when propranolol given with ●chlorpromazine; increased risk of ventricular arrhythmias when sotalol given with ●amisulpride, ●phenothiazines, ●pimozide or ●sulpiride; enhanced hypotensive effect when beta-blockers given with phenothiazines; possible increased risk of ventricular arrhythmias when sotalol given with ●risperidone
- Antivirals: increased risk of ventricular arrhythmias when sotalol given with ●saquinavir—avoid concomitant use; avoidance of sotalol advised by manufacturer of ●telaprevir (risk of ventricular arrhythmias); avoidance of metoprolol for heart failure advised by manufacturer of ●tipranavir

Anxiolytics and Hypnotics: enhanced hypotensive effect when beta-blockers given with anxiolytics and hypnotics

- Atomoxetine: increased risk of ventricular arrhythmias when sotalol given with ●atomoxetine
- Calcium-channel Blockers: enhanced hypotensive effect when beta-blockers given with calcium-channel blockers; possible severe hypotension and heart failure when beta-blockers given with ●nifedipine; increased risk of AV block and bradycardia when beta-blockers given with ●diltiazem; asystole, severe hypotension and heart failure when beta-blockers given with ●verapamil (see p. 138)

Cardiac Glycosides: increased risk of AV block and bradycardia when beta-blockers given with cardiac glycosides

- Ciclosporin: carvedilol increases plasma concentration of ●ciclosporin
- Clonidine: increased risk of withdrawal hypertension when beta-blockers given with ●clonidine (withdraw beta-blockers several days before slowly withdrawing clonidine)

Corticosteroids: hypotensive effect of beta-blockers antagonised by corticosteroids

- Cytotoxics: possible increased risk of ventricular arrhythmias when sotalol given with ●bosutinib; possible increased risk of bradycardia when beta-blockers given with crizotinib; possible increased risk of ventricular arrhythmias when sotalol given with ●vandetanib—avoid concomitant use; increased risk of ventricular arrhythmias when sotalol given with ●arsenic trioxide

Diazoxide: enhanced hypotensive effect when beta-blockers given with diazoxide

- Diuretics: enhanced hypotensive effect when beta-blockers given with diuretics; risk of ventricular arrhythmias with sotalol increased by hypokalaemia caused by ●loop diuretics or ●thiazides and related diuretics

Dopaminergics: enhanced hypotensive effect when beta-blockers given with levodopa

Ergot Alkaloids: increased peripheral vasoconstriction when beta-blockers given with ergotamine

- Fingolimod: possible increased risk of bradycardia when beta-blockers given with ●fingolimod

Hormone Antagonists: possible increased risk of bradycardia when carteolol, metoprolol, propranolol or sotalol given with pasireotide

5HT₁-receptor Agonists: propranolol increases plasma concentration of rizatriptan (manufacturer of rizatriptan advises halve dose and avoid within 2 hours of propranolol)

- Ivabradine: increased risk of ventricular arrhythmias when sotalol given with ●ivabradine

Beta-blockers *(continued)*

Methyldopa: enhanced hypotensive effect when beta-blockers given with methyldopa

Mirabegron: plasma concentration of metoprolol increased by mirabegron

- Moxisylyte: possible severe postural hypotension when beta-blockers given with ●moxisylyte

Moxonidine: enhanced hypotensive effect when beta-blockers given with moxonidine

Muscle Relaxants: propranolol enhances effects of muscle relaxants; enhanced hypotensive effect when beta-blockers given with baclofen; possible enhanced hypotensive effect and bradycardia when beta-blockers given with tizanidine

Nitrates: enhanced hypotensive effect when beta-blockers given with nitrates

Oestrogens: hypotensive effect of beta-blockers antagonised by oestrogens

Parasympathomimetics: propranolol antagonises effects of neostigmine and pyridostigmine; increased risk of arrhythmias when beta-blockers given with pilocarpine

Prostaglandins: enhanced hypotensive effect when beta-blockers given with alprostadil

- Ranolazine: avoidance of sotalol advised by manufacturer of ●ranolazine
- Sympathomimetics: increased risk of severe hypertension and bradycardia when non-cardioselective beta-blockers given with ●adrenaline (epinephrine), also reponse to adrenaline (epinephrine) may be reduced; increased risk of severe hypertension and bradycardia when non-cardioselective beta-blockers given with ●dobutamine; possible increased risk of severe hypertension and bradycardia when non-cardioselective beta-blockers given with ●noradrenaline (norepinephrine)

Thyroid Hormones: metabolism of propranolol accelerated by levothyroxine

Ulcer-healing Drugs: plasma concentration of labetalol, metoprolol and propranolol increased by cimetidine; plasma concentration of *oral* timolol possibly increased by cimetidine

Vasodilator Antihypertensives: enhanced hypotensive effect when beta-blockers given with hydralazine, minoxidil or sodium nitroprusside

Betahistine

Antihistamines: effect of betahistine theoretically antagonised by antihistamines

Betamethasone *see* Corticosteroids

Betaxolol *see* Beta-blockers

Bethanechol *see* Parasympathomimetics

Bevacizumab

- Antipsychotics: avoid concomitant use of cytotoxics with ●clozapine (increased risk of agranulocytosis)
- Vaccines: avoid concomitant use of monoclonal antibodies with live ●vaccines (see p. 842)

Bexarotene

- Antipsychotics: avoid concomitant use of cytotoxics with ●clozapine (increased risk of agranulocytosis)
- Lipid-regulating Drugs: plasma concentration of bexarotene increased by ●gemfibrozil—avoid concomitant use

Bezafibrate *see* Fibrates

Bicalutamide

Anticoagulants: bicalutamide possibly enhances anticoagulant effect of coumarins

Biguanides *see* Antidiabetics

Bilastine *see* Antihistamines

Bile Acid Sequestrants *see* Colesevelam, Colestipol, and Colestyramine

Bile Acids

Antacids: absorption of bile acids possibly reduced by antacids

- Ciclosporin: ursodeoxycholic acid increases absorption of ●ciclosporin

Bile Acids *(continued)*

Lipid-regulating Drugs: absorption of bile acids possibly reduced by colestipol and colestyramine

Bisoprolol *see Beta-blockers*

Bisphosphonates

Antacids: absorption of bisphosphonates reduced by antacids

Antibacterials: increased risk of hypocalcaemia when bisphosphonates given with aminoglycosides

Calcium Salts: absorption of bisphosphonates reduced by calcium salts

- Cytotoxics: sodium clodronate increases plasma concentration of ●estramustine

Iron: absorption of bisphosphonates reduced by *oral* iron

Bivalirudin

- Analgesics: increased risk of haemorrhage when anticoagulants given with *intravenous* ●diclofenac (avoid concomitant use, including low-dose heparins); increased risk of haemorrhage when anticoagulants given with ●ketorolac (avoid concomitant use, including low-dose heparins)
- Anticoagulants: increased risk of haemorrhage when other anticoagulants given with ●apixaban, ●dabigatran and ●rivaroxaban (avoid concomitant use except when switching with other anticoagulants or using heparin to maintain catheter patency)

Bleomycin

- Antipsychotics: avoid concomitant use of cytotoxics with ●clozapine (increased risk of agranulocytosis)

Cardiac Glycosides: bleomycin possibly reduces absorption of digoxin *tablets*

- Cytotoxics: increased risk of pulmonary toxicity when bleomycin given with ●brentuximab vedotin—avoid concomitant use; increased pulmonary toxicity when bleomycin given with ●cisplatin

Boceprevir

Alpha-blockers: boceprevir possibly increases plasma concentration of doxazosin and tamsulosin—manufacturer of boceprevir advises avoid concomitant use

Analgesics: possible increased risk of prolonged sedation and respiratory depression when boceprevir given with buprenorphine; boceprevir possibly affects plasma concentration of methadone

- Antibacterials: manufacturer of boceprevir advises avoid concomitant use with ●rifampicin (plasma concentration of boceprevir possibly reduced)

Anticoagulants: avoidance of boceprevir advised by manufacturer of apixaban

- Antiepileptics: manufacturer of boceprevir advises avoid concomitant use with ●carbamazepine, ●phenobarbital and ●phenytoin (plasma concentration of boceprevir possibly reduced)
- Antimalarials: manufacturer of boceprevir advises avoid concomitant use with ●artemether with lumefantrine
- Antipsychotics: boceprevir possibly increases plasma concentration of ●lurasidone—avoid concomitant use; manufacturer of boceprevir advises avoid concomitant use with ●pimozide; boceprevir possibly increases plasma concentration of ●quetiapine—manufacturer of quetiapine advises avoid concomitant use
- Antivirals: boceprevir reduces plasma concentration of ●atazanavir; boceprevir possibly increases the plasma concentration of ●daclatasvir—reduce dose of daclatasvir (see Dose under Daclatasvir, p. 438); avoid concomitant use of boceprevir with ●darunavir; effects of both drugs reduced when boceprevir given with etravirine; avoidance of boceprevir advised by manufacturer of ●fosamprenavir, nevirapine and tipranavir; manufacturers advise avoid concomitant use of boceprevir with ●lopinavir; boceprevir increases plasma concentration of maraviroc (consider reducing dose of maraviroc);

Boceprevir

- Antivirals *(continued)*

plasma concentration of both drugs reduced when boceprevir given with ●ritonavir

- Anxiolytics and Hypnotics: boceprevir increases plasma concentration of *oral* ●midazolam—manufacturer of boceprevir advises avoid concomitant use

Cardiac Glycosides: boceprevir possibly increases side-effects of digoxin

- Ciclosporin: boceprevir increases plasma concentration of ●ciclosporin
- Cilostazol: boceprevir possibly increases plasma concentration of ●cilostazol (see Dose under Cilostazol, p. 141)

Cobicistat: avoidance of boceprevir advised by manufacturer of cobicistat

- Cytotoxics: boceprevir possibly increases the plasma concentration of ●bosutinib—manufacturer of bosutinib advises avoid or consider reducing dose of bosutinib; manufacturer of boceprevir advises avoid concomitant use with ●dasatinib, ●erlotinib, ●gefitinib, ●imatinib, ●lapatinib, ●nilotinib, ●pazopanib, ●sorafenib and ●sunitinib; manufacturer of ruxolitinib advises dose reduction when boceprevir given with ●ruxolitinib—consult ruxolitinib product literature
- Domperidone: possible increased risk of ventricular arrhythmias when boceprevir given with ●domperidone—avoid concomitant use
- Ergot Alkaloids: manufacturer of boceprevir advises avoid concomitant use with ●ergot alkaloids
- Lipid-regulating Drugs: boceprevir increases plasma concentration of atorvastatin (reduce dose of atorvastatin); boceprevir increases plasma concentration of pravastatin; manufacturers advise avoid concomitant use of boceprevir with ●simvastatin

Progestogens: boceprevir increases plasma concentration of drospirenone (increased risk of toxicity)

- Sirolimus: boceprevir increases plasma concentration of ●sirolimus (increased risk of toxicity—reduce sirolimus dose)
- Tacrolimus: boceprevir increases plasma concentration of ●tacrolimus (reduce dose of tacrolimus)

Bortezomib

- Antibacterials: plasma concentration of bortezomib reduced by ●rifampicin—manufacturer of bortezomib advises avoid concomitant use

Antidepressants: plasma concentration of bortezomib possibly reduced by St John's wort—manufacturer of bortezomib advises avoid concomitant use

Antiepileptics: plasma concentration of bortezomib possibly reduced by carbamazepine, phenobarbital and phenytoin—manufacturer of bortezomib advises avoid concomitant use

- Antipsychotics: avoid concomitant use of cytotoxics with ●clozapine (increased risk of agranulocytosis)

Bosentan

- Antibacterials: plasma concentration of bosentan reduced by ●rifampicin—avoid concomitant use

Anticoagulants: manufacturer of bosentan recommends monitoring anticoagulant effect of coumarins

- Antidiabetics: increased risk of hepatotoxicity when bosentan given with ●glibenclamide—avoid concomitant use
- Antifungals: plasma concentration of bosentan possibly increased by ●fluconazole—avoid concomitant use; plasma concentration of bosentan possibly increased by itraconazole
- Antivirals: avoidance of bosentan advised by manufacturer of elvitegravir and tipranavir; bosentan possibly reduces plasma concentration of indinavir; plasma concentration of bosentan increased by ●lopinavir and ●ritonavir (consider reducing dose of bosentan); bosentan possibly reduces plasma con-

Bosentan

- Antivirals *(continued)*
  centration of telaprevir, also plasma concentration of bosentan possibly increased
  Avanafil: bosentan possibly reduces plasma concentration of avanafil—manufacturer of avanafil advises avoid concomitant use
- Ciclosporin: plasma concentration of bosentan increased by ●ciclosporin (also plasma concentration of ciclosporin reduced—avoid concomitant use)
  Cobicistat: avoidance of bosentan advised by manufacturer of cobicistat
- Cytotoxics: bosentan possibly reduces plasma concentration of ●bosutinib—manufacturer of bosutinib advises avoid concomitant use
  Lipid-regulating Drugs: bosentan reduces plasma concentration of simvastatin
- Oestrogens: bosentan possibly causes contraceptive failure of hormonal contraceptives containing ●oestrogens (alternative contraception recommended)
- Progestogens: bosentan possibly causes contraceptive failure of hormonal contraceptives containing ●progestogens (alternative contraception recommended)
  Riociguat: bosentan reduces plasma concentration of riociguat
  Sildenafil: bosentan reduces plasma concentration of sildenafil, also plasma concentration of bosentan increased
  Tadalafil: bosentan reduces plasma concentration of tadalafil

Bosutinib

- Analgesics: possible increased risk of ventricular arrhythmias when bosutinib given with ●methadone
  Antacids: manufacturer of bosutinib advises separating administration with antacids by about 12 hours
- Anti-arrhythmics: possible increased risk of ventricular arrhythmias when bosutinib given with ●amiodarone and ●disopyramide; plasma concentration of bosutinib possibly increased by ●dronedarone—manufacturer of bosutinib advises avoid or consider reducing dose of bosutinib
- Antibacterials: plasma concentration of bosutinib possibly increased by ●ciprofloxacin, ●clarithromycin, ●erythromycin and ●telithromycin—manufacturer of bosutinib advises avoid or consider reducing dose of bosutinib; possible increased risk of ventricular arrhythmias when bosutinib given with ●moxifloxacin; plasma concentration of bosutinib possibly reduced by ●rifabutin—manufacturer of bosutinib advises avoid concomitant use; plasma concentration of bosutinib reduced by ●rifampicin—manufacturer of bosutinib advises avoid concomitant use
- Antidepressants: plasma concentration of bosutinib possibly reduced by ●St John's wort—manufacturer of bosutinib advises avoid concomitant use
- Antiepileptics: plasma concentration of bosutinib possibly reduced by ●carbamazepine, ●phenobarbital and ●phenytoin—manufacturer of bosutinib advises avoid concomitant use
- Antifungals: plasma concentration of bosutinib possibly increased by ●fluconazole, ●itraconazole, ●posaconazole and ●voriconazole—manufacturer of bosutinib advises avoid or consider reducing dose of bosutinib
- Antimalarials: possible increased risk of ventricular arrhythmias when bosutinib given with ●chloroquine and hydroxychloroquine
- Antipsychotics: possible increased risk of ventricular arrhythmias when bosutinib given with ●haloperidol; avoid concomitant use of cytotoxics with ●clozapine (increased risk of agranulocytosis)
- Antivirals: plasma concentration of bosutinib possibly increased by ●atazanavir, ●boceprevir, ●darunavir, ●fosamprenavir, ●indinavir, ●ritonavir, ●saquinavir

Bosutinib

- Antivirals *(continued)*
  and ●telaprevir—manufacturer of bosutinib advises avoid or consider reducing dose of bosutinib; plasma concentration of bosutinib possibly reduced by ●efavirenz and ●etravirine—manufacturer of bosutinib advises avoid concomitant use
- Aprepitant: plasma concentration of bosutinib possibly increased by ●aprepitant—manufacturer of bosutinib advises avoid or consider reducing dose of bosutinib
- Beta-blockers: possible increased risk of ventricular arrhythmias when bosutinib given with ●sotalol
- Bosentan: plasma concentration of bosutinib possibly reduced by ●bosentan—manufacturer of bosutinib advises avoid concomitant use
- Calcium-channel Blockers: plasma concentration of bosutinib possibly increased by ●diltiazem and ●verapamil—manufacturer of bosutinib advises avoid or consider reducing dose of bosutinib
- Cytotoxics: plasma concentration of bosutinib possibly increased by ●imatinib—manufacturer of bosutinib advises avoid or consider reducing dose of bosutinib
- Domperidone: manufacturer of bosutinib advises avoid concomitant use with ●domperidone (risk of ventricular arrhythmias)
- Grapefruit Juice: plasma concentration of bosutinib possibly increased by ●grapefruit juice—manufacturer of bosutinib advises avoid or consider reducing dose of bosutinib
- Modafinil: plasma concentration of bosutinib possibly reduced by ●modafinil—manufacturer of bosutinib advises avoid concomitant use
  Ulcer-healing Drugs: plasma concentration of bosutinib reduced by lansoprazole

Brentuximab vedotin

  Antibacterials: effects of brentuximab vedotin possibly reduced by rifampicin
- Antipsychotics: avoid concomitant use of cytotoxics with ●clozapine (increased risk of agranulocytosis)
- Cytotoxics: increased risk of pulmonary toxicity when brentuximab vedotin given with ●bleomycin—avoid concomitant use
- Vaccines: avoid concomitant use of monoclonal antibodies with live ●vaccines (see p. 842)

Brimonidine

  Antidepressants: manufacturer of brimonidine advises avoid concomitant use with MAOIs, tricyclic-related antidepressants and tricyclics

Brinzolamide *see* Diuretics

Bromocriptine

  Alcohol: tolerance of bromocriptine reduced by alcohol
  Antibacterials: plasma concentration of bromocriptine increased by erythromycin (increased risk of toxicity); plasma concentration of bromocriptine possibly increased by macrolides (increased risk of toxicity)
  Antipsychotics: hypoprolactinaemic and antiparkinsonian effects of bromocriptine antagonised by antipsychotics
  Domperidone: hypoprolactinaemic effect of bromocriptine possibly antagonised by domperidone
  Hormone Antagonists: plasma concentration of bromocriptine increased by octreotide
  Memantine: effects of dopaminergics possibly enhanced by memantine
  Methyldopa: antiparkinsonian effect of dopaminergics antagonised by methyldopa
  Metoclopramide: hypoprolactinaemic effect of bromocriptine antagonised by metoclopramide
- Sympathomimetics: risk of toxicity when bromocriptine given with ●isometheptene

Buclizine *see* Antihistamines
Budesonide *see* Corticosteroids

Bumetanide *see* Diuretics

Bupivacaine

Anti-arrhythmics: increased myocardial depression when bupivacaine given with anti-arrhythmics

- Beta-blockers: increased risk of bupivacaine toxicity when given with ●propranolol

Buprenorphine *see* Opioid Analgesics

Bupropion

- Antidepressants: bupropion possibly increases plasma concentration of citalopram; manufacturer of bupropion advises avoid for 2 weeks after stopping ●MAOIs; manufacturer of bupropion advises avoid concomitant use with ●moclobemide; bupropion possibly increases plasma concentration of tricyclics (possible increased risk of convulsions)

Antiepileptics: plasma concentration of bupropion reduced by carbamazepine and phenytoin; metabolism of bupropion inhibited by valproate

Antivirals: metabolism of bupropion accelerated by efavirenz (reduced plasma concentration); plasma concentration of bupropion reduced by ritonavir

Atomoxetine: possible increased risk of convulsions when bupropion given with atomoxetine

Dopaminergics: increased risk of side-effects when bupropion given with amantadine or levodopa

- Hormone Antagonists: bupropion possibly inhibits metabolism of ●tamoxifen to active metabolite (avoid concomitant use)
- Methylthioninium: possible risk of CNS toxicity when bupropion given with ●methylthioninium—avoid concomitant use (if avoidance not possible, use lowest possible dose of methylthioninium and observe patient for up to 4 hours after administration)

Buspirone *see* Anxiolytics and Hypnotics

Busulfan

Analgesics: metabolism of *intravenous* busulfan possibly inhibited by paracetamol (manufacturer of *intravenous* busulfan advises caution within 72 hours of paracetamol)

- Antibacterials: plasma concentration of busulfan increased by ●metronidazole (increased risk of toxicity)

Antiepileptics: plasma concentration of busulfan possibly reduced by phenytoin

Antifungals: metabolism of busulfan inhibited by itraconazole (increased risk of toxicity)

- Antipsychotics: avoid concomitant use of cytotoxics with ●clozapine (increased risk of agranulocytosis)

Cytotoxics: increased risk of hepatotoxicity when busulfan given with tioguanine

Butyrophenones *see* Antipsychotics

Cabazitaxel

- Antibacterials: plasma concentration of cabazitaxel possibly increased by ●clarithromycin and ●telithromycin—manufacturer of cabazitaxel advises avoid or consider reducing dose of cabazitaxel; manufacturer of cabazitaxel advises avoid concomitant use with ●rifabutin; plasma concentration of cabazitaxel reduced by ●rifampicin—manufacturer of cabazitaxel advises avoid concomitant use
- Antidepressants: manufacturer of cabazitaxel advises avoid concomitant use with ●St John's wort
- Antiepileptics: manufacturer of cabazitaxel advises avoid concomitant use with ●carbamazepine, ●phenobarbital and ●phenytoin
- Antifungals: plasma concentration of cabazitaxel possibly increased by ●itraconazole and ●voriconazole—manufacturer of cabazitaxel advises avoid or consider reducing dose of cabazitaxel
- Antipsychotics: avoid concomitant use of cytotoxics with ●clozapine (increased risk of agranulocytosis)
- Antivirals: manufacturer of cabazitaxel advises avoid concomitant use with ●atazanavir; plasma concentration of cabazitaxel possibly increased by ●indinavir, ●ritonavir and ●saquinavir—manufac-

Cabazitaxel

- Antivirals *(continued)*

turer of cabazitaxel advises avoid or consider reducing dose of cabazitaxel

Cabergoline

Antibacterials: plasma concentration of cabergoline increased by erythromycin (increased risk of toxicity); plasma concentration of cabergoline possibly increased by macrolides (increased risk of toxicity)

Antipsychotics: hypoprolactinaemic and anti-parkinsonian effects of cabergoline antagonised by antipsychotics

Domperidone: hypoprolactinaemic effect of cabergoline possibly antagonised by domperidone

Memantine: effects of dopaminergics possibly enhanced by memantine

Methyldopa: antiparkinsonian effect of dopaminergics antagonised by methyldopa

Metoclopramide: hypoprolactinaemic effect of cabergoline antagonised by metoclopramide

Cabozantinib

- Antibacterials: plasma concentration of cabozantinib possibly increased by clarithromycin and erythromycin; plasma concentration of cabozantinib reduced by ●rifampicin—avoid concomitant use

Antidepressants: plasma concentration of cabozantinib possibly reduced by St John's wort—manufacturer of cabozantinib advises avoid concomitant use

- Antiepileptics: plasma concentration of cabozantinib possibly reduced by ●carbamazepine, ●phenobarbital and ●phenytoin—avoid concomitant use

Antifungals: plasma concentration of cabozantinib possibly increased by itraconazole

- Antipsychotics: avoid concomitant use of cytotoxics with ●clozapine (increased risk of agranulocytosis)

Antivirals: plasma concentration of cabozantinib possibly increased by ritonavir

Corticosteroids: plasma concentration of cabozantinib possibly reduced by dexamethasone—manufacturer of cabozantinib advises avoid concomitant use

Grapefruit Juice: plasma concentration of cabozantinib possibly increased by grapefruit juice

Caffeine citrate

Anti-arrhythmics: caffeine citrate antagonises anti-arrhythmic effect of adenosine—manufacturer of adenosine advises avoid caffeine citrate for at least 12 hours before adenosine

Antiepileptics: caffeine citrate possibly antagonises effects of phenobarbital; plasma concentration of caffeine citrate reduced by phenytoin

Theophylline: manufacturer of caffeine citrate advises avoid concomitant use with theophylline

Ulcer-healing Drugs: plasma concentration of caffeine citrate increased by cimetidine

Calcitriol *see* Vitamins

Calcium Salts

Note *see also* Antacids

Antibacterials: calcium salts reduce absorption of ciprofloxacin and tetracycline

Antivirals: calcium salts reduce absorption of dolutegravir—manufacturer of dolutegravir advises give at least 2 hours before or 6 hours after calcium salts; manufacturer of rilpivirine advises give calcium salts 2 hours before or 4 hours after rilpivirine

Bisphosphonates: calcium salts reduce absorption of bisphosphonates

Cardiac Glycosides: large *intravenous* doses of calcium salts can precipitate arrhythmias when given with cardiac glycosides

Corticosteroids: absorption of calcium salts reduced by corticosteroids

Cytotoxics: calcium salts reduce absorption of estramustine (manufacturer of estramustine advises avoid concomitant administration)

Diuretics: increased risk of hypercalcaemia when calcium salts given with thiazides and related diuretics

Calcium Salts (continued)

Eltrombopag: calcium salts possibly reduce absorption of eltrombopag (give at least 4 hours apart)

Fluorides: calcium salts reduce absorption of fluorides

Iron: calcium salts reduce absorption of *oral* iron

Thyroid Hormones: calcium salts reduce absorption of levothyroxine

Zinc: calcium salts reduce absorption of zinc

Calcium-channel Blockers

Note Dihydropyridine calcium-channel blockers include amlodipine, felodipine, isradipine, lacidipine, lercanidipine, nicardipine, nifedipine, and nimodipine

ACE Inhibitors: enhanced hypotensive effect when calcium-channel blockers given with ACE inhibitors

Adrenergic Neurone Blockers: enhanced hypotensive effect when calcium-channel blockers given with adrenergic neurone blockers

Alcohol: enhanced hypotensive effect when calcium-channel blockers given with alcohol; verapamil possibly increases plasma concentration of alcohol

Aldesleukin: enhanced hypotensive effect when calcium-channel blockers given with aldesleukin

Aliskiren: verapamil increases plasma concentration of aliskiren

• Alpha-blockers: verapamil increases plasma concentration of tamsulosin; enhanced hypotensive effect when calcium-channel blockers given with ●alpha-blockers, also increased risk of first-dose hypotension with post-synaptic alpha-blockers such as prazosin

• Anaesthetics, General: enhanced hypotensive effect when calcium-channel blockers given with general anaesthetics or isoflurane; hypotensive effect of verapamil enhanced by ●general anaesthetics (also AV delay)

Analgesics: hypotensive effect of calcium-channel blockers antagonised by NSAIDs; diltiazem inhibits metabolism of alfentanil (risk of prolonged or delayed respiratory depression)

Angiotensin-II Receptor Antagonists: enhanced hypotensive effect when calcium-channel blockers given with angiotensin-II receptor antagonists

• Anti-arrhythmics: increased risk of bradycardia, AV block and myocardial depression when diltiazem or verapamil given with ●amiodarone; increased risk of myocardial depression and asystole when verapamil given with ●disopyramide or ●flecainide; increased risk of bradycardia and myocardial depression when diltiazem and verapamil given with ●dronedarone; nifedipine increases plasma concentration of ●dronedarone

• Antibacterials: metabolism of calcium-channel blockers possibly inhibited by ●clarithromycin, ●erythromycin and ●telithromycin (increased risk of side-effects); manufacturer of lercanidipine advises avoid concomitant use with erythromycin; metabolism of diltiazem, nifedipine, nimodipine and verapamil accelerated by ●rifampicin (plasma concentration significantly reduced); metabolism of isradipine and nicardipine possibly accelerated by ●rifampicin (possible significantly reduced plasma concentration); plasma concentration of felodipine possibly reduced by rifampicin

• Anticoagulants: verapamil possibly increases plasma concentration of ●dabigatran (see Dose under Dabigatran, p. 156)

• Antidepressants: metabolism of nifedipine possibly inhibited by fluoxetine (increased plasma concentration); diltiazem and verapamil increase plasma concentration of imipramine; enhanced hypotensive effect when calcium-channel blockers given with MAOIs; plasma concentration of amlodipine and felodipine possibly reduced by St John's wort; plasma concentration of verapamil significantly reduced by ●St John's wort; plasma concentration of nifedipine reduced by St John's wort; diltiazem

Calcium-channel Blockers

• Antidepressants (continued)

and verapamil possibly increase plasma concentration of tricyclics

Antidiabetics: glucose tolerance occasionally impaired when nifedipine given with insulin

• Antiepileptics: effects of dihydropyridines, nicardipine and nifedipine probably reduced by carbamazepine; effects of felodipine and isradipine reduced by carbamazepine; diltiazem and verapamil enhance effects of ●carbamazepine; manufacturer of nimodipine advises avoid concomitant use with carbamazepine and phenytoin (plasma concentration of nimodipine possibly reduced); effects of calcium-channel blockers probably reduced by ●phenobarbital; manufacturer of nimodipine advises avoid concomitant use with ●phenobarbital (plasma concentration of nimodipine reduced); manufacturer of isradipine advises avoid concomitant use with phenobarbital and phenytoin; effects of felodipine and verapamil reduced by phenytoin; diltiazem increases plasma concentration of ●phenytoin but also effect of diltiazem reduced

• Antifungals: negative inotropic effect possibly increased when calcium-channel blockers given with itraconazole; metabolism of dihydropyridines possibly inhibited by itraconazole (increased plasma concentration); metabolism of felodipine inhibited by ●itraconazole (increased plasma concentration); manufacturer of lercanidipine advises avoid concomitant use with itraconazole; plasma concentration of nifedipine increased by micafungin

Antimalarials: possible increased risk of bradycardia when calcium-channel blockers given with mefloquine

Antimuscarinics: avoidance of verapamil advised by manufacturer of darifenacin; verapamil increases plasma concentration of solifenacin

• Antipsychotics: enhanced hypotensive effect when calcium-channel blockers given with antipsychotics; verapamil possibly increases the plasma concentration of ●lurasidone (see Dose under Lurasidone, p. 243); diltiazem increases the plasma concentration of ●lurasidone (see Dose under Lurasidone, p. 243)

• Antivirals: plasma concentration of diltiazem increased by ●atazanavir (reduce dose of diltiazem); plasma concentration of verapamil possibly increased by atazanavir; plasma concentration of diltiazem reduced by efavirenz; manufacturer of lercanidipine advises avoid concomitant use with ritonavir; plasma concentration of calcium-channel blockers possibly increased by ●ritonavir; caution with diltiazem, felodipine, nicardipine, nifedipine and verapamil advised by manufacturer of telaprevir; plasma concentration of amlodipine increased by telaprevir (consider reducing dose of amlodipine)

Anxiolytics and Hypnotics: enhanced hypotensive effect when calcium-channel blockers given with anxiolytics and hypnotics; diltiazem and verapamil inhibit metabolism of midazolam (increased plasma concentration with increased sedation); absorption of lercanidipine increased by midazolam; diltiazem and verapamil increase plasma concentration of buspirone (reduce dose of buspirone)

Aprepitant: plasma concentration of both drugs may increase when diltiazem given with aprepitant

Avanafil: diltiazem and verapamil possibly increase plasma concentration of ●avanafil—see Dose under Avanafil, p. 571

• Beta-blockers: enhanced hypotensive effect when calcium-channel blockers given with beta-blockers; increased risk of AV block and bradycardia when diltiazem given with ●beta-blockers; asystole, severe hypotension and heart failure when verapamil given with ●beta-blockers (see p. 138); possible severe

Calcium-channel Blockers

- Beta-blockers *(continued)*
  hypotension and heart failure when nifedipine given with ●beta-blockers
  Calcium-channel Blockers: plasma concentration of both drugs may increase when diltiazem given with nifedipine
- Cardiac Glycosides: diltiazem, lercanidipine and nicardipine increase plasma concentration of ●digoxin; verapamil increases plasma concentration of ●digoxin, also increased risk of AV block and bradycardia; nifedipine possibly increases plasma concentration of ●digoxin
- Ciclosporin: diltiazem, nicardipine and verapamil increase plasma concentration of ●ciclosporin; combination of lercanidipine with ●ciclosporin may increase plasma concentration of either drug (or both)—avoid concomitant use; plasma concentration of nifedipine possibly increased by ciclosporin (increased risk of toxicity including gingival hyperplasia)
  Cilostazol: diltiazem increases plasma concentration of cilostazol (consider reducing dose of cilostazol)
  Clonidine: enhanced hypotensive effect when calcium-channel blockers given with clonidine
- Colchicine: diltiazem and verapamil possibly increase risk of ●colchicine toxicity—suspend or reduce dose of colchicine (avoid concomitant use in hepatic or renal impairment)
  Corticosteroids: hypotensive effect of calcium-channel blockers antagonised by corticosteroids; diltiazem increases plasma concentration of methylprednisolone
- Cytotoxics: verapamil possibly increases plasma concentration of doxorubicin; verapamil possibly increases the plasma concentration of afatinib—manufacturer of afatinib advises separating administration of verapamil by 6 to 12 hours; diltiazem and verapamil possibly increase the plasma concentration of ●bosutinib—manufacturer of bosutinib advises avoid or consider reducing dose of bosutinib; possible increased risk of bradycardia when diltiazem or verapamil given with crizotinib; plasma concentration of both drugs may increase when verapamil given with ●everolimus (consider reducing the dose of everolimus —consult everolimus product literature); diltiazem and verapamil possibly increase the plasma concentration of ●ibrutinib—reduce dose of ibrutinib (see Dose under Ibrutinib, p. 615); nifedipine possibly inhibits metabolism of vincristine
  Dapoxetine: manufacturer of dapoxetine advises dose reduction when diltiazem and verapamil given with dapoxetine (see Dose under Dapoxetine, p. 572)
  Diazoxide: enhanced hypotensive effect when calcium-channel blockers given with diazoxide
  Diuretics: enhanced hypotensive effect when calcium-channel blockers given with diuretics; diltiazem and verapamil increase plasma concentration of eplerenone (reduce dose of eplerenone)
  Dopaminergics: enhanced hypotensive effect when calcium-channel blockers given with levodopa
  Fidaxomicin: avoidance of verapamil advised by manufacturer of fidaxomicin
  Fingolimod: possible increased risk of bradycardia when diltiazem or verapamil given with ●fingolimod
  Grapefruit Juice: plasma concentration of felodipine, isradipine, lacidipine, lercanidipine, nicardipine, nifedipine, nimodipine and verapamil increased by grapefruit juice; plasma concentration of amlodipine possibly increased by grapefruit juice
  Hormone Antagonists: diltiazem and verapamil increase plasma concentration of dutasteride; possible increased risk of bradycardia when diltiazem or verapamil given with pasireotide

Calcium-channel Blockers *(continued)*

- Ivabradine: diltiazem and verapamil increase plasma concentration of ●ivabradine—avoid concomitant use
- Lenalidomide: verapamil possibly increases plasma concentration of ●lenalidomide (increased risk of toxicity)
- Lipid-regulating Drugs: diltiazem increases plasma concentration of atorvastatin—possible increased risk of myopathy; plasma concentration of verapamil increased by ●atorvastatin, also possible increased risk of myopathy (consider reducing dose of atorvastatin); possible increased risk of myopathy when amlodipine and diltiazem given with ●simvastatin (see Dose under Simvastatin, p. 177); increased risk of myopathy when verapamil given with ●simvastatin (see Dose under Simvastatin, p. 177); avoidance of diltiazem and verapamil advised by manufacturer of ●lomitapide (plasma concentration of lomitapide possibly increased)
  Lithium: neurotoxicity may occur when diltiazem or verapamil given with lithium without increased plasma concentration of lithium
- Magnesium (parenteral): profound hypotension reported with concomitant use of nifedipine and ●parenteral magnesium in pre-eclampsia
  Methyldopa: enhanced hypotensive effect when calcium-channel blockers given with methyldopa
  Moxisylyte: enhanced hypotensive effect when calcium-channel blockers given with moxisylyte
  Moxonidine: enhanced hypotensive effect when calcium-channel blockers given with moxonidine
  Muscle Relaxants: verapamil enhances effects of non-depolarising muscle relaxants and suxamethonium; enhanced hypotensive effect when calcium-channel blockers given with baclofen or tizanidine; possible increased risk of ventricular arrhythmias when diltiazem given with *intravenous* dantrolene—manufacturer of diltiazem advises avoid concomitant use; manufacturer of verapamil advises avoid concomitant use of *intravenous* dantrolene; calcium-channel blockers possibly enhance effects of non-depolarising muscle relaxants
  Nitrates: enhanced hypotensive effect when calcium-channel blockers given with nitrates
  Oestrogens: hypotensive effect of calcium-channel blockers antagonised by oestrogens
  Prostaglandins: enhanced hypotensive effect when calcium-channel blockers given with alprostadil
  Ranolazine: diltiazem and verapamil increase plasma concentration of ranolazine (consider reducing dose of ranolazine)
  Sildenafil: enhanced hypotensive effect when amlodipine given with sildenafil
- Sirolimus: diltiazem increases plasma concentration of ●sirolimus; plasma concentration of both drugs increased when verapamil given with ●sirolimus
  Sulfinpyrazone: plasma concentration of verapamil reduced by sulfinpyrazone
- Tacrolimus: diltiazem and nifedipine increase plasma concentration of ●tacrolimus; felodipine, nicardipine and verapamil possibly increase plasma concentration of tacrolimus
- Theophylline: calcium-channel blockers possibly increase plasma concentration of ●theophylline (enhanced effect); diltiazem increases plasma concentration of theophylline; verapamil increases plasma concentration of ●theophylline (enhanced effect)
  Ticagrelor: diltiazem increases plasma concentration of ticagrelor
  Ulcer-healing Drugs: metabolism of calcium-channel blockers possibly inhibited by cimetidine (increased plasma concentration); plasma concentration of isradipine increased by cimetidine (halve dose of isradipine)

Calcium-channel Blockers *(continued)*

  Ulipristal: avoidance of verapamil advised by manufacturer of *low-dose* ulipristal

  Vardenafil: enhanced hypotensive effect when nifedipine given with vardenafil

  Vasodilator Antihypertensives: enhanced hypotensive effect when calcium-channel blockers given with hydralazine, minoxidil or sodium nitroprusside

Calcium-channel Blockers (dihydropyridines) *see* Calcium-channel Blockers

Canagliflozin *see* Antidiabetics

Canakinumab

- Antipsychotics: avoid concomitant use of cytotoxics with ●clozapine (increased risk of agranulocytosis)
- Vaccines: avoid concomitant use of monoclonal antibodies with live ●vaccines (see p. 842)

Candesartan *see* Angiotensin-II Receptor Antagonists

Cannabis Extract

- Antibacterials: plasma concentration of cannabis extract reduced by ●rifampicin—manufacturer of cannabis extract advises avoid concomitant use
- Antidepressants: plasma concentration of cannabis extract possibly reduced by ●St John's wort—manufacturer of cannabis extract advises avoid concomitant use; possible increased risk of hypertension and tachycardia when cannabis extract given with tricyclics
- Antiepileptics: plasma concentration of cannabis extract possibly reduced by ●carbamazepine, ●phenobarbital and ●phenytoin—manufacturer of cannabis extract advises avoid concomitant use

Capecitabine *see* Fluorouracil

Capreomycin

  Antibacterials: increased risk of nephrotoxicity when capreomycin given with colistimethate sodium or polymyxins; increased risk of nephrotoxicity and ototoxicity when capreomycin given with aminoglycosides or vancomycin

  Cytotoxics: increased risk of nephrotoxicity and ototoxicity when capreomycin given with platinum compounds

  Vaccines: antibacterials inactivate oral typhoid vaccine—see p. 864

Captopril *see* ACE Inhibitors

Carbamazepine

  Alcohol: CNS side-effects of carbamazepine possibly increased by alcohol

- Analgesics: effects of carbamazepine enhanced by ●dextropropoxyphene; carbamazepine possibly accelerates metabolism of fentanyl (reduced effect); carbamazepine reduces plasma concentration of methadone; carbamazepine reduces effects of tramadol; carbamazepine possibly accelerates metabolism of paracetamol (also isolated reports of hepatotoxicity)
- Anti-arrhythmics: carbamazepine possibly reduces plasma concentration of ●dronedarone—avoid concomitant use
- Antibacterials: plasma concentration of carbamazepine increased by ●clarithromycin (consider reducing dose of carbamazepine); plasma concentration of carbamazepine increased by ●erythromycin; plasma concentration of carbamazepine reduced by ●rifabutin; carbamazepine accelerates metabolism of doxycycline (reduced effect); carbamazepine possibly reduces plasma concentration of ●bedaquiline—manufacturer of bedaquiline advises avoid concomitant use; avoidance of carbamazepine advised by manufacturer of delamanid; plasma concentration of carbamazepine increased by ●isoniazid (also possibly increased isoniazid hepatotoxicity); carbamazepine reduces plasma concentration of ●telithromycin (avoid during and for 2 weeks after carbamazepine)
- Anticoagulants: carbamazepine possibly reduces plasma concentration of ●apixaban—manufacturer

Carbamazepine

- Anticoagulants *(continued)*
of apixaban advises avoid concomitant use when given for treatment of deep-vein thrombosis or pulmonary embolism; carbamazepine accelerates metabolism of ●coumarins (reduced anticoagulant effect); carbamazepine possibly reduces plasma concentration of dabigatran—manufacturer of dabigatran advises avoid concomitant use; carbamazepine possibly reduces plasma concentration of ●rivaroxaban—manufacturer of rivaroxaban advises monitor for signs of thrombosis
- Antidepressants: carbamazepine possibly reduces plasma concentration of reboxetine; plasma concentration of carbamazepine increased by ●fluoxetine and ●fluvoxamine; carbamazepine reduces plasma concentration of ●mianserin, mirtazapine and trazodone; manufacturer of carbamazepine advises avoid for 2 weeks after stopping ●MAOIs, also antagonism of anticonvulsant effect; anticonvulsant effect of antiepileptics possibly antagonised by MAOIs and ●tricyclic-related antidepressants (convulsive threshold lowered); anticonvulsant effect of antiepileptics antagonised by ●SSRIs and ●tricyclics (convulsive threshold lowered); plasma concentration of carbamazepine possibly reduced by St John's wort; carbamazepine accelerates metabolism of ●tricyclics (reduced plasma concentration and reduced effect)
- Antiepileptics: carbamazepine possibly reduces plasma concentration of eslicarbazepine but risk of side-effects increased; carbamazepine possibly reduces plasma concentration of ethosuximide and retigabine; carbamazepine often reduces plasma concentration of lamotrigine, also plasma concentration of an active metabolite of carbamazepine sometimes raised (but evidence is conflicting); possible increased risk of carbamazepine toxicity when given with levetiracetam; plasma concentration of carbamazepine sometimes reduced by oxcarbazepine (but concentration of an active metabolite of carbamazepine may be increased), also plasma concentration of an active metabolite of oxcarbazepine often reduced; carbamazepine reduces plasma concentration of ●perampanel (see Dose under Perampanel, p. 313); carbamazepine possibly increases plasma concentration of phenobarbital, plasma concentration of both drugs often reduced when carbamazepine given with phenytoin, also plasma concentration of phenytoin may be increased; plasma concentration of both drugs possibly reduced when carbamazepine given with rufinamide; plasma concentration of carbamazepine increased by ●stiripentol; carbamazepine reduces plasma concentration of tiagabine and zonisamide; carbamazepine often reduces plasma concentration of topiramate; carbamazepine reduces plasma concentration of valproate, also plasma concentration of active metabolite of carbamazepine increased
- Antifungals: plasma concentration of carbamazepine possibly increased by fluconazole and miconazole; carbamazepine possibly reduces plasma concentration of itraconazole and ●posaconazole; carbamazepine possibly reduces plasma concentration of ●voriconazole—avoid concomitant use; carbamazepine possibly reduces plasma concentration of caspofungin—consider increasing dose of caspofungin
- Antimalarials: avoidance of carbamazepine advised by manufacturer of piperaquine with artenimol; anticonvulsant effect of antiepileptics antagonised by ●mefloquine
- Antipsychotics: anticonvulsant effect of antiepileptics antagonised by ●antipsychotics (convulsive threshold lowered); carbamazepine accelerates metabolism of haloperidol, olanzapine, quetiapine and risperidone (reduced plasma concentration);

Carbamazepine

- Antipsychotics *(continued)*
  carbamazepine reduces plasma concentration of
  ●aripiprazole (avoid concomitant use or consider
  increasing the dose of aripiprazole —consult aripiprazole product literature); carbamazepine accelerates metabolism of ●clozapine (reduced plasma
  concentration), also avoid concomitant use of drugs
  with substantial potential for causing agranulocytosis; carbamazepine possibly reduces plasma concentration of ●lurasidone—avoid concomitant use;
  carbamazepine reduces plasma concentration of
  paliperidone
- Antivirals: avoidance of carbamazepine advised by
  manufacturer of ●boceprevir and ●rilpivirine
  (plasma concentration of boceprevir and rilpivirine
  possibly reduced); carbamazepine possibly reduces
  plasma concentration of ●daclatasvir and ●simepre-
  vir—manufacturer of daclatasvir and simeprevir
  advises avoid concomitant use; carbamazepine possibly reduces plasma concentration of darunavir,
  fosamprenavir, lopinavir, saquinavir and tipranavir;
  avoidance of carbamazepine advised by manufacturer of ●dolutegravir, ●elvitegravir, etravirine, sofosbuvir and ●telaprevir; plasma concentration of both
  drugs reduced when carbamazepine given with efavirenz; carbamazepine possibly reduces plasma
  concentration of ●indinavir, also plasma concentration of carbamazepine possibly increased; carbamazepine reduces plasma concentration of nevirapine; plasma concentration of carbamazepine
  possibly increased by ●ritonavir
  Anxiolytics and Hypnotics: carbamazepine often
  reduces plasma concentration of clonazepam;
  carbamazepine reduces plasma concentration of
  midazolam
  Aprepitant: carbamazepine possibly reduces plasma
  concentration of aprepitant
  Avanafil: carbamazepine possibly reduces plasma concentration of avanafil—manufacturer of avanafil
  advises avoid concomitant use
  Bupropion: carbamazepine reduces plasma concentration of bupropion
- Calcium-channel Blockers: carbamazepine reduces
  effects of felodipine and isradipine; carbamazepine
  probably reduces effects of dihydropyridines, nicardipine and nifedipine; avoidance of carbamazepine
  advised by manufacturer of nimodipine (plasma
  concentration of nimodipine possibly reduced);
  effects of carbamazepine enhanced by ●diltiazem
  and ●verapamil
- Cannabis Extract: carbamazepine possibly reduces
  plasma concentration of ●cannabis extract—manufacturer of cannabis extract advises avoid concomitant use
- Ciclosporin: carbamazepine accelerates metabolism of
  ●ciclosporin (reduced plasma concentration)
- Clopidogrel: carbamazepine possibly reduces antiplatelet effect of ●clopidogrel
- Cobicistat: carbamazepine possibly reduces plasma
  concentration of ●cobicistat—manufacturer of cobicistat advises avoid concomitant use
- Corticosteroids: carbamazepine accelerates metabolism of ●corticosteroids (reduced effect)
- Cytotoxics: carbamazepine possibly decreases plasma
  concentration of axitinib (increase dose of axitinib—consult axitinib product literature); carbamazepine possibly reduces plasma concentration of bortezomib, ●bosutinib, crizotinib, ●ibrutinib, ●idelalisib
  and ponatinib—manufacturer of bortezomib, bosutinib, crizotinib, ibrutinib, idelalisib and ponatinib
  advises avoid concomitant use; carbamazepine possibly reduces plasma concentration of ●cabozanti-
  nib—avoid concomitant use; avoidance of carbamazepine advised by manufacturer of ●cabazitaxel,
  dabrafenib, gefitinib and vemurafenib; carbamaze-

Carbamazepine

- Cytotoxics *(continued)*
  pine reduces plasma concentration of ●imatinib and
  ●lapatinib—avoid concomitant use; avoidance of
  carbamazepine advised by manufacturer of vandetanib and ●vismodegib (plasma concentration of
  vandetanib and vismodegib possibly reduced);
  carbamazepine possibly reduces plasma concentration of eribulin; carbamazepine reduces plasma concentration of irinotecan and its active metabolite;
  manufacturer of procarbazine advises possible
  increased risk of hypersensitivity reactions when
  carbamazepine given with procarbazine
- Diuretics: increased risk of hyponatraemia when
  carbamazepine given with diuretics; plasma concentration of carbamazepine increased by ●acetazol-
  amide; carbamazepine reduces plasma concentration of ●eplerenone—avoid concomitant use
  Fingolimod: carbamazepine reduces plasma concentration of fingolimod
- Hormone Antagonists: carbamazepine possibly
  reduces plasma concentration of ●abiraterone—
  manufacturer of abiraterone advises avoid concomitant use; metabolism of carbamazepine inhibited by
  ●danazol (increased risk of toxicity); carbamazepine
  possibly accelerates metabolism of toremifene
  (reduced plasma concentration)
  5HT$_3$-receptor Antagonists: carbamazepine accelerates
  metabolism of ondansetron (reduced effect)
- Ivacaftor: carbamazepine possibly reduces plasma
  concentration of ●ivacaftor—manufacturer of ivacaftor advises avoid concomitant use
- Lipid-regulating Drugs: carbamazepine reduces plasma
  concentration of ●simvastatin—consider increasing
  dose of simvastatin
  Lithium: neurotoxicity may occur when carbamazepine given with lithium without increased plasma
  concentration of lithium
  Macitentan: avoidance of carbamazepine advised by
  manufacturer of ●macitentan
  Muscle Relaxants: carbamazepine antagonises muscle
  relaxant effect of non-depolarising muscle relaxants
  (accelerated recovery from neuromuscular blockade)
- Oestrogens: carbamazepine accelerates metabolism of
  ●oestrogens (reduced contraceptive effect—see
  p. 548)
- Orlistat: possible increased risk of convulsions when
  antiepileptics given with ●orlistat
- Progestogens: carbamazepine accelerates metabolism
  of ●progestogens (reduced contraceptive effect—
  see p. 548)
  Retinoids: plasma concentration of carbamazepine
  possibly reduced by isotretinoin
  Roflumilast: carbamazepine possibly inhibits effects of
  roflumilast (manufacturer of roflumilast advises
  avoid concomitant use)
  Theophylline: carbamazepine accelerates metabolism
  of theophylline (reduced effect)
  Thyroid Hormones: carbamazepine accelerates metabolism of thyroid hormones (may increase requirements for thyroid hormones in hypothyroidism)
  Tibolone: carbamazepine accelerates metabolism of
  tibolone (reduced plasma concentration)
  Ticagrelor: carbamazepine possibly reduces plasma
  concentration of ticagrelor
- Ulcer-healing Drugs: metabolism of carbamazepine
  inhibited by ●cimetidine (increased plasma concentration)
- Ulipristal: avoidance of carbamazepine advised by
  manufacturer of ●ulipristal (contraceptive effect of
  ulipristal possibly reduced)
  Vitamins: carbamazepine possibly increases requirements for vitamin D

Carbapenems see Ertapenem, Imipenem with Cilastatin, and Meropenem

Carbonic Anhydrase Inhibitors *see* Diuretics
Carboplatin *see* Platinum Compounds
Carboprost *see* Prostaglandins
Cardiac Glycosides
ACE Inhibitors: plasma concentration of digoxin possibly increased by captopril
Alpha-blockers: plasma concentration of digoxin increased by prazosin
Aminosalicylates: absorption of digoxin possibly reduced by sulfasalazine
Analgesics: plasma concentration of cardiac glycosides possibly increased by NSAIDs, also possible exacerbation of heart failure and reduction of renal function
Antacids: absorption of digoxin possibly reduced by antacids
- Anti-arrhythmics: plasma concentration of digoxin increased by ●amiodarone, ●dronedarone and ●propafenone (halve dose of digoxin)
Antibacterials: plasma concentration of digoxin possibly increased by gentamicin, telithromycin and trimethoprim; absorption of digoxin reduced by neomycin; plasma concentration of digoxin possibly reduced by rifampicin; plasma concentration of digoxin increased by macrolides (increased risk of toxicity)
- Antidepressants: plasma concentration of digoxin reduced by ●St John's wort—avoid concomitant use
Antidiabetics: plasma concentration of digoxin possibly reduced by acarbose; plasma concentration of digoxin increased by canagliflozin and sitagliptin
Antiepileptics: plasma concentration of digoxin possibly reduced by phenytoin
- Antifungals: increased cardiac toxicity with cardiac glycosides if hypokalaemia occurs with ●amphotericin; plasma concentration of digoxin increased by ●itraconazole
- Antimalarials: plasma concentration of digoxin possibly increased by ●chloroquine and hydroxychloroquine; possible increased risk of bradycardia when digoxin given with mefloquine; plasma concentration of digoxin increased by ●quinine
Antimuscarinics: plasma concentration of digoxin possibly increased by darifenacin
- Antivirals: side-effects of digoxin possibly increased by boceprevir; plasma concentration of digoxin increased by ●daclatasvir, etravirine, simeprevir and telaprevir; plasma concentration of digoxin possibly increased by ritonavir
Anxiolytics and Hypnotics: plasma concentration of digoxin increased by alprazolam (increased risk of toxicity)
Beta-blockers: increased risk of AV block and bradycardia when cardiac glycosides given with beta-blockers
Calcium Salts: arrhythmias can be precipitated when cardiac glycosides given with large *intravenous* doses of calcium salts
- Calcium-channel Blockers: plasma concentration of digoxin increased by ●diltiazem, ●lercanidipine and ●nicardipine; plasma concentration of digoxin possibly increased by ●nifedipine; plasma concentration of digoxin increased by ●verapamil, also increased risk of AV block and bradycardia
- Ciclosporin: plasma concentration of digoxin increased by ●ciclosporin (increased risk of toxicity)
Cobicistat: plasma concentration of digoxin possibly increased by cobicistat—reduce initial dose of digoxin
- Colchicine: possible increased risk of myopathy when digoxin given with ●colchicine
Corticosteroids: increased risk of hypokalaemia when cardiac glycosides given with corticosteroids
Cytotoxics: absorption of digoxin *tablets* possibly reduced by bleomycin, carmustine, cyclophosph-

Cardiac Glycosides
Cytotoxics *(continued)*
amide, cytarabine, doxorubicin, melphalan, methotrexate, procarbazine and vincristine; possible increased risk of bradycardia when digoxin given with crizotinib; manufacturer of digoxin advises give ibrutinib at least 6 hours before or after ibrutinib; plasma concentration of digoxin increased by vandetanib—possible increased risk of bradycardia
- Diuretics: increased cardiac toxicity with cardiac glycosides if hypokalaemia occurs with ●acetazolamide, ●loop diuretics or ●thiazides and related diuretics; plasma concentration of digoxin possibly increased by potassium canrenoate; plasma concentration of digoxin increased by ●spironolactone
Ivacaftor: plasma concentration of digoxin increased by ivacaftor
Lenalidomide: plasma concentration of digoxin possibly increased by lenalidomide
Lipid-regulating Drugs: absorption of cardiac glycosides possibly reduced by colestipol and colestyramine; plasma concentration of digoxin possibly increased by atorvastatin
Mirabegron: plasma concentration of digoxin increased by mirabegron—reduce initial dose of digoxin
Muscle Relaxants: risk of ventricular arrhythmias when cardiac glycosides given with suxamethonium; possible increased risk of bradycardia when cardiac glycosides given with tizanidine
Penicillamine: plasma concentration of digoxin possibly reduced by penicillamine
Ranolazine: plasma concentration of digoxin increased by ranolazine
Sympathomimetics, Beta$_2$: plasma concentration of digoxin possibly reduced by salbutamol
- Ticagrelor: plasma concentration of digoxin increased by ●ticagrelor
Tolvaptan: plasma concentration of digoxin increased by tolvaptan (increased risk of toxicity)
Ulcer-healing Drugs: plasma concentration of digoxin possibly slightly increased by proton pump inhibitors; absorption of cardiac glycosides possibly reduced by sucralfate
Ulipristal: manufacturer of ulipristal advises give digoxin at least 1.5 hours before or after ulipristal
Carmustine
- Antipsychotics: avoid concomitant use of cytotoxics with ●clozapine (increased risk of agranulocytosis)
Cardiac Glycosides: carmustine possibly reduces absorption of digoxin *tablets*
Ulcer-healing Drugs: myelosuppressive effects of carmustine possibly enhanced by cimetidine
Carteolol *see* Beta-blockers
Carvedilol *see* Beta-blockers
Caspofungin
Antibacterials: plasma concentration of caspofungin initially increased and then reduced by rifampicin (consider increasing dose of caspofungin)
Antiepileptics: plasma concentration of caspofungin possibly reduced by carbamazepine and phenytoin—consider increasing dose of caspofungin
Antivirals: plasma concentration of caspofungin possibly reduced by efavirenz and nevirapine—consider increasing dose of caspofungin
- Ciclosporin: plasma concentration of caspofungin increased by ●ciclosporin (manufacturer of caspofungin recommends monitoring liver enzymes)
Corticosteroids: plasma concentration of caspofungin possibly reduced by dexamethasone—consider increasing dose of caspofungin
- Tacrolimus: caspofungin reduces plasma concentration of ●tacrolimus

Catumaxomab

- Antipsychotics: avoid concomitant use of cytotoxics with ●clozapine (increased risk of agranulocytosis)
- Vaccines: avoid concomitant use of monoclonal antibodies with live ●vaccines (see p. 842)

Cefaclor *see* Cephalosporins

Cefadroxil *see* Cephalosporins

Cefalexin *see* Cephalosporins

Cefixime *see* Cephalosporins

Cefotaxime *see* Cephalosporins

Cefradine *see* Cephalosporins

Ceftaroline *see* Cephalosporins

Ceftazidime *see* Cephalosporins

Ceftriaxone *see* Cephalosporins

Cefuroxime *see* Cephalosporins

Celecoxib *see* NSAIDs

Celiprolol *see* Beta-blockers

Cephalosporins

Antacids: absorption of cefaclor reduced by antacids
Antibacterials: possible increased risk of nephrotoxicity when cephalosporins given with aminoglycosides
- Anticoagulants: cephalosporins possibly enhance anticoagulant effect of ●coumarins
Teriflunomide: plasma concentration of cefaclor increased by teriflunomide
Vaccines: antibacterials inactivate oral typhoid vaccine—see p. 864

Certolizumab pegol

- Abatacept: avoid concomitant use of certolizumab pegol with ●abatacept
- Anakinra: avoid concomitant use of certolizumab pegol with ●anakinra
- Antipsychotics: avoid concomitant use of cytotoxics with ●clozapine (increased risk of agranulocytosis)
- Vaccines: avoid concomitant use of monoclonal antibodies with live ●vaccines (see p. 842)

Cetirizine *see* Antihistamines

Cetuximab

- Antipsychotics: avoid concomitant use of cytotoxics with ●clozapine (increased risk of agranulocytosis)
- Vaccines: avoid concomitant use of monoclonal antibodies with live ●vaccines (see p. 842)

Chenodeoxycholic Acid *see* Bile Acids

Chloral *see* Anxiolytics and Hypnotics

Chloramphenicol

Antibacterials: metabolism of chloramphenicol accelerated by rifampicin (reduced plasma concentration)
- Anticoagulants: chloramphenicol enhances anticoagulant effect of ●coumarins
- Antidiabetics: chloramphenicol enhances effects of ●sulfonylureas
- Antiepileptics: metabolism of chloramphenicol possibly accelerated by ●phenobarbital (reduced plasma concentration); chloramphenicol increases plasma concentration of ●phenytoin (increased risk of toxicity)
- Antipsychotics: avoid concomitant use of chloramphenicol with ●clozapine (increased risk of agranulocytosis)
- Ciclosporin: chloramphenicol possibly increases plasma concentration of ●ciclosporin
- Clopidogrel: chloramphenicol possibly reduces antiplatelet effect of ●clopidogrel
Hydroxocobalamin: chloramphenicol reduces response to hydroxocobalamin
- Tacrolimus: chloramphenicol possibly increases plasma concentration of ●tacrolimus
Vaccines: antibacterials inactivate oral typhoid vaccine—see p. 864

Chlordiazepoxide *see* Anxiolytics and Hypnotics

Chloroprocaine

- Antibacterials: chloroprocaine possibly inhibits effects of ●sulfonamides (manufacturer of chloroprocaine advises avoid concomitant use)

Chloroquine and Hydroxychloroquine

Adsorbents: absorption of chloroquine and hydroxychloroquine reduced by kaolin
Agalsidase Alfa and Beta: chloroquine and hydroxychloroquine possibly inhibit effects of agalsidase alfa and beta (manufacturers of agalsidase alfa and beta advise avoid concomitant use)
Antacids: absorption of chloroquine and hydroxychloroquine reduced by antacids
- Anti-arrhythmics: increased risk of ventricular arrhythmias when chloroquine and hydroxychloroquine given with ●amiodarone—avoid concomitant use
- Antibacterials: increased risk of ventricular arrhythmias when chloroquine and hydroxychloroquine given with ●moxifloxacin—avoid concomitant use
- Antidepressants: avoidance of antimalarials advised by manufacturer of ●citalopram and ●escitalopram (risk of ventricular arrhythmias)
- Antimalarials: avoidance of antimalarials advised by manufacturer of ●artemether with lumefantrine; increased risk of convulsions when chloroquine and hydroxychloroquine given with ●mefloquine
- Antipsychotics: increased risk of ventricular arrhythmias when chloroquine and hydroxychloroquine given with ●droperidol—avoid concomitant use
- Cardiac Glycosides: chloroquine and hydroxychloroquine possibly increase plasma concentration of ●digoxin
- Ciclosporin: chloroquine and hydroxychloroquine increase plasma concentration of ●ciclosporin (increased risk of toxicity)
- Cytotoxics: possible increased risk of ventricular arrhythmias when chloroquine and hydroxychloroquine given with ●bosutinib
Histamine: avoidance of antimalarials advised by manufacturer of histamine
Lanthanum: absorption of chloroquine and hydroxychloroquine possibly reduced by lanthanum (give at least 2 hours apart)
Laronidase: chloroquine and hydroxychloroquine possibly inhibit effects of laronidase (manufacturer of laronidase advises avoid concomitant use)
Parasympathomimetics: chloroquine and hydroxychloroquine have potential to increase symptoms of myasthenia gravis and thus diminish effect of neostigmine and pyridostigmine
Ulcer-healing Drugs: metabolism of chloroquine and hydroxychloroquine inhibited by cimetidine (increased plasma concentration)
Vaccines: antimalarials inactivate oral typhoid vaccine—see p. 864

Chlorothiazide *see* Diuretics

Chlorphenamine *see* Antihistamines

Chlorpromazine *see* Antipsychotics

Chlortalidone *see* Diuretics

Cholera vaccine *see* Vaccines

Ciclesonide *see* Corticosteroids

Ciclosporin

- ACE Inhibitors: increased risk of hyperkalaemia when ciclosporin given with ●ACE inhibitors
- Aliskiren: ciclosporin increases plasma concentration of ●aliskiren—avoid concomitant use
Allopurinol: plasma concentration of ciclosporin possibly increased by allopurinol (risk of nephrotoxicity)
- Ambrisentan: ciclosporin increases plasma concentration of ●ambrisentan (see Dose under Ambrisentan, p. 111)
- Analgesics: increased risk of nephrotoxicity when ciclosporin given with ●NSAIDs; ciclosporin increases plasma concentration of ●diclofenac (halve dose of diclofenac)

Ciclosporin *(continued)*
- Angiotensin-II Receptor Antagonists: increased risk of hyperkalaemia when ciclosporin given with ●angiotensin-II receptor antagonists
  Anti-arrhythmics: plasma concentration of ciclosporin possibly increased by amiodarone and propafenone
- Antibacterials: metabolism of ciclosporin inhibited by ●clarithromycin and ●erythromycin (increased plasma concentration); metabolism of ciclosporin accelerated by ●rifampicin (reduced plasma concentration); plasma concentration of ciclosporin possibly reduced by ●sulfadiazine; increased risk of nephrotoxicity when ciclosporin given with ●aminoglycosides, ●polymyxins, ●quinolones, ●sulfonamides or ●vancomycin; plasma concentration of ciclosporin possibly increased by ●chloramphenicol and ●telithromycin; increased risk of myopathy when ciclosporin given with ●daptomycin (preferably avoid concomitant use); metabolism of ciclosporin possibly inhibited by ●macrolides (increased plasma concentration); increased risk of nephrotoxicity when ciclosporin given with ●trimethoprim, also plasma concentration of ciclosporin reduced by *intravenous* trimethoprim
- Anticoagulants: ciclosporin possibly increases plasma concentration of ●dabigatran—manufacturer of dabigatran advises avoid concomitant use
- Antidepressants: plasma concentration of ciclosporin reduced by ●St John's wort—avoid concomitant use
  Antidiabetics: ciclosporin possibly enhances hypoglycaemic effect of repaglinide
- Antiepileptics: metabolism of ciclosporin accelerated by ●carbamazepine, ●phenobarbital and ●phenytoin (reduced plasma concentration); plasma concentration of ciclosporin possibly reduced by oxcarbazepine
- Antifungals: metabolism of ciclosporin possibly inhibited by ●miconazole (increased plasma concentration); increased risk of nephrotoxicity when ciclosporin given with ●amphotericin; metabolism of ciclosporin inhibited by ●fluconazole, ●itraconazole, ●posaconazole and ●voriconazole (increased plasma concentration); ciclosporin increases plasma concentration of ●caspofungin (manufacturer of caspofungin recommends monitoring liver enzymes); plasma concentration of ciclosporin possibly reduced by griseofulvin and terbinafine; plasma concentration of ciclosporin possibly increased by micafungin
- Antimalarials: plasma concentration of ciclosporin increased by ●chloroquine and hydroxychloroquine (increased risk of toxicity)
  Antimuscarinics: avoidance of ciclosporin advised by manufacturer of darifenacin
- Antivirals: increased risk of nephrotoxicity when ciclosporin given with aciclovir; plasma concentration of ciclosporin possibly increased by ●atazanavir and ●ritonavir; plasma concentration of ciclosporin increased by ●boceprevir, ●fosamprenavir and ●indinavir; plasma concentration of ciclosporin possibly reduced by ●efavirenz; plasma concentration of both drugs increased when ciclosporin given with ●saquinavir; plasma concentration of both drugs increased when ciclosporin given with ●telaprevir (reduce dose of ciclosporin)
- Beta-blockers: plasma concentration of ciclosporin increased by ●carvedilol
- Bile Acids: absorption of ciclosporin increased by ●ursodeoxycholic acid
- Bosentan: ciclosporin increases plasma concentration of ●bosentan (also plasma concentration of ciclosporin reduced—avoid concomitant use)
- Calcium-channel Blockers: combination of ciclosporin with ●lercanidipine may increase plasma concentration of either drug (or both)—avoid concomitant

Ciclosporin
- Calcium-channel Blockers *(continued)*
  use; plasma concentration of ciclosporin increased by ●diltiazem, ●nicardipine and ●verapamil; ciclosporin possibly increases plasma concentration of nifedipine (increased risk of toxicity including gingival hyperplasia)
- Cardiac Glycosides: ciclosporin increases plasma concentration of ●digoxin (increased risk of toxicity)
- Colchicine: possible increased risk of nephrotoxicity and myotoxicity when ciclosporin given with ●colchicine—suspend or reduce dose of colchicine (avoid concomitant use in hepatic or renal impairment)
  Colestilan: manufacturer of colestilan advises give ciclosporin at least 1 hour before or 3 hours after colestilan
- Corticosteroids: plasma concentration of ciclosporin increased by high-dose ●methylprednisolone (risk of convulsions); ciclosporin increases plasma concentration of prednisolone
- Cytotoxics: increased risk of nephrotoxicity when ciclosporin given with ●melphalan; increased risk of neurotoxicity when ciclosporin given with ●doxorubicin; ciclosporin increases plasma concentration of ●epirubicin and ●idarubicin; ciclosporin reduces excretion of mitoxantrone (increased plasma concentration); risk of toxicity when ciclosporin given with ●methotrexate; ciclosporin possibly increases the plasma concentration of afatinib—manufacturer of afatinib advises separating administration of ciclosporin by 6 to 12 hours; caution with ciclosporin advised by manufacturer of ●crizotinib; ciclosporin increases plasma concentration of ●everolimus (consider reducing the dose of everolimus —consult everolimus product literature); plasma concentration of ciclosporin possibly increased by imatinib; *in vitro* studies suggest a possible interaction between ciclosporin and docetaxel (consult docetaxel product literature); ciclosporin possibly increases plasma concentration of etoposide (increased risk of toxicity)
  Dexrazoxane: increased risk of immunosupression with ciclosporin advised by manufacturer of dexrazoxane
- Diuretics: plasma concentration of ciclosporin possibly increased by ●acetazolamide; increased risk of hyperkalaemia when ciclosporin given with ●potassium-sparing diuretics and aldosterone antagonists; increased risk of nephrotoxicity and possibly hypermagnesaemia when ciclosporin given with thiazides and related diuretics
  Fidaxomicin: avoidance of ciclosporin advised by manufacturer of fidaxomicin
- Grapefruit Juice: plasma concentration of ciclosporin increased by ●grapefruit juice (increased risk of toxicity)
- Hormone Antagonists: metabolism of ciclosporin inhibited by ●danazol (increased plasma concentration); plasma concentration of ciclosporin reduced by lanreotide and ●octreotide; plasma concentration of ciclosporin possibly reduced by ●pasireotide
- Lenalidomide: ciclosporin possibly increases plasma concentration of ●lenalidomide (increased risk of toxicity)
- Lipid-regulating Drugs: absorption of ciclosporin reduced by ●colesevelam; increased risk of renal impairment when ciclosporin given with bezafibrate or fenofibrate; increased risk of myopathy when ciclosporin given with ●atorvastatin (see Dose under Atorvastatin, p. 175); increased risk of myopathy when ciclosporin given with ●fluvastatin or ●pravastatin; increased risk of myopathy when ciclosporin given with ●rosuvastatin or ●simvastatin (avoid concomitant use); plasma concentration of

Ciclosporin
- **Lipid-regulating Drugs** *(continued)*
  both drugs may increase when ciclosporin given with ●ezetimibe
  Mannitol: possible increased risk of nephrotoxicity when ciclosporin given with mannitol
- **Metoclopramide**: plasma concentration of ciclosporin increased by ●metoclopramide
  Mifamurtide: avoidance of ciclosporin advised by manufacturer of mifamurtide
- **Modafinil**: plasma concentration of ciclosporin reduced by ●modafinil
  Oestrogens: plasma concentration of ciclosporin possibly increased by oestrogens
- **Orlistat**: absorption of ciclosporin possibly reduced by ●orlistat
- **Potassium Salts**: increased risk of hyperkalaemia when ciclosporin given with ●potassium salts
  Progestogens: plasma concentration of ciclosporin possibly increased by progestogens
  Ranolazine: plasma concentration of both drugs may increase when ciclosporin given with ranolazine
  Sevelamer: plasma concentration of ciclosporin possibly reduced by sevelamer
  Sirolimus: ciclosporin increases plasma concentration of sirolimus
- **Sulfinpyrazone**: plasma concentration of ciclosporin reduced by ●sulfinpyrazone
- **Tacrolimus**: plasma concentration of ciclosporin increased by ●tacrolimus (increased risk of nephrotoxicity)—avoid concomitant use
  Ticagrelor: ciclosporin increases plasma concentration of ticagrelor
- **Ulcer-healing Drugs**: plasma concentration of ciclosporin possibly increased by ●cimetidine; plasma concentration of ciclosporin possibly affected by omeprazole
  Vitamins: plasma concentration of ciclosporin possibly affected by vitamin E

Cilostazol
- **Anagrelide**: avoidance of cilostazol advised by manufacturer of ●anagrelide
- **Antibacterials**: plasma concentration of cilostazol possibly increased by ●clarithromycin (see Dose under Cilostazol, p. 141); plasma concentration of cilostazol increased by ●erythromycin (see Dose under Cilostazol, p. 141)
- **Antifungals**: plasma concentration of cilostazol possibly increased by ●itraconazole (see Dose under Cilostazol, p. 141)
- **Antivirals**: plasma concentration of cilostazol possibly increased by ●boceprevir, ●ritonavir and ●telaprevir (see Dose under Cilostazol, p. 141)
  Calcium-channel Blockers: plasma concentration of cilostazol increased by diltiazem (consider reducing dose of cilostazol)
- **Ulcer-healing Drugs**: plasma concentration of cilostazol increased by ●omeprazole (see Dose under Cilostazol, p. 141)

Cimetidine *see* Histamine H₂-antagonists

Cinacalcet
- **Hormone Antagonists**: cinacalcet possibly inhibits metabolism of ●tamoxifen to active metabolite (avoid concomitant use)

Cinnarizine *see* Antihistamines
Ciprofibrate *see* Fibrates
Ciprofloxacin *see* Quinolones
Cisatracurium *see* Muscle Relaxants
Cisplatin *see* Platinum Compounds
Citalopram *see* Antidepressants, SSRI

Cladribine
- **Antipsychotics**: avoid concomitant use of cytotoxics with ●clozapine (increased risk of agranulocytosis)
- **Antivirals**: avoidance of cladribine advised by manufacturer of ●lamivudine

Clarithromycin *see* Macrolides
Clemastine *see* Antihistamines

Clindamycin
- **Muscle Relaxants**: clindamycin enhances effects of ●non-depolarising muscle relaxants and ●suxamethonium
  Parasympathomimetics: clindamycin antagonises effects of neostigmine and pyridostigmine
  Vaccines: antibacterials inactivate oral typhoid vaccine—see p. 864

Clobazam *see* Anxiolytics and Hypnotics

Clofazimine
- **Antibacterials**: possible increased risk of ventricular arrhythmias when clofazimine given with ●bedaquiline
  Vaccines: antibacterials inactivate oral typhoid vaccine—see p. 864

Clomethiazole *see* Anxiolytics and Hypnotics
Clomipramine *see* Antidepressants, Tricyclic
Clonazepam *see* Anxiolytics and Hypnotics

Clonidine
  ACE Inhibitors: enhanced hypotensive effect when clonidine given with ACE inhibitors; previous treatment with clonidine possibly delays antihypertensive effect of captopril
  Adrenergic Neurone Blockers: enhanced hypotensive effect when clonidine given with adrenergic neurone blockers
  Alcohol: enhanced hypotensive effect when clonidine given with alcohol
  Aldesleukin: enhanced hypotensive effect when clonidine given with aldesleukin
  Alpha-blockers: enhanced hypotensive effect when clonidine given with alpha-blockers
  Anaesthetics, General: enhanced hypotensive effect when clonidine given with general anaesthetics
  Analgesics: hypotensive effect of clonidine antagonised by NSAIDs
  Angiotensin-II Receptor Antagonists: enhanced hypotensive effect when clonidine given with angiotensin-II receptor antagonists
- **Antidepressants**: enhanced hypotensive effect when clonidine given with MAOIs; hypotensive effect of clonidine possibly antagonised by mirtazapine; hypotensive effect of clonidine antagonised by ●tricyclics, also increased risk of hypertension on clonidine withdrawal
  Antipsychotics: enhanced hypotensive effect when clonidine given with phenothiazines
  Anxiolytics and Hypnotics: enhanced hypotensive effect when clonidine given with anxiolytics and hypnotics
- **Beta-blockers**: increased risk of withdrawal hypertension when clonidine given with ●beta-blockers (withdraw beta-blockers several days before slowly withdrawing clonidine)
  Calcium-channel Blockers: enhanced hypotensive effect when clonidine given with calcium-channel blockers
  Corticosteroids: hypotensive effect of clonidine antagonised by corticosteroids
  Cytotoxics: possible increased risk of bradycardia when clonidine given with crizotinib
  Diazoxide: enhanced hypotensive effect when clonidine given with diazoxide
  Diuretics: enhanced hypotensive effect when clonidine given with diuretics
  Dopaminergics: enhanced hypotensive effect when clonidine given with levodopa
  Histamine: avoidance of clonidine advised by manufacturer of histamine
  Methyldopa: enhanced hypotensive effect when clonidine given with methyldopa
  Moxisylyte: enhanced hypotensive effect when clonidine given with moxisylyte

Clonidine *(continued)*

  Moxonidine: enhanced hypotensive effect when clonidine given with moxonidine

  Muscle Relaxants: enhanced hypotensive effect when clonidine given with baclofen or tizanidine

  Nitrates: enhanced hypotensive effect when clonidine given with nitrates

  Oestrogens: hypotensive effect of clonidine antagonised by oestrogens

  Prostaglandins: enhanced hypotensive effect when clonidine given with alprostadil

- Sympathomimetics: possible risk of hypertension when clonidine given with adrenaline (epinephrine) or noradrenaline (norepinephrine); serious adverse events reported with concomitant use of clonidine and ●methylphenidate (causality not established)

  Vasodilator Antihypertensives: enhanced hypotensive effect when clonidine given with hydralazine, minoxidil or sodium nitroprusside

Clopamide *see* Diuretics

Clopidogrel

  Analgesics: increased risk of bleeding when clopidogrel given with NSAIDs or aspirin

- Antibacterials: antiplatelet effect of clopidogrel possibly reduced by ●chloramphenicol, ●ciprofloxacin and ●erythromycin

- Anticoagulants: manufacturer of clopidogrel advises avoid concomitant use with ●warfarin; antiplatelet action of clopidogrel enhances anticoagulant effect of ●coumarins and ●phenindione; increased risk of bleeding when clopidogrel given with heparins

- Antidepressants: antiplatelet effect of clopidogrel possibly reduced by ●fluoxetine, ●fluvoxamine and ●moclobemide

- Antiepileptics: antiplatelet effect of clopidogrel possibly reduced by ●carbamazepine and ●oxcarbazepine

- Antifungals: antiplatelet effect of clopidogrel possibly reduced by ●fluconazole, ●itraconazole and ●voriconazole

- Antivirals: antiplatelet effect of clopidogrel possibly reduced by ●etravirine

  Dipyridamole: increased risk of bleeding when clopidogrel given with dipyridamole

  Iloprost: increased risk of bleeding when clopidogrel given with iloprost

- Lipid-regulating Drugs: clopidogrel increases plasma concentration of ●rosuvastatin—adjust dose of rosuvastatin (consult product literature)

  Prasugrel: possible increased risk of bleeding when clopidogrel given with prasugrel

- Ulcer-healing Drugs: antiplatelet effect of clopidogrel possibly reduced by ●cimetidine, lansoprazole, pantoprazole and rabeprazole; antiplatelet effect of clopidogrel reduced by ●esomeprazole and ●omeprazole

Clozapine *see* Antipsychotics

Co-amoxiclav *see* Penicillins

Co-beneldopa *see* Levodopa

Cobicistat

- Alpha-blockers: cobicistat possibly increases plasma concentration of ●alfuzosin—manufacturer of cobicistat advises avoid concomitant use

- Anti-arrhythmics: cobicistat possibly increases plasma concentration of ●amiodarone—manufacturer of cobicistat advises avoid concomitant use

- Antibacterials: plasma concentration of cobicistat reduced by ●rifabutin (adjust dose—consult product literature); plasma concentration of cobicistat possibly reduced by ●rifampicin—manufacturer of cobicistat advises avoid concomitant use

- Anticoagulants: avoidance of cobicistat advised by manufacturer of apixaban; cobicistat possibly enhances anticoagulant effect of ●rivaroxaban—avoid concomitant use

Cobicistat *(continued)*

- Antidepressants: plasma concentration of cobicistat possibly reduced by ●St John's wort—manufacturer of cobicistat advises avoid concomitant use

- Antiepileptics: plasma concentration of cobicistat possibly reduced by ●carbamazepine, ●phenobarbital and ●phenytoin—manufacturer of cobicistat advises avoid concomitant use

  Antifungals: cobicistat possibly increases plasma concentration of itraconazole—manufacturer of cobicistat advises reduce dose of itraconazole

- Antipsychotics: cobicistat possibly increases plasma concentration of ●lurasidone—avoid concomitant use; cobicistat possibly increases plasma concentration of ●pimozide—manufacturer of cobicistat advises avoid concomitant use

- Antivirals: manufacturer of cobicistat advises avoid concomitant use with boceprevir; cobicistat possibly increases the plasma concentration of ●daclatasvir—reduce dose of daclatasvir (see Dose under Daclatasvir, p. 438); cobicistat possibly increases plasma concentration of ●maraviroc (reduce dose of maraviroc); avoidance of cobicistat advised by manufacturer of nevirapine; cobicistat possibly increases plasma concentration of ●simeprevir—manufacturer of simeprevir advises avoid concomitant use; plasma concentration of both drugs reduced when cobicistat given with ●tipranavir (avoid concomitant use)

- Anxiolytics and Hypnotics: manufacturer of cobicistat advises avoid concomitant use with *oral* ●midazolam

  Bosentan: manufacturer of cobicistat advises avoid concomitant use with bosentan

  Cardiac Glycosides: cobicistat possibly increases plasma concentration of digoxin—reduce initial dose of digoxin

- Cytotoxics: cobicistat possibly increases the plasma concentration of ●ibrutinib—reduce dose of ibrutinib (see Dose under Ibrutinib, p. 615)

- Domperidone: possible increased risk of ventricular arrhythmias when cobicistat given with ●domperidone—avoid concomitant use

- Ergot Alkaloids: cobicistat possibly increases plasma concentration of ●ergot alkaloids—manufacturer of cobicistat advises avoid concomitant use

- Lipid-regulating Drugs: cobicistat possibly increases plasma concentration of atorvastatin—manufacturer of cobicistat advises reduce dose of atorvastatin; manufacturer of cobicistat advises avoid concomitant use with ●simvastatin

- Oestrogens: cobicistat accelerates metabolism of ●oestrogens (reduced contraceptive effect—see p. 548)

  Progestogens: cobicistat increases plasma concentration of norgestimate

- Sildenafil: cobicistat possibly increases plasma concentration of ●sildenafil—manufacturer of cobicistat advises avoid concomitant use of sildenafil for pulmonary arterial hypertension or reduce dose of sildenafil for erectile dysfunction—consult cobicistat product literature

  Sympathomimetics, Beta$_2$: manufacturer of cobicistat advises avoid concomitant use with salmeterol

- Tadalafil: cobicistat possibly increases plasma concentration of ●tadalafil—manufacturer of cobicistat advises reduce dose of tadalafil (consult cobicistat product literature)

- Vardenafil: cobicistat possibly increases plasma concentration of ●vardenafil—manufacturer of cobicistat advises reduce dose of vardenafil (consult cobicistat product literature)

Co-careldopa *see* Levodopa

Codeine *see* Opioid Analgesics

Co-fluampicil *see* Penicillins

Colchicine

- Anti-arrhythmics: possible increased risk of colchicine toxicity when given with ●amiodarone
- Antibacterials: possible increased risk of colchicine toxicity when given with ●azithromycin, ●clarithromycin, ●erythromycin and ●telithromycin—suspend or reduce dose of colchicine (avoid concomitant use in hepatic or renal impairment)
- Antifungals: possible increased risk of colchicine toxicity when given with ●itraconazole—suspend or reduce dose of colchicine (avoid concomitant use in hepatic or renal impairment)
- Antivirals: possible increased risk of colchicine toxicity when given with ●atazanavir, ●indinavir, ●ritonavir and ●telaprevir—suspend or reduce dose of colchicine (avoid concomitant use in hepatic or renal impairment)
- Calcium-channel Blockers: possible increased risk of colchicine toxicity when given with ●diltiazem and ●verapamil—suspend or reduce dose of colchicine (avoid concomitant use in hepatic or renal impairment)
- Cardiac Glycosides: possible increased risk of myopathy when colchicine given with ●digoxin
- Ciclosporin: possible increased risk of nephrotoxicity and myotoxicity when colchicine given with ●ciclosporin—suspend or reduce dose of colchicine (avoid concomitant use in hepatic or renal impairment)
- Grapefruit Juice: possible increased risk of colchicine toxicity when given with ●grapefruit juice
- Lipid-regulating Drugs: possible increased risk of myopathy when colchicine given with ●fibrates or ●statins

Colesevelam

Note Other drugs should be taken at least 4 hours before or after colesevelam to reduce possible interference with absorption

Antidiabetics: colesevelam reduces absorption of glibenclamide and glipizide; colesevelam reduces absorption of glimepiride—manufacturer of glimepiride advises give at least 4 hours before colesevelam; manufacturer of canagliflozin advises give bile acid sequestrants at least 1 hour after or 4–6 before canagliflozin

Antiepileptics: colesevelam possibly reduces absorption of phenytoin

- Ciclosporin: colesevelam reduces absorption of ●ciclosporin

Lipid-regulating Drugs: bile acid sequestrants possibly reduce absorption of lomitapide (give at least 4 hours apart)

Oestrogens: colesevelam reduces absorption of ethinylestradiol

Thyroid Hormones: colesevelam reduces absorption of levothyroxine

Colestilan

Note Other drugs should be taken at least 1 hour before or 3 hours after colestilan to reduce possible interference with absorption

Ciclosporin: manufacturer of colestilan advises give ciclosporin at least 1 hour before or 3 hours after colestilan

Mycophenolate: manufacturer of colestilan advises give mycophenolate at least 1 hour before or 3 hours after colestilan

Tacrolimus: manufacturer of colestilan advises give tacrolimus at least 1 hour before or 3 hours after colestilan

Thyroid Hormones: manufacturer of colestilan advises give levothyroxine at least 1 hour before or 3 hours after colestilan

Colestipol

Note Other drugs should be taken at least 1 hour before or 4–6 hours after colestipol to reduce possible interference with absorption

Colestipol (continued)

Antibacterials: colestipol possibly reduces absorption of tetracycline

Antidiabetics: manufacturer of canagliflozin advises give bile acid sequestrants at least 1 hour after or 4–6 before canagliflozin

Bile Acids: colestipol possibly reduces absorption of bile acids

Cardiac Glycosides: colestipol possibly reduces absorption of cardiac glycosides

Diuretics: colestipol reduces absorption of thiazides and related diuretics (give at least 2 hours apart)

Lipid-regulating Drugs: bile acid sequestrants possibly reduce absorption of lomitapide (give at least 4 hours apart)

Thyroid Hormones: colestipol reduces absorption of thyroid hormones

Colestyramine

Note Other drugs should be taken at least 1 hour before or 4–6 hours after colestyramine to reduce possible interference with absorption

Analgesics: colestyramine increases the excretion of meloxicam; colestyramine reduces absorption of paracetamol

Antibacterials: colestyramine possibly reduces absorption of tetracycline; colestyramine antagonises effects of *oral* vancomycin

- Anticoagulants: colestyramine may enhance or reduce anticoagulant effect of ●coumarins and ●phenindione

Antidiabetics: colestyramine possibly enhances hypoglycaemic effect of acarbose; manufacturer of canagliflozin advises give bile acid sequestrants at least 1 hour after or 4–6 before canagliflozin

Antiepileptics: colestyramine possibly reduces absorption of valproate

Bile Acids: colestyramine possibly reduces absorption of bile acids

Cardiac Glycosides: colestyramine possibly reduces absorption of cardiac glycosides

Diuretics: colestyramine reduces absorption of thiazides and related diuretics (give at least 2 hours apart)

Leflunomide: colestyramine significantly decreases effect of leflunomide (enhanced elimination)—avoid unless drug elimination desired

Lipid-regulating Drugs: bile acid sequestrants possibly reduce absorption of lomitapide (give at least 4 hours apart)

Mycophenolate: colestyramine reduces absorption of mycophenolate

Raloxifene: colestyramine reduces absorption of raloxifene (manufacturer of raloxifene advises avoid concomitant administration)

Teriflunomide: colestyramine significantly decreases effect of teriflunomide (enhanced elimination)—avoid unless drug elimination desired

Thyroid Hormones: colestyramine reduces absorption of thyroid hormones

Vitamins: colestyramine possibly reduces absorption of calcitriol (give at least 1 hour before or 4 to 6 hours after colestyramine)

Colistimethate Sodium see Polymyxins

Contraceptives, oral see Oestrogens and Progestogens

Corticosteroids

Note Interactions do not generally apply to corticosteroids used for topical action (including inhalation) unless specified

ACE Inhibitors: corticosteroids antagonise hypotensive effect of ACE inhibitors

Adrenergic Neurone Blockers: corticosteroids antagonise hypotensive effect of adrenergic neurone blockers

- Aldesleukin: avoidance of corticosteroids advised by manufacturer of ●aldesleukin

Alpha-blockers: corticosteroids antagonise hypotensive effect of alpha-blockers

Corticosteroids (continued)

Analgesics: increased risk of gastro-intestinal bleeding and ulceration when corticosteroids given with NSAIDs; increased risk of gastro-intestinal bleeding and ulceration when corticosteroids given with aspirin, also corticosteroids reduce plasma concentration of salicylate

Angiotensin-II Receptor Antagonists: corticosteroids antagonise hypotensive effect of angiotensin-II receptor antagonists

Antacids: absorption of deflazacort reduced by antacids

• Antibacterials: plasma concentration of methylprednisolone possibly increased by clarithromycin; metabolism of corticosteroids possibly inhibited by erythromycin; metabolism of methylprednisolone inhibited by erythromycin; corticosteroids possibly reduce plasma concentration of isoniazid; metabolism of corticosteroids accelerated by •rifamycins (reduced effect)

• Anticoagulants: corticosteroids may enhance or reduce anticoagulant effect of •coumarins (highdose corticosteroids enhance anticoagulant effect); corticosteroids may enhance or reduce anticoagulant effect of phenindione

Antidiabetics: corticosteroids antagonise hypoglycaemic effect of antidiabetics

• Antiepileptics: metabolism of corticosteroids accelerated by •carbamazepine, •phenobarbital and •phenytoin (reduced effect)

• Antifungals: increased risk of hypokalaemia when corticosteroids given with •amphotericin—avoid concomitant use unless corticosteroids needed to control reactions; metabolism of corticosteroids and methylprednisolone possibly inhibited by itraconazole; plasma concentration of inhaled and oral (and possibly also intranasal and rectal) budesonide increased by •itraconazole; plasma concentration of inhaled fluticasone increased by itraconazole; dexamethasone possibly reduces plasma concentration of caspofungin—consider increasing dose of caspofungin

• Antivirals: dexamethasone possibly reduces plasma concentration of daclatasvir and simeprevir—manufacturer of daclatasvir and simeprevir advises avoid concomitant use; dexamethasone possibly reduces plasma concentration of indinavir, lopinavir, saquinavir and telaprevir; avoidance of dexamethasone (except when given as a single dose) advised by manufacturer of •rilpivirine; plasma concentration of budesonide (including inhaled, intranasal, and rectal budesonide) possibly increased by •ritonavir—increased risk of adrenal suppresion; plasma concentration of corticosteroids possibly increased by •ritonavir—increased risk of adrenal suppression; plasma concentration of inhaled and intranasal fluticasone increased by •ritonavir—increased risk of adrenal suppression; plasma concentration of inhaled and intranasal budesonide and fluticasone possibly increased by telaprevir

Aprepitant: metabolism of dexamethasone and methylprednisolone inhibited by aprepitant (reduce dose of dexamethasone and methylprednisolone)

Beta-blockers: corticosteroids antagonise hypotensive effect of beta-blockers

Calcium Salts: corticosteroids reduce absorption of calcium salts

Calcium-channel Blockers: corticosteroids antagonise hypotensive effect of calcium-channel blockers; plasma concentration of methylprednisolone increased by diltiazem

Cardiac Glycosides: increased risk of hypokalaemia when corticosteroids given with cardiac glycosides

• Ciclosporin: high-dose methylprednisolone increases plasma concentration of •ciclosporin (risk of con-

Corticosteroids

• Ciclosporin (continued)
vulsions); plasma concentration of prednisolone increased by ciclosporin

Clonidine: corticosteroids antagonise hypotensive effect of clonidine

Cytotoxics: possible increased risk of hepatoxicity when dexamethasone given with high-dose methotrexate; dexamethasone possibly decreases plasma concentration of axitinib (increase dose of axitinib—consult axitinib product literature); dexamethasone possibly reduces plasma concentration of cabozantinib—manufacturer of cabozantinib advises avoid concomitant use

Diazoxide: corticosteroids antagonise hypotensive effect of diazoxide

Diuretics: corticosteroids antagonise diuretic effect of diuretics; increased risk of hypokalaemia when corticosteroids given with acetazolamide, loop diuretics or thiazides and related diuretics

Histamine: avoidance of corticosteroids advised by manufacturer of histamine

Methyldopa: corticosteroids antagonise hypotensive effect of methyldopa

Mifamurtide: avoidance of corticosteroids advised by manufacturer of mifamurtide

Mifepristone: effect of corticosteroids (including inhaled corticosteroids) may be reduced for 3–4 days after mifepristone

Moxonidine: corticosteroids antagonise hypotensive effect of moxonidine

Muscle Relaxants: corticosteroids possibly antagonise effects of pancuronium and vecuronium

Nitrates: corticosteroids antagonise hypotensive effect of nitrates

Oestrogens: plasma concentration of corticosteroids increased by oral contraceptives containing oestrogens

Sodium Benzoate: corticosteroids possibly reduce effects of sodium benzoate

Sodium Phenylbutyrate: corticosteroids possibly reduce effects of sodium phenylbutyrate

Somatropin: corticosteroids may inhibit growth-promoting effect of somatropin

Sympathomimetics: metabolism of dexamethasone accelerated by ephedrine

Sympathomimetics, Beta$_2$: increased risk of hypokalaemia when corticosteroids given with high doses of beta$_2$ sympathomimetics—see Hypokalaemia, p. 189

Theophylline: increased risk of hypokalaemia when corticosteroids given with theophylline

• Vaccines: high doses of corticosteroids impair immune response to •vaccines, avoid concomitant use with live vaccines (see p. 842)

Vasodilator Antihypertensives: corticosteroids antagonise hypotensive effect of hydralazine, minoxidil and sodium nitroprusside

Co-trimoxazole see Trimethoprim and Sulfamethoxazole

Coumarins

Note Change in patient's clinical condition, particularly associated with liver disease, intercurrent illness, or drug administration, necessitates more frequent testing. Major changes in diet (especially involving salads and vegetables) and in alcohol consumption may also affect anticoagulant control

• Alcohol: anticoagulant control with coumarins may be affected by major changes in consumption of •alcohol

Allopurinol: anticoagulant effect of coumarins possibly enhanced by allopurinol

• Anabolic Steroids: anticoagulant effect of coumarins enhanced by •anabolic steroids

• Analgesics: anticoagulant effect of coumarins possibly enhanced by •NSAIDs; increased risk of haemorr-

Coumarins

- **Analgesics** *(continued)*
  hage when anticoagulants given with *intravenous*
  ●diclofenac (avoid concomitant use, including low-
  dose heparins); increased risk of haemorrhage when
  anticoagulants given with ●ketorolac (avoid concomitant use, including low-dose heparins); anticoagulant effect of coumarins enhanced by ●trama-
  dol; increased risk of bleeding when coumarins
  given with ●aspirin (due to antiplatelet effect); anticoagulant effect of coumarins possibly enhanced by
  prolonged regular use of paracetamol
- **Anti-arrhythmics:** metabolism of coumarins inhibited
  by ●amiodarone (enhanced anticoagulant effect);
  anticoagulant effect of warfarin may be enhanced
  or reduced by disopyramide; anticoagulant effect of
  coumarins possibly enhanced by ●dronedarone;
  anticoagulant effect of coumarins enhanced by
  ●propafenone
- **Antibacterials:** experience in anticoagulant clinics suggests that INR possibly altered when coumarins are
  given with ●neomycin (given for local action on
  gut); anticoagulant effect of coumarins possibly
  enhanced by ●azithromycin, ●aztreonam,
  ●cephalosporins, ciprofloxacin, levofloxacin,
  ●tetracyclines, tigecycline and trimethoprim; anticoagulant effect of coumarins enhanced by
  ●chloramphenicol, ●clarithromycin, ●erythromycin,
  ●metronidazole, ●nalidixic acid, ●norfloxacin,
  ●ofloxacin and ●sulfonamides; an interaction
  between coumarins and broad-spectrum penicillins
  has not been demonstrated in studies, but common
  experience in anticoagulant clinics is that INR can
  be altered; metabolism of coumarins accelerated by
  ●rifamycins (reduced anticoagulant effect)
- **Anticoagulants:** increased risk of haemorrhage when
  other anticoagulants given with ●apixaban, ●dabiga-
  tran and ●rivaroxaban (avoid concomitant use
  except when switching with other anticoagulants or
  using heparin to maintain catheter patency)
- **Antidepressants:** anticoagulant effect of warfarin possibly enhanced by ●venlafaxine; anticoagulant effect
  of warfarin may be enhanced or reduced by
  trazodone; anticoagulant effect of coumarins possibly enhanced by ●SSRIs; anticoagulant effect of
  coumarins reduced by ●St John's wort (avoid concomitant use); anticoagulant effect of warfarin
  enhanced by mirtazapine; anticoagulant effect of
  coumarins may be enhanced or reduced by ●tricyc-
  lics
- **Antidiabetics:** anticoagulant effect of warfarin possibly
  enhanced by exenatide; coumarins possibly
  enhance hypoglycaemic effect of ●sulfonylureas,
  also possible changes to anticoagulant effect
- **Antiepileptics:** metabolism of coumarins accelerated
  by ●carbamazepine and ●phenobarbital (reduced
  anticoagulant effect); plasma concentration of warfarin reduced by eslicarbazepine; metabolism of
  coumarins accelerated by ●phenytoin (possibility of
  reduced anticoagulant effect, but enhancement also
  reported); anticoagulant effect of coumarins possibly enhanced by valproate
- **Antifungals:** anticoagulant effect of coumarins
  enhanced by ●miconazole (miconazole oral gel and
  possibly vaginal and topical formulations absorbed);
  anticoagulant effect of coumarins enhanced by
  ●fluconazole, ●itraconazole and ●voriconazole; anticoagulant effect of coumarins reduced by ●griseo-
  fulvin
  Antimalarials: isolated reports that anticoagulant
  effect of warfarin may be enhanced by proguanil;
  plasma concentration of both drugs increased when
  warfarin given with quinine
- **Antivirals:** anticoagulant effect of warfarin may be
  enhanced or reduced by atazanavir, ●nevirapine
  and ●ritonavir; plasma concentration of coumarins

Coumarins

- **Antivirals** *(continued)*
  possibly affected by ●efavirenz; anticoagulant effect
  of coumarins may be enhanced or reduced by
  fosamprenavir; anticoagulant effect of coumarins
  possibly enhanced by ●ritonavir; anticoagulant
  effect of warfarin possibly enhanced by saquinavir;
  plasma concentration of warfarin possibly affected
  by ●telaprevir
  Anxiolytics and Hypnotics: anticoagulant effect of
  coumarins may be transiently enhanced by chloral
  Aprepitant: anticoagulant effect of warfarin possibly
  reduced by aprepitant
- **Azathioprine:** anticoagulant effect of coumarins possibly reduced by ●azathioprine
  Bosentan: monitoring anticoagulant effect of coumarins recommended by manufacturer of bosentan
- **Clopidogrel:** anticoagulant effect of coumarins
  enhanced due to antiplatelet action of ●clopidogrel;
  avoidance of warfarin advised by manufacturer of
  ●clopidogrel
- **Corticosteroids:** anticoagulant effect of coumarins
  may be enhanced or reduced by ●corticosteroids
  (high-dose corticosteroids enhance anticoagulant
  effect)
- **Cranberry Juice:** anticoagulant effect of coumarins possibly enhanced by ●cranberry juice—avoid concomitant use
- **Cytotoxics:** anticoagulant effect of coumarins possibly
  enhanced by ●etoposide, ●ifosfamide and ●sorafe-
  nib; anticoagulant effect of coumarins enhanced by
  ●fluorouracil; anticoagulant effect of warfarin possibly enhanced by ●gefitinib, gemcitabine and
  ●vemurafenib; anticoagulant effect of coumarins
  possibly reduced by ●mercaptopurine and ●mito-
  tane; plasma concentration of warfarin reduced by
  dabrafenib; increased risk of bleeding when coumarins given with ●erlotinib; avoidance of coumarins
  advised by manufacturer of ibrutinib; replacement
  of warfarin with a heparin advised by manufacturer
  of imatinib (possibility of enhanced warfarin effect);
  increased risk of bleeding when warfarin given with
  ●regorafenib
- **Dipyridamole:** anticoagulant effect of coumarins
  enhanced due to antiplatelet action of ●dipyrid-
  amole
- **Disulfiram:** anticoagulant effect of coumarins
  enhanced by ●disulfiram
- **Dopaminergics:** anticoagulant effect of warfarin
  enhanced by ●entacapone
- **Enteral Foods:** anticoagulant effect of coumarins
  antagonised by vitamin K (present in some ●enteral
  feeds)
- **Glucosamine:** anticoagulant effect of warfarin
  enhanced by ●glucosamine (avoid concomitant use)
- **Hormone Antagonists:** anticoagulant effect of coumarins possibly enhanced by bicalutamide and ●tore-
  mifene; metabolism of coumarins inhibited by ●dan-
  azol (enhanced anticoagulant effect); plasma
  concentration of coumarins possibly reduced by
  ●enzalutamide; anticoagulant effect of coumarins
  enhanced by ●flutamide and ●tamoxifen
  Iloprost: anticoagulant effect of coumarins possibly
  enhanced by iloprost
  Lactulose: anticoagulant effect of coumarins possibly
  enhanced by lactulose
  Leflunomide: anticoagulant effect of warfarin possibly
  enhanced by leflunomide
  Leukotriene Receptor Antagonists: anticoagulant effect
  of warfarin enhanced by zafirlukast
- **Levamisole:** anticoagulant effect of warfarin possibly
  enhanced by ●levamisole
  Levocarnitine: anticoagulant effect of coumarins possibly enhanced by levocarnitine
- **Lipid-regulating Drugs:** anticoagulant effect of coumarins may be enhanced or reduced by ●colestyra-

Coumarins

- Lipid-regulating Drugs (continued)
  mine; anticoagulant effect of warfarin may be transiently reduced by atorvastatin; anticoagulant effect of coumarins enhanced by •fibrates, •fluvastatin and simvastatin; anticoagulant effect of coumarins possibly enhanced by ezetimibe and •rosuvastatin; anticoagulant effect of warfarin possibly enhanced by lomitapide
  Memantine: anticoagulant effect of warfarin possibly enhanced by memantine
  Oestrogens: anticoagulant effect of coumarins may be enhanced or reduced by oestrogens
  Orlistat: monitoring anticoagulant effect of coumarins recommended by manufacturer of orlistat
  Prasugrel: possible increased risk of bleeding when coumarins given with prasugrel
  Progestogens: anticoagulant effect of coumarins may be enhanced or reduced by progestogens
  Raloxifene: anticoagulant effect of coumarins antagonised by raloxifene
- Retinoids: anticoagulant effect of coumarins possibly reduced by •acitretin
- Sulfinpyrazone: anticoagulant effect of coumarins enhanced by •sulfinpyrazone
- Sympathomimetics: anticoagulant effect of coumarins possibly enhanced by •methylphenidate
- Testolactone: anticoagulant effect of coumarins enhanced by •testolactone
- Testosterone: anticoagulant effect of coumarins enhanced by •testosterone
- Thyroid Hormones: anticoagulant effect of coumarins enhanced by •thyroid hormones
  Ubidecarenone: anticoagulant effect of warfarin may be enhanced or reduced by ubidecarenone
- Ulcer-healing Drugs: metabolism of coumarins inhibited by •cimetidine (enhanced anticoagulant effect); anticoagulant effect of coumarins possibly enhanced by •esomeprazole and •omeprazole; anticoagulant effect of coumarins might be enhanced by pantoprazole; absorption of coumarins possibly reduced by •sucralfate (reduced anticoagulant effect)
  Vaccines: anticoagulant effect of warfarin possibly enhanced by influenza vaccine
- Vitamins: anticoagulant effect of coumarins possibly enhanced by •vitamin E; anticoagulant effect of coumarins antagonised by •vitamin K

Cranberry Juice

- Anticoagulants: cranberry juice possibly enhances anticoagulant effect of •coumarins—avoid concomitant use

Crizotinib

- Analgesics: manufacturer of crizotinib advises caution with •alfentanil and •fentanyl
- Antibacterials: plasma concentration of crizotinib possibly increased by •clarithromycin and •telithromycin—manufacturer of crizotinib advises avoid concomitant use; plasma concentration of crizotinib possibly reduced by rifabutin—manufacturer of crizotinib advises avoid concomitant use; plasma concentration of crizotinib reduced by •rifampicin—manufacturer of crizotinib advises avoid concomitant use
  Antidepressants: plasma concentration of crizotinib possibly reduced by St John's wort—manufacturer of crizotinib advises avoid concomitant use
  Antiepileptics: plasma concentration of crizotinib possibly reduced by carbamazepine, phenobarbital and phenytoin—manufacturer of crizotinib advises avoid concomitant use
- Antifungals: plasma concentration of crizotinib possibly increased by •itraconazole and •voriconazole—manufacturer of crizotinib advises avoid concomitant use
  Antimalarials: possible increased risk of bradycardia when crizotinib given with mefloquine

Crizotinib (continued)

- Antipsychotics: avoid concomitant use of cytotoxics with •clozapine (increased risk of agranulocytosis); manufacturer of crizotinib advises caution with •pimozide
- Antivirals: plasma concentration of crizotinib possibly increased by •atazanavir, •indinavir, •ritonavir and •saquinavir—manufacturer of crizotinib advises avoid concomitant use
- Anxiolytics and Hypnotics: crizotinib increases plasma concentration of •midazolam
  Beta-blockers: possible increased risk of bradycardia when crizotinib given with beta-blockers
  Calcium-channel Blockers: possible increased risk of bradycardia when crizotinib given with diltiazem or verapamil
  Cardiac Glycosides: possible increased risk of bradycardia when crizotinib given with digoxin
- Ciclosporin: manufacturer of crizotinib advises caution with •ciclosporin
  Clonidine: possible increased risk of bradycardia when crizotinib given with clonidine
- Cytotoxics: crizotinib possibly increases the plasma concentration of •ibrutinib—reduce dose of ibrutinib (see Dose under Ibrutinib, p. 615)
- Ergot Alkaloids: manufacturer of crizotinib advises caution with •ergot alkaloids
- Grapefruit Juice: plasma concentration of crizotinib possibly increased by •grapefruit juice—manufacturer of crizotinib advises avoid concomitant use
- Oestrogens: manufacturer of crizotinib advises contraceptive effect of •oestrogens possibly reduced
  Parasympathomimetics: possible increased risk of bradycardia when crizotinib given with pilocarpine
- Progestogens: manufacturer of crizotinib advises contraceptive effect of •progestogens possibly reduced
- Sirolimus: manufacturer of crizotinib advises caution with •sirolimus
- Tacrolimus: manufacturer of crizotinib advises caution with •tacrolimus

Cyclizine see Antihistamines

Cyclopenthiazide see Diuretics

Cyclopentolate see Antimuscarinics

Cyclophosphamide

Antifungals: side-effects of cyclophosphamide possibly increased by fluconazole and itraconazole

- Antipsychotics: avoid concomitant use of cytotoxics with •clozapine (increased risk of agranulocytosis)
  Cardiac Glycosides: cyclophosphamide possibly reduces absorption of digoxin tablets
- Cytotoxics: increased toxicity when high-dose cyclophosphamide given with •pentostatin—avoid concomitant use
  Muscle Relaxants: cyclophosphamide enhances effects of suxamethonium

Cycloserine

- Alcohol: increased risk of convulsions when cycloserine given with •alcohol
  Antibacterials: increased risk of CNS toxicity when cycloserine given with isoniazid
  Vaccines: antibacterials inactivate oral typhoid vaccine—see p. 864

Cyproheptadine see Antihistamines

Cytarabine

Antifungals: cytarabine possibly reduces plasma concentration of flucytosine

- Antipsychotics: avoid concomitant use of cytotoxics with •clozapine (increased risk of agranulocytosis)
  Cardiac Glycosides: cytarabine possibly reduces absorption of digoxin tablets
  Cytotoxics: intracellular concentration of cytarabine increased by fludarabine

Cytotoxics see individual drugs

Dabigatran

- Analgesics: possible increased risk of bleeding when dabigatran given with •NSAIDs; increased risk of

Dabigatran

- Analgesics *(continued)*
  haemorrhage when anticoagulants given with *intravenous* ●diclofenac (avoid concomitant use, including low-dose heparins); increased risk of haemorrhage when anticoagulants given with ●ketorolac (avoid concomitant use, including low-dose heparins)
- Anti-arrhythmics: plasma concentration of dabigatran increased by ●amiodarone (see Dose under Dabigatran, p. 156); plasma concentration of dabigatran increased by ●dronedarone—avoid concomitant use
- Antibacterials: possible increased risk of bleeding when dabigatran given with clarithromycin; plasma concentration of dabigatran reduced by ●rifampicin—manufacturer of dabigatran advises avoid concomitant use
- Anticoagulants: increased risk of haemorrhage when dabigatran given with other ●anticoagulants (avoid concomitant use except when switching with other anticoagulants or using heparin to maintain catheter patency); increased risk of haemorrhage when other anticoagulants given with ●apixaban and ●rivaroxaban (avoid concomitant use except when switching with other anticoagulants or using heparin to maintain catheter patency)
- Antidepressants: possible increased risk of bleeding when dabigatran given with ●SSRI-related antidepressants or ●SSRIs; plasma concentration of dabigatran possibly reduced by St John's wort—manufacturer of dabigatran advises avoid concomitant use
  Antiepileptics: plasma concentration of dabigatran possibly reduced by carbamazepine and phenytoin—manufacturer of dabigatran advises avoid concomitant use
  Antifungals: manufacturer of dabigatran advises avoid concomitant use with itraconazole
  Antivirals: plasma concentration of dabigatran possibly increased by rilpivirine and telaprevir
- Calcium-channel Blockers: plasma concentration of dabigatran possibly increased by ●verapamil (see Dose under Dabigatran, p. 156)
- Ciclosporin: plasma concentration of dabigatran possibly increased by ●ciclosporin—manufacturer of dabigatran advises avoid concomitant use
- Sulfinpyrazone: possible increased risk of bleeding when dabigatran given with ●sulfinpyrazone
- Tacrolimus: plasma concentration of dabigatran possibly increased by ●tacrolimus—manufacturer of dabigatran advises avoid concomitant use
- Ticagrelor: plasma concentration of dabigatran increased by ●ticagrelor
  Ulipristal: manufacturer of ulipristal advises give dabigatran at least 1.5 hours before or after ulipristal

Dabrafenib

  Antibacterials: manufacturer of dabrafenib advises avoid concomitant use with rifampicin
  Anticoagulants: dabrafenib reduces plasma concentration of warfarin
  Antidepressants: manufacturer of dabrafenib advises avoid concomitant use with St John's wort
  Antiepileptics: manufacturer of dabrafenib advises avoid concomitant use with carbamazepine, phenobarbital and phenytoin
- Antipsychotics: avoid concomitant use of cytotoxics with ●clozapine (increased risk of agranulocytosis)
  Lipid-regulating Drugs: plasma concentration of dabrafenib increased by gemfibrozil
- Oestrogens: manufacturer of dabrafenib advises contraceptive effect of hormonal contraceptives containing ●oestrogens possibly reduced (alternative contraceptive recommended)
- Progestogens: manufacturer of dabrafenib advises contraceptive effect of hormonal contraceptives

Dabrafenib

- Progestogens *(continued)*
  containing ●progestogens possibly reduced (alternative contraceptive recommended)
  Ulcer-healing Drugs: manufacturer of dabrafenib advises avoid concomitant use with proton pump inhibitors (plasma concentration of dabrafenib possibly reduced)

Dacarbazine

- Aldesleukin: avoidance of dacarbazine advised by manufacturer of ●aldesleukin
- Antipsychotics: avoid concomitant use of cytotoxics with ●clozapine (increased risk of agranulocytosis)

Daclatasvir

- Antibacterials: plasma concentration of daclatasvir possibly increased by ●clarithromycin and ●telithromycin—reduce dose of daclatasvir (see Dose under Daclatasvir, p. 438); plasma concentration of daclatasvir possibly reduced by ●rifabutin—manufacturer of daclatasvir advises avoid concomitant use; plasma concentration of daclatasvir reduced by ●rifampicin—avoid concomitant use
  Antidepressants: plasma concentration of daclatasvir possibly reduced by St John's wort—manufacturer of daclatasvir advises avoid concomitant use
- Antiepileptics: plasma concentration of daclatasvir possibly reduced by ●carbamazepine, ●oxcarbazepine, ●phenobarbital and ●phenytoin—manufacturer of daclatasvir advises avoid concomitant use
- Antifungals: plasma concentration of daclatasvir possibly increased by ●itraconazole, ●posaconazole and ●voriconazole—reduce dose of daclatasvir (see Dose under Daclatasvir, p. 438)
- Antivirals: plasma concentration of daclatasvir increased by ●atazanavir and ●telaprevir—reduce dose of daclatasvir (see Dose under Daclatasvir, p. 438); plasma concentration of daclatasvir possibly increased by ●boceprevir—reduce dose of daclatasvir (see Dose under Daclatasvir, p. 438); manufacturer of daclatasvir advises avoid concomitant use with darunavir and lopinavir (plasma concentration of daclatasvir possibly increased); plasma concentration of daclatasvir reduced by ●efavirenz—increase dose of daclatasvir (see Dose under Daclatasvir, p. 438); manufacturer of daclatasvir advises avoid concomitant use with etravirine and nevirapine (plasma concentration of daclatasvir possibly reduced)
- Cardiac Glycosides: daclatasvir increases plasma concentration of ●digoxin
- Cobicistat: plasma concentration of daclatasvir possibly increased by ●cobicistat—reduce dose of daclatasvir (see Dose under Daclatasvir, p. 438)
  Corticosteroids: plasma concentration of daclatasvir possibly reduced by dexamethasone—manufacturer of daclatasvir advises avoid concomitant use
  Lipid-regulating Drugs: daclatasvir increases plasma concentration of rosuvastatin

Dactinomycin

- Antipsychotics: avoid concomitant use of cytotoxics with ●clozapine (increased risk of agranulocytosis)
  Vitamins: dactinomycin possibly reduces effects of vitamin D

Dairy Products

  Antibacterials: dairy products reduce absorption of ciprofloxacin and norfloxacin; dairy products reduce absorption of tetracyclines (except doxycycline and minocycline)
  Cytotoxics: dairy products possibly reduce plasma concentration of mercaptopurine—manufacturer of mercaptopurine advises give at least 1 hour before or 2 hours after dairy products
  Eltrombopag: dairy products possibly reduce absorption of eltrombopag (give at least 4 hours apart)

Dalteparin *see* Heparins

Danaparoid

- Analgesics: increased risk of haemorrhage when anti-coagulants given with *intravenous* ●diclofenac (avoid concomitant use, including low-dose heparins); increased risk of haemorrhage when anticoagulants given with ●ketorolac (avoid concomitant use, including low-dose heparins)
- Anticoagulants: increased risk of haemorrhage when other anticoagulants given with ●apixaban, ●dabigatran and ●rivaroxaban (avoid concomitant use except when switching with other anticoagulants or using heparin to maintain catheter patency)

Danazol

- Anticoagulants: danazol inhibits metabolism of ●coumarins (enhanced anticoagulant effect)
- Antiepileptics: danazol inhibits metabolism of ●carbamazepine (increased risk of toxicity)
- Ciclosporin: danazol inhibits metabolism of ●ciclosporin (increased plasma concentration)
- Lipid-regulating Drugs: possible increased risk of myopathy when danazol given with ●simvastatin—avoid concomitant use
  Tacrolimus: danazol possibly increases plasma concentration of tacrolimus

Dantrolene *see* Muscle Relaxants

Dapagliflozin *see* Antidiabetics

Dapoxetine

- Alcohol: increased sedative effect when dapoxetine given with ●alcohol
- Analgesics: possible increased risk of serotonergic effects when dapoxetine given with ●tramadol (manufacturer of dapoxetine advises tramadol should not be started until 1 week after stopping dapoxetine, avoid dapoxetine for 2 weeks after stopping tramadol)
- Antibacterials: manufacturer of dapoxetine advises dose reduction when dapoxetine given with clarithromycin and erythromycin (see Dose under Dapoxetine, p. 572); manufacturer of dapoxetine advises avoid concomitant use with ●telithromycin (increased risk of toxicity)
- Antidepressants: possible increased risk of serotonergic effects when dapoxetine given with ●SSRIs, ●St John's wort, ●duloxetine, ●tricyclics and ●venlafaxine (manufacturer of dapoxetine advises SSRIs, St John's wort, duloxetine, tricyclics and venlafaxine should not be started until 1 week after stopping dapoxetine, avoid dapoxetine for 2 weeks after stopping SSRIs, St John's wort, duloxetine, tricyclics and venlafaxine); increased risk of serotonergic effects when dapoxetine given with ●MAOIs (MAOIs should not be started until 1 week after stopping dapoxetine, avoid dapoxetine for 2 weeks after stopping MAOIs)
- Antifungals: manufacturer of dapoxetine advises dose reduction when dapoxetine given with fluconazole (see Dose under Dapoxetine, p. 572); manufacturer of dapoxetine advises avoid concomitant use with ●itraconazole (increased risk of toxicity)
- Antivirals: manufacturer of dapoxetine advises avoid concomitant use with ●atazanavir, ●ritonavir and ●saquinavir (increased risk of toxicity); manufacturer of dapoxetine advises dose reduction when dapoxetine given with fosamprenavir (see Dose under Dapoxetine, p. 572)
  Aprepitant: manufacturer of dapoxetine advises dose reduction when dapoxetine given with aprepitant (see Dose under Dapoxetine, p. 572)
  Calcium-channel Blockers: manufacturer of dapoxetine advises dose reduction when dapoxetine given with diltiazem and verapamil (see Dose under Dapoxetine, p. 572)
- 5HT₁-receptor Agonists: possible increased risk of serotonergic effects when dapoxetine given with ●5HT₁ agonists (manufacturer of dapoxetine advises 5HT₁ agonists should not be started until

Dapoxetine

- 5HT₁-receptor Agonists *(continued)*
  1 week after stopping dapoxetine, avoid dapoxetine for 2 weeks after stopping 5HT₁ agonists)
- Lithium: possible increased risk of serotonergic effects when dapoxetine given with ●lithium (manufacturer of dapoxetine advises lithium should not be started until 1 week after stopping dapoxetine, avoid dapoxetine for 2 weeks after stopping lithium)
  Sildenafil: manufacturer of dapoxetine advises avoid concomitant use with sildenafil
  Tadalafil: manufacturer of dapoxetine advises avoid concomitant use with tadalafil
  Vardenafil: manufacturer of dapoxetine advises avoid concomitant use with vardenafil

Dapsone

  Antibacterials: plasma concentration of dapsone reduced by rifamycins; plasma concentration of both drugs may increase when dapsone given with trimethoprim
- Antivirals: increased risk of ventricular arrhythmias when dapsone given with ●saquinavir—avoid concomitant use
  Vaccines: antibacterials inactivate oral typhoid vaccine—see p. 864

Daptomycin

- Ciclosporin: increased risk of myopathy when daptomycin given with ●ciclosporin (preferably avoid concomitant use)
- Lipid-regulating Drugs: increased risk of myopathy when daptomycin given with ●fibrates or ●statins (preferably avoid concomitant use)
  Vaccines: antibacterials inactivate oral typhoid vaccine—see p. 864

Darifenacin *see* Antimuscarinics

Darunavir

  Anti-arrhythmics: darunavir possibly increases plasma concentration of lidocaine—avoid concomitant use
- Antibacterials: darunavir increases plasma concentration of ●rifabutin (reduce dose of rifabutin); plasma concentration of darunavir significantly reduced by ●rifampicin—avoid concomitant use
  Anticoagulants: avoidance of darunavir advised by manufacturer of apixaban and rivaroxaban
- Antidepressants: darunavir possibly reduces plasma concentration of paroxetine and sertraline; plasma concentration of darunavir reduced by ●St John's wort—avoid concomitant use
  Antiepileptics: plasma concentration of darunavir possibly reduced by carbamazepine, phenobarbital and phenytoin
- Antimalarials: darunavir increases plasma concentration of lumefantrine; darunavir possibly increases plasma concentration of ●quinine (increased risk of toxicity)
- Antipsychotics: darunavir possibly increases plasma concentration of ●aripiprazole (reduce dose of aripiprazole—consult aripiprazole product literature); darunavir possibly increases plasma concentration of ●quetiapine—manufacturer of quetiapine advises avoid concomitant use
- Antivirals: avoid concomitant use of darunavir with ●boceprevir or ●telaprevir; avoidance of darunavir advised by manufacturer of daclatasvir (plasma concentration of daclatasvir possibly increased); manufacturer of darunavir advises take didanosine 1 hour before or 2 hours after darunavir; plasma concentration of darunavir reduced by ●efavirenz (adjust dose—consult product literature); plasma concentration of both drugs increased when darunavir given with indinavir; plasma concentration of darunavir reduced by ●lopinavir, also plasma concentration of lopinavir increased (avoid concomitant use); darunavir increases plasma concentration of ●maraviroc (consider reducing dose of maraviroc); increased risk of rash when darunavir given with

Darunavir

- **Antivirals** *(continued)*
  raltegravir; plasma concentration of darunavir
  reduced by saquinavir; plasma concentration of
  both drugs increased when darunavir given with
  •simeprevir—manufacturer of simeprevir advises
  avoid concomitant use
- **Cytotoxics**: darunavir possibly increases the plasma
  concentration of •bosutinib—manufacturer of bosutinib advises avoid or consider reducing dose of
  bosutinib; darunavir possibly increases plasma concentration of •everolimus—manufacturer of everolimus advises avoid concomitant use; darunavir possibly increases the plasma concentration of
  •ibrutinib—reduce dose of ibrutinib (see Dose
  under Ibrutinib, p. 615)
- **Ergot Alkaloids**: increased risk of ergotism when darunavir given with •ergot alkaloids—manufacturer of
  darunavir advises avoid concomitant use
- **Lipid-regulating Drugs**: possible increased risk of myopathy when darunavir given with atorvastatin; darunavir possibly increases plasma concentration of
  pravastatin; darunavir increases plasma concentration of •rosuvastatin—adjust dose of rosuvastatin
  (consult product literature); avoidance of darunavir
  advised by manufacturer of •lomitapide (plasma
  concentration of lomitapide possibly increased)
- **Orlistat**: absorption of darunavir possibly reduced by
  •orlistat
- **Ranolazine**: darunavir possibly increases plasma concentration of •ranolazine—manufacturer of ranolazine advises avoid concomitant use

Dasatinib

- **Antibacterials**: metabolism of dasatinib accelerated by
  •rifampicin (reduced plasma concentration—avoid
  concomitant use)
- **Antipsychotics**: avoid concomitant use of cytotoxics
  with •clozapine (increased risk of agranulocytosis)
- **Antivirals**: avoidance of dasatinib advised by manufacturer of •boceprevir
  Lipid-regulating Drugs: dasatinib possibly increases
  plasma concentration of simvastatin
  Ulcer-healing Drugs: plasma concentration of dasatinib
  possibly reduced by famotidine

Decitabine

- **Antipsychotics**: avoid concomitant use of cytotoxics
  with •clozapine (increased risk of agranulocytosis)

Deferasirox

Antacids: absorption of deferasirox possibly reduced
by antacids containing aluminium (manufacturer of
deferasirox advises avoid concomitant use)
Antibacterials: plasma concentration of deferasirox
reduced by rifampicin
Antidiabetics: deferasirox increases plasma concentration of repaglinide
Antipsychotics: manufacturer of deferasirox advises
avoid concomitant use with clozapine
Anxiolytics and Hypnotics: deferasirox possibly
reduces plasma concentration of midazolam
Muscle Relaxants: manufacturer of deferasirox advises
avoid concomitant use with tizanidine
- **Theophylline**: deferasirox increases plasma concentration of •theophylline (consider reducing dose of
  theophylline)

Deferiprone

Antacids: absorption of deferiprone possibly reduced
by antacids containing aluminium (manufacturer of
deferiprone advises avoid concomitant use)

Deflazacort *see* Corticosteroids

Delamanid

- **Analgesics**: increased risk of ventricular arrhythmias
  when delamanid given with •methadone
- **Anti-arrhythmics**: increased risk of ventricular arrhythmias when delamanid given with •amiodarone or
  •disopyramide

Delamanid *(continued)*

- **Antibacterials**: possible increased risk of ventricular
  arrhythmias when delamanid given with •clarithro-
  mycin and •erythromycin; increased risk of ventricular arrhythmias when delamanid given with
  •moxifloxacin; plasma concentration of delamanid
  reduced by •rifampicin; delamanid increases plasma
  concentration of ethambutol
- **Antidepressants**: possible increased risk of ventricular
  arrhythmias when delamanid given with •tricyclics
  that prolong the QT interval
  Antiepileptics: manufacturer of delamanid advises
  avoid concomitant use with carbamazepine
- **Antipsychotics**: increased risk of ventricular arrhythmias when delamanid given with •droperidol,
  •haloperidol or •pimozide; increased risk of ventricular arrhythmias when delamanid given with
  •phenothiazines that prolong the QT interval
- **Antivirals**: plasma concentration of delamanid
  increased by lopinavir and ritonavir; increased risk
  of ventricular arrhythmias when delamanid given
  with •saquinavir
- **Beta-blockers**: increased risk of ventricular arrhythmias when delamanid given with •sotalol
- **Cytotoxics**: increased risk of ventricular arrhythmias
  when delamanid given with •arsenic trioxide or
  •vinflunine; possible increased risk of ventricular
  arrhythmias when delamanid given with
  •vinblastine, •vincristine, •vindesine and •vinorel-
  bine
- **Domperidone**: possible increased risk of ventricular
  arrhythmias when delamanid given with •domperi-
  done
- **Pentamidine Isetionate**: increased risk of ventricular
  arrhythmias when delamanid given with •pent-
  amidine isetionate
  Vaccines: antibacterials inactivate oral typhoid
  vaccine—see p. 864

Demeclocycline *see* Tetracyclines

Desferrioxamine

Antipsychotics: avoidance of desferrioxamine advised
by manufacturer of levomepromazine; manufacturer
of desferrioxamine advises avoid concomitant use
with prochlorperazine

Desflurane *see* Anaesthetics, General

Desloratadine *see* Antihistamines

Desmopressin

Analgesics: effects of desmopressin enhanced by
indometacin
Loperamide: plasma concentration of *oral* desmopressin increased by loperamide

Desogestrel *see* Progestogens

Dexamethasone *see* Corticosteroids

Dexamfetamine *see* Sympathomimetics

Dexibuprofen *see* NSAIDs

Dexketoprofen *see* NSAIDs

Dexrazoxane

- **Antiepileptics**: absorption of dexrazoxane possibly
  reduced by •phenytoin
  Ciclosporin: manufacturer of dexrazoxane advises
  increased risk of immunosuppression with ciclosporin
  Tacrolimus: manufacturer of dexrazoxane advises
  increased risk of immunosuppression with tacrolimus
- **Vaccines**: avoid concomitant use of dexrazoxane with
  live •vaccines (see p. 842)

Dextromethorphan *see* Opioid Analgesics

Dextropropoxyphene *see* Opioid Analgesics

Diamorphine *see* Opioid Analgesics

Diazepam *see* Anxiolytics and Hypnotics

Diazoxide

ACE Inhibitors: enhanced hypotensive effect when
diazoxide given with ACE inhibitors

Diazoxide *(continued)*

Adrenergic Neurone Blockers: enhanced hypotensive effect when diazoxide given with adrenergic neurone blockers

Alcohol: enhanced hypotensive effect when diazoxide given with alcohol

Aldesleukin: enhanced hypotensive effect when diazoxide given with aldesleukin

Alpha-blockers: enhanced hypotensive effect when diazoxide given with alpha-blockers

Anaesthetics, General: enhanced hypotensive effect when diazoxide given with general anaesthetics

Analgesics: hypotensive effect of diazoxide antagonised by NSAIDs

Angiotensin-II Receptor Antagonists: enhanced hypotensive effect when diazoxide given with angiotensin-II receptor antagonists

Antidepressants: enhanced hypotensive effect when diazoxide given with MAOIs or tricyclic-related antidepressants

Antidiabetics: diazoxide antagonises hypoglycaemic effect of antidiabetics

Antiepileptics: diazoxide reduces plasma concentration of phenytoin, also effect of diazoxide may be reduced

Antipsychotics: enhanced hypotensive effect when diazoxide given with phenothiazines

Anxiolytics and Hypnotics: enhanced hypotensive effect when diazoxide given with anxiolytics and hypnotics

Beta-blockers: enhanced hypotensive effect when diazoxide given with beta-blockers

Calcium-channel Blockers: enhanced hypotensive effect when diazoxide given with calcium-channel blockers

Clonidine: enhanced hypotensive effect when diazoxide given with clonidine

Corticosteroids: hypotensive effect of diazoxide antagonised by corticosteroids

Diuretics: enhanced hypotensive and hyperglycaemic effects when diazoxide given with diuretics

Dopaminergics: enhanced hypotensive effect when diazoxide given with levodopa

Methyldopa: enhanced hypotensive effect when diazoxide given with methyldopa

Moxisylyte: enhanced hypotensive effect when diazoxide given with moxisylyte

Moxonidine: enhanced hypotensive effect when diazoxide given with moxonidine

Muscle Relaxants: enhanced hypotensive effect when diazoxide given with baclofen or tizanidine

Nitrates: enhanced hypotensive effect when diazoxide given with nitrates

Prostaglandins: enhanced hypotensive effect when diazoxide given with alprostadil

Vasodilator Antihypertensives: enhanced hypotensive effect when diazoxide given with hydralazine, minoxidil or sodium nitroprusside

Diclofenac *see* NSAIDs

Dicycloverine *see* Antimuscarinics

Didanosine

Note Antacids in tablet formulation might affect absorption of other drugs—give at least 2 hours apart

- Allopurinol: plasma concentration of didanosine increased by ●allopurinol (risk of toxicity)—avoid concomitant use

Analgesics: plasma concentration of didanosine possibly reduced by methadone

Antibacterials: manufacturer of norfloxacin advises give didanosine at least 2 hours before or after norfloxacin

- Antivirals: didanosine *tablets* reduce absorption of atazanavir (give at least 2 hours before or 1 hour after didanosine *tablets*); manufacturer of darunavir advises take didanosine 1 hour before or 2 hours after darunavir; plasma concentration of didanosine

Didanosine

- Antivirals *(continued)*
  possibly increased by ganciclovir; didanosine *tablets* reduce absorption of indinavir (give at least 1 hour apart); increased risk of side-effects when didanosine given with ●ribavirin—avoid concomitant use; manufacturer of rilpivirine advises give didanosine 2 hours before or 4 hours after rilpivirine; manufacturer of ritonavir advises didanosine and ritonavir should be taken 2.5 hours apart; increased risk of side-effects when didanosine given with ●stavudine; plasma concentration of didanosine increased by ●tenofovir (increased risk of toxicity)—avoid concomitant use; plasma concentration of didanosine reduced by tipranavir—manufacturer of tipranavir advises tipranavir and didanosine *capsules* should be taken at least 2 hours apart

- Cytotoxics: increased risk of toxicity when didanosine given with ●hydroxycarbamide—avoid concomitant use

- Orlistat: absorption of didanosine possibly reduced by ●orlistat

Dienogest *see* Progestogens

Digoxin *see* Cardiac Glycosides

Dihydrocodeine *see* Opioid Analgesics

Diltiazem *see* Calcium-channel Blockers

Dimethyl sulfoxide

- Analgesics: avoid concomitant use of dimethyl sulfoxide with ●sulindac

Dinoprostone *see* Prostaglandins

Diphenoxylate *see* Opioid Analgesics

Diphtheria vaccines *see* Vaccines

Dipipanone *see* Opioid Analgesics

Dipyridamole

Antacids: absorption of dipyridamole possibly reduced by antacids

- Anti-arrhythmics: dipyridamole enhances and extends effect of ●adenosine (important risk of toxicity)—reduce dose of adenosine, see Dose under Adenosine, p. 96

- Anticoagulants: antiplatelet action of dipyridamole enhances anticoagulant effect of ●coumarins and ●phenindione; dipyridamole enhances anticoagulant effect of heparins

Clopidogrel: increased risk of bleeding when dipyridamole given with clopidogrel

Cytotoxics: dipyridamole possibly reduces effects of fludarabine

Disopyramide

Anaesthetics, Local: increased myocardial depression when anti-arrhythmics given with bupivacaine, levobupivacaine, prilocaine or ropivacaine

- Anti-arrhythmics: increased myocardial depression when anti-arrhythmics given with other ●anti-arrhythmics; increased risk of ventricular arrhythmias when disopyramide given with ●amiodarone or ●dronedarone—avoid concomitant use

- Antibacterials: plasma concentration of disopyramide possibly increased by ●azithromycin (increased risk of toxicity); plasma concentration of disopyramide possibly increased by ●clarithromycin (increased risk of ventricular arrhythmias); plasma concentration of disopyramide increased by ●erythromycin (increased risk of toxicity); increased risk of ventricular arrhythmias when disopyramide given with ●moxifloxacin—avoid concomitant use; increased risk of ventricular arrhythmias when disopyramide given with ●delamanid; metabolism of disopyramide accelerated by ●rifamycins (reduced plasma concentration); possible increased risk of ventricular arrhythmias when disopyramide given with ●telithromycin

Anticoagulants: disopyramide may enhance or reduce anticoagulant effect of warfarin

Appendix 1: Interactions

Disopyramide *(continued)*

- Antidepressants: avoidance of disopyramide advised by manufacturer of ●citalopram and ●escitalopram (risk of ventricular arrhythmias); increased risk of ventricular arrhythmias when disopyramide given with ●tricyclics

  Antidiabetics: disopyramide possibly enhances hypoglycaemic effect of gliclazide, insulin and metformin

  Antiepileptics: metabolism of disopyramide accelerated by phenobarbital (reduced plasma concentration); plasma concentration of disopyramide reduced by phenytoin

- Antifungals: avoidance of disopyramide advised by manufacturer of ●itraconazole

- Antihistamines: increased risk of ventricular arrhythmias when disopyramide given with ●mizolastine—avoid concomitant use

- Antimalarials: avoidance of disopyramide advised by manufacturer of ●piperaquine with artenimol (possible risk of ventricular arrhythmias); avoidance of disopyramide advised by manufacturer of ●artemether with lumefantrine (risk of ventricular arrhythmias)

- Antimuscarinics: increased risk of antimuscarinic side-effects when disopyramide given with antimuscarinics; increased risk of ventricular arrhythmias when disopyramide given with ●tolterodine

- Antipsychotics: increased risk of ventricular arrhythmias when anti-arrhythmics that prolong the QT interval given with ●antipsychotics that prolong the QT interval; increased risk of ventricular arrhythmias when disopyramide given with ●amisulpride, ●droperidol, ●pimozide or ●zuclopenthixol—avoid concomitant use; possible increased risk of ventricular arrhythmias when disopyramide given with ●haloperidol—avoid concomitant use; increased risk of ventricular arrhythmias when disopyramide given with ●phenothiazines or ●sulpiride

- Antivirals: plasma concentration of disopyramide possibly increased by ●ritonavir (increased risk of toxicity); increased risk of ventricular arrhythmias when disopyramide given with ●saquinavir—avoid concomitant use; avoidance of disopyramide advised by manufacturer of ●telaprevir (risk of ventricular arrhythmias)

- Atomoxetine: increased risk of ventricular arrhythmias when disopyramide given with ●atomoxetine

- Beta-blockers: increased myocardial depression when anti-arrhythmics given with ●beta-blockers; increased risk of ventricular arrhythmias when disopyramide given with ●sotalol—avoid concomitant use

- Calcium-channel Blockers: increased risk of myocardial depression and asystole when disopyramide given with ●verapamil

- Cytotoxics: possible increased risk of ventricular arrhythmias when disopyramide given with ●bosutinib; possible increased risk of ventricular arrhythmias when disopyramide given with ●vandetanib—avoid concomitant use; increased risk of ventricular arrhythmias when disopyramide given with ●arsenic trioxide

- Diuretics: increased cardiac toxicity with disopyramide if hypokalaemia occurs with ●acetazolamide, ●loop diuretics or ●thiazides and related diuretics

- Fingolimod: possible increased risk of bradycardia when disopyramide given with ●fingolimod

- Ivabradine: increased risk of ventricular arrhythmias when disopyramide given with ●ivabradine

  Nitrates: disopyramide reduces effects of sublingual tablets of nitrates (failure to dissolve under tongue owing to dry mouth)

- Pentamidine Isetionate: possible increased risk of ventricular arrhythmias when disopyramide given with ●pentamidine isetionate

Disopyramide *(continued)*

- Ranolazine: avoidance of disopyramide advised by manufacturer of ●ranolazine

  Sildenafil: manufacturer of disopyramide advises avoid concomitant use with sildenafil (risk of ventricular arrhythmias)

  Tadalafil: manufacturer of disopyramide advises avoid concomitant use with tadalafil (risk of ventricular arrhythmias)

  Vardenafil: manufacturer of disopyramide advises avoid concomitant use with vardenafil (risk of ventricular arrhythmias)

Disulfiram

Alcohol: disulfiram reaction when disulfiram given with alcohol (see p. 339)

Antibacterials: psychotic reaction reported when disulfiram given with metronidazole; CNS effects of disulfiram possibly increased by isoniazid

- Anticoagulants: disulfiram enhances anticoagulant effect of ●coumarins

  Antidepressants: increased disulfiram reaction with alcohol reported with concomitant amitriptyline; disulfiram inhibits metabolism of tricyclics (increased plasma concentration)

- Antiepileptics: disulfiram inhibits metabolism of ●phenytoin (increased risk of toxicity)

  Anxiolytics and Hypnotics: disulfiram increases risk of temazepam toxicity; disulfiram inhibits metabolism of benzodiazepines (increased sedative effects)

- Paraldehyde: risk of toxicity when disulfiram given with ●paraldehyde

  Theophylline: disulfiram inhibits metabolism of theophylline (increased risk of toxicity)

Diuretics

Note Since systemic absorption may follow topical application of brinzolamide to the eye, the possibility of interactions should be borne in mind

Note Since systemic absorption may follow topical application of dorzolamide to the eye, the possibility of interactions should be borne in mind

- ACE Inhibitors: enhanced hypotensive effect when diuretics given with ●ACE inhibitors; increased risk of severe hyperkalaemia when potassium-sparing diuretics and aldosterone antagonists given with ●ACE inhibitors

  Adrenergic Neurone Blockers: enhanced hypotensive effect when diuretics given with adrenergic neurone blockers

  Alcohol: enhanced hypotensive effect when diuretics given with alcohol

  Aldesleukin: enhanced hypotensive effect when diuretics given with aldesleukin

  Aliskiren: plasma concentration of furosemide reduced by aliskiren; increased risk of hyperkalaemia when potassium-sparing diuretics and aldosterone antagonists given with aliskiren

  Allopurinol: increased risk of hypersensitivity when thiazides and related diuretics given with allopurinol especially in renal impairment

- Alpha-blockers: enhanced hypotensive effect when diuretics given with ●alpha-blockers, also increased risk of first-dose hypotension with post-synaptic alpha-blockers such as prazosin

  Anaesthetics, General: enhanced hypotensive effect when diuretics given with general anaesthetics

- Analgesics: possible increased risk of hyperkalaemia when potassium-sparing diuretics and aldosterone antagonists given with NSAIDs; diuretics increase risk of nephrotoxicity of NSAIDs, also antagonism of diuretic effect; diuretic effect of potassium canrenoate possibly antagonised by NSAIDs; furosemide possibly increases the excretion of acemetacin; effects of diuretics antagonised by indometacin and ketorolac; increased risk of hyperkalaemia when potassium-sparing diuretics and aldosterone antagonists given with indometacin; occasional

Diuretics

- **Analgesics** *(continued)*

  reports of reduced renal function when triamterene given with ●indometacin—avoid concomitant use; diuretic effect of spironolactone antagonised by aspirin; possible increased risk of toxicity when loop diuretics given with high-dose aspirin (also possible reduced effect of loop diuretics); increased risk of toxicity when acetazolamide given with high-dose ●aspirin

- **Angiotensin-II Receptor Antagonists:** enhanced hypotensive effect when diuretics given with ●angiotensin-II receptor antagonists; increased risk of hyperkalaemia when potassium-sparing diuretics and aldosterone antagonists given with ●angiotensin-II receptor antagonists

- **Anti-arrhythmics:** plasma concentration of eplerenone increased by amiodarone (reduce dose of eplerenone); hypokalaemia caused by acetazolamide, loop diuretics or thiazides and related diuretics increases cardiac toxicity with amiodarone; hypokalaemia caused by acetazolamide, loop diuretics or thiazides and related diuretics increases cardiac toxicity with ●disopyramide; hypokalaemia caused by acetazolamide, loop diuretics or thiazides and related diuretics increases cardiac toxicity with ●flecainide; hypokalaemia caused by acetazolamide, loop diuretics or thiazides and related diuretics antagonises action of ●lidocaine

- **Antibacterials:** plasma concentration of eplerenone increased by ●clarithromycin and ●telithromycin—avoid concomitant use; plasma concentration of eplerenone increased by erythromycin (reduce dose of eplerenone); plasma concentration of eplerenone reduced by ●rifampicin—avoid concomitant use; avoidance of diuretics advised by manufacturer of lymecycline; increased risk of otoxicity when loop diuretics given with ●aminoglycosides, ●polymyxins or ●vancomycin; acetazolamide antagonises effects of ●methenamine; possible increased risk of hyperkalaemia when spironolactone given with trimethoprim; increased risk of hyperkalaemia when eplerenone given with trimethoprim

- **Antidepressants:** possible increased risk of hypokalaemia when loop diuretics or thiazides and related diuretics given with reboxetine; enhanced hypotensive effect when diuretics given with MAOIs; plasma concentration of eplerenone reduced by ●St John's wort—avoid concomitant use; increased risk of postural hypotension when diuretics given with tricyclics

  Antidiabetics: loop diuretics and thiazides and related diuretics antagonise hypoglycaemic effect of antidiabetics; diuretic effect of diuretics possibly enhanced by canagliflozin; avoidance of loop diuretics advised by manufacturer of canagliflozin; diuretic effect of loop diuretics and thiazides and related diuretics possibly enhanced by dapagliflozin

- **Antiepileptics:** plasma concentration of eplerenone reduced by ●carbamazepine, ●phenobarbital and ●phenytoin—avoid concomitant use; increased risk of hyponatraemia when diuretics given with carbamazepine; acetazolamide increases plasma concentration of ●carbamazepine; increased risk of osteomalacia when carbonic anhydrase inhibitors given with phenobarbital or phenytoin; effects of furosemide antagonised by phenytoin; acetazolamide possibly increases plasma concentration of ●phenytoin; hydrochlorothiazide possibly increases plasma concentration of topiramate; avoidance of carbonic anhydrase inhibitors in children advised by manufacturer of zonisamide

- **Antifungals:** increased risk of hypokalaemia when loop diuretics or thiazides and related diuretics given with amphotericin; hydrochlorothiazide increases plasma concentration of fluconazole;

Diuretics

- **Antifungals** *(continued)*

  plasma concentration of eplerenone increased by fluconazole (reduce dose of eplerenone); plasma concentration of eplerenone increased by ●itraconazole—avoid concomitant use

- **Antipsychotics:** hypokalaemia caused by diuretics increases risk of ventricular arrhythmias with ●amisulpride; enhanced hypotensive effect when diuretics given with phenothiazines; hypokalaemia caused by diuretics increases risk of ventricular arrhythmias with ●pimozide (avoid concomitant use)

- **Antivirals:** plasma concentration of eplerenone increased by ●ritonavir—avoid concomitant use; plasma concentration of eplerenone increased by saquinavir (reduce dose of eplerenone)

  Anxiolytics and Hypnotics: enhanced hypotensive effect when diuretics given with anxiolytics and hypnotics; administration of *parenteral* furosemide with chloral may displace thyroid hormone from binding sites

- **Atomoxetine:** hypokalaemia caused by diuretics increases risk of ventricular arrhythmias with ●atomoxetine

- **Beta-blockers:** enhanced hypotensive effect when diuretics given with beta-blockers; hypokalaemia caused by loop diuretics or thiazides and related diuretics increases risk of ventricular arrhythmias with ●sotalol

  Calcium Salts: increased risk of hypercalcaemia when thiazides and related diuretics given with calcium salts

  Calcium-channel Blockers: enhanced hypotensive effect when diuretics given with calcium-channel blockers; plasma concentration of eplerenone increased by diltiazem and verapamil (reduce dose of eplerenone)

- **Cardiac Glycosides:** hypokalaemia caused by acetazolamide, loop diuretics or thiazides and related diuretics increases cardiac toxicity with ●cardiac glycosides; potassium canrenoate possibly increases plasma concentration of digoxin; spironolactone increases plasma concentration of ●digoxin

- **Ciclosporin:** increased risk of nephrotoxicity and possibly hypermagnesaemia when thiazides and related diuretics given with ciclosporin; increased risk of hyperkalaemia when potassium-sparing diuretics and aldosterone antagonists given with ●ciclosporin; acetazolamide possibly increases plasma concentration of ●ciclosporin

  Clonidine: enhanced hypotensive effect when diuretics given with clonidine

  Corticosteroids: diuretic effect of diuretics antagonised by corticosteroids; increased risk of hypokalaemia when acetazolamide, loop diuretics or thiazides and related diuretics given with corticosteroids

- **Cytotoxics:** alkaline urine due to acetazolamide increases exceretion of methotrexate; hypokalaemia caused by acetazolamide, loop diuretics or thiazides and related diuretics increases risk of ventricular arrhythmias with ●arsenic trioxide; avoidance of spironolactone advised by manufacturer of mitotane (antagonism of effect); increased risk of nephrotoxicity and ototoxicity when diuretics given with platinum compounds

  Diazoxide: enhanced hypotensive and hyperglycaemic effects when diuretics given with diazoxide

  Diuretics: increased risk of hypokalaemia when loop diuretics or thiazides and related diuretics given with acetazolamide; profound diuresis possible when metolazone given with furosemide; increased risk of hypokalaemia when thiazides and related diuretics given with loop diuretics

  Dopaminergics: enhanced hypotensive effect when diuretics given with levodopa

Diuretics *(continued)*

Hormone Antagonists: increased risk of hypercalcaemia when thiazides and related diuretics given with toremifene

Lipid-regulating Drugs: absorption of thiazides and related diuretics reduced by colestipol and colestyramine (give at least 2 hours apart)

- Lithium: loop diuretics and thiazides and related diuretics reduce excretion of ●lithium (increased plasma concentration and risk of toxicity)—loop diuretics safer than thiazides; potassium-sparing diuretics and aldosterone antagonists reduce excretion of ●lithium (increased plasma concentration and risk of toxicity); acetazolamide increases the excretion of ●lithium

Methyldopa: enhanced hypotensive effect when diuretics given with methyldopa

Moxisylyte: enhanced hypotensive effect when diuretics given with moxisylyte

Moxonidine: enhanced hypotensive effect when diuretics given with moxonidine

Muscle Relaxants: enhanced hypotensive effect when diuretics given with baclofen or tizanidine

Nitrates: enhanced hypotensive effect when diuretics given with nitrates

Oestrogens: diuretic effect of diuretics antagonised by oestrogens

- Potassium Salts: increased risk of hyperkalaemia when potassium-sparing diuretics and aldosterone antagonists given with ●potassium salts

Progestogens: risk of hyperkalaemia when potassium-sparing diuretics and aldosterone antagonists given with drospirenone (monitor serum potassium during first cycle)

Prostaglandins: enhanced hypotensive effect when diuretics given with alprostadil

Sympathomimetics, Beta$_2$: increased risk of hypokalaemia when acetazolamide, loop diuretics or thiazides and related diuretics given with high doses of beta$_2$ sympathomimetics—see Hypokalaemia, p. 189

- Tacrolimus: increased risk of hyperkalaemia when potassium-sparing diuretics and aldosterone antagonists given with ●tacrolimus

Theophylline: increased risk of hypokalaemia when acetazolamide, loop diuretics or thiazides and related diuretics given with theophylline

Vasodilator Antihypertensives: enhanced hypotensive effect when diuretics given with hydralazine, minoxidil or sodium nitroprusside

Vitamins: increased risk of hypercalcaemia when thiazides and related diuretics given with vitamin D

Diuretics, Loop *see* Diuretics

Diuretics, Potassium-sparing and Aldosterone Antagonists *see* Diuretics

Diuretics, Thiazide and related *see* Diuretics

Dobutamine *see* Sympathomimetics

Docetaxel

- Antibacterials: plasma concentration of docetaxel possibly increased by ●clarithromycin and ●telithromycin—manufacturer of docetaxel advises avoid concomitant use or consider reducing docetaxel dose

- Antifungals: plasma concentration of docetaxel possibly increased by ●itraconazole and ●voriconazole—manufacturer of docetaxel advises avoid concomitant use or consider reducing docetaxel dose

- Antipsychotics: avoid concomitant use of cytotoxics with ●clozapine (increased risk of agranulocytosis)

- Antivirals: plasma concentration of docetaxel possibly increased by ●indinavir, ●ritonavir and ●saquinavir—manufacturer of docetaxel advises avoid concomitant use or consider reducing docetaxel dose

Ciclosporin: *in vitro* studies suggest a possible interaction between docetaxel and ciclosporin (consult docetaxel product literature)

Docetaxel *(continued)*

Cytotoxics: possible increased risk of neutropenia when docetaxel given with lapatinib; plasma concentration of docetaxel increased by sorafenib

Dolutegravir

Antacids: absorption of dolutegravir reduced by aluminium hydroxide and oral magnesium salts—manufacturer of dolutegravir advises give at least 2 hours before or 6 hours after aluminium hydroxide and oral magnesium salts

- Antibacterials: plasma concentration of dolutegravir reduced by ●rifampicin (see Dose under Dolutegravir, p. 429)

Antidepressants: manufacturer of dolutegravir advises avoid concomitant use with St John's wort

Antiepileptics: manufacturer of dolutegravir advises avoid concomitant use with carbamazepine, oxcarbazepine, phenobarbital and phenytoin

- Antivirals: plasma concentration of dolutegravir reduced by ●efavirenz and ●tipranavir (see Dose under Dolutegravir, p. 429); plasma concentration of dolutegravir reduced by ●etravirine (see Cautions under Dolutegravir, p. 429); plasma concentration of dolutegravir reduced by ●fosamprenavir; plasma concentration of dolutegravir possibly reduced by ●nevirapine (see Dose under Dolutegravir, p. 429)

Calcium Salts: absorption of dolutegravir reduced by calcium salts—manufacturer of dolutegravir advises give at least 2 hours before or 6 hours after calcium salts

Iron: absorption of dolutegravir reduced by *oral* iron—manufacturer of dolutegravir advises give at least 2 hours before or 6 hours after *oral* iron

Domperidone

Analgesics: effects of domperidone on gastro-intestinal activity antagonised by opioid analgesics

- Antibacterials: possible increased risk of ventricular arrhythmias when domperidone given with ●clarithromycin or ●telithromycin—avoid concomitant use; plasma concentration of domperidone increased by ●erythromycin (increased risk of ventricular arrhythmias—avoid concomitant use); possible increased risk of ventricular arrhythmias when domperidone given with ●delamanid

- Antifungals: possible increased risk of ventricular arrhythmias when domperidone given with ●itraconazole or ●voriconazole—avoid concomitant use

- Antimalarials: avoidance of domperidone advised by manufacturer of ●piperaquine with artenimol (possible risk of ventricular arrhythmias)

Antimuscarinics: effects of domperidone on gastrointestinal activity antagonised by antimuscarinics

- Antivirals: possible increased risk of ventricular arrhythmias when domperidone given with ●boceprevir, ●ritonavir, ●saquinavir or ●telaprevir—avoid concomitant use

- Cobicistat: possible increased risk of ventricular arrhythmias when domperidone given with ●cobicistat—avoid concomitant use

- Cytotoxics: avoidance of domperidone advised by manufacturer of ●bosutinib (risk of ventricular arrhythmias)

Dopaminergics: domperidone possibly antagonises hypoprolactinaemic effects of bromocriptine and cabergoline

Donepezil *see* Parasympathomimetics

Dopamine *see* Sympathomimetics

Dopaminergics *see* Amantadine, Apomorphine, Bromocriptine, Cabergoline, Entacapone, Levodopa, Pergolide, Pramipexole, Quinagolide, Rasagiline, Ropinirole, Rotigotine, Selegiline, and Tolcapone

Dopexamine *see* Sympathomimetics

Dorzolamide *see* Diuretics

Dosulepin *see* Antidepressants, Tricyclic

Doxapram

- Anaesthetics, General: increased risk of arrhythmias when doxapram given with ●volatile liquid general anaesthetics (avoid doxapram for at least 10 minutes after volatile liquid general anaesthetics)

  Antidepressants: effects of doxapram enhanced by MAOIs

  Sympathomimetics: increased risk of hypertension when doxapram given with sympathomimetics

  Theophylline: increased CNS stimulation when doxapram given with theophylline

Doxazosin *see* Alpha-blockers

Doxepin *see* Antidepressants, Tricyclic

Doxorubicin

- Antipsychotics: avoid concomitant use of cytotoxics with ●clozapine (increased risk of agranulocytosis)

  Antivirals: doxorubicin possibly inhibits effects of stavudine

  Calcium-channel Blockers: plasma concentration of doxorubicin possibly increased by verapamil

  Cardiac Glycosides: doxorubicin possibly reduces absorption of digoxin *tablets*

- Ciclosporin: increased risk of neurotoxicity when doxorubicin given with ●ciclosporin

  Cytotoxics: plasma concentration of doxorubicin increased by sorafenib

  Ulcer-healing Drugs: plasma concentration of doxorubicin reduced by cimetidine

- Vaccines: avoid concomitant use of doxorubicin with live ●vaccines (see p. 842)

Doxycycline *see* Tetracyclines

Dronedarone

Anaesthetics, Local: increased myocardial depression when anti-arrhythmics given with bupivacaine, levobupivacaine, prilocaine or ropivacaine

- Anti-arrhythmics: increased myocardial depression when anti-arrhythmics given with other ●anti-arrhythmics; increased risk of ventricular arrhythmias when dronedarone given with ●amiodarone or ●disopyramide—avoid concomitant use

- Antibacterials: manufacturer of dronedarone advises avoid concomitant use with ●clarithromycin (risk of ventricular arrhythmias); plasma concentration of dronedarone increased by ●erythromycin (increased risk of ventricular arrhythmias—avoid concomitant use); plasma concentration of dronedarone reduced by ●rifampicin—avoid concomitant use; increased risk of ventricular arrhythmias when dronedarone given with ●telithromycin—avoid concomitant use

- Anticoagulants: dronedarone possibly enhances anticoagulant effect of ●coumarins and ●phenindione; dronedarone increases plasma concentration of ●dabigatran—avoid concomitant use; avoidance of dronedarone advised by manufacturer of rivaroxaban

- Antidepressants: avoidance of dronedarone advised by manufacturer of ●citalopram and ●escitalopram (risk of ventricular arrhythmias); plasma concentration of dronedarone possibly reduced by ●St John's wort—avoid concomitant use; manufacturer of dronedarone advises avoid concomitant use with ●tricyclics (risk of ventricular arrhythmias)

- Antiepileptics: plasma concentration of dronedarone possibly reduced by ●carbamazepine, ●phenobarbital and ●phenytoin—avoid concomitant use

- Antifungals: manufacturer of dronedarone advises avoid concomitant use with ●itraconazole, ●posaconazole and ●voriconazole

- Antipsychotics: increased risk of ventricular arrhythmias when anti-arrhythmics that prolong the QT interval given with ●antipsychotics that prolong the QT interval; manufacturer of dronedarone advises avoid concomitant use with ●phenothiazines (risk of ventricular arrhythmias)

- Antivirals: manufacturer of dronedarone advises avoid concomitant use with ●ritonavir; increased risk of

Dronedarone

- Antivirals *(continued)*

  ventricular arrhythmias when dronedarone given with ●saquinavir—avoid concomitant use

- Beta-blockers: increased myocardial depression when anti-arrhythmics given with ●beta-blockers; dronedarone possibly increases plasma concentration of metoprolol and propranolol; increased risk of ventricular arrhythmias when dronedarone given with ●sotalol—avoid concomitant use

- Calcium-channel Blockers: plasma concentration of dronedarone increased by ●nifedipine; increased risk of bradycardia and myocardial depression when dronedarone given with ●diltiazem and ●verapamil

- Cardiac Glycosides: dronedarone increases plasma concentration of ●digoxin (halve dose of digoxin)

- Cytotoxics: dronedarone possibly increases the plasma concentration of ●bosutinib—manufacturer of bosutinib advises avoid or consider reducing dose of bosutinib; dronedarone possibly increases the plasma concentration of ●ibrutinib—reduce dose of ibrutinib (see Dose under Ibrutinib, p. 615)

  Fidaxomicin: avoidance of dronedarone advised by manufacturer of fidaxomicin

- Fingolimod: possible increased risk of bradycardia when dronedarone given with ●fingolimod

- Grapefruit Juice: plasma concentration of dronedarone increased by ●grapefruit juice—avoid concomitant use

- Lipid-regulating Drugs: dronedarone possibly increases plasma concentration of atorvastatin; dronedarone increases plasma concentration of ●rosuvastatin—adjust dose of rosuvastatin (consult product literature); increased risk of myopathy when dronedarone given with ●simvastatin; avoidance of dronedarone advised by manufacturer of ●lomitapide (plasma concentration of lomitapide possibly increased)

  Sirolimus: manufacturer of dronedarone advises caution with sirolimus

  Tacrolimus: manufacturer of dronedarone advises caution with tacrolimus

Droperidol *see* Antipsychotics

Drospirenone *see* Progestogens

Duloxetine

Analgesics: possible increased serotonergic effects when SSRI-related antidepressants given with fentanyl; possible increased serotonergic effects when duloxetine given with pethidine or tramadol

- Antibacterials: metabolism of duloxetine inhibited by ●ciprofloxacin—avoid concomitant use

- Anticoagulants: possible increased risk of bleeding when SSRI-related antidepressants given with ●dabigatran

- Antidepressants: metabolism of duloxetine inhibited by ●fluvoxamine—avoid concomitant use; possible increased serotonergic effects when duloxetine given with SSRIs, St John's wort, amitriptyline, clomipramine, ●moclobemide or venlafaxine; duloxetine should not be started until 2 weeks after stopping ●MAOIs, also MAOIs should not be started until at least 5 days after stopping duloxetine; after stopping SSRI-related antidepressants do not start ●moclobemide for at least 1 week

- Antimalarials: avoidance of antidepressants advised by manufacturer of ●artemether with lumefantrine and ●piperaquine with artenimol

  Atomoxetine: possible increased risk of convulsions when antidepressants given with atomoxetine

- Dapoxetine: possible increased risk of serotonergic effects when duloxetine given with ●dapoxetine (manufacturer of dapoxetine advises duloxetine should not be started until 1 week after stopping dapoxetine, avoid dapoxetine for 2 weeks after stopping duloxetine)

Duloxetine *(continued)*

5HT$_1$-receptor Agonists: possible increased serotonergic effects when duloxetine given with 5HT$_1$ agonists

5HT$_3$-receptor Antagonists: possible increased serotonergic effects when SSRI-related antidepressants given with 5HT$_3$ antagonists

- Methylthioninium: risk of CNS toxicity when SSRI-related antidepressants given with ●methylthioninium—avoid concomitant use (if avoidance not possible, use lowest possible dose of methylthioninium and observe patient for up to 4 hours after administration)

Dutasteride

Calcium-channel Blockers: plasma concentration of dutasteride increased by diltiazem and verapamil

Dydrogesterone *see* Progestogens

Efavirenz

Analgesics: efavirenz reduces plasma concentration of methadone

Antibacterials: efavirenz reduces plasma concentration of clarithromycin, also plasma concentration of active metabolite of clarithromycin increased; efavirenz reduces plasma concentration of rifabutin—increase dose of rifabutin; plasma concentration of efavirenz reduced by rifampicin—increase dose of efavirenz; efavirenz possibly reduces plasma concentration of bedaquiline—manufacturer of bedaquiline advises avoid concomitant use

- Anticoagulants: efavirenz possibly affects plasma concentration of ●coumarins

- Antidepressants: plasma concentration of efavirenz reduced by ●St John's wort—avoid concomitant use

Antiepileptics: plasma concentration of both drugs reduced when efavirenz given with carbamazepine

- Antifungals: efavirenz reduces plasma concentration of itraconazole and ●posaconazole; efavirenz reduces plasma concentration of ●voriconazole, also plasma concentration of efavirenz increased (increase voriconazole dose and reduce efavirenz dose); efavirenz possibly reduces plasma concentration of caspofungin—consider increasing dose of caspofungin

- Antimalarials: efavirenz reduces plasma concentration of ●artemether with lumefantrine; efavirenz possibly affects plasma concentration of proguanil

- Antipsychotics: efavirenz possibly reduces plasma concentration of ●aripiprazole (avoid concomitant use or consider reducing the dose of aripiprazole—consult aripiprazole product literature); efavirenz possibly increases plasma concentration of ●pimozide (increased risk of ventricular arrhythmias—avoid concomitant use)

- Antivirals: avoidance of efavirenz advised by manufacturer of ●atazanavir (plasma concentration of atazanavir reduced); efavirenz reduces the plasma concentration of ●daclatasvir—increase dose of daclatasvir (see Dose under Daclatasvir, p. 438); efavirenz reduces plasma concentration of ●darunavir (adjust dose—consult product literature); efavirenz reduces the plasma concentration of ●dolutegravir (see Dose under Dolutegravir, p. 429); avoidance of efavirenz advised by manufacturer of elvitegravir; efavirenz possibly reduces plasma concentration of ●etravirine—avoid concomitant use; efavirenz reduces plasma concentration of indinavir and simeprevir; efavirenz reduces plasma concentration of ●lopinavir—consider increasing dose of lopinavir; efavirenz possibly reduces plasma concentration of ●maraviroc—consider increasing dose of maraviroc; plasma concentration of efavirenz reduced by ●nevirapine—avoid concomitant use; toxicity of efavirenz increased by ●ritonavir, monitor liver function tests —manufacturer of *Atripla*® advises avoid concomitant use with high-dose ritona-

Efavirenz

- Antivirals *(continued)*

vir; efavirenz significantly reduces plasma concentration of saquinavir; efavirenz reduces plasma concentration of ●telaprevir—increase dose of telaprevir

- Anxiolytics and Hypnotics: increased risk of prolonged sedation when efavirenz given with ●midazolam—avoid concomitant use

- Atovaquone: efavirenz reduces plasma concentration of ●atovaquone—avoid concomitant use

Avanafil: efavirenz possibly reduces plasma concentration of avanafil—manufacturer of avanafil advises avoid concomitant use

Bupropion: efavirenz accelerates metabolism of bupropion (reduced plasma concentration)

Calcium-channel Blockers: efavirenz reduces plasma concentration of diltiazem

- Ciclosporin: efavirenz possibly reduces plasma concentration of ●ciclosporin

- Cytotoxics: efavirenz possibly reduces plasma concentration of ●bosutinib—manufacturer of bosutinib advises avoid concomitant use

- Ergot Alkaloids: increased risk of ergotism when efavirenz given with ●ergot alkaloids—avoid concomitant use

Grapefruit Juice: plasma concentration of efavirenz possibly increased by grapefruit juice

Lipid-regulating Drugs: efavirenz reduces plasma concentration of atorvastatin, pravastatin and simvastatin

- Orlistat: absorption of efavirenz possibly reduced by ●orlistat

- Progestogens: efavirenz possibly reduces contraceptive effect of ●progestogens

- Tacrolimus: efavirenz possibly affects plasma concentration of ●tacrolimus

Eletriptan *see* 5HT$_1$-receptor Agonists (under HT)

Eltrombopag

Antacids: absorption of eltrombopag reduced by antacids (give at least 4 hours apart)

Antivirals: plasma concentration of eltrombopag possibly reduced by lopinavir

Calcium Salts: absorption of eltrombopag possibly reduced by calcium salts (give at least 4 hours apart)

Dairy Products: absorption of eltrombopag possibly reduced by dairy products (give at least 4 hours apart)

Iron: absorption of eltrombopag possibly reduced by *oral* iron (give at least 4 hours apart)

- Lipid-regulating Drugs: eltrombopag increases plasma concentration of ●rosuvastatin—adjust dose of rosuvastatin (consult product literature)

Selenium: absorption of eltrombopag possibly reduced by selenium (give at least 4 hours apart)

Zinc: absorption of eltrombopag possibly reduced by zinc (give at least 4 hours apart)

Elvitegravir

Antacids: absorption of elvitegravir reduced by antacids (give at least 4 hours apart)

- Antibacterials: plasma concentration of elvitegravir reduced by ●rifabutin, also plasma concentration of active metabolite of rifabutin increased—reduce dose of rifabutin; manufacturer of elvitegravir advises avoid concomitant use with ●rifampicin

- Antidepressants: manufacturer of elvitegravir advises avoid concomitant use with ●St John's wort

- Antiepileptics: manufacturer of elvitegravir advises avoid concomitant use with ●carbamazepine, ●phenobarbital and ●phenytoin

- Antivirals: plasma concentration of elvitegravir increased by ●atazanavir and ●lopinavir boosted with ritonavir (reduce dose of elvitegravir); manufacturer of elvitegravir advises avoid concomitant use with efavirenz and nevirapine

Elvitegravir *(continued)*
　Bosentan: manufacturer of elvitegravir advises avoid concomitant use with bosentan
● Orlistat: absorption of elvitegravir possibly reduced by ●orlistat
　Progestogens: elvitegravir increases plasma concentration of norgestimate
Empagliflozin *see* Antidiabetics
Emtricitabine
　Antivirals: manufacturer of emtricitabine advises avoid concomitant use with lamivudine
● Orlistat: absorption of emtricitabine possibly reduced by ●orlistat
Enalapril *see* ACE Inhibitors
Enfuvirtide
● Orlistat: absorption of enfuvirtide possibly reduced by ●orlistat
Enoxaparin *see* Heparins
Enoximone *see* Phosphodiesterase Inhibitors
Entacapone
● Anticoagulants: entacapone enhances anticoagulant effect of ●warfarin
● Antidepressants: manufacturer of entacapone advises caution with moclobemide, tricyclics and venlafaxine; avoid concomitant use of entacapone with non-selective ●MAOIs
　Dopaminergics: entacapone possibly enhances effects of apomorphine; entacapone possibly reduces plasma concentration of rasagiline; manufacturer of entacapone advises max. dose of 10 mg selegiline if used concomitantly
　Iron: absorption of entacapone reduced by *oral* iron
　Memantine: effects of dopaminergics possibly enhanced by memantine
　Methyldopa: entacapone possibly enhances effects of methyldopa; antiparkinsonian effect of dopaminergics antagonised by methyldopa
　Sympathomimetics: entacapone possibly enhances effects of adrenaline (epinephrine), dobutamine, dopamine and noradrenaline (norepinephrine)
Enteral Foods
● Anticoagulants: the presence of vitamin K in some enteral feeds can antagonise the anticoagulant effect of ●coumarins and ●phenindione
　Antiepileptics: enteral feeds possibly reduce absorption of phenytoin
Enzalutamide
　Antibacterials: manufacturer of enzalutamide advises avoid concomitant use with rifampicin
● Anticoagulants: enzalutamide possibly reduces plasma concentration of ●coumarins
● Lipid-regulating Drugs: plasma concentration of enzalutamide increased by ●gemfibrozil—manufacturer of enzalutamide advises avoid concomitant use or halve dose of enzalutamide
Ephedrine *see* Sympathomimetics
Epinephrine (adrenaline) *see* Sympathomimetics
Epirubicin
● Antipsychotics: avoid concomitant use of cytotoxics with ●clozapine (increased risk of agranulocytosis)
● Ciclosporin: plasma concentration of epirubicin increased by ●ciclosporin
● Ulcer-healing Drugs: plasma concentration of epirubicin increased by ●cimetidine
Eplerenone *see* Diuretics
Eprosartan *see* Angiotensin-II Receptor Antagonists
Eptifibatide
　Iloprost: increased risk of bleeding when eptifibatide given with iloprost
Ergometrine *see* Ergot Alkaloids
Ergot Alkaloids
● Antibacterials: increased risk of ergotism when ergometrine given with ●clarithromycin or ●erythromycin—avoid concomitant use; increased risk of ergotism when ergotamine given with

Ergot Alkaloids
● Antibacterials *(continued)*
　　●macrolides or ●telithromycin—avoid concomitant use; increased risk of ergotism when ergotamine given with tetracyclines
　Antidepressants: possible risk of hypertension when ergotamine given with reboxetine
● Antifungals: avoidance of ergometrine advised by manufacturer of ●itraconazole (increased risk of ergotism); increased risk of ergotism when ergometrine given with ●voriconazole—avoid concomitant use; increased risk of ergotism when ergotamine given with ●imidazoles or ●triazoles—avoid concomitant use
　Antipsychotics: plasma concentration of ergot alkaloids possibly increased by lurasidone (increased risk of toxicity)
● Antivirals: plasma concentration of ergot alkaloids possibly increased by ●atazanavir—avoid concomitant use; avoidance of ergot alkaloids advised by manufacturer of ●boceprevir and ●telaprevir; increased risk of ergotism when ergot alkaloids given with ●darunavir—manufacturer of darunavir advises avoid concomitant use; increased risk of ergotism when ergot alkaloids given with ●efavirenz—avoid concomitant use; increased risk of ergotism when ergotamine given with ●fosamprenavir, ●indinavir, ●ritonavir or ●saquinavir—avoid concomitant use; increased risk of ergotism when ergometrine given with ●indinavir or ●ritonavir—avoid concomitant use
　Beta-blockers: increased peripheral vasoconstriction when ergotamine given with beta-blockers
● Cobicistat: plasma concentration of ergot alkaloids possibly increased by ●cobicistat—manufacturer of cobicistat advises avoid concomitant use
● Cytotoxics: caution with ergot alkaloids advised by manufacturer of ●crizotinib; avoidance of ergotamine advised by manufacturer of idelalisib
● 5HT₁-receptor Agonists: increased risk of vasospasm when ergotamine given with ●almotriptan, ●rizatriptan, ●sumatriptan or ●zolmitriptan (avoid ergotamine for 6 hours after almotriptan, rizatriptan, sumatriptan or zolmitriptan, avoid almotriptan, rizatriptan, sumatriptan or zolmitriptan for 24 hours after ergotamine); increased risk of vasospasm when ergotamine given with ●eletriptan, ●frovatriptan or ●naratriptan (avoid ergotamine for 24 hours after eletriptan, frovatriptan or naratriptan, avoid eletriptan, frovatriptan or naratriptan for 24 hours after ergotamine)
　Sympathomimetics: increased risk of ergotism when ergotamine given with sympathomimetics
● Ticagrelor: plasma concentration of ergot alkaloids possibly increased by ●ticagrelor
● Ulcer-healing Drugs: increased risk of ergotism when ergotamine given with ●cimetidine—avoid concomitant use
Ergotamine *see* Ergot Alkaloids
Eribulin
　Antibacterials: plasma concentration of eribulin possibly reduced by rifampicin
　Antidepressants: plasma concentration of eribulin possibly reduced by St John's wort
　Antiepileptics: plasma concentration of eribulin possibly reduced by carbamazepine and phenytoin
● Antipsychotics: avoid concomitant use of cytotoxics with ●clozapine (increased risk of agranulocytosis)
Erlotinib
● Analgesics: increased risk of bleeding when erlotinib given with ●NSAIDs
● Antacids: plasma concentration of erlotinib possibly reduced by ●antacids—give antacids at least 4 hours before or 2 hours after erlotinib
　Antibacterials: plasma concentration of erlotinib increased by ciprofloxacin; metabolism of erlotinib

Erlotinib

Antibacterials *(continued)*
accelerated by rifampicin (reduced plasma concentration)
- Anticoagulants: increased risk of bleeding when erlotinib given with ●coumarins
- Antipsychotics: avoid concomitant use of cytotoxics with ●clozapine (increased risk of agranulocytosis)
- Antivirals: avoidance of erlotinib advised by manufacturer of ●boceprevir
Cytotoxics: plasma concentration of erlotinib possibly increased by capecitabine
- Ulcer-healing Drugs: manufacturer of erlotinib advises avoid concomitant use with ●cimetidine, ●esomeprazole, ●famotidine, ●lansoprazole, ●nizatidine, ●pantoprazole and ●rabeprazole; plasma concentration of erlotinib reduced by ●ranitidine—manufacturer of erlotinib advises give at least 2 hours before or 10 hours after ranitidine; plasma concentration of erlotinib reduced by ●omeprazole—manufacturer of erlotinib advises avoid concomitant use

Ertapenem

- Antiepileptics: carbapenems reduce plasma concentration of ●valproate—avoid concomitant use
Vaccines: antibacterials inactivate oral typhoid vaccine—see p. 864

Erythromycin *see* Macrolides

Escitalopram *see* Antidepressants, SSRI

Eslicarbazepine

Anticoagulants: eslicarbazepine reduces plasma concentration of warfarin
- Antidepressants: anticonvulsant effect of antiepileptics possibly antagonised by MAOIs and ●tricyclic-related antidepressants (convulsive threshold lowered); anticonvulsant effect of antiepileptics antagonised by ●SSRIs and ●tricyclics (convulsive threshold lowered)
Antiepileptics: plasma concentration of eslicarbazepine possibly reduced by carbamazepine but risk of side-effects increased; manufacturer of eslicarbazepine advises avoid concomitant use with oxcarbazepine; plasma concentration of eslicarbazepine reduced by phenytoin, also plasma concentration of phenytoin increased
- Antimalarials: anticonvulsant effect of antiepileptics antagonised by ●mefloquine
- Antipsychotics: anticonvulsant effect of antiepileptics antagonised by ●antipsychotics (convulsive threshold lowered)
Lipid-regulating Drugs: eslicarbazepine reduces plasma concentration of rosuvastatin; eslicarbazepine reduces plasma concentration of simvastatin—consider increasing dose of simvastatin
- Oestrogens: eslicarbazepine accelerates metabolism of ●oestrogens (reduced contraceptive effect—see p. 548)
- Orlistat: possible increased risk of convulsions when antiepileptics given with ●orlistat
- Progestogens: eslicarbazepine accelerates metabolism of ●progestogens (reduced contraceptive effect—see p. 548)

Esmolol *see* Beta-blockers

Esomeprazole *see* Proton Pump Inhibitors

Estradiol *see* Oestrogens

Estramustine

Antacids: absorption of estramustine possibly reduced by aluminium hydroxide and oral magnesium salts—manufacturer of estramustine advises avoid concomitant administration
- Antipsychotics: avoid concomitant use of cytotoxics with ●clozapine (increased risk of agranulocytosis)
- Bisphosphonates: plasma concentration of estramustine increased by ●sodium clodronate

Estramustine *(continued)*

Calcium Salts: absorption of estramustine reduced by calcium salts (manufacturer of estramustine advises avoid concomitant administration)

Estriol *see* Oestrogens

Estrone *see* Oestrogens

Etanercept

- Abatacept: avoid concomitant use of etanercept with ●abatacept
- Anakinra: avoid concomitant use of etanercept with ●anakinra
- Vaccines: avoid concomitant use of etanercept with live ●vaccines (see p. 842)

Ethambutol

Antibacterials: plasma concentration of ethambutol increased by delamanid
Vaccines: antibacterials inactivate oral typhoid vaccine—see p. 864

Ethinylestradiol *see* Oestrogens

Ethosuximide

- Antibacterials: metabolism of ethosuximide inhibited by ●isoniazid (increased plasma concentration and risk of toxicity)
- Antidepressants: anticonvulsant effect of antiepileptics possibly antagonised by MAOIs and ●tricyclic-related antidepressants (convulsive threshold lowered); anticonvulsant effect of antiepileptics antagonised by ●SSRIs and ●tricyclics (convulsive threshold lowered)
- Antiepileptics: plasma concentration of ethosuximide possibly reduced by carbamazepine and phenobarbital; plasma concentration of ethosuximide possibly reduced by ●phenytoin, also plasma concentration of phenytoin possibly increased; plasma concentration of ethosuximide possibly increased by valproate
- Antimalarials: anticonvulsant effect of antiepileptics antagonised by ●mefloquine
- Antipsychotics: anticonvulsant effect of antiepileptics antagonised by ●antipsychotics (convulsive threshold lowered)
- Orlistat: possible increased risk of convulsions when antiepileptics given with ●orlistat

Etidronate Disodium *see* Bisphosphonates

Etodolac *see* NSAIDs

Etomidate *see* Anaesthetics, General

Etonogestrel *see* Progestogens

Etoposide

- Anticoagulants: etoposide possibly enhances anticoagulant effect of ●coumarins
Antiepileptics: plasma concentration of etoposide possibly reduced by phenobarbital and phenytoin
- Antipsychotics: avoid concomitant use of cytotoxics with ●clozapine (increased risk of agranulocytosis)
Atovaquone: plasma concentration of etoposide possibly increased by atovaquone
Ciclosporin: plasma concentration of etoposide possibly increased by ciclosporin (increased risk of toxicity)

Etoricoxib *see* NSAIDs

Etravirine

- Antibacterials: etravirine reduces plasma concentration of ●clarithromycin (but concentration of an active metabolite increased), also plasma concentration of etravirine increased; plasma concentration of both reduced when etravirine given with ●rifabutin; manufacturer of etravirine advises avoid concomitant use with rifampicin; etravirine possibly reduces plasma concentration of bedaquiline—manufacturer of bedaquiline advises avoid concomitant use
Antidepressants: manufacturer of etravirine advises avoid concomitant use with St John's wort

Etravirine *(continued)*

Antiepileptics: manufacturer of etravirine advises avoid concomitant use with carbamazepine, phenobarbital and phenytoin

Antimalarials: etravirine reduces plasma concentration of artemether with lumefantrine

- Antivirals: effects of both drugs possibly reduced when etravirine given with boceprevir; avoidance of etravirine advised by manufacturer of daclatasvir (plasma concentration of daclatasvir possibly reduced); etravirine reduces the plasma concentration of ●dolutegravir (see Cautions under Dolutegravir, p. 429); plasma concentration of etravirine possibly reduced by ●efavirenz and ●nevirapine—avoid concomitant use; etravirine increases plasma concentration of ●fosamprenavir (consider reducing dose of fosamprenavir); etravirine possibly reduces plasma concentration of ●indinavir—avoid concomitant use; etravirine possibly reduces plasma concentration of maraviroc; avoidance of etravirine advised by manufacturer of simeprevir; plasma concentration of etravirine reduced by ●tipranavir, also plasma concentration of tipranavir increased (avoid concomitant use)

Cardiac Glycosides: etravirine increases plasma concentration of digoxin

- Clopidogrel: etravirine possibly reduces antiplatelet effect of ●clopidogrel
- Cytotoxics: etravirine possibly reduces plasma concentration of ●bosutinib—manufacturer of bosutinib advises avoid concomitant use

Lipid-regulating Drugs: etravirine possibly reduces plasma concentration of atorvastatin

- Orlistat: absorption of etravirine possibly reduced by ●orlistat

Sildenafil: etravirine reduces plasma concentration of sildenafil

Everolimus

- ACE Inhibitors: increased risk of angioedema when everolimus given with ●ACE inhibitors
- Antibacterials: plasma concentration of everolimus possibly increased by ●clarithromycin and ●telithromycin—manufacturer of everolimus advises avoid concomitant use; plasma concentration of everolimus increased by ●erythromycin (consider reducing the dose of everolimus —consult everolimus product literature); plasma concentration of everolimus reduced by ●rifampicin (avoid concomitant use or consider increasing the dose of everolimus —consult everolimus product literature)

Antidepressants: plasma concentration of everolimus possibly reduced by St John's wort—manufacturer of everolimus advises avoid concomitant use

- Antifungals: plasma concentration of everolimus possibly increased by ●itraconazole, ●posaconazole and ●voriconazole—manufacturer of everolimus advises avoid concomitant use
- Antipsychotics: avoid concomitant use of cytotoxics with ●clozapine (increased risk of agranulocytosis)
- Antivirals: plasma concentration of everolimus possibly increased by ●atazanavir, ●darunavir, ●indinavir, ●ritonavir and ●saquinavir—manufacturer of everolimus advises avoid concomitant use
- Calcium-channel Blockers: plasma concentration of both drugs may increase when everolimus given with ●verapamil (consider reducing the dose of everolimus —consult everolimus product literature)
- Ciclosporin: plasma concentration of everolimus increased by ●ciclosporin (consider reducing the dose of everolimus —consult everolimus product literature)
- Cytotoxics: plasma concentration of everolimus increased by ●imatinib (consider reducing the dose of everolimus —consult everolimus product literature)

Everolimus *(continued)*

Grapefruit Juice: manufacturer of everolimus advises avoid concomitant use with grapefruit juice

Exemestane

Antibacterials: plasma concentration of exemestane possibly reduced by rifampicin

Exenatide *see* Antidiabetics

Ezetimibe

Anticoagulants: ezetimibe possibly enhances anticoagulant effect of coumarins

- Ciclosporin: plasma concentration of both drugs may increase when ezetimibe given with ●ciclosporin
- Lipid-regulating Drugs: ezetimibe increases plasma concentration of ●rosuvastatin—adjust dose of rosuvastatin (consult product literature); increased risk of cholelithiasis and gallbladder disease when ezetimibe given with fibrates—discontinue if suspected

Famotidine *see* Histamine H$_2$-antagonists

Fampridine

- Ulcer-healing Drugs: manufacturer of fampridine advises avoid concomitant use with ●cimetidine

Febuxostat

- Azathioprine: manufacturer of febuxostat advises avoid concomitant use with ●azathioprine
- Cytotoxics: manufacturer of febuxostat advises avoid concomitant use with ●mercaptopurine

Felodipine *see* Calcium-channel Blockers

Fenofibrate *see* Fibrates

Fenoprofen *see* NSAIDs

Fentanyl *see* Opioid Analgesics

Ferrous Salts *see* Iron

Fesoterodine *see* Antimuscarinics

Fexofenadine *see* Antihistamines

Fibrates

- Antibacterials: increased risk of myopathy when fibrates given with ●daptomycin (preferably avoid concomitant use)
- Anticoagulants: fibrates enhance anticoagulant effect of ●coumarins and ●phenindione
- Antidiabetics: fibrates may improve glucose tolerance and have an additive effect with insulin or sulfonylureas; gemfibrozil possibly enhances hypoglycaemic effect of nateglinide; increased risk of severe hypoglycaemia when gemfibrozil given with ●repaglinide—avoid concomitant use

Ciclosporin: increased risk of renal impairment when bezafibrate or fenofibrate given with ciclosporin

- Colchicine: possible increased risk of myopathy when fibrates given with ●colchicine
- Cytotoxics: gemfibrozil increases plasma concentration of dabrafenib; gemfibrozil increases plasma concentration of ●bexarotene (avoid concomitant use)
- Hormone Antagonists: gemfibrozil increases plasma concentration of ●enzalutamide—manufacturer of enzalutamide advises avoid concomitant use or halve dose of enzalutamide

Leukotriene Receptor Antagonists: gemfibrozil increases plasma concentration of montelukast

- Lipid-regulating Drugs: increased risk of myopathy when gemfibrozil given with ●atorvastatin, ●fluvastatin or ●pravastatin (preferably avoid concomitant use); increased risk of myopathy when fibrates given with ●rosuvastatin (see Dose under Rosuvastatin, p. 176); possible increased risk of myopathy when bezafibrate and ciprofibrate given with ●simvastatin (see Dose under Simvastatin, p. 177); increased risk of myopathy when gemfibrozil given with ●simvastatin (avoid concomitant use); increased risk of cholelithiasis and gallbladder disease when fibrates given with ezetimibe—discontinue if suspected; increased risk of myopathy when fibrates given with ●statins; reduce maximum dose of fenofibrate when given with statins—see Dose under Fenofibrate, p. 179

Fidaxomicin

Anti-arrhythmics: manufacturer of fidaxomicin advises avoid concomitant use with amiodarone and drone-darone

Antibacterials: manufacturer of fidaxomicin advises avoid concomitant use with clarithromycin and erythromycin

Calcium-channel Blockers: manufacturer of fidaxomicin advises avoid concomitant use with verapamil

Ciclosporin: manufacturer of fidaxomicin advises avoid concomitant use with ciclosporin

Fidaxomicin

Vaccines: antibacterials inactivate oral typhoid vaccine—see p. 864

Filgrastim

Note Pegfilgrastim interactions as for filgrastim

Cytotoxics: neutropenia possibly exacerbated when filgrastim given with fluorouracil

Fingolimod

- Anti-arrhythmics: possible increased risk of brady-cardia when fingolimod given with ●amiodarone, ●disopyramide or ●dronedarone

Antidepressants: plasma concentration of fingolimod possibly reduced by St John's wort—manufacturer of fingolimod advises avoid concomitant use

Antiepileptics: plasma concentration of fingolimod reduced by carbamazepine

- Beta-blockers: possible increased risk of bradycardia when fingolimod given with ●beta-blockers
- Calcium-channel Blockers: possible increased risk of bradycardia when fingolimod given with ●diltiazem or ●verapamil

Flavoxate see Antimuscarinics

Flecainide

Anaesthetics, Local: increased myocardial depression when anti-arrhythmics given with bupivacaine, levobupivacaine, prilocaine or ropivacaine

- Anti-arrhythmics: increased myocardial depression when anti-arrhythmics given with other ●anti-arrhythmics; plasma concentration of flecainide increased by ●amiodarone (halve dose of flecainide)
- Antidepressants: plasma concentration of flecainide increased by fluoxetine; increased risk of ventricular arrhythmias when flecainide given with ●tricyclics
- Antihistamines: increased risk of ventricular arrhythmias when flecainide given with ●mizolastine—avoid concomitant use
- Antimalarials: avoidance of flecainide advised by manufacturer of ●artemether with lumefantrine (risk of ventricular arrhythmias); plasma concentration of flecainide increased by ●quinine
- Antimuscarinics: increased risk of ventricular arrhythmias when flecainide given with ●tolterodine
- Antipsychotics: increased risk of ventricular arrhythmias when anti-arrhythmics that prolong the QT interval given with ●antipsychotics that prolong the QT interval; increased risk of arrhythmias when flecainide given with ●clozapine
- Antivirals: plasma concentration of flecainide possibly increased by ●fosamprenavir, ●indinavir, ●lopinavir and ●ritonavir (increased risk of ventricular arrhythmias—avoid concomitant use); increased risk of ventricular arrhythmias when flecainide given with ●saquinavir—avoid concomitant use; caution with flecainide advised by manufacturer of ●telaprevir (risk of ventricular arrhythmias)
- Beta-blockers: increased risk of myocardial depression and bradycardia when flecainide given with ●beta-blockers; increased myocardial depression when anti-arrhythmics given with ●beta-blockers
- Calcium-channel Blockers: increased risk of myocardial depression and asystole when flecainide given with ●verapamil
- Diuretics: increased cardiac toxicity with flecainide if hypokalaemia occurs with ●acetazolamide, ●loop diuretics or ●thiazides and related diuretics

Flecainide (continued)

Ulcer-healing Drugs: metabolism of flecainide inhibited by cimetidine (increased plasma concentration)

Flucloxacillin see Penicillins

Fluconazole see Antifungals, Triazole

Flucytosine

Antifungals: renal excretion of flucytosine decreased and cellular uptake increased by amphotericin (toxicity possibly increased)

Cytotoxics: plasma concentration of flucytosine possibly reduced by cytarabine

Fludarabine

- Antipsychotics: avoid concomitant use of cytotoxics with ●clozapine (increased risk of agranulocytosis)
- Cytotoxics: fludarabine increases intracellular concentration of cytarabine; increased pulmonary toxicity when fludarabine given with ●pentostatin (unacceptably high incidence of fatalities)

Dipyridamole: effects of fludarabine possibly reduced by dipyridamole

Fludrocortisone see Corticosteroids

Fluorides

Calcium Salts: absorption of fluorides reduced by calcium salts

Fluorouracil

Note Capecitabine is a prodrug of fluorouracil

Note Tegafur is a prodrug of fluorouracil

- Allopurinol: manufacturer of capecitabine advises avoid concomitant use with ●allopurinol

Antibacterials: metabolism of fluorouracil inhibited by metronidazole (increased toxicity)

- Anticoagulants: fluorouracil enhances anticoagulant effect of ●coumarins

Antiepileptics: fluorouracil possibly inhibits metabolism of phenytoin (increased risk of toxicity)

- Antipsychotics: avoid concomitant use of cytotoxics with ●clozapine (increased risk of agranulocytosis)

Cytotoxics: capecitabine possibly increases plasma concentration of erlotinib

Filgrastim: neutropenia possibly exacerbated when fluorouracil given with filgrastim

- Folates: toxicity of fluorouracil increased by ●folic acid—avoid concomitant use
- Temoporfin: increased skin photosensitivity when topical fluorouracil used with ●temoporfin

Ulcer-healing Drugs: metabolism of fluorouracil inhibited by cimetidine (increased plasma concentration)

Fluoxetine see Antidepressants, SSRI

Flupentixol see Antipsychotics

Fluphenazine see Antipsychotics

Flurazepam see Anxiolytics and Hypnotics

Flurbiprofen see NSAIDs

Flutamide

- Anticoagulants: flutamide enhances anticoagulant effect of ●coumarins

Fluticasone see Corticosteroids

Fluvastatin see Statins

Fluvoxamine see Antidepressants, SSRI

Folates

Aminosalicylates: absorption of folic acid possibly reduced by sulfasalazine

Antacids: absorption of folic acid possibly reduced by antacids (manufacturer of folic acid advises give at least 2 hours apart)

Antiepileptics: folates possibly reduce plasma concentration of phenobarbital and phenytoin

- Cytotoxics: folic acid increases toxicity of ●fluorouracil—avoid concomitant use; avoidance of folates advised by manufacturer of ●raltitrexed

Folic Acid see Folates

Folinic Acid see Folates

Fondaparinux

- Analgesics: increased risk of haemorrhage when anti-coagulants given with intravenous ●diclofenac (avoid concomitant use, including low-dose heparins);

Fondaparinux

- Analgesics *(continued)*
  increased risk of haemorrhage when anticoagulants given with ●ketorolac (avoid concomitant use, including low-dose heparins)
- Anticoagulants: increased risk of haemorrhage when other anticoagulants given with ●apixaban, ●dabigatran and ●rivaroxaban (avoid concomitant use except when switching with other anticoagulants or using heparin to maintain catheter patency)

Formoterol *see* Sympathomimetics, Beta$_2$

Fosamprenavir

Note Fosamprenavir is a prodrug of amprenavir

Analgesics: fosamprenavir reduces plasma concentration of methadone

- Anti-arrhythmics: fosamprenavir possibly increases plasma concentration of ●amiodarone, ●flecainide and ●propafenone (increased risk of ventricular arrhythmias—avoid concomitant use); fosamprenavir possibly increases plasma concentration of ●lidocaine—avoid concomitant use
- Antibacterials: fosamprenavir increases plasma concentration of ●rifabutin (reduce dose of rifabutin); plasma concentration of fosamprenavir significantly reduced by ●rifampicin—avoid concomitant use; avoidance of concomitant fosamprenavir in severe renal and hepatic impairment advised by manufacturer of ●telithromycin

Anticoagulants: avoidance of fosamprenavir advised by manufacturer of apixaban and rivaroxaban; fosamprenavir may enhance or reduce anticoagulant effect of coumarins

- Antidepressants: plasma concentration of fosamprenavir reduced by ●St John's wort—avoid concomitant use

Antiepileptics: plasma concentration of fosamprenavir possibly reduced by carbamazepine and phenobarbital

Antifungals: plasma concentration of both drugs may increase when fosamprenavir given with itraconazole; fosamprenavir possibly reduces plasma concentration of posaconazole

- Antimalarials: caution with fosamprenavir advised by manufacturer of artemether with lumefantrine; fosamprenavir possibly increases plasma concentration of ●quinine (increased risk of toxicity)

Antimuscarinics: avoidance of fosamprenavir advised by manufacturer of darifenacin and tolterodine

- Antipsychotics: fosamprenavir possibly increases plasma concentration of ●aripiprazole (reduce dose of aripiprazole—consult aripiprazole product literature); fosamprenavir increases plasma concentration of ●pimozide (increased risk of ventricular arrhythmias—avoid concomitant use); fosamprenavir possibly increases plasma concentration of ●quetiapine—manufacturer of quetiapine advises avoid concomitant use
- Antivirals: manufacturer of fosamprenavir advises avoid concomitant use with ●boceprevir and ●raltegravir; fosamprenavir reduces plasma concentration of ●dolutegravir; plasma concentration of fosamprenavir increased by ●etravirine (consider reducing dose of fosamprenavir); plasma concentration of fosamprenavir reduced by lopinavir, effect on lopinavir plasma concentration not predictable—avoid concomitant use; plasma concentration of fosamprenavir reduced by ●maraviroc—avoid concomitant use; plasma concentration of fosamprenavir possibly reduced by nevirapine—avoid unboosted fosamprenavir; manufacturers advise avoid concomitant use of fosamprenavir with ●telaprevir; plasma concentration of fosamprenavir reduced by ●tipranavir
- Anxiolytics and Hypnotics: fosamprenavir possibly increases plasma concentration of ●midazolam (risk

Fosamprenavir

- Anxiolytics and Hypnotics *(continued)*
  of prolonged sedation—avoid concomitant use of *oral* midazolam)
- Avanafil: fosamprenavir possibly increases plasma concentration of ●avanafil—see Dose under Avanafil, p. 571
- Ciclosporin: fosamprenavir increases plasma concentration of ●ciclosporin
- Cytotoxics: fosamprenavir possibly increases the plasma concentration of ●bosutinib—manufacturer of bosutinib advises avoid or consider reducing dose of bosutinib; fosamprenavir possibly increases the plasma concentration of ●ibrutinib—reduce dose of ibrutinib (see Dose under Ibrutinib, p. 615)

Dapoxetine: manufacturer of dapoxetine advises dose reduction when fosamprenavir given with dapoxetine (see Dose under Dapoxetine, p. 572)

- Ergot Alkaloids: increased risk of ergotism when fosamprenavir given with ●ergotamine—avoid concomitant use
- Lipid-regulating Drugs: possible increased risk of myopathy when fosamprenavir given with atorvastatin; possible increased risk of myopathy when fosamprenavir given with ●rosuvastatin—manufacturer of rosuvastatin advises avoid concomitant use; possible increased risk of myopathy when fosamprenavir given with ●simvastatin—avoid concomitant use; avoidance of fosamprenavir advised by manufacturer of ●lomitapide (plasma concentration of lomitapide possibly increased)
- Orlistat: absorption of fosamprenavir possibly reduced by ●orlistat
- Ranolazine: fosamprenavir possibly increases plasma concentration of ●ranolazine—manufacturer of ranolazine advises avoid concomitant use

Sildenafil: fosamprenavir possibly increases plasma concentration of sildenafil

- Tacrolimus: fosamprenavir increases plasma concentration of ●tacrolimus

Tadalafil: fosamprenavir possibly increases plasma concentration of tadalafil

Vardenafil: fosamprenavir possibly increases plasma concentration of vardenafil

Fosaprepitant *see* Aprepitant

Foscarnet

- Pentamidine Isetionate: increased risk of hypocalcaemia when foscarnet given with *parenteral* ●pentamidine isetionate

Fosfomycin

Metoclopramide: plasma concentration of fosfomycin reduced by metoclopramide

Vaccines: antibacterials inactivate oral typhoid vaccine—see p. 864

Fosinopril *see* ACE Inhibitors

Fosphenytoin *see* Phenytoin

Frovatriptan *see* 5HT$_1$-receptor Agonists (under HT)

Furosemide *see* Diuretics

Fusidic Acid

- Antivirals: plasma concentration of both drugs increased when fusidic acid given with ●ritonavir—avoid concomitant use; plasma concentration of both drugs may increase when fusidic acid given with saquinavir
- Lipid-regulating Drugs: risk of myopathy and rhabdomyolysis when fusidic acid given with ●statins—avoid concomitant use and for 7 days after last fusidic acid dose

Sugammadex: fusidic acid possibly reduces response to sugammadex

Vaccines: antibacterials inactivate oral typhoid vaccine—see p. 864

Gabapentin

Analgesics: bioavailability of gabapentin increased by morphine

Gabapentin *(continued)*

Antacids: absorption of gabapentin reduced by antacids

- Antidepressants: anticonvulsant effect of antiepileptics possibly antagonised by MAOIs and •tricyclic-related antidepressants (convulsive threshold lowered); anticonvulsant effect of antiepileptics antagonised by •SSRIs and •tricyclics (convulsive threshold lowered)
- Antimalarials: anticonvulsant effect of antiepileptics antagonised by •mefloquine
- Antipsychotics: anticonvulsant effect of antiepileptics antagonised by •antipsychotics (convulsive threshold lowered)
- Orlistat: possible increased risk of convulsions when antiepileptics given with •orlistat

Galantamine *see* Parasympathomimetics

Ganciclovir

Note Increased risk of myelosuppression with other myelosuppressive drugs—consult product literature

Note Valganciclovir interactions as for ganciclovir

- Antibacterials: increased risk of convulsions when ganciclovir given with •imipenem with cilastatin
- Antivirals: ganciclovir possibly increases plasma concentration of didanosine; profound myelosuppression when ganciclovir given with •zidovudine (if possible avoid concomitant administration, particularly during initial ganciclovir therapy)

Mycophenolate: plasma concentration of ganciclovir possibly increased by mycophenolate, also plasma concentration of inactive metabolite of mycophenolate possibly increased

Tacrolimus: possible increased risk of nephrotoxicity when ganciclovir given with tacrolimus

Gefitinib

- Antibacterials: plasma concentration of gefitinib reduced by •rifampicin—avoid concomitant use
- Anticoagulants: gefitinib possibly enhances anticoagulant effect of •warfarin

Antidepressants: manufacturer of gefitinib advises avoid concomitant use with St John's wort

Antiepileptics: manufacturer of gefitinib advises avoid concomitant use with carbamazepine, phenobarbital and phenytoin

Antifungals: plasma concentration of gefitinib increased by itraconazole

- Antipsychotics: avoid concomitant use of cytotoxics with •clozapine (increased risk of agranulocytosis)
- Antivirals: avoidance of gefitinib advised by manufacturer of •boceprevir
- Ulcer-healing Drugs: plasma concentration of gefitinib reduced by •ranitidine

Gemcitabine

Anticoagulants: gemcitabine possibly enhances anticoagulant effect of warfarin

- Antipsychotics: avoid concomitant use of cytotoxics with •clozapine (increased risk of agranulocytosis)

Gemeprost *see* Prostaglandins

Gemfibrozil *see* Fibrates

Gentamicin *see* Aminoglycosides

Gestodene *see* Progestogens

Glibenclamide *see* Antidiabetics

Gliclazide *see* Antidiabetics

Glimepiride *see* Antidiabetics

Glipizide *see* Antidiabetics

Glucosamine

- Anticoagulants: glucosamine enhances anticoagulant effect of •warfarin (avoid concomitant use)

Glyceryl Trinitrate *see* Nitrates

Glycopyrronium *see* Antimuscarinics

Gold *see* Sodium Aurothiomalate

Golimumab

- Abatacept: avoid concomitant use of golimumab with •abatacept

Golimumab *(continued)*

- Anakinra: avoid concomitant use of golimumab with •anakinra
- Antipsychotics: avoid concomitant use of cytotoxics with •clozapine (increased risk of agranulocytosis)
- Vaccines: avoid concomitant use of monoclonal antibodies with live •vaccines (see p. 842)

Granisetron *see* 5HT$_3$-receptor Antagonists (under HT)

Grapefruit Juice

- Aliskiren: grapefruit juice reduces plasma concentration of •aliskiren—avoid concomitant use
- Anti-arrhythmics: grapefruit juice increases plasma concentration of amiodarone; grapefruit juice increases plasma concentration of •dronedarone—avoid concomitant use

Antidepressants: grapefruit juice possibly increases plasma concentration of sertraline

- Antihistamines: grapefruit juice reduces plasma concentration of bilastine; grapefruit juice increases plasma concentration of •rupatadine—avoid concomitant use

Antimalarials: avoidance of grapefruit juice advised by manufacturer of piperaquine with artenimol; grapefruit juice possibly increases plasma concentration of artemether with lumefantrine

- Antipsychotics: avoidance of grapefruit juice advised by manufacturer of lurasidone; grapefruit juice possibly increases plasma concentration of •quetiapine—manufacturer of quetiapine advises avoid concomitant use

Antivirals: grapefruit juice possibly increases plasma concentration of efavirenz

Anxiolytics and Hypnotics: grapefruit juice possibly increases plasma concentration of *oral* midazolam; grapefruit juice increases plasma concentration of buspirone

Avanafil: grapefruit juice possibly increases plasma concentration of avanafil— manufacturer of avanafil advises avoid grapefruit juice for 24 hours before avanafil

Calcium-channel Blockers: grapefruit juice possibly increases plasma concentration of amlodipine; grapefruit juice increases plasma concentration of felodipine, isradipine, lacidipine, lercanidipine, nicardipine, nifedipine, nimodipine and verapamil

- Ciclosporin: grapefruit juice increases plasma concentration of •ciclosporin (increased risk of toxicity)
- Colchicine: grapefruit juice possibly increases risk of •colchicine toxicity
- Cytotoxics: grapefruit juice possibly increases plasma concentration of axitinib, cabozantinib and ponatinib; grapefruit juice possibly increases the plasma concentration of •bosutinib—manufacturer of bosutinib advises avoid or consider reducing dose of bosutinib; grapefruit juice possibly increases plasma concentration of •crizotinib and vinflunine—manufacturer of crizotinib and vinflunine advises avoid concomitant use; avoidance of grapefruit juice advised by manufacturer of everolimus, ibrutinib, •lapatinib, •nilotinib and •pazopanib

Ivabradine: grapefruit juice increases plasma concentration of ivabradine

Ivacaftor: grapefruit juice possibly increases plasma concentration of ivacaftor—manufacturer of ivacaftor advises avoid concomitant use

- Lipid-regulating Drugs: grapefruit juice possibly increases plasma concentration of atorvastatin; grapefruit juice increases plasma concentration of •simvastatin—avoid concomitant use; avoidance of grapefruit juice advised by manufacturer of lomitapide

Pirfenidone: avoidance of grapefruit juice advised by manufacturer of pirfenidone

- Ranolazine: grapefruit juice possibly increases plasma concentration of •ranolazine—manufacturer of ranolazine advises avoid concomitant use

Grapefruit Juice *(continued)*

Sildenafil: grapefruit juice possibly increases plasma concentration of sildenafil
- Sirolimus: grapefruit juice increases plasma concentration of ●sirolimus—avoid concomitant use
- Tacrolimus: grapefruit juice increases plasma concentration of ●tacrolimus

Tadalafil: grapefruit juice possibly increases plasma concentration of tadalafil
- Tolvaptan: grapefruit juice increases plasma concentration of ●tolvaptan—avoid concomitant use

Uliprestal: avoidance of grapefruit juice advised by manufacturer of *low-dose* uliprestal
- Vardenafil: grapefruit juice possibly increases plasma concentration of ●vardenafil—avoid concomitant use

Griseofulvin

Alcohol: griseofulvin possibly enhances effects of alcohol
- Anticoagulants: griseofulvin reduces anticoagulant effect of ●coumarins

Antiepileptics: absorption of griseofulvin reduced by phenobarbital (reduced effect)

Ciclosporin: griseofulvin possibly reduces plasma concentration of ciclosporin

Oestrogens: anecdotal reports of contraceptive failure and menstrual irregularities when griseofulvin given with oestrogens

Progestogens: anecdotal reports of contraceptive failure and menstrual irregularities when griseofulvin given with progestogens

Guanethidine *see* Adrenergic Neurone Blockers

Haemophilus vaccine *see* Vaccines

Haloperidol *see* Antipsychotics

Heparin *see* Heparins

Heparins

ACE Inhibitors: increased risk of hyperkalaemia when heparins given with ACE inhibitors

Aliskiren: increased risk of hyperkalaemia when heparins given with aliskiren
- Analgesics: possible increased risk of bleeding when heparins given with NSAIDs; increased risk of haemorrhage when anticoagulants given with *intravenous* ●diclofenac (avoid concomitant use, including low-dose heparins); increased risk of haemorrhage when anticoagulants given with ●ketorolac (avoid concomitant use, including low-dose heparins); anticoagulant effect of heparins enhanced by ●aspirin

Angiotensin-II Receptor Antagonists: increased risk of hyperkalaemia when heparins given with angiotensin-II receptor antagonists
- Anticoagulants: increased risk of haemorrhage when other anticoagulants given with ●apixaban, ●dabigatran and ●rivaroxaban (avoid concomitant use except when switching with other anticoagulants or using heparin to maintain catheter patency)

Clopidogrel: increased risk of bleeding when heparins given with clopidogrel

Dipyridamole: anticoagulant effect of heparins enhanced by dipyridamole

Iloprost: anticoagulant effect of heparins possibly enhanced by iloprost
- Nitrates: anticoagulant effect of heparins reduced by *infusion* of ●glyceryl trinitrate

Hepatitis vaccines *see* Vaccines

Histamine

Antidepressants: manufacturer of histamine advises avoid concomitant use with MAOIs; effects of histamine theoretically antagonised by tricyclics—manufacturer of histamine advises avoid concomitant use

Antihistamines: effects of histamine theoretically antagonised by antihistamines—manufacturer of histamine advises avoid concomitant use

Histamine *(continued)*

Antimalarials: manufacturer of histamine advises avoid concomitant use with antimalarials

Antipsychotics: effects of histamine theoretically antagonised by antipsychotics—manufacturer of histamine advises avoid concomitant use

Atovaquone: manufacturer of histamine advises avoid concomitant use with atovaquone

Clonidine: manufacturer of histamine advises avoid concomitant use with clonidine

Corticosteroids: manufacturer of histamine advises avoid concomitant use with corticosteroids

Ulcer-healing Drugs: effects of histamine theoretically antagonised by histamine H_2-antagonists—manufacturer of histamine advises avoid concomitant use

Histamine H_2-antagonists

- Alpha-blockers: cimetidine and ranitidine antagonise effects of ●tolazoline

Analgesics: cimetidine inhibits metabolism of opioid analgesics (increased plasma concentration)
- Anti-arrhythmics: cimetidine increases plasma concentration of amiodarone and ●propafenone; cimetidine inhibits metabolism of flecainide (increased plasma concentration); cimetidine increases plasma concentration of ●lidocaine (increased risk of toxicity)

Antibacterials: cimetidine increases plasma concentration of erythromycin (increased risk of toxicity, including deafness); cimetidine inhibits metabolism of metronidazole (increased plasma concentration); metabolism of cimetidine accelerated by rifampicin (reduced plasma concentration)
- Anticoagulants: cimetidine inhibits metabolism of ●coumarins (enhanced anticoagulant effect)

Antidepressants: cimetidine increases plasma concentration of citalopram, escitalopram, mirtazapine and sertraline; cimetidine inhibits metabolism of amitriptyline, doxepin, imipramine and nortriptyline (increased plasma concentration); cimetidine increases plasma concentration of moclobemide (halve dose of moclobemide); cimetidine possibly increases plasma concentration of tricyclics

Antidiabetics: cimetidine reduces excretion of metformin (increased plasma concentration); cimetidine enhances hypoglycaemic effect of sulfonylureas
- Antiepileptics: cimetidine inhibits metabolism of ●carbamazepine, ●phenytoin and ●valproate (increased plasma concentration)
- Antifungals: histamine H_2-antagonists reduce absorption of itraconazole; cimetidine reduces plasma concentration of ●posaconazole—manufacturer of posaconazole *suspension* advises avoid concomitant use; famotidine, nizatidine and ranitidine possibly reduce plasma concentration of ●posaconazole—manufacturer of posaconazole *suspension* advises avoid concomitant use; cimetidine increases plasma concentration of terbinafine

Antihistamines: manufacturer of loratadine advises cimetidine possibly increases plasma concentration of loratadine; cimetidine increases plasma concentration of hydroxyzine
- Antimalarials: avoidance of cimetidine advised by manufacturer of ●artemether with lumefantrine; cimetidine inhibits metabolism of chloroquine and hydroxychloroquine and quinine (increased plasma concentration)

Antipsychotics: cimetidine possibly enhances effects of antipsychotics, chlorpromazine and clozapine
- Antivirals: manufacturer of atazanavir advises adjust doses of both drugs when cimetidine and nizatidine given with atazanavir—consult atazanavir product literature; famotidine and ranitidine reduce the plasma concentration of ●atazanavir (adjust doses of both drugs—consult atazanavir product literature); famotidine increases plasma concentration of raltegravir; avoidance of histamine H_2-antagonists for 12 hours before or 4 hours after

Histamine H₂-antagonists

- **Antivirals** *(continued)*
  rilpivirine advised by manufacturer of rilpivirine—consult product literature; cimetidine possibly increases plasma concentration of saquinavir

  Anxiolytics and Hypnotics: cimetidine inhibits metabolism of benzodiazepines, clomethiazole and zaleplon (increased plasma concentration); cimetidine increases plasma concentration of melatonin

  Beta-blockers: cimetidine increases plasma concentration of labetalol, metoprolol and propranolol; cimetidine possibly increases plasma concentration of *oral* timolol

  Caffeine citrate: cimetidine increases plasma concentration of caffeine citrate

  Calcium-channel Blockers: cimetidine possibly inhibits metabolism of calcium-channel blockers (increased plasma concentration); cimetidine increases plasma concentration of isradipine (halve dose of isradipine)

- Ciclosporin: cimetidine possibly increases plasma concentration of ●ciclosporin

- Clopidogrel: cimetidine possibly reduces antiplatelet effect of ●clopidogrel

- Cytotoxics: cimetidine possibly enhances myelosuppressive effects of carmustine and lomustine; cimetidine reduces plasma concentration of doxorubicin; cimetidine increases plasma concentration of ●epirubicin; cimetidine inhibits metabolism of fluorouracil (increased plasma concentration); famotidine possibly reduces plasma concentration of dasatinib; avoidance of cimetidine, famotidine and nizatidine advised by manufacturer of ●erlotinib; ranitidine reduces plasma concentration of ●erlotinib—manufacturer of erlotinib advises give at least 2 hours before or 10 hours after ranitidine; ranitidine reduces plasma concentration of ●gefitinib; histamine H₂-antagonists possibly reduce absorption of lapatinib; histamine H₂-antagonists possibly reduce absorption of pazopanib—manufacturer of pazopanib advises give at least 2 hours before or 10 hours after histamine H₂-antagonists

  Dopaminergics: cimetidine reduces excretion of pramipexole (increased plasma concentration)

- Ergot Alkaloids: increased risk of ergotism when cimetidine given with ●ergotamine—avoid concomitant use

- Fampridine: avoidance of cimetidine advised by manufacturer of ●fampridine

  Histamine: histamine H₂-antagonists theoretically antagonise effects of histamine—manufacturer of histamine advises avoid concomitant use

  Hormone Antagonists: absorption of cimetidine possibly delayed by octreotide

  5HT₁-receptor Agonists: cimetidine inhibits metabolism of zolmitriptan (reduce dose of zolmitriptan)

  Lipid-regulating Drugs: manufacturer of lomitapide advises dose reduction when cimetidine given with lomitapide (see Dose under Lomitapide, p. 180)

  Mebendazole: cimetidine possibly inhibits metabolism of mebendazole (increased plasma concentration)

  Roflumilast: cimetidine inhibits the metabolism of roflumilast

  Sildenafil: cimetidine increases plasma concentration of sildenafil—consider reducing dose of sildenafil for erectile dysfunction

  Sympathomimetics: cimetidine possibly inhibits metabolism of dobutamine

- Theophylline: cimetidine inhibits metabolism of ●theophylline (increased plasma concentration)

  Thyroid Hormones: cimetidine reduces absorption of levothyroxine

Homatropine *see* Antimuscarinics

Hormone Antagonists *see* Abiraterone, Bicalutamide, Danazol, Dutasteride, Enzalutamide, Exemestane,

Hormone Antagonists *(continued)*

Flutamide, Lanreotide, Octreotide, Pasireotide, Tamoxifen, and Toremifene

5HT₁-receptor Agonists

- Antibacterials: plasma concentration of eletriptan increased by ●clarithromycin and ●erythromycin (risk of toxicity)—avoid concomitant use; metabolism of zolmitriptan possibly inhibited by quinolones (reduce dose of zolmitriptan)

- Antidepressants: increased risk of CNS toxicity when 5HT₁ agonists given with ●citalopram (manufacturer of citalopram advises avoid concomitant use); increased risk of CNS toxicity when sumatriptan given with ●citalopram, ●escitalopram, ●fluoxetine, ●fluvoxamine or ●paroxetine; metabolism of frovatriptan inhibited by fluvoxamine; metabolism of zolmitriptan possibly inhibited by fluvoxamine (reduce dose of zolmitriptan); CNS toxicity reported when sumatriptan given with sertraline; possible increased serotonergic effects when 5HT₁ agonists given with duloxetine or venlafaxine; risk of CNS toxicity when zolmitriptan given with ●MAOIs or ●moclobemide (reduce dose of zolmitriptan); risk of CNS toxicity when rizatriptan or sumatriptan given with ●MAOIs (avoid rizatriptan or sumatriptan for 2 weeks after MAOIs); risk of CNS toxicity when rizatriptan or sumatriptan given with ●moclobemide (avoid rizatriptan or sumatriptan for 2 weeks after moclobemide); possible increased serotonergic effects when naratriptan given with SSRIs; increased serotonergic effects when 5HT₁ agonists given with ●St John's wort—avoid concomitant use

- Antifungals: plasma concentration of eletriptan increased by ●itraconazole (risk of toxicity)—avoid concomitant use

- Antivirals: plasma concentration of eletriptan increased by ●indinavir and ●ritonavir (risk of toxicity)—avoid concomitant use

  Beta-blockers: plasma concentration of rizatriptan increased by propranolol (manufacturer of rizatriptan advises halve dose and avoid within 2 hours of propranolol)

- Dapoxetine: possible increased risk of serotonergic effects when 5HT₁ agonists given with ●dapoxetine (manufacturer of dapoxetine advises 5HT₁ agonists should not be started until 1 week after stopping dapoxetine, avoid dapoxetine for 2 weeks after stopping 5HT₁ agonists)

  Dopaminergics: avoidance of 5HT₁ agonists advised by manufacturer of selegiline

- Ergot Alkaloids: increased risk of vasospasm when almotriptan, rizatriptan, sumatriptan or zolmitriptan given with ●ergotamine (avoid ergotamine for 6 hours after almotriptan, rizatriptan, sumatriptan or zolmitriptan, avoid almotriptan, rizatriptan, sumatriptan or zolmitriptan for 24 hours after ergotamine); increased risk of vasospasm when eletriptan, frovatriptan or naratriptan given with ●ergotamine (avoid ergotamine for 24 hours after eletriptan, frovatriptan or naratriptan, avoid eletriptan, frovatriptan or naratriptan for 24 hours after ergotamine)

  Lithium: possible risk of toxicity when sumatriptan given with lithium

  Ulcer-healing Drugs: metabolism of zolmitriptan inhibited by cimetidine (reduce dose of zolmitriptan)

5HT₃-receptor Antagonists

  Analgesics: ondansetron possibly antagonises effects of tramadol

  Antibacterials: metabolism of ondansetron accelerated by rifampicin (reduced effect)

  Antidepressants: possible increased serotonergic effects when 5HT₃ antagonists given with SSRI-related antidepressants or SSRIs

  Antiepileptics: metabolism of ondansetron accelerated by carbamazepine and phenytoin (reduced effect)

5HT$_3$-receptor Antagonists *(continued)*
- Cytotoxics: increased risk of ventricular arrhythmias when ondansetron given with ●vandetanib—avoid concomitant use
- Dopaminergics: possible increased hypotensive effect when ondansetron given with ●apomorphine—avoid concomitant use

Human papillomavirus vaccine *see* Vaccines

Hydralazine *see* Vasodilator Antihypertensives

Hydrochlorothiazide *see* Diuretics

Hydrocortisone *see* Corticosteroids

Hydroflumethiazide *see* Diuretics

Hydromorphone *see* Opioid Analgesics

Hydrotalcite *see* Antacids

Hydroxocobalamin
- Antibacterials: response to hydroxocobalamin reduced by chloramphenicol

Hydroxycarbamide
- Antipsychotics: avoid concomitant use of cytotoxics with ●clozapine (increased risk of agranulocytosis)
- Antivirals: increased risk of toxicity when hydroxycarbamide given with ●didanosine and ●stavudine—avoid concomitant use

Hydroxychloroquine *see* Chloroquine and Hydroxychloroquine

Hydroxyzine *see* Antihistamines

Hyoscine *see* Antimuscarinics

Ibandronic Acid *see* Bisphosphonates

Ibrutinib
- Anti-arrhythmics: plasma concentration of ibrutinib possibly increased by ●amiodarone and ●dronedarone—reduce dose of ibrutinib (see Dose under Ibrutinib, p. 615)
- Antibacterials: plasma concentration of ibrutinib possibly increased by ●ciprofloxacin, ●clarithromycin, ●erythromycin and ●telithromycin—reduce dose of ibrutinib (see Dose under Ibrutinib, p. 615); plasma concentration of ibrutinib reduced by ●rifampicin—avoid concomitant use
  Anticoagulants: manufacturer of ibrutinib advises avoid concomitant use with coumarins and phenindione
- Antidepressants: plasma concentration of ibrutinib possibly reduced by ●St John's wort—manufacturer of ibrutinib advises avoid concomitant use
- Antiepileptics: plasma concentration of ibrutinib possibly reduced by ●carbamazepine and ●phenytoin—manufacturer of ibrutinib advises avoid concomitant use
- Antifungals: plasma concentration of ibrutinib possibly increased by ●fluconazole, ●itraconazole and ●voriconazole—reduce dose of ibrutinib (see Dose under Ibrutinib, p. 615)
- Antipsychotics: avoid concomitant use of cytotoxics with ●clozapine (increased risk of agranulocytosis)
- Antivirals: plasma concentration of ibrutinib possibly increased by ●atazanavir, ●darunavir, ●fosamprenavir, ●indinavir, ●ritonavir and ●saquinavir—reduce dose of ibrutinib (see Dose under Ibrutinib, p. 615)
- Aprepitant: plasma concentration of ibrutinib possibly increased by ●aprepitant—reduce dose of ibrutinib (see Dose under Ibrutinib, p. 615)
- Calcium-channel Blockers: plasma concentration of ibrutinib possibly increased by ●diltiazem and ●verapamil—reduce dose of ibrutinib (see Dose under Ibrutinib, p. 615)
  Cardiac Glycosides: manufacturer of ibrutinib advises give digoxin at least 6 hours before or after ibrutinib
- Cobicistat: plasma concentration of ibrutinib possibly increased by ●cobicistat—reduce dose of ibrutinib (see Dose under Ibrutinib, p. 615)

Ibrutinib *(continued)*
- Cytotoxics: plasma concentration of ibrutinib possibly increased by ●crizotinib and ●imatinib—reduce dose of ibrutinib (see Dose under Ibrutinib, p. 615)
  Grapefruit Juice: manufacturer of ibrutinib advises avoid concomitant use with grapefruit juice
  Vitamins: manufacturer of ibrutinib advises avoid concomitant use with vitamin E

Ibuprofen *see* NSAIDs

Idarubicin
- Antipsychotics: avoid concomitant use of cytotoxics with ●clozapine (increased risk of agranulocytosis)
- Ciclosporin: plasma concentration of idarubicin increased by ●ciclosporin

Idelalisib
  Alpha-blockers: manufacturer of idelalisib advises avoid concomitant use with alfuzosin
  Anti-arrhythmics: manufacturer of idelalisib advises avoid concomitant use with amiodarone
- Antibacterials: plasma concentration of idelalisib reduced by ●rifampicin—avoid concomitant use
- Antidepressants: plasma concentration of idelalisib possibly reduced by ●St John's wort—manufacturer of idelalisib advises avoid concomitant use
- Antiepileptics: plasma concentration of idelalisib possibly reduced by ●carbamazepine and ●phenytoin—manufacturer of idelalisib advises avoid concomitant use
- Antipsychotics: avoid concomitant use of cytotoxics with ●clozapine (increased risk of agranulocytosis); manufacturer of idelalisib advises avoid concomitant use with pimozide and quetiapine
  Anxiolytics and Hypnotics: manufacturer of idelalisib advises avoid concomitant use of *oral* midazolam
  Ergot Alkaloids: manufacturer of idelalisib advises avoid concomitant use with ergotamine
  Lipid-regulating Drugs: manufacturer of idelalisib advises avoid concomitant use with simvastatin
  Sildenafil: manufacturer of idelalisib advises avoid concomitant use of sildenafil for pulmonary arterial hypertension
  Sympathomimetics, Beta$_2$: manufacturer of idelalisib advises avoid concomitant use with salmeterol

Ifosfamide
- Anticoagulants: ifosfamide possibly enhances anticoagulant effect of ●coumarins
- Antipsychotics: avoid concomitant use of cytotoxics with ●clozapine (increased risk of agranulocytosis)
  Cytotoxics: increased risk of otoxicity when ifosfamide given with cisplatin

Iloprost
  Analgesics: increased risk of bleeding when iloprost given with NSAIDs or aspirin
  Anticoagulants: iloprost possibly enhances anticoagulant effect of coumarins and heparins; increased risk of bleeding when iloprost given with phenindione
  Clopidogrel: increased risk of bleeding when iloprost given with clopidogrel
  Eptifibatide: increased risk of bleeding when iloprost given with eptifibatide
  Tirofiban: increased risk of bleeding when iloprost given with tirofiban

Imatinib
  Analgesics: manufacturer of imatinib advises caution with paracetamol
- Antibacterials: plasma concentration of imatinib reduced by ●rifampicin—avoid concomitant use
  Anticoagulants: manufacturer of imatinib advises replacement of warfarin with a heparin (possibility of enhanced warfarin effect)
- Antidepressants: plasma concentration of imatinib reduced by ●St John's wort—avoid concomitant use

Imatinib *(continued)*
- Antiepileptics: plasma concentration of imatinib reduced by ●carbamazepine, ●oxcarbazepine and ●phenytoin—avoid concomitant use
- Antipsychotics: avoid concomitant use of cytotoxics with ●clozapine (increased risk of agranulocytosis)
- Antivirals: avoidance of imatinib advised by manufacturer of ●boceprevir

  Ciclosporin: imatinib possibly increases plasma concentration of ciclosporin
- Cytotoxics: imatinib possibly increases the plasma concentration of ●bosutinib—manufacturer of bosutinib advises avoid or consider reducing dose of bosutinib; imatinib increases plasma concentration of ●everolimus (consider reducing the dose of everolimus —consult everolimus product literature); imatinib possibly increases the plasma concentration of ●ibrutinib—reduce dose of ibrutinib (see Dose under Ibrutinib, p. 615)

  Lipid-regulating Drugs: imatinib increases plasma concentration of simvastatin

  Tacrolimus: imatinib increases plasma concentration of tacrolimus

  Thyroid Hormones: imatinib possibly reduces plasma concentration of levothyroxine

Imidapril *see* ACE Inhibitors

Imipenem with Cilastatin
- Antiepileptics: carbapenems reduce plasma concentration of ●valproate—avoid concomitant use
- Antivirals: increased risk of convulsions when imipenem with cilastatin given with ●ganciclovir

  Vaccines: antibacterials inactivate oral typhoid vaccine—see p. 864

Imipramine *see* Antidepressants, Tricyclic

Immunoglobulins

Note For advice on immunoglobulins and live virus vaccines, see under Normal Immunoglobulin, p. 867

Indacaterol *see* Sympathomimetics, Beta$_2$

Indapamide *see* Diuretics

Indinavir

Aldesleukin: plasma concentration of indinavir possibly increased by aldesleukin
- Anti-arrhythmics: indinavir possibly increases plasma concentration of ●amiodarone—avoid concomitant use; indinavir possibly increases plasma concentration of ●flecainide (increased risk of ventricular arrhythmias—avoid concomitant use)
- Antibacterials: indinavir increases plasma concentration of ●rifabutin (also plasma concentration of indinavir reduced)—reduce rifabutin dose; metabolism of indinavir accelerated by ●rifampicin (reduced plasma concentration—avoid concomitant use); avoidance of concomitant indinavir in severe renal and hepatic impairment advised by manufacturer of ●telithromycin

  Anticoagulants: avoidance of indinavir advised by manufacturer of apixaban and rivaroxaban
- Antidepressants: plasma concentration of indinavir reduced by ●St John's wort—avoid concomitant use
- Antiepileptics: plasma concentration of indinavir possibly reduced by ●carbamazepine and ●phenytoin, also plasma concentration of carbamazepine and phenytoin possibly increased; plasma concentration of indinavir possibly reduced by ●phenobarbital
- Antifungals: plasma concentration of indinavir increased by ●itraconazole (consider reducing dose of indinavir)
- Antimalarials: caution with indinavir advised by manufacturer of artemether with lumefantrine; indinavir possibly increases plasma concentration of ●quinine (increased risk of toxicity)

  Antimuscarinics: avoidance of indinavir advised by manufacturer of darifenacin and tolterodine; manufacturer of fesoterodine advises dose reduction

Indinavir

Antimuscarinics *(continued)*
  when indinavir given with fesoterodine—consult fesoterodine product literature
- Antipsychotics: indinavir possibly increases plasma concentration of ●aripiprazole (reduce dose of aripiprazole—consult aripiprazole product literature); indinavir possibly increases plasma concentration of ●lurasidone—avoid concomitant use; indinavir possibly increases plasma concentration of ●pimozide (increased risk of ventricular arrhythmias—avoid concomitant use); indinavir possibly increases plasma concentration of ●quetiapine—manufacturer of quetiapine advises avoid concomitant use
- Antivirals: avoid concomitant use of indinavir with ●atazanavir; plasma concentration of both drugs increased when indinavir given with darunavir; absorption of indinavir reduced by didanosine *tablets* (give at least 1 hour apart); plasma concentration of indinavir reduced by efavirenz and nevirapine; plasma concentration of indinavir possibly reduced by ●etravirine—avoid concomitant use; indinavir increases plasma concentration of ●maraviroc (consider reducing dose of maraviroc); plasma concentration of indinavir increased by ritonavir; indinavir increases plasma concentration of saquinavir
- Anxiolytics and Hypnotics: increased risk of prolonged sedation when indinavir given with ●alprazolam—avoid concomitant use; indinavir possibly increases plasma concentration of ●midazolam (risk of prolonged sedation—avoid concomitant use of *oral* midazolam)

  Atovaquone: plasma concentration of indinavir possibly reduced by atovaquone
- Avanafil: indinavir possibly increases plasma concentration of ●avanafil—manufacturer of avanafil advises avoid concomitant use

  Bosentan: plasma concentration of indinavir possibly reduced by bosentan
- Ciclosporin: indinavir increases plasma concentration of ●ciclosporin
- Colchicine: indinavir possibly increases risk of ●colchicine toxicity—suspend or reduce dose of colchicine (avoid concomitant use in hepatic or renal impairment)

  Corticosteroids: plasma concentration of indinavir possibly reduced by dexamethasone
- Cytotoxics: indinavir possibly increases plasma concentration of axitinib (reduce dose of axitinib—consult axitinib product literature); indinavir possibly increases the plasma concentration of ●bosutinib and ●cabazitaxel—manufacturer of bosutinib and cabazitaxel advises avoid or consider reducing dose of bosutinib and cabazitaxel; indinavir possibly increases plasma concentration of ●crizotinib and ●everolimus—manufacturer of crizotinib and everolimus advises avoid concomitant use; indinavir possibly increases the plasma concentration of ●ibrutinib—reduce dose of ibrutinib (see Dose under Ibrutinib, p. 615); indinavir possibly increases plasma concentration of ●pazopanib (reduce dose of pazopanib); indinavir possibly increases plasma concentration of ●ponatinib—consider reducing initial dose of ponatinib (see Dose under Ponatinib, p. 618); manufacturer of ruxolitinib advises dose reduction when indinavir given with ●ruxolitinib—consult ruxolitinib product literature; indinavir possibly increases plasma concentration of ●docetaxel—manufacturer of docetaxel advises avoid concomitant use or consider reducing docetaxel dose
- Ergot Alkaloids: increased risk of ergotism when indinavir given with ●ergometrine or ●ergotamine—avoid concomitant use

Indinavir *(continued)*

- 5HT$_1$-receptor Agonists: indinavir increases plasma concentration of ●eletriptan (risk of toxicity)—avoid concomitant use
- Lipid-regulating Drugs: possible increased risk of myopathy when indinavir given with atorvastatin; possible increased risk of myopathy when indinavir given with ●rosuvastatin—manufacturer of rosuvastatin advises avoid concomitant use; increased risk of myopathy when indinavir given with ●simvastatin (avoid concomitant use); avoidance of indinavir advised by manufacturer of ●lomitapide (plasma concentration of lomitapide possibly increased)
- Orlistat: absorption of indinavir possibly reduced by ●orlistat
- Ranolazine: indinavir possibly increases plasma concentration of ●ranolazine—manufacturer of ranolazine advises avoid concomitant use
- Sildenafil: indinavir increases plasma concentration of ●sildenafil—reduce initial dose of sildenafil
  Tadalafil: indinavir possibly increases plasma concentration of tadalafil
- Vardenafil: indinavir increases plasma concentration of ●vardenafil—avoid concomitant use

Indometacin *see* NSAIDs

Indoramin *see* Alpha-blockers

Infliximab

- Abatacept: avoid concomitant use of infliximab with ●abatacept
- Anakinra: avoid concomitant use of infliximab with ●anakinra
- Antipsychotics: avoid concomitant use of cytotoxics with ●clozapine (increased risk of agranulocytosis)
- Vaccines: avoid concomitant use of monoclonal antibodies with live ●vaccines (see p. 842)

Influenza Vaccine *see* Vaccines

Insulin *see* Antidiabetics

Interferon Alfa *see* Interferons

Interferon Gamma *see* Interferons

Interferons

  Note Peginterferon alfa interactions as for interferon alfa

- Antivirals: caution with peginterferon alfa advised by manufacturer of adefovir; increased risk of peripheral neuropathy when interferon alfa given with ●telbivudine
- Theophylline: interferon alfa inhibits metabolism of ●theophylline (consider reducing dose of theophylline)
  Vaccines: manufacturer of interferon gamma advises avoid concomitant use with vaccines

Ipilimumab

- Antipsychotics: avoid concomitant use of cytotoxics with ●clozapine (increased risk of agranulocytosis)
  Cytotoxics: manufacturer of ipilimumab advises avoid concomitant use with vemurafenib
- Vaccines: avoid concomitant use of monoclonal antibodies with live ●vaccines (see p. 842)

Ipratropium *see* Antimuscarinics

Irbesartan *see* Angiotensin-II Receptor Antagonists

Irinotecan

- Antidepressants: metabolism of irinotecan accelerated by ●St John's wort (reduced plasma concentration—avoid concomitant use)
  Antiepileptics: plasma concentration of irinotecan and its active metabolite reduced by carbamazepine, phenobarbital and phenytoin
- Antifungals: increased risk of toxicity when irinotecan given with ●itraconazole—avoid concomitant use
- Antipsychotics: avoid concomitant use of cytotoxics with ●clozapine (increased risk of agranulocytosis)
- Antivirals: metabolism of irinotecan possibly inhibited by ●atazanavir (increased risk of toxicity)
- Cytotoxics: plasma concentration of active metabolite of irinotecan increased by ●lapatinib—consider reducing dose of irinotecan; plasma concentration

Irinotecan

- Cytotoxics *(continued)*
  of irinotecan increased by regorafenib; plasma concentration of irinotecan possibly increased by sorafenib

Iron

  Antacids: absorption of *oral* iron reduced by oral magnesium salts (as magnesium trisilicate)

- Antibacterials: *oral* iron reduces absorption of ciprofloxacin, levofloxacin, moxifloxacin and ofloxacin; *oral* iron reduces absorption of norfloxacin (give at least 2 hours apart); *oral* iron reduces absorption of tetracyclines, also absorption of *oral* iron reduced by tetracyclines
  Antivirals: *oral* iron reduces absorption of dolutegravir—manufacturer of dolutegravir advises give at least 2 hours before or 6 hours after *oral* iron
  Bisphosphonates: *oral* iron reduces absorption of bisphosphonates
  Calcium Salts: absorption of *oral* iron reduced by calcium salts
  Dopaminergics: *oral* iron reduces absorption of entacapone; *oral* iron possibly reduces absorption of levodopa
  Eltrombopag: *oral* iron possibly reduces absorption of eltrombopag (give at least 4 hours apart)
  Methyldopa: *oral* iron antagonises hypotensive effect of methyldopa
  Mycophenolate: *oral* iron reduces absorption of mycophenolate
  Penicillamine: *oral* iron reduces absorption of penicillamine
  Thyroid Hormones: *oral* iron reduces absorption of levothyroxine (give at least 2 hours apart)
  Trientine: absorption of *oral* iron reduced by trientine
  Zinc: *oral* iron reduces absorption of zinc, also absorption of *oral* iron reduced by zinc

Isocarboxazid *see* MAOIs

Isoflurane *see* Anaesthetics, General

Isometheptene *see* Sympathomimetics

Isoniazid

  Anaesthetics, General: increased risk of hepatotoxicity when isoniazid given with isoflurane
  Analgesics: avoidance of isoniazid advised by manufacturer of pethidine
  Antacids: absorption of isoniazid reduced by antacids

- Antibacterials: increased risk of hepatotoxicity when isoniazid given with ●rifampicin; increased risk of CNS toxicity when isoniazid given with cycloserine
- Antiepileptics: isoniazid increases plasma concentration of ●carbamazepine (also possibly increased isoniazid hepatotoxicity); isoniazid inhibits metabolism of ●ethosuximide (increased plasma concentration and risk of toxicity); isoniazid possibly inhibits metabolism of phenytoin (increased risk of toxicity)
  Anxiolytics and Hypnotics: isoniazid inhibits the metabolism of diazepam
  Corticosteroids: plasma concentration of isoniazid possibly reduced by corticosteroids
  Disulfiram: isoniazid possibly increases CNS effects of disulfiram
  Dopaminergics: isoniazid possibly reduces effects of levodopa
  Theophylline: isoniazid possibly increases plasma concentration of theophylline
  Vaccines: antibacterials inactivate oral typhoid vaccine—see p. 864

Isosorbide Dinitrate *see* Nitrates

Isosorbide Mononitrate *see* Nitrates

Isotretinoin *see* Retinoids

Isradipine *see* Calcium-channel Blockers

Itraconazole *see* Antifungals, Triazole

Ivabradine

- Anti-arrhythmics: increased risk of ventricular arrhythmias when ivabradine given with ●amiodarone or ●disopyramide
- Antibacterials: plasma concentration of ivabradine possibly increased by ●clarithromycin and ●telithromycin—avoid concomitant use; increased risk of ventricular arrhythmias when ivabradine given with ●erythromycin—avoid concomitant use

  Antidepressants: plasma concentration of ivabradine reduced by St John's wort—avoid concomitant use
- Antifungals: plasma concentration of ivabradine increased by fluconazole—reduce initial dose of ivabradine; plasma concentration of ivabradine possibly increased by ●itraconazole—avoid concomitant use
- Antimalarials: increased risk of ventricular arrhythmias when ivabradine given with ●mefloquine
- Antipsychotics: increased risk of ventricular arrhythmias when ivabradine given with ●pimozide
- Antivirals: plasma concentration of ivabradine possibly increased by ●ritonavir—avoid concomitant use
- Beta-blockers: increased risk of ventricular arrhythmias when ivabradine given with ●sotalol
- Calcium-channel Blockers: plasma concentration of ivabradine increased by ●diltiazem and ●verapamil—avoid concomitant use

  Grapefruit Juice: plasma concentration of ivabradine increased by grapefruit juice
- Pentamidine Isetionate: increased risk of ventricular arrhythmias when ivabradine given with ●pentamidine isetionate

Ivacaftor

- Antibacterials: plasma concentration of ivacaftor possibly increased by ●clarithromycin, ●erythromycin and ●telithromycin (see Dose under Ivacaftor, p. 220); plasma concentration of ivacaftor possibly reduced by ●rifabutin—manufacturer of ivacaftor advises avoid concomitant use; plasma concentration of ivacaftor reduced by ●rifampicin—manufacturer of ivacaftor advises avoid concomitant use
- Antidepressants: plasma concentration of ivacaftor possibly reduced by ●St John's wort—manufacturer of ivacaftor advises avoid concomitant use
- Antiepileptics: plasma concentration of ivacaftor possibly reduced by ●carbamazepine, ●phenobarbital and ●phenytoin—manufacturer of ivacaftor advises avoid concomitant use
- Antifungals: plasma concentration of ivacaftor increased by ●fluconazole (see Dose under Ivacaftor, p. 220); plasma concentration of ivacaftor possibly increased by ●itraconazole, ●posaconazole and ●voriconazole (see Dose under Ivacaftor, p. 220)

  Anxiolytics and Hypnotics: ivacaftor increases plasma concentration of midazolam

  Cardiac Glycosides: ivacaftor increases plasma concentration of digoxin

  Grapefruit Juice: plasma concentration of ivacaftor possibly increased by grapefruit juice—manufacturer of ivacaftor advises avoid concomitant use

Japanese encephalitis vaccine *see* Vaccines

Kaolin

Analgesics: kaolin possibly reduces absorption of aspirin

Antibacterials: kaolin possibly reduces absorption of tetracyclines

Antimalarials: kaolin reduces absorption of chloroquine and hydroxychloroquine

Antipsychotics: kaolin possibly reduces absorption of phenothiazines

Ketamine *see* Anaesthetics, General
Ketoprofen *see* NSAIDs
Ketorolac *see* NSAIDs
Ketotifen *see* Antihistamines
Labetalol *see* Beta-blockers
Lacidipine *see* Calcium-channel Blockers

Lacosamide

- Antidepressants: anticonvulsant effect of antiepileptics possibly antagonised by MAOIs and ●tricyclic-related antidepressants (convulsive threshold lowered); anticonvulsant effect of antiepileptics antagonised by ●SSRIs and ●tricyclics (convulsive threshold lowered)
- Antimalarials: anticonvulsant effect of antiepileptics antagonised by ●mefloquine
- Antipsychotics: anticonvulsant effect of antiepileptics antagonised by ●antipsychotics (convulsive threshold lowered)
- Orlistat: possible increased risk of convulsions when antiepileptics given with ●orlistat

Lactulose

Anticoagulants: lactulose possibly enhances anticoagulant effect of coumarins

Lamivudine

Antibacterials: plasma concentration of lamivudine increased by trimethoprim (as co-trimoxazole)—avoid concomitant use of high-dose co-trimoxazole

Antivirals: avoidance of lamivudine advised by manufacturer of emtricitabine
- Cytotoxics: manufacturer of lamivudine advises avoid concomitant use with ●cladribine
- Orlistat: absorption of lamivudine possibly reduced by ●orlistat

Lamotrigine

- Antibacterials: plasma concentration of lamotrigine reduced by ●rifampicin
- Antidepressants: anticonvulsant effect of antiepileptics possibly antagonised by MAOIs and ●tricyclic-related antidepressants (convulsive threshold lowered); anticonvulsant effect of antiepileptics antagonised by ●SSRIs and ●tricyclics (convulsive threshold lowered)
- Antiepileptics: plasma concentration of lamotrigine often reduced by carbamazepine, also plasma concentration of an active metabolite of carbamazepine sometimes raised (but evidence is conflicting); plasma concentration of lamotrigine reduced by phenobarbital and phenytoin; plasma concentration of lamotrigine increased by ●valproate (increased risk of toxicity—reduce lamotrigine dose)
- Antimalarials: anticonvulsant effect of antiepileptics antagonised by ●mefloquine
- Antipsychotics: anticonvulsant effect of antiepileptics antagonised by ●antipsychotics (convulsive threshold lowered)

  Antivirals: plasma concentration of lamotrigine possibly reduced by ritonavir
- Oestrogens: plasma concentration of lamotrigine reduced by ●oestrogens—consider increasing dose of lamotrigine
- Orlistat: possible increased risk of convulsions when antiepileptics given with ●orlistat

  Progestogens: plasma concentration of lamotrigine possibly increased by desogestrel

Lanreotide

Antidiabetics: lanreotide possibly reduces requirements for antidiabetics

Ciclosporin: lanreotide reduces plasma concentration of ciclosporin

Lansoprazole *see* Proton Pump Inhibitors

Lanthanum

Antibacterials: lanthanum possibly reduces absorption of quinolones (give at least 2 hours before or 4 hours after lanthanum)

Antimalarials: lanthanum possibly reduces absorption of chloroquine and hydroxychloroquine (give at least 2 hours apart)

Thyroid Hormones: lanthanum reduces absorption of levothyroxine (give at least 2 hours apart)

Lapatinib

- Antibacterials: manufacturer of lapatinib advises avoid concomitant use with ●rifabutin, ●rifampicin and ●telithromycin
- Antidepressants: manufacturer of lapatinib advises avoid concomitant use with ●St John's wort
- Antidiabetics: manufacturer of lapatinib advises avoid concomitant use with ●repaglinide
- Antiepileptics: plasma concentration of lapatinib reduced by ●carbamazepine—avoid concomitant use; manufacturer of lapatinib advises avoid concomitant use with ●phenytoin
- Antifungals: manufacturer of lapatinib advises avoid concomitant use with ●itraconazole, ●posaconazole and ●voriconazole
- Antipsychotics: avoid concomitant use of cytotoxics with ●clozapine (increased risk of agranulocytosis); manufacturer of lapatinib advises avoid concomitant use with ●pimozide
- Antivirals: avoidance of lapatinib advised by manufacturer of ●boceprevir; manufacturer of lapatinib advises avoid concomitant use with ●ritonavir and ●saquinavir
- Cytotoxics: lapatinib increases plasma concentration of pazopanib; possible increased risk of neutropenia when lapatinib given with docetaxel; increased risk of neutropenia when lapatinib given with ●paclitaxel; lapatinib increases plasma concentration of active metabolite of ●irinotecan—consider reducing dose of irinotecan
- Grapefruit Juice: manufacturer of lapatinib advises avoid concomitant use with ●grapefruit juice

Ulcer-healing Drugs: absorption of lapatinib possibly reduced by histamine H_2-antagonists and proton pump inhibitors

Laronidase

Antimalarials: effects of laronidase possibly inhibited by chloroquine and hydroxychloroquine (manufacturer of laronidase advises avoid concomitant use)

Leflunomide

Note Increased risk of toxicity with other haematotoxic and hepatotoxic drugs

Antibacterials: plasma concentration of active metabolite of leflunomide possibly increased by rifampicin

Anticoagulants: leflunomide possibly enhances anticoagulant effect of warfarin

Antidiabetics: leflunomide possibly enhances hypoglycaemic effect of tolbutamide

Antiepileptics: leflunomide possibly increases plasma concentration of phenytoin

- Cytotoxics: risk of toxicity when leflunomide given with ●methotrexate

Lipid-regulating Drugs: the effect of leflunomide is significantly decreased by colestyramine (enhanced elimination)—avoid unless drug elimination desired

- Vaccines: avoid concomitant use of leflunomide with live ●vaccines (see p. 842)

Lenalidomide

- Antibacterials: plasma concentration of lenalidomide possibly increased by ●clarithromycin (increased risk of toxicity)
- Antifungals: plasma concentration of lenalidomide possibly increased by ●itraconazole (increased risk of toxicity)
- Calcium-channel Blockers: plasma concentration of lenalidomide possibly increased by ●verapamil (increased risk of toxicity)

Cardiac Glycosides: lenalidomide possibly increases plasma concentration of digoxin

- Ciclosporin: plasma concentration of lenalidomide possibly increased by ●ciclosporin (increased risk of toxicity)

Lercanidipine *see* Calcium-channel Blockers

Leukotriene Receptor Antagonists

Analgesics: plasma concentration of zafirlukast increased by aspirin

Antibacterials: plasma concentration of zafirlukast reduced by erythromycin

Anticoagulants: zafirlukast enhances anticoagulant effect of warfarin

Antiepileptics: plasma concentration of montelukast reduced by phenobarbital

Antifungals: plasma concentration of zafirlukast increased by fluconazole

Lipid-regulating Drugs: plasma concentration of montelukast increased by gemfibrozil

Theophylline: zafirlukast possibly increases plasma concentration of theophylline, also plasma concentration of zafirlukast reduced

Levamisole

Alcohol: possibility of disulfiram-like reaction when levamisole given with alcohol

- Anticoagulants: levamisole possibly enhances anticoagulant effect of ●warfarin

Antiepileptics: levamisole possibly increases plasma concentration of phenytoin

Levetiracetam

- Antidepressants: anticonvulsant effect of antiepileptics possibly antagonised by MAOIs and ●tricyclic-related antidepressants (convulsive threshold lowered); anticonvulsant effect of antiepileptics antagonised by ●SSRIs and ●tricyclics (convulsive threshold lowered)

Antiepileptics: levetiracetam possibly increases risk of carbamazepine toxicity

- Antimalarials: anticonvulsant effect of antiepileptics antagonised by ●mefloquine
- Antipsychotics: anticonvulsant effect of antiepileptics antagonised by ●antipsychotics (convulsive threshold lowered)
- Orlistat: possible increased risk of convulsions when antiepileptics given with ●orlistat

Levobunolol *see* Beta-blockers

Levobupivacaine

Anti-arrhythmics: increased myocardial depression when levobupivacaine given with anti-arrhythmics

Levocarnitine

Anticoagulants: levocarnitine possibly enhances anticoagulant effect of coumarins

Levocetirizine *see* Antihistamines

Levodopa

ACE Inhibitors: enhanced hypotensive effect when levodopa given with ACE inhibitors

Adrenergic Neurone Blockers: enhanced hypotensive effect when levodopa given with adrenergic neurone blockers

Alpha-blockers: enhanced hypotensive effect when levodopa given with alpha-blockers

- Anaesthetics, General: increased risk of arrhythmias when levodopa given with ●volatile liquid general anaesthetics

Angiotensin-II Receptor Antagonists: enhanced hypotensive effect when levodopa given with angiotensin-II receptor antagonists

Antibacterials: effects of levodopa possibly reduced by isoniazid

- Antidepressants: risk of hypertensive crisis when levodopa given with ●MAOIs, avoid levodopa for at least 2 weeks after stopping MAOIs; increased risk of side-effects when levodopa given with moclobemide

Antiepileptics: effects of levodopa possibly reduced by phenytoin

Antimuscarinics: absorption of levodopa possibly reduced by antimuscarinics

Antipsychotics: effects of levodopa antagonised by antipsychotics; avoidance of levodopa advised by manufacturer of amisulpride (antagonism of effect)

Levodopa *(continued)*

Anxiolytics and Hypnotics: effects of levodopa possibly antagonised by benzodiazepines

Beta-blockers: enhanced hypotensive effect when levodopa given with beta-blockers

Bupropion: increased risk of side-effects when levodopa given with bupropion

Calcium-channel Blockers: enhanced hypotensive effect when levodopa given with calcium-channel blockers

Clonidine: enhanced hypotensive effect when levodopa given with clonidine

Diazoxide: enhanced hypotensive effect when levodopa given with diazoxide

Diuretics: enhanced hypotensive effect when levodopa given with diuretics

Dopaminergics: enhanced effects and increased toxicity of levodopa when given with selegiline (reduce dose of levodopa)

Iron: absorption of levodopa possibly reduced by *oral* iron

Memantine: effects of dopaminergics possibly enhanced by memantine

Methyldopa: enhanced hypotensive effect when levodopa given with methyldopa; antiparkinsonian effect of dopaminergics antagonised by methyldopa

Moxonidine: enhanced hypotensive effect when levodopa given with moxonidine

Muscle Relaxants: possible agitation, confusion and hallucinations when levodopa given with baclofen

Nitrates: enhanced hypotensive effect when levodopa given with nitrates

Vasodilator Antihypertensives: enhanced hypotensive effect when levodopa given with hydralazine, minoxidil or sodium nitroprusside

Vitamins: effects of levodopa reduced by pyridoxine when given without dopa-decarboxylase inhibitor

Levofloxacin *see* Quinolones

Levofolinic Acid *see* Folates

Levomepromazine *see* Antipsychotics

Levonorgestrel *see* Progestogens

Levothyroxine *see* Thyroid Hormones

Lidocaine

Note Interactions less likely when lidocaine used topically

Anaesthetics, Local: increased myocardial depression when anti-arrhythmics given with bupivacaine, levobupivacaine, prilocaine or ropivacaine

• Anti-arrhythmics: increased myocardial depression when anti-arrhythmics given with other ●anti-arrhythmics

• Antipsychotics: increased risk of ventricular arrhythmias when anti-arrhythmics that prolong the QT interval given with ●antipsychotics that prolong the QT interval

• Antivirals: plasma concentration of lidocaine possibly increased by ●atazanavir and lopinavir; plasma concentration of lidocaine possibly increased by darunavir and ●fosamprenavir—avoid concomitant use; increased risk of ventricular arrhythmias when lidocaine given with ●saquinavir—avoid concomitant use; caution with *intravenous* lidocaine advised by manufacturer of telaprevir

• Beta-blockers: increased myocardial depression when anti-arrhythmics given with ●beta-blockers; possible increased risk of lidocaine toxicity when given with nadolol; increased risk of lidocaine toxicity when given with ●propranolol

• Diuretics: action of lidocaine antagonised by hypokalaemia caused by ●acetazolamide, ●loop diuretics or ●thiazides and related diuretics

Muscle Relaxants: neuromuscular blockade enhanced and prolonged when lidocaine given with suxamethonium

• Ulcer-healing Drugs: plasma concentration of lidocaine increased by ●cimetidine (increased risk of toxicity)

Linagliptin *see* Antidiabetics

Linezolid

Note Linezolid is a reversible, non-selective MAO inhibitor—see interactions of MAOIs

Antibacterials: plasma concentration of linezolid reduced by rifampicin (possible therapeutic failure of linezolid)

Vaccines: antibacterials inactivate oral typhoid vaccine—see p. 864

Liothyronine *see* Thyroid Hormones

Lipid-regulating Drugs *see* Colesevelam, Colestipol, Colestyramine, Ezetimibe, Fibrates, Lomitapide, Nicotinic Acid, and Statins

Liraglutide *see* Antidiabetics

Lisdexamfetamine *see* Sympathomimetics

Lisinopril *see* ACE Inhibitors

Lithium

• ACE Inhibitors: excretion of lithium reduced by ●ACE inhibitors (increased plasma concentration)

• Analgesics: excretion of lithium reduced by ●NSAIDs (increased risk of toxicity); excretion of lithium reduced by ●ketorolac (increased risk of toxicity)—avoid concomitant use

• Angiotensin-II Receptor Antagonists: excretion of lithium reduced by ●angiotensin-II receptor antagonists (increased plasma concentration)

Antacids: excretion of lithium increased by sodium bicarbonate (reduced plasma concentration)

• Anti-arrhythmics: avoidance of lithium advised by manufacturer of ●amiodarone (risk of ventricular arrhythmias)

Antibacterials: increased risk of lithium toxicity when given with metronidazole

• Antidepressants: possible increased serotonergic effects when lithium given with venlafaxine; increased risk of CNS effects when lithium given with ●SSRIs (lithium toxicity reported); risk of toxicity when lithium given with tricyclics

Antiepileptics: neurotoxicity may occur when lithium given with carbamazepine or phenytoin without increased plasma concentration of lithium; plasma concentration of lithium possibly affected by topiramate

• Antipsychotics: increased risk of extrapyramidal side-effects and possibly neurotoxicity when lithium given with clozapine, flupentixol, haloperidol, phenothiazines, ●risperidone or zuclopenthixol; possible risk of toxicity when lithium given with olanzapine; lithium possibly increases extrapyramidal side-effects of quetiapine; increased risk of extrapyramidal side-effects when lithium given with sulpiride

Anxiolytics and Hypnotics: increased risk of neurotoxicity when lithium given with clonazepam

Calcium-channel Blockers: neurotoxicity may occur when lithium given with diltiazem or verapamil without increased plasma concentration of lithium

• Cytotoxics: increased risk of ventricular arrhythmias when lithium given with ●arsenic trioxide

• Dapoxetine: possible increased risk of serotonergic effects when lithium given with ●dapoxetine (manufacturer of dapoxetine advises lithium should not be started until 1 week after stopping dapoxetine, avoid dapoxetine for 2 weeks after stopping lithium)

• Diuretics: excretion of lithium increased by ●acetazolamide; excretion of lithium reduced by ●loop diuretics and ●thiazides and related diuretics (increased plasma concentration and risk of toxicity)—loop diuretics safer than thiazides; excretion of lithium reduced by ●potassium-sparing diuretics and aldosterone antagonists (increased plasma concentration and risk of toxicity)

5HT₁-receptor Agonists: possible risk of toxicity when lithium given with sumatriptan

• Methyldopa: neurotoxicity may occur when lithium given with ●methyldopa without increased plasma concentration of lithium

Lithium *(continued)*

Muscle Relaxants: lithium enhances effects of muscle relaxants; hyperkinesis caused by lithium possibly aggravated by baclofen

Parasympathomimetics: lithium antagonises effects of neostigmine

Theophylline: excretion of lithium increased by theophylline (reduced plasma concentration)

Lixisenatide *see* Antidiabetics

Lofepramine *see* Antidepressants, Tricyclic

Lofexidine

Alcohol: increased sedative effect when lofexidine given with alcohol

Anxiolytics and Hypnotics: increased sedative effect when lofexidine given with anxiolytics and hypnotics

Lomitapide

Alcohol: manufacturer of lomitapide advises avoid concomitant use with alcohol

● Anti-arrhythmics: manufacturer of lomitapide advises avoid concomitant use with ●dronedarone (plasma concentration of lomitapide possibly increased)

● Antibacterials: manufacturer of lomitapide advises avoid concomitant use with ●clarithromycin, ●erythromycin and ●telithromycin (plasma concentration of lomitapide possibly increased)

Anticoagulants: lomitapide possibly enhances anticoagulant effect of warfarin

● Antifungals: manufacturer of lomitapide advises avoid concomitant use with ●triazoles (plasma concentration of lomitapide possibly increased)

● Antivirals: manufacturer of lomitapide advises avoid concomitant use with ●darunavir, ●fosamprenavir, ●indinavir, ●lopinavir, ●ritonavir, ●saquinavir, ●telaprevir and ●tipranavir (plasma concentration of lomitapide possibly increased)

Aprepitant: manufacturer of lomitapide advises dose reduction when lomitapide given with fosaprepitant (see Dose under Lomitapide, p. 180)

● Calcium-channel Blockers: manufacturer of lomitapide advises avoid concomitant use with ●diltiazem and ●verapamil (plasma concentration of lomitapide possibly increased)

Grapefruit Juice: manufacturer of lomitapide advises avoid concomitant use with grapefruit juice

● Lipid-regulating Drugs: lomitapide increases plasma concentration of atorvastatin; lomitapide increases plasma concentration of ●simvastatin (see Dose under Simvastatin, p. 177); absorption of lomitapide possibly reduced by bile acid sequestrants (give at least 4 hours apart)

Ranolazine: manufacturer of lomitapide advises dose reduction when lomitapide given with ranolazine (see Dose under Lomitapide, p. 180)

Ulcer-healing Drugs: manufacturer of lomitapide advises dose reduction when lomitapide given with cimetidine (see Dose under Lomitapide, p. 180)

Lomustine

● Antipsychotics: avoid concomitant use of cytotoxics with ●clozapine (increased risk of agranulocytosis)

Ulcer-healing Drugs: myelosuppressive effects of lomustine possibly enhanced by cimetidine

Loperamide

Desmopressin: loperamide increases plasma concentration of *oral* desmopressin

Lopinavir

Note In combination with ritonavir as *Kaletra*® (ritonavir is present to inhibit lopinavir metabolism and increase plasma-lopinavir concentration)—see also Ritonavir

● Anti-arrhythmics: lopinavir possibly increases plasma concentration of ●flecainide (increased risk of ventricular arrhythmias—avoid concomitant use); lopinavir possibly increases plasma concentration of lidocaine

● Antibacterials: plasma concentration of lopinavir reduced by ●rifampicin—avoid concomitant use;

Lopinavir

● Antibacterials *(continued)*

lopinavir increases plasma concentration of delamanid; avoidance of concomitant lopinavir in severe renal and hepatic impairment advised by manufacturer of ●telithromycin

Anticoagulants: avoidance of lopinavir advised by manufacturer of apixaban; manufacturers advise avoid concomitant use of lopinavir with rivaroxaban

● Antidepressants: plasma concentration of lopinavir reduced by ●St John's wort—avoid concomitant use

● Antiepileptics: plasma concentration of lopinavir possibly reduced by carbamazepine, ●phenobarbital and phenytoin

Antihistamines: lopinavir possibly increases plasma concentration of chlorphenamine

Antimalarials: caution with lopinavir advised by manufacturer of artemether with lumefantrine

Antimuscarinics: avoidance of lopinavir advised by manufacturer of darifenacin and tolterodine

● Antipsychotics: lopinavir possibly increases plasma concentration of ●aripiprazole (reduce dose of aripiprazole—consult aripiprazole product literature); lopinavir possibly increases plasma concentration of ●quetiapine—manufacturer of quetiapine advises avoid concomitant use

● Antivirals: manufacturers advise avoid concomitant use of lopinavir with ●boceprevir and ●telaprevir; avoidance of lopinavir advised by manufacturer of daclatasvir (plasma concentration of daclatasvir possibly increased); lopinavir reduces plasma concentration of ●darunavir, also plasma concentration of lopinavir increased (avoid concomitant use); plasma concentration of lopinavir reduced by ●efavirenz—consider increasing dose of lopinavir; lopinavir boosted with ritonavir increases plasma concentration of ●elvitegravir (reduce dose of elvitegravir); lopinavir reduces plasma concentration of fosamprenavir, effect on lopinavir plasma concentration not predictable—avoid concomitant use; lopinavir increases plasma concentration of ●maraviroc (consider reducing dose of maraviroc); plasma concentration of lopinavir possibly reduced by ●nevirapine—consider increasing dose of lopinavir; increased risk of ventricular arrhythmias when lopinavir given with ●saquinavir—avoid concomitant use; lopinavir increases plasma concentration of tenofovir; plasma concentration of lopinavir reduced by ●tipranavir

● Bosentan: lopinavir increases plasma concentration of ●bosentan (consider reducing dose of bosentan)

Corticosteroids: plasma concentration of lopinavir possibly reduced by dexamethasone

● Cytotoxics: manufacturer of ruxolitinib advises dose reduction when lopinavir given with ●ruxolitinib—consult ruxolitinib product literature

Eltrombopag: lopinavir possibly reduces plasma concentration of eltrombopag

● Lipid-regulating Drugs: possible increased risk of myopathy when lopinavir given with atorvastatin; lopinavir increases plasma concentration of ●rosuvastatin—adjust dose of rosuvastatin (consult product literature); possible increased risk of myopathy when lopinavir given with ●simvastatin—avoid concomitant use; avoidance of lopinavir advised by manufacturer of ●lomitapide (plasma concentration of lomitapide possibly increased)

● Orlistat: absorption of lopinavir possibly reduced by ●orlistat

● Ranolazine: lopinavir possibly increases plasma concentration of ●ranolazine—manufacturer of ranolazine advises avoid concomitant use

Sirolimus: lopinavir possibly increases plasma concentration of sirolimus

Appendix 1: Interactions

Lopinavir (continued)

Sympathomimetics, Beta$_2$: manufacturer of lopinavir advises avoid concomitant use with salmeterol

Loprazolam see Anxiolytics and Hypnotics

Loratadine see Antihistamines

Lorazepam see Anxiolytics and Hypnotics

Lormetazepam see Anxiolytics and Hypnotics

Losartan see Angiotensin-II Receptor Antagonists

Lumefantrine see Artemether with Lumefantrine

Lurasidone see Antipsychotics

Lymecycline see Tetracyclines

Macitentan

- Antibacterials: plasma concentration of macitentan reduced by ●rifampicin—avoid concomitant use
  Antidepressants: manufacturer of macitentan advises avoid concomitant use with St John's wort
  Antiepileptics: manufacturer of macitentan advises avoid concomitant use with carbamazepine and phenytoin

Macrogols

Note Some manufacturers suggest taking other oral medication 1 hour before or 1 hour after macrogols to reduce possible interference with absorption

Macrolides

Note See also Telithromycin

Note Interactions do not apply to small amounts of erythromycin used topically

Analgesics: erythromycin increases plasma concentration of alfentanil; clarithromycin possibly increases plasma concentration of fentanyl

Antacids: absorption of azithromycin reduced by antacids

- Anti-arrhythmics: increased risk of ventricular arrhythmias when *parenteral* erythromycin given with ●amiodarone—avoid concomitant use; azithromycin possibly increases plasma concentration of ●disopyramide (increased risk of toxicity); erythromycin increases plasma concentration of ●disopyramide (increased risk of toxicity); clarithromycin possibly increases plasma concentration of ●disopyramide (increased risk of ventricular arrhythmias); erythromycin increases plasma concentration of ●dronedarone (increased risk of ventricular arrhythmias—avoid concomitant use); avoidance of clarithromycin advised by manufacturer of ●dronedarone (risk of ventricular arrhythmias)

- Antibacterials: increased risk of ventricular arrhythmias when *parenteral* erythromycin given with ●moxifloxacin—avoid concomitant use; increased risk of side-effects including neutropenia when azithromycin given with ●rifabutin; clarithromycin increases plasma concentration of ●rifabutin (increased risk of toxicity—reduce rifabutin dose); erythromycin possibly increases plasma concentration of ●rifabutin (increased risk of toxicity—reduce rifabutin dose); clarithromycin and erythromycin possibly increase plasma concentration of bedaquiline—avoid concomitant use if clarithromycin and erythromycin given for more than 14 days; possible increased risk of ventricular arrhythmias when clarithromycin and erythromycin given with ●delamanid; plasma concentration of clarithromycin reduced by rifamycins

- Anticoagulants: avoidance of clarithromycin advised by manufacturer of apixaban; clarithromycin and erythromycin enhance anticoagulant effect of ●coumarins; azithromycin possibly enhances anticoagulant effect of ●coumarins; possible increased risk of bleeding when clarithromycin given with dabigatran

- Antidepressants: avoidance of macrolides advised by manufacturer of ●reboxetine; avoidance of *intravenous* erythromycin advised by manufacturer of ●citalopram and ●escitalopram (risk of ventricular arrhythmias); clarithromycin possibly increases plasma concentration of trazodone

Macrolides (continued)

Antidiabetics: clarithromycin enhances effects of repaglinide

- Antiepileptics: erythromycin increases plasma concentration of ●carbamazepine; clarithromycin increases plasma concentration of ●carbamazepine (consider reducing dose of carbamazepine); clarithromycin inhibits metabolism of phenytoin (increased plasma concentration); erythromycin possibly inhibits metabolism of valproate (increased plasma concentration)
  Antifungals: avoidance of erythromycin advised by manufacturer of fluconazole; clarithromycin increases plasma concentration of itraconazole

- Antihistamines: manufacturer of loratadine advises erythromycin possibly increases plasma concentration of loratadine; macrolides possibly inhibit metabolism of ●mizolastine (avoid concomitant use); erythromycin inhibits metabolism of ●mizolastine—avoid concomitant use; erythromycin increases plasma concentration of rupatadine

- Antimalarials: avoidance of macrolides advised by manufacturer of ●piperaquine with artenimol (possible risk of ventricular arrhythmias); avoidance of macrolides advised by manufacturer of ●artemether with lumefantrine
  Antimuscarinics: erythromycin possibly increases plasma concentration of darifenacin; manufacturer of fesoterodine advises dose reduction when clarithromycin given with fesoterodine—consult fesoterodine product literature; avoidance of clarithromycin and erythromycin advised by manufacturer of tolterodine

- Antipsychotics: avoidance of macrolides advised by manufacturer of ●droperidol (risk of ventricular arrhythmias); increased risk of ventricular arrhythmias when *parenteral* erythromycin given with ●zuclopenthixol—avoid concomitant use; increased risk of ventricular arrhythmias when erythromycin given with ●amisulpride—avoid concomitant use; erythromycin possibly increases plasma concentration of ●clozapine (possible increased risk of convulsions); erythromycin possibly increases the plasma concentration of ●lurasidone (see Dose under Lurasidone, p. 243); clarithromycin possibly increases plasma concentration of ●lurasidone—avoid concomitant use; possible increased risk of ventricular arrhythmias when erythromycin given with ●pimozide—avoid concomitant use; increased risk of ventricular arrhythmias when clarithromycin given with ●pimozide—avoid concomitant use; erythromycin increases plasma concentration of ●quetiapine—manufacturer of quetiapine advises avoid concomitant use; clarithromycin possibly increases plasma concentration of ●quetiapine—manufacturer of quetiapine advises avoid concomitant use; increased risk of ventricular arrhythmias when *parenteral* erythromycin given with ●sulpiride

- Antivirals: plasma concentration of both drugs increased when clarithromycin given with atazanavir; clarithromycin possibly increases the plasma concentration of ●daclatasvir—reduce dose of daclatasvir (see Dose under Daclatasvir, p. 438); plasma concentration of clarithromycin reduced by efavirenz, also plasma concentration of active metabolite of clarithromycin increased; plasma concentration of clarithromycin reduced by ●etravirine and nevirapine (but concentration of an active metabolite increased), also plasma concentration of etravirine and nevirapine increased; clarithromycin possibly increases plasma concentration of ●maraviroc (consider reducing dose of maraviroc); avoidance of clarithromycin and erythromycin advised by manufacturer of ●rilpivirine (plasma concentration of rilpivirine possibly increased); plasma concentration of azithromycin and erythromycin possibly

Macrolides

- **Antivirals** *(continued)*
increased by ritonavir; plasma concentration of clarithromycin increased by •ritonavir (reduce dose of clarithromycin in renal impairment); plasma concentration of both drugs possibly increased when clarithromycin given with •saquinavir and •telaprevir (increased risk of ventricular arrhythmias); increased risk of ventricular arrhythmias when erythromycin given with •saquinavir—avoid concomitant use; clarithromycin possibly increases plasma concentration of •simeprevir—manufacturer of simeprevir advises avoid concomitant use; plasma concentration of both drugs increased when erythromycin given with •simeprevir—manufacturer of simeprevir advises avoid concomitant use; plasma concentration of both drugs possibly increased when erythromycin given with •telaprevir (increased risk of ventricular arrhythmias); plasma concentration of clarithromycin increased by •tipranavir (reduce dose of clarithromycin in renal impairment), also clarithromycin increases plasma concentration of tipranavir; clarithromycin tablets reduce absorption of zidovudine (give at least 2 hours apart)
- **Anxiolytics and Hypnotics**: clarithromycin and erythromycin inhibit metabolism of •midazolam (increased plasma concentration with increased sedation); erythromycin increases plasma concentration of buspirone (reduce dose of buspirone); erythromycin inhibits the metabolism of zopiclone
Aprepitant: clarithromycin possibly increases plasma concentration of aprepitant
- **Atomoxetine**: increased risk of ventricular arrhythmias when *parenteral* erythromycin given with •atomoxetine
- **Avanafil**: clarithromycin possibly increases plasma concentration of •avanafil—manufacturer of avanafil advises avoid concomitant use; erythromycin increases plasma concentration of •avanafil—see Dose under Avanafil, p. 571
- **Calcium-channel Blockers**: clarithromycin and erythromycin possibly inhibit metabolism of •calcium-channel blockers (increased risk of side-effects); avoidance of erythromycin advised by manufacturer of lercanidipine
Cardiac Glycosides: macrolides increase plasma concentration of digoxin (increased risk of toxicity)
- **Ciclosporin**: macrolides possibly inhibit metabolism of •ciclosporin (increased plasma concentration); clarithromycin and erythromycin inhibit metabolism of •ciclosporin (increased plasma concentration)
- **Cilostazol**: clarithromycin possibly increases plasma concentration of •cilostazol (see Dose under Cilostazol, p. 141); erythromycin increases plasma concentrations of •cilostazol (see Dose under Cilostazol, p. 141)
- **Clopidogrel**: erythromycin possibly reduces antiplatelet effect of •clopidogrel
- **Colchicine**: azithromycin, clarithromycin and erythromycin possibly increase risk of •colchicine toxicity—suspend or reduce dose of colchicine (avoid concomitant use in hepatic or renal impairment)
Corticosteroids: erythromycin possibly inhibits metabolism of corticosteroids; clarithromycin possibly increases plasma concentration of methylprednisolone; erythromycin inhibits the metabolism of methylprednisolone
- **Cytotoxics**: erythromycin possibly increases the plasma concentration of afatinib—manufacturer of afatinib advises separating administration of erythromycin by 6 to 12 hours; clarithromycin and erythromycin possibly increase plasma concentration of axitinib (reduce dose of axitinib—consult axitinib product literature); clarithromycin and erythromycin possibly increase the plasma concen-

Macrolides

- **Cytotoxics** *(continued)*
tration of •bosutinib—manufacturer of bosutinib advises avoid or consider reducing dose of bosutinib; clarithromycin and erythromycin possibly increase plasma concentration of cabozantinib; clarithromycin possibly increases plasma concentration of •crizotinib and •everolimus—manufacturer of crizotinib and everolimus advises avoid concomitant use; erythromycin increases plasma concentration of •everolimus (consider reducing the dose of everolimus —consult everolimus product literature); clarithromycin and erythromycin possibly increase the plasma concentration of •ibrutinib—reduce dose of ibrutinib (see Dose under Ibrutinib, p. 615); avoidance of clarithromycin advised by manufacturer of •nilotinib; clarithromycin possibly increases plasma concentration of •pazopanib (reduce dose of pazopanib); clarithromycin possibly increases plasma concentration of ponatinib—consider reducing initial dose of ponatinib (see Dose under Ponatinib, p. 618); manufacturer of ruxolitinib advises dose reduction when clarithromycin given with •ruxolitinib—consult ruxolitinib product literature; possible increased risk of ventricular arrhythmias when *parenteral* erythromycin given with •vandetanib—avoid concomitant use; clarithromycin possibly increases the plasma concentration of •cabazitaxel—manufacturer of cabazitaxel advises avoid or consider reducing dose of cabazitaxel; clarithromycin possibly increases plasma concentration of •docetaxel—manufacturer of docetaxel advises avoid concomitant use or consider reducing docetaxel dose; increased risk of ventricular arrhythmias when erythromycin given with •arsenic trioxide; erythromycin increases toxicity of •vinblastine—avoid concomitant use; possible increased risk of neutropenia when clarithromycin given with •vinorelbine
Dapoxetine: manufacturer of dapoxetine advises dose reduction when clarithromycin and erythromycin given with dapoxetine (see Dose under Dapoxetine, p. 572)
- **Diuretics**: clarithromycin increases plasma concentration of •eplerenone—avoid concomitant use; erythromycin increases plasma concentration of eplerenone (reduce dose of eplerenone)
- **Domperidone**: possible increased risk of ventricular arrhythmias when clarithromycin given with •domperidone—avoid concomitant use; erythromycin increases plasma concentration of •domperidone (increased risk of ventricular arrhythmias—avoid concomitant use)
Dopaminergics: macrolides possibly increase plasma concentration of bromocriptine and cabergoline (increased risk of toxicity); erythromycin increases plasma concentration of bromocriptine and cabergoline (increased risk of toxicity)
- **Ergot Alkaloids**: increased risk of ergotism when clarithromycin or erythromycin given with •ergometrine—avoid concomitant use; increased risk of ergotism when macrolides given with •ergotamine—avoid concomitant use
Fidaxomicin: avoidance of clarithromycin and erythromycin advised by manufacturer of fidaxomicin
- **5HT$_1$-receptor Agonists**: clarithromycin and erythromycin increase plasma concentration of •eletriptan (risk of toxicity)—avoid concomitant use
- **Ivabradine**: clarithromycin possibly increases plasma concentration of •ivabradine—avoid concomitant use; increased risk of ventricular arrhythmias when erythromycin given with •ivabradine—avoid concomitant use
- **Ivacaftor**: clarithromycin and erythromycin possibly increase plasma concentration of •ivacaftor (see Dose under Ivacaftor, p. 220)

Macrolides *(continued)*

- Lenalidomide: clarithromycin possibly increases plasma concentration of ●lenalidomide (increased risk of toxicity)

  Leukotriene Receptor Antagonists: erythromycin reduces plasma concentration of zafirlukast

- Lipid-regulating Drugs: clarithromycin increases plasma concentration of ●atorvastatin and pravastatin; possible increased risk of myopathy when erythromycin given with atorvastatin; erythromycin increases plasma concentration of pravastatin; erythromycin reduces plasma concentration of rosuvastatin; increased risk of myopathy when clarithromycin or erythromycin given with ●simvastatin (avoid concomitant use); avoidance of clarithromycin and erythromycin advised by manufacturer of ●lomitapide (plasma concentration of lomitapide possibly increased)

  Mirabegron: when given with clarithromycin avoid or reduce dose of mirabegron in hepatic or renal impairment—see Mirabegron, p. 564

  Oestrogens: erythromycin increases plasma concentration of estradiol

  Parasympathomimetics: erythromycin increases plasma concentration of galantamine

- Pentamidine Isetionate: increased risk of ventricular arrhythmias when *parenteral* erythromycin given with ●pentamidine isetionate

  Progestogens: erythromycin increases plasma concentration of dienogest

- Ranolazine: clarithromycin possibly increases plasma concentration of ●ranolazine—manufacturer of ranolazine advises avoid concomitant use

- Sildenafil: clarithromycin increases the plasma concentration of ●sildenafil—consider reducing initial dose of sildenafil for erectile dysfunction or reduce sildenafil dose frequency to once daily for pulmonary hypertension; erythromycin increases plasma concentration of sildenafil—reduce initial dose of sildenafil for erectile dysfunction or reduce sildenafil dose frequency to twice daily for pulmonary hypertension

- Sirolimus: clarithromycin increases plasma concentration of ●sirolimus—avoid concomitant use; plasma concentration of both drugs increased when erythromycin given with ●sirolimus

- Tacrolimus: clarithromycin and erythromycin increase plasma concentration of ●tacrolimus

  Tadalafil: clarithromycin and erythromycin possibly increase plasma concentration of tadalafil

- Theophylline: clarithromycin possibly increases plasma concentration of theophylline; erythromycin increases plasma concentration of ●theophylline (also theophylline may reduce absorption of *oral* erythromycin)

- Ticagrelor: clarithromycin possibly increases plasma concentration of ●ticagrelor—manufacturer of ticagrelor advises avoid concomitant use; erythromycin possibly increases plasma concentration of ticagrelor

  Ulcer-healing Drugs: plasma concentration of erythromycin increased by cimetidine (increased risk of toxicity, including deafness); plasma concentration of both drugs increased when clarithromycin given with omeprazole

  Ulipristal: avoidance of clarithromycin advised by manufacturer of *low-dose* ulipristal; erythromycin increases plasma concentration of *low-dose* ulipristal—manufacturer of *low-dose* ulipristal advises avoid concomitant use

  Vaccines: antibacterials inactivate oral typhoid vaccine—see p. 864

  Vardenafil: clarithromycin possibly increases plasma concentration of vardenafil (consider reducing initial dose of vardenafil); erythromycin increases plasma

Macrolides

Vardenafil *(continued)*

  concentration of vardenafil (reduce dose of vardenafil)

Magnesium (parenteral)

- Calcium-channel Blockers: profound hypotension reported with concomitant use of parenteral magnesium and ●nifedipine in pre-eclampsia

  Muscle Relaxants: parenteral magnesium enhances effects of non-depolarising muscle relaxants and suxamethonium

Magnesium Salts (oral) *see* Antacids

Mannitol

  Antibacterials: avoidance of mannitol advised by manufacturer of tobramycin

  Ciclosporin: possible increased risk of nephrotoxicity when mannitol given with ciclosporin

MAOIs

Note For interactions of reversible MAO-A inhibitors (RIMAs) see Moclobemide, and for interactions of MAO-B inhibitors see Rasagiline and Selegiline; the antibacterial Linezolid is a reversible, non-selective MAO inhibitor

ACE Inhibitors: MAOIs possibly enhance hypotensive effect of ACE inhibitors

Adrenergic Neurone Blockers: enhanced hypotensive effect when MAOIs given with adrenergic neurone blockers

- Alcohol: MAOIs interact with tyramine found in some beverages containing ●alcohol and some dealcoholised beverages (hypertensive crisis)—if no tyramine, enhanced hypotensive effect

  Alpha$_2$-adrenoceptor Stimulants: avoidance of MAOIs advised by manufacturer of apraclonidine and brimonidine

- Alpha-blockers: avoidance of MAOIs advised by manufacturer of ●indoramin; enhanced hypotensive effect when MAOIs given with alpha-blockers

- Analgesics: possible increased serotonergic effects when MAOIs given with fentanyl; CNS excitation or depression (hypertension or hypotension) when MAOIs given with ●pethidine—avoid concomitant use and for 2 weeks after stopping MAOIs; possible increased serotonergic effects and increased risk of convulsions when MAOIs given with ●tramadol—some manufacturers advise avoid concomitant use and for 2 weeks after stopping MAOIs; avoidance of MAOIs advised by manufacturer of ●nefopam; possible CNS excitation or depression (hypertension or hypotension) when MAOIs given with ●opioid analgesics—some manufacturers advise avoid concomitant use and for 2 weeks after stopping MAOIs

  Angiotensin-II Receptor Antagonists: MAOIs possibly enhance hypotensive effect of angiotensin-II receptor antagonists

- Antidepressants: increased risk of hypertension and CNS excitation when MAOIs given with ●reboxetine (MAOIs should not be started until 1 week after stopping reboxetine, avoid reboxetine for 2 weeks after stopping MAOIs); after stopping MAOIs do not start ●citalopram, ●escitalopram, ●fluvoxamine, ●paroxetine or ●sertraline for 2 weeks, also MAOIs should not be started until at least 1 week after stopping citalopram, escitalopram, fluvoxamine, paroxetine or sertraline; after stopping MAOIs do not start ●fluoxetine for 2 weeks, also MAOIs should not be started until at least 5 weeks after stopping fluoxetine; after stopping MAOIs do not start ●duloxetine for 2 weeks, also MAOIs should not be started until at least 5 days after stopping duloxetine; enhanced CNS effects and toxicity when MAOIs given with ●venlafaxine (venlafaxine should not be started until 2 weeks after stopping MAOIs, avoid MAOIs for 1 week after stopping venlafaxine); increased risk of hypertension and CNS excitation when MAOIs given with other ●MAOIs (avoid for at least 2

MAOIs

- **Antidepressants** *(continued)*
  weeks after stopping previous MAOIs and then start at a reduced dose); after stopping MAOIs do not start ●moclobemide for at least 1 week; MAOIs increase CNS effects of ●SSRIs (risk of serious toxicity); after stopping MAOIs do not start ●mirtazapine for 2 weeks, also MAOIs should not be started until at least 2 weeks after stopping mirtazapine; after stopping MAOIs do not start ●tricyclic-related antidepressants for 2 weeks, also MAOIs should not be started until at least 1–2 weeks after stopping tricyclic-related antidepressants; increased risk of hypertension and CNS excitation when MAOIs given with ●tricyclics, tricyclics should not be started until 2 weeks after stopping MAOIs (3 weeks if starting clomipramine or imipramine), also MAOIs should not be started for at least 1–2 weeks after stopping tricyclics (3 weeks in the case of clomipramine or imipramine)

  Antidiabetics: MAOIs possibly enhance hypoglycaemic effect of antidiabetics; MAOIs enhance hypoglycaemic effect of insulin, metformin and sulfonylureas

- **Antiepileptics**: MAOIs possibly antagonise anticonvulsant effect of antiepileptics (convulsive threshold lowered); avoidance for 2 weeks after stopping MAOIs advised by manufacturer of ●carbamazepine, also antagonism of anticonvulsant effect

  Antihistamines: avoidance of MAOIs advised by manufacturer of hydroxyzine; avoidance of promethazine for 2 weeks after stopping MAOIs advised by manufacturer of promethazine; increased antimuscarinic and sedative effects when MAOIs given with antihistamines

- **Antimalarials**: avoidance of antidepressants advised by manufacturer of ●artemether with lumefantrine and ●piperaquine with artenimol

  Antimuscarinics: increased risk of antimuscarinic side-effects when MAOIs given with antimuscarinics

- **Antipsychotics**: CNS effects of MAOIs possibly increased by ●clozapine
- **Anxiolytics and Hypnotics**: avoidance of MAOIs advised by manufacturer of buspirone; manufacturer of tranylcypromine advises avoid ●buspirone for 14 days after stopping tranylcypromine
- **Atomoxetine**: after stopping MAOIs do not start ●atomoxetine for 2 weeks, also MAOIs should not be started until at least 2 weeks after stopping atomoxetine; possible increased risk of convulsions when antidepressants given with atomoxetine

  Beta-blockers: enhanced hypotensive effect when MAOIs given with beta-blockers

- **Bupropion**: avoidance of bupropion for 2 weeks after stopping MAOIs advised by manufacturer of ●bupropion

  Calcium-channel Blockers: enhanced hypotensive effect when MAOIs given with calcium-channel blockers

  Clonidine: enhanced hypotensive effect when MAOIs given with clonidine

- **Dapoxetine**: increased risk of serotonergic effects when MAOIs given with ●dapoxetine (MAOIs should not be started until at least 1 week after stopping dapoxetine, avoid dapoxetine for 2 weeks after stopping MAOIs)

  Diazoxide: enhanced hypotensive effect when MAOIs given with diazoxide

  Diuretics: enhanced hypotensive effect when MAOIs given with diuretics

- **Dopaminergics**: avoid concomitant use of non-selective MAOIs with ●entacapone; risk of hypertensive crisis when MAOIs given with ●levodopa, avoid levodopa for at least 2 weeks after stopping MAOIs; risk of hypertensive crisis when MAOIs given with

MAOIs

- **Dopaminergics** *(continued)*
  ●rasagiline, avoid MAOIs for at least 2 weeks after stopping rasagiline; enhanced hypotensive effect when MAOIs given with ●selegiline—manufacturer of selegiline advises avoid concomitant use; avoid concomitant use of MAOIs with tolcapone

  Doxapram: MAOIs enhance effects of doxapram

  Histamine: avoidance of MAOIs advised by manufacturer of histamine

- **5HT₁-receptor Agonists**: risk of CNS toxicity when MAOIs given with ●rizatriptan or ●sumatriptan (avoid rizatriptan or sumatriptan for 2 weeks after MAOIs); risk of CNS toxicity when MAOIs given with ●zolmitriptan (reduce dose of zolmitriptan)
- **Methyldopa**: avoidance of MAOIs advised by manufacturer of ●methyldopa

  Moxonidine: enhanced hypotensive effect when MAOIs given with moxonidine

  Muscle Relaxants: phenelzine enhances effects of suxamethonium

  Nicorandil: enhanced hypotensive effect when MAOIs given with nicorandil

  Nitrates: enhanced hypotensive effect when MAOIs given with nitrates

  Pholcodine: avoidance of pholcodine for 2 weeks after stopping MAOIs advised by manufacturer of pholcodine

- **Sympathomimetics**: risk of hypertensive crisis when MAOIs given with ●adrenaline (epinephrine), ●dobutamine, ●dopamine, ●noradrenaline (norepinephrine) or ●xylometazoline; risk of hypertensive crisis when MAOIs given with ●dexamfetamine, ●ephedrine, ●isometheptene, ●lisdexamfetamine, ●metaraminol, ●methylphenidate, ●phenylephrine or ●pseudoephedrine, avoid dexamfetamine, ephedrine, isometheptene, lisdexamfetamine, metaraminol, methylphenidate, phenylephrine or pseudoephedrine for at least 2 weeks after stopping MAOIs; risk of hypertensive crisis when MAOIs given with ●oxymetazoline, some manufacturers advise avoid oxymetazoline for at least 2 weeks after stopping MAOIs
- **Tetrabenazine**: risk of CNS toxicity when MAOIs given with ●tetrabenazine (avoid tetrabenazine for 2 weeks after MAOIs)

  Vasodilator Antihypertensives: enhanced hypotensive effect when MAOIs given with hydralazine, minoxidil or sodium nitroprusside

MAOIs, reversible *see* Moclobemide

Maraviroc

- **Antibacterials**: plasma concentration of maraviroc possibly increased by ●clarithromycin and ●telithromycin (consider reducing dose of maraviroc); plasma concentration of maraviroc reduced by ●rifampicin—consider increasing dose of maraviroc
- **Antidepressants**: plasma concentration of maraviroc possibly reduced by ●St John's wort—avoid concomitant use
- **Antivirals**: plasma concentration of maraviroc increased by ●atazanavir, boceprevir, ●darunavir, ●indinavir, ●lopinavir, ●saquinavir and telaprevir (consider reducing dose of maraviroc); plasma concentration of maraviroc possibly reduced by ●efavirenz—consider increasing dose of maraviroc; plasma concentration of maraviroc possibly reduced by etravirine; maraviroc reduces plasma concentration of ●fosamprenavir—avoid concomitant use; plasma concentration of maraviroc increased by ritonavir
- **Cobicistat**: plasma concentration of maraviroc possibly increased by ●cobicistat (reduce dose of maraviroc)
- **Orlistat**: absorption of maraviroc possibly reduced by ●orlistat

Mebendazole

Ulcer-healing Drugs: metabolism of mebendazole possibly inhibited by cimetidine (increased plasma concentration)

Medroxyprogesterone see Progestogens

Mefenamic Acid see NSAIDs

Mefloquine

- Anti-arrhythmics: increased risk of ventricular arrhythmias when mefloquine given with ●amiodarone—avoid concomitant use
- Antibacterials: increased risk of ventricular arrhythmias when mefloquine given with ●moxifloxacin—avoid concomitant use; plasma concentration of mefloquine reduced by ●rifampicin—avoid concomitant use
- Antidepressants: avoidance of antimalarials advised by manufacturer of ●citalopram and ●escitalopram (risk of ventricular arrhythmias)
- Antiepileptics: mefloquine antagonises anticonvulsant effect of ●antiepileptics
- Antimalarials: avoidance of antimalarials advised by manufacturer of ●artemether with lumefantrine; increased risk of convulsions when mefloquine given with ●chloroquine and hydroxychloroquine; increased risk of convulsions when mefloquine given with ●quinine (but should not prevent the use of *intravenous* quinine in severe cases)
- Antipsychotics: possible increased risk of ventricular arrhythmias when mefloquine given with ●haloperidol—avoid concomitant use; avoidance of mefloquine advised by manufacturer of amisulpride; increased risk of ventricular arrhythmias when mefloquine given with ●pimozide—avoid concomitant use; manufacturer of risperidone advises possible risk of ventricular arrhythmias when mefloquine given with ●risperidone

  Antivirals: mefloquine possibly reduces plasma concentration of ritonavir
- Atomoxetine: increased risk of ventricular arrhythmias when mefloquine given with ●atomoxetine

  Beta-blockers: increased risk of bradycardia when mefloquine given with beta-blockers

  Calcium-channel Blockers: possible increased risk of bradycardia when mefloquine given with calcium-channel blockers

  Cardiac Glycosides: possible increased risk of bradycardia when mefloquine given with digoxin

  Cytotoxics: possible increased risk of bradycardia when mefloquine given with crizotinib

  Histamine: avoidance of antimalarials advised by manufacturer of histamine
- Ivabradine: increased risk of ventricular arrhythmias when mefloquine given with ●ivabradine

  Vaccines: antimalarials inactivate oral typhoid vaccine—see p. 864

Megestrol see Progestogens

Melatonin see Anxiolytics and Hypnotics

Meloxicam see NSAIDs

Melphalan

Antibacterials: increased risk of melphalan toxicity when given with nalidixic acid
- Antipsychotics: avoid concomitant use of cytotoxics with ●clozapine (increased risk of agranulocytosis)

  Cardiac Glycosides: melphalan possibly reduces absorption of digoxin *tablets*
- Ciclosporin: increased risk of nephrotoxicity when melphalan given with ●ciclosporin

Memantine

- Anaesthetics, General: increased risk of CNS toxicity when memantine given with ●ketamine (manufacturer of memantine advises avoid concomitant use)
- Analgesics: increased risk of CNS toxicity when memantine given with ●dextromethorphan (manufacturer of memantine advises avoid concomitant use)

  Anticoagulants: memantine possibly enhances anticoagulant effect of warfarin

Memantine *(continued)*

Antimuscarinics: memantine possibly enhances effects of antimuscarinics

Antipsychotics: memantine possibly reduces effects of antipsychotics
- Dopaminergics: memantine possibly enhances effects of dopaminergics and selegiline; increased risk of CNS toxicity when memantine given with ●amantadine (manufacturer of memantine advises avoid concomitant use)

  Muscle Relaxants: memantine possibly modifies effects of baclofen and dantrolene

Meningococcal vaccines see Vaccines

Mepacrine

Antimalarials: mepacrine increases plasma concentration of primaquine (increased risk of toxicity)

Meprobamate see Anxiolytics and Hypnotics

Meptazinol see Opioid Analgesics

Mercaptopurine

- Allopurinol: enhanced effects and increased toxicity of mercaptopurine when given with ●allopurinol (reduce dose of mercaptopurine to one quarter of usual dose)
- Antibacterials: increased risk of haematological toxicity when mercaptopurine given with ●sulfamethoxazole (as co-trimoxazole); increased risk of haematological toxicity when mercaptopurine given with ●trimethoprim (also with co-trimoxazole)
- Anticoagulants: mercaptopurine possibly reduces anticoagulant effect of ●coumarins
- Antipsychotics: avoid concomitant use of cytotoxics with ●clozapine (increased risk of agranulocytosis)

  Dairy Products: plasma concentration of mercaptopurine possibly reduced by dairy products—manufacturer of mercaptopurine advises give at least 1 hour before or 2 hours after dairy products
- Febuxostat: avoidance of mercaptopurine advised by manufacturer of ●febuxostat

Meropenem

- Antiepileptics: carbapenems reduce plasma concentration of ●valproate—avoid concomitant use

  Vaccines: antibacterials inactivate oral typhoid vaccine—see p. 864

Mestranol see Oestrogens

Metaraminol see Sympathomimetics

Metformin see Antidiabetics

Methadone see Opioid Analgesics

Methenamine

Antacids: avoid concomitant use of methenamine with antacids
- Antibacterials: increased risk of crystalluria when methenamine given with ●sulfonamides
- Diuretics: effects of methenamine antagonised by ●acetazolamide

  Potassium Salts: avoid concomitant use of methenamine with potassium citrate

  Sodium Citrate: avoid concomitant use of methenamine with sodium citrate

  Vaccines: antibacterials inactivate oral typhoid vaccine—see p. 864

Methocarbamol see Muscle Relaxants

Methotrexate

- Anaesthetics, General: antifolate effect of methotrexate increased by ●nitrous oxide—avoid concomitant use
- Analgesics: excretion of methotrexate probably reduced by ●NSAIDs (increased risk of toxicity)—but for concomitant use in rheumatic disease see p. 732; excretion of methotrexate reduced by ●aspirin, ●diclofenac, ●ibuprofen, ●indometacin, ●ketoprofen, ●meloxicam and ●naproxen (increased risk of toxicity)—but for concomitant use in rheumatic disease see p. 732
- Antibacterials: absorption of methotrexate possibly reduced by neomycin; excretion of methotrexate

Methotrexate

- Antibacterials *(continued)*
  possibly reduced by ciprofloxacin (increased risk of toxicity); increased risk of haematological toxicity when methotrexate given with ●sulfamethoxazole (as co-trimoxazole); increased risk of methotrexate toxicity when given with doxycycline, sulfonamides or tetracycline; excretion of methotrexate reduced by penicillins (increased risk of toxicity); increased risk of haematological toxicity when methotrexate given with ●trimethoprim (also with co-trimoxazole)
  Antiepileptics: antifolate effect of methotrexate increased by phenytoin
- Antimalarials: antifolate effect of methotrexate increased by ●pyrimethamine
- Antipsychotics: avoid concomitant use of cytotoxics with ●clozapine (increased risk of agranulocytosis)
  Cardiac Glycosides: methotrexate possibly reduces absorption of digoxin *tablets*
- Ciclosporin: risk of toxicity when methotrexate given with ●ciclosporin
  Corticosteroids: possible increased risk of hepatoxicity when *high-dose* methotrexate given with dexamethasone
- Cytotoxics: increased pulmonary toxicity when methotrexate given with ●cisplatin
  Diuretics: excretion of methotrexate increased by alkaline urine due to acetazolamide
- Leflunomide: risk of toxicity when methotrexate given with ●leflunomide
- Retinoids: plasma concentration of methotrexate increased by ●acitretin (also increased risk of hepatotoxicity)—avoid concomitant use
  Theophylline: methotrexate possibly increases plasma concentration of theophylline
  Ulcer-healing Drugs: excretion of methotrexate possibly reduced by proton pump inhibitors (increased risk of toxicity)

Methyldopa

ACE Inhibitors: enhanced hypotensive effect when methyldopa given with ACE inhibitors
Adrenergic Neurone Blockers: enhanced hypotensive effect when methyldopa given with adrenergic neurone blockers
Alcohol: enhanced hypotensive effect when methyldopa given with alcohol
Aldesleukin: enhanced hypotensive effect when methyldopa given with aldesleukin
Alpha-blockers: enhanced hypotensive effect when methyldopa given with alpha-blockers
Anaesthetics, General: enhanced hypotensive effect when methyldopa given with general anaesthetics
Analgesics: hypotensive effect of methyldopa antagonised by NSAIDs
Angiotensin-II Receptor Antagonists: enhanced hypotensive effect when methyldopa given with angiotensin-II receptor antagonists
- Antidepressants: manufacturer of methyldopa advises avoid concomitant use with ●MAOIs
  Antipsychotics: enhanced hypotensive effect when methyldopa given with antipsychotics (also increased risk of extrapyramidal effects)
  Anxiolytics and Hypnotics: enhanced hypotensive effect when methyldopa given with anxiolytics and hypnotics
  Beta-blockers: enhanced hypotensive effect when methyldopa given with beta-blockers
  Calcium-channel Blockers: enhanced hypotensive effect when methyldopa given with calcium-channel blockers
  Clonidine: enhanced hypotensive effect when methyldopa given with clonidine
  Corticosteroids: hypotensive effect of methyldopa antagonised by corticosteroids
  Diazoxide: enhanced hypotensive effect when methyldopa given with diazoxide

Methyldopa *(continued)*

Diuretics: enhanced hypotensive effect when methyldopa given with diuretics
Dopaminergics: methyldopa antagonises antiparkinsonian effect of dopaminergics; increased risk of extrapyramidal side-effects when methyldopa given with amantadine; effects of methyldopa possibly enhanced by entacapone; enhanced hypotensive effect when methyldopa given with levodopa
Iron: hypotensive effect of methyldopa antagonised by *oral* iron
- Lithium: neurotoxicity may occur when methyldopa given with ●lithium without increased plasma concentration of lithium
  Moxisylyte: enhanced hypotensive effect when methyldopa given with moxisylyte
  Moxonidine: enhanced hypotensive effect when methyldopa given with moxonidine
  Muscle Relaxants: enhanced hypotensive effect when methyldopa given with baclofen or tizanidine
  Nitrates: enhanced hypotensive effect when methyldopa given with nitrates
  Oestrogens: hypotensive effect of methyldopa antagonised by oestrogens
  Prostaglandins: enhanced hypotensive effect when methyldopa given with alprostadil
- Sympathomimetics, Beta$_2$: acute hypotension reported when methyldopa given with *infusion* of ●salbutamol
  Vasodilator Antihypertensives: enhanced hypotensive effect when methyldopa given with hydralazine, minoxidil or sodium nitroprusside

Methylphenidate *see* Sympathomimetics

Methylprednisolone *see* Corticosteroids

Methylthioninium

- Antidepressants: risk of CNS toxicity when methylthioninium given with ●SSRI-related antidepressants, ●SSRIs and ●clomipramine—avoid ●concomitant use (if avoidance not possible, use lowest possible dose of methylthioninium and observe patient for up to 4 hours after administration); possible risk of CNS toxicity when methylthioninium given with ●mirtazapine—avoid concomitant use (if avoidance not possible, use lowest possible dose of methylthioninium and observe patient for up to 4 hours after administration)
- Anxiolytics and Hypnotics: possible risk of CNS toxicity when methylthioninium given with ●buspirone—avoid concomitant use (if avoidance not possible, use lowest possible dose of methylthioninium and observe patient for up to 4 hours after administration)
- Bupropion: possible risk of CNS toxicity when methylthioninium given with ●bupropion—avoid concomitant use (if avoidance not possible, use lowest possible dose of methylthioninium and observe patient for up to 4 hours after administration)

Metoclopramide

Alcohol: metoclopramide possibly increases absorption of alcohol
Anaesthetics, General: metoclopramide enhances effects of thiopental
Analgesics: metoclopramide increases rate of absorption of aspirin (enhanced effect); effects of metoclopramide on gastro-intestinal activity antagonised by opioid analgesics; metoclopramide increases rate of absorption of paracetamol
Antibacterials: metoclopramide reduces plasma concentration of fosfomycin
Antidepressants: CNS toxicity reported when metoclopramide given with SSRIs
Antimuscarinics: effects of metoclopramide on gastro-intestinal activity antagonised by antimuscarinics
Antipsychotics: increased risk of extrapyramidal side-effects when metoclopramide given with antipsychotics

Metoclopramide *(continued)*

Atovaquone: metoclopramide reduces plasma concentration of atovaquone—avoid concomitant use

- Ciclosporin: metoclopramide increases plasma concentration of ●ciclosporin

Dopaminergics: metoclopramide antagonises hypoprolactinaemic effects of bromocriptine and cabergoline; metoclopramide antagonises antiparkinsonian effect of pergolide; avoidance of metoclopramide advised by manufacturer of ropinirole and rotigotine (antagonism of effect)

Muscle Relaxants: metoclopramide enhances effects of suxamethonium

Tetrabenazine: increased risk of extrapyramidal side-effects when metoclopramide given with tetrabenazine

Metolazone *see* Diuretics

Metoprolol *see* Beta-blockers

Metronidazole

Note Interactions do not apply to topical metronidazole preparations

Alcohol: disulfiram-like reaction when metronidazole given with alcohol

- Anticoagulants: metronidazole enhances anticoagulant effect of ●coumarins

Antiepileptics: metabolism of metronidazole accelerated by phenobarbital (reduced effect); metronidazole possibly inhibits metabolism of phenytoin (increased plasma concentration)

- Cytotoxics: metronidazole increases plasma concentration of ●busulfan (increased risk of toxicity); metronidazole inhibits metabolism of fluorouracil (increased toxicity)

Disulfiram: psychotic reaction reported when metronidazole given with disulfiram

Lithium: metronidazole increases risk of lithium toxicity

Mycophenolate: metronidazole possibly reduces bioavailability of mycophenolate

Ulcer-healing Drugs: metabolism of metronidazole inhibited by cimetidine (increased plasma concentration)

Vaccines: antibacterials inactivate oral typhoid vaccine—see p. 864

Mianserin *see* Antidepressants, Tricyclic (related)

Micafungin

Antifungals: micafungin possibly increases plasma concentration of amphotericin; micafungin increases plasma concentration of itraconazole (consider reducing dose of itraconazole)

Calcium-channel Blockers: micafungin increases plasma concentration of nifedipine

Ciclosporin: micafungin possibly increases plasma concentration of ciclosporin

Sirolimus: micafungin increases plasma concentration of sirolimus

Miconazole *see* Antifungals, Imidazole

Midazolam *see* Anxiolytics and Hypnotics

Mifamurtide

Analgesics: manufacturer of mifamurtide advises avoid concomitant use with high doses of NSAIDs

Ciclosporin: manufacturer of mifamurtide advises avoid concomitant use with ciclosporin

Corticosteroids: manufacturer of mifamurtide advises avoid concomitant use with corticosteroids

Tacrolimus: manufacturer of mifamurtide advises avoid concomitant use with tacrolimus

Mifepristone

Corticosteroids: mifepristone may reduce effect of corticosteroids (including *inhaled* corticosteroids) for 3–4 days

Milrinone *see* Phosphodiesterase Inhibitors

Minocycline *see* Tetracyclines

Minoxidil *see* Vasodilator Antihypertensives

Mirabegron

Antibacterials: avoid or reduce dose of mirabegron in hepatic or renal impairment when given with clarithromycin—see Mirabegron, p. 564

Antifungals: avoid or reduce dose of mirabegron in hepatic or renal impairment when given with itraconazole—see Mirabegron, p. 564

Antivirals: avoid or reduce dose of mirabegron in hepatic or renal impairment when given with ritonavir—see Mirabegron, p. 564

Beta-blockers: mirabegron increases plasma concentration of metoprolol

Cardiac Glycosides: mirabegron increases plasma concentration of digoxin—reduce initial dose of digoxin

Mirtazapine

- Alcohol: increased sedative effect when mirtazapine given with ●alcohol

Analgesics: possible increased serotonergic effects when mirtazapine given with tramadol

Anticoagulants: mirtazapine enhances anticoagulant effect of warfarin

- Antidepressants: possible increased serotonergic effects when mirtazapine given with fluoxetine, fluvoxamine or venlafaxine; mirtazapine should not be started until 2 weeks after stopping ●MAOIs, also MAOIs should not be started until at least 2 weeks after stopping mirtazapine; after stopping mirtazapine do not start ●moclobemide for at least 1 week

Antiepileptics: plasma concentration of mirtazapine reduced by carbamazepine and phenytoin

- Antimalarials: avoidance of antidepressants advised by manufacturer of ●artemether with lumefantrine and ●piperaquine with artenimol

Anxiolytics and Hypnotics: increased sedative effect when mirtazapine given with anxiolytics and hypnotics

Atomoxetine: possible increased risk of convulsions when antidepressants given with atomoxetine

Clonidine: mirtazapine possibly antagonises hypotensive effect of clonidine

- Methylthioninium: possible risk of CNS toxicity when mirtazapine given with ●methylthioninium—avoid concomitant use (if avoidance not possible, use lowest possible dose of methylthioninium and observe patient for up to 4 hours after administration)

Ulcer-healing Drugs: plasma concentration of mirtazapine increased by cimetidine

Mitomycin

- Antipsychotics: avoid concomitant use of cytotoxics with ●clozapine (increased risk of agranulocytosis)

Mitotane

- Anticoagulants: mitotane possibly reduces anticoagulant effect of ●coumarins
- Antipsychotics: avoid concomitant use of cytotoxics with ●clozapine (increased risk of agranulocytosis)

Diuretics: manufacturer of mitotane advises avoid concomitant use of spironolactone (antagonism of effect)

Mitoxantrone

- Antipsychotics: avoid concomitant use of cytotoxics with ●clozapine (increased risk of agranulocytosis)

Ciclosporin: excretion of mitoxantrone reduced by ciclosporin (increased plasma concentration)

Mivacurium *see* Muscle Relaxants

Mizolastine *see* Antihistamines

MMR vaccine *see* Vaccines

Moclobemide

- Analgesics: possible CNS excitation or depression (hypertension or hypotension) when moclobemide given with ●dextromethorphan or ●pethidine—avoid concomitant use; possible CNS excitation or depression (hypertension or hypotension) when moclobemide given with ●opioid analgesics—manufacturer of moclobemide advises consider reducing dose of opioid analgesics

Moclobemide *(continued)*
- Antidepressants: moclobemide should not be started for at least 1 week after stopping ●MAOIs, ●SSRI-related antidepressants, ●citalopram, ●fluvoxamine, ●mirtazapine, ●paroxetine, ●sertraline, ●tricyclic-related antidepressants or ●tricyclics; increased risk of CNS toxicity when moclobemide given with ●escitalopram, preferably avoid concomitant use; moclobemide should not be started until 5 weeks after stopping ●fluoxetine; possible increased serotonergic effects when moclobemide given with ●duloxetine
- Antimalarials: avoidance of antidepressants advised by manufacturer of ●artemether with lumefantrine and ●piperaquine with artenimol
  Atomoxetine: possible increased risk of convulsions when antidepressants given with atomoxetine
- Bupropion: avoidance of moclobemide advised by manufacturer of ●bupropion
- Clopidogrel: moclobemide possibly reduces antiplatelet effect of ●clopidogrel
- Dopaminergics: caution with moclobemide advised by manufacturer of entacapone; increased risk of side-effects when moclobemide given with levodopa; avoid concomitant use of moclobemide with ●selegiline
- 5HT₁-receptor Agonists: risk of CNS toxicity when moclobemide given with ●rizatriptan or ●sumatriptan (avoid rizatriptan or sumatriptan for 2 weeks after moclobemide); risk of CNS toxicity when moclobemide given with ●zolmitriptan (reduce dose of zolmitriptan)
- Sympathomimetics: risk of hypertensive crisis when moclobemide given with ●sympathomimetics
  Ulcer-healing Drugs: plasma concentration of moclobemide increased by cimetidine (halve dose of moclobemide)

Modafinil
  Antiepileptics: modafinil possibly increases plasma concentration of phenytoin
- Ciclosporin: modafinil reduces plasma concentration of ●ciclosporin
- Cytotoxics: modafinil possibly reduces plasma concentration of ●bosutinib—manufacturer of bosutinib advises avoid concomitant use
- Oestrogens: modafinil accelerates metabolism of ●oestrogens (reduced contraceptive effect—see p. 548)

Moexipril *see* ACE Inhibitors
Mometasone *see* Corticosteroids
Monobactams *see* Aztreonam
Monoclonal antibodies *see* individual drugs
Montelukast *see* Leukotriene Receptor Antagonists
Morphine *see* Opioid Analgesics
Moxifloxacin *see* Quinolones

Moxisylyte
  ACE Inhibitors: enhanced hypotensive effect when moxisylyte given with ACE inhibitors
  Adrenergic Neurone Blockers: enhanced hypotensive effect when moxisylyte given with adrenergic neurone blockers
- Alpha-blockers: possible severe postural hypotension when moxisylyte given with ●alpha-blockers
  Angiotensin-II Receptor Antagonists: enhanced hypotensive effect when moxisylyte given with angiotensin-II receptor antagonists
- Beta-blockers: possible severe postural hypotension when moxisylyte given with ●beta-blockers
  Calcium-channel Blockers: enhanced hypotensive effect when moxisylyte given with calcium-channel blockers
  Clonidine: enhanced hypotensive effect when moxisylyte given with clonidine
  Diazoxide: enhanced hypotensive effect when moxisylyte given with diazoxide

Moxisylyte *(continued)*
  Diuretics: enhanced hypotensive effect when moxisylyte given with diuretics
  Methyldopa: enhanced hypotensive effect when moxisylyte given with methyldopa
  Moxonidine: enhanced hypotensive effect when moxisylyte given with moxonidine
  Nitrates: enhanced hypotensive effect when moxisylyte given with nitrates
  Vasodilator Antihypertensives: enhanced hypotensive effect when moxisylyte given with hydralazine, minoxidil or sodium nitroprusside

Moxonidine
  ACE Inhibitors: enhanced hypotensive effect when moxonidine given with ACE inhibitors
  Adrenergic Neurone Blockers: enhanced hypotensive effect when moxonidine given with adrenergic neurone blockers
  Alcohol: enhanced hypotensive effect when moxonidine given with alcohol
  Aldesleukin: enhanced hypotensive effect when moxonidine given with aldesleukin
  Alpha-blockers: enhanced hypotensive effect when moxonidine given with alpha-blockers
  Anaesthetics, General: enhanced hypotensive effect when moxonidine given with general anaesthetics
  Analgesics: hypotensive effect of moxonidine antagonised by NSAIDs
  Angiotensin-II Receptor Antagonists: enhanced hypotensive effect when moxonidine given with angiotensin-II receptor antagonists
  Antidepressants: enhanced hypotensive effect when moxonidine given with MAOIs; hypotensive effect of moxonidine possibly antagonised by tricyclics (manufacturer of moxonidine advises avoid concomitant use)
  Antipsychotics: enhanced hypotensive effect when moxonidine given with phenothiazines
  Anxiolytics and Hypnotics: enhanced hypotensive effect when moxonidine given with anxiolytics and hypnotics; sedative effects possibly increased when moxonidine given with benzodiazepines
  Beta-blockers: enhanced hypotensive effect when moxonidine given with beta-blockers
  Calcium-channel Blockers: enhanced hypotensive effect when moxonidine given with calcium-channel blockers
  Clonidine: enhanced hypotensive effect when moxonidine given with clonidine
  Corticosteroids: hypotensive effect of moxonidine antagonised by corticosteroids
  Diazoxide: enhanced hypotensive effect when moxonidine given with diazoxide
  Diuretics: enhanced hypotensive effect when moxonidine given with diuretics
  Dopaminergics: enhanced hypotensive effect when moxonidine given with levodopa
  Methyldopa: enhanced hypotensive effect when moxonidine given with methyldopa
  Moxisylyte: enhanced hypotensive effect when moxonidine given with moxisylyte
  Muscle Relaxants: enhanced hypotensive effect when moxonidine given with baclofen or tizanidine
  Nitrates: enhanced hypotensive effect when moxonidine given with nitrates
  Oestrogens: hypotensive effect of moxonidine antagonised by oestrogens
  Prostaglandins: enhanced hypotensive effect when moxonidine given with alprostadil
  Vasodilator Antihypertensives: enhanced hypotensive effect when moxonidine given with hydralazine, minoxidil or sodium nitroprusside

Muscle Relaxants
  ACE Inhibitors: enhanced hypotensive effect when baclofen or tizanidine given with ACE inhibitors

Muscle Relaxants (continued)

Adrenergic Neurone Blockers: enhanced hypotensive effect when baclofen or tizanidine given with adrenergic neurone blockers

Alcohol: increased sedative effect when baclofen, methocarbamol or tizanidine given with alcohol

Alpha-blockers: enhanced hypotensive effect when baclofen or tizanidine given with alpha-blockers

• Anaesthetics, General: effects of atracurium enhanced by ketamine; increased risk of myocardial depression and bradycardia when suxamethonium given with •propofol; effects of non-depolarising muscle relaxants and suxamethonium enhanced by volatile liquid general anaesthetics

Analgesics: excretion of baclofen possibly reduced by NSAIDs (increased risk of toxicity); excretion of baclofen reduced by ibuprofen (increased risk of toxicity); increased sedative effect when baclofen given with fentanyl or morphine

Angiotensin-II Receptor Antagonists: enhanced hypotensive effect when baclofen or tizanidine given with angiotensin-II receptor antagonists

Anti-arrhythmics: neuromuscular blockade enhanced and prolonged when suxamethonium given with lidocaine

• Antibacterials: effects of non-depolarising muscle relaxants and suxamethonium enhanced by piperacillin; plasma concentration of tizanidine increased by •ciprofloxacin (increased risk of toxicity)—avoid concomitant use; plasma concentration of tizanidine possibly increased by norfloxacin (increased risk of toxicity); plasma concentration of tizanidine possibly reduced by rifampicin; effects of non-depolarising muscle relaxants and suxamethonium enhanced by •aminoglycosides; effects of non-depolarising muscle relaxants and suxamethonium enhanced by •clindamycin; effects of non-depolarising muscle relaxants and suxamethonium enhanced by •polymyxins; effects of suxamethonium enhanced by •vancomycin

• Antidepressants: plasma concentration of tizanidine increased by •fluvoxamine (increased risk of toxicity)—avoid concomitant use; effects of suxamethonium enhanced by phenelzine; muscle relaxant effect of baclofen enhanced by tricyclics

• Antiepileptics: muscle relaxant effect of non-depolarising muscle relaxants antagonised by carbamazepine (accelerated recovery from neuromuscular blockade); effects of non-depolarising muscle relaxants reduced by long-term use of •phenytoin (but effects of non-depolarising muscle relaxants might be increased by acute use of phenytoin)

Antimalarials: effects of suxamethonium possibly enhanced by quinine

Antipsychotics: effects of suxamethonium possibly enhanced by promazine

Anxiolytics and Hypnotics: increased sedative effect when baclofen or tizanidine given with anxiolytics and hypnotics

Beta-blockers: enhanced hypotensive effect when baclofen given with beta-blockers; possible enhanced hypotensive effect and bradycardia when tizanidine given with beta-blockers; effects of muscle relaxants enhanced by propranolol

Calcium-channel Blockers: enhanced hypotensive effect when baclofen or tizanidine given with calcium-channel blockers; effects of non-depolarising muscle relaxants possibly enhanced by calcium-channel blockers; possible increased risk of ventricular arrhythmias when intravenous dantrolene given with diltiazem—manufacturer of diltiazem advises avoid concomitant use; effects of non-depolarising muscle relaxants and suxamethonium enhanced by verapamil; avoidance of intravenous dantrolene advised by manufacturer of verapamil

Muscle Relaxants (continued)

Cardiac Glycosides: possible increased risk of bradycardia when tizanidine given with cardiac glycosides; risk of ventricular arrhythmias when suxamethonium given with cardiac glycosides

Clonidine: enhanced hypotensive effect when baclofen or tizanidine given with clonidine

Corticosteroids: effects of pancuronium and vecuronium possibly antagonised by corticosteroids

Cytotoxics: effects of suxamethonium enhanced by cyclophosphamide and thiotepa

Deferasirox: avoidance of tizanidine advised by manufacturer of deferasirox

Diazoxide: enhanced hypotensive effect when baclofen or tizanidine given with diazoxide

Diuretics: enhanced hypotensive effect when baclofen or tizanidine given with diuretics

Dopaminergics: possible agitation, confusion and hallucinations when baclofen given with levodopa

Lithium: effects of muscle relaxants enhanced by lithium; baclofen possibly aggravates hyperkinesis caused by lithium

Magnesium (parenteral): effects of non-depolarising muscle relaxants and suxamethonium enhanced by parenteral magnesium

Memantine: effects of baclofen and dantrolene possibly modified by memantine

Methyldopa: enhanced hypotensive effect when baclofen or tizanidine given with methyldopa

Metoclopramide: effects of suxamethonium enhanced by metoclopramide

Moxonidine: enhanced hypotensive effect when baclofen or tizanidine given with moxonidine

Nitrates: enhanced hypotensive effect when baclofen or tizanidine given with nitrates

Oestrogens: plasma concentration of tizanidine possibly increased by oestrogens (increased risk of toxicity)

Parasympathomimetics: effects of non-depolarising muscle relaxants possibly antagonised by donepezil; effects of suxamethonium possibly enhanced by donepezil; effects of suxamethonium enhanced by galantamine, neostigmine, pyridostigmine and rivastigmine; effects of non-depolarising muscle relaxants antagonised by neostigmine, pyridostigmine and rivastigmine

Progestogens: plasma concentration of tizanidine possibly increased by progestogens (increased risk of toxicity)

Sympathomimetics, Beta$_2$: effects of suxamethonium enhanced by bambuterol

Vasodilator Antihypertensives: enhanced hypotensive effect when baclofen or tizanidine given with hydralazine; enhanced hypotensive effect when baclofen or tizanidine given with minoxidil; enhanced hypotensive effect when baclofen or tizanidine given with sodium nitroprusside

Muscle Relaxants, depolarising see Muscle Relaxants

Muscle Relaxants, non-depolarising see Muscle Relaxants

Mycophenolate

Antacids: absorption of mycophenolate reduced by antacids

• Antibacterials: plasma concentration of mycophenolate possibly reduced by co-amoxiclav; bioavailability of mycophenolate possibly reduced by metronidazole and norfloxacin; plasma concentration of active metabolite of mycophenolate reduced by •rifampicin

Antivirals: mycophenolate increases plasma concentration of aciclovir, also plasma concentration of inactive metabolite of mycophenolate increased; mycophenolate possibly increases plasma concentration of ganciclovir, also plasma concentration of

Mycophenolate

Antivirals *(continued)*
inactive metabolite of mycophenolate possibly
increased

Colestilan: manufacturer of colestilan advises give
mycophenolate at least 1 hour before or 3 hours
after colestilan

Iron: absorption of mycophenolate reduced by *oral
iron*

Lipid-regulating Drugs: absorption of mycophenolate
reduced by colestyramine

Sevelamer: plasma concentration of mycophenolate
possibly reduced by sevelamer

Mycophenolate Mofetil *see* Mycophenolate

Mycophenolate Sodium *see* Mycophenolate

Mycophenolic Acid *see* Mycophenolate

Nabumetone *see* NSAIDs

Nadolol *see* Beta-blockers

Nalidixic Acid *see* Quinolones

Nalmefene

● Analgesics: manufacturer of nalmefene advises avoid
concomitant use with ●opioid analgesics

Nandrolone *see* Anabolic Steroids

Naproxen *see* NSAIDs

Naratriptan *see* 5HT$_1$-receptor Agonists (under HT)

Natalizumab

● Antipsychotics: avoid concomitant use of cytotoxics
with ●clozapine (increased risk of agranulocytosis)

● Vaccines: avoid concomitant use of monoclonal antibodies with live ●vaccines (see p. 842)

Nateglinide *see* Antidiabetics

Nebivolol *see* Beta-blockers

Nefopam

● Antidepressants: manufacturer of nefopam advises
avoid concomitant use with ●MAOIs; side-effects
possibly increased when nefopam given with tricyclics

Antimuscarinics: increased risk of antimuscarinic side-
effects when nefopam given with antimuscarinics

Neomycin *see* Aminoglycosides

Neostigmine *see* Parasympathomimetics

Nevirapine

Analgesics: nevirapine possibly reduces plasma concentration of methadone

● Antibacterials: nevirapine reduces plasma concentration of clarithromycin (but concentration of an
active metabolite increased), also plasma concentration of nevirapine increased; nevirapine possibly
increases plasma concentration of rifabutin; plasma
concentration of nevirapine reduced by ●rif-
ampicin—avoid concomitant use

● Anticoagulants: nevirapine may enhance or reduce
anticoagulant effect of ●warfarin

● Antidepressants: plasma concentration of nevirapine
reduced by ●St John's wort—avoid concomitant
use

Antiepileptics: plasma concentration of nevirapine
reduced by carbamazepine

● Antifungals: plasma concentration of nevirapine
increased by ●fluconazole; nevirapine possibly
reduces plasma concentration of caspofungin and
itraconazole—consider increasing dose of caspofungin and itraconazole

● Antipsychotics: nevirapine possibly reduces plasma
concentration of ●aripiprazole (avoid concomitant
use or consider increasing the dose of aripiprazole—consult aripiprazole product literature)

● Antivirals: nevirapine possibly reduces plasma concentration of ●atazanavir and ●etravirine—avoid
concomitant use; manufacturer of nevirapine
advises avoid concomitant use with boceprevir and
rilpivirine; avoidance of nevirapine advised by manufacturer of daclatasvir (plasma concentration of
daclatasvir possibly reduced); nevirapine possibly
reduces the plasma concentration of

Nevirapine

● Antivirals *(continued)*
●dolutegravir (see Dose under Dolutegravir, p. 429);
nevirapine reduces plasma concentration of ●efavir-
enz—avoid concomitant use; avoidance of nevirapine advised by manufacturer of elvitegravir; nevirapine possibly reduces plasma concentration of
fosamprenavir—avoid unboosted fosamprenavir;
nevirapine reduces plasma concentration of indinavir; nevirapine possibly reduces plasma concentration of ●lopinavir and telaprevir—consider increasing dose of lopinavir and telaprevir; nevirapine
possibly reduces plasma concentration of ●simepre-
vir—manufacturer of simeprevir advises avoid concomitant use; increased risk of granulocytopenia
when nevirapine given with ●zidovudine

Cobicistat: manufacturer of nevirapine advises avoid
concomitant use with cobicistat

● Oestrogens: nevirapine accelerates metabolism of
●oestrogens (reduced contraceptive effect—see
p. 548)

● Orlistat: absorption of nevirapine possibly reduced by
●orlistat

● Progestogens: nevirapine accelerates metabolism of
●progestogens (reduced contraceptive effect—see
p. 548)

Nicardipine *see* Calcium-channel Blockers

Nicorandil

Alcohol: hypotensive effect of nicorandil possibly
enhanced by alcohol

Antidepressants: enhanced hypotensive effect when
nicorandil given with MAOIs; hypotensive effect of
nicorandil possibly enhanced by tricyclics

● Avanafil: hypotensive effect of nicorandil significantly
enhanced by ●avanafil (avoid concomitant use)

● Sildenafil: hypotensive effect of nicorandil significantly enhanced by ●sildenafil (avoid concomitant
use)

● Tadalafil: hypotensive effect of nicorandil significantly
enhanced by ●tadalafil (avoid concomitant use)

● Vardenafil: possible increased hypotensive effect
when nicorandil given with ●vardenafil—avoid concomitant use

Vasodilator Antihypertensives: possible enhanced
hypotensive effect when nicorandil given with
hydralazine, minoxidil or sodium nitroprusside

Nicotine

Anti-arrhythmics: nicotine possibly enhances effects of
adenosine

Nicotinic Acid

Note Interactions apply to lipid-regulating doses of nicotinic
acid

● Lipid-regulating Drugs: increased risk of myopathy
when nicotinic acid given with ●statins (applies to
lipid regulating doses of nicotinic acid)

Nifedipine *see* Calcium-channel Blockers

Nilotinib

● Antibacterials: manufacturer of nilotinib advises avoid
concomitant use with ●clarithromycin and ●telithro-
mycin; plasma concentration of nilotinib reduced by
●rifampicin—avoid concomitant use

● Antifungals: manufacturer of nilotinib advises avoid
concomitant use with ●itraconazole and ●voricona-
zole

● Antipsychotics: avoid concomitant use of cytotoxics
with ●clozapine (increased risk of agranulocytosis)

● Antivirals: avoidance of nilotinib advised by manufacturer of ●boceprevir; plasma concentration of nilotinib possibly increased by ritonavir—manufacturer
of nilotinib advises avoid concomitant use

Anxiolytics and Hypnotics: nilotinib increases plasma
concentration of midazolam

● Grapefruit Juice: manufacturer of nilotinib advises
avoid concomitant use with ●grapefruit juice

Nimodipine *see* Calcium-channel Blockers

Appendix 1: Interactions

Nitrates

ACE Inhibitors: enhanced hypotensive effect when nitrates given with ACE inhibitors

Adrenergic Neurone Blockers: enhanced hypotensive effect when nitrates given with adrenergic neurone blockers

Alcohol: enhanced hypotensive effect when nitrates given with alcohol

Aldesleukin: enhanced hypotensive effect when nitrates given with aldesleukin

Alpha-blockers: enhanced hypotensive effect when nitrates given with alpha-blockers

Anaesthetics, General: enhanced hypotensive effect when nitrates given with general anaesthetics

Analgesics: hypotensive effect of nitrates antagonised by NSAIDs

Angiotensin-II Receptor Antagonists: enhanced hypotensive effect when nitrates given with angiotensin-II receptor antagonists

Anti-arrhythmics: effects of sublingual tablets of nitrates reduced by disopyramide (failure to dissolve under tongue owing to dry mouth)

• Anticoagulants: *infusion* of glyceryl trinitrate reduces anticoagulant effect of •heparins

Antidepressants: enhanced hypotensive effect when nitrates given with MAOIs; effects of sublingual tablets of nitrates possibly reduced by tricyclic-related antidepressants (failure to dissolve under tongue owing to dry mouth); effects of sublingual tablets of nitrates reduced by tricyclics (failure to dissolve under tongue owing to dry mouth)

Antimuscarinics: effects of sublingual tablets of nitrates possibly reduced by antimuscarinics (failure to dissolve under tongue owing to dry mouth)

Antipsychotics: enhanced hypotensive effect when nitrates given with phenothiazines

Anxiolytics and Hypnotics: enhanced hypotensive effect when nitrates given with anxiolytics and hypnotics

• Avanafil: hypotensive effect of nitrates significantly enhanced by •avanafil (avoid concomitant use)

Beta-blockers: enhanced hypotensive effect when nitrates given with beta-blockers

Calcium-channel Blockers: enhanced hypotensive effect when nitrates given with calcium-channel blockers

Clonidine: enhanced hypotensive effect when nitrates given with clonidine

Corticosteroids: hypotensive effect of nitrates antagonised by corticosteroids

Diazoxide: enhanced hypotensive effect when nitrates given with diazoxide

Diuretics: enhanced hypotensive effect when nitrates given with diuretics

Dopaminergics: enhanced hypotensive effect when nitrates given with levodopa

Methyldopa: enhanced hypotensive effect when nitrates given with methyldopa

Moxisylyte: enhanced hypotensive effect when nitrates given with moxisylyte

Moxonidine: enhanced hypotensive effect when nitrates given with moxonidine

Muscle Relaxants: enhanced hypotensive effect when nitrates given with baclofen or tizanidine

Oestrogens: hypotensive effect of nitrates antagonised by oestrogens

Prostaglandins: enhanced hypotensive effect when nitrates given with alprostadil

• Riociguat: possible enhanced hypotensive effect when nitrates given with •riociguat—avoid concomitant use

• Sildenafil: hypotensive effect of nitrates significantly enhanced by •sildenafil (avoid concomitant use)

• Tadalafil: hypotensive effect of nitrates significantly enhanced by •tadalafil (avoid concomitant use)

Nitrates *(continued)*

• Vardenafil: possible increased hypotensive effect when nitrates given with •vardenafil—avoid concomitant use

Vasodilator Antihypertensives: enhanced hypotensive effect when nitrates given with hydralazine, minoxidil or sodium nitroprusside

Nitrazepam *see* Anxiolytics and Hypnotics

Nitrofurantoin

Antacids: absorption of nitrofurantoin reduced by oral magnesium salts (as magnesium trisilicate)

Antibacterials: nitrofurantoin possibly antagonises effects of nalidixic acid

Sulfinpyrazone: excretion of nitrofurantoin reduced by sulfinpyrazone (increased risk of toxicity)

Vaccines: antibacterials inactivate oral typhoid vaccine—see p. 864

Nitroimidazoles *see* Metronidazole and Tinidazole

Nitrous Oxide *see* Anaesthetics, General

Nizatidine *see* Histamine H$_2$-antagonists

Nomegestrol *see* Progestogens

Noradrenaline (norepinephrine) *see* Sympathomimetics

Norelgestromin *see* Progestogens

Norepinephrine (noradrenaline) *see* Sympathomimetics

Norethisterone *see* Progestogens

Norfloxacin *see* Quinolones

Norgestimate *see* Progestogens

Norgestrel *see* Progestogens

Nortriptyline *see* Antidepressants, Tricyclic

NSAIDs

Note *See also* Aspirin. Interactions do not generally apply to topical NSAIDs

ACE Inhibitors: increased risk of renal impairment when NSAIDs given with ACE inhibitors, also hypotensive effect antagonised

Adrenergic Neurone Blockers: NSAIDs antagonise hypotensive effect of adrenergic neurone blockers

Aliskiren: NSAIDs possibly antagonise hypotensive effect of aliskiren

Alpha-blockers: NSAIDs antagonise hypotensive effect of alpha-blockers

• Analgesics: avoid concomitant use of NSAIDs with •NSAIDs or •aspirin (increased side-effects); avoid concomitant use of NSAIDs with •ketorolac (increased side-effects and haemorrhage); ibuprofen possibly reduces antiplatelet effect of aspirin

Angiotensin-II Receptor Antagonists: increased risk of renal impairment when NSAIDs given with angiotensin-II receptor antagonists, also hypotensive effect antagonised

Antacids: absorption of acemetacin possibly reduced by antacids

• Antibacterials: indometacin possibly increases plasma concentration of amikacin and gentamicin in neonates; plasma concentration of celecoxib, diclofenac and etoricoxib reduced by rifampicin; possible increased risk of convulsions when NSAIDs given with •quinolones

• Anticoagulants: increased risk of haemorrhage when *intravenous* diclofenac given with •anticoagulants (avoid concomitant use, including low-dose heparins); increased risk of haemorrhage when ketorolac given with •anticoagulants (avoid concomitant use, including low-dose heparins); NSAIDs possibly enhance anticoagulant effect of •coumarins and •phenindione; possible increased risk of bleeding when NSAIDs given with •dabigatran or heparins

• Antidepressants: increased risk of bleeding when NSAIDs given with •SSRIs or •venlafaxine

• Antidiabetics: NSAIDs possibly enhance effects of •sulfonylureas

Antiepileptics: acemetacin possibly reduces excretion of phenytoin (increased risk of toxicity)

NSAIDs *(continued)*

Antifungals: plasma concentration of parecoxib increased by fluconazole (reduce dose of parecoxib); plasma concentration of celecoxib increased by fluconazole (halve dose of celecoxib); plasma concentration of flurbiprofen and ibuprofen increased by fluconazole; plasma concentration of diclofenac and ibuprofen increased by voriconazole

Antipsychotics: possible severe drowsiness when acemetacin or indometacin given with haloperidol

- Antivirals: plasma concentration of NSAIDs possibly increased by ritonavir; plasma concentration of piroxicam increased by •ritonavir (risk of toxicity)—avoid concomitant use; increased risk of haematological toxicity when NSAIDs given with zidovudine

Beta-blockers: NSAIDs antagonise hypotensive effect of beta-blockers

Calcium-channel Blockers: NSAIDs antagonise hypotensive effect of calcium-channel blockers

Cardiac Glycosides: NSAIDs possibly increase plasma concentration of cardiac glycosides, also possible exacerbation of heart failure and reduction of renal function

- Ciclosporin: increased risk of nephrotoxicity when NSAIDs given with •ciclosporin; plasma concentration of diclofenac increased by •ciclosporin (halve dose of diclofenac)

Clonidine: NSAIDs antagonise hypotensive effect of clonidine

Clopidogrel: increased risk of bleeding when NSAIDs given with clopidogrel

Corticosteroids: increased risk of gastro-intestinal bleeding and ulceration when NSAIDs given with corticosteroids

- Cytotoxics: NSAIDs probably reduce excretion of •methotrexate (increased risk of toxicity)—but for concomitant use in rheumatic disease see p. 732; diclofenac, ibuprofen, indometacin, ketoprofen, meloxicam and naproxen reduce excretion of •methotrexate (increased risk of toxicity)—but for concomitant use in rheumatic disease see p. 732; NSAIDs possibly reduce renal excretion of pemetrexed—consult product literature; increased risk of bleeding when NSAIDs given with •erlotinib; avoidance of mefenamic acid advised by manufacturer of regorafenib

Desmopressin: indometacin enhances effects of desmopressin

Diazoxide: NSAIDs antagonise hypotensive effect of diazoxide

- Dimethyl sulfoxide: avoid concomitant use of sulindac with •dimethyl sulfoxide

- Diuretics: risk of nephrotoxicity of NSAIDs increased by diuretics, also antagonism of diuretic effect; indometacin and ketorolac antagonise effects of diuretics; excretion of acemetacin possibly increased by furosemide; NSAIDs possibly antagonise diuretic effect of potassium canrenoate; occasional reports of reduced renal function when indometacin given with •triamterene—avoid concomitant use; increased risk of hyperkalaemia when indometacin given with potassium-sparing diuretics and aldosterone antagonists; possible increased risk of hyperkalaemia when NSAIDs given with potassium-sparing diuretics and aldosterone antagonists

Iloprost: increased risk of bleeding when NSAIDs given with iloprost

Lipid-regulating Drugs: excretion of meloxicam increased by colestyramine

- Lithium: NSAIDs reduce excretion of •lithium (increased risk of toxicity); ketorolac reduces excretion of •lithium (increased risk of toxicity)—avoid concomitant use

NSAIDs *(continued)*

Methyldopa: NSAIDs antagonise hypotensive effect of methyldopa

Mifamurtide: avoidance of high doses of NSAIDs advised by manufacturer of mifamurtide

Moxonidine: NSAIDs antagonise hypotensive effect of moxonidine

Muscle Relaxants: ibuprofen reduces excretion of baclofen (increased risk of toxicity); NSAIDs possibly reduce excretion of baclofen (increased risk of toxicity)

Nitrates: NSAIDs antagonise hypotensive effect of nitrates

Oestrogens: etoricoxib increases plasma concentration of ethinylestradiol

Penicillamine: possible increased risk of nephrotoxicity when NSAIDs given with penicillamine

- Pentoxifylline: possible increased risk of bleeding when NSAIDs given with pentoxifylline; increased risk of bleeding when ketorolac given with •pentoxifylline (avoid concomitant use)

Prasugrel: possible increased risk of bleeding when NSAIDs given with prasugrel

- Tacrolimus: possible increased risk of nephrotoxicity when NSAIDs given with tacrolimus; increased risk of nephrotoxicity when ibuprofen given with •tacrolimus

Vasodilator Antihypertensives: NSAIDs antagonise hypotensive effect of hydralazine, minoxidil and sodium nitroprusside

Obinutuzumab

- Antipsychotics: avoid concomitant use of cytotoxics with •clozapine (increased risk of agranulocytosis)
- Vaccines: avoid concomitant use of monoclonal antibodies with live •vaccines (see p. 842)

Octreotide

Antidiabetics: octreotide possibly reduces requirements for antidiabetics

- Ciclosporin: octreotide reduces plasma concentration of •ciclosporin

Dopaminergics: octreotide increases plasma concentration of bromocriptine

Ulcer-healing Drugs: octreotide possibly delays absorption of cimetidine

Oestrogens

Note Interactions of combined oral contraceptives may also apply to combined contraceptive patches and vaginal rings, see p. 548

ACE Inhibitors: oestrogens antagonise hypotensive effect of ACE inhibitors

Adrenergic Neurone Blockers: oestrogens antagonise hypotensive effect of adrenergic neurone blockers

Alpha-blockers: oestrogens antagonise hypotensive effect of alpha-blockers

Analgesics: plasma concentration of ethinylestradiol increased by etoricoxib

Angiotensin-II Receptor Antagonists: oestrogens antagonise hypotensive effect of angiotensin-II receptor antagonists

- Antibacterials: plasma concentration of estradiol increased by erythromycin; metabolism of oestrogens accelerated by •rifamycins (reduced contraceptive effect—see p. 548)

- Anticoagulants: oestrogens may enhance or reduce anticoagulant effect of coumarins; oestrogens antagonise anticoagulant effect of •phenindione

- Antidepressants: contraceptive effect of oestrogens reduced by •St John's wort (avoid concomitant use); oestrogens antagonise antidepressant effect of tricyclics (but side-effects of tricyclics possibly increased due to increased plasma concentration)

Antidiabetics: oestrogens antagonise hypoglycaemic effect of antidiabetics

- Antiepileptics: metabolism of oestrogens accelerated by •carbamazepine, •eslicarbazepine, •oxcarbazepine, •phenobarbital, •phenytoin,

Oestrogens

- **Antiepileptics** *(continued)*
  •rufinamide and •topiramate (reduced contraceptive effect—see p. 548); oestrogens reduce plasma concentration of •lamotrigine—consider increasing dose of lamotrigine; ethinylestradiol possibly reduces plasma concentration of valproate

  Antifungals: oestrogens increase plasma concentration of voriconazole; anecdotal reports of contraceptive failure and menstrual irregularities when oestrogens given with griseofulvin; anecdotal reports of contraceptive failure when oestrogens given with imidazoles; occasional reports of breakthrough bleeding when oestrogens (used for contraception) given with terbinafine

- **Antivirals:** plasma concentration of ethinylestradiol increased by atazanavir; metabolism of oestrogens accelerated by •nevirapine and •ritonavir (reduced contraceptive effect—see p. 548); plasma concentration of ethinylestradiol possibly reduced by •telaprevir—manufacturer of telaprevir advises additional contraceptive precautions

  Anxiolytics and Hypnotics: oestrogens possibly increase plasma concentration of chlordiazepoxide, diazepam and nitrazepam; oestrogens possibly reduce plasma concentration of lorazepam, oxazepam and temazepam; oestrogens increase plasma concentration of melatonin

- **Aprepitant:** possible contraceptive failure of hormonal contraceptives containing oestrogens when given with •aprepitant (alternative contraception recommended)

  Beta-blockers: oestrogens antagonise hypotensive effect of beta-blockers

- **Bosentan:** possible contraceptive failure of hormonal contraceptives containing oestrogens when given with •bosentan (alternative contraception recommended)

  Calcium-channel Blockers: oestrogens antagonise hypotensive effect of calcium-channel blockers

  Ciclosporin: oestrogens possibly increase plasma concentration of ciclosporin

  Clonidine: oestrogens antagonise hypotensive effect of clonidine

- **Cobicistat:** metabolism of oestrogens accelerated by •cobicistat (reduced contraceptive effect—see p. 548)

  Corticosteroids: oral contraceptives containing oestrogens increase plasma concentration of corticosteroids

- **Cytotoxics:** possible reduction in contraceptive effect of oestrogens advised by manufacturer of •crizotinib and •vemurafenib; possible reduced contraceptive effect of hormonal contraceptives containing oestrogens advised by manufacturer of •dabrafenib (alternative contraception recommended)

  Diuretics: oestrogens antagonise diuretic effect of diuretics

- **Dopaminergics:** oestrogens increase plasma concentration of ropinirole; oestrogens increase plasma concentration of •selegiline—manufacturer of selegiline advises avoid concomitant use

  Lipid-regulating Drugs: absorption of ethinylestradiol reduced by colesevelam; plasma concentration of ethinylestradiol increased by atorvastatin and rosuvastatin

  Methyldopa: oestrogens antagonise hypotensive effect of methyldopa

- **Modafinil:** metabolism of oestrogens accelerated by •modafinil (reduced contraceptive effect—see p. 548)

  Moxonidine: oestrogens antagonise hypotensive effect of moxonidine

  Muscle Relaxants: oestrogens possibly increase plasma concentration of tizanidine (increased risk of toxicity)

Oestrogens *(continued)*

Nitrates: oestrogens antagonise hypotensive effect of nitrates

Somatropin: oestrogens (when used as oral replacement therapy) may increase dose requirements of somatropin

Tacrolimus: ethinylestradiol possibly increases plasma concentration of tacrolimus

Teriflunomide: plasma concentration of ethinylestradiol increased by teriflunomide

Theophylline: oestrogens increase plasma concentration of theophylline (consider reducing dose of theophylline)

Thyroid Hormones: oestrogens may increase requirements for thyroid hormones in hypothyroidism

Vasodilator Antihypertensives: oestrogens antagonise hypotensive effect of hydralazine, minoxidil and sodium nitroprusside

Oestrogens, conjugated *see* Oestrogens

Ofatumumab

- **Antipsychotics:** avoid concomitant use of cytotoxics with •clozapine (increased risk of agranulocytosis)
- **Vaccines:** avoid concomitant use of monoclonal antibodies with live •vaccines (see p. 842)

Ofloxacin *see* Quinolones

Olanzapine *see* Antipsychotics

Olmesartan *see* Angiotensin-II Receptor Antagonists

Olodaterol *see* Sympathomimetics, Beta$_2$

Omeprazole *see* Proton Pump Inhibitors

Ondansetron *see* 5HT$_3$-receptor Antagonists (under HT)

Opioid Analgesics

Alcohol: enhanced hypotensive and sedative effects when opioid analgesics given with alcohol

Anaesthetics, General: fentanyl inhibits metabolism of etomidate (consider reducing dose of etomidate); opioid analgesics possibly enhance effects of intravenous general anaesthetics and volatile liquid general anaesthetics

Analgesics: avoidance of buprenorphine advised by manufacturer of fentanyl; manufacturer of fentanyl advises avoid concomitant use with pentazocine

- **Antibacterials:** plasma concentration of fentanyl possibly increased by clarithromycin; plasma concentration of alfentanil increased by erythromycin; metabolism of alfentanil, codeine, fentanyl, methadone and morphine accelerated by rifampicin (reduced effect); metabolism of oxycodone possibly accelerated by rifampicin; increased risk of ventricular arrhythmias when methadone given with •delamanid; manufacturer of pethidine advises avoid concomitant use with isoniazid; possible increased risk of ventricular arrhythmias when methadone given with •telithromycin; metabolism of oxycodone inhibited by telithromycin

- **Anticoagulants:** tramadol enhances anticoagulant effect of •coumarins

- **Antidepressants:** plasma concentration of methadone possibly increased by fluoxetine, fluvoxamine, paroxetine and sertraline; possible increased serotonergic effects when pethidine or tramadol given with duloxetine; possible increased serotonergic effects when tramadol given with mirtazapine or venlafaxine; possible increased serotonergic effects and increased risk of convulsions when tramadol given with •MAOIs—some manufacturers advise avoid concomitant use and for 2 weeks after stopping MAOIs; CNS excitation or depression (hypertension or hypotension) when pethidine given with •MAOIs—avoid concomitant use and for 2 weeks after stopping MAOIs; possible increased serotonergic effects when fentanyl given with MAOIs, SSRI-related antidepressants or SSRIs; possible CNS excitation or depression (hypertension or hypotension) when opioid analgesics given with •MAOIs—some manufacturers advise avoid conco-

Opioid Analgesics

- Antidepressants *(continued)*

  mitant use and for 2 weeks after stopping MAOIs; possible CNS excitation or depression (hypertension or hypotension) when opioid analgesics given with ●moclobemide—manufacturer of moclobemide advises consider reducing dose of opioid analgesics; possible CNS excitation or depression (hypertension or hypotension) when dextromethorphan or pethidine given with ●moclobemide—avoid concomitant use; increased risk of CNS toxicity when tramadol given with ●SSRIs or ●tricyclics; plasma concentration of methadone possibly reduced by St John's wort; sedative effects possibly increased when opioid analgesics given with tricyclics

- Antiepileptics: plasma concentration of methadone reduced by carbamazepine and phenobarbital; metabolism of fentanyl possibly accelerated by carbamazepine and phenytoin (reduced effect); dextropropoxyphene enhances effects of ●carbamazepine; effects of tramadol reduced by carbamazepine; morphine increases bioavailability of gabapentin; possible increased risk of pethidine toxicity when given with ●phenytoin; metabolism of methadone accelerated by phenytoin (reduced effect and risk of withdrawal effects)

- Antifungals: metabolism of alfentanil inhibited by fluconazole (risk of prolonged or delayed respiratory depression); plasma concentration of methadone increased by fluconazole; metabolism of alfentanil possibly inhibited by itraconazole; plasma concentration of methadone possibly increased by ●itraconazole (increased risk of ventricular arrhythmias); plasma concentration of oxycodone increased by itraconazole and ●voriconazole; plasma concentration of alfentanil and methadone increased by ●voriconazole (consider reducing dose of alfentanil and methadone); plasma concentration of fentanyl possibly increased by ●triazoles

- Antihistamines: sedative effects possibly increased when opioid analgesics given with ●sedating antihistamines

- Antimalarials: avoidance of methadone advised by manufacturer of ●piperaquine with artenimol (possible risk of ventricular arrhythmias)

  Antimuscarinics: possible increased risk of antimuscarinic side-effects when codeine given with antimuscarinics

- Antipsychotics: enhanced hypotensive and sedative effects when opioid analgesics given with antipsychotics; increased risk of ventricular arrhythmias when methadone given with ●antipsychotics that prolong the QT interval; increased risk of convulsions when tramadol given with antipsychotics; increased risk of ventricular arrhythmias when methadone given with ●amisulpride—avoid concomitant use

- Antivirals: plasma concentration of methadone possibly reduced by abacavir, nevirapine and rilpivirine; possible increased risk of prolonged sedation and respiratory depression when buprenorphine given with boceprevir; plasma concentration of methadone possibly affected by boceprevir; methadone possibly reduces plasma concentration of didanosine; plasma concentration of methadone reduced by efavirenz, fosamprenavir and ritonavir; plasma concentration of buprenorphine possibly increased by ritonavir; plasma concentration of alfentanil and fentanyl increased by ●ritonavir; plasma concentration of pethidine reduced by ●ritonavir, but plasma concentration of toxic pethidine metabolite increased (avoid concomitant use); plasma concentration of morphine possibly reduced by ritonavir; plasma concentration of dextropropoxyphene increased by ●ritonavir (risk of toxicity)—avoid concomitant use; increased risk of ventricular arrhyth-

Opioid Analgesics

- Antivirals *(continued)*

  mias when alfentanil, fentanyl or methadone given with ●saquinavir—avoid concomitant use; caution with methadone advised by manufacturer of ●telaprevir (risk of ventricular arrhythmias); buprenorphine possibly reduces plasma concentration of tipranavir; methadone possibly increases plasma concentration of zidovudine

  Anxiolytics and Hypnotics: increased sedative effect when opioid analgesics given with anxiolytics and hypnotics; fentanyl possibly inhibits metabolism of midazolam

- Atomoxetine: increased risk of ventricular arrhythmias when methadone given with ●atomoxetine; possible increased risk of convulsions when tramadol given with atomoxetine

  Beta-blockers: morphine possibly increases plasma concentration of esmolol

  Calcium-channel Blockers: metabolism of alfentanil inhibited by diltiazem (risk of prolonged or delayed respiratory depression)

- Cytotoxics: possible increased risk of ventricular arrhythmias when methadone given with ●bosutinib; caution with alfentanil and fentanyl advised by manufacturer of ●crizotinib; possible increased risk of ventricular arrhythmias when methadone given with ●vandetanib—avoid concomitant use

- Dapoxetine: possible increased risk of serotonergic effects when tramadol given with ●dapoxetine (manufacturer of dapoxetine advises tramadol should not be started until 1 week after stopping dapoxetine, avoid dapoxetine for 2 weeks after stopping tramadol)

  Domperidone: opioid analgesics antagonise effects of domperidone on gastro-intestinal activity

- Dopaminergics: risk of CNS toxicity when pethidine given with ●rasagiline (avoid pethidine for 2 weeks after rasagiline); avoid concomitant use of dextromethorphan with ●rasagiline; hyperpyrexia and CNS toxicity reported when pethidine given with ●selegiline (avoid concomitant use); avoidance of opioid analgesics advised by manufacturer of selegiline

  Hormone Antagonists: plasma concentration of dextromethorphan increased by abiraterone

  5HT$_3$-receptor Antagonists: effects of tramadol possibly antagonised by ondansetron

- Memantine: increased risk of CNS toxicity when dextromethorphan given with ●memantine (manufacturer of memantine advises avoid concomitant use)

  Metoclopramide: opioid analgesics antagonise effects of metoclopramide on gastro-intestinal activity

  Muscle Relaxants: increased sedative effect when fentanyl or morphine given with baclofen

- Nalmefene: avoidance of opioid analgesics advised by manufacturer of ●nalmefene

- Sodium Oxybate: opioid analgesics enhance effects of ●sodium oxybate (avoid concomitant use)

  Ulcer-healing Drugs: metabolism of opioid analgesics inhibited by cimetidine (increased plasma concentration)

Orlistat

  Anti-arrhythmics: orlistat possibly reduces plasma concentration of amiodarone

  Anticoagulants: manufacturer of orlistat recommends monitoring anticoagulant effect of coumarins

  Antidiabetics: manufacturer of orlistat advises avoid concomitant use with acarbose

- Antiepileptics: possible increased risk of convulsions when orlistat given with ●antiepileptics

- Antivirals: orlistat possibly reduces absorption of ●abacavir, ●atazanavir, ●darunavir, ●didanosine, ●efavirenz, ●elvitegravir, ●emtricitabine, ●enfuvirtide, ●etravirine, ●fosamprenavir,

Orlistat
- *Antivirals (continued)*
  - ●indinavir, ●lamivudine, ●lopinavir, ●maraviroc, ●nevirapine, ●raltegravir, ●rilpivirine, ●ritonavir, ●saquinavir, ●stavudine, ●tenofovir, ●tipranavir and ●zidovudine
- Ciclosporin: orlistat possibly reduces absorption of ●ciclosporin
  Thyroid Hormones: possible increased risk of hypothyroidism when orlistat given with levothyroxine

Orphenadrine *see* Antimuscarinics

Oxaliplatin *see* Platinum Compounds

Oxandrolone *see* Anabolic Steroids

Oxazepam *see* Anxiolytics and Hypnotics

Oxcarbazepine
- Antidepressants: anticonvulsant effect of antiepileptics possibly antagonised by MAOIs and ●tricyclic-related antidepressants (convulsive threshold lowered); anticonvulsant effect of antiepileptics antagonised by ●SSRIs and ●tricyclics (convulsive threshold lowered)
- Antiepileptics: oxcarbazepine sometimes reduces plasma concentration of carbamazepine (but concentration of an active metabolite of carbamazepine may be increased), also plasma concentration of an active metabolite of oxcarbazepine often reduced; avoidance of oxcarbazepine advised by manufacturer of eslicarbazepine; oxcarbazepine reduces plasma concentration of ●perampanel (see Dose under Perampanel, p. 313); oxcarbazepine increases plasma concentration of phenobarbital and phenytoin, also plasma concentration of an active metabolite of oxcarbazepine reduced; plasma concentration of an active metabolite of oxcarbazepine sometimes reduced by valproate
- Antimalarials: anticonvulsant effect of antiepileptics antagonised by ●mefloquine
- Antipsychotics: anticonvulsant effect of antiepileptics antagonised by ●antipsychotics (convulsive threshold lowered)
- Antivirals: oxcarbazepine possibly reduces plasma concentration of ●daclatasvir and ●simeprevir—manufacturer of daclatasvir and simeprevir advises avoid concomitant use; avoidance of oxcarbazepine advised by manufacturer of dolutegravir and sofosbuvir; avoidance of oxcarbazepine advised by manufacturer of ●rilpivirine (plasma concentration of rilpivirine possibly reduced)
  Ciclosporin: oxcarbazepine possibly reduces plasma concentration of ciclosporin
- Clopidogrel: oxcarbazepine possibly reduces antiplatelet effect of ●clopidogrel
- Cytotoxics: oxcarbazepine reduces plasma concentration of ●imatinib—avoid concomitant use
- Oestrogens: oxcarbazepine accelerates metabolism of ●oestrogens (reduced contraceptive effect—see p. 548)
- Orlistat: possible increased risk of convulsions when antiepileptics given with ●orlistat
- Progestogens: oxcarbazepine accelerates metabolism of ●progestogens (reduced contraceptive effect—see p. 548)

Oxprenolol *see* Beta-blockers

Oxybutynin *see* Antimuscarinics

Oxycodone *see* Opioid Analgesics

Oxymetazoline *see* Sympathomimetics

Oxytetracycline *see* Tetracyclines

Oxytocin
  Anaesthetics, General: oxytocic effect possibly reduced, also enhanced hypotensive effect and risk of arrhythmias when oxytocin given with volatile liquid general anaesthetics
  Prostaglandins: uterotonic effect of oxytocin potentiated by prostaglandins

Oxytocin *(continued)*
  Sympathomimetics: risk of hypertension when oxytocin given with vasoconstrictor sympathomimetics (due to enhanced vasopressor effect)

Paclitaxel
- Antipsychotics: avoid concomitant use of cytotoxics with ●clozapine (increased risk of agranulocytosis)
  Antivirals: plasma concentration of paclitaxel increased by ritonavir
- Cytotoxics: increased risk of neutropenia when paclitaxel given with ●lapatinib

Paliperidone *see* Antipsychotics

Pamidronate Disodium *see* Bisphosphonates

Pancreatin
  Antidiabetics: pancreatin antagonises hypoglycaemic effect of acarbose

Pancuronium *see* Muscle Relaxants

Panitumumab
- Antipsychotics: avoid concomitant use of cytotoxics with ●clozapine (increased risk of agranulocytosis)
- Vaccines: avoid concomitant use of monoclonal antibodies with live ●vaccines (see p. 842)

Pantoprazole *see* Proton Pump Inhibitors

Papaveretum *see* Opioid Analgesics

Paracetamol
  Anticoagulants: prolonged regular use of paracetamol possibly enhances anticoagulant effect of coumarins
  Antidiabetics: absorption of paracetamol possibly reduced when given 1 to 4 hours after lixisenatide
  Antiepileptics: metabolism of paracetamol possibly accelerated by carbamazepine, phenobarbital and phenytoin (also isolated reports of hepatotoxicity)
  Cytotoxics: paracetamol possibly inhibits metabolism of *intravenous* busulfan (manufacturer of *intravenous* busulfan advises caution within 72 hours of paracetamol); caution with paracetamol advised by manufacturer of imatinib
  Lipid-regulating Drugs: absorption of paracetamol reduced by colestyramine
  Metoclopramide: rate of absorption of paracetamol increased by metoclopramide

Paraldehyde
- Alcohol: increased sedative effect when paraldehyde given with ●alcohol
- Disulfiram: risk of toxicity when paraldehyde given with ●disulfiram

Parasympathomimetics
  Anti-arrhythmics: effects of neostigmine and pyridostigmine possibly antagonised by propafenone
- Antibacterials: plasma concentration of galantamine increased by erythromycin; effects of neostigmine and pyridostigmine antagonised by ●aminoglycosides; effects of neostigmine and pyridostigmine antagonised by clindamycin; effects of neostigmine and pyridostigmine antagonised by ●polymyxins
  Antidepressants: plasma concentration of galantamine increased by paroxetine
  Antimalarials: effects of neostigmine and pyridostigmine may be diminished because of potential for chloroquine and hydroxychloroquine to increase symptoms of myasthenia gravis
  Antimuscarinics: effects of parasympathomimetics antagonised by antimuscarinics
  Beta-blockers: increased risk of arrhythmias when pilocarpine given with beta-blockers; effects of neostigmine and pyridostigmine antagonised by propranolol
  Cytotoxics: possible increased risk of bradycardia when pilocarpine given with crizotinib
  Lithium: effects of neostigmine antagonised by lithium
  Muscle Relaxants: donepezil possibly enhances effects of suxamethonium; galantamine, neostigmine, pyridostigmine and rivastigmine enhance effects of suxamethonium; neostigmine, pyridostigmine and rivastigmine antagonise effects of non-depolarising

Parasympathomimetics
Muscle Relaxants *(continued)*
muscle relaxants; donepezil possibly antagonises effects of non-depolarising muscle relaxants
Parecoxib *see* NSAIDs
Paricalcitol *see* Vitamins
Paroxetine *see* Antidepressants, SSRI
Pasireotide
Antidiabetics: pasireotide possibly reduces requirements for antidiabetics
Antimuscarinics: possible increased risk of bradycardia when pasireotide given with ipratropium or oxybutynin
Beta-blockers: possible increased risk of bradycardia when pasireotide given with carteolol, metoprolol, propranolol or sotalol
Calcium-channel Blockers: possible increased risk of bradycardia when pasireotide given with diltiazem or verapamil
- Ciclosporin: pasireotide possibly reduces plasma concentration of ●ciclosporin
Pazopanib
- Antibacterials: plasma concentration of pazopanib possibly increased by ●clarithromycin and ●telithromycin (reduce dose of pazopanib); plasma concentration of pazopanib possibly reduced by ●rifampicin
- Antifungals: plasma concentration of pazopanib possibly increased by ●itraconazole and ●voriconazole (reduce dose of pazopanib)
- Antipsychotics: avoid concomitant use of cytotoxics with ●clozapine (increased risk of agranulocytosis)
- Antivirals: plasma concentration of pazopanib possibly increased by ●atazanavir, ●indinavir and ●ritonavir (reduce dose of pazopanib); avoidance of pazopanib advised by manufacturer of ●boceprevir; increased risk of ventricular arrhythmias when pazopanib given with ●saquinavir—avoid concomitant use
Cytotoxics: plasma concentration of pazopanib increased by lapatinib
- Grapefruit Juice: manufacturer of pazopanib advises avoid concomitant use with ●grapefruit juice
Ulcer-healing Drugs: absorption of pazopanib possibly reduced by histamine H₂-antagonists—manufacturer of pazopanib advises give at least 2 hours before or 10 hours after histamine H₂-antagonists; absorption of pazopanib possibly reduced by proton pump inhibitors—manufacturer of pazopanib advises give at the same time as proton pump inhibitors
Pegfilgrastim *see* Filgrastim
Peginterferon Alfa *see* Interferons
Pemetrexed
Analgesics: renal excretion of pemetrexed possibly reduced by NSAIDs and aspirin—consult product literature
- Antimalarials: antifolate effect of pemetrexed increased by ●pyrimethamine
- Antipsychotics: avoid concomitant use of cytotoxics with ●clozapine (increased risk of agranulocytosis)
Penicillamine
Analgesics: possible increased risk of nephrotoxicity when penicillamine given with NSAIDs
Antacids: absorption of penicillamine reduced by antacids
- Antipsychotics: avoid concomitant use of penicillamine with ●clozapine (increased risk of agranulocytosis)
Cardiac Glycosides: penicillamine possibly reduces plasma concentration of digoxin
Gold: manufacturer of penicillamine advises avoid concomitant use with sodium aurothiomalate (increased risk of toxicity)
Iron: absorption of penicillamine reduced by *oral* iron
Zinc: penicillamine reduces absorption of zinc, also absorption of penicillamine reduced by zinc

Penicillins
Allopurinol: increased risk of rash when amoxicillin or ampicillin given with allopurinol
Antibacterials: absorption of phenoxymethylpenicillin reduced by neomycin; effects of penicillins possibly antagonised by tetracyclines
Anticoagulants: an interaction between broad-spectrum penicillins and coumarins and phenindione has not been demonstrated in studies, but common experience in anticoagulant clinics is that INR can be altered
- Antiepileptics: manufacturer of pivmecillinam advises avoid concomitant use with ●valproate
Cytotoxics: penicillins reduce excretion of methotrexate (increased risk of toxicity)
Muscle Relaxants: piperacillin enhances effects of non-depolarising muscle relaxants and suxamethonium
Mycophenolate: co-amoxiclav possibly reduces plasma concentration of mycophenolate
Sulfinpyrazone: excretion of penicillins reduced by sulfinpyrazone
Vaccines: antibacterials inactivate oral typhoid vaccine—see p. 864
Pentamidine Isetionate
- Anti-arrhythmics: increased risk of ventricular arrhythmias when pentamidine isetionate given with ●amiodarone—avoid concomitant use; possible increased risk of ventricular arrhythmias when pentamidine isetionate given with ●disopyramide
- Antibacterials: increased risk of ventricular arrhythmias when pentamidine isetionate given with *parenteral* ●erythromycin; increased risk of ventricular arrhythmias when pentamidine isetionate given with ●moxifloxacin—avoid concomitant use; increased risk of ventricular arrhythmias when pentamidine isetionate given with ●delamanid; possible increased risk of ventricular arrhythmias when *parenteral* pentamidine isetionate given with ●telithromycin
- Antidepressants: avoidance of pentamidine isetionate advised by manufacturer of ●citalopram and ●escitalopram (risk of ventricular arrhythmias); increased risk of ventricular arrhythmias when pentamidine isetionate given with ●tricyclics
Antifungals: possible increased risk of nephrotoxicity when pentamidine isetionate given with amphotericin
- Antimalarials: avoidance of pentamidine isetionate advised by manufacturer of ●piperaquine with artenimol (possible risk of ventricular arrhythmias)
- Antipsychotics: increased risk of ventricular arrhythmias when pentamidine isetionate given with ●amisulpride or ●droperidol—avoid concomitant use; increased risk of ventricular arrhythmias when pentamidine isetionate given with ●phenothiazines
- Antivirals: increased risk of hypocalcaemia when *parenteral* pentamidine isetionate given with ●foscarnet; increased risk of ventricular arrhythmias when pentamidine isetionate given with ●saquinavir—avoid concomitant use
- Cytotoxics: possible increased risk of ventricular arrhythmias when pentamidine isetionate given with ●vandetanib—avoid concomitant use
- Ivabradine: increased risk of ventricular arrhythmias when pentamidine isetionate given with ●ivabradine
Pentazocine *see* Opioid Analgesics
Pentostatin
- Antipsychotics: avoid concomitant use of cytotoxics with ●clozapine (increased risk of agranulocytosis)
- Cytotoxics: increased toxicity when pentostatin given with high-dose ●cyclophosphamide—avoid concomitant use; increased pulmonary toxicity when pentostatin given with ●fludarabine (unacceptably high incidence of fatalities)

Pentoxifylline

- Analgesics: possible increased risk of bleeding when pentoxifylline given with NSAIDs; increased risk of bleeding when pentoxifylline given with •ketorolac (avoid concomitant use)
  Theophylline: pentoxifylline increases plasma concentration of theophylline

Perampanel

- Antidepressants: anticonvulsant effect of antiepileptics possibly antagonised by MAOIs and •tricyclic-related antidepressants (convulsive threshold lowered); anticonvulsant effect of antiepileptics antagonised by •SSRIs and •tricyclics (convulsive threshold lowered)
- Antiepileptics: plasma concentration of perampanel reduced by •carbamazepine, •oxcarbazepine and •phenytoin (see Dose under Perampanel, p. 313); plasma concentration of perampanel reduced by topiramate
- Antimalarials: anticonvulsant effect of antiepileptics antagonised by •mefloquine
- Antipsychotics: anticonvulsant effect of antiepileptics antagonised by •antipsychotics (convulsive threshold lowered)
  Anxiolytics and Hypnotics: perampanel reduces plasma concentration of midazolam
- Orlistat: possible increased risk of convulsions when antiepileptics given with •orlistat
- Progestogens: perampanel accelerates metabolism of •progestogens (reduced contraceptive effect—see p. 548)

Pergolide

Antipsychotics: effects of pergolide antagonised by antipsychotics
Memantine: effects of dopaminergics possibly enhanced by memantine
Methyldopa: antiparkinsonian effect of dopaminergics antagonised by methyldopa
Metoclopramide: antiparkinsonian effect of pergolide antagonised by metoclopramide

Pericyazine *see* Antipsychotics

Perindopril *see* ACE Inhibitors

Perphenazine *see* Antipsychotics

Pertuzumab

- Antipsychotics: avoid concomitant use of cytotoxics with •clozapine (increased risk of agranulocytosis)
- Vaccines: avoid concomitant use of monoclonal antibodies with live •vaccines (see p. 842)

Pethidine *see* Opioid Analgesics

Phenelzine *see* MAOIs

Phenindione

Note Change in patient's clinical condition particularly associated with liver disease, intercurrent illness, or drug administration, necessitates more frequent testing. Major changes in diet (especially involving salads and vegetables) and in alcohol consumption may also affect anticoagulant control

- Alcohol: anticoagulant control with phenindione may be affected by major changes in consumption of •alcohol
- Anabolic Steroids: anticoagulant effect of phenindione enhanced by •anabolic steroids
- Analgesics: anticoagulant effect of phenindione possibly enhanced by •NSAIDs; increased risk of haemorrhage when anticoagulants given with *intravenous* •diclofenac (avoid concomitant use, including low-dose heparins); increased risk of haemorrhage when anticoagulants given with •ketorolac (avoid concomitant use, including low-dose heparins); increased risk of bleeding when phenindione given with •aspirin (due to antiplatelet effect)
- Anti-arrhythmics: metabolism of phenindione inhibited by •amiodarone (enhanced anticoagulant effect); anticoagulant effect of phenindione possibly enhanced by •dronedarone

Phenindione *(continued)*

- Antibacterials: experience in anticoagulant clinics suggests that INR possibly altered when phenindione is given with •neomycin (given for local action on gut); anticoagulant effect of phenindione possibly enhanced by levofloxacin and •tetracyclines; an interaction between phenindione and broad-spectrum penicillins has not been demonstrated in studies, but common experience in anticoagulant clinics is that INR can be altered; metabolism of phenindione possibly inhibited by sulfonamides
- Anticoagulants: increased risk of haemorrhage when other anticoagulants given with •apixaban, •dabigatran and •rivaroxaban (avoid concomitant use except when switching with other anticoagulants or using heparin to maintain catheter patency)
- Antivirals: anticoagulant effect of phenindione possibly enhanced by •ritonavir
- Clopidogrel: anticoagulant effect of phenindione enhanced due to antiplatelet action of •clopidogrel
  Corticosteroids: anticoagulant effect of phenindione may be enhanced or reduced by corticosteroids
  Cytotoxics: avoidance of phenindione advised by manufacturer of ibrutinib
- Dipyridamole: anticoagulant effect of phenindione enhanced due to antiplatelet action of •dipyridamole
- Enteral Foods: anticoagulant effect of phenindione antagonised by vitamin K (present in some •enteral feeds)
  Iloprost: increased risk of bleeding when phenindione given with iloprost
- Lipid-regulating Drugs: anticoagulant effect of phenindione may be enhanced or reduced by •colestyramine; anticoagulant effect of phenindione possibly enhanced by •rosuvastatin; anticoagulant effect of phenindione enhanced by •fibrates
- Oestrogens: anticoagulant effect of phenindione antagonised by •oestrogens
  Prasugrel: possible increased risk of bleeding when phenindione given with prasugrel
- Progestogens: anticoagulant effect of phenindione antagonised by •progestogens
- Testolactone: anticoagulant effect of phenindione enhanced by •testolactone
- Testosterone: anticoagulant effect of phenindione enhanced by •testosterone
- Thyroid Hormones: anticoagulant effect of phenindione enhanced by •thyroid hormones
- Vitamins: anticoagulant effect of phenindione antagonised by •vitamin K

Phenobarbital

Note Primidone interactions as for phenobarbital
Alcohol: increased sedative effect when phenobarbital given with alcohol
Analgesics: phenobarbital reduces plasma concentration of methadone; phenobarbital possibly accelerates metabolism of paracetamol (also isolated reports of hepatotoxicity)
Anti-arrhythmics: phenobarbital accelerates metabolism of disopyramide (reduced plasma concentration); phenobarbital possibly reduces plasma concentration of •dronedarone—avoid concomitant use; phenobarbital possibly accelerates metabolism of propafenone

- Antibacterials: phenobarbital accelerates metabolism of metronidazole (reduced effect); phenobarbital possibly reduces plasma concentration of rifampicin; phenobarbital accelerates metabolism of doxycycline (reduced plasma concentration); phenobarbital possibly accelerates metabolism of •chloramphenicol (reduced plasma concentration); phenobarbital reduces plasma concentration of •telithromycin (avoid during and for 2 weeks after phenobarbital)

Phenobarbital *(continued)*

- Anticoagulants: phenobarbital possibly reduces plasma concentration of ●apixaban; phenobarbital accelerates metabolism of ●coumarins (reduced anticoagulant effect); phenobarbital possibly reduces plasma concentration of ●rivaroxaban—manufacturer of rivaroxaban advises monitor for signs of thrombosis

- Antidepressants: phenobarbital possibly reduces plasma concentration of reboxetine; phenobarbital reduces plasma concentration of paroxetine; phenobarbital accelerates metabolism of ●mianserin (reduced plasma concentration); anticonvulsant effect of antiepileptics possibly antagonised by MAOIs and ●tricyclic-related antidepressants (convulsive threshold lowered); anticonvulsant effect of antiepileptics antagonised by ●SSRIs and ●tricyclics (convulsive threshold lowered); plasma concentration of phenobarbital possibly reduced by ●St John's wort—avoid concomitant use; phenobarbital possibly accelerates metabolism of ●tricyclics (reduced plasma concentration)

- Antiepileptics: plasma concentration of phenobarbital possibly increased by carbamazepine; phenobarbital possibly reduces plasma concentration of ethosuximide, rufinamide and topiramate; phenobarbital reduces plasma concentration of lamotrigine, tiagabine and zonisamide; plasma concentration of phenobarbital increased by oxcarbazepine, also plasma concentration of an active metabolite of oxcarbazepine reduced; plasma concentration of phenobarbital often increased by phenytoin, plasma concentration of phenytoin often reduced but may be increased; plasma concentration of phenobarbital increased by ●stiripentol; plasma concentration of phenobarbital increased by valproate (also plasma concentration of valproate reduced)

- Antifungals: phenobarbital possibly reduces plasma concentration of itraconazole and ●posaconazole; phenobarbital possibly reduces plasma concentration of ●voriconazole—avoid concomitant use; phenobarbital reduces absorption of griseofulvin (reduced effect)

- Antimalarials: avoidance of phenobarbital advised by manufacturer of piperaquine with artenimol; anticonvulsant effect of antiepileptics antagonised by ●mefloquine

- Antipsychotics: anticonvulsant effect of antiepileptics antagonised by ●antipsychotics (convulsive threshold lowered); phenobarbital accelerates metabolism of haloperidol (reduced plasma concentration); plasma concentration of both drugs reduced when phenobarbital given with chlorpromazine; phenobarbital possibly reduces plasma concentration of ●aripiprazole (avoid concomitant use or consider increasing the dose of aripiprazole—consult aripiprazole product literature); phenobarbital possibly reduces plasma concentration of clozapine; phenobarbital possibly reduces plasma concentration of ●lurasidone—avoid concomitant use

- Antivirals: phenobarbital possibly reduces plasma concentration of abacavir, darunavir, fosamprenavir, ●indinavir, ●lopinavir and ●saquinavir; avoidance of phenobarbital advised by manufacturer of ●boceprevir and ●rilpivirine (plasma concentration of boceprevir and rilpivirine possibly reduced); phenobarbital possibly reduces plasma concentration of ●daclatasvir and ●simeprevir—manufacturer of daclatasvir and simeprevir advises avoid concomitant use; avoidance of phenobarbital advised by manufacturer of dolutegravir, ●elvitegravir, etravirine, sofosbuvir and ●telaprevir

Anxiolytics and Hypnotics: increased sedative effect when phenobarbital given with anxiolytics and hypnotics; phenobarbital often reduces plasma concentration of clonazepam

Phenobarbital *(continued)*

Aprepitant: phenobarbital possibly reduces plasma concentration of aprepitant

Avanafil: phenobarbital possibly reduces plasma concentration of avanafil—manufacturer of avanafil advises avoid concomitant use

Beta-blockers: phenobarbital possibly reduces plasma concentration of propranolol

Caffeine citrate: effects of phenobarbital possibly antagonised by caffeine citrate

- Calcium-channel Blockers: phenobarbital probably reduces effects of ●calcium-channel blockers; avoidance of phenobarbital advised by manufacturer of isradipine; avoidance of phenobarbital advised by manufacturer of ●nimodipine (plasma concentration of nimodipine reduced)

- Cannabis Extract: phenobarbital possibly reduces plasma concentration of ●cannabis extract—manufacturer of cannabis extract advises avoid concomitant use

- Ciclosporin: phenobarbital accelerates metabolism of ●ciclosporin (reduced plasma concentration)

- Cobicistat: phenobarbital possibly reduces plasma concentration of ●cobicistat—manufacturer of cobicistat advises avoid concomitant use

- Corticosteroids: phenobarbital accelerates metabolism of ●corticosteroids (reduced effect)

- Cytotoxics: phenobarbital possibly decreases plasma concentration of axitinib (increase dose of axitinib—consult axitinib product literature); phenobarbital possibly reduces plasma concentration of bortezomib, ●bosutinib, crizotinib and ponatinib—manufacturer of bortezomib, bosutinib, crizotinib and ponatinib advises avoid concomitant use; phenobarbital possibly reduces plasma concentration of ●cabozantinib—avoid concomitant use; avoidance of phenobarbital advised by manufacturer of ●cabazitaxel, dabrafenib and gefitinib; avoidance of phenobarbital advised by manufacturer of vandetanib (plasma concentration of vandetanib possibly reduced); phenobarbital possibly reduces plasma concentration of etoposide; phenobarbital reduces plasma concentration of irinotecan and its active metabolite; manufacturer of procarbazine advises possible increased risk of hypersensitivity reactions when phenobarbital given with procarbazine

- Diuretics: phenobarbital reduces plasma concentration of ●eplerenone—avoid concomitant use; increased risk of osteomalacia when phenobarbital given with carbonic anhydrase inhibitors

Folates: plasma concentration of phenobarbital possibly reduced by folates

- Hormone Antagonists: phenobarbital possibly reduces plasma concentration of ●abiraterone—manufacturer of abiraterone advises avoid concomitant use; phenobarbital accelerates metabolism of toremifene (reduced plasma concentration)

- Ivacaftor: phenobarbital possibly reduces plasma concentration of ●ivacaftor—manufacturer of ivacaftor advises avoid concomitant use

Leukotriene Receptor Antagonists: phenobarbital reduces plasma concentration of montelukast

- Oestrogens: phenobarbital accelerates metabolism of ●oestrogens (reduced contraceptive effect—see p. 548)

- Orlistat: possible increased risk of convulsions when antiepileptics given with ●orlistat

- Progestogens: phenobarbital accelerates metabolism of ●progestogens (reduced contraceptive effect—see p. 548)

Roflumilast: phenobarbital possibly inhibits effects of roflumilast (manufacturer of roflumilast advises avoid concomitant use)

Sodium Oxybate: avoidance of phenobarbital advised by manufacturer of sodium oxybate

Phenobarbital *(continued)*
  Sympathomimetics: plasma concentration of phenobarbital possibly increased by methylphenidate
- Tacrolimus: phenobarbital reduces plasma concentration of •tacrolimus
- Theophylline: phenobarbital accelerates metabolism of
  •theophylline (reduced effect)
  Thyroid Hormones: phenobarbital accelerates metabolism of thyroid hormones (may increase requirements for thyroid hormones in hypothyroidism)
  Ticagrelor: phenobarbital possibly reduces plasma
  concentration of ticagrelor
- Ulipristal: avoidance of phenobarbital advised by
  manufacturer of •ulipristal (contraceptive effect of
  ulipristal possibly reduced)
  Vitamins: phenobarbital possibly increases requirements for vitamin D

Phenothiazines *see* Antipsychotics

Phenoxybenzamine *see* Alpha-blockers

Phenoxymethylpenicillin *see* Penicillins

Phentolamine *see* Alpha-blockers

Phenylephrine *see* Sympathomimetics

Phenytoin
  Note Fosphenytoin interactions as for phenytoin
  Alcohol: plasma concentration of phenytoin possibly
  reduced by chronic heavy consumption of alcohol
- Analgesics: excretion of phenytoin possibly reduced
  by acemetacin (increased risk of toxicity); phenytoin
  possibly accelerates metabolism of fentanyl
  (reduced effect); phenytoin accelerates metabolism
  of methadone (reduced effect and risk of withdrawal
  effects); phenytoin possibly increases risk of •pethi-
  dine toxicity; effects of phenytoin enhanced by
  aspirin; phenytoin possibly accelerates metabolism
  of paracetamol (also isolated reports of hepatotoxicity)
  Antacids: absorption of phenytoin reduced by
  antacids
- Anti-arrhythmics: metabolism of phenytoin inhibited
  by •amiodarone (increased plasma concentration);
  phenytoin reduces plasma concentration of disopyramide; phenytoin possibly reduces plasma concentration of •dronedarone—avoid concomitant use
- Antibacterials: metabolism of phenytoin inhibited by
  clarithromycin (increased plasma concentration);
  metabolism of phenytoin possibly inhibited by
  metronidazole (increased plasma concentration);
  plasma concentration of phenytoin increased or
  decreased by ciprofloxacin; phenytoin accelerates
  metabolism of doxycycline (reduced plasma concentration); phenytoin possibly reduces plasma concentration of •bedaquiline—manufacturer of bedaquiline advises avoid concomitant use; plasma
  concentration of phenytoin increased by •chloram-
  phenicol (increased risk of toxicity); metabolism of
  phenytoin possibly inhibited by isoniazid (increased
  risk of toxicity); metabolism of phenytoin accelerated by •rifamycins (reduced plasma concentration); plasma concentration of phenytoin possibly
  increased by sulfonamides; phenytoin reduces
  plasma concentration of •telithromycin (avoid during and for 2 weeks after phenytoin); plasma concentration of phenytoin increased by •trimethoprim
  (also increased antifolate effect)
- Anticoagulants: phenytoin possibly reduces plasma
  concentration of •apixaban; phenytoin accelerates
  metabolism of •coumarins (possibility of reduced
  anticoagulant effect, but enhancement also
  reported); phenytoin possibly reduces plasma concentration of dabigatran—manufacturer of dabigatran advises avoid concomitant use; phenytoin possibly reduces plasma concentration of
  •rivaroxaban—manufacturer of rivaroxaban advises
  monitor for signs of thrombosis
- Antidepressants: plasma concentration of phenytoin
  increased by •fluoxetine and •fluvoxamine; pheny-

Phenytoin
- Antidepressants *(continued)*
  toin reduces plasma concentration of •mianserin,
  mirtazapine and paroxetine; plasma concentration
  of phenytoin possibly increased by sertraline, also
  plasma concentration of sertraline possibly reduced;
  anticonvulsant effect of antiepileptics possibly
  antagonised by MAOIs and •tricyclic-related antidepressants (convulsive threshold lowered); anticonvulsant effect of antiepileptics antagonised by
  •SSRIs and •tricyclics (convulsive threshold lowered); plasma concentration of phenytoin possibly
  reduced by •St John's wort—avoid concomitant
  use; phenytoin possibly reduces plasma concentration of •tricyclics
  Antidiabetics: plasma concentration of phenytoin
  transiently increased by tolbutamide (possibility of
  toxicity)
- Antiepileptics: plasma concentration of both drugs
  often reduced when phenytoin given with carbamazepine, also plasma concentration of phenytoin
  may be increased; phenytoin reduces plasma concentration of eslicarbazepine, also plasma concentration of phenytoin increased; plasma concentration of phenytoin possibly increased by
  •ethosuximide, also plasma concentration of ethosuximide possibly reduced; phenytoin reduces
  plasma concentration of lamotrigine, tiagabine and
  zonisamide; plasma concentration of phenytoin
  increased by oxcarbazepine, also plasma concentration of an active metabolite of oxcarbazepine
  reduced; phenytoin reduces plasma concentration
  of •perampanel (see Dose under Perampanel,
  p. 313); phenytoin often increases plasma concentration of phenobarbital, plasma concentration of
  phenytoin often reduced but may be increased;
  phenytoin possibly reduces plasma concentration of
  retigabine; phenytoin possibly reduces plasma concentration of rufinamide, also plasma concentration
  of phenytoin possibly increased; plasma concentration of phenytoin increased by •stiripentol; plasma
  concentration of phenytoin increased by •topira-
  mate (also plasma concentration of topiramate
  reduced); plasma concentration of phenytoin
  increased or possibly reduced when given with valproate, also plasma concentration of valproate
  reduced; plasma concentration of phenytoin
  reduced by vigabatrin
- Antifungals: anticonvulsant effect of phenytoin
  enhanced by •miconazole (plasma concentration of
  phenytoin increased); plasma concentration of
  phenytoin increased by •fluconazole (consider reducing dose of phenytoin); phenytoin reduces plasma
  concentration of •itraconazole—avoid concomitant
  use; phenytoin reduces plasma concentration of
  •posaconazole; plasma concentration of phenytoin
  increased by •voriconazole, also phenytoin reduces
  plasma concentration of voriconazole (increase
  dose of voriconazole and also monitor for phenytoin toxicity); phenytoin possibly reduces plasma
  concentration of caspofungin—consider increasing
  dose of caspofungin
- Antimalarials: avoidance of phenytoin advised by
  manufacturer of piperaquine with artenimol; anticonvulsant effect of antiepileptics antagonised by
  •mefloquine; anticonvulsant effect of phenytoin
  antagonised by •pyrimethamine, also increased
  antifolate effect
- Antipsychotics: anticonvulsant effect of antiepileptics
  antagonised by •antipsychotics (convulsive threshold lowered); phenytoin reduces plasma concentration of haloperidol; plasma concentration of phenytoin possibly increased or decreased by
  chlorpromazine; phenytoin possibly reduces plasma
  concentration of •aripiprazole (avoid concomitant
  use or consider increasing the dose of aripipra-

Phenytoin

- Antipsychotics *(continued)*

    zole—consult aripiprazole product literature); phenytoin accelerates metabolism of clozapine and quetiapine (reduced plasma concentration); phenytoin possibly reduces plasma concentration of •lurasidone—avoid concomitant use

- Antivirals: phenytoin possibly reduces plasma concentration of abacavir, darunavir, lopinavir and saquinavir; avoidance of phenytoin advised by manufacturer of •boceprevir and •rilpivirine (plasma concentration of boceprevir and rilpivirine possibly reduced); phenytoin possibly reduces plasma concentration of •daclatasvir and •simeprevir—manufacturer of daclatasvir and simeprevir advises avoid concomitant use; avoidance of phenytoin advised by manufacturer of dolutegravir, •elvitegravir, etravirine, sofosbuvir and •telaprevir; phenytoin possibly reduces plasma concentration of •indinavir, also plasma concentration of phenytoin possibly increased; phenytoin possibly reduces plasma concentration of ritonavir, also plasma concentration of phenytoin possibly affected; plasma concentration of phenytoin increased or decreased by zidovudine

    Anxiolytics and Hypnotics: phenytoin often reduces plasma concentration of clonazepam; plasma concentration of phenytoin increased or decreased by diazepam; plasma concentration of phenytoin possibly increased or decreased by benzodiazepines

    Aprepitant: phenytoin possibly reduces plasma concentration of aprepitant

    Bupropion: phenytoin reduces plasma concentration of bupropion

    Caffeine citrate: phenytoin reduces plasma concentration of caffeine citrate

- Calcium-channel Blockers: phenytoin reduces effects of felodipine and verapamil; avoidance of phenytoin advised by manufacturer of isradipine; avoidance of phenytoin advised by manufacturer of nimodipine (plasma concentration of nimodipine possibly reduced); plasma concentration of phenytoin increased by •diltiazem but also effect of diltiazem reduced

- Cannabis Extract: phenytoin possibly reduces plasma concentration of •cannabis extract—manufacturer of cannabis extract advises avoid concomitant use

- Cardiac Glycosides: phenytoin possibly reduces plasma concentration of digoxin

- Ciclosporin: phenytoin accelerates metabolism of •ciclosporin (reduced plasma concentration)

- Cobicistat: phenytoin possibly reduces plasma concentration of •cobicistat—manufacturer of cobicistat advises avoid concomitant use

- Corticosteroids: phenytoin accelerates metabolism of •corticosteroids (reduced effect)

- Cytotoxics: phenytoin possibly reduces plasma concentration of busulfan, eribulin and etoposide; metabolism of phenytoin possibly inhibited by fluorouracil (increased risk of toxicity); phenytoin increases antifolate effect of methotrexate; plasma concentration of phenytoin possibly reduced by cisplatin; phenytoin possibly decreases plasma concentration of axitinib (increase dose of axitinib—consult axitinib product literature); phenytoin possibly reduces plasma concentration of bortezomib, •bosutinib, crizotinib, •ibrutinib, •idelalisib and ponatinib—manufacturer of bortezomib, bosutinib, crizotinib, ibrutinib, idelalisib and ponatinib advises avoid concomitant use; phenytoin possibly reduces plasma concentration of •cabozantinib—avoid concomitant use; avoidance of phenytoin advised by manufacturer of •cabazitaxel, dabrafenib, gefitinib, •lapatinib and vemurafenib; phenytoin reduces plasma concentration of •imatinib—avoid concomitant use; phenytoin reduces plasma concentration of irinotecan and its active metabolite; manufac-

Phenytoin

- Cytotoxics *(continued)*

    turer of procarbazine advises possible increased risk of hypersensitivity reactions when phenytoin given with procarbazine; avoidance of phenytoin advised by manufacturer of •vismodegib (plasma concentration of vismodegib possibly reduced)

- Dexrazoxane: phenytoin possibly reduces absorption of •dexrazoxane

    Diazoxide: plasma concentration of phenytoin reduced by diazoxide, also effect of diazoxide may be reduced

- Disulfiram: metabolism of phenytoin inhibited by •disulfiram (increased risk of toxicity)

- Diuretics: plasma concentration of phenytoin possibly increased by •acetazolamide; phenytoin antagonises effects of furosemide; phenytoin reduces plasma concentration of •eplerenone—avoid concomitant use; increased risk of osteomalacia when phenytoin given with carbonic anhydrase inhibitors

    Dopaminergics: phenytoin possibly reduces effects of levodopa

    Enteral Foods: absorption of phenytoin possibly reduced by enteral feeds

    Folates: plasma concentration of phenytoin possibly reduced by folates

- Hormone Antagonists: phenytoin possibly reduces plasma concentration of •abiraterone—manufacturer of abiraterone advises avoid concomitant use; phenytoin possibly accelerates metabolism of toremifene

    5HT$_3$-receptor Antagonists: phenytoin accelerates metabolism of ondansetron (reduced effect)

- Ivacaftor: phenytoin possibly reduces plasma concentration of •ivacaftor—manufacturer of ivacaftor advises avoid concomitant use

    Leflunomide: plasma concentration of phenytoin possibly increased by leflunomide

    Levamisole: plasma concentration of phenytoin possibly increased by levamisole

    Lipid-regulating Drugs: absorption of phenytoin possibly reduced by colesevelam; combination of phenytoin with fluvastatin may increase plasma concentration of either drug (or both)

    Lithium: neurotoxicity may occur when phenytoin given with lithium without increased plasma concentration of lithium

    Macitentan: avoidance of phenytoin advised by manufacturer of macitentan

    Modafinil: plasma concentration of phenytoin possibly increased by modafinil

- Muscle Relaxants: *long-term use* of phenytoin reduces effects of •non-depolarising muscle relaxants (but *acute use* of phenytoin might increase effects of non-depolarising muscle relaxants)

- Oestrogens: phenytoin accelerates metabolism of •oestrogens (reduced contraceptive effect—see p. 548)

- Orlistat: possible increased risk of convulsions when antiepileptics given with •orlistat

- Progestogens: phenytoin accelerates metabolism of •progestogens (reduced contraceptive effect—see p. 548)

    Roflumilast: phenytoin possibly inhibits effects of roflumilast (manufacturer of roflumilast advises avoid concomitant use)

- Sulfinpyrazone: plasma concentration of phenytoin increased by •sulfinpyrazone

    Sympathomimetics: plasma concentration of phenytoin increased by methylphenidate

    Tacrolimus: phenytoin reduces plasma concentration of tacrolimus, also plasma concentration of phenytoin possibly increased

- Theophylline: plasma concentration of both drugs reduced when phenytoin given with •theophylline

Appendix 1: Interactions

Phenytoin *(continued)*

Thyroid Hormones: phenytoin accelerates metabolism of thyroid hormones (may increase requirements in hypothyroidism), also plasma concentration of phenytoin possibly increased

Tibolone: phenytoin accelerates metabolism of tibolone

Ticagrelor: phenytoin possibly reduces plasma concentration of ticagrelor

- Ulcer-healing Drugs: metabolism of phenytoin inhibited by ●cimetidine (increased plasma concentration); effects of phenytoin enhanced by ●esomeprazole; effects of phenytoin possibly enhanced by omeprazole; absorption of phenytoin reduced by ●sucralfate
- Ulipristal: avoidance of phenytoin advised by manufacturer of ●ulipristal (contraceptive effect of ulipristal possibly reduced)

Vaccines: effects of phenytoin enhanced by influenza vaccine

Vitamins: phenytoin possibly increases requirements for vitamin D

Pholcodine

Antidepressants: manufacturer of pholcodine advises avoid for 2 weeks after stopping MAOIs

Phosphodiesterase Type-3 Inhibitors

- Anagrelide: avoidance of enoximone and milrinone advised by manufacturer of ●anagrelide

Pilocarpine *see* Parasympathomimetics

Pimozide *see* Antipsychotics

Pindolol *see* Beta-blockers

Pioglitazone *see* Antidiabetics

Piperacillin *see* Penicillins

Piperaquine *see* Piperaquine with Artenimol

Piperaquine with Artenimol

Note Piperaquine has a long half-life; there is a potential for drug interactions to occur for up to 3 months after treatment has been stopped

- Analgesics: manufacturer of piperaquine with artenimol advises avoid concomitant use with ●methadone (possible risk of ventricular arrhythmias)
- Anti-arrhythmics: manufacturer of piperaquine with artenimol advises avoid concomitant use with ●amiodarone and ●disopyramide (possible risk of ventricular arrhythmias)
- Antibacterials: manufacturer of piperaquine with artenimol advises avoid concomitant use with ●macrolides and ●moxifloxacin (possible risk of ventricular arrhythmias); manufacturer of piperaquine with artenimol advises avoid concomitant use with rifampicin
- Antidepressants: avoidance of antimalarials advised by manufacturer of ●citalopram and ●escitalopram (risk of ventricular arrhythmias); manufacturer of piperaquine with artenimol advises avoid concomitant use with ●antidepressants

Antiepileptics: manufacturer of piperaquine with artenimol advises avoid concomitant use with carbamazepine, phenobarbital and phenytoin

- Antifungals: manufacturer of piperaquine with artenimol advises avoid concomitant use with ●imidazoles and ●triazoles (possible risk of ventricular arrhythmias)
- Antihistamines: manufacturer of piperaquine with artenimol advises avoid concomitant use with ●mizolastine (possible risk of ventricular arrhythmias)
- Antimalarials: avoidance of antimalarials advised by manufacturer of ●artemether with lumefantrine
- Antipsychotics: manufacturer of piperaquine with artenimol advises avoid concomitant use with ●droperidol, ●haloperidol, ●phenothiazines and ●pimozide (possible risk of ventricular arrhythmias)
- Antivirals: manufacturer of piperaquine with artenimol advises avoid concomitant use with ●saquinavir (possible risk of ventricular arrhythmias)

Piperaquine with Artenimol *(continued)*

- Beta-blockers: manufacturer of piperaquine with artenimol advises avoid concomitant use with ●sotalol (possible risk of ventricular arrhythmias)
- Cytotoxics: manufacturer of piperaquine with artenimol advises avoid concomitant use with ●arsenic trioxide (possible risk of ventricular arrhythmias); manufacturer of piperaquine with artenimol advises avoid concomitant use with ●vinblastine, ●vincristine, ●vinflunine and ●vinorelbine
- Domperidone: manufacturer of piperaquine with artenimol advises avoid concomitant use with ●domperidone (possible risk of ventricular arrhythmias)

Grapefruit Juice: manufacturer of piperaquine with artenimol advises avoid concomitant use with grapefruit juice

Histamine: avoidance of antimalarials advised by manufacturer of histamine

- Pentamidine Isetionate: manufacturer of piperaquine with artenimol advises avoid concomitant use with ●pentamidine isetionate (possible risk of ventricular arrhythmias)

Vaccines: antimalarials inactivate oral typhoid vaccine—see p. 864

Pipotiazine *see* Antipsychotics

Pirfenidone

- Antibacterials: plasma concentration of pirfenidone increased by ●ciprofloxacin—see Cautions under Pirfenidone, p. 223
- Antidepressants: plasma concentration of pirfenidone increased by ●fluvoxamine—manufacturer of pirfenidone advises avoid concomitant use

Grapefruit Juice: manufacturer of pirfenidone advises avoid concomitant use with grapefruit juice

Piroxicam *see* NSAIDs

Pivmecillinam *see* Penicillins

Pixantrone

- Antipsychotics: avoid concomitant use of cytotoxics with ●clozapine (increased risk of agranulocytosis)
- Vaccines: avoid concomitant use of pixantrone with live ●vaccines (see p. 842)

Pizotifen

Adrenergic Neurone Blockers: pizotifen antagonises hypotensive effect of adrenergic neurone blockers

Platinum Compounds

- Aldesleukin: avoidance of cisplatin advised by manufacturer of ●aldesleukin
- Antibacterials: increased risk of nephrotoxicity and possibly of ototoxicity when platinum compounds given with ●aminoglycosides or ●polymyxins; increased risk of nephrotoxicity and ototoxicity when platinum compounds given with capreomycin; increased risk of nephrotoxicity and possibly of ototoxicity when cisplatin given with vancomycin

Antiepileptics: cisplatin possibly reduces plasma concentration of phenytoin

- Antipsychotics: avoid concomitant use of cytotoxics with ●clozapine (increased risk of agranulocytosis)
- Cytotoxics: increased risk of otoxicity when cisplatin given with ifosfamide; increased pulmonary toxicity when cisplatin given with ●bleomycin and ●methotrexate

Diuretics: increased risk of nephrotoxicity and ototoxicity when platinum compounds given with diuretics

Pneumococcal vaccine *see* Vaccines

Poliomyelitis vaccine *see* Vaccines

Polymyxin B *see* Polymyxins

Polymyxins

Antibacterials: increased risk of nephrotoxicity when colistimethate sodium or polymyxins given with aminoglycosides; increased risk of nephrotoxicity when colistimethate sodium or polymyxins given with capreomycin; increased risk of nephrotoxicity when polymyxins given with vancomycin; increased risk of nephrotoxicity and ototoxicity when colistimethate sodium given with vancomycin

Polymyxins (continued)

  Antifungals: increased risk of nephrotoxicity when polymyxins given with amphotericin

- Ciclosporin: increased risk of nephrotoxicity when polymyxins given with ●ciclosporin
- Cytotoxics: increased risk of nephrotoxicity and possibly of ototoxicity when polymyxins given with ●platinum compounds
- Diuretics: increased risk of otoxicity when polymyxins given with ●loop diuretics
- Muscle Relaxants: polymyxins enhance effects of ●non-depolarising muscle relaxants and ●suxamethonium
- Parasympathomimetics: polymyxins antagonise effects of ●neostigmine and ●pyridostigmine

  Vaccines: antibacterials inactivate oral typhoid vaccine—see p. 864

Polystyrene Sulfonate Resins

  Antacids: risk of intestinal obstruction when polystyrene sulfonate resins given with aluminium hydroxide; risk of metabolic alkalosis when polystyrene sulfonate resins given with oral magnesium salts

  Thyroid Hormones: polystyrene sulfonate resins reduce absorption of levothyroxine

Pomalidomide

- Antidepressants: plasma concentration of pomalidomide increased by ●fluvoxamine

Ponatinib

- Antibacterials: plasma concentration of ponatinib possibly increased by clarithromycin and telithromycin—consider reducing initial dose of ponatinib (see Dose under Ponatinib, p. 618); plasma concentration of ponatinib possibly reduced by rifabutin—manufacturer of ponatinib advises avoid concomitant use; plasma concentration of ponatinib reduced by ●rifampicin—manufacturer of ponatinib advises avoid concomitant use

  Antidepressants: plasma concentration of ponatinib possibly reduced by St John's wort—manufacturer of ponatinib advises avoid concomitant use

  Antiepileptics: plasma concentration of ponatinib possibly reduced by carbamazepine, phenobarbital and phenytoin—manufacturer of ponatinib advises avoid concomitant use

  Antifungals: plasma concentration of ponatinib possibly increased by itraconazole and voriconazole—consider reducing initial dose of ponatinib (see Dose under Ponatinib, p. 618)

- Antipsychotics: avoid concomitant use of cytotoxics with ●clozapine (increased risk of agranulocytosis)

  Antivirals: plasma concentration of ponatinib possibly increased by indinavir, ritonavir and saquinavir—consider reducing initial dose of ponatinib (see Dose under Ponatinib, p. 618)

  Grapefruit Juice: plasma concentration of ponatinib possibly increased by grapefruit juice

Posaconazole see Antifungals, Triazole

Potassium Canrenoate see Diuretics

Potassium Aminobenzoate

  Antibacterials: potassium aminobenzoate inhibits effects of sulfonamides

Potassium Bicarbonate see Potassium Salts

Potassium Chloride see Potassium Salts

Potassium Citrate see Potassium Salts

Potassium Salts

  Note Includes salt substitutes

- ACE Inhibitors: increased risk of severe hyperkalaemia when potassium salts given with ●ACE inhibitors

  Aliskiren: increased risk of hyperkalaemia when potassium salts given with aliskiren

- Angiotensin-II Receptor Antagonists: increased risk of hyperkalaemia when potassium salts given with ●angiotensin-II receptor antagonists

  Antibacterials: avoid concomitant use of potassium citrate with methenamine

Potassium Salts (continued)

- Ciclosporin: increased risk of hyperkalaemia when potassium salts given with ●ciclosporin
- Diuretics: increased risk of hyperkalaemia when potassium salts given with ●potassium-sparing diuretics and aldosterone antagonists
- Tacrolimus: increased risk of hyperkalaemia when potassium salts given with ●tacrolimus

  Ulcer-healing Drugs: avoidance of potassium citrate advised by manufacturer of sucralfate

Pramipexole

  Antipsychotics: manufacturer of pramipexole advises avoid concomitant use of antipsychotics (antagonism of effect)

  Memantine: effects of dopaminergics possibly enhanced by memantine

  Methyldopa: antiparkinsonian effect of dopaminergics antagonised by methyldopa

  Ulcer-healing Drugs: excretion of pramipexole reduced by cimetidine (increased plasma concentration)

Prasugrel

  Analgesics: possible increased risk of bleeding when prasugrel given with NSAIDs

  Anticoagulants: possible increased risk of bleeding when prasugrel given with coumarins or phenindione

  Clopidogrel: possible increased risk of bleeding when prasugrel given with clopidogrel

Pravastatin see Statins

Prazosin see Alpha-blockers

Prednisolone see Corticosteroids

Prednisone see Corticosteroids

Pregabalin

- Antidepressants: anticonvulsant effect of antiepileptics possibly antagonised by MAOIs and ●tricyclic-related antidepressants (convulsive threshold lowered); anticonvulsant effect of antiepileptics antagonised by ●SSRIs and ●tricyclics (convulsive threshold lowered)
- Antimalarials: anticonvulsant effect of antiepileptics antagonised by ●mefloquine
- Antipsychotics: anticonvulsant effect of antiepileptics antagonised by ●antipsychotics (convulsive threshold lowered)
- Orlistat: possible increased risk of convulsions when antiepileptics given with ●orlistat

Prilocaine

  Anti-arrhythmics: increased myocardial depression when prilocaine given with anti-arrhythmics

  Antibacterials: increased risk of methaemoglobinaemia when prilocaine given with sulfonamides

Primaquine

- Antidepressants: avoidance of antimalarials advised by manufacturer of ●citalopram and ●escitalopram (risk of ventricular arrhythmias)
- Antimalarials: avoidance of antimalarials advised by manufacturer of ●artemether with lumefantrine

  Histamine: avoidance of antimalarials advised by manufacturer of histamine

  Mepacrine: plasma concentration of primaquine increased by mepacrine (increased risk of toxicity)

  Vaccines: antimalarials inactivate oral typhoid vaccine—see p. 864

Primidone see Phenobarbital

Procarbazine

  Alcohol: disulfiram-like reaction when procarbazine given with alcohol

  Antiepileptics: manufacturer of procarbazine advises possible increased risk of hypersensitivity reactions when given with carbamazepine, phenobarbital and phenytoin

- Antipsychotics: avoid concomitant use of cytotoxics with ●clozapine (increased risk of agranulocytosis)

  Cardiac Glycosides: procarbazine possibly reduces absorption of digoxin *tablets*

Prochlorperazine see Antipsychotics

Procyclidine *see* Antimuscarinics
Progesterone *see* Progestogens
Progestogens

Note Interactions of combined oral contraceptives may also apply to combined contraceptive patches and vaginal rings, see p. 548. For further information on interactions of oral progestogen-only contraceptives, see also p. 551; parenteral progestogen-only contraceptives, see also p. 555; the intra-uterine progestogen-only device, see also p. 556; hormonal emergency contraception, see also p. 559

- Antibacterials: plasma concentration of dienogest increased by erythromycin; metabolism of progestogens accelerated by ●rifamycins (reduced contraceptive effect—see p. 548)
- Anticoagulants: progestogens may enhance or reduce anticoagulant effect of coumarins; progestogens antagonise anticoagulant effect of ●phenindione
- Antidepressants: contraceptive effect of progestogens reduced by ●St John's wort (avoid concomitant use)

  Antidiabetics: progestogens antagonise hypoglycaemic effect of antidiabetics
- Antiepileptics: metabolism of progestogens accelerated by ●carbamazepine, ●eslicarbazepine, ●oxcarbazepine, ●perampanel, ●phenobarbital, ●phenytoin, ●rufinamide and ●topiramate (reduced contraceptive effect—see p. 548); desogestrel possibly increases plasma concentration of lamotrigine

  Antifungals: progestogens possibly increase plasma concentration of voriconazole; anecdotal reports of contraceptive failure and menstrual irregularities when progestogens given with griseofulvin; occasional reports of breakthrough bleeding when progestogens (used for contraception) given with terbinafine
- Antivirals: plasma concentration of norethisterone increased by atazanavir; plasma concentration of drospirenone increased by boceprevir (increased risk of toxicity); contraceptive effect of progestogens possibly reduced by ●efavirenz; plasma concentration of norgestimate increased by elvitegravir; metabolism of progestogens accelerated by ●nevirapine (reduced contraceptive effect—see p. 548)

  Anxiolytics and Hypnotics: progestogens possibly increase plasma concentration of chlordiazepoxide, diazepam and nitrazepam; progestogens possibly reduce plasma concentration of lorazepam, oxazepam and temazepam
- Aprepitant: possible contraceptive failure of hormonal contraceptives containing progestogens when given with ●aprepitant (alternative contraception recommended)
- Bosentan: possible contraceptive failure of hormonal contraceptives containing progestogens when given with ●bosentan (alternative contraception recommended)

  Ciclosporin: progestogens possibly increase plasma concentration of ciclosporin

  Cobicistat: plasma concentration of norgestimate increased by cobicistat
- Cytotoxics: possible reduction in contraceptive effect of progestogens advised by manufacturer of ●crizotinib and ●vemurafenib; possible reduced contraceptive effect of hormonal contraceptives containing progestogens advised by manufacturer of ●dabrafenib (alternative contraception recommended)

  Diuretics: risk of hyperkalaemia when drospirenone given with potassium-sparing diuretics and aldosterone antagonists (monitor serum potassium during first cycle)
- Dopaminergics: progestogens increase plasma concentration of ●selegiline—manufacturer of selegiline advises avoid concomitant use

  Lipid-regulating Drugs: plasma concentration of norethisterone increased by atorvastatin; plasma concentration of active metabolite of norgestimate

Progestogens
  Lipid-regulating Drugs *(continued)*
    increased by rosuvastatin; plasma concentration of norgestrel increased by rosuvastatin

  Muscle Relaxants: progestogens possibly increase plasma concentration of tizanidine (increased risk of toxicity)

  Sugammadex: plasma concentration of progestogens possibly reduced by sugammadex—manufacturer of sugammadex advises additional contraceptive precautions

  Teriflunomide: plasma concentration of levonorgestrel increased by teriflunomide
- Ulipristal: contraceptive effect of progestogens possibly reduced by ●ulipristal

Proguanil
  Antacids: absorption of proguanil reduced by oral magnesium salts (as magnesium trisilicate)

  Anticoagulants: isolated reports that proguanil may enhance anticoagulant effect of warfarin
- Antidepressants: avoidance of antimalarials advised by manufacturer of ●citalopram and ●escitalopram (risk of ventricular arrhythmias)
- Antimalarials: avoidance of antimalarials advised by manufacturer of ●artemether with lumefantrine; increased antifolate effect when proguanil given with pyrimethamine

  Antivirals: plasma concentration of proguanil possibly affected by efavirenz

  Histamine: avoidance of antimalarials advised by manufacturer of histamine

  Vaccines: antimalarials inactivate oral typhoid vaccine—see p. 864

Promazine *see* Antipsychotics
Promethazine *see* Antihistamines
Propafenone
  Anaesthetics, Local: increased myocardial depression when anti-arrhythmics given with bupivacaine, levobupivacaine, prilocaine or ropivacaine
- Anti-arrhythmics: increased myocardial depression when anti-arrhythmics given with other ●anti-arrhythmics
- Antibacterials: metabolism of propafenone accelerated by ●rifampicin (reduced effect)
- Anticoagulants: propafenone enhances anticoagulant effect of ●coumarins
- Antidepressants: metabolism of propafenone possibly inhibited by fluoxetine and paroxetine; increased risk of arrhythmias when propafenone given with ●tricyclics

  Antiepileptics: metabolism of propafenone possibly accelerated by phenobarbital

  Antihistamines: avoidance of propafenone advised by manufacturer of mizolastine (possible risk of ventricular arrhythmias)
- Antipsychotics: increased risk of ventricular arrhythmias when anti-arrhythmics that prolong the QT interval given with ●antipsychotics that prolong the QT interval
- Antivirals: plasma concentration of propafenone possibly increased by ●fosamprenavir (increased risk of ventricular arrhythmias—avoid concomitant use); plasma concentration of propafenone increased by ●ritonavir (increased risk of ventricular arrhythmias—avoid concomitant use); increased risk of ventricular arrhythmias when propafenone given with ●saquinavir—avoid concomitant use; caution with propafenone advised by manufacturer of ●telaprevir (risk of ventricular arrhythmias)
- Beta-blockers: increased myocardial depression when anti-arrhythmics given with ●beta-blockers; propafenone increases plasma concentration of metoprolol and propranolol
- Cardiac Glycosides: propafenone increases plasma concentration of ●digoxin (halve dose of digoxin)

Propafenone *(continued)*

Ciclosporin: propafenone possibly increases plasma concentration of ciclosporin

Parasympathomimetics: propafenone possibly antagonises effects of neostigmine and pyridostigmine

Theophylline: propafenone increases plasma concentration of theophylline

- Ulcer-healing Drugs: plasma concentration of propafenone increased by ●cimetidine

Propantheline *see* Antimuscarinics

Propiverine *see* Antimuscarinics

Propofol *see* Anaesthetics, General

Propranolol *see* Beta-blockers

Prostaglandins

ACE Inhibitors: enhanced hypotensive effect when alprostadil given with ACE inhibitors

Adrenergic Neurone Blockers: enhanced hypotensive effect when alprostadil given with adrenergic neurone blockers

Alpha-blockers: enhanced hypotensive effect when alprostadil given with alpha-blockers

Angiotensin-II Receptor Antagonists: enhanced hypotensive effect when alprostadil given with angiotensin-II receptor antagonists

Beta-blockers: enhanced hypotensive effect when alprostadil given with beta-blockers

Calcium-channel Blockers: enhanced hypotensive effect when alprostadil given with calcium-channel blockers

Clonidine: enhanced hypotensive effect when alprostadil given with clonidine

Diazoxide: enhanced hypotensive effect when alprostadil given with diazoxide

Diuretics: enhanced hypotensive effect when alprostadil given with diuretics

Methyldopa: enhanced hypotensive effect when alprostadil given with methyldopa

Moxonidine: enhanced hypotensive effect when alprostadil given with moxonidine

Nitrates: enhanced hypotensive effect when alprostadil given with nitrates

Oxytocin: prostaglandins potentiate uterotonic effect of oxytocin

Vasodilator Antihypertensives: enhanced hypotensive effect when alprostadil given with hydralazine, minoxidil or sodium nitroprusside

Protein Kinase Inhibitors *see* individual drugs

Proton Pump Inhibitors

Antacids: absorption of lansoprazole possibly reduced by antacids

Antibacterials: plasma concentration of both drugs increased when omeprazole given with clarithromycin

- Anticoagulants: esomeprazole and omeprazole possibly enhance anticoagulant effect of ●coumarins; pantoprazole might enhance the anticoagulant effect of coumarins

Antidepressants: omeprazole increases plasma concentration of escitalopram; plasma concentration of lansoprazole possibly increased by fluvoxamine; plasma concentration of omeprazole possibly reduced by St John's wort

- Antiepileptics: esomeprazole enhances effects of ●phenytoin; omeprazole possibly enhances effects of phenytoin

- Antifungals: proton pump inhibitors reduce absorption of itraconazole; esomeprazole reduces plasma concentration of ●posaconazole—manufacturer of posaconazole *suspension* advises avoid concomitant use; lansoprazole, omeprazole, pantoprazole and rabeprazole possibly reduce plasma concentration of ●posaconazole—manufacturer of posaconazole *suspension* advises avoid concomitant use; plasma concentration of esomeprazole possibly increased by voriconazole; plasma concentration of ome-

Proton Pump Inhibitors

- Antifungals *(continued)*

prazole increased by voriconazole (consider reducing dose of omeprazole)

Antipsychotics: omeprazole possibly reduces plasma concentration of clozapine

- Antivirals: proton pump inhibitors reduce plasma concentration of ●atazanavir—avoid or adjust dose of both drugs (consult product literature); omeprazole increases plasma concentration of raltegravir; avoidance of esomeprazole, lansoprazole, pantoprazole and rabeprazole advised by manufacturer of rilpivirine (plasma concentration of rilpivirine possibly reduced); omeprazole reduces plasma concentration of ●rilpivirine—avoid concomitant use; esomeprazole, lansoprazole, pantoprazole and rabeprazole possibly increase plasma concentration of ●saquinavir—manufacturer of saquinavir advises avoid concomitant use; omeprazole increases plasma concentration of ●saquinavir—manufacturer of saquinavir advises avoid concomitant use; plasma concentration of esomeprazole and omeprazole reduced by ●tipranavir

Anxiolytics and Hypnotics: esomeprazole and omeprazole possibly inhibit metabolism of diazepam (increased plasma concentration)

Cardiac Glycosides: proton pump inhibitors possibly slightly increase plasma concentration of digoxin

Ciclosporin: omeprazole possibly affects plasma concentration of ciclosporin

- Cilostazol: omeprazole increases plasma concentrations of ●cilostazol (see Dose under Cilostazol, p. 141)

- Clopidogrel: esomeprazole and omeprazole reduce antiplatelet effect of ●clopidogrel; lansoprazole, pantoprazole and rabeprazole possibly reduce antiplatelet effect of clopidogrel

- Cytotoxics: proton pump inhibitors possibly reduce excretion of methotrexate (increased risk of toxicity); lansoprazole reduces plasma concentration of bosutinib; avoidance of proton pump inhibitors advised by manufacturer of dabrafenib (plasma concentration of dabrafenib possibly reduced); avoidance of esomeprazole, lansoprazole, pantoprazole and rabeprazole advised by manufacturer of ●erlotinib; omeprazole reduces plasma concentration of ●erlotinib—manufacturer of erlotinib advises avoid concomitant use; proton pump inhibitors possibly reduce absorption of lapatinib; proton pump inhibitors possibly reduce absorption of pazopanib—manufacturer of pazopanib advises give at the same time as proton pump inhibitors

Tacrolimus: omeprazole possibly increases plasma concentration of tacrolimus

Ulcer-healing Drugs: absorption of lansoprazole possibly reduced by sucralfate

Pseudoephedrine *see* Sympathomimetics

Pyrazinamide

Sulfinpyrazone: pyrazinamide antagonises effects of sulfinpyrazone

Vaccines: antibacterials inactivate oral typhoid vaccine—see p. 864

Pyridostigmine *see* Parasympathomimetics

Pyridoxine *see* Vitamins

Pyrimethamine

- Antibacterials: increased antifolate effect when pyrimethamine given with ●sulfonamides or ●trimethoprim

- Antidepressants: avoidance of antimalarials advised by manufacturer of ●citalopram and ●escitalopram (risk of ventricular arrhythmias)

- Antiepileptics: pyrimethamine antagonises anticonvulsant effect of ●phenytoin, also increased antifolate effect

- Antimalarials: avoidance of antimalarials advised by manufacturer of ●artemether with lumefantrine;

Pyrimethamine

- **Antimalarials** *(continued)*
  increased antifolate effect when pyrimethamine
  given with proguanil
  Antivirals: increased antifolate effect when pyrimethamine given with zidovudine
- **Cytotoxics:** pyrimethamine increases antifolate effect
  of ●methotrexate and ●pemetrexed
  Histamine: avoidance of antimalarials advised by
  manufacturer of histamine
  Vaccines: antimalarials inactivate oral typhoid
  vaccine—see p. 864

Quetiapine *see* Antipsychotics

Quinagolide

Memantine: effects of dopaminergics possibly
enhanced by memantine
Methyldopa: antiparkinsonian effect of dopaminergics
antagonised by methyldopa

Quinapril *see* ACE Inhibitors

Quinine

- **Anti-arrhythmics:** increased risk of ventricular arrhythmias when quinine given with ●amiodarone—avoid
  concomitant use; quinine increases plasma concentration of ●flecainide
- **Antibacterials:** increased risk of ventricular arrhythmias when quinine given with ●moxifloxacin—
  avoid concomitant use; plasma concentration of
  quinine reduced by ●rifampicin
  Anticoagulants: plasma concentration of both drugs
  increased when quinine given with warfarin
  Antidepressants: avoidance of antimalarials advised
  by manufacturer of ●citalopram and ●escitalopram
  (risk of ventricular arrhythmias)
- **Antimalarials:** avoidance of antimalarials advised by
  manufacturer of ●artemether with lumefantrine;
  increased risk of ventricular arrhythmias when quinine given with ●artemether with lumefantrine;
  increased risk of convulsions when quinine given
  with ●mefloquine (but should not prevent the use of
  intravenous quinine in severe cases)
- **Antipsychotics:** increased risk of ventricular arrhythmias when quinine given with ●droperidol or
  ●pimozide—avoid concomitant use; possible
  increased risk of ventricular arrhythmias when quinine given with ●haloperidol—avoid concomitant
  use; possible increased risk of ventricular arrhythmias when quinine given with ●risperidone
- **Antivirals:** plasma concentration of quinine possibly
  increased by ●atazanavir, ●darunavir,
  ●fosamprenavir, ●indinavir and ●tipranavir
  (increased risk of toxicity); plasma concentration of
  quinine increased by ●ritonavir (increased risk of
  toxicity); increased risk of ventricular arrhythmias
  when quinine given with ●saquinavir—avoid concomitant use
- **Cardiac Glycosides:** quinine increases plasma concentration of ●digoxin
  Dopaminergics: quinine possibly increases plasma
  concentration of amantadine
  Histamine: avoidance of antimalarials advised by
  manufacturer of histamine
  Muscle Relaxants: quinine possibly enhances effects
  of suxamethonium
  Ulcer-healing Drugs: metabolism of quinine inhibited
  by cimetidine (increased plasma concentration)
  Vaccines: antimalarials inactivate oral typhoid
  vaccine—see p. 864

Quinolones

- **Analgesics:** possible increased risk of convulsions
  when quinolones given with ●NSAIDs
  Antacids: absorption of ciprofloxacin, levofloxacin,
  moxifloxacin, norfloxacin and ofloxacin reduced by
  antacids
- **Anti-arrhythmics:** increased risk of ventricular arrhythmias when levofloxacin or moxifloxacin given with
  ●amiodarone—avoid concomitant use; increased

Quinolones

- **Anti-arrhythmics** *(continued)*
  risk of ventricular arrhythmias when moxifloxacin
  given with ●disopyramide—avoid concomitant use
- **Antibacterials:** increased risk of ventricular arrhythmias when moxifloxacin given with *parenteral*
  ●erythromycin—avoid concomitant use; avoidance
  of moxifloxacin advised by manufacturer of bedaquiline; ciprofloxacin possibly increases plasma concentration of bedaquiline—avoid concomitant use if
  ciprofloxacin given for more than 14 days;
  increased risk of ventricular arrhythmias when moxifloxacin given with ●delamanid; effects of nalidixic
  acid possibly antagonised by nitrofurantoin; possible increased risk of ventricular arrhythmias when
  moxifloxacin given with ●telithromycin
- **Anticoagulants:** ciprofloxacin and levofloxacin possibly enhance anticoagulant effect of coumarins; nalidixic acid, norfloxacin and ofloxacin enhance anticoagulant effect of ●coumarins; levofloxacin
  possibly enhances anticoagulant effect of phenindione
- **Antidepressants:** avoidance of moxifloxacin advised
  by manufacturer of ●citalopram and ●escitalopram
  (risk of ventricular arrhythmias); ciprofloxacin inhibits metabolism of ●duloxetine—avoid concomitant
  use; avoidance of ciprofloxacin advised by manufacturer of ●agomelatine; increased risk of ventricular
  arrhythmias when moxifloxacin given with ●tricyc-
  lics—avoid concomitant use
  Antidiabetics: norfloxacin possibly enhances effects of
  glibenclamide
  Antiepileptics: ciprofloxacin increases or decreases
  plasma concentration of phenytoin
- **Antihistamines:** increased risk of ventricular arrhythmias when moxifloxacin given with ●mizolastine—
  avoid concomitant use
- **Antimalarials:** avoidance of moxifloxacin advised by
  manufacturer of ●piperaquine with artenimol (possible risk of ventricular arrhythmias); avoidance of
  quinolones advised by manufacturer of ●artemether
  with lumefantrine; increased risk of ventricular
  arrhythmias when moxifloxacin given with ●chloro-
  quine and hydroxychloroquine, ●mefloquine or
  ●quinine—avoid concomitant use
- **Antipsychotics:** increased risk of ventricular arrhythmias when moxifloxacin given with ●benperidol—
  manufacturer of benperidol advises avoid concomitant use; increased risk of ventricular arrhythmias
  when moxifloxacin given with ●droperidol,
  ●haloperidol, ●phenothiazines, ●pimozide or
  ●zuclopenthixol—avoid concomitant use; ciprofloxacin increases plasma concentration of clozapine;
  ciprofloxacin possibly increases plasma concentration of olanzapine
- **Antivirals:** manufacturer of norfloxacin advises give
  didanosine at least 2 hours before or after norfloxacin; increased risk of ventricular arrhythmias when
  moxifloxacin given with ●saquinavir—avoid concomitant use
  Anxiolytics and Hypnotics: avoidance of ciprofloxacin
  advised by manufacturer of zolpidem
- **Atomoxetine:** increased risk of ventricular arrhythmias
  when moxifloxacin given with ●atomoxetine
- **Beta-blockers:** increased risk of ventricular arrhythmias when moxifloxacin given with ●sotalol—avoid
  concomitant use
  Calcium Salts: absorption of ciprofloxacin reduced by
  calcium salts
- **Ciclosporin:** increased risk of nephrotoxicity when
  quinolones given with ●ciclosporin
- **Clopidogrel:** ciprofloxacin possibly reduces antiplatelet
  effect of ●clopidogrel
- **Cytotoxics:** nalidixic acid increases risk of melphalan
  toxicity; ciprofloxacin possibly reduces excretion of
  methotrexate (increased risk of toxicity); possible

Quinolones

- **Cytotoxics** *(continued)*
  increased risk of ventricular arrhythmias when moxifloxacin given with ●bosutinib; ciprofloxacin possibly increases the plasma concentration of ●bosutinib—manufacturer of bosutinib advises avoid or consider reducing dose of bosutinib; ciprofloxacin increases plasma concentration of erlotinib; ciprofloxacin possibly increases the plasma concentration of ●ibrutinib—reduce dose of ibrutinib (see Dose under Ibrutinib, p. 615); possible increased risk of ventricular arrhythmias when moxifloxacin given with ●vandetanib—avoid concomitant use; increased risk of ventricular arrhythmias when levofloxacin or moxifloxacin given with ●arsenic trioxide

  Dairy Products: absorption of ciprofloxacin and norfloxacin reduced by dairy products

  Dopaminergics: ciprofloxacin increases plasma concentration of rasagiline; ciprofloxacin inhibits metabolism of ropinirole (increased plasma concentration)

  5HT₁-receptor Agonists: quinolones possibly inhibit metabolism of zolmitriptan (reduce dose of zolmitriptan)

  Iron: absorption of ciprofloxacin, levofloxacin, moxifloxacin and ofloxacin reduced by *oral* iron; absorption of norfloxacin reduced by *oral* iron (give at least 2 hours apart)

  Lanthanum: absorption of quinolones possibly reduced by lanthanum (give at least 2 hours before or 4 hours after lanthanum)

- **Muscle Relaxants:** norfloxacin possibly increases plasma concentration of tizanidine (increased risk of toxicity); ciprofloxacin increases plasma concentration of ●tizanidine (increased risk of toxicity)—avoid concomitant use

  Mycophenolate: norfloxacin possibly reduces bioavailability of mycophenolate

- **Pentamidine Isetionate:** increased risk of ventricular arrhythmias when moxifloxacin given with ●pentamidine isetionate—avoid concomitant use

- **Pirfenidone:** ciprofloxacin increases plasma concentration of ●pirfenidone—see Cautions under Pirfenidone, p. 223

  Sevelamer: bioavailability of ciprofloxacin reduced by sevelamer

  Strontium Ranelate: absorption of quinolones reduced by strontium ranelate (manufacturer of strontium ranelate advises avoid concomitant use)

- **Theophylline:** possible increased risk of convulsions when quinolones given with ●theophylline; ciprofloxacin and norfloxacin increase plasma concentration of ●theophylline

  Ulcer-healing Drugs: absorption of ciprofloxacin, levofloxacin, moxifloxacin and ofloxacin reduced by sucralfate; absorption of norfloxacin reduced by sucralfate (give at least 2 hours apart)

  Vaccines: antibacterials inactivate oral typhoid vaccine—see p. 864

  Zinc: absorption of ciprofloxacin, levofloxacin, moxifloxacin and ofloxacin reduced by zinc; absorption of norfloxacin reduced by zinc (give at least 2 hours apart)

Rabeprazole *see* Proton Pump Inhibitors

Rabies vaccine *see* Vaccines

Raloxifene

  Anticoagulants: raloxifene antagonises anticoagulant effect of coumarins

  Lipid-regulating Drugs: absorption of raloxifene reduced by colestyramine (manufacturer of raloxifene advises avoid concomitant administration)

Raltegravir

  Antacids: absorption of raltegravir possibly reduced by antacids (give at least 2 hours apart)

Raltegravir *(continued)*

- Antibacterials: plasma concentration of raltegravir reduced by ●rifampicin—consider increasing dose of raltegravir

- Antivirals: increased risk of rash when raltegravir given with darunavir; avoidance of raltegravir advised by manufacturer of ●fosamprenavir

- Orlistat: absorption of raltegravir possibly reduced by ●orlistat

  Ulcer-healing Drugs: plasma concentration of raltegravir increased by famotidine and omeprazole

Raltitrexed

- Antipsychotics: avoid concomitant use of cytotoxics with ●clozapine (increased risk of agranulocytosis)

- Folates: manufacturer of raltitrexed advises avoid concomitant use with ●folates

Ramipril *see* ACE Inhibitors

Ranitidine *see* Histamine H₂-antagonists

Ranolazine

- Anti-arrhythmics: manufacturer of ranolazine advises avoid concomitant use with ●disopyramide

- Antibacterials: plasma concentration of ranolazine possibly increased by ●clarithromycin and ●telithromycin—manufacturer of ranolazine advises avoid concomitant use; plasma concentration of ranolazine reduced by ●rifampicin—manufacturer of ranolazine advises avoid concomitant use

  Antidepressants: plasma concentration of ranolazine increased by paroxetine

- Antifungals: plasma concentration of ranolazine possibly increased by ●itraconazole, ●posaconazole and ●voriconazole—manufacturer of ranolazine advises avoid concomitant use

- Antivirals: plasma concentration of ranolazine possibly increased by ●atazanavir, ●darunavir, ●fosamprenavir, ●indinavir, ●lopinavir, ●ritonavir, ●saquinavir and ●tipranavir—manufacturer of ranolazine advises avoid concomitant use

- Beta-blockers: manufacturer of ranolazine advises avoid concomitant use with ●sotalol

  Calcium-channel Blockers: plasma concentration of ranolazine increased by diltiazem and verapamil (consider reducing dose of ranolazine)

  Cardiac Glycosides: ranolazine increases plasma concentration of digoxin

  Ciclosporin: plasma concentration of both drugs may increase when ranolazine given with ciclosporin

- Grapefruit Juice: plasma concentration of ranolazine possibly increased by ●grapefruit juice—manufacturer of ranolazine advises avoid concomitant use

- Lipid-regulating Drugs: ranolazine increases plasma concentration of ●simvastatin (see Dose under Simvastatin, p. 177); manufacturer of lomitapide advises dose reduction when ranolazine given with lomitapide (see Dose under Lomitapide, p. 180)

- Tacrolimus: ranolazine increases plasma concentration of ●tacrolimus

Rasagiline

  Note Rasagiline is a MAO-B inhibitor

- Analgesics: avoid concomitant use of rasagiline with ●dextromethorphan; risk of CNS toxicity when rasagiline given with ●pethidine (avoid pethidine for 2 weeks after rasagiline)

  Antibacterials: plasma concentration of rasagiline increased by ciprofloxacin

- Antidepressants: after stopping rasagiline do not start ●fluoxetine for 2 weeks, also rasagiline should not be started until at least 5 weeks after stopping fluoxetine; after stopping rasagiline do not start ●fluvoxamine for 2 weeks; risk of hypertensive crisis when rasagiline given with ●MAOIs, avoid MAOIs for at least 2 weeks after stopping rasagiline; increased risk of CNS toxicity when rasagiline given with ●SSRIs or ●tricyclics

  Dopaminergics: plasma concentration of rasagiline possibly reduced by entacapone

Rasagiline *(continued)*

Memantine: effects of dopaminergics possibly enhanced by memantine

Methyldopa: antiparkinsonian effect of dopaminergics antagonised by methyldopa

- Sympathomimetics: avoid concomitant use of rasagiline with ●sympathomimetics

Reboxetine

- Antibacterials: manufacturer of reboxetine advises avoid concomitant use with ●macrolides
- Antidepressants: manufacturer of reboxetine advises avoid concomitant use with ●fluvoxamine; increased risk of hypertension and CNS excitation when reboxetine given with ●MAOIs (MAOIs should not be started until 1 week after stopping reboxetine, avoid reboxetine for 2 weeks after stopping MAOIs)

Antiepileptics: plasma concentration of reboxetine possibly reduced by carbamazepine and phenobarbital

- Antifungals: manufacturer of reboxetine advises avoid concomitant use with ●imidazoles and ●triazoles
- Antimalarials: avoidance of antidepressants advised by manufacturer of ●artemether with lumefantrine and ●piperaquine with artenimol

Atomoxetine: possible increased risk of convulsions when antidepressants given with atomoxetine

Diuretics: possible increased risk of hypokalaemia when reboxetine given with loop diuretics or thiazides and related diuretics

Ergot Alkaloids: possible risk of hypertension when reboxetine given with ergotamine

Regorafenib

Analgesics: manufacturer of regorafenib advises avoid concomitant use with mefenamic acid

- Antibacterials: plasma concentration of regorafenib reduced by ●rifampicin—manufacturer of regorafenib advises avoid concomitant use
- Anticoagulants: increased risk of bleeding when regorafenib given with ●warfarin
- Antipsychotics: avoid concomitant use of cytotoxics with ●clozapine (increased risk of agranulocytosis)

Cytotoxics: regorafenib increases plasma concentration of irinotecan

Remifentanil *see* Opioid Analgesics

Repaglinide *see* Antidiabetics

Retigabine

Alcohol: increased risk of blurred vision when retigabine given with alcohol

- Antidepressants: anticonvulsant effect of antiepileptics possibly antagonised by MAOIs and ●tricyclic-related antidepressants (convulsive threshold lowered); anticonvulsant effect of antiepileptics antagonised by ●SSRIs and ●tricyclics (convulsive threshold lowered)

Antiepileptics: plasma concentration of retigabine possibly reduced by carbamazepine and phenytoin

- Antimalarials: anticonvulsant effect of antiepileptics antagonised by ●mefloquine
- Antipsychotics: anticonvulsant effect of antiepileptics antagonised by ●antipsychotics (convulsive threshold lowered)
- Orlistat: possible increased risk of convulsions when antiepileptics given with ●orlistat

Retinoids

- Alcohol: etretinate formed from acitretin in presence of ●alcohol (increased risk of teratogenicity in women of child-bearing potential)
- Antibacterials: possible increased risk of benign intracranial hypertension when retinoids given with ●tetracyclines (avoid concomitant use)
- Anticoagulants: acitretin possibly reduces anticoagulant effect of ●coumarins

Antiepileptics: isotretinoin possibly reduces plasma concentration of carbamazepine

Retinoids *(continued)*

- Antifungals: possible increased risk of tretinoin toxicity when given with ●fluconazole and ●voriconazole
- Cytotoxics: acitretin increases plasma concentration of ●methotrexate (also increased risk of hepatotoxicity)—avoid concomitant use

Lipid-regulating Drugs: alitretinoin reduces plasma concentration of simvastatin

- Vitamins: risk of hypervitaminosis A when retinoids given with ●vitamin A—avoid concomitant use

Ribavirin

- Antivirals: effects of ribavirin possibly reduced by ●abacavir; increased risk of side-effects when ribavirin given with ●didanosine—avoid concomitant use; increased risk of toxicity when ribavirin given with ●stavudine; increased risk of anaemia when ribavirin given with ●zidovudine—avoid concomitant use
- Azathioprine: ribavirin possibly enhances myelosuppressive effects of ●azathioprine

Rifabutin *see* Rifamycins

Rifampicin *see* Rifamycins

Rifamycins

Note Interactions do not apply to rifaximin

ACE Inhibitors: rifampicin reduces plasma concentration of active metabolite of imidapril (reduced antihypertensive effect)

Aliskiren: rifampicin reduces plasma concentration of aliskiren

Ambrisentan: rifampicin possibly increases plasma concentration of ambrisentan

Analgesics: rifampicin reduces plasma concentration of celecoxib, diclofenac and etoricoxib; rifampicin accelerates metabolism of alfentanil, codeine, fentanyl, methadone and morphine (reduced effect); rifampicin possibly accelerates metabolism of oxycodone

Angiotensin-II Receptor Antagonists: rifampicin reduces plasma concentration of losartan and its active metabolite

Antacids: absorption of rifampicin reduced by antacids

- Anti-arrhythmics: rifamycins accelerate metabolism of ●disopyramide (reduced plasma concentration); rifampicin reduces plasma concentration of ●dronedarone—avoid concomitant use; rifampicin accelerates metabolism of ●propafenone (reduced effect)
- Antibacterials: increased risk of side-effects including neutropenia when rifabutin given with ●azithromycin; rifamycins reduce plasma concentration of clarithromycin and dapsone; plasma concentration of rifabutin increased by ●clarithromycin (increased risk of toxicity—reduce rifabutin dose); plasma concentration of rifabutin possibly increased by ●erythromycin (increased risk of toxicity—reduce rifabutin dose); rifampicin possibly reduces plasma concentration of tinidazole and trimethoprim; rifampicin reduces plasma concentration of doxycycline—consider increasing dose of doxycycline; rifabutin possibly reduces plasma concentration of bedaquiline—manufacturer of bedaquiline advises avoid concomitant use; rifampicin reduces plasma concentration of ●bedaquiline—manufacturer of bedaquiline advises avoid concomitant use; rifampicin accelerates metabolism of chloramphenicol (reduced plasma concentration); rifampicin reduces plasma concentration of ●delamanid; increased risk of hepatotoxicity when rifampicin given with ●isoniazid; rifampicin reduces plasma concentration of linezolid (possible therapeutic failure of linezolid); rifampicin reduces plasma concentration of ●telithromycin (avoid during and for 2 weeks after rifampicin)
- Anticoagulants: rifampicin possibly reduces plasma concentration of ●apixaban—manufacturer of apixa-

Rifamycins

- **Anticoagulants** *(continued)*

  ban advises avoid concomitant use when given for treatment of deep-vein thrombosis or pulmonary embolism; rifamycins accelerate metabolism of ●coumarins (reduced anticoagulant effect); rifampicin reduces plasma concentration of ●dabigatran—manufacturer of dabigatran advises avoid concomitant use; rifampicin reduces plasma concentration of ●rivaroxaban—manufacturer of rivaroxaban advises monitor for signs of thrombosis

- **Antidiabetics:** rifamycins accelerate metabolism of ●tolbutamide (reduced effect); rifampicin reduces plasma concentration of ●canagliflozin and nateglinide; rifampicin possibly reduces effects of linagliptin; rifampicin possibly antagonises hypoglycaemic effect of repaglinide; rifamycins possibly accelerate metabolism of ●sulfonylureas (reduced effect)

- **Antiepileptics:** rifabutin reduces plasma concentration of ●carbamazepine; rifampicin reduces plasma concentration of ●lamotrigine; plasma concentration of rifampicin possibly reduced by phenobarbital; rifamycins accelerate metabolism of ●phenytoin (reduced plasma concentration)

- **Antifungals:** plasma concentration of rifabutin increased by ●fluconazole (increased risk of uveitis—reduce rifabutin dose); rifampicin accelerates metabolism of ●fluconazole (reduced plasma concentration); rifabutin and rifampicin reduce plasma concentration of ●itraconazole—manufacturer of itraconazole advises avoid concomitant use; plasma concentration of rifabutin increased by ●posaconazole (also plasma concentration of posaconazole reduced); rifampicin reduces plasma concentration of ●posaconazole and ●terbinafine; plasma concentration of rifabutin increased by ●voriconazole, also rifabutin reduces plasma concentration of voriconazole (increase dose of voriconazole and also monitor for rifabutin toxicity); rifampicin reduces plasma concentration of ●voriconazole—avoid concomitant use; rifampicin initially increases and then reduces plasma concentration of caspofungin (consider increasing dose of caspofungin); plasma concentration of rifabutin possibly increased by ●triazoles (increased risk of uveitis—reduce rifabutin dose)

  Antihistamines: rifampicin possibly reduces effects of fexofenadine

- **Antimalarials:** avoidance of rifampicin advised by manufacturer of piperaquine with artenimol; rifampicin reduces plasma concentration of ●mefloquine—avoid concomitant use; rifampicin reduces plasma concentration of ●quinine

  Antimuscarinics: rifampicin reduces plasma concentration of active metabolite of fesoterodine

- **Antipsychotics:** rifampicin accelerates metabolism of ●haloperidol (reduced plasma concentration); rifabutin and rifampicin possibly reduce plasma concentration of ●aripiprazole (avoid concomitant use or consider increasing the dose of aripiprazole—consult aripiprazole product literature); rifampicin possibly reduces plasma concentration of clozapine; rifampicin reduces plasma concentration of ●lurasidone—avoid concomitant use

- **Antivirals:** rifampicin possibly reduces plasma concentration of abacavir; plasma concentration of rifabutin increased by ●atazanavir, ●darunavir, ●fosamprenavir and ●tipranavir (reduce dose of rifabutin); rifampicin reduces plasma concentration of ●atazanavir, ●daclatasvir, ●lopinavir, ●nevirapine and ●rilpivirine—avoid concomitant use; avoidance of rifampicin advised by manufacturer of ●boceprevir (plasma concentration of boceprevir possibly reduced); rifampicin possibly reduces plasma concentration of ●daclatasvir and simeprevir—manufacturer of daclatasvir and simeprevir advises avoid concomitant use; rifampicin significantly reduces

Rifamycins

- **Antivirals** *(continued)*

  plasma concentration of ●darunavir, ●fosamprenavir and ●telaprevir—avoid concomitant use; rifampicin reduces the plasma concentration of ●dolutegravir (see Dose under Dolutegravir, p. 429); rifampicin reduces plasma concentration of efavirenz—increase dose of efavirenz; plasma concentration of rifabutin reduced by efavirenz—increase dose of rifabutin; avoidance of rifampicin advised by manufacturer of ●elvitegravir, etravirine, sofosbuvir and zidovudine; rifabutin reduces plasma concentration of ●elvitegravir also plasma concentration of active metabolite of rifabutin increased—reduce dose of rifabutin; plasma concentration of both drugs reduced when rifabutin given with ●etravirine; plasma concentration of rifabutin increased by ●indinavir and ●saquinavir (also plasma concentration of indinavir and saquinavir reduced)—reduce rifabutin dose; rifampicin accelerates metabolism of ●indinavir (reduced plasma concentration—avoid concomitant use); rifampicin reduces plasma concentration of ●maraviroc and ●raltegravir—consider increasing dose of maraviroc and raltegravir; plasma concentration of rifabutin possibly increased by nevirapine; rifabutin decreases plasma concentration of ●rilpivirine (increase dose of rilpivirine—consult rilpivirine product literature); rifampicin reduces plasma concentration of ritonavir; plasma concentration of rifabutin increased by ●ritonavir (increased risk of toxicity—reduce rifabutin dose); rifampicin significantly reduces plasma concentration of ●saquinavir, also risk of hepatotoxicity—avoid concomitant use; rifampicin reduces plasma concentration of ●simeprevir—manufacturer of simeprevir advises avoid concomitant use; avoidance of rifabutin advised by manufacturer of sofosbuvir and ●telaprevir; rifampicin possibly reduces plasma concentration of ●tipranavir—avoid concomitant use

  Anxiolytics and Hypnotics: rifampicin accelerates metabolism of diazepam and zaleplon (reduced plasma concentration); rifampicin possibly accelerates metabolism of benzodiazepines (reduced plasma concentration); rifampicin possibly accelerates metabolism of buspirone; rifampicin accelerates metabolism of zolpidem (reduced plasma concentration and reduced effect); rifampicin significantly reduces plasma concentration of zopiclone

  Aprepitant: rifampicin reduces plasma concentration of aprepitant

- **Atovaquone:** avoidance of concomitant rifabutin advised by manufacturer of atovaquone (plasma concentration of both drugs reduced); rifampicin reduces plasma concentration of ●atovaquone (and concentration of rifampicin increased)—avoid concomitant use

  Avanafil: rifampicin possibly reduces plasma concentration of avanafil—manufacturer of avanafil advises avoid concomitant use

  Beta-blockers: rifampicin accelerates metabolism of bisoprolol and propranolol (plasma concentration significantly reduced); rifampicin reduces plasma concentration of carvedilol, celiprolol and metoprolol; rifampicin possibly reduces plasma concentration of *oral* timolol

- **Bosentan:** rifampicin reduces plasma concentration of ●bosentan—avoid concomitant use

- **Calcium-channel Blockers:** rifampicin possibly reduces plasma concentration of felodipine; rifampicin possibly accelerates metabolism of ●isradipine and ●nicardipine (possible significantly reduced plasma concentration); rifampicin accelerates metabolism of ●diltiazem, ●nifedipine, ●nimodipine and ●verapamil (plasma concentration significantly reduced)

Rifamycins (continued)

- Cannabis Extract: rifampicin reduces plasma concentration of ●cannabis extract—manufacturer of cannabis extract advises avoid concomitant use
- Cardiac Glycosides: rifampicin possibly reduces plasma concentration of digoxin
- Ciclosporin: rifampicin accelerates metabolism of ●ciclosporin (reduced plasma concentration)
- Cobicistat: rifabutin reduces plasma concentration of ●cobicistat (adjust dose—consult product literature); rifampicin possibly reduces plasma concentration of ●cobicistat—manufacturer of cobicistat advises avoid concomitant use
- Corticosteroids: rifamycins accelerate metabolism of ●corticosteroids (reduced effect)
- Cytotoxics: rifampicin possibly reduces effects of brentuximab vedotin; rifampicin reduces plasma concentration of afatinib, ruxolitinib, sorafenib and ●trabectedin; rifabutin possibly decreases plasma concentration of axitinib (increase dose of axitinib—consult axitinib product literature); rifampicin decreases plasma concentration of axitinib (increase dose of axitinib—consult axitinib product literature); rifabutin possibly reduces plasma concentration of ●bosutinib, crizotinib and ponatinib—manufacturer of bosutinib, crizotinib and ponatinib advises avoid concomitant use; rifampicin reduces plasma concentration of ●bortezomib, ●bosutinib, ●cabazitaxel, ●crizotinib, ●ponatinib, ●regorafenib and ●vandetanib—manufacturer of bortezomib, bosutinib, cabazitaxel, crizotinib, ponatinib, regorafenib and vandetanib advises avoid concomitant use; rifampicin reduces plasma concentration of ●cabozantinib, ●gefitinib, ●ibrutinib, ●idelalisib, ●imatinib and ●nilotinib—avoid concomitant use; avoidance of rifampicin advised by manufacturer of dabrafenib, ●lapatinib and vemurafenib; rifampicin accelerates metabolism of ●dasatinib (reduced plasma concentration—avoid concomitant use); rifampicin accelerates metabolism of erlotinib and sunitinib (reduced plasma concentration); rifampicin reduces plasma concentration of ●everolimus (avoid concomitant use or consider increasing the dose of everolimus —consult everolimus product literature); avoidance of rifabutin advised by manufacturer of ●cabazitaxel, ●lapatinib and vemurafenib; rifampicin possibly reduces plasma concentration of eribulin and ●pazopanib; rifampicin reduces plasma concentration of active metabolite of ●temsirolimus—avoid concomitant use; rifampicin possibly reduces plasma concentration of ●vinflunine—manufacturer of vinflunine advises avoid concomitant use; avoidance of rifampicin advised by manufacturer of ●vismodegib (plasma concentration of vismodegib possibly reduced)
- Deferasirox: rifampicin reduces plasma concentration of deferasirox
- Diuretics: rifampicin reduces plasma concentration of ●eplerenone—avoid concomitant use
- Hormone Antagonists: rifampicin reduces plasma concentration of ●abiraterone—manufacturer of abiraterone advises avoid concomitant use; rifabutin possibly reduces plasma concentration of ●abiraterone—manufacturer of abiraterone advises avoid concomitant use; avoidance of rifampicin advised by manufacturer of enzalutamide; rifampicin possibly reduces plasma concentration of exemestane; rifampicin accelerates metabolism of tamoxifen (reduced plasma concentration)
- 5HT₃-receptor Antagonists: rifampicin accelerates metabolism of ondansetron (reduced effect)
- Ivacaftor: rifabutin possibly reduces plasma concentration of ●ivacaftor—manufacturer of ivacaftor advises avoid concomitant use; rifampicin reduces plasma concentration of ●ivacaftor—manufacturer of ivacaftor advises avoid concomitant use

Rifamycins (continued)

- Leflunomide: rifampicin possibly increases plasma concentration of active metabolite of leflunomide
- Lipid-regulating Drugs: rifampicin possibly reduces plasma concentration of atorvastatin and simvastatin; rifampicin accelerates metabolism of fluvastatin (reduced effect)
- Macitentan: rifampicin reduces plasma concentration of ●macitentan—avoid concomitant use
- Muscle Relaxants: rifampicin possibly reduces plasma concentration of tizanidine
- Mycophenolate: rifampicin reduces plasma concentration of active metabolite of ●mycophenolate
- Oestrogens: rifamycins accelerate metabolism of ●oestrogens (reduced contraceptive effect—see p. 548)
- Progestogens: rifamycins accelerate metabolism of ●progestogens (reduced contraceptive effect—see p. 548)
- Ranolazine: rifampicin reduces plasma concentration of ●ranolazine—manufacturer of ranolazine advises avoid concomitant use
- Roflumilast: rifampicin inhibits effects of ●roflumilast (manufacturer of roflumilast advises avoid concomitant use)
- Sirolimus: rifabutin and rifampicin reduce plasma concentration of ●sirolimus—avoid concomitant use
- Tacrolimus: rifabutin possibly reduces plasma concentration of tacrolimus; rifampicin reduces plasma concentration of ●tacrolimus
- Tadalafil: rifampicin reduces plasma concentration of ●tadalafil—manufacturer of tadalafil advises avoid concomitant use
- Teriflunomide: rifampicin reduces plasma concentration of teriflunomide
- Theophylline: rifampicin accelerates metabolism of theophylline (reduced plasma concentration)
- Thyroid Hormones: rifampicin accelerates metabolism of levothyroxine (may increase requirements for levothyroxine in hypothyroidism)
- Tibolone: rifampicin accelerates metabolism of tibolone (reduced plasma concentration)
- Ticagrelor: rifampicin reduces plasma concentration of ●ticagrelor
- Tolvaptan: rifampicin reduces plasma concentration of tolvaptan
- Ulcer-healing Drugs: rifampicin accelerates metabolism of cimetidine (reduced plasma concentration)
- Ulipristal: avoidance of rifampicin advised by manufacturer of ●ulipristal (contraceptive effect of ulipristal possibly reduced)
- Vaccines: antibacterials inactivate oral typhoid vaccine—see p. 864

Rilpivirine

- Analgesics: rilpivirine possibly reduces plasma concentration of methadone
- Antacids: manufacturer of rilpivirine advises give antacids 2 hours before or 4 hours after rilpivirine
- Antibacterials: manufacturer of rilpivirine advises avoid concomitant use with ●clarithromycin and ●erythromycin (plasma concentration of rilpivirine possibly increased); plasma concentration of rilpivirine decreased by ●rifabutin (increase dose of rilpivirine—consult rilpivirine product literature); plasma concentration of rilpivirine reduced by ●rifampicin—avoid concomitant use
- Anticoagulants: rilpivirine possibly increases plasma concentration of dabigatran
- Antidepressants: manufacturer of rilpivirine advises avoid concomitant use with ●St John's wort (plasma concentration of rilpivirine possibly reduced)
- Antiepileptics: manufacturer of rilpivirine advises avoid concomitant use with ●carbamazepine, ●oxcarbazepine, ●phenobarbital and

Rilpivirine

- Antiepileptics *(continued)*
  - ●phenytoin (plasma concentration of rilpivirine possibly reduced)
  - Antivirals: manufacturer of rilpivirine advises give didanosine 2 hours before or 4 hours after rilpivirine; avoidance of rilpivirine advised by manufacturer of nevirapine
  - Calcium Salts: manufacturer of rilpivirine advises give calcium salts 2 hours before or 4 hours after rilpivirine
- Corticosteroids: manufacturer of rilpivirine advises avoid concomitant use with ●dexamethasone (except when given as a single dose)
- Orlistat: absorption of rilpivirine possibly reduced by ●orlistat
- Ulcer-healing Drugs: manufacturer of rilpivirine advises avoid concomitant use with esomeprazole, lansoprazole, pantoprazole and rabeprazole (plasma concentration of rilpivirine possibly reduced); plasma concentration of rilpivirine reduced by ●omeprazole—avoid concomitant use; manufacturer of rilpivirine advises avoid histamine H₂-antagonists for 12 hours before or 4 hours after rilpivirine—consult product literature

Riociguat

- Antacids: absorption of riociguat reduced by antacids (give at least 2 hours before or 1 hour after riociguat)
- Antifungals: manufacturer of riociguat advises avoid concomitant use with itraconazole and voriconazole
- Antivirals: manufacturer of riociguat advises avoid concomitant use with ritonavir
- Avanafil: possible enhanced hypotensive effect when riociguat given with ●avanafil—avoid concomitant use
- Bosentan: plasma concentration of riociguat reduced by bosentan
- Nitrates: possible enhanced hypotensive effect when riociguat given with ●nitrates—avoid concomitant use
- Sildenafil: enhanced hypotensive effect when riociguat given with ●sildenafil—avoid concomitant use
- Tadalafil: possible enhanced hypotensive effect when riociguat given with ●tadalafil—avoid concomitant use
- Vardenafil: possible enhanced hypotensive effect when riociguat given with ●vardenafil—avoid concomitant use

Risedronate Sodium *see* Bisphosphonates
Risperidone *see* Antipsychotics
Ritonavir

- Alpha-blockers: ritonavir possibly increases plasma concentration of ●alfuzosin—avoid concomitant use
- Analgesics: ritonavir possibly increases plasma concentration of NSAIDs and buprenorphine; ritonavir increases plasma concentration of ●dextropropoxyphene and ●piroxicam (risk of toxicity)—avoid concomitant use; ritonavir increases plasma concentration of ●alfentanil and ●fentanyl; ritonavir reduces plasma concentration of methadone; ritonavir possibly reduces plasma concentration of morphine; ritonavir reduces plasma concentration of ●pethidine, but increases plasma concentration of toxic metabolite of pethidine (avoid concomitant use)
- Anti-arrhythmics: ritonavir increases plasma concentration of ●amiodarone and ●propafenone (increased risk of ventricular arrhythmias—avoid concomitant use); ritonavir possibly increases plasma concentration of ●disopyramide (increased risk of toxicity); avoidance of ritonavir advised by manufacturer of ●dronedarone; ritonavir possibly increases plasma concentration of ●flecainide (increased risk of ventricular arrhythmias—avoid concomitant use)

Ritonavir *(continued)*

- Antibacterials: ritonavir possibly increases plasma concentration of azithromycin and erythromycin; ritonavir increases plasma concentration of ●clarithromycin (reduce dose of clarithromycin in renal impairment); ritonavir increases plasma concentration of ●rifabutin (increased risk of toxicity—reduce rifabutin dose); plasma concentration of ritonavir reduced by rifampicin; ritonavir possibly increases plasma concentration of bedaquiline—avoid concomitant use if ritonavir given for more than 14 days; ritonavir increases plasma concentration of delamanid; plasma concentration of both drugs increased when ritonavir given with ●fusidic acid—avoid concomitant use; avoidance of concomitant ritonavir in severe renal and hepatic impairment advised by manufacturer of ●telithromycin
- Anticoagulants: ritonavir may enhance or reduce anticoagulant effect of ●warfarin; avoidance of ritonavir advised by manufacturer of apixaban; ritonavir possibly enhances anticoagulant effect of ●coumarins and ●phenindione; ritonavir increases plasma concentration of ●rivaroxaban—avoid concomitant use
- Antidepressants: ritonavir possibly reduces plasma concentration of paroxetine; ritonavir increases plasma concentration of ●trazodone (increased risk of toxicity); ritonavir possibly increases plasma concentration of ●SSRIs and ●tricyclics; plasma concentration of ritonavir reduced by ●St John's wort—avoid concomitant use
  - Antidiabetics: ritonavir possibly increases plasma concentration of tolbutamide
- Antiepileptics: ritonavir possibly increases plasma concentration of ●carbamazepine; ritonavir possibly reduces plasma concentration of lamotrigine and valproate; plasma concentration of ritonavir possibly reduced by phenytoin, also plasma concentration of phenytoin possibly affected
- Antifungals: plasma concentration of ritonavir increased by fluconazole; combination of ritonavir with ●itraconazole may increase plasma concentration of either drug (or both); ritonavir reduces plasma concentration of ●voriconazole—avoid concomitant use
  - Antihistamines: ritonavir possibly increases plasma concentration of non-sedating antihistamines
- Antimalarials: caution with ritonavir advised by manufacturer of artemether with lumefantrine; plasma concentration of ritonavir possibly reduced by mefloquine; ritonavir increases plasma concentration of ●quinine (increased risk of toxicity)
- Antimuscarinics: avoidance of ritonavir advised by manufacturer of darifenacin and tolterodine; manufacturer of fesoterodine advises dose reduction when ritonavir given with fesoterodine—consult fesoterodine product literature; ritonavir possibly increases plasma concentration of ●solifenacin—see Dose under Solifenacin, p. 565
- Antipsychotics: ritonavir possibly increases plasma concentration of ●antipsychotics; ritonavir possibly increases plasma concentration of ●aripiprazole (reduce dose of aripiprazole—consult aripiprazole product literature); manufacturer of ritonavir advises avoid concomitant use with ●clozapine (increased risk of toxicity); ritonavir possibly increases plasma concentration of ●lurasidone—avoid concomitant use; ritonavir reduces plasma concentration of olanzapine—consider increasing dose of olanzapine; ritonavir increases plasma concentration of ●pimozide (increased risk of ventricular arrhythmias—avoid concomitant use); ritonavir possibly increases plasma concentration of ●quetiapine—manufacturer of quetiapine advises avoid concomitant use
- Antivirals: plasma concentration of both drugs reduced when ritonavir given with ●boceprevir;

Ritonavir

- Antivirals *(continued)*
  manufacturer of ritonavir advises ritonavir and didanosine should be taken 2.5 hours apart; ritonavir
  increases the toxicity of ●efavirenz, monitor liver
  function tests —manufacturer of *Atripla*® advises
  avoid concomitant use with *high-dose* ritonavir; ritonavir increases plasma concentration of indinavir,
  maraviroc and ●saquinavir; ritonavir increases
  plasma concentration of ●simeprevir—manufacturer
  of simeprevir advises avoid concomitant use; ritonavir possibly reduces plasma concentration of telaprevir

- Anxiolytics and Hypnotics: ritonavir possibly increases
  plasma concentration of ●anxiolytics and hypnotics;
  ritonavir possibly increases plasma concentration of
  ●alprazolam, ●diazepam, ●flurazepam and ●zolpi-
  dem (risk of extreme sedation and respiratory
  depression—avoid concomitant use); ritonavir possibly increases plasma concentration of ●midazolam
  (risk of prolonged sedation—avoid concomitant use
  of *oral* midazolam); ritonavir increases plasma concentration of buspirone (increased risk of toxicity)
  Aprepitant: ritonavir possibly increases plasma concentration of aprepitant
  Atovaquone: ritonavir possibly reduces plasma concentration of atovaquone—manufacturer of atovaquone advises avoid concomitant use

- Avanafil: ritonavir significantly increases plasma concentration of ●avanafil—avoid concomitant use

- Bosentan: ritonavir increases plasma concentration of
  ●bosentan (consider reducing dose of bosentan)
  Bupropion: ritonavir reduces plasma concentration of
  bupropion

- Calcium-channel Blockers: ritonavir possibly increases
  plasma concentration of ●calcium-channel blockers;
  avoidance of ritonavir advised by manufacturer of
  lercanidipine
  Cardiac Glycosides: ritonavir possibly increases
  plasma concentration of digoxin

- Ciclosporin: ritonavir possibly increases plasma concentration of ●ciclosporin

- Cilostazol: ritonavir possibly increases plasma concentration of ●cilostazol (see Dose under Cilostazol,
  p. 141)

- Colchicine: ritonavir possibly increases risk of ●colchi-
  cine toxicity—suspend or reduce dose of colchicine
  (avoid concomitant use in hepatic or renal impairment)

- Corticosteroids: ritonavir possibly increases plasma
  concentration of ●corticosteroids—increased risk of
  adrenal supression; ritonavir possibly increases
  plasma concentration of ●budesonide (including
  inhaled, intranasal, and *rectal* budesonide)—
  increased risk of adrenal supression; ritonavir
  increases plasma concentration of *inhaled* and *intranasal* ●fluticasone—increased risk of adrenal suppression

- Cytotoxics: ritonavir increases the plasma concentration of afatinib—manufacturer of afatinib advises
  separating administration of ritonavir by 6 to 12
  hours; ritonavir possibly increases plasma concentration of axitinib (reduce dose of axitinib—consult
  axitinib product literature); ritonavir possibly
  increases the plasma concentration of ●bosutinib
  and ●cabazitaxel—manufacturer of bosutinib and
  cabazitaxel advises avoid or consider reducing dose
  of bosutinib and cabazitaxel; ritonavir possibly
  increases plasma concentration of cabozantinib and
  vinblastine; ritonavir possibly increases plasma
  concentration of ●crizotinib, ●everolimus, nilotinib and
  ●vinflunine—manufacturer of crizotinib, everolimus,
  nilotinib and vinflunine advises avoid concomitant
  use; ritonavir possibly increases the plasma concentration of ●ibrutinib—reduce dose of ibrutinib (see
  Dose under Ibrutinib, p. 615); avoidance of ritonavir

Ritonavir

- Cytotoxics *(continued)*
  advised by manufacturer of ●lapatinib; ritonavir
  possibly increases plasma concentration of ●pazo-
  panib (reduce dose of pazopanib); ritonavir possibly
  increases plasma concentration of ponatinib—consider reducing initial dose of ponatinib (see Dose
  under Ponatinib, p. 618); manufacturer of ruxolitinib
  advises dose reduction when ritonavir given with
  ●ruxolitinib—consult ruxolitinib product literature;
  ritonavir possibly increases plasma concentration of
  ●docetaxel—manufacturer of docetaxel advises
  avoid concomitant use or consider reducing docetaxel dose; ritonavir increases plasma concentration
  of paclitaxel

- Dapoxetine: avoidance of ritonavir advised by manufacturer of ●dapoxetine (increased risk of toxicity)

- Diuretics: ritonavir increases plasma concentration of
  ●eplerenone—avoid concomitant use

- Domperidone: possible increased risk of ventricular
  arrhythmias when ritonavir given with ●domperi-
  done—avoid concomitant use

- Ergot Alkaloids: increased risk of ergotism when ritonavir given with ●ergometrine or ●ergotamine—
  avoid concomitant use

- 5HT₁-receptor Agonists: ritonavir increases plasma
  concentration of ●eletriptan (risk of toxicity)—avoid
  concomitant use

- Ivabradine: ritonavir possibly increases plasma concentration of ●ivabradine—avoid concomitant use

- Lipid-regulating Drugs: possible increased risk of myopathy when ritonavir given with atorvastatin; possible increased risk of myopathy when ritonavir given
  with ●rosuvastatin—manufacturer of rosuvastatin
  advises avoid concomitant use; increased risk of
  myopathy when ritonavir given with ●simvastatin
  (avoid concomitant use); avoidance of ritonavir
  advised by manufacturer of ●lomitapide (plasma
  concentration of lomitapide possibly increased)
  Mirabegron: when given with ritonavir avoid or
  reduce dose of mirabegron in hepatic or renal
  impairment—see Mirabegron, p. 564

- Oestrogens: ritonavir accelerates metabolism of
  ●oestrogens (reduced contraceptive effect—see
  p. 548)

- Orlistat: absorption of ritonavir possibly reduced by
  ●orlistat

- Ranolazine: ritonavir possibly increases plasma concentration of ●ranolazine—manufacturer of ranolazine advises avoid concomitant use
  Riociguat: avoidance of ritonavir advised by manufacturer of riociguat

- Sildenafil: ritonavir significantly increases plasma concentration of ●sildenafil—avoid concomitant use
  Sympathomimetics: ritonavir possibly increases
  plasma concentration of dexamfetamine
  Sympathomimetics, Beta₂: manufacturer of ritonavir
  advises avoid concomitant use with salmeterol

- Tacrolimus: ritonavir possibly increases plasma concentration of ●tacrolimus

- Tadalafil: ritonavir increases plasma concentration of
  ●tadalafil—manufacturer of tadalafil advises avoid
  concomitant use

- Theophylline: ritonavir accelerates metabolism of
  ●theophylline (reduced plasma concentration)

- Ticagrelor: ritonavir possibly increases plasma concentration of ●ticagrelor—manufacturer of ticagrelor
  advises avoid concomitant use

- Ulipristal: avoidance of ritonavir advised by manufacturer of ●ulipristal (contraceptive effect of ulipristal
  possibly reduced)

- Vardenafil: ritonavir increases plasma concentration
  of ●vardenafil—avoid concomitant use

Rituximab

- Antipsychotics: avoid concomitant use of cytotoxics
  with ●clozapine (increased risk of agranulocytosis)

Rituximab *(continued)*
- Vaccines: avoid concomitant use of monoclonal antibodies with live ●vaccines (see p. 842)

Rivaroxaban
- Analgesics: increased risk of haemorrhage when anticoagulants given with *intravenous* ●diclofenac (avoid concomitant use, including low-dose heparins); increased risk of haemorrhage when anticoagulants given with ●ketorolac (avoid concomitant use, including low-dose heparins)
  Anti-arrhythmics: manufacturer of rivaroxaban advises avoid concomitant use with dronedarone
- Antibacterials: plasma concentration of rivaroxaban reduced by ●rifampicin—manufacturer of rivaroxaban advises monitor for signs of thrombosis
- Anticoagulants: increased risk of haemorrhage when rivaroxaban given with other ●anticoagulants (avoid concomitant use except when switching with other anticoagulants or using heparin to maintain catheter patency); increased risk of haemorrhage when other anticoagulants given with ●apixaban and ●dabigatran (avoid concomitant use except when switching with other anticoagulants or using heparin to maintain catheter patency)
- Antidepressants: plasma concentration of rivaroxaban possibly reduced by ●St John's wort—manufacturer of rivaroxaban advises monitor for signs of thrombosis
- Antiepileptics: plasma concentration of rivaroxaban possibly reduced by ●carbamazepine, ●phenobarbital and ●phenytoin—manufacturer of rivaroxaban advises monitor for signs of thrombosis
  Antifungals: manufacturer of rivaroxaban advises avoid concomitant use with itraconazole, posaconazole and voriconazole
- Antivirals: manufacturer of rivaroxaban advises avoid concomitant use with atazanavir, darunavir, fosamprenavir, indinavir, saquinavir and tipranavir; manufacturers advise avoid concomitant use of rivaroxaban with lopinavir; plasma concentration of rivaroxaban increased by ●ritonavir—avoid concomitant use
- Cobicistat: anticoagulant effect of rivaroxaban possibly enhanced by ●cobicistat—avoid concomitant use

Rivastigmine *see* Parasympathomimetics
Rizatriptan *see* 5HT$_1$-receptor Agonists (under HT)
Rocuronium *see* Muscle Relaxants
Roflumilast
- Antibacterials: effects of roflumilast inhibited by ●rifampicin (manufacturer of roflumilast advises avoid concomitant use)
  Antidepressants: metabolism of roflumilast inhibited by fluvoxamine
  Antiepileptics: effects of roflumilast possibly inhibited by carbamazepine, phenobarbital and phenytoin (manufacturer of roflumilast advises avoid concomitant use)
  Theophylline: manufacturer of roflumilast advises avoid concomitant use with theophylline
  Ulcer-healing Drugs: metabolism of roflumilast inhibited by cimetidine

Ropinirole
  Antibacterials: metabolism of ropinirole inhibited by ciprofloxacin (increased plasma concentration)
  Antipsychotics: manufacturer of ropinirole advises avoid concomitant use of antipsychotics (antagonism of effect)
  Memantine: effects of dopaminergics possibly enhanced by memantine
  Methyldopa: antiparkinsonian effect of dopaminergics antagonised by methyldopa
  Metoclopramide: manufacturer of ropinirole advises avoid concomitant use of metoclopramide (antagonism of effect)

Ropinirole *(continued)*
  Oestrogens: plasma concentration of ropinirole increased by oestrogens

Ropivacaine
  Anti-arrhythmics: increased myocardial depression when ropivacaine given with anti-arrhythmics
  Antidepressants: metabolism of ropivacaine inhibited by fluvoxamine—avoid prolonged administration of ropivacaine

Rosuvastatin *see* Statins
Rotavirus vaccine *see* Vaccines
Rotigotine
  Antipsychotics: manufacturer of rotigotine advises avoid concomitant use of antipsychotics (antagonism of effect)
  Memantine: effects of dopaminergics possibly enhanced by memantine
  Methyldopa: antiparkinsonian effect of dopaminergics antagonised by methyldopa
  Metoclopramide: manufacturer of rotigotine advises avoid concomitant use of metoclopramide (antagonism of effect)

Rufinamide
- Antidepressants: anticonvulsant effect of antiepileptics possibly antagonised by MAOIs and ●tricyclic-related antidepressants (convulsive threshold lowered); anticonvulsant effect of antiepileptics antagonised by ●SSRIs and ●tricyclics (convulsive threshold lowered)
  Antiepileptics: plasma concentration of both drugs possibly reduced when rufinamide given with carbamazepine; plasma concentration of rufinamide possibly reduced by phenobarbital; plasma concentration of rufinamide possibly reduced by phenytoin, also plasma concentration of phenytoin possibly increased; plasma concentration of rufinamide possibly increased by valproate (reduce dose of rufinamide)
- Antimalarials: anticonvulsant effect of antiepileptics antagonised by ●mefloquine
- Antipsychotics: anticonvulsant effect of antiepileptics antagonised by ●antipsychotics (convulsive threshold lowered)
- Oestrogens: rufinamide accelerates metabolism of ●oestrogens (reduced contraceptive effect—see p. 548)
- Orlistat: possible increased risk of convulsions when antiepileptics given with ●orlistat
- Progestogens: rufinamide accelerates metabolism of ●progestogens (reduced contraceptive effect—see p. 548)

Rupatadine *see* Antihistamines
Ruxolitinib
- Antibacterials: manufacturer of ruxolitinib advises dose reduction when ruxolitinib given with ●clarithromycin and ●telithromycin—consult ruxolitinib product literature; plasma concentration of ruxolitinib reduced by rifampicin
- Antifungals: manufacturer of ruxolitinib advises dose reduction when ruxolitinib given with ●fluconazole, ●itraconazole, ●posaconazole and ●voriconazole—consult ruxolitinib product literature
- Antipsychotics: avoid concomitant use of cytotoxics with ●clozapine (increased risk of agranulocytosis)
- Antivirals: manufacturer of ruxolitinib advises dose reduction when ruxolitinib given with ●boceprevir, ●indinavir, ●lopinavir, ●ritonavir, ●saquinavir and ●telaprevir—consult ruxolitinib product literature

St John's Wort
  Analgesics: St John's wort possibly reduces plasma concentration of methadone
- Anti-arrhythmics: St John's wort possibly reduces plasma concentration of ●dronedarone—avoid concomitant use
- Antibacterials: St John's wort possibly reduces plasma concentration of bedaquiline—manufacturer of

St John's Wort

- Antibacterials *(continued)*
  bedaquiline advises avoid concomitant use; St John's wort reduces plasma concentration of •telithromycin (avoid during and for 2 weeks after St John's wort)
- Anticoagulants: St John's wort possibly reduces plasma concentration of •apixaban—manufacturer of apixaban advises avoid concomitant use when given for treatment of deep-vein thrombosis or pulmonary embolism; St John's wort reduces anticoagulant effect of •coumarins (avoid concomitant use); St John's wort possibly reduces plasma concentration of dabigatran—manufacturer of dabigatran advises avoid concomitant use; St John's wort possibly reduces plasma concentration of •rivaroxaban—manufacturer of rivaroxaban advises monitor for signs of thrombosis
- Antidepressants: possible increased serotonergic effects when St John's wort given with duloxetine or venlafaxine; St John's wort reduces plasma concentration of amitriptyline; increased serotonergic effects when St John's wort given with •SSRIs—avoid concomitant use
- Antiepileptics: St John's wort possibly reduces plasma concentration of carbamazepine; St John's wort possibly reduces plasma concentration of •phenobarbital and •phenytoin—avoid concomitant use
- Antifungals: St John's wort reduces plasma concentration of •voriconazole—avoid concomitant use
- Antimalarials: avoidance of antidepressants advised by manufacturer of •artemether with lumefantrine and •piperaquine with artenimol
- Antipsychotics: St John's wort possibly reduces plasma concentration of •aripiprazole (avoid concomitant use or consider increasing the dose of aripiprazole—consult aripiprazole product literature); St John's wort possibly reduces plasma concentration of •lurasidone—avoid concomitant use
- Antivirals: St John's wort reduces plasma concentration of •atazanavir, •darunavir, •efavirenz, •fosamprenavir, •indinavir, •lopinavir, •nevirapine, •ritonavir and •saquinavir—avoid concomitant use; St John's wort possibly reduces plasma concentration of daclatasvir and •simeprevir—manufacturer of daclatasvir and simeprevir advises avoid concomitant use; avoidance of St John's wort advised by manufacturer of dolutegravir, •elvitegravir, etravirine, sofosbuvir and •telaprevir; St John's wort possibly reduces plasma concentration of •maraviroc and •tipranavir—avoid concomitant use; avoidance of St John's wort advised by manufacturer of •rilpivirine (plasma concentration of rilpivirine possibly reduced)
  Anxiolytics and Hypnotics: St John's wort possibly reduces plasma concentration of *oral* midazolam
- Aprepitant: avoidance of St John's wort advised by manufacturer of •aprepitant
  Atomoxetine: possible increased risk of convulsions when antidepressants given with atomoxetine
- Calcium-channel Blockers: St John's wort possibly reduces plasma concentration of amlodipine and felodipine; St John's wort reduces plasma concentration of nifedipine; St John's wort significantly reduces plasma concentration of •verapamil
- Cannabis Extract: St John's wort possibly reduces plasma concentration of •cannabis extract—manufacturer of cannabis extract advises avoid concomitant use
- Cardiac Glycosides: St John's wort reduces plasma concentration of •digoxin—avoid concomitant use
- Ciclosporin: St John's wort reduces plasma concentration of •ciclosporin—avoid concomitant use
- Cobicistat: St John's wort possibly reduces plasma concentration of •cobicistat—manufacturer of cobicistat advises avoid concomitant use

St John's Wort *(continued)*

- Cytotoxics: St John's wort possibly reduces plasma concentration of axitinib—consider increasing dose of axitinib; St John's wort possibly reduces plasma concentration of bortezomib, •bosutinib, cabozantinib, crizotinib, everolimus, •ibrutinib, •idelalisib, ponatinib and •vinflunine—manufacturer of bortezomib, bosutinib, cabozantinib, crizotinib, everolimus, ibrutinib, idelalisib, ponatinib and vinflunine advises avoid concomitant use; avoidance of St John's wort advised by manufacturer of •cabazitaxel, dabrafenib, gefitinib, •lapatinib and vemurafenib; St John's wort reduces plasma concentration of •imatinib—avoid concomitant use; avoidance of St John's wort advised by manufacturer of vandetanib and •vismodegib (plasma concentration of vandetanib and vismodegib possibly reduced); St John's wort possibly reduces plasma concentration of •eribulin; St John's wort accelerates metabolism of •irinotecan (reduced plasma concentration—avoid concomitant use)
- Dapoxetine: possible increased risk of serotonergic effects when St John's wort given with •dapoxetine (manufacturer of dapoxetine advises St John's wort should not be started until 1 week after stopping dapoxetine, avoid dapoxetine for 2 weeks after stopping St John's wort)
- Diuretics: St John's wort reduces plasma concentration of •eplerenone—avoid concomitant use
  Fingolimod: St John's wort possibly reduces plasma concentration of fingolimod—manufacturer of fingolimod advises avoid concomitant use
- Hormone Antagonists: St John's wort possibly reduces plasma concentration of •abiraterone—manufacturer of abiraterone advises avoid concomitant use
- 5HT$_1$-receptor Agonists: increased serotonergic effects when St John's wort given with •5HT$_1$ agonists—avoid concomitant use
  Ivabradine: St John's wort reduces plasma concentration of ivabradine—avoid concomitant use
- Ivacaftor: St John's wort possibly reduces plasma concentration of •ivacaftor—manufacturer of ivacaftor advises avoid concomitant use
  Lipid-regulating Drugs: St John's wort reduces plasma concentration of simvastatin
  Macitentan: avoidance of St John's wort advised by manufacturer of macitentan
- Oestrogens: St John's wort reduces contraceptive effect of •oestrogens (avoid concomitant use)
- Progestogens: St John's wort reduces contraceptive effect of •progestogens (avoid concomitant use)
- Tacrolimus: St John's wort reduces plasma concentration of •tacrolimus—avoid concomitant use
  Theophylline: St John's wort possibly reduces plasma concentration of theophylline
  Ulcer-healing Drugs: St John's wort possibly reduces plasma concentration of omeprazole
- Uliprial: avoidance of St John's wort advised by manufacturer of •ulipristal (contraceptive effect of ulipristal possibly reduced)

Salbutamol *see* Sympathomimetics, Beta$_2$
Salmeterol *see* Sympathomimetics, Beta$_2$
Saquinavir

- Analgesics: increased risk of ventricular arrhythmias when saquinavir given with •alfentanil, •fentanyl or •methadone—avoid concomitant use
- Anti-arrhythmics: increased risk of ventricular arrhythmias when saquinavir given with •amiodarone, •disopyramide, •dronedarone, •flecainide, •lidocaine or •propafenone—avoid concomitant use
- Antibacterials: plasma concentration of both drugs possibly increased when saquinavir given with •clarithromycin (increased risk of ventricular arrhythmias); increased risk of ventricular arrhythmias when saquinavir given with •dapsone, •erythromycin or •moxifloxacin—avoid concomitant use;

Saquinavir

- Antibacterials *(continued)*

  saquinavir increases plasma concentration of •rifa-butin (also plasma concentration of saquinavir reduced)—reduce rifabutin dose; plasma concentration of saquinavir significantly reduced by •rif-ampicin, also risk of hepatotoxicity—avoid concomitant use; increased risk of ventricular arrhythmias when saquinavir given with •delamanid; plasma concentration of both drugs may increase when saquinavir given with fusidic acid; avoidance of saquinavir advised by manufacturer of •telithromy-cin (risk of ventricular arrhythmias)

  Anticoagulants: saquinavir possibly enhances anticoagulant effect of warfarin; avoidance of saquinavir advised by manufacturer of apixaban and rivaroxaban

- Antidepressants: increased risk of ventricular arrhythmias when saquinavir given with •trazodone or •tricyclics—avoid concomitant use; plasma concentration of saquinavir reduced by •St John's wort—avoid concomitant use

- Antiepileptics: plasma concentration of saquinavir possibly reduced by carbamazepine, •phenobarbital and phenytoin

  Antifungals: plasma concentration of saquinavir possibly increased by imidazoles and triazoles

- Antihistamines: increased risk of ventricular arrhythmias when saquinavir given with •mizolastine—avoid concomitant use

- Antimalarials: avoidance of saquinavir advised by manufacturer of •piperaquine with artenimol (possible risk of ventricular arrhythmias); caution with saquinavir advised by manufacturer of artemether with lumefantrine; increased risk of ventricular arrhythmias when saquinavir given with •quinine—avoid concomitant use

  Antimuscarinics: avoidance of saquinavir advised by manufacturer of darifenacin and tolterodine; manufacturer of fesoterodine advises dose reduction when saquinavir given with fesoterodine—consult fesoterodine product literature

- Antipsychotics: increased risk of ventricular arrhythmias when saquinavir given with •clozapine, •haloperidol or •phenothiazines—avoid concomitant use; saquinavir possibly increases plasma concentration of •aripiprazole (reduce dose of aripiprazole—consult aripiprazole product literature); saquinavir possibly increases plasma concentration of •lurasi-done—avoid concomitant use; saquinavir possibly increases plasma concentration of •pimozide (increased risk of ventricular arrhythmias—avoid concomitant use); saquinavir possibly increases plasma concentration of •quetiapine—manufacturer of quetiapine advises avoid concomitant use

- Antivirals: increased risk of ventricular arrhythmias when saquinavir given with •atazanavir or •lopinavir—avoid concomitant use; saquinavir reduces plasma concentration of darunavir; plasma concentration of saquinavir significantly reduced by efavirenz; plasma concentration of saquinavir increased by indinavir and •ritonavir; saquinavir increases plasma concentration of •maraviroc (consider reducing dose of maraviroc); plasma concentration of saquinavir reduced by •tipranavir

- Anxiolytics and Hypnotics: saquinavir increases plasma concentration of •midazolam (risk of prolonged sedation—avoid concomitant use of *oral* midazolam)

- Avanafil: saquinavir possibly increases plasma concentration of •avanafil—manufacturer of avanafil advises avoid concomitant use

- Beta-blockers: increased risk of ventricular arrhythmias when saquinavir given with •sotalol—avoid concomitant use

Saquinavir *(continued)*

- Ciclosporin: plasma concentration of both drugs increased when saquinavir given with •ciclosporin

  Corticosteroids: plasma concentration of saquinavir possibly reduced by dexamethasone

- Cytotoxics: saquinavir possibly increases the plasma concentration of afatinib—manufacturer of afatinib advises separating administration of saquinavir by 6 to 12 hours; saquinavir possibly increases plasma concentration of axitinib (reduce dose of axitinib—consult axitinib product literature); saquinavir possibly increases the plasma concentration of •bosutinib and •cabazitaxel—manufacturer of bosutinib and cabazitaxel advises avoid or consider reducing dose of bosutinib and cabazitaxel; saquinavir possibly increases plasma concentration of •crizotinib and •everolimus—manufacturer of crizotinib and everolimus advises avoid concomitant use; saquinavir possibly increases the plasma concentration of •ibrutinib—reduce dose of ibrutinib (see Dose under Ibrutinib, p. 615); avoidance of saquinavir advised by manufacturer of •lapatinib; increased risk of ventricular arrhythmias when saquinavir given with •pazopanib—avoid concomitant use; saquinavir possibly increases plasma concentration of ponatinib—consider reducing initial dose of ponatinib (see Dose under Ponatinib, p. 618); manufacturer of ruxolitinib advises dose reduction when saquinavir given with •ruxolitinib—consult ruxolitinib product literature; saquinavir possibly increases plasma concentration of •docetaxel—manufacturer of docetaxel advises avoid concomitant use or consider reducing docetaxel dose

- Dapoxetine: avoidance of saquinavir advised by manufacturer of •dapoxetine (increased risk of toxicity)

  Diuretics: saquinavir increases plasma concentration of eplerenone (reduce dose of eplerenone)

- Domperidone: possible increased risk of ventricular arrhythmias when saquinavir given with •domperidone—avoid concomitant use

- Ergot Alkaloids: increased risk of ergotism when saquinavir given with •ergotamine—avoid concomitant use

- Lipid-regulating Drugs: possible increased risk of myopathy when saquinavir given with atorvastatin; possible increased risk of myopathy when saquinavir given with •rosuvastatin—manufacturer of rosuvastatin advises avoid concomitant use; increased risk of myopathy when saquinavir given with •simvastatin (avoid concomitant use); avoidance of saquinavir advised by manufacturer of •lomitapide (plasma concentration of lomitapide possibly increased)

- Orlistat: absorption of saquinavir possibly reduced by •orlistat

- Pentamidine Isetionate: increased risk of ventricular arrhythmias when saquinavir given with •pentamidine isetionate—avoid concomitant use

- Ranolazine: saquinavir possibly increases plasma concentration of •ranolazine—manufacturer of ranolazine advises avoid concomitant use

- Sildenafil: increased risk of ventricular arrhythmias when saquinavir given with •sildenafil—avoid concomitant use

- Tacrolimus: saquinavir increases plasma concentration of •tacrolimus (consider reducing dose of tacrolimus)

- Tadalafil: increased risk of ventricular arrhythmias when saquinavir given with •tadalafil—avoid concomitant use

- Ulcer-healing Drugs: plasma concentration of saquinavir possibly increased by cimetidine; plasma concentration of saquinavir possibly increased by •esomeprazole, •lansoprazole, •pantoprazole and •rabeprazole—manufacturer of saquinavir advises avoid concomitant use; plasma concentration of

Saquinavir
- Ulcer-healing Drugs *(continued)*
  saquinavir increased by ●omeprazole—manufacturer of saquinavir advises avoid concomitant use
- Vardenafil: increased risk of ventricular arrhythmias when saquinavir given with ●vardenafil—avoid concomitant use

Saxagliptin *see* Antidiabetics
Selegiline
Note Selegiline is a MAO-B inhibitor
- Analgesics: hyperpyrexia and CNS toxicity reported when selegiline given with ●pethidine (avoid concomitant use); manufacturer of selegiline advises avoid concomitant use with opioid analgesics
- Antidepressants: manufacturer of selegiline advises avoid concomitant use with citalopram and escitalopram; increased risk of hypertension and CNS excitation when selegiline given with ●fluoxetine (selegiline should not be started until 5 weeks after stopping fluoxetine, avoid fluoxetine for 2 weeks after stopping selegiline); increased risk of hypertension and CNS excitation when selegiline given with ●fluvoxamine, ●sertraline or ●venlafaxine (selegiline should not be started until 1 week after stopping fluvoxamine, sertraline or venlafaxine, avoid fluvoxamine, sertraline or venlafaxine for 2 weeks after stopping selegiline); increased risk of hypertension and CNS excitation when selegiline given with ●paroxetine (selegiline should not be started until 2 weeks after stopping paroxetine, avoid paroxetine for 2 weeks after stopping selegiline); enhanced hypotensive effect when selegiline given with ●MAOIs—manufacturer of selegiline advises avoid concomitant use; avoid concomitant use of selegiline with ●moclobemide; CNS toxicity reported when selegiline given with ●tricyclics
Dopaminergics: max. dose of 10 mg selegiline advised by manufacturer of entacapone if used concomitantly; selegiline enhances effects and increases toxicity of levodopa (reduce dose of levodopa)
5HT₁-receptor Agonists: manufacturer of selegiline advises avoid concomitant use with 5HT₁ agonists
Memantine: effects of dopaminergics and selegiline possibly enhanced by memantine
Methyldopa: antiparkinsonian effect of dopaminergics antagonised by methyldopa
- Oestrogens: plasma concentration of selegiline increased by ●oestrogens—manufacturer of selegiline advises avoid concomitant use
- Progestogens: plasma concentration of selegiline increased by ●progestogens—manufacturer of selegiline advises avoid concomitant use
- Sympathomimetics: manufacturer of selegiline advises avoid concomitant use with sympathomimetics; risk of hypertensive crisis when selegiline given with ●dopamine

Selenium
Eltrombopag: selenium possibly reduces absorption of eltrombopag (give at least 4 hours apart)
Vitamins: absorption of selenium possibly reduced by ascorbic acid (give at least 4 hours apart)

Sertraline *see* Antidepressants, SSRI
Sevelamer
Antibacterials: sevelamer reduces bioavailability of ciprofloxacin
Ciclosporin: sevelamer possibly reduces plasma concentration of ciclosporin
Mycophenolate: sevelamer possibly reduces plasma concentration of mycophenolate
Tacrolimus: sevelamer possibly reduces plasma concentration of tacrolimus
Thyroid Hormones: sevelamer possibly reduces absorption of levothyroxine
Vitamins: sevelamer reduces absorption of calcitriol (give at least 1 hour before or 3 hours after sevelamer)

Sevoflurane *see* Anaesthetics, General
Sildenafil
- Alpha-blockers: enhanced hypotensive effect when sildenafil given with ●alpha-blockers (avoid alpha-blockers for 4 hours after sildenafil)—see also p. 570
Anti-arrhythmics: avoidance of sildenafil advised by manufacturer of disopyramide (risk of ventricular arrhythmias)
- Antibacterials: plasma concentration of sildenafil increased by ●clarithromycin—consider reducing initial dose of sildenafil for erectile dysfunction or reduce sildenafil dose frequency to once daily for pulmonary hypertension; plasma concentration of sildenafil increased by erythromycin—reduce initial dose of sildenafil for erectile dysfunction or reduce sildenafil dose frequency to twice daily for pulmonary hypertension; plasma concentration of sildenafil possibly increased by ●telithromycin—consider reducing initial dose of sildenafil for erectile dysfunction or reduce sildenafil dose frequency to once daily for pulmonary hypertension
Antifungals: plasma concentration of sildenafil increased by itraconazole—reduce initial dose of sildenafil
- Antivirals: side-effects of sildenafil possibly increased by ●atazanavir; plasma concentration of sildenafil reduced by etravirine; plasma concentration of sildenafil possibly increased by fosamprenavir; plasma concentration of sildenafil increased by ●indinavir—reduce initial dose of sildenafil; plasma concentration of sildenafil significantly increased by ●ritonavir—avoid concomitant use; increased risk of ventricular arrhythmias when sildenafil given with ●saquinavir—avoid concomitant use; avoidance of sildenafil advised by manufacturer of ●telaprevir; avoidance of sildenafil for pulmonary arterial hypertension advised by manufacturer of tipranavir
Bosentan: plasma concentration of sildenafil reduced by bosentan, also plasma concentration of bosentan increased
Calcium-channel Blockers: enhanced hypotensive effect when sildenafil given with amlodipine
- Cobicistat: plasma concentration of sildenafil possibly increased by ●cobicistat—manufacturer of cobicistat advises avoid concomitant use of sildenafil for pulmonary arterial hypertension or reduce dose of sildenafil for erectile dysfunction—consult cobicistat product literature
Cytotoxics: avoidance of sildenafil for pulmonary arterial hypertension advised by manufacturer of idelalisib
Dapoxetine: avoidance of sildenafil advised by manufacturer of dapoxetine
Grapefruit Juice: plasma concentration of sildenafil possibly increased by grapefruit juice
- Nicorandil: sildenafil significantly enhances hypotensive effect of ●nicorandil (avoid concomitant use)
- Nitrates: sildenafil significantly enhances hypotensive effect of ●nitrates (avoid concomitant use)
- Riociguat: enhanced hypotensive effect when sildenafil given with ●riociguat—avoid concomitant use
Ulcer-healing Drugs: plasma concentration of sildenafil increased by cimetidine—consider reducing dose of sildenafil for erectile dysfunction

Siltuximab
- Antipsychotics: avoid concomitant use of cytotoxics with ●clozapine (increased risk of agranulocytosis)
- Vaccines: avoid concomitant use of monoclonal antibodies with live ●vaccines (see p. 842)

Simeprevir
- Antibacterials: plasma concentration of simeprevir possibly increased by ●clarithromycin and ●telithromycin—manufacturer of simeprevir advises avoid concomitant use; plasma concentration of both drugs increased when simeprevir given with

Simeprevir
- Antibacterials *(continued)*
  - •erythromycin—manufacturer of simeprevir advises avoid concomitant use; plasma concentration of simeprevir possibly reduced by rifabutin—manufacturer of simeprevir advises avoid concomitant use; plasma concentration of simeprevir reduced by •rifampicin—manufacturer of simeprevir advises avoid concomitant use
- Antidepressants: plasma concentration of simeprevir possibly reduced by •St John's wort—manufacturer of simeprevir advises avoid concomitant use
- Antiepileptics: plasma concentration of simeprevir possibly reduced by •carbamazepine, •oxcarbazepine, •phenobarbital and •phenytoin—manufacturer of simeprevir advises avoid concomitant use
- Antifungals: plasma concentration of simeprevir possibly increased by •fluconazole, •itraconazole, •posaconazole and •voriconazole—manufacturer of simeprevir advises avoid concomitant use
- Antivirals: plasma concentration of both drugs increased when simeprevir given with •darunavir—manufacturer of simeprevir advises avoid concomitant use; plasma concentration of simeprevir reduced by efavirenz; manufacturer of simeprevir advises avoid concomitant use with etravirine; plasma concentration of simeprevir possibly reduced by •nevirapine—manufacturer of simeprevir advises avoid concomitant use; plasma concentration of simeprevir increased by •ritonavir—manufacturer of simeprevir advises avoid concomitant use

  Anxiolytics and Hypnotics: simeprevir increases plasma concentration of *oral* midazolam

  Cardiac Glycosides: simeprevir increases plasma concentration of digoxin
- Cobicistat: plasma concentration of simeprevir possibly increased by •cobicistat—manufacturer of simeprevir advises avoid concomitant use

  Corticosteroids: plasma concentration of simeprevir possibly reduced by dexamethasone—manufacturer of simeprevir advises avoid concomitant use

  Lipid-regulating Drugs: simeprevir increases plasma concentration of atorvastatin, rosuvastatin and simvastatin (consider reducing dose of atorvastatin, rosuvastatin and simvastatin)

Simvastatin *see* Statins
Sirolimus
  Anti-arrhythmics: caution with sirolimus advised by manufacturer of dronedarone
- Antibacterials: plasma concentration of sirolimus increased by •clarithromycin and •telithromycin—avoid concomitant use; plasma concentration of both drugs increased when sirolimus given with •erythromycin; plasma concentration of sirolimus reduced by •rifabutin and •rifampicin—avoid concomitant use
- Antifungals: plasma concentration of sirolimus increased by micafungin and •miconazole; plasma concentration of sirolimus possibly increased by fluconazole and posaconazole; plasma concentration of sirolimus increased by •itraconazole and •voriconazole—avoid concomitant use
- Antivirals: plasma concentration of sirolimus possibly increased by •atazanavir and lopinavir; plasma concentration of sirolimus increased by •boceprevir (increased risk of toxicity—reduce sirolimus dose); plasma concentration of both drugs increased when sirolimus given with •telaprevir (reduce dose of sirolimus)
- Calcium-channel Blockers: plasma concentration of sirolimus increased by •diltiazem; plasma concentration of both drugs increased when sirolimus given with •verapamil

Sirolimus *(continued)*
  Ciclosporin: plasma concentration of sirolimus increased by ciclosporin
- Cytotoxics: caution with sirolimus advised by manufacturer of •crizotinib
- Grapefruit Juice: plasma concentration of sirolimus increased by •grapefruit juice—avoid concomitant use

Sitagliptin *see* Antidiabetics
Smallpox vaccine *see* Vaccines
Sodium Aurothiomalate
- ACE Inhibitors: flushing and hypotension reported when sodium aurothiomalate given with •ACE inhibitors

  Penicillamine: avoidance of sodium aurothiomalate advised by manufacturer of penicillamine (increased risk of toxicity)

Sodium Benzoate
  Antiepileptics: effects of sodium benzoate possibly reduced by valproate

  Antipsychotics: effects of sodium benzoate possibly reduced by haloperidol

  Corticosteroids: effects of sodium benzoate possibly reduced by corticosteroids

Sodium Bicarbonate *see* Antacids
Sodium Citrate
  Antibacterials: avoid concomitant use of sodium citrate with methenamine

  Ulcer-healing Drugs: avoidance of sodium citrate advised by manufacturer of sucralfate

Sodium Clodronate *see* Bisphosphonates
Sodium Nitroprusside *see* Vasodilator Antihypertensives
Sodium Oxybate
- Analgesics: effects of sodium oxybate enhanced by •opioid analgesics (avoid concomitant use)

  Antidepressants: increased risk of side-effects when sodium oxybate given with tricyclics
- Antiepileptics: manufacturer of sodium oxybate advises avoid concomitant use with phenobarbital; plasma concentration of sodium oxybate increased by •valproate (see Dose under Sodium Oxybate, p. 230)

  Antipsychotics: effects of sodium oxybate possibly enhanced by antipsychotics
- Anxiolytics and Hypnotics: effects of sodium oxybate enhanced by •benzodiazepines (avoid concomitant use)

Sodium Phenylbutyrate
  Antiepileptics: effects of sodium phenylbutyrate possibly reduced by valproate

  Antipsychotics: effects of sodium phenylbutyrate possibly reduced by haloperidol

  Corticosteroids: effects of sodium phenylbutyrate possibly reduced by corticosteroids

Sodium Stibogluconate
- Antifungals: possible increased risk of arrhythmias when sodium stibogluconate given before •amphotericin—manufacturer of sodium stibogluconate advises giving 14 days apart

Sodium Valproate *see* Valproate
Sofosbuvir
  Antibacterials: manufacturer of sofosbuvir advises avoid concomitant use with rifabutin and rifampicin

  Antidepressants: manufacturer of sofosbuvir advises avoid concomitant use with St John's wort

  Antiepileptics: manufacturer of sofosbuvir advises avoid concomitant use with carbamazepine, oxcarbazepine, phenobarbital and phenytoin

Solifenacin *see* Antimuscarinics
Somatropin
  Corticosteroids: growth-promoting effect of somatropin may be inhibited by corticosteroids

Appendix 1: Interactions

Somatropin *(continued)*

Oestrogens: increased doses of somatropin may be needed when given with oestrogens (when used as oral replacement therapy)

Sorafenib

Antibacterials: bioavailability of sorafenib reduced by neomycin; plasma concentration of sorafenib reduced by rifampicin

- Anticoagulants: sorafenib possibly enhances anticoagulant effect of ●coumarins
- Antipsychotics: avoid concomitant use of cytotoxics with ●clozapine (increased risk of agranulocytosis)
- Antivirals: avoidance of sorafenib advised by manufacturer of ●boceprevir

Cytotoxics: sorafenib increases plasma concentration of docetaxel and doxorubicin; sorafenib possibly increases plasma concentration of irinotecan

Sotalol *see* Beta-blockers

Spironolactone *see* Diuretics

Statins

Antacids: absorption of rosuvastatin reduced by antacids

- Anti-arrhythmics: increased risk of myopathy when simvastatin given with ●amiodarone (see Dose under Simvastatin, p. 177); increased risk of myopathy when simvastatin given with ●dronedarone; plasma concentration of atorvastatin possibly increased by dronedarone; plasma concentration of rosuvastatin increased by ●dronedarone—adjust dose of rosuvastatin (consult product literature)
- Antibacterials: plasma concentration of atorvastatin and pravastatin increased by ●clarithromycin; increased risk of myopathy when simvastatin given with ●clarithromycin, ●erythromycin or ●telithromycin (avoid concomitant use); plasma concentration of rosuvastatin reduced by erythromycin; possible increased risk of myopathy when atorvastatin given with erythromycin; plasma concentration of pravastatin increased by erythromycin; plasma concentration of atorvastatin and simvastatin possibly reduced by rifampicin; metabolism of fluvastatin accelerated by rifampicin (reduced effect); increased risk of myopathy when statins given with ●daptomycin (preferably avoid concomitant use); risk of myopathy and rhabdomyolysis when statins given with ●fusidic acid—avoid concomitant use and for 7 days after last fusidic acid dose; increased risk of myopathy when atorvastatin given with ●telithromycin (avoid concomitant use); possible increased risk of myopathy when pravastatin given with telithromycin
- Anticoagulants: atorvastatin may transiently reduce anticoagulant effect of warfarin; fluvastatin and simvastatin enhance anticoagulant effect of ●coumarins; rosuvastatin possibly enhances anticoagulant effect of ●coumarins and ●phenindione

Antidepressants: plasma concentration of simvastatin reduced by St John's wort

Antidiabetics: fluvastatin possibly increases plasma concentration of glibenclamide

- Antiepileptics: plasma concentration of simvastatin reduced by ●carbamazepine and eslicarbazepine—consider increasing dose of simvastatin; plasma concentration of rosuvastatin reduced by eslicarbazepine; combination of fluvastatin with phenytoin may increase plasma concentration of either drug (or both)
- Antifungals: possible increased risk of myopathy when simvastatin given with ●fluconazole or ●miconazole; possible increased risk of myopathy when atorvastatin given with ●fluconazole or imidazoles; plasma concentration of fluvastatin increased by fluconazole—possible increased risk of myopathy; plasma concentration of rosuvastatin increased by ●itraconazole—adjust dose of rosuvastatin (consult product literature); increased risk of myopathy when ator-

Statins

- Antifungals *(continued)*

vastatin given with ●itraconazole, ●posaconazole or ●voriconazole; increased risk of myopathy when simvastatin given with ●itraconazole or ●posaconazole (avoid concomitant use); increased risk of myopathy when simvastatin given with ●voriconazole

- Antivirals: plasma concentration of rosuvastatin increased by ●atazanavir, ●darunavir, ●lopinavir and ●tipranavir—adjust dose of rosuvastatin (consult product literature); increased risk of myopathy when simvastatin given with ●atazanavir, ●indinavir, ●ritonavir or ●saquinavir (avoid concomitant use); possible increased risk of myopathy when atorvastatin or pravastatin given with ●atazanavir; plasma concentration of atorvastatin increased by boceprevir (reduce dose of atorvastatin); manufacturers advise avoid concomitant use of simvastatin with ●boceprevir and ●telaprevir; plasma concentration of pravastatin increased by boceprevir; plasma concentration of rosuvastatin increased by daclatasvir; plasma concentration of pravastatin possibly increased by darunavir; possible increased risk of myopathy when atorvastatin given with darunavir, fosamprenavir, indinavir, lopinavir, ritonavir or saquinavir; plasma concentration of atorvastatin, pravastatin and simvastatin reduced by efavirenz; plasma concentration of atorvastatin possibly reduced by etravirine; possible increased risk of myopathy when rosuvastatin given with ●fosamprenavir, ●indinavir, ●ritonavir and ●saquinavir—manufacturer of rosuvastatin advises avoid concomitant use; possible increased risk of myopathy when simvastatin given with ●fosamprenavir or ●lopinavir—avoid concomitant use; plasma concentration of atorvastatin, rosuvastatin and simvastatin increased by simeprevir (consider reducing dose of atorvastatin, rosuvastatin and simvastatin); avoidance of atorvastatin advised by manufacturer of ●telaprevir; plasma concentration of simvastatin possibly increased by ●tipranavir—avoid concomitant use; increased risk of myopathy when atorvastatin given with ●tipranavir (see Dose under Atorvastatin, p. 175)

Anxiolytics and Hypnotics: atorvastatin possibly increases plasma concentration of midazolam

Bosentan: plasma concentration of simvastatin reduced by bosentan

- Calcium-channel Blockers: possible increased risk of myopathy when simvastatin given with ●amlodipine and diltiazem (see Dose under Simvastatin, p. 177); plasma concentration of atorvastatin increased by diltiazem—possible increased risk of myopathy; atorvastatin increases plasma concentration of ●verapamil, also possible increased risk of myopathy (consider reducing dose of atorvastatin); increased risk of myopathy when simvastatin given with ●verapamil (see Dose under Simvastatin, p. 177)

Cardiac Glycosides: atorvastatin possibly increases plasma concentration of digoxin

- Ciclosporin: increased risk of myopathy when rosuvastatin or simvastatin given with ●ciclosporin (avoid concomitant use); increased risk of myopathy when atorvastatin given with ●ciclosporin (see Dose under Atorvastatin, p. 175); increased risk of myopathy when fluvastatin or pravastatin given with ●ciclosporin
- Clopidogrel: plasma concentration of rosuvastatin increased by ●clopidogrel—adjust dose of rosuvastatin (consult product literature)
- Cobicistat: plasma concentration of atorvastatin possibly increased by cobicistat—manufacturer of cobicistat advises reduce dose of atorvastatin; avoidance of simvastatin advised by manufacturer of ●cobicistat

Statins *(continued)*

- Colchicine: possible increased risk of myopathy when statins given with ●colchicine

  Cytotoxics: plasma concentration of simvastatin possibly increased by dasatinib; avoidance of simvastatin advised by manufacturer of idelalisib; plasma concentration of simvastatin increased by imatinib

- Eltrombopag: plasma concentration of rosuvastatin increased by ●eltrombopag—adjust dose of rosuvastatin (consult product literature)

- Grapefruit Juice: plasma concentration of atorvastatin possibly increased by grapefruit juice; plasma concentration of simvastatin increased by ●grapefruit juice—avoid concomitant use

- Hormone Antagonists: possible increased risk of myopathy when simvastatin given with ●danazol—avoid concomitant use

- Lipid-regulating Drugs: possible increased risk of myopathy when simvastatin given with ●bezafibrate and ●ciprofibrate (see Dose under Simvastatin, p. 177); when given with statins reduce maximum dose of fenofibrate—see Dose under Fenofibrate, p. 179; increased risk of myopathy when atorvastatin, fluvastatin or pravastatin given with ●gemfibrozil (preferably avoid concomitant use); increased risk of myopathy when simvastatin given with ●gemfibrozil (avoid concomitant use); plasma concentration of rosuvastatin increased by ●ezetimibe—adjust dose of rosuvastatin (consult product literature); increased risk of myopathy when statins given with ●fibrates; increased risk of myopathy when rosuvastatin given with ●fibrates (see Dose under Rosuvastatin, p. 176); plasma concentration of atorvastatin increased by lomitapide; plasma concentration of simvastatin increased by ●lomitapide (see Dose under Simvastatin, p. 177); increased risk of myopathy when statins given with ●nicotinic acid (applies to lipid regulating doses of nicotinic acid)

  Oestrogens: atorvastatin **and** rosuvastatin increase plasma concentration of ethinylestradiol

  Progestogens: atorvastatin increases plasma concentration of norethisterone; rosuvastatin increases plasma concentration of active metabolite of norgestimate; rosuvastatin increases plasma concentration of norgestrel

- Ranolazine: plasma concentration of simvastatin increased by ●ranolazine (see Dose under Simvastatin, p. 177)

  Retinoids: plasma concentration of simvastatin reduced by alitretinoin

- Teriflunomide: plasma concentration of rosuvastatin increased by ●teriflunomide (consider reducing dose of rosuvastatin)

- Ticagrelor: plasma concentration of simvastatin increased by ●ticagrelor (increased risk of toxicity)

Stavudine

- Antivirals: increased risk of side-effects when stavudine given with ●didanosine; increased risk of toxicity when stavudine given with ●ribavirin; effects of stavudine possibly inhibited by ●zidovudine (manufacturers advise avoid concomitant use)

- Cytotoxics: effects of stavudine possibly inhibited by doxorubicin; increased risk of toxicity when stavudine given with ●hydroxycarbamide—avoid concomitant use

- Orlistat: absorption of stavudine possibly reduced by ●orlistat

Stiripentol

- Antidepressants: anticonvulsant effect of antiepileptics possibly antagonised by MAOIs and ●tricyclic-related antidepressants (convulsive threshold lowered); anticonvulsant effect of antiepileptics antagonised by ●SSRIs and ●tricyclics (convulsive threshold lowered)

Stiripentol *(continued)*

- Antiepileptics: stiripentol increases plasma concentration of ●carbamazepine, ●phenobarbital and ●phenytoin

- Antimalarials: anticonvulsant effect of antiepileptics antagonised by ●mefloquine

- Antipsychotics: anticonvulsant effect of antiepileptics antagonised by ●antipsychotics (convulsive threshold lowered)

  Anxiolytics and Hypnotics: stiripentol increases plasma concentration of clobazam

- Orlistat: possible increased risk of convulsions when antiepileptics given with ●orlistat

Streptomycin *see* Aminoglycosides

Strontium Ranelate

  Antibacterials: strontium ranelate reduces absorption of quinolones and tetracyclines (manufacturer of strontium ranelate advises avoid concomitant use)

Sucralfate

  Antibacterials: sucralfate reduces absorption of ciprofloxacin, levofloxacin, moxifloxacin, ofloxacin and tetracyclines; sucralfate reduces absorption of norfloxacin (give at least 2 hours apart)

- Anticoagulants: sucralfate possibly reduces absorption of ●coumarins (reduced anticoagulant effect)

- Antiepileptics: sucralfate reduces absorption of ●phenytoin

  Antipsychotics: sucralfate reduces absorption of sulpiride

  Cardiac Glycosides: sucralfate possibly reduces absorption of cardiac glycosides

  Potassium Salts: manufacturer of sucralfate advises avoid concomitant use with potassium citrate

  Sodium Citrate: manufacturer of sucralfate advises avoid concomitant use with sodium citrate

  Theophylline: sucralfate possibly reduces absorption of theophylline (give at least 2 hours apart)

  Thyroid Hormones: sucralfate reduces absorption of levothyroxine

  Ulcer-healing Drugs: sucralfate possibly reduces absorption of lansoprazole

Sugammadex

  Antibacterials: response to sugammadex possibly reduced by fusidic acid

  Progestogens: sugammadex possibly reduces plasma concentration of progestogens—manufacturer of sugammadex advises additional contraceptive precautions

Sulfadiazine *see* Sulfonamides

Sulfadoxine *see* Sulfonamides

Sulfamethoxazole *see* Sulfonamides

Sulfasalazine

  Cardiac Glycosides: sulfasalazine possibly reduces absorption of digoxin

  Folates: sulfasalazine possibly reduces absorption of folic acid

Sulfinpyrazone

  Analgesics: effects of sulfinpyrazone antagonised by aspirin

  Antibacterials: sulfinpyrazone reduces excretion of nitrofurantoin (increased risk of toxicity); sulfinpyrazone reduces excretion of penicillins; effects of sulfinpyrazone antagonised by pyrazinamide

- Anticoagulants: increased risk of bleeding when sulfinpyrazone given with apixaban; sulfinpyrazone enhances anticoagulant effect of ●coumarins; possible increased risk of bleeding when sulfinpyrazone given with ●dabigatran

- Antidiabetics: sulfinpyrazone enhances effects of ●sulfonylureas

- Antiepileptics: sulfinpyrazone increases plasma concentration of ●phenytoin

  Calcium-channel Blockers: sulfinpyrazone reduces plasma concentration of verapamil

- Ciclosporin: sulfinpyrazone reduces plasma concentration of ●ciclosporin

Sulfinpyrazone *(continued)*
Theophylline: sulfinpyrazone reduces plasma concentration of theophylline

Sulfonamides
Anaesthetics, General: sulfonamides enhance effects of thiopental
- Anaesthetics, Local: effects of sulfonamides possibly inhibited by ●chloroprocaine (manufacturer of chloroprocaine advises avoid concomitant use); increased risk of methaemoglobinaemia when sulfonamides given with prilocaine
Anti-arrhythmics: possible increased risk of ventricular arrhythmias when sulfamethoxazole (as co-trimoxazole) given with amiodarone—manufacturer of amiodarone advises avoid concomitant use of co-trimoxazole
- Antibacterials: increased risk of crystalluria when sulfonamides given with ●methenamine
- Anticoagulants: sulfonamides enhance anticoagulant effect of ●coumarins; sulfonamides possibly inhibit metabolism of phenindione
Antidiabetics: sulfonamides rarely enhance the effects of sulfonylureas
Antiepileptics: sulfonamides possibly increase plasma concentration of phenytoin
- Antimalarials: increased antifolate effect when sulfonamides given with ●pyrimethamine
- Antipsychotics: avoid concomitant use of sulfonamides with ●clozapine (increased risk of agranulocytosis)
- Azathioprine: increased risk of haematological toxicity when sulfamethoxazole (as co-trimoxazole) given with ●azathioprine
- Ciclosporin: increased risk of nephrotoxicity when sulfonamides given with ●ciclosporin; sulfadiazine possibly reduces plasma concentration of ●ciclosporin
- Cytotoxics: increased risk of haematological toxicity when sulfamethoxazole (as co-trimoxazole) given with ●mercaptopurine or ●methotrexate; sulfonamides increase risk of methotrexate toxicity
Potassium Aminobenzoate: effects of sulfonamides inhibited by potassium aminobenzoate
Vaccines: antibacterials inactivate oral typhoid vaccine—see p. 864

Sulfonylureas *see* Antidiabetics
Sulindac *see* NSAIDs
Sulpiride *see* Antipsychotics
Sumatriptan *see* 5HT$_1$-receptor Agonists (under HT)
Sunitinib
Antibacterials: metabolism of sunitinib accelerated by rifampicin (reduced plasma concentration)
- Antipsychotics: avoid concomitant use of cytotoxics with ●clozapine (increased risk of agranulocytosis)
- Antivirals: avoidance of sunitinib advised by manufacturer of ●boceprevir

Suxamethonium *see* Muscle Relaxants
Sympathomimetics
- Adrenergic Neurone Blockers: ephedrine, isometheptene, metaraminol, methylphenidate, noradrenaline (norepinephrine), oxymetazoline, phenylephrine, pseudoephedrine and xylometazoline antagonise hypotensive effect of ●adrenergic neurone blockers; dexamfetamine and lisdexamfetamine antagonise hypotensive effect of ●guanethidine; increased risk of hypertension when adrenaline (epinephrine) given with ●guanethidine
Alcohol: effects of methylphenidate possibly enhanced by alcohol
Alpha$_2$-adrenoceptor Stimulants: avoidance of sympathomimetics advised by manufacturer of apraclonidine
- Alpha-blockers: avoid concomitant use of adrenaline (epinephrine) or dopamine with ●tolazoline
- Anaesthetics, General: avoidance of sympathomimetics advised by manufacturer of ●isoflurane (risk of ventricular arrhythmias); increased risk of

Sympathomimetics
- Anaesthetics, General *(continued)*
arrhythmias when adrenaline (epinephrine) or noradrenaline (norepinephrine) given with ●volatile liquid general anaesthetics; increased risk of hypertension when methylphenidate given with ●volatile liquid general anaesthetics
Antacids: absorption of pseudoephedrine possibly increased by aluminium hydroxide
- Anticoagulants: methylphenidate possibly enhances anticoagulant effect of ●coumarins
- Antidepressants: risk of hypertensive crisis when dexamfetamine, ephedrine, isometheptene, lisdexamfetamine, metaraminol, methylphenidate, phenylephrine or pseudoephedrine given with ●MAOIs, avoid dexamfetamine, ephedrine, isometheptene, lisdexamfetamine, metaraminol, methylphenidate, phenylephrine or pseudoephedrine for at least 2 weeks after stopping MAOIs; risk of hypertensive crisis when adrenaline (epinephrine), dobutamine, dopamine, noradrenaline (norepinephrine) or xylometazoline given with ●MAOIs; risk of hypertensive crisis when oxymetazoline given with ●MAOIs, some manufacturers advise avoid oxymetazoline for at least 2 weeks after stopping MAOIs; risk of hypertensive crisis when sympathomimetics given with ●moclobemide; methylphenidate possibly inhibits metabolism of SSRIs and tricyclics; increased risk of hypertension and arrhythmias when noradrenaline (norepinephrine) or phenylephrine given with ●tricyclics; increased risk of hypertension and arrhythmias when adrenaline (epinephrine) given with ●tricyclics (but local anaesthetics with adrenaline appear to be safe)
Antiepileptics: methylphenidate possibly increases plasma concentration of phenobarbital; methylphenidate increases plasma concentration of phenytoin
Antipsychotics: hypertensive effect of sympathomimetics antagonised by antipsychotics; effects of lisdexamfetamine possibly reduced by chlorpromazine; dexamfetamine possibly antagonises antipsychotic effects of chlorpromazine; methylphenidate possibly increases side-effects of risperidone
Antivirals: plasma concentration of dexamfetamine possibly increased by ritonavir
- Beta-blockers: increased risk of severe hypertension and bradycardia when adrenaline (epinephrine) given with non-cardioselective ●beta-blockers, also response to adrenaline (epinephrine) may be reduced; increased risk of severe hypertension and bradycardia when dobutamine given with non-cardioselective ●beta-blockers; possible increased risk of severe hypertension and bradycardia when noradrenaline (norepinephrine) given with non-cardioselective ●beta-blockers
- Clonidine: possible risk of hypertension when adrenaline (epinephrine) or noradrenaline (norepinephrine) given with clonidine; serious adverse events reported with concomitant use of methylphenidate and ●clonidine (causality not established)
Corticosteroids: ephedrine accelerates metabolism of dexamethasone
- Dopaminergics: risk of toxicity when isometheptene given with ●bromocriptine; effects of adrenaline (epinephrine), dobutamine, dopamine and noradrenaline (norepinephrine) possibly enhanced by entacapone; avoid concomitant use of sympathomimetics with ●rasagiline; risk of hypertensive crisis when dopamine given with ●selegiline; avoidance of sympathomimetics advised by manufacturer of selegiline
Doxapram: increased risk of hypertension when sympathomimetics given with doxapram
Ergot Alkaloids: increased risk of ergotism when sympathomimetics given with ergotamine

Sympathomimetics *(continued)*

Oxytocin: risk of hypertension when vasoconstrictor sympathomimetics given with oxytocin (due to enhanced vasopressor effect)

- Sympathomimetics: effects of adrenaline (epinephrine) possibly enhanced by ●dopexamine; dopexamine possibly enhances effects of ●noradrenaline (norepinephrine)

Theophylline: avoidance of ephedrine in children advised by manufacturer of theophylline

Ulcer-healing Drugs: metabolism of dobutamine possibly inhibited by cimetidine

Sympathomimetics, Beta$_2$

- Antivirals: avoidance of salmeterol advised by manufacturer of lopinavir, ritonavir and tipranavir; avoidance of salmeterol advised by manufacturer of ●telaprevir (risk of ventricular arrhythmias)

Atomoxetine: Increased risk of cardiovascular side-effects when *parenteral* salbutamol given with atomoxetine

Cardiac Glycosides: salbutamol possibly reduces plasma concentration of digoxin

Cobicistat: avoidance of salmeterol advised by manufacturer of cobicistat

Corticosteroids: increased risk of hypokalaemia when high doses of beta$_2$ sympathomimetics given with corticosteroids—see Hypokalaemia, p. 189

Cytotoxics: avoidance of salmeterol advised by manufacturer of idelalisib

Diuretics: increased risk of hypokalaemia when high doses of beta$_2$ sympathomimetics given with acetazolamide, loop diuretics or thiazides and related diuretics—see Hypokalaemia, p. 189

- Methyldopa: acute hypotension reported when *infusion* of salbutamol given with ●methyldopa

Muscle Relaxants: bambuterol enhances effects of suxamethonium

Theophylline: increased risk of hypokalaemia when high doses of beta$_2$ sympathomimetics given with theophylline—see Hypokalaemia, p. 189

Tacrolimus

Note Interactions do not generally apply to tacrolimus used topically; risk of facial flushing and skin irritation with alcohol consumption (p. 818) does not apply to tacrolimus taken systemically

- Analgesics: possible increased risk of nephrotoxicity when tacrolimus given with NSAIDs; increased risk of nephrotoxicity when tacrolimus given with ●ibuprofen

Angiotensin-II Receptor Antagonists: increased risk of hyperkalaemia when tacrolimus given with angiotensin-II receptor antagonists

Anti-arrhythmics: caution with tacrolimus advised by manufacturer of dronedarone

- Antibacterials: plasma concentration of tacrolimus increased by ●clarithromycin and ●erythromycin; plasma concentration of tacrolimus possibly reduced by rifabutin; plasma concentration of tacrolimus reduced by ●rifampicin; increased risk of nephrotoxicity when tacrolimus given with ●aminoglycosides; plasma concentration of tacrolimus possibly increased by ●chloramphenicol and ●telithromycin; possible increased risk of nephrotoxicity when tacrolimus given with vancomycin

- Anticoagulants: tacrolimus possibly increases plasma concentration of ●dabigatran—manufacturer of dabigatran advises avoid concomitant use

- Antidepressants: plasma concentration of tacrolimus reduced by ●St John's wort—avoid concomitant use

- Antiepileptics: plasma concentration of tacrolimus reduced by ●phenobarbital; plasma concentration of tacrolimus reduced by phenytoin, also plasma concentration of phenytoin possibly increased

- Antifungals: plasma concentration of tacrolimus possibly increased by ●miconazole *oral gel*; increased

Tacrolimus

- Antifungals *(continued)*
  risk of nephrotoxicity when tacrolimus given with ●amphotericin; plasma concentration of tacrolimus increased by ●fluconazole, ●itraconazole, ●posaconazole and ●voriconazole (consider reducing dose of tacrolimus); plasma concentration of tacrolimus reduced by ●caspofungin

- Antipsychotics: avoidance of tacrolimus advised by manufacturer of ●droperidol (risk of ventricular arrhythmias)

- Antivirals: possible increased risk of nephrotoxicity when tacrolimus given with aciclovir or ganciclovir; plasma concentration of tacrolimus possibly increased by ●atazanavir and ●ritonavir; plasma concentration of tacrolimus increased by ●boceprevir (reduce dose of tacrolimus); plasma concentration of tacrolimus possibly affected by ●efavirenz; plasma concentration of tacrolimus increased by ●fosamprenavir; plasma concentration of tacrolimus increased by ●saquinavir (consider reducing dose of tacrolimus); plasma concentration of both drugs increased when tacrolimus given with ●telaprevir (reduce dose of tacrolimus)

- Calcium-channel Blockers: plasma concentration of tacrolimus possibly increased by felodipine, nicardipine and verapamil; plasma concentration of tacrolimus increased by ●diltiazem and ●nifedipine

- Ciclosporin: tacrolimus increases plasma concentration of ●ciclosporin (increased risk of nephrotoxicity)—avoid concomitant use

Colestilan: manufacturer of colestilan advises give tacrolimus at least 1 hour before or 3 hours after colestilan

- Cytotoxics: tacrolimus possibly increases the plasma concentration of afatinib—manufacturer of afatinib advises separating administration of tacrolimus by 6 to 12 hours; caution with tacrolimus advised by manufacturer of ●crizotinib; plasma concentration of tacrolimus increased by imatinib

Dexrazoxane: increased risk of immunosupression with tacrolimus advised by manufacturer of dexrazoxane

- Diuretics: increased risk of hyperkalaemia when tacrolimus given with ●potassium-sparing diuretics and aldosterone antagonists

- Grapefruit Juice: plasma concentration of tacrolimus increased by ●grapefruit juice

Hormone Antagonists: plasma concentration of tacrolimus possibly increased by danazol

Mifamurtide: avoidance of tacrolimus advised by manufacturer of mifamurtide

Oestrogens: plasma concentration of tacrolimus possibly increased by ethinylestradiol

- Potassium Salts: increased risk of hyperkalaemia when tacrolimus given with ●potassium salts

- Ranolazine: plasma concentration of tacrolimus increased by ●ranolazine

Sevelamer: plasma concentration of tacrolimus possibly reduced by sevelamer

Ulcer-healing Drugs: plasma concentration of tacrolimus possibly increased by omeprazole

Tadalafil

- Alpha-blockers: enhanced hypotensive effect when tadalafil given with ●doxazosin—manufacturer of tadalafil advises avoid concomitant use; enhanced hypotensive effect when tadalafil given with ●alpha-blockers—see also p. 570

Anti-arrhythmics: avoidance of tadalafil advised by manufacturer of disopyramide (risk of ventricular arrhythmias)

- Antibacterials: plasma concentration of tadalafil possibly increased by clarithromycin and erythromycin; plasma concentration of tadalafil reduced by ●rifampicin—manufacturer of tadalafil advises avoid concomitant use

Tadalafil *(continued)*

Antifungals: plasma concentration of tadalafil possibly increased by itraconazole

- Antivirals: plasma concentration of tadalafil possibly increased by fosamprenavir and indinavir; plasma concentration of tadalafil increased by ●ritonavir—manufacturer of tadalafil advises avoid concomitant use; increased risk of ventricular arrhythmias when tadalafil given with ●saquinavir—avoid concomitant use; avoidance of high doses of tadalafil advised by manufacturer of ●telaprevir—consult product literature

Bosentan: plasma concentration of tadalafil reduced by bosentan

- Cobicistat: plasma concentration of tadalafil possibly increased by ●cobicistat—manufacturer of cobicistat advises reduce dose of tadalafil (consult cobicistat product literature)

Dapoxetine: avoidance of tadalafil advised by manufacturer of dapoxetine

Grapefruit Juice: plasma concentration of tadalafil possibly increased by grapefruit juice

- Nicorandil: tadalafil significantly enhances hypotensive effect of ●nicorandil (avoid concomitant use)
- Nitrates: tadalafil significantly enhances hypotensive effect of ●nitrates (avoid concomitant use)
- Riociguat: possible enhanced hypotensive effect when tadalafil given with ●riociguat—avoid concomitant use

Tamoxifen

Antibacterials: metabolism of tamoxifen accelerated by rifampicin (reduced plasma concentration)

- Anticoagulants: tamoxifen enhances anticoagulant effect of ●coumarins
- Antidepressants: metabolism of tamoxifen to active metabolite possibly inhibited by ●fluoxetine and ●paroxetine (avoid concomitant use)
- Antipsychotics: avoidance of tamoxifen advised by manufacturer of ●droperidol (risk of ventricular arrhythmias)
- Bupropion: metabolism of tamoxifen to active metabolite possibly inhibited by ●bupropion (avoid concomitant use)
- Cinacalcet: metabolism of tamoxifen to active metabolite possibly inhibited by ●cinacalcet (avoid concomitant use)

Tamsulosin *see* Alpha-blockers

Tapentadol *see* Opioid Analgesics

Taxanes *see* Cabazitaxel, Docetaxel, and Paclitaxel

Tegafur *see* Fluorouracil

Teicoplanin

Vaccines: antibacterials inactivate oral typhoid vaccine—see p. 864

Telaprevir

- Alpha-blockers: manufacturer of telaprevir advises avoid concomitant use with ●alfuzosin
- Analgesics: manufacturer of telaprevir advises caution with ●methadone (risk of ventricular arrhythmias)
- Anti-arrhythmics: manufacturer of telaprevir advises avoid concomitant use with ●amiodarone and ●disopyramide (risk of ventricular arrhythmias); manufacturer of telaprevir advises caution with ●flecainide and ●propafenone (risk of ventricular arrhythmias); manufacturer of telaprevir advises caution with *intravenous* lidocaine
- Antibacterials: plasma concentration of both drugs possibly increased when telaprevir given with ●clarithromycin, ●erythromycin and ●telithromycin (increased risk of ventricular arrhythmias); manufacturer of telaprevir advises avoid concomitant use with ●rifabutin; plasma concentration of telaprevir significantly reduced by ●rifampicin—avoid concomitant use
- Anticoagulants: telaprevir possibly affects plasma concentration of ●warfarin; avoidance of telaprevir advised by manufacturer of apixaban; telaprevir

Telaprevir

- Anticoagulants *(continued)*

possibly increases plasma concentration of dabigatran

- Antidepressants: telaprevir possibly increases plasma concentration of trazodone; manufacturer of telaprevir advises avoid concomitant use with ●St John's wort

Antidiabetics: telaprevir increases plasma concentration of metformin (consider reducing dose of metformin)

- Antiepileptics: manufacturer of telaprevir advises avoid concomitant use with ●carbamazepine, ●phenobarbital and ●phenytoin
- Antifungals: telaprevir possibly increases plasma concentration of itraconazole; telaprevir possibly increases plasma concentration of ●posaconazole (increased risk of ventricular arrhythmias); telaprevir possibly affects plasma concentration of ●voriconazole (possible increased risk of ventricular arrhythmias)
- Antipsychotics: telaprevir possibly increases plasma concentration of ●lurasidone—avoid concomitant use; manufacturer of telaprevir advises avoid concomitant use with ●pimozide; telaprevir possibly increases plasma concentration of ●quetiapine—manufacturer of quetiapine advises avoid concomitant use
- Antivirals: plasma concentration of telaprevir possibly reduced by atazanavir, also plasma concentration of atazanavir possibly increased; telaprevir increases the plasma concentration of ●daclatasvir—reduce dose of daclatasvir (see Dose under Daclatasvir, p. 438); avoid concomitant use of telaprevir with ●darunavir; plasma concentration of telaprevir reduced by ●efavirenz—increase dose of telaprevir; manufacturers advise avoid concomitant use of telaprevir with ●fosamprenavir and ●lopinavir; telaprevir increases plasma concentration of maraviroc (consider reducing dose of maraviroc); plasma concentration of telaprevir possibly reduced by nevirapine—consider increasing dose of telaprevir; plasma concentration of telaprevir possibly reduced by ritonavir; telaprevir increases plasma concentration of tenofovir; avoidance of telaprevir advised by manufacturer of tipranavir
- Anxiolytics and Hypnotics: telaprevir possibly increases plasma concentration of ●midazolam (risk of prolonged sedation—avoid concomitant use of *oral* midazolam)
- Beta-blockers: manufacturer of telaprevir advises avoid concomitant use with ●sotalol (risk of ventricular arrhythmias)

Bosentan: plasma concentration of telaprevir possibly reduced by bosentan, also plasma concentration of bosentan possibly increased

Calcium-channel Blockers: telaprevir increases plasma concentration of amlodipine (consider reducing dose of amlodipine); manufacturer of telaprevir advises caution with diltiazem, felodipine, nicardipine, nifedipine and verapamil

Cardiac Glycosides: telaprevir increases plasma concentration of digoxin

- Ciclosporin: plasma concentration of both drugs increased when telaprevir given with ●ciclosporin (reduce dose of ciclosporin)
- Cilostazol: telaprevir possibly increases plasma concentration of ●cilostazol (see Dose under Cilostazol, p. 141)
- Colchicine: telaprevir possibly increases risk of ●colchicine toxicity—suspend or reduce dose of colchicine (avoid concomitant use in hepatic or renal impairment)

Corticosteroids: telaprevir possibly increases plasma concentration of *inhaled* and *intranasal*

Telaprevir

Corticosteroids *(continued)*
budesonide and fluticasone; plasma concentration of telaprevir possibly reduced by dexamethasone
- Cytotoxics: telaprevir possibly increases the plasma concentration of ●bosutinib—manufacturer of bosutinib advises avoid or consider reducing dose of bosutinib; manufacturer of ruxolitinib advises dose reduction when telaprevir given with ●ruxolitinib—consult ruxolitinib product literature
- Domperidone: possible increased risk of ventricular arrhythmias when telaprevir given with ●domperidone—avoid concomitant use
- Ergot Alkaloids: manufacturer of telaprevir advises avoid concomitant use with ●ergot alkaloids
- Lipid-regulating Drugs: manufacturer of telaprevir advises avoid concomitant use with ●atorvastatin; manufacturers advise avoid concomitant use of telaprevir with ●simvastatin; avoidance of telaprevir advised by manufacturer of ●lomitapide (plasma concentration of lomitapide possibly increased)
- Oestrogens: telaprevir possibly reduces plasma concentration of ●ethinylestradiol—manufacturer of telaprevir advises additional contraceptive precautions
- Sildenafil: manufacturer of telaprevir advises avoid concomitant use with ●sildenafil
- Sirolimus: plasma concentration of both drugs increased when telaprevir given with ●sirolimus (reduce dose of sirolimus)
- Sympathomimetics, Beta$_2$: manufacturer of telaprevir advises avoid concomitant use with ●salmeterol (risk of ventricular arrhythmias)
- Tacrolimus: plasma concentration of both drugs increased when telaprevir given with ●tacrolimus (reduce dose of tacrolimus)
- Tadalafil: manufacturer of telaprevir advises avoid concomitant use with high doses of ●tadalafil—consult product literature
- Vardenafil: manufacturer of telaprevir advises avoid concomitant use with ●vardenafil

Telavancin

Vaccines: antibacterials inactivate oral typhoid vaccine—see p. 864

Telbivudine

- Interferons: increased risk of peripheral neuropathy when telbivudine given with ●interferon alfa

Telithromycin

- Analgesics: possible increased risk of ventricular arrhythmias when telithromycin given with ●methadone; telithromycin inhibits the metabolism of oxycodone
- Anti-arrhythmics: possible increased risk of ventricular arrhythmias when telithromycin given with ●amiodarone and ●disopyramide; increased risk of ventricular arrhythmias when telithromycin given with ●dronedarone—avoid concomitant use
- Antibacterials: possible increased risk of ventricular arrhythmias when telithromycin given with ●moxifloxacin; plasma concentration of telithromycin reduced by ●rifampicin (avoid during and for 2 weeks after rifampicin)

Anticoagulants: avoidance of telithromycin advised by manufacturer of apixaban
- Antidepressants: possible increased risk of ventricular arrhythmias when telithromycin given with ●citalopram and ●tricyclics; plasma concentration of telithromycin reduced by ●St John's wort (avoid during and for 2 weeks after St John's wort)
- Antiepileptics: plasma concentration of telithromycin reduced by ●carbamazepine, ●phenobarbital and ●phenytoin (avoid during and for 2 weeks after carbamazepine, phenobarbital and phenytoin)

Antimuscarinics: manufacturer of fesoterodine advises dose reduction when telithromycin given with fesoterodine—consult fesoterodine product literature

Telithromycin *(continued)*

- Antipsychotics: possible increased risk of ventricular arrhythmias when telithromycin given with ●chlorpromazine; telithromycin possibly increases plasma concentration of ●lurasidone—avoid concomitant use; increased risk of ventricular arrhythmias when telithromycin given with ●pimozide—avoid concomitant use; telithromycin possibly increases plasma concentration of quetiapine
- Antivirals: manufacturer of telithromycin advises avoid concomitant use with ●atazanavir, ●fosamprenavir, ●indinavir, ●lopinavir, ●ritonavir and ●tipranavir in severe renal and hepatic impairment; telithromycin possibly increases the plasma concentration of ●daclatasvir—reduce dose of daclatasvir (see Dose under Daclatasvir, p. 438); telithromycin possibly increases plasma concentration of ●maraviroc (consider reducing dose of maraviroc); manufacturer of telithromycin advises avoid concomitant use with ●saquinavir (risk of ventricular arrhythmias); telithromycin possibly increases plasma concentration of ●simeprevir—manufacturer of simeprevir advises avoid concomitant use; plasma concentration of both drugs possibly increased when telithromycin given with ●telaprevir (increased risk of ventricular arrhythmias)
- Anxiolytics and Hypnotics: telithromycin inhibits metabolism of ●midazolam (increased plasma concentration with increased sedation)

Aprepitant: telithromycin possibly increases plasma concentration of aprepitant
- Avanafil: telithromycin possibly increases plasma concentration of ●avanafil—manufacturer of avanafil advises avoid concomitant use
- Calcium-channel Blockers: telithromycin possibly inhibits metabolism of ●calcium-channel blockers (increased risk of side-effects)

Cardiac Glycosides: telithromycin possibly increases plasma concentration of digoxin
- Ciclosporin: telithromycin possibly increases plasma concentration of ●ciclosporin
- Colchicine: telithromycin possibly increases risk of ●colchicine toxicity—suspend or reduce dose of colchicine (avoid concomitant use in hepatic or renal impairment)
- Cytotoxics: telithromycin possibly increases plasma concentration of axitinib (reduce dose of axitinib—consult axitinib product literature); telithromycin possibly increases the plasma concentration of ●bosutinib and ●cabazitaxel—manufacturer of bosutinib and cabazitaxel advises avoid or consider reducing dose of bosutinib and cabazitaxel; telithromycin possibly increases plasma concentration of ●crizotinib and ●everolimus—manufacturer of crizotinib and everolimus advises avoid concomitant use; telithromycin possibly increases the plasma concentration of ●ibrutinib—reduce dose of ibrutinib (see Dose under Ibrutinib, p. 615); avoidance of telithromycin advised by manufacturer of ●lapatinib and ●nilotinib; telithromycin possibly increases plasma concentration of ●pazopanib (reduce dose of pazopanib); telithromycin possibly increases plasma concentration of ●ponatinib—consider reducing initial dose of ponatinib (see Dose under Ponatinib, p. 618); manufacturer of ruxolitinib advises dose reduction when telithromycin given with ●ruxolitinib—consult ruxolitinib product literature; telithromycin possibly increases plasma concentration of ●docetaxel—manufacturer of docetaxel advises avoid concomitant use or consider reducing docetaxel dose
- Dapoxetine: avoidance of telithromycin advised by manufacturer of ●dapoxetine (increased risk of toxicity)
- Diuretics: telithromycin increases plasma concentration of ●eplerenone—avoid concomitant use

Appendix 1: Interactions

Telithromycin *(continued)*

- Domperidone: possible increased risk of ventricular arrhythmias when telithromycin given with ●domperidone—avoid concomitant use
- Ergot Alkaloids: increased risk of ergotism when telithromycin given with ●ergotamine—avoid concomitant use
- Ivabradine: telithromycin possibly increases plasma concentration of ●ivabradine—avoid concomitant use
- Ivacaftor: telithromycin possibly increases plasma concentration of ●ivacaftor (see Dose under Ivacaftor, p. 220)
- Lipid-regulating Drugs: increased risk of myopathy when telithromycin given with ●atorvastatin or ●simvastatin (avoid concomitant use); possible increased risk of myopathy when telithromycin given with pravastatin; avoidance of telithromycin advised by manufacturer of ●lomitapide (plasma concentration of lomitapide possibly increased)
- Pentamidine Isetionate: possible increased risk of ventricular arrhythmias when telithromycin given with *parenteral* ●pentamidine isetionate
- Ranolazine: telithromycin possibly increases plasma concentration of ●ranolazine—manufacturer of ranolazine advises avoid concomitant use
- Sildenafil: telithromycin possibly increases plasma concentration of ●sildenafil—consider reducing initial dose of sildenafil for erectile dysfunction or reduce sildenafil dose frequency to once daily for pulmonary hypertension
- Sirolimus: telithromycin increases plasma concentration of ●sirolimus—avoid concomitant use
- Tacrolimus: telithromycin possibly increases plasma concentration of ●tacrolimus

  Ulipristal: avoidance of telithromycin advised by manufacturer of *low-dose* ulipristal

  Vaccines: antibacterials inactivate oral typhoid vaccine—see p. 864

Telmisartan *see* Angiotensin-II Receptor Antagonists

Temazepam *see* Anxiolytics and Hypnotics

Temocillin *see* Penicillins

Temoporfin

- Cytotoxics: increased skin photosensitivity when temoporfin given with *topical* ●fluorouracil

Temozolomide

  Antiepileptics: plasma concentration of temozolomide increased by valproate
- Antipsychotics: avoid concomitant use of cytotoxics with ●clozapine (increased risk of agranulocytosis)

Temsirolimus

  Note The main active metabolite of temsirolimus is sirolimus—*see also* interactions of sirolimus and consult product literature
- Antibacterials: plasma concentration of active metabolite of temsirolimus reduced by ●rifampicin—avoid concomitant use
- Antifungals: manufacturer of temsirolimus advises avoid concomitant use with ●itraconazole (plasma concentration of temsirolimus possibly increased)
- Antipsychotics: avoid concomitant use of cytotoxics with ●clozapine (increased risk of agranulocytosis)

Tenofovir

- Antivirals: manufacturer of tenofovir advises avoid concomitant use with adefovir, tenofovir reduces plasma concentration of atazanavir, also plasma concentration of tenofovir possibly increased; tenofovir increases plasma concentration of ●didanosine (increased risk of toxicity)—avoid concomitant use; plasma concentration of tenofovir increased by lopinavir and telaprevir
- Orlistat: absorption of tenofovir possibly reduced by ●orlistat

Tenoxicam *see* NSAIDs

Terazosin *see* Alpha-blockers

Terbinafine

- Antibacterials: plasma concentration of terbinafine reduced by ●rifampicin

  Antidepressants: terbinafine possibly increases plasma concentration of paroxetine and tricyclics

  Antifungals: terbinafine increases plasma concentration of fluconazole

  Ciclosporin: terbinafine possibly reduces plasma concentration of ciclosporin

  Oestrogens: occasional reports of breakthrough bleeding when terbinafine given with oestrogens (when used for contraception)

  Progestogens: occasional reports of breakthrough bleeding when terbinafine given with progestogens (when used for contraception)

  Ulcer-healing Drugs: plasma concentration of terbinafine increased by cimetidine

Terbutaline *see* Sympathomimetics, Beta₂

Teriflunomide

  Antibacterials: teriflunomide increases plasma concentration of cefaclor, plasma concentration of teriflunomide reduced by rifampicin

  Antidiabetics: teriflunomide increases plasma concentration of repaglinide
- Lipid-regulating Drugs: the effect of teriflunomide is significantly decreased by colestyramine (enhanced elimination)—avoid unless drug elimination desired; teriflunomide increases plasma concentration of ●rosuvastatin (consider reducing dose of rosuvastatin)

  Oestrogens: teriflunomide increases plasma concentration of ethinylestradiol

  Progestogens: teriflunomide increases plasma concentration of levonorgestrel
- Vaccines: avoid concomitant use of teriflunomide with live ●vaccines (see p. 842)

Testolactone

- Anticoagulants: testolactone enhances anticoagulant effect of ●coumarins and ●phenindione

Testosterone

- Anticoagulants: testosterone enhances anticoagulant effect of ●coumarins and ●phenindione

  Antidiabetics: testosterone possibly enhances hypoglycaemic effect of antidiabetics

Tetrabenazine

- Antidepressants: risk of CNS toxicity when tetrabenazine given with ●MAOIs (avoid tetrabenazine for 2 weeks after MAOIs)

  Antipsychotics: increased risk of extrapyramidal side-effects when tetrabenazine given with antipsychotics

  Dopaminergics: increased risk of extrapyramidal side-effects when tetrabenazine given with amantadine

  Metoclopramide: increased risk of extrapyramidal side-effects when tetrabenazine given with metoclopramide

Tetracosactide *see* Corticosteroids

Tetracycline *see* Tetracyclines

Tetracyclines

  ACE Inhibitors: absorption of tetracyclines reduced by quinapril tablets (quinapril tablets contain magnesium carbonate)

  Adsorbents: absorption of tetracyclines possibly reduced by kaolin

  Antacids: absorption of tetracyclines reduced by antacids

  Antibacterials: plasma concentration of doxycycline reduced by rifampicin—consider increasing dose of doxycycline; tetracyclines possibly antagonise effects of penicillins
- Anticoagulants: tetracyclines possibly enhance anticoagulant effect of ●coumarins and ●phenindione

  Antidiabetics: tetracyclines possibly enhance hypoglycaemic effect of sulfonylureas

  Antiepileptics: metabolism of doxycycline accelerated by carbamazepine (reduced effect); metabolism of

Tetracyclines

Antiepileptics (continued)
doxycycline accelerated by phenobarbital and phenytoin (reduced plasma concentration)

Atovaquone: tetracycline reduces plasma concentration of atovaquone

Calcium Salts: absorption of tetracycline reduced by calcium salts

Cytotoxics: doxycycline or tetracycline increase risk of methotrexate toxicity

Dairy Products: absorption of tetracyclines (except doxycycline and minocycline) reduced by dairy products

Diuretics: manufacturer of lymecycline advises avoid concomitant use with diuretics

Ergot Alkaloids: increased risk of ergotism when tetracyclines given with ergotamine

Iron: absorption of tetracyclines reduced by *oral* iron, also absorption of *oral* iron reduced by tetracyclines

Lipid-regulating Drugs: absorption of tetracycline possibly reduced by colestipol and colestyramine

• **Retinoids:** possible increased risk of benign intracranial hypertension when tetracyclines given with ●retinoids (avoid concomitant use)

Strontium Ranelate: absorption of tetracyclines reduced by strontium ranelate (manufacturer of strontium ranelate advises avoid concomitant use)

Ulcer-healing Drugs: absorption of tetracyclines reduced by sucralfate and tripotassium dicitratobismuthate

Vaccines: antibacterials inactivate oral typhoid vaccine—see p. 864

Zinc: absorption of tetracyclines reduced by zinc, also absorption of zinc reduced by tetracyclines

Theophylline

Allopurinol: plasma concentration of theophylline possibly increased by allopurinol

Anaesthetics, General: increased risk of convulsions when theophylline given with ketamine

Anti-arrhythmics: theophylline antagonises anti-arrhythmic effect of adenosine—manufacturer of adenosine advises avoid theophylline for 24 hours before adenosine; plasma concentration of theophylline increased by propafenone

• **Antibacterials:** plasma concentration of theophylline possibly increased by clarithromycin and isoniazid; plasma concentration of theophylline increased by ●erythromycin (also theophylline may reduce absorption of *oral* erythromycin); plasma concentration of theophylline increased by ●ciprofloxacin and ●norfloxacin; metabolism of theophylline accelerated by rifampicin (reduced plasma concentration); possible increased risk of convulsions when theophylline given with ●quinolones

• **Antidepressants:** plasma concentration of theophylline increased by ●fluvoxamine (concomitant use should usually be avoided, but where not possible halve theophylline dose and monitor plasma-theophylline concentration); plasma concentration of theophylline possibly reduced by St John's wort

• **Antiepileptics:** metabolism of theophylline accelerated by carbamazepine and ●phenobarbital (reduced effect); plasma concentration of both drugs reduced when theophylline given with ●phenytoin

• **Antifungals:** plasma concentration of theophylline possibly increased by ●fluconazole

• **Antivirals:** plasma concentration of theophylline possibly increased by aciclovir; metabolism of theophylline accelerated by ●ritonavir (reduced plasma concentration)

Anxiolytics and Hypnotics: theophylline possibly reduces effects of benzodiazepines

Caffeine citrate: avoidance of theophylline advised by manufacturer of caffeine citrate

• **Calcium-channel Blockers:** plasma concentration of theophylline possibly increased by ●calcium-

Theophylline

• **Calcium-channel Blockers** (continued)
channel blockers (enhanced effect); plasma concentration of theophylline increased by diltiazem; plasma concentration of theophylline increased by ●verapamil (enhanced effect)

Corticosteroids: increased risk of hypokalaemia when theophylline given with corticosteroids

Cytotoxics: plasma concentration of theophylline possibly increased by methotrexate

• **Deferasirox:** plasma concentration of theophylline increased by ●deferasirox (consider reducing dose of theophylline)

Disulfiram: metabolism of theophylline inhibited by disulfiram (increased risk of toxicity)

Diuretics: increased risk of hypokalaemia when theophylline given with acetazolamide, loop diuretics or thiazides and related diuretics

Doxapram: increased CNS stimulation when theophylline given with doxapram

• **Interferons:** metabolism of theophylline inhibited by ●interferon alfa (consider reducing dose of theophylline)

Leukotriene Receptor Antagonists: plasma concentration of theophylline possibly increased by zafirlukast, also plasma concentration of zafirlukast reduced

Lithium: theophylline increases excretion of lithium (reduced plasma concentration)

Oestrogens: plasma concentration of theophylline increased by oestrogens (consider reducing dose of theophylline)

Pentoxifylline: plasma concentration of theophylline increased by pentoxifylline

Roflumilast: avoidance of theophylline advised by manufacturer of roflumilast

Sulfinpyrazone: plasma concentration of theophylline reduced by sulfinpyrazone

Sympathomimetics: manufacturer of theophylline advises avoid concomitant use with ephedrine in children

Sympathomimetics, Beta₂: increased risk of hypokalaemia when theophylline given with high doses of beta₂ sympathomimetics—see Hypokalaemia, p. 189

• **Ulcer-healing Drugs:** metabolism of theophylline inhibited by ●cimetidine (increased plasma concentration); absorption of theophylline possibly reduced by sucralfate (give at least 2 hours apart)

Vaccines: plasma concentration of theophylline possibly increased by influenza vaccine

Thiazolidinediones *see* Antidiabetics

Thiopental *see* Anaesthetics, General

Thiotepa

• **Antipsychotics:** avoid concomitant use of cytotoxics with ●clozapine (increased risk of agranulocytosis)

Muscle Relaxants: thiotepa enhances effects of suxamethonium

Thioxanthenes *see* Antipsychotics

Thyroid Hormones

Antacids: absorption of levothyroxine possibly reduced by antacids

Anti-arrhythmics: for concomitant use of thyroid hormones and amiodarone see p. 98

Antibacterials: metabolism of levothyroxine accelerated by rifampicin (may increase requirements for levothyroxine in hypothyroidism)

• **Anticoagulants:** thyroid hormones enhance anticoagulant effect of ●coumarins and ●phenindione

Antidepressants: thyroid hormones enhance effects of amitriptyline and imipramine; thyroid hormones possibly enhance effects of tricyclics

Antiepileptics: metabolism of thyroid hormones accelerated by carbamazepine and phenobarbital (may increase requirements for thyroid hormones in hypothyroidism); metabolism of thyroid hormones

Thyroid Hormones

Antiepileptics *(continued)*
accelerated by phenytoin (may increase requirements in hypothyroidism), also plasma concentration of phenytoin possibly increased

Beta-blockers: levothyroxine accelerates metabolism of propranolol

Calcium Salts: absorption of levothyroxine reduced by calcium salts

Colestilan: manufacturer of colestilan advises give levothyroxine at least 1 hour before or 3 hours after colestilan

Cytotoxics: plasma concentration of levothyroxine possibly reduced by imatinib

Iron: absorption of levothyroxine reduced by *oral* iron (give at least 2 hours apart)

Lanthanum: absorption of levothyroxine reduced by lanthanum (give at least 2 hours apart)

Lipid-regulating Drugs: absorption of levothyroxine reduced by colesevelam; absorption of thyroid hormones reduced by colestipol and colestyramine

Oestrogens: requirements for thyroid hormones in hypothyroidism may be increased by oestrogens

Orlistat: possible increased risk of hypothyroidism when levothyroxine given with orlistat

Polystyrene Sulfonate Resins: absorption of levothyroxine reduced by polystyrene sulfonate resins

Sevelamer: absorption of levothyroxine possibly reduced by sevelamer

Ulcer-healing Drugs: absorption of levothyroxine reduced by cimetidine and sucralfate

Tiagabine

- **Antidepressants:** anticonvulsant effect of antiepileptics possibly antagonised by MAOIs and ●tricyclic-related antidepressants (convulsive threshold lowered); anticonvulsant effect of antiepileptics antagonised by ●SSRIs and ●tricyclics (convulsive threshold lowered)

Antiepileptics: plasma concentration of tiagabine reduced by carbamazepine, phenobarbital and phenytoin

- **Antimalarials:** anticonvulsant effect of antiepileptics antagonised by ●mefloquine

- **Antipsychotics:** anticonvulsant effect of antiepileptics antagonised by ●antipsychotics (convulsive threshold lowered)

- **Orlistat:** possible increased risk of convulsions when antiepileptics given with ●orlistat

Tiaprofenic Acid *see* NSAIDs

Tibolone

Antibacterials: metabolism of tibolone accelerated by rifampicin (reduced plasma concentration)

Antiepileptics: metabolism of tibolone accelerated by carbamazepine (reduced plasma concentration); metabolism of tibolone accelerated by phenytoin

Ticagrelor

- **Antibacterials:** plasma concentration of ticagrelor possibly increased by ●clarithromycin—manufacturer of ticagrelor advises avoid concomitant use; plasma concentration of ticagrelor possibly increased by erythromycin; plasma concentration of ticagrelor reduced by ●rifampicin

- **Anticoagulants:** ticagrelor increases plasma concentration of ●dabigatran

Antidepressants: possible increased risk of bleeding when ticagrelor given with citalopram, paroxetine or sertraline

Antiepileptics: plasma concentration of ticagrelor possibly reduced by carbamazepine, phenobarbital and phenytoin

- **Antivirals:** plasma concentration of ticagrelor possibly increased by ●atazanavir and ●ritonavir—manufacturer of ticagrelor advises avoid concomitant use

Calcium-channel Blockers: plasma concentration of ticagrelor increased by diltiazem

Ticagrelor *(continued)*
- **Cardiac Glycosides:** ticagrelor increases plasma concentration of ●digoxin

Ciclosporin: plasma concentration of ticagrelor increased by ciclosporin

- **Ergot Alkaloids:** ticagrelor possibly increases plasma concentration of ●ergot alkaloids

- **Lipid-regulating Drugs:** ticagrelor increases plasma concentration of ●simvastatin (increased risk of toxicity)

Ticarcillin *see* Penicillins

Tick-borne encephalitis vaccine *see* Vaccines

Tigecycline

Anticoagulants: tigecycline possibly enhances anticoagulant effect of coumarins

Vaccines: antibacterials inactivate oral typhoid vaccine—see p. 864

Timolol *see* Beta-blockers

Tinidazole

Alcohol: possibility of disulfiram-like reaction when tinidazole given with alcohol

Antibacterials: plasma concentration of tinidazole possibly reduced by rifampicin

Vaccines: antibacterials inactivate oral typhoid vaccine—see p. 864

Tinzaparin *see* Heparins

Tioguanine

- **Antipsychotics:** avoid concomitant use of cytotoxics with ●clozapine (increased risk of agranulocytosis)

Cytotoxics: increased risk of hepatotoxicity when tioguanine given with busulfan

Tiotropium *see* Antimuscarinics

Tipranavir

Analgesics: plasma concentration of tipranavir possibly reduced by buprenorphine

Antacids: absorption of tipranavir reduced by antacids (give at least 2 hours apart)

- **Antibacterials:** tipranavir increases plasma concentration of ●clarithromycin (reduce dose of clarithromycin in renal impairment), also plasma concentration of tipranavir increased by clarithromycin; tipranavir increases plasma concentration of ●rifabutin (reduce dose of rifabutin); plasma concentration of tipranavir possibly reduced by ●rifampicin—avoid concomitant use; avoidance of concomitant tipranavir in severe renal and hepatic impairment advised by manufacturer of ●telithromycin

Anticoagulants: avoidance of tipranavir advised by manufacturer of apixaban and rivaroxaban

- **Antidepressants:** plasma concentration of tipranavir possibly reduced by ●St John's wort—avoid concomitant use

Antiepileptics: plasma concentration of tipranavir possibly reduced by carbamazepine

Antifungals: plasma concentration of tipranavir increased by fluconazole

- **Antimalarials:** caution with tipranavir advised by manufacturer of artemether with lumefantrine; tipranavir possibly increases plasma concentration of ●quinine (increased risk of toxicity)

Antimuscarinics: avoidance of tipranavir advised by manufacturer of darifenacin

- **Antipsychotics:** tipranavir possibly increases plasma concentration of ●aripiprazole (reduce dose of aripiprazole—consult aripiprazole product literature); tipranavir possibly increases plasma concentration of ●quetiapine—manufacturer of quetiapine advises avoid concomitant use

- **Antivirals:** tipranavir reduces plasma concentration of ●abacavir, ●fosamprenavir, ●lopinavir, ●saquinavir and ●zidovudine; plasma concentration of tipranavir increased by atazanavir (also plasma concentration of atazanavir reduced); manufacturer of tipranavir advises avoid concomitant use with boceprevir and telaprevir; tipranavir reduces plasma concentration of didanosine—manufacturer of tipranavir advises

Tipranavir

- Antivirals *(continued)*
  tipranavir and didanosine *capsules* should be taken at least 2 hours apart; tipranavir reduces the plasma concentration of ●dolutegravir (see Dose under Dolutegravir, p. 429); tipranavir reduces plasma concentration of ●etravirine, also plasma concentration of tipranavir increased (avoid concomitant use)
- Beta-blockers: manufacturer of tipranavir advises avoid concomitant use with ●metoprolol for heart failure
  Bosentan: manufacturer of tipranavir advises avoid concomitant use with bosentan
- Cobicistat: plasma concentration of both drugs reduced when tipranavir given with ●cobicistat (avoid concomitant use)
- Lipid-regulating Drugs: increased risk of myopathy when tipranavir given with ●atorvastatin (see Dose under Atorvastatin, p. 175); tipranavir increases plasma concentration of ●rosuvastatin—adjust dose of rosuvastatin (consult product literature); tipranavir possibly increases plasma concentration of ●simvastatin—avoid concomitant use; avoidance of tipranavir advised by manufacturer of ●lomitapide (plasma concentration of lomitapide possibly increased)
- Orlistat: absorption of tipranavir possibly reduced by ●orlistat
- Ranolazine: tipranavir possibly increases plasma concentration of ●ranolazine—manufacturer of ranolazine advises avoid concomitant use
  Sildenafil: manufacturer of tipranavir advises avoid concomitant use of sildenafil for pulmonary arterial hypertension
  Sympathomimetics, Beta$_2$: manufacturer of tipranavir advises avoid concomitant use with salmeterol
- Ulcer-healing Drugs: tipranavir reduces plasma concentration of ●esomeprazole and ●omeprazole
  Vardenafil: manufacturer of tipranavir advises caution with vardenafil
  Vitamins: increased risk of bleeding when tipranavir given with high doses of vitamin E

Tirofiban
  Iloprost: increased risk of bleeding when tirofiban given with iloprost

Tizanidine *see* Muscle Relaxants
Tobramycin *see* Aminoglycosides

Tocilizumab

- Antipsychotics: avoid concomitant use of cytotoxics with ●clozapine (increased risk of agranulocytosis)
- Vaccines: avoid concomitant use of monoclonal antibodies with live ●vaccines (see p. 842)

Tolazoline *see* Alpha-blockers
Tolbutamide *see* Antidiabetics

Tolcapone
  Antidepressants: avoid concomitant use of tolcapone with MAOIs
  Memantine: effects of dopaminergics possibly enhanced by memantine
  Methyldopa: antiparkinsonian effect of dopaminergics antagonised by methyldopa

Tolfenamic Acid *see* NSAIDs
Tolterodine *see* Antimuscarinics

Tolvaptan
  Antibacterials: plasma concentration of tolvaptan reduced by rifampicin
  Cardiac Glycosides: tolvaptan increases plasma concentration of digoxin (increased risk of toxicity)
- Grapefruit Juice: plasma concentration of tolvaptan increased by ●grapefruit juice—avoid concomitant use

Topiramate
- Antidepressants: anticonvulsant effect of antiepileptics possibly antagonised by MAOIs and ●tricyclic-related antidepressants (convulsive threshold low-

Topiramate
- Antidepressants *(continued)*
  ered); anticonvulsant effect of antiepileptics antagonised by ●SSRIs and ●tricyclics (convulsive threshold lowered)
  Antidiabetics: topiramate possibly increases plasma concentration of metformin; topiramate possibly reduces plasma concentration of glibenclamide
- Antiepileptics: plasma concentration of topiramate often reduced by carbamazepine; topiramate reduces plasma concentration of perampanel; plasma concentration of topiramate possibly reduced by phenobarbital; topiramate increases plasma concentration of ●phenytoin (also plasma concentration of topiramate reduced); hyperammonaemia and CNS toxicity reported when topiramate given with valproate
- Antimalarials: anticonvulsant effect of antiepileptics antagonised by ●mefloquine
- Antipsychotics: anticonvulsant effect of antiepileptics antagonised by ●antipsychotics (convulsive threshold lowered)
  Diuretics: plasma concentration of topiramate possibly increased by hydrochlorothiazide
  Lithium: topiramate possibly affects plasma concentration of lithium
- Oestrogens: topiramate accelerates metabolism of ●oestrogens (reduced contraceptive effect—see p. 548)
- Orlistat: possible increased risk of convulsions when antiepileptics given with ●orlistat
- Progestogens: topiramate accelerates metabolism of ●progestogens (reduced contraceptive effect—see p. 548)

Torasemide *see* Diuretics

Toremifene
- Anticoagulants: toremifene possibly enhances anticoagulant effect of ●coumarins
  Antiepileptics: metabolism of toremifene possibly accelerated by carbamazepine (reduced plasma concentration); metabolism of toremifene accelerated by phenobarbital (reduced plasma concentration); metabolism of toremifene possibly accelerated by phenytoin
- Cytotoxics: possible increased risk of ventricular arrhythmias when toremifene given with ●vandetanib—avoid concomitant use
  Diuretics: increased risk of hypercalcaemia when toremifene given with thiazides and related diuretics

Trabectedin
- Alcohol: manufacturer of trabectedin advises avoid concomitant use with ●alcohol
- Antibacterials: plasma concentration of trabectedin reduced by ●rifampicin
- Antipsychotics: avoid concomitant use of cytotoxics with ●clozapine (increased risk of agranulocytosis)
- Vaccines: avoid concomitant use of trabectedin with live ●vaccines (see p. 842)

Tramadol *see* Opioid Analgesics
Trandolapril *see* ACE Inhibitors
Tranylcypromine *see* MAOIs

Trastuzumab
- Antipsychotics: avoid concomitant use of cytotoxics with ●clozapine (increased risk of agranulocytosis)
- Vaccines: avoid concomitant use of monoclonal antibodies with live ●vaccines (see p. 842)

Trazodone *see* Antidepressants, Tricyclic (related)
Tretinoin *see* Retinoids
Triamcinolone *see* Corticosteroids
Triamterene *see* Diuretics

Trientine
  Iron: trientine reduces absorption of *oral* iron
  Zinc: trientine reduces absorption of zinc, also absorption of trientine reduced by zinc

Trifluoperazine *see* Antipsychotics

Trihexyphenidyl *see* Antimuscarinics

Trimethoprim

ACE Inhibitors: possible increased risk of hyperkalaemia when trimethoprim given with ACE inhibitors

Angiotensin-II Receptor Antagonists: possible increased risk of hyperkalaemia when trimethoprim given with angiotensin-II receptor antagonists

Anti-arrhythmics: possible increased risk of ventricular arrhythmias when trimethoprim (as co-trimoxazole) given with amiodarone—manufacturer of amiodarone advises avoid concomitant use of co-trimoxazole

Antibacterials: plasma concentration of trimethoprim possibly reduced by rifampicin; plasma concentration of both drugs may increase when trimethoprim given with dapsone

Anticoagulants: trimethoprim possibly enhances anticoagulant effect of coumarins

Antidiabetics: trimethoprim possibly enhances hypoglycaemic effect of repaglinide—manufacturer advises avoid concomitant use; trimethoprim rarely enhances the effects of sulfonylureas

- Antiepileptics: trimethoprim increases plasma concentration of ●phenytoin (also increased antifolate effect)

- Antimalarials: increased antifolate effect when trimethoprim given with ●pyrimethamine

Antivirals: trimethoprim (as co-trimoxazole) increases plasma concentration of lamivudine—avoid concomitant use of high-dose co-trimoxazole

- Azathioprine: increased risk of haematological toxicity when trimethoprim (also with co-trimoxazole) given with ●azathioprine

Cardiac Glycosides: trimethoprim possibly increases plasma concentration of digoxin

- Ciclosporin: increased risk of nephrotoxicity when trimethoprim given with ●ciclosporin, also plasma concentration of ciclosporin reduced by *intravenous* trimethoprim

- Cytotoxics: increased risk of haematological toxicity when trimethoprim (also with co-trimoxazole) given with ●mercaptopurine or ●methotrexate

Diuretics: increased risk of hyperkalaemia when trimethoprim given with eplerenone; possible increased risk of hyperkalaemia when trimethoprim given with spironolactone

Vaccines: antibacterials inactivate oral typhoid vaccine—see p. 864

Trimipramine *see* Antidepressants, Tricyclic

Tripotassium Dicitratobismuthate

Antibacterials: tripotassium dicitratobismuthate reduces absorption of tetracyclines

Tropicamide *see* Antimuscarinics

Trospium *see* Antimuscarinics

Typhoid Vaccine (oral) *see* Vaccines

Typhoid Vaccine (parenteral) *see* Vaccines

Ubidecarenone

Anticoagulants: ubidecarenone may enhance or reduce anticoagulant effect of warfarin

Ulcer-healing Drugs *see* Histamine H$_2$-antagonists, Proton Pump Inhibitors, Sucralfate, and Tripotassium Dicitratobismuthate

Ulipristal

- Antibacterials: manufacturer of *low-dose* ulipristal advises avoid concomitant use with clarithromycin and telithromycin; plasma concentration of *low-dose* ulipristal increased by erythromycin—manufacturer of *low-dose* ulipristal advises avoid concomitant use; manufacturer of ulipristal advises avoid concomitant use with ●rifampicin (contraceptive effect of ulipristal possibly reduced)

Anticoagulants: manufacturer of ulipristal advises give dabigatran at least 1.5 hours before or after ulipristal

Ulipristal *(continued)*

- Antidepressants: manufacturer of ulipristal advises avoid concomitant use with ●St John's wort (contraceptive effect of ulipristal possibly reduced)

- Antiepileptics: manufacturer of ulipristal advises avoid concomitant use with ●carbamazepine, ●phenobarbital and ●phenytoin (contraceptive effect of ulipristal possibly reduced)

Antifungals: manufacturer of ulipristal advises avoid concomitant use with itraconazole

Antihistamines: manufacturer of ulipristal advises give fexofenadine at least 1.5 hours before or after ulipristal

- Antivirals: manufacturer of ulipristal advises avoid concomitant use with ●ritonavir (contraceptive effect of ulipristal possibly reduced)

Calcium-channel Blockers: manufacturer of *low-dose* ulipristal advises avoid concomitant use with verapamil

Cardiac Glycosides: manufacturer of ulipristal advises give digoxin at least 1.5 hours before or after ulipristal

Grapefruit Juice: manufacturer of *low-dose* ulipristal advises avoid concomitant use with grapefruit juice

- Progestogens: ulipristal possibly reduces contraceptive effect of ●progestogens

Umeclidinium *see* Antimuscarinics

Ursodeoxycholic Acid *see* Bile Acids

Ustekinumab

- Antipsychotics: avoid concomitant use of cytotoxics with ●clozapine (increased risk of agranulocytosis)

- Vaccines: avoid concomitant use of monoclonal antibodies with live ●vaccines (see p. 842)

Vaccines

Note For a general warning on live vaccines and high doses of corticosteroids or other immunosuppressive drugs, see p. 842 ; for advice on live vaccines and immunoglobulins, see under Normal Immunoglobulin, p. 867

- Abatacept: avoid concomitant use of live vaccines with ●abatacept (see p. 842)

- Anakinra: avoid concomitant use of live vaccines with ●anakinra (see p. 842)

Antibacterials: oral typhoid vaccine inactivated by antibacterials—see p. 864

Anticoagulants: influenza vaccine possibly enhances anticoagulant effect of warfarin

Antiepileptics: influenza vaccine enhances effects of phenytoin

Antimalarials: oral typhoid vaccine inactivated by antimalarials—see p. 864

- Corticosteroids: immune response to vaccines impaired by high doses of ●corticosteroids, avoid concomitant use with live vaccines (see p. 842)

- Cytotoxics: avoid concomitant use of live vaccines with ●doxorubicin, ●monoclonal antibodies, ●pixantrone or ●trabectedin (see p. 842)

- Dexrazoxane: avoid concomitant use of live vaccines with ●dexrazoxane (see p. 842)

- Etanercept: avoid concomitant use of live vaccines with ●etanercept (see p. 842)

Interferons: avoidance of vaccines advised by manufacturer of interferon gamma

- Leflunomide: avoid concomitant use of live vaccines with ●leflunomide (see p. 842)

- Teriflunomide: avoid concomitant use of live vaccines with ●teriflunomide (see p. 842)

Theophylline: influenza vaccine possibly increases plasma concentration of theophylline

Valaciclovir *see* Aciclovir

Valganciclovir *see* Ganciclovir

Valproate

Analgesics: effects of valproate enhanced by aspirin

- Antibacterials: metabolism of valproate possibly inhibited by erythromycin (increased plasma concentration); avoidance of valproate advised by manufacturer of ●pivmecillinam; plasma concentration of

Valproate

- Antibacterials *(continued)*
  valproate reduced by ●carbapenems—avoid concomitant use
  Anticoagulants: valproate possibly enhances anticoagulant effect of coumarins
- Antidepressants: anticonvulsant effect of antiepileptics possibly antagonised by MAOIs and ●tricyclic-related antidepressants (convulsive threshold lowered); anticonvulsant effect of antiepileptics antagonised by ●SSRIs and ●tricyclics (convulsive threshold lowered)
- Antiepileptics: plasma concentration of valproate reduced by carbamazepine, also plasma concentration of active metabolite of carbamazepine increased; valproate possibly increases plasma concentration of ethosuximide; valproate increases plasma concentration of ●lamotrigine (increased risk of toxicity—reduce lamotrigine dose); valproate sometimes reduces plasma concentration of an active metabolite of oxcarbazepine; valproate increases plasma concentration of phenobarbital (also plasma concentration of valproate reduced); valproate increases or possibly decreases plasma concentration of phenytoin, also plasma concentration of valproate reduced; valproate possibly increases plasma concentration of rufinamide (reduce dose of rufinamide); hyperammonaemia and CNS toxicity reported when valproate given with topiramate
- Antimalarials: anticonvulsant effect of antiepileptics antagonised by ●mefloquine
- Antipsychotics: anticonvulsant effect of antiepileptics antagonised by ●antipsychotics (convulsive threshold lowered); valproate possibly increases or decreases plasma concentration of clozapine; increased risk of side-effects including neutropenia when valproate given with ●olanzapine
  Antivirals: plasma concentration of valproate possibly reduced by ritonavir; valproate possibly increases plasma concentration of zidovudine (increased risk of toxicity)
  Anxiolytics and Hypnotics: plasma concentration of valproate possibly increased by clobazam; increased risk of side-effects when valproate given with clonazepam; valproate possibly increases plasma concentration of diazepam and lorazepam
  Bupropion: valproate inhibits the metabolism of bupropion
  Cytotoxics: valproate increases plasma concentration of temozolomide
  Lipid-regulating Drugs: absorption of valproate possibly reduced by colestyramine
  Oestrogens: plasma concentration of valproate possibly reduced by ethinylestradiol
- Orlistat: possible increased risk of convulsions when antiepileptics given with ●orlistat
  Sodium Benzoate: valproate possibly reduces effects of sodium benzoate
  Sodium Oxybate: valproate increases the plasma concentration of ●sodium oxybate (see Dose under Sodium Oxybate, p. 230)
  Sodium Phenylbutyrate: valproate possibly reduces effects of sodium phenylbutyrate
- Ulcer-healing Drugs: metabolism of valproate inhibited by cimetidine (increased plasma concentration)

Valsartan *see* Angiotensin-II Receptor Antagonists

Vancomycin

Anaesthetics, General: hypersensitivity-like reactions can occur when *intravenous* vancomycin given with general anaesthetics
- Antibacterials: increased risk of nephrotoxicity and ototoxicity when vancomycin given with ●aminoglycosides, capreomycin or colistimethate sodium; increased risk of nephrotoxicity when vancomycin given with polymyxins

Vancomycin *(continued)*

Antifungals: possible increased risk of nephrotoxicity when vancomycin given with amphotericin
- Ciclosporin: increased risk of nephrotoxicity when vancomycin given with ●ciclosporin
  Cytotoxics: increased risk of nephrotoxicity and possibly of ototoxicity when vancomycin given with cisplatin
- Diuretics: increased risk of ototoxicity when vancomycin given with ●loop diuretics
  Lipid-regulating Drugs: effects of *oral* vancomycin antagonised by colestyramine
- Muscle Relaxants: vancomycin enhances effects of ●suxamethonium
  Tacrolimus: possible increased risk of nephrotoxicity when vancomycin given with tacrolimus
  Vaccines: antibacterials inactivate oral typhoid vaccine—see p. 864

Vandetanib

- Analgesics: possible increased risk of ventricular arrhythmias when vandetanib given with ●methadone—avoid concomitant use
- Anti-arrhythmics: possible increased risk of ventricular arrhythmias when vandetanib given with ●amiodarone or ●disopyramide—avoid concomitant use
- Antibacterials: possible increased risk of ventricular arrhythmias when vandetanib given with *parenteral* ●erythromycin—avoid concomitant use; possible increased risk of ventricular arrhythmias when vandetanib given with ●moxifloxacin—avoid concomitant use; plasma concentration of vandetanib reduced by ●rifampicin—manufacturer of vandetanib advises avoid concomitant use
  Antidepressants: manufacturer of vandetanib advises avoid concomitant use with St John's wort (plasma concentration of vandetanib possibly reduced)
  Antidiabetics: vandetanib possibly increases plasma concentration of metformin (consider reducing dose of metformin)
  Antiepileptics: manufacturer of vandetanib advises avoid concomitant use with carbamazepine and phenobarbital (plasma concentration of vandetanib possibly reduced)
- Antihistamines: possible increased risk of ventricular arrhythmias when vandetanib given with ●mizolastine—avoid concomitant use
- Antimalarials: possible increased risk of ventricular arrhythmias when vandetanib given with ●artemether with lumefantrine—avoid concomitant use
- Antipsychotics: possible increased risk of ventricular arrhythmias when vandetanib given with ●amisulpride, ●chlorpromazine, ●haloperidol, ●pimozide, ●sulpiride or ●zuclopenthixol—avoid concomitant use; avoid concomitant use of cytotoxics with ●clozapine (increased risk of agranulocytosis)
- Beta-blockers: possible increased risk of ventricular arrhythmias when vandetanib given with ●sotalol—avoid concomitant use
  Cardiac Glycosides: vandetanib increases plasma concentration of digoxin—possible increased risk of bradycardia
- Cytotoxics: possible increased risk of ventricular arrhythmias when vandetanib given with ●arsenic trioxide—avoid concomitant use
- Hormone Antagonists: possible increased risk of ventricular arrhythmias when vandetanib given with ●toremifene—avoid concomitant use
- 5HT₃-receptor Antagonists: increased risk of ventricular arrhythmias when vandetanib given with ●ondansetron—avoid concomitant use
- Pentamidine Isetionate: possible increased risk of ventricular arrhythmias when vandetanib given with ●pentamidine isetionate—avoid concomitant use

Vardenafil

- Alpha-blockers: enhanced hypotensive effect when vardenafil given with ●alpha-blockers—separate doses by 6 hours (except with tamsulosin)—see also p. 570

  Anti-arrhythmics: avoidance of vardenafil advised by manufacturer of disopyramide (risk of ventricular arrhythmias)

  Antibacterials: plasma concentration of vardenafil possibly increased by clarithromycin (consider reducing initial dose of vardenafil); plasma concentration of vardenafil increased by erythromycin (reduce dose of vardenafil)

- Antifungals: plasma concentration of vardenafil possibly increased by ●itraconazole—avoid concomitant use

- Antivirals: plasma concentration of vardenafil possibly increased by fosamprenavir; plasma concentration of vardenafil increased by ●indinavir and ●ritonavir—avoid concomitant use; increased risk of ventricular arrhythmias when vardenafil given with ●saquinavir—avoid concomitant use; avoidance of vardenafil advised by manufacturer of ●telaprevir; caution with vardenafil advised by manufacturer of tipranavir

  Calcium-channel Blockers: enhanced hypotensive effect when vardenafil given with nifedipine

- Cobicistat: plasma concentration of vardenafil possibly increased by ●cobicistat—manufacturer of cobicistat advises reduce dose of vardenafil (consult cobicistat product literature)

  Dapoxetine: avoidance of vardenafil advised by manufacturer of dapoxetine

- Grapefruit Juice: plasma concentration of vardenafil possibly increased by ●grapefruit juice—avoid concomitant use

- Nicorandil: possible increased hypotensive effect when vardenafil given with ●nicorandil—avoid concomitant use

- Nitrates: possible increased hypotensive effect when vardenafil given with ●nitrates—avoid concomitant use

- Riociguat: possible enhanced hypotensive effect when vardenafil given with ●riociguat—avoid concomitant use

Varicella-zoster Vaccine see Vaccines

Vasodilator Antihypertensives

ACE Inhibitors: enhanced hypotensive effect when hydralazine, minoxidil or sodium nitroprusside given with ACE inhibitors

Adrenergic Neurone Blockers: enhanced hypotensive effect when hydralazine, minoxidil or sodium nitroprusside given with adrenergic neurone blockers

Alcohol: enhanced hypotensive effect when hydralazine, minoxidil or sodium nitroprusside given with alcohol

Aldesleukin: enhanced hypotensive effect when hydralazine, minoxidil or sodium nitroprusside given with aldesleukin

Alpha-blockers: enhanced hypotensive effect when hydralazine, minoxidil or sodium nitroprusside given with alpha-blockers

Anaesthetics, General: enhanced hypotensive effect when hydralazine, minoxidil or sodium nitroprusside given with general anaesthetics

Analgesics: hypotensive effect of hydralazine, minoxidil and sodium nitroprusside antagonised by NSAIDs

Angiotensin-II Receptor Antagonists: enhanced hypotensive effect when hydralazine, minoxidil or sodium nitroprusside given with angiotensin-II receptor antagonists

Antidepressants: enhanced hypotensive effect when hydralazine, minoxidil or sodium nitroprusside given with MAOIs; enhanced hypotensive effect

Vasodilator Antihypertensives

Antidepressants *(continued)*

when hydralazine or sodium nitroprusside given with tricyclic-related antidepressants

Antipsychotics: enhanced hypotensive effect when hydralazine, minoxidil or sodium nitroprusside given with phenothiazines

Anxiolytics and Hypnotics: enhanced hypotensive effect when hydralazine, minoxidil or sodium nitroprusside given with anxiolytics and hypnotics

Beta-blockers: enhanced hypotensive effect when hydralazine, minoxidil or sodium nitroprusside given with beta-blockers

Calcium-channel Blockers: enhanced hypotensive effect when hydralazine, minoxidil or sodium nitroprusside given with calcium-channel blockers

Clonidine: enhanced hypotensive effect when hydralazine, minoxidil or sodium nitroprusside given with clonidine

Corticosteroids: hypotensive effect of hydralazine, minoxidil and sodium nitroprusside antagonised by corticosteroids

Diazoxide: enhanced hypotensive effect when hydralazine, minoxidil or sodium nitroprusside given with diazoxide

Diuretics: enhanced hypotensive effect when hydralazine, minoxidil or sodium nitroprusside given with diuretics

Dopaminergics: enhanced hypotensive effect when hydralazine, minoxidil or sodium nitroprusside given with levodopa

Methyldopa: enhanced hypotensive effect when hydralazine, minoxidil or sodium nitroprusside given with methyldopa

Moxisylyte: enhanced hypotensive effect when hydralazine, minoxidil or sodium nitroprusside given with moxisylyte

Moxonidine: enhanced hypotensive effect when hydralazine, minoxidil or sodium nitroprusside given with moxonidine

Muscle Relaxants: enhanced hypotensive effect when hydralazine, minoxidil or sodium nitroprusside given with baclofen; enhanced hypotensive effect when hydralazine, minoxidil or sodium nitroprusside given with tizanidine

Nicorandil: possible enhanced hypotensive effect when hydralazine, minoxidil or sodium nitroprusside given with nicorandil

Nitrates: enhanced hypotensive effect when hydralazine, minoxidil or sodium nitroprusside given with nitrates

Oestrogens: hypotensive effect of hydralazine, minoxidil and sodium nitroprusside antagonised by oestrogens

Prostaglandins: enhanced hypotensive effect when hydralazine, minoxidil or sodium nitroprusside given with alprostadil

Vasodilator Antihypertensives: enhanced hypotensive effect when hydralazine given with minoxidil or sodium nitroprusside; enhanced hypotensive effect when minoxidil given with sodium nitroprusside

Vecuronium see Muscle Relaxants

Vedolizumab

- Antipsychotics: avoid concomitant use of cytotoxics with ●clozapine (increased risk of agranulocytosis)

- Vaccines: avoid concomitant use of monoclonal antibodies with live ●vaccines (see p. 842)

Vemurafenib

Antibacterials: manufacturer of vemurafenib advises avoid concomitant use with rifabutin and rifampicin

- Anticoagulants: vemurafenib possibly enhances anticoagulant effect of ●warfarin

Antidepressants: manufacturer of vemurafenib advises avoid concomitant use with St John's wort

Vemurafenib *(continued)*

Antiepileptics: manufacturer of vemurafenib advises avoid concomitant use with carbamazepine and phenytoin

- Antipsychotics: avoid concomitant use of cytotoxics with ●clozapine (increased risk of agranulocytosis)

Cytotoxics: avoidance of vemurafenib advised by manufacturer of ipilimumab

- Oestrogens: manufacturer of vemurafenib advises contraceptive effect of ●oestrogens possibly reduced
- Progestogens: manufacturer of vemurafenib advises contraceptive effect of ●progestogens possibly reduced

Venlafaxine

- Analgesics: increased risk of bleeding when venlafaxine given with ●NSAIDs or ●aspirin; possible increased serotonergic effects when SSRI-related antidepressants given with fentanyl; possible increased serotonergic effects when venlafaxine given with tramadol
- Anticoagulants: venlafaxine possibly enhances anticoagulant effect of ●warfarin; possible increased risk of bleeding when SSRI-related antidepressants given with ●dabigatran
- Antidepressants: possible increased serotonergic effects when venlafaxine given with St John's wort, duloxetine or mirtazapine; enhanced CNS effects and toxicity when venlafaxine given with ●MAOIs (venlafaxine should not be started until 2 weeks after stopping MAOIs, avoid MAOIs for 1 week after stopping venlafaxine); after stopping SSRI-related antidepressants do not start ●moclobemide for at least 1 week
- Antimalarials: avoidance of antidepressants advised by manufacturer of ●artemether with lumefantrine and ●piperaquine with artenimol

Antipsychotics: venlafaxine increases plasma concentration of haloperidol

Atomoxetine: possible increased risk of convulsions when antidepressants given with atomoxetine

- Dapoxetine: possible increased risk of serotonergic effects when venlafaxine given with ●dapoxetine (manufacturer of dapoxetine advises venlafaxine should not be started until 1 week after stopping dapoxetine, avoid dapoxetine for 2 weeks after stopping venlafaxine)
- Dopaminergics: caution with venlafaxine advised by manufacturer of entacapone; increased risk of hypertension and CNS excitation when venlafaxine given with ●selegiline (selegiline should not be started until 1 week after stopping venlafaxine, avoid venlafaxine for 2 weeks after stopping selegiline)

5HT₁-receptor Agonists: possible increased serotonergic effects when venlafaxine given with 5HT₁ agonists

5HT₃-receptor Antagonists: possible increased serotonergic effects when SSRI-related antidepressants given with 5HT₃ antagonists

Lithium: possible increased serotonergic effects when venlafaxine given with lithium

- Methylthioninium: risk of CNS toxicity when SSRI-related antidepressants given with ●methylthioninium—avoid concomitant use (if avoidance not possible, use lowest possible dose of methylthioninium and observe patient for up to 4 hours after administration)

Verapamil *see* Calcium-channel Blockers

Vigabatrin

- Antidepressants: anticonvulsant effect of antiepileptics possibly antagonised by MAOIs and ●tricyclic-related antidepressants (convulsive threshold lowered); anticonvulsant effect of antiepileptics antagonised by ●SSRIs and ●tricyclics (convulsive threshold lowered)

Vigabatrin *(continued)*

Antiepileptics: vigabatrin reduces plasma concentration of phenytoin

- Antimalarials: anticonvulsant effect of antiepileptics antagonised by ●mefloquine
- Antipsychotics: anticonvulsant effect of antiepileptics antagonised by ●antipsychotics (convulsive threshold lowered)
- Orlistat: possible increased risk of convulsions when antiepileptics given with ●orlistat

Vilanterol *see* Sympathomimetics, Beta₂

Vildagliptin *see* Antidiabetics

Vinblastine

- Aldesleukin: avoidance of vinblastine advised by manufacturer of ●aldesleukin
- Antibacterials: toxicity of vinblastine increased by ●erythromycin—avoid concomitant use; possible increased risk of ventricular arrhythmias when vinblastine given with ●delamanid
- Antifungals: possible increased risk of vinblastine toxicity when given with ●itraconazole; metabolism of vinblastine possibly inhibited by ●posaconazole (increased risk of neurotoxicity)
- Antimalarials: avoidance of vinblastine advised by manufacturer of ●piperaquine with artenimol
- Antipsychotics: avoid concomitant use of cytotoxics with ●clozapine (increased risk of agranulocytosis)

Antivirals: plasma concentration of vinblastine possibly increased by ritonavir

Vincristine

- Antibacterials: possible increased risk of ventricular arrhythmias when vincristine given with ●delamanid
- Antifungals: increased risk of vincristine toxicity when given with ●itraconazole; metabolism of vincristine possibly inhibited by ●posaconazole (increased risk of neurotoxicity)
- Antimalarials: avoidance of vincristine advised by manufacturer of ●piperaquine with artenimol
- Antipsychotics: avoid concomitant use of cytotoxics with ●clozapine (increased risk of agranulocytosis)

Calcium-channel Blockers: metabolism of vincristine possibly inhibited by nifedipine

Cardiac Glycosides: vincristine possibly reduces absorption of digoxin *tablets*

Vindesine

- Antibacterials: possible increased risk of ventricular arrhythmias when vindesine given with ●delamanid
- Antifungals: possible increased risk of vindesine toxicity when given with ●itraconazole
- Antipsychotics: avoid concomitant use of cytotoxics with ●clozapine (increased risk of agranulocytosis)

Vinflunine

- Antibacterials: plasma concentration of vinflunine possibly reduced by ●rifampicin—manufacturer of vinflunine advises avoid concomitant use; increased risk of ventricular arrhythmias when vinflunine given with ●delamanid
- Antidepressants: plasma concentration of vinflunine possibly reduced by ●St John's wort—manufacturer of vinflunine advises avoid concomitant use
- Antifungals: possible increased risk of vinflunine toxicity when given with ●itraconazole
- Antimalarials: avoidance of vinflunine advised by manufacturer of ●piperaquine with artenimol
- Antipsychotics: avoid concomitant use of cytotoxics with ●clozapine (increased risk of agranulocytosis)
- Antivirals: plasma concentration of vinflunine possibly increased by ●ritonavir—manufacturer of vinflunine advises avoid concomitant use

Grapefruit Juice: plasma concentration of vinflunine possibly increased by grapefruit juice—manufacturer of vinflunine advises avoid concomitant use

Vinorelbine

- Antibacterials: possible increased risk of neutropenia when vinorelbine given with ●clarithromycin; possi-

Vinorelbine
- Antibacterials *(continued)*
  ble increased risk of ventricular arrhythmias when
  vinorelbine given with ●delamanid
- Antifungals: possible increased risk of vinorelbine
  toxicity when given with ●itraconazole
- Antimalarials: avoidance of vinorelbine advised by
  manufacturer of ●piperaquine with artenimol
- Antipsychotics: avoid concomitant use of cytotoxics
  with ●clozapine (increased risk of agranulocytosis)

Vismodegib
- Antibacterials: manufacturer of vismodegib advises
  avoid concomitant use with ●rifampicin (plasma
  concentration of vismodegib possibly reduced)
- Antidepressants: manufacturer of vismodegib advises
  avoid concomitant use with ●St John's wort
  (plasma concentration of vismodegib possibly
  reduced)
- Antiepileptics: manufacturer of vismodegib advises
  avoid concomitant use with ●carbamazepine and
  ●phenytoin (plasma concentration of vismodegib
  possibly reduced)
- Antipsychotics: avoid concomitant use of cytotoxics
  with ●clozapine (increased risk of agranulocytosis)

Vitamin A *see* Vitamins
Vitamin D *see* Vitamins
Vitamin E *see* Vitamins
Vitamin K (Phytomenadione) *see* Vitamins
Vitamins
- Antibacterials: absorption of vitamin A possibly
  reduced by neomycin
- Anticoagulants: vitamin K antagonises anticoagulant
  effect of ●coumarins and ●phenindione; vitamin E
  possibly enhances anticoagulant effect of ●coum-
  arins
- Antiepileptics: vitamin D requirements possibly
  increased when given with carbamazepine, phenobarbital or phenytoin
- Antifungals: effects of vitamin D possibly reduced by
  miconazole
- Antivirals: increased risk of bleeding when high doses
  of vitamin E given with tipranavir
- Ciclosporin: vitamin E possibly affects plasma concentration of ciclosporin
- Cytotoxics: effects of vitamin D possibly reduced by
  dactinomycin; avoidance of vitamin E advised by
  manufacturer of ibrutinib
- Diuretics: increased risk of hypercalcaemia when vitamin D given with thiazides and related diuretics
- Dopaminergics: pyridoxine reduces effects of levodopa when given without dopa-decarboxylase inhibitor
- Lipid-regulating Drugs: absorption of calcitriol possibly
  reduced by colestyramine (give at least 1 hour
  before or 4 to 6 hours after colestyramine)
- Retinoids: risk of hypervitaminosis A when vitamin A
  given with ●retinoids—avoid concomitant use
- Selenium: ascorbic acid possibly reduces absorption
  of selenium (give at least 4 hours apart)
- Sevelamer: absorption of calcitriol reduced by sevelamer (give at least 1 hour before or 3 hours after
  sevelamer)

Voriconazole *see* Antifungals, Triazole
Warfarin *see* Coumarins
Xipamide *see* Diuretics
Xylometazoline *see* Sympathomimetics
Yellow fever vaccine *see* Vaccines
Zafirlukast *see* Leukotriene Receptor Antagonists
Zaleplon *see* Anxiolytics and Hypnotics
Zidovudine
Note Increased risk of toxicity with nephrotoxic and
myelosuppressive drugs—for further details consult product
literature
Analgesics: increased risk of haematological toxicity
when zidovudine given with NSAIDs; plasma con-

Zidovudine
Analgesics *(continued)*
centration of zidovudine possibly increased by
methadone
Antibacterials: absorption of zidovudine reduced by
clarithromycin tablets (give at least 2 hours apart);
manufacturer of zidovudine advises avoid concomitant use with rifampicin
Antiepileptics: zidovudine increases or decreases
plasma concentration of phenytoin; plasma concentration of zidovudine possibly increased by valproate (increased risk of toxicity)
- Antifungals: plasma concentration of zidovudine
  increased by ●fluconazole (increased risk of toxicity)
Antimalarials: increased antifolate effect when zidovudine given with pyrimethamine
- Antivirals: profound myelosuppression when zidovudine given with ●ganciclovir (if possible avoid
  concomitant administration, particularly during initial ganciclovir therapy); increased risk of granulocytopenia when zidovudine given with ●nevirapine;
  increased risk of anaemia when zidovudine given
  with ●ribavirin—avoid concomitant use; zidovudine
  possibly inhibits effects of ●stavudine (manufacturers advise avoid concomitant use); plasma concentration of zidovudine reduced by ●tipranavir
Atovaquone: plasma concentration of zidovudine
increased by atovaquone (increased risk of toxicity)
- Orlistat: absorption of zidovudine possibly reduced by
  ●orlistat

Zinc
Antibacterials: zinc reduces absorption of ciprofloxacin, levofloxacin, moxifloxacin and ofloxacin; zinc
reduces absorption of norfloxacin (give at least 2
hours apart); zinc reduces absorption of tetracyclines, also absorption of zinc reduced by tetracyclines
Calcium Salts: absorption of zinc reduced by calcium
salts
Eltrombopag: zinc possibly reduces absorption of
eltrombopag (give at least 4 hours apart)
Iron: absorption of zinc reduced by *oral* iron, also
absorption of *oral* iron reduced by zinc
Penicillamine: absorption of zinc reduced by penicillamine, also absorption of penicillamine reduced by
zinc
Trientine: absorption of zinc reduced by trientine, also
absorption of trientine reduced by zinc

Zoledronic Acid *see* Bisphosphonates
Zolmitriptan *see* 5HT$_1$-receptor Agonists (under HT)
Zolpidem *see* Anxiolytics and Hypnotics
Zonisamide
- Antidepressants: anticonvulsant effect of antiepileptics
  possibly antagonised by MAOIs and ●tricyclic-
  related antidepressants (convulsive threshold lowered); anticonvulsant effect of antiepileptics antagonised by ●SSRIs and ●tricyclics (convulsive threshold lowered)
Antiepileptics: plasma concentration of zonisamide
reduced by carbamazepine, phenobarbital and
phenytoin
- Antimalarials: anticonvulsant effect of antiepileptics
  antagonised by ●mefloquine
- Antipsychotics: anticonvulsant effect of antiepileptics
  antagonised by ●antipsychotics (convulsive threshold lowered)
Diuretics: manufacturer of zonisamide advises avoid
concomitant use with carbonic anhydrase inhibitors
in children
- Orlistat: possible increased risk of convulsions when
  antiepileptics given with ●orlistat

Zopiclone *see* Anxiolytics and Hypnotics
Zuclopenthixol *see* Antipsychotics

A2 Borderline substances

In certain conditions some foods (and toilet preparations) have characteristics of drugs and the Advisory Committee on Borderline Substances (ACBS) advises as to the circumstances in which such substances may be regarded as drugs. Prescriptions issued in accordance with the Committee's advice and endorsed 'ACBS' will normally not be investigated.

General Practitioners are reminded that the ACBS recommends products on the basis that they may be regarded as drugs for the management of specified conditions. Doctors should satisfy themselves that the products can safely be prescribed, that patients are adequately monitored and that, where necessary, expert hospital supervision is available.

Foods which may be prescribed on FP10, GP10 (Scotland), or WP10 (Wales) All the food products listed in this appendix have ACBS approval. The clinical condition for which the product has been approved is included with each entry.

Note Foods included in this appendix may contain cariogenic sugars and patients should be advised to take appropriate oral hygiene measures.

Enteral feeds and supplements For most enteral feeds and nutritional supplements, the main source of **carbohydrate** is either maltodextrin or glucose syrup; other carbohydrate sources are listed in the relevant table, below. Feeds containing residual lactose (less than 1 g lactose/100 mL formula) are described as 'clinically lactose-free' or 'lactose-free' by some manufacturers. The presence of lactose (including residual lactose) in feeds is indicated in the relevant table, below. The primary sources of **protein** or **amino acids** are included with each product entry. The **fat** or **oil** content is derived from a variety of sources such as vegetables, soya bean, corn, palm nuts, and seeds; where the fat content is derived from animal or fish sources, this information is included in the relevant table, below. The presence of medium chain triglycerides (MCT) is also noted where the quantity exceeds 30% of the fat content.

Enteral feeds and nutritional supplements can contain varying amounts of **vitamins**, **minerals**, and **trace elements**—the manufacturer's product literature should be consulted for more detailed information. For further information on enteral nutrition, see section 9.4.2. Feeds containing vitamin K may affect the INR in patients receiving warfarin; see **interactions**: Appendix 1 (vitamins).

The suitability of food products for patients requiring a vegan, kosher, halal, or other compliant diet should be confirmed with individual manufacturers.

For details of enteral feeds, nutritional supplements, and specialised formulas suitable for infants and children under 12 years see *BNF for Children*.

Note Feeds containing more than 6 g/100 mL protein or 2 g/100 mL fibre should be avoided in children unless recommended by an appropriate specialist or dietician.

> **Standard ACBS indications**
> Disease-related malnutrition, intractable malabsorption, pre-operative preparation of malnourished patients, dysphagia, proven inflammatory bowel disease, following total gastrectomy, short-bowel syndrome, bowel fistula

Prices quoted in Appendix 2 are basic NHS net prices; for further information see Prices in the BNF.

Appendix 2: Borderline substances

Appendix 2: Borderline substances

A2.1 Enteral feeds (non-disease specific)

A2.1.1 Enteral feeds (non-disease specific): less than 5 g protein/100 mL

A2.1.1.1 Enteral feeds: 1 kcal/mL and less than 5 g protein/100 mL
Not suitable for use in child under 1 year unless otherwise stated; not recommended for child 1–6 years

Product	Formulation	Energy	Protein	Carbohydrate	Fat	Fibre	Special Characteristics	ACBS Indications	Presentation & Flavour
Fresubin® Original (Fresenius Kabi)	Liquid (sip or tube feed) per 100 mL	420 kJ (100 kcal)	3.8 g cows' milk soya	13.8 g (sugars 3.5 g¹)	3.4 g	Nil	Gluten-free Residual lactose Contains fish gelatin Feed in flexible pack contains fish oil and fish gelatin	Standard, p. 1017	Bottle: 200 mL = £2.07 Black currant, chocolate, nut, peach, vanilla Flexible pack: 500 mL = £4.02 1000 mL = £7.96 1500 mL = £11.95
Fresubin® Original Fibre (Fresenius Kabi)	Liquid (tube feed) per 100 mL	420 kJ (100 kcal)	3.8 g cows' milk soya	13 g (sugars 0.9 g)	3.4 g	1.5 g	Gluten-free Residual lactose Contains fish oil	Standard, p. 1017 except bowel fistula and pre-operative preparation of malnourished patients. Not suitable for child under 2 years	Flexible pack: 500 mL = £4.55 1000 mL = £9.08
Fresubin® 1500 Complete (Fresenius Kabi)	Liquid (tube feed) per 100 mL	420 kJ (100 kcal)	3.8 g cows' milk soya	13 g (sugars 0.9 g)	3.4 g	1.5 g	Gluten-free Residual lactose Contains fish oil	Standard, p. 1017 except bowel fistula and pre-operative preparation of malnourished patients. Not suitable for child under 2 years	Flexible pack: 1500 mL = £12.81
Jevity® (Abbott)	Liquid (tube feed) per 100 mL	449 kJ (107 kcal)	4 g caseinates	14.1 g (sugars 470 mg)	3.47 g	1.76 g	Gluten-free Residual lactose	Standard, p. 1017 except bowel fistula. Not suitable for child under 2 years	Flexible pack: 500 mL = £4.80 1000 mL = £9.02 1500 mL = £13.55
Novasource® GI Control (Nestlé)	Liquid (tube feed) per 100 mL	444 kJ (106 kcal)	4.1 g cows' milk	14.4 g (sugars 500 mg)	3.5 g (MCT 40 %)	2.2 g	Gluten-free Residual lactose	Standard, p. 1017	Flexible pack: 500 mL = £5.43
Nutrison® (Nutricia Clinical)	Liquid (tube feed) per 100 mL	420 kJ (100 kcal)	4 g cows' milk	12.3 g (sugars 1 g)	3.9 g	Nil	Gluten-free Residual lactose	Standard, p. 1017	Bottle: 500 mL = £4.23 Flexible pack: 500 mL = £4.70 1000 mL = £8.25 1500 mL = £12.35

1. Sugar content varies with flavour

Product	Formulation	Energy	Protein	Carbohydrate	Fat		Characteristics	Indications	Presentations
Nutrison® Multi Fibre (Nutricia Clinical)	Liquid (tube feed) per 100 mL	420 kJ (100 kcal)	4 g cows' milk	12.3 g (sugars 1 g)	3.9 g	1.5 g	Gluten-free Residual lactose	Standard, p. 1017 except bowel fistula	Bottle: 500 mL = £4.77 Flexible pack: 500 mL = £5.08 1000 mL = £9.54 1500 mL = £14.31
Osmolite® (Abbott)	Liquid (tube feed) per 100 mL	424 kJ (100 kcal)	4 g caseinates soy isolate	13.6 g (sugars 630 mg)	3.4 g	Nil	Gluten-free Residual lactose	Standard, p. 1017	Can: 250 mL = £2.17 Bottle: 500 mL = £4.12 1000 mL = £7.76 1500 mL = £11.63

Soya protein formula

Product	Formulation	Energy	Protein	Carbohydrate	Fat		Characteristics	Indications	Presentations
Fresubin® Soya Fibre (Fresenius Kabi)	Liquid (tube feed) per 100 mL	420 kJ (100 kcal)	3.8 g soya protein	13.3 g (sugars 4.1 g)	3.6 g	2 g	Gluten-free Lactose-free Contains fish oil	Standard, p. 1017; *also* cows' milk protein intolerance, lactose intolerance	Flexible pack: 500 mL = £4.71
Nutrison® Soya (Nutricia Clinical)	Liquid (tube feed) per 100 mL	420 kJ (100 kcal)	4 g soy isolate	12.3 g (sugars 1 g)	3.9 g	Nil	Gluten-free Residual lactose Milk protein-free	Standard, p. 1017; *also* cows' milk protein and lactose intolerance	Bottle: 500 mL = £5.07 Flexible pack: 1000 mL = £10.15
Nutrison® Soya Multi Fibre (Nutricia Clinical)	Liquid (tube feed) per 100 mL	420 kJ (100 kcal)	4 g soy isolate	12.3 g (sugars 700 mg)	3.9 g	1.5 g	Gluten-free Residual lactose Milk protein-free	Standard, p. 1017 except bowel fistula; *also* cows' milk protein and lactose intolerance	Flexible pack: 1500 mL = £16.88

Peptide-based formula

Product	Formulation	Energy	Protein	Carbohydrate	Fat		Characteristics	Indications	Presentations
Peptamen® (Nestlé)	Liquid (sip or tube feed) per 100 mL	420 kJ (100 kcal)	4 g whey peptides	12.7 g (sugars 480 mg[*])	3.7 g (MCT 70%)	Nil	Gluten-free Residual lactose	Short bowel syndrome, intractable malabsorption, proven inflammatory bowel disease, bowel fistula	Bottle: 200 mL = £2.97 Vanilla Flexible pack: 500 mL = £6.66 1000 mL = £12.50
Peptisorb® (Nutricia Clinical)	Liquid (tube feed) per 100 mL	425 kJ (100 kcal)	4 g whey protein hydrolysate	17.6 g (sugars 1.7 g)	1.7 g (MCT 47%)	Nil	Gluten-free Residual lactose	Short bowel syndrome, intractable malabsorption, proven inflammatory bowel disease, bowel fistula	Bottle: 500 mL = £6.73 Flexible pack: 500 mL = £7.38 1000 mL = £13.32
Survimed® OPD (Fresenius Kabi)	Liquid (tube feed) per 100 mL	420 kJ (100 kcal)	4.5 g whey protein hydrolysate	14.3 g (sugars 1.1 g)	2.8 g (MCT 51%)	100 mg	Gluten-free Residual lactose Contains fish oil	Standard, p. 1017; *also* growth failure	Flexible pack: 500 mL = £6.71 1000 mL = £13.42

1. Sugar content varies with flavour

Appendix 2: Borderline substances

Appendix 2: Borderline substances

A2.1.1.2 Enteral feeds: Less than 1 kcal/mL and less than 5 g protein/100 mL

Not suitable for use in child under 1 year unless otherwise stated; not recommended for child 1–6 years

Amino acid formula (essential and non-essential amino acids)

Product	Formulation	Energy	Protein	Carbohydrate	Fat	Fibre	Special Characteristics	ACBS Indications	Presentation & Flavour
Elemental 028® Extra (Nutricia Clinical)	Liquid (sip feed) **per 100 mL**	360 kJ (86 kcal)	2.5 g (protein equivalent)	11 g (sugars 4.7 g)	3.5 g (MCT 35%)	Nil		Short bowel syndrome, intractable malabsorption, proven inflammatory bowel disease, bowel fistula	Carton: 250 mL = £3.50 Grapefruit, orange-pineapple, summer fruits
	Standard dilution (20% of powder (sip or tube feed) **per 100 mL**	374 kJ (89 kcal)[1]	2.5 g (protein equivalent)	11.8 g (sugars 1.1 g)	3.5 g (MCT 35%)	Nil		Short bowel syndrome, intractable malabsorption, proven inflammatory bowel disease, bowel fistula	Sachet: 100 g = £6.81 Banana, citrus, orange, unflavoured[2]

Powder provides protein equivalent 12.5 g, carbohydrate 59 g, fat 17.45 g, energy 1871 kJ (443 kcal)/100 g

1. Nutritional values vary with flavour—consult product literature
2. Flavouring: see *Modjul® Flavour System*, p. 1041

A2.1.2.2 Enteral feeds (non-disease specific): 5 g (or more) protein/100 mL

A2.1.2.2.1 Enteral feeds: 1.5 kcal/mL and 5 g (or more) protein/100 mL

Not suitable for use in child under 1 year unless otherwise stated; not recommended for child 1–6 years

Product	Formulation	Energy	Protein	Carbohydrate	Fat	Fibre	Special Characteristics	ACBS Indications	Presentation & Flavour
Fresubin® 2250 Complete (Fresenius Kabi)	Liquid (tube feed) **per 100 mL**	630 kJ (150 kcal)	5.6 g cows' milk	18.8 g (sugars 1.5 g)	5.8 g	2 g	Gluten-free Residual lactose Contains fish oil and fish gelatin	Standard, p. 1017	Flexible pack: 1500 mL = £14.29
Fresubin® Energy (Fresenius Kabi)	Liquid (sip feed) **per 100 mL**	630 kJ (150 kcal)	5.6 g cows' milk	18.8 g (sugars[1])	5.8 g	Nil	Gluten-free[2] Residual lactose Contains fish gelatin	Standard, p. 1017	Bottle: 200 mL = £1.48 Banana, black currant, cappuccino, chocolate, lemon, neutral, strawberry, tropical fruits, vanilla
	Liquid (tube feed) **per 100 mL**	630 kJ (150 kcal)	5.6 g cows' milk	18.8 g (sugars 1.4 g)	5.8 g	Nil	Gluten-free Residual lactose Contains fish oil and fish gelatin	Standard, p. 1017	Flexible pack: 500 mL = £4.92 1000 mL = £9.67 1500 mL = £12.96

1. Sugar content varies with flavour
2. Strawberry flavour may contain traces of wheat, starch and egg

Product	Form	Energy	Protein	Carbohydrate	Fat	Fibre	Special characteristics	Standard/suitability	Presentation
Fresubin® Energy Fibre (Fresenius Kabi)	Liquid (sip feed) **per 100 mL**	630 kJ (150 kcal)	5.6 g cows' milk	18.8 g (sugars¹)	5.8 g	2 g	Gluten-free, Residual lactose, Contains fish gelatin	Standard, p. 1017	Bottle: 200 mL = £1.98, Banana, caramel, cherry, chocolate, strawberry, vanilla
	Liquid (tube feed) **per 100 mL**	630 kJ (150 kcal)	5.6 g cows' milk	18.8 g (sugars 1.5 g)	5.8 g	2 g	Gluten-free, Residual lactose, Contains fish oil and fish gelatin	Standard, p. 1017	Flexible pack: 500 mL = £5.40, 1000 mL = £10.29
Fresubin® HP Energy (Fresenius Kabi)	Liquid (tube feed) **per 100 mL**	630 kJ (150 kcal)	7.5 g cows' milk	17 g (sugars 1 g)	5.8 g (MCT 57%)	Nil	Gluten-free, Residual lactose, Contains fish oil and fish gelatin	Standard, p. 1017; *also* CAPD and haemodialysis	Flexible pack: 500 mL = £5.01, 1000 mL = £10.03
Jevity® 1.5 kcal (Abbott)	Liquid (tube feed) **per 100 mL**	649 kJ (154 kcal)	6.38 g caseinates soy isolate	20.1 g (sugars 1.47 g)	4.9 g	2.2 g	Gluten-free, Residual lactose	Standard, p. 1017, Not suitable for child under 2 years; not recommended for child 2–10 years	Flexible pack: 500 mL = £5.68, 1000 mL = £10.86, 1500 mL = £16.63
Novasource® GI Forte (Nestlé)	Liquid (tube feed) **per 100 mL**	631 kJ (150 kcal)	6 g cows' milk	18.3 g (sugars 1.8 g)	5.9 g	2.2 g	Gluten-free, Residual lactose	Standard, p. 1017	Flexible pack: 500 mL = £5.39, 1000 mL = £10.44
Nutrison® Energy (Nutricia Clinical)	Liquid (tube feed) **per 100 mL**	630 kJ (150 kcal)	6 g cows' milk	18.5 g (sugars 1.5 g)	5.8 g	Nil	Gluten-free, Residual lactose	Standard, p. 1017	Bottle: 500 mL = £5.12, Flexible pack: 500 mL = £5.47, 1000 mL = £10.29, 1500 mL = £15.39
Nutrison® Energy Multi Fibre (Nutricia Clinical)	Liquid (tube feed) **per 100 mL**	630 kJ (150 kcal)	6 g cows' milk	18.5 g (sugars 1.5 g)	5.8 g	1.5 g	Gluten-free, Residual lactose	Standard, p. 1017	Bottle: 500 mL = £5.72, Flexible pack: 500 mL = £6.07, 1000 mL = £11.42, 1500 mL = £17.63
Osmolite® 1.5 kcal (Abbott)	Liquid (tube feed) **per 100 mL**	632 kJ (150 kcal)	6.25 g cows' milk soya protein isolate	20 g (sugars 4.9 g)	5 g	Nil	Gluten-free, Residual lactose	Standard, p. 1017	Flexible pack: 500 mL = £5.05, 1000 mL = £9.68, 1500 mL = £14.49
Resource® Energy (Nestlé)	Liquid (sip feed) **per 100 mL**	630 kJ (150 kcal)	5.6 g cows' milk	21 g (sugars 5.2 g¹)	5 g	less than 500 mg	Gluten-free, Residual lactose	Standard, p. 1017, Not suitable for child under 3 years	Bottle: 4 × 200 mL = £7.67, Apricot, banana, chocolate, coffee, strawberry-raspberry, vanilla
Vital® 1.5 kcal (Abbott)	Liquid (sip or tube feed) **per 100 mL**	631 kJ (150 kcal)	6.75 g caseinate whey protein hydrolysate	18.4 g (sugars 3.6 g)	5.5 g (MCT 64%)	Nil	Gluten-free, Residual lactose	Standard, p. 1017; except proven inflammatory bowel disease and following total gastrectomy; not recommended for use in children	Bottle: 200 mL = £2.98, Vanilla, Flexible pack: 1000 mL = £14.60

1. Sugar content varies with flavour

Appendix 2: Borderline substances

Appendix 2: Borderline substances

A2.1.2.2 Enteral feeds: Less than 1.5 kcal/mL and 5 g (or more) protein/100 mL

Not suitable for use in child under 1 year unless otherwise stated; not recommended for child 1–6 years

Product	Formulation	Energy	Protein	Carbohydrate	Fat	Fibre	Special Characteristics	ACBS Indications	Presentation & Flavour
Fresubin® 1000 Complete (Fresenius Kabi)	Liquid (tube feed) **per 100 mL**	420 kJ (100 kcal)	5.5 g cows' milk	12.5 g (sugars 1.1 g)	3.1 g	2 g	Gluten-free Residual lactose Contains fish oil	Standard, 1017	Flexible pack: 1000 mL = £10.29
Fresubin® 1200 Complete (Fresenius Kabi)	Liquid (tube feed) **per 100 mL**	500 kJ (120 kcal)	6 g cows' milk	15 g (sugars 1.22 g)	4.1 g	2 g	Gluten-free Residual lactose Contains fish oil	Standard, p. 1017	Flexible pack: 1000 mL = £13.11
Fresubin® 1800 Complete (Fresenius Kabi)	Liquid (tube feed) **per 100 mL**	500 kJ (120 kcal)	6 g cows' milk	15 g (sugars 1.22 g)	4.1 g	2 g	Gluten-free Residual lactose Contains fish oil	Standard, p. 1017	Flexible pack: 1500 mL = £13.11
Jevity® Plus (Abbott)	Liquid (tube feed) **per 100 mL**	514 kJ (122 kcal)	5.5 g caseinates soy isolates	15.1 g (sugars 890 mg)	3.93 g	2.2 g	Gluten-free Residual lactose	Standard, p. 1017 Not suitable for child under 2 years; not recommended for child 2–10 years	Flexible pack: 500 mL = £5.24 1000 mL = £10.58 1500 mL = £15.88
Jevity® Plus HP (Abbott)	Liquid (tube feed) **per 100 mL**	551 kJ (131 kcal)	8.13 g cows' milk soy isolates	14.2 g (sugars 950 mg)	4.33 g	1.5 g	Gluten-free Residual lactose	Standard, p. 1017; *also* CAPD, haemodialysis Not suitable for child under 2 years; not recommended for child 2–10 years	Flexible pack: 500 mL = £5.28
Jevity® Promote (Abbott)	Liquid (tube feed) **per 100 mL**	434 kJ (103 kcal)	5.55 g caseinates soy isolates	12 g (sugars 670 mg)	3.32 g	1.7 g	Gluten-free Residual lactose	Standard, p. 1017 Not suitable for child under 2 years; not recommended for child 2–10 years	Flexible pack: 1000 mL = £10.34
Nutrison® MCT (Nutricia Clinical)	Liquid (tube feed) **per 100 mL**	420 kJ (100 kcal)	5 g cows' milk	12.6 g (sugars 1 g)	3.3 g (MCT 61%)	Nil	Gluten-free Residual lactose	Standard, p. 1017	Flexible pack: 1000 mL = £9.53
Nutrison® Protein Plus (Nutricia Clinical)	Liquid (tube feed) **per 100 mL**	525 kJ (125 kcal)	6.3 g cows' milk	14.2 g (sugars 1.1 g)	4.9 g	Nil	Gluten-free Residual lactose	Standard, p. 1017	Flexible pack: 1000 mL = £9.80
Nutrison® Protein Plus Multi Fibre (Nutricia Clinical)	Liquid (tube feed) **per 100 mL**	525 kJ (125 kcal)	6.3 g cow's milk	14.1 g (sugars 1.1 g)	4.9 g	1.5 g	Gluten-free Residual lactose	Disease-related malnutrition	Flexible pack: 1000 mL = £10.91
Nutrison® 800 Complete Multi Fibre (Nutricia Clinical)	Liquid (tube feed) **per 100 mL**	345 kJ (83 kcal)	5.5 g cows' milk soya protein pea protein	8.8 g (sugars 600 mg)	2.5 g	1.5 g	Gluten-free Residual lactose Contains fish oil	Standard, p. 1017 except bowel fistula Not suitable for child under 6 years; not recommended for child 6–12 years	Flexible pack: 1000 mL = £9.99

Product	Formulation	Energy	Protein	Carbohydrate	Fat	Fibre	Special Characteristics	ACBS Indications	Presentation & Flavour
Nutrison® 1000 Complete Multi Fibre (Nutricia Clinical)	Liquid (tube feed) per 100 mL	420 kJ (100 kcal)	5.5 g cows' milk	11.3 g (sugars 700 mg)	3.7 g	2 g	Gluten-free Residual lactose	Disease-related malnutrition in patients with low energy and/or low fluid requirements	Flexible pack: 1000 mL = £10.58
Nutrison® 1200 Complete Multi Fibre (Nutricia Clinical)	Liquid (tube feed) per 100 mL	505 kJ (120 kcal)	5.5 g cows' milk	15 g (sugars 1.2 g)	4.3 g	2 g	Gluten-free Residual lactose	Standard, p. 1017 except bowel fistula	Flexible pack: 1000 mL = £11.21; 1500 mL = £16.83
Osmolite® Plus (Abbott)	Liquid (tube feed) per 100 mL	508 kJ (121 kcal)	5.55 g caseinates	15.8 g (sugars 730 mg)	3.93 g	Nil	Gluten-free Residual lactose	Standard, p. 1017 Not recommended for child under 10 years	Flexible pack: 500 mL = £4.83; 1000 mL = £9.31; 1500 mL = £13.94
Peptamen® HN (Nestlé)	Liquid (tube feed) per 100 mL	556 kJ (133 kcal)	6.6 g whey protein hydrolysates	15.6 g (sugars 1.4 g)	4.9 g (MCT 70%)	Nil	Gluten-free Residual lactose Hydrolysed with pork trypsin	Short bowel syndrome, intractable malabsorption, proven inflammatory bowel disease, bowel fistula Not suitable for child under 3 years	Flexible pack: 500 mL = £7.17
Perative® (Abbott)	Liquid (tube feed) per 100 mL	552 kJ (131 kcal)	6.7 g caseinate whey protein hydrolysates	17.7 g (sugars 660 mg)	3.7 g (MCT 42%)	Nil	Gluten-free Residual lactose	Standard, p. 1017 Not suitable for child under 5 years	Flexible pack: 500 mL = £6.73; 1000 mL = £13.45

A2.1.2.3 Enteral feeds: More than 1.5 kcal/mL and 5 g (or more) protein/100 mL

Not suitable for use in child under 1 year unless otherwise stated; not recommended for child 1–6 years

Product	Formulation	Energy	Protein	Carbohydrate	Fat	Fibre	Special Characteristics	ACBS Indications	Presentation & Flavour
Ensure® Twocal (Abbott)	Liquid (sip or tube feed) per 100 mL	838 kJ (200 kcal)	8.4 g cows' milk	21 g (sugars 4.5 g)	8.9 g	1 g	Gluten-free Residual lactose	Standard, p. 1017, also haemodialysis, CAPD	Bottle: 200 mL = £2.22. Banana, neutral, strawberry, vanilla
TwoCal® (Abbott)	Liquid (tube feed) per 100 mL	837 kJ (200 kcal)	8.4 g cows' milk caseinates	21 g (sugars 4.5 g)	8.9 g	1 g	Gluten-free Residual lactose	Adults with or at risk of disease-related malnutrition, catabolic or fluid-restricted patients, and other patients requiring a 2 kcal/mL feed	Bottle: 1000 mL = £13.22

Appendix 2: Borderline substances

Appendix 2: Borderline substances

A2.1.3 Enteral feeds (non-disease specific): Child under 12 years
see *BNF for Children*

A2.2 Nutritional supplements (non-disease specific)

A2.2.1 Nutritional supplements: less than 5 g protein/100 mL

A2.2.1.1 Nutritional supplements: 1 kcal/mL and less than 5 g protein/100 mL
Not suitable for use in child under 1 year; use with caution in child 1–5 years unless otherwise stated

Product	Formulation	Energy	Protein	Carbohydrate	Fat	Fibre	Special Characteristics	ACBS Indications	Presentation & Flavour
Ensure® (Abbott)	Liquid (sip or tube feed) **per 100 mL**	423 kJ (100 kcal)[1]	4 g caseinates soy isolate	13.6 g (sugars 3.93 g)	3.36 g	Nil	Gluten-free Residual lactose	Standard, p. 1017	Can: 250 mL = £2.26 Chocolate, coffee, vanilla

1. Nutritional values vary with flavour—consult product literature

A2.2.1.2 Nutritional supplements: More than 1 kcal/mL and less than 5 g protein/100 mL
Not suitable for use in child under 1 year; use with caution in child 1–5 years unless otherwise stated

Product	Formulation	Energy	Protein	Carbohydrate	Fat	Fibre	Special Characteristics	ACBS Indications	Presentation & Flavour
AYMES® Shake (AYMES)	Standard dilution of powder (57 g in 200 mL water) (sip feed) **per 100 mL**	530.5 kJ (126 kcal)[1]	4.5 g cows' milk	17.5 g (sugars 8.4 g)	4.2 g	Nil	Gluten-free Contains lactose	Standard, p. 1017. Use with caution in child 1–6 years	Sachets: 7 × 57 g = £5.46 Banana, chocolate, neutral, strawberry, vanilla Sample pack (mixed): 5 × 57 g = £4.78
Powder 57 g reconstituted with 200 mL whole milk provides: protein 15.8 g, carbohydrate 44.1 g, fat 16.4 g, energy 1625 kJ (388 kcal)									
Ensure® Plus Juce (Abbott)	Liquid (sip feed) **per 100 mL**	638 kJ (150 kcal)	4.8 g whey protein isolate	32.7 g (sugars 9.4 g[2])	Nil	Nil	Gluten-free Residual lactose Non-milk taste	Standard, p. 1017	Bottle: 220 mL = £1.97 Apple, fruit punch, lemon-lime, orange, peach, strawberry
Fortijuce® (Nutricia Clinical)	Liquid (sip feed) **per 100 mL**	640 kJ (150 kcal)	4 g cows' milk	33.5 g (sugars 13.1 g[2])	Nil	Nil	Gluten-free Residual lactose Non-milk taste	Standard, p. 1017 Not suitable for child under 3 years	Bottle: 200 mL = £2.02 Apple, black currant, forest fruits, lemon, orange, strawberry, tropical Starter pack (mixed): 4 × 200 mL = £8.08

1. Nutritional values vary with flavour—consult product literature
2. Sugar content varies with flavour

Product	Formulation	Energy	Protein	Carbohydrate	Fat	Fibre	Special Characteristics	ACBS Indications	Presentation & Flavour
Fresubin® Jucy Drink (Fresenius Kabi)	Liquid (sip feed) **per 100 mL**	630 kJ (150 kcal)	4 g whey protein	33.5 g (sugars 8 g)	Nil	Nil	Gluten-free, Residual lactose	Standard, p. 1017; *also* CAPD, haemodialysis	Bottle: 4 × 200 mL = £7.52; Apple, black currant, cherry, orange, pineapple
ProvideXtra® Juice Drink (Fresenius Kabi)	Liquid (sip feed) **per 100 mL**	630 kJ (150 kcal)	4 g pea and soya protein hydrolysates	33.5 g[1]	Nil	Nil[2]	Gluten-free, Lactose-free, Non-milk taste	Standard, p. 1017	Bottle: 200 mL = £1.82; Apple, black currant, cherry, lemon-lime, orange-pineapple
Resource® Dessert Energy (Nestlé)	Semi-solid **per 100 g**	671 kJ (160 kcal)	4.8 g cows' milk	21.2 g (sugars 9.9 g[1])	6.2 g	Nil	Gluten-free, Contains lactose	Standard, p. 1017; *also* CAPD, haemodialysis	Cup: 125 g = £1.59; Caramel, chocolate, vanilla
Resource® Fruit (Nestlé)	Liquid (sip feed) **per 100 mL**	520 kJ (125 kcal)	4 g whey protein hydrolysate	27 g (sugars 9.5 g[1])	less than 200 mg	less than 200 mg[2]	Gluten-free, Residual lactose, Non-milk taste	Standard, p. 1017; Not suitable for child under 3 years	Bottle: 4 × 200 mL = £7.35; Apple, orange, pear-cherry, raspberry-black currant

1. Sugar content varies with flavour
2. Fibre content varies with flavour

A2.2.2 Nutritional supplements: 5 g (or more) protein/100 mL

A2.2.2.1 Nutritional supplements: 1.5 kcal/mL and 5 g (or more) protein/100 mL
Not suitable for use in child under 1 year; use with caution in child 1–5 years unless otherwise stated

Product	Formulation	Energy	Protein	Carbohydrate	Fat	Fibre	Special Characteristics	ACBS Indications	Presentation & Flavour
Ensure® Plus Fibre (Abbott)	Liquid (sip or tube feed) **per 100 mL**	652 kJ (155 kcal)[1]	6.25 g cows' milk soya protein isolate	20.2 g (sugars 5.5 g)	4.92 g	2.5 g	Gluten-free, Residual lactose	Standard, p. 1017; *also* CAPD, haemodialysis	Bottle: 200 mL = £2.02; Banana, chocolate, raspberry, strawberry, vanilla
Ensure® Plus Milkshake style (Abbott)	Liquid (sip or tube feed) **per 100 mL**	632 kJ (150 kcal)[1]	6.25 g cows' milk soya protein isolate	20.2 g (sugars 6.89 g)	4.92 g	Nil	Gluten-free, Residual lactose	Standard, p. 1017; *also* CAPD, haemodialysis	Bottle: 220 mL = £2.02; Banana, chocolate, coffee, fruits of the forest, orange, peach, raspberry, strawberry, vanilla, neutral
Ensure® Plus Savoury (Abbott)	Liquid (sip or tube feed) **per 100 mL**	632 kJ (150 kcal)[1]	6.25 g cows' milk soy protein isolate	20.2 g (sugars 1.13 g)	4.92 g	Nil	Gluten-free, Residual lactose	Standard, p. 1017; *also* CAPD, haemodialysis	Bottle: 220 mL = £2.02; Chicken, mushroom
Ensure® Plus Yoghurt style (Abbott)	Liquid (sip feed) **per 100 mL**	632 kJ (150 kcal)[1]	6.25 g cows' milk	20.2 g (sugars 11.7 g)	4.92 g	Nil	Gluten-free, Residual lactose	Standard, p. 1017; *also* CAPD, haemodialysis	Bottle: 220 mL = £2.02; Peach, strawberry

1. Nutritional values vary with flavour—consult product literature

Appendix 2: Borderline substances

Appendix 2: Borderline substances

A2.2.2.1 Nutritional supplements: 1.5 kcal/mL and 5 g (or more) protein/100 mL (product list continued)

Not suitable for use in child under 1 year; use with caution in child 1–5 years unless otherwise stated

Product	Formulation	Energy	Protein	Carbohydrate	Fat	Fibre	Special Characteristics	ACBS Indications	Presentation & Flavour
Ensure® Plus Commence (Abbott)	Starter pack (5–10 day's supply), contains: Ensure® Plus Milkshake Style (various flavours), 1 pack (10 × 220-mL) = £20.23.								
Fortisip® Bottle (Nutricia Clinical)	Liquid (sip feed) **per 100 mL**	630 kJ (150 kcal)	6 g cows' milk	18.4 g[1]	5.8 g	Nil	Gluten-free Residual lactose	Standard, p. 1017 Not suitable for child under 3 years	Bottle: 200 mL = £2.06 Banana, chocolate, neutral, orange, strawberry, toffee, tropical fruits, vanilla
Fortisip® Multi Fibre (Nutricia Clinical)	Liquid (sip feed) **per 100 mL**	630 kJ (150 kcal)	6 g cows' milk	18.4 g (sugars 7.0 g)	5.8 g	2.3 g	Gluten-free Residual lactose	Standard, p. 1017 Not suitable for child under 3 years	Bottle: 200 mL = £2.09 Vanilla
Fortisip® Savoury Multi Fibre (Nutricia Clinical)	Liquid (sip feed) **per 100 mL**	625 kJ (150 kcal)	7.5 g cows' milk	12.8 g (sugars 900 mg)	7 g	2.3 g	Gluten-free Residual lactose	Standard, p. 1017 except bowel fistula Not suitable for child under 3 years; use with caution in child 3–6 years	Bottle: 2 × 200 mL = £4.32 Chicken
Fortisip® Yogurt Style (Nutricia Clinical)	Liquid (sip feed) **per 100 mL**	630 kJ (150 kcal)	6 g cows' milk	18.7 g (sugars 10.8 g)	5.8 g	200 mg	Gluten-free Contains lactose	Standard, p. 1017 Not suitable for child under 3 years	Bottle: 200 mL = £2.02 Peach-orange, raspberry, vanilla-lemon
Fortisip® Range (Nutricia Clinical)	Starter pack contains 4 × Fortisip® Bottle, 4 × Fortijuce®, 2 × Fortisip® Yogurt Style, 1 pack (10 × 200 mL) = £20.20.								
Fresubin® Protein Energy Drink (Fresenius Kabi)	Liquid (sip feed) **per 100 mL**	630 kJ (150 kcal)	10 g cows' milk	12.4 g (sugars 6.4 g[1])	6.7 g	Nil[2]	Gluten-free Residual lactose Contains fish gelatin	Standard, p. 1017; also CAPD, haemodialysis	Bottle: 200 mL = £1.97 Cappuccino, chocolate, strawberry, tropical fruits, vanilla
Fresubin® Thickened (Fresenius Kabi)	Liquid (sip feed) **per 100 mL**	630 kJ (150 kcal)	10 g cows' milk	12.2 g (sugars 7.1 g[3])	6.7 g	480 mg[4]	Gluten-free Residual lactose	Dysphagia or disease-related malnutrition Not suitable for child under 3 years; use with caution in child 3–4 years	Bottle: 200 mL = £2.10 Syrup (Stage 1) and custard (Stage 2) consistencies Strawberry, vanilla
Fresubin® YOCrème (Fresenius Kabi)	Semi-solid **per 100 g**	630 kJ (150 kcal)	7.5 g whey protein	19.5 g (sugars 16.8 g)	4.7 g	Nil	Gluten-free Contains lactose	Dysphagia, or presence or risk of malnutrition Not suitable for child under 3 years	Pot: 4 × 125 g = £7.72 Apricot-peach, biscuit, lemon, raspberry
Nutriplen® Protein (Nualtra)	Liquid (sip feed) **per 100 mL**	632 kJ (150 kcal)	10 g cows' milk soya protein	15 g (sugars 4.6 g)	5.6 g	Nil	Gluten-free Residual lactose	Standard, p. 1017 Not suitable for child under 3 years; use with caution in child 3–6 years	Bottle: 4 × 200 mL = £5.80 Strawberry, vanilla

1. Sugar content varies with flavour
3. Sugar content varies with consistency
4. Fibre content varies with consistency

A2.2.2.2 Nutritional supplements: Less than 1.5 kcal/mL and 5 g (or more) protein/100 mL

Not suitable for use in child under 1 year; use with caution in child 1–5 years unless otherwise stated

Product	Formulation	Energy	Protein	Carbohydrate	Fat	Fibre	Special Characteristics	ACBS Indications	Presentation & Flavour
Clinutren® Dessert (Nestlé)	Semi-solid **per 100 g**	520 kJ (125 kcal)	9.5 g cows' milk	15.5 g (sugars 14 g[1])	2.6 g	500 mg[2]	Gluten-free Contains lactose	Standard, p. 1017; *also* CAPD, haemodialysis Not suitable for child under 3 years	Pot: 4 × 125 g = £5.88 Caramel, chocolate, peach, vanilla
Ensure® Plus Crème (Abbott)	Semi-solid **per 100 g**	574 kJ (137 kcal)[3]	5.68 g cows' milk soy protein isolates	18.4 g (sugars 12.4 g)	4.47 g	Nil	Gluten-free Residual lactose Contains soya	Standard, p. 1017; *also* CAPD, haemodialysis Not suitable for child under 3 years	Pot: 125 g = £1.76 Banana, chocolate, neutral, vanilla
Fortimel® Regular (Nutricia Clinical)	Liquid (sip feed) **per 100 mL**	420 kJ (100 kcal)	10 g cows' milk	10.3 g (sugars 8.1 g[1])	2.1 g	Nil	Gluten-free Contains lactose	Standard, p. 1017 Not suitable for child under 3 years	Bottle: 200 mL = £1.57 Chocolate, forest fruits, strawberry, vanilla
Nutilis® Fruit Stage 3 (Nutricia Clinical)	Semi-Solid **per 100 g**	560 kJ (133 kcal)	7 g whey isolate	16.7 g (sugars 11.3 g[1])	4 g	2.6 g	Residual lactose Gluten-free	Standard, p. 1017 except bowel fistula; *also* CAPD, haemodialysis Not suitable for child under 3 years	Pot: 3 × 150 g = £7.08 Apple, strawberry
Oral Impact® (Nestlé)	Standard dilution of powder (74 g in 250 mL water) (sip feed) **per 100 mL**	425 kJ (101 kcal)[3]	5.6 g cows' milk	13.4 g (sugars 7.4 g)	2.8 g	1 g	Residual lactose Contains fish oil	Preoperative nutritional supplement for malnourished patients or patients at risk of malnourishment Not suitable for child under 3 years	Sachet: 5 × 74 g = £16.93 Citrus, coffee, tropical
	Powder provides: protein 16.8 g, carbohydrate 40.2 g, fat 8.3 g, fibre 3 g, energy 1276 kJ (303 kcal)/74 g								
Resource® Protein (Nestlé)	Liquid (sip feed) **per 100 mL**	530 kJ (125 kcal)[3]	9.4 g cows' milk	14 g (sugars 4.5 g)	3.5 g	Nil	Gluten-free Contains lactose	Standard, p. 1017 Not suitable for child under 3 years	Bottle: 200 mL = £1.52 Apricot, chocolate, forest fruits, strawberry, vanilla

1. Sugar content varies with flavour
2. Fibre content varies with flavour
3. Nutritional values vary with flavour—consult product literature

Appendix 2: Borderline substances

Appendix 2: Borderline substances

A2.2.3 Nutritional supplements: More than 1.5 kcal/mL and 5 g (or more) protein/100 mL

Not suitable for use in child under 1 year; use with caution in child 1–5 years unless otherwise stated

Product	Formulation	Energy	Protein	Carbohydrate	Fat	Fibre	Special Characteristics	ACBS Indications	Presentation & Flavour
Complan® Shake (Complan Foods)	Powder per 57 g	1057 kJ (251 kcal)[1]	8.8 g cows' milk	35.2 g (sugars 22.7 g)	8.4 g	Trace	Gluten-free Contains lactose	Standard, p. 1017	Sachet: 4 × 57 g = £3.40 Banana, chocolate, original, strawberry, vanilla Starter pack: 5 × 57 g = £4.79

Powder 57 g reconstituted with 200 mL whole milk provides: protein 15.6 g, carbohydrate 44.5 g, fat 16.4 g, energy 1621 kJ (387 kcal)

Product	Formulation	Energy	Protein	Carbohydrate	Fat	Fibre	Special Characteristics	ACBS Indications	Presentation & Flavour
Foodlink® Complete (Foodlink)	Powder per 100 g	1826 kJ (434 kcal)[1]	21.3g cows' milk	56.7 g	13.5 g	Nil	Contains lactose	Standard, p. 1017	Carton: 450 g = £3.25 Banana, chocolate, natural, strawberry

Recommended serving = 4 heaped dessertspoonfuls in 200 mL full cream milk provides: protein 18.9 g, carbohydrate 41.8 g, fat 15.7 g, energy 1605 kJ (383 kcal)

Product	Formulation	Energy	Protein	Carbohydrate	Fat	Fibre	Special Characteristics	ACBS Indications	Presentation & Flavour
Foodlink® Complete with Fibre (Foodlink)	Powder per 100 g	1683 kJ (400 kcal)[1]	19.4 g cows' milk	52.7 g (sugars 27.3 g)	12.4 g	7.2 g	Contains lactose	Standard, p. 1017	Sachet: 10 × 63 g = £6.70 Carton: 450 g = £3.25 Vanilla + fibre

Recommended serving = 4 heaped dessertspoonfuls (or the contents of a 63-g sachet) in 200 mL full cream milk provides: protein 19.0, carbohydrate 42.7 g, fat 15.8 g, fibre 4.5 g, energy 1624 kJ (388 kcal)

Product	Formulation	Energy	Protein	Carbohydrate	Fat	Fibre	Special Characteristics	ACBS Indications	Presentation & Flavour
Forticreme® Complete (Nutricia Clinical)	Semi-solid per 100 g	675 kJ (160 kcal)	9.5 g cows' milk	19.2 g (sugars 10.6 g)	5 g	100 mg[2]	Gluten-free Residual lactose	Standard, p. 1017; *also* CAPD, haemodialysis Not suitable for child under 3 years	Pot: 4 × 125 g = £7.84 Banana, chocolate, forest fruits, vanilla
Fortisip® Compact (Nutricia Clinical)	Liquid (sip feed) per 100 mL	1010 kJ (240 kcal)	9.6 g cows' milk	29.7 g (sugars 15 g)	9.3 g	Nil	Residual lactose	Standard, p. 1017 Not suitable for child under 3 years	Bottle: 125 mL = £1.85 Apricot, banana, chocolate, forest fruits, mocha, strawberry, vanilla Starter pack: 6 × 125 mL = £12.12
Fortisip® Compact Fibre (Nutricia Clinical)	Liquid (sip feed) per 100 mL	1000 kJ (240 kcal)	9.4 g cows' milk	25.2 g (sugars 13.9 g)	10.4 g	3.6 g	Gluten-free Residual lactose	Standard, p. 1017 Not suitable for child under 3 years	Bottle: 125 mL = £1.85 Mocha, strawberry, vanilla Starter pack: 4 × 125 mL = £8.36
Fortisip® Compact Protein (Nutricia Clinical)	Liquid (sip feed) per 100 mL	1010 kJ (240 kcal)[1]	14.4 g cows' milk	24.4 g (sugars 13.3 g)	9.4 g	Nil	Gluten-free Residual lactose	Standard, p. 1017 Not suitable for child under 3 years	Bottle: 4 × 125 mL = £8.00 Banana, mocha, strawberry, vanilla
Fortisip® Extra (Nutricia Clinical)	Liquid (sip feed) per 100 mL	675 kJ (160 kcal)	10 g cows' milk	18.1 g (sugars 9 g)	5.3 g	Nil[2]	Gluten-free Contains lactose	Standard, p. 1017 Not suitable for child under 3 years	Bottle: 200 mL = £2.08 Chocolate, forest fruits, mocha, strawberry, vanilla Starter pack: 4 × 200 mL = £8.32

1. Nutritional values vary with flavour, consult product literature

Product	Form	Energy	Protein source	Carbohydrate	Fat	Fibre	Characteristics	Indications	Presentation / flavours
Fresubin® 2 kcal Drink (Fresenius Kabi)	Liquid (sip feed) **per 100 mL**	840 kJ (200 kcal)	10 g cows' milk	22.5 g (sugars 5.8 g¹)	7.8 g	Nil	Gluten-free Residual lactose	Standard, p. 1017; *also* CAPD, haemodialysis	Bottle: 200 mL = £1.91 Apricot-peach, cappuccino, fruits of the forest, neutral, toffee, vanilla
Fresubin® 2 kcal Fibre Drink (Fresenius Kabi)	Liquid (sip feed) **per 100 mL**	840 kJ (200 kcal)²	10 g cows' milk	22.5 g (sugars 5.8 g)	7.8 g	1.6 g	Gluten-free Residual lactose	Standard, p. 1017; *also* CAPD, haemodialysis	Bottle: 200 mL = £1.91 Apricot-peach, cappuccino, chocolate, lemon, neutral, vanilla
Fresubin® Crème (Fresenius Kabi)	Semi-solid **per 100 g**	775 kJ (185 kcal)²	10 g cows' milk	19 g (sugars 14.4 g)	7.2 g	2 g	Gluten-free Residual lactose	Standard, p. 1017; *also* CAPD, haemodialysis Not suitable for child under 3 years	Pot: 4 × 125 g = £7.72 Cappuccino, chocolate, praline, strawberry, vanilla
Fresubin® Powder Extra (Fresenius Kabi)	Powder **per 100 g**	1764 kJ (420 kcal)²	17.5 g cows' milk whey protein	63 g (sugars 24.7 g)	10.9 g	Nil	Gluten-free Contains lactose	Standard, p. 1017	Sachet: 7 × 62 g = £5.60 Chocolate, neutral, strawberry, vanilla

Powder 62 g reconstituted with 200 mL whole milk provides: protein 17.7 g, carbohydrate 48.5 g, fat 14.8 g, energy 1658 kJ (397 kcal)

Product	Form	Energy	Protein source	Carbohydrate	Fat	Fibre	Characteristics	Indications	Presentation / flavours
Nutilis® Complete Stage 1 (Nutricia Clinical)	Liquid (pre-thickened) **per 100 mL**	1010 kJ (240 kcal)	9.6 g cows' milk	29.1 g (sugars 5.4 g)	9.3 g	3.2 g	Gluten-free Residual lactose	Standard, p. 1017 Not suitable for child under 3 years	Bottle: 125 mL = £2.10 Strawberry, vanilla
Nutilis® Complete Stage 2 (Nutricia Clinical)	Semi-solid **per 100 g**	1030 kJ (245 kcal)²	9.6 g cows' milk	29.1 g (sugars 11.8 g)	9.4 g	3.2 g	Gluten-free Residual lactose	Standard, p. 1017 Not suitable for child under 3 years; use with caution in child 3–6 years	Pot: 4 × 125 g = £8.84 Strawberry, vanilla
Nutricrem® (Nualtra)	Semi-solid **per 100 g**	756 kJ (180 kcal)	10 g cows' milk soya protein	18.8 g (sugars 9.7 g)	7.2 g	Nil	Gluten-free Residual lactose	Standard, p. 1017 Not suitable for child under 3 years; use with caution in child 3–6 years	Pot: 4 × 125 g = £5.60 Strawberry, vanilla
Nutriplen® (Nualtra)	Liquid (sip feed) **per 100 mL**	1008 kJ (240 kcal)	9.6 g cows' milk soya protein	28.8 g (sugars 11.6 g)¹	9.6 g	Nil	Gluten-free Residual lactose	Standard, p. 1017 Not suitable for child under 3 years; use with caution in child 3–6 years	Bottle: 4 × 125 mL = £5.80 Strawberry, vanilla
Renilon® 7.5 (Nutricia Clinical)	Liquid (sip feed) **per 100 mL**	840 kJ (200 kcal)	7.5 g cows' milk	20 g (sugars 4.8 g)	10 g	Nil	Gluten-free Residual lactose	Standard, p. 1017 Not suitable for child under 3 years	Bottle: 4 × 125 mL = £8.24 Apricot, caramel
Resource® 2.0 Fibre (Nestlé)	Liquid (sip feed) **per 100 mL**	836 kJ (200 kcal)²	9 g cows' milk	21.4 g (sugars 5.5 g)	8.7 g	2.5 g	Gluten-free Residual lactose	Standard, p. 1017 Not suitable for child under 6 years; use with caution in child 6–10 years	Carton: 200 mL = £1.88 Apricot, coffee, neutral, strawberry, summer fruits, vanilla

1. Sugar content varies with flavour
2. Nutritional values vary with flavour—consult product literature

Appendix 2: Borderline substances

Appendix 2: Borderline substances

A2.2.2.3 Nutritional supplements: More than 1.5 kcal/mL and 5 g (or more) protein/100 mL (product list continued)

Not suitable for use in child under 1 year; use with caution in child 1–5 years unless otherwise stated

Product	Formulation	Energy	Protein	Carbohydrate	Fat	Fibre	Special Characteristics	ACBS Indications	Presentation & Flavour
Resource® Dessert Fruit (Nestlé)	Semi-solid per 100 g	678 kJ (160 kcal)[1]	5 g cows' milk	24 g (sugars 16.4 g)	5 g	1.4 g	Gluten-free Residual lactose	Standard, p. 1017; also CAPD, haemodialysis	Cup: 3 × 125 g = £4.77 Apple, apple-peach, apple-strawberry[2]
Vegenat®-med Balanced Protein (Vegenat)	Powder per 110 g serving	1924 kJ (458 kcal)[1]	18 g cows' milk	62 g	15.35 g	5.8 g	Gluten-free Residual lactose	Standard, p. 1017 except bowel fistula Not suitable for child under 14 years	Sachet: 12 × 110 g = £36.26 Apple, chocolate, honey, orange
Vegenat®-med High Protein (Vegenat)	Powder per 110 g serving	1940 kJ (463 kcal)[1]	23.3 g cows' milk	57.2 g	15.6 g	6 g	Gluten-free Residual lactose	Standard, p. 1017 except bowel fistula Not suitable for child under 14 years	Sachet: 12 × 110 g = £50.76 Chicken, chickpea, fish, fish-vegetable, ham, lentil, veal, vegetable, winter vegetable 12 × 110 g = £48.95 Curry chicken 12 × 110 g = £48.22 Lemon, rice with lemon 24 × 55 g = £46.50 Rice with apple

1. Nutritional values vary with flavour—consult product literature
2. Flavour not suitable for child under 3 years

A2.3 Specialised formulas

A2.3.1 Specialised formulas: Infant and child
see BNF for Children

A2.3.2 Specialised formulas for specific clinical conditions

Product	Formulation	Energy	Protein	Carbohydrate	Fat	Fibre	Special Characteristics	ACBS Indications	Presentation & Flavour
Alicalm® (SHS)	Standard dilution (30%) of powder per 100 mL	567 kJ (135 kcal)	4.5 g caseinate whey	17.4 g (sugars 3.2 g)	5.3 g	Nil	Residual lactose	Crohn's disease Not suitable for child under 1 year; use as nutritional supplement only in children 1–6 years.	Powder: 400 g = £20.48 Vanilla

Powder provides: protein 15 g, carbohydrate 58 g, fat 17.5 g, energy 1889 kJ (450 kcal)/100 g

Product	Formulation	Energy	Protein	Carbohydrate	Fat	Fibre	Special characteristics	Indications	Presentation & price
Forticare® (Nutricia Clinical)	Liquid (sip feed) **per 100 mL**	675 kJ (160 kcal)	9 g cows' milk	19.1 g (sugars 13.6 g)	5.3 g	2.1 g	Gluten-free, Residual lactose, Contains fish oil	Nutritional supplement in patients with lung cancer undergoing chemotherapy, or with pancreatic cancer. Not suitable in child under 3 years	Bottle: 4 × 125 mL = £8.84, Cappuccino, orange-lemon, peach-ginger
Generaid® (SHS)	Powder **per 100 g**	1586 kJ (374 kcal)	76 g protein equivalent (whey protein, plus branched chain amino acids)	5 g (sugars 5 g)	5.5 g	Nil	Electrolytes/100 g: Na$^+$ 6.1 mmol, K$^+$ 10.8 mmol, Ca^{2+} 6.5 mmol, P* 6.45 mmol	Nutritional supplement for use in chronic liver disease and/or porto-hepatic encephalopathy	Tub: 400 g = £58.32, Unflavoured[1]
Generaid® Plus (SHS)	Standard dilution (22%) of powder **per 100 mL**	428 kJ (102 kcal)	2.4 g protein equivalent (whey protein, branched chain amino acids)	13.6 g (sugars 1.4 g)	4.2 g (MCT 32%)	Nil	Electrolytes/100 mL: Na$^+$ 0.7 mmol, K$^+$ 2.7 mmol, Ca^{2+} 1.72 mmol, P* 1.67 mmol	Enteral feed or nutritional supplement in children over 1 year with hepatic disorders	Can: 400 g = £20.86, Unflavoured[1] (5-g measuring scoop provided)

Powder provides: protein equivalent 11 g, carbohydrate 62 g, fat 19 g, energy 1944 kJ (463 kcal)/100 g

Product	Formulation	Energy	Protein	Carbohydrate	Fat	Fibre	Special characteristics	Indications	Presentation & price
Heparon® Junior (SHS)	Standard dilution (18%) of powder **per 100 mL**	363 kJ (86 kcal)	2 g cows' milk	11.6 g (sugars 2.9 g)	3.6 g	Nil	Contains lactose, Electrolytes/100 mL: Na$^+$ 0.56 mmol, K$^+$ 1.9 mmol, Ca^{2+} 2.3 mmol, P* 1.6 mmol	Enteral feed or nutritional supplement for children with acute or chronic liver failure	Can: 400 g = £20.63 (4.5-g measuring scoop provided)

Powder provides: protein 11.1 g, carbohydrate 64.2 g, fat 19.9 g, energy 2016 kJ (480 kcal)/100 g

Product	Formulation	Energy	Protein	Carbohydrate	Fat	Fibre	Special characteristics	Indications	Presentation & price
KetoCal® (SHS)	Standard dilution (20%) of powder **per 100 mL**	602 kJ (146 kcal)	3.1 g cows' milk with additional amino acids	600 mg (sugars 120 mg)	14.6 g (LCT 100%)	Nil	Electrolytes/100 mL: Na$^+$ 4.3 mmol, K$^+$ 4.1 mmol, Ca^{2+} 2.15 mmol, P* 2.77 mmol	Enteral feed or nutritional supplement as part of ketogenic diet in management of epilepsy resistant to drug therapy, in children over 1 year, only on the advice of secondary care physician with experience of ketogenic diet	Can: 300 g = £29.04, Vanilla, Unflavoured

Powder provides: protein 15.25 g, carbohydrate 3 g, fat 73 g, energy 3011 kJ (730 kcal)/100 g

1. Flavouring: see *Modjul® Flavour System*, p. 1041

Appendix 2: Borderline substances

Appendix 2: Borderline substances

A2.3.2 Specialised formulas for specific clinical conditions (product list continued)

Product	Formulation	Energy	Protein	Carbohydrate	Fat	Fibre	Special Characteristics	ACBS Indications	Presentation & Flavour
KetoCal® 3:1 (SHS)	Standard dilution (9.5%) of powder **per 100 mL**	276 kJ (66 kcal)	1.5 g	680 mg (sugars 570 mg)	6.4 g	Nil	Electrolytes/100 mL: Na⁺ 1.3 mmol K⁺ 2.4 mmol Ca²⁺ 2 mmol P⁺ 1.7 mmol	Enteral feed or nutritional supplement as part of ketogenic diet in management of drug resistant epilepsy or other conditions for which a ketogenic diet is indicated in children from birth to 6 years; as a nutritional supplement in children over 6 years	Can: 300 g = £28.11 Unflavoured
Powder provides: protein 15.3 g, carbohydrate 7.2 g, fat 67.7 g, energy 2927 kJ (699 kcal)/100 g									
KetoCal® 4:1 LQ (SHS)	Liquid (sip or tube feed) **per 100 mL**	620 kJ (150 kcal)	3.09 g casein and whey with additional amino acids	610 mg (sugars 230 mg)	14.8 g (LCT 100%)	1.12 g	Residual lactose Electrolytes/100 mL: Na⁺ 4.7 mmol K⁺ 4.9 mmol Ca²⁺ 2.4 mmol P⁺ 3.1 mmol	Enteral feed or nutritional supplement as part of ketogenic diet in management of drug resistant epilepsy or other conditions for which a ketogenic diet is indicated in children 1–10 years; as a nutritional supplement in children over 10 years	Carton: 237 mL = £4.76 Vanilla
Kindergen® (SHS)	Standard dilution (20%) of powder **per 100 mL**	421 kJ (101 kcal)	1.5 g whey protein	11.8 mg (sugars 1.2 g)	5.3 g (LCT 93%)	Nil	Electrolytes/100 mL: Na⁺ 2 mmol K⁺ 0.6 mmol Ca²⁺ 2.8 mmol P 3 mmol Low Vitamin A	Enteral feed or nutritional supplement for children with chronic renal failure receiving peritoneal rapid overnight dialysis	Tub: 400 g = £27.69 (5-g measuring scoop provided)
Powder provides: protein 7.5 g, carbohydrate 59 g, fat 26.3 g, energy 2104 kJ (504 kcal)/100 g									
Modulen IBD® (Nestlé)	Standard dilution (20%) of powder (sip or tube feed) **per 100 mL**	420 kJ (100 kcal)	3.6 g casein	11 g (sugars 3.98 g)	4.7 g	Nil	Gluten-free Residual lactose	Crohn's disease active phase, and in remission if malnourished	Can: 400 g = £15.06 Unflavoured¹ (8.3-g measuring scoop provided)
Powder provides: protein 18 g, carbohydrate 54 g, fat 23 g, energy 2070 kJ (500 kcal)/100 g									

1. Flavouring: see *Flavour Mix*, p. 1041

Product	Formulation	Energy	Protein (source)	Carbohydrate	Fat		Special characteristics	Standard indication (ACBS)	Presentation
Nepro® (Abbott)	Liquid (sip or tube feed) **per 100 mL**	838 kJ (200 kcal)[1]	7 g cows' milk	20.6 g (sugars 3.26 g)	9.6 g	1.56 g	Gluten-free, Residual lactose, Electrolytes/100 mL: Na⁺ 3.67 mmol, K⁺ 2.72 mmol, Ca²⁺ 3.43 mmol, P* 2.23 mmol	Enteral feed or nutritional supplement in patients with chronic renal failure who are on haemodialysis or CAPD, or with cirrhosis, or other conditions requiring a high energy, low fluid, low electrolyte diet. Not suitable for child under 1 year; use with caution in child 1–5 years	Carton: 200 mL = £2.69 Strawberry, vanilla; Flexible pack: 500 mL = £5.84 Vanilla
ProSure® (Abbott)	Liquid (sip or tube feed) **per 100 mL**	536 kJ (127 kcal)[1]	6.65 g cows' milk	18.3 g (sugars 2.95 g)	2.56 g	2.07 g	Gluten-free, Residual lactose, Contains fish oil	Nutritional supplement for patients with pancreatic cancer. Not suitable for child under 1 year; use with caution in child 1–4 years	Carton: 240 mL = £3.29 Vanilla
Renamil® (KoRa)	Powder (sip or tube feed when reconstituted) **per 100 g**	2003 kJ (477 kcal)	4.6 g cows' milk	70.8 g	19.3 g	Nil	Contains lactose, Gluten-free, Electrolytes/100 g: Na⁺ 1.04 mmol, K⁺ 0.13 mmol, Ca²⁺ 10.22 mmol, P* 1.06 mmol, Contains no vitamin A or vitamin D	Enteral feed or nutritional supplement for adults and children over 1 year with chronic renal failure	Sachet: 10 × 100 g = £25.40
Renapro® (KoRa)	Powder **per 100 g**	1580 kJ (372 kcal)	90 g whey protein	800 mg	1 g	Nil	Gluten-free, Residual lactose, Electrolytes/100 g: Na⁺ 23 mmol, K⁺ 2 mmol, Ca²⁺ 4.99 mmol, P* 4.84 mmol	Nutritional supplement for biochemically proven hypoproteinaemia and patients undergoing dialysis. Not suitable for child under 1 year	Sachet: 30 × 20 g = £69.60

Powder provides: protein 18 g, energy 316 kJ (74 kcal)/20 g sachet

Product	Formulation	Energy	Protein (source)	Carbohydrate	Fat		Special characteristics	Standard indication (ACBS)	Presentation
Renastart® (Vitaflo)	Standard dilution (20%) of powder **per 100 mL**	414 kJ (99 kcal)	1.5 g cows' milk, soya	12.5 g (sugars 1.3 g)	4.8 g	Nil	Contains lactose, Electrolytes/100 mL: Na⁺ 2.1 mmol, K⁺ 0.6 mmol, Ca²⁺ 0.6 mmol, P* 0.6 mmol	Dietary management of renal failure in child from birth to 10 years	Can: 400 g = £25.42 Unflavoured (7-g measuring scoop provided)

Powder provides: protein 7.5 g, carbohydrate 62.5 g, fat 23.8 g, energy 2071 kJ (494 kcal)/100 g

1. Nutritional values vary with flavour—consult product literature

Appendix 2: Borderline substances

Appendix 2: Borderline substances

A2.3.2 Specialised formulas for specific clinical conditions (product list continued)

Product	Formulation	Energy	Protein	Carbohydrate	Fat	Fibre	Special Characteristics	ACBS Indications	Presentation & Flavour
Respifor® (Nutricia Clinical)	Liquid (sip feed) **per 100 mL**	633 kJ (150 kcal)	7.5 g cows' milk	22.5 g (sugars 6.4 g[1])	3.3 g	Nil[2]	Contains lactose	Nutritional supplement for dietary management of disease-related malnutrition in patients with chronic obstructive pulmonary disease and body-mass index less than 20.	Bottle: 125 mL = £1.85 Chocolate, strawberry, vanilla
Suplena® (Abbott)	Liquid (sip or tube feed) **per 100 mL**	840 kJ (200 kcal)	3 g caseinates	25.5 g (sugars 2.7 g)	9.6 g	Nil	Gluten-free Residual lactose Electrolytes/100 mL: Na⁺ 3.39 mmol K⁺ 2.87 mmol Ca²⁺ 3.48 mmol P⁻ 2.39 mmol	Enteral feed or nutritional supplement in patients with chronic or acute renal failure who are not undergoing dialysis, or with chronic or acute liver disease with fluid restriction; other conditions requiring high energy, low protein, low electrolyte, low volume enteral feed Not suitable for child under 1 year; use with caution in child 1–5 years	Can: 237 mL = £2.85 Vanilla
Supportan® (Fresenius Kabi)	Liquid (sip feed) **per 100 mL**	630 kJ (150 kcal)	10 g cows' milk	12.4 g (sugars 7.5 g)	6.7 g	1.5 g	Gluten-free Residual lactose Contains fish oil	Nutritional supplement in patients with pancreatic cancer or with lung cancer undergoing chemotherapy Not suitable for child under 1 year; use with caution in child 1–4 years	Bottle: 200 mL = £2.30 Cappuccino, tropical fruits

1. Sugar content varies with flavour
2. Fibre content varies with flavour

A2.4 Feed supplements

A2.4.1 High-energy supplements

A2.4.1.1 High-energy supplements: carbohydrate

Flavoured carbohydrate supplements are not suitable for use in child under 1 year; liquid supplements should be diluted before use in child under 5 years

ACBS Indications: disease-related malnutrition, malabsorption states, or other conditions requiring fortification with a high or readily available carbohydrate supplement

Product	Formulation	Energy	Protein	Carbohydrate	Fat	Fibre	Special Characteristics	ACBS Indications	Presentation & Flavour
Caloreen® (Nestlé)	Powder per 100 g	1640 kJ (390 kcal)	Nil	96 g Maltodextrin	Nil	Nil	Gluten-free Lactose-free	See above Not suitable for child under 3 years	Powder: 500 g = £3.69 Unflavoured (10-g measuring scoop provided)
Maxijul® Super Soluble (SHS)	Powder per 100 g	1615 kJ (380 kcal)	Nil	95 g Glucose polymer (sugars 8.6 g)	Nil	Nil	Gluten-free Lactose-free	See above	Sachets: 4 × 132 g = £6.16 Can: 200 g = £2.48 2.5 kg = £19.25 25 kg = £148.21 Unflavoured
Polycal® (Nutricia Clinical)	Powder per 100 g	1630 kJ (384 kcal)	Nil	96 g Maltodextrin (sugars 6 g)	Nil	Nil	Gluten-free Lactose-free	See above	Can: 400 g = £4.09 Neutral (5-g measuring scoop provided)
	Liquid per 100 mL	1050 kJ (247 kcal)	Nil	61.9 g Maltodextrin (sugars 12.2 g)	Nil	Nil	Gluten-free Lactose-free	See above; liquid not suitable for child under 3 years	Bottle: 200 mL = £1.64 Neutral, orange
S.O.S.® (Vitaflo)	Powder per 100 g	1590 kJ (380 kcal)	Nil	95 g (sugars 9 g)	Nil	Nil		For use as an emergency regimen in the dietary management of inborn errors of metabolism in adults and children from birth	Sachets[1] : 30 × 21 g (S.O.S. 10) = £7.05; 30 × 31 g (S.O.S. 15) = £10.40; 30 × 42 g (S.O.S. 20) = £14.09; 30 × 52 g (S.O.S. 25) = £17.44

Contents of each sachet should be reconstituted with water to a total volume of 200 mL

Vitajoule® (Vitaflo)	Powder per 100 g	1590 kJ (380 kcal)	Nil	95 g Dried glucose syrup (sugars 9 g)	Nil	Nil	Gluten-free Lactose-free	See above	Can: 500 g = £4.22 2.5 kg = £20.54 25 kg = £123.70 (10-g measuring scoop provided)

1. S.O.S. products are age-range specific—consult product literature

Appendix 2: Borderline substances

Appendix 2: Borderline substances

A2.4.1.2 High-energy supplements: fat

Liquid supplements should be diluted before use in child under 5 years

ACBS indications: disease-related malnutrition, malabsorption states, or other conditions requiring fortification with a high fat (or fat and carbohydrate) supplement

Product	Formulation	Energy	Protein	Carbohydrate	Fat	Fibre	Special Characteristics	ACBS Indications	Presentation & Flavour
Calogen® (Nutricia Clinical)	Liquid (emulsion) per 100 mL	1850 kJ (450 kcal)[1]	Nil	100 mg	50 g (LCT 100%)	Nil	Gluten-free Lactose-free	See above	Bottle: 200 mL = £4.36 500 mL = £10.72 Banana[2], neutral, strawberry[2]
Fresubin® 5 kcal Shot (Fresenius Kabi)	Liquid (emulsion) per 100 mL	2100 kJ (500 kcal)	Nil	4.0 g (sucrose)	53.8 g	400 mg	Gluten-free Lactose-free	See above Not suitable for child under 3 years	Bottle: 120 mL = £2.55 Lemon, neutral
Liquigen® (SHS)	Liquid (emulsion) per 100 mL	1850 kJ (450 kcal)	Nil	Nil	50 g (MCT 97%) Fractionated coconut oil	Nil	Gluten-free Lactose-free	Steatorrhoea associated with cystic fibrosis of the pancreas, intestinal lymphangiectasia, intestinal surgery, chronic liver disease, liver cirrhosis, other proven malabsorption syndromes, ketogenic diet in epilepsy, and in type 1 lipoproteinaemia Not suitable for child under 1 year	Bottle: 250 mL = £8.83
Medium-chain Triglyceride (MCT) Oil (Nutricia Clinical)	Liquid per 100 mL	3515 kJ (855 kcal)	Nil	Nil	MCT 100 %	Nil		Nutritional supplement for steatorrhoea associated with cystic fibrosis of the pancreas, intestinal lymphangiectasia, intestinal surgery, chronic liver disease and liver cirrhosis, other proven malabsorption syndromes, ketogenic diet in management of epilepsy, type 1 hyperlipoproteinaemia	Bottle: 500 mL = £13.99
Fat and Carbohydrate									
Duocal® Super Soluble (SHS)	Powder per 100 g	2061 kJ (492 kcal)	Nil	72.7 g (sugars 6.5 g)	22.3 g (MCT 35%)	Nil	Gluten-free Lactose-free	See above	Can: 400 g = £17.23 (5-g measuring scoop provided)

1. Nutritional values vary with flavour—consult product literature
2. Flavour not suitable for child under 3 years

Product	Formulation	Energy	Protein	Carbohydrate	Fat	Fibre	Special Characteristics	ACBS Indications	Presentation & Flavour
Energivit® (SHS)	Standard dilution (15%) of powder **per 100 mL**	309 kJ (74 kcal)	Nil	10 g (sugars 900 mg)	3.75 g	Nil	Lactose-free With vitamins, minerals, and trace elements	For children requiring additional energy, vitamins, minerals, and trace elements following a protein-restricted diet	Can: 400 g = £20.95 (5-g measuring scoop provided)
MCT Duocal® (SHS)	Powder **per 100 g**	2082 kJ (497 kcal)	Nil	72 g (sugars 10.1 g)	23.2 g (MCT 83%)	Nil		See above	Can: 400 g = £20.47

Powder provides: carbohydrate 66.7 g, fat 25 g, energy 2059 kJ (492 kcal)/100 g

A2.4.1.3 High-energy supplements: protein

ACBS indications: disease-related malnutrition, malabsorption states, or other conditions requiring fortification with a high fat or carbohydrate (with protein) supplement

Product	Formulation	Energy	Protein	Carbohydrate	Fat	Fibre	Special Characteristics	ACBS Indications	Presentation & Flavour
ProSource® Jelly (Nutrinovo)	Semi-solid **per 100 mL**	315 kJ (75 kcal)	16.9 g collagen protein hydrolysate whey protein isolate	Less than 1 g	Nil	less than 1 g	Gluten-free Lactose-free Contains porcine derivatives	Hypoproteinaemia Not recommended for child under 3 years	Cup: 118 mL = £1.78 Fruit punch, orange
Protifar® (Nutricia Clinical)	Powder **per 100 g**	1580 kJ (373 kcal)	88.5 g cows' milk	less than 1.5 g	1.6 g	Nil	Gluten-free Residual lactose Electrolytes/100 mL: Na⁺ 1.3 mmol K⁺ 1.28 mmol Ca²⁺ 33.75 mmol P⁺ 22.58 mmol	Nutritional supplement for use in biochemically proven hypoproteinaemia	Can: 225 g = £8.31 Unflavoured (2.5-g measuring scoop provided)

Powder provides: protein 2.2 g per 2.5-g scoopful

Vitapro® (Vitaflo)	Powder **per 100 g**	1632 kJ (390 kcal)	75 g whey protein isolate	9 g (sugars 9 g)	6 g	Nil	Contains lactose	Biochemically proven hypoproteinaemia	Tub: 250 g = £8.60 2 kg = £67.60 (5-g measuring scoop provided)

Appendix 2: Borderline substances

A2.4.1.3 High-energy supplements: protein (product list continued)

ACBS indications: disease-related malnutrition, malabsorption states, or other conditions requiring fortification with a high fat or carbohydrate (with protein) supplement

Product	Formulation	Energy	Protein	Carbohydrate	Fat	Fibre	Special Characteristics	ACBS Indications	Presentation & Flavour
Protein and carbohydrate									
Dialamine® (SHS)	Standard dilution (20%) of powder per 100 mL	264 kJ (62 kcal)	4.3 g protein equivalent (essential and non-essential amino acids)	11.2 g (sugars 10.2 g)	Nil	Nil	Contains vitamin C	Hypoproteinaemia, chronic renal failure, wound fistula leakage with excessive protein loss, conditions requiring a controlled nitrogen intake, and haemodialysis Not suitable for child under 6 months	Can: 400 g = £69.99 Orange
Powder provides: protein equivalent 25 g, carbohydrate 65 g, vitamin C 125 mg, energy 1530 kJ (360 kcal)/100 g									
ProSource® Liquid (Nutrinovo)	Liquid per 30 mL	420 kJ (100 kcal)	10 g collagen protein whey protein isolate	15 g (sugars 8 g)	Nil	Nil	Gluten-free Lactose-free May contain porcine derivatives	Biochemically proven hypoproteinaemia Not recommended for child under 3 years	Sachet: 100 × 30 mL = £96.17 Citrus-berry, lemon, neutral, orange creme
ProSource® Plus (Nutrinovo)	Liquid per 30 mL	420 kJ (100 kcal)	15 g collagen protein whey protein isolate	11 g (sugars 10 g)	Nil	Nil	Gluten-free Lactose-free May contain porcine derivatives	Hypoproteinaemia Not recommended for child under 3 years	Sachet: 100 × 30 mL = £139.00 Unflavoured
Protein, fat, and carbohydrate									
Calogen® Extra (Nutricia Clinical)	Liquid per 100 mL	1650 kJ (400 kcal)[1]	5 g cows' milk	4.5 g (sugars 3.5 g)	40.3 g	Nil	Gluten-free Residual lactose With vitamins and minerals	See above Not suitable for child under 3 years; use with caution in child 3–6 years May require dilution for child 3–5 years	Bottle: 200 mL = £4.98 Neutral, strawberry
Calogen® Extra Shots (Nutricia Clinical)	Liquid per 100 mL	1650 kJ (400 kcal)[1]	5 g cows' milk	4.5 g (sugars 3.5 g)	40.3 g	Nil	Gluten-free Residual lactose With vitamins and minerals	See above Not suitable for child under 3 years; use with caution in child 3–6 years May require dilution for child 3–5 years	Pot: 6 × 40 mL = £5.75 Neutral, strawberry
Calshake® (Fresenius Kabi)	Powder per 87 g	1841 kJ (439 kcal)[1]	4.1 g cows' milk	56.4 g (sugars 20 g)	22 g	Nil	Contains lactose Gluten-free	See above Not suitable for child under 1 year	Sachet: 87 g = £2.10 Banana, neutral, strawberry, vanilla 90 g = £2.10 Chocolate

Powder: one sachet reconstituted with 240 mL whole milk provides approx. 2 kcal/mL and protein 12 g

Product	Form	Energy	Protein (source)	Carbohydrate	Fat	Fibre	Residual lactose / With vitamins and minerals	Suitability	Presentation and flavour
Enshake® (Abbott)	Powder **per 100 g**	1893 kJ (450 kcal)[1]	8.4 g cows' milk, soy protein isolate	69 g (sugars 14.5 g)	15.6 g	Nil	With vitamins and minerals	See above; Not suitable for child under 1 year; use with caution in child 1–6 years	Sachet: 96.5 g = £2.02 Banana, chocolate, strawberry, vanilla
		Powder: one sachet reconstituted with 240 mL whole milk provides approx. 2 kcal/mL and protein 16 g							
MCT Procal® (Vitaflo)	Powder **per 100 g**	2742 kJ (657 kcal)	12.5 g cows' milk	20.6 g (sugars 3.1 g)	63.1 g (MCT 99%)	Nil	Contains lactose	Dietary management of disorders of long-chain fatty acid oxidation, fat malabsorption, and other disorders requiring a low LCT, high MCT supplement. Not suitable for child under 1 year	Sachet: 30 × 16 g = £22.91
		Powder 16 g provides: protein 2 g, carbohydrate 3.3 g, fat 10.1 g, energy 439 kJ (105 kcal)							
Pro-Cal® (Vitaflo)	Powder **per 100 g**	2787 kJ (667 kcal)	13.6 g cows' milk	28.2 g (sugars 16 g)	55.5 g	Nil	Contains lactose Gluten-free	See above; Not suitable for child under 1 year; use with caution in child 1–5 years	Sachets: 25 × 15 g = £15.26 Tub: 510 g = £14.14 1.5 kg = £28.81 12.5 kg = £204.74 25 kg = £315.52 (15-g measuring scoop provided)
		Powder 15 g provides: protein 2 g, carbohydrate 4.2 g, fat 8.3 g, energy 418 kJ (100 kcal)							
Pro-Cal® Shot (Vitaflo)	Liquid **per 100 mL**	1385 kJ (334 kcal)	6.7 g cows' milk	13.4 g (sugars 13.3 g)	28.2 g	Nil	Gluten-free Contains lactose Contains soya	See above; Not suitable for child under 3 years	Bottle: 6 × 250 mL = £27.06 Banana, neutral, strawberry Starter pack (mixed) 3 × 250 mL = £14.67
Pro-Cal® Singles (Vitaflo)	Liquid **per 100 mL**	1385 kJ (334 kcal)[1]	6.7 g cows' milk soya	13.4 g (sugars 13.3 g)	28.2 g	Nil	Contains lactose Gluten-free	See above; Not suitable for child under 3 years	Pot: 60 × 30 mL = £39.22 Neutral, strawberry Starter pack (mixed): 16 × 30 mL = £10.25
Scandishake® Mix (Nutricia Clinical)	Powder **per 100 g**	2099 kJ (500 kcal)[1]	4.7 g cows' milk	65 g (sugars 14.3 g)	24.7 g	Nil	Gluten-free Contains lactose	See above; Not suitable for child under 3 years	Sachet: 85 g = £2.08 Banana, caramel, chocolate, strawberry, vanilla, unflavoured
		Powder: 85 g reconstituted with 240 mL whole milk provides: protein 11.7 g, carbohydrate 66.8 g, fat 30.4 g, energy 2457 kJ (588 kcal)							
Vitasavoury® (Vitaflo)	Powder **per 100 g**	2562 kJ (619 kcal)[1]	12 g cows' milk	52 g (sugars 1.4 g)	22.5 g	6.4 g	Contains lactose Contains soya (chicken flavour)	See above; Not suitable for child under 3 years	Cup (200 kcal): 24 × 33 g = £29.97 Sachet (300 kcal) 10 × 50 g = £18.29 Chicken, leek and potato, mushroom, vegetable Starter pack (mixed): 4 × 33-g cups and 4 × 50-g sachets = £11.93

1. Nutritional values vary with flavour—consult product literature

Appendix 2: Borderline substances

Appendix 2: Borderline substances

A2.4.2 Fibre, vitamin, and mineral supplements

Product	Formulation	Energy	Protein	Carbohydrate	Fat	Fibre	Special Characteristics	ACBS Indications	Presentation & Flavour
High-fibre supplements									
Resource® Optifibre® (Nestlé)	Powder per 100 g	323 kJ (76 kcal)	Nil	19 g guar gum, partially hydrolysed	Nil	78 g	Gluten-free Lactose-free	Standard, p. 1017 except dysphagia Not suitable for child under 5 years	Sachets 16 x 10 g = £8.35 Can: 250 g = £10.28 (5-g measuring scoop provided)
Vitamin and Mineral supplements									
FruitiVits® (Vitaflo)	Powder per 100 g	133 kJ (33 kcal)	Nil	8.3 g (sugars 400 mg)	less than 100 mg	3.3 g		Vitamin, mineral, and trace element supplement in children 3–10 years with restrictive therapeutic diets	Sachets: 30 × 6 g = £61.92 Orange
Paediatric Seravit® (SHS)	Powder per 100 g	1275 kJ (300 kcal)	Nil	75 g (sugars 6.75 g[1])	Nil	Nil		Vitamin, mineral, and trace element supplement in infants and children with restrictive therapeutic diets	Tub: 200 g = £17.07 Unflavoured[2] 200 g = £18.17 Pineapple[3] (5-g measuring scoop provided)
Renavit® (Stanningley)	Tablet per 450 mg	3.15 kJ (0.75 kcal)	Nil	170 mg	Nil	Nil		Dietary management of water-soluble vitamin deficiency in adults with renal failure on dialysis	100 × 450-mg tablets = £12.50

1. Sugar content varies with flavour
2. Flavouring: see *Modjul® Flavour System*, p. 1041
3. Flavour not suitable for child under 6 months

Appendix 2: Borderline substances

A2.5 Feed additives

A2.5.1 Special additives for conditions of intolerance

Colief® (Forum)

Liquid, lactase 50 000 units/g, Net price 7-mL dropper bottle = £8.40

For the relief of symptoms associated with lactose intolerance in infants, provided that lactose intolerance is confirmed by the presence of reducing substances and/or excessive acid in stools, a low concentration of the corresponding disaccharide enzyme on intestinal biopsy or by breath hydrogen test or lactose intolerance test. For dosage and administration details, consult product literature

Fructose

(Laevulose)

For proven glucose/galactose intolerance

Glucose

(Dextrose monohydrate)

Net price 500 g = £1.53

For use as an energy supplement in sucrase-isomaltase deficiency

VSL#3® (Ferring)

Powder, containing 8 strains of live, freeze-dried, lactic acid bacteria. Contains traces of soya, gluten, and lactose. Net price 30 × 4.4-g sachets = £41.66

Nutritional supplement for use under the supervision of a physician, for the maintenance of remission of ileoanal pouchitis induced by antibacterials in adults. For dosage and administration details, consult product literature

A2.5.2 Feed thickeners and pre-thickened drinks

For pre-thickened infant feeds see *BNF for Children*.

Carobel, Instant® (Cow & Gate)

Powder, carob seed flour. Net price 135 g = £2.80

For thickening feeds in the treatment of vomiting

Multi-thick® (Abbott)

Powder, modified maize starch, gluten- and lactose-free, net price 250 g = £4.83

For thickening of liquids and foods in dysphagia. Not suitable for children under 1 year except in cases of failure to thrive

Nutilis® Clear (Nutricia Clinical)

Powder, maltodextrin, xanthan gum, guar gum, gluten- and lactose-free, net price 175 g = £8.46

For thickening of liquids or foods in dysphagia. Not suitable for children under 3 years

Nutilis® Powder (Nutricia Clinical)

Powder, modified maize starch, gluten- and lactose-free, net price 20 × 12-g sachets = £6.40; 300 g = £4.92.

For thickening of foods in dysphagia. Not suitable for children under 3 years

Resource® Thickened Drink (Nestlé)

Liquid, carbohydrate 22 g, energy: orange 382 kJ (90 kcal); apple 375 kJ (89 kcal)/100 mL. Syrup and custard consistencies. Gluten- and lactose-free, net price 12 × 114-mL cups = £7.80

For dysphagia. Not suitable for children under 1 year

Resource® ThickenUp® (Nestlé)

Powder, modified maize starch. Gluten- and lactose-free, net price 227 g = £4.55; 75 × 4.5-g sachet = £17.44

For thickening of foods in dysphagia. Not suitable for children under 1 year

Resource® ThickenUp Clear (Nestlé)

Powder, maltodextrin, xanthan gum, gluten- and lactose-free, net price 125 g = £8.46; 24 x 1.2-g sachets = £5.28

For thickening of liquids or foods in dysphagia. Not suitable for children under 3 years

SLO Drinks® (SLO Drinks)

Powder, carbohydrate content varies with flavour and chosen consistency (3 consistencies available), see product literature. Flavours: black currant, lemon, orange; (hot drinks) chocolate, white coffee, white tea, net price 25 × 115 mL = £7.50.

Nutritional supplement for patient hydration in the dietary management of dysphagia. Not suitable for children under 3 years

Thick and Easy® (Fresenius Kabi)

Powder, modified maize starch, net price 225-g can = £4.93; 100 × 9-g sachets = £30.00; 4.54 kg = £82.56.

For thickening of foods in dysphagia. Not suitable for children under 1 year except in cases of failure to thrive

Thicken Aid® (M & A Pharmachem)

Powder, modified maize starch, maltodextrin, gluten- and lactose-free, net price 225 g = £3.71; 100 × 9-g sachets = £22.40

For thickening of foods in dysphagia. Not suitable for children under 1 year

Thixo-D® (Sutherland)

Powder, modified maize starch, gluten-free. Net price 375-g tub = £7.15.

For thickening of foods in dysphagia. Not suitable for children under 1 year except in cases of failure to thrive

Vitaquick® (Vitaflo)

Powder. Modified maize starch. Net price 300 g = £6.87; 2 kg = £37.93; 6 kg = £98.22.

For thickening of foods in dysphagia. Not suitable for children under 1 year except in cases of failure to thrive

A2.5.3 Flavouring preparations

Flavour Mix® (Nestlé)

Powder, flavours: banana, chocolate, coffee, lemon-lime, strawberry. Net price 60 g = £7.17

FlavourPac® (Vitaflo)

Powder, flavours: black currant, lemon, orange, tropical or raspberry, net price 30 × 4-g sachets = £13.29

For use with Vitaflo's range of unflavoured protein substitutes for metabolic diseases; not suitable for child under 1 year

Modjul® Flavour System (SHS)

Powder, flavours: black currant, orange, pineapple, 100 g = £11.60; cherry-vanilla, grapefruit, lemon-lime, 20 × 5-g sachets = £11.60

For use with unflavoured SHS products based on peptides or amino acids; not suitable for child under 6 months

A2.6 Foods for special diets

A2.6.1 Gluten-free foods

> **ACBS indications:** established gluten-sensitive enteropathies including steatorrhoea due to gluten sensitivity, coeliac disease, and dermatitis herpetiformis.

Bread

◢Loaves

Barkat® (Gluten Free Foods Ltd)
Gluten-free. Loaf, multigrain 500 g = £5.73. Loaf, sliced, wholemeal 500 g = £3.98. Loaf, sliced, part-baked, country-style 250 g = £4.35. Loaf, sliced, part-baked, white 300 g = £4.13, 550 g = £5.78. Rice bread, brown 500 g = £5.73; white 500 g = £5.73

Dietary Specials® (Nutrition Point)
Gluten-free. Loaf, sliced, multigrain, brown 400 g = £3.10; white 400 g = £3.10.

Ener-G® (General Dietary)
Gluten-free. Loaf, sliced Seattle brown 600 g = £6.04. Rice bread, sliced, brown 474 g = £5.41; white 456 g = £5.41. Rice loaf, sliced 612 g = £5.41. Tapioca bread, sliced 480 g = £5.41

Genius Gluten Free® (Genius Foods)
Gluten-free. Loaf, unsliced, brown 400 g = £2.67; white 400 g = £2.67. Loaf, sliced, brown 400 g = £2.77; white 400 g = £2.77. Sandwich bread, sliced, brown 535 g = £3.59; white 535 g = £3.59

Glutafin® (Nutrition Point)
Gluten-free. Loaf, sliced, fibre 400 g = £3.85; white 400 g = £3.85

Glutafin® Select (Nutrition Point)
Gluten-free. Loaf, sliced, fresh, brown 400 g = £3.43; white 400 g = £3.43. Loaf, sliced, fibre 400 g = £3.43; white 400 g = £3.43. Loaf, seeded 400 g = £3.72.

Juvela® (Juvela)
Gluten-free. Loaf, sliced, fresh, fibre 400 g = £3.39; white 400 g = £3.69. Loaf, sliced, white 400 g = £3.59; fibre 400 g = £3.54. Loaf, white 400 g = £3.54; fibre 400 g = £3.54. Loaf, part-baked, fibre 400 g = £3.80; white 400 g = £3.95

Lifestyle® (Ultrapharm)
Gluten-free. Loaf, sliced, brown 400 g = £2.82; high fibre 400 g = £2.82; white 400 g = £2.82. Loaf, brown 400 g = £2.82; high fibre 400 g = £2.82; white 400 g = £2.82

Livwell® (Livwell)
Gluten-free. Loaf, sliced, brown (seeded) 200 g = £2.25; white 200 g = £2.25

Proceli® (Proceli)
Gluten-free. Loaf, sliced, white 165 g = £2.30; sandwich 155 g = £2.32. Rice bread, brown 220 g = £2.30; sandwich 220 g = £2.30.

Ultra® (Ultrapharm)
Gluten-free. Loaf, white 400 g = £2.46; high fibre 500 g = £3.35

Warburtons® (Warburtons)
Gluten free. Loaf, sliced, brown 400 g = £2.99; white 400 g = £2.99

Wellfoods® (Wellfoods)
Gluten-free. Loaf, sliced 600 g = £4.95; unsliced 600 g = £4.85

◢Baguettes, buns and rolls

Barkat® (Gluten Free Foods Ltd)
Gluten-free. Baguette, part-baked 200 g = £4.35. Rolls, part-baked 2 x 100 g = £3.98; 6 x 50 g = £4.35

Ener-G® (General Dietary)
Gluten-free. Rolls, dinner × 6 = £3.67; white, long 4 × 55 g = £2.95; round 4 × 55 g = £2.95

Glutafin® (Nutrition Point)
Gluten-free. Baguette 2 × 175 g = £3.51. Rolls, fibre 4 × 50 g = £3.68; white 4 × 50 g = £3.68

Glutafin® Select (Nutrition Point)
Gluten-free. Rolls, part-baked, white 4 × 50 g = £3.68; long 2 × 75 g = £2.81

Juvela® (Juvela)
Gluten-free. Rolls, fresh, fibre 5 × 85 g = £4.42; white 5 × 85 g = £4.42. Rolls, fibre 5 × 85 g = £4.77; white 5 × 85 g = £4.77. Rolls, part-baked, fibre 5 × 75 g = £4.94; white 5 × 75 g = £4.94

Lifestyle® (Ultrapharm)
Gluten-free. Rolls, brown 5 × 80 g = £2.82; high fibre 5 × 80 g = £2.82; white 5 × 80 g = £2.82

Livwell® (Livwell)
Gluten-free. Baguette, white 140 g = £2.15. Buns, toasting 4 × 45 g = £2.40. Rolls, white 4 = £2.25. Rolls, part-baked, circle (bagel) 2 × 70 g = £2.30; dinner (square) 2 × 80 g = £2.09

Proceli® (Proceli)
Gluten-free. Baguette, part-baked 2 × 125 g = £3.24. Buns 4 × 50 g = £3.41. Lunch rolls, white 8 × 34 g = £3.26. Rolls, hotdog 3 × 35 g = £2.24

Warburtons® (Warburtons)
Gluten-free. Baguette, 2 × 75 g = £2.79. Rolls, brown 3 × 100 g = £2.49; white 3 × 100 g = £2.49

Wellfoods® (Wellfoods)
Gluten-free. Burger buns 4 × 75 g = £3.95. Rolls 4 × 70 g = £3.65

◢Speciality breads

Livwell® (Livwell)
Gluten-free. Flat bread (pitta) 4 = £3.00. Tear-drop shape (naan) 2 × 90 g = £3.00

Cereals

Juvela® (Juvela)
Gluten-free. Fibre flakes 300 g = £2.78; flakes 300 g = £2.78; pure oats 500 g = £2.78

Nairns® (Nairns)
Gluten-free. Oat porridge 500 g = £3.05

Cookies and biscuits

Barkat® (Gluten Free Foods Ltd)
Gluten-free. Biscuits, coffee-style 200 g = £3.38;
digestive 175 g = £2.61

Ener-G® (General Dietary)
Gluten-free. Cookies, vanilla 435 g = £6.16

Glutafin® (Nutrition Point)
Gluten-free. Biscuits, plain 200 g = £4.14; digestive
150 g = £2.13; savoury shorts 130 g = £2.80;
shortbread 100 g = £1.73; sweet (without chocolate
or sultanas) 150 g = £2.13; tea 150 g = £2.09

Juvela® (Juvela)
Gluten-free. Biscuits, digestive 150 g = £3.05;
savoury 150 g = £3.82; sweet 150 g = £2.88, tea
150 g = £3.05

Crackers, crispbreads, and breadsticks

Barkat® (Gluten Free Foods Ltd)
Gluten-free. Crackers, round (matzo) 200 g = £3.52

Dietary Specials® (Nutrition Point)
Gluten-free. Cracker bread 150 g = £2.09

Glutafin® (Nutrition Point)
Gluten-free. Crackers, high fibre 200 g = £2.90; plain
200 g = £3.46; mini 175 g = £2.96.

Juvela® (Juvela)
Gluten-free. Crispbread, plain 200 g = £4.64

Ultra® (Ultrapharm)
Gluten-free. Crackerbread 200 g = £1.77

Warburtons® (Warburtons)
Gluten-free. Crackers, bran 150 g = £2.29

Flour mixes and xanthan gum

◢Flour mixes

Barkat® (Gluten Free Foods Ltd)
Gluten-free. Flour mix, bread 500 g = £6.81. Plain
750 g = £6.98

Finax® (Drossa)
Gluten-free. Flour mix, bread, fibre 1 kg = £9.92.
Flour mix 900 g = £8.66; coarse 900 g = £8.66

Glutafin® (Nutrition Point)
Gluten-free. Flour mix, fibre 500 g = £6.66; white
500 g = £6.66

Glutafin Select® (Nutrition Point)
Gluten-free. Flour mix, bread, fibre 500 g = £6.66;
white 500 g = £6.66. Fibre 500 g = £6.66; white
500 g = £6.66

Heron Foods® (Gluten Free Foods Ltd)
Gluten-free. Flour mix, organic, bread, standard
500 g = £8.96; high fibre 500 g = £8.96

Juvela® (Juvela)
Gluten-free. Flour mix, fibre 500 g = £7.35; plain
500 g = £7.35; harvest 500 g = £7.35

Mrs Crimbles® (Stiletto Foods)
Gluten-free. Bread mix, net price 275 g = £1.04.
Pastry mix, net price 200 g = £1.04

Orgran® (Community)
Gluten-free. Flour mix, bread 450 g = £3.10. Self-
raising 500 g = £3.10. Pastry and pizza 375 g =
£3.80

Proceli® (Proceli)
Gluten-free. Flour mix, white 1 kg = £9.95

Pure® (Innovative)
Gluten-free. Flour mix, blended 1 kg = £4.35. Potato
starch 500 g = £1.73. Rice, brown 500 g = £1.63;
white 500 g = £1.73. Tapioca starch 500 g = £2.33.
Teff, brown 1 kg = £4.91; white 1 kg = £4.91

Tobia® (Tobia Teff)
Gluten-free. Flour mix, teff, brown 1 kg = £3.30;
white 1 kg = £3.30

Tritamyl® (Gluten Free Foods Ltd)
Gluten-free. Flour mix, bread, brown 1 kg = £7.10;
white 2 kg = £14.26. Plain 2 kg = £14.26

Wellfoods® (Wellfoods)
Gluten-free. Flour mix, plain 1 kg = £7.65

◢Xanthan gum

Ener-G® (General Dietary)
Gluten-free. Xanthan gum 170 g = £8.53

Pure® (Innovative)
Gluten-free. Xanthan gum 100 g = £6.85

Pasta

Barkat® (Gluten Free Foods Ltd)
Gluten-free. Pasta, animal shapes 500 g = £5.88;
macaroni 500 g = £5.88; spaghetti 500 g = £5.88;
spirals 500 g = £5.88; tagliatelle 500 g = £5.88.
Buckwheat, penne 250 g = £2.93; spirals 250 g =
£2.93

BiAlimenta® (Drossa)
Gluten-free. Pasta, acini di pepe 500 g = £5.97;
formati misti 500 g = £5.97; penne 500 g = £5.97;
sagnette 500 g = £5.97; spirali 500 g = £5.97; tubetti
500 g = £5.90; potato-based, gnocchi 500 g = £5.59;
perle di gnocchi 500 g = £5.60.

Dietary Specials® (Nutrition Point)
Gluten-free. Pasta, fusilli 500 g = £3.54; penne 500 g
= £3.54; spaghetti 500 g = £3.54

Ener-G® (General Dietary)
Gluten-free. Pasta, rice-based, lasagne 454 g =
£5.03; macaroni 454 g = £5.03; shells, small 454 g =
£5.03; spaghetti 454 g = £5.03; vermicelli 300 g =
£5.03

Glutafin® (Nutrition Point)
Gluten-free. Pasta, lasagne 250 g = £3.53; macaroni
penne 500 g = £6.73; shells 500 g = £6.73; spirals
500 g = £6.73; spaghetti, long 500 g = £6.73;
tagliatelle 250 g = £3.53

Juvela® (Juvela)
Gluten-free. Pasta, fusilli 500 g = £7.21; lasagne
250 g = £3.68; macaroni 500 g = £7.21; spaghetti
500 g = £7.21; tagliatelle 250 g = £3.47. Fibre, penne
500 g = £6.61

Orgran® (Community)
Gluten-free. Pasta, rice and corn, lasagne 200 g = £3.13; macaroni 250 g = £2.42. Spirals, buckwheat 250 g = £2.42; corn 250 g = £2.42; brown rice 250 g = £2.42; rice and corn 250 g = £2.42; rice and millet 250 g = £2.42

Proceli® (Proceli)
Gluten-free. Pasta, macaroni penne 250 g = £2.95; spirals 250 g = £2.59

Rizopia® (PGR Health Foods)
Gluten-free. Pasta, brown rice, fusilli 500 g = £2.72; lasagne 375 g = £2.72; penne 500 g = £2.72; spaghetti 500 g = £2.72

Ultra® (Ultrapharm)
Gluten-free. Pasta, fusilli 250 g = £2.95; penne 250 g = £2.95; spaghetti 250 g = £2.95

Pizza bases

Barkat® (Gluten Free Foods Ltd)
Gluten-free. Pizza crust, rice, brown 150 g = £5.00; white 150 g = £5.00

Dietary Specials® (Nutrition Point)
Gluten-free. Pizza base 2 × 150 g = £5.68

Glutafin® (Nutrition Point)
Gluten-free. Pizza base 2 × 150 g = £6.56

Juvela® (Juvela)
Gluten-free. Pizza base 2 × 180 g = £8.78

Proceli® (Proceli)
Gluten-free. Pizza base 2 × 250 g = £3.90

Ultra® (Ultrapharm)
Gluten-free. Pizza base 2 × 200 g = £2.65

Wellfoods® (Wellfoods)
Gluten-free. Pizza base 2 × 300 g = £8.95

A2.6.1.1 Gluten- and wheat-free foods

ACBS indications: established gluten-sensitive enteropathies with coexisting established wheat sensitivity only.

Ener-G® (General Dietary)
Gluten-free, wheat-free. Bread loaf, six flour 576 g = £4.54. Rolls, Seattle brown, round (hamburger) 4 × 119 g = £3.96; long (hot dog) 4 × 119 g = £3.96. Pizza base, 3 × 124 g = £4.74

Glutafin® (Nutrition Point)
Gluten-free, wheat-free. Flour mix, bread 500 g = £6.66; fibre 500 g = £6.66. Crispbread 150 g = £3.25

Heron Foods® (Gluten Free Foods Ltd)
Gluten-free, wheat-free. Flour mix, organic, bread, fibre 500 g = £8.96. Bread and cake mix 500 g = £8.96

A2.6.2 Low-protein foods

ACBS indications: inherited metabolic disorders, renal or liver failure, requiring a low-protein diet

Bread

Ener-G® (General Dietary)
Low protein, Rice bread, 600 g = £5.54

Juvela® (Juvela)
Low protein. Loaf, sliced 400 g = £3.64. Rolls 5 × 70 g = £4.52

Loprofin® (SHS)
Low protein. Loaf, part-baked, sliced 400 g = £3.80. Rolls, part-baked 4 × 65 g = £4.00

PK Foods® (Gluten Free Foods Ltd)
Low protein. Loaf, white, sliced 550 g = £4.75

Cake, biscuits, and snacks

Harifen® (Ultrapharm)
Low protein. Cracker toast, 200 g = £2.75

Juvela® (Juvela)
Low-protein. Cookies, cinnamon 125 g = £7.62; chocolate chip 110 g = £7.62; orange 125 g = £7.62

Loprofin® (SHS)
Low-protein. Wafers, chocolate 100 g = £2.46; vanilla 100 g = £2.46. Crackers 150 g = £3.45, herb 150 g = £3.45

PK Foods® (Gluten Free Foods Ltd)
Low-protein. *Aminex®* biscuits 200 g = £5.04; cookies 150 g = £5.04. Cookies, chocolate chip 150 g = £5.04; cinnamon 150 g = £5.04; orange 150 g = £5.04. Rusks 200 g = £5.04. Cripsbread 75 g = £2.42

Promin® (Firstplay Dietary)
Low-protein. Fried maize and potato starch 'Snax', cheese and onion 12 x 25 g = £9.84; jalapeno 12 x 25 g = £9.84; ready-salted 12 x 25 g = £9.84; salt and vinegar 12 x 25 g = £9.84

Taranis® (Firstplay Dietary)
Low-protein. Cake bars, apricot 6 × 40 g = £5.91, lemon 6 × 40 g = £5.91, pear 6 × 40 g = £5.91

Vita Bite® (Vitaflo)
Low protein. Bar, protein 30 mg (less than 2.5 mg phenylalanine), carbohydrate 15.35 g, fat 8.4 g, energy 572 kJ (137 kcal)/25 g. Chocolate flavoured, 25 g = £1.06.
Not recommended for any child under 1 year

Vitaflo Choices® (Vitaflo)
Low-protein. Mini crackers, 40 g = £0.82
Not suitable for child under 3 years

Cereals

Loprofin® (SHS)
Low-protein. Breakfast cereal flakes, apple 375 g = £7.60; chocolate 375 g = £7.60; strawberry 375 g = £7.60. Cereal loops 375 g = £7.88

Promin® (Firstplay Dietary)
Low-protein. Hot breakfast (powder sachets), apple and cinnamon 6 × 57 g = £7.87, banana 6 × 57 g = £7.87, chocolate 6 × 57 g = £7.87; original 6 × 56 g = £7.87

Desserts

Loprofin® (SHS)
Low-protein. Powder, chocolate 150 g = £4.65; strawberry 150 g = £4.65; vanilla 150 g = £4.65

PK Foods® (Gluten Free Foods Ltd)
Low-protein. Jelly, orange 4 × 80 g = £8.03, cherry 4 × 80 g = £8.03

Promin® (Firstplay Dietary)
Low-protein. Dessert mix, caramel 6 × 36.5 g = £6.18; custard 6 × 36.5 g = £6.18; chocolate and banana 6 × 36.5 g = £6.18; strawberry and vanilla 6 × 36.5 g = £6.18. Rice pudding imitation, apple 4 × 69 g = £6.18; banana 4 × 69 g = £6.18; original 4 × 69 g = £6.18; strawberry 4 × 69 g = £6.18

Flour mixes and egg substitutes

Ener-G® (General Dietary)
Low-protein. Egg replacer 454 g = £5.11

Fate® (Fate)
Low protein. All purpose mix 500 g = £6.97. Cake mix, 2 × 250 g = £6.97; chocolate-flavour 2 × 250 g = £6.97

Juvela® (Juvela)
Low-protein. Mix 500 g = £7.79

Loprofin® (SHS)
Low-protein. Mix, plain 500 g = £8.03; chocolate 500 g = £8.50; lemon 500 g = £8.50. Egg replacer 2 × 250 g = £14.78. Egg-white replacer 100 g = £9.50

PK Foods® (Gluten Free Foods Ltd)
Low-protein. Flour mix 750 g = £10.71. Egg replacer 350 g = £5.04

Pasta

Loprofin® (SHS)
Low-protein. Pasta, animal shapes 500 g = £8.09; spirals 500 g = £8.41; lasagne 250 g = £4.09; macaroni elbows 250 g = £4.04; penne 500 g = £8.41; spaghetti 500 g = £8.41; tagliatelle 250 g = £4.04; vermicelli 250 g = £4.17. Rice, imitation 500 g = £8.16

Promin® (Firstplay Dietary)
Low-protein. Pasta, alphabet shapes 500 g = £6.80; lasagne sheets 200 g = £2.95; macaroni 500 g = £6.80; noodles, flat 500 g = £6.80; shells 500 g = £6.80; spaghetti, short-cut 500 g = £6.80; spirals 500 g = £6.80. Rice, imitation 500 g = £6.80. Tricolour pasta, alphabet shapes 500 g = £6.80; shells 500 g = £6.80; spirals 500 g = £6.80.

Pizza bases

Juvela® (Juvela)
Low-protein. Pizza base 2 × 180 g = £8.61

Savoury meals and mixes

Promin® (Firstplay Dietary)
Low-protein. Burger mix 2 × 62 g = £6.18; lamb & mint 2 × 62 g = £6.18. Couscous 500 g = £6.80. Pasta elbows in cheese and broccoli sauce 4 × 66 g = £8.08. Pasta meal 500 g = £6.80. Pasta shells in tomato, pepper, and herb sauce 4 × 72 g = £8.08. Pasta spirals in Moroccan sauce 4 × 72 g = £8.08. Sausage mix, apple & sage 4 × 30 g = £6.95; original 4 × 30 g = £6.95; tomato & basil 4 × 30 g = £6.95. Mac pot, cheese 4 × 61 g = £18.60; tomato 4 × 61 g = £18.60. Potato pot, cabbage and bacon 4 × 50 g = £15.95; onion 4 × 50 g = £15.95; sausage 4 × 50 g = £15.95. Xpot, all day scramble 4 × 60 g = £20.36; beef and tomato 4 × 60 g = £20.36; chip shop curry 4 × 60 g = £20.36; rogan style curry 4 × 60 g = £20.36

Spreads

Taranis® (Firstplay Dietary)
Low-protein. Spread, hazelnut 230 g = £7.65

A2.7 Nutritional supplements for metabolic diseases

◢Glutaric aciduria (type 1)

GA1 Anamix® Infant (SHS)
Powder, protein equivalent (essential and non-essential amino acids except lysine, and low tryptophan) 13.1 g, carbohydrate 49.5 g, fat 23 g, fibre 5.3 g, energy 1915 kJ (457 kcal)/100 g, with vitamins, minerals, and trace elements; *standard dilution* (15%) provides protein equivalent 2 g, carbohydrate 7.4 g, fat 3.5 g, fibre 800 mg, energy 287 kJ (69 kcal)/100 mL. Unflavoured, net price 400 g = £37.07 (5-g measuring scoop provided)
Nutritional supplement for the dietary management of proven glutaric aciduria (type 1) in children from birth to 3 years

GA Gel® (Vitaflo)
Gel, protein equivalent (essential and non-essential amino acids except lysine, and low tryptophan) 10 g, carbohydrate 10.3 g, fat trace, energy 339 kJ (81 kcal)/24 g, with vitamins, minerals, and trace elements. Unflavoured (flavouring: see *FlavourPac®*, p. 1041), net price 30 × 24-g sachets = £204.80
Nutritional supplement for dietary management of type 1 glutaric aciduria in children 6 months–10 years

¹XLYS, Low TRY, Maxamaid® (SHS)
Powder, protein equivalent (essential and non-essential amino acids except lysine, and low tryptophan) 25 g, carbohydrate 51 g, fat less than 500 mg, energy 1311 kJ (309 kcal)/100 g, with vitamins, minerals, and trace elements. Unflavoured, (flavouring: see *Modjul® Flavour System*, p. 1041), net price 500 g = £93.59
Nutritional supplement for the dietary management of type 1 glutaric aciduria

XLYS, TRY Glutaridon® (SHS)
Powder, protein equivalent (essential and non-essential amino acids except lysine and tryptophan)

---

1. Maxamaid products are generally intended for use in children 1–8 years

79 g, carbohydrate 4 g, energy 1411 kJ (332 kcal)/100 g. Unflavoured (flavouring: see *Modjul® Flavour System*, p. 1041), net price 2 × 500 g = £312.84

Nutritional supplement for the dietary management of type 1 glutaric aciduria in children and adults; requires additional source of vitamins, minerals, and trace elements

◀Glycogen storage disease

Corn flour and corn starch
For glycogen storage disease

Glycosade® (Vitaflo)
Powder, protein 200 mg, carbohydrate (maize starch) 47.6 g, fat 100 mg, fibre less than 600 mg, energy 803 kJ (192 kcal)/60 g, net price 30 × 60-g sachets = £107.64

Nutritional supplement for use in the dietary management of glycogen storage disease and other metabolic conditions where a constant supply of glucose is essential. Not suitable for children under 2 years

◀Homocystinuria or hypermethioninaemia

HCU Anamix® Infant (SHS)
Powder, protein equivalent (essential and non-essential amino acids except methionine) 13.1 g, carbohydrate 49.5 g, fat 23 g, fibre 5.3 g, energy 1915 kJ (457 kcal)/100 g, with vitamins, minerals, and trace elements; *standard dilution* (15%) provides protein equivalent 2 g, carbohydrate 7.4 g, fat 3.5 g, fibre 800 mg, energy 287 kJ (69 kcal)/100 mL. Unflavoured, net price 400 g = £37.07 (5-g measuring scoop provided)

Nutritional supplement for the dietary management of proven vitamin B_6 non-responsive homocystinuria or hypermethioninaemia in children from birth to 3 years

HCU cooler® 15 (Vitaflo)
Liquid, protein (essential and non-essential amino acids except methionine) 15 g, carbohydrate 7 g, fat 500 mg, energy 393 kJ (92 kcal)/130 mL, with vitamins, minerals, and trace elements. Orange or red flavour, net price 30 × 130-mL pouch = £289.80

A methionine-free protein substitute for use as a nutritional supplement in patients over 3 years of age with homocystinuria

HCU Express® 15 (Vitaflo)
Powder, protein (essential and non-essential amino acids except methionine) 15 g, carbohydrate 3.8 g, fat 30 mg, energy 315 kJ (75.3 kcal)/25 g with vitamins, minerals, and trace elements. Unflavoured (flavouring: see *FlavourPac®*, p. 1041), net price 30 × 25-g sachets = £318.03

A methionine-free protein substitute for use as a nutritional supplement in patients over 8 years of age with homocystinuria

HCU Express® 20 (Vitaflo)
Powder, protein (essential and non-essential amino acids except methionine) 20 g, carbohydrate 4.7 g, fat 70 mg, energy 416 kJ (99 kcal)/34 g with vitamins, minerals, and trace elements. Unflavoured (flavouring: see *FlavourPac®*, p. 1041), net price 30 × 34-g sachets = £410.89

A methionine-free protein substitute for use as a nutritional supplement in patients over 8 years with homocystinuria

HCU gel® (Vitaflo)
Powder, protein (essential and non-essential amino acids except methionine) 10 g, carbohydrate 10.3 g, fat 20 mg, energy 339 kJ (81 kcal)/24 g with vitamins, minerals, and trace elements. Unflavoured (flavouring: see *FlavourPac®*, p. 1041), net price 30 × 24-g sachets = £204.75

A methionine-free protein substitute for use as a nutritional supplement for the dietary management of children 1–10 years with homocystinuria

HCU Lophlex® LQ 20 (Nutricia Clinical)
Liquid, protein equivalent (essential and non-essential amino acids except methionine) 20 g, carbohydrate 8.8 g, fat 440 mg, energy 509 kJ (120 kcal)/125 mL, with vitamins, minerals, and trace elements. Juicy berries flavour, net price 125 mL = £15.29

Nutritional supplement for the dietary management of homocystinuria in patients over 3 years

HCU LV® (SHS)
Powder, protein (essential and non-essential amino acids except methionine) 20 g, carbohydrate 2.5 g, fat 190 mg, energy 390 kJ (92 kcal)/27.8-g sachet, with vitamins, minerals and trace elements. Unflavoured (flavouring: see *Modjul® Flavour System*, p. 1041) or tropical flavour (formulation varies slightly), net price 30 × 27.8-g sachets = £469.80

A nutritional supplement for the dietary management of hypermethioninaemia or vitamin B_6 non-responsive homocystinuria in patients over 8 years.

XMET Homidon® (SHS)
Powder, protein equivalent (essential and non-essential amino acids except methionine) 77 g, carbohydrate 4.5 g, fat nil, energy 1386 kJ (326 kcal)/100 g. Unflavoured (flavouring: see *Modjul® Flavour system*, p. 1041), net price 500 g = £171.63

Nutritional supplement for the dietary management of hypermethioninaemia or homocystinuria in children and adults

[1]XMET Maxamaid® (SHS)
Powder, protein equivalent (essential and non-essential amino acids except methionine) 25 g, carbohydrate 51 g, fat less than 500 mg, energy 1311 kJ (309 kcal)/100 g, with vitamins, minerals, and trace elements. Unflavoured (flavouring: see *Modjul® Flavour Sytem*, p. 1041), net price 500 g = £93.59

Nutritional supplement for the dietary management of hypermethioninaemia or homocystinuria

[2]XMET Maxamum® (SHS)
Powder, protein equivalent (essential and non-essential amino acids except methionine) 39 g, carbohydrate 34 g, fat less than 500 mg, energy 1260 kJ (297 kcal)/100 g, with vitamins, minerals, and trace elements. Unflavoured (flavouring: see *Modjul® Flavour System*, p. 1041), net price 500 g = £150.02

Nutritional supplement for the dietary management of hypermethioninaemia or homocystinuria

---

1. Maxamaid products are generally intended for use in children 1–8 years
2. Maxamum products are generally intended for use in children over 8 years and adults

◢Hyperlysinaemia

HYPER LYS Anamix® Infant (SHS)
Powder, protein equivalent (essential and non-essential amino acids except lysine) 13.1 g, carbohydrate 49.5 g, fat 23 g, fibre 5.3 g, energy 1915 kJ (457 kcal)/100 g, with vitamins, minerals, and trace elements; *standard dilution* (15%) provides protein equivalent 2 g, carbohydrate 7.4 g, fat 3.5 g, fibre 800 mg, energy 287 kJ (69 kcal)/100 mL. Unflavoured, net price 400 g = £37.07 (5-g measuring scoop provided)
Nutritional supplement for the dietary management of proven hyperlysinaemia in children from birth to 3 years

¹XLYS Maxamaid® (SHS)
Powder, protein equivalent (essential and non-essential amino acids except lysine) 25 g, carbohydrate 51 g, fat less than 500 mg, energy 1311 kJ (309 kcal)/100 g, with vitamins, minerals, and trace elements. Unflavoured (flavouring: see *Modjul® Flavour System*, p. 1041), net price 500 g = £93.59
Nutritional supplement for the dietary management of hyperlysinaemia

◢Isovaleric acidaemia

IVA Anamix® Infant (SHS)
Powder, protein equivalent (essential and non-essential amino acids except leucine) 13.1 g, carbohydrate 49.5 g, fat 23 g, fibre 5.3 g, energy 1915 kJ (457 kcal)/100 g, with vitamins, minerals, and trace elements; *standard dilution* (15%) provides protein equivalent 2 g, carbohydrate 7.4 g, fat 3.5 g, fibre 800 mg, energy 287 kJ (69 kcal)/100 mL. Unflavoured, net price 400 g = £37.07 (5-g measuring scoop provided)
Nutritional supplement for the dietary management of proven isovaleric acidaemia or other proven disorders of leucine metabolism in children from birth to 3 years

XLEU Faladon® (SHS)
Powder, protein equivalent (essential and non-essential amino acids except leucine) 25 g, carbohydrate 4.5 g, fat nil, energy 1386 kJ (326 kcal)/100 g. Unflavoured (flavouring: see *Modjul® Flavour System*, p. 1041), net price 200 g = £70.91
Nutritional supplement for the dietary management of isovaleric acidaemia

¹XLEU Maxamaid® (SHS)
Powder, protein equivalent (essential and non-essential amino acids except leucine) 25 g, carbohydrate 51 g, fat less than 500 mg, energy 1311 kJ (309 kcal)/100 g, with vitamins, minerals, and trace elements. Unflavoured (flavouring: see *Modjul® Flavour System*, p. 1041), net price 500 g = £93.59
Nutritional supplement for the dietary management of isovaleric acidaemia

1. Maxamaid products are generally intended for use in children 1–8 years

◢Maple syrup urine disease

MSUD Aid III® (SHS)
Powder, protein equivalent (essential and non-essential amino acids except isoleucine, leucine, and valine) 77 g, carbohydrate 4.5 g, energy 1386 kJ (326 kcal)/100 g. Unflavoured, (flavouring: see *Modjul® Flavour System*, p. 1041), net price 500 g = £177.29
Nutritional supplement for the dietary management of maple syrup urine disease and related conditions in children and adults where it is necessary to limit the intake of branched chain amino acids

MSUD Anamix® Infant (SHS)
Powder, protein equivalent (essential and non-essential amino acids except isoleucine, leucine, and valine) 13.1 g, carbohydrate 49.5 g, fat 23 g, fibre 5.3 g, energy 1915 kJ (457 kcal)/100 g, with vitamins, minerals, and trace elements; *standard dilution* (15%) provides protein equivalent 2 g, carbohydrate 7.4 g, fat 3.5 g, fibre 800 mg, energy 287 kJ (69 kcal)/100 mL. Unflavoured, net price 400 g = £37.07 (5-g measuring scoop provided)
Nutritional supplement for the dietary management of proven maple syrup urine disease in children from birth to 3 years

MSUD Anamix® Junior (SHS)
Powder, protein equivalent (essential and non-essential amino acids except isoleucine, leucine, and valine) 8.4 g, carbohydrate 11 g, fat 3.9 g, energy 474 kJ (113 kcal)/29-g sachet, with vitamins, minerals, and trace elements. Unflavoured (flavouring: see *Modjul® Flavour System*, p. 1041), net price 30 × 29-g sachets = £198.00.
Nutritional supplement for the dietary management of maple syrup urine disease in children 1–10 years

MSUD Anamix® Junior LQ (SHS)
Liquid, protein equivalent (essential and non-essential amino acids except isoleucine, leucine, and valine) 10 g, carbohydrate 8.8 g, fat 4.8 g, fibre 310 mg, energy 497 kJ (118 kcal)/125 mL, with vitamins, minerals, and trace elements. Lactose-free. Orange flavour, net price 125-mL carton = £8.59
Nutritional supplement for the dietary management of maple syrup urine disease in children 1–10 years

MSUD cooler® 15 (Vitaflo)
Liquid, protein equivalent (essential and non-essential amino acids except leucine, isoleucine, and valine) 15 g, carbohydrate 7 g, fat 500 mg, energy 393 kJ (92 kcal)/130-mL pouch, with vitamins, minerals, and trace elements. Orange or red flavour, net price 30 × 130-mL = £289.80
Nutritional supplement for the dietary management of maple syrup urine disease in children over 3 years and adults

MSUD express® 15 (Vitaflo)
Powder, protein equivalent (essential and non-essential amino acids except leucine, isoleucine, and valine) 15 g, carbohydrate 3.8 g, fat less than 100 mg, energy 315 kJ (75 kcal)/25 g with vitamins, minerals, and trace elements. Unflavoured (flavouring: see *FlavourPac®*, p. 1041), net price 30 × 25-g sachets = £318.03.
Nutritional supplement for the dietary management of maple syrup urine disease in children over 8 years and adults

Appendix 2: Borderline substances

MSUD express® 20 (Vitaflo)

Powder, protein equivalent (essential and non-essential amino acids except leucine, isoleucine, and valine) 20 g, carbohydrate 4.7 g, fat less than 100 mg, energy 416 kJ (99 kcal)/34 g, with vitamins, minerals, and trace elements. Unflavoured (flavouring: see *FlavourPac®*, p. 1041), net price 30 × 34-g sachets = £410.89

Nutritional supplement for the dietary management of maple syrup urine disease in children over 8 years and adults

MSUD Gel® (Vitaflo)

Powder, protein equivalent (essential and non-essential amino acids except leucine, isoleucine, and valine) 10 g, carbohydrate 10.3 g, fat less than 100 mg, energy 339 kJ (81 kcal)/24 g with vitamins, minerals, and trace elements. Unflavoured (flavouring: see *FlavourPac®*, p. 1041), net price 30 × 24-g sachets = £207.15

Nutritional supplement for the dietary management of maple syrup urine disease in children 1–10 years

MSUD Lophlex® LQ 20 (Nutricia Clinical)

Liquid, protein equivalent (essential and non-essential amino acids except isoleucine, leucine, and valine) 20 g, carbohydrate 8.8 g, fat less than 500 mg, energy 509 kJ (120 kcal)/125 mL, with vitamins, minerals, and trace elements. Juicy berries flavour, net price 125 mL = £15.29

Nutritional supplement for the dietary management of maple syrup urine disease in children over 3 years and adults

[1]MSUD Maxamaid® (SHS)

Powder, protein equivalent (essential and non-essential amino acids except isoleucine, leucine, and valine) 25 g, carbohydrate 51 g, fat less than 500 mg, energy 1311 kJ (309 kcal)/100 g, with vitamins, minerals, and trace elements. Unflavoured, (flavouring: see *Modjul® Flavour System*, p. 1041), net price 500 g = £93.59

Nutritional supplement for the dietary management of maple syrup urine disease

[2]MSUD Maxamum® (SHS)

Powder, protein equivalent (essential and non-essential amino acids except isoleucine, leucine, and valine) 39 g, carbohydrate 34 g, fat less than 500 mg, energy 1260 kJ (297 kcal)/100 g, with vitamins, minerals, and trace elements. Orange flavour or unflavoured (flavouring: see *Modjul® Flavour System*, p. 1041), net price 500 g = £150.02

Nutritional supplement for the dietary management of maple syrup urine disease

1. Maxamaid products are generally intended for use in children 1–8 years
2. Maxamum products are generally intended for use in children over 8 years and adults

◢ **Methylmalonic or propionic acidaemia**

MMA/PA Anamix® Infant (SHS)

Powder, protein equivalent (essential and non-essential amino acids except methionine, threonine, and valine, and low isoleucine) 13.1 g, carbohydrate 49.5 g, fat 23 g, fibre 5.3 g, energy 1915 kJ (457 kcal)/100 g, with vitamins, minerals, and trace elements; *standard dilution* (15%) provides protein equivalent 2 g, carbohydrate 7.4 g, fat 3.5 g, fibre 800 mg, energy 287 kJ (69 kcal)/100 mL. Unflavoured, net price 400 g = £37.07 (5-g measuring scoop provided)

Nutritional supplement for the dietary management of proven methylmalonic acidaemia or propionic acidaemia in children from birth to 3 years

XMTVI Asadon® (SHS)

Powder, protein equivalent (essential and non-essential amino acids except methionine, threonine, and valine, and low isoleucine) 77 g, carbohydrate 4.5 g, fat nil, energy 1386 kJ (326 kcal)/100 g. Unflavoured, (flavouring: see *Modjul® Flavour System*, p. 1041), net price 200 g = £70.91

Nutritional supplement for the dietary management of methylmalonic acidaemia or propionic acidaemia in children and adults

[1]XMTVI Maxamaid® (SHS)

Powder, protein equivalent (essential and non-essential amino acids except methionine, threonine, and valine, and low isoleucine) 25 g, carbohydrate 51 g, fat less than 500 mg, energy 1311 kJ (309 kcal)/100 g, with vitamins, minerals, and trace elements. Unflavoured, (flavouring: see *Modjul® Flavour System*, p. 1041), net price 500 g = £93.59

Nutritional supplement for the dietary management of methylmalonic acidaemia or propionic acidaemia

[2]XMTVI Maxamum® (SHS)

Powder, protein equivalent (essential and non-essential amino acids except methionine, threonine, and valine, and low isoleucine) 39 g, carbohydrate 34 g, fat less than 500 mg, energy 1260 kJ (297 kcal)/100 g, with vitamins, minerals, and trace elements. Unflavoured (flavouring: see *Modjul® Flavour System*, p. 1041), net price 500 g = £150.02

Nutritional supplement for the dietary management of methylmalonic acidaemia or propionic acidaemia

◢ **Other inborn errors of metabolism**

Cystine500® (Vitaflo)

Powder, cystine 500 mg, carbohydrate 3.3 g, fat nil, energy 63 kJ (15 kcal)/4 g, net price 30 x 4-g sachets = £52.03

Nutritional supplement for the dietary management of inborn errors of amino acid metabolism in adults and children from birth

DocOmega® (Vitaflo)

Powder, protein (cows' milk, soya protein) 100 mg, carbohydrate 3.2 g, fat 500 mg (of which docosahexaenoic acid 200 mg), fibre nil, energy 74 kJ (18 kcal)/4 g, with minerals, net price 30 × 4-g sachets = £37.66

Nutritional supplement for the dietary management of inborn errors of metabolism for adults and children from birth

EAA®️ Supplement (Vitaflo)

Powder, protein equivalent (essential amino acids) 5 g, carbohydrate 4 g, fat nil, energy 151 kJ (36 kcal)/12.5 g, with vitamins, minerals, and trace elements. Tropical flavour, net price 50 x 12.5-g sachets = £196.32

Nutritional supplement for the dietary management of disorders of protein metabolism including urea cycle disorders. Not suitable for children under 3 years

Isoleucine50®️ (Vitaflo)

Powder, isoleucine 50 mg, carbohydrate 3.8 g, fat nil, energy 63 kJ (15 kcal)/4 g, net price 30 × 4-g sachets = £52.03

Nutritional supplement for the dietary management of inborn errors of amino acid metabolism in adults and children from birth

KeyOmega®️ (Vitaflo)

Powder, protein (cows' milk, soya) 170 mg, carbohydrate 2.8 g, fat 800 mg (of which arachidonic acid 200 mg, docosahexaenoic acid 100 mg), energy 80 kJ (19 kcal)/4 g, net price 30 × 4-g sachet = £38.50

A nutritional supplement for the dietary management of inborn errors of metabolism

Leucine100®️ (Vitaflo)

Powder, leucine 100 mg, carbohydrate 3.7 g, fat nil, energy 63 kJ (15 kcal)/4 g, net price 30 × 4-g sachets = £52.03

Nutritional supplement for the dietary management of inborn errors of amino acid metabolism in adults and children from birth

Low protein drink (Milupa)

Powder, protein (cows' milk) 4.5 g (phenylalanine 100 mg), carbohydrate 59.5 g, fat 29.9 g, fibre nil, energy 2194 kJ (528 kcal)/100 g, with vitamins, minerals, and trace elements. Contains lactose. Net price 400 g = £8.80 (5-g measuring scoop provided)

Nutritional supplement for the dietary management of inborn errors of amino acid metabolism in adults and children over 1 year

Note Termed *Milupa®️ lp-drink* by manufacturer

Phenylalanine50®️ (Vitaflo)

Powder, phenylalanine 50 mg, carbohydrate 3.8 g, fat nil, energy 63 kJ (15 kcal)/4 g, net price 30 × 4-g sachets = £50.52

Nutritional supplement for use in the dietary management of inborn errors of metabolism in adults and children from birth

ProZero®️ (Vitaflo)

Liquid, carbohydrate 8.1 g (of which sugars 3.5 g), fat 3.8 g, energy 278 kJ (66 kcal)/100 mL. Contains lactose. Net price 18 × 250 mL = £22.68; 6 × 1 litre = £30.30

A protein-free nutritional supplement for the dietary management of inborn errors of metabolism in children over 6 months and adults

Tyrosine1000®️ (Vitaflo)

Powder, tyrosine 1 g, carbohydrate 2.9 g, fat nil, energy 63 kJ (15 kcal)/4-g sachet, net price 30 × 4-g sachets = £4.77

Nutritional supplement for the dietary management of inborn errors of amino acid metabolism in adults and children from birth

Valine50®️ (Vitaflo)

Powder, valine 50 mg, carbohydrate 3.8 g, fat nil, energy 63 kJ (15 kcal)/4 g, net price 30 × 4-g sachets = £52.03

Nutritional supplement for the dietary management of inborn errors of amino acid metabolism in adults and children from birth

◢ **Phenylketonuria**

Add-Ins®️ (SHS)

Powder, protein equivalent (containing essential and non-essential amino acids except phenylalanine) 10 g, carbohydrate nil, fat 5.1 g, energy 359 kJ (86 kcal)/18.2-g sachet, with vitamins, minerals, and trace elements. Unflavoured (flavouring: see *Modjul®️ Flavour System*, p. 1041), net price 60 × 18.2-g sachets = £357.60.

Nutritional supplement for the dietary management of proven phenylketonuria. Not suitable for children under 4 years

Easiphen®️ (SHS)

Liquid, protein equivalent (containing essential and non-essential amino acids except phenylalanine) 6.7 g, carbohydrate 5.1 g, fat 2 g, energy 275 kJ (65 kcal)/100 mL with vitamins, minerals, and trace elements. Flavours: forest berries, orange, or tropical fruit, net price 250-mL carton = £9.19.

Nutritional supplement for the dietary management of proven phenylketonuria. Not suitable for children under 8 years

Lophlex®️ (SHS)

Powder, protein equivalent (containing essential and non-essential amino acids except phenylalanine) 20 g, carbohydrate 2.5 g, fat 60 mg, fibre 220 mg, energy[1] 385 kJ (91 kcal)/27.8-g sachet, with vitamins, minerals, and trace elements. Flavours: berry, orange or unflavoured, net price 30 × 27.8-g sachets = £276.00

Nutritional supplement for the dietary management of proven phenylketonuria in children over 8 years and adults including pregnant women

Loprofin®️ PKU Drink (SHS)

Liquid, protein (cows' milk) 400 mg (phenylalanine 10 mg), lactose 9.4 g, fat 2 g, energy 165 kJ (40 kcal)/100 mL. Net price 200-mL carton = 72p.

Nutritional supplement for the dietary management of phenylketonuria in children over 1 year and adults

Loprofin®️ Sno-Pro (SHS)

Liquid, protein (cows' milk) 220 mg (phenylalanine 12.5 mg), carbohydrate 8 g, fat 3.8 g, energy 273 kJ (65 kcal)/100 mL. Contains lactose. Net price 200 mL= £1.19p

Nutritional supplement for the dietary management of phenylketonuria, chronic renal failure, and other inborn errors of amino acid metabolism

Milupa PKU 2-prima®️ (Milupa)

Powder, protein equivalent (essential and non-essential amino acids except phenylalanine) 60 g, carbohydrate 10 g, fat nil, energy 1190 kJ (280 kcal)/100 g, with vitamins, minerals, and trace elements. Vanilla flavour, net price 500 g = £149.25

Nutritional supplement for the dietary management of phenylketonuria in children 1–8 years

1. Nutritional values vary with flavour—consult product literature

Appendix 2: Borderline substances

Milupa PKU 2-secunda® (Milupa)

Powder, protein equivalent (essential and non-essential amino acids except phenylalanine) 70 g, carbohydrate 6.8 g, fat nil, energy 1306 kJ (307 kcal)/100 g, with vitamins, minerals, and trace elements. Vanilla flavour, net price 500 g = £174.12

Nutritional supplement for the dietary management of phenylketonuria in children 9–14 years

Milupa PKU 3-advanta® (Milupa)

Powder, protein equivalent (essential and non-essential amino acids except phenylalanine) 70 g, carbohydrate 4.7 g, fat nil, energy 1270 kJ (299 kcal)/100 g, with vitamins, minerals, and trace elements. Vanilla flavour, net price 500 g = £174.12

Nutritional supplement for the dietary management of phenylketonuria in patients 15 years and over

Phlexy-10® Exchange System (SHS)

Capsules, protein equivalent (essential and non-essential amino acids except phenylalanine) 416.5 mg/capsule, net price 200-cap pack = £40.55

Tablets, protein equivalent (essential and non-essential amino acids except phenylalanine), 833 mg/tablet, net price 75-tab pack = £26.26

Drink Mix, powder, protein equivalent (essential and non-essential amino acids except phenylalanine) 8.33 g, carbohydrate 8.8 g/20-g sachet. Apple-black currant, citrus, or tropical flavour, net price 30 × 20-g sachet = £122.40

Nutritional supplement for the dietary management of phenylketonuria

Phlexy-Vits® (SHS)

Powder, vitamins, minerals, and trace elements, net price 30 × 7-g sachets = £68.10

Tablets, vitamins, minerals, and trace elements, net price 180-tab pack = £77.35

For use as a vitamin and mineral component of restricted therapeutic diets in children 11 years and over and adults with phenylketonuria and similar amino acid abnormalities

PK Aid-4® (SHS)

Powder, protein equivalent (essential and non-essential amino acids except phenylalanine) 79 g, carbohydrate 4.5 g, fat nil, energy 1420 kJ (334 kcal)/100 g. Unflavoured, (flavouring: see *Modjul® Flavour System*, p. 1041), net price 500 g = £136.28 (5-g measuring scoop provided).

Nutritional supplement for the dietary management of phenylketonuria in children and adults

PKU Anamix® Infant (SHS)

Powder, protein equivalent (essential and non-essential amino acids except phenylalanine) 13.1 g, carbohydrate 49.5 g, fat 23 g, fibre 5.3 g, energy 1915 kJ (457 kcal)/100 g, with vitamins, minerals, and trace elements; *standard dilution* (15%) provides protein equivalent 2 g, carbohydrate 7.4 g, fat 3.5 g, fibre 800 mg, energy 287 kJ (69 kcal)/100 mL. Unflavoured, net price 400 g = £33.69 (5-g measuring scoop provided)

Nutritional supplement for the dietary management of proven phenylketonuria in children from birth to 3 years

PKU Anamix® Junior (SHS)

Powder, protein equivalent (essential and non-essential amino acids except phenylalanine) 8.4 g, carbohydrate 9.9 g, fat 3.9 g, energy 455 (108 kcal)/29-g sachet, with vitamins, minerals, and trace elements. Chocolate, pineapple-vanilla. Unflavoured (carbohydrate 11 g, energy 474 kJ (113 kcal)/29-g sachet), net price 30 × 29-g sachets = £120.30

Nutritional supplement for the dietary management of phenylketonuria in children 1–10 years

PKU Anamix® Junior LQ (SHS)

Liquid, protein equivalent (essential and non-essential amino acids except phenylalanine) 10 g, carbohydrate 8.8 g, fat 4.8 g, fibre 310 mg, energy 497 kJ (118 kcal)/125 mL, with vitamins, minerals, and trace elements. Lactose-free. Flavours: Berry, orange, or unflavoured, net price 125-mL carton = £5.35

Nutritional supplement for the dietary management of phenylketonuria in children 1–10 years

PKU cooler10® (Vitaflo)

Liquid, protein equivalent (essential and non-essential amino acids except phenylalanine) 10 g, carbohydrate 5.1 g, energy 258 kJ (62 kcal)/87-mL pouch, with vitamins, minerals, and trace elements. Unflavoured (white) or flavoured (orange, purple, or red), net price 30 × 87 mL = £117.90.

Nutritional supplement for the dietary management of phenylketonuria. Not recommended for children under 3 years

PKU cooler15® (Vitaflo)

Liquid, protein equivalent (essential and non-essential amino acids except phenylalanine) 15 g, carbohydrate 7.8 g, energy 386 kJ (92 kcal)/130-mL pouch, with vitamins, minerals, and trace elements. Unflavoured (white) or flavoured (orange, purple, or red), net price 30 x 130 mL = £175.80.

Nutritional supplement for the dietary management of phenylketonuria, not recommended for children under 3 years

PKU cooler20® (Vitaflo)

Liquid, protein equivalent (essential and non-essential amino acids except phenylalanine) 20 g, carbohydrate 10.2 g, energy 517 kJ (124 kcal)/174-mL pouch, with vitamins, minerals, and trace elements. Unflavoured (white) or flavoured (orange, purple, or red), net price 30 × 174 mL = £236.10

Nutritional supplement for the dietary management of phenylketonuria. Not recommended for children under 3 years

PKU express15® (Vitaflo)

Powder, protein equivalent (essential and non-essential amino acids except phenylalanine) 15 g, carbohydrate 2.4 g, energy 293 kJ (70 kcal)/25-g sachet, with vitamins, minerals, and trace elements. Lemon, orange, tropical or unflavoured (carbohydrate 3.4 g, energy 310 kJ (74 kcal)/25 g), (flavouring: see *FlavourPac®*, p. 1041), net price 30 x 25-g sachets = £192.81

Nutritional supplement for the dietary management of phenylketonuria. Not recommended for children under 3 years

PKU express20® (Vitaflo)

Powder, protein equivalent (essential and non-essential amino acids except phenylalanine) 20 g, carbohydrate 3.3 g, energy 389 kJ (93 kcal)/34-g sachet, with vitamins, minerals, and trace elements. Lemon, orange, tropical, or unflavoured (carbohydrate 4.7 g, energy 416 kJ (99 kcal)/34 g), (flavouring: see *FlavourPac®*, p. 1041), net price 30 × 34-g sachets = £249.10

Nutritional supplement for the dietary management of phenylketonuria. Not recommended for children under 3 years

PKU gel® (Vitaflo)

Powder, protein equivalent (essential and non-essential amino acids except phenylalanine) 10 g, carbohydrate 8.9 g, fat less than 100 mg, energy 318 kJ (76 kcal)/24-g sachet, with vitamins, minerals, and trace elements. Orange, raspberry, or unflavoured (carbohydrate 10.3 g, energy 339 kJ (81 kcal)/24 g), (flavouring: see *FlavourPac®*, p. 1041), net price 30 × 24-g sachets = £133.39

Nutritional supplement for use as part of the low-protein dietary management of phenylketonuria in children 1–10 years

PKU Lophlex® LQ 10 (SHS)

Liquid, protein equivalent (containing essential and non-essential amino acids except phenylalanine) 10 g, carbohydrate 4.4 g, fibre 250 mg, energy 245 kJ (58 kcal)/62.5 mL, with vitamins, minerals, and trace elements. Flavours: berry, citrus, orange, or tropical, net price 62.5-mL carton = £4.93; juicy berries, juicy orange (energy 246 kJ (58 kcal)/62.5 mL), 62.5-mL carton = £4.93

Nutritional supplement for the dietary management of phenylketonuria in children over 4 years and adults including pregnant women

PKU Lophlex® LQ 20 (SHS)

Liquid, protein equivalent (containing essential and non-essential amino acids except phenylalanine) 20 g, carbohydrate 8.8 g, fibre 340 mg, energy 490 kJ (115 kcal)/125 mL, with vitamins, minerals, and trace elements. Flavours: berry, citrus, orange, or tropical, net price 125-mL carton = £9.84; juicy berries, juicy orange (fibre 500 mg, energy 493 kJ (116 kcal)/125 mL), 125-mL carton = £9.84

Nutritional supplement for the dietary management of phenylketonuria in children over 4 years and adults including pregnant women

PKU Lophlex® Sensation 20 (SHS)

Semi-solid, protein equivalent (containing essential and non-essential amino acids except phenylalanine) 20 g, carbohydrate 20.2 g, fibre 1 g, energy 706 kJ (166 kcal)/109 g, with vitamins, minerals, and trace elements. Flavours: berry or orange, net price 3 × 109-g pot = £31.44

Nutritional supplement for the dietary management of phenylketonuria in children over 4 years and adults including pregnant women

PKU squeezie® (Vitaflo)

Liquid, protein equivalent (essential and non-essential amino acids except phenylalanine) 10 g, carbohydrate 22.5 g, fat 500 mg, energy 565 kJ (135 kcal)/85 g, with vitamins, minerals, and trace elements. Flavour: apple-banana, net price 30 × 85-g pouch = £127.52

Nutritional supplement for the dietary management of phenylketonuria in children from 6 months to 10 years

PKU Start® (Vitaflo)

Liquid, protein equivalent (essential and non-essential amino acids except phenylalanine) 2 g, carbohydrate 8.3 g, fat 2.9 g, energy 286 kJ (68 kcal)/100 mL with vitamins, minerals, and trace elements. Contains lactose and fish oil. Net price 500-mL bottle = £6.53

Nutritional supplement for the dietary management of phenylketonuria in children under 1 year

L-Tyrosine (SHS)

Powder, L-tyrosine 20 g, carbohydrate 76.8 g, fat nil, energy 1612 kJ (379 kcal)/100 g, net price 100 g = £20.87

Nutritional supplement for the dietary management of phenylketonuria in pregnant women with low plasma tyrosine concentrations

[1]XP Maxamaid® (SHS)

Powder, protein equivalent (essential and non-essential amino acids except phenylalanine) 25 g, carbohydrate 51 g, fat less than 500 mg, energy 1311 kJ (309 kcal)/100 g, with vitamins, minerals, and trace elements. Orange flavour or unflavoured (flavouring: see *Modjul® Flavour System*, p. 1041), net price 500 g = £55.37

Nutritional supplement for the dietary management of phenylketonuria in children 1–8 years

[2]XP Maxamum® (SHS)

Powder, protein equivalent (essential and non-essential amino acids except phenylalanine) 39 g, carbohydrate 34 g, fat less than 500 mg, energy 1260 kJ (297 kcal)/100 g, with vitamins, minerals, and trace elements. Flavours: orange, unflavoured (flavouring: see *Modjul® Flavour System*, p. 1041). Net price 30 × 50-g sachets = £256.80, 500 g = £85.63

Nutritional supplement for the dietary management of phenylketonuria in children over 8 years and adults

◢Tyrosinaemia

Methionine-free TYR Anamix® Infant (SHS)

Powder, protein equivalent (essential and non-essential amino acids except methionine, phenylalanine, and tyrosine) 13.1 g, carbohydrate 49.5 g, fat 23 g, fibre 5.3 g, energy 1915 kJ (457 kcal)/100 g, with vitamins, minerals, and trace elements; *standard dilution* (15%) provides protein equivalent 2 g, carbohydrate 7.4 g, fat 3.5 g, fibre 800 mg, energy 287 kJ (69 kcal)/100 mL. Unflavoured, net price 400 g = £37.07 (5-g measuring scoop provided)

Nutritional supplement for the dietary management of proven tyrosinaemia type 1 in children from birth to 3 years

TYR Anamix® Infant (SHS)

Powder, protein equivalent (essential and non-essential amino acids except phenylalanine, and tyrosine) 13.1 g, carbohydrate 49.5 g, fat 23 g, fibre 5.3 g, energy 1915 kJ (457 kcal)/100 g, with vitamins, minerals, and trace elements; *standard dilution* (15%) provides protein equivalent 2 g, carbohydrate 7.4 g, fat 3.5 g, fibre 800 mg, energy 287 kJ (69 kcal)/100 mL. Unflavoured, net price

---

1. Maxamaid products are generally intended for use in children 1–8 years
2. Maxamum products are generally intended for use in children over 8 years and adults

400 g = £37.07 (5-g measuring scoop provided)
Nutritional supplement for the dietary management of
proven tyrosinaemia where plasma-methionine
concentrations are normal in children from birth to 3 years

TYR Anamix® Junior (SHS)

Powder, protein equivalent (essential and non-
essential amino acids except phenylalanine and
tyrosine) 8.4 g, carbohydrate 11 g, fat 3.9 g, energy
475 kJ (113 kcal)/29-g sachet, with vitamins,
minerals, and trace elements. Unflavoured, net price
30 x 29-g sachets = £196.50
Nutritional supplement for the dietary management of
proven tyrosinaemia in children 1–10 years

TYR Anamix® Junior LQ (SHS)

Liquid, protein equivalent (essential and non-
essential amino acids except phenylalanine and
tyrosine) 10 g, carbohydrate 8.8 g, fat 4.8 g, fibre
310 mg, energy 500 kJ (119 kcal)/125 mL, with
vitamins, minerals, and trace elements. Orange
flavour, net price 36 × 125-mL bottle = £272.79
Nutritional supplement for the dietary management of
tyrosinaemia type 1 (when nitisinone (NTBC) is used, see
section 9.8.1), type II, and type III, in children over 1 year

TYR cooler® 15 (Vitaflo)

Liquid, protein equivalent (essential and non-
essential amino acids except tyrosine and
phenylalanine) 15 g, carbohydrate 7 g, fat 500 mg,
energy 393 kJ (92 kcal)/130 mL, with vitamins,
minerals, and trace elements. Orange or red flavour,
net price 30 x 130-mL pouch = £289.80
Nutritional supplement for the dietary management of
tyrosinaemia in children over 3 years and adults

TYR express15® (Vitaflo)

Powder, protein equivalent (essential and non-
essential amino acids except tyrosine and
phenylalanine) 15 g, carbohydrate 3.4 g, fat less than
100 mg, energy 310 kJ (74 kcal)/25 g, with vitamins,
minerals, and trace elements. Unflavoured
(flavouring: see FlavourPac®, p. 1041), net price 30
× 25-g sachets = £318.03
Nutritional supplement for the dietary management of
tyrosinaemia in children over 8 years and adults

TYR express20® (Vitaflo)

Powder, protein equivalent (essential and non-
essential amino acids except tyrosine and
phenylalanine) 20 g, carbohydrate 4.7 g, fat less than
100 mg, energy 416 kJ (99 kcal)/34 g, with vitamins,
minerals, and trace elements. Unflavoured
(flavouring: see FlavourPac®, p. 1041), net price 30
× 34-g sachets = £410.89
Nutritional supplement for the dietary management of
tyrosinaemia. Not recommended for children under 8
years

TYR Gel® (Vitaflo)

Gel, protein equivalent (essential and non-essential
amino acids except tyrosine and phenylalanine)
10 g, carbohydrate 10.3 g, fat less than 100 mg,
energy 339 kJ (81 kcal)/24 g, with vitamins,
minerals, and trace elements. Unflavoured
(flavouring: see FlavourPac®, p. 1041), net price 30
× 24-g sachets = £204.75
Nutritional supplement for the dietary management of
tyrosinaemia in children 1–10 years

TYR Lophlex® LQ 20 (Nutricia Clinical)

Liquid, protein equivalent (essential and non-
essential amino acids except phenylalanine and
tyrosine) 20 g, carbohydrate 8.8 g, fat less than
500 mg, fibre 500 mg, energy 509 kJ (120 kcal)/
125 mL, with vitamins, minerals, and trace elements.
Juicy berries flavour, net price 125 mL = £15.29
Nutritional supplement for the dietary management of
tyrosinaemia in children over 3 years and adults

[1]XPHEN TYR Maxamaid® (SHS)

Powder, protein equivalent (essential and non-
essential amino acids except phenylalanine and
tyrosine) 25 g, carbohydrate 51 g, fat less than
500 mg, energy 1311 kJ (309 kcal)/100 g with
vitamins, minerals, and trace elements. Unflavoured
(flavouring: see Modjul® Flavour System, p. 1041).
Net price 500 g = £93.59
Nutritional supplement for the dietary management of
tyrosinaemia in children 1–8 years

XPHEN TYR Tyrosidon® (SHS)

Powder, protein equivalent (essential and non-
essential amino acids except phenylalanine and
tyrosine) 77 g, carbohydrate 4.5 g, fat nil, energy
1386 kJ (326 kcal)/100 g. Unflavoured (flavouring:
see Modjul® Flavour System, p. 1041). Net price
500 g = £177.29
Nutritional supplement for the dietary management of
tyrosinaemia in children and adults where plasma-
methionine concentrations are normal

XPTM Tyrosidon® (SHS)

Powder, protein equivalent (essential and non-
essential amino acids except phenylalanine,
tyrosine, and methionine) 77 g, carbohydrate 4.5 g,
fat nil, energy 1386 kJ (326 kcal)/100 g. Unflavoured
(flavouring: see Modjul® Flavour System, p. 1041).
Net price 500 g = £88.65
Nutritional supplement for the dietary management of
tyrosinaemia type 1 in children and adults where plasma-
methionine concentrations are above normal

Conditions for which ACBS products can be prescribed

Birthmarks   See Disfiguring skin lesions, below

Dermatitis   Aveeno® Bath Oil; Aveeno® Cream;
Aveeno® Lotion; E45® Emollient Bath Oil; E45® Emollient Wash Cream; E45® Lotion

For details of preparations see section 13.2.1, p. 795

Dermatitis herpetiformis   See also Gluten-free
foods, p. 1042

**Disfiguring skin lesions (birthmarks, mutilat-
ing lesions, scars, vitiligo)**   Covermark® classic
foundation and finishing powder; Dermablend® Ultra
corrective foundation; Dermacolor® Camouflage cream
and fixing powder; Keromask® masking cream and
finishing powder; Veil® Cover cream and Finishing
Powder. (Cleansing Creams, Cleansing Milks, and
Cleansing Lotions are excluded)

For details of preparations see section 13.8.2, p. 828

Disinfectants (antiseptics)   May be prescribed on
an FP10 only when ordered in such quantities and with

---

1. Maxamaid products are generally intended for use in
   children 1–8 years

such directions as are appropriate for the treatment of patients, but not for general hygenic purposes.

Dry mouth (xerostomia) For patients suffering from dry mouth as a result of having (or having undergone) radiotherapy, or sicca syndrome.

Biotène Oralbalance®; *BioXtra®*; *Glandosane®*; *Saliveze®*.

For details of preparations see section 12.3.5, p. 792

Eczema See Dermatitis, above

Photodermatoses (skin protection in) *Anthelios®* XL SPF 50+ Melt-in cream; *Sunsense®* Ultra; *Uvistat®* Lipscreen SPF 50, *Uvistat®* Suncream SPF 30 and 50.

For details of preparations see section 13.8.1, p. 826

Pruritus See Dermatitis, above

A3 Cautionary and advisory labels for dispensed medicines

Numbers following the preparation entries in the BNF correspond to the code numbers of the cautionary labels that pharmacists are recommended to add when dispensing. It is also expected that pharmacists will counsel patients when necessary.

Counselling needs to be related to the age, experience, background, and understanding of the individual patient. The pharmacist should ensure that the patient understands how to take or use the medicine and how to follow the correct dosage schedule. Any effects of the medicine on driving or work, any foods or medicines to be avoided, and what to do if a dose is missed should also be explained. Other matters, such as the possibility of staining of the clothes or skin by a medicine should also be mentioned.

For some preparations there is a special need for counselling, such as an unusual method or time of administration or a potential interaction with a common food or domestic remedy, and this is indicated where necessary.

Original packs   Most preparations are dispensed in unbroken original packs that include further advice for the patient in the form of patient information leaflets. Label 10 may be of value where appropriate. More general leaflets advising on the administration of preparations such as eye drops, eye ointments, inhalers, and suppositories are also available.

Scope of labels   In general no label recommendations have been made for injections on the assumption that they will be administered by a healthcare professional or a well-instructed patient. The labelling is not exhaustive and pharmacists are recommended to use their professional discretion in labelling new preparations and those for which no labels are shown.

Individual labelling advice is not given on the administration of the large variety of antacids. In the absence of instructions from the prescriber, and if on enquiry the patient has had no verbal instructions, the directions given under 'Dose' should be used on the label.

It is recognised that there may be occasions when pharmacists will use their knowledge and professional discretion and decide to omit one or more of the recommended labels for a particular patient. In this case counselling is of the utmost importance. There may also be an occasion when a prescriber does not wish additional cautionary labels to be used, in which case the prescription should be endorsed 'NCL' (no cautionary labels). The exact wording that is required instead should then be specified on the prescription.

Pharmacists label medicines with various wordings in addition to those directions specified on the prescription. Such labels include 'Shake the bottle', 'For external use only', and 'Store in a cool place', as well as 'Discard .

. . . days after opening' and 'Do not use after . . . .', which apply particularly to antibiotic mixtures, diluted liquid and topical preparations, and to eye-drops. Although not listed in the BNF these labels should continue to be used when appropriate; indeed, 'For external use only' is a legal requirement on external liquid preparations, while 'Keep out of the reach of children' is a legal requirement on all dispensed medicines. Care should be taken not to obscure other relevant information with adhesive labelling.

It is the usual practice for patients to take standard tablets with water or other liquid and for this reason no separate label has been recommended.

The label wordings recommended by the BNF apply to medicines dispensed against a prescription. Patients should be aware that a dispensed medicine should never be taken by, or shared with, anyone other than for whom the prescriber intended it. Therefore, the BNF does not include warnings against the use of a dispensed medicine by persons other than for whom it was specifically prescribed.

The label or labels for each preparation are recommended after careful consideration of the information available. However, it is recognised that in some cases this information may be either incomplete or open to a different interpretation. The BNF will therefore be grateful to receive any constructive comments on the labelling suggested for any preparation.

Recommended label wordings

> For BNF 61 (March 2011), a revised set of cautionary and advisory labels were introduced. All of the existing labels were user-tested, and the revised wording selected reflects terminology that is better understood by patients.

Wordings which can be given as separate warnings are labels 1–19, 29–30, and 32. Wordings which can be incorporated in an appropriate position in the directions for dosage or administration are labels 21–28. A label has been omitted for number 20; labels 31 and 33 no longer apply to any medicines in the BNF and have therefore been deleted.

If separate labels are used it is recommended that the wordings be used without modification. If changes are made to suit computer requirements, care should be taken to retain the sense of the original.

1   **Warning: This medicine may make you sleepy**
To be used on *preparations for children* containing antihistamines, or other preparations given to children where the warnings of label 2 on driving or alcohol would not be appropriate.

2 **Warning: This medicine may make you sleepy. If this happens, do not drive or use tools or machines. Do not drink alcohol**

To be used on *preparations for adults that can cause drowsiness*, thereby affecting coordination and the ability to drive and operate hazardous machinery; label 1 is more appropriate for children. *It is an offence to drive while under the influence of drink or drugs.*

Some of these preparations only cause drowsiness in the first few days of treatment and some only cause drowsiness in higher doses.

In such cases the patient should be told that the advice applies until the effects have worn off. However many of these preparations can produce a slowing of reaction time and a loss of mental concentration that can have the same effects as drowsiness.

Avoidance of alcoholic drink is recommended because the effects of CNS depressants are enhanced by alcohol. Strict prohibition however could lead to some patients not taking the medicine. Pharmacists should therefore explain the risk and encourage compliance, particularly in patients who may think they already tolerate the effects of alcohol (see also label 3). Queries from patients with epilepsy regarding fitness to drive should be referred back to the patient's doctor.

Side-effects unrelated to drowsiness that may affect a patient's ability to drive or operate machinery safely include *blurred vision, dizziness, or nausea*. In general, no label has been recommended to cover these cases, but the patient should be suitably counselled.

3 **Warning: This medicine may make you sleepy. If this happens, do not drive or use tools or machines**

To be used on *preparations containing monoamine-oxidase inhibitors*; the warning to avoid alcohol and dealcoholised (low alcohol) drink is covered by the patient information leaflet.

Also to be used as for label 2 but where alcohol is not an issue.

4 **Warning: Do not drink alcohol**

To be used on *preparations where a reaction such as flushing may occur if alcohol is taken* (e.g. metronidazole). Alcohol may also enhance the hypoglycaemia produced by some oral antidiabetic drugs but routine application of a warning label is not considered necessary.

Patients should be advised not to drink alcohol for as long as they are receiving/using a course of medication, and in some cases for a period of time after the course is finished.

5 **Do not take indigestion remedies 2 hours before or after you take this medicine**

To be used with label 25 on *preparations coated to resist gastric acid* (e.g. enteric-coated tablets). This is to avoid the possibility of premature dissolution of the coating in the presence of an alkaline pH.

Label 5 also applies to drugs such as gabapentin *where the absorption is significantly affected by antacids*. Pharmacists will be aware (from a knowledge of physiology) that the usual time during which indigestion remedies should be avoided is at least 2 hours before and after the majority of medicines have been taken; when a manufacturer advises a different time period, this can be followed, and should be explained to the patient.

6 **Do not take indigestion remedies, or medicines containing iron or zinc, 2 hours before or after you take this medicine**

To be used on *preparations containing ofloxacin and some other quinolones, doxycycline, lymecycline, minocycline, and penicillamine*. These drugs chelate calcium, iron, and zinc and are less well absorbed when taken with calcium-containing antacids or preparations containing iron or zinc. Pharmacists will be aware (from a knowledge of physiology) that these incompatible preparations should be taken at least 2 hours apart for the majority of medicines; when a manufacturer advises a different time period, this can be followed, and should be explained to the patient.

7 **Do not take milk, indigestion remedies, or medicines containing iron or zinc, 2 hours before or after you take this medicine**

To be used on *preparations containing ciprofloxacin, norfloxacin, or tetracyclines that chelate calcium, iron, magnesium, and zinc*, and are thus less available for absorption. Pharmacists will be aware (from a knowledge of physiol-

ogy) that these incompatible preparations should be taken at least 2 hours apart for the majority of medicines; when a manufacturer advises a different time period, this can be followed, and should be explained to the patient. Doxycycline, lymecycline, and minocycline are less liable to form chelates and therefore only require label 6 (see above).

8 **Warning: Do not stop taking this medicine unless your doctor tells you to stop**

To be used on *preparations that contain a drug which is required to be taken over long periods without the patient necessarily perceiving any benefit* (e.g. antituberculous drugs).

Also to be used on *preparations that contain a drug whose withdrawal is likely to be a particular hazard* (e.g. clonidine for hypertension). Label 10 (see below) is more appropriate for corticosteroids.

9 **Space the doses evenly throughout the day. Keep taking this medicine until the course is finished, unless you are told to stop**

To be used on *preparations where a course of treatment should be completed* to reduce the incidence of relapse or failure of treatment.

The preparations are antimicrobial drugs given by mouth. Very occasionally, some may have severe side-effects (e.g. diarrhoea in patients receiving clindamycin) and in such cases the patient may need to be advised of reasons for stopping treatment quickly and returning to the doctor.

10 **Warning: Read the additional information given with this medicine**

To be used particularly on *preparations containing anticoagulants, lithium, and oral corticosteroids*. The appropriate treatment card should be given to the patient and any necessary explanations given.

This label may also be used on other preparations to remind the patient of the instructions that have been given.

11 **Protect your skin from sunlight—even on a bright but cloudy day. Do not use sunbeds**

To be used on *preparations that may cause phototoxic or photoallergic reactions* if the patient is exposed to ultra-violet radiation. Many drugs other than those listed in Appendix 3 (e.g. phenothiazines and sulfonamides) may, on rare occasions, cause reactions in susceptible patients. Exposure to high intensity ultraviolet radiation from sun-ray lamps and sunbeds is particularly likely to cause reactions.

12 **Do not take anything containing aspirin while taking this medicine**

To be used on *preparations containing sulfinpyrazone* whose activity is reduced by aspirin.

Label 12 should not be used for anticoagulants since label 10 is more appropriate.

13 **Dissolve or mix with water before taking**

To be used on *preparations that are intended to be dissolved in water* (e.g. soluble tablets) or *mixed with water* (e.g. powders, granules) before use. In a few cases other liquids such as fruit juice or milk may be used.

14 **This medicine may colour your urine. This is harmless**

To be used on *preparations that may cause the patient's urine to turn an unusual colour*. These include triamterene (blue under some lights), levodopa (dark reddish), and rifampicin (red).

15 **Caution: flammable. Keep your body away from fire or flames after you have put on the medicine**

To be used on *preparations containing sufficient flammable solvent to render them flammable if exposed to a naked flame*.

16 **Dissolve the tablet under your tongue—do not swallow. Store the tablets in this bottle with the cap tightly closed. Get a new supply 8 weeks after opening**

To be used on *glyceryl trinitrate tablets* to remind the patient not to transfer the tablets to plastic or less suitable containers.

17 **Do not take more than . . . in 24 hours**

To be used on *preparations for the treatment of acute migraine* except those containing ergotamine, for which label 18 is used. The dose form should be specified, e.g.

tablets or capsules.
It may also be used on preparations for which no dose has been specified by the prescriber.

18   **Do not take more than . . . in 24 hours. Also, do not take more than . . . in any one week**
To be used on preparations containing ergotamine. The dose form should be specified, e.g. tablets or suppositories.

19   **Warning: This medicine makes you sleepy. If you still feel sleepy the next day, do not drive or use tools or machines. Do not drink alcohol**
To be used on *preparations containing hypnotics (or some other drugs with sedative effects) prescribed to be taken at night.* On the rare occasions when hypnotics are prescribed for daytime administration (e.g. nitrazepam in epilepsy), this label would clearly not be appropriate. Also to be used as an *alternative to the label 2 wording* (the choice being at the discretion of the pharmacist) *for anxiolytics prescribed to be taken at night.*
It is hoped that this wording will convey adequately the problem of residual morning sedation after taking 'sleeping tablets'.

21   **Take with or just after food, or a meal**
To be used on *preparations that are liable to cause gastric irritation, or those that are better absorbed with food.*
Patients should be advised that a *small amount of food is sufficient.*

22   **Take 30 to 60 minutes before food**
To be used on *some preparations whose absorption is thereby improved.*
Most oral antibacterials require label 23 instead (see below).

23   **Take this medicine when your stomach is empty. This means an hour before food or 2 hours after food**
To be used on *oral antibacterials whose absorption may be reduced by the presence of food and acid in the stomach.*

24   **Suck or chew this medicine**
To be used on *preparations that should be sucked or chewed.* The pharmacist should use discretion as to which of these words is appropriate.

25   **Swallow this medicine whole. Do not chew or crush**
To be used on *preparations that are enteric-coated or designed for modified-release.*

Also to be used on *preparations that taste very unpleasant or may damage the mouth* if not swallowed whole.
Patients should be advised (where relevant) that some modified-release preparations can be broken in half, but that the halved tablet should still be swallowed whole, and not chewed or crushed.

26   **Dissolve this medicine under your tongue**
To be used on *preparations designed for sublingual use.* Patients should be advised to hold under the tongue and avoid swallowing until dissolved. The buccal mucosa between the gum and cheek is occasionally specified by the prescriber.

27   **Take with a full glass of water**
To be used on *preparations that should be well diluted* (e.g. chloral hydrate), *where a high fluid intake is required* (e.g. sulfonamides), or *where water is required to aid the action* (e.g. methylcellulose). The patient should be advised that 'a full glass' means at least 150 mL. In most cases fruit juice, tea, or coffee may be used.

28   **Spread thinly on the affected skin only**
To be used on *external preparations that should be applied sparingly* (e.g. corticosteroids, dithranol).

29   **Do not take more than 2 at any one time. Do not take more than 8 in 24 hours**
To be used on containers of dispensed *solid dose preparations containing paracetamol for adults when the instruction on the label indicates that the dose can be taken on an 'as required' basis.* The dose form should be specified, e.g. tablets or capsules.
This label has been introduced because of the serious consequences of overdosage with paracetamol.

30   **Contains paracetamol. Do not take anything else containing paracetamol while taking this medicine. Talk to a doctor at once if you take too much of this medicine, even if you feel well**
To be used on all containers of dispensed *preparations containing paracetamol.*

32   **Contains aspirin. Do not take anything else containing aspirin while taking this medicine**
To be used on containers of dispensed *preparations containing aspirin when the name on the label does not include the word 'aspirin'.*

Products and their labels

Proprietary names are in *italic.*
C = counselling advised; see BNF = consult product entry in BNF

Alfuzosin m/r, 21, 25, C, initial dose, driving, see BNF

Alimemazine, 2

Aliskiren, 21

Alitretinoin, 10, patient information leaflet, 11, 21

Allegron, 2

Allopurinol, 8, 21, 27

Almogran, 3

Almotriptan, 3

Alphaderm, 28, C, application, see BNF

Alprazolam, 2

Altargo, 28

Alvesco, 8, C, administration

Amantadine, C, driving

Amifampridine, 3, 21

Aminophylline m/r, see preps

Aminosalicylic acid, 9, 25, C, administration, see BNF

Amiodarone, 11

Amisulpride, 2

Amitiza, 21

Amitriptyline, 2

Amorolfine, 10, patient information leaflet

Amoxicillin, 9

Amoxicillin dispersible sachets, 9, 13

Amoxil, 9

Amoxil dispersible sachets, 9, 13

Amoxil paed susp, 9, C, use of pipette

Ampicillin, 9, 23

Anafranil m/r, 2, 25

Anagrelide, C, driving

Anakinra, C, blood disorder symptoms

Androcur, 21

Angitil SR, 25

Angitil XL, 25

Anhydrol Forte, 15

Anoro Ellipta, C, administration

Anquil, 2

Antabuse, 2, C, alcohol reaction, see BNF

Antacids, see BNF dose statements

Antepsin, 5

Anticoagulants, oral, 10, anticoagulant card

Antihistamines, (see individual preparations)

APO-go, 10, C, driving, see BNF

Apomorphine, 10, C, driving, see BNF

Aptivus caps, 5, 21

Aptivus oral solution, 5, 21, C, crystallisation

Arava, 4

Aricept Evess, C, administration

Aripiprazole, 2

Aripiprazole orodispersible tabs, 2, C, administration, see BNF

Arlevert, 2

Aromasin, 21

Arpicolin, C, driving

Artemether with lumefantrine, 21, C, driving

Arthrotec, 21, 25

Arythmol, 21, 25, C, driving

Asacol enema and supps, C, blood disorder symptoms, see BNF

Asacol MR tabs, 5, 25, C, blood disorder symptoms, see BNF

Asasantin Retard, 21, 25, 32

Ascorbic acid tabs (500 mg), 24

Asenapine, 2, 26, C, administration

Asmabec preps, 8, C, administration; with high doses, 10, steroid card

Asmanex, 8, 10, steroid card, C, administration

Asmasal, C, administration

Aspirin dispersible tabs, 13, 21, also 32 (if 'aspirin' not on label)

Aspirin e/c, 5, 25, also 32 (if 'aspirin' not on label)

Aspirin m/r, 25, also 32 (if 'aspirin' not on label)

Aspirin supps, 32, (if 'aspirin' not on label)

Aspirin tabs, 21, also 32 (if 'aspirin' not on label)

Atarax, 2

Atazanavir, 5, 21

Atenolol, 8

Atimos Modulite, C, administration

Atomoxetine, 3

Atorvastatin chewable tabs, 24, C, muscle effects, see BNF

Atorvastatin tabs, C, muscle effects, see BNF

Atovaquone, 21

Atripla, 23, 25

Atrovent inhalations, C, administration

Augmentin Duo, 9

Augmentin susp and tabs, 9

Aureocort, 28, C, application, see BNF

Avelox, 6, 9, C, driving

Avloclor, 5, C, malaria prophylaxis, see BNF

Avodart, 25

Avomine, 2

Axitinib, 21

Axorid, 21, 25

Azathioprine, 21

Azithromycin caps, 5, 9, 23

Azithromycin susp and tabs, 5, 9

Azzalure, C, side-effects, see BNF

Baclofen, 2, 8, 21

Balsalazide, 21, 25

Baraclude, C, administration

Beclometasone external preps, 28, C, application, see BNF

Beclometasone inhalations, 8, C, administration; with high doses, 10, steroid card

Bedaquiline, 4, 8, 21, C, driving

Benemid, 12, 21, 27

Benperidol, 2

Benzoin tincture, compound, 15

Besavar XL, 21, 25, C, initial dose, driving, see BNF

Beta-Adalat, 8, 25

Betacap, 15, 28, C, application, see BNF

Beta-Cardone, 8

Betahistine, 21

Betamethasone external preps, 28, C, application, see BNF

Betamethasone inj, 10, steroid card

Betamethasone plaster, C, application, see BNF

Betamethasone scalp application, 15, 28, C, application, see BNF

Betamethasone soluble tab, 10, steroid card, 13, 21, (when used as a mouthwash, Label: 10, 13, C, administration)

Betesil, C, application, see BNF

Bethanechol, 22

Betmiga, 25

Betnesol injection, 10, steroid card

Betnovate external preps, 28, C, application, see BNF

Betnovate scalp application, 15, 28, C, application, see BNF

Betnovate-RD, 28, C, application, see BNF

Bettamousse, 28, C, application, see BNF

Bezafibrate, 21

Bezafibrate m/r, 21, 25

Bezalip, 21

Bezalip-Mono, 21, 25

Bimatoprost, C, see BNF

Bilastine, 23, C, administration

BindRen gran, 21, C, avoid other drugs at the same time, see BNF

BindRen tabs, 21, 25, C, avoid other drugs at the same time, see BNF

Biorphen, C, driving

Bisacodyl tabs, 5, 25

Bisoprolol, 8

Boceprevir, 21

Bocouture, C, side-effects, see BNF

Bondronat tabs, C, administration, see BNF

Bonefos caps and tabs, C, food and calcium, see BNF

Bonviva tabs, C, administration, see BNF

Bosulif, 21

Bosutinib, 21

Botox, C, side-effects, see BNF

Botulinum toxin type A, C, side-effects, see BNF

Botulinum toxin type B, C, side-effects, see BNF

Breakyl, 2, C, administration, see BNF

Brexidol, 21

Bricanyl inhalations, C, administration

Brimonidine tartrate gel, 28

Britlofex, 2

Bromocriptine, 10, 21, C, driving, see BNF

Bronchitol, C, administration

Brufen, 21

Brufen gran, 13, 21

Brufen Retard, 25, 27

Buccastem, 2, C, administration, see BNF

Buccolam, 2, C, administration

Budelin Novolizer, 8, C, administration; with high doses, 10, steroid card

Budenofalk caps, 5, 10, steroid card, 22, 25

Budenofalk gran, 5, 10, steroid card, 22, 25, C, administration

Budesonide caps, 5, 10, steroid card, 22, 25

Budesonide gran, 5, 10, steroid card, 22, 25, C, administration

Budesonide inhalations, 8, C, administration; with high doses, 10, steroid card

Budesonide nebs, 8, 10, steroid card, C, administration

Budesonide m/r caps, 5, 10, steroid card, 25

Buprenorphine patches, 2

Buprenorphine tabs, 2, 26

Bupropion, 25, C, driving

Buserelin nasal spray, C, nasal decongestants, see BNF

Buspirone, C, driving

BuTrans, 2

Bydureon, 10, C, administration, see BNF

Byetta, 10, C, administration, see BNF

Cabaser, 10, 21, C, driving, see BNF

Cabergoline, 10, 21, C, driving, see BNF

Cabozantinib, 25, C, driving, see BNF

Cacit, 13

Cacit D3, 13

Calceos, 24

Calcichew-D₃ tabs, chewable, 24

Calcichew tabs, chewable, 24

Calcium-500, 25

Calcium acetate caps, C, with meals

Calcium acetate tabs, 25, C, with meals, see BNF

Calcium carbonate tabs, chewable, 24

Calcium carbonate tabs and gran effervescent, 13

Calcium gluconate effervescent tabs, 13

Calcium phosphate sachets, 13

Calcium Resonium, 13

Calcium and ergocalciferol tabs, C, administration, see BNF

Calcort, 5, 10, steroid card

Calfovit D3, 13, 21

Calmurid HC, 28, C, application, see BNF

Camcolit 250 tabs, 10, lithium card, C, driving, fluid and salt intake, toxicity symptoms, see BNF

Camcolit 400 tabs, 10, lithium card, 25, C, driving, fluid and salt intake, toxicity symptoms, see BNF

Campral EC, 21, 25

Canagliflozin, C, volume depletion, see BNF

Canesten HC, 28, C, application, see BNF

Canesten spray, 15

Cannabis sativa extract, C, driving, see BNF

Capecitabine, 21

Capexion, 23, C, driving, see BNF

Capimune, C, administration, see BNF

Caprelsa, Alert card

Caprin, 5, 25, 32

Capsorin, C, administration, see BNF

Caramet CR, 10, 14, 25, C, driving, see BNF

Carbaglu, 13

Carbamazepine chewable, 3, 8, 21, 24, C, blood, hepatic or skin disorder symptoms, driving, see BNF

Carbamazepine liq, supps and tabs, 3, 8, C, blood, hepatic or skin disorder symptoms, driving, see BNF

Carbamazepine m/r, 3, 8, 25, C, blood, hepatic or skin disorder symptoms, driving, see BNF

Carbimazole, C, blood disorder symptoms, see BNF

Cardene SR, 25

Cardura, C, initial dose, driving

Cardura XL, 25, C, initial dose, driving

Carglumic acid, 13

Carvedilol, 8

Catapres, 3, 8

Cefaclor, 9

Cefaclor m/r, 9, 21, 25

Cefadroxil, 9

Cefalexin, 9

Cefixime, 9

Cefradine, 9

Cefuroxime susp, 9, 21

Cefuroxime tab, 9, 21, 25

Celectol, 8, 22

Celevac (constipation or diarrhoea), C, administration, see BNF

Celiprolol, 8, 22

Ceporex, 9

Certolizumab pegol, 10, Alert card, C, tuberculosis, blood disorders

Cetirizine, C, driving

Champix, 3

Chemydur 60XL, 25

Chloral hydrate, 19, 27

Chloral mixt, 19, 27

Chloral paed elixir, 1, 27

Chlordiazepoxide, 2

Chloroquine, 5, C, malaria prophylaxis, see BNF

Chlorphenamine, 2

Chlorpromazine solution, supps and tabs, 2, 11

Cholera vaccine (oral), C, administration

Cholestagel, 21, C, avoid other drugs at same time, see BNF

Ciclesonide, 8, C, administration

Ciclosporin, C, administration, see BNF

Cilostazol, C, blood disorders, see BNF

Cimzia, 10, Alert card, C, tuberculosis, blood disorders

Cinacalcet, 21

Cinnarizine, 2

Cipralex drops, C, driving, administration

Cipralex tabs, C, driving

Cipramil drops, C, driving, administration

Cipramil tabs, C, driving

Ciprofloxacin, 7, 9, 25, C, driving

Ciproxin susp and tabs, 7, 9, 25, C, driving

Circadin, 2, 21, 25

Citalopram drops, C, driving, administration

Citalopram tabs, C, driving

CitraFleet, 10, patient information leaflet, 13, C, administration

Citramag, 10, patient information leaflet, 13, C, administration

Clarelux, 15, 28, C, application, see BNF

Clarithromycin, 9

Clarithromycin m/r, 9, 21, 25

Clarithromycin sachets, 9, 13

Clasteon, C, food and calcium, see BNF

Clemastine, 2

Clenil Modulite, 8, C, administration; with high doses, 10, steroid card

Clindamycin, 9, 27, C, diarrhoea, see BNF

Clipper, 25

Clobazam, 2 or 19, 8, C, driving, see BNF

Clobetasol external preps, 28, C, application, see BNF

Clobetasol scalp application, 15, 28, C, application, see BNF

Clobetasone butyrate, 28, C, application, see BNF

Clofazimine, 8, 14, (urine red), 21

Clomethiazole, 19

Clomipramine, 2

DHC Continus, 2, 25
Diamicron MR, 25
Diamorphine preps, 2
Diamox SR, 3, 25
Diamox tabs, 3
Diazepam, 2 or 19
Diclofenac diethylammonium gel, C, photosensitivity, see BNF
Diclofenac epolamine gel patch, C, photosensitivity, see BNF
Diclofenac potassium, 21
Diclofenac sodium dispersible tabs, 13, 21
Diclofenac sodium e/c, 5, 25
Diclofenac sodium m/r, 21, 25
Diclofenac sodium spray, C, photosensitivity, see BNF
Diclomax 75 mg SR and Retard, 21, 25
Didanosine e/c caps, 25, C, administration
Didanosine tabs, 23, C, administration
Didronel, C, food and calcium, see BNF
Differin, 11
Diflclir, 9
Diflucan 50 and 200 mg, 9
Diflucan susp, 9
Diflucortolone external preps, 28, C, application, see BNF
Digoxin elixir, C, use of pipette
Dihydrocodeine, 2
Dihydrocodeine m/r, 2, 25
Dilcardia SR, 25
Diloxanide, 9
Diltiazem, 25
Dilzem preps, 25
Dimethyl fumarate, 21, 25
Dioderm, 28, C, application, see BNF
Dipentum, 21, C, blood disorder symptoms, see BNF
Diprosalic, 28, C, application, see BNF
Diprosone, 28, C, application, see BNF
Dipyridamole, 22
Dipyridamole m/r, 21, 25
Disipal, C, driving
Disopyramide m/r, 25
Distaclor, 9
Distaclor MR, 9, 21, 25
Distamine, 6, 22, C, blood disorder symptoms, see BNF
Disulfiram, 2, C, alcohol reaction, see BNF
Dithranol preps, 28
Dithrocream preps, 28
Dithrolan, 28
Ditropan, 3
Diumide-K Continus, 25, 27
Dolmatil, 2
Dolocodon PR, 2, 25
Dolutegravir, C, antacids
Domperidone, 22, C, arrhythmias
Donepezil orodispersible tabs, C, administration

Doralese, 2
Dostinex, 10, 21, C, driving, see BNF
Dosulepin, 2
Dovobet, 28
Doxazosin, C, initial dose, driving
Doxazosin m/r, 25, C, initial dose, driving
Doxepin, 2
Doxepin topical, 2, 10, patient information leaflet
Doxycycline caps, 6, 9, 11, 27, C, posture, see BNF
Doxycycline caps m/r, 6, 11, 27, C, posture, see BNF
Doxycycline dispersible tabs, 6, 9, 11, 13
Doxycycline tabs, 6, 11, 27, C, posture, see BNF
Dozic, 2
Driclor, 15
Dronedarone, 21, C, hepatic disorders, heart failure, see BNF
Dukoral, C, administration
Duloxetine, 2
Duodopa, 10, 14, (urine reddish), C, driving, see BNF
Duofilm, 15
DuoTrav, C, see BNF
Duraphat toothpaste, C, administration
Durogesic DTrans, 2, C, administration
Dutasteride, 25
Dyazide, 14, (urine blue in some lights), 21
Dysport, C, side-effects, see BNF

Easyhaler Salbutamol, C, administration
Eculizumab, C, meningococcal infection, patient information card
Edronax, C, driving
Edurant, 21, 25, C, antacids
Efavirenz caps and tabs, 23
Efcortesol, 10, steroid card
Efexor XL, 3, 21, 25, C, driving
Effentora, 2, C, administration, see BNF
Efracea, 6, 11, 27, C, posture, see BNF
Eklira Genuair, C, administration
Elantan LA, 25
Eldepryl, C, driving, see BNF
Eletriptan tabs, 3
Elidel, 4, 11, 28
Elleste Solo MX patches, C, administration, see BNF
Elocon, 28, C, application, see BNF
Eltrombopag, C, other drugs, see BNF
Elvanse, 3, 25, C, administration, driving, see BNF
Elvitegravir, see preps
Emeside, 8, C, blood disorder symptoms, driving, see BNF
Emflex, 21, C, driving

Emozul, C, administration
Emselex, 3, 25
Enbrel, 10, Alert card, C, tuberculosis, blood disorders, see BNF
En-De-Kay mouthwash, C, food and drink, see BNF
Enfuvirtide, C, hypersensitivity reactions, see BNF
Entacapone, 14, (urine reddishbrown), C, driving, avoid iron-containing preparations at the same time of day
Entecavir, C, administration
Entocort CR, 5, 10, steroid card, 25
Enzalutamide, 25
Epanutin Infatabs, 8, 24, C, blood or skin disorder symptoms, driving, see BNF
Epanutin susp, 8, C, administration, blood or skin disorder symptoms, driving, see BNF
Epiduo, 11
Epilim Chrono, 8, 21, 25, C, pancreatitis, blood, or hepatic disorder symptoms, pregnancy, driving, see BNF
Epilim Chronosphere, 8, 21, 25, C, administration, pancreatitis, blood, or hepatic disorder symptoms, pregnancy, driving, see BNF
Epilim crushable tabs, liquid and syrup, 8, 21, C, pancreatitis, blood, or hepatic disorder symptoms, pregnancy, driving, see BNF
Epilim e/c tabs, 5, 8, 25, C, pancreatitis, blood, or hepatic disorder symptoms, pregnancy, driving, see BNF
Episenta, 8, 21, 25, C, administration, pancreatitis, blood, or hepatic disorder symptoms, pregnancy, driving, see BNF
Epival, 8, 21, 25, C, pancreatitis, blood, or hepatic disorder symptoms, pregnancy, driving, see BNF
Eprosartan, 21
Equasym XL, 25, C, driving
Ergotamine, 18, C, dosage
Erivedge, 25, C, pregnancy and contraception
Erlotinib, 23
Erymax, 5, 9, 25
Erythrocin, 9
Erythromycin caps, 5, 9, 25
Erythromycin ethyl succinate, 9
Erythromycin stearate tabs, 9
Erythromycin tabs, 5, 9, 25
Erythroped, 9
Erythroped A tabs, 9
Esbriet, 21, 25, C, driving
Escitalopram drops, C, driving, administration
Escitalopram tabs, C, driving
Eslicarbazepine, 8, C, driving

Esomeprazole caps, C, administration

Esomeprazole granules, 25, C, administration

Esomeprazole tabs, C, administration

Estracyt, 5, 23, C, administration, see BNF

Estraderm MX, C, administration, see BNF

Estraderm TTS, C, administration, see BNF

Estradot, C, administration, see BNF

Estramustine, 5, 23, C, administration, see BNF

Estring, 10, patient information leaflet

Etanercept, 10, Alert card, C, tuberculosis, blood disorders, see BNF

Ethambutol, 8

Ethibide XL, 25

Ethosuximide, 8, C, blood disorder symptoms, driving, see BNF

Etidronate disodium, C, food and calcium, see BNF

Etodolac m/r, 25

Etonogestrel implant, C, see patient information leaflet

Etoposide caps, 23

Etravirine, 21, C, rash and hypersensitivity reactions

Etrivex, 28, C, application, see BNF

Eucreas, 21

Eumovate external preps, 28, C, application, see BNF

Eurartesim, C, administration

Everolimus, 25, C, pneumonitis, see BNF

Eviplera, 21, 25, C, antacids

Evorel preps, C, administration, see BNF

Exelon caps, 21, 25

Exelon patches, C, administration, see BNF

Exelon solution, 21

Exemestane, 21

Exenatide, 10, C, administration, see BNF

Exjade, 13, 22, C, administration, see BNF

Famciclovir, 9

Fampridine, 23, 25

Fampyra, 23, 25

Famvir, 9

Fasigyn, 4, 9, 21, 25

Faverin, C, driving, see BNF

Fefol, 25

Felbinac foam, 15, C, photosensitivity, see BNF

Felbinac gel, C, photosensitivity, see BNF

Feldene caps, 21

Feldene gel, C, photosensitivity, see BNF

Feldene Melt, 10, patient information leaflet, 21

Felodipine m/r, 25

FemSeven, C, administration, see BNF

Fenbid Forte gel, C, photosensitivity, see BNF

Fenofibrate, 21

Fenoprofen, 21

Fenopron, 21

Fentanyl buccal films, 2, C, administration, see BNF

Fentanyl buccal tablets, 2, C, administration, see BNF

Fentanyl lozenges, 2

Fentanyl nasal spray, 2, C, administration, see BNF

Fentanyl patches, 2, C, administration

Fentanyl sublingual tablets, 2, 26

Fentazin, 2

Feospan, 25

Ferriprox, 14, C, blood disorders

Ferrograd, 25

Ferrograd C, 25

Ferrograd Folic, 25

Ferrous salts m/r, see preps

Fesoterodine, 3, 25

Fexofenadine, 5, C, driving

Fidaxomicin, 9

Filnarine SR, 2, 25

Firdapse, 3, 21

Flagyl supps, 4, 9

Flagyl tabs, 4, 9, 21, 25, 27

Flamasacard, 25, 32

Flavoxate, 3

Flecainide m/r, 25

Fleet Phospho-soda, 10, patient information leaflet, C, administration

Flixotide, 8, C, administration; with high doses, 10, steroid card

Flomaxtra XL, 25, C, driving, see BNF

Florinef, 10, steroid card

Flotros, 23

Floxapen, 9, 23

Fluanxol, 2, C, administration, driving, see BNF

Flucloxacillin, 9, 23

Fluconazole 50 and 200 mg, 9

Fluconazole susp, 9

Fludrocortisone, 10, steroid card

Fludroxycortide external preps, 28, C, application, see BNF

Fluocinolone external preps, 28, C, application, see BNF

Fluocinonide external preps, 28, C, application, see BNF

Fluocortolone external preps, 28, C, application, see BNF

Fluorigard mouthwash, C, food and drink, see BNF

Fluoxetine, C, driving, see BNF

Fluoxetine dispersible tablets, 10, C, administration, driving, see BNF

Flupentixol, see preps

Flurazepam, 19

Flurbiprofen, 21

Fluticasone external preps, 28, C, application, see BNF

Fluticasone inhalations, 8, C, administration; with high doses, 10, steroid card

Flutiform, 8, C, administration; with high doses, 10, steroid card

Fluvastatin, C, muscle effects, see BNF

Fluvastatin m/r, 25, C, muscle effects, see BNF

Fluvoxamine, C, driving, see BNF

Foradil, C, administration

Forceval caps, 25

Formoterol fumarate, C, administration

Fortipine LA 40, 21, 25

Fortral caps and tabs, 2, 21

Fosamax, C, administration, see BNF

Fosamprenavir susp, C, administration, see BNF

Fosavance, C, administration, see BNF

Fosfomycin granules, 9, 13, 23

Fosrenol powder, 21, C, administration, see BNF

Fosrenol tabs, 21, C, to be chewed

Fostair, 8, C, administration; with high doses, 10, steroid card

Frisium, 2 or 19, 8, C, driving, see BNF

Froben, 21

Frovatriptan, 3

Frusene, 14, (urine blue in some lights)

Fucibet, 28, C, application, see BNF

Fucidin H, 28, C, application, see BNF

Fucidin susp, 9, 21

Fucidin tabs, 9

Fuzeon, C, hypersensitivity reactions, see BNF

Fybogel, 13, C, administration, see BNF

Fybogel Mebeverine, 13, 22, C, administration, see BNF

Fycompa, 3, 8, 25, C, driving, see BNF

Gabapentin, 3, 5, 8, C, driving, see BNF

Gabitril, 21

Galantamine, 3, 21

Galantamine m/r, 3, 21, 25

Galsya m/r, 3, 21, 25

Ganciclovir, 21

Ganfort, C, see BNF

Gatalin XL, 3, 21, 25

Gemfibrozil, 22

Giotrif, 25, C, administration, driving, see BNF

Gliclazide m/r, 25

Glivec, 21, 27

Klaricid, 9
Klaricid sachets, 9, 13
Klaricid XL, 9, 21, 25
Klean-Prep, 10, patient information leaflet, 13, C, administration
Komboglyze, 21
Kuvan, 13, 21, C, administration, see BNF
Kwells, 2

Labetalol, 8, 21
Lacosamlde tabs, 8, C, driving, see BNF
Lamictal dispersible tabs, 8, 13, C, driving, skin reactions, see BNF
Lamictal tabs, 8, C, driving, skin reactions, see BNF
Lamisil, 9
Lamotrigine dispersible tabs, 8, 13, C, driving, skin reactions, see BNF
Lamotrigine tabs, 8, C, driving, skin reactions, see BNF
Lanoxin-PG elixir, C, use of pipette
Lansoprazole caps, 5, 22, 25
Lansoprazole oro-dispersible tabs, 5, 22, C, administration, see BNF
Lanthanum powder, 21, C, administration, see BNF
Lanthanum tabs, 21, C, to be chewed
Lapatinib, C, see BNF
Largactil, 2, 11
Lariam, 21, 27, C, driving, malaria prophylaxis, see BNF
Latanoprost, C, see BNF
Latuda, 2, 21, 25
Laxido Orange, 13
Leflunomide, 4
Lenalidomide, 25, C, pregnancy and contraception, symptoms of thromboembolism, neutropenia, and thrombocytopenia, see BNF
Lercanidipine, 22
Lescol, C, muscle effects, see BNF
Lescol XL, 25, C, muscle effects, see BNF
Levetiracetam, 8
Levocetirizine, C, driving
Levofloxacin, 6, 9, 25, C, driving
Levomepromazine, 2
Li-Liquid, 10, lithium card, C, driving, fluid and salt intake, toxicity symptoms, see BNF
Linaclotide, 22
Linezolid susp and tabs, 9, 10, patient information leaflet
Lioresal, 2, 8, 21
Lipantil, 21
Lipitor chewable tablets, 24, C, muscle effects, see BNF
Lipitor tabs, C, muscle effects, see BNF

Lipostat, C, muscle effects, see BNF
Liquid paraffin, C, administration, see BNF
Liraglutide, C, administration
Lisdexamfetamine, 3, 25, C, administration, driving, see BNF
Liskonum, 10, lithium card, 25, C, driving, fluid and salt intake, toxicity symptoms, see BNF
Lithium carbonate, 10, lithium card, C, driving, fluid and salt intake, toxicity symptoms, see BNF
Lithium carbonate m/r, 10, lithium card, 25, C, driving, fluid and salt intake, toxicity symptoms, see BNF
Lithium citrate liq, 10, lithium card, C, driving, fluid and salt intake, toxicity symptoms, see BNF
Lithonate, 10, lithium card, 25, C, driving, fluid and salt intake, toxicity symptoms, see BNF
Lixisenatide, 10, C, administration, see BNF
Loceryl, 10, patient information leaflet
Locoid cream, oint, and topical emulsion, 28, C, application, see BNF
Locoid scalp lotion, 15, 28, C, application, see BNF
Lodotra, 10, steroid card, 21, 25
Lofepramine, 2
Lofexidine, 2
Longtec, 2, 25
Lopid, 22
Loprazolam, 19
Lopresor, 8
Lopresor SR, 8, 25
Loramyc C, 10, C, administration, see BNF
Loratadine, C, driving
Lorazepam, 2 or 19
Lormetazepam, 19
Loron tabs, 10, patient information leaflet, C, food and calcium, see BNF
Losec, C, administration, see BNF
Lotprosin XL, 3, 21, 25
Lotriderm, 28, C, application, see BNF
Lubiprostone, 21
Lugol's solution, 27
Lumigan, C, see BNF
Lurasidone, 2, 21, 25
Lustral, C, driving, see BNF
Lyclear Dermal cream, 10, patient information leaflet
Lymecycline, 6, 9
Lyrica, 3, 8, C, driving
Lysodren, 2, 10, 21, C, driving, adrenal suppression
Lysovir, C, driving

Lyxumia, 10, C, administration, see BNF

Macitentan, C, hepatotoxicity, patient card, see BNF
Macrobid, 9, 14, (urine yellow or brown), 21, 25
Macrogol oral concentrate, 13, C, administration
Macrogols oral powder, see preps
Madopar, 10, 14, (urine reddish), 21, C, driving, see BNF
Madopar CR, 5, 10, 14, (urine reddish), 25, C, driving, see BNF
Madopar dispersible tabs, 10, 14, (urine reddish), 21, C, administration, driving, see BNF
Magnapen, 9, 22
Magnesium citrate effervescent pdr, 10, patient information leaflet, 13, C, administration
Magnesium sulphate, 13, 23
Malarivon, 5, C, malaria prophylaxis
Malarone preps, 21, C, malaria prophylaxis
Manerix, 10, patient information leaflet, 21
Manevac, 25, 27
Mannitol inhalation, C, administration
Marevan, 10, anticoagulant card
Maxalt, 3
Maxalt Melt, 3, C, administration
Maxepa, 21
Maxolon SR, 25
Mebeverine, C, administration, see BNF
Mecasermin, C, administration, see BNF
Medikinet XL, 25, C, driving, see BNF
Medrone tabs, 10, steroid card, 21
Mefenamic acid caps, paed susp, and tabs, 21
Mefloquine, 21, 27, C, driving, malaria prophylaxis, see BNF
Melatonin, 2, 21, 25
Meloxicam tabs, 21
Mepacrine, 4, 9, 14, 21
Meprobamate, 2
Meptazinol, 2
Meptid, 2
Mercaptamine, 21
Mesalazine e/c, see preps
Mesalazine enema and supps, C, blood disorder symptoms, see BNF
Mesalazine gran, see preps
Mesalazine m/r, see preps
Metformin m/r, 21, 25
Metformin solution and tabs, 21
Methadone, 2
Methadose, 2
Methenamine, 9

Methocarbamol, 2

Methotrexate tabs, C, dose, treatment booklet, NSAIDs, see BNF

Methylcellulose (constipation or diarrhoea), C, administration, see BNF

Methyldopa, 3, 8

Methylphenidate, C, driving, see BNF

Methylphenidate m/r, 25, C, driving, see BNF

Methylprednisolone inj, 10, steroid card

Methylprednisolone tabs, 10, steroid card, 21

Metirosine, 2

Metoclopramide m/r, 25

Metoclopramide oral solution, C, use of pipette

Metopirone, 21, C, driving

Metoprolol, 8

Metoprolol m/r, 8, 25

Metosyn cream and oint, 28, C, application, see BNF

Metrolyl supps, 4, 9

Metronidazole mixt, 4, 9

Metronidazole supps, 4, 9

Metronidazole tabs, 4, 9, 21, 25, 27

Metyrapone, 21, C, driving

Mezavant XL, 21, 25, C, blood disorder symptoms, see BNF

Mianserin, 2, 25

Micanol, 28

Miconazole buccal tabs, 10, C, administration, see BNF

Miconazole oral gel, 9, C, hold in mouth, after food

Miconazole spray powder, 15

Midazolam oromucosal solution, 2, C, administration

Midrid, 30, C, dosage

Mifegyne, 10, patient information leaflet

Mifepristone, 10, patient information leaflet

Migard, 3

Migraleve, 2, (pink tablets), 17, 30

Migril, 2, 18, C, dosage

Mildison, 28, C, application, see BNF

Mimpara, 21

Minocin MR, 6, 25

Minocycline, 6, 9, C, posture, see BNF

Minocycline m/r, 6, 25

Mintec, 5, 22, 25

Mirabegron, 25

Mirapexin, 10, C, driving, see BNF

Mirapexin Prolonged Release, 10, 25, C, driving, see BNF

Mirtazapine oral solution, 2

Mirtazapine orodispersible tablets, 2, C, administration, see BNF

Mirtazapine tabs, 2, 25

Mirvaso, 28

Misofen, 21, 25

Misoprostol, 21

Mitotane, 2, 10, 21, C, driving, adrenal suppression

Mizolastine, 25, C, driving

Mizollen, 25, C, driving

Mobiflex, 21

Moclobemide, 10, patient information leaflet, 21

Modigraf, 13, 23, C, driving, see BNF

Modisal XL, 25

Modrasone, 28, C, application, see BNF

Molaxole, 13

Molipaxin, 2, 21

Mometasone external preps, 28, C, application, see BNF

Mometasone inhaler, 8, 10, steroid card, C, administration

Monomax SR, 25

Monomax XL, 25

Monomil XL, 25

Monopost, C, see BNF

Monosorb XL, 25

Montelukast chewable tabs, 23, 24

Montelukast granules, C, administration

Morphgesic SR, 2, 25

Morphine m/r caps and tabs, see preps

Morphine m/r susp, 2, 13

Morphine preps, 2

Motifene, 25

Motilium, 22, C, arrhythmias

Movicol oral concentrate, 13, C, administration

Movicol oral powder preps, 13, C, administration

Moviprep, 10, patient information leaflet, 13, C, administration

Moxifloxacin, 6, 9, C, driving

Moxisylyte, 21

Moxonidine, 3

MST Continus susp, 2, 13

MST Continus tabs, 2, 25

Multaq, 21, C, hepatic disorders, heart failure, see BNF

MXL, 2, C, administration, see BNF

Mycobutin, 8, 14, (urine orange-red), C, soft lenses

Mycophenolic acid, 25

Myfortic, 25

Myocrisin inj, 11, C, blood disorder symptoms, see BNF

Myotonine Chloride, 22

Nabilone, 2, C, behavioural effects, see BNF

Nabumetone, 21

Nabumetone susp, 21

Nadolol, 8

Nafarelin spray, 10, patient information leaflet, C, nasal decongestants, see BNF

Naftidrofuryl, 25, 27

Nalcrom, 22, C, administration, see BNF

Nalidixic acid, 9, 11

Nalmefene, 25

Napratec, 21

Naprosyn EC, 5, 25

Naprosyn tabs, 21

Naproxen e/c, 5, 25

Naproxen tabs, 21

Naramig, 3

Naratriptan, 3

Nardil, 3, 10, patient information leaflet

Natecal D3, 24

Natrilix SR, 25

Navelbine caps, 21, 25

Nebilet, 8

Nebivolol, 8

Nedocromil sodium inhalation, 8, C, administration

Nefopam, 2, 14, (urine pink)

Neoclarityn, C, driving

Neoral, C, administration, see BNF

Neotigason, 10, patient information leaflet, 11, 21

Nerisone, 28, C, application, see BNF

Nerisone Forte, 28, application, see BNF

Neulactil, 2

Neupro, 10, C, driving

NeuroBloc, C, side-effects, see BNF

Neurontin, 3, 5, 8, C, driving, see BNF

Nevirapine, C, hypersensitivity reactions

Nevirapine m/r, 25, C, hypersensitivity reactions

Nexavar, 23

Nexium granules, 25, C, administration

Nexium tabs, C, administration

Niaspan, 21, 25

Nicardipine m/r, 25

Nicorette gum, C, administration, see BNF

Nicorette Inhalator, C, administration, see BNF

Nicorette lozenge, C, administration, see BNF

Nicorette Microtab, 26, C, administration, see BNF

Nicorette nasal spray, C, administration, see BNF

Nicorette patches, C, administration, see BNF

Nicorette Quickmist oral spray, C, administration, see BNF

Nicotine (inhaled), C, administration, see BNF

Nicotine (lozenges), C, administration, see BNF

Nicotine (patches), C, administration, see BNF

Nicotine (sublingual), 26, C, administration, see BNF

Physiotens, 3

Picolax, 10, patient information leaflet, 13, C, solution, see BNF

Pilocarpine tabs, 21, 27, C, driving

Pimecrolimus, 4, 11, 28

Pimozide, 2

Pindolol, 8

Piperaquine with artenimol, C, administration

Piracetam, 3

Pirfenidone, 21, 25, C, driving

Piriton, 2

Piroxicam caps and tabs, 21

Piroxicam dispersible tabs, 13, 21

Piroxicam gel, C, photosensitivity, see BNF

Pivmecillinam, 9, 21, 27, C, posture, see BNF

Pizotifen, 2

Plaquenil, 21, C, antacids, see BNF

Plenadren, 10, steroid card, 22, 25

Plendil, 25

Pletal, C, blood disorders, see BNF

Podophyllin paint cpd, 15, C, application, see BNF

Pomalidomide, 3, 25, C, pregnancy and contraception, symptoms of thromboembolism, neutropenia, and thrombocytopenia, see BNF

Ponatinib, 3, 25

Ponstan, 21

Posaconazole susp, 3, 9, 21

Posaconazole e/c tabs, 3, 9, 25

Potaba caps, 21

Potaba Envules, 13, 21

Potassium chloride m/r, see preps

Potassium citrate mixt, 27

Potassium effervescent tabs, 13, 21

Powergel, C, photosensitivity, see BNF

Pradaxa, 25

Pramipexole, 10, C, driving, see BNF

Pramipexole m/r, 10, 25, C, driving, see BNF

Pravastatin, C, muscle effects, see BNF

Praxilene, 25, 27

Prazosin, C, initial dose, driving, see BNF

Prednisolone e/c, 5, 10, steroid card, 25

Prednisolone inj, 10, steroid card

Prednisone m/r, 10, steroid card, 21, 25

Prednisolone soluble, 10, steroid card, 13, 21

Prednisolone tabs, 10, steroid card, 21

Pregabalin, 3, 8, C, driving

Preservex, 21

Prestim, 8

Prestylon, 21

Prezista, 21, C, missed dose, see BNF

Priadel liq, 10, lithium card, C, driving, fluid and salt intake, toxicity symptoms, see BNF

Priadel tabs, 10, lithium card, 25, C, driving, fluid and salt intake, toxicity symptoms, see BNF

Priligy, 2, 25, C, postural hypotension, see BNF

Primidone, 2, 8, C, driving, see BNF

Pro-Banthine, 23

Procarbazine, 4

Prochlorperazine, 2

Prochlorperazine buccal tabs, 2, C, administration, see BNF

Procyclidine, C, driving

Progesterone (micronised), C, administration, see BNF

Prograf, 23, C, driving, see BNF

Proguanil, 21, C, malaria prophylaxis, see BNF

Progynova TS preps, C, administration, see BNF

Promazine, 2

Promethazine, 2

Propafenone, 21, 25, C, driving

Propantheline, 23

Propiverine hydrochloride, 3

Propiverine hydrochloride m/r, 3, 25

Propranolol m/r, 8, 25

Propranolol oral solution and tabs, 8

Protelos, 5, 13, C, administration, see BNF

Prothiaden, 2

Protopic, 4, 11, 28

Prozac, C, driving, see BNF

Psorin, 28

Pulmicort, 8, C, administration; with high doses, 10, steroid card

Pulmicort Respules, 8, 10, steroid card, C, dose

Pulvinal Salbutamol, C, administration

Pyrazinamide, 8

Questran preps, 13, C, avoid other drugs at same time, see BNF

Quetiapine, 2

Quetiapine m/r, 2, 23, 25

Quinagolide, 10, 21, C, driving, see BNF

Qvar preps, 8, C, administration; with high doses, 10, steroid card

Rabeprazole, 25

Racecadotril gran, C, administration

Raltegravir chewable, 24

Raltegravir tabs, 25

Ranexa, 25, patient alert card

Ranitidine effervescent tabs, 13

Ranolazine, 25, patient alert card

Rapamune, C, administration

Rasilez, 21

Rebetol, 21

Recivit, 2, 26, C, administration, see BNF

Reboxetine, C, driving

Regorafenib, 21, C, administration, see BNF

Regulan, 13, C, administration, see BNF

Regurin, 23

Regurin XL, 23, 25

Relifex, 21

Relifex susp, 21

Relpax, 3

Relvar Ellipta, 8, C, administration, 10, steroid card

Remedeine, 2, 29, 30

Remicade, 10, Alert card, C, tuberculosis, blood disorders, and hypersensitivity reactions

Reminyl, 3, 21

Reminyl XL, 3, 21, 25

Renacet, 25, C, with meals, avoid other drugs at the same time, see BNF

Renagel, 25, C, with meals

Renvela sachets, 13, C, with meals

Renvela tabs, 25, C, with meals

Repinex XL, 10, 25, C, driving, see BNF

Requip, 10, 21, C, driving, see BNF

Requip XL, 10, 25, C, driving, see BNF

Resonium A, 13

Restandol, 21, 25

Retapamulin, 28

Retigabine, 8, 14, 25 C, driving, see BNF

Retrovir oral solution, C, use of oral syringe

Revlimid, 25, C, pregnancy and contraception, symptoms of thromboembolism, neutropenia, and thrombocytopenia, see BNF

Revolade, C, other drugs, see BNF

Reyataz, 5, 21

Riamet, 21, C, driving

Ribavirin caps, tabs, and solution, 21

Rifabutin, 8, 14, (urine orange-red), C, soft lenses

Rifadin, 8, 14, (urine orange-red), 22, C, soft lenses

Rifampicin caps and syrup, 8, 14, (urine orange-red), 22, C, soft lenses

Rifater, 8, 14, (urine orange-red), 22, C, soft lenses

Rifaximin, see individual preparations

Rifinah, 8, 14, (urine orange-red), 22, C, soft lenses

Rilutek, C, blood disorders, driving

Rilpivirine, 21, 25, C, antacids

Rimactane, 8, 14, (urine orange-red), 22, C, soft lenses

Risedronate sodium, C, administration, food and calcium, see BNF

Risperdal liquid, 2, C, use of dose syringe

Risperdal orodispersible tabs, 2, C, administration, see BNF

Risperdal tabs, 2

Risperidone liquid, 2, C, use of dose syringe

Risperidone orodispersible tabs, 2, C, administration, see BNF

Risperidone tabs, 2

Ritalin, C, driving, see BNF

Ritonavir oral solution, 21, C, administration, see BNF

Ritonavir tabs, 21, 25

Rivastigmine caps, 21, 25

Rivastigmine oral solution, 21

Rivastigmine patches, C, administration, see BNF

Rizatriptan tabs, 3

Rizatriptan orodispersible tabs, 3, C, administration

Rizatriptan wafers, 3, C, administration

Roaccutane, 10, patient information leaflet, 11, 21

RoActemra, alert card, C, diverticular perforation, infection, see BNF

Robaxin, 2

Roflumilast, C, patient card

Romiplostim, C, driving

Ropinirole, 10, 21, C, driving, see BNF

Ropinirole m/r, 10, 25, C, driving, see BNF

Rosuvastatin, C, muscle effects, see BNF

Rotigotine, 10, C, driving

Rowachol, 22

Rowatinex caps, 25

Rufinamide, 8, 21, C, driving, see BNF

Rupafin, C, driving

Rupatadine, C, driving

Rythmodan Retard, 25

Sabril sachets, 3, 8, 13, C, driving, see BNF

Sabril tabs, 3, 8, C, driving, see BNF

Saflutan, C, see BNF

Salactol, 15

Salagen, 21, 27, C, driving

Salamol Easi-Breathe, C, administration

Salatac, 15

Salazopyrin, 14, (urine orange-yellow), C, blood disorder symptoms and soft lenses, see BNF

Salazopyrin EN-tabs, 5, 14, (urine orange-yellow), 25, C, blood disorder symptoms and soft lenses, see BNF

Salbulin Novolizer, C, administration

Salbutamol inhalations, C, administration

Salbutamol m/r, 25

Salicylic acid collodion, 15

Salmeterol, C, administration

Salofalk enema and supps, C, blood disorder symptoms, see BNF

Salofalk gran, 25, C, administration, blood disorder symptoms, see BNF

Salofalk tabs, 5, 25, C, blood disorder symptoms, see BNF

Sancuso, C, administration

Sandocal, 13

Sando-K, 13, 21

Sandrena, C, administration, see BNF

Sanomigran, 2

Sapropterin, 13, 21, C, administration, see BNF

Saquinavir, 21, C, arrhythmias

Sativex, C, driving, see BNF

Scopoderm TTS, 19, C, administration, see BNF

Sebivo, C, muscle effects

Sebomin MR, 6, 25

Sectral, 8

Securon SR, 25

Seebri Breezhaler, C, administration

Selegiline, C, driving, see BNF

Selegiline (freeze-dried tablets), C, administration, driving, see BNF

Selexid, 9, 21, 27, C, posture, see BNF

Selincro, 25

Septrin susp and tabs, 9

Seractil, 21

Serc, 21

Serenace, 2

Seretide 100 Accuhaler, 8, C, administration

Seretide 250- and 500-Accuhaler, 8, 10, steroid card, C, administration

Seretide 50 Evohaler, 8, C, administration

Seretide 125- and 250-Evohaler, 8, C, administration, 10, steroid card

Serevent, C, administration

Seroquel, 2

Seroquel XL, 2, 23, 25

Seroxat susp, 5, 21, C, driving

Seroxat tabs, 21, C, driving

Sertraline, C, driving, see BNF

Sevelamer carbonate sachets, 13, C, with meals

Sevelamer carbonate tabs, 25, C, with meals

Sevelamer hydrochloride, 25, C, with meals

Sevredol, 2

Sildenafil chewable tabs, 24

Simeprevir, 11, 21

Simeticone, see paediatric prep

Simponi, 10, Alert card, C, tuberculosis, blood disorders

Simvastatin, C, muscle effects, see BNF

Sinemet CR, 10, 14, (urine reddish), 25, C, driving, see BNF

Sinemet, 10, 14, (urine reddish), C, driving, see BNF

Sinepin, 2

Singulair chewable tabs, 23, 24

Singulair granules, C, administration

Sinthrome, 10, anticoagulant card

Sirolimus, C, administration

Sirturo, 4, 8, 21, C, driving

Slo-Phyllin, 25 or C, administration, see BNF

Sloprolol, 8, 25

Slow-Fe, 25

Slow-Fe Folic, 25

Slow-K, 25, 27, C, posture, see BNF

Slow Sodium, 25

Slow-Trasicor, 8, 25

Slozem, 25

Sodium aurothiomalate, 11, C, blood disorder symptoms, see BNF

Sodium chloride m/r, 25

Sodium chloride and glucose oral pdr, cpd, 13

Sodium clodronate, C, food and calcium, see BNF

Sodium cromoglicate (oral), 22, C, administration, see BNF

Sodium cromoglicate inhalation, 8, C, administration

Sodium fusidate susp, 9, 21

Sodium fusidate tabs, 9

Sodium oxybate, 13, 19, C, administration, driving, see BNF

Sodium picosulfate pdr, 10, patient information leaflet, 13, C, see BNF

Sodium valproate crushable tabs, liquid and syrup, 8, 21, C, pancreatitis, blood, or hepatic disorder symptoms, pregnancy, driving, see BNF

Sodium valproate e/c, 5, 8, 25, C, pancreatitis, blood, or hepatic disorder symptoms, pregnancy, driving, see BNF

Sodium valproate m/r and granules, 8, 21, 25, C, pancreatitis, blood, or hepatic disorder symptoms, pregnancy, driving, see BNF

Sofosbuvir, 21, 25

Solian, 2

Solifenacin, 3

Soliris, C, meningococcal infection, patient information card
Solpadol caps and caplets, 2, 29, 30
Solpadol Effervescent, 2, 13, 29, 30
Solu-Cortef, 10, steroid card
Solu-Medrone, 10, steroid card
Solvazinc, 13, 21
Sonata, 2
Sorafenib, 23
Sorbisterit, 13, 21
Sotacor, 8
Sotalol, 8
Sovaldi, 21, 25
Spiriva inhalations, C, administration
Spironolactone, 21
Sporanox caps, 5, 9, 21, 25, C, hepatotoxicity
Sporanox liq, 9, 23, C, administration, hepatotoxicity
Sprycel, 25
Stalevo, 10, 14, (urine reddish-brown), C, driving, see BNF
Stavudine, 23
Stelara, 10, C, tuberculosis, see BNF
Stelazine, 2
Stemetil, 2
Sterculia, C, administration, see BNF
Stilnoct, 19
Stivarga, 21, C, administration, see BNF
Strattera, 3
Striant SR, C, administration, see BNF
Stribild, 21, C, antacids
Striverdi Respimat, C, administration
Strontium, 5, 13, C, administration, see BNF
Stugeron, 2
Suboxone, 2, 26
Subutex, 2, 26
Sucralfate, 5
Sulfadiazine, 9, 27
Sulfasalazine, 14, (urine orange-yellow), C, blood disorder symptoms and soft lenses, see BNF
Sulfasalazine e/c, 5, 14, (urine orange-yellow), 25, C, blood disorder symptoms and soft lenses, see BNF
Sulfinpyrazone, 12, 21
Sulindac, 21
Sulpiride, 2
Sulpor, 2
Sumatriptan, 3, 10, patient information leaflet
Sunitinib, 14
Supralip, 21
Suprax, 9
Suprecur, C, nasal decongestants, see BNF
Suprefact nasal spray, C, nasal decongestants, see BNF

Surgam tabs, 21
Surgical spirit, 15
Surmontil, 2
Sustiva caps and tabs, 23
Sutent, 14
Sycrest, 2, 26, C, administration
Symbicort, 8, C, administration; with high doses, 10, steroid card
Symmetrel, C, driving
Synalar external preps, 28, C, application, see BNF
Synarel, 10, patient information leaflet, C, nasal decongestants, see BNF

Tacni, 23, C, driving, see BNF
Tacrolimus caps, 23, C, driving, see BNF
Tacrolimus granules, 13, 23, C, driving, see BNF
Tacrolimus topical, 4, 11, 28
Tafamidis, 25
Tafinlar, 23, 25, C, driving, see BNF
Tafluprost, C, see BNF
Tambocor XL, 25
Tamiflu, 9
Tamsulosin m/r, 25, C, driving, see BNF
Tapclob, 2, or 19, 8, C, driving, see BNF
Tapentadol, 2
Tapentadol m/r, 2, 25
Tarceva, 23
Targaxan, 14 (urine red)
Targinact, 2, 25
Tarivid, 6, 9, 11, C, driving
Tasigna, 23, 25, 27
Tasmar, 14, 25
Tavanic, 6, 9, 25, C, driving
Tavegil, 2
Tecfidera, 21, 25
Tegretol Chewtabs, 3, 8, 21, 24, C, blood, hepatic or skin disorder symptoms, driving, see BNF
Tegretol liq, supps and tabs, 3, 8, C, blood, hepatic or skin disorder symptoms, driving, see BNF
Tegretol Prolonged Release, 3, 8, 25, C, blood, hepatic or skin disorder symptoms, driving, see BNF
Telaprevir, 21, C, rash
Telbivudine, C, muscle effects
Telfast, 5, C, driving
Telithromycin, 9, C, driving, hepatic disorders
Telzir susp, C, administration, see BNF
Temazepam, 19
Temgesic, 2, 26
Temodal, 23, 25
Temozolomide, 23, 25
Tenif, 8, 25
Tenofovir granules, 21, C, administration

Tenofovir tabs, 21
Tenoret 50, 8
Tenoretic, 8
Tenormin, 8
Tenoxicam tabs, 21
Tensaid XL, 25
Tensipine MR, 25
Terazosin, C, initial dose, driving, see BNF
Terbinafine, 9
Terbutaline inhalations, C, administration
Terbutaline m/r, 25
Terra-Cortril, 28, C, application, see BNF
Testim, C, administration, see BNF
Testogel, C, administration, see BNF
Testosterone buccal tablets, C, administration, see BNF
Testosterone gel, C, administration, see BNF
Testosterone patch, C, administration, see BNF
Testosterone undecanoate caps, 21, 25
Tetrabenazine, 2
Tetracycline, 7, 9, 23, C, posture
Tetralysal preps, 6, 9
Teveten, 21
Teysuno, 23
Thalidomide, 2, C, pregnancy and contraception, symptoms of peripheral neuropathy, thromboembolism, neutropenia and thrombocytopenia, see BNF
Thalidomide Celgene, 2, C, pregnancy and contraception, symptoms of peripheral neuropathy and thromboembolism, neutropenia and thrombocytopenia, see BNF
Theophylline m/r, see preps
Tiagabine, 21
Tiaprofenic acid tabs, 21
Tilade, 8, C, administration
Tildiem preps, 25
Timodine, 28, C, application, see BNF
Timolol, 8
Tinidazole tabs, 4, 9, 21, 25
Tiotropium inhalations, C, administration
Tipranavir caps, 5, 21
Tipranavir oral solution, 5, 21, C, crystallisation
Tivicay, C, antacids
Tizanidine, 2, 8
Tobi Podhaler, C, administration
Tobramycin dry powder for inhalation, C, administration
Tocilizumab, alert card, C, diverticular perforation, infection, see BNF
Toctino, 10, patient information leaflet, 11, 21
Tolcapone, 14, 25
Tolfenamic acid, 21

Tolterodine, 3
Tolterodine m/r, 3, 25
Topamax Sprinkle, 3, 8, C, administration, driving, see BNF
Topamax tabs, 3, 8, C, driving, see BNF
Topiramate caps, 3, 8, C, driving, see BNF
Topiramate *Sprinkle* caps, 3, 8, C, administration, driving, see BNF
Topiramate tabs, 3, 8, C, driving, see BNF
Topotecan, 25
Tostran, C, administration
Toviaz, 3, 25
Tramacet, 2, 25, 29, 30
Tramacet effervescent tabs, 2, 13, 29, 30
Tramadol caps, 2
Tramadol m/r, 2, 25
Tramadol oral drops, 2, 13
Tramadol orodispersible tabs, 2, C, administration
Tramadol soluble, 2, 13
Tramake, 2
Trandate, 8, 21
Transtec, 2
Tranylcypromine, 3, 10, patient information leaflet
Travatan, C, see BNF
Travoprost, C, see BNF
Traxam foam, 15, C, photosensitivity, see BNF
Traxam gel, C, photosensitivity, see BNF
Trazodone, 2, 21
Treclin, 11
Trental m/r, 21, 25
Treosulfan, 25
Tretinoin caps, 21, 25
Tretinoin external preps, 11
Triamcinolone inj, 10, steroid card
Triamterene, 14, (urine blue in some lights), 21
Triapin preps, 25
Trientine, 6, 22
Trifluoperazine, 2
Trihexyphenidyl syrup, C, driving, see BNF
Trihexyphenidyl tabs, C, with or after food, driving, see BNF
Trileptal, 3, 8, C, see BNF
Trimethoprim susp and tabs, 9
Trimipramine, 2
Trimopan, 9
Trimovate, 28, C, application, see BNF
Tripotassium dicitratobismuthate, C, administration, see BNF
Triptafen, 2
Triumeq, C, hypersensitivity reactions, see BNF
Trizivir, C, hypersensitivity reactions, see BNF
Trobalt, 8, 14, 25, C, driving, see BNF

Trospium chloride, 23
Trospium chloride m/r, 23, 25
Truvada, 21, C, administration, see BNF
Tybost, 21
Tylex caps, 2, 29, 30
Tylex effervescent tabs, 2, 13, 29, 30
Typhoid vaccine, oral, 25, C, administration, see BNF
Tyverb, C, see BNF

Ucerax, 2
Ultralanum Plain, 28, C, application, see BNF
Umeclidinium, C, administration
Uniphyllin Continus, 25
Univer, 25
Urispas, 3
Ursodeoxycholic acid, 21
Ursofalk, 21
Ursogal, 21
Ustekinumab, 10, C, tuberculosis, see BNF
Utrogestan, C, administration, see BNF

Valaciclovir, 9
Valcyte, 21
Valganciclovir, 21
Vallergan, 2
Valni XL, 25
Valproic acid, see individual preparations
Valtrex, 9
Vancocin caps, 9
Vancomycin caps, 9
Vandetanib, Alert card
Varenicline, 3
Vasran XL, 21, 25, C, initial dose, driving, see BNF
Vemurafenib, 25, C, administration, see BNF
Venlafaxine, 3, C, driving
Venlafaxine m/r, 3, 21, 25, C, driving
Ventmax SR, 25
Ventolin inhalations, C, administration
Vepesid caps, 23
Verapamil m/r, 25
Verapress, 25
Vertab SR, 25
Vesanoid, 21, 25
Vesicare, 3
Vesomni, 3, 25
Vfend, 9, 11, 23, C, hepatotoxicity, phototoxicity
Viazem XL, 25
Vibramycin-D, 6, 9, 11, 13
Victoza, C, administration
Victrelis, 21
Videx e/c caps, 25, C, administration, see BNF
Videx tabs, 23, C, administration, see BNF
Vigabatrin sachets, 3, 8, 13, C, driving, see BNF

Vigabatrin tabs, 3, 8, C, driving, see BNF
Vimovo, 22, 25
Vimpat tabs, 8, C, driving, see BNF
Vinorelbine caps, 21, 25
Vipdomet, 21
Viramune, C, hypersensitivity reactions
Viramune Prolonged Release, 25, C, hypersensitivity reactions
Viread granules, 21, C, administration
Viread tabs, 21
Viskaldix, 8
Visken, 8
Vismodegib, 25, C, pregnancy and contraception
Vistabel, C, side-effects, see BNF
Vistide, 21, C, administration, see BNF
Vivotif, 25, C, administration, see BNF
Vokanamet, 21, C, volume depletion, see BNF
Voltarol dispersible tabs, 13, 21
Voltarol Emulgel, C, photosensitivity, see BNF
Voltarol Gel Patch, C, photosensitivity, see BNF
Voltarol Rapid, 21
Voltarol 75 mg SR and Retard, 21, 25
Voltarol tabs, 5, 25
Voractiv, 8, 14, (urine orange-red), 22, C, soft lenses
Voriconazole, 9, 11, 23, C, hepatotoxicity, phototoxicity
Votrient, 23, 25, C, antacids, see BNF
Votubia, 25, C, pneumonitis, see BNF
Vyndaqel, 25

Warfarin, 10, anticoagulant card
Warticon, 15
Welldorm, 19, 27
Wellvone, 21
Wilzin, 23

Xagrid, C, driving
Xalacom, C, see BNF
Xalatan, C, see BNF
Xalkori, 25
Xanax, 2
Xatral, C, initial dose, driving, see BNF
Xatral XL, 21, 25, C, initial dose, driving, see BNF
Xeloda, 21
Xeomin, C, side-effects, see BNF
Xepin, 2, 10, patient information leaflet
Xifaxanta, 9
Xigduo, 21
Xismox XL, 25
Xtandi, 25
Xultophy, C, administration, see BNF
Xyzal, C, driving

A4 Intravenous additives

Intravenous additives policies A local policy on the addition of drugs to intravenous fluids should be drawn up by a multi-disciplinary team in each Strategic Health Authority (or equivalent) and issued as a document to the members of staff concerned.

Centralised additive services are provided in a number of hospital pharmacy departments and should be used in preference to making additions on wards.

The information that follows should be read in conjunction with local policy documents.

Guidelines

1. Drugs should only be added to infusion containers when constant plasma concentrations are needed or when the administration of a more concentrated solution would be harmful.

2. In general, only one drug should be added to any infusion container and the components should be compatible. Ready-prepared solutions should be used whenever possible. Drugs should not normally be added to blood products, mannitol, or sodium bicarbonate. Only specially formulated additives should be used with fat emulsions or amino-acid solutions (section 9.3).

3. Solutions should be thoroughly mixed by shaking and checked for absence of particulate matter before use.

4. Strict asepsis should be maintained throughout and in general the giving set should not be used for more than 24 hours (for drug admixtures).

5. The infusion container should be labelled with the patient's name, the name and quantity of additives, and the date and time of addition (and the new expiry date or time). Such additional labelling should not interfere with information on the manufacturer's label that is still valid. When possible, containers should be retained for a period after use in case they are needed for investigation.

6. It is good practice to examine intravenous infusions from time to time while they are running. If cloudiness, crystallisation, change of colour, or any other sign of interaction or contamination is observed the infusion should be discontinued.

Problems

Microbial contamination The accidental entry and subsequent growth of micro-organisms converts the infusion fluid pathway into a potential vehicle for infection with micro-organisms, particularly species of Candida, Enterobacter, and Klebsiella. Ready-prepared infusions containing the additional drugs, or infusions prepared by an additive service (when available) should therefore be used in preference to making extemporaneous additions to infusion containers on wards etc. However, when this is necessary strict aseptic procedure should be followed.

Incompatibility Physical and chemical incompatibilities may occur with loss of potency, increase in toxicity, or other adverse effect. The solutions may become opalescent or precipitation may occur, but in many instances there is no visual indication of incompatibility. Interaction may take place at any point in the infusion fluid pathway, and the potential for incompatibility is increased when more than one substance is added to the infusion fluid.

Common incompatibilities Precipitation reactions are numerous and varied and may occur as a result of pH, concentration changes, 'salting-out' effects, complexation or other chemical changes. Precipitation or other particle formation must be avoided since, apart from lack of control of dosage on administration, it may initiate or exacerbate adverse effects. This is particularly important in the case of drugs which have been implicated in either thrombophlebitis (e.g. diazepam) or in skin sloughing or necrosis caused by extravasation (e.g. sodium bicarbonate and certain cytotoxic drugs). It is also especially important to effect solution of colloidal drugs and to prevent their subsequent precipitation in order to avoid a pyrogenic reaction (e.g. amphotericin).

It is considered undesirable to mix beta-lactam antibiotics, such as semi-synthetic penicillins and cephalosporins, with proteinaceous materials on the grounds that immunogenic and allergenic conjugates could be formed.

A number of preparations undergo significant loss of potency when added singly or in combination to large volume infusions. Examples include ampicillin in infusions that contain glucose or lactates. The breakdown products of dacarbazine have been implicated in adverse effects.

Blood Because of the large number of incompatibilities, drugs should not normally be added to blood and blood products for infusion purposes. Examples of incompatibility with blood include hypertonic mannitol solutions (irreversible crenation of red cells), dextrans (rouleaux formation and interference with cross-matching), glucose (clumping of red cells), and oxytocin (inactivated).

If the giving set is not changed after the administration of blood, but used for other infusion fluids, a fibrin clot may form which, apart from blocking the set, increases the likelihood of microbial growth.

Intravenous fat emulsions These may break down with coalescence of fat globules and separation of phases when additions such as antibacterials or electrolytes are made, thus increasing the possibility of embolism. Only specially formulated products such as *Vitlipid N*® (section 9.3) may be added to appropriate intravenous fat emulsions.

Other infusions Infusions that frequently give rise to incompatibility include amino acids, mannitol, and sodium bicarbonate.

Bactericides Bactericides such as chlorocresol 0.1% or phenylmercuric nitrate 0.001% are present in some injection solutions. The total volume of such solutions added to a container for infusion on one occasion should not exceed 15 mL.

Method

Ready-prepared infusions should be used whenever available. **Potassium chloride** is usually available in concentrations of 20, 27, and 40 mmol/litre in sodium chloride intravenous infusion (0.9%), glucose intravenous infusion (5%) or sodium chloride and glucose intravenous infusion. **Lidocaine hydrochloride** is usually available in concentrations of 0.1 or 0.2% in glucose intravenous infusion (5%).

When addition is required to be made extemporaneously, any product reconstitution instructions such as those relating to concentration, vehicle, mixing, and handling precautions should be strictly followed using an aseptic technique throughout. Once the product has been reconstituted, addition to the infusion fluid should be made immediately in order to minimise microbial contamination and, with certain products, to prevent degradation or other formulation change which may occur; e.g. reconstituted ampicillin injection degrades rapidly on standing, and also may form polymers which could cause sensitivity reactions.

It is also important in certain instances that an infusion fluid of specific pH be used (e.g. **furosemide** injection requires dilution in infusions of pH greater than 5.5).

When drug additions are made it is important to mix thoroughly; additions should not be made to an infusion container that has been connected to a giving set, as mixing is hampered. If the solutions are not thoroughly mixed a concentrated layer of the additive may form owing to differences in density. **Potassium chloride** is particularly prone to this 'layering' effect when added without adequate mixing to infusions packed in non-rigid infusion containers; if such a mixture is administered it may have a serious effect on the heart.

A time limit between addition and completion of administration must be imposed for certain admixtures to guarantee satisfactory drug potency and compatibility. For admixtures in which degradation occurs without the formation of toxic substances, an acceptable limit is the time taken for 10% decomposition of the drug. When toxic substances are produced stricter limits may be imposed. Because of the risk of microbial contamination a maximum time limit of 24 hours may be appropriate for additions made elsewhere than in hospital pharmacies offering central additive service.

Certain injections must be protected from light during continuous infusion to minimise oxidation, e.g. dacarbazine and sodium nitroprusside.

Dilution with a small volume of an appropriate vehicle and administration using a motorised infusion pump is advocated for preparations such as unfractionated heparin where strict control over administration is required. In this case the appropriate dose may be dissolved in a convenient volume (e.g. 24–48 mL) of sodium chloride intravenous infusion (0.9%).

Use of table

The table lists preparations given by three methods:

- continuous infusion;
- intermittent infusion;
- addition via the drip tubing.

Drugs for **continuous infusion** must be diluted in a large volume infusion. Penicillins and cephalosporins are not usually given by continuous infusion because of stability problems and because adequate plasma and tissue concentrations are best obtained by intermittent infusion. Where it is necessary to administer them by continuous infusion, detailed literature should be consulted.

Drugs that are both compatible and clinically suitable may be given by **intermittent infusion** in a relatively small volume of infusion over a short period of time, e.g. 100 mL in 30 minutes. The method is used if the product is incompatible or unstable over the period necessary for continuous infusion; the limited stability of ampicillin or amoxicillin in large volume glucose or lactate infusions may be overcome in this way.

Intermittent infusion is also used if adequate plasma and tissue concentrations are not produced by continuous infusion as in the case of drugs such as dacarbazine, gentamicin, and ticarcillin.

An in-line burette may be used for intermittent infusion techniques in order to achieve strict control over the time and rate of administration, especially for infants and children and in intensive care units. Intermittent infusion may also make use of the 'piggy-back' technique provided that no additions are made to the primary infusion. In this method the drug is added to a small secondary container connected to a Y-type injection site on the primary infusion giving set; the secondary solution is usually infused within 30 minutes.

Addition *via* **the drip tubing** is indicated for a number of cytotoxic drugs in order to minimise extravasation. The preparation is added aseptically *via* the rubber septum of the injection site of a fast-running infusion. In general, drug preparations intended for a bolus effect should be given directly into a separate vein where possible. Failing this, administration may be made *via* the drip tubing provided that the preparation is compatible with the infusion fluid when given in this manner.

Table of drugs given by intravenous infusion

Covers addition to *Glucose intravenous infusion* 5 and 10%, and *Sodium chloride intravenous infusion* 0.9%. Compatibility with glucose 5% and with sodium chloride 0.9% indicates compatibility with *Sodium chloride and glucose intravenous infusion*. Infusion of a large volume of hypotonic solution should be avoided therefore care should be taken if water for injections is used. The information in the Table relates to the proprietary preparations indicated; for other preparations suitability should be checked with the manufacturer

Abatacept (*Orencia*®)

Intermittent *in* Sodium chloride 0.9%
Reconstitute each vial with 10 mL water for injections using the silicone-free syringe provided; dilute requisite dose in infusion fluid to 100 mL (using the same silicone-free syringe); give over 30 minutes through a low protein-binding filter (pore size 0.2–1.2 micron)

Abciximab (*ReoPro*®)

Continuous *in* Glucose 5% *or* Sodium chloride 0.9%
Dilute requisite dose in infusion fluid and give *via* infusion pump; filter upon dilution with infusion fluid through a non-pyrogenic low protein-binding 0.2, 0.22, or 5 micron filter *or* upon administration through an in-line non-pyrogenic low protein-binding 0.2 or 0.22 micron filter

Acetylcysteine (*Parvolex®*)
Continuous *in* Glucose 5% or Sodium chloride 0.9%
Glucose 5% is preferable—see Emergency Treatment of Poisoning

Aciclovir (as sodium salt) (*Zovirax IV®*; *Aciclovir IV*, Hospira; *Aciclovir IV*, Genus; *Aciclovir Sodium*, Zurich)
Intermittent *in* Sodium chloride 0.9% *or* Sodium chloride and glucose
For *Zovirax IV®*, *Aciclovir IV* (Genus) initially reconstitute to 25 mg/mL in water for injections or sodium chloride 0.9% then dilute to not more than 5 mg/mL with the infusion fluid; to be given over 1 hour; alternatively, may be administered in a concentration of 25 mg/mL using a suitable infusion pump and given over 1 hour; for *Aciclovir IV* (Hospira) dilute to not more than 5 mg/mL with infusion fluid; give over 1 hour

Agalsidase alfa (*Replagal®*)
Intermittent *in* Sodium chloride 0.9%
Dilute requisite dose with 100 mL infusion fluid and give over 40 minutes using an in-line filter; use within 3 hours of dilution

Agalsidase beta (*Fabrazyme®*)
Intermittent *in* Sodium chloride 0.9%
Reconstitute with water for injections (35 mg in 7.2 mL, 5 mg in 1.1 mL) to produce a solution containing 5 mg/mL; dilute with infusion fluid (for doses less than 35 mg dilute with at least 50 mL; doses 35–70 mg dilute with at least 100 mL; doses 70–100 mg dilute with at least 250 mL; doses greater than 100 mg dilute with 500 mL) and give through an in-line low protein-binding 0.2 micron filter at an initial rate of no more than 15 mg/hour; for subsequent infusions, infusion rate may be increased gradually once tolerance has been established

Alfentanil (as hydrochloride) (*Rapifen®*)
Continuous *or* intermittent *in* Glucose 5% *or* Sodium chloride 0.9%

Alglucosidase alfa (*Myozyme®*)
Intermittent *in* Sodium chloride 0.9%
Reconstitute 50 mg with 10.3 mL water for injections to produce 5 mg/mL solution; gently rotate vial without shaking; dilute requisite dose with infusion fluid to give a final concentration of 0.5–4 mg/mL; give through a low protein-binding in-line filter (0.2 micron) at an initial rate of 1 mg/kg/hour increased by 2 mg/kg/hour every 30 minutes to max. 7 mg/kg/hour

Alteplase (*Actilyse®*)
Continuous *or* intermittent *in* Sodium chloride 0.9%
Dissolve in water for injections to a concentration of 1 mg/mL or 2 mg/mL and infuse intravenously; alternatively dilute the solution further in the infusion fluid to a concentration of not less than 200 micrograms/mL; not to be infused in glucose solution

Amikacin sulfate (*Amikin®*)
Intermittent *in* Glucose 5% *or* Sodium chloride 0.9%
To be given over 30 minutes

Aminophylline Continuous *in* Glucose 5% *or* Sodium chloride 0.9%

Amiodarone hydrochloride (*Cordarone X®*)
Continuous *or* intermittent *in* Glucose 5%
Suggested initial infusion volume 250 mL given over 20–120 minutes; for repeat infusions up to 1.2 g in max. 500 mL; infusion in extreme emergency see section 2.7.3; should not be diluted to less than 600 micrograms/mL; incompatible with sodium chloride solutions; avoid equipment containing the plasticizer di-2-ethylhexyphthalate (DEHP)

Amoxicillin (as sodium salt) (*Amoxil®*)
Intermittent *in* Glucose 5% *or* Sodium chloride 0.9%
Reconstituted solutions diluted and given without delay; suggested volume 100 mL given over 30–60 minutes *via* drip tubing *in* Glucose 5% *or* Sodium chloride 0.9%
Continuous infusion not usually recommended

Amphotericin (lipid complex) (*Abelcet®*)
Intermittent *in* Glucose 5%
Allow suspension to reach room temperature, shake gently to ensure no yellow settlement, withdraw requisite dose (using 17–19 gauge needle) into one or more 20-mL syringes; replace needle on syringe with a 5-micron filter needle provided (fresh needle for each syringe) and dilute to a concentration of 1 mg/mL (2 mg/mL can be used in fluid restriction and in children); preferably give *via* an infusion pump at a rate of 2.5 mg/kg/hour (initial test dose of 1 mg given over 15 minutes); an in-line filter (pore size no less than 15 micron) may be used; do not use sodium chloride or other electrolyte solutions, flush existing intravenous line with glucose 5% or use separate line

Amphotericin (liposomal) (*AmBisome®*)
Intermittent *in* Glucose 5% or 10%
Reconstitute each vial with 12 mL water for injections and shake vigorously to produce a preparation containing 4 mg/mL; withdraw requisite dose from vial and introduce into infusion fluid through the 5 micron filter provided to produce a final concentration of 0.2–2 mg/mL; infuse over 30–60 minutes, or if non-anaphylactic infusion-related reactions occur infuse over 2 hours (initial test dose 1 mg over 10 minutes); an in-line filter (pore size no less than 1 micron) may be used; incompatible with sodium chloride solutions, flush existing intravenous line with glucose 5% or 10%, or use separate line

Amphotericin (as sodium deoxycholate complex) (*Fungizone®*)
Intermittent *in* Glucose 5%
Reconstitute each vial with 10 mL water for injections and shake immediately to produce a 5 mg/mL colloidal solution; dilute further in infusion fluid to a concentration of 100 micrograms/mL; pH of the glucose must not be below 4.2 (check each container—consult product literature for details of buffer); infuse over 2–4 hours, or longer if not tolerated (initial test dose 1 mg over 20–30 minutes); begin infusion immediately after dilution and protect from light; incompatible with sodium chloride solutions, flush existing intravenous line with glucose 5% or use separate line; an in-line filter (pore size no less than 1 micron) may be used

Ampicillin sodium (*Penbritin®*)
Intermittent *in* Glucose 5% *or* Sodium chloride 0.9%
Reconstituted solutions diluted and given without delay; suggested volume 100 mL given over 30–60 minutes *via* drip tubing *in* Glucose 5% *or* Sodium chloride 0.9%
Continuous infusion not usually recommended

Anidulafungin (*Ecalta®*)
Intermittent *in* Glucose 5% *or* Sodium chloride 0.9%
Reconstitute each 100 mg with 30 mL water for injections, allow up to 5 minutes for reconstitution; dilute dose in infusion fluid to a concentration of 770 micrograms/mL; give at a rate not exceeding 1.1 mg/minute
Note Follow product information if using stock supplied with ethanol solvent

Antithymocyte immunoglobulin (*Thymoglobuline®*)
Continuous *in* Glucose 5% *or* Sodium chloride 0.9%
Reconstitute each vial with 5 mL water for injections to produce a solution of 5 mg/mL; gently rotate to dissolve. Dilute requisite dose with infusion fluid to a total volume of 50–500 mL (usually 50 mL/vial); begin infusion immediately after dilution; give through an in-line filter (pore size 0.22 micron); not to be given with unfractionated heparin and hydrocortisone in glucose infusion as precipitation reported

Argatroban monohydrate (*Exembol®*)
Continuous *in* Glucose 5% *or* Sodium chloride 0.9%
Dilute each 2.5-mL vial with 250 mL infusion fluid

Atenolol (*Tenormin®*)
Intermittent *in* Glucose 5% *or* Sodium chloride 0.9%
Suggested infusion time 20 minutes

Appendix 4: Intravenous additives

Atosiban (*Tractocile*® concentrate for intravenous infusion)

Continuous *in* Glucose 5% *or* Sodium chloride 0.9%
Withdraw 10 mL infusion fluid from 100-mL bag and replace with 10 mL atosiban concentrate (7.5 mg/mL) to produce a final concentration of 750 micrograms/mL

Atracurium besilate (*Tracrium*®; *Atracurium besilate injection*, Hospira; *Atracurium injection/infusion*, Genus)

Continuous *in* Glucose 5% *or* Sodium chloride 0.9%
Stability varies with diluent; dilute requisite dose with infusion fluid to a concentration of 0.5–5 mg/mL

Azathioprine (as sodium salt) (*Imuran*®)

Intermittent *in* Glucose 5% *or* Sodium chloride 0.9%
Reconstitute 50 mg with 5–15 mL water for injections; dilute requisite dose to a volume of 20–200 mL with infusion fluid

Azithromycin (*Zedbac*®)

Intermittent *in* Glucose 5% *or* Sodium chloride 0.9%
Reconstitute 500 mg with 4.8 mL water for injections to produce a 100 mg/mL solution, then dilute 5 mL of solution with infusion fluid to a final concentration of 1 or 2 mg/mL; give the 1 mg/mL solution over 3 hours *or* give the 2 mg/mL solution over 1 hour

Aztreonam (*Azactam*®)

Intermittent *in* Glucose 5% *or* Sodium chloride 0.9%
Dissolve initially in water for injections (1 g per 3 mL) then dilute to a concentration of less than 20 mg/mL; to be given over 20–60 minutes

Basiliximab (*Simulect*®)

Intermittent *in* Glucose 5% *or* Sodium chloride 0.9%
Reconstitute 10 mg with 2.5 mL water for injections then dilute to at least 25 mL with infusion fluid; reconstitute 20 mg with 5 mL water for injections then dilute to at least 50 mL with infusion fluid; give over 20–30 minutes

Belimumab (*Benlysta*®)

Intermittent *in* Sodium chloride 0.9%
Reconstitute with water for injections (120 mg in 1.5 mL, 400 mg in 4.8 mL) to produce a solution containing 80 mg/mL; gently swirl vial for 60 seconds, then allow to stand; swirl vial (without shaking) for 60 seconds every 5 minutes until dissolved; dilute requisite dose with infusion fluid to a final volume of 250 mL and give over 1 hour

Benzylpenicillin sodium (*Crystapen*®)

Intermittent *in* Glucose 5% *or* Sodium chloride 0.9%
Suggested volume 100 mL given over 30–60 minutes
Continuous infusion not usually recommended

Betamethasone (as sodium phosphate) (*Betnesol*®)

Continuous *or* intermittent *or via* drip tubing *in* Glucose 5% *or* Sodium chloride 0.9%

Bivalirudin (*Angiox*®)

Continuous *in* Glucose 5% *or* Sodium chloride 0.9%
Reconstitute each 250-mg vial with 5 mL water for injections then withdraw 5 mL and dilute to 50 mL with infusion fluid

Bumetanide

Intermittent *in* Glucose 5% *or* Sodium chloride 0.9%
Suggested volume 500 mL given over 30–60 minutes; concentrations above 25 micrograms/mL may cause precipitation

Calcitonin (salmon) (*Miacalcic*®)

Intermittent *in* Sodium chloride 0.9%
Diluted solution given without delay; dilute in 500 mL and give over at least 6 hours; glass or hard plastic containers should not be used; some loss of potency on dilution and administration

Calcium gluconate Continuous *in* Glucose 5% *or* Sodium chloride 0.9%
Avoid bicarbonates, phosphates, or sulfates

Caspofungin (*Cancidas*®)

Intermittent *in* Sodium chloride 0.9%
Allow vial to reach room temperature; initially reconstitute each vial with 10.5 mL water for injections, mixing gently to dissolve then dilute requisite dose in 250 mL infusion fluid (35- or 50-mg doses may be diluted in 100 mL infusion fluid if necessary); give over 60 minutes; incompatible with glucose solutions

Cefotaxime (as sodium salt) Intermittent *in* Glucose 5% *or* Sodium chloride 0.9%
Suggested volume 40–100 mL given over 20–60 minutes; incompatible with alkaline solutions

Ceftaroline fosamil (*Zinforo*®)

Intermittent *in* Glucose 5% *or* Sodium chloride 0.9%
Reconstitute 600 mg with 20 mL water for injections, then dilute with 250 mL infusion fluid (in fluid restriction, may be diluted with 50–100 mL infusion fluid); give over 60 minutes

Ceftazidime (as pentahydrate) (*Fortum*®, *Kefadim*®)

Intermittent *or via* drip tubing *in* Glucose 5% or 10% *or* Sodium chloride 0.9%
Dissolve 2 g initially in 10 mL (3 g in 15 mL) infusion fluid; for *Fortum*® dilute further to a concentration of 40 mg/mL; for *Kefadim*® dilute further to a concentration of 20 mg/mL; give over up to 30 minutes

Ceftriaxone (as sodium salt) (*Rocephin*®; *Ceftriaxone Injection*, Genus)

Intermittent *or via* drip tubing *in* Glucose 5% or 10% *or* Sodium chloride 0.9%
Reconstitute 2-g vial with 40 mL infusion fluid; give intermittent infusion over at least 30 minutes (60 minutes in neonates); not to be given simultaneously with total parenteral nutrition or infusion fluids containing calcium, even by different infusion lines; may be infused sequentially with infusion fluids containing calcium if flush with sodium chloride 0.9% between infusions or give infusions by different infusion lines at different sites

Cefuroxime (as sodium salt) (*Zinacef*®)

Intermittent *or via* drip tubing *in* Glucose 5% *or* Sodium chloride 0.9%
Dissolve initially in water for injections (at least 2 mL for each 250 mg, 15 mL for 1.5 g); suggested volume 50–100 mL given over 30 minutes

Chloramphenicol (as sodium succinate) (*Kemicetine*®)

Intermittent *or via* drip tubing *in* Glucose 5% *or* Sodium chloride 0.9%

Ciclosporin (*Sandimmun*®)

Intermittent *or* continuous *in* Glucose 5% *or* Sodium chloride 0.9%
Dilute to a concentration of 50 mg in 20–100 mL; give intermittent infusion over 2–6 hours; not to be used with PVC equipment

Cisatracurium (*Nimbex*®, *Nimbex Forte*®)

Continuous *in* Glucose 5% *or* Sodium chloride 0.9%
Solutions of 2 mg/mL and 5 mg/mL may be infused undiluted; alternatively dilute with infusion fluid to a concentration of 0.1–2 mg/mL

Clarithromycin (*Klaricid*® I.V.)

Intermittent *in* Glucose 5% *or* Sodium chloride 0.9%
Dissolve initially in water for injections (500 mg in 10 mL) then dilute to a concentration of 2 mg/mL; give over 60 minutes

Clindamycin (as phosphate) (*Dalacin*® C Phosphate)

Continuous *or* intermittent *in* Glucose 5% *or* Sodium chloride 0.9%
Dilute to not more than 18 mg/mL and give over 10–60 minutes at a rate not exceeding 30 mg/minute (1.2 g over at least 60 minutes; higher doses by continuous infusion)

Co-amoxiclav (*Augmentin*®)
Intermittent *in* Sodium chloride 0.9%
Reconstitute 600 mg initially with 10 mL water for injections, then dilute with 50 mL infusion fluid; reconstitute 1.2 g initially with 20 mL water for injections, then dilute with 100 mL infusion fluid; give over 30–40 minutes
via drip tubing *in* Sodium chloride 0.9%

Co-fluampicil (as sodium salts) (*Magnapen*®)
Intermittent *in* Glucose 5% *or* Sodium chloride 0.9%
Reconstituted solutions diluted and given without delay; suggested volume 100 mL given over 30–60 minutes
via drip tubing *in* Glucose 5% *or* Sodium chloride 0.9%

Colistimethate sodium (*Colomycin*®, *Promixin*®)
Intermittent *in* Sodium chloride 0.9% (*or* Glucose 5% for *Promixin*® brand only)
Dilute with 50 mL infusion fluid and give over 30 minutes

Co-trimoxazole (*Septrin*® for infusion)
Intermittent *in* Glucose 5% or 10% *or* Sodium chloride 0.9%
Dilute contents of 1 ampoule (5 mL) to 125 mL, 2 ampoules (10 mL) to 250 mL or 3 ampoules (15 mL) to 500 mL; suggested duration of infusion 60–90 minutes (but may be adjusted according to fluid requirements); if fluid restriction necessary, 1 ampoule (5 mL) may be diluted with 75 mL glucose 5% and infused over max. 60 minutes

Cyclophosphamide (*Cyclophosphamide injection*, Baxter)
via drip tubing *in* Glucose 5% *or* Sodium chloride 0.9%
Reconstitute 500 mg with 25 mL sodium chloride 0.9%; reconstitute 1 g with 50 mL sodium chloride 0.9%

Danaparoid sodium (*Orgaran*®)
Continuous *in* Glucose 5% *or* Sodium chloride 0.9%

Daptomycin (*Cubicin*®)
Intermittent *in* Sodium chloride 0.9%
Reconstitute with sodium chloride 0.9% (350 mg in 7 mL, 500 mg in 10 mL); gently rotate vial without shaking; allow to stand for at least 10 minutes then rotate gently to dissolve; dilute requisite dose in 50 mL infusion fluid and give over 30 minutes

Desferrioxamine mesilate (*Desferal*®)
Continuous *or* intermittent *in* Glucose 5% *or* Sodium chloride 0.9%
Reconstitute with water for injections to a concentration of 100 mg/mL; dilute with infusion fluid

Desmopressin (*DDAVP*®, *Octim*®)
Intermittent *in* Sodium chloride 0.9%
Dilute with 50 mL and give over 20 minutes

Dexamethasone sodium phosphate (*Dexamethasone*, Hospira)
Continuous *or* intermittent *or via* drip tubing *in* Glucose 5% *or* Sodium chloride 0.9%

Dexmedetomidine (as hydrochloride) (*Dexdor*®)
Continuous *in* Glucose 5% *or* Sodium chloride 0.9%
Dilute to a concentration of 4 micrograms/mL

Dexrazoxane (*Cardioxane*®)
Intermittent *in* Compound sodium lactate
Reconstitute each vial with 25 mL water for injections and dilute each vial with 25–100 mL infusion fluid; give requisite dose over 15 minutes

Dexrazoxane (*Savene*®)
Intermittent *in* *Savene*® diluent
Reconstitute each 500-mg vial with 25 mL of *Savene*® diluent; dilute requisite dose further in remaining *Savene*® diluent, and give over 1–2 hours into a large vein, in an area other than the one affected

Diamorphine hydrochloride (*Diamorphine Injection*, Wockhardt)
Continuous *in* Glucose 5% *or* Sodium chloride 0.9%
Glucose is preferred as infusion fluid

Diazepam (solution) (*Diazepam*, Wockhardt)
Continuous *in* Glucose 5% *or* Sodium chloride 0.9%
Dilute to a concentration of not more than 10 mg in 200 mL; adsorbed to some extent by the plastics of bags and infusion sets

Diazepam (emulsion) (*Diazemuls*®)
Continuous *in* Glucose 5% or 10%
May be diluted to a max. concentration of 200 mg in 500 mL; max. 6 hours between addition and completion of administration; adsorbed to some extent by the plastics of the infusion set
via drip tubing *in* Glucose 5% or 10% *or* Sodium chloride 0.9%
Adsorbed to some extent by the plastics of the infusion set

Diclofenac sodium (*Voltarol*®)
Continuous *or* intermittent *in* Glucose 5% *or* Sodium chloride 0.9%
Dilute 75 mg with 100–500 mL infusion fluid (previously buffered with 0.5 mL sodium bicarbonate 8.4% solution *or* with 1 mL sodium bicarbonate 4.2% solution); for intermittent infusion give 25–50 mg over 15–60 minutes or 75 mg over 30–120 minutes; for continuous infusion give at a rate of 5 mg/hour

Digoxin (*Lanoxin*®)
Intermittent *in* Glucose 5% *or* Sodium chloride 0.9%
Dilute to a concentration of not more than 62.5 micrograms/mL. To be given over at least 2 hours

Digoxin-specific antibody fragments (*DigiFab*®)
Intermittent *in* Sodium chloride 0.9%
Reconstitute with water for injections (4 mL/vial), then dilute with infusion fluid and give over 30 minutes

Dinoprostone (*Prostin E2*®)
Continuous *or* intermittent *in* Glucose 5% *or* Sodium chloride 0.9%

Disopyramide (as phosphate) (*Rythmodan*®)
Continuous *or* intermittent *in* Glucose 5% *or* Sodium chloride 0.9%
Max. rate by continuous infusion 20–30 mg/hour (or 400 micrograms/kg/hour)

Dobutamine (as hydrochloride) Continuous *in* Glucose 5% *or* Sodium chloride 0.9%
Dilute to a concentration of 0.5–1 mg/mL and give *via* an infusion pump; give higher concentration (max. 5 mg/mL) through central venous catheter; incompatible with bicarbonate and other strong alkaline solutions

Dopamine hydrochloride
Continuous *in* Glucose 5% *or* Sodium chloride 0.9%
Dilute to max. concentration of 3.2 mg/mL; incompatible with bicarbonate

Dopexamine hydrochloride (*Dopacard*®)
Continuous *in* Glucose 5% *or* Sodium chloride 0.9%
Dilute to a concentration of 400 or 800 micrograms/mL; max. concentration *via* large peripheral vein 1 mg/mL, concentrations up to 4 mg/mL may be infused *via* central vein; give *via* infusion pump or other device which provides accurate control of rate; contact with metal should be minimised; incompatible with bicarbonate

Eculizumab (*Soliris*®)
Intermittent *in* Glucose 5% *or* Sodium chloride 0.9%
Dilute requisite dose to a concentration of 5 mg/mL and mix gently; give over 25–45 minutes (infusion time may be increased to 2 hours if infusion-related reactions occur)

Enoximone (*Perfan*®)
Continuous *or* intermittent *in* Sodium chloride 0.9% *or* Water for injections
Dilute to a concentration of 2.5 mg/mL; incompatible with glucose solutions; use only plastic containers or syringes

Epoprostenol (*Flolan*®, *Veletri*®)
Continuous in Sodium chloride 0.9% (but see also below)
For *Flolan*®, reconstitute using the filter and solvent (glycine buffer diluent) provided to make a concentrate; may be diluted further (consult product literature); for *pulmonary hypertension* dilute further with glycine buffer diluent only and administer via a central venous catheter (can give via peripheral vein until central venous access established), for *renal dialysis* may be diluted further with sodium chloride 0.9%; protect infusion from light
For *Veletri*®, reconstitute each vial with 5 mL sodium chloride 0.9% then dilute to required concentration with sodium chloride 0.9% (consult product literature); administer through an in-line 0.22 micron filter; for *pulmonary hypertension*, administer via a central venous catheter (can give via peripheral vein until central venous access established); protect infusion from direct sunlight

Ertapenem (*Invanz*®)
Intermittent *in* Sodium chloride 0.9%
Reconstitute 1 g with 10 mL water for injections or sodium chloride 0.9%; dilute requisite dose in infusion fluid to a final concentration not exceeding 20 mg/mL; give over 30 minutes; incompatible with glucose solutions

Erythromycin (as lactobionate) Intermittent *in* Glucose 5% (neutralised with sodium bicarbonate) *or* Sodium chloride 0.9%
Dissolve initially in water for injections (1 g in 20 mL) then dilute to a concentration of 1–5 mg/mL; give over 20–60 minutes

Esomeprazole (as sodium salt) (*Nexium*®)
Continuous *or* intermittent *in* Sodium chloride 0.9%
Reconstitute 40–80 mg with up to 100 mL infusion fluid; for intermittent infusion, give requisite dose over 10–30 minutes; stable for 12 hours in sodium chloride 0.9%

Ethanol Continuous *in* Glucose 5% *or* Sodium chloride 0.9%
Dilute to a concentration of 5–10%

Fentanyl (*Sublimaze*®)
Continuous *or* intermittent *in* Glucose 5% *or* Sodium chloride 0.9%

Ferric carboxymaltose (*Ferinject*®)
Intermittent *in* Sodium chloride 0.9%
Dilute 200–500 mg in up to 100 mL infusion fluid and give over at least 6 minutes; dilute 0.5–1 g in up to 250 mL infusion fluid and give over at least 15 minutes

Ferumoxytol (*Rienso*®)
Intermittent *in* Glucose 5% *or* Sodium chloride 0.9%
Dilute each vial with 50–250 mL infusion fluid and give over at least 15 minutes; if second dose required administer 2–8 days after first dose

Filgrastim (*Neupogen*®; *Nivestim*®; *Ratiograstim*®; *Zarzio*®)
Continuous *or* intermittent *in* Glucose 5%
For a filgrastim concentration of less than 1 500 000 units/mL (15 micrograms/mL) albumin solution (human albumin solution) is added to produce a final albumin concentration of 2 mg/mL; should not be diluted to a filgrastim concentration of less than 200 000 units/mL (2 micrograms/mL) and should not be diluted with sodium chloride solution

Flecainide acetate (*Tambocor*®)
Continuous *or* intermittent *in* Glucose 5% *or* Sodium chloride 0.9%
Minimum volume in infusion fluids containing chlorides 500 mL

Flucloxacillin (as sodium salt) (*Floxapen*®)
Intermittent *in* Glucose 5% *or* Sodium chloride 0.9%
Suggested volume 100 mL given over 30–60 minutes *via* drip tubing *in* Glucose 5% *or* Sodium chloride 0.9%
Continuous infusion not usually recommended

Flumazenil
Continuous *in* Glucose 5% *or* Sodium chloride 0.9%

Fondaparinux (*Arixtra*®)
Intermittent *in* Sodium chloride 0.9%
For ST-segment elevation myocardial infarction, add requisite dose to 25–50 mL infusion fluid and give over 1–2 minutes

Fosaprepitant (*Ivemend*®)
Intermittent *in* Sodium chloride 0.9%
Reconstitute each 150-mg vial with 5 mL sodium chloride 0.9% gently without shaking to avoid foaming, then dilute in 145 mL infusion fluid; give over 20–30 minutes

Foscarnet sodium (*Foscavir*®)
Intermittent *in* Glucose 5% *or* Sodium chloride 0.9%
Dilute to a concentration of 12 mg/mL for infusion into peripheral vein (undiluted solution *via* central venous line only); infuse over at least 1 hour (infuse doses greater than 60 mg/kg over 2 hours)

Fosfomycin (*Fomicyt*®)
Intermittent *in* Glucose 5% or 10% *or* Water for Injections
Reconstitute each 2-g vial with 50 mL infusion fluid; give 2 g over 15 minutes

Fosphenytoin Sodium (*Pro-Epanutin*®)
Intermittent *in* Glucose 5% *or* Sodium chloride 0.9%
Dilute to a concentration of 1.5–25 mg (phenytoin sodium equivalent)/mL

Furosemide (as sodium salt) (*Lasix*®)
Continuous *in* Sodium chloride 0.9%
Infusion pH must be above 5.5 and rate should not exceed 4 mg/minute; glucose solutions are unsuitable

Galsulfase (*Naglazyme*®)
Intermittent *in* Sodium chloride 0.9%
Dilute requisite dose with infusion fluid to final volume of 250 mL and mix gently; infuse through a 0.2 micron in-line filter; give approx. 2.5% of the total volume over 1 hour, then infuse remaining volume over next 3 hours; if body-weight under 20 kg and at risk of fluid overload, dilute requisite dose in 100 mL infusion fluid and give over at least 4 hours

Ganciclovir (as sodium salt) (*Cymevene*®)
Intermittent *in* Glucose 5% *or* Sodium chloride 0.9%
Reconstitute initially in water for injections (500 mg/10 mL) then dilute to not more than 10 mg/mL with infusion fluid (usually 100 mL); give over 1 hour

Gentamicin (as sulfate) (*Cidomycin*®; Gentamicin Paediatric Injection, Beacon; Gentamicin Injection, Hospira)
Intermittent *or via* drip tubing *in* Glucose 5% *or* Sodium chloride 0.9%
Suggested volume for intermittent infusion 50–100 mL given over 20–30 minutes (given over 60 minutes for once daily dose regimen)

Glyceryl trinitrate (*Nitrocine*®, *Nitronal*®)
Continuous *in* Glucose 5% *or* Sodium chloride 0.9%
For *Nitrocine*® suggested infusion concentration 100 micrograms/mL; incompatible with polyvinyl chloride infusion containers such as *Viaflex*® or *Steriflex*®; use glass or polyethylene containers or give *via* a syringe pump

Granisetron (as hydrochloride)
Intermittent *in* Glucose 5% *or* Sodium chloride 0.9%
Dilute up to 3 mL in 20–50 mL infusion fluid (up to 3 mL in a total volume of 10–30 mL for children); give over 5 minutes

Haem arginate (*Normosang*®)

Intermittent *in* Sodium chloride 0.9%

Dilute requisite dose in 100 mL infusion fluid in glass bottle and give over at least 30 minutes through a filter *via* large antebrachial or central vein; administer within 1 hour after dilution

Heparin sodium Continuous *in* Glucose 5% *or* Sodium chloride 0.9%

Administration with a motorised pump advisable

Hydralazine hydrochloride (*Apresoline*®)

Continuous *in* Sodium chloride 0.9%

Suggested infusion volume 500 mL

Hydrocortisone (as sodium phosphate) (*Efcortesol*®)

Continuous *or* intermittent *or via* drip tubing *in* Glucose 5% *or* Sodium chloride 0.9%

Hydrocortisone (as sodium succinate) (*SoluCortef*®)

Continuous *or* intermittent *or via* drip tubing *in* Glucose 5% *or* Sodium chloride 0.9%

Hydroxocobalamin (*Cyanokit*®)

Intermittent *in* Sodium chloride 0.9%

Reconstitute each 5-g vial with 200 mL infusion fluid; gently invert vial for at least 1 minute to mix; do not shake

Ibandronic acid (*Bondronat*®)

Intermittent *in* Glucose 5% *or* Sodium chloride 0.9%

Dilute requisite dose in 500 mL infusion fluid and give over 1–2 hours

Idursulfase (*Elaprase*®)

Intermittent *in* Sodium chloride 0.9%

Dilute requisite dose in 100 mL infusion fluid and mix gently (do not shake); give over 3 hours (gradually reduced to 1 hour if no infusion-related reactions)

Imiglucerase (*Cerezyme*®)

Intermittent *in* Sodium chloride 0.9%

Initially reconstitute with water for injections (200 units in 5.1 mL, 400 units in 10.2 mL) to give 40 units/mL solution; dilute requisite dose with infusion fluid to a final volume of 100–200 mL and give initial dose at a rate not exceeding 0.5 units/kg/minute, subsequent doses to be given at a rate not exceeding 1 unit/kg/minute; administer within 3 hours after reconstitution

Imipenem with cilastatin (as sodium salt) (*Primaxin*®)

Intermittent *in* Sodium chloride 0.9%

Dilute to a concentration of 5 mg (as imipenem)/mL; infuse 500 mg (as imipenem) over 20–30 minutes, dose greater than 500 mg (as imipenem) over 40–60 minutes

Infliximab (*Remicade*®)

Intermittent *in* Sodium chloride 0.9%

Reconstitute each 100-mg vial with 10 mL water for injections using a 21-gauge or smaller needle; gently swirl vial without shaking to dissolve; allow to stand for 5 minutes; dilute requisite dose with infusion fluid to a final volume of 250 mL and give through a low protein-binding filter (1.2 micron or less) over at least 2 hours (adults over 18 years who have tolerated 3 initial 2-hour infusions may be given subsequent infusions of up to 6 mg/kg over at least 1 hour); start infusion within 3 hours of reconstitution

Insulin (soluble) Continuous *in* Sodium chloride 0.9%

Adsorbed to some extent by plastics of infusion set; see also section 6.1.3; ensure insulin is not injected into 'dead space' of injection port of the infusion bag

Insulin aspart Continuous *in* Glucose 5% *or* Sodium chloride 0.9%

Dilute to 0.05–1 unit/mL with infusion fluid; adsorbed to some extent by plastics of infusion set

Insulin glulisine (*Apidra*®)

Continuous in Sodium chloride 0.9%

Dilute to 1 unit/mL with infusion fluid; use a co-extruded polyolefin/polyamide plastic infusion bag with a dedicated infusion line

Insulin lispro Continuous *in* Glucose 5% *or* Sodium chloride 0.9%

Adsorbed to some extent by plastics of infusion set

Iron dextran (*Cosmofer*®)

Intermittent *in* Glucose 5% *or* Sodium chloride 0.9%

Dilute 100–200 mg in 100 mL infusion fluid; give 25 mg over 15 minutes initially, then give at a rate not exceeding 6.67 mg/minute; *total dose infusion* diluted in 500 mL infusion fluid and given over 4–6 hours (initial dose 25 mg over 15 minutes)

Iron isomaltoside 1000 (*Monofer*®)

Intermittent *in* Sodium chloride 0.9%

For details consult product literature

Iron sucrose (*Venofer*®)

Intermittent *in* Sodium chloride 0.9%

Dilute 100 mg in up to 100 mL infusion fluid; give 25 mg over 15 minutes initially, then give at a rate not exceeding 3.33 mg/minute

Isosorbide dinitrate (*Isoket 0.05%*®, *Isoket 0.1%*®)

Continuous *in* Glucose 5% *or* Sodium chloride 0.9%

Adsorbed to some extent by polyvinyl chloride infusion containers; preferably use glass or polyethylene containers or give *via* a syringe pump; *Isoket 0.05%*® can alternatively be administered undiluted using a syringe pump with a glass or rigid plastic syringe

Itraconazole (*Sporanox*®)

Intermittent *in* Sodium chloride 0.9%

Dilute 250 mg in 50 mL infusion fluid and infuse only 60 mL through an in-line filter (0.2 micron) over 60 minutes

Ketamine (as hydrochloride) (*Ketalar*®)

Continuous *in* Glucose 5% *or* Sodium chloride 0.9%

Dilute to 1 mg/mL; microdrip infusion for maintenance of anaesthesia

Labetalol hydrochloride

Intermittent *in* Glucose 5% *or* Sodium chloride and glucose

Dilute to a concentration of 1 mg/mL; suggested volume 200 mL; adjust rate with in-line burette

Lacosamide (*Vimpat*®)

Intermittent *in* Glucose 5% *or* Sodium chloride 0.9%

May be administered undiluted

Laronidase (*Aldurazyme*®)

Intermittent *in* Sodium chloride 0.9%

Body-weight under 20 kg, use 100 mL infusion fluid; body-weight over 20 kg use 250 mL infusion fluid; withdraw volume of infusion fluid equivalent to volume of laronidase concentrate being added; give through an in-line filter (0.22 micron) at an initial rate of 2 units/kg/hour then increasing gradually every 15 minutes to max. 43 units/kg/hour

Lenograstim (*Granocyte*®)

Intermittent *in* Sodium chloride 0.9%

Initially reconstitute with 1 mL water for injection provided (do not shake vigorously) then dilute with up to 50 mL infusion fluid for each vial of *Granocyte-13* or up to 100 mL infusion fluid for *Granocyte-34*; give over 30 minutes

Levetiracetam (*Keppra*®)

Intermittent *in* Glucose 5% *or* Sodium chloride 0.9%

Dilute requisite dose with at least 100 mL of infusion fluid; give over 15 minutes

Magnesium sulfate injection, BP Continuous *in* Glucose 5% *or* Sodium chloride 0.9%

Suggested concentration up to 200 mg/mL (20%) (0.8 mmol/mL Mg²⁺) magnesium sulfate heptahydrate; max. rate 150 mg/minute (0.6 mmol/minute Mg²⁺)

Meropenem (*Meronem*®) Intermittent *in* Glucose 5% *or* Sodium chloride 0.9%

Dilute dose in infusion fluid to a final concentration of 1–20 mg/mL; give over 15–30 minutes

Metaraminol (as tartrate) (*Aramine*®) Continuous *or via* drip tubing *in* Glucose 5% *or* Sodium chloride 0.9%

Suggested volume 500 mL

Methylprednisolone (as sodium succinate) (*Solu-Medrone*®)

Continuous *or* intermittent *or via* drip tubing *in* Glucose 5% *or* Sodium chloride 0.9%

Reconstitute initially with water for injections; doses up to 250 mg should be given over at least 5 minutes, high doses over at least 30 minutes

Micafungin (*Mycamine*®) Intermittent *in* Glucose 5% *or* Sodium chloride 0.9%

Reconstitute each vial with 5 mL infusion fluid; gently rotate vial, without shaking, to dissolve; dilute requisite dose with infusion fluid to 100 mL (final concentration 0.5–2 mg/mL); protect infusion from light; give over 60 minutes

Midazolam (*Hypnovel*®) Continuous *in* Glucose 5% *or* Sodium chloride 0.9%

For neonates and children under 15 kg dilute to a max. concentration of 1 mg/mL

Milrinone (*Primacor*®) Continuous *in* Glucose 5% *or* Sodium chloride 0.9%

Dilute to a suggested concentration of 200 micrograms/mL

Mivacurium (as chloride) (*Mivacron*®) Continuous *in* Glucose 5% *or* Sodium chloride 0.9%

Dilute to a concentration of 500 micrograms/mL; may also be given undiluted

Mycophenolate mofetil (as hydrochloride) (*CellCept*®) Intermittent *in* Glucose 5%

Reconstitute each 500-mg vial with 14 mL glucose 5% and dilute the contents of 2 vials in 140 mL infusion fluid; give over 2 hours

Naloxone (*Minijet*® *Naloxone Hydrochloride*) Continuous *in* Glucose 5% *or* Sodium chloride 0.9%

Dilute to a concentration of up to 200 micrograms/mL and administer via an infusion pump, see Emergency Treatment of Poisoning

Natalizumab (*Tysabri*®) Intermittent *in* Sodium chloride 0.9%

Dilute 300 mg in 100 mL infusion fluid; gently invert to mix, do not shake. Use within 8 hours of dilution and give over 1 hour

Nicardipine hydrochloride Continuous *in* Glucose 5%

Dilute dose in infusion fluid to a final concentration of 100–200 micrograms/mL (undiluted solution *via* central venous line only) and give *via* volumetric infusion pump or syringe driver; protect from light; to minimise peripheral venous irritation, change site of infusion every 12 hours; risk of adsorption on to plastic of infusion set in the presence of saline solutions; incompatible with bicarbonate or alkaline solutions—consult product literature

Nimodipine (*Nimotop*®) *via* drip tubing *in* Glucose 5% *or* Sodium chloride 0.9%

Not to be added to infusion container; administer *via* an infusion pump through a Y-piece into a central venous catheter; incompatible with polyvinyl chloride giving sets or containers; protect infusion from light

Nizatidine (*Axid*®) Continuous *or* intermittent *in* Glucose 5% *or* Sodium chloride 0.9%

For continuous infusion, dilute 300 mg in 150 mL and give at a rate of 10 mg/hour; for intermittent infusion, dilute 100 mg in 50 mL and give over 15 minutes

Noradrenaline/Norepinephrine Continuous *in* Glucose 5% *or* Sodium chloride and glucose

Give *via* controlled infusion device; for administration *via* syringe pump, dilute 2 mg (2 mL of solution) noradrenaline base with 48 mL infusion fluid; for administration *via* drip counter dilute 20 mg (20 mL of solution) noradrenaline base with 480 mL infusion fluid; give through a central venous catheter; incompatible with alkalis.

1 mg of noradrenaline base is equivalent to 2 mg noradrenaline acid tartrate

Omeprazole (as sodium salt) (*Losec*®) Intermittent *or* continuous *in* Glucose 5% *or* Sodium chloride 0.9%

Reconstitute each 40 mg vial with infusion fluid and dilute to 100 mL; for intermittent infusion, give 40 mg over 20–30 minutes; stable for 3 hours in glucose 5% *or* 12 hours in sodium chloride 0.9%

Ondansetron (as hydrochloride) (*Zofran*®) Continuous *or* intermittent *in* Glucose 5% *or* Glucose 5% with potassium chloride 0.3% *or* Sodium chloride 0.9% *or* Sodium chloride 0.9% with potassium chloride 0.3% *or* Mannitol 10% *or* Ringers solution

For intermittent infusion, dilute the required dose in 50–100 mL of infusion fluid and give over at least 15 minutes

Oxycodone hydrochloride (*OxyNorm*®) Continuous *or* intermittent *in* Glucose 5% *or* Sodium chloride 0.9%

Dilute to a concentration of 1 mg/mL

Oxytocin (*Syntocinon*®) Continuous *in* Glucose 5% *or* Sodium chloride 0.9%

Preferably given *via* a variable-speed infusion pump in a concentration appropriate to the pump; if given by drip infusion for *induction or enhancement of labour*, dilute 5 units in 500 mL infusion fluid or for higher doses, 10 units in 500 mL; for *treatment of postpartum uterine haemorrhage* dilute 40 units in 500 mL; if high doses given for prolonged period (e.g. for inevitable or missed abortion or for postpartum haemorrhage), use low volume of an electrolyte-containing infusion fluid (not Glucose 5%) given at higher concentration than for induction or enhancement of labour; close attention to patient's fluid and electrolyte status essential

Pamidronate disodium (*Aredia*®; *Pamidronate disodium*, Hospira, Medac, Wockhardt) Intermittent *in* Glucose 5% *or* Sodium chloride 0.9%

For *Aredia*®, reconstitute initially with water for injections (15 mg in 5 mL, 30 mg or 90 mg in 10 mL); for *Pamidronate disodium* (Wockhardt), dilute with infusion fluid to a concentration of not more than 60 mg in 250 mL; for *Aredia*®, *Pamidronate disodium* (Medac, Hospira) dilute with infusion fluid to a concentration of not more than 90 mg in 250 mL; give at a rate not exceeding 1 mg/minute; not to be given with infusion fluids containing calcium

Pantoprazole (as sodium sesquihydrate) (*Protium*®) Intermittent *in* Glucose 5% *or* Sodium chloride 0.9%

Reconstitute 40 mg with 10 mL sodium chloride 0.9% and dilute with 100 mL of infusion fluid; give 40 mg over 15 minutes

Paracetamol (*Perfalgan*®) Intermittent *in* Glucose 5% *or* Sodium chloride 0.9%

Dilute to a concentration of not less than 1 mg/mL and use within 1 hour; may also be given undiluted

Pentamidine isetionate (*Pentacarinat*®) Intermittent *in* Glucose 5% *or* Sodium chloride 0.9%

Dissolve initially in water for injections (300 mg in 3–5 mL) then dilute in 50–250 mL; give over at least 60 minutes

Phenoxybenzamine hydrochloride Intermittent *in* Sodium chloride 0.9%
Dilute in 200–500 mL infusion fluid; give over at least 2 hours; max. 4 hours between dilution and completion of administration

Phenylephrine hydrochloride Intermittent *in* Glucose 5% *or* Sodium chloride 0.9%
Dilute 10 mg in 500 mL infusion fluid

Phenytoin sodium (*Epanutin*®)
Intermittent *in* Sodium chloride 0.9%
Flush intravenous line with Sodium chloride 0.9% before and after infusion; dilute in 50–100 mL infusion fluid (final concentration not to exceed 10 mg/mL) and give into a large vein through an in-line filter (0.22–0.50 micron) at a rate not exceeding 1 mg/kg/minute (max. 50 mg/minute); complete administration within 1 hour of preparation

Phytomenadione (In mixed micelles vehicle) (*Konakion*® *MM*)
Intermittent *in* Glucose 5%
Dilute with 55 mL; may be injected into lower part of infusion apparatus

Piperacillin with tazobactam (as sodium salts) Intermittent *in* Glucose 5% *or* Sodium chloride 0.9%
Reconstitute initially (2.25 g in 10 mL, 4.5 g in 20 mL) with water for injections, or glucose 5% (*Tazocin*® brand only), or sodium chloride 0.9%, then dilute to 50–150 mL with infusion fluid; give over 30 minutes

Potassium chloride Continuous *in* Glucose 5% *or* Sodium chloride 0.9%
Dilute in a large-volume infusion; mix thoroughly to avoid 'layering', especially in non-rigid infusion containers; use ready-prepared solutions when possible

Propofol (emulsion) (*Diprivan*®; *Propofol-Lipuro*®)
Shake before use; microbiological filter not recommended; may be administered via a Y-piece close to injection site co-administered with Glucose 5% *or* Sodium chloride 0.9%
0.5% emulsion
Intermittent
May be administered undiluted, or diluted with Glucose 5% or Sodium chloride 0.9%; dilute to a concentration not less than 1 mg/mL
1% emulsion
Continuous *or* intermittent
May be administered undiluted, or diluted with Sodium Chloride 0.9% (*Propofol-Lipuro*® only) or Glucose 5%; dilute to a concentration not less than 2 mg/mL; use within 6 hours of preparation
2% emulsion
Continuous
Do not dilute

Quinine dihydrochloride Continuous *In* Glucose 5% *or* Sodium chloride 0.9%
To be given over 4 hours; see also section 5.4.1

Ranitidine (as hydrochloride) (*Zantac*®)
Intermittent *in* Glucose 5% *or* Sodium chloride 0.9%

Rasburicase (*Fasturtec*®)
Intermittent *in* Sodium chloride 0.9%
Reconstitute with solvent provided; gently swirl vial without shaking to dissolve; dilute requisite dose to 50 mL with infusion fluid and give over 30 minutes

Remifentanil (*Ultiva*®)
Continuous *in* Glucose 5% *or* Sodium chloride 0.9% *or* Water for injections
Reconstitute with infusion fluid to a concentration of 1 mg/ mL then dilute further to a concentration of 20–250 micrograms/mL (50 micrograms/mL recommended for general anaesthesia, 20–25 micrograms/mL recommended for children 1–12 years; 20–50 micrograms/mL recommended when used with target controlled infusion (TCI) device)

Rifampicin (*Rifadin*®)
Intermittent *in* Glucose 5% *or* Sodium chloride 0.9%
Reconstitute with solvent provided then dilute with 500 mL infusion fluid; give over 2–3 hours

Rituximab (*MabThera*®)
Intermittent *in* Glucose 5% *or* Sodium chloride 0.9%
Dilute to 1–4 mg/mL and gently invert bag to avoid foaming

Rocuronium bromide (*Esmeron*®)
Continuous *or via* drip tubing *in* Glucose 5% *or* Sodium chloride 0.9%

Salbutamol (as sulfate) (*Ventolin*® For Intravenous Infusion)
Continuous *in* Glucose 5%
For *bronchodilatation* dilute to a concentration of 200 micrograms/mL with glucose 5% or sodium chloride 0.9%; for *premature labour* dilute with glucose 5% to a concentration of 200 micrograms/mL for use in a syringe pump *or* for other infusion methods (preferably *via* controlled infusion device), dilute to a concentration of 20 micrograms/mL; close attention to patient's fluid and electrolyte status essential

Siltuximab (*Sylvant*®)
Intermittent *in* Glucose 5%
Allow vials to reach room temperature over approximately 30 minutes, then reconstitute each 100 mg vial with 5.2 mL of water for injection, and each 400 mg vial with 20 mL of water for injection, to produce a 20 mg/mL solution. Gently swirl without shaking to dissolve. Further dilute to 250 mL with glucose 5% and gently mix. Use within 6 hours of dilution and give over 60 minutes using an administration set lined with polyvinyl chloride or polyurethane, through a low-protein binding in-line 0.2 micron filter

Sodium nitroprusside Continuous *in* Glucose 5%
Infuse *via* infusion device to allow precise control; protect infusion from light. For further details consult product literature

Sodium valproate (*Epilim*®, *Episenta*®)
Continuous *or* intermittent *in* Glucose 5% *or* Sodium chloride 0.9%
Reconstitute *Epilim*® with solvent provided then dilute with infusion fluid

Streptokinase (*Streptase*®)
Continuous *or* intermittent *in* Glucose 5% *or* Sodium chloride 0.9%
Reconstitute with sodium chloride 0.9%, then dilute further with infusion fluid

Tacrolimus (*Prograf*®)
Continuous *in* Glucose 5% *or* Sodium chloride 0.9%
Dilute concentrate in infusion fluid to a final concentration of 4–100 micrograms/mL; give over 24 hours; incompatible with PVC

Teicoplanin (*Targocid*®)
Intermittent *in* Glucose 5% *or* Sodium chloride 0.9%
Reconstitute initially with water for injections provided; infuse over 30 minutes
Continuous infusion not usually recommended

Telavancin (*Vibativ*®)
Intermittent *in* Glucose 5% *or* Sodium chloride 0.9%
Reconstitute each 750 mg with 45 mL glucose 5%, sodium chloride 0.9%, or water for injections to produce a 15 mg/ mL solution; for doses of 150–800 mg, dilute requisite dose in 100 to 250 mL infusion fluid; for doses outside this range, dilute to a final concentration of 0.6–8 mg/mL; give over at least 60 minutes

Temocillin (*Negaban*®)
Intermittent *in* Glucose 5% or 10% *or* Sodium chloride 0.9%
Reconstitute 1 g with 10 mL water for injections then dilute with 50–150 mL infusion fluid; give over 30–40 minutes

Terbutaline sulfate (*Bricanyl®*)
Continuous *in* Glucose 5%
For *bronchodilatation* dilute 1.5–2.5 mg with 500 mL glucose 5% or sodium chloride 0.9% and give over 8–10 hours; for *premature labour* dilute in glucose 5% and give *via* controlled infusion device preferably a syringe pump; if syringe pump available dilute to a concentration of 100 micrograms/mL; if syringe pump not available dilute to a concentration of 10 micrograms/mL; close attention to patient's fluid and electrolyte status essential

Ticarcillin sodium with clavulanic acid (*Timentin®*)
Intermittent *in* Glucose 5%
Suggested volume (depending on dose) 100–150 mL; give over 30–40 minutes

Tigecycline (*Tygacil®*)
Intermittent *in* Glucose 5% *or* Sodium chloride 0.9%
Reconstitute each vial with 5.3 mL infusion fluid to produce a 10 mg/mL solution; dilute requisite dose in 100 mL infusion fluid; give over 30–60 minutes

Tirofiban (*Aggrastat®*)
Continuous *in* Glucose 5% *or* Sodium chloride 0.9%
Withdraw 50 mL infusion fluid from 250-mL bag and replace with 50 mL tirofiban concentrate (250 micrograms/mL) to give a final concentration of 50 micrograms/mL

Tobramycin (as sulfate) (*Nebcin®*)
Intermittent *or via* drip tubing *in* Glucose 5% *or* Sodium chloride 0.9%
For adult intermittent infusion suggested volume 50–100 mL (children proportionately smaller volume) given over 20–60 minutes

Tocilizumab (*RoActemra®*)
Intermittent *in* Sodium chloride 0.9%
Dilute requisite dose to a volume of 100 mL with infusion fluid and give over 1 hour

Tramadol hydrochloride (*Zydol®*)
Continuous *or* intermittent *in* Glucose 5% *or* Sodium chloride 0.9%

Tranexamic acid (*Cyklokapron®*)
Continuous *or* intermittent *in* Glucose 5% *or* Sodium chloride 0.9%

Urokinase (*Syner-KINASE®*)
Continuous *or* intermittent *in* Sodium chloride 0.9%

Vancomycin (as hydrochloride) (*Vancocin®*)
Intermittent *in* Glucose 5% *or* Sodium chloride 0.9%
Reconstitute each 500 mg with 10 mL water for injections and dilute with infusion fluid to a concentration of up to 5 mg/mL (10 mg/mL in fluid restriction but increased risk of infusion-related effects); give over at least 60 minutes (rate not to exceed 10 mg/minute for doses over 500 mg); use continuous infusion only if intermittent not feasible

Vasopressin, synthetic (argipressin)
Intermittent *in* Glucose 5%
Suggested concentration 20 units/100 mL given over 15 minutes

Vecuronium bromide (*Norcuron®*)
Continuous *or via* drip tubing *in* Glucose 5% *or* Sodium chloride 0.9%
Reconstitute each vial with 5 mL water for injections to give 2 mg/mL solution; *alternatively* reconstitute with up to 10 mL glucose 5% *or* sodium chloride 0.9% *or* water for injections—unsuitable for further dilution if not reconstituted with water for injections. For *continuous intravenous infusion*, dilute to a concentration up to 40 micrograms/mL

Vedolizumab (*Entyvio®*)
Intermittent *in* Sodium chloride 0.9%
Allow vial to reach room temperature then reconstitute with 4.8 mL of water for injection (using a syringe with a 21–25 gauge needle); gently swirl vial for at least 15 seconds, do not shake vigorously or invert; allow to stand for up to 20 minutes (gently swirl vial if needed), leave for an additional 10 minutes if not dissolved; gently invert vial three times, withdraw 5 mL of reconstituted solution (using a syringe with a 21–25 gauge needle), and add to 250 mL of infusion fluid; gently mix and give over 30 minutes

Velaglucerase alfa (*VPRIV®*)
Intermittent *in* Sodium chloride 0.9%
Reconstitute each 400–unit vial with 4.3 mL water for injections to produce a 100 units/mL solution; dilute requisite dose in 100 mL infusion fluid; give over 60 minutes through a 0.22 micron filter; start infusion within 24 hours of reconstitution

Verteporfin (*Visudyne®*)
Intermittent *in* Glucose 5%
Reconstitute each 15 mg with 7 mL water for injections to produce a 2 mg/mL solution then dilute requisite dose with infusion fluid to a final volume of 30 mL and give over 10 minutes; protect infusion from light and administer within 4 hours of reconstitution. Incompatible with sodium chloride infusion

Vitamins B & C (*Pabrinex® I/V High potency*)
Intermittent *or via* drip tubing *in* Glucose 5% *or* Sodium chloride 0.9%
Ampoule contents should be mixed, diluted, and administered without delay; give over 30 minutes (see MHRA/CHM advice, section 9.6.2)

Vitamins, multiple
(*Cernevit®*)
Intermittent *in* Glucose 5% *or* Sodium chloride 0.9%
Dissolve initially in 5 mL water for injections (or infusion fluid)
(*Solivito N®*)
Intermittent *in* Glucose 5 and 10%
Suggested volume 500–1000 mL given over 2–3 hours; see also section 9.3

Voriconazole (*Vfend®*)
Intermittent *in* Glucose 5% *or* Sodium chloride 0.9%
Reconstitute each 200 mg with 19 mL water for injections or sodium chloride 0.9% to produce a 10 mg/mL solution; dilute dose in infusion fluid to concentration of 0.5–5 mg/mL; give at a rate not exceeding 3 mg/kg/hour

Zidovudine (*Retrovir®*)
Intermittent *in* Glucose 5%
Dilute to a concentration of 2 mg/mL or 4 mg/mL and give over 1 hour

Zoledronic acid (*Zometa®*)
Intermittent *in* Glucose 5% *or* Sodium chloride 0.9%
Dilute requisite dose according to product literature; infuse over at least 15 minutes; administer as a single intravenous solution in a separate infusion line

A5 Wound management products and elasticated garments

Wound dressings   The correct dressing for wound management depends not only on the type of wound but also on the stage of the healing process. The principal stages of healing are:

- cleansing, removal of debris;
- granulation, vascularisation;
- epithelialisation.

The ideal dressing for moist wound healing needs to ensure that the wound remains:

- moist with exudate, but not macerated;
- free of clinical infection and excessive slough;
- free of toxic chemicals, particles or fibres;
- at the optimum temperature for healing;
- undisturbed by the need for frequent changes;
- at the optimum pH value.

As wound healing passes through its different stages, different types of dressings may be required to satisfy better one or other of these requirements. Under normal circumstances, a moist environment is a necessary part of the wound healing process; exudate provides a moist environment and promotes healing, but excessive exudate can cause maceration of the wound and surrounding healthy tissue. The volume and viscosity of exudate changes as the wound heals. There are certain circumstances when moist wound healing is not appropriate (e.g. gangrenous toes associated with vascular disease).

Advanced wound dressings, (section A5.2) are designed to control the environment for wound healing, for example to donate fluid (**hydrogels**), maintain hydration (**hydrocolloids**), or to absorb wound exudate (**alginates, foams**).

Practices such as the use of irritant cleansers and desloughing agents may be harmful and are largely obsolete; removal of debris and dressing remnants should need minimal irrigation with lukewarm sterile sodium chloride 0.9% solution or water.

Hydrogel, hydrocolloid, and medical grade honey dressings can be used to deslough wounds by promoting autolytic debridement; there is insufficient evidence to support any particular method of debridement for difficult-to-heal surgical wounds. Sterile larvae (maggots) are also available for biosurgical removal of wound debris.

There have been few clinical trials able to establish a clear advantage for any particular product. The choice between different dressings depends not only on the type and stage of the wound, but also on patient preference or tolerance, site of the wound, and cost. For further information, see *Buyers' Guide: Advanced wound dressings* (October 2008); NHS Purchasing and Supply Agency, Centre for Evidence-based Purchasing.

Prices quoted in Appendix 5 are basic NHS net prices; for further information see Prices in the BNF.

The table below gives suggestions for choices of primary dressing depending on the type of wound (a secondary dressing may be needed in some cases).

A5.1 Basic wound contact dressings

A5.1.1 Low adherence dressings

Low adherence dressings are used as interface layers under secondary absorbent dressings. Placed directly on the wound bed, non-absorbent, low adherence dressings are suitable for clean, granulating, lightly exuding wounds without necrosis, and protect the wound bed from direct contact with secondary dressings. Care must be taken to avoid granulation tissue growing into the weave of these dressings.

Tulle dressings are manufactured from cotton or viscose fibres which are impregnated with white or yellow soft paraffin to prevent the fibres from sticking, but this

Wound contact material for different types of wounds

Wound PINK (Epithelialising)

Low Exudate	Moderate Exudate
Low adherence A5.1.1	Soft polymer A5.2.3
Vapour-permeable film A5.2.2	Foam, low absorbent A5.2.5
Soft polymer A.5.2.3	Alginate A5.2.6
Hydrocolloid A5.2.4	

Wound RED (Granulating)
Symptoms or signs of infection, see **Wounds with signs of infection**

Low Exudate	Moderate Exudate	Heavy Exudate
Low adherence A5.1.1	Hydrocolloid-fibrous A5.2.4	Foam with extra absorbency A5.2.5
Soft polymer A5.2.3	Foam A5.2.5	Hydrocolloid-fibrous A5.2.4
Hydrocolloid A5.2.4	Alginate A5.2.6	Alginate A5.2.6
Foam, low absorbent A5.2.5		

Wound YELLOW (Sloughy)
Symptoms or signs of infection, see **Wounds with signs of infection**

Low Exudate	Moderate Exudate	Heavy Exudate
Hydrogel A5.2.1	Hydrocolloid-fibrous A5.2.4	Hydrocolloid-fibrous A5.2.4
Hydrocolloid A5.2.4	Alginate A5.2.6	Alginate A5.2.6
		Capillary-action A5.2.7

Wound BLACK (Necrotic/Eschar)
Consider mechanical debridement alongside autolytic debridement

Low Exudate or Dry	Moderate Exudate	Heavy Exudate
Hydrogel A5.2.1	Hydrocolloid A5.2.4	Seek advice from wound care specialist
Hydrocolloid A5.2.4	Hydrocolloid-fibrous A5.2.4	
	Foam A5.2.5	

Wounds with signs of infection
Consider systemic antibacterials if appropriate; also consider odour-absorbent dressings (section A5.2.8)
For malodourous wounds with slough or necrotic tissue, consider mechanical or autolytic debridement

Low Exudate	Moderate Exudate	Heavy Exudate
Low adherence with honey A5.3.1	Hydrocolloid-fibrous with silver A5.3.3	Hydrocolloid-fibrous with silver A5.3.3
Low adherence with iodine A5.3.2	Foam with silver A5.3.3	Foam, extra absorbent, with silver A5.3.3
Low adherence with silver A5.3.3	Alginate with silver A5.3.3	Alginate with honey A5.3.1
Hydrocolloid with silver A5.3.3	Honey—topical A5.3.1	Alginate with silver A5.3.3
Honey—topical A5.3.1	Cadexomer—iodine A5.3.2	

Note In each section of this table the dressings are listed in order of increasing absorbency.
Some wound contact (primary) dressings require a secondary dressing

is only partly successful and it may be necessary to change the dressings frequently. The paraffin reduces absorbency of the dressing. Dressings with a reduced content (light loading) of soft paraffin are less liable to interfere with absorption; dressings with 'normal loading' (such as *Jelonet*®) have been used for skin graft transfer.

Knitted viscose primary dressing is an alternative to tulle dressings for exuding wounds; it can be used as the initial layer of multi-layer compression bandaging in the treatment of venous leg ulcers.

Knitted Viscose Primary Dressing, BP 1993
Warp knitted fabric manufactured from a bright viscose monofilament.
N-A Dressing®, 9.5 cm × 9.5 cm = 35p, 9.5 cm × 19 cm = 67p (Systagenix)
N-A Ultra® (silicone-coated), 9.5 cm × 9.5 cm = 33p, 9.5 cm × 19 cm = 63p (Systagenix)
Profore®, 14 cm × 20 cm = 30p (S&N Hlth.)
Tricotex®, 9.5 cm × 9.5 cm = 32p (S&N Hlth.)

Paraffin Gauze Dressing, BP 1993
(Tulle Gras). Fabric of leno weave, weft and warp threads of cotton and/or viscose yarn, impregnated with white or yellow soft paraffin, 10 cm × 10 cm, (light loading) = 25p; (normal loading) = 37p (most suppliers including Synergy Healthcare—*Paranet*® (light loading); BSN Medical—*Cuticell*® *Classic* (normal loading); S&N Hlth.—*Jelonet*® (normal loading); Neomedic—*Neotulle*® (normal loading); C D Medical—*Paragauze*® (normal loading))

Atrauman® (Hartmann)
Non-adherent knitted polyester primary dressing impregnated with neutral triglycerides, 5 cm × 5 cm = 24p, 7.5 cm × 10 cm = 26p, 10 cm × 20 cm = 59p, 20 cm × 30 cm = £1.63

A5.1.2   Absorbent dressings

Perforated film absorbent dressings are suitable only for wounds with mild to moderate amounts of exudate; they are **not** appropriate for leg ulcers or for other lesions that produce large quantities of viscous exudate. Dressings with an absorbent cellulose or polymer wadding layer are suitable for use on moderately to heavily exuding wounds.

◀ **For lightly exuding wounds**

Absorbent Perforated Dressing with Adhesive Border
Low-adherence primary dressing consisting of viscose and rayon absorbent pad with adhesive border.
Adpore®, 7 cm × 8 cm = 8p, 10 cm × 10 cm = 10p, 10 cm × 15 cm = 16p, 10 cm × 20 cm = 30p, 10 cm × 25 cm = 34p, 10 cm × 30 cm = 42p, 10 cm × 35 cm = 50p (Medicareplus International)
Cosmopor E®, 5 cm × 7.2 cm = 8p, 8 cm × 10 cm = 16p, 8 cm × 15 cm = 26p, 10 cm × 20 cm = 43p, 10 cm × 25 cm = 53p, 10 cm × 35 cm = 74p (Hartmann)
Cutiplast® Steril, 5 cm × 7.2 cm = 5p, 8 cm × 10 cm = 10p, 8 cm × 15 cm = 23p, 10 cm × 20 cm = 29p, 10 cm × 25 cm = 30p, 10 cm × 30 cm = 40p (S&N Hlth.)

Leukomed®, 7.2 cm × 5 cm = 8p, 8 cm × 10 cm = 17p, 8 cm × 15 cm = 30p, 10 cm × 20 cm = 40p, 10 cm × 25 cm = 46p, 10 cm × 30 cm = 59p, 10 cm × 35 cm = 68p (BSN Medical)
Medipore® + Pad, 5 cm × 7.2 cm = 7p, 10 cm × 10 cm = 15p, 10 cm × 15 cm = 24p, 10 cm × 20 cm = 36p, 10 cm × 25 cm = 45p, 10 cm × 35 cm = 62p (3M)
Medisafe®, 6 cm × 8 cm = 8p, 8 cm × 10 cm = 13p, 8 cm × 12 cm = 23p, 9 cm × 15 cm = 29p, 9 cm × 20 cm = 34p, 9 cm × 25 cm = 36p (Neomedic)
Mepore®, 7 cm × 8 cm = 10p, 10 cm × 11 cm = 21p, 11 cm × 15 cm = 34p, 9 cm × 20 cm = 42p, 9 cm × 25 cm = 58p, 9 cm × 30 cm = 67p, 9 cm × 35 cm = 73p (Mölnlycke)
PremierPore®, 5 cm × 7 cm = 5p, 10 cm × 10 cm = 12p, 10 cm × 15 cm = 18p, 10 cm × 20 cm = 32p, 10 cm × 25 cm = 36p, 10 cm × 30 cm = 45p, 10 cm × 35 cm = 52p (Shermond)
Primapore®, 6 cm × 8.3 cm = 17p, 8 cm × 10 cm = 18p, 8 cm × 15 cm = 31p, 10 cm × 20 cm = 41p, 10 cm × 25 cm = 47p, 10 cm × 30 cm = 59p, 10 cm × 35 cm = 91p (S&N Hlth)
Softpore®, 6 cm × 7 cm = 6p, 10 cm × 10 cm = 13p, 10 cm × 15 cm = 20p, 10 cm × 20 cm = 35p, 10 cm × 25 cm = 40p, 10 cm × 30 cm = 49p, 10 cm × 35 cm = 58p (Richardson)
Sterifix®, 5 cm × 7 cm = 19p, 7 cm × 10 cm = 31p, 10 cm × 14 cm = 55p (Hartmann)
Telfa® Island, 5 cm × 10 cm = 8p, 10 cm × 12.5 cm = 27p, 10 cm × 20 cm = 35p, 10 cm × 25.5 cm = 44p, 10 cm × 35 cm = 61p (Covidien)

Absorbent Perforated Plastic Film Faced Dressing
Low-adherence primary dressing consisting of 3 layers—perforated polyester film wound contact layer, absorbent cotton pad, and hydrophobic backing. Where no size specified by the prescriber, the 5 cm size to be supplied
Absopad®, 5 cm × 5 cm = 7p, 10 cm × 10 cm = 13p, 20 cm × 10 cm = 28p, (Medicareplus International)
Askina® Pad, 10 cm × 10 cm = 20p, (B. Braun)
Cutisorb® LA, 5 cm × 5 cm = 8p, 10 cm × 10 cm = 14p, 10 cm × 20 cm = 29p (BSN Medical)
Interpose®, 5 cm × 5 cm = 9p, 10 cm × 10 cm = 15p, 10 cm × 20 cm = 32p (Frontier)
Melolin®, 5 cm × 5 cm = 16p, 10 cm × 10 cm = 26p, 20 cm × 10 cm = 51p (S&N Hlth)
Release®, 5 cm × 5 cm = 14p, 10 cm × 10 cm = 23p, 20 cm × 10 cm = 44p (Systagenix)
Skintact®, 5 cm × 5 cm = 10p, 10 cm × 10 cm = 17p, 20 cm × 10 cm = 34p (Robinson)
Solvaline N®, 5 cm × 5 cm = 9p, 10 cm × 10 cm = 17p, 10 cm × 20 cm = 34p (Activa)
Telfa®, 5 cm × 7.5 cm = 12p, 10 cm × 10 cm = 7.5 cm = 15p, 15 cm × 7.5 cm = 17p, 20 cm × 7.5 cm = 29p (Covidien)

◀ **For moderately to heavily exuding wounds**

Absorbent Cellulose Dressing with Fluid Repellent Backing
CelluDress®, 10 cm × 10 cm = 19p, 10 cm × 15 cm = 20p, 10 cm × 20 cm = 22p, 15 cm × 20 cm = 30p, 20 cm × 25 cm = 40p, 20 cm × 30 cm = 85p (Medicareplus International)

Eclypse®, 15 cm × 15 cm = 97p, 20 cm × 30 cm =
£2.14, 60 cm × 40 cm = £8.15, 60 cm × 70 cm
(boot-shape) = £13.78 (Advancis)
Exu-Dry®, 10 cm × 15 cm = £1.06, 15 cm × 23 cm
= £2.17, 23 cm × 38 cm = £5.04 (S&N Hlth.)
Mesorb®, cellulose wadding pad with gauze wound
contact layer and non-woven repellent backing,
10 cm × 10 cm = 59p, 10 cm × 15 cm = 77p,
10 cm × 20 cm = 95p, 15 cm × 20 cm = £1.36,
20 cm × 25 cm = £2.14, 20 cm × 30 cm = £2.43
(Mölnlycke)
Telfa Max®, 22.8 cm × 38 cm = £4.62, 38 cm ×
45.7 cm = £5.61, 38 cm × 60.9 cm = £8.16
(Covidien)
Zetuvit® E, non-sterile, 10 cm × 10 cm = 6p, 10 cm
× 20 cm = 8p, 20 cm × 20 cm = 14p, 20 cm ×
40 cm = 26p; sterile, 10 cm × 10 cm = 20p, 10 cm
× 20 cm = 23p, 20 cm × 20 cm = 37p, 20 cm ×
40 cm = £1.04 (Hartmann)

◀For heavily exuding wounds

Curea® (Bullen)
Super absorbent cellulose and polymer primary
dressing.
Curea P1®, 7.5 cm × 7.5 cm = £1.68, 10 cm ×
10 cm = £2.10, 10 cm × 20 cm = £3.56, 10 cm ×
30 cm = £5.09, 20 cm × 20 cm = £6.74, 20 cm ×
30 cm = £9.81, 12 cm × 12 cm (drain) = £2.59
Curea P2®, (non-adherent) 10 cm × 20 cm = £9.52,
11 cm × 11 cm = £5.70, 20 cm × 20 cm = £16.51,
20 cm × 30 cm = 24.77

Cutisorb® Ultra (BSN Medical)
Super absorbent cellulose and polymer primary
dressing, 10 cm × 10 cm = £2.01, 20 cm × 20 cm =
£6.32, 10 cm × 20 cm = £3.37, 20 cm × 30 cm =
£9.53

Drawtex® (Martindale)
Super absorbent hydroconductive dressing with
absorbent, cross-action structures of viscose,
polyester and cotton, 5 cm × 5 cm = 95p, 7.5 cm ×
7.5 cm = £1.77, 10 cm × 10 cm = £2.24, 15 cm ×
20 cm = £6.00, 20 cm × 20 cm = £6.98, 7.5 cm ×
1 m = £15.50, 10 cm × 1 m = £16.00, 10 cm ×
1.3 m = £16.00, 20 cm × 1 m = £25.00

DryMax® Extra (Aspen Medical)
Super absorbent cellulose and polymer primary
dressing, 10 cm × 10 cm = £1.80, 20 cm × 20 cm =
£4.20, 10 cm × 20 cm = £2.38, 20 cm × 30 cm =
£4.80

ELECT Superabsorber® (S&N)
Super absorbent cellulose and polymer primary
dressing, 10 cm × 10 cm = 93p, 10 cm × 20 cm =
£1.10, 20 cm × 20 cm = £1.96, 20 cm × 30 cm =
£2.47

Zetuvit® Plus (Hartmann)
Super absorbent cellulose primary dressing, 10 cm
× 10 cm = 60p, 10 cm × 20 cm = 83p, 15 cm ×
20 cm = 95p, 20 cm × 25 cm = £1.30, 20 cm ×
40 cm = £2.00

Appendix 5: Wound Management

A5.2 Advanced wound dressings

Advanced wound dressings can be used for both acute
and chronic wounds. Categories for dressings in this
section (A5.2) start with the least absorptive, moisture-
donating hydrogel dressings, followed by increasingly
more absorptive dressings. These dressings are classified according to their primary component; some dressings are comprised of several components.

A5.2.1 Hydrogel dressings

Hydrogel dressings are most commonly supplied as an
amorphous, cohesive topical application that can take
up the shape of a wound. A secondary, non-absorbent
dressing is needed. These dressings are generally used
to donate liquid to dry sloughy wounds and facilitate
autolytic debridement of necrotic tissue; some also have
the ability to absorb very small amounts of exudate.
Hydrogel products that do not contain propylene glycol
should be used if the wound is to be treated with larval
therapy.

Hydrogel sheets have a fixed structure and limited fluid-
handling capacity; hydrogel sheet dressings are best
avoided in the presence of infection, and are unsuitable
for heavily exuding wounds.

◀Hydrogel sheet dressings

ActiFormCool® (Activa)
Hydrogel dressing, 5 cm × 6.5 cm = £1.70, 10 cm
× 10 cm = £2.49, 20 cm × 20 cm = £7.51, 10 cm
× 15 cm = £3.58

Aquaflo® (Covidien)
Hydrogel dressing, 7.5 cm diameter = £2.55, 12 cm
diameter = £5.26

Coolie® (Zeroderma)
Hydrogel dressing (without adhesive border), disc
7 cm diameter = £1.96

Gel FX® (Synergy Healthcare)
Hydrogel dressing (without adhesive border) 10 cm
× 10 cm = £1.60, 15 cm × 15 cm = £3.20

Geliperm® (Geistlich)
Hydrogel sheets, 10 cm × 10 cm = £2.48

Hydrosorb® (Hartmann)
Absorbent, transparent, hydrogel sheets containing
polyurethane polymers covered with a semi-
permeable film, 5 cm × 7.5 cm = £1.49; 10 cm ×
10 cm = £2.12; 20 cm × 20 cm = £6.37
Hydrosorb® Comfort (with adhesive border,
waterproof), 4.5 cm × 6.5 cm = £1.76; 7.5 cm × 10
cm = £2.33; 12.5 cm × 12.5 cm = £3.40

Intrasite Conformable® (S&N Hlth.)
Soft non-woven dressing impregnated with
Intrasite® gel, 10 cm × 10 cm = £1.70; 10 cm ×
20 cm = £2.30; 10 cm × 40 cm = £4.10

Novogel® (Ford)
Glycerol-based hydrogel sheets, 10 cm × 10 cm =
£3.07; 30 cm × 30 cm, standard = £13.00, thin =
£12.27; 5 cm × 7.5 cm = £1.95; 15 cm × 20 cm =
£5.86; 20 cm × 40 cm = £11.16; 7.5 cm diameter =
£2.79

SanoSkin® NET (SanoMed)
Hydrogel sheet (without adhesive border), 8.5 cm × 12 cm = £2.28

Vacunet® (Protex)
Non-adherent, hydrogel coated polyester net dressing, 10 cm × 10 cm = £1.93, 10 cm × 15 cm = £2.86

◢**Hydrogel application (amorphous)**

ActivHeal® Hydrogel (MedLogic)
Hydrogel containing guar gum and propylene glycol, 8 g = £1.23, 15 g = £1.41

Aquaform® (Aspen Medical)
Hydrogel containing modified starch copolymer, 8 g = £1.61, 15 g = £1.96

Askina® Gel (B. Braun)
Hydrogel containing modified starch and glycerol, 15 g = £1.92

Cutimed® (BSN Medical)
Hydrogel, 8 g = £1.58, 15 g = £1.92, 25 g = £2.83

Flexigran® (A1 Pharmaceuticals)
Hydrogel containing starch polymer and glycerol, 15 g = £1.90

GranuGel® (ConvaTec)
Hydrogel containing carboxymethylcellulose, pectin, and propylene glycol, 15 g = £2.19

Intrasite® Gel (S&N Hlth.)
Hydrogel containing modified carmellose polymer and propylene glycol, 8-g sachet = £1.70, 15-g sachet = £2.28, 25-g sachet = £3.38

Nu-Gel® (Systagenix)
Hydrogel containing alginate and propylene glycol, 15 g = £2.09

Purilon® Gel (Coloplast)
Hydrogel containing carboxymethylcellulose and calcium alginate, 8 g = £1.64, 15 g = £2.14

A5.2.1.1   Sodium hyaluronate dressings

The hydrating properties of sodium hyaluronate promote wound healing, and dressings can be applied directly to the wound, or to a primary dressing (a secondary dressing should also be applied). The iodine and potassium iodide in these dressings prevent the bacterial decay of sodium hyaluronate in the wound.

Hyiodine® (H&R)
Sodium hyaluronate 1.5%, potassium iodide 0.15%, iodine 0.1%, in a viscous solution, 22-g = £19.95, 50-g = £35.00
Cautions thyroid disorders

A5.2.2   Vapour-permeable films and membranes

Vapour-permeable films and membranes allow the passage of water vapour and oxygen but are impermeable to water and micro-organisms, and are suitable for lightly exuding wounds. They are highly conformable, provide protection, and a moist healing environment; transparent film dressings permit constant observation of the wound. Water vapour loss can occur at a slower rate than exudate is generated, so that fluid accumulates under the dressing, which can lead to tissue maceration and to wrinkling at the adhesive contact site (with risk of bacterial entry). Newer versions of these dressings have increased moisture vapour permeability. Despite these advances, vapour-permeable films and membranes are unsuitable for infected, large heavily exuding wounds, and chronic leg ulcers.

Vapour-permeable films and membranes are suitable for partial-thickness wounds with minimal exudate, or wounds with eschar. Most commonly, they are used as a secondary dressing over alginates or hydrogels; film dressings can also be used to protect the fragile skin of patients at risk of developing minor skin damage caused by friction or pressure.

◢**Vapour-permeable Adhesive Film Dressing (Semi-permeable Adhesive Dressing)**
Extensible, waterproof, water vapour-permeable polyurethane film coated with synthetic adhesive mass; transparent. Supplied in single-use pieces.

Askina® Derm (B.Braun)
Film dressing, 6 cm × 7 cm = 36p, 10 cm × 12 cm = £1.04, 10 cm × 20 cm = £1.97, 15 cm × 20 cm = £2.39, 20 cm × 30 cm = £4.27

Bioclusive® (Systagenix)
Film dressing, 10.2 cm × 12.7 cm = £1.54

C-View® (Aspen Medical)
Film dressing, 6 cm × 7 cm = 38p, 10 cm × 12 cm = £1.02, 12 cm × 12 cm = £1.09, 15 cm × 20 cm = £2.36

Dressfilm® (St George's Medical)
Film dressing, 6 cm × 7 cm = 30p, 12 cm × 12 cm = 93p, 15 cm × 20 cm = £1.90

Hydrofilm® (Hartmann)
Film dressing, 6 cm × 7 cm = 21p, 10 cm × 12.5 cm = 40p, 10 cm × 15 cm = 50p, 10 cm × 25 cm = 77p, 12 cm × 25 cm = 81p, 15 cm × 20 cm = 92p, 20 cm × 30 cm = £1.52

Hypafix® Transparent (BSN Medical)
Film dressing, 10 cm × 2 m = £8.24

Leukomed T® (BSN Medical)
Film dressing, 7.2 cm × 5 cm = 35p, 8 cm × 10 cm = 66p, 10 cm × 12.5 cm = 96p, 11 cm × 14 cm = £1.16, 15 cm × 20 cm = £2.23, 15 cm × 25 cm = £2.38

Mepitel® Film (Mölnlycke)
Film dressing, 6.5 cm × 7 cm = 49p, 10.5 cm × 12 cm = £1.31, 10.5 cm × 25 cm = £2.55, 15.5 cm × 20 cm = £3.24

Mepore® Film (Mölnlycke)
Film dressing, 6 cm × 7 cm = 44p, 10 cm × 12 cm = £1.18, 10 cm × 25 cm = £2.29, 15 cm × 20 cm = £2.91

OpSite® Flexifix (S&N Hlth.)
Film dressing, 5 cm × 1 m = £3.69, 10 cm × 1 m = £6.22; *OpSite® Flexigrid*, 6 cm × 7 cm = 37p, 12 cm × 12 cm = £1.06, 15 cm × 20 cm = £2.69

Polyskin® II (Covidien)
Film dressing, 4 cm × 4 cm = 36p, 5 cm × 7 cm = 39p, 10 cm × 12 cm = £1.01, 10 cm × 20 cm = £2.00, 15 cm × 20 cm = £2.31, 20 cm × 25 cm = £4.03

ProtectFilm® (Wallace Cameron)
Film dressing, 6 cm × 7 cm = 11p, 10 cm × 12 cm
= 20p, 15 cm × 20 cm = 40p

Suprasorb F® (Activa)
Film dressing, 5 cm × 7 cm = 32p, 10 cm × 12
cm = 76p, 15 cm × 20 cm = £2.37

Tegaderm® (3M)
Film dressing, 6 cm × 7 cm = 38p, 12 cm × 12 cm
= £1.09, 15 cm × 20 cm = £2.37
Tegaderm® diamond, film dressing, 6 cm × 7 cm =
£0.44, 10 cm × 12 cm = £1.19

Vacuskin® (Protex)
Film dressing, 6 cm × 7 cm = 40p, 10 cm × 12 cm
= £1.06, 10 cm × 25 cm = £2.06, 15 cm × 20 cm =
£2.19

Vellafilm® (Advancis)
Film dressing, 12 cm × 12 cm = £1.10, 12 cm ×
35 cm = £2.75, 15 cm × 20 cm = £2.10

◢**Vapour-permeable Adhesive Film Dressing with
absorbent pad**

Adpore® **Ultra** (Medicare)
Film dressing, with absorbent pad, 7 cm × 8 cm =
12p, 10 cm × 10 cm = 14p, 10 cm × 15 cm = 22p,
10 cm × 20 cm = 33p, 10 cm × 25 cm = 35p,
10 cm × 30 cm = 52p

Alldress® (Mölnlycke)
Film dressing, with absorbent pad, 10 cm × 10 cm
= 91p, 15 cm × 15 cm = £1.98, 15 cm × 20 cm =
£2.44

Clearpore® (Richardson)
Film dressing, with absorbent pad, 6 cm × 7 cm =
12p, 6 cm × 10 cm = 15p, 10 cm × 10 cm = 20p,
10 cm × 30 cm = 65p, 15 cm × 10 cm = 24p,
20 cm × 10 cm = 36p, 25 cm × 10 cm = 40p

C-View® **Post-Op** (Aspen Medical)
Film dressing, with absorbent pad, 6 cm × 7 cm =
£0.40, 10 cm × 12 cm = £1.10, 10 cm × 25 cm =
£1.60, 10 cm × 35 cm = £2.60

Hydrofilm® **Plus** (Hartmann)
Film dressing, with absorbent pad, 5 cm × 7.2 cm =
15p, 9 cm × 10 cm = 20p, 9 cm × 15 cm = 22p,
10 cm × 20 cm = 35p, 10 cm × 25 cm = 37p,
10 cm × 30 cm = 54p

Leukomed T® **Plus** (BSN Medical)
Film dressing, with absorbent pad, 7.2 cm × 5 cm =
25p, 8 cm x 10 cm = 51p, 8 cm x 15 cm = 76p,
10 cm x 20 cm = £1.26, 10 cm x 25 cm = £1.42,
10 cm x 30 cm = £2.38, 10 cm x 35 cm = £2.88

Mepore® (Mölnlycke)
Mepore® Film & Pad, film dressing, with absorbent
pad, 4 cm × 5 cm = 24p, 5 cm × 7 cm = 24p, 9 cm
× 10 cm = 62p, 9 cm × 15 cm = 92p, 9 cm ×
20 cm = £1.36, 9 cm × 25 cm = £1.50, 9 cm ×
30 cm = £2.00, 9 cm × 35 cm = £2.49
Mepore® Ultra, film dressing, with absorbent pad,
7 cm × 8 cm = 40p, 9 cm × 20 cm = £1.50, 9 cm
× 25 cm = £1.65, 9 cm × 30 cm = £2.73, 10 cm ×
11 cm = 79p, 11 cm × 15 cm = £1.16

OpSite® (S&N Hlth.)
OpSite® Plus, film dressing, with absorbent pad,
6.5 cm × 5 cm = 30p, 9.5 cm × 8.5 cm = 83p,
10 cm × 12 cm = £1.13, 10 cm × 20 cm = £1.90,
35 cm × 10 cm = £3.15
OpSite® Post-op, film dressing, with absorbent pad,
8.5 cm × 9.5 cm = 82p, 8.5 cm × 15.5 cm = £1.13,
10 cm × 12 cm = £1.11, 10 cm × 20 cm = £1.86,
10 cm × 25 cm = £2.35, 10 cm × 30 cm = £2.78,
10 cm × 35 cm = £3.09

Pharmapore-PU® (Wallace Cameron)
Film dressing, with absorbent pad, 8.5 cm ×
15.5 cm = 20p, 10 cm × 25 cm = 38p, 10 cm ×
30 cm = 58p

PremierPore VP® (Shermond)
Film dressing, with absorbent pad, 5 cm × 7 cm =
13p, 10 cm × 10 cm = 16p, 10 cm × 15 cm = 24p,
10 cm × 20 cm = 36p, 10 cm × 25 cm = 38p,
10 cm × 30 cm = 57p, 10 cm × 35 cm = 69p

Tegaderm® (3M)
Film dressing, with absorbent pad, 5 cm × 7 cm =
25p, 9 cm × 10 cm = 63p, 9 cm × 15 cm = 93p,
9 cm × 20 cm = £1.36, 9 cm × 25 cm = £1.53, 9 cm
× 35 cm = £2.53
Tegaderm® Absorbent Clear, film dressing, with
clear acrylic polymer oval-shaped pad, 7.6 cm ×
9.5 cm = £3.02, 11.1 cm × 12.7 cm = £3.91, 14.2 cm
× 15.8 cm = £5.51; rectangular, 14.9 cm ×
15.2 cm = £8.26, 20 cm × 20.3 cm = £13.26;
16.8 cm × 19 cm (sacral) = £9.89

◢**For intravenous and subcutaneous catheter sites**

Central Gard® (Unomedical)
Vapour–permeable transparent film dressing with
adhesive foam border, 16 cm × 7 cm (central
venous catheter) = 94p, 16 cm × 8.8 cm (central
venous catheter) = £1.03

Easi-V® (ConvaTec)
Vapour–permeable transparent film dressing with
adhesive foam border, 7 cm × 7.5 cm (intravenous
peripheral cannula) = 38p

Hydrofilm® **I.V. Control** (Hartmann)
Vapour-permeable, transparent, adhesive film
dressing, 7 cm x 9 cm = 29p

IV3000® (S&N Hlth.)
Vapour–permeable, transparent, adhesive film
dressing, 5 cm × 6 cm (1-hand) = 40p, 6 cm ×
7 cm (non-winged peripheral catheter) = 52p, 7 cm
× 9 cm (ported peripheral catheter) = 69p, 9 cm ×
12 cm (PICC line) = £1.37, 10 cm × 12 cm (central
venous catheter) = £1.32

Mepore® **IV** (Mölnlycke)
Vapour–permeable, transparent, adhesive film
dressing, 5 cm × 5.5 cm = 29p, 8 cm × 9 cm =
38p, 10 cm × 11 cm = 99p

Niko Fix® (Unomedical)
Non-woven fabric dressing with viscose-rayon pad,
7 cm × 8.5 cm (intravenous ported peripheral
catheter) = 19p

Pharmapore-PU® **IV** (Wallace Cameron)
Vapour–permeable, transparent, adhesive film
dressing, 8.5 cm × 7 cm = 7p, 6 cm × 7 cm (ported
peripheral cannula) = 8p, 7 cm × 9 cm (peripheral
cannula, hand) = 17p

Tegaderm® IV (3M)

Vapour–permeable, transparent, adhesive film dressing, 7 cm × 8.5 cm (peripheral catheter) = 58p, 8.5 cm × 10.5 cm (central venous catheter) = £1.12, 10 cm × 15.5 cm (peripherally inserted central venous catheter) = £1.62

A5.2.3 Soft polymer dressings

Dressings with soft polymer, often a soft silicone polymer, in a non-adherent or gently adherent layer are suitable for use on lightly to moderately exuding wounds. For moderately to heavily exuding wounds, an absorbent secondary dressing can be added, or a soft polymer dressing with an absorbent pad can be used.

Wound contact dressings coated with soft silicone have gentle adhesive properties and can be used on fragile skin areas or where it is beneficial to reduce the frequency of primary dressing changes.

Soft polymer dressings should not be used on heavily bleeding wounds; blood clots can cause the dressing to adhere to the wound surface.

For *silicone keloid dressings* see section A5.4.2.

◄**Without absorbent pad**

Adaptic® Touch (Systagenix)

Non-adherent soft silicone wound contact dressing, 5 cm x 7.6 cm = £1.13, 7.6 cm x 11 cm = £2.25, 12.7 cm x 15 cm = £4.65, 20 cm x 32 cm = £12.50

Askina® SilNet (B. Braun)

Soft silicone-coated wound contact dressing, 5 cm x 7.5 cm = £1.09, 7.5 cm x 10 cm = £2.20, 10 cm x 18 cm = £4.80, 20 cm x 30 cm = £11.75

Mepitel® (Mölnlycke)

Soft silicone, semi-transparent wound contact dressing. 5 cm × 7 cm = £1.57, 8 cm × 10 cm = £3.13, 12 cm × 15 cm = £6.34, 20 cm × 30 cm = £16.61

Mepitel® One, soft silicone, thin, transparent wound contact dressing, 6 cm × 7 cm = £1.79, 9 cm × 10 cm = £3.36, 13 cm × 15 cm = £6.54, 24 cm × 27.5 cm = £16.79

Physiotulle® (Coloplast)

Non-adherent soft polymer wound contact dressing, 10 cm × 10 cm = £2.13, 15 cm × 20 cm = £6.50

Silflex® (Advancis)

Soft silicone-coated polyester wound contact dressing, 5 cm × 7 cm = £1.25, 8 cm × 10 cm = £2.55, 12 cm × 15 cm = £5.15, 20 cm × 30 cm = £13.25, 35 cm × 60 cm = £39.54

Silon-TSR® (Jobskin)

Soft silicone polymer wound contact dressing, 13 cm × 13 cm = £3.52, 13 cm × 25 cm = £5.47, 28 cm × 30 cm = £7.37

Sorbion® Contact (H&R)

Non-adherent soft polymer wound contact dressing, 7.5 cm × 7.5 cm = £1.49, 10 cm × 10 cm = £1.99, 10 cm × 20 cm = £3.99, 20 cm × 20 cm = £6.99, 20 cm × 30 cm = £9.99

Tegaderm® Contact (3M)

Non-adherent soft polymer wound contact dressing, 7.5 cm × 10 cm = £2.17, 7.5 cm × 20 cm = £4.25, 20 cm × 25 cm = £10.35

Urgotul® (Urgo)

Non-adherent soft polymer wound contact dressing, 5 cm × 5cm = £1.50, 10 cm × 10 cm = £3.00, 10 cm × 40 cm = £10.08, 15 cm × 15 cm = £6.45, 15 cm × 20 cm = £8.49, 20 cm × 30 cm = £13.65

◄**With absorbent pad**

Advazorb® Border (Advancis)

Soft silicone wound contact dressing, with polyurethane foam film backing and adhesive border, 7.5 cm × 7.5 cm = £1.19, 10 cm × 10 cm = £2.10, 10 cm × 20 cm = £2.90, 10 cm × 30 cm = £4.25, 12.5 cm × 12.5 cm = £2.58, 15 cm × 15 cm = £3.15, 20 cm × 20 cm = £5.46

Advazorb® Border Lite, soft silicone wound contact dressing, with polyurethane foam film backing and adhesive border, 7.5 cm × 7.5 cm = £1.07, 10 cm × 10 cm = £1.89, 10 cm × 20 cm = £2.61, 10 cm × 30 cm = £3.83, 12.5 cm × 12.5 cm = £2.32, 15 cm × 15 cm = £2.84, 20 cm × 20 cm = £4.91

Advazorb® Silfix (Advancis)

Soft silicone wound contact dressing, with polyurethane foam film backing, 7.5 cm × 7.5 cm = £0.99, 10 cm × 10 cm = £1.85, 10 cm × 20 cm = £3.18, 12.5 cm × 12.5 cm = £2.59, 15 cm × 15 cm = £3.36, 20 cm × 20 cm = £4.98

Advazorb® Silfix Lite, soft silicone wound contact dressing, with polyurethane foam film backing, 7.5 cm × 7.5 cm = £0.89, 10 cm × 10 cm = £1.67, 10 cm × 20 cm = £2.86, 12.5 cm × 12.5 cm = £2.33, 15 cm × 15 cm = £3.02, 20 cm × 20 cm = £4.48

Allevyn® Gentle (S&N Hlth.)

Soft gel wound contact dressing, with polyurethane foam film backing, 5 cm × 5 cm = £1.21, 10 cm × 10 cm = £2.40, 10 cm × 20 cm = £3.86, 15 cm × 15 cm = £4.03, 20 cm × 20 cm = £6.44

Allevyn® Gentle Border, silicone gel wound contact dressing, with polyurethane foam film backing, 7.5 cm × 7.5 cm = £1.43, 10 cm × 10 cm = £2.10, 12.5 cm × 12.5 cm = £2.57, 17.5 cm × 17.5 cm = £5.07, 23 cm × 23.2 cm (heel) = £9.24

Allevyn® Gentle Border Lite, silicone gel wound contact dressing, with polyurethane foam film backing, 5 cm x 5 cm = 86p, 5.5 cm x 12 cm = £1.77, 7.5 cm x 7.5 cm = £1.33, 8 cm x 15 cm = £3.29, 10 cm x 10 cm = £2.07, 15 cm x 15 cm = £3.65

Allevyn® Life (S&N Hlth)

Soft silicone wound contact dressing, with central mesh screen, polyurethane foam film backing and adhesive border, 10.3 cm × 10.3 cm = £1.65, 12.9 cm × 12.9 cm = £2.42, 15.4 cm × 15.4 cm = £2.96, 21 cm × 21 cm = £5.83

Cutimed® Siltec (BSN Medical)
Soft silicone wound contact dressing, with polyurethane foam film backing, 5 cm × 6 cm = £1.24, 10 cm × 10 cm = £2.33, 10 cm × 20 cm = £3.84, 15 cm × 15 cm = £4.35, 20 cm × 20 cm = £6.59, 16 cm × 24 cm (heel) = £6.77; *with adhesive border*, 17.5 cm × 17.5 cm (sacrum) = £4.31, 23 cm x 23 cm (sacrum) = £7.02
Cutimed® Siltec B, with adhesive border, for lightly to moderately exuding wounds, 7.5 cm × 7.5 cm = £1.45, 12.5 cm × 12.5 cm = £3.06, 15 cm × 15 cm = £4.71, 17.5 cm × 17.5 cm = £4.97, 22.5 cm x 22.5 cm = £8.16
Cutimed® Siltec L, for lightly to moderately exuding wounds, 5 cm × 6 cm = 99p, 10 cm × 10 cm = £2.00, 15 cm × 15 cm = £3.30

Eclypse® Adherent (Advancis)
Soft silicone wound contact layer with absorbent pad and film-backing, 10 cm × 10 cm = £2.99, 10 cm × 20 cm = £3.75, 15 cm × 15 cm = £4.99, 20 cm × 30 cm = £9.99, 17 cm × 19 cm (sacral) = £3.76, 22 cm × 23 cm (sacral) = £6.23

Flivasorb® (Activa)
Absorbent polymer dressing with non-adherent wound contact layer, 10 cm × 10 cm = £2.16, 20 cm × 20 cm = £6.80, 10 cm × 20 cm = £3.61, 20 cm × 30 cm = £9.62
Flivasorb® Adhesive, absorbent polymer dressing with non-adherent wound contact layer and adhesive border, 12 cm × 12 cm = £3.25, 15 cm × 15 cm = £4.45

Mepilex® (Mölnlycke)
Absorbent soft silicone dressing with polyurethane foam film backing, 5 cm × 5 cm = £1.21, 10 cm × 11 cm = £2.66, 11 cm × 20 cm = £4.39, 15 cm × 16 cm = £4.82, 20 cm × 21 cm = £7.28, 20 cm × 50 cm = £28.74, 13 cm × 20 cm (heel) = £5.41, 15 cm × 22 cm (heel) = £6.22
Mepilex® Border, absorbent soft silicone dressing with polyurethane foam and adhesive border, 7 cm × 7.5 cm = £1.39, 10 cm × 12.5 cm = £2.72, 10 cm × 20 cm = £3.69, 10 cm × 30 cm = £5.55, 15 cm × 17.5 cm = £4.74, 17 cm × 20 cm = £6.07, 15 cm × 15 cm (sacrum) = £3.34, 18 cm × 18 cm (sacrum) = £4.85, 23 cm × 23 cm (sacrum) = £7.91, 18.5 cm × 24 cm (heel) = £6.63
Mepilex® Border Lite, thin absorbent soft silicone dressing with polyurethane foam and adhesive border, 4 cm × 5 cm = 92p, 7.5 cm × 7.5 cm = £1.39, 5 cm × 12.5 cm = £2.01, 10 cm × 10 cm = £2.53, 15 cm × 15 cm = £4.13
Mepilex® Lite, thin absorbent soft silicone dressing with polyurethane foam, 6 cm × 8.5 cm = £1.82, 10 cm × 10 cm = £2.17, 15 cm × 15 cm = £4.22, 20 cm × 50 cm = £26.66
Mepilex® Transfer, soft silicone exudate transfer dressing, 7.5 cm × 8.5 cm = £2.23, 10 cm × 12 cm = £3.51, 15 cm × 20 cm = £10.64, 20 cm × 50 cm = £27.20

Sorbion® Sana (H&R)
Non-adherent polyethylene wound contact dressing with absorbent core, 8.5 cm × 8.5 cm = £5.00, 12 cm × 12 cm = £6.78, 12 cm × 22 cm = £12.56, 22 cm × 22 cm = £20.14

Urgotul® Duo (Urgo)
Non-adherent, soft polymer wound contact dressing with absorbent pad, 5 cm × 10 cm = £2.33, 10 cm × 12 cm = £3.61, 15 cm × 20 cm = £8.38
Urgotul® Duo Border, soft polymer wound contact dressing with absorbent pad and adhesive polyurethane film backing, 8 cm × 8 cm = £2.27, 10 cm × 12 cm = £3.52, 15 cm × 20 cm = £8.17

◀**Cellulose dressings**

Sorbion® Sachet (H&R)
Sorbion® Sachet Border, absorbent polymers in cellulose matrix, hypoallergenic polypropylene envelope, with adhesive border (for moderately to heavily exuding wounds), 10 cm × 10 cm = £2.95, 15 cm × 15 cm = £4.49, 15 cm × 25 cm = £6.99, 25 cm × 25 cm = £11.99
Sorbion® Sachet Drainage, absorbent polymers in cellulose matrix, hypoallergenic polypropylene envelope ('v' shaped dressing), 10 cm × 10 cm = £2.64
Sorbion® Sachet EXTRA, absorbent polymers in cellulose matrix, hypoallergenic polypropylene envelope (for moderately to heavily exuding wounds), 5 cm × 5 cm =£1.45, 7.5 cm × 7.5 cm = £1.78, 10 cm × 10 cm = £2.25, 10 cm × 20 cm = £3.73, 20 cm × 20 cm = £7.00, 30 cm × 20 cm = £9.99
Sorbion® Sachet Multi Star, absorbent polymers in cellulose matrix, hypoallergenic polypropylene envelope (for moderately to heavily exuding wounds), 8 cm × 8 cm = £2.99, 14 cm × 14 cm = £4.89

Suprasorb® X (Activa)
Biosynthetic cellulose fibre dressing (for lightly to moderately exuding wounds), 5 cm × 5 cm = £1.93, 9 cm × 9 cm = £4.02, 14 cm × 20 cm = £7.96; 2 cm × 21 cm (rope) = £6.19

A5.2.4 Hydrocolloid dressings

Hydrocolloid dressings are usually presented as a hydrocolloid layer on a vapour-permeable film or foam pad. Semi-permeable to water vapour and oxygen, these dressings form a gel in the presence of exudate to facilitate rehydration in lightly to moderately exuding wounds and promote autolytic debridement of dry, sloughy, or necrotic wounds; they are also suitable for promoting granulation.

Hydrocolloid-fibrous dressings made from modified carmellose fibres resemble alginate dressings; hydrocolloid-fibrous dressings are more absorptive and suitable for moderately to heavily exuding wounds.

◀**Without adhesive border**

ActivHeal® Hydrocolloid (MedLogic)
Semi-permeable polyurethane film backing, hydrocolloid wound contact layer, 5 cm × 7.5 cm = 76p, 10 cm × 10 cm = £1.55, 15 cm × 15 cm = £3.37, 15 cm × 18 cm (sacral) = £3.91; *with polyurethane foam layer*, 5 cm × 7.5 cm = 96p, 10 cm × 10 cm = £1.52, 15 cm × 15 cm = £2.86, 15 cm × 18 cm (sacral) = £3.30

Askina® Biofilm Transparent (B. Braun)
Semi-permeable, polyurethane film dressing with hydrocolloid adhesive, 10 cm × 10 cm = £1.02, 20 cm × 20 cm = £3.02

Biatain® Super (Coloplast)
Semi–permeable hydrocolloid dressing without adhesive border, 10 cm × 10 cm = £3.12, 12.5 cm × 12.5 cm = £4.29, 12 cm × 20 cm = £5.63, 15 cm × 15 cm = £5.43, 20 cm × 20 cm = £8.10

Comfeel® Plus (Coloplast)
Hydrocolloid dressings containing carmellose sodium and calcium alginate. *contour*, 6 cm × 8 cm = £2.08, 9 cm × 11 cm = £3.61; *ulcer*, 4 cm × 6 cm = 90p, 10 cm × 10 cm = £2.29, 15 cm × 15 cm = £4.91, 18 cm × 20 cm (triangular) = £5.35, 20 cm × 20 cm = £7.08; *transparent*, 5 cm × 7 cm = 63p, 5 cm × 15 cm = £1.48, 5 cm × 25 cm = £2.41, 9 cm × 14 cm = £2.28, 9 cm × 25 cm = £3.24, 10 cm × 10 cm = £1.20, 15 cm × 15 cm = £3.12, 15 cm × 20 cm = £3.17, 20 cm × 20 cm = £3.19; *pressure relieving*, 7 cm diameter = £3.24, 10 cm diameter = £4.34, 15 cm diameter = £6.54

DuoDERM® Extra Thin (ConvaTec)
Semi-permeable hydrocolloid dressing, 5 cm × 10 cm = 72p, 7.5 cm × 7.5 cm = 75p, 10 cm × 10 cm = £1.24, 9 cm × 15 cm = £1.66, 9 cm × 25 cm = £2.66, 9 cm × 35 cm = £3.72, 15 cm × 15 cm = £2.68

DuoDERM® Signal, hydrocolloid dressing with 'Time to change' indicator, 10 cm × 10 cm = £2.00, 14 cm × 14 cm = £3.52, 20 cm × 20 cm = £6.99, 11 cm × 19 cm (oval) = £3.05, 18.5 cm × 19.5 cm (heel) = £4.92, 22.5 cm × 20 cm (sacral) = £5.74

Flexigran® (A1 Pharmaceuticals)
Semi-permeable hydrocolloid dressing without adhesive border, 10 cm × 10 cm = £2.19; *thin*, 10 cm × 10 cm = £1.08

Granuflex® (ConvaTec)
Hydrocolloid wound contact layer bonded to plastic foam layer, with outer semi-permeable polyurethane film, 10 cm × 10 cm = £2.64, 15 cm × 15 cm = £5.00, 15 cm × 20 cm = £5.42, 20 cm × 20 cm = £7.52

Hydrocoll® Basic (Hartmann)
Hydrocolloid dressing with absorbent wound contact pad, 10 cm × 10 cm = £2.32; *thin*, 7.5 cm × 7.5 cm = 66p, 10 cm × 10 cm = £1.09, 15 cm × 15 cm = £2.46

NU DERM® (Systagenix)
Semi-permeable hydrocolloid dressing, 5 cm × 5 cm = 85p, 10 cm × 10 cm = £1.56, 15 cm × 15 cm = £3.18, 20 cm × 20 cm = £6.36, 8 cm × 12 cm (heel/elbow) = £3.18, 15 cm × 18 cm (sacral) = £4.45; *thin*, 10 cm × 10 cm = £1.06

Tegaderm® Hydrocolloid (3M)
Hydrocolloid dressing without adhesive border, 10 cm × 10 cm = £2.30, 15 cm × 15 cm = £4.46; *thin*, semi-permeable, clear film dressing with hydrocolloid, 10 cm × 10 cm = £1.51

Ultec Pro® (Covidien)
Semi-permeable hydrocolloid dressing; without adhesive border 10 cm × 10 cm = £2.23, 15 cm × 15 cm = £4.36, 20 cm × 20 cm = £6.56

◀**With adhesive border**

Biatain® Super (Coloplast)
Semi-permeable hydrocolloid dressing with adhesive border, 10 cm × 10 cm = £3.12, 12.5 cm × 12.5 cm = £4.29, 12 cm × 20 cm = £5.63, 15 cm × 15 cm = £5.43, 20 cm × 20 cm = £8.10

Granuflex® Bordered (ConvaTec)
Hydrocolloid wound contact layer bonded to plastic foam layer, with outer semi-permeable polyurethane film, 6 cm × 6 cm = £1.66, 10 cm × 10 cm = £3.14, 15 cm × 15 cm = £5.99, 10 cm × 13 cm (triangular) = £3.71, 15 cm × 18 cm (triangular) = £5.78

Hydrocoll® Border (Hartmann)
Hydrocolloid dressing with adhesive border and absorbent wound contact layer, 5 cm × 5 cm = 95p, 7.5 cm × 7.5 cm = £1.57, 10 cm × 10 cm = £2.29, 15 cm × 15 cm = £4.30; 8 cm × 12 cm (concave) = £2.01; 12 cm × 18 cm (sacral) = £3.42

Tegaderm® Hydrocolloid (3M)
Hydrocolloid dressing with adhesive border, 10 cm × 12 cm (oval) = £2.26, 13 cm × 15 cm (oval) = £4.22; 17.1 cm × 16.1 cm (sacral) = £4.71; *thin*, semi-permeable, clear film dressing with hydrocolloid, 10 cm × 12 cm (oval) = £1.50; 13 cm × 15 cm (oval) = £2.81

Ultec Pro® (Covidien)
Semi-permeable hydrocolloid dressing with adhesive border, 21 cm × 21 cm = £4.58, 15 cm × 18 cm (sacral) = £3.23, 19.5 cm × 23 cm (sacral) = £4.88

◀**Hydrocolloid-fibrous dressings**

Aquacel® (ConvaTec)
Soft non-woven pad containing hydrocolloid-fibres, 4 cm × 10 cm = £1.40, 4 cm × 20 cm = £2.07, 4 cm × 30 cm = £3.11, 5 cm × 5 cm = £1.10; 10 cm × 10 cm = £2.61; 15 cm × 15 cm = £4.91; 1 cm × 45 cm (ribbon) = £1.76, 2 cm × 45 cm (ribbon) = £2.64

Aquacel® Foam, soft non-woven pad containing hydrocolloid-fibres with foam layer, without adhesive border, 5 cm × 5 cm = £1.31, 10 cm × 10 cm = £2.48, 15 cm × 15 cm = £4.17, 15 cm × 20 cm = £5.70, 20 cm × 20 cm = £6.80, *with adhesive border*, 8 cm × 8 cm = £1.37, 10 cm × 10 cm = £2.10, 12.5 cm × 12.5 cm = £2.60, 17.5 cm × 17.5 cm = £5.20, 21 cm × 21 cm = £7.61, 25 cm × 30 cm = £9.85, 19.8 cm × 14 cm (heel) = £5.32, 20 cm × 16.9 cm (sacral) = £4.77

UrgoClean® (Urgo)
Pad, hydrocolloid fibres coated with soft-adherent lipo-colloidal wound contact layer, 6 cm × 6 cm = £0.94, 10 cm × 10 cm = £2.09, 15 cm × 20 cm = £3.93

Rope, non-woven rope containing hydrocolloid fibres, 2.5 cm × 40 cm = £2.35, 5 cm × 40 cm = £3.11

Versiva® XC (ConvaTec)
Hydrocolloid gelling foam dressing, without adhesive border, 7.5 cm × 7.5 cm = £1.39, 11 cm × 11 cm = £2.31, 15 cm × 15 cm = £4.26, 20 cm × 20 cm = £6.37; *with adhesive border*, 10 cm × 10 cm = £2.36, 14 cm × 14 cm = £3.19, 19 cm × 19 cm = £5.09, 22 cm × 22 cm = £5.65, 18.5 cm × 20.5 cm (heel) = £5.65, 21 cm × 25 cm (sacral) = £6.06

Appendix 5: Wound Management

◢Polyurethane matrix dressing

Cutinova® Hydro (S&N Hlth.)
Polyurethane matrix with absorbent particles and waterproof polyurethane film, 5 cm × 6 cm = £1.19, 10 cm × 10 cm = £2.40, 15 cm × 20 cm = £5.07

A5.2.5   Foam dressings

Dressings containing hydrophilic polyurethane foam (adhesive or non-adhesive), with or without plastic film-backing, are suitable for all types of exuding wounds, but not for dry wounds; some foam dressings have a moisture-sensitive film backing with variable permeability dependant on the level of exudate

Foam dressings vary in their ability to absorb exudate; some are suitable only for lightly to moderately exuding wounds, others have greater fluid-handing capacity and are suitable for heavily exuding wounds. Saturated foam dressings can cause maceration of healthy skin if left in contact with the wound.

Foam dressings can be used in combination with other primary wound contact dressings. If used under compression bandaging or compression garments, the fluid-handling capacity of the foam dressing may be reduced. Foam dressings can also be used to provide a protective cushion for fragile skin. A foam dressing containing ibuprofen is available and may be useful for treating painful exuding wounds.

◢For lightly exuding wounds

Polyurethane Foam Film Dressing with Adhesive Border
PolyMem®, 5 cm × 5 cm = 50p (Aspen Medical)
Tielle® Lite, 11 cm × 11 cm = £2.28; 7 cm × 9 cm = £1.21; 8 cm × 15 cm = £2.81; 8 cm × 20 cm = £2.97 (Systagenix)

◢For lightly to moderately exuding wounds

Polyurethane Foam Dressing, BP 1993
Lyofoam®, 7.5 cm × 7.5 cm = £1.05, 10 cm × 10 cm = £1.20, 10 cm × 17.5 cm = £1.94, 15 cm × 20 cm = £2.61 (Mölnlycke)

Polyurethane Foam Film Dressing with Adhesive Border
Tielle®, 11 cm × 11 cm = £2.38; 15 cm × 15 cm = £3.89, 18 cm × 18 cm = £4.95, 7 cm × 9 cm = £1.28, 15 cm × 20 cm = £4.87, 18 cm × 18 cm (sacral) = £3.60 (Systagenix)

Polyurethane Foam Film Dressing without Adhesive Border
Advazorb® Lite, 7.5 cm × 7.5 cm = £0.70, 10 cm × 10 cm = £0.97, 10 cm × 20 cm = £3.02, 12.5 cm × 12.5 cm = £1.43, 15 cm × 15 cm = £1.89, 20 cm × 20 cm = £3.38 (Advancis)
Allevyn® Lite, 5 cm × 5 cm = £1.11; 10 cm × 10 cm = £2.02; 10 cm × 20 cm = £3.46; 15 cm × 20 cm = £4.32 (S&N Hlth.)
Allevyn® Thin, self-adhesive, 5 cm × 6 cm = £1.05, 10 cm × 10 cm = £2.13, 15 cm × 15 cm = £3.51, 15 cm × 20 cm = £4.26 (S&N Hlth)
Kerraheel®, non-adhesive, 12 cm × 20 cm (heel) = £4.56 (Crawford)

PolyMem®, 7 cm × 7 cm (tube) = £1.70, 9 cm × 9 cm (tube) = £2.15, size 1 (finger/toe) = £2.50, size 2 (finger/toe) = £2.50, size 3 (finger/toe) = £2.50 (Aspen Medical)
Transorbent®, self-adhesive, 5 cm × 7 cm = £1.04; 10 cm × 10 cm = £1.96; 15 cm × 15 cm = £3.60; 20 cm × 20 cm = £5.75 (B. Braun)
UrgoCell® TLC, soft-adherent, 6 cm × 6 cm = £1.82, 10 cm × 10 cm = £2.65, 15 cm × 20 cm = £6.01, 12 cm × 19 cm (heel) = £4.73 (Urgo)

◢For moderately to heavily exuding wounds

Polyurethane Foam Dressing
Cutimed® Cavity, 5 cm × 6 cm = £1.76, 10 cm × 10 cm = £2.92, 15 cm × 2 cm = £1.63, 15 cm × 15 cm = £4.39 (BSN Medical)
Kendall®, 5 cm × 5 cm = £0.71, 7.5 cm × 7.5 cm = £1.21, 10 cm × 10 cm = £1.06, 12.5 cm × 12.5 cm = £1.80, 15 cm × 15 cm = £2.60, 20 cm × 20 cm = £3.01, 10 cm × 20 cm = £2.05, 8.5 cm × 7.5 cm (fenestrated) = £0.91 (Covidien)

Polyurethane Foam Film Dressing with Adhesive Border
ActivHeal® Foam Adhesive, 7.5 cm × 7.5 cm = £1.18, 10 cm × 10 cm = £1.60, 12.5 cm × 12.5 cm = £1.68, 15 cm × 15 cm = £2.15, 20 cm × 20 cm = £4.42 (MedLogic)
Allevyn® Adhesive, 7.5 cm × 7.5 cm = £1.43, 10 cm × 10 cm = £2.10, 12.5 cm × 12.5 cm = £2.57, 17.5 cm × 17.5 cm = £5.07, 12.5 cm × 22.5 cm = £4.00, 22.5 cm × 22.5 cm = £7.38; (sacral) 17 cm x 17 cm = £3.80, 22 cm x 22 cm = £5.47 (S&N Hlth.)
Allevyn® Plus Adhesive, 12.5 cm × 12.5 cm = £3.16; 17.5 cm × 17.5 cm = £6.10; 12.5 cm × 22.5 cm = £5.60; (sacral) 17 cm x 17 cm = £4.61, 22 cm x 22 cm = £6.67 (S&N Hlth)
Biatain® Adhesive, 10 cm × 10 cm = £1.65 12.5 cm × 12.5 cm = £2.41, 18 cm × 18 cm = £4.86, 18 cm × 28 cm = £7.20, 23 cm × 23 cm (sacral) = £4.16, 19 cm × 20 cm (heel) = £4.85; 17 cm diameter (contour) = £4.67 (Coloplast)
Biatain® Silicone, 7.5 cm × 7.5 cm = £1.41, 10 cm × 10 cm = £2.27, 12.5 cm × 12.5 cm = £2.90, 15 cm × 15 cm = £3.98, 17.5 cm × 17.5 cm = £5.49 (Coloplast)
Kendall® Island, 10 cm × 10 cm = £1.51, 15 cm × 15 cm = £2.84, 20 cm × 20 cm = £5.36 (Coviden)
PermaFoam®, 16.5 cm × 18 cm (concave) = £ 3.82; 18 cm × 18 cm (sacral) = £3.14; 22 cm × 22 cm (sacral) = £3.61; *PermaFoam Comfort®* 8 cm × 8 cm = £1.06, 10 cm × 20 cm = £3.18, 11 cm × 11 cm = £2.02, 15 cm × 15 cm = £3.29, 20 cm × 20 cm = £4.78 (Hartmann)
PolyMem®, 5 cm × 7.6 cm = £1.12, 8.8 cm × 12.7 cm = £1.99, 10 cm × 13 cm = £2.11, 15 cm × 15 cm = £2.84, 16.5 cm × 20.9 cm = £6.54, 18.4 cm × 20 cm (sacral) = £4.39 (Aspen Medical)
Tegaderm® Foam Adhesive, 6.9 cm × 7.6 cm = £1.42, 10 cm × 11 cm = £2.33, 14.3 cm × 14.3 cm = £3.44, 14.3 cm × 15.6 cm = £4.12, 19 cm × 22.5 cm = £6.76, 6.9 cm x 6.9 cm (soft cloth border) = £1.66, 13.9 cm × 13.9 cm (heel) = £4.14 (3M)
Tielle® Plus, 11 cm × 11 cm = £2.63; 15 cm × 15 cm = £4.30; 15 cm × 20 cm = £5.39; 15 cm × 15 cm (sacrum) = £3.13; 20 cm × 26.5 cm (heel) = £4.45 (Systagenix)

Trufoam®, 11 cm × 11 cm = £2.18, 15 cm × 15 cm = £3.64, 7 cm × 9 cm = £1.14, 15 cm × 20 cm = £4.57 (Aspen Medical)

Polyurethane Foam Film Dressing without Adhesive Border

ActivHeal® Foam Non-Adhesive, 5 cm × 5 cm = £0.75, 10 cm × 10 cm = £1.13, 10 cm × 17.8 cm = £2.34, 10 cm × 20 cm =£2.34, 20 cm × 20 cm = £3.92, 18 cm × 12 cm (heel) = £3.48 (MedLogic)

Advazorb®, 5 cm × 5 cm = £0.65, 7.5 cm × 7.5 cm = £0.78, 10 cm × 10 cm = £1.08, 10 cm × 20 cm = £3.35, 12.5 cm × 12.5 cm £1.59, 15 cm × 15 cm = £2.10, 20 cm × 20 cm = £3.75, 17 cm × 21 cm (heel) =£4.75 (Advancis)

Allevyn® Cavity, circular, 5 cm diameter = £3.97, 10 cm diameter = £9.46; tubular, 9 cm × 2.5 cm = £3.85, 12 cm × 4 cm = £6.78 (S&N Hlth.)

Allevyn® Compression, 5 cm × 6 cm = £1.18; 10 cm × 10 cm = £2.43; 15 cm × 15 cm = £4.12, 15 cm × 20 cm = £4.62 (S&N Hlth.)

Allevyn® Non-Adhesive, 5 cm × 5 cm = £1.21, 10 cm × 10 cm = £2.40, 10 cm × 20 cm = £3.86, 20 cm × 20 cm = £6.44, 10.5 cm × 13.5 cm (heel) = £4.81 (S&N Hlth.)

Allevyn® Plus Cavity, 5 cm × 6 cm = £1.78, 10 cm × 10 cm = £2.97, 15 cm × 20 cm = £5.95 (S&N Hlth.)

Askina® Foam, 10 cm × 10 cm = £2.10, 10 cm × 20 cm = £3.31, 20 cm × 20 cm = £5.53, 12 cm × 20 cm (heel) = £4.48; cavity dressing, 2.4 cm × 40 cm = £2.34 (B. Braun)

Biatain® -Ibu Non-Adhesive, impregnated with ibuprofen 0.5 mg/cm², 5 cm × 7 cm = £1.62, 10 cm x 12 cm = £3.12, 10 cm x 22.5 cm = £4.91, 15 cm x 15 cm = £4.91, 20 cm x 20 cm = £8.34 (Coloplast)
Note for cautions and contra-indications of ibuprofen see section 10.1.1

Biatain® -Ibu Soft-Hold, impregnated with ibuprofen 0.5 mg/cm², 10 cm x 12 cm = £3.12, 10 cm x 22.5 cm = £4.91, 15 cm x 15 cm = £4.91 (Coloplast)
Note for cautions and contra-indications of ibuprofen see section 10.1.1

Biatain® Non-Adhesive, 10 cm × 10 cm = £2.24, 10 cm × 20 cm = £3.70, 15 cm × 15 cm = £4.13, 20 cm × 20 cm = £6.13; 5 cm × 7 cm = £1.23; Biatain® Soft-Hold, 10 cm × 10 cm = £2.44, 15 cm × 15 cm = £4.05, 5 cm × 7 cm = £1.22, 10 cm × 20 cm = £3.70 (Coloplast)

Kendall® Plus, 5 cm × 5 cm = 80p, 7.5 cm × 7.5 cm = £1.39, 10 cm × 10 cm = £1.44, 15 cm × 15 cm = £3.32, 20 cm × 20 cm = £3.96, 10 cm × 20 cm = £2.64, 8.5 cm × 7.5 cm (fenestrated) = £1.22 (Covidien)

Kerraboot®, (clear or white), foot-shaped, extra small = £14.54, small = £14.83, large = £14.83, extra large = £14.54 (Crawford)

Lyofoam® Extra, 10 cm × 10 cm = £2.08, 17.5 cm × 10 cm = £3.52, 20 cm × 15 cm = £4.56 (Mölnlycke)

Lyofoam® Max, 7.5 cm × 8.5 cm = £1.05, 10 cm × 10 cm = £1.10, 10 cm × 20 cm = £1.94, 15 cm × 15 cm = £2.07, 15 cm × 20 cm = £2.61, 20 cm × 20 cm = £3.84 (Mölnlycke)

PermaFoam®, 10 cm × 10 cm = £2.02, 10 cm × 20 cm = £3.45, 15 cm × 15 cm = £3.82, 20 cm × 20 cm = £5.84; 6 cm diameter = £1.04, 8 cm × 8 cm (fenestrated) = £1.19; cavity dressing, 10 cm × 10 cm = £1.91 (Hartmann)

PolyMem®, 8 cm × 8 cm = £1.54, 10 cm × 10 cm = £2.39, 13 cm × 13 cm = £3.99, 17 cm × 19 cm = £5.90, 10 cm × 61 cm = £12.70, 20 cm × 60 cm = £30.55; PolyMem®WIC 8 cm × 8 cm (cavity) = £3.58; PolyMem®Max 11 cm × 11 cm = £2.88, 20 cm × 20 cm = £11.55 (Aspen Medical)

Tegaderm® Foam, 8.8 cm × 8.8 cm (fenestrated) = £2.17, 10 cm × 10 cm = £2.13, 10 cm × 20 cm = £3.61, 20 cm × 20 cm = £5.76, 10 cm × 60 cm = £12.19 (3M)

Tielle® Plus Borderless, 11 cm × 11 cm = £3.04; 15 cm × 20 cm = £5.51 (Systagenix)

Tielle® Xtra, 11 cm × 11 cm = £2.24; 15 cm × 15 cm = £3.37, 15 cm × 20 cm = £5.51 (Systagenix)

Trufoam® NA, 5 cm × 5 cm = £1.09, 10 cm × 10 cm = £2.07, 15 cm × 15 cm = £3.81 (Aspen Medical)

Cavi-Care® (S&N Hlth.)

Soft, conforming cavity wound dressing prepared by mixing thoroughly for 15 seconds immediately before use and allowing to expand its volume within the cavity. 20 g = £18.62

A5.2.6 Alginate dressings

Non-woven or fibrous, non-occlusive, alginate dressings, made from calcium alginate, or calcium sodium alginate, derived from brown seaweed, form a soft gel in contact with wound exudate.

Alginate dressings are highly absorbent and suitable for use on exuding wounds, and for the promotion of autolytic debridement of debris in very moist wounds. Alginate dressings also act as a haemostatic, but caution is needed because blood clots can cause the dressing to adhere to the wound surface. Alginate dressings should not be used if bleeding is heavy and extreme caution is needed if used for tumours with friable tissue.

Alginate sheets are suitable for use as a wound contact dressing for moderately to heavily exuding wounds and can be layered into deep wounds; alginate rope can be used in sinus and cavity wounds to improve absorption of exudate and prevent maceration. If the dressing does not have an adhesive border or integral adhesive plastic film backing, a secondary dressing will be required.

ActivHeal® (MedLogic)

Activheal® Alginate, calcium sodium alginate dressing, 5 cm × 5 cm = 58p, 10 cm × 10 cm = £1.13, 10 cm × 20 cm = £2.78; cavity dressing, 2 cm × 30 cm = £2.09

ActivHeal Aquafiber®, non-woven, calcium sodium alginate dressing, 5 cm × 5 cm = 74p, 10 cm × 10 cm = £1.77, 15 cm × 15 cm = £3.34; cavity dressing, 2 cm × 42 cm = £1.78

Algisite® M (S&N Hlth.)

Calcium alginate fibre, non-woven dressing, 5 cm × 5 cm = 87p, 10 cm × 10 cm = £1.80, 15 cm × 20 cm = £4.84; cavity dressing, 2 cm × 30 cm = £3.27

Algosteril® (S&N Hlth.)

Calcium alginate dressing. 5 cm × 5 cm = 87p, 10 cm × 10 cm = £1.98, 10 cm × 20 cm = £3.34; cavity dressing, 2 g, 30 cm = £3.57

Appendix 5: Wound Management

Biatain® Alginate (Coloplast)
Alginate and carboxymethylcellulose dressing, highly absorbent, gelling dressing, 5 cm × 5 cm = 96p, 10 cm × 10 cm = £2.28, 15 cm × 15 cm = £4.32; gelling filler, 44 cm = £2.69

Cutimed® Alginate (BSN Medical)
Calcium sodium alginate dressing, 5 cm × 5 cm = 73p, 10 cm × 10 cm = £1.54, 10 cm × 20 cm = £2.89

Kaltostat® (ConvaTec)
Calcium alginate fibre, non-woven, 5 cm × 5 cm, = 90p, 7.5 cm × 12 cm = £1.96, 10 cm × 20 cm = £3.84, 15 cm × 25 cm = £6.61; cavity dressing, 2 g = £3.60

Kendall® (Covidien)
Calcium alginate dressing, 5 cm × 5 cm = 70p, 10 cm × 10 cm = £1.49, 10 cm × 14 cm = £2.41, 10 cm × 20 cm = £2.93, 15 cm × 25 cm = £5.15, 30 cm × 61 cm = £27.03; cavity dressing, 30 cm = £2.84, 61 cm = £4.98, 91 cm = £5.36

Kendall® Plus, calcium alginate dressing, 10 cm × 10 cm = £2.04

Kendall® Zn, calcium alginate and zinc dressing, 5 cm × 5 cm = 80p, 10 cm × 10 cm = £1.68, 10 cm × 20 cm = £3.30

Melgisorb® (Mölnlycke)
Calcium sodium alginate fibre, highly absorbent, gelling dressing, non-woven, 5 cm × 5 cm = 86p, 10 cm × 10 cm = £1.79, 10 cm × 20 cm = £3.36; cavity dressing, 32 cm × 2.2 cm, (2 g) = £3.39

Sorbalgon® (Hartmann)
Calcium alginate dressing, 5 cm × 5 cm = 77p, 10 cm × 10 cm = £1.62; *Sorbalgon® T*, cavity dressing, 2 g, 30 cm = £3.30

Sorbsan® (Aspen Medical)
Sorbsan® Flat, calcium alginate fibre, highly absorbent, flat non-woven pads, 5 cm × 5 cm = 80p, 10 cm × 10 cm = £1.68, 10 cm × 20 cm = £3.15

Sorbsan® Plus, alginate dressing bonded to a secondary absorbent viscose pad, 7.5 cm × 10 cm = £1.70, 10 cm × 15 cm = £3.01, 10 cm × 20 cm = £3.84, 15 cm × 20 cm = £5.33

Sorbsan® Ribbon, 40 cm (with probe) = £2.04
Sorbsan® Surgical Packing, 30 cm (2 g, with probe) = £3.47

Suprasorb® A (Activa)
Calcium alginate dressing, 5 cm × 5 cm = 59p, 10 cm × 10 cm = £1.16; cavity dressing, 30 cm (2 g) = £2.15

Tegaderm® Alginate (3M)
Calcium alginate dressing, 5 cm × 5 cm = 78p, 10 cm × 10 cm = £1.64; cavity dressing, 2 cm × 30.4 cm = £2.74

Urgosorb® (Urgo)
Alginate and carboxymethylcellulose dressing without adhesive border, 5 cm × 5 cm = 83p, 10 cm × 10 cm = £1.99, 10 cm × 20 cm = £3.64; cavity dressing, 30 cm = £2.65

Capillary-action dressings consist of an absorbent core of hydrophilic fibres sandwiched between two low-adherent wound-contact layers to ensure no fibres are shed on to the wound surface. Wound exudate is taken up by the dressing and retained within the highly absorbent central layer.

The dressing may be applied intact to relatively superficial areas, but for deeper wounds or cavities it may be cut to shape to ensure good contact with the wound base. Multiple layers may be applied to heavily exuding wounds to further increase the fluid-absorbing capacity of the dressing. A secondary adhesive dressing is necessary.

Capillary-action dressings are suitable for use on all types of exuding wounds, but particularly on sloughy wounds where removal of fluid from the wound aids debridement; capillary-action dressings are contra-indicated for heavily bleeding wounds or arterial bleeding.

Advadraw® (Advancis)
Non-adherent dressing consisting of a soft viscose and polyester absorbent pad with central wicking layer between two perforated permeable wound contact layers. 5 cm × 7.5 cm = 57p, 10 cm × 10 cm = 88p, 10 cm × 15 cm = £1.19, 15 cm × 20 cm = £1.57

Advadraw Spiral®, 0.5 cm × 40 cm = 82p

Cerdak® Basic (CliniMed)
Non-adhesive wound contact sachet containing ceramic spheres, 5 cm × 5 cm = 70p, 10 cm × 10 cm = £1.56, 10 cm × 15 cm = £2.08; cavity dressing, 10 cm × 10 cm = £2.10, 10 cm × 15 cm = £2.63

Cerdak® Aerocloth, non-adhesive wound contact sachet containing ceramic spheres, with non-woven fabric adhesive backing, 5 cm × 5 cm = £1.37, 5 cm × 10 cm = £1.94

Cerdak® Aerofilm, non-adhesive wound contact sachet containing ceramic spheres, with waterproof transparent adhesive film backing, 5 cm × 5 cm = £1.51, 5 cm × 10 cm = £2.07

Sumar® (Lantor)
Sumar® Lite, for light to moderately exuding wounds and cavities, 5 cm × 5 cm = 93p, 10 cm × 10 cm = £1.59, 10 cm × 15 cm = £2.12

Sumar® Max, for heavily exuding wounds, 5 cm × 5 cm = 95p, 10 cm × 10 cm = £1.61, 10 cm × 15 cm = £2.15

Sumar®Spiral, 0.5 cm × 40 cm = £1.57

Vacutex® (Protex)
Low-adherent dressing consisting of two external polyester wound contact layers with central wicking polyester/cotton mix absorbent layer. 5 cm × 5 cm = 94p, 10 cm × 10 cm = £1.66, 10 cm × 15 cm = £2.23, 10 cm × 20 cm = £2.68, 15 cm × 20 cm = £3.14, 20 cm × 20 cm = £4.28

A5.2.8   Odour absorbent dressings

Dressings containing activated charcoal are used to absorb odour from wounds. The underlying cause of wound odour should be identified. Wound odour is most effectively reduced by debridement of slough, reduction in bacterial levels, and frequent dressing changes.

Fungating wounds and chronic infected wounds produce high volumes of exudate which can reduce the effectiveness of odour absorbent dressings. Many odour absorbent dressings are intended for use in combination with other dressings; odour absorbent dressings with a suitable wound contact layer can be used as a primary dressing.

Askina® Carbosorb (B. Braun)
> Activated charcoal and non-woven viscose rayon dressing, 10 cm × 10 cm = £2.77, 10 cm × 20 cm = £5.34

CarboFLEX® (ConvaTec)
> Dressing in 5 layers: wound-facing absorbent layer containing alginate and hydrocolloid; water-resistant second layer; third layer containing activated charcoal; non-woven absorbent fourth layer; water-resistant backing layer. 10 cm × 10 cm = £3.01, 8 cm × 15 cm = £3.61, 15 cm × 20 cm = £6.85

Carbopad® VC (Synergy Healthcare)
> Activated charcoal non-absorbent dressing, 10 cm × 10 cm = £1.59, 10 cm × 20 cm = £2.15

CliniSorb® Odour Control Dressings (CliniMed)
> Activated charcoal cloth enclosed in viscose rayon with outer polyamide coating. 10 cm × 10 cm = £1.78, 10 cm × 20 cm = £2.37, 15 cm × 25 cm = £3.81

Sorbsan® Plus Carbon (Aspen Medical)
> Alginate dressing with activated carbon, 7.5 cm × 10 cm = £2.48, 10 cm × 15 cm = £4.81, 10 cm × 20 cm = £5.76, 15 cm × 20 cm = £6.63

A5.3 Antimicrobial dressings

Spreading infection at the wound site requires treatment with systemic antibacterials.

For local wound infection, a topical antimicrobial dressing can be used to reduce the level of bacteria at the wound surface but will not eliminate a spreading infection. Some dressings are designed to release the antimicrobial into the wound, others act upon the bacteria after absorption from the wound. The amount of exudate present and the level of infection should be taken into account when selecting an antimicrobial dressing.

Medical grade honey (section A5.3.1), has antimicrobial and anti-inflammatory properties. Dressings impregnated with **iodine** (section A5.3.2), can be used to treat clinically infected wounds. Dressings containing **silver** (section A5.3.3), should be used only when clinical signs or symptoms of infection are present.

Dressings containing other **antimicrobials** (section A5.3.4) such as polihexanide (polyhexamethylene biguanide) or dialkylcarbamoyl chloride are available for use on infected wounds. Although hypersensitivity is unlikely with chlorhexidine impregnated tulle dressing, the antibacterial efficacy of these dressings has not been established.

A5.3.1 Honey

Medical grade honey has antimicrobial and anti-inflammatory properties and can be used for acute or chronic wounds. Medical grade honey has osmotic properties, producing an environment that promotes autolytic debridement; it can help control wound malodour. Honey dressings should not be used on patients with extreme sensitivity to honey, bee stings or bee products. Patients with diabetes should be monitored for changes in blood-glucose concentrations during treatment with topical honey or honey-impregnated dressings.

◢**Sheet dressing**

Actilite® (Advancis)
> Knitted viscose impregnated with medical grade manuka honey and manuka oil, 10 cm × 10 cm = 97p, 10 cm × 20 cm = £1.88

Activon Tulle® (Advancis)
> Knitted viscose impregnated with medical grade manuka honey, 5 cm × 5 cm = £1.82, 10 cm × 10 cm = £3.06
> Where no size stated by the prescriber the 5 cm size to be supplied

Algivon® (Advancis)
> Absorbent, non-adherent calcium alginate dressing impregnated with medical grade manuka honey, 5 cm × 5 cm = £2.13, 10 cm × 10 cm = £3.59
> Algivon® Plus, reinforced calcium alginate dressing impregnated with medical grade manuka honey, 5 cm × 5 cm = £1.96, 10 cm × 10 cm = £3.36, 2.5 cm × 20 cm (ribbon with with probe) = £3.36

Medihoney® (Derma Sciences Europe)
> Antibacterial Honey Tulle, woven fabric impregnated with medical grade manuka honey, 10 cm × 10 cm = £2.98
> Gel sheet, sodium alginate dressing impregnated with medical grade honey, 5 cm × 5 cm = £1.75, 10 cm × 10 cm = £4.20
> Antibacterial Honey Apinate®, non-adherent calcium alginate dressing, impregnated with medical grade honey, 5 cm × 5 cm =£2.00, 10 cm × 10 cm = £3.40, 1.9 cm × 30 cm (rope) = £4.20

Melladerm® Plus Tulle (Danetre)
> Knitted viscose impregnated with medical grade honey (Bulgarian, mountain flower) 45% in a basis containing polyethylene glycol, 10 cm × 10 cm = £2.10

MelMax® (CliniMed)
> Acetate wound contact layer impregnated with buckwheat honey 75% in ointment basis, 5 cm × 6 cm = £4.82, 8 cm × 10 cm = £9.90, 8 cm × 20 cm = £19.79

Mesitran® (Aspen Medical)
> Hydrogel, semi-permeable dressing impregnated with medical grade honey, 10 cm × 10 cm = £2.55, 15 cm × 20 cm = £5.31; *with adhesive border*, 10 cm × 10 cm = £2.66, 15 cm × 13 cm (sacral) = £4.50, 15 cm × 15 cm = £4.70
> Mesitran® Mesh, hydrogel, non-adherent wound contact layer, without adhesive border, 10 cm × 10 cm = £2.45

◢Honey-based topical application

Medical grade honey is applied directly to the wound and covered with a primary low adherence wound dressing; an additional secondary dressing may be required for exuding wounds.

Activon® (Advancis)
Honey, (medical grade, manuka), 25-g tube = £2.02

MANUKApli® (Manuka Medical)
Honey, (medical grade, manuka), 15-g tube = £2.95

Medihoney® (Derma Sciences Europe)
Antibacterial Medical Honey, honey (medical grade, *Leptospermum* sp.), 20-g tube = £3.96, 50-g tube = £9.90

Antibacterial Wound Gel, honey (medical grade, *Leptospermum* sp.), 80% in natural waxes and oils, 10-g tube = £2.69, 20-g tube = £4.02
Note *Antibacterial Wound Gel* is not recommended for use in deep wounds or body cavities where removal of waxes may be difficult

Melladerm® Plus (SanoMed)
Honey, (medical grade; Bulgarian, mountain flower) 45% in basis containing polyethylene glycol, 20-g tube = £3.98, 50-g tube = £8.50

Mesitran® (Aspen Medical)
Ointment, honey (medical grade) 47%, 15-g tube = £3.47, 50-g tube = £9.55
Excipients include lanolin

Ointment S, honey (medical grade) 40%, 15-g tube = £3.46
Excipients include lanolin

A5.3.2 Iodine

Cadexomer–iodine, like povidone–iodine, releases free iodine when exposed to wound exudate. The free iodine acts as an antiseptic on the wound surface, the cadexomer absorbs wound exudate and encourages de-sloughing.

Two-component hydrogel dressings containing glucose oxidase and iodide ions generate a low level of free iodine in the presence of moisture and oxygen.

Povidone–iodine fabric dressing is a knitted viscose dressing with povidone–iodine incorporated in a hydrophilic polyethylene glycol basis; this facilitates diffusion of the iodine into the wound and permits removal of the dressing by irrigation. The iodine has a wide spectrum of antimicrobial activity but it is rapidly deactivated by wound exudate.

Systemic absorption of iodine may occur, particularly from large wounds or with prolonged use.

Iodoflex® (S&N Hlth.)
Paste, iodine 0.9% as cadexomer–iodine in a paste basis with gauze backing, 5-g unit = £3.88; 10 g = £7.76; 17 g = £12.29
Uses for treatment of chronic exuding wounds; max. single application 50 g, max. weekly application 150 g; max. duration up to 3 months in any single course of treatment
Cautions iodine may be absorbed, particularly from large wounds or during prolonged use; severe renal impairment; history of thyroid disorder
Contra-indications children; patients receiving lithium; thyroid disorders; pregnancy and breast-feeding

Iodosorb® (S&N Hlth.)
Ointment, iodine 0.9% as cadexomer–iodine in an ointment basis, 10 g = £4.29; 20 g = £8.58

Powder, iodine 0.9% as cadexomer–iodine microbeads, 3-g sachet = £1.84
Uses for treatment of chronic exuding wounds; max. single application 50 g, max. weekly application 150 g; max. duration up to 3 months in any single course of treatment
Cautions iodine may be absorbed, particularly from large wounds or during prolonged use; severe renal impairment; history of thyroid disorder
Contra-indications children; patients receiving lithium; thyroid disorders; pregnancy and breast-feeding

Iodozyme® (Archimed)
Hydrogel (two-component dressing containing glucose oxidase and iodide ions), 6.5 cm × 5 cm = £7.50, 10 cm × 10 cm = £12.50
Uses antimicrobial dressing for lightly to moderately exuding wounds
Cautions children; pregnancy and breast-feeding
Contra-indications thyroid disorders; patients receiving lithium

Oxyzyme® (Archimed)
Hydrogel (two-component dressing containing glucose oxidase and iodide ions), 6.5 cm × 5 cm = £6.00, 10 cm × 10 cm = £10.00
Uses non-infected, dry to moderately exuding wounds
Cautions children; pregnancy and breast-feeding
Contra-indications thyroid disorders; patients receiving lithium

Povidone–iodine Fabric Dressing

(Drug Tariff specification 43). Knitted viscose primary dressing impregnated with povidone–iodine ointment 10%, 5 cm × 5 cm = 32p; 9.5 cm × 9.5 cm = 48p (Systagenix—*Inadine®*)
Uses wound contact layer for abrasions and superficial burns
Cautions iodine may be absorbed particularly if large wounds treated; children under 6 months; thyroid disease
Contra-indications severe renal impairment; pregnancy; breast-feeding

A5.3.3 Silver

Antimicrobial dressings containing **silver** should be used only when infection is suspected as a result of clinical signs or symptoms (see also p. 1093). Silver ions exert an antimicrobial effect in the presence of wound exudate; the volume of wound exudate as well as the presence of infection should be considered when selecting a silver-containing dressing. Silver-impregnated dressings should not be used routinely for the management of uncomplicated ulcers. It is recommended that these dressings should not be used on acute wounds as there is some evidence to suggest they delay wound healing.

Dressings impregnated with silver sulfadiazine have broad antimicrobial activity; if silver sulfadiazine is applied to large areas, or used for prolonged periods, there is a risk of blood disorders and skin discoloration (see section 13.10.1.1). The use of silver sulfadiazine-impregnated dressings is contra-indicated in neonates, in pregnancy, and in patients with significant renal or hepatic impairment, sensitivity to sulfonamides, or G6PD deficiency. Large amounts of silver sulfadiazine applied topically may interact with other drugs—see Appendix 1 (sulfonamides).

◢ Low adherence dressings

Acticoat® (S&N Hlth.)
Three-layer antimicrobial barrier dressing consisting of a polyester core between low adherent silver-coated high density polyethylene mesh (for 3-day wear), 5 cm × 5 cm = £3.30, 10 cm × 10 cm = £8.07, 10 cm × 20 cm = £12.62, 20 cm × 40 cm = £43.18

Acticoat® 7 five-layer antimicrobial barrier dressing consisting of a polyester core between low adherent silver-coated high density polyethylene mesh (for 7-day wear), 5 cm × 5 cm = £5.74, 10 cm × 12.5 cm = £17.11, 15 cm × 15 cm = £30.76

Acticoat® Flex 3, conformable antimicrobial barrier dressing consisting of a polyester core between low adherent silver-coated high density polyethylene mesh (for 3-day wear), 5 cm × 5 cm = £3.32, 10 cm × 10 cm = £8.10, 10 cm × 20 cm = £12.66, 20 cm × 40 cm = £43.34

Acticoat® Flex 7, conformable antimicrobial barrier dressing consisting of a polyester core between low adherent silver-coated high density polyethylene mesh (for 7-day wear), 5 cm × 5 cm = £5.77, 15 cm × 15 cm = £30.88, 10 cm × 12.5 cm = £17.18

Atrauman® Ag (Hartmann)
Non-adherent polyamide fabric impregnated with silver and neutral triglycerides, 5 cm × 5 cm = 49p, 10 cm × 10 cm = £1.19, 10 cm × 20 cm = £2.32

◢ With charcoal

Actisorb® Silver 220 (Systagenix)
Knitted fabric of activated charcoal, with one-way stretch, with silver residues, within spun-bonded nylon sleeve. 6.5 cm × 9.5 cm = £1.64, 10.5 cm × 10.5 cm = £2.58, 10.5 cm × 19 cm = £4.70

◢ Soft polymer dressings

Allevyn® Ag Gentle (S&N Hlth.)
Soft polymer wound contact dressing, with silver sulfadiazine impregnated polyurethane foam layer, *with adhesive border*, 7.5 cm × 7.5 cm = £3.99, 10 cm × 10 cm = £5.99, 12.5 cm × 12.5 cm = £7.71, 17.5 cm × 17.5 cm = £14.69; *without adhesive border*, 5 cm × 5 cm = £3.12, 10 cm × 10 cm = £5.82, 10 cm × 20 cm = £9.62, 15 cm × 15 cm = £10.83, 20 cm × 20 cm = £16.04
Contra-indications   see notes above

Mepilex® Ag (Mölnlycke)
Soft silicone wound contact dressing with polyurethane foam film backing, with silver, *with adhesive border*, 7 cm × 7.5 cm = £3.30, 10 cm × 12.5 cm = £5.97, 10 cm × 20 cm = £8.69, 10 cm × 25 cm = £10.88, 10 cm × 30 cm = £13.04, 15 cm × 17.5 cm = £10.96, 17 cm × 20 cm = £14.20, 18 cm × 18 cm (sacral) = £11.46, 20 cm × 20 cm (sacral) = £13.93, 23 cm × 23 cm = £18.30; *without adhesive border*, 10 cm × 10 cm = £5.91, 10 cm × 20 cm = £9.75, 15 cm × 15 cm = £10.98, 20 cm × 20 cm = £16.27, 20 cm × 50 cm = £61.22, 13 cm × 20 cm (heel) = £12.38, 15 cm × 22 cm = £13.87

Urgotul® Silver (Urgo)
Non-adherent soft polymer wound contact dressing, with silver, 10 cm × 12 cm = £3.34, 15 cm × 20 cm = £9.09

Urgotul® Duo Silver, non-adherent, soft polymer wound contact dressing, with silver, 5 cm × 7 cm = £1.95, 11 cm × 11 cm = £3.87, 15 cm × 20 cm = £9.35

Urgotul® SSD (Urgo)
Non-adherent, soft polymer wound contact dressing, with silver sulfadiazine, 11 cm × 11 cm = £2.99, 16 cm × 21 cm = £8.48
Contra-indications   see notes above

◢ Hydrocolloid dressings

Aquacel® Ag (ConvaTec)
Soft non-woven pad containing hydrocolloid fibres, (silver impregnated), 4 cm × 10 cm = £2.70, 4 cm × 20 cm = £3.52, 4 cm × 30 cm = £5.27, 5 cm × 5 cm = £1.86, 10 cm × 10 cm = £4.44, 15 cm × 15 cm = £8.36, 20 cm × 30 cm = £20.73; 1 cm × 45 cm (ribbon) = £2.97, 2 cm × 45 cm (ribbon) = £4.46

Physiotulle® Ag (Coloplast)
Non-adherent polyester fabric with hydrocolloid and silver sulfadiazine, 10 cm × 10 cm = £2.14
Contra-indications   see notes above

◢ Foam dressings

Acticoat® Moisture Control (S&N Hlth.)
Three layer polyurethane dressing consisting of a silver coated layer, a foam layer, and a waterproof layer, 5 cm × 5 cm = £6.76, 10 cm × 10 cm = £15.82, 10 cm × 20 cm = £30.82

Allevyn® Ag (S&N Hlth.)
Silver sulfadiazine impregnated polyurethane foam film dressing *with adhesive border*, 7.5 cm × 7.5 cm = £3.27, 10 cm × 10 cm = £5.16, 12.5 cm × 12.5 cm = £6.78, 17.5 cm × 17.5 cm = £13.03, 17 cm × 17 cm (sacral) = £10.18, 22 cm × 22 cm (sacral) = £13.64; *without adhesive border*, 5 cm × 5 cm = £3.06, 10 cm × 10 cm = £5.76, 15 cm × 15 cm = £10.91, 20 cm × 20 cm = £15.99, 10.5 cm × 13.5 cm (heel) = £10.09
Contra-indications   see notes above

Biatain® Ag (Coloplast)
Silver impregnated polyurethane foam film dressing *with adhesive border*, 12.5 cm × 12.5 cm = £8.71, 18 cm × 18 cm = £17.47, 19 cm × 20 cm (heel) = £17.23, 23 cm × 23 cm (sacral) = £18.31; *without adhesive border*, 10 cm × 10 cm = £7.61, 5 cm × 7 cm = £3.13, 10 cm × 20 cm = £13.99, 15 cm × 15 cm = £15.28, 20 cm × 20 cm = £21.55; 5 cm × 8 cm (cavity) = £3.79

PolyMem® Silver (Aspen Medical)
Silver impregnated polyurethane foam film dressing, *with adhesive border*, 5 cm × 7.6 cm (oval) = £2.20, 12.7 cm × 8.8 cm (oval) = £5.43; *without adhesive border*, 10.8 cm × 10.8 cm = £8.60, 17 cm × 19 cm = £17.22; 8 cm × 8 cm (cavity) = £6.84

UrgoCell® Silver (Urgo)
Non-adherent, polyurethane foam film dressing with silver in wound contact layer, 6 cm × 6 cm = £4.11, 10 cm × 10 cm = £5.65, 15 cm × 20 cm = £10.17

◢ **Alginate dressings**

Acticoat® Absorbent (S&N Hlth.)
Calcium alginate dressing with a silver coated antimicrobial barrier, 5 cm × 5 cm = £5.04, 10 cm × 12.5 cm = £12.11; 2 cm × 30 cm (cavity) = £12.18

Algisite® Ag (S&N Hlth.)
Calcium alginate dressing, with silver, 5 cm × 5 cm = £1.56, 10 cm × 10 cm = £3.90, 10 cm × 20 cm = £7.17; 2 g, 30 cm (cavity) = £5.38

Askina® Calgitrol (B. Braun)
Askina® Calgitrol Ag, Calcium alginate and silver alginate dressing with polyurethane foam backing, 10 cm × 10 cm = £3.14, 15 cm × 15 cm = £6.08, 20 cm × 20 cm = £14.19

Askina® Calgitrol Thin, Calcium alginate and silver alginate matrix, for use with absorptive secondary dressings, 5 cm × 5 cm = £1.94, 10 cm × 10 cm = £4.03, 15 cm × 15 cm = £9.04, 20 cm × 20 cm = £15.97

Melgisorb® Ag (Mölnlycke)
Alginate and carboxymethylcellulose dressing, with ionic silver, 5 cm × 5 cm = £1.71, 10 cm × 10 cm = £3.43, 15 cm × 15 cm = £7.25; 3 cm × 44 cm (cavity) = £4.32

Seasorb® Ag (Coloplast)
Alginate and carboxymethylcellulose dressing, with ionic silver, 5 cm × 5 cm = £1.53, 10 cm × 10 cm = £3.74, 15 cm × 15 cm = £6.12; 3 cm × 44 cm (cavity) = £4.05

Silvercel® (Systagenix)
Alginate and carboxymethylcellulose dressing impregnated with silver, 2.5 cm × 30.5 cm = £4.45, 5 cm × 5 cm = £1.68, 10 cm × 20 cm = £7.68, 11 cm × 11 cm = £4.14

Silvercel® Non-adherent, alginate and carboxymethylcellulose dressing with film wound contact layer, impregnated with silver, 5 cm × 5 cm = £1.62, 11 cm × 11 cm = £3.89, 10 cm × 20 cm = £7.25; 2.5 cm × 30.5 cm (cavity) = £3.94

Sorbsan® Silver (Aspen Medical)
Sorbsan® Silver Flat, calcium alginate fibre, highly absorbent, flat non-woven pads, with silver, 5 cm × 5 cm = £1.57, 10 cm × 10 cm = £3.97, 10 cm × 20 cm = £7.26

Sorbsan® Silver Plus, calcium alginate dressing with absorbent backing, with silver, 7.5 cm × 10 cm = £3.31, 10 cm × 15 cm = £5.50, 10 cm × 20 cm = £6.69, 15 cm × 20 cm = £8.98

Sorbsan® Silver Plus SA, calcium alginate dressing with absorbent backing and adhesive border, with silver, 11.5 cm × 14 cm = £5.38, 14 cm × 19 cm = £7.73, 14 cm × 24 cm = £8.51, 19 cm × 24 cm = £9.49

Sorbsan® Silver Ribbon, with silver, 40 cm (with probe) = £4.15

Sorbsan® Silver Surgical Packing, with silver, 30 cm (2 g, with probe) = £5.76

Suprasorb® A + Ag (Activa)
Calcium alginate dressing, with silver, 5 cm × 5 cm = £1.54, 10 cm × 10 cm = £3.87, 10 cm × 20 cm = £7.14; cavity dressing, 30 cm (2 g) = £5.72

Tegaderm® Alginate Ag (3M)
Calcium alginate and carboxymethylcellulose dressing, with silver, 5 cm × 5 cm = £1.35, 10 cm × 10 cm = £3.15; cavity dressing 3 cm × 30 cm = £3.60

Urgosorb® Silver (Urgo)
Alginate and carboxymethylcellulose dressing, impregnated with silver, 5 cm × 5 cm = £1.44, 10 cm × 10 cm = £3.44, 10 cm × 20 cm = £6.48; cavity dressing, 2.5 cm × 30 cm = £3.46

A5.3.4 Other antimicrobials

Chlorhexidine Gauze Dressing, BP 1993 ◢
Fabric of leno weave, weft and warp threads of cotton and/or viscose yarn, impregnated with ointment containing chlorhexidine acetate, 5 cm × 5 cm = 28p; 10 cm × 10 cm = 58p (S&N Hlth.— *Bactigras®*)

Cutimed® Sorbact (BSN Medical)
Low adherence acetate tissue impregnated with dialkylcarbamoyl chloride, (dressing pad) 7 cm × 9 cm = £3.42, 10 cm × 10 cm = £5.34, 10 cm × 20 cm = £8.33; (swabs) 4 cm × 6 cm = £1.60, 7 cm × 9 cm = £2.67, (round swabs) 3 cm, 5 pad pack = £3.20; (ribbon gauze, cotton) 2 cm × 50 cm = £3.92, 5 cm × 2 m = £7.72
Gel, hydrogel dressing impregnated with dialkylcarbamoyl chloride, 7.5 cm × 7.5 cm = £2.58, 7.5 cm × 15 cm = £4.35
Cutimed® Sorbact Hydroactive, non-adhesive gel dressing with hydropolymer matrix and acetate fabric coated with dialkylcarbamoyl chloride, 7 cm × 8.5 cm = £3.57, 14 cm × 14 cm = £5.21, 14 cm × 24 cm = £8.35, 19 cm × 19 cm = £9.81, 24 cm × 24 cm = £14.87
Cutimed® Sorbact Hydroactive B, gel dressing with hydropolymer matrix and acetate fabric coated with dialkylcarbamoyl chloride, with adhesive border, 5 cm × 6.5 cm = £3.86, 10 cm × 10 cm =£6.88, 10 cm × 20 cm = £11.02, 15 cm × 15 cm = £12.95, 20 cm × 20 cm = £19.63
Cutimed® Siltec Sorbact, polyurethane foam dressing with acetate fabric coated with dialkylcarbamoyl chloride, with adhesive border, 7.5 cm × 7.5 cm = £2.47, 12.5 cm × 12.5 cm = £6.33, 15 cm × 15 cm = £7.84, 17.5 cm × 17.5 cm = £10.97, 22.5 cm × 22.5 cm = £16.69, 17.5 cm × 17.5 cm (sacral) = £7.93, 23 cm × 23 cm (sacral) = £11.92

Flaminal® (Crawford)
Forte gel, alginate with glucose oxidase and lactoperoxidase, for moderately to heavily exuding wounds, 15 g = £7.26, 50 g = £24.04

Hydro gel, alginate with glucose oxidase and lactoperoxidase, for lightly to moderately exuding wounds, 15 g = £7.26, 50 g = £24.04

Kendall AMD® (Covidien)
Foam dressing with polihexanide, *without adhesive border*, 5 cm × 5 cm = £2.45, 10 cm × 10 cm = £4.62, 15 cm × 15 cm = £8.75, 20 cm × 20 cm = £12.82, 8.8 cm × 7.5 cm (fenestrated) = £4.15, 10 cm × 20 cm = £8.75
Kendall AMD® Plus 10 cm × 10 cm = £4.85, 8.8 cm × 7.5 cm (fenestrated) = £4.35

Octenilin® (Schülke)
Wound gel, hydroxyethylcellulose and propylene glycol, with octenidine hydrochloride, 20 mL = £4.78

Prontosan® Wound Gel (B. Braun)
Hydrogel containing betaine surfactant and polihexanide, 30 mL = £6.12

Suprasorb® X + PHMB (Activa)
Biosynthetic cellulose fibre dressing with polihexanide, 5 cm × 5 cm = £2.42, 9 cm × 9 cm = £4.81, 14 cm × 20 cm = £10.95; 2 cm × 21 cm (rope) = £6.82

Telfa® AMD (Covidien)
Low adherence absorbent perforated plastic film faced dressing with polihexanide, 7.5 cm × 10 cm = 17p, 7.5 cm × 20 cm = 28p
Telfa® AMD Island, low adherence dressing with adhesive border and absorbent pad, with polihexanide, 10 cm × 12.5 cm = 58p, 10 cm × 20 cm = 85p, 10 cm × 25.5 cm = 96p, 10 cm × 35 cm = £1.19

◢**Irrigation fluids**

Octenilin® (Schülke)
Wound irrigation solution, aqueous solution containing glycerol, ethylhexylglycerin and octenidine hydrochloride, 350 mL = £4.60

Prontosan® Wound Irrigation Solution (B.Braun)
Aqueous solution containing betaine surfactant and polihexanide, 40 mL = £0.58, 350 mL = £4.66

A5.4 Specialised dressings

A5.4.1 Protease-modulating matrix dressings

Protease-modulating matrix dressings alter the activity of *proteolytic enzymes* in chronic wounds; the clinical significance of this approach is yet to be demonstrated.

Cadesorb® (S&N Hlth.)
Ointment, starch-based, 20 g = £9.18

Catrix® (Cranage)
Powder, collagen matrix (cartilage, bovine), 1-g sachet = £3.80

Promogran® (Systagenix)
Collagen and oxidised regenerated cellulose matrix, applied directly to wound and covered with suitable dressing, 28 cm² (hexagonal) = £5.19, 123 cm² (hexagonal) = £15.62
Promogran® Prisma® Matrix, collagen, silver and oxidised regenerated cellulose matrix, applied directly to wound and covered with suitable dressing, 28 cm² (hexagonal) = £6.31, 123 cm² (hexagonal) = £17.98

Suprasorb® C (Activa)
Collagen, 4 cm × 6 cm = £4.56, 6 cm × 8 cm = £7.04, 8 cm × 12 cm = £12.72

Tegaderm® Matrix (3M)
Cellulose acetate matrix, impregnated with polyhydrated ionogens ointment in polyethylene glycol basis, 5 cm × 6 cm = £4.94, 8 cm × 10 cm = £10.14

UrgoStart® (Urgo)
Soft adherent polymer matrix containing nano-oligosaccharide factor (NOSF), with polyurethane foam film backing, 6 cm × 6 cm = £4.39, 10 cm × 10 cm = £6.07, 15 cm × 20 cm = £10.92, 12 cm × 19 cm (heel) = £8.36

UrgoStart® Contact (Urgo)
Non-adherent soft polymer wound contact dressing containing nano-oligosaccharide factor (NOSF), 5 cm × 7 cm = £2.96, 10 cm × 10 cm = £4.17, 15 cm × 20 cm = £9.95

A5.4.2 Silicone keloid dressings

Silicone gel and gel sheets are used to reduce or prevent hypertrophic and keloid scarring. They should not be used on open wounds. Application times should be increased gradually. Silicone sheets can be washed and reused.

◢**Silicone sheets**

Advasil® Conform (Advancis)
Self-adhesive silicone gel sheet with polyurethane film backing, 10 cm × 10 cm = £5.20, 10 cm × 15 cm = £9.17

BAP Scar Care T® (BAP)
Self-adhesive silicone gel sheet, 5 cm × 7 cm = £3.15, 5 cm × 30 cm = £9.00, 10 cm × 15 cm = £9.00

Cica-Care® (S&N Hlth.)
Soft, self-adhesive, semi-occlusive silicone gel sheet with backing. 6 cm × 12 cm = £13.79; 15 cm × 12 cm = £26.89

Ciltech® (Su-Med)
Silicone gel sheet, 10 cm × 10 cm = £7.50, 15 cm × 15 cm = £14.00, 10 cm × 20 cm = £12.50

Dermatix® (Meda)
Self-adhesive silicone gel sheet (clear- or fabric-backed), 4 cm × 13 cm = £6.69, 13 cm × 13 cm = £15.34, 13 cm × 25 cm = £27.73, 20 cm × 30 cm = £50.49

Mepiform® (Mölnlycke)
Self-adhesive silicone gel sheet with polyurethane film backing, 5 cm × 7 cm = £3.26, 9 cm × 18 cm = £12.76, 4 cm × 31 cm = £10.31

Scar FX® (Jobskin)
Self-adhesive, transparent, silicone gel sheet, 10 cm × 20 cm = £16.00, 25.5 cm × 30.5 cm = £60.00, 3.75 cm × 22.5 cm = £12.00, 7.5 cm diameter = £8.50, 22.5 cm × 14.5 cm = £12.00

Silgel® (Nagor)
Silicone gel sheet, 10 cm × 10 cm = £13.50; 20 cm × 20 cm = £40.00; 40 cm × 40 cm = £144.00; 10 cm × 5 cm = £7.50; 15 cm x 10 cm = £19.50; 30 cm × 5 cm = £19.50; 10 cm × 30 cm = £31.50; 25 cm × 15 cm (submammary) = £21.12; 46 cm × 8.5 cm (abdominal) = £39.46; 5.5 cm diameter (circular) = £4.00

◢ **Silicone gel**

BAP Scar Care® (BAP)
Silicone gel, 20 g = £17.00

Ciltech® (Su-Med)
Silicone gel, 15 g = £17.50, 60 g = £50.00

Dermatix® (Meda)
Silicone gel, 15 g = £16.18, 60 g = £58.81

Kelo-cote® (Sinclair IS)
Silicone gel, 15 g = £17.88, 60 g = £51.00
Silicone spray, 100 mL = £51.00
Kelo-cote® UV, Silicone gel with SPF 30 UV protection, 15 g = £17.88

NewGel+®E (Advantech Surgical)
Silicone gel with vitamin E, 15 g = £17.70

ScarSil® (Jobskin)
Silicone gel, 30 g = £15.00

Silgel® STC-SE (Nagor)
Silicone gel, 20-mL tube = £19.00

A5.5 Adjunct dressings and appliances

A5.5.1 Surgical absorbents

Surgical absorbents applied directly to the wound have many disadvantages—dehydration of and adherence to the wound, shedding of fibres, and the leakage of exudate ('strike through') with an associated risk of infection. Gauze and cotton absorbent dressings can be used as secondary layers in the management of heavily exuding wounds (but see also Capillary-action dressings, section A5.2.7). Absorbent cotton gauze fabric can be used for swabbing and cleaning skin. Ribbon gauze can be used post-operatively to pack wound cavities, but adherence to the wound bed will cause bleeding and tissue damage on removal of the dressing—an advanced wound dressing (e.g. hydrocolloid-fibrous (section A5.2.4), foam (section A5.2.5), or alginate (section A5.2.6)) layered into the cavity is often more suitable.

◢ **Cotton**

Absorbent Cotton, BP
Carded cotton fibres of not less than 10 mm average staple length, available in rolls and balls, 25 g = 72p; 100 g = £1.64; 500 g = £5.53 (most suppliers).
Drug Tariff specifies 25-g pack to be supplied when weight not stated

Absorbent Cotton, Hospital Quality
As for absorbent cotton but lower quality materials, shorter staple length etc. 100 g = £1.14; 500 g = £3.60 (most suppliers)
Drug Tariff specifies to be supplied only where specifically ordered
Note Not suitable for wound cleansing

◢ **Gauze and tissue**

Absorbent Cotton Gauze, BP 1988
Cotton fabric of plain weave, in rolls and as swabs (see below), usually Type 13 light, sterile, 90 cm (all) × 1 m = £1.08; 3 m = £2.26; 5 m = £3.52; 10 m = £6.73 (most suppliers). 1-m packet supplied when no size stated
Note Drug Tariff also includes unsterilised absorbent cotton gauze, 25 m roll = £15.42

Absorbent Cotton and Viscose Ribbon Gauze, BP 1988
Woven fabric in ribbon form with fast selvedge edges, warp threads of cotton, weft threads of viscose or combined cotton and viscose yarn, sterile. 5 m (both) × 1.25 cm = 81p; 2.5 cm = 90p

Gauze and Cotton Tissue, BP 1988
Consists of absorbent cotton enclosed in absorbent cotton gauze type 12 or absorbent cotton and viscose gauze type 2. 500 g = £7.01 (most suppliers, including Robinsons—*Gamgee Tissue®* (blue label))

Gauze and Cotton Tissue
(Drug Tariff specification 14). Similar to above.
500 g = £5.12 (most suppliers, including Robinsons—*Gamgee Tissue®* (pink label))
Drug Tariff specifies to be supplied only where specifically ordered

◢ **Lint**

Absorbent Lint, BPC ◢
Cotton cloth of plain weave with nap raised on one side from warp yarns. 25 g = 89p; 100 g = £2.74; 500 g = £11.52 (most suppliers).
Drug Tariff specifies 25-g pack supplied where no quantity stated
Note Not recommended for wound management

◢ **Pads**

Absorbent Dressing Pads, Sterile
Drisorb®, 10 cm × 20 cm = 17p (Synergy Healthcare)
PremierPad®, 10 cm × 20 cm = 18p, 20 cm × 20 cm = 25p (Shermond)
Xupad®, 10 cm × 20 cm = 17p, 20 cm × 20 cm = 28p, 20 cm × 40 cm = 40p (Richardson)

A5.5.2 Wound drainage pouches

Wound drainage pouches can be used in the management of wounds and fistulas with significant levels of exudate.

Biotrol® (B. Braun)
Draina S Fistula, wound drainage pouch, mini (cut to 20 mm), 150-mL capacity = £2.44; medium (cut to 50 mm), 350-mL capacity = £3.64; large (cut to 88 mm), 500-mL capacity = £4.48
Draina S Vision, wound drainage pouch, (cut to 50 mm), 150-mL capacity = £9.39; (cut to 88 mm), 250-mL capacity = £9.92; (cut to 100 mm), 300-mL capacity = £11.51

Eakin® (Eakin)

Wound pouch, *fold and tuck closure*, small (wound size up to 45 mm × 30 mm) = £4.50; medium (wound size up to 110 mm × 75 mm) = £6.50; large (wound size up to 175 mm × 110 mm) = £8.50; extra large (horizontal wound up to 245 mm × 160 mm) = £15.00

Wound pouch, *bung closure*, small (wound size up to 45 mm × 30 mm) = £5.00; medium (wound size up to 110 mm × 75 mm) = £7.00; large (wound size up to 175 mm × 110 mm) = £9.50; extra large (horizontal or vertical wound up to 245 mm × 160 mm) = £17.00, (vertical incision wound up to 290 mm × 130 mm) = £17.00; (horizontal wound up to 245 mm × 160 mm), *with access window* = £19.00

Access window, for use with *Eakin®* pouches = £7.00

Wound Drainage Collector (Hollister)

Pouch, drainable, small (wound size up to 76 mm) = £7.45, medium (wound size up to 95 mm) = £8.13, large (wound size up to 100 mm × 200 mm) = £16.10

Oakmed® Option (OakMed)

Wound Manager, extra small (wound size up to 90 mm × 180 mm) = £11.00; small (horizontal wound size up to 245 mm × 160 mm) = £12.23; medium (vertical wound size up to 90 mm × 260 mm) = £12.50; large (wound size up to 160 mm × 260 mm) = £14.90; square (vertical wound up to 160 mm × 200 mm) = £13.05

Wound Manager, *with access port*, extra small (wound size up to 90 mm × 180 mm) = £12.02; small (horizontal wound size up to 245 mm × 160 mm) = £12.77; medium (vertical wound size up to 90 mm × 260 mm) = £13.05; large (wound size up to 160 mm × 260 mm) = £15.93; square (vertical wound size up to 160 mm × 200 mm) = £13.59

Wound Manager, *cut-to-fit*, small (10–30 mm) = £2.25, medium (10–50 mm) = £2.49, large (10–50 mm) = £2.61

Welland® (CliniMed)

Fistula bag, wound manager, *cut-to-fit* (wound size up to 40 mm × 70 mm) = £2.54

A5.5.3 Physical debridement pads

DebriSoft® is a pad that is used for the debridement of superficial wounds containing loose slough and debris, and for the removal of hyperkeratosis from the skin. *DebriSoft®* must be fully moistened with a wound cleansing solution before use and is not appropriate for use as a wound dressing.

DebriSoft® (Activa)

Pad, polyester fibres with bound edges and knitted outer surface coated with polyacrylate, 10 cm × 10 cm = £6.19

A5.6 Complex adjunct therapies

Topical negative pressure (or vacuum-assisted) therapy requires specific wound dressings for use with the vacuum-pump equipment.

Other complex adjunct therapies include sterile larvae (maggots).

A5.6.1 Topical negative pressure therapy

◢Vacuum assisted closure products

Exsu-Fast® (Synergy Healthcare)

Dressing kit, Kit 1 (small wound, low exudate) = £28.04; Kit 2 (large wound, heavy exudate) = £35.83; Kit 3 (large wound, medium to low exudate) = £35.83; Kit 4 (small wound, heavy exudate) = £28.04

Renasys® F/P (S&N Hlth.)

Dressing kit, foam dressing with round drain (plus port, drapes and fixation film), small = £19.49, medium = £22.64, large = £26.85, extra large = £45.28

Renasys® G (S&N Hlth.)

Dressing kit, non-adherent gauze and transparent film dressing, with flat drain, small = £16.64, medium = £20.86, large = £26.48; round drain, small = £16.64, large = £26.48; channel drain, medium = £20.86

V.A.C.® (KCI Medical)

GranuFoam® dressing kit, polyurethane foam dressing (with adhesive drapes and pad connector), 10 cm × 7.5 cm × 3.3 cm (small) = £21.73, 18 cm × 12.5 cm × 3.3 cm (medium) = £25.87, 26 cm × 15 cm × 3.3 cm (large) = £30.01; bridge dressing kit (for diabetic foot wound) = £30.63; *with silver*, small = £31.86, medium = £36.96

Simplace® dressing kit, spiral-cut polyurethane foam dressings, vapour-permeable adhesive film dressings (with adhesive drapes and pad connector), small = £25.43, medium = £29.23

WhiteFoam®, polyvinyl alcohol foam dressing 10 cm × 7.5 cm (small) = £10.18, 10 cm × 15 cm (large) = £16.29; dressing kit (with adhesive drape and pad connector), 10 cm × 7.5 cm (small) = £24.77, 10 cm × 15 cm (large) = £32.06

Venturi® (Talley)

Wound sealing kit, flat drain, standard = £15.00, large = £17.50; channel drain = £15.00

WoundASSIST® (Huntleigh)

Wound pack, small–medium = £20.81, medium–large = £23.85, extra large = £34.05; channel drain, small–medium = £20.81, medium–large = £23.85

◢Wound drainage collection devices

ActiV.A.C.® (KCI Medical)

Canister (with gel), 300 mL = £26.91

Renasys® Go (S&N Hlth.)

Canister kit (with solidifier), 300 mL = £18.77, 750 mL = £25.88

S-Canister® (S&N Hlth.)

Canister kit, 250 mL (with solidifier) = £19.00

V.A.C Freedom® (KCI Medical)

Canister (with gel), 300 mL = £27.58

Venturi® (Talley)

Canister kit, (with solidifier) = £12.50; *Compact* canister kit (with solidifier) = £12.50

WoundASSIST® (Huntleigh)

Canister, 500 mL = £20.30

Appendix 5: Wound Management

◢Accessories

Renasys® (S&N Hlth.)
Port for foam dressing = £9.31, Y-connector = £3.10

V.A.C.® (KCI Medical)
Drape = £8.97. Gel for canister = £3.59. Sensa T.R.
A.C. pad = £10.29. T.R.A.C. Y-connector = £2.94

Venturi® (Talley)
Gel patches, adhesive, pack of 5 = £15.00. Y-connector, pack of 5 = £15.00

WoundASSIST® (Huntleigh)
Gel strip = £3.37

A5.7 Wound care accessories

A5.7.1 Dressing packs

The role of dressing packs is very limited. They are used to provide a clean or sterile working surface; some packs shown below include cotton wool balls, which are not recommended for use on wounds.

Multiple Pack Dressing No. 1
(Drug Tariff). Contains absorbent cotton, absorbent cotton gauze type 13 light (sterile), open-wove bandages (banded). 1 pack = £4.09

Non-Drug Tariff Specification Sterile Dressing Pack
Dressit® contains vitrex gloves, large apron, disposable bag, paper towel, softswabs, adsorbent pad, sterile field = 60p (Richardson)
Nurse It® contains latex-free, powder-free nitrile gloves, sterile laminated paper sheet, large apron, non-woven swabs, paper towel, disposable bag, compartmentation tray, disposable forceps, paper measuring tape = 52p (Medicare)
Polyfield® Nitrile Patient Pack contains powder-free nitrile gloves, laminate sheet, non-woven swabs, towel, polythene disposable bag, apron = 52p (Shermond)
Propax® SDP contains paper towel, disposable bag, gauze swabs, dressing pad, sterile field = 46p (BSN Medical)
Woundcare® contains nitrile gloves, sterile field, compartmentation tray, large apron, disposable bag, non-woven swabs, drape = 44p (Frontier)

Sterile Dressing Pack
(Drug Tariff specification 10). Contains gauze and cotton tissue pad, gauze swabs, absorbent cotton wool balls, absorbent paper towel, water repellent inner wrapper. 1 pack = 51p (Synergy Healthcare—Vernaid®)

Sterile Dressing Pack with Non-woven Pads
(Drug Tariff specification 35). Contains non-woven fabric covered dressing pad, non-woven fabric swabs, absorbent cotton wool balls, absorbent paper towel, water repellent inner wrapper. 1 pack = 50p (Synergy Healthcare—Vernaid®)

A5.7.2 Woven and fabric swabs

Gauze Swab, BP 1988
Consists of absorbent cotton gauze type 13 light or absorbent cotton and viscose gauze type 1 folded into squares or rectangles of 8-ply with no cut edges exposed, sterile, 7.5 cm × 7.5 cm 5-pad packet = 39p; non-sterile, 10 cm × 10 cm, 100-pad packet = £1.37 (most suppliers)

Filmated Gauze Swab, BP 1988
As for Gauze Swab, but with thin layer of Absorbent Cotton enclosed within, non-sterile, 10 cm × 10 cm, 100-pad packet = £3.67 (Synergy Healthcare—Cotfil®)

Non-woven Fabric Swab
(Drug Tariff specification 28). Consists of non-woven fabric folded 4-ply; alternative to gauze swabs, type 13 light, sterile, 7.5 cm × 7.5 cm, 5-pad packet = 25p; non-sterile, 10 cm × 10 cm, 100-pad packet = 79p

Filmated Non-woven Fabric Swab
(Drug Tariff specification 29). Film of viscose fibres enclosed within non-woven viscose fabric folded 8-ply, non-sterile, 10 cm × 10 cm, 100-pad packet = £3.55 (Systagenix—Regal®)

A5.7.3 Surgical adhesive tapes

Adhesive tapes are useful for retaining dressings on joints or awkward body parts. These tapes, particularly those containing rubber, can cause irritant and allergic reactions in susceptible patients; synthetic adhesives have been developed to overcome this problem, but they, too, may sometimes be associated with reactions. Synthetic adhesive, or silicon adhesive, tapes can be used for patients with skin reactions to plasters and strapping containing rubber, or undergoing prolonged treatment.

Adhesive tapes that are occlusive may cause skin maceration. Care is needed not to apply these tapes under tension, to avoid creating a tourniquet effect. If applied over joints they need to be orientated so that the area of maximum extensibility of the fabric is in the direction of movement of the limb.

◢Permeable adhesive tapes

Elastic Adhesive Tape, BP 1988
(Elastic Adhesive Plaster). Woven fabric, elastic in warp (crepe-twisted cotton threads), weft of cotton and/or viscose threads, spread with adhesive mass containing zinc oxide. 4.5 m stretched × 2.5 cm = £1.71 (S&N—Elastoplast®)
For 5 cm width, see Elastic Adhesive Bandage

Permeable, Apertured Non-Woven Synthetic Adhesive Tape, BP 1988
Non-woven fabric with a polyacrylate adhesive. Chemifix®, 2.5 cm × 5 m = 90p, 5 cm × 5 m = £1.25, 10 cm × 5 m = £2.10, 2.5 cm × 10 m = £1.00, 5 cm × 10 m = £1.40, 10 cm × 10 m = £2.10 (Medicareplus International)
Hypafix®, 5 cm × 5 m = £1.36, 10 cm × 5 m = £2.28, 10 m (all): 2.5 cm = £1.58, 5 cm = £2.51, 10 cm = £4.38, 15 cm = £6.49, 20 cm = £8.61, 30 cm = £12.45 (BSN Medical)

Mefix®, 5 m (all): 2.5 cm = 98p, 5 cm = £1.72; 10 cm = £2.76, 15 cm = £3.76, 20 cm = £4.82, 30 cm = £6.91 (Mölnlycke)

Omnifix®, 10 m (all): 5 cm = £2.28, 10 cm = £3.84, 15 cm = £5.66 (Hartmann)

Primafix®, 5 cm × 10 m = £1.50, 10 cm × 10 m = £2.20, 15 cm × 10 m = £3.25, 20 cm × 10 m = £4.00 (S&N Hlth.)

Permeable Non-woven Synthetic Adhesive Tape, BP 1988

Backing of paper-based or non-woven textile material spread with a polymeric adhesive mass:

Chemipore®, 5 m (all) 1.25 cm = 27p, 2.5 cm = 45p, 5 cm = 95p; 2.5 cm × 10 m = 70p (Medicareplus International)

Clinipore®, 5 m (all) 1.25 cm = 35p, 2.5 cm = 59p, 5 cm = 99p; 2.5 cm × 10 m = 73p (Clinisupplies)

Leukofix®, 5 m (all) 1.25 cm = 52p, 2.5 cm = 84p, 5 cm = £1.47 (BSN Medical)

Leukopor®, 5 m (all) 1.25 cm = 46p, 2.5 cm = 72p, 5 cm = £1.27 (BSN Medical)

Mediplast®, 5 m (all) 1.25 cm = 30p, 2.5 cm = 50p (Neomedic)

Micropore®, 5 m (all) 1.25 cm = 60p, 2.5 cm = 89p, 5 cm = £1.57 (3M)

Scanpor®, 5 m (all) 1.25 cm = 41p, 2.5 cm = 66p, 5 cm = £1.14; 10 m (all), 1.25 cm = 53p, 2.5 cm = 88p, 5 cm = £1.68, 7.5 cm = £2.46 (BioDiagnostics)

Transpore®, 5 m (all) 1.25 cm = 51p, 2.5 cm = 82p, 5 cm = £1.44 (3M)

Where no brand stated by prescriber, net price of tape supplied not to exceed 35p (1.25 cm), 59p (2.5 cm), 99p (5 cm)

Silicone adhesive tape

Soft silicone, water-resistant, knitted fabric, polyurethane film adhesive tape

3M® Kind Removal Silicone Tape, 5 m (all), 2.5 cm = £3.52, 5 cm = £6.38 (3M)

Insil®, 2 cm × 3 m = £5.77, 4 cm × 1.5 m = £5.77 (Insight)

Mepitac®, 2 cm × 3 m = £6.87, 4 cm × 1.5 m = £6.87 (Mölnlycke)

OpSite® Flexifix Gentle, 5 m (all), 2.5 cm = £10.00, 5 cm = £18.75 (S&N)

Siltape®, 2 cm × 3 m = £5.60, 4 cm × 1.5 m = £5.60 (Advancis)

Zinc Oxide Adhesive Tape, BP 1988

(Zinc Oxide Plaster). Fabric, plain weave, warp and weft of cotton and / or viscose, spread with an adhesive containing zinc oxide. 5 m (all): 1.25 cm = 97p; 2.5 cm = £1.40; 5 cm = £2.37; 7.5 cm = £3.57 (most suppliers)

Zinc Oxide Adhesive Tape

Mediplast®, 5 m (all), 1.25 cm = 82p, 2.5 cm = £1.19, 5 cm = £1.99, 7.5 cm = £2.99 (Neomedic)

Strappal®, 5 m (all): 2.5 cm = £1.30, 5 cm = £2.20, 7.5 cm = £3.31 (BSN Medical)

◢Occlusive adhesive tapes

Impermeable Plastic Adhesive Tape, BP 1988

Extensible water-impermeable plastic film spread with an adhesive mass. 2.5 cm × 3 m = £1.36; 2.5 cm × 5 m = £2.03; 5 cm × 5 m = £2.57; 7.5 cm × 5 m = £3.74 (BSN Medical—*Sleek*®)

Impermeable Plastic Synthetic Adhesive Tape, BP 1988

Extensible water-impermeable plastic film spread with a polymeric adhesive mass. 5 m (both): 2.5 cm = £1.72; 5 cm = £3.27 (3M—*Blenderm*®)

A5.7.4 Adhesive dressings

Adhesive dressings (also termed 'island dressings') have a limited role for minor wounds only. The inclusion of an antiseptic is not particularly useful and may cause skin irritation in susceptible subjects.

◢Vapour permeable adhesive dressings

Vapour-permeable Waterproof Plastic Wound Dressing, BP 1993

(former Drug Tariff title: Semipermeable Waterproof Plastic Wound Dressing). Consists of absorbent pad, may be dyed and impregnated with suitable antiseptic (see under Elastic Adhesive Dressing), attached to piece of semi-permeable waterproof surgical adhesive tape, to leave suitable adhesive margin; both pad and margin covered with suitable protector (S&N Hlth—*Elastoplast Airstrip*®)

A5.7.5 Skin closure dressings

Skin closure strips are used as an alternative to sutures for minor cuts and lacerations. Skin tissue adhesive (section 13.10.5) can be used for closure of minor skin wounds and for additional suture support.

Skin closure strips, sterile

Leukostrip®, 6.4 mm × 76 mm, 3 strips per envelope. 10 envelopes = £5.95 (S&N Hlth.)

Omnistrip®, 6 mm × 76 mm, 3 strips per envelope. 50 envelopes = £22.89 (Hartmann)

Steri-strip®, 6 mm × 76 mm, 3 strips per envelope. 12 envelopes = £8.52 (3M)

Drug Tariff specifies that these are specifically for personal administration by the prescriber

A5.8 Bandages

According to their structure and performance bandages are used for dressing retention, for support, and for compression.

A5.8.1 Non-extensible bandages

Bandages made from non-extensible, woven fabrics have generally been replaced by more conformable products, therefore their role is now extremely limited. Triangular calico bandage has a role as a sling.

Open-wove Bandage, Type 1 BP 1988

Cotton cloth, plain weave, warp of cotton, weft of cotton, viscose, or combination, one continuous length. 5 m (all): 2.5 cm = 31p; 5 cm = 53p; 7.5 cm = 75p; 10 cm = 98p (most suppliers)

Triangular Calico Bandage, BP 1980

Unbleached calico right-angled triangle, 90 cm × 90 cm × 1.27 m = £1.17 (most suppliers)

Appendix 5: Wound Management

A5.8.2   Light-weight conforming bandages

Lightweight conforming bandages are used for dressing retention, with the aim of keeping the dressing close to the wound without inhibiting movement or restricting blood flow. The elasticity of **conforming-stretch bandages** (also termed contour bandages) is greater than that of **cotton conforming bandages**.

Conforming Bandage (Synthetic)
Fabric, plain weave, warp of polyamide, weft of viscose. 4 m stretched (all):
Hospiform®, 6 cm = 13p, 8 cm = 16p, 10 cm = 18p, 12 cm = 22p (Hartmann)

Cotton Conforming Bandage, BP 1988
Cotton fabric, plain weave, treated to impart some elasticity to warp and weft. 3.5 m (all): type A, 5 cm = 64p, 7.5 cm = 78p, 10 cm = 97p, 15 cm = £1.32 (BSN Medical—*Easifix Crinx*®)

Knitted Polyamide and Cellulose Contour Bandage, BP 1988
Fabric, knitted warp of polyamide filament, weft of cotton or viscose, fast edges, one continuous length. 4 m stretched (all):
Easifix K®, 2.5 cm = 9p, 5 cm = 10p, 7.5 cm = 15p, 10 cm = 17p, 15 cm = 30p (BSN Medical)
K-Band®, 5 cm = 19p, 7 cm = 24p, 10 cm = 27p, 15 cm = 47p (Urgo)
Knit-Band®, 5 cm = 10p, 7 cm = 15p, 10 cm = 17p, 15 cm = 30p (CliniMed)
Knit Fix®, 5 cm = 12p, 7 cm = 17p, 10 cm = 17p, 15 cm = 33p (Steraid)

Polyamide and Cellulose Contour Bandage
Peha-haft®, cohesive, latex-free, 4 m (all) 2.5 cm = 69p, 4 cm = 45p, 6 cm = 53p, 8 cm = 63p, 10 cm = 72p, 12 cm = 85p (Hartmann)
PremierBand®, 4 m (all); 5 cm = 12p, 7.5 cm = 14p, 10 cm = 17p, 15 cm = 25p (Shermond)

Polyamide and Cellulose Contour Bandage, BP 1988
(Nylon and Viscose Stretch Bandage)
Fabric, plain weave, warp of polyamide filament, weft of cotton or viscose, fast edges, one continuous length, 4 m stretched (all):
Acti-Wrap®, cohesive, latex-free, 6 cm = 44p, 8 cm = 64p, 10 cm = 76p (Activa)
Easifix®, 2.5 cm = 9p, 5 cm = 33p, 7.5 cm = 40p, 10 cm = 48p, 15 cm = 81p (BSN Medical)
Kontour®, cohesive, 5 cm = 28p, 7.5 cm = 35p, 10 cm = 40p, 15 cm = 66p (Easigrip)
Mollelast®, latex-free, 4 cm = 28p (Activa)
Slinky®, 7.5 cm = 57p, 10 cm = 68p, 15 cm = 98p (Mölnlycke)
Stayform®, 5 cm = 29p, 7.5 cm = 36p, 10 cm = 40p, 15 cm = 68p (Robinsons)

A5.8.3   Tubular bandages and garments

Tubular bandages are available in different forms, according to the function required of them. Some are used under orthopaedic casts and some are suitable for protecting areas to which creams or ointments (other than those containing potent corticosteroids) have been

applied. The conformability of the elasticated versions makes them particularly suitable for retaining dressings on difficult parts of the body or for soft tissue injury, but their use as the only means of applying pressure to an oedematous limb or to a varicose ulcer is not appropriate, since the pressure they exert is inadequate.

Compression hosiery (section A5.9.1) reduces the recurrence of venous leg ulcers and should be considered for use after wound healing.

Silk clothing is available as an alternative to elasticated viscose stockinette garments, for use in the management of severe eczema and allergic skin conditions (see below).

◢ Elasticated

Elasticated Surgical Tubular Stockinette, Foam padded
(Drug Tariff specification 25). Fabric as for Elasticated Tubular Bandage with polyurethane foam lining. Heel, elbow, knee, small = £3.00, medium = £3.23, large = £3.46; sacral, medium, and large (all) = £15.28 (Mölnlycke—*Tubipad*®)
Uses   relief of pressure and elimination of friction in relevant area; porosity of foam lining allows normal water loss from skin surface

Elasticated Tubular Bandage, BP 1993
(formerly Elasticated Surgical Tubular Stockinette). Knitted fabric, elasticated threads of rubber-cored polyamide or polyester with cotton or cotton and viscose yarn, tubular. Lengths 50 cm and 1 m, widths 6.25 cm, 6.75 cm, 7.5 cm, 8.75 cm, 10 cm, 12 cm; Synergy—*Comfigrip*®; Easigrip—*EasiGRIP*®; Sallis—*Eesiban*®; Mölnlycke—*Tubigrip*®. Where no size stated by prescriber the 50 cm length should be supplied and width endorsed

Elasticated Viscose Stockinette
(Drug Tariff specification 46). Lightweight plain-knitted elasticated tubular bandage.
Acti-Fast®, 3.5 cm red line (small limb), length 1 m = 62p; 5 cm green line (medium limb), length 1 m = 65p, 3 m = £1.90, 5 m = £3.30; 7.5 cm blue line (large limb), length 1 m = 90p, 3 m = £2.50, 5 m = £4.40; 10.75 cm yellow line (child trunk), length 1 m = £1.45, 3 m = £4.10, 5 m = £7.10; 17.5 cm beige line (adult trunk), length 1 m = £2.15; 20 cm purple line (large adult trunk), length 1 m = £3.20, 5 m = £16.15 (Activa)
CliniFast®, 3.5 cm red line (small limb), length 1 m = 56p; 5 cm green line (medium limb), length 1 m = 58p, 3 m = £1.62, 5 m = £2.81; 7.5 cm blue line (large limb), length 1 m = 77p, 3 m = £2.13, 5 m = £3.74; 10.75 cm yellow line (child trunk), length 1 m = £1.20, 3 m = £3.49, 5 m = £6.04; 17.5 cm beige line (adult trunk), length 1 m = £1.83; vest (long-sleeved), 6–24 months = £7.13, 2–5 years = £9.50, 5–8 years = £10.69, 8–11 years = £11.88, 11–14 years = £11.88, adult, small, = £12.75, medium = £14.54, large = £16.58; vest (short-sleeved), adult, small = £12.50, medium = £14.25, large = £16.25; tights (pair) 6–24 months = £7.13; leggings (pair) 2–5 years = £9.50, 5–8 years = £10.69, 8–11 years = £11.88, 11–14 years = £11.88, adult, small, = £12.75, medium = £14.54, large = £16.58; cycle shorts, adult, small = £12.50, medium = £14.25, large = £16.25; socks (pair) up to 8 years = £2.97, 8–14 years = £2.97; mittens (pair) up to 24 months = £2.97, 2–8 years = £2.97, 8–14 years = £2.97; gloves,

child, small, medium, large = £4.99, adult, small, medium, large = £4.99; *clava*, 6 months–5 years = £5.85, 5–14 years = £6.75 (Clinisupplies)
Comfifast®, 3.5 cm red line (small limb), length 1 m = 56p; 5 cm green line (medium limb), length 1 m = 58p, 3 m = £1.62, 5 m = £2.81; 7.5 cm blue line (large limb), length 1 m = 77p, 3 m = £2.13, 5 m = £3.74; 10.75 cm yellow line (child trunk), length 1 m = £1.20, 3 m = £3.49, 5 m = £6.04; 17.5 cm beige line (adult trunk), length 1 m = £1.83 (Synergy)
Comfifast® Easy Wrap, *vest (long-sleeved)*, 6–24 months = £7.13, 2–5 years = £9.50, 5–8 years = £10.69, 8–11 years = £11.88, 11–14 years = £11.88, adult, small = £12.75, medium = £14.54, large = £16.58; *tights (pair)*, 6–24 months = £7.13; *leggings (pair)*, 2–5 years = £9.50, 5–8 years = £10.69, 8–11 years = £11.88, 11–14 years = £11.88, adult, small = £12.75, medium = £14.54, large = £16.58; *socks (pair)*, up to 8 years = £2.97, 8–14 = £2.97; *mittens (pair)*, up to 24 months = £2.97, 2–8 years = £2.97, 8–14 years = £2.97; *clava*, 6 months–5 years = £5.85, 5–14 years = £6.75 (Synergy)
Comfifast® Multistretch, 3.5 cm red line (small limb), length 1 m = 72p; 5 cm green line (medium limb), length 1 m = 78p, 3 m = £2.23, 5 m = £3.82; 7.5 cm blue line (large limb), length 1 m = £1.05, 3 m = £2.93, 5 m = £5.12; 10.75 cm yellow line (child trunk), length 1 m = £1.67, 3 m = £4.78, 5 m = £8.21; 17.5 cm beige line (adult trunk), length 1 m = £2.49 (Synergy Healthcare)
Coverflex®, 3.5 cm red line (small limb), length 1 m = 78p; 5 cm green line (medium limb), length 1 m = 81p, 3 m = £2.38, 5 m = £4.10; 7.5 cm blue line (large limb), length 1 m = £1.13, 3 m = £2.70, 5 m = £5.35; 10.75 cm yellow line (child trunk), length 1 m = £1.78, 3 m = £5.13, 5 m = £9.02; 17.5 cm beige line (adult trunk), length 1 m = £2.38 (Hartmann)
Easifast®, 3.5 cm red line (small limb), length 1 m = 65p; 5 cm green line (medium limb), length 1 m = 69p, 3 m = £1.95, 5 m = £3.40; 7.5 cm blue line (large limb), length 1 m = 94p, 3 m = £2.60, 5 m = £4.50; 10.75 cm yellow line (child trunk), length 1 m = £1.50, 3 m = £4.25, 5 m = £7.20; 17.5 cm beige line (adult trunk), length 1 m = £1.90 (Easigrip)
Skinnies®, *body-suit*, premature, 0–3 months, or 3–6 months = £15.90, 6–12 months = £17.90; *clava*, 6 months–5 years = £6.62, 5–14 years = £7.60; *gloves* child (small) = £5.20, (medium or large) = £5.25, adult (small) = £5.20, (medium or large) = £5.25; *leggings (pair)*, 6–24 months = £10.30, 2–5 years = £13.50, 5–8 years = £15.25, 8–11 years or 11–14 years = £16.90, adult (small) = £20.90, (medium) = £22.80, (large) = £24.70; *mittens*, 0–24 months, 2–8 years, or 8–14 years = £3.80; *socks, ankle (pair)*, 6 months–8 years or 8–14 years = £4.20; *socks, knee (pair)*, child (small, medium, or large, up to shoe size 4) = £13.70, adult (shoe size 4–6, 6–8, 8–11, or size 11+) = £13.70; *vest (long-sleeved)*, 6–24 months = £10.30, 2–5 years = £13.50, 5–8 years = £15.25, 8–11 years or 11–14 years = £16.90, adult (small) = £20.90, (medium) = £22.80, (large) = £24.70; *vest (short-sleeved)*, 6–24 months = £10.20, 2–5 years = £13.40, 5–8 years = £15.10, 8–11 years or 11–14 years = £16.80, adult (small) = £20.80, (medium) = £22.70, (large) = £24.60; *vest (sleeveless)*, 6–24 months = £10.20, 2–5 years = £13.40, 5–8 years = £15.15, 8–11 years = £16.80, 11–14 years = £16.80, adult (small) = £20.80, (medium) = £22.70, (large) = £24.60 (Skinnies)

Tubifast® 2-way stretch, 3.5 cm red line (small limb), length 1 m = 88p; 5 cm green line (medium limb), length 1 m = 95p, 3 m = £2.70, 5 m = £4.61; 7.5 cm blue line (large limb), length 1 m = £1.26, 3 m = £3.55, 5 m = £6.19; 10.75 cm yellow line (child trunk), length 1 m = £2.02, 3 m = £5.78, 5 m = £9.92; 20 cm purple line (large adult trunk), length 1 m = £3.27, 5 m = £16.00; *vest (long-sleeved)*, 6–24 months = £10.97, 2–5 years = £14.63, 5–8 years = £16.46, 8–11 years = £18.28, 11–14 years = £18.28; *tights (pair)*, 6–24 months = £10.97; *leggings (pair)*, 2–5 years = £14.63, 5–8 years = £16.46, 8–11 years = £18.28, 11–14 years = £18.28; *socks (pair)*, one-size = £4.58; *gloves*, (small-medium or medium-large adult, extra small or small child) = £5.50 (Mölnlycke)

◢**Non-elasticated**

Cotton Stockinette, Bleached, BP 1988
Knitted fabric, cotton yarn, tubular length, 1 m (all), 2.5 cm = 37p; 5 cm = 58p; 7.5 cm = 69p; 6 m × 10 cm = £4.75 (Sallis—*Eesiban*®)
Uses 1 m lengths, basis (with wadding) for Plaster of Paris bandages etc.; 6 m length, compression bandage

Ribbed Cotton and Viscose Surgical Tubular Stockinette, BP 1988
Knitted fabric of 1:1 ribbed structure, singles yarn spun from blend of two-thirds cotton and one-third viscose fibres, tubular. Length 5 m (all):
Type A (lightweight): arm/leg (child), arm (adult) 5 cm = £2.45; arm (OS adult), leg (adult) 7.5 cm = £3.22; leg (OS adult) 10 cm = £4.27; trunk (child) 15 cm = £6.15; trunk (adult) 20 cm = £7.11; trunk (OS adult) 25 cm = £8.50 (Mölnlycke)
Type B (heavyweight): sizes as for Type A, net price £2.55–£8.83 (Sallis—*Eesiban*®)
Drug Tariff specifies various combinations of sizes to provide sufficient material for part or full body coverage
Uses protective dressings with tar-based and other non-steroid ointments

◢**Silk Clothing**

Knitted, medical grade silk clothing can be used as an adjunct to normal treatment for severe eczema and allergic skin conditions. When used in combination with medical creams and ointments, care should be taken to ensure that the medication is fully absorbed into the skin before the silk clothing is worn; silk garments are not suitable for use in direct contact with emollients used in 'wet wrapping techniques'.

DermaSilk® (Espere)
Knitted silk fabric, hypoallergenic, sericin-free, *body suit*, child 0–3 months (height 62 cm) = £36.18, 3–6 months (height 68 cm) = £36.82, 6–9 months (height 74 cm) = £37.87, 9–12 months (height 74 cm) = 38.25, 12–18 months (height 86 cm) = £38.92, 18–24 months (height 92 cm) = £39.29, 2–3 years (height 98 cm) = £38.71, 3–4 years (height 110 cm) = £41.03; *boxer shorts*, adult (male), small–XXXL = £39.95; *briefs*, 3–4 years = £20.95, 5–6 years = £20.95, 7–8 years = £20.95, 10–12 years = £20.95, adult (female), small–XXL = £29.39; *facial mask*, child (head circumference up to 47 cm) = £15.80, child (head circumference up to 50 cm) = £15.80, teen or adult = £20.19; *gloves*, adult (small, medium, large, or extra large) = £19.96, child (small or medium) = £14.22; *leggings*, child 0–3 months (height 62 cm) = £25.83, 3–6 months (height 68 cm) = £26.28, 6–9 months (height 74 cm) = £27.34, 9–12

months (height 74 cm) = £27.90, 12–18 months (height 86 cm) = £28.39, 18–24 months (height 92 cm) = £28.94, 2–3 years (height 98 cm) = £28.51, 3–4 years (height 110 cm) = £30.50, adult (male), small–XXL = £75.60, adult (female), small–XXL = £75.60; *pyjamas*, child 3–4 years (height 110 cm) = £68.42, 5–6 years (height 120 cm) = £72.63, 7–8 years (height 135 cm) = £75.79, 10–12 years (height 150 cm) = £78.95; *shirt, roll-neck*, 3–4 years = £45.56, 5–6 years = £48.49, 7–8 years = £50.51, 10–12 years = £52.54, adult, small–XXL = £74.72; *shirt, round-neck*, adult (male), small–XXL = £74.72, adult (female), small–XXL = £74.72; *sleeves (tubular)*, length 33 cm = £26.28, 50 cm = £32.50; *undersocks, (heel-less)*, 2 pairs standard or longer length = £23.39; *undersocks*, adult shoe-size 5½–6½, 7–8½, 9–10½, 11–13, child shoe-size 3–8, 9–1, 2–5, 2 pairs = £17.78

DreamSkin® (Dreamskin)

Knitted silk fabric, hypoallergenic, sericin-free, with methyacrylate copolymer and zinc-based antibacterial, *body suit (with foldaway mitts)*, child 0–3 months = £35.15, 0–6 months = £35.65, 3–6 months = £35.65, 6–9 months = £36.67, 9–12 months = £37.20, 12–18 months = £37.69, 18–24 months = £38.20, 2–3 years = £38.71, 3–4 years = £39.73; *briefs or fitted boxers*, 3–4 years = £20.95, 5–6 years = £20.95, 7–8 years = £20.95, 9–10 years = £20.95, 11–12 years = £20.95, adult (male) small–XXL = £32.95, adult (female) small–XXL = £30.95; *eye mask*, one size = £9.95; *gloves*, child (small or medium) = £13.98, adult (small, medium, large, or extra large) = £19.62; *head mask*, child up to 1 year (head circumference 39–45cm) = £15.30, child 1–8 years (head circumference 48–50cm) = £15.30, child 12–18 years = £19.96, adult = £19.96; *baby leggings (with foldaway feet)*, child 0–3 months = £24.95, 0–6 months = £25.45, 3–6 months = £25.45, 6–9 months = £26.47, 9–12 months = £26.98, 12–18 months = £27.49, 18–24 months = £28.00, 2–3 years = £28.51, 3–4 years = £29.53; *leggings (without feet; male or female styles)*, 3–4 years = £29.53, 5–6 years = £30.99, 7–8 years = £31.49, 9–10 years = £31.99, 11–12 years = £32.49, adult small–XXL = £74.74; *pyjamas (male or female styles)*, 3–4 years = £66.25, 5–6 years = £70.33, 7–8 years = £73.39, 9–10 years = £74.95, 11–12 years = £76.45; *shirt, polo-neck, long-sleeved (male or female styles)*, 3–4 years = £44.94, 5–6 years = £47.94, 7–8 years = £49.94, 9–10 years = £50.94, 11–12 years = £51.94, adult small–XXL = £73.87; *shirt, round-neck, long-sleeved (male or female styles)*, 3–4 years = £44.95, 5–6 years = £46.95, 7–8 years = £48.95, 9–10 years = £49.95, 11–12 years = £50.95, adult small–XXL = £73.87; *sleeves, (tubular)*, pair, length 33 cm = £25.83, 50 cm = £32.13; *tights*, adult (female) small–XL = £22.95; *undersocks, (liner socks)*, 2 pairs, child shoe-size 3–5½, 6–8½, 9–12, 12½–3½, 4–5½, = £17.58, adult (male) shoe-size 6–8½, 9–11 = £17.58, adult (female) shoe-size 4–5½, 6–8½ = £17.58; *undersocks (heel-less)*, one size = £23.12

A5.8.4 Support bandages

Light support bandages, which include the various forms of crepe bandage, are used in the prevention of oedema; they are also used to provide support for mild

sprains and joints but their effectiveness has not been proven for this purpose. Since they have limited extensibility, they are able to provide light support without exerting undue pressure. For a warning against injudicious compression see section A5.8.7.

Crepe Bandage, BP 1988

Fabric, plain weave, warp of wool threads and crepe-twisted cotton threads, weft of cotton threads; stretch bandage. 4.5 m stretched (all): 5 cm = 93p; 7.5 cm = £1.31; 10 cm = £1.71; 15 cm = £2.48 (most suppliers)

Cotton Crepe Bandage

Light support bandage, 4.5 m stretched (all) 5 cm = 44p; 7.5 cm = 62p; 10 cm = 80p; 15 cm = £1.17 (Hartmann—*Hospicrepe*® 239) 4.5 m stretched (all), 5 cm = 44p, 7.5 cm = 61p, 10 cm = 79p, 15 cm = £1.16 (Hartmann—*Hospicrepe*® 229)

Cotton Crepe Bandage, BP 1988

Fabric, plain weave, warp of crepe-twisted cotton threads, weft of cotton and/or viscose threads; stretch bandage. 4.5 m stretched (both): 7.5 cm = £2.93; 10 cm = £3.76 (most suppliers)

Cotton, Polyamide and Elastane Bandage

Fabric, cotton, polyamide, and elastane; light support bandage (Type 2), 4.5 m stretched (all) Hospilite®, 5 cm = 35p, 7.5 cm = 48p, 10 cm = 58p, 15 cm = 85p (Hartmann) Neosport®, 5 cm = 54p, 7.5 cm = 73p, 10 cm = 91p, 15 cm = £1.12 (Neomedic) Profore® #2, 10 cm = £1.27, latex-free = £1.35 (S&N Hlth) Setocrepe®, 10 cm = £1.13 (Mölnlycke) Soffcrepe®, 5 cm = 65p, 7.5 cm = 92p, 10 cm = £1.16, 15 cm = £1.69 (BSN Medical)

Cotton Stretch Bandage, BP 1988

Fabric, plain weave, warp of crepe-twisted cotton threads, weft of cotton threads; stretch bandage, lighter than cotton crepe, 4.5 m stretched (all): Hospicrepe® 233, 5 cm = 52p; 7.5 cm = 72p; 10 cm = 96p; 15 cm = £1.36 (Steraid) PremierBand®, 5 cm = 45p, 7.5 cm = 63p, 10 cm = 79p, 15 cm = £1.18 (Shermond)

Cotton Suspensory Bandage

(Drug Tariff). Type 1: cotton net bag with draw tapes and webbing waistband; small, medium, and large (all) = £1.62, extra large = £1.71. Type 2: cotton net bag with elastic edge and webbing waistband; small = £1.79, medium = £1.84, large = £1.91, extra large = £1.98. Type 3: cotton net bag with elastic edge and webbing waistband with elastic insertion; small, medium, and large (all) = £1.93; extra large = £2.00. Type supplied to be endorsed

Knitted Elastomer and Viscose Bandage

Knitted fabric, viscose and elastomer yarn. *Type 2 (light support bandage)* CliniLite®, 4.5 m (all), 5 cm = 44p, 7.5 cm = 61p, 10 cm = 80p, 15 cm = £1.16 (Clinisupplies) K-Lite®, 4.5 m stretched, 5 cm = 52p, 7 cm = 73p, 10 cm = 95p, 15 cm = £1.38; 5.2 m stretched, 10 cm = £1.09 (Urgo) Knit-Firm®, 4.5 m stretched, 5 cm = 36p, 7 cm = 51p, 10 cm = 66p, 15 cm = 96p (Steraid) *Type 3a (light compression bandage)*: CliniPlus®, 8.7 m × 10 cm = £1.80 (Clinisupplies)

Elset®, 6 m stretched, 10 cm = £2.46, 15 cm = £2.66;
8 m stretched, 10 cm = £3.14; 12 m stretched, 15 cm
= £5.27 (Mölnlycke)

K-Plus®, 8.7 m stretched, 10 cm = £2.14; long,
10.25 m stretched, 10 cm = £2.47 (Urgo)

Profore® #3, 8.7 m stretched, 10 cm = £3.70, latex-
free = £4.02 (S&N Hlth.)

L3, 8.6 m stretched, 10 cm = £2.07 (S&N Hlth.)

A5.8.5 Adhesive bandages

Elastic adhesive bandages are used to provide compression in the treatment of varicose veins and for the
support of injured joints; they should no longer be used
for the support of fractured ribs and clavicles. They have
also been used with **zinc paste bandage** in the treatment of venous ulcers, but they can cause skin reactions
in susceptible patients and may not produce sufficient
pressures for healing (significantly lower than those
provided by other compression bandages).

Elastic Adhesive Bandage, BP 1993
   Woven fabric, elastic in warp (crepe-twisted cotton
   threads), weft of cotton and/or viscose threads
   spread with adhesive mass containing zinc oxide.
   4.5 m stretched (all): 5 cm = £3.56; 7.5 cm = £5.15;
   10 cm = £6.85
   Drug Tariff specifies 7.5 cm width supplied when size not
   stated

A5.8.6 Cohesive bandages

Cohesive bandages adhere to themselves, but not to
the skin, and are useful for providing support for sports
use where ordinary stretch bandages might become
displaced and adhesive bandages are inappropriate.
Care is needed in their application, however, since the
loss of ability for movement between turns of the
bandage to equalise local areas of high tension carries
the potential for creating a tourniquet effect. Cohesive
bandages can be used to support sprained joints and as
an outer layer for multi-layer compression bandaging;
they should not be used if arterial disease is suspected.

◢Cohesive extensible bandages

Coban® (3M)
   Bandage, 6 m (stretched), 10 cm = £2.79

K-Press® (Urgo)
   Bandage, 6.5 m × 10 cm (0, short) = £2.78; 7.5 m,
   18–25 cm ankle circumference, 8 cm = £3.06, 10 cm
   = £3.25, 12 cm = £4.09; 10.5 m, 25–32 cm ankle
   circumference, 8 cm = £3.33, 10 cm = £3.55, 12 cm
   = £4.48

Profore® #4 (S&N Hlth.)
   Bandage, 2.5 m (unstretched) = £3.06, latex-free =
   £3.32

Ultra Fast® (Robinsons)
   Bandage, 6.3 m (stretched), 10 cm = £2.59

A5.8.7 Compression bandages

High compression products are used to provide the high
compression needed for the management of gross varices, post-thrombotic venous insufficiency, venous leg

ulcers, and gross oedema in average-sized limbs. Their
use calls for an expert knowledge of the elastic properties of the products and experience in the technique of
providing careful graduated compression. Incorrect
application can lead to uneven and inadequate pressures or to hazardous levels of pressure. In particular,
injudicious use of compression in limbs with arterial
disease has been reported to cause severe skin and
tissue necrosis (in some instances calling for amputation). Doppler testing is required before treatment with
compression. Oral pentoxifylline (section 2.6.4) can be
used as adjunct therapy if a chronic venous leg ulcer
does not respond to compression bandaging [unli-
censed indication].

◢High compression bandages

PEC High Compression Bandage
   Polyamide, elastane, and cotton compression (high)
   extensible bandage, 3.5 m unstretched, 10 cm =
   £3.34 (Mölnlycke—*Setopress®*)

VEC High Compression Bandage
   Viscose, elastane, and cotton compression (high)
   extensible bandage, 3 m unstretched (both); 7.5 cm
   = £2.56; 10 cm = £3.29 (S&N—*Tensopress®*)

High Compression Bandage
   Cotton, viscose, nylon, and Lycra® extensible
   bandage, 3 m (unstretched), 10 cm = £3.42
   (ConvaTec— *SurePress®*); 3 m (unstretched), 10 cm
   = £2.66 (Urgo—*K-ThreeC®*)

◢Short stretch compression bandage

Short stretch bandages help to reduce oedema and
promote healing of venous leg ulcers. They are also
used to reduce swelling associated with lymphoedema.
They are applied at full stretch over padding (*see* Sub-
compression Wadding Bandage below) which protects
areas of high pressure and sites at high risk of pressure
damage.

Actico® (Activa)
   Bandage, cohesive, 6 m (all), 4 cm = £2.25, 6 cm =
   £2.64, 8 cm = £3.03, 10 cm = £3.15, 12 cm = £4.02

Comprilan® (BSN Medical)
   Bandage, 5 m (all), 6 cm = £2.55; 8 cm = £2.99;
   10 cm = £3.22; 12 cm = £3.92

Rosidal K® (Activa)
   Bandage, 5 m (all), 4cm = £1.79, 6cm = £2.50, 8 cm
   = £2.98, 10 cm = £3.26, 12 cm = £3.95; 10m x 10cm
   = £5.67

Silkolan® (Urgo)
   Bandage, 5 m (all), 8 cm = £3.00; 10 cm = £3.39

◢Sub-compression wadding bandage

Cellona® Undercast Padding (Activa)
   Padding, 2.75 m unstretched (all): 5 cm = 29p;
   7.5 cm = 36p; 10 cm = 44p; 15 cm = 57p

Flexi-Ban® (Activa)
   Padding, 3.5 m unstretched, 10cm = 47p

K-Soft® (Urgo)
   Padding, absorbent, 3.5 m unstretched, 10 cm = 43p;
   4.5 m unstretched, 10 cm = 53p

Appendix 5: Wound Management

K-Tech® (Urgo)
Padding, 5 m × 10 cm (0, short) = £3.76; 6 m, 18–25 cm ankle circumference, 8 cm = £4.26, 10 cm = £4.51, 12 cm = £5.69; 7.3 m, 25–32 cm ankle circumference, 8 cm = £4.64, 10 cm = £4.92, 12 cm = £6.21
Note *K-Tech®* also includes a short stretch compressive fabric component

K-Tech® Reduced (Urgo)
Padding, 6 m x 10 cm, 18–25 cm ankle circumference = £4.51; 7.3 m x 10 cm, 25–32 cm ankle circumference = £4.92
Note *K-Tech® Reduced* also includes a short stretch compressive fabric component

Ortho-Band Plus® (Steraid)
Padding, 10 cm × 3.5 cm unstretched = 37p

Profore® #1 (S&N Hlth.)
Padding, viscose fleece, 3.5 m unstretched, 10 cm = 66p, latex-free = 72p

Softexe® (Mölnlycke)
Padding, absorbent, 3.5 m unstretched, 10 cm = 60p

SurePress® (ConvaTec)
Padding, absorbent, 3 m unstretched, 10 cm = 56p

Ultra Soft® (Robinsons)
Padding, absorbent, 3.5 m unstretched, 10 cm = 39p

Velband® (BSN Medical)
Padding, absorbent, 4.5 m unstretched, 10 cm = 68p

A5.8.8 Multi-layer compression bandaging

Multi-layer compression bandaging systems are an alternative to High Compression Bandages (section A5.8.7) for the treatment of venous leg ulcers. Compression is achieved by the combined effects of two or three extensible bandages applied over a layer of orthopaedic wadding and a wound contact dressing.

◢ Four layer systems

K-Four® (Urgo)
K-Four® # 1 (*K-Soft®*—see Sub-compression Wadding Bandage, p. 1105); *K-Four®* # 2 (*K-Lite®*—see Knitted Elastomer and Viscose Bandage, p. 1104); *K-Four®* # 3 (*K-Plus®*—see Knitted Elastomer and Viscose Bandage, p. 1104); *K-Three C®*—see High compression bandages, p. 1105; *K-Four®* # 4 (*Ko-Flex®*), 6 m (stretched), 10 cm = £2.84; 7 m (stretched), 10 cm = £3.25
Multi-layer compression bandaging kit, four layer system, for ankle circumference up to 18 cm = £6.73, 18–25 cm = £6.44, 25–30 cm = £6.44, above 30 cm = £8.87; *reduced compression*, 18 cm and above = £4.21

Profore® (S&N Hlth.)
Profore® wound contact layer (see Knitted Viscose Primary Dressing, p. 1083); *Profore®* #1 (see Sub-compression Wadding Bandage, p. 1106); *Profore®* #2 (see Cotton, Polyamide and Elastane Bandage, p. 1104); *Profore®* #3 (see Knitted Elastomer and Viscose Bandage, p. 1104); *Profore®* #4 (see Cohesive bandages, p. 1105); *Profore® Plus* 3 m (unstretched), 10 cm = £3.46, latex-free = £3.70

Multi-layer compression bandaging kit, four layer system, for ankle circumference up to 18 cm = £9.58, 18–25 cm = £8.92, 25–30 cm = £7.41, above 30 cm = £11.09, latex-free, 18–25 cm = £9.53; *Profore Lite®* above 18 cm = £5.15, latex-free = £5.60

System 4® (Mölnlycke)
System 4® #1 (*Softexe®*—see Sub-compression Wadding Bandage, p. 1106); *System 4®* #2 (*Setocrepe®*—see Cotton, Polyamide and Elastane Bandage, p. 1104); *System 4®* #3 (*Elset®*—see Knitted Elastomer and Viscose Bandage, p. 1104); *System 4®* #4 (*Meban®*)
Multi-layer compression bandaging kit, four layer system, for ankle circumference 18–25 cm = £7.46

Ultra Four® (Robinsons)
Ultra Four® #1 (*Ultra Soft®*—see Sub-compression Wadding Bandage, p. 1106); *Ultra Four®* #2 (*Ultra Lite®*) 10 cm × 4.5 cm (stretched) = 85p; *Ultra Four®* #3 (*Ultra Plus®*) 10 cm × 8.7 cm (stretched) = £1.89; *Ultra Four®* #4 (*Ultra Fast®*—see Cohesive Bandages, p. 1105)
Multi-layer compression bandaging kit, four layer system, for ankle circumference up to 18 cm = £6.41, 18–25 cm = £5.67; *Ultra Four® RC* (reduced compression) 18–25 cm = £4.14

◢ Two layer systems

Coban® 2 (3M)
Multi-layer compression bandaging kit, two layer system (latex-free, foam bandage and cohesive compression bandage), one size = £8.08; *Coban® 2 Lite* (reduced compression), one size = £8.08

K-Two® (Urgo)
K-Tech® (see Sub-compression Wadding Bandages, p. 1106); *K-Press®* (see Cohesive bandages, p. 1105)
Multi-layer compression bandaging kit, two layer system, size 0 (short) = £6.55; 18–25 cm ankle circumference, 8 cm = £7.32, 10 cm = £7.76, 12 cm = £9.78; 25–32 cm ankle circumference, 8 cm = £7.96, 10 cm = £8.48, 12 cm = £10.69
K-Two® Latex Free, *K-Tech®* (see Sub-compression Wadding Bandages, above); *K-Press®* Latex Free
Multi-layer compression bandaging kit, two layer system, for ankle circumference 18–25 cm = £8.38; 25–32 cm = £9.16
K-Two® Reduced, *K-Tech®* Reduced (see Sub-compression Wadding Bandages, above); *K-Press®* (see Cohesive Bandages, p. 1105)
Multi-layer compression bandaging kit, two layer system, for ankle circumference 18–25 cm = £7.76; 25–32 cm = £8.48
K-Two® Reduced Latex Free, *K-Tech®* (see Sub-compression Wadding Bandages, above); *K-Press®* Reduced Latex Free
Multi-layer compression bandaging kit, two layer system, for ankle circumference 18–25 cm = £8.38; 25–32 cm = £9.16
K-Two® Start, *UgoStart®* Contact (see Protease-modulating matrix, p. 1097); *K-Tech®* (see Sub-compression Wadding Bandages, p. 1106); *K-Press®* (see Cohesive Bandages, p. 1105)
Multi-layer compression bandaging kit, two-layer system, for ankle circumference 18–25cm = £9.68; 25–32cm = £10.33

A5.8.9 Medicated bandages

Zinc Paste Bandage has been used with compression bandaging for the treatment of venous leg ulcers. However, paste bandages are associated with hypersensitivity reactions and should be used with caution.

Zinc paste bandages are also used with **coal tar** or **ichthammol** in chronic lichenified skin conditions such as chronic eczema (ichthammol often being preferred since its action is considered to be milder). They are also used with **calamine** in milder eczematous skin conditions.

Zinc Paste Bandage, BP 1993
Cotton fabric, plain weave, impregnated with suitable paste containing zinc oxide; requires additional bandaging, 6 m × 7.5 cm = £3.44 (S&N Hlth.—*Viscopaste PB7*® (10%), *excipients: include* cetostearyl alcohol, hydroxybenzoates)

Zinc Paste and Ichthammol Bandage, BP 1993
Cotton fabric, plain weave, impregnated with suitable paste containing zinc oxide and ichthammol; requires additional bandaging, 6 m × 7.5 cm = £3.47 S&N Hlth.—*Ichthopaste*® (6/2%), *excipients: include* cetostearyl alcohol
Uses see section 13.5

Steripaste® (Mölnlycke)
Cotton fabric, selvedge weave impregnated with paste containing zinc oxide (requires additional bandaging), 6 m × 7.5 cm = £3.24
Excipients include polysorbate 80

◢Medicated stocking

Zipzoc® (S&N Hlth.)
Sterile rayon stocking impregnated with ointment containing zinc oxide 20%. 4-pouch carton = £12.52; 10-pouch carton = £31.30
Note Can be used under appropriate compression bandages or hosiery in chronic venous insufficiency

A5.9 Compression hosiery and garments

Compression (elastic) hosiery is used to treat conditions associated with chronic venous insufficiency, to prevent recurrence of thrombosis, or to reduce the risk of further venous ulceration after treatment with compression bandaging (section A5.8.7). Doppler testing to confirm arterial sufficiency is required before recommending the use of compression hosiery.

Before elastic hosiery can be dispensed, the quantity (single or pair), article (including accessories), and compression class must be specified by the prescriber. There are different compression values for graduated compression hosiery and lymphoedema garments (see table below). All dispensed elastic hosiery articles must state on the packaging that they conform with Drug Tariff technical specification No. 40, for further details see Drug Tariff.
Note Graduated compression tights are ⒩⒣⒮.

Compression values for hosiery and lymphoedema garments

Compression class	Compression hosiery (British standard)	Lymphoedema garments (European classification)
Class 1	14–17 mmHg	18–21 mmHg
Class 2	18–24 mmHg	23–32 mmHg
Class 3	25–35 mmHg	34–46 mmHg
Class 4	Not available	49–70 mmHg
Class 4 super	Not available	60–90 mmHg

A5.9.1 Graduated compression hosiery

Class 1 Light Support
Hosiery, compression at ankle 14–17 mmHg, thigh length or below knee with knitted in heel. 1 pair, circular knit (standard), thigh length = £7.61, below knee = £6.95, (made-to-measure), thigh length = £37.79, below knee = £23.64; lightweight elastic net (made-to-measure), thigh length = £20.38, below knee = £15.91
Uses superficial or early varices, varicosis during pregnancy

Class 2 Medium Support
Hosiery, compression at ankle 18–24 mmHg, thigh length or below knee with knitted in heel. 1 pair, circular knit (standard), thigh length = £11.31, below knee = £10.16, (made-to-measure), thigh length = £37.79, below knee = £23.64; net (made-to-measure), thigh length = £20.38, below knee = £15.91; flat bed (made-to-measure, only with closed heel and open toe), thigh length = £37.79, below knee = £23.64
Uses varices of medium severity, ulcer treatment and prophylaxis, mild oedema, varicosis during pregnancy

Class 3 Strong Support
Hosiery, compression at ankle 25–35 mmHg, thigh length or below knee with open or knitted in heel. 1 pair, circular knit (standard), thigh length = £13.40, below knee = £11.52, (made-to-measure) thigh length = £37.79, below knee = £23.64; flat bed (made-to-measure, only with open heel and open toe), thigh length = £37.79, below knee = £23.64
Uses gross varices, post thrombotic venous insufficiency, gross oedema, ulcer treatment and prophylaxis

◢Accessories

In addition to the product listed below, accessories such as application aids for hosiery are available, see Drug Tariff for details

Suspender
Suspender, for thigh stockings = 67p, belt (specification 13), = £5.16, fitted (additional price) = 62p

◢Anklets

Class 2 Medium Support
Anklets, compression 18–24 mmHg, circular knit (standard and made-to-measure), 1 pair = £6.66; flat bed (standard and made-to-measure) = £13.84; net (made-to-measure) = £13.09

Appendix 5: Wound Management

Class 3 Strong Support

Anklets, compression 25–35 mmHg, circular knit (standard and made-to-measure), 1 pair = £9.09; flat bed (standard) = £9.29, (made-to-measure) = £13.84

◀ **Knee caps**

Class 2 Medium Support

Kneecaps, compression 18–24 mmHg, circular knit (standard and made-to-measure), 1 pair = £6.66; flat bed (standard and made-to-measure) = £13.84; net (made-to-measure) = £10.87

Class 3 Strong Support

Kneecaps, compression 25–35 mmHg, circular knit (standard and made-to-measure), 1 pair = £8.88; flat bed (standard) = £8.88, (made-to-measure) = £13.84

A5.9.2 Lymphoedema garments

Lymphoedema compression garments are used to maintain limb shape and prevent additional fluid retention. Either flat-bed or circular knitting methods are used in the manufacture of elasticated compression garments. Seamless, circular-knitted garments (in standard sizes) can be used to prevent swelling if the lymphoedema is well controlled and if the limb is in good shape and without skin folds. Flat-knitted garments (usually made-to-measure) with a seam, provide greater rigidity and stiffness to maintain reduction of lymphoedema following treatment with compression bandages.

A standard range of light, medium, or high compression garments are available, as well as low compression (12–16 mmHg) armsleeves, made-to-measure garments up to compression 90 mmHg, and accessories—see Drug Tariff for details.

Note There are different compression values for lymphoedema garments and graduated compression hosiery, see table, p. 1107.

Dental Practitioners' Formulary

List of Dental Preparations

The following list has been approved by the appropriate Secretaries of State, and the preparations therein may be prescribed by dental practitioners on form FP10D (GP14 in Scotland, WP10D in Wales).

Licensed **sugar-free** versions, where available, are preferred.

Licensed **alcohol-free** mouthwashes, where available, are preferred.

Aciclovir Cream, BP
Aciclovir Oral Suspension, BP, 200 mg/5 mL
Aciclovir Tablets, BP, 200 mg
Aciclovir Tablets, BP, 800 mg
Amoxicillin Capsules, BP
Amoxicillin Oral Powder, DPF
Amoxicillin Oral Suspension, BP
Artificial Saliva Gel, DPF
Artificial Saliva Oral Spray, DPF
Artificial Saliva Pastilles, DPF
Artificial Saliva Protective Spray, DPF
[1]Artificial Saliva Substitutes as listed below (to be prescribed only for indications approved by ACBS):
    BioXtra® Gel Mouthspray
    BioXtra® Moisturising Gel
    Glandosane®
    Saliveze®
Artificial Saliva Substitute Spray, DPF
[2]Aspirin Tablets, Dispersible, BP
Azithromycin Capsules, 250 mg, DPF
Azithromycin Oral Suspension, 200 mg/5 mL, DPF
Azithromycin Tablets, 250 mg, DPF
Azithromycin Tablets, 500 mg, DPF
Beclometasone Pressurised Inhalation, BP, 50 micrograms/metered inhalation, CFC-free, as:
    Clenil Modulite®
Benzydamine Mouthwash, BP 0.15%
Benzydamine Oromucosal Spray, BP 0.15%
Betamethasone Soluble Tablets, 500 micrograms, DPF
Carbamazepine Tablets, BP
Cefalexin Capsules, BP
Cefalexin Oral Suspension, BP
Cefalexin Tablets, BP
Cefradine Capsules, BP
Cetirizine Oral Solution, BP, 5 mg/5 mL
Cetirizine Tablets, BP, 10 mg
Chlorhexidine Gluconate Gel, BP
Chlorhexidine Mouthwash, BP
Chlorhexidine Oral Spray, DPF
Chlorphenamine Oral Solution, BP
Chlorphenamine Tablets, BP
Choline Salicylate Dental Gel, BP
Clarithromycin Oral Suspension, 125 mg/5 mL, DPF
Clarithromycin Oral Suspension, 250 mg/5 mL, DPF
Clarithromycin Tablets, BP
Clindamycin Capsules, BP

Co-amoxiclav Tablets, BP, 250/125 (amoxicillin 250 mg as trihydrate, clavulanic acid 125 mg as potassium salt)
Co-amoxiclav Oral Suspension, BP, 125/31 (amoxicillin 125 mg as trihydrate, clavulanic acid 31.25 mg as potassium salt)/5 mL
Co-amoxiclav Oral Suspension, BP, 250/62 (amoxicillin 250 mg as trihydrate, clavulanic acid 62.5 mg as potassium salt)/5 mL
Diazepam Oral Solution, BP, 2 mg/5 mL
Diazepam Tablets, BP
Diclofenac Sodium Tablets, Gastro-resistant, BP
Dihydrocodeine Tablets, BP, 30 mg
Doxycycline Tablets, Dispersible, BP
Doxycycline Capsules, BP, 100 mg
[3]Doxycycline Tablets, 20 mg, DPF
Ephedrine Nasal Drops, BP
Erythromycin Ethyl Succinate Oral Suspension, BP
Erythromycin Ethyl Succinate Tablets, BP
Erythromycin Stearate Tablets, BP
Erythromycin Tablets, Gastro-resistant, BP
Fluconazole Capsules, 50 mg, DPF
Fluconazole Oral Suspension, 50 mg/5 mL, DPF
Hydrocortisone Cream, BP, 1%
Hydrocortisone Oromucosal Tablets, BP
Hydrogen Peroxide Mouthwash, BP, 6%
Ibuprofen Oral Suspension, BP, sugar-free
Ibuprofen Tablets, BP
Lansoprazole Capsules, Gastro-resistant, BP
Lidocaine Ointment, BP, 5%
Lidocaine Spray 10%, DPF
Loratadine Syrup, 5 mg/5 mL, DPF
Loratadine Tablets, BP, 10 mg
[4]Menthol and Eucalyptus Inhalation, BP 1980
Metronidazole Oral Suspension, BP
Metronidazole Tablets, BP
Miconazole Cream, BP
Miconazole Oromucosal Gel, BP
Miconazole and Hydrocortisone Cream, BP
Miconazole and Hydrocortisone Ointment, BP
Nystatin Oral Suspension, BP
Omeprazole Capsules, Gastro-resistant, BP
Oxytetracycline Tablets, BP
[5]Paracetamol Oral Suspension, BP
Paracetamol Tablets, BP
Paracetamol Tablets, Soluble, BP
Phenoxymethylpenicillin Oral Solution, BP
Phenoxymethylpenicillin Tablets, BP
Promethazine Hydrochloride Tablets, BP
Promethazine Oral Solution, BP
Saliva Stimulating Tablets, DPF
Sodium Chloride Mouthwash, Compound, BP
Sodium Fluoride Mouthwash, BP
Sodium Fluoride Oral Drops, BP
Sodium Fluoride Tablets, BP

Dental Practitioners' Formulary

---

1. Indications approved by the ACBS are: patients suffering from dry mouth as a result of having (or having undergone) radiotherapy or sicca syndrome
2. The BP directs that when soluble aspirin tablets are prescribed, dispersible aspirin tablets should be dispensed

3. May be difficult to obtain
4. This preparation does not appear in subsequent editions of the BP
5. The BP directs that when Paediatric Paracetamol Oral Suspension or Paediatric Paracetamol Mixture is prescribed and no strength stated Paracetamol Oral Suspension 120 mg/5 mL should be dispensed

Sodium Fluoride Toothpaste 0.619%, DPF
Sodium Fluoride Toothpaste 1.1%, DPF
Sodium Fusidate Ointment, BP
Temazepam Oral Solution, BP
Temazepam Tablets, BP
Tetracycline Tablets, BP

> Preparations in this list which are not included in the
> BP or BPC are described under Details of DPF
> preparations, p. 1110.
>
> For details of preparations that can be prescribed,
> see individual entries under the relevant drug mono-
> graphs throughout the BNF.

Details of DPF preparations

Preparations on the List of Dental Preparations which
are specified as DPF are described as follows in the
DPF.

Although brand names have sometimes been included
for identification purposes preparations on the list
should be prescribed by non-proprietary name.

Amoxicillin Oral Powder [PoM]
amoxicillin (as trihydrate) 3 g sachet

Artificial Saliva Gel
(proprietary product: *Biotene Oralbalance*), lactoperoxidase, lactoferrin, lysozyme, glucose oxidase, xylitol in a gel basis

Artificial Saliva Oral Spray
(proprietary product: *Xerotin*) consists of water,
sorbitol, carmellose (carboxymethylcellulose), potassium chloride, sodium chloride, potassium phosphate, magnesium chloride, calcium chloride and
other ingredients, pH neutral

Artificial Saliva Pastilles
(proprietary product: *Salivix*), consists of acacia,
malic acid, and other ingredients

Artificial Saliva Protective Spray
(proprietary product: *Aquoral*) consists of oxidised
glycerol triesters, silicon dioxide, flavouring agents,
aspartame (section 9.4.1)

Artificial Saliva Substitute Spray
(proprietary product: *AS Saliva Orthana Spray*) consists of mucin, methylparaben, benzalkonium chloride, EDTA, xylitol, peppermint oil, spearmint oil,
mineral salts

Azithromycin Capsules [PoM]
azithromycin 250 mg

Azithromycin Oral Suspension 200 mg/5 mL [PoM]
azithromycin 200 mg/5 mL when reconstituted with
water

Azithromycin Tablets [PoM]
azithromycin 250 mg and 500 mg

**Betamethasone Soluble Tablets
500 micrograms** [PoM]
betamethasone (as sodium phosphate) 500 micrograms

Chlorhexidine Oral Spray
(proprietary product: *Corsodyl Oral Spray*), chlorhexidine gluconate 0.2%

Clarithromycin Oral Suspension 125 mg/5 mL [PoM]
clarithromycin 125 mg/5 mL when reconstituted
with water

Clarithromycin Oral Suspension 250 mg/5 mL [PoM]
clarithromycin 250 mg/5 mL when reconstituted
with water

Doxycycline Tablets 20 mg [PoM]
(proprietary product: *Periostat*), doxycycline (as
hyclate) 20 mg

Fluconazole Capsules 50 mg [PoM]
fluconazole 50 mg

Fluconazole Oral Suspension 50 mg/5 mL [PoM]
(proprietary product: *Diflucan*), fluconazole 50 mg/
5 mL when reconstituted with water

Lidocaine Spray 10%
(proprietary product: *Xylocaine Spray*), lidocaine
10% supplying 10 mg lidocaine/spray

Loratadine Syrup 5 mg/5 mL
loratadine 5 mg/5 mL

Saliva Stimulating Tablets
(proprietary product: *SST*), citric acid, malic acid
and other ingredients in a sorbitol base

Sodium Fluoride Toothpaste 0.619% [PoM]
(proprietary product: *Duraphat '2800 ppm' Toothpaste*), sodium fluoride 0.619%

Sodium Fluoride Toothpaste 1.1% [PoM]
(proprietary product: *Duraphat '5000 ppm' Toothpaste*), sodium fluoride 1.1%

Changes to Dental Practitioners' Formulary since September 2014

Additions

Artificial Saliva Substitute Spray, DPF

Deletions

Penciclovir Cream, DPF

Changes of title

None

Dental Practitioners' Formulary

Nurse Prescribers' Formulary

Nurse Prescribers' Formulary for Community Practitioners

Nurse Prescribers' Formulary Appendix (Appendix NPF). List of preparations approved by the Secretary of State which may be prescribed on form FP10P (form HS21(N) in Northern Ireland, form GP10(N) in Scotland, forms WP10CN and WP10PN in Wales) by Nurses for National Health Service patients.

Community practitioners who have completed the necessary training may only prescribe items appearing in the nurse prescribers' list set out below. Community Practitioner Nurse Prescribers are recommended to prescribe generically, except where this would not be clinically appropriate or where there is no approved generic name.

Medicinal Preparations

> Preparations on this list which are not included in the BP or BPC are described on p. 1112

Almond Oil Ear Drops, BP
Arachis Oil Enema, NPF
[1]Aspirin Tablets, Dispersible, 300 mg, BP
Bisacodyl Suppositories, BP (includes 5-mg and 10-mg strengths)
Bisacodyl Tablets, BP
Catheter Maintenance Solution, Sodium Chloride, NPF
Catheter Maintenance Solution, 'Solution G', NPF
Catheter Maintenance Solution, 'Solution R', NPF
Chlorhexidine Gluconate Alcoholic Solutions containing at least 0.05%
Chlorhexidine Gluconate Aqueous Solutions containing at least 0.05%
Choline Salicylate Dental Gel, BP
Clotrimazole Cream 1%, BP
Co-danthramer Capsules, NPF
Co-danthramer Capsules, Strong, NPF
Co-danthramer Oral Suspension, NPF
Co-danthramer Oral Suspension, Strong, NPF
Co-danthrusate Capsules, BP
Co-danthrusate Oral Suspension, NPF
Crotamiton Cream, BP
Crotamiton Lotion, BP
Dimeticone barrier creams containing at least 10%
Dimeticone Lotion, NPF
Docusate Capsules, BP
Docusate Enema, NPF
Docusate Oral Solution, BP
Docusate Oral Solution, Paediatric, BP
Econazole Cream 1%, BP
Emollients as listed below:
  Aquadrate® 10% w/w Cream
  Arachis Oil, BP
  Balneum® Plus Cream
  Cetraben® Emollient Cream
  Dermamist®
  Diprobase® Cream

Diprobase® Ointment
Doublebase®
Doublebase® Dayleve Gel
E45® Cream
E45® Itch Relief Cream
Emulsifying Ointment, BP
Eucerin® Intensive 10% w/w Urea Treatment Cream
Eucerin® Intensive 10% w/w Urea Treatment Lotion
Hydromol® Cream
Hydromol® Intensive
Hydrous Ointment, BP
Lipobase®
Liquid and White Soft Paraffin Ointment, NPF
Neutrogena® Norwegian Formula Dermatological Cream
Nutraplus® Cream
Oilatum® Cream
Oilatum® Junior Cream
Paraffin, White Soft, BP
Paraffin, Yellow Soft, BP
Ultrabase®
Unguentum M®
Emollient Bath and Shower Preparations as listed below:
  Aqueous Cream, BP
  [2]Balneum®
  [2]Balneum Plus® Bath Oil
  Cetraben® Emollient Bath Additive
  Dermalo® Bath Emollient
  Doublebase® Emollient Bath Additive
  Doublebase® Emollient Shower Gel
  Doublebase® Emollient Wash Gel
  Hydromol® Bath and Shower Emollient
  Oilatum® Emollient
  Oilatum® Gel
  Oilatum® Junior Bath Additive
  Zerolatum® Emollient Medicinal Bath Oil
Folic Acid Tablets 400 micrograms, BP
Glycerol Suppositories, BP
[3]Ibuprofen Oral Suspension, BP
[3]Ibuprofen Tablets, BP
Ispaghula Husk Granules, BP
Ispaghula Husk Granules, Effervescent, BP
Ispaghula Husk Oral Powder, BP
Lactulose Solution, BP
Lidocaine Ointment, BP
Lidocaine and Chlorhexidine Gel, BP
Macrogol Oral Liquid, Compound, NPF
Macrogol Oral Powder, Compound, NPF
Macrogol Oral Powder, Compound, Half-strength, NPF
Magnesium Hydroxide Mixture, BP
Magnesium Sulfate Paste, BP
Malathion aqueous lotions containing at least 0.5%
Mebendazole Oral Suspension, NPF
Mebendazole Tablets, NPF
Methylcellulose Tablets, BP

---

1. Max. 96 tablets; max. pack size 32 tablets
2. Except pack sizes that are not to be prescribed under the NHS (see Part XVIIIA of the Drug Tariff, Part XI of the Northern Ireland Drug Tariff)
3. Except for indications and doses that are PoM

Miconazole Cream 2%, BP
Miconazole Oromucosal Gel, BP
Mouthwash Solution-tablets, NPF
Nicotine Inhalation Cartridge for Oromucosal Use, NPF
Nicotine Lozenge, NPF
Nicotine Medicated Chewing Gum, NPF
Nicotine Nasal Spray, NPF
Nicotine Oral Spray, NPF
Nicotine Sublingual Tablets, NPF
Nicotine Transdermal Patches, NPF
Nystatin Oral Suspension, BP
Olive Oil Ear Drops, BP
Paracetamol Oral Suspension, BP (includes 120 mg/
5 mL and 250 mg/5 mL strengths—both of which are
available as sugar-free formulations)
[1]Paracetamol Tablets, BP
[1]Paracetamol Tablets, Soluble, BP (includes 120-mg
and 500-mg tablets)
Permethrin Cream, NPF
Phosphates Enema, BP
Povidone–Iodine Solution, BP
Senna Oral Solution, NPF
Senna Tablets, BP
Senna and Ispaghula Granules, NPF
Sodium Chloride Solution, Sterile, BP
Sodium Citrate Compound Enema, NPF
Sodium Picosulfate Capsules, NPF
Sodium Picosulfate Elixir, NPF
Spermicidal contraceptives as listed below:
    Gygel® Contraceptive Jelly
Sterculia Granules, NPF
Sterculia and Frangula Granules, NPF
Titanium Ointment, BP
Water for Injections, BP
Zinc and Castor Oil Ointment, BP
Zinc Oxide and Dimeticone Spray, NPF
Zinc Oxide Impregnated Medicated Bandage, NPF
Zinc Oxide Impregnated Medicated Stocking, NPF
Zinc Paste Bandage, BP 1993
Zinc Paste and Ichthammol Bandage, BP 1993

Appliances and Reagents (including Wound Management Products)

Community Practitioner Nurse Prescribers in England, Wales and Northern Ireland can prescribe any appliance or reagent in the relevant Drug Tariff. In the Scottish Drug Tariff, Appliances and Reagents which may **not** be prescribed by Nurses are annotated **Nx**.

Appliances (including Contraceptive Devices[2]) as listed in Part IXA of the Drug Tariff (Part III of the Northern Ireland Drug Tariff, Part 3 (Appliances) and Part 2 (Dressings) of the Scottish Drug Tariff)

Incontinence Appliances as listed in Part IXB of the Drug Tariff (Part III of the Northern Ireland Drug Tariff, Part 5 of the Scottish Drug Tariff)

Stoma Appliances and Associated Products as listed in Part IXC of the Drug Tariff (Part III of the Northern Ireland Drug Tariff, Part 6 of the Scottish Drug Tariff)

1. Max. 96 tablets; max. pack size 32 tablets
2. Nurse Prescribers in Family Planning Clinics—where it is not appropriate for nurse prescribers in family planning clinics to prescribe contraceptive devices using form FP10(P) (forms WP10CN and WP10PN in Wales), they may prescribe using the same system as doctors in the clinic

Chemical Reagents as listed in Part IXR of the Drug Tariff (Part II of the Northern Ireland Drug Tariff, Part 9 of the Scottish Drug Tariff)

> The Drug Tariffs can be accessed online at:
> National Health Service Drug Tariff for England and Wales: www.ppa.org.uk/ppa/edt_intro.htm
> Health and Personal Social Services for Northern Ireland Drug Tariff: www.dhsspsni.gov.uk/pas-tariff
> Scottish Drug Tariff: www.isdscotland.org/Health-topics/Prescribing-and-Medicines/Scottish-Drug-Tariff/

Details of NPF preparations

Preparations on the Nurse Prescribers' Formulary which are not included in the BP or BPC are described as follows in the Nurse Prescribers' Formulary.

Although brand names have sometimes been included for identification purposes, it is recommended that non-proprietary names should be used for prescribing medicinal preparations in the NPF except where a non-proprietary name is not available.

Arachis Oil Enema
arachis oil 100%

Catheter Maintenance Solution, Sodium Chloride
(proprietary products: *OptiFlo S*; *Uro-Tainer Sodium Chloride*; *Uriflex-S*), sodium chloride 0.9%

Catheter Maintenance Solution, 'Solution G'
(proprietary products: *OptiFlo G*; *Uro-Tainer Suby G*; *Uriflex G*), citric acid 3.23%, magnesium oxide 0.38%, sodium bicarbonate 0.7%, disodium edetate 0.01%

Catheter Maintenance Solution, 'Solution R'
(proprietary products: *OptiFlo R*; *Uro-Tainer Solution R*; *Uriflex R*), citric acid 6%, gluconolactone 0.6%, magnesium carbonate 2.8%, disodium edetate 0.01%

Chlorhexidine gluconate alcoholic solutions
(proprietary products: *ChloraPrep*; *Hydrex Solution*; *Hydrex spray*), chlorhexidine gluconate in alcoholic solution

Chlorhexidine gluconate aqueous solutions
(proprietary product: *Unisept*) chlorhexidine gluconate in aqueous solution

Co-danthramer Capsules (PoM)
co-danthramer 25/200 (dantron 25 mg, poloxamer '188' 200 mg)

Co-danthramer Capsules, Strong (PoM)
co-danthramer 37.5/500 (dantron 37.5 mg, poloxamer '188' 500 mg)

Co-danthramer Oral Suspension (PoM)
(proprietary product: *Codalax*), co-danthramer 25/200 in 5 mL (dantron 25 mg, poloxamer '188' 200 mg/5 mL)

Co-danthramer Oral Suspension, Strong (PoM)
(proprietary product: *Codalax Forte*), co-danthramer 75/1000 in 5 mL (dantron 75 mg, poloxamer '188' 1 g/5 mL)

Co-danthrusate Oral Suspension (PoM)
(proprietary product: *Normax*), co-danthrusate 50/60 (dantron 50 mg, docusate sodium 60 mg/5 mL)

Dimeticone barrier creams
(proprietary products: *Conotrane Cream*, dimeticone '350' 22%; *Siopel Barrier Cream*, dimeticone '1000' 10%), dimeticone 10–22%

Dimeticone Lotion
(proprietary product: *Hedrin*), dimeticone 4%

Docusate Enema
(proprietary product: *Norgalax Micro-enema*) docusate sodium 120 mg in 10 g

Liquid and White Soft Paraffin Ointment
liquid paraffin 50%, white soft paraffin 50%

Macrogol Oral Liquid, Compound
(proprietary product: *Movicol Liquid*), macrogol '3350' (polyethylene glycol '3350') 13.125 g, sodium bicarbonate 178.5 mg, sodium chloride 350.7 mg, potassium chloride 46.6 mg/25 mL

Macrogol Oral Powder, Compound
(proprietary products: *Laxido Orange, Molaxole, Movicol*) macrogol '3350' (polyethylene glycol '3350') 13.125 g, sodium bicarbonate 178.5 mg, sodium chloride 350.7 mg, potassium chloride 46.6 mg/sachet
Note Amount of potassium chloride varies according to flavour of *Movicol*® as follows: plain-flavour (sugar-free) = 50.2 mg/sachet; lime and lemon flavour = 46.6 mg/sachet; chocolate flavour = 31.7 mg/sachet. 1 sachet when reconstituted with 125 mL water provides K⁺ 5.4 mmol/litre

Macrogol Oral Powder, Compound, Half-strength
(proprietary product: *Movicol-Half*), macrogol '3350' (polyethylene glycol '3350') 6.563 g, sodium bicarbonate 89.3 g, sodium chloride 175.4 mg, potassium chloride 23.3 mg/sachet

Malathion aqueous lotions
(proprietary products: *Derbac-M Liquid*), malathion 0.5% in an aqueous basis

Mebendazole Oral Suspension (PoM)
(proprietary product: *Vermox*), mebendazole 100 mg/5 mL

¹Mebendazole Tablets (PoM)
(proprietary products: *Ovex, Vermox*), mebendazole 100 mg

Mouthwash Solution-tablets
consist of tablets which may contain antimicrobial, colouring and flavouring agents in a suitable soluble effervescent basis to make a mouthwash

²Nicotine Inhalation Cartridge for Oromucosal Use
(proprietary products: *NicAssist Inhalator, Nicorette Inhalator*), nicotine 10 mg or 15 mg

Nicotine Lozenge
nicotine (as bitartrate) 1 mg or 2 mg (proprietary product: *Nicorette Mint Lozenge, Nicotinell Mint Lozenge*), or nicotine (as resinate) 1.5 mg, 2mg, or 4 mg (proprietary product: *NiQuitin Lozenges, NiQuitin Minis, NiQuitin Pre-quit*)

Nicotine Medicated Chewing Gum
(proprietary products: *NicAssist Gum, Nicorette Gum, Nicotinell Gum, NiQuitin Gum*), nicotine 2 mg or 4 mg

Nicotine Nasal Spray
(proprietary product: *NicAssist Nasal Spray, Nicorette Nasal Spray*), nicotine 500 micrograms/metered spray

Nicotine Oral Spray
(proprietary product: *Nicorette Quickmist*), nicotine 1 mg/metered spray

³Nicotine Sublingual Tablets
(proprietary product: *NicAssist Microtab, Nicorette Microtab*), nicotine (as a cyclodextrin complex) 2 mg

⁴Nicotine Transdermal Patches
releasing in each 16 hours, nicotine approx. 5 mg, 10 mg, or 15 mg (proprietary products: *Boots NicAssist Patch, Nicorette Patch*) or releasing in each 16 hours approx. 10 mg, 15 mg, or 25 mg (proprietary products: *NicAssist Translucent Patch, Nicorette Invisi Patch*), or releasing in each 24 hours nicotine approx. 7 mg, 14 mg, or 21 mg (proprietary products: *Nicopatch, Nicotinell TTS, NiQuitin, NiQuitin Clear*)

Permethrin Cream
(proprietary product: *Lyclear Dermal Cream*), permethrin 5%

Senna Oral Solution
(proprietary product: *Senokot Syrup*), sennosides 7.5 mg/5 mL

Senna and Ispaghula Granules
(proprietary product: *Manevac Granules*), senna fruit 12.4%, ispaghula 54.2%

Sodium Citrate Compound Enema
(proprietary products: *Micolette Micro-enema; Micralax Micro-enema, Relaxit Micro-enema*), sodium citrate 450 mg with glycerol, sorbitol and an anionic surfactant

Sodium Picosulfate Capsules
(proprietary products: *Dulcolax Perles*), sodium picosulfate 2.5 mg

Sodium Picosulfate Elixir
(proprietary products: *Dulcolax Liquid*), sodium picosulfate 5 mg/5 mL

Sterculia Granules
(proprietary product: *Normacol Granules*), sterculia 62%

Sterculia and Frangula Granules
(proprietary product: *Normacol Plus Granules*), sterculia 62%, frangula (standardised) 8%

Zinc Oxide and Dimeticone Spray
(proprietary product: *Sprilon*), dimeticone 1.04%, zinc oxide 12.5% in a pressurised aerosol unit

Zinc Oxide Impregnated Medicated Bandage
(proprietary product: *Steripaste*), sterile cotton bandage impregnated with paste containing zinc oxide 15%

Zinc Oxide Impregnated Medicated Stocking
(proprietary product: *Zipzoc*), sterile rayon stocking impregnated with ointment containing zinc oxide 20%

---

1. For (PoM) exemption, see p. 461
2. For use with inhalation mouthpiece; to be prescribed as either a starter pack (6 cartridges with inhalator device and holder) or refill pack (42 cartridges with inhalator device)

3. To be prescribed as either a starter pack (2 x 15-tablet discs with dispenser) or refill pack (7 x 15-tablet discs)
4. Prescriber should specify the brand to be dispensed

Nurse Prescribers' Formulary

Non-medical prescribing

A range of non-medical healthcare professionals can prescribe medicines for patients as either Independent or Supplementary Prescribers.

Independent prescribers are practitioners responsible and accountable for the assessment of patients with previously undiagnosed or diagnosed conditions and for decisions about the clinical management required, including prescribing. They are recommended to prescribe generically, except where this would not be clinically appropriate or where there is no approved non-proprietary name.

Supplementary prescribing is a partnership between an independent prescriber (a doctor or a dentist) and a supplementary prescriber to implement an agreed Clinical Management Plan for an individual patient with that patient's agreement.

Independent and Supplementary Prescribers are identified by an annotation next to their name in the relevant professional register.

Information and guidance on non-medical prescribing is available on the Department of Health website at www.dh.gov.uk/health/2012/04/prescribing-change.

For information on the mixing of medicines by Independent and Supplementary Prescribers, see *Mixing of medicines prior to administration in clinical practice—responding to legislative changes*, National Prescribing Centre, May 2010 (available at www.npc.nhs.uk/improving_safety/mixing_meds/resources/mixing_of_medicines.pdf).

For information on the supply and administration of medicines to groups of patients using Patient Group Directions, see p. 4.

Nurses

Nurse Independent Prescribers (formerly known as Extended Formulary Nurse Prescribers) are able to prescribe any medicine for any medical condition.

Nurse Independent Prescribers are able to prescribe, administer, and give directions for the administration of Schedule 2, 3, 4, and 5 Controlled Drugs. This extends to diamorphine, dipipanone, or cocaine for treating organic disease or injury, but not for treating addiction.

Nurse Independent Prescribers must work within their own level of professional competence and expertise.

For information on prescribing from the Nurse Prescribers' Formulary for Community Practitioners, see Nurse Prescribers' Formulary for Community Practitioners p. 1111

Pharmacists

Pharmacist Independent Prescribers can prescribe any medicine for any medical condition.

They are also able to prescribe, administer, and give directions for the administration of Schedule 2, 3, 4, and 5 Controlled Drugs. This extends to diamorphine, dipipanone, or cocaine for treating organic disease or injury, but not for treating addiction.

Pharmacist Independent Prescribers must work within their own level of professional competence and expertise.

Optometrists

Optometrist Independent Prescribers can prescribe any licensed medicine for ocular conditions affecting the eye and the tissues surrounding the eye, except Controlled Drugs or medicines for parenteral administration. Optometrist Independent Prescribers must work within their own level of professional competence and expertise.

Index of manufacturers

The following is an alphabetical list of manufacturers and other companies referenced in the BNF, with their medicines information or general contact details. For information on 'special-order' manufacturers and specialist importing companies see p. 1124.

3M
3M Health Care Ltd
Tel: (01509) 611 611

A&H
Allen & Hanburys Ltd
 See GSK

A1 Pharmaceuticals
A1 Pharmaceuticals Plc
Tel: (01708) 528 900
sales@a1plc.co.uk

Abbott
(01628) 773 355

Abbott Healthcare
Abbott Healthcare Products Ltd
Tel: (01628) 773 355
medinfo.shl@abbott.com

AbbVie
AbbVie Ltd
Tel: (01628) 561 090
ukmedinfo@abbvie.com

Abraxis
Abraxis BioScience Ltd
Tel: (020) 7081 0850
abraxismedical@idispharma.com

Acorus
Acorus Therapeutics Ltd
Tel: (01244) 625 152

Actavis
Actavis UK Ltd
Tel: (01271) 311 257
medinfo@actavis.co.uk

Actelion
Actelion Pharmaceuticals UK Ltd
Tel: (020) 8987 3333
medinfo_uk@actelion.com

Activa
Activa Healthcare
Tel: 0845 060 6707
advice@activahealthcare.co.uk

Adienne
Adienne Pharma and Biotech
Tel: 0039 (0) 335 873 8731

ADI Medical
ADI Medical UK
Tel: (01628) 485159
info@adimedical.co.uk

Advanced Medical Solutions
Advanced Medical Solutions Group Plc
Tel: (01606) 863 500

Advancis
Advancis Medical Ltd
Tel: (01623) 751 500
info@advancis.co.uk

Advantech Surgical
Advantech Surgical Ltd
Tel: 0845 130 5866
customerservice@newgel.co.uk

Aegerion
Aegerion Pharmaceuticals Ltd
Tel: 00800 2343 7466
medinfo.emea@aegerion.com

AgaMatrix
AgaMatrix Europe Ltd
Tel: (01235) 838 639
info@wavesense.co.uk

Agepha
Agepha GmbH
Tel: (020) 3239 6241
uk@agepha.com

Aguettant
Aguettant Ltd
Tel: (01934) 835 694
info@aguettant.co.uk

Air Products
Air Products plc
Tel: 0800 373 580

Alan Pharmaceuticals
Alan Pharmaceuticals
Tel: (020) 7284 2887
info@alanpharmaceuticals.com

Alcon
Alcon Laboratories (UK) Ltd
Tel: 0345 266 9363
gbmedicaldepartment@alcon.com

Alexion
Alexion Pharma UK Ltd
Tel: (01932) 359 220
alexion.uk@alxn.com

Alimera
Alimera Sciences Limited
Tel: 0800 019 1253
medicalinformation@alimerasciences.com

Alissa
Alissa Healthcare
Tel: (01489) 780 759
enquiries@alissahealthcare.com

ALK-Abelló
ALK-Abelló (UK) Ltd
Tel: (0118) 903 7940
info@uk.alk-abello.com

Alkopharma
Alkopharma Sarl
Tel: (0041) 277 206 969
regulatory@alkopharma.com

Allergan
Allergan Ltd
Tel: (01628) 494 026

Allergy
Allergy Therapeutics Ltd
Tel: (01903) 844 702

Alliance
Alliance Pharmaceuticals Ltd
Tel: (01249) 466 966
info@alliancepharma.co.uk

Almirall
Almirall Ltd
Tel: 0800 008 7399
medinfouk@almirall.com

Altacor
Altacor Ltd
Tel: (01223) 421 411
info@altacor-pharma.com

AMCo
Amdipharm Mercury Company Ltd
Tel: 08700 70 30 33
medicalinformation@amcolimited.com

Amgen
Amgen Ltd
Tel: (01223) 420 305
gbinfoline@amgen.com

AMO
Abbot Medical Optics
Tel: 0800 376 7950

Amred
Amred Healthcare Ltd
Tel: (0330) 333 0079
info@amredhealthcare.com

Apollo Medical
Apollo Medical Technologies Ltd
Tel: (01636) 831 201
supercheck2@btinternet.com

Archimed
Archimed
Tel: 0800 756 9951
enquiries@archimed.co.uk

Archimedes
Archimedes Pharma UK Ltd
Tel: (0118) 931 5094
medicalinformationuk@archimede-spharma.com

Arctic Medical
Arctic Medical Ltd
Tel: (01303) 277 751
sales@arcticmedical.co.uk

Ardana
Ardana Bioscience Ltd
Tel: (0131) 226 8550

ARIAD
ARIAD Pharma UK Ltd
Tel: 0800 0002 7423
eumedinfo@ariad.com

Ark Therapeutics
Ark Therapeutics Group Plc
Tel: (020) 7388 7722
info@arktherapeutics.com

Aspen
Aspen
Tel: 0800 008 7392
aspenmedinfo@professionalinformation.co.uk

Aspen Medical
Aspen Medical Europe Ltd
Tel: (01527) 587 728
customers@aspenmedicaleurope.com

AS Pharma
AS Pharma Ltd
Tel: 0870 066 4117
info@aspharma.co.uk

Aspire
Aspire Pharma Ltd
Tel: (01730) 231 148
info@aspirepharma.co.uk

Astellas
Astellas Pharma Ltd
Tel: (020) 3379 8000
medinfo.gb@astellas.com

AstraZeneca
AstraZeneca UK Ltd
Tel: 0800 783 0033
medical.informationuk@astrazeneca.com

Auden Mckenzie
Auden Mckenzie (Pharma Division) Ltd
Tel: (01895) 627 420

Auxilium
Auxilium
Tel: 0845 017 2315
auxilium@pilglobal.com

Axcan
Axcan Pharma SA
Tel: (0033) 130 461 900

AYMES
AYMES International Ltd
Tel: 0845 6805 496
info@aymes.com

Ayrton Saunders
Ayrton Saunders Ltd
Tel: (0151) 709 2074
info@ayrtons.com

BAP
BAP Medical UK Ltd
Tel: 0844 879 7689

Bard
Bard Ltd
Tel: (01293) 527 888

Basilea
Basilea Pharmaceuticals Ltd
Tel: (01483) 790 023
ukmedinfo@basilea.com

Bausch & Lomb
Bausch & Lomb UK Ltd
Tel: (01748) 828 864
medicalinformationuk@bausch.com

Baxter
Baxter Healthcare Ltd
Tel: (01635) 206 345
surecall@baxter.com

Bayer
Bayer Healthcare Pharmaceuticals
Tel: (01635) 563 000
medical.information@bayer.co.uk

Bayer Consumer Care
 See Bayer

Bayer Diabetes Care
 See Bayer

Bayer Diagnostics
 See Bayer

BBI Healthcare
BBI Healthcare
Tel: (01792) 229 333
info@bbihealthcare.com

B. Braun
B. Braun Medical Ltd
Tel: (0114) 225 9000
info.bbmuk@bbraun.com

Beacon
Beacon Pharmaceuticals Ltd
Tel: (01892) 600 930
info@beaconpharma.co.uk

Beiersdorf
Beiersdorf UK Ltd
Tel: (0121) 329 8800

Besins
Besins Healthcare (UK) Ltd
Tel: (01748) 828 789
information@besins-healthcare.com

BHR
BHR Pharmaceuticals Ltd
Tel: (024) 7637 7210
info@bhr.co.uk

Biogen
Biogen Idec Ltd
Tel: 0800 008 7401

Biolitec
Biolitec Pharma Ltd
Tel: (00353) 1463 7415

BioMarin
BioMarin Europe Ltd
Tel: (020) 7420 0800
biomarin-europe@bmrn.com

BioMonde
BioMonde
Tel: 0845 230 1810
info@biomonde.com

Biotest UK
Biotest (UK) Ltd
Tel: (0121) 733 3393
medicinesinformation@biotestuk.com

Blackwell
Blackwell Supplies Ltd
Tel: (01634) 877 620

BOC
BOC Medical
Tel: 0800 111 333

Boehringer Ingelheim
Boehringer Ingelheim Ltd
Tel: (01344) 424 600
medinfo@bra.boehringer-ingelheim.com

Boots
The Boots Company PLC
Tel: (0115) 959 5165

BPC 100
BPC 100 Ltd
Tel: 01942 852085

BPL
Bio Products Laboratory Ltd
Tel: (020) 8957 2255
medinfo@bpl.co.uk

Bray
Bray Healthcare
Tel: (01367) 240 736
info@bray-healthcare.com

Bristol-Myers Squibb
Bristol-Myers Squibb Pharmaceuticals Ltd
Tel: (01895) 523 000
medical.information@bms.com

Britannia
Britannia Pharmaceuticals
Tel: 0870 851 0207
enquiries@medinformation.co.uk

BSN Medical
BSN Medical Ltd
Tel: 0845 122 3600

BTG
BTG International Ltd
Tel: (0207) 575 0000
medical.services@btgplc.com

Bullen
Bullen Healthcare
Tel: 0800 269 327

Cambridge Medical Aesthetics
Cambridge Medical Aesthetics Ltd
Tel: (01733) 396171
info@cambridgemedicalaesthetics.com

Cambridge Sensors
Cambridge Sensors Ltd
Tel: (01480) 482 920
sales-orders@cs-limited.co.uk

CareFusion
CareFusion UK 244 Ltd
Tel: 0800 043 7546
enquiries@chloraprep.co.uk

Casen-Fleet
Casen-Fleet
Tel: (0034) 913 518 800

C D Medical
C D Medical Ltd
Tel: (01942) 816 184

Celgene
Celgene Ltd
Tel: 0844 801 0045
medinfo.uk.ire@celgene.com

Chanelle Medical
Chanelle Medical UK Ltd
Tel: (01233) 822 297

Chattem UK
Chattem UK Ltd
Tel: (01256) 844 144

Chefaro UK
Chefaro UK Ltd
Tel: (01748) 828 860
info@omegapharma.co.uk

Chemidex
Chemidex Pharma Ltd
Tel: (01784) 477 167
info@chemidex.co.uk

Chiesi
Chiesi Ltd
Tel: (0161) 488 5555
medinfo.uk@chiesi.com

CHS
Cambridge Healthcare Supplies Ltd
Tel: (01953) 607 856
customerservices@cambridge-health-care.co.uk

Chugai
Chugai Pharma UK Ltd
Tel: (020) 8987 5680

Clement Clarke
Clement Clarke International Ltd
Tel: (01279) 414 969
resp@clement-clarke.com

Clinigen
Clinigen Group Plc
Tel: (01748) 828 375
clinigeneu@professionalinformation.
co.uk

CliniMed
CliniMed Ltd
Tel: (01628) 535 250

Clinisupplies
Clinisupplies Ltd
Tel: (020) 8863 4168
info@clinisupplies.co.uk

Colgate-Palmolive
Colgate-Palmolive Ltd
Tel: (01483) 302 222

Coloplast
Coloplast Ltd
Tel: (01733) 392 000

Community
Community Foods Ltd
Tel: (020) 8450 9411
email@communityfoods.co.uk

Complan Foods
Complan Foods Ltd
Tel: (020) 7395 7565

Consilient
Consilient Health UK Ltd
Tel: (020) 8956 2310
drugsafety@consilienthealth.com

ConvaTec
ConvaTec Ltd
Tel: (01895) 628 400

Co-Pharma
Co-Pharma Ltd
Tel: 0870 851 0207

Correvio
Correvio GmbH
Tel: (020) 3002 8114
info@correvio.com

Covidien
Covidien UK Commercial Ltd
Tel: (01329) 224 226

Cow & Gate
Cow & Gate
Tel: 0845 762 3624

Cranage
Cranage Healthcare Ltd
Tel: (01477) 549 392
db@cranagehealth.com

Crawford
Crawford Healthcare Ltd
Tel: (01565) 654 920

Crescent
Crescent Pharma
Tel: (01256) 772 730
info@crescentpharma.com

Crucell
Crucell (UK) Ltd
Tel: 0844 800 3907
info@crucell.co.uk

CSL Behring
CSL Behring UK Ltd
Tel: (01444) 447 400
medinfo@cslbehring.com

CTI
CTI Life Sciences Ltd
Tel: (01628) 643 974

Daiichi Sankyo
Daiichi Sankyo UK Ltd
Tel: (01753) 482 771
medinfo@daiichi-sankyo.co.uk

Danetre
Danetre Health Products Ltd
Tel: (01327) 310 909
enquiries@danetrehealthproducts.com

DDD
DDD Ltd
Tel: (01923) 229 251

Dee
Dee Pharmaceuticals Ltd
Tel: (01978) 661993
enquiries@deepharmaceuticalsltd.co.
uk

Dental Health
Dental Health Products Ltd
Tel: (01622) 749 222

Dentsply
Dentsply Ltd
Tel: (01932) 837 279

Dermal
Dermal Laboratories Ltd
Tel: (01462) 458 866

Dermato Logical
Dermato Logical Ltd
Tel: (0208) 449 2931
enquiries@aqua-max.co.uk

Dermatonics
Dermatonics Ltd
Tel: (01480) 462 910
sales@dermatonics.co.uk

Derma Sciences Europe
Derma Sciences Europe Ltd
Tel: (01628) 625 916
cs@dermasciences.com

Derma UK
Derma UK Ltd
Tel: (01462) 733 500
info@dermauk.co.uk

Desitin
Desitin Pharma Ltd
Tel: (01483) 688 240
medinfo@desitin.co.uk

DeVilbiss
DeVilbiss Healthcare UK Ltd
Tel: (01384) 446 688

Dexcel
Dexcel-Pharma Ltd
Tel: (01327) 312 266
office@dexcelpharma.co.uk

DHP Healthcare
DHP Healthcare Ltd
Tel: (01622) 749 222
sales@dhphealthcare.co.uk

DiME
DiME
Tel: (01483) 715 008
info@dime-med.com

Dreamskin
Dreamskin Health Ltd
Tel: (01707) 228 688

Dr Falk
Dr Falk Pharma UK Ltd
Tel: (01628) 536 600

Drossa
Drossa Ltd
Tel: (020) 3393 0859
info@drossa.co.uk

Durbin
Durbin plc
Tel: (020) 8869 6500
info@durbin.co.uk

Eakin
T G Eakin
Tel: (028) 9187 1000
mail@eakin.co.uk

Easigrip
Easigrip Ltd
Tel: (01926) 497 108
enquiry@easigrip.co.uk

Ecolab
Ecolab UK
Tel: (0113) 232 0066
info.healthcare@ecolab.co.uk

Egis
Egis Pharmaceuticals UK Ltd
Tel: (020) 7266 2669
enquiries@medimpexuk.com

Eisai
Eisai Ltd
Tel: (020) 8600 1400
eumedinfo@eisai.net

Encysive
Encysive (UK) Ltd
Tel: (01895) 876 168

Entra Health
Entra Health Systems
Tel: (0113) 815 5108

Espere
Espere Healthcare Ltd
Tel: (01462) 346 100
info@esperehealth.co.uk

Essential
Essential Pharmaceuticals Ltd
Tel: (01784) 477 167
info@essentialpharmaceuticals.com

Ethicon
Ethicon Ltd
Tel: (01506) 594 500

Eumedica
Eumedica S.A.
Tel: (020) 8444 3377
enquiries@eumedica.com

European Pharma
European Pharma Group
Tel: 0031 (0) 20 316 0140
info@insujet.com

EUSA Pharma
EUSA Pharma (Europe) Ltd
Tel: (01438) 740 720
medinfo-uk@eusapharma.com

Fabre
Pierre Fabre Ltd
Tel: (01962) 874 435
medicalinformation@pierre-fabre.co.uk

Fate
Fate Special Foods
Tel: (01215) 224 433

Fenton
Fenton Pharmaceuticals Ltd
Tel: (020) 7224 1388
mail@fent-pharm.co.uk

Ferndale
Ferndale Pharmaceuticals Ltd
Tel: (01937) 541 122
info@ferndalepharma.co.uk

Ferring
Ferring Pharmaceuticals (UK)
Tel: 0844 931 0050
medical@ferring.com

Firstplay Dietary
Firstplay Dietary Foods Ltd
Tel: (0161) 474 7576

Flynn
Flynn Pharma Ltd
Tel: (01438) 727 822
medinfo@flynnpharma.com

Focus
Focus Pharmaceuticals Ltd
Tel: (01283) 495 280
medinfo@focuspharma.co.uk

Foodlink
Foodlink (UK) Ltd
Tel: (01752) 344 544
info@foodlinkltd.co.uk

Ford
Ford Medical Associates Ltd
Tel: (01233) 633 224
enquiries@fordmedical.co.uk

Forest
Forest Laboratories UK Ltd
Tel: (01322) 421 800
medinfo@forest-labs.co.uk

Forum
Forum Health Products Ltd
Tel: (01737) 857 700
enquiries@forumgroup.co.uk

Fox
C. H. Fox Ltd
Tel: (020) 7240 3111

Fresenius Biotech
Fresenius Biotech GmbH
Tel: 0049 (0) 893 065 9311
med.info@fresenius-biotech.com

Fresenius Kabi
Fresenius Kabi Ltd
Tel: (01928) 533 533
med.info-uk@fresenius-kabi.com

Fresenius Medical Care
Fresenius Medical Care UK Ltd
Tel: (01623) 445 171
medinfo-uk@fmc-ag.com

Frontier
Frontier Multigate
Tel: (01495) 233 050
multigate@frontier-group.co.uk

Fyne Dynamics
Fyne Dynamics Ltd
Tel: (01279) 423 423
info@fyne-dynamics.com

Galderma
Galderma (UK) Ltd
Tel: (01923) 208 950
medinfo.uk@galderma.com

Galen
Galen Ltd
Tel: (028) 3833 4974
customer.services@galen.co.uk

Gedeon Richter
Gedeon Richter UK Ltd
Tel: (020) 7604 8806
drugsafety.uk@gedeonrichter.eu

GE Healthcare
GE Healthcare
Tel: (01494) 544 000

Geistlich
Geistlich Pharma
Tel: (01244) 347 534

General Dietary
General Dietary Ltd
Tel: (0203) 044 2933
info@generaldietary.com

Generics
See Mylan

Genius Foods
Genius Foods Ltd
Tel: 0845 874 4000
info@geniusglutenfree.com

Genopharm
Laboratoires Genopharm
Tel: (0808) 234 2664
info@genopharm.eu

Genus
Genus Pharmaceuticals
Tel: (01635) 568 400
info@genuspharma.com

Genzyme
Genzyme Therapeutics
Tel: (01865) 405 200
ukmedinfo@genzyme.com

GFF Trade
GF Foods Ltd
Tel: (01757) 289 207
admin@gffdirect.co.uk

Gilead
Gilead Sciences Ltd
Tel: (01223) 897 555
ukmedinfo@gilead.com

Glenwood
Glenwood GmbH
Tel: (0049) 815 199 8790
info@glenwood.de

GlucoRx
GlucoRx Ltd
Tel: (01483) 755 133
info@glucorx.co.uk

Gluten Free Foods Ltd
Gluten Free Foods Ltd
Tel: (020) 8953 4444
info@glutenfree-foods.co.uk

Goldshield
See Mercury

GP Pharma
See Derma UK

Grifols
Grifols UK Ltd
Tel: (01223) 395 700
reception.uk@grifols.com

Grünenthal
Grünenthal Ltd
Tel: 0870 351 8960
medicalinformationuk@grunenthal.
com

GSK
GlaxoSmithKline
Tel: 0800 221 441
customercontactuk@gsk.com

GSK Consumer Healthcare
GlaxoSmithKline Consumer Healthcare
Tel: (020) 8047 2500
customer.relations@gsk.com

H&R
H&R Healthcare Ltd
Tel: (01482) 631 606
info@hrhealthcare.co.uk

Hartmann
Paul Hartmann Ltd
Tel: (01706) 363 200
info@uk.hartmann.info

Henleys
Henleys Medical Supplies Ltd
Tel: (01707) 333 164

Hennig Arzneimittel
Hennig Arzneimittel GmbH & Co.
Tel: 0844 504 0866

HFA Healthcare
HFA Healthcare Ltd
Tel: 0844 335 8270

HK Pharma
HK Pharma Ltd
Tel: 0845 519 1609

Hollister
Hollister Ltd
Tel: (0118) 989 5000

Hospira
Hospira UK Ltd
Tel: (01926) 834 400
medinfouk@hospira.com

HRA Pharma
HRA Pharma UK & Ireland Ltd
Tel: 0800 917 9548
med.info.uk@hra-pharma.com

Huntleigh
Huntleigh Healthcare Ltd
Tel: (01582) 413 104

Huxley
Huxley Europe Ltd
Tel: (0161) 773 0485

Idis
Idis Ltd
Tel: (01932) 824 000
mi@idispharma.com

iMed
iMed Systems Ltd
Tel: (0203) 397 8020
emerade@imed-systems.com

INCA-Pharm
INCA-Pharm UK
Tel: (01748) 828 812
info@inca-pharm.com

Infai
Infai UK Ltd
Tel: (01904) 435 228
info@infai.co.uk

Injex UK
Injex UK Ltd
Tel: 0845 126 8900
enquiries@injexuk.com

Innovative
Innovative Solutions UK Ltd
Tel: (01706) 746 713
enquiries@innovative-solutions.org.uk

Insight
Insight Medical Products Ltd
Tel: (01666) 500 055
info@insightmedical.net

InterMune
InterMune
Tel: (03308) 080 960
med-info@intermune.co.uk

Internis
Internis Pharmaceuticals Ltd
Tel: (020) 8346 5588
regulatory@jensongroup.com

Intrapharm
Intrapharm Laboratories Ltd
Tel: (01628) 771 800
sales@intrapharmlabs.com

Ipsen
Ipsen Ltd
Tel: (01753) 627 777
medical.information.uk@ipsen.com

Iroko
Iroko Cardio GmbH
Tel: (020) 3002 8114
info@irokocardio.com

IS Pharmaceuticals
See Sinclair IS

IVAX
See TEVA UK

J&J
Johnson & Johnson Ltd
Tel: (01628) 822 222
medinfo@congb.jnj.com

Janssen
Janssen-Cilag Ltd
Tel: 0800 731 8450
medinfo@its.jnj.com

Jobskin
Jobskin Ltd
Tel: (0115) 973 4300
dw@jobskin.co.uk

Juvela
Juvela (Hero UK) Ltd
Tel: (0151) 432 5300
info@juvela.co.uk

K/L
K/L Pharmaceuticals Ltd
Tel: (01294) 215 951

KCI Medical
KCI Medical Ltd
Tel: (01865) 840 600

Kestrel Ophthalmics
Kestrel Ophthalmics Ltd
Tel: (01202) 658 444
info@kestrelophthalmics.co.uk

King
King Pharmaceuticals Ltd
Tel: (01438) 356 924

KoRa
KoRa Healthcare Ltd
Tel: 0845 303 8631
info@kora.ie

Labopharm
Labopharm Europe Ltd
Tel: 0800 028 0037
medinfo@paladin-labs.com

LaCorium
LaCorium Health (UK) Ltd
Tel: 0800 158 8233
ukinfo@flexitol.com

Lantor
Lantor UK Ltd
Tel: (01204) 855 000
help@lantor.co.uk

LEO
LEO Laboratories Ltd
Tel: (01844) 347 333
medical-info.uk@leo-pharma.com

LifeScan
LifeScan
Tel: 0800 001 210

Lilly
Eli Lilly & Co Ltd
Tel: (01256) 315 000
ukmedinfo@lilly.com

Lincoln Medical
Lincoln Medical Ltd
Tel: (01722) 742 900
info@lincolnmedical.co.uk

Linderma
Linderma Ltd
Tel: (01942) 816 184
linderma@virgin.net

Lipomed
Lipomed GmbH
Tel: (0041) 6170 20200
save@lipomed.com

Livwell
Livwell Ltd
Tel: 0845 120 0038
info@livwell.eu

LogixX
LogixX Pharma Solutions Ltd
Tel: (01189) 011 747
medinfo@logixxpharma.com

Lornamead
Lornamead UK Ltd
Tel: (01276) 674000
lornamead@dhl.com

LPC
LPC Pharmaceuticals Ltd
Tel: (01582) 560 393
info@lpcpharma.com

Lucane
Lucane Pharma
Tel: 0033 (0) 153 868 750
info@lucanepharma.com

Lundbeck
Lundbeck Ltd
Tel: (01908) 649 966
ukmedicalinformation@lundbeck.com

L'Oréal Active
L'Oréal Active Cosmetics UK
Tel: 0800 055 6822

M & A Pharmachem
M & A Pharmachem Ltd
Tel: (01942) 816 184

Manuka Medical
Manuka Medical Ltd
Tel: (01623) 600 669

Manx
Manx Healthcare
Tel: (01926) 482 511
info@manxhealthcare.com

Marlborough
Marlborough Pharmaceuticals
Tel: (01279) 406 759
info@marlborough-pharma.co.uk

Martindale
Martindale Pharma
Tel: (01277) 266 600
medinfo@martindalepharma.com

MASTA
MASTA
Tel: (0113) 238 7500
medical@masta.org

McNeil
McNeil Products Ltd
Tel: (01628) 822 222

MDE
Medical Diagnostics Europe Ltd
Tel: 0845 370 8077
info@mdediagnostic.co.uk

Mead Johnson
Mead Johnson Nutritionals
Tel: (01895) 523 764

Meadow
Meadow Laboratories Ltd
Tel: (020) 8597 1203

Meda
Meda Pharmaceuticals Ltd
Tel: (01748) 828 810
meda@professionalinformation.co.uk

Medac
Medac (UK)
Tel: (01786) 458 086
info@medac-uk.co.uk

Medical Developments
Medical Developments UK Ltd
Tel: 0870 850 1234
enquiries@ashfieldin2focus.com

Medicare
Medicare Plus International Ltd
Tel: (020) 8810 8811
info@medicare-plus.com

Medicom
Medicom Healthcare Ltd
Tel: (01489) 574 119
info@medicomhealthcare.com

Medihoney
Medihoney (Europe) Ltd
Tel: 0800 071 3912

Medisana
Medisana
Tel: +49 (0) 2131/36 68 0

Medlock
Medlock Medical Ltd
Tel: (0161) 621 2100

MedLogic
MedLogic Global Ltd
Tel: (01752) 209 955
enquiries@mlgl.co.uk

Menarini
A. Menarini Farmaceutica Internazionale SRL
Tel: (01628) 856 400
menarini@medinformation.co.uk

Menarini Diagnostics
A. Menarini Diagnostics
Tel: (0118) 944 4100

Merck Serono
Merck Serono Ltd
Tel: (020) 8818 7200
medinfo.uk@merckserono.net

Merus
Merus Labs
Tel: 00352 (0) 2637 5878
qchs.mi@quintiles.com

Merz
Merz Pharma UK Ltd
Tel: (020) 8236 0000
info@merzpharma.co.uk

Micro Medical
Micro Medical Ltd
Tel: (01634) 893 500

Milupa
Milupa Aptamil
Tel: 0845 762 3676
careline@aptamil4hcps.co.uk

Mitsubishi
Mitsubishi Pharma
Tel: (0207) 382 9000
medinfo@mitsubishi-pharma.eu

Mölnlycke
Mölnlycke Health Care Ltd
Tel: (0161) 777 2628
info.uk@molnlycke.net

Moorfields
Moorfields Pharmaceuticals
Tel: (020) 7684 9090

Morningside
Morningside Healthcare Ltd
Tel: (0116) 204 5950

Movianto
Movianto UK
Tel: (01234) 248 500
movianto.uk@movianto.com

MSD
Merck Sharp & Dohme Ltd
Tel: (01992) 467 272
medicalinformationuk@merck.com

Mylan
Mylan
Tel: (01707) 853 000
info@mylan.co.uk

Nagor
Nagor Ltd
Tel: (01624) 625 556
enquiries@nagor.com

Nairns
Nairn's Oatcakes Ltd
Tel: (0131) 620 7000

Napp
Napp Pharmaceuticals Ltd
Tel: (01223) 424 444

Neoceuticals
Neoceuticals Ltd
Tel: (01748) 828 865

Neolab
Neolab Ltd
Tel: (01256) 704 110
info@neolab.co.uk

Neomedic
Neomedic Ltd
Tel: (01923) 836 379
marketing@neomedic.co.uk

Neon Diagnostics
Neon Diagnostics Ltd
Tel: (01376) 500 720

Nestlé
Nestlé Nutrition
Tel: 00800 6887 4846
nestlehealthcarenutrition@uk.nestle.
com

Newport
Newport Pharmaceuticals Ltd
Tel: (00353) 1890 3011

NIBTS
Northern Ireland Blood Transfusion
Service
Tel: (028) 9032 1414
inet@nibts.hscni.net

Nipro Diagnostics
Nipro Diagnostics (UK) Ltd
Tel: (01489) 569 469
info@homediagnostics-uk.com

Nordic
Nordic Pharma UK Ltd
Tel: (0118) 929 8233
info@nordicpharma.co.uk

Norgine
Norgine Pharmaceuticals Ltd
Tel: (01895) 826 600
medinfo@norgine.com

Nova
Nova Laboratories Ltd
Tel: 08707 120 655
xaluprine@aptivsolutions.com

Novartis
Novartis Pharmaceuticals UK Ltd
Tel: (01276) 698 370
medinfo.uk@novartis.com

Novartis Consumer Health
Novartis Consumer Health
Tel: (01276) 687 202
medicalaffairs.uk@novartis.com

Novartis Vaccines
Novartis Vaccines Ltd
Tel: 0845 745 1500
service.uk@novartis.com

Novo Nordisk
Novo Nordisk Ltd
Tel: (01293) 613 555

nSPIRE Health
nSPIRE Health Ltd
Tel: (01992) 526 300
info@nspirehealth.com

Nualtra
Nualtra Ltd
Tel: 0808 101 0926
support@nualtra.co.uk

Nutricia
Nutricia
Tel: (01225) 751 098
resourcecentre@nutricia.com

Nutrinovo
Nutrinovo Ltd
Tel: (01304) 829 068
info@nutrinovo.com

Nutrition Point
Nutrition Point Ltd
Tel: (07041) 544 044
info@nutritionpoint.co.uk

Nycomed
Nycomed UK Ltd
Tel: (01628) 646 4397
medinfo@nycomed.com

OakMed
OakMed Ltd
Tel: 0800 592 786
orders@oakmed.co.uk

Octapharma
Octapharma Ltd
Tel: (0161) 837 3770
octapharma@octapharma.co.uk

Omega Pharma
Omega Pharma
Tel: (01748) 828 860
omega@professionalinformation.co.uk

Omron
Omron Healthcare (UK) Ltd
Tel: 0870 750 2771
info.omronhealthcare.uk@eu.omron.
com

Organon
See MSD

Orion
Orion Pharma (UK) Ltd
Tel: (01635) 520 300
medicalinformation@orionpharma.
com

Orphan Europe
Orphan Europe (UK) Ltd
Tel: (01491) 414 333
infouk@orphan-europe.com

Otsuka
Otsuka Pharmaceuticals (UK) Ltd
Tel: (020) 3747 5300
ukmedinfo@otsuka.co.uk

Otsuka Novel
Otsuka Novel Products GmbH
Tel: (0049) 892 0602 0500
medical@otsuka-onpg.com

Ovation
Ovation Healthcare International Ltd
Tel: (00353) 1613 9707

Owen Mumford
Owen Mumford Ltd
Tel: (01993) 812 021
customerservices@owenmumford.co.
uk

Oxbridge
Oxbridge Pharma Ltd
Tel: (020) 8335 4110
enquiries@oxbridgepharma.com

Oxford Nutrition
Oxford Nutrition Ltd
Tel: (01626) 832 067
info@nutrinox.com

Pari
PARI Medical Ltd
Tel: (01932) 341 122
infouk@pari.de

Parkside
Parkside Healthcare
Tel: (0161) 795 2792

Peckforton
Peckforton Pharmaceuticals Ltd
Tel: (01270) 582 255
info@peckforton.com

Penn
Penn Pharmaceuticals Services Ltd
Tel: (01495) 711 222
penn@pennpharm.co.uk

Pfizer
Pfizer Ltd
Tel: (01304) 616 161
eumedinfo@pfizer.com

PGR Health Foods
PGR Health Foods Ltd
Tel: (01992) 581 715
info@pgrhealthfoods.co.uk

Pharmacia
See Pfizer

Pharmacosmos
Pharmacosmos UK Ltd
Tel: (01844) 269 007
info@vitalineuk.co.uk

Pharma Mar
See Idis

Pharma Nord
Pharma Nord (UK) Ltd
Tel: (01670) 519 989
uksales@pharmanord.co.uk

Pharmasure
Pharmasure Ltd
Tel: (01923) 233 466
info@pharmasure.co.uk

Pharmaxis
Pharmaxis Pharmaceuticals Ltd
Tel: (01628) 902 053
med.info@pharmaxis.com.au

PharSafer
PharSafer Associates Ltd
Tel: 01483 212151
medinfoenquiries@pharsafer.com

Phoenix
Phoenix Labs
Tel: (00353) 1468 8917
medicalinformation@phoenixlabs.ie

Pinewood
Pinewood Healthcare
Tel: (00353) 523 6253
info@pinewood.ie

Pinnacle
Pinnacle Biologics Inc.
Tel: 1-866-248-2039
pinnaclemedinfo@optum.com

Potters
Potters Herbal Medicines
Tel: (01942) 219 960

Proceli
Proceli
Tel: (01226) 713 044
admin@proceli.co.uk

Procter & Gamble
Procter & Gamble (Health and Beauty
Care) Ltd
Tel: (0191) 297 5000

Profile
Profile Pharma Ltd
Tel: 0800 1300 855
info@profilepharma.com

ProStrakan
ProStrakan Ltd
Tel: (01896) 664 000
medinfo@prostrakan.com

Protex
Protex Healthcare (UK) Ltd
Tel: 0870 011 4112
orders@protexhealthcare.co.uk

Qdem
Qdem
Tel: (01223) 426 929
medicalinformationukqdem@qdem.co.
uk

Ranbaxy
Ranbaxy UK Ltd
Tel: (020) 8280 1986
medinfoeurope@ranbaxy.com

Ransom
Ransom Consumer Healthcare
Tel: (01462) 437 615
info@williamransom.com

Ratiopharm UK
Ratiopharm UK Ltd
Tel: (023) 9231 3592
info@ratiopharm.co.uk

Reckitt Benckiser
Reckitt Benckiser Healthcare
Tel: (01482) 326 151
info.miu@reckittbenckiser.com

Recordati
Recordati Pharmaceuticals Ltd
Tel: (01491) 576 336
medinfo@recordati.co.uk

ReSource Medical
ReSource Medical UK Ltd
Tel: (01484) 531 489
info@resource-medical.co.uk

Respironics
Philips Respironics (UK) Ltd
Tel: 0800 130 0840
rukmarketing@respironics.com

RF Medical
RF Medical Supplies Ltd
Tel: (0151) 493 1473
enquiries@rfmedicalsupplies.co.uk

Richardson
Richardson Healthcare Ltd
Tel: 0800 170 1126
info@richardsonhealthcare.com

Riemser
Riemser Arzneimittel AG
Tel: (0049) 383 517 6679
info@riemser.de

RIS Products
RIS Products Ltd
Tel: (01438) 840 135

Robinsons
Robinson Healthcare Ltd
Tel: (01909) 735 064
enquiry@robinsonhealthcare.com

Roche
Roche Products Ltd
Tel: 0800 328 1629
medinfo.uk@roche.com

Roche Diagnostics
Roche Diagnostics Ltd
Tel: (01444) 256 000

Rosemont
Rosemont Pharmaceuticals Ltd
Tel: 0800 919 312
infodesk@rosemontpharma.com

Rowa
Rowa Pharmaceuticals Ltd
Tel: (00353) 275 0077
rowa@rowa-pharma.ie

RPH
RPH Pharmaceuticals
Tel: (01483) 212 151
medinfoenquiries@pharsafer.com

S&N Hlth.
Smith & Nephew Healthcare Ltd
Tel: (01482) 222 200
advice@smith-nephew.com

Sallis
Sallis Healthcare Ltd
Tel: (0115) 978 7841

Sandoz
Sandoz Ltd
Tel: (01276) 698 020
sandoz@professionalinformation.co.uk

Sanochemia
Sanochemia Diagnostics UK Ltd
Tel: (0117) 906 3562

Sanofi-Aventis
Sanofi-Aventis Ltd
Tel: 0845 372 7101
uk-medicalinformation@sanofi-aventis.
com

Sanofi Pasteur
Sanofi Pasteur MSD Ltd
Tel: (01628) 785 291

SanoMed
SanoMed Manufacturing bv
Tel: +32 503 93627
info@sanomed.nl

Schering-Plough
See MSD

Schuco
Schuco International Ltd
Tel: (020) 8368 1642
sales@schuco.co.uk

Schülke
Schülke UK
Tel: (0114) 254 3500
mail.uk@schuelke.com

Scope Ophthalmics
Scope Ophthamics Ltd
Tel: (01293) 897 209
info@scopeophthalmics.com

SD Biosensor
SD Biosensor, Inc.
Tel: 0082 31 300 0475
sales@sdbiosensor.com

SD Healthcare
SD Healthcare
Tel: (0161) 776 7626
sales@sdhealthcare.com

Seahorse
Seahorse Laboratories Ltd
Tel: (020) 8257 8412
info@seahorse-labs.com

Septodont
Septodont Ltd
Tel: (01622) 695 520

Servier
Servier Laboratories Ltd
Tel: (01753) 666 409
medical.information@uk.netgrs.com

Seven Seas
Seven Seas Ltd
Tel: (01482) 375 234

Shermond
Shermond
Tel: 0870 242 7701
sales@shermond.com

Shire
Shire Pharmaceuticals Ltd
Tel: 0800 055 6614
medinfouk@shire.com

Shire HGT
Shire Human Genetic Therapies
Tel: (01256) 894 000
hgtmedcomm@shire.com

SHS
SHS International Ltd
Tel: (0151) 228 8161

Siemens
Siemens Healthcare Diagnostics Ltd
Tel: 0845 600 1966
dx-diag_sales-uk.med@siemens.com

Sigma-Tau
Sigma-Tau Pharma Ltd (UK)
Tel: 0800 043 1268
medical.information@sigma-tau.co.uk

SilDerm
SilDerm Ltd
Tel: (01260) 271 666

Index of manufacturers

Sinclair IS
Sinclair IS Pharma
Tel: (01244) 625 152
enquiries@ispharma.plc.uk

Skin Camouflage Co.
The Skin Camouflage Company Ltd
Tel: (01507) 343 091
smjcovermark@aol.com

Skinnies
Skinnies UK
Tel: (01562) 546 123
info@skinniesuk.com

SLO Drinks
SLO Drinks Ltd
Tel: 0845 222 2205
info@slodrinks.com

SMA Nutrition
See Wyeth

SNBTS
Scottish National Blood Transfusion
Service
Tel: (0131) 536 5700
contact.pfc@snbts.csa.scot.nhs.uk

Sound Opinion
Sound Opinion
Tel: 0870 192 3283
enquiries@medinformation.co.uk

Speciality European
Speciality European Pharma Ltd
Tel: (020) 7421 7400
info@spepharma.com

Spectrum Thea
Spectrum Thea Pharmaceuticals
Tel: 0870 192 3283
theasupport@spectrum-thea.co.uk

SpePharm
SpePharm UK Ltd
Tel: 0844 800 7579
medinfo.uk@spepharm.com

Spirit
Spirit Healthcare Ltd
Tel: 0800 881 5423
cs@spirit-healthcare.co.uk

Squibb
See Bristol-Myers Squibb

SSL
SSL International plc
Tel: 0870 122 2690
medical.information@ssl-international.
com

Stanningley
Stanningley Pharma Ltd
Tel: (01159) 124 253
medinfo@stanningleypharma.co.uk

STD Pharmaceutical
STD Pharmaceutical Products Ltd
Tel: (01432) 373 555
enquiries@stdpharm.co.uk

Steraid
Steraid (Gainsborough) Ltd
Tel: (01427) 677 559

St George's Medical
St George's Medical
Tel: (020) 7582 1015

Stiefel
Stiefel Laboratories (UK) Ltd
Tel: (01628) 612 000

Stiletto Foods
Stiletto Foods UK Ltd
Tel: 0845 130 0869

Stragen
Stragen UK Ltd
Tel: 0870 351 8744
info@stragenuk.com

Sucampo
Sucampo Pharma
Tel: 0800 756 3416
infoeu@sucampo.com

Su-Med
Su-Med International UK Ltd
Tel: (01457) 890 980
sales@sumed.co.uk

Sunovion
Sunovion Pharmaceuticals Europe Ltd
Tel: (020) 7821 2840
medinfo@sunovion.eu

Sutherland
Sutherland Health Ltd
Tel: (01635) 874 488

Swedish Orphan
Swedish Orphan Biovitrum Ltd
Tel: (01638) 722 380
medical.info@sobi.com

Synergy Healthcare
Synergy Healthcare (UK) Ltd
Tel: (0161) 624 5641
healthcaresolutions@synergyhealthplc.
com

Syner-Med
Syner-Med (Pharmaceutical Products)
Ltd
Tel: 0845 634 2100
mail@syner-med.com

Systagenix
Systagenix Wound Management
Tel: (01344) 871 000

Takeda
Takeda UK Ltd
Tel: (01628) 537 900
medinfo@takeda.co.uk

Talley
Talley Group Ltd
Tel: (01794) 503 500

Taro
Taro Pharmaceuticals (UK) Ltd
Tel: 0870 736 9544
customerservice@taropharma.co.uk

Teoforma
Teoforma S.r.l.
serviziocclienti@teoforma.it

Teva
See TEVA UK

TEVA UK
TEVA UK Ltd
Tel: 0870 502 0304
medinfo@tevauk.com

The Medicines Company
The Medicines Company
Tel: 00800 8436 3326
medical.information@themedco.com

Therabel
Therabel Pharma UK Ltd
Tel: 0800 066 5446
info@therabel.co.uk

The Urology Co.
The Urology Company Ltd
Tel: (020) 3077 5411
info@theurologyco.com

Thomas Blake
Thomas Blake Cosmetic Creams Ltd
Tel: (01207) 279 432
sales@veilcover.com

Thornton & Ross
Thornton & Ross Ltd
Tel: (01484) 842 217

Tillomed
Tillomed Laboratories Ltd
Tel: (01480) 402 400
info@tillomed.co.uk

Tillotts
Tillotts Pharma UK Ltd
Tel: 0845 034 4476

TMC
TMC Pharma Services Ltd
Tel: (01252) 842 255
info@tmcpharma.com

Tobia Teff
Tobia Teff UK Ltd
Tel: (020) 7328 2045
info@tobiateff.co.uk

Torbet
Torbet Laboratories Ltd
Tel: (01953) 607 856
customerservices@cambridge-health-
care.co.uk

Transdermal
Transdermal Ltd
Tel: (020) 8654 2251
info@transdermal.co.uk

TRB Chemedica
TRB Chemedica (UK) Ltd
Tel: 0845 330 7556

Typharm
Typharm Ltd
Tel: (01603) 722 480
customerservices@typharm.com

UCB Pharma
UCB Pharma Ltd
Tel: (01753) 534 655
medicalinformationuk@ucb.com

Ultrapharm
Ultrapharm Ltd
Tel: (01491) 578 016

Univar
Univar Ltd
Tel: (01908) 362 200
trientine@univareurope.com

Unomedical
Unomedical Ltd
Tel: (01527) 587 700

Urgo
Urgo Ltd
Tel: (01509) 502 051
woundcare@uk.urgo.com

Vegenat
c/o Archaelis Ltd
Tel: 0870 803 2484

Vertex
Vertex Pharmaceuticals (UK) Ltd
Tel: 0800 028 2616
eumedicalinfo@vrtx.com

Vifor
Vifor Pharma UK Ltd
Tel: (01276) 853 633
medicalinfo_uk@viforpharma.com

ViiV
ViiV Healthcare UK Ltd
See GSK

Viridian
Viridian Pharma Ltd
Tel: (01633) 400 335
info@viridianpharma.co.uk

ViroPharma
ViroPharma Ltd
Tel: (020) 7572 1222

Vitaflo
Vitaflo International Ltd
Tel: (0151) 709 9020
vitaflo@vitaflo.co.uk

Vitalograph
Vitalograph Ltd
Tel: (01280) 827 110
sales@vitalograph.co.uk

Wallace Cameron
Wallace Cameron Ltd
Tel: (01698) 354 600
sales@wallacecameron.com

Wallace Mfg
Wallace Manufacturing Chemists Ltd
Tel: (01235) 538 700
info@alinter.co.uk

Warburtons
Warburtons
Tel: (01204) 513 004

Warner Chilcott
Warner Chilcott UK Ltd
Tel: (01932) 824 700

WBS
Welsh Blood Service
Tel: (01443) 622 000
donor.care@wales.nhs.uk

Wellfoods
Wellfoods Ltd
Tel: (01226) 381 712
wellfoods@wellfoods.co.uk

Williams
Williams Medical Supplies Ltd
Tel: (01685) 844 739

Wockhardt
Wockhardt UK Ltd
Tel: (01978) 661 261

Wyeth
Wyeth Pharmaceuticals
Tel: (01628) 604 377
eumedinfo@pfizer.com

Wynlit
Wynlit Laboratories
Tel: (07903) 370 130

Wyvern
Wyvern Medical Ltd
Tel: (01531) 631 105

Zentiva
Zentiva
(01483) 554 101
gb-zentivamedicalinformation@sanofi.
com

Zeroderma
Zeroderma Ltd
Tel: (01858) 525 643

Special-order Manufacturers

Unlicensed medicines are available from 'special-order' manufacturers and specialist-importing companies; the MHRA maintains a register of these companies at http://tinyurl.com/cdslke

Licensed **hospital manufacturing units** also manufacture 'special-order' products as unlicensed medicines, the principal NHS units are listed below. A database (*Pro-File*; www.pro-file.nhs.uk) provides information on medicines manufactured in the NHS; access is restricted to NHS pharmacy staff.

The Association of Pharmaceutical Specials Manufacturers may also be able to provide further information about commercial companies (www.apsm-uk.com).

> The MHRA recommends that an unlicensed medicine should only be used when a patient has special requirements that cannot be met by use of a licensed medicine

As well as being available direct from the hospital manufacturer(s) concerned, many NHS-manufactured Specials may be bought from the Oxford Pharmacy Store, owned and operated by Oxford Health NHS Foundation Trust.

England

London

Barts and the London NHS Trust
Mr J. Singh
Head of PMU
Barts Health NHS Trust
Pathology and Pharmacy Building
Royal London Hospital
80 Newark St
Whitechapel
London, E1 2ES
Tel: (020) 3246 0274 (order)
Tel: (020) 3246 0399 (enquiry)
jasdeep.singh@bartshealth.nhs.uk

Guy's and St. Thomas' NHS Foundation Trust
Mr P. Forsey
Associate Chief Pharmacist
Guy's and St. Thomas' NHS Foundation Trust
Pharmacy Department
Guy's Hospital
Great Maze Pond
London, SE1 9RT
Tel: (020) 7188 4992 (order)
Tel: (020) 7188 5003 (enquiry)
Fax: (020) 7188 5013
paul.forsey@gstt.nhs.uk

Moorfields Pharmaceuticals
Mr N. Precious
Technical Director
Moorfields Pharmaceuticals
34 Nile St
London, N1 7TP
Tel: (020) 7684 9090 (order)
Tel: (020) 7684 8574 (enquiry)
Fax: (020) 7502 2332
nick.precious@moorfields.nhs.uk

North West London Hospitals NHS Trust
Dr K. Middleton
North West London Hospitals NHS Trust
Northwick Park Hospital
Watford Rd
Harrow
Middlesex, HA1 3UJ
Tel: (020) 8869 2295 (order)
Tel: (020) 8869 2204/2223 (enquiry)
keith.middleton@nwlh.nhs.uk

Royal Free Hampstead NHS Trust
Ms C. Trehane
Production Manager
Royal Free
Pond St
London, NW3 2QG
Tel: (020) 7830 2424 (order)
Tel: (020) 7830 2282 (enquiry)
Fax: (020) 7794 1875
christine.trehane@nhs.net

St George's Healthcare NHS Trust
Mr V. Kumar
Assistant Chief Pharmacist
Technical Services
St George's Hospital
Blackshaw Rd
Tooting
London, SW17 0QT
Tel: (020) 8725 1770/1768
Fax: (020) 8725 3947
vinodh.kumar@stgeorges.nhs.uk

University College Hospital NHS Foundation Trust
Mr T. Murphy
Production Manager
University College Hospital
235 Euston Rd
London, NW1 2BU
Tel: (020) 7380 9723 (order)
Tel: (020) 7380 9472 (enquiry)
Fax: (020) 7380 9726
tony.murphy@uclh.nhs.uk

Midlands and Eastern

Barking, Havering and Redbridge University Trust
Mr N. Fisher
Senior Principal Pharmacist
Pharmacy Department
Queen's Hospital
Romford
Essex, RM7 0AG
Tel: (01708) 435 463 (order)
Tel: (01708) 435 042 (enquiry)
neil.fisher@bhrhospitals.nhs.uk

Burton Hospitals NHS Trust
Mr P. Williams
Pharmacy Technical and Support Services Manager
Pharmacy Manufacturing Unit
Queens Hospital
Burton Hospitals NHS Trust
Belvedere Rd
Burton-on-Trent, DE13 0RB
Tel: (01283) 511 511 (or 566 333) ext: 5115 (order) 5138 (enquiry)
Fax: (01283) 593 036
paul.williams@burtonh-tr.wmids.nhs.uk

Colchester Hospital University NHS Foundation Trust
Mrs A. Reynolds
Pharmacy Business Manager
Pharmacy Support Unit
Colchester General Hospital
Turner Rd
Colchester, C04 5JL
Tel: (01206) 742 007 (order)
Tel: (01206) 746 148 (enquiry)
Fax: (01206) 841 249
pharmacy.stores@colchesterhospital.nhs.uk (order)
psuenquiries@colchesterhospital.nhs.uk (enquiries)

Ipswich Hospital NHS Trust
Dr J. Harwood
Production Manager
Pharmacy Manufacturing Unit
Ipswich Hospital NHS Trust
Heath Rd
Ipswich, IP4 5PD
Tel: (01473) 703 440 (order)
Tel: (01473) 703 603 (enquiry)
Fax: (01473) 703 609
john.harwood@ipswichhospital.nhs.uk

Nottingham University Hospitals NHS Trust
Ms J. Kendall
Assistant Head of Pharmacy, Technical and Logistical Services
Pharmacy Production Units
Nottingham University Hospitals NHS Trust
Queens Medical Centre Campus
Nottingham, NG7 2UH
Tel: (0115) 875 4521 (order)
Tel: (0115) 924 9924 ext: 64177 (enquiry)
Fax: (0115) 970 9780
jeanette.kendall@nuh.nhs.uk

University Hospital of North Staffordshire NHS Trust
Ms K. Ferguson
Chief Technician
Pharmacy Technical Services
University Hospital of North Staffordshire NHS Trust
City General Site
Stoke-on-Trent, ST4 6QG
Tel: (01782) 674 568 (order)
Tel: (01782) 674 568 (enquiry)
Fax: (01782) 674 575
caroline.ferguson@uhns.nhs.uk

North East

The Newcastle upon Tyne Hospitals NHS Foundation Trust
Mr Y. Hunter-Blair
Production Manager
Newcastle Specials
Pharmacy Production Unit
Royal Victoria Infirmary
Queen Victoria Rd
Newcastle-upon-Tyne, NE1 4LP
Tel: (0191) 282 0395 (order)
Tel: (0191) 282 0389 (enquiry)
Fax: (0191) 282 0469
yan.hunter-blair@nuth.nhs.uk

North West

Preston Pharmaceuticals
Ms A. Nutman
Assistant Director of Pharmacy
Preston Pharmaceuticals
Royal Preston Hospital
Fulwood
Preston, PR2 9HT
Tel: (01772) 523 617 (order)
Tel: (01772) 522 593 (enquiry)
Fax: (01772) 523 645
angela.nutman@lthtr.nhs.uk

Stockport Pharmaceuticals
Mrs S. Miller
Production Manager
Stockport Pharmaceuticals
Pharmacy Department
Stepping Hill Hospital
Stockport, SK2 7JE
Tel: (0161) 419 5666 (order)
Tel: (0161) 419 5657 (enquiry)
Fax: (0161) 419 5426
sally.miller@stockport.nhs.uk

South

Portsmouth Hospitals NHS Trust
Mr R. Lucas
Product Development Manager
Pharmacy Manufacturing Unit
Portsmouth Hospitals NHS Trust
Unit D2, Railway Triangle Industrial Estate
Walton Road
Farlington, Portsmouth, PO6 1TF
Tel: (02392) 389 078 (order)
Tel: (02392) 316 312 (enquiry)
Fax: (02392) 316 316
robert.lucas@porthosp.nhs.uk

South East

East Sussex Healthcare NHS Trust
Mr P. Keen
Business Manager
Eastbourne Pharmaceuticals
Eastbourne District General Hospital
East Sussex Hospitals NHS Trust
Kings Drive, Eastbourne, BN21 2UD
Tel: (01323) 414 906 (order)
Tel: (01323) 417 400 ext: 3076 (enquiry)
Fax: (01323) 414 931
paul.keen@esht.nhs.uk

South West

Torbay PMU
Mr P. Bendell
Pharmacy Manufacturing Services Manager
Torbay PMU
South Devon Healthcare NHS Foundation Trust
Kemmings Close, Long Rd
Paignton, TQ4 7TW
Tel: (01803) 664 707
Fax: (01803) 664 354
phil.bendell@nhs.net

Yorkshire

Calderdale and Huddersfield NHS Foundation Trust
Dr S. Langford
Pharmacy Production Director
Pharmacy Manufacturing Unit
Huddersfield Royal Infirmary
Gate 2-Acre Mills, School St
Lindley
Huddersfield, HD3 3ET
Tel: (01484) 355 388 (order)
Tel: (01484) 355 371 (enquiry)
Fax: (01484) 355 377
stephen.langford@cht.nhs.uk

Northern Ireland

Victoria Pharmaceuticals
Ms C. McBride
Production Manager
Victoria Pharmaceuticals
Plenum Building
Royal Hospitals
Grosvenor Road
Belfast, BT12 6BA
Tel: (028) 9263 0070 (order/enquiry)
Fax: (028) 9063 5282 (order/enquiry)
colettemcbride@belfasttrust.hscni.net

Scotland

NHS Greater Glasgow and Clyde
Mr G. Conkie
Production Manager
Western Infirmary
Dumbarton Rd
Glasgow, G11 6NT
Tel: (0141) 211 2754 (order)
Tel: (0141) 211 2882 (enquiry)
Fax: (0141) 211 1967
graham.conkie@ggc.scot.nhs.uk

Tayside Pharmaceuticals
Dr B. Millar
General Manager
Tayside Pharmaceuticals
Ninewells Hospital
Dundee, DD1 9SY
Tel: (01382) 632 052 (order)
Tel: (01382) 632 183 (enquiry)
Fax: (01382) 632 060
baxter.millar@nhs.net

Wales

Cardiff and Vale University Health Board
Mr P. Spark
Principal Pharmacist (Production)
Cardiff and Vale University Health Board
20 Fieldway
Cardiff, CF14 4HY
Tel: (029) 2074 8120
Fax: (029) 2074 8130
paul.spark@wales.nhs.uk

Index

Principal page references are printed in **bold** type. Proprietary (trade) names and names of organisms are printed in *italic* type; where the BNF does not include a full entry for a branded product, the non-proprietary name is shown in brackets

Index

Index

Index

Index

Index

Index

Index

Index

Index

Index

Index

Index

Index

Index

Index

Index

Index

Index

ADULT ADVANCED LIFE SUPPORT ALGORITHM

Unresponsive?
Not breathing or only occasional gasps

⟷ Call Resuscitation Team

CPR 30:2
Attach defibrillator/monitor
Minimise interruptions

Assess rhythm

Shockable
(VF/pulseless VT)

Non-shockable
(PEA/Asystole)

Return of spontaneous circulation

1 Shock

Immediately resume
CPR for 2 min
Minimise interruptions

Immediate post cardiac arrest treatment
- Use ABCDE approach
- Controlled oxygenation and ventilation
- 12-lead ECG
- Treat precipitating cause
- Temperature control / therapeutic hypothermia

Immediately resume
CPR for 2 min
Minimise interruptions

During CPR
- Ensure high-quality CPR: rate, depth, recoil
- Plan actions before interrupting CPR
- Give oxygen
- Consider advanced airway and capnography
- Continuous chest compressions when advanced airway in place
- Vascular access (intravenous, intraosseous)
- Give adrenaline every 3-5 min
- Correct reversible causes

Reversible causes
- Hypoxia
- Hypovolaemia
- Hypo- / hyperkalaemia / metabolic
- Hypothermia

- Thrombosis - coronary or pulmonary
- Tamponade - cardiac
- Toxins
- Tension pneumothorax

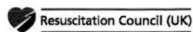 Resuscitation Council (UK)

Medical emergencies in the community

Drug treatment outlined below is intended for use by appropriately qualified healthcare professionals. Only drugs that are used for immediate relief are shown; advice on supporting care is not given. Where the patient's condition requires investigation and further treatment, the patient should be transferred to hospital promptly.

Anaphylaxis
(section 3.4.3)

Adrenaline injection (1 mg/mL (1 in 1000))

- By intramuscular injection
  CHILD UNDER 6 YEARS 150 micrograms (0.15 mL), repeated every 5 minutes if necessary
  CHILD 6–12 YEARS 300 micrograms (0.3 mL), repeated every 5 minutes if necessary
  CHILD 12–18 YEARS 500 micrograms (0.5 mL), repeated every 5 minutes if necessary; 300 micrograms (0.3 mL) if CHILD is small or prepubertal
  ADULT 500 micrograms (0.5 mL), repeated every 5 minutes if necessary

High-flow **oxygen** (section 3.6) and **intravenous fluids** should be given as soon as available.

Chlorphenamine injection by intramuscular or intravenous injection (section 3.4.1) may help counter histamine-mediated vasodilation and bronchoconstriction.

Hydrocortisone (preferably as sodium succinate) by intravenous injection (section 6.3.2) has delayed action but should be given to severely affected patients to prevent further deterioration.

Angina: unstable
(section 2.10.1)

Aspirin dispersible tablets (75 mg, 300 mg)

- By mouth (dispersed in water or chewed)
  ADULT 300 mg

Plus

either **Glyceryl trinitrate aerosol spray** (400 micrograms/metered dose)

- Sublingually
  ADULT 1–2 sprays, repeated as required

or **Glyceryl trinitrate tablets** (300 micrograms, 500 micrograms, 600 micrograms)

- Sublingually
  ADULT 0.3–1 mg, repeated as required

Asthma: acute
(section 3.1)

Regard each emergency consultation as being for **severe acute asthma** until shown otherwise; failure to respond adequately **at any time** requires immediate transfer to hospital

Either **salbutamol aerosol inhaler** (100 micrograms/metered inhalation)

- By aerosol inhalation via large-volume spacer (and a close-fitting face mask if child under 3 years)
  ADULT and CHILD 2–10 puffs each inhaled separately, repeated every 10–20 minutes or as necessary

or **salbutamol nebuliser solution** (1 mg/mL, 2 mg/mL)

- By inhalation of nebulised solution (via oxygen-driven nebuliser if available)
  CHILD UNDER 5 YEARS 2.5 mg every 20–30 minutes or as necessary
  CHILD 5–12 YEARS 2.5–5 mg every 20–30 minutes or as necessary
  ADULT 5 mg every 20–30 minutes or as necessary

or **terbutaline nebuliser solution** (2.5 mg/mL)

- By inhalation of nebulised solution (via oxygen-driven nebuliser if available)
  CHILD UNDER 5 YEARS 5 mg every 20–30 minutes or as necessary
  CHILD 5–12 YEARS 5–10 mg every 20–30 minutes or as necessary
  ADULT 10 mg every 20–30 minutes or as necessary

Plus (in all cases)

either **prednisolone tablets** (*or* **prednisolone** soluble tablets) (5 mg)

- By mouth
  CHILD UNDER 12 YEARS 1–2 mg/kg (max. 40 mg) once daily for up to 3 days or longer if necessary; if child has been taking an oral corticosteroid for more than a few days, give prednisolone 2 mg/kg (max. 60 mg) once daily
  ADULT 40–50 mg once daily for at least 5 days

or **hydrocortisone (preferably as sodium succinate)**

- By intravenous injection
  CHILD UNDER 12 YEARS 4 mg/kg (max. 100 mg) every 6 hours until conversion to oral prednisolone is possible; alternative dose if weight unavailable, CHILD UNDER 2 YEARS 25 mg, 2–5 YEARS 50 mg, 5–12 YEARS 100 mg
  ADULT 100 mg every 6 hours until conversion to oral prednisolone is possible

High-flow **oxygen** (section 3.6) if available (via face mask in children)

Monitor response 15 to 30 minutes after nebulisation; if any signs of acute asthma persist, arrange hospital admission. While awaiting ambulance, repeat **nebulised beta$_2$ agonist** (as above) and give with

ipratropium nebuliser solution (250 micrograms/mL)

- By inhalation of nebulised solution (via oxygen-driven nebuliser if available)
  CHILD UNDER 12 YEARS 250 micrograms, repeated every 20–30 minutes for the first 2 hours, then every 4–6 hours as necessary
  ADULT 500 micrograms every 4–6 hours as necessary

Convulsive (including febrile) seizures lasting longer than 5 minutes
(section 4.8.2 and section 4.8.3)

Either **diazepam** rectal solution (2 mg/mL, 4 mg/mL)

- By rectum
  NEONATE 1.25–2.5 mg, repeated once after 10–15 minutes if necessary
  CHILD 1 MONTH–2 YEARS 5 mg, repeated once after 10–15 minutes if necessary
  CHILD 2–12 YEARS 5–10 mg, repeated once after 10–15 minutes if necessary
  ADULT and CHILD OVER 12 YEARS 10–20 mg (ELDERLY 10 mg), repeated once after 10–15 minutes if necessary

or **midazolam** oromucosal solution

- By buccal administration, repeated once after 10 minutes if necessary
  NEONATE 300 micrograms/kg [unlicensed]
  CHILD 1–3 MONTHS 300 micrograms/kg (max. 2.5 mg) [unlicensed]
  CHILD 3 MONTHS–1 YEAR 2.5 mg
  CHILD 1–5 YEARS 5 mg
  CHILD 5–10 YEARS 7.5 mg
  CHILD 10–18 YEARS 10 mg
  ADULT OVER 18 YEARS 10 mg [unlicensed]

Croup
(section 3.1)

Dexamethasone oral solution (2 mg/5 mL)

- By mouth
  CHILD 1 MONTH–2 YEARS 150 micrograms/kg as a single dose

Diabetic hypoglycaemia
(section 6.1.4)

Glucose or **sucrose**

- By mouth
  ADULT and CHILD OVER 2 YEARS approx. 10–20 g (55–110 mL *Lucozade®* *Energy Original* or 100–200 mL *Coca-Cola®*—both non-diet versions *or* 2–4 teaspoonfuls of sugar *or* 3–6 sugar lumps) repeated after 10–15 minutes if necessary

or **if hypoglycaemia unresponsive** *or* **if oral route cannot be used**

Glucagon injection (1 mg/mL)

- By subcutaneous or intramuscular injection
  CHILD BODY-WEIGHT UNDER 25 KG 500 micrograms (0.5 mL)
  CHILD BODY-WEIGHT OVER 25 KG 1 mg (1 mL)
  ADULT 1 mg (1 mL)

or **if hypoglycaemia prolonged** *or* **unresponsive to glucagon after 10 minutes**

Glucose intravenous infusion (10%)

- By intravenous injection into large vein
  CHILD 1 MONTH–18 YEARS 5 mL/kg (glucose 500 mg/kg)

Glucose intravenous infusion (20%)

- By intravenous injection into large vein
  ADULT 50 mL

Meningococcal disease
(Table 1, section 5.1)

Benzylpenicillin sodium injection (600 mg, 1.2 g)

- By intravenous injection (or by intramuscular injection if venous access not available)
  NEONATE 300 mg
  CHILD 1 MONTH–1 YEAR 300 mg
  CHILD 1–10 YEARS 600 mg
  CHILD 10–18 YEARS 1.2 g
  ADULT 1.2 g
  Note A single dose should be given before urgent transfer to hospital, so long as this does not delay the transfer

or **if history of allergy to penicillin**

Cefotaxime injection (1 g)

- By intravenous injection (or by intramuscular injection if venous access not available)
  NEONATE 50 mg/kg
  CHILD 1 MONTH–12 YEARS 50 mg/kg (max. 1 g)
  CHILD 12–18 YEARS 1 g
  ADULT 1 g
  Note A single dose can be given before urgent transfer to hospital, so long as this does not delay the transfer

or **if history of immediate hypersensitivity reaction (including anaphylaxis, angioedema, urticaria, or rash immediately after administration) to penicillin or to cephalosporins**

Chloramphenicol injection (1 g)

- By intravenous injection
  CHILD 1 MONTH–18 YEARS 12.5–25 mg/kg
  ADULT 12.5–25 mg/kg
  Note A single dose can be given before urgent transfer to hospital, so long as this does not delay the transfer

Myocardial infarction: ST-segment elevation
(section 2.10.1)

Aspirin dispersible tablets (75 mg, 300 mg)

- By mouth (dispersed in water or chewed)
  ADULT 300 mg

Glyceryl trinitrate aerosol spray (400 micrograms/metered dose)

- Sublingually
  ADULT 1–2 sprays, repeated as required

or **Glyceryl trinitrate** tablets (300 micrograms, 500 micrograms, 600 micrograms)

- Sublingually
  ADULT 0.3–1 mg, repeated as required

Metoclopramide injection (5 mg/mL)

- By intravenous injection
  ADULT (UNDER 60 KG) 18–19 YEARS 5 mg
  ADULT (OVER 60 KG) 18–19 YEARS 10 mg
  ADULT OVER 19 YEARS 10 mg

Diamorphine injection (5 mg powder for reconstitution)

- By slow intravenous injection (1–2 mg/minute)
  ADULT 5 mg followed by a further 2.5–5 mg if
  necessary; ELDERLY or FRAIL patients, reduce dose by
  half

or **Morphine sulphate** injection (10 mg/mL)

- By slow intravenous injection (1–2 mg/minute)
  ADULT 5–10 mg followed by a further 5–10 mg if
  necessary; ELDERLY or FRAIL patients, reduce dose by
  half

Oxygen, if appropriate

Myocardial infarction: non-ST-segment elevation

Treat as for *Angina: unstable*, above

Approximate conversions and units

lb	kg	stones	kg	mL	fl oz
1	0.45	1	6.35	50	1.8
2	0.91	2	12.70	100	3.5
3	1.36	3	19.05	150	5.3
4	1.81	4	25.40	200	7.0
5	2.27	5	31.75	500	17.6
6	2.72	6	38.10	1000	35.2
7	3.18	7	44.45		
8	3.63	8	50.80		
9	4.08	9	57.15		
10	4.54	10	63.50		
11	4.99	11	69.85		
12	5.44	12	76.20		
13	5.90	13	82.55		
14	6.35	14	88.90		
		15	95.25		

Length

1 metre (m)	= 1000 millimetres (mm)
1 centimetre (cm)	= 10 mm
1 inch (in)	= 25.4 mm
1 foot (ft)	= 12 inches
12 inches	= 304.8 mm

Mass

1 kilogram (kg)	= 1000 grams (g)
1 gram (g)	= 1000 milligrams (mg)
1 milligram (mg)	= 1000 micrograms
1 microgram	= 1000 nanograms
1 nanogram	= 1000 picograms

Volume

1 litre	= 1000 millilitres (mL)
1 millilitre (1 mL)	= 1000 microlitres
1 pint	≈ 568 mL

Other units

1 kilocalorie (kcal)	= 4186.8 joules (J)
1000 kilocalories (kcal)	= 4.1868 megajoules (MJ)
1 megajoule (MJ)	= 238.8 kilocalories (kcal)
1 millimetre of mercury (mmHg)	= 133.3 pascals (Pa)
1 kilopascal (kPa)	= 7.5 mmHg (pressure)

> **Plasma-drug concentrations** in the BNF are expressed in mass units per litre (e.g. mg/litre). The approximate equivalent in terms of amount of substance units (e.g. micromol/litre) is given in brackets.

Prescribing for children

Weight, height, and gender

The table below shows the **mean values** for weight, height, and gender by age; these values have been derived from the UK-WHO growth charts 2009 and UK1990 standard centile charts, by extrapolating the 50th centile, and may be used to calculate doses in the absence of measurements. However, an individual's weight and height might vary considerably from the values in the table and it is important to ensure that the value chosen is appropriate. In most cases the actual measurement should be obtained as soon as possible and the dose re-calculated.

Age	Weight	Height
	kg	cm
Full-term neonate	3.5	51
1 month	4.3	55
2 months	5.4	58
3 months	6.1	61
4 months	6.7	63
6 months	7.6	67
1 year	9	75
3 years	14	96
5 years	18	109
7 years	23	122
10 years	32	138
12 years	39	149
14 year-old boy	49	163
14 year-old girl	50	159
Adult male	68	176
Adult female	58	164

Recommended wording of cautionary and advisory labels

For details see Appendix 3

1. Warning: This medicine may make you sleepy
2. Warning: This medicine may make you sleepy. If this happens, do not drive or use tools or machines. Do not drink alcohol
3. Warning: This medicine may make you sleepy. If this happens, do not drive or use tools or machines
4. Warning: Do not drink alcohol
5. Do not take indigestion remedies 2 hours before or after you take this medicine
6. Do not take indigestion remedies, or medicines containing iron or zinc, 2 hours before or after you take this medicine
7. Do not take milk, indigestion remedies, or medicines containing iron or zinc, 2 hours before or after you take this medicine
8. Warning: Do not stop taking this medicine unless your doctor tells you to stop
9. Space the doses evenly throughout the day. Keep taking this medicine until the course is finished, unless you are told to stop
10. Warning: Read the additional information given with this medicine
11. Protect your skin from sunlight—even on a bright but cloudy day. Do not use sunbeds
12. Do not take anything containing aspirin while taking this medicine
13. Dissolve or mix with water before taking
14. This medicine may colour your urine. This is harmless
15. Caution: flammable. Keep your body away from fire or flames after you have put on the medicine
16. Dissolve the tablet under your tongue—do not swallow. Store the tablets in this bottle with the cap tightly closed. Get a new supply 8 weeks after opening
17. Do not take more than... in 24 hours
18. Do not take more than... in 24 hours. Also, do not take more than... in any one week
19. Warning: This medicine makes you sleepy. If you still feel sleepy the next day, do not drive or use tools or machines. Do not drink alcohol
21. Take with or just after food, or a meal
22. Take 30 to 60 minutes before food
23. Take this medicine when your stomach is empty. This means an hour before food or 2 hours after food
24. Suck or chew this medicine
25. Swallow this medicine whole. Do not chew or crush
26. Dissolve this medicine under your tongue
27. Take with a full glass of water
28. Spread thinly on the affected skin only
29. Do not take more than 2 at any one time. Do not take more than 8 in 24 hours
30. Contains paracetamol. Do not take anything else containing paracetamol while taking this medicine. Talk to a doctor at once if you take too much of this medicine, even if you feel well
32. Contains aspirin. Do not take anything else containing aspirin while taking this medicine